W0258969

HANDBUCH DER MEDIZINISCHEN RADIOLOGIE

ENCYCLOPEDIA OF MEDICAL RADIOLOGY

HERAUSGEGEBEN VON · EDITED BY

L. DIETHELM
MAINZ

O. OLSSON
LUND

F. STRNAD
FRANKFURT/M.

H. VIETEN
DÜSSELDORF

A. ZUPPINGER
BERN

BAND / VOLUME IV
TEIL / PART 1

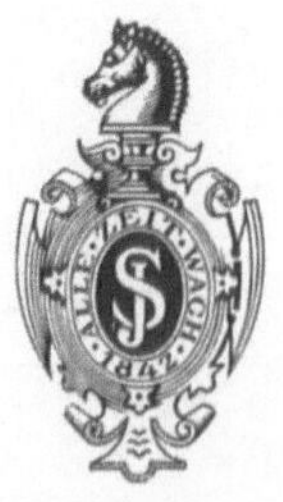

SPRINGER-VERLAG BERLIN · HEIDELBERG · NEW YORK · 1970

SKELETANATOMIE (RÖNTGENDIAGNOSTIK)

TEIL 1

ANATOMY OF THE SKELETAL SYSTEM (ROENTGEN DIAGNOSIS)

PART 1

VON · BY

R. AMPRINO · H.-J. DULCE · A. ENGSTRÖM · K. HAASCH · F. HEUCK
A. HULTH · A. IBALL · K. H. KNESE · R. MAATZ

REDIGIERT VON · EDITED BY

L. DIETHELM
MAINZ

MIT 559 ABBILDUNGEN
WITH 559 FIGURES

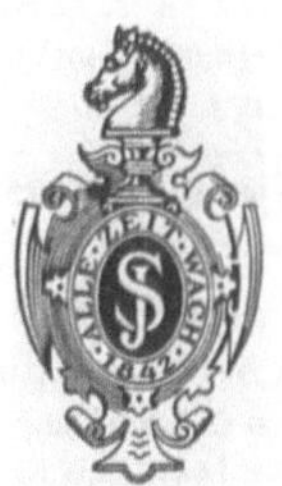

SPRINGER-VERLAG BERLIN · HEIDELBERG · NEW YORK 1970

Das Werk ist urheberrechtlich geschützt. Die dadurch begründeten Rechte, insbesondere die der Übersetzung, des Nachdruckes, der Entnahme von Abbildungen, der Funksendung, der Wiedergabe auf photomechanischem oder ähnlichem Wege und der Speicherung in Datenverarbeitungsanlagen bleiben, auch bei nur auszugsweiser Verwertung, vorbehalten.

Bei Vervielfältigungen für gewerbliche Zwecke ist gemäß § 54 UrhG eine Vergütung an den Verlag zu zahlen, deren Höhe mit dem Verlag zu vereinbaren ist.

ISBN-13: 978-3-642-95148-0 e-ISBN-13: 978-3-642-95147-3
DOI: 10.1007/978-3-642-95147-3

© by Springer-Verlag Berlin · Heidelberg 1970. Library of Congress Catalog Card Number 68—26459.
Softcover reprint of the hardcover 1st edition 1970

Die Wiedergabe von Gebrauchsnamen, Handelsnamen, Warenbezeichnungen usw. in diesem Werk berechtigt auch ohne besondere Kennzeichnung nicht zu der Annahme, daß solche Namen im Sinne der Warenzeichen- und Markenschutz-Gesetzgebung als frei zu betrachten wären und daher von jedermann benutzt werden dürften.

Titel-Nr. 5827

Vorwort

Unsere Kenntnisse über das Skelet als Organ und seine Veränderungen unter physiologischen und pathologischen Bedingungen sind noch lückenhaft. Neuere Forschungen haben sich intensiver mit morphologischen, chemischen und biologischen Vorgängen beschäftigt, deren Kenntnis zum Verständnis des Knochens als Stützorgan sowie als Speicherorgan für Mineralien, aber auch zum Verständnis der Bruchheilung, Pseudarthrosenentstehung und der Knochentransplantationsfolgen unerläßlich ist.

Dem Radiologen fällt bei der Beurteilung nicht nur die Feststellung eines gerade eben vorhandenen Zustandes als Aufgabe zu, sondern auch die Einordnung dieses Zustandes in einen biologischen Geschehensablauf. Hierzu werden neben Verlaufsbeobachtungen in zunehmendem Maße auch zusätzliche Untersuchungsverfahren herangezogen werden müssen, wie die radiologische Bestimmung des Mineralgehaltes, die Klärung der Durchblutungsverhältnisse oder Studien mit Isotopen.

Aus diesen Gründen erschien es notwendig, in einem allgemeinen Teil diese Grundlagen zusammenzufassen und dem speziellen Teil, den Skeleterkrankungen und den speziellen Skeletbänden über Wirbelsäule und Schädel, vorausgehen zu lassen. Hier ist noch vieles im Fluß — eine Zusammenfassung des derzeitigen Wissens-Standes, aber auch der offenen Probleme kann daher nur Anregungen zu weiterer Forschung geben.

Mainz, Februar 1970

L. Diethelm

Preface

There are still gaps in our knowledge of the skeletal system and the changes induced by physiological and pathological stress. Recent research has been much more concerned with the morphological, chemical and biological processes which we have to understand before we can appreciate the function of bone as a supporting structure or as a reservoir of minerals, not to mention understanding how fractures heal, what causes pseudoarthroses and how bone transplantation works.

It is part of the radiologist's job to determine the condition which is present and then to give an opinion as to where it fits into the sequence of biological events. This calls for an increasing range of auxiliary examination techniques in addition to observing the course of the disease, including radiological determination of the mineral content of the bones, tracing the blood circulation, or studies with radioactive tracers.

For these reasons it seemed expedient to collect such data in a general section to precede the special sections on bone diseases and the volumes dealing with the spine and the skull. The situation here is still very fluid, so a summary both of the state of the art and the remaining problems may help to stimulate further research.

Mainz, February 1970

L. Diethelm

Inhaltsverzeichnis

Mitarbeiter von Band IV/1 — Contributors to volume IV/1

Professor Dr. Rodolfo Amprino, Istituto di Anatomia Umana, Università di Bari, Policlinico, Bari (Italien)

Professor Dr. Hans-Joachim Dulce, Institut für Klinische Chemie und Klinische Biochemie der Freien Universität, 1 Berlin 45, Hindenburgdamm 30

Professor Dr. Arne Engström, Karolinska Institutet, Institutionen för Medicinsk Fysik, Stockholm 60 (Schweden)

Dr. K. Haasch, 1 Berlin 49, Kronbergstraße 17

Professor Dr. Friedrich Heuck, Röntgeninstitut, Katharinenhospital, 7 Stuttgart 1, Kriegsbergstraße 60

Professor Dr. A. Hulth, Orthopädische Abteilung des Allmänna Sjukhuset, Malmö (Schweden)

Dr. John Iball, Chemistry Department, University of Dundee, Dundee (Scotland)

Professor Dr. Karl-Heinrich Knese, Institut für Histologie und Embryologie der Universität Hohenheim, 7 Stuttgart-Hohenheim, Fruwirthstraße 16

Professor Dr. Richard Maatz, Chirurgische Abteilung des Städtischen Auguste-Viktoria-Krankenhauses, 1 Berlin 41, Rubensstraße 125

Inhaltsübersicht zu Band IV/2

A. The mineralogy of bone

By

John Iball

With 3 figures

1. Introduction

In this article the word "bone" is used in its everyday sense and excludes the other calcified tissues in the body and excludes teeth. Much of the discussion however will have a close bearing on the structure of these other tissues.

Bones consist normally of three main constituents (i) fibres (collagen) which are organic; (ii) ground substance, or cement, the nature of which is not well understood but contains mucopolysaccharides; (iii) inorganic salts in the form of minute crystals which consist of calcium phosphate complexes. There are in addition traces of a large number of other substances and the rôle of these is probably underestimated. As with many other structures the whole is very much greater than the sum of the parts. One of the chief characteristics of bones is their strength and this is closely linked with the inorganic part of the tissue though how the calcium salts produce such strength is far from being clearly understood. What is perhaps more surprising is the fact that so far it has been impossible to show any quantitative, or for that matter any qualitative, correlation between the profound changes in strength (e.g. in rickets) which take place in bones and the molecular structure of the bones. In normal bone some 65% of the dry weight is inorganic material but this varies over quite a wide range under different conditions, in different bones and even in different parts of the same bone. This is one of the reasons why it is so difficult to get a clear, unambiguous picture of the physical and chemical structure of bones. In addition, the composition of the mineral varies and even apparently mild treatment can produce changes in it. Bones are living tissues just as any other tissue in the body and although the mineral part may be regarded as inanimate it is produced as a part of the living process. Even when it is present as crystals it is by no means static but is an essential component of the living bone. It is not therefore surprising that there are conflicting opinions about its exact nature. The situation is further complicated by the fact that two investigators rarely study the same material. It is not therefore surprising that there are conflicting opinions about its exact nature.

2. Chemical investigations

a) The chemical composition of bone minerals. The elements present

The main elements, apart from carbon and oxygen, are calcium and phosphorus with much smaller quantities of sodium, fluorine, magnesium. Other elements which can, and on occasion do, appear in bone are strontium, barium, potassium. It is clear from roentgen ray diffraction studies (see below) that the crystals of the inorganic material have a structure which resembles the mineral apatite and in this kind of structure it is possible to substitute one element for another without altering the basic structural lattice in an appreciable manner. This is why the chemical composition of an apparently homogeneous substance can vary.

b) Different theories of the composition of bone mineral

The earliest suggestion was that the salts consisted of $Ca_3(PO_4)_2$ with smaller quantities of $CaCO_3$, $Mg_2(PO_4)_2$. BERZELIUS (1845) suggested $Ca_5H_2(PO_4)_2$ as the main constituent while HOPPE-SEYLER (1862) put forward a much more complicated substance $Ca[(O \cdot PO_3Ca)_2Ca]_3CO_3$. Over the years many such formulae have been suggested and this shows that the substance does not have a fixed composition and that the attempt to define the mineral component of bone by a single chemical formula is doomed to failure. In recent years the general view is that there are only three theories worth consideration. These claim that the main component of bone mineral consists of crystals which have a composition resembling,

(a) α-tricalcium phosphate (hydrated) $[3\,Ca_3(PO_4)_2 \cdot H_2(OH)_2]$ mixed with $CaCO_3$ (as a separate phase),

(b) carbonate apatite (in this case the carbonate ions are an integral part of the crystal lattice) $[Ca_6OH_2\{(P \cdot C)O_4\}_6(Ca \cdot C)_4]$,

(c) hydroxyapatite with $CaCO_3$ adsorbed on the surface of the apatite crystals $[Ca_{10}(PO_4)_6(OH)_2]$.

The reasons for adopting one or other of the above theories are partly chemical and partly based on the evidence from roentgen ray diffraction. It will be more convenient to discuss them later when the methods and results of roentgen ray diffraction have been described.

3. Roentgen ray diffraction

a) Techniques

There are several different techniques available for the study of crystalline and para-crystalline substances by roentgen ray diffraction. The method of choice depends on the kind of material available and on the kind of information required. However, the basic principle is the same in all methods. This is simply that when atoms or molecules or groups of molecules arranged in a periodic repeating system are irradiated by a beam of roentgen rays the roentgen rays are diffracted and the diffracted beam has, in certain directions, intensity maxima and minima which are related to the periodic arrangement within the diffracting substance. The phenomenon is exactly analogous to interference in optics but because of the short wavelength of roentgen rays the scale of the periodicity which can be detected is in the region of 1.0 Å i.e. on the atomic scale. Interference in optics is usually a two-dimensional phenomenon, that is the periodicity in the diffracting substance (e.g. a diffraction grating) extends over a plane. With diffraction of roentgen rays by crystals we are usually dealing with periodicity over three-dimensions.

The simplest way of regarding three-dimensional diffraction is to consider a crystal to be a regular arrangement of parallel planes of atoms each plane being a constant distance d from its neighbours (Fig. 1). If a beam of roentgen rays of wavelength λ is incident on these planes at an angle Θ we get "reflection" from each plane, the reflected beam also making an angle Θ with the planes. The path difference between a beam reflected from one plane and a beam reflected from a neighbouring plane is ABC. From the geometry of the construction it can be seen that $ABC = 2d \sin \Theta$ and if this path difference is a whole number of wavelengths then the beams reflected from each successive layer are in phase and their intensities reinforce each other and the total reflected beam has an intensity maximum. On the other hand if the separation of the planes is such that $2d \sin \Theta$ is equal to one half of a wavelength the reflected beams are out-of-phase and destructive interference occurs giving an intensity minimum in the total beam. In an actual crystal the separation of the planes is of course a constant but we can vary the angle Θ at will. Thus by changing the angle of the roentgen ray beam it is found that maxima in the diffracted beam are observed when $n\,\lambda = 2d \sin \Theta$ (n = a whole number). This is known as BRAGG's Law. In a true crystal the constituent atoms or molecules are arranged on a three dimensional lattice with the periodicity of the lattice extending in all directions throughout the crystal. In this case the diffraction pattern extends over three dimensions. However some materials of a para-crystalline nature may have a periodic arrangement extending, in the main, only in one direction (e.g. fibres) and the diffraction pattern from such materials has a correspondingly restricted periodicity. We can therefore by examining the roentgen ray diffraction pattern from a substance determine whether it is crystalline and the degree of crystallinity present. By careful measurement of the angles which the diffracted beams make with the incident beam ($2\,\Theta$) we can determine the spacing (d) of the crystal planes (the periodicity) and we can in fact obtain the shape and size of the unit of the crystal lattice. By measuring the intensities of the diffracted beams it is possible with suitable crystals to determine the position of each atom in the crystal lattice.

α) The powder method

If the substance to be studied is in the form of microscopic crystals as in metals (in bone the inorganic crystals are too small to be seen by an optical microscope) then they are usually arranged in a random orientation to one another and to the roentgen ray beam. This means that each crystal plane is, in some crystals, at the correct angle to the roentgen ray beam for BRAGG's Law to be satisfied. If therefore we have a narrow pencil of roentgen rays of uniform wavelength striking a small mass of randomly orientated crystallites the diffracted beams, for each crystal plane, form a cone of rays with the primary beam as the axis of the cone and the semi-angle of the cone equal to $2\,\Theta$. If a photographic film is arranged to receive these cones of rays the picture consists of a series of concentric rings (Fig. 3). If a short cylindrical film is arranged with the crystal mass on the axis the picture will consist of short lines corresponding to the intersection of a cone with a cylinder. From the position of the lines on the film and the geometry of the apparatus it is possible to calculate the spacing of the planes which gave rise to each line. If the lattice unit-cell is small and cubic, hexagonal or tetragonal it is possible to identify each diffraction line since the total number will be small and each line will be clearly resolved. However, if the unit-cell is large and/or belongs to the orthorhombic, monoclinic or triclinic systems then in general the number of lines will be large and it will not be possible to identify each diffraction line. A further complication arises when the crystallites are very small (e.g. less than 1,000 Å diameter). In this case the diffraction lines are rather diffuse and weak lines tend to merge into the background. This is the situation in the case of bone mineral. Untreated normal bone contains crystals which are probably not more than 200 Å maximum dimension and so although the crystals are hexagonal it is not possible to determine the spacings with a high accuracy and many of the weaker diffraction lines are not measurable at all. As mentioned above if a flat film is arranged perpendicular to the incident beam the diffraction pattern consists of a series of concentric rings. The uniformity of the density around each ring is an indication of the *randomness* of the crystallite orientation. If the crystallites are completely random the rings will be perfectly uniform. On the other hand if the crystallites tend to orient themselves parallel to some preferred direction (as the crystallites in a metal wire when the wire is subjected to mechanical drawing) then the rings will not be uniform but will

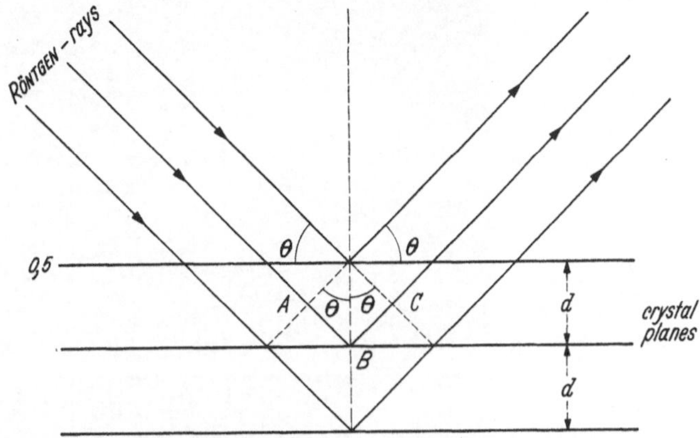

Fig. 1. Diagram of roentgen ray reflection from a set of equidistant parallel planes (BRAGG's Law)

have arcs of high density, perpendicular to the preferred orientation, and consequently arcs of low density at right angles to this direction. The crystals may be orientated with one crystal direction approximately parallel to a preferred direction but randomly orientated in the plane perpendicular to the preferred direction. This also occurs in bones, e.g. the shafts of long bones, and so while some diffraction rings are of uniform density others are not.

Since each crystalline material has, with very few exceptions, a different size of lattice unit-cell the powder diffraction pattern is unique for that substance. Thus the pattern can be used to identify the substance. Even when the pattern is too complicated for the structure to be determined it is usually possible to identify the substance. If

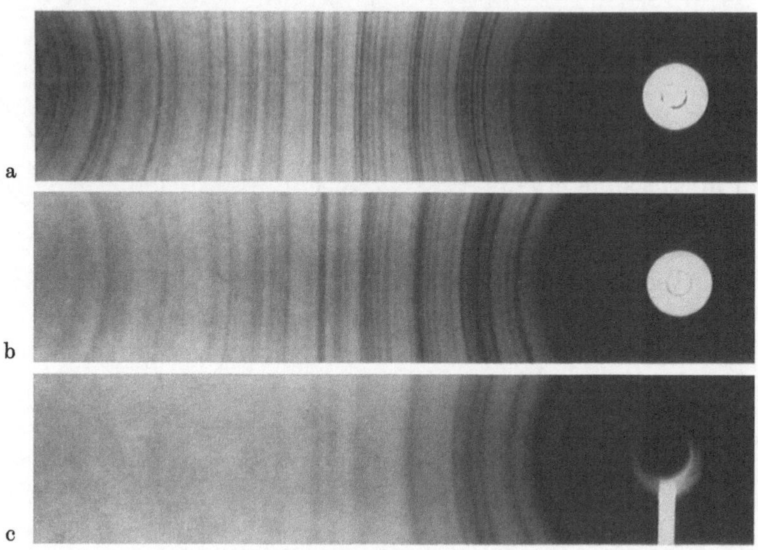

Fig. 2a—c. Roentgen ray powder photographs of a powdered fluorapatite, b precipitated hydroxyapatite, c powdered bone (rat femur)

two samples give identical diffraction patterns it is most unlikely that they are different substances. Unfortunately, in the case of bone mineral there are two main difficulties which prevent an unequivocal identification by the roentgen ray powder method. The diffraction lines are diffuse because the crystallites are so small and the structure of apatites is such that small changes in composition can take place without causing changes in the crystal lattice which can be detected by any normal techniques.

In Fig. 2 powder photographs are reproduced of

a fluorapetite, obtained by grinding a single crystal of the mineral in a mortar, note the sharp lines extending to the end of the film.

b Hydroxyapatite prepared chemically as a fine precipitate. The same arrangement of lines as in a but they are not quite so sharp.

c Powdered bone (rat femur). The strong lines of a and b are present but they are much more diffuse and there are only a few lines compared to a and b.

β) *Single crystal method*

If the substance under investigation can be obtained in the form of a single crystal (which need not be larger than a few micrograms) then the individual beams diffracted from each set of parallel planes in the crystal can be recorded and their intensities can be measured. This is by far the most powerful method of structure determination and even with very complicated molecules it is possible to obtain not only accurate values for the shape and size of the crystal unit cell but in many cases the position of each atom in the lattice can be fixed with high precision. The mineral fluorapatite which is very similar in structure to bone mineral has been studied with this method. The general layout of the structure was described by NARAY-SZABO (1930) and this was confirmed and accurate atomic positions determined by BEEVERS and MCINTYRE (1946).

When using this technique the small single crystal is mounted in a narrow beam of monochromatic roentgen rays and rotated about a principle lattice direction. As the crystal rotates each lattice plane in turn comes into position so that the Bragg Law is satisfied and a diffracted beam can be observed at the angle appropriate to the spacing of the planes and the wavelength of the radiation. These diffraction beams can be recorded on photographic film or detected by GEIGER-MÜLLER counters. With a moderately sized unit-cell there may be several thousand independent diffracted beams. The task of recording and measuring their intensities is therefore considerable.

γ) *Fibre diagrams*

Many substances (e.g. collagen) appear to be far removed from the normal crystalline form and yet they possess some of the characteristics of crystals in so far as roentgen ray diffraction is concerned. They are certainly not single crystals nor are they composed of randomly oriented microcrystals. Their diffraction pattern however has some of the characteristics both of crystalline powders and of single crystals. A good example is provided by a metal wire which when annealed gives a diffraction pattern of a crystalline powder, that is, of continuous uniform rings on a photographic plate. If the wire is

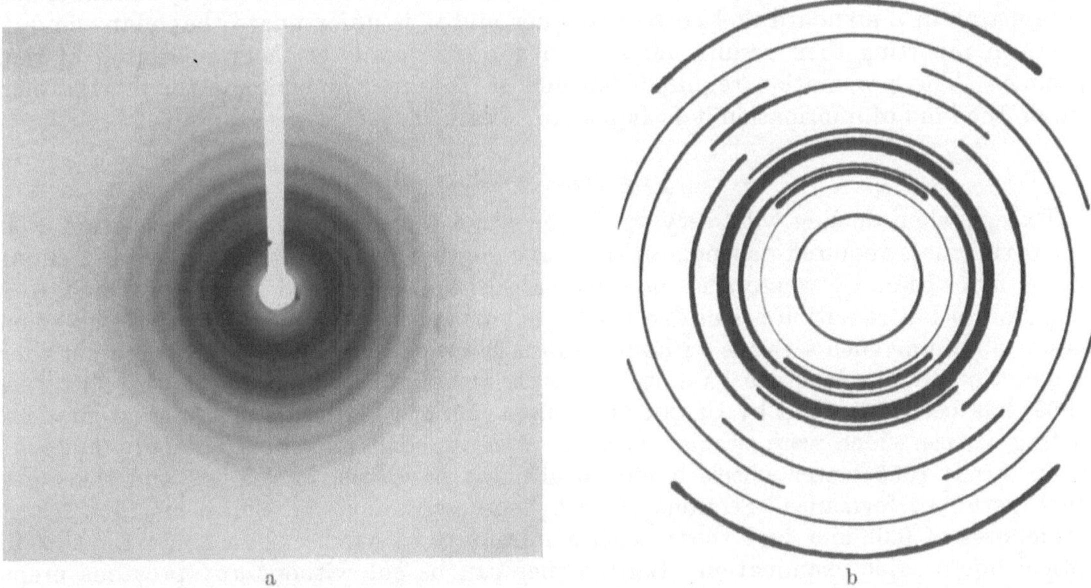

Fig. 3. a Roentgen ray diffraction pattern from a section of rat femur cut parallel to the long axis of the bone. b Drawing from original film of a on a slightly enlarged scale to show the "arcing" of the circles

drawn out by applying mechanical force the diffraction pattern changes and the rings instead of being uniform and continuous, show arcs of high density separated by regions of low density. This shows that the minute crystals which were formerly in a random arrangement in the wire have been orientated by the mechanical stress so that most of them have one lattice direction parallel to the direction of drawing. They are said to have a "preferred orientation" and in respect of one axis they are behaving as a single crystal but a "single" crystal made up of a large number of units each having one crystal direction approximately parallel to the axis of the wire but randomly orientated about this axis. We have much the same phenomenon in bone, in the case of long bones for example the sub-microscopic crystals of bone salt tend to orientate themselves with one direction parallel to the long axis of the bone. In this case, however, there is no mechanical stress imposing orientation but presumably the presence of organic fibres induces the growth of the crystals preferentially parallel to the fibre axis, which in turn is parallel to the long axis of the bone. This is discussed later.

Collagen and similar substances give a "fibre" diffraction diagram but the reason is slightly different. Here there are very long protein chains with units repeated at regular intervals along the chain and each chain is separated from its neighbours by a fixed distance determined by the length of the side chains. The pattern produced shows the effect of the chain spacing as a set of arcs parallel to the chain and a set of arcs in the perpendicular direction. There is no true three-dimensional crystalline lattice even on a submicroscopic scale but rather a series of repeating units in certain directions. Consequently the diffraction diagrams are of poor quality compared with ordinary crystalline material but in spite of this they have provided valuable information.

The roentgen ray diffraction pattern obtained by placing a flat film behind a section of a rat femur cut parallel to the long axis of the bone is shown in Fig. 3 (a). Since it is difficult to reproduce this kind of photograph to show the detail, a drawing is given in 3 (b). Many of the rings are incomplete because of the preferential orientation of the crystallites with respect to the axis of the bone.

b) Preparation of specimens for roentgen ray diffraction

It is most important with such a variable material as bone that the specimen should be prepared in a standard and correct manner and it is unfortunate that many investigators in reporting their results have failed to give details of the preparation of their specimen. The preparation required depends on the kind of bone, on the pretreatment and on the kind of information it is hoped to obtain.

α) Bone sections

Except when dealing with very small bones it is necessary to obtain a section. The actual thickness required depends on the wavelength of the roentgen rays but it should not be more than $1/\gamma$ where μ is the linear absorption coefficient for the wavelength in use. For such a radiation a suitable thickness of bone is 0.1 mm. The most convenient way of obtaining such sections without losing a large part of the specimen is to cut them on a section cutting machine. A suitable simple machine based on a design by Atkinson (1950) has been described by Clark and Iball (1955). The latter machine at first had cutting wheels which were circular discs of rubber bonded silicon-carbide only 0.075 mm thick. Since 1955 newer wheels based on alumina have been developed and these give much better performance. Sections of hard bone can be cut on such a machine having a thickness of 0.02 mm and these, with a minimum of hand finishing, are suitable for optical microscopic examination. Large bones can be cut without any previous preparation but small bones must first be embedded in some suitable medium e.g. methylmethacrylate. Some of the other softer embedding media have advantages for certain specimens. With such a machine it is possible to cut sections with known orientation to the macroscopic shape of the whole bone and from a definite location on the bone. It is, in addition, possible to use the same section, or a serial section, for examination with the light microscope and for micro-radiography.

β) Bone powder

Ground bone can be mounted in the form of a rod by mixing with an adhesive such as gum tragacanth and rolling on a glass slide. For this purpose it is best to make the rod about 0.3 mm diameter and to use the gum to dilute the bone powder so that the linear absorption coefficient is reduced. The gum itself produces no appreciable roentgen ray diffraction. The earliest workers calcined the bone before grinding but it was realised even then (DE JONG 1926) that the substance thus obtained is probably different from the mineral in untreated bone.

γ) Pre-treatment of bone

Because the diffraction pattern from whole untreated bone is so poor in comparison with normal crystalline substances various methods have been adopted in order to obtain an improvement. As mentioned above, calcining at high temperatures was used in the early days to remove the organic portion of bone. However although this is very effective in improving the sharpness of the diffraction lines and consequently in increasing the number of lines which can be observed it does not really assist in solving the problem of the constitution of the mineral of normal bone. In the first place heating to a high temperature (900° C) causes the sub-microscopic crystals to grow in size. This can happen only when *some* crystals grow at the expense of others. With a substance similar in structure to apatite this growth can mean substitution in the lattice of one kind of atom by another. But a more serious objections is that the heating can cause a complete transformation of the chemical nature of the mineral.

Milder methods of treatment have been tried with moderate success. DAWSON (1946) found that the diffraction pattern could be improved if the bone was first boiled in water for 24 hours and then digested with trypsin at p_H 8 for 4 or 5 days. It was pointed out however by BEAULIEU et al. (1950) that the improvement in the pattern was almost entirely due to the boiling alone and this was confirmed by CLARK and IBALL (1957). The effect of boiling may be partly due to slight growth of the crystallites but probably this is not the whole explanation. The manner in which the crystals are formed in the living tissue is not at all understood and it may be that they are to some extent "incomplete" and the lattice may consequently be "strained". The effect of boiling may be to give the atoms considerable mobility and that this strain may be removed. A similar effect is produced when strains in microscopic metal crystals are removed by annealing.

c) Early results obtained by roentgen ray diffraction

The earliest roentgen ray diffraction study of bone salts was carried out by DE JONG (1926). He showed that the pattern given by powdered bone was very similar to that given by the mineral fluorapatite. This established the fact that whatever the exact nature of bone salts the main constituent was a calcium phosphate complex which was crystalline and that the crystals had an apatite-like structure. TAYLOR and SHEARD (1929), who used both optical and roentgen ray diffraction methods, made a systematic comparison between several mineral apatites such as fluorapatite, dahllite and podolite on the one hand and normal bone, dental enamel, rachitic bone and several pathological calcified tissues on the other hand. Very similar diffraction patterns were obtained from all these substances. They showed that the substance $CaHPO_4 2\,H_2O$ (Brushite) gives a different diffraction pattern and thus removed *one* calcium phosphate from the list of those which had been suggested as constituents of bone.

The question as to whether carbonate, which is undoubtedly present in bone, is there as free calcium carbonate or whether the carbonate ion is incorporated in the apatite lattice continues to be debated up to the present time. One group of workers takes one view and the opposite view is held by another group.

d) More recent results obtained by roentgen ray diffraction

α) The nature of the crystals

There can be no doubt that the main inorganic constituent of bone is a calcium-phosphate with a crystal lattice which if not an apatite is almost indistinguishable from it. However of the many suggestions put forward as to the *exact* nature of this elusive structure only three need now be considered seriously. They are: (i) α-tricalcium phosphate with some free calcium carbonate; (ii) carbonate-apatite, in which the carbonate ion is an intrinsic part of an apatite lattice such as occurs in the mineral dahllite; (iii) hydroxyapatite with calcium carbonate adsorbed on the surface of the apatite crystals. These suggestions will now be discussed in turn.

(i) The main supporter of the α-tricalcium phosphate theory is Dallemagne (Brasseur, Dallemagne and Melon 1946). He claims that the roentgen ray diffraction pattern of bone is identical with that of α-tricalcium phosphate. This is not of great importance because of the poor quality of the bone diffraction patterns and because of the close similarity of the patterns of apatites and α-tricalcium phosphate. Strong support from chemical evidence is given by Cartier (1948a, 1948b, 1951) and by Barrand and Cartier (1951). According to these studies bone salt is supposed to consist of:

	%
α-tricalcium phosphate	74.6
Calcium carbonate	10.4
Disodium phosphate	2.46
Calcium citrate	2.0
Magnesium carbonate	1.03
Tricalcium phosphate	0.93
Ca^{++}, PO_4^{---} } Protein	8.76

Other evidence supporting Dallemagne's theory comes from refractive index measurements. Dallemagne and Melon (1944) and Dallemagne (1945) reported that the refractive indices of bone salts and of dentine were the same as that of a mixture of 90% α-tricalcium phosphate, 10% calcium carbonate viz. 1.590. When bone and dentine are calcined the refractive indices are 1.649 which is the value found for carbonate-apatite. Many workers have disagreed with the conclusions of Dallemagne but his theories are far from being disproved.

(ii) McConnell (1938, 1952) is perhaps the strongest advocate of the theory that bone salt is mainly an apatite in which the carbonate ion is an inherent constituent of the apatite lattice. It was Roseberry, Hastings and Morse (1931) who first stated that the roentgen ray diffraction pattern from bone salts resembled the mineral dahllite and Gruner, McConnell and Armstrong (1937) showed how carbon atoms could take the place of calcium and phosphorus in an apatite lattice.

(iii) The most widely held view is that bone salt consists mainly of hydroxyapatite, that is a calcium-phosphate complex which has crystallised in a lattice almost identical in size and shape to that of the mineral fluorapatite but with the fluorine sites occupied by oxygen atoms (chemically the F^- ions are replaced by $(OH)^-$ ions). This suggestion first made by Klement (1929) has been followed by many investigators since then (e.g. Carlström 1955) but it is very difficult to find any conclusive evidence to prove that this is the correct view.

It seems to be that although other substances are consistent with most of the experimental data hydroxyapatite is the most probable. This does however raise two important questions regarding calcium carbonate and water. $CaCO_3$ is generally supposed to be adsorbed on the surface of the hydroxyapatite crystals. It is not so easy, however, to explain how the water which is firmly bound to bone salt, is incorporated in the hydroxyapatite. On these two points and on the importance of surface reactions in bone mineralisation the recent book by Neuman and Neuman (1958) is most informative. These authors discuss also the most recent and certainly the most novel suggestion put forward to describe bone mineral. The suggestion made by Ascenzi (1952, 1956) is that the bone mineral forms a continuous honeycomb structure with organic material occupying the spaces in the honeycomb. Neuman and Neuman point out many of the obvious criticisms which can be made of such a structure but such a semicontinuous or micellar structure is an attractive idea when considering the inability of present theories of structure to explain mechanical properties of bone.

β) *The size of the bone crystals*

It is not possible to see the crystals of bone salt with an optical microscope and it is only with difficulty that they are observed with the electron microscope. The difficulty with the electron microscope may not be entirely due to the smallness of the crystals but because of the difficulty of preparing suitable specimens. It is not easy to cut sufficiently thin sections of such a hard material as bone and even when they can be produced there is the possibility that the cutting process may have caused changes which alter or mask the original structure. However electron-microscopy is the only satisfactory method for determining the size and shape of the crystals. Modern microscopes are capable of a resolution down to 10 Å and so we may expect that at least one problem will be solved satisfactorily in the near future. At the present time the evidence provided by the electron microscope suggests that the crystals are approximately 250 Å in length and 20—50 Å thick. It is unlikely that they are all the same size since in living bone inorganic material is continually being laid down and removed. There should therefore be crystals of all sizes up to some indeterminate maximum with a majority having some optinum size. No-one has yet produced an electron micrograph of a well formed crystal of bone salt so it seems safe to conclude that either they do not exist as distinct separate crystals as ASCENZI claims or they *never* grow to a size more than a few hundred Ångströms.

Roentgen ray diffraction gives some information on crystal size which in general supports the figures obtained from electron-microscopy. The diffraction lines of an roentgen ray pattern tend to broaden as the crystal size decreases from a certain value. This is an optical interference effect due to the decreasing number of repeating units. It is possible by measuring the width of the roentgen ray lines to estimate how large the crystals are. Another phenomenon "low angle scattering" also appears when the crystals are very small. In addition to the diffraction "lines" which normally appear the roentgen rays are scattered at a small angle (in the range 1 or 2 degress) to the primary beam in a continuous streak or hand. The extent of this scattering, which is similar to light scattering by a colloidal solution, gives an indication of the crystal or particle size. Both line-broadening and low-angle scatter experiments suggest that the bone crystals are approximately 200 × 65 Å (e.g. CARLSTRÖM and FINEAN 1954).

Since the crystals are so small the total surface area of all the crystals in a bone must be very large, perhaps 300 square metres per gram (NEUMAN and NEUMAN 1958). It is not surprising that surface reactions should be regarded as of extreme importance in the process of crystallisation and in the process of ion exchange.

γ) *The orientation of bone crystals*

It is necessary to define what is meant by orientation because a certain amount of unnecessary argument has taken place in the past and this would have been avoided if the different investigators had explained what they meant by orientation.

Some authors mean by "orientation" that a particular direction, or lattice axis, of the crystals is approximately parallel to some obvious direction of the bone. A good example is provided by the femur in which the crystals are usually arranged so that a majority of them have the hexagonal, or "c" axis nearly parallel to the "long" axis of the bone. This is clearly shown in an roentgen ray diffraction diagram of a section cut parallel to the long axis of the bone. Instead of the diffraction rings being uniform they are in the form of arcs. The arcs due to the (001) planes of the crystals appear on the photographic film along the line parallel to the line in the specimen which was parallel to the long axis of the bone from which it was cut. This means that the (001) planes are perpendicular to this direction. Because of the kind of hexagonal lattice in bone crystals the odd orders of diffraction from this plane are absent and so on the photographs we see only the even orders, usually indicated by the indices 002, 004 etc.

On the other hand other authors refer only to orientation of the crystals with respect to the collagen fibres in the bone. It is possible therefore for two investigators to say, of exactly the same specimen, that orientation does exist or that it does not exist and for *both* to be correct.

As regards orientation with respect to the whole bone it is well established that in adult long bones the minute inorganic crystals are arranged preferentially with their hexagonal axes parallel to the long direction of the bone. It so happens of course that the organic collagen fibres are in this case also parallel to the long axis of the bone and the crystals are therefore parallel to the fibres. It has been shown (Clark and Iball 1957) that in very young bones there is no evidence, from roentgen ray diffraction, of preferred orientation with respect to the shape of the whole bone. In the femur of rats it is only after about 3 days from birth that this orientation appears. In human bones orientation is present at birth but is absent in foetal bones until approximately 4 months' development has taken place. With the roentgen ray diffraction technique the pattern obtained is an average over the volume irradiated by the roentgen ray beam. It is usual to use sections of 0.1 mm thickness and the cross section of the roentgen ray beam is often 0.1 mm diameter. There is therefore no orientation, with respect to the shape of the whole bone, within this small volume of these immature bones. It may still be true, as is claimed by investigators using the electron-microscope (Glimcher 1959) that on a still smaller scale the crystals appear to be orientated parallel to individual collagen fibres. However it would seem to follow that if this is the case then the collagen fibres must be randomly arranged within this small volume ($0.1 \times 0.1 \times 0.1$ mm) of these young bones. Furthermore, since the pressure or absence of orientation, as demonstrated by roentgen ray diffraction, in the case of young rat bones covers only a few days of life this very profound change in the organisation of the structure of the *whole* bone must take place at an astonishing rate. There is still a great deal to be learnt about the changes which take place in the mineralisation of bone during the earliest stages of growth.

4. The mineral constituent in pathological bones

Many investigators have tried to find a correlation between the structure of the mineral constituent of bone and various pathological conditions. The results have been disappointing and it is probably true to say that no reliable evidence is available which would suggest that there is any significant difference between normal bones and diseased bones either as regards their constitution or their orientation within the tissue (Clark and Iball 1957). Bell et al. (1957) demonstrated a great change in the strength of bones from lathyritic rats. However there was no appreciable change in the percentage ash of the bones as compared with normal control rats nor was there any difference in the roentgen ray diffraction pattern. This absence of any apparent change in the mineral component of bone when such gross changes take place in the strength is difficult to understand. It has been suggested recently (Khogali 1960; Bell and Sharma 1960) that some of the differences in strength between normal and pathological bones are due to differences in the distribution of the bone material (e.g. sponginess) rather than to changes in the composition or structure of the bone material. In this field it is probable that the big advances being made in electron-microscope techniques will provide some much needed knowledge of the relation of the inorganic crystal with the organic fibres and ground substance.

I wish to thank Professor G. H. Bell for his valuable advice during the preparation of this chapter.

References

ASCENZI, A.: Structure of bone tissue as studied in electron microscope. Sci. med. ital. 3, 670—709 (1955).

ATKINSON, H. F.: A high speed section cutting machine. Brit. dent. J. 88, 29—31 (1950).

— Ground sections of enamel. Brit. dent. Ann. 144—149 (1952).

BARRAND, J., and P. CARTIER: Étude radiocristallographique de la demineralisation de l'os. C. R. Acad. Sci. (Paris) 232, 417—419 (1951).

BEAULIEU, M., H. BRASSEUR, M. J. DALLEMAGNE and J. MELON: Critique des méthods de minéralisation de l'os. Arch. int. Physiol. 57, 411—418 (1950).

BEEVERS, C. A., and D. B. MCINTYRE: The atomic structure of fluor-apatite and its relation to that of tooth and bone material. Min. Mag. 27, 254—257 (1946).

BELL, G. H., O. DUNBAR, J. A. GILLESPIE, J. IBALL and J. OLIVER: Effect of sweet-pea poisoning on strength of bone and skin. J. Physiol. (Lond.) 139, 17—18 (1957).

—, and D. N. SHARMA: Quantitative effects of β-aminopropionitrite on bone growth. J. Physiol. (Lond.) 154, 46P. (1960).

BERZELIUS, J.: Über basische phosphorsaure Kalkerde. Justus Liebigs Ann. Chem. 53, 286—288 (1845).

BRASSEUR, H., M. J. DALLEMAGNE and J. MELON: Chemical nature of salts from bones and teeth and of tricalcium phosphate precipitates. Nature (Lond.) 157, 453 (1946).

CAGLIOTI, V., A. ASCENZI and A. SANTORO: On the interpretation of the low-angle scatter of X-rays from bone tissue. Experientia (Basel) 12, 305—306 (1956).

CARLSTRÖM, D.: X-ray crystallographic studies on apatites and calcified structures. Acta radiol. (Stockh.) Suppl. A 7—59, 121—124 (1955).

—, and J. B. FINEAN: X-ray diffraction studies on the ultrastructure of bone. Biochem. biophys. Acta 13, 183—191 (1954).

CARTIER, P.: Les constituants minéraux des tissus calcifiés. I. La structure minérale de l'os, de la dentine et du cément. Bull. Soc. Chem. biol. 30, 65—73 (1948a).

— Les constituants minéraux des tissus calcifiés. II. La structure moléculaire du selt de l'os. Bull. Soc. Chem. biol. 30, 73—81 (1948b).

— Les constituants minéraux des tissus calcifiés; les premiers stades de l'ossification. Bull. Soc. Chem. biol. 33, 155—160 (1951).

CLARK, S. M., and J. IBALL: The preparation of thin bone sections. J. sci. Instrum. 32, 366—367 (1955).

CLARK, S. M., and J. IBALL: The X-ray crystal analysis of bone. Progr. Biophysics 7, 225—253 (1957).

DALLEMAGNE, M. J.: Données récentes sur la nature et le métabolisme de l'os actualitiés biochemiques, Part 2, p. 1—68. Paris: Masson, Liège: Desoer 1945.

—, and J. MELON: La proportion des éléments minéraux et organiques dans les différentes régions du système Haversien de l'os. C. R. Soc. Biol. 138, 1031—1034 (1944).

DAWSON, J. M.: X-ray diffraction pattern of bone: evidence of reflections due to organic constituent. Nature (Lond.) 157, 660—661 (1946).

GLIMCHER, M. J.: Molecular biology of mineralized tissues with particular reference to bone. Rev. mod. Phys. 31, 359—393 (1959).

— Calcification in biological systems (Edit. R. F. SOGNNAES). Amer. Assoc. Adv. Sci., Washinton, D. C., U.S.A. 421—487, 1960.

GRUNER, J. W., D. MCCONNELL and W. D. ARMSTRONG: The relationship between crystal structure and chemical composition of enamel and dentin. J. biol. Chem. 121, 771—781 (1937).

HOPPE-SEYLER, F.: Untersuchungen über die Constitution des Zahnschmelzes. Arch. path. Anat. u. Physiol. 24, 13—32 (1862).

JONG, W. F. DE: Le substance mineral dans les os. Rec. Trav. chim. Pays-Bas 45, 445—448 (1926).

KHOGALI, A.: Bone strength and calcium retention of rats in hypervitaminosis. J. Physiol. (Lond.) 154, 45—46 (1960).

KLEMENT, R.: Die Zusammensetzung der Knochenstützsubstanz. Hoppe-Seylers Z. physiol. Chem. 184, 132—142 (1929).

MCCONNELL, D.: A structural investigation of the isomorphism of the apatite group. Amer. Mineralogist 23, 1—19 (1938).

— The crystal chemistry of francolite and its relationship to calcified animal tissues. Trans. Macy Conf. on Metabol. Interrel. 4, 169—184 (1952).

NARAY-SZABO, ST.: Structure of fluorapatite. Z. Kristallogr. 75, 387—398 (1930).

NEUMAN, W. F., and M. W. NEUMAN: The chemical dynamics of bone mineral. Chicago: University Chicago Press 1958.

ROSEBERRY, H. H., A. B. HASTINGS and J. K. MORSE: X-ray analysis of bone and teeth. J. biol. Chem. 90, 395—407 (1931).

TAYLOR, N. W., and C. SHEARD: Microscopic and X-ray investigations on the calcification of tissue. J. biol. Chem. 81, 479—493 (1929).

B. Biochemie des Knochens

Von

H.-J. Dulce

Mit 13 Abbildungen

Das Knochengewebe ist die wichtigste Stützsubstanz des menschlichen Organismus. Vom Wachstum des Knochens hängt das Längenwachstum des Menschen ab. Ca. 10% des Körpergewichtes entfallen auf das Knochengewebe. Unter diesem Gewebe versteht man im strengen biochemischen Sinne den periost-, mark- und blutfreien Knochen. Er läßt sich für die Analyse am besten als Corticalis der Diaphysen oder als Flachknochen, etwa Calvaria, gewinnen.

Bausteine des Knochens

I. Quantitative Zusammensetzung des Knochens

1. Fett-, Wasser-, Mineral-, Matrix-Anteile

Kompakter Knochen besteht beim Erwachsenen anteilig aus ca. 4 % Fett, ca. 12 % Wasser, ca. 24 % organischer Matrix und ca. 60 % Mineral. Typische spongiöse Teile des Skelets lassen sich nur selten von Mark und Blut so vollständig befreien, daß die Analyse der Frischsubstanz mit der der Corticalis-Frischsubstanz unmittelbar vergleichbar wird. Epiphysen oder andere spongiosahaltige Knochenabschnitte, die beim Erwachsenen mehr Fettmark enthalten, haben ca. 35% Fett, ca. 25% Wasser, ca. 20% Matrix und ca. 20% Mineralanteil. Spongiosaknochen, wie z.B. Wirbelkörper, die mehr blutbildendes Mark enthalten, besitzen ca. 10% Fett, aber ca. 45% Wasser, ca. 20% Mineral und ca. 25% organische Matrix. Zahnschmelz besteht dagegen zu ca. 4,3% aus Wasser, zu ca. 0,7% aus Matrix und zu ca. 95% aus Mineral. Dentin ist etwa wie Knochencorticalis zusammengesetzt.

Tabelle 1. *Altersabhängige Zusammensetzung von Knochencorticalis des Menschen* (H. Brubacher, 1890; Z. Ruiz-Gijon, 1941)

	Femur Corticalis Fetus	Femur Corticalis Kind 4 J. alt	Tibia Corticalis Erwachsener
Mineralgehalt in % FG	39	48	62
Organische Matrix in % FG	24	25	25
Wassergehalt in % FG	37	27	13

Analysen auf fettfreie Frischsubstanz bezogen.

Um Analysen von Knochen verschiedener Skeletabschnitte und Entwicklungsstadien untereinander vergleichen zu können, muß man auf die entfettete Frischsubstanz oder die entfettete Trockensubstanz beziehen. In einem derartigen Bezugssystem sieht man, daß sich jugendlicher und embryonaler Knochen vom reifen Knochen unterscheidet (Tabelle 1). Der Anteil der organischen Matrix an der fettfreien Knochencorticalis bleibt aber ziemlich konstant. In stärker spongiosahaltigen Knochenabschnitten nimmt dagegen im Laufe des Wachstums der Matrixanteil erheblich zu (Tabelle 2). Gleichzeitig erkennt man in höheren Lebensaltern die Abnahme des Wassergehaltes und die gleichzeitige Zunahme des Mineralgehaltes.

Grundsätzlich ist Knochencompacta mineralisierter als die Spongiosa, was sich auf die Zusammensetzung von Röhrenknochen, Flachknochen und Wirbelkörpern besonders auswirkt. In der Compacta finden wir ein Verhältnis von Matrix zu Mineral von ca. 1 : 2,5, in der Spongiosa von ca. 1,2 : 1,0. Auf diese Weise sind bei den einzelnen Knochen die verschiedenen Anteile an der fettfreien Trockensubstanz zu erklären.

Knochen von Frauen ist offensichtlich etwas weniger mineralisiert als der von Männern (Tabelle 3).

Die Dichte des Knochens ist ein weiteres Maß für seinen Mineralisationsgrad. Frischer Knochen des erwachsenen Menschen hat eine Dichte von 1,86—1,9 g/ml (R. A. ROBINSON,

Tabelle 2. *Altersabhängige Zusammensetzung fettfreier, spongiosahaltiger Knochen-Frischsubstanz*

	Wassergehalt % FG	% Matrix	% Mineral	
			a)	b)
Gesamtfemur				
Fetus, 12—14 Wochen	77,8	8,9	6,6	9,0
Fetus, 30—34 Wochen	63,8	12,9	15,2	15,5
Neugeborenes	63,9	15,0	16,4	17,0
Kind, 1—2 Jahre	55,4	18,9	18,8	19,5
Kind, 11—12 Jahre	36,4	21	37,3	37,5
Erwachsener, 18—35 Jahre	22,7	22,1	52,4	49,8
Femur, Epiphyse				
Fetus, 12—14 Wochen	85,6	6,9	0,2	0,8
Fetus, 30—34 Wochen	83,7	10,5	0,3	0,5
Neugeborenes	79,2	13,2	0,7	0,8
Kind, 1—2 Jahre	72,5	18	3,3	3,2
Kind, 11—12 Jahre	50,1	22,1	20,9	21,4

Die Tabelle beruht auf Analysen des Wassergehaltes, Gesamtstickstoffgehaltes, Ca- und P-Gehaltes von DICKERSON (1962). Als mittlerer Umrechnungsfaktor von N in organische Matrix wurde 5,5 verwendet (Umrechnungsfaktor N in Kollagen = 5,4). Der Mineralgehalt wurde unter a durch Multiplikation des Calciumgehalts mit 2,7 und unter b durch Multiplikation des Phosphatgehalts mit 6,0 ermittelt.

1955; H. Q. WOODARD, 1962; B. E. KEANE, 1959). Aus Corticalis isoliertes Knochenmineral hat eine Dichte von 2,93—3,06 g/ml (R. A. ROBINSON, 1957; H. STEGEMANN, 1960; J. MUENDEZ, 1960), aus Spongiosa isoliertes von 2,72 g/ml. Die Dichte des synthetischen Hydroxylapatits beträgt 3,18 g/ml, die der organischen Matrix 1,45 g/ml und die des

Tabelle 3. *Aschegehalt der Knochen in % fettfreier Trockensubstanz (FTS)*

	Aschegehalt in % FTS Männer	Aschegehalt in % FTS Frauen
Mandibula	69,53	68,80
Humerus	67,04	66,44
Tibia	67,25	66,33
Patella	67,02	65,44
Sternum	63,02	61,57
Sacrum	63,92	62,55

Die angegebenen Zahlen sind Mittelwerte der Analysen von Knochen bei 60 Personen (M. TROTTER, 1962).

Tabelle 4. *Analysen der Corticalis von Tibiaknochen des Hundes* (nach R. A. ROBINSON, 1957)

Dichte g/ml	H_2O-Gehalt % FG	Aschegehalt (600°) % FG	CO_2-Raum[1] % FG	Matrixgehalt % FG
2,10	8,1	60,9	8,5	22,5
2,00	12,2	58,1	8,1	21,6
1,80	21,7	51,5	7,1	19,7
1,60	33,6	43,2	6,0	17,2
1,40	49	32,5	4,5	14,0
1,30	58,4	26,0	3,5	12,1

[1] Berechnet als Glühverlust bei 105—600° abzüglich Matrixgehalt. (FG = Frischgewicht)

CO_2-Raumes 2,08 g/ml (R. A. ROBINSON, 1957). Tierexperimentelle Analysen haben gezeigt, daß sich Matrix und Mineralgehalt konstant proportional und der Wassergehalt konstant umgekehrt proportional zur Dichte verhalten (R. A. ROBINSON, 1957) (Tabelle 4).

Es ist deshalb in gewissen Grenzen zulässig, aus der Dichte, also einer volumenbezogenen Gewichtsangabe, auf den Mineralisationsgrad eines Knochens zu schließen, wenn das Knochenmark entfernt ist.

Vielfach wird aber der Mineralisationsgrad des Knochens aufgrund einer Messung der Röntgendichte als mg Hydroxylapatit/ml Knochen angegeben. Dieser Wert läßt keine direkte Aussage über die Mineralisation der Matrix zu, weil hierbei in das Volumen der gesamte Markraum eingeht. Man bestimmt vielmehr in vivo den Apatitanteil am Knochen und am vom Knochen umschlossenen Markraum. Er beträgt beim Erwachsenen:

Tabelle 5. *Analysenwerte*

Femur, Humerus, Ulna, Radius, Wirbel, Handknochen	250—400 mg/ml	F. HEUCK (1960, 1960a), E. KROKOWSKI (1959), H. OESER (1963), B. E. KEANE (1959), K. M. MAYO (1961), P. STRUG (1964)
Scapula, Rippe, Calcaneus	170—250 mg/ml	F. HEUCK (1960, 1960a), E. KROKOWSKI (1959), W. GRASSMANN (1952)
Calvaria	bis 980 mg/ml	F. HEUCK (1960, 1960a)
Knochen- Compacta	600—800 mg/ml	F. HEUCK (1960, 1960a)

In Knochen der rechten Körperhälfte findet man ca. 9% mehr Mineral/Volumen als in denen der linken Körperhälfte (P. VIRTAMA, 1957). Im Säuglingsalter ist der Apatitgehalt im Calcaneus geringer [93 mg/ml (F. HEUCK, 1960, 1960a)]. Die größte Röntgendichte der Knochen wird zwischen 20 und 40 Jahren erreicht (F. HEUCK, 1960, 1960a; E. KROKOWSKI, 1959). Im höheren Lebensalter nimmt die Röntgendichte bis zu 20% ab (E. KROKOWSKI, 1959).

a) Bestimmungsmethodik

Methodisch ermittelt man im Knochen:
den Fettgehalt
 durch mehrmalige Aceton-Ätherextraktion;
den Wassergehalt
 durch Gefriertrocknung,
 durch Trocknung bei 105°;
den Mineralgehalt
 durch Formamidaufschluß (H. STEGEMANN, 1960),
 durch *Autoclavieren* (R. A. ROBINSON, 1955),
 durch Veraschung bei 500°,
 durch Röntgendichtemessung,
 durch KOH-Glycerin-Aufschluß nach GABRIEL (1894);
den Matrixgehalt einschließlich Zellgehalt
 durch Entkalkung mit Äthylendiamintetraessigsäure (ÄDTE) (10% pH 7,5),
 durch Säureentkalkung (1n HCl, 7,5%ige Essigsäure),
 durch Differenz: fettfreie Trockensubstanz — Mineralgehalt;
die Dichte
 durch Wägung eines Volumens (R. A. ROBINSON, 1957).

Der als Aschegehalt bestimmte Mineralanteil liegt um ca. 6% niedriger als der Tatsache entspricht, weil beim Glühen zwischen 105—600° CO_2 und Kristallwasser aus dem Knochenmineral verdampfen.

2. Zellanteile

Im Anteil der organischen Matrix ist ein kleiner Prozentsatz Zelltrockensubstanz enthalten, der bei den meisten Analysen vernachlässigt wird. Analytische Aussagen über an Knochenzellen gebundene Stoffwechselfunktionen (Enzymaktivitäten u.a.) werden aber manchmal auf den Zell- oder Desoxyribonucleinsäuregehalt bezogen. Der Gehalt an Zelltrockensubstanz beträgt beim Erwachsenen im kompakten Knochen der Corticalis und in fettmarkreichen spongiösen Epiphysenabschnitten ca. 1% des Frischgewichtes, beim Kind in der Compacta ca. 2,4% und in der Spongiosa ca. 4%, beim Feten in der Compacta bis zu 8% und in der Spongiosa ca. 4% des Frischgewichtes. Spongiosaknochen, die mehr blutbildendes Mark enthalten, haben einen Zellgehalt um ca. 5% des Frischgewichtes. Die Werte wurden aufgrund der Analysen von DICKERSON (1962) vom Verfasser errechnet. Die höheren Zellanteile bei jugendlichen und embryonalen Knochen gehen mit einem geringen Fettgehalt, im Fall der embryonalen Compacta auch mit einem geringeren Mineralgehalt einher.

a) Bestimmungsmethodik

Der Zellgehalt wird methodisch ermittelt durch Bestimmung der Desoxyribonucleinsäure (DNS) (F. KÖRBER, 1964; J. D. BIGGERS, 1961; G. M. VAES, 1963, 1962) und durch Bestimmung des Nichtkollagen Stickstoffs (DICKERSON, 1962; A. B. BORLE, 1960).

II. Struktur der Knochenbausteine

1. Das Knochenmineral

Das Knochenmineral gehört in die Gruppe der Calciumphosphate und setzt sich aus folgenden Bausteinen zusammen:

Calcium ca. 34—37%
anorganisches Phosphat ca. 48—51%
Carbonat ca. 6—7%
Natrium 0,4—0,8%
Magnesium 0,4—0,6%
Kalium 0,2%
Fluor ca. 0,01—0,3% (ISAAK, 1958)
Chlor ca. 0,1%
Blei ca. 0,001% (GOSSMANN, 1967)
Wasserstoff ca. 0,2%
Hydroxylionen ca. 3%
Citrat ca. 1%.

Dentinmineral unterscheidet sich vom übrigen Knochenmineral durch einen geringeren Calciumgehalt von ca. 34% und den höheren Magnesiumgehalt von ca. 0,9% (C. D. CROWELL, 1934). Zahnschmelz zeigt dagegen einen bedeutend geringeren Gehalt an Magnesium (0,2%), Carbonat (ca. 4%) und Citrat (0,1%), aber einen etwas höheren Phosphatgehalt von ca. 53%. HENDRICKS und HILLS (1942) geben die molare Zusammensetzung isolierter anorganischer Knochensubstanz pro Kilogramm an:

Ca 8,5 Mol	PO_4 5,07 Mol
Mg 0,25 Mol	CO_3 1,24 Mol
Na 0,19 Mol	OH 2 Mol
H 2 Mol.	

Das Citrat wird häufig auf der Seite der organischen Matrix erfaßt, obwohl es als Coprecipitat eigentlich zum Knochenmineral gehört. Im Dentin kommt Citrat als stabiler Citrat-Peptid-Komplex vor, der sich mit dem Mineral über polare Carboxylgruppen verbinden soll (A. G. LEAVER, 1960; R. L. HARTLES, 1960).

Der molare oder der gewichtsmäßige Ca/P-Quotient läßt unabhängig vom Bezugssystem der verwerteten Calcium- und Phosphor-Analysen Aussagen über die Art des Knochenminerals zu, solange nicht größere Anteile von organischen Phosphaten oder chelatgebundenem Calcium vorliegen. Will man diesen Fehler bei Calcium- und Phosphatanalysen ausschalten, muß man die Knochentrockensubstanz schonend von Matrix durch Formamidaufschluß oder KOH-Glycerinextraktion befreien. Der Ca/P-Quotient zeigt, daß Knochen- und Zahnmineral tertiärem Calciumphosphat nahestehen (Tabelle 6).

Weiteren Aufschluß über die kristallchemische Struktur des Knochenminerals geben Röntgenbeugungsdiagramme nach DEBYE-SCHERRER. Das Knochenmineral zeigt etwa dieselben Beugungslinien und Längen der kristallographischen Axen wie ein synthetischer, bei 360° unter 200 Atmosphären Druck aus β-Tricalciumphosphat, Calciumcarbonat und Wasser hergestellter Hydroxylapatit (O. R. TRAUTZ, 1955).

Durch Erhitzen auf 900° wird das Beugungsdiagramm von Knochenmineral und Carbonat angereichertem Hydroxylapatit in das eines reinen Hydroxylapatits umgewandelt. Da im Knochenmineral, Schmelzmineral und im synthetischen Carbonat angereicherten Hydroxylapatit der Carbonatgehalt nicht zu einer Verkürzung der a-Achse wie

Tabelle 6

	Ca/P-Gewichts-quotient	Molarer Ca/P-Quotient
Knochenmineral	2,16—2,35	1,67—1,81
Dentinmineral	2,13	1,65
Schmelzmineral	2,09	1,59
$Ca_{10}(PO_4, CO_3)_6 ((OH)_2)$	2,21—2,59	1,60—2,0
$Ca_{10}(PO_4)_6(OH)_2$ / $Ca_{10}(PO_4)_6CO_3$ / $Ca_{10}(PO_4)_6F_2$	2,16	1,67
$C_9H_2(PO_4)_6 \cdot (OH)_2$ / $Ca_3(PO_4)_2$	1,94	1,5
$Ca_8H_2(PO_4)_6 \cdot 5H_2O$	1,71	1,33
$CaHPO_4 \cdot 2H_2O$	1,29	1,0

im Dahlit führt, muß ein großer Teil des Carbonats außerhalb des eigentlichen Kristallgitters gebunden sein. Der im Kristallgitter gebundene Carbonatanteil von ca. $^1/_5$ des Gesamtcarbonats ersetzt teilweise wahrscheinlich Phosphat (D. McCONNELL, 1955), teilweise aber OH, wodurch Gitterunregelmäßigkeiten auftreten. Für diese Vorstellung spricht, daß sich Knochenmineral beim Erhitzen von 600 auf 900° wie Dahlit verhält und CO_2 abgibt, sowie bei 878/72 cm^{-2} eine Deformationsschwingung im Infrarotspektrum auftritt (M. GADE, 1963). Die CO_2-Abgabe beträgt ca. 1% (M. J. DALLEMAGNE, 1956). Eine

Tabelle 7. *Längen der kristallographischen a- und c-Achsen von verschiedenen synthetischen Apatiten und Knochenmineral* (O. R. TRAUTZ, 1955)

	a-Achse	b-Achse	% CO_2
Francolit, F-haltiger Carbonatapatit	9,340 Å	6,890 Å	3,36
Fluorapatit	9,373	6,882	0
Dahlit, Carbonatapatit	9,394	6,890	ca. 5
OH-Apatit	9,421	6,881	0
Synthetischer CO_3-angereicherter OH-Apatit	9,448	6,881	1,3
Knochenmineral	9,43	6,88	ca. 6
Schmelzmineral	9,441	6,884	ca. 3

selbständige kristalline Phase von Calciumcarbonat konnte bisher, von einer Ausnahme abgesehen (C. HENSCHEN, 1932), in Röntgenbeugungsdiagrammen von Knochen- und Zahnmineral nicht erkannt werden (C. HUGGINS, 1937; S. MORGULIS, 1931; H. H. ROSEBERRY, 1931; O. R. TRAUTZ, 1955). Auch Löslichkeitsversuche mit Knochenmineral sprechen gegen ein selbständiges Calciumcarbonat (M. J. DALLEMAGNE, 1956; J. RAAFLAUB, 1961). Lediglich im Malleus und Incus des Menschen und in Otolithen von Salamandern konnte man röntgenographisch ein selbständig kristallines Calciumcarbonat nachweisen (W. F. NEUMAN, 1950). Anscheinend ist Carbonat im Knochenmineral zusammen mit anderen Ionen, eventuell auch noch mit Calcium amorph copräcipitiert und an den Oberflächen adsorbiert (S. B. HENDRICKS, 1950; O. R. TRAUTZ, 1955; R. KLEMENT, 1929, 1932; W. F. BALE, 1936). Das erklärt, weshalb Knochenmineral beim Erhitzen auf 600° ca.

4,3 % CO_2 verliert. Dieses CO_2, entsprechend $^4/_5$ der Gesamtmenge, kann nur aus leicht mobilisierbarem Carbonat stammen (M. J. DALLEMAGNE, 1956). Neuerdings konnte EANES (1966) durch quantitative Röntgenstrukturanalyse von Rinder- und Rattenknochen nachweisen, daß ca. 60 % des Knochenminerals in kristalliner und ca. 40 % in metastabiler amorpher oder besser mikrokristalliner Phase vorliegen. Magnesium- und Carbonationen stabilisieren diese mikrokristalline Phase, die sonst leicht in die stabile kristalline übergeht. Es ist zu vermuten, daß diese amorphe Phase beim Kristallisationsvorgang eine besondere Bedeutung hat.

Aufgrund dieser Befunde sollte man das Knochenmineral als ein mit amorphen Phasen durchsetztes carbonathaltiges apatitisches Calciumphosphat von unregelmäßigem Gitterbau bezeichnen. BAUD (1964) spricht von einem Gemisch aus Carbonatohydroxylapatit und Carbonatofluorapatit. In dem unregelmäßigen, hexagonalen Kristallgitter sind neben den Einheitszellen

des Hydroxylapatits $Ca_{10}(PO_4)_6 \cdot (OH)_2$,
des Carbonatapatits $Ca_{10}(PO_4)_6 \cdot CO_3$,
des carbonatsubstituierten Hydroxylapatits $Ca_{10}(PO_4CO_3)_6 \cdot (OH)_2$
und des Fluorapatits $Ca_{10}(PO_4)_6F_2$

auch Einheitszellen, die im Infrarotspektrum eine für H-Brücken charakteristische Absorption bei 3400 cm^{-1} zeigen, vertreten. (W. E. BROWN, 1962; D. TAVES, 1963). Zu diesen Einheitszellen gehören:

α-Tricalciumphosphathydrat = Defektapatit $Ca_9H_2(PO_4)_6 \cdot (OH)_2$,
Octacalciumphosphat $Ca_8H_2(PO_4)_6 \cdot 5\,H_2O$.

Defektapatit besitzt ein dem Hydroxylapatit isomorphes Kristallgitter mit den Achslängen 9,42—9,44 Å = a-Achse und 6,88 Å = c-Achse (A. S. POSNER, 1964; O. R. TRAUTZ, 1955; D. CARLSTROEM, 1956). Octacalciumphosphat hat dagegen ein anderes hexagonales Gitter mit den Achslängen a = 19,87 Å, b = 9,63 Å und c = 6,88 Å (W.E. BROWN, 1962). Octacalciumphosphat geht durch Hydrolyse insbesondere in Gegenwart von Fluoridionen leicht in Hydroxylapatit über. Die Netzebenenabstände (dhkl-Werte) der Apatite und verwandter Calciumphosphate im Vergleich zum unveraschten Knochenmineral zeigt Tabelle 8.

Isomorphe Substitution von Hydroxyl durch F bewirkt eine Vergrößerung der Apatitkristalle in Richtung der a-Achsen (H. SCHRAER, 1962; J. MENZEL, 1962; I. ZIPKIN, 1962). Dabei werden die spezifischen Oberflächen geringer und die Löslichkeit schlechter. Gleichzeitig verringert sich der Citratgehalt des Knochenminerals.

Ca. 40 % des Knochennatriums haben Calcium im Gitter isomorph ersetzt (T. G. TAYLOR, 1960; W. F. NEUMAN, 1962). Nach neueren Untersuchungen vermag auch Magnesium, das mit 0,065 *nm* einen kleineren Ionenradius als Natrium hat (0,098 *nm*), anstelle von Calcium in das Gitter einzutreten. Sechs Calciumatome des Apatitgitters sind leichter substituierbar als die anderen vier (O. R. TRAUTZ, 1955).

Alle anderen Mineralbausteine wie Cl, K, Citrat, sowie ein großer Teil des Na, Mg und CO_3 sind an der Oberfläche der Kristalle adsorbiert, Citrat und Carbonat offensichtlich als Copräcipitat besonders fest (T. G. TAYLOR, 1960a; A. C. KUYPER, 1938).

Eine einheitliche Formel für die kristalline Phase des Knochenminerals und eine statistische Verteilung der im Knochenmineral vorliegenden Kristallgitter kann man nicht angeben. In beiden Kristallgittern sind, wie gezeigt werden konnte, nicht stöchiometrische Substitutionen nach dem Prinzip:

$$(Ca, H., Na. Mg)_{10}(PO_4CO_3)_6(OH, F, CO_3)_2$$
$$\text{und} \quad (Ca, Na)_8H_2(PO_4CO_3)_6 \cdot 5\,H_2O$$

möglich. Im Knochenmineral des Erwachsenen ist der Bautyp des apatitischen Calciumphosphats fast ausschließlich vertreten. Das Gitter des Octacalciumphosphats findet man im Knochenmineral jüngerer Individuen (QUICKER, 1968).

Tabelle 8. *d_{hkl}-Werte von den Verbindungen Fluorapatit, Hydroxylapatit, Octacalciumphosphat, Calciumhydrogenphosphat, Calcit, Aragonit, Whitlockit*

$Ca_{10}(PO_4)_6F_2$ ASTM 3—0736		$Ca_{10}(PO_4)_6(OH)_2$ ASTM 9—432		$Ca_8H_2(PO_4)_6 5H_2O$ ASTM 11—184		$CaHPO_4$ ASTM 9—80		Calcit ASTM 5—0586		Aragonit ASTM 5—0453		Whitlockit ASTM 9—169	
d_{hkl}	I/I_1	d_{hkl}	I/I_1	d_{hkl}	I/I_1	d_{hkl}	I/I_1	d_{hkl}	I/I_1	d_{hkl}	I/I_1	d_{hkl}	I/I_1
				18,6	100								
				9,46	70								
				9,07	70								
		8,17	11									8,15	11
						6,74	13						
				5,52	60							6,49	15
						5,43	3					6,22	5
		5,26	5									5,21	20
				5,08	50								
						4,99	5						
												4,80	1
		4,72	3										
				4,46	50	4,48	1						
						4,38	3					4,39	7
				4,27	40	4,27	3			4,21	2		
		4,07	9			4,03	5					4,06	15
												4,00	3
				3,91	50								
		3,88	9	3,85	50			3,86	12				
				3,74	60	3,70	3						
				3,65	80								
		3,51	1										
				3,48	50	3,48	13						
3,44	20	3,44	40	3,43	100							3,45	25
										3,396	100	3,40	3
				3,38	50	3,37	70						
						3,35	75					3,36	9
				3,32	50	3,33	17						
						3,30	9						
				3,27	50					3,273	52	3,25	7
				3,22	50							3,21	55
		3,17	11	3,17	50								
						3,13	20					3,11	1
						3,10	5						
3,07	30	3,08	17										
				3,05	60			3,035	100				
				3,02	50								
				2,99	40	2,986	3						
				2,95	40	2,958	100						
						2,93	35						
						2,91	5						
						2,881	9			2,871	4	2,88	100
				2,85	50	2,867	3						
				2,84	100	2,843	1	2,845	3				
				2,83	100								
2,81	100	2,814	100										
2,78	40	2,778	60	2,77	60	2,763	9						
				2,75	60	2,754	20					2,757	20
2,71	60	2,72	60			2,721	35			2,73	9		
										2,70	46	2,71	9
				2,69	30								
				2,67	70							2,67	7
2,63	30	2,63	25	2,64	60								
				2,60	60							2,607	65
						2,581	3						
												2,562	5
				2,55	50							2,553	7

d_{hkl} = Netzebenenabstand. ASTM = American Society for Testing Materials.

Tabelle 8. (Fortsetzung)

$Ca_{10}(PO_4)_6F_2$ ASTM 3—0736		$Ca_{10}(PO_4)_6(OH)_2$ ASTM 9—432		$Ca_8H_2(PO_4)_6 5H_2O$ ASTM 11—184		$CaHPO_4$ ASTM 9—80		Calcit ASTM 5—0586		Aragonit ASTM 5—0453		Whitlockit ASTM 9—169	
d_{hkl}	I/I_1	d_{hkl}	I/I_1	d_{hkl}	I/I_1	d_{hkl}	I/I_1	d_{hkl}	I/I_1	d_{hkl}	I/I_1	d_{hkl}	I/I_1
2,53	5	2,528	5			2,532	3					2,520	11
						2,499	15	2,495	14			2,499	5
						2,489	1			2,481	33		
				2,45	50	2,443	1						
						2,411	1			2,409	14	2,407	9
										2,372	38	2,375	5
						2,351	3			2,341	31		
				2,33	100	2,305	9			2,328	6		
2,30	5	2,296	7	2,29	50	2,287	3	2,285	18				
2,26	20	2,262	20	2,26	40	2,251	15					2,263	9
						2,242	5					2,249	3
						2,234	9					2,241	1
		2,28	1	2,21	60	2,216	3						
						2,199	13					2,195	13
						2,189	3			2,188	11		
						2,160	11					2,165	11
2,14	10	2,148	9	2,15	60	2,139	7						
						2,117	7						
				2,10	50	2,105	3			2,106	23	2,103	3
				2,08	50	2,089	7	2,095	18			2,076	7
		2,065	7			2,070	5					2,068	3
2,06	10											2,061	5
		2,04	1			2,032	7					2,033	9
												2,023	5
				2,01	50	2,013	1					2,017	3
2,000	5	2,000	5			1,996	7					2,000	7
						1,986	5			1,977	65	1,970	1
				1,95	50	1,959	3						
1,94	40	1,943	30	1,95	50							1,946	3
						1,936	1	1,927	5			1,433	20
						1,915	17						
1,89	10	1,89	15			1,885	1			1,882	32	1,895	15
		1,871	5	1,86	100	1,869	7	1,875	17	1,877	25	1,879	13
1,84	60	1,841	40	1,84	60	1,850	20					1,830	11
1,80	30	1,806	20			1,799	7			1,814	23	1,812	5
1,77	30	1,78	11			1,772	5					1,781	5
1,75	30	1,754	15			1,755	5			1,759	4	1,774	7
						1,725	20			1,728	15	1,728	25
1,72	30	1,722	20									1,711	7
						1,703	1						
						1,690	5			1,698	3		
		1,684	3			1,684	5					1,685	7
						1,679	5						
						1,667	5					1,665	3
						1,652	7						
1,64	10	1,644	9			1,643	5					1,637	5
						1,620	1	1,626	4			1,625	5
1,61	5	1,611	7			1,609	7	1,604	8			1,603	5
		1,587	3					1,587	2				
1,54	5	1,542	5							1,557	4	1,552	11
1,52	5	1,53	5					1,525	5	1,535	2	1,532	3
1,50	10	1,503	9					1,510	4	1,499	4	1,505	3
1,47	20	1,474	11					1,473	2	1,475	3		
1,46	10	1,465	3							1,460	5	1,465	5
1,45	10												
1,43	10							1,44	5			1,44	3
								1,422	3			1,429	3
										1,411	5	1,414	3
								1,339	2	1,328	2		

Tabelle 8. (Fortsetzung)

$Ca_{10}(PO_4)_6F_2$ ASTM 3—0736		$Ca_{10}(PO_4)_6(OH)_2$ ASTM 9—432		$Ca_8H_2(PO_4)_6 5H_2O$ ASTM 11—184		$CaHPO_4$ ASTM 9—80		Calcit ASTM 5—0586		Aragonit ASTM 5—0453		Whitlockit ASTM 9—169	
d_{hkl}	I/I_1	d_{hkl}	I/I_1	d_{hkl}	I/I_1	d_{hkl}	I/I_1	d_{hkl}	I/I_1	d_{hkl}	I/I_1	d_{hkl}	I/I_1
								1,297	2				
								1,284	1				
										1,261	6		
								1,247	1	1,240	7		
								1,235	2	1,224	5		
										1,205	6		
								1,179	3	1,171	6		
								1,153	3	1,159	3		
								1,143	1				
								1,124	1				

Tabelle 9. *d_{hkl}-Werte von Zahnschmelz, Dentin und Knochen*

Zahnschmelz nach R. QUICKER und H. J. DULCE (1967)	Dentin nach ROSEBERRY (1931)	Knochen nach ROSEBERRY (1931)	Zahnschmelz nach R. QUICKER und H. J. DULCE (1967)	Dentin nach ROSEBERRY (1931)	Knochen nach ROSEBERRY (1931)
18,6			1,892		
9,09			1,8717		
8,16			1,8406	1,83	1,83
5,27			1,806		
4,70			1,781		
4,37			1,755		
4,09			1,720	1,71	1,71
3,87			1,645		
3,71			1,61		
3,61			1,587		
3,528			1,568		
3,43			1,545		
	3,35	3,35	1,53		
3,318			1,505		
3,178			1,475		
3,095			1,453		
3,008	3,02	3,02	1,434	1,43	1,43
2,887			1,4092		
2,822			1,3493		
2,817			1,319		
2,718	2,72	2,72	1,307		
2,63			1,282		
2,578			1,266		
2,549			1,254		
2,525			1,237		
2,302			1,223	1,21	1,21
2,260	2,25	2,25	1,199		
2,148			1,178		
2,062			1,159		
2,04			1,147	1,14	
1,997			1,133		
1,946			1,115	1,10	1,10
	1,93	1,93	1,103		

2. Die organische Matrix

Die sog. organische Matrix setzt sich aus Kollagen verschiedener Reifestufen, aus Mucoproteiden und aus einem wasserbeständigen Protein zusammen. Alle drei Komponenten sind stickstoffhaltig. Man kann deshalb über den gesamten Stickstoffgehalt der fettfreien Trockensubstanz den Matrixanteil näherungsweise bestimmen. Als Umrechnungsfaktor ermittelte J. E. EASTOE (1954) 5,5. Nur ca. 6—12% des Gesamt-N der Matrix entfallen bei reifen Corticalisknochen auf Nichtkollagen-Komponenten, während ca. 88—94% Kollagen-N darstellen (J. W. DICKERSON,1962). Bei Matrix embryonaler Corticalis sind Nichtkollagen-Komponenten zu ca. 25—50% am Gesamt-N-Gehalt beteiligt. Die Matrix des menschlichen Femurknochens besteht zu ca. 92% aus Kollagen, zu ca. 4% aus Mucoproteiden und zu ca. 4% aus wasserbeständigem Protein (H. J. ROGERS, 1952, 1949), die Matrix des Dentins zu ca. 94% aus Kollagen, zu 4% aus Mucoproteid und zu ca. 2% aus wasserbeständigem Protein. Vergleiche mit Matrix von Rinderknochen lassen erwarten, daß die Mucoproteidfraktion zu ca. 50% aus Mucopolysacchariden besteht und auch dem Kollagen noch ca. 1% Mucopolysaccharide bzw. Polysaccharide anhaften (J. E. EASTOE, 1954). Demgegenüber setzt sich die Schmelzmatrix zu je ein Drittel aus sog. Eukeratin, löslichem Mucoproteid und löslichen Peptiden zusammen.

a) Kollagen

Man unterscheidet lösliches und unlösliches Kollagen. Unlösliches Kollagen verschiedener Gewebe hat einen Stickstoffgehalt von ca. 18,5% (J. E. EASTOE, 1955). Das lösliche Kollagen wird auch als Prokollagen bezeichnet. Es ist in einer säurelöslichen (pH 3,5—3,7), in einer neutralsalzlöslichen (0,15 und 0,45 molar NaCl) und in einer guanidinlöslichen Fraktion aus nativem Kollagen darstellbar. Sein N-Gehalt beträgt ca. 17% (W. GRASSMANN, 1960). Haut und Knorpel besitzen ca. 3—15% säurelösliches Kollagen [W. GRASSMANN, 1956; K. KÜHN, 1959; J. S. BRAUN (unveröffentlichte Untersuchungen)], Knochen ca. 2% (H. J. ROGERS, 1952). Während aus der Haut 7—30% neutralsalzlösliches Kollagen extrahiert werden können (K. H. GUSTAVSON, 1956), ist das aus Knorpelkollagen unmöglich (BRAUN). Knochenkollagen ist bisher in dieser Weise quantitativ nicht fraktioniert worden, wir wissen nur, daß Anteile im sauren Bereich gelöst werden können.

Kollagen besitzt je nach Trocknungsverfahren eine Dichte von 1,28—2 g/ml (E. HEIDEMANN, 1963), Prokollagen dagegen von 0,56—0,83 g/ml. Demnach ist Kollagen außerordentlich stark verformbar.

Dem Aufbau des nativen Knochenkollagens (A. COURTS, 1960) liegt ähnlich, wie beim übrigen Bindegewebe (J. GROSS, 1954, 1955), das Tropokollagen mit einem Molekulargewicht von ca. 350000 zugrunde (K. KÜHN, 1960; J. ENGEL, 1963). Die Tropokollagenmolekel hat eine Länge von ca. 2600—2800 Å und eine Dicke von ca. 15 Å (H. BOEDTKER, 1956; W. GRASSMANN, 1961). Sie besteht aus ca. 3000 Aminosäureresten, die in der Primärstruktur zu drei gleich langen Ketten peptidartig verbunden sind. Die unverknüpfte einzelne Kette von ca. 1000 Aminosäuren mit einem Molekulargewicht von ca. 115000 bezeichnet man als α-Komponente. Zwei α-Komponenten können sich zu einer β-Komponente und 3 α-Komponenten zu einer γ-Komponente intramolekular verknüpft haben. An den intramolekularen Bindungen sind Wasserstoffbrücken zwischen den Keto- und Imidgruppen beteiligt (K. H. GUSTAVSON, 1956; A. RICH, 1955; K. PIEZ, 1960). Auf diese Weise entsteht die Tertiärstruktur der Tropokollagenmolekel. Das aus drei α-Komponenten bestehende Tropokollagen I bildet keine Fibrillen. Eine Mischung von einer α- und einer β-Komponente, der Tropokollagentyp II (J. ENGEL, 1963; R. HAFTER, 1963), bildet am leichtesten Fibrillen (G. C. WOOD, 1962) und stellt die Hauptkomponente des nativen Kollagens dar. Die reine γ-Komponente, das Tropokollagen III, ist zum Aufbau der regelmäßigen Helixstruktur des Kollagens besonders befähigt.

Die Tropokollagenmolekel besitzt polare Eigenschaften aufgrund der primären Aminosäurezusammensetzung seiner drei Ketten. Man hat die Aminosäurezusammensetzung des unlöslichen Kollagens verschiedener Gewebe gut untersucht. Das Kollagen zeichnet sich gegenüber anderen Proteinen durch seinen Gehalt an Hydroxyprolin (12—14%) und Hydroxylysin und seinen hohen Gehalt an Prolin und polaren basischen Aminsoäuren, sowie durch das Fehlen von Tryptophan und Cystin aus. Ca. $^1/_3$ der Dicarbonsäuren sind zu Säureamiden verbunden. Das reife säureunlösliche Kollagen der Knochencompacta stimmt in seiner Aminosäurezusammensetzung mit dem der Haut gut überein (Tabelle 10).

Tabelle 10. *Quantitative Aminosäurezusammensetzung von Kollagen*

	g/100 g fettfreie Protein-Trockensubstanz		Mol/1000 Mol Aminosäuren			
	Kollagen, Ochsenhaut a)	Kollagen, Femur, Compacta, Mensch b)	Kollagen, Ochsenhaut a)	Kollagen, Femur, Compacta, Mensch b)	Kollagen Fetus, Dentin, Schwein, c)	säureunlösliches Schmelzprotein Mensch, Erwachsener d)
Glykokoll	27,2	25,8	337	319	329	304
Alanin	9,5	10,9	100	114	112	111
Valin	3,4	2,97	27	24	25	33,8
Leucin	} 5,6	3,6	} 40	25	24	41,9
Isoleucin		1,88		13	9,3	16,3
Prolin	15,1	15,3	122	124	116	47,0
OH-Prolin	14,0	14,1	100	100	99	47,3
Phenylalanin	2,5	2,49	14	14	16	45,8
Tyrosin	1,0	0,86	5,1	4,4	6,4	6,9
Serin	3,37	4,06	30	36	33	75,5
Threonin	2,28	2,35	18	18	17	44,8
Methionin	0,8	0,84	5	5,3	5,3	8,3
Lysin	4,47	4,4	28	28	22	31,2
OH-Lysin	1,1	0,62	6,3	3,5	9,6	
Histidin	0,74	0,96	4,4	5,8	4,7	9
Arginin	8,59	8,8	46	47	52,0	47,0
Asparaginsäure	6,3	6,7	44	47	46,0	45,8
Glutaminsäure	11,3	11,4	71	72	74	78,0
Cystin						3,0
Tryptophan						
Gesamt-N	18,6	18,45				
Amid		0,64		(37)		

a) G.R. TRISTRAM (1953), b) J. E. EASTOE (1955), c) K. A. PIEZ (1961), d) J. E. EASTOE (1960).

Vollständige Aminosäureanalysen von Prokollagen des Knochens existieren nicht. EASTOE (1956) gibt an, daß es mehr Hydroxyprolin als reines Kollagen enthält. Die aus Haut isolierten α- und β-Komponenten sollen sich in ihrem Aminosäuregehalt unterscheiden (K. PIEZ, 1960).

Untersuchungen über Aminosäuresequenzen sind am Knochenkollagen nicht durchgeführt worden. Man weiß nur, daß beim Demineralisieren des Knochens mit Säure ein Kollagen verbleibt, daß N-terminal Glykokoll zu stehen hat (A. COURTS, 1960). Vom nativen unbehandelten Kollagen sind dagegen keine N-terminalen Aminosäuren bekannt (J. H. BOWES, 1951). Durch Abbau und Sequenzanalyse von Hautkollagen sind polare und apolare Aminosäuresequenzen als Bausteine der Peptidketten nachgewiesen worden. Als apolare Anteile treten Tripeptidsequenzen wie Glycin-Prolin-Hydroxyprolin, Glycin-Prolin-Alanin und Glycin-Prolin-Glycin auf. Durch die Glycin-Prolin-Bindung konnten bereits 21,8 % aller Aminosäuren des Kollagens erfaßt werden. Ca. 40 % des gesamten Hydroxyprolins liegen in apolaren Bereichen (W. GRASSMANN, 1963). An polaren Peptidsequenzen wurden zwei isoliert (W. GRASSMANN, 1960), innerhalb dieser Sequenzen sind ca. 30 % des Hydroxyprolins an Lysin oder Arginin gebunden.

Dem Kollagen des Knochens haftet ebenso wie dem der Haut eine Kohlenhydratkomponente zu ca. 1 % der Trockensubstanz (K.-Y. T. KAO, 1962; W. GRASSMANN, 1935; R. CONSDEN, 1953; J. BEEK, 1941; L. E. GLYNN, 1956) an, im Dentinkollagen sind es ca. 3,5 % der Trockensubstanz (M. V. STACK, 1955; H. J. ROGERS, 1949; W. C. HESS, 1952).

Ein Teil dieses Kohlenhydrates sind saure, Hexosamin und Estersulfat enthaltende Mucopolysaccharide, die aber ohne die Kollagenstruktur zu beeinflussen, entfernt werden können (K. KÜHN, 1961; K. KÜHN, 1959). Ein anderer Teil ist ein Oligosaccharid aus Glucose, Galaktose, Mannose und Fucose, (I. ONESON, 1960; J. MOSS, 1955; R. E. GLEGG, 1953), das an intermolekularen Ester- oder Glykosidbindungen bei der Alterung des Kollagens und damit an seinem Unlöslichwerden beteiligt ist (F. VERZAR, 1963). Solange intermolekulare Esterbindungen dieser Art fehlen, bleibt das Kollagen säurelöslich (R. HAFTER, 1963). Durch intermolekulare Esterbindungen verliert es anscheinend diese Eigenschaft und quillt nur noch.

An das Dentinkollagen sind 0,4% der Trockensubstanz Phosphorsäure gebunden (A. VEIS, 1963). Kollagen weicher Bindegewebe ist Phosphorsäure-frei. Man schließt aus dem chemischen Verhalten dieser Phosphorsäurereste, daß sie ester- oder amidartig mit der Polypeptidkette verbunden sind. Es werden 12 intermolekulare P-Brücken pro Tropokollagenmolekel vermutet. VEIS (1963) zeigte, daß auch nach Überführen in Gelatine $^{2}/_{3}$ der Phosphorsäure proteingebunden bleibt. Durch die Phosphatbindung wird die Denaturierbarkeit und Quellungsfähigkeit des Kollagens geringer. Es muß geprüft werden, ob in der Kollagen-Phosphatbindung ein charakteristischer Unterschied zwischen mineralisiertem und nicht mineralisiertem Bindegewebe zu suchen ist.

Wie wir aus der Morphologie wissen, treten innerhalb der Kollagenfibrillen des Knochens, wie auch des übrigen Bindegewebes, dunkle Querstreifungen im Abstand von ca. 640 Å auf. Untersuchungen von GRASSMANN (1961) am Hautkollagen führten zu der Vorstellung, daß die Querstreifungen durch Überlappen von aufgrund ihrer Ladungsschwerpunkte kettenförmig angeordneten Tropokollagenmolekeln zustande kommen (Abb. 1).

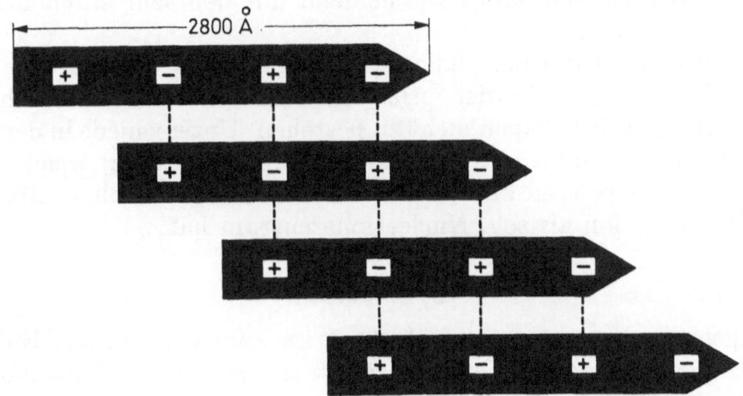

Abb. 1. Aufbau einer Kollagenfibrille aus Tropokollagenmolekülen in gestaffelter Anordnung jeweils um ein Viertel ihrer Länge versetzt. Stabilisierung durch elektrostatische Anziehungskräfte (W. GRASSMANN, 1961)

(Tropo-)Kollagen-„Molekül", drei Peptidketten in seilartiger Verwindung
[+] [−] vorwiegend positiv oder negativ aufgeladene (saure bzw. basische) Bereiche
----- elektrostatische Anziehung

GRASSMANN (1963, 1962) und KÜHN (1959, 1961a) konnten derartige quergestreifte Fibrillen aus säurelöslichem Kollagen rekonstituieren. Den hellen 45 Å langen kristallinen Interbanden der Fibrillen liegen wahrscheinlich die apolaren Sequenzbereiche zugrunde, während in den dunklen amorphen Querbanden die polaren Peptidsequenzen vorzustellen wären. Sowohl die intermolekularen Salzbindungen zwischen den polaren Gruppen, als auch die intermolekularen Ester- oder Glykosidbindungen (P. M. GALLOP, 1959; J. BELLO, 1960; W. GRASSMANN, 1957) führen neben Wasserbrückenbindungen (R. D. B. FRASER, 1959; W. F. HARRINGTON, 1961) und Wasserstoffionenbrückenbindungen (K. H. GUSTAVSON, 1956) durch Verknüpfen von Tropokollagenmolekeln zur Quartärstruktur der Fibrillen. Für ihre Querstreifung, die auch unabhängig vom Kohlenhydratanteil auftritt (K. KÜHN, 1959), sind anscheinend die intermolekularen Salzbindungen allein verantwortlich. Saure Mucopolysaccharide und 0,5 molare Neutralsalzlösungen können durch ihre eigene Ladung (K. KÜHN, 1959) das Entstehen solcher Salzbindungen hemmen und die Querstreifung einer Fibrille verhindern, sie fördern aber die End-zu-End-Anlagerung von bereits quergestreiften Kollagensegmenten (K. KÜHN, 1961).

Durch Vorbehandeln von nativen Kollagenen mit Alkali werden Säureamidbindungen und intramolekulare H-Brückenbindungen gespalten (K. Kühn, 1963). Es entsteht der neutralsalzlösliche Tropokollagentyp I mit drei α-Komponenten. Man bezeichnet dieses Kollagen auch als Eukollagen (A. Courts, 1960). Es hat ein Molekulargewicht von 62000—130000 und ist eine Vorstufe der Gelatine. Es enthält wenig Tyrosin und N-terminal treten neben Glykokoll Serin, Threonin, Alanin und Dicarbonsäuren auf.

Eine andere Kollagenform ist die Gelatine, die durch Autoclavieren oder Heißwasserextraktion entsteht. Gelatinen können Molekulargewichte von 62000—1,2 Mill. aufweisen. Ihre Aminosäurenzusammensetzung entspricht der des Eukollagens. Man kann Gelatine als unorientierte Form des Eukollagens auffassen (A. Courts, 1960, 1961). Höhermolekulare Gelatine kann im Gegensatz zu niedermolekularer Gelatine und Eukollagen unter geeigneten Bedingungen wieder zu quergestreiften Fibrillen rekonstituieren (M. Veis, 1961; M. Drake, 1964).

Der isoelektrische Punkt des nativen Kollagens liegt bei pH 9,4 (Eastoe, 1956), der des säurelöslichen Prokollagens bei pH 5,8, der des Eukollagens bei pH 4,8 (A. Courts, 1960).

Die thermische Stabilität des Kollagens scheint seinem Hydroxyprolingehalt proportional zu sein. (F. Verzar, 1963; K. H. Gustavson, 1956; K. A. Piez, 1960a). Die Gummielastizität nach dem Erhitzen hängt anscheinend mit den sehr stabilen Esterbindungen zusammen.

Die Kollagenfibrille ist das morphologische Grundgerüst, an dem sich die Mineralisation orientiert. Unterschiede in der primären Aminosäurestruktur scheinen zwischen Knochen- und Bindegewebskollagen nicht zu bestehen. Unterschiede in der Tertiärstruktur müssen heute diskutiert werden. Insbesondere bleibt zu prüfen, welche Bedeutung die chemische Struktur der polaren und apolaren Abschnitte der Kollagenfibrille im Primärstadium der Mineralisation als sog. Nucleationszentrum hat.

b) Eukeratin

Dem Kollagen des Knochens äquivalent ist im Zahnschmelz das Eukeratin, das als säureunlösliches Schmelzprotein beim Erwachsenen eine dem Dentinkollagen ähnliche Aminosäurezusammensetzung hat (Tabelle 10).

Im Eukeratin fehlt lediglich Hydroxylysin, dafür tritt aber Cystin auf. Der N-Gehalt des Eukeratins beträgt ca. 13% der Trockensubstanz (M. V. Stack, 1955). Mit zunehmender Reife und Alterung nimmt das Eukeratin wie Keratin fibrilläre Strukturen mit Periodizität an und bildet eine α-Helix (F. G. Pautard, 1963). Im fetalen Stadium hindert anscheinend der hohe Prolingehalt das Ausbilden einer stabilen α-Helix (H. R. Wilson, 1960).

Dem Eukeratin haften ebenso wie dem Kollagen Kohlenhydrate an. Man findet ca. 3% der Trockensubstanz Glucose und ca. 0,5% Hexosamin (M. V. Stack, 1955), wahrscheinlich Galaktosamin (H. J. Glimcher, 1961).

c) Wasserbeständige Proteinfraktion

Nach Autoclavieren oder Heißwasserextraktion verbleibt im Knochen ein Proteinrückstand. Diese Fraktion enthält zu ca. 14,6% der Trockensubstanz Stickstoff (J. E. Eastoe, 1955), stammt sie aus dem Dentin nur ca. 12% Stickstoff (M. V. Stack, 1955). Ca. 0,1% der Trockensubstanz des wasserbeständigen Proteins sind Hexosamin als Baustein eines sulfathaltigen, uronsäurefreien Mucopolysaccharids (M. V. Stack, 1955). Papierchromatographisch ist das Protein in seiner Aminosäurezusammensetzung kollagenunähnlich, aber den Serumproteiden ähnlich. Es besitzt viel Tyrosin (5%) und kaum Hydroxyprolin (0,3—0,6%) (M. V. Stack, 1955; J. E. Eastoe, 1954). Man vermutet (J. E. Eastoe, 1956), daß diese Proteinfraktion aus Capillarwänden der Gefäße des Knochens stammt.

d) Mucoproteidfraktion (Osseomucoid)

Durch basische Calciumchloridlösung oder Basen von pH 9,0 läßt sich aus Knochen (J. E. EASTOE, 1954) eine Fraktion extrahieren, die zu ca. 30% aus Mucopolysacchariden und zu ca. 70% aus Proteinen besteht. Ca. 12% der 30% sind Hexosamin, überwiegend Galaktosamin, und ca. 18% Galaktose, Mannose und Glucuronsäure. Außerdem können ca. 1,6% Sulfatschwefel innerhalb dieser Fraktion nachgewiesen werden. Das Mucoproteid kann man durch Fällen mit 1%iger Essigsäure in zwei Komponenten zerlegen (H. HISAMURA, 1938; R. E. GLEGG, 1955), deren eine Chondroitinschwefelsäure ist.

Tabelle 11. *Analyse der zwei von* HISAMURA (1938) *dargestellten Mucoproteidkomponenten der Knochenmatrix*

	% der Gesamttrockensubstanz	% TS-Komponente A	% TS-Komponente B
N-Gehalt	13,28	3,06	12,55
SO_4-S	1,07	5,85	0,56
Galaktosamin	11,2	26,81	7,53
Glucuronsäure	6,6	26,85	0,54
Galaktose	4,8		6,9

TS = Trockensubstanz.

Die Komponente B ist ein neutrales Mucoproteid, das nach GLEGG (1955) noch Mannose, Fucose und Glucosamin enthält.

Menschliche Knochenmatrix besitzt zu ca. 0,6% Hexosamin (H. J. ROGERS, 1949), das der Mucoproteidfraktion angehört. Chondroitinschwefelsäure wurde in Alkaliextrakten der Knochen aufgrund ihrer Metachromasie direkt colorimetrisch nachgewiesen (G. DILLMANN, 1956). MEYER (1956) und ROGERS (1951) beobachteten bei Rinderknochen als

Tabelle 12. *Aminosäurezusammensetzung der Mucoproteide aus Knochen und Zahnschmelz*

	Schmelzprotein[1] Mol/1000 Mol	Mucoproteidfraktion[2] Mol/1000 Mol		Schmelzprotein[1] Mol/1000 Mol	Mucoproteidfraktion[2] Mol/1000 Mol
Alanin	20,3	74	Threonin	38,1	62
Glykokoll	65	63	Cystin	2	8,3
Valin	39,6	68	Methionin	42,3	9,9
Leucin	91,3	99	Arginin	23,3	39
Isoleucin	32,7	50	Histidin	64,5	30
Prolin	251	65	Lysin	17,7	52
Phenylalanin	23,4	31	Asparaginsäure	30,3	128
Tyrosin	53,4	19	Glutaminsäure	142,0	140
Serin	62,5	61			

[1] Mensch, Fetus (J. E. EASTOE, 1960).
[2] $CaCl_2$-lösliche Fraktion Rinderknochen (J. E. EASTOE, 1954).
Die Zahlenangaben in Mol/1000 Mol wurden für den Rinderknochen nach Analysen von EASTOE (1954) umgerechnet.

einziges Mucopolysaccharid Chondroitinschwefelsäure (Poly-β-glucuronido-1,3 N-acetylgalaktosamin-6-Sulfat) zu 0,25% der Matrixtrockensubstanz, während MEYER (1956) in der Matrix von Kälberknochen auch Hyaluronsäure (Poly-β-Glucuronido-1,3 N-acetylglucosamin) und Keratosulfat (Poly-Galakto-N-acetylglucosamin-Sulfat) fand. Lösliche Schmelzproteine bestehen zu ca. 10% der Trockensubstanz aus Glucose und zu ca. 2% aus Galaktosamin (M. V. STACK, 1955; H. J. GLIMCHER, 1961).

Die Proteinkomponente der Mucoproteidfraktion ist hydroxyprolin- und hydroxylysinfrei (J. E. EASTOE, 1954, 1960) und kollagenunähnlich. Man findet wie beim Serumalbumin mehr aromatische Aminosäuren. Auch das lösliche Mucoproteid des fetalen Zahnschmelzes ist hydroxyprolin- und hydroxylysinfrei. Erst im reifen Schmelz treten ca. 2% Hydroxyprolin auf (M. V. STACK, 1955).

Alle Bausteine der Mucoproteidfraktion findet man auch im permanenten Knorpel. Innerhalb der Mucoproteidfraktion der Knochenmatrix gibt es außerdem ein Sialoproteid (G. HERRING, 1963, 1964), das sich in der Zusammensetzung und elektrophoretischen Beweglichkeit vom Orosomucoid des Plasmas deutlich unterscheidet. Sein Molekulargewicht beträgt ca. 30000 (Tabelle 13).

Tabelle 13. *Zusammensetzung des Sialoproteids aus Knochen* (G. HERRING, 1963, 1964)

	% TS	% TS
Hexose	10,3	
Methylpentose	2,3	(0,8)
Glucosamin	3,5	
Galaktosamin	3,8	(0,7)
Sialinsäure	17,1	
Phosphat	1,8	(0,2)

( ) = Gehalt im Orosomucoid des Serums. TS = Trockensubstanz

Man nimmt an, daß das Sialoproteid im Knochen gebildet wird. Ein ähnliches Sialoproteid findet man auch im permanenten Knorpel (A. J. ANDERSON, 1962).

Die Mucoproteide der organischen Knochenmatrix sind morphologisch hauptsächlich in den osteoiden Säumen der Trabekel und der Auskleidung der Haversschen Kanäle gelegen (H. J. ROGERS, 1949). In der zentralen Zone der Osteone sollen mehr neutrale Mucopolysaccharide vorkommen, in der peripheren mehr saure (K. H. KNESE, 1959). Ein für verknöcherndes Gewebe typisches Mucopolysaccharid ist noch nicht bekannt. Die Verflechtung der Mucoproteide mit dem Kollagen ist in der Knochenmatrix bedeutend fester als in der Knorpelmatrix.

Stoffwechsel des Knochengewebes

Stoffwechselleistungen von Geweben müssen vergleichend betrachtet werden, um typische Merkmale zu erkennen. Man hat darauf zu achten, daß diese Vergleiche in demselben Bezugssystem erfolgen. Da es sich beim Stoffwechsel größtenteils um celluläre Leistungen handelt, muß dem Zellanteil der Gewebe in diesem Falle Rechnung getragen werden, wenn man zellarme und zellreiche Gewebeabschnitte gegenüberstellt. Beim Knochen müssen insbesondere die Mineralanteile durch das Bezugssystem ausgeschaltet werden. Die Untersuchungen über den Stoffwechsel des Knochengewebes sind meistens tierexperimentell in vitro oder in vivo durchgeführt. Es wird angenommen, daß die Ergebnisse grundsätzlich auf menschliches Knochengewebe übertragbar sind.

Wir unterscheiden auch beim Knochen den Betriebs- und den Baustoffwechsel. Zum Betriebsstoffwechsel gehören Atmung und Glykolyse, zum Baustoffwechsel Kollagen-, Mucoproteid- und Mineralumsatz.

I. Betriebsstoffwechsel und seine Regulation

1. Atmung im Knochengewebe

Die Atmung der Knochenzellen ist bedeutend geringer als die der Parenchym- oder Knorpelzellen. Metaphysenschnitte Parathormon-vorbehandelter Kaninchen zeigen eine reduzierte Atmung, gleichgültig ob Glucose, Succinat, Pyruvat oder Citrat veratmet wurden (Tabelle 14). Auf mg Trockensubstanz bezogene Angaben sind bei diesen Vergleichen weniger aussagekräftig. Trotzdem schließen BOYD und NEUMAN aufgrund ihrer Untersuchungen bei embryonalem Knorpelgewebe auf eine leberzellähnliche Atmungsgröße (E. S. BOYD, W. F. NEUMAN, 1954). Nach Befunden von A. B. BORLE (1960a), G. M. VAES (1963) und F. KÖRBER (1964) errechnet sich die Atmung der Knochenzellen auf 3—4 μl O_2/mg Zell-TS/Stunde, die der Knochenmarkszellen auf ca. 3,5, die der Leberzellen auf ca. 9,5 μl O_2/mg Zell-TS/Stunde. Im Vitamin D-Mangelzustand nimmt der Q_{O_2} ab. Sowohl im Knorpel (G. M. HILLS, 1940; A. FINE, 1963; M. S. BURSTONE, 1960) als auch im hypertrophen Säulenknorpel (A. FINE, 1963: M. S. BURSTONE, 1960; T. F. DIXON, 1952) und im Knochen (G. M. VAES, 1964; M. S. BURSTONE, 1960; D. M. LASKIN, 1956; A. G. PEARSE, 1966; D. G. WALKER, 1961; K. BALOGH, 1961, 1963) sind die Enzyme der Atmungskette mehr oder weniger lückenlos und einzelne Substrate (C. LUTWAK-MANN, 1940) nachgewiesen worden. Im Knochengewebe wird Adenosintriphosphat (ATP) gebildet (E. BARBIERI, 1957; H. G. ALBAUM 1952). Permanenter Knorpel besitzt keine ATPaseaktivität, hypertropher Säulenknorpel (H. J. DULCE, 1960a; J. D. CIPERA, 1963) und Knochen (H. J. DULCE, 1960a) wohl.

Tabelle 14

	Q_{O_2} µl O_2/mg DNS/Std	
Leberschnitte, Kaninchen	−1320	D. M. LASKIN (1956)
Knorpelschnitte, Kaninchen (permanenter Knorpel)	−273	D. M. LASKIN (1952, 1956)
Metaphysenschnitte	−57 bis −74	D. M. LASKIN (1956)
Kaninchen, Ratte		G. M. VAES (1963)
Metaphysenschnitte Parathyreoidenextrakt-vorbehandelter Tiere	−33	D. M. LASKIN (1956), G. M. VAES (1963)

Q_{O_2} = Meßgröße für den O_2-Verbrauch von Zellen.

2. Anaerobe Glykolyse

Die anaerobe Glykolyse im Knochengewebe ist auf DNS bezogen deutlich geringer als im Knorpel und in der Leber (Tabelle 15). Vergleicht man im Bezugssystem der Trockensubstanz, dann sind die Meßwerte untereinander ähnlicher (Tabelle 16).

Embryonales Knorpelgewebe (E. G. BYWATERS, 1937, 1936, 1936a) zeigt dagegen $Q\frac{N_2}{G}$-Werte zwischen 3,0—4,5 µl CO_2/mg TS/Stunde. Als Substrat der Glykolyse dient im Knorpel hauptsächlich diffundierte Glucose. Glykogen der Knorpelzellen wird anscheinend nicht direkt dem Embden-Meyerhof-Weg zugeführt, weil im permanenten Knorpel anaerob keine Phosphorylase nachzuweisen ist (H. J. DULCE, 1960a; A. B. GUTMAN, 1941).

Tabelle 15. (LASKIN, 1956)

Kaninchen	$Q\frac{N_2}{G}$ µl CO_2/mg DNS/Std
Leber	+275
Permanenter Knorpel	+467
Metaphysenknochen	+33

$Q\frac{N_2}{G}$ = Meßgröße für die Milchsäurebildung aus Glucose (G) unter N_2-Begasung.

Tabelle 16

	$Q\frac{N_2}{G}$ µl CO_2/mg TS/Std	
Leber, Ratte	3,4	E. G. BYWATERS (1937)
Permanenter Knorpel		
Ratte	1,36	F. DICKENS (1936)
Mensch	1,8	R. F. HAGERTY (1960)
Kaninchen	0,64	E. G. BYWATERS (1937)
Hypertropher Knorpel		
Ratte	2,46	N. EGG-LARSEN (1956)
Osteoblastenkulturen	48—78	H. A. KREBS, L. KIESOW (1959)
Metaphysenknochen		
Ratte	0,5	G. M. VAES (1962a)
Maus	3,06	A. B. BORLE (1960)

An Stelle einer Phosphorylase findet man aber im Knorpel eine Diastase (C. LUTWAK-MANN, 1940), die Glykogen abbauen kann. Einige Enzyme (Glycerinaldehyd-6-Phosphat Dehydrogenase, Lactat Dehydrogenase, Pyruvatkinase) und Zwischenstoffe (Brenztraubensäure, Fructose-1-6-Diphosphat, Dioxyacetonphosphat) der Glykolyse sind im Gelenkknorpel des Menschen von VIERENSTEIN (1959) histochemisch nachgewiesen worden.

Hypertropher verknöcherungsfähiger Knorpel der Epiphysenplatten hat den höchsten Glykogengehalt in der Verknöcherungszone (A. HOFFMAN, 1928) (Tabelle 17). Man muß annehmen, daß diese Zellen Milchsäure in erhöhtem Maße zur Glykoneogenese verwenden. Im Gegensatz zum permanenten Knorpel vermag verknöcherungsfähiger Knorpel Glucose über die Hexokinase und Glykogen über die Phosphorylasereaktion als Substrate in die Glykolyse einzuführen (A. B. GUTMAN, 1941; H. J. DULCE, 1960a; D. G. WALKER, 1961) und in Milchsäure anaerob umzuwandeln (N. EGG-LARSEN, 1956). Die wichtigsten Enzyme dieses Zwischenstoffwechsels sind im verknöcherungsfähigen Knorpel nachgewiesen worden (H. G. ALBAUM, 1952a; A. B. GUTMAN, 1951, 1941).

Tabelle 17. *Glykogengehalt in Schichten des Humeruskopfes von Rinderfeten* (A. HOFFMAN, 1928)

	% FG
Hyaliner Knorpel	0,05
Verknöcherungsfähige Knorpelzone	0,25
Knochenkernanlage	0,115

FG = Frischgewicht.

Im Knochengewebe läuft die Glykolyse sowohl mit Glykogen als auch mit Glucose als Substrat ab. Die Phosphorylase ist im Knochen nahezu von gleicher Aktivität wie in den Leberzellen (A. B. GUTMAN, 1941). Parathormonvorbehandlung in vivo senkt den $Q\frac{N_2}{G}$, die Lactatbildung und den Glucoseverbrauch von Metaphysenschnitten um 20% (A. B. BORLE, 1960a; D. M. LASKIN, 1956). Östradiolvorbehandlung senkte die Lactatbildung um 60% und erhöhte den Glucoseverbrauch, wie vom Insulin her bekannt, um ca. 30%. In vitro Knochenschnitten zugegebenes Parathormon steigerte dagegen die Milchsäurebildung bei gleichzeitiger Abnahme des Glucoseverbrauches (L. RAISZ, 1961).

3. Aerobe Glykolyse

Eine aerobe Glykolyse, d.h. eine Milchsäurebildung aus Glucose unter Sauerstoffzufuhr beobachtet man im besonderen Maße im permanenten Knorpel mit einem $Q\frac{O_2}{G}$ von 1,22 µl CO_2/mg TS/Stunde (F. DICKENS, 1936) und im verknöcherungsfähigen Knorpel mit einem $Q\frac{O_2}{G}$ von 2,46 µl CO_2/mg TS/Stunde; das entspricht maximal 110 µ Mol Lactat/g TS/Stunde bei einem Glucoseverbrauch von 60—95 µ Mol/g TS/Stunde (N. EGG-LARSEN, 1956). Beim Vergleich mit Werten der anaeroben Glykolyse von 1,36 µl/mg TS/Stunde bzw. 2,46 µl/mg TS/Stunde sieht man, daß ca. 0,3 mm dünne Schnitte dieser Gewebe unter Beatmung mit 95% O_2/5% CO_2 keinen Pasteureffekt zeigen.

Knochenschnitte haben eine deutliche aerobe Glykolyse und einen Pasteureffekt, wobei die Werte der anaeroben Glykolyse um ca. 50% gesenkt werden (A. B. BORLE, 1960; G. M. VAES, 1962a; A. D. KENNY, 1962) (Tabelle 18 und 19).

Unter aeroben Bedingungen wird in Metaphysenschnitten Glucose zu 54% in Milchsäure, zu 10% in CO_2 und zu ca. 36% in Proteine verwandelt (B. FLANAGAN, 1964). Osteoblasten zeigen in der Zellkultur ebenfalls eine aerobe Glykolyse und ein $Q\frac{O_2}{G}$ von ca. 24 µl CO_2/mg TS/Stunde (H. A. KREBS, L. KIESOW).). Es wäre zu prüfen, ob die aerobe Glykolyse der Knochenschnitte tatsächlich besteht, oder ob sie durch schlechte Diffusion des O_2 vorgetäuscht wird. In Knorpelschnitten sollte man ein solches Diffusionshindernis weniger erwarten.

Parathormon steigert in Metaphysenschnitten die aerobe Glykolyse (A. B. BORLE, 1960a; G. M. VAES, 1962; L. RAISZ, 1961) und verringert den Pasteureffekt (Tabelle 20). Der letzte Schritt der Glykolyse, die Milchsäurebildung aus Brenztraubensäure, wird durch Parathormon nicht beeinflußt (G. M. VAES, 1961). Die Wirkung des Parathormons kann einerseits durch einen hemmenden Einfluß im Krebscyclus, andererseits aber auch durch einen aktivierenden Einfluß in der Glykolyse erklärt werden.

Adrenalin-Vorbehandlung aktiviert die aerobe Glykolyse innerhalb von 6 Stunden (A. D. KENNY, 1962). In dieser Zeit wirkt sich eine Parathormoninjektion auf die Milchsäurebildung von entnommenen Knochenschnitten noch nicht aus.

Tabelle 18. *Aerobe Glykolyse von Knochenschnitten*

	Lactatbildung µ Mol/g TS/Std	$Q\frac{O_2}{G}$* µl CO_2/mg TS/Std
Calvaria, Maus, 1—2 Wochen alt (A. D. KENNY, 1962)	6—11	0,13—0,25
Metaphyse, Maus 8 Wochen alt (A. B. BORLE, 1960)	64	1,4
Metaphyse, Ratte, 2 Monate alt (G. M. VAES, 1962a)	12	0,34

Tabelle 19. *Anaerobe Glykolyse von Knochenschnitten*

	Lactatbildung µ Mol/g TS/Std	$Q\frac{N_2}{G}$* µl CO_2/mg TS/Std
Calvaria, Maus, 1—2 Wochen alt (A. D. KENNY, 1962)	9—24	0,21—0,55
Metaphyse, Maus, 8 Wochen alt (A. B. BORLE, 1960a)	136	3,06
Metaphyse, Ratte, 8 Wochen alt (G. M. VAES, 1962a)	22	0,5

* Errechnete Werte.

Tabelle 20. *Einfluß von Parathyreoideaextrakt und Oestradiol auf die aerobe Glykolyse von Metaphysenschnitten von Mäusen* (A. B. BORLE, 1960)

	Laktatbildung µMol/Std/mg Zell-N	Glucoseverbrauch µMol/Std/mg Zell-N
Metaphysenschnitte, Kontrolle	2,56	1,52
Metaphysenschnitte von mit Parathyreoideaextrakt vorbehandelten Mäusen	3,44	1,48
Metaphysenschnitte von mit Oestradiol vorbehandelten Mäusen	2,07	1,14

4. CO_2-Bildung

Verknöcherungsfähiger hypertropher Knorpel (D. S. BERNSTEIN, 1961) und Knochengewebe (B. FLANAGAN, 1964) verbrennen Glucose aerob zu CO_2 und H_2O. Metaphysenschnitte von Ratten wandeln Glucose aerob zu 10% in CO_2 um (B. FLANAGAN, 1964). Bei Metaphysenschnitten von Mäusen beträgt der Glucoseumsatz in CO_2 0,18 µ Mol/mg DNS/Stunde (G. M. VAES, 1962). Unter anaeroben Bedingungen wird Glucose durch Knochenschnitte nur zu einem Bruchteil in CO_2 umgewandelt (G. M. VAES, 1962a).

a) Citronensäurecyclus

An Hand einer ^{14}C-Markierung erkennt man im in vitro-Versuch mit Epiphysenplatten rachitischer Ratten alle wesentlichen Zwischenstoffe des Citronensäurecyclus (A. W. NOR-

MAN, 1964 (Tabelle 21). Man erkennt an der großen Menge ^{14}C — aktiver Milchsäure, daß auch hier eine deutliche aerobe Glykolyse abläuft. Hinter der Bernsteinsäure scheint ein langsamer Reaktionsschritt zu liegen, ebenso nach der transaminierenden Seitenreaktion.

Tabelle 21. *Incorporation von ^{14}C in Zwischenstoffe des Citronensäurecyclus nach Inkubation von Schnitten verknöcherungsfähigen Epiphysenknorpels rachitischer Ratten mit 1-^{14}C-Acetat* (A. W. NORMAN, 1964)

	^{14}C Imp./min/g FG
Milchsäure	6020
Citronensäure	1460
α-Ketoglutarsäure	1490
Glutaminsäure	3020
Bernsteinsäure	4770
Äpfelsäure	910

FG = Frischgewicht.

An Enzymen fanden DIXON u. Mitarb. (1952) in verknöcherungsfähigen Epiphysenplatten von Kaninchen mit chemischen Methoden das condensing enzyme, die Aconitase, die Isocitricodehydrogenase und bei Ratten auch die Bernsteinsäuredehydrogenase. Einige Enzyme des Citratcyclus konnte man histochemisch in die hypertrophen Knorpelzellen lokalisieren (D. G. WALKER, 1961; K. BALOGH, 1961).

Vitamin D steigert den Citratgehalt verknöcherungsfähiger Epiphysenplatten (P. K. DIKSHIT, 1961) wahrscheinlich deshalb, weil einerseits die Synthese von Thiamin-Pyrophosphat (C. E. RAEIHA, 1954, 1952) und so die oxydative Decarboxylierung von Pyruvat (A. W. NORMAN, 1964; P. G. TULPULE, 1954) aktiviert wird und andererseits der Umbau von Citrat in α-Ketoglutarat gehemmt wird (A. W. NORMAN, 1964) (Tabelle 22).

Tabelle 22. *Einbau von ^{14}C aus 1-^{14}C-Acetat in organische Säuren von verknöcherungsfähigen Epiphysen rachitischer Ratten. Meßwerte ^{14}C Imp./min/g FG* (A. W. NORMAN, 1964)

Organische Säuren	Verknöcherungsfähige Epiphyse		Verknöcherungsfähige Epiphysenlinie		Metaphyse	
	rach.	rach. + Vit. D	rach.	rach. + Vit. D	rach.	rach. + Vit. D
Citronensäure	1460	3910	1790	2340	2110	5210
α-Ketoglutarsäure	1490	890	1470	680	2830	1580
Glutaminsäure	3020	1600	700	950	460	300

Tabelle 23. *Umwandlung von 6-^{14}C-Glucose in $^{14}CO_2$ durch Metaphysenschnitte* (D. COHN, 1962)

0,5 m Molar 6-^{14}C-Glucose + 500 mg Metaphysenschnitte pro Ansatz	μMol verbrauchte Glucose	μMol gebildetes Lactat	$^{14}CO_2$ Imp./min aus 6-^{14}C-Glucose
Kontrolle	1,5	2,3	6100
Metaphysenschnitte von mit Parathormon vorbehandelten Kaninchen	1,7	2,6	11300

Tabelle 24. *CO_2-Bildung in Calvariahomogenaten von mit Parathyreoideaextrakt behandelten 5 Tage alten Mäusen* (C. MECCA, 1964)

Substrat	$^{14}CO_2$ Imp./min
1,5 ^{14}C-Citrat-Kontrollhomogenat	415
Homogenat von mit Parathyreoideaextrakt vorbehandelten Tieren	229
5,6 ^{14}C-Isocitrat-Kontrollhomogenat	10266
Homogenat von mit Parathyreoideaextrakt vorbehandelten Tieren	9544

Parathormonvorbehandlung steigert die aerobe Bildung von $^{14}CO_2$ in vitro aus 6-^{14}C-Glucose in Knochen- und Nierengewebe, in Leber- und Muskelzellen dagegen nicht (D. V. COHN, 1962) (Tabelle 23). Metaphysenschnitte von mit Parathyreoideaextrakt vorbehandelten Kaninchen veratmen im Vergleich zu unbehandelten Kontrollen ^{14}C-Pyruvat stärker als ^{14}C-Citrat zu $^{14}CO_2$ (D. V. COHN, 1962; 1964). Parathormon hemmt anscheinend die Umwandlung von Citrat in Isocitrat, nicht aber die Weiteroxydation von Isocitrat (C. MECCA, 1964) (Tabelle 24).

Diese Befunde lassen annehmen, daß Parathormon die oxydative Decarboxylierung der Brenztraubensäure oder die ersten Schritte der Gluconeogenese aktiviert und die Aconitase hemmt. Die verstärkte CO_2-Bildung aus Pyruvat wäre allerdings auch erklärbar, wenn bei unbeeinflußter Gluconeogenese Parathyreoideaextrakt den Horeckercyclus aktiviert. Daß Parathormon die Umwandlung von Substraten in CO_2 in Knochenschnitten steigert, tritt bei der Oxydation des gesamten Citrats im Körper der Ratte nicht in Erscheinung (J. L. SPRATT, 1963).

Tabelle 25. *Incorporation von ^{14}C in Zwischenstoffe des Citronensäurecyclus nach Inkubation von Knochenschnitten mit 1-^{14}C-Acetat bei 60 g schweren Ratten* (A. W. NORMAN, 1964)

Organische Säure	^{14}C Imp./min/g FG		
	verknöchernde Epiphyse	Metaphyse und Spongiosa	Diaphyse
Milchsäure	2320	1950	1280
Citronensäure	15000	15600	2820
α-Ketoglutarsäure	5660	8860	700
Glutaminsäure	2550	900	130
Bernsteinsäure	7070	5400	—
Fumarsäure	2690	3500	—
Äpfelsäure	4860	2780	1610

FG = Frischgewicht.

Im verknöchernden Gewebe und im hypertrophen Säulenknorpel steigern Vitamin D (L. TESSARI, 1960; C. E. RAEIHA, 1954, 1952) und Insulin (E. BARBIERI, 1957a) wahrscheinlich durch Thiaminkinaseaktivierung die Codecarboxylaseaktivität. Man darf deshalb vermuten, daß unter Vitamin D neben Pyruvat auch α-Ketogluturat schneller decarboxyliert wird und α-Ketogluturat als Zwischenstoff abnimmt (A. W. NORMAN, 1964).

Die Citronensäure ist in Knochenschnitten nach Inkubation mit 1-^{14}C-Acetat unter aeroben Bedingungen der bevorzugt gebildete Zwischenstoff (Tabelle 25). Trotzdem beträgt ihre absolute Menge nur ca. $^1/_{70}$ der Menge gebildeter Milchsäure. Metaphysenschnitte von Ratten (G. M. VAES, 1963) oder Mäusen (G. M. VAES, 1961) bilden aerob in Gegenwart von Fluoracetat 0,022—0,08 μMol Citrat/mg Zell-N/Stunde (G. M. VAES, 1961) (1 mg Zell-N = 0,6 mg DNS). Mit Glucose als Substrat bilden Metaphysenschnitte 0,035 μMol Citrat/mg Zell-N/Stunde (A. B. BORLE, 1960). Die Aktivität des condensing enzyme ist in der Metaphyse höher als in Leber und Diaphyse (T. F. DIXON, 1952) (Tabelle 26).

Tabelle 26. *Enzymaktivitäten in Knochengeweben von Kaninchen* (T. F. DIXON, 1952)

	Condensing enzyme mg gebildete Citronensäure /g FG/Std	Aconitase mg gebildete Citronensäure /g FG/Std
Leber	1,27	54
Knochenmark	0,26	8,6
Metaphyse	0,51	11,9
Diaphyse	0,04	0,61

Tabelle 27. *Einfluß von Parathyreoideaextrakt und Oestradiol in vivo auf Citratbildung und -umsatz von Metaphysenschnitten erwachsener Mäuse in vitro* (G. M. VAES, 1961)

	Citratproduktion		Citratoxydation		α-Ketosäurebildung	
	μMol/Std/mg Zell-N = 0,6 mg DNS					
	Kontrolle	Experiment	Kontrolle	Experiment	Kontrolle	Experiment
Mit Parathyreoideaextrakt vorbehandelte Tiere (4 Einh./g, 3 Tage lang)	0,0217	0,0342	0,161	0,149	0,225	0,192
Mit Oestradiol vorbehandelte Tiere (2 mg in 3 Tagen)	0,0198	0,0308	0,162	0,240	0,191	0,239

Parathormon und Oestradiol in vivo verabfolgt, erhöhen die aerobe Citratproduktion in Knochenschnitten in vitro aus Glucose oder Pyruvat um ca. 60% (G. M. VAES, 1961; D. M. LASKIN, 1960; A. B. BORLE, 1960a) (Tabelle 27).

Der sehr hohe Citratgehalt verknöchernder Gewebe mit ca. 1—7 mg/g FG (T. F. Dixon, 1952; D. M. Laskin, 1960; H. J. Dulce, 1960; R. E. Ranney, 1960) ist auf den hohen extracellulären, mineraladsorbierten, Stoffwechsel-inaktiven Citrat-Anteil zurückzuführen. Er ist durch Parathyreoideaextrakt, Oestradiol und am stärksten durch Vitamin D-Gaben noch zu steigern (Tabelle 28 und 29). Die citratanstauende Wirkung des Vitamins D_2 und auch des AT 10 hat man versucht durch die in vitro beobachtete Hemmung der Aconitase zu erklären (E. Bruchmann, 1961).

Die Citratoxydation überwiegt grundsätzlich die Citratproduktion nach Zugabe aller Cofaktoren (G. M. Vaes, 1961). Parathormon senkt die Citratoxydation und die α-Ketosäurebildung nur wenig, während Oestradiol beide Reaktionen aktiviert. Die Isocitricodehydrogenase ist ein im Knochen sehr aktives Enzym, aktiver als die Aconitase (R. van Reen, 1959), die ebenfalls extrahiert werden kann (J. W. Hekkelmann, 1964 (Tabelle 30).

Tabelle 28. *Citratgehalt von Tibia und Femur erwachsener Mäuse* (R. E. Ranney, 1960)

	mg Citrat/g TS Kontrolle	mg Citrat/g TS Experiment
Mit Parathyreoideaextrakt vorbehandelte Tiere (230 E/kg)	7,17	8,81
Mit Oestron vorbehandelte Tiere (2 mg/kg)	7,17	13,0

Tabelle 29. *Citratgehalt des Humerusknochens von Ratten* (H. Steenbock, 1953)

	mg Citrat/g TS
Normalkost	3,39
Normalkost + Vitamin D	5,23
Rachitische Kost	4,4
Rachitische Kost + Vitamin D	6,05

Die Isocitricodehydrogenase ist an Partikel der Knochenzellen gebunden und unter Nicotinsäureamid-adenin-dinucleotidphosphat (NADP) und NADPH-Zusatz besonders gut zu extrahieren (J. W. Hekkelmann, 1964). Histochemisch fand man Isocitricodehydrogenase bevorzugt in Osteoblasten und Odontoblasten, weniger in Osteocyten und Osteoclasten (D. G. Walker, 1961; K. Balogh, 1961, 1963; A. G. Pearse, 1966). Nach Parathormonvorbehandlung konnte Hekkelmann (1964) aus Kaninchenknochen eine um 20% inaktivierte, NADP-abhängige Isocitricodehydrogenase und gleichzeitig eine unbeeinflußte Aconitase extrahieren. Dieser Befund widerspricht zwar den Beobachtungen von Mecca (1964), es bleibt aber wahrscheinlich, daß die Citratanhäufung im Knochenstoffwechsel nach Parathormongaben durch langsameren Citratabbau und eventuell zusätzliche Aktivierung der Pyruvatdecarboxylase zustande kommt. Weitere Untersuchungen von Hekkelmann (1964 und 1966) und De Voogd (1963) zeigen, daß Parathormon den NADP-Gehalt der Knochenzellen durch Aktivieren einer NADP-Phosphatase herabsetzt und dadurch die Isocitricodehydrogenase hemmt. Knochen besitzt in seinem Stoffwechsel bezogen auf die Cytochrom-C-Reduktaseaktivität eine höhere NADP-Transhydrogenaseaktivität als Leber, Niere und Gehirn (J. W. Hekkelmann, 1964). Demnach scheint der NADP-Gehalt des Knochens in verschiedenen Richtungen an Bedeutung zu gewinnen.

Tabelle 30. *Aconitase und Isocitricodehydrogenaseaktivität in Knochen von 8—9 Wochen alten jungen Kaninchen* (R. van Reen, 1959)

	Aconitaseaktivität in μ Mol gebildete Isocitronensäure/Std		Isocitricodehydrogenaseaktivität in μ Mol oxydierter Isocitronensäure/Std	
	je mg Protein	je g FG	je mg Protein	je g FG
Knochenmark	0,387	12,55	3,6	115,3
Epiphyse	0,395	6,6	5,73	92,4
Epi-Metaphyse	0,391	7,09	4,4	76,8
Diaphyse	0,228	0,41	5,66	9,6

α-Ketoglutarsäuredehydrogenase hat man bisher nur in Osteoclasten nachgewiesen (D. G. Walker, 1961).

In sämtlichen Knochenzellen fand man mitochondriale NADH- und NADPH-Diaphoraseaktivität (D. G. WALKER, 1961; K. BALOGH, 1961, 1963; A. G. PEARSE, 1966) (NAD = Nicotinsäureamid-adenin-dinucleotid).

Die in Knochenschnitten mitochondrial gebunden (A. G. PEARSE, 1966) und quantitativ chemisch nachgewiesene Bernsteinsäuredehydrogenase (D. M. LASKIN, 1956) stammt wahrscheinlich bevorzugt aus Osteoclasten (D. G. WALKER, 1961; K. BALOGH, 1961; M. S. BURSTONE, 1960, 1960a; F. SCHAJOWICZ, 1960). Histochemisch wird sie in das Cytoplasma lokalisiert. Parathormon soll in Metaphysen von Kaninchen die Bernsteinsäuredehydrogenase hemmen (D. M. LASKIN, 1956) und dadurch den Q_{O_2} herabsetzen. Bei Ratten fand man im Gegensatz dazu eine Aktivierung des Enzyms durch Parathormon (B. MILLS, 1965). Schließlich ist Malatdehydrogenase in allen Knochenzellen (A. G. PEARSE, 1966) nach histochemischen Untersuchungen, besonders aber in Osteoclasten, vertreten (D. G. WALKER, 1961; K. BALOGH, 1961).

b) Horeckercyclus

Im permanenten Knorpel hat man bisher keine CO_2-Bildung über den Horeckercyclus nachgewiesen. Es fehlt möglicherweise das Zwischenferment (K. VIERENSTEIN, 1959).

Hypertropher verknöcherungsfähiger Knorpel vermag aber anscheinend CO_2 über den Horeckercyclus zu bilden. Im in vitro Versuch (D. S. BERNSTEIN, 1961) mit Schnitten von Epiphysenplatten rachitischer Ratten wurde mehr $^{14}CO_2$ aus 1-^{14}C-Glucose als aus 6-^{14}C-Glucose gebildet. Insulin steigerte sogar in vitro die Oxydation von 1-^{14}C-Glucose in $^{14}CO_2$. Das Zwischenferment konnte histochemisch in den hypertrophen Knorpelzellen nachgewiesen werden (K. BALOGH, 1961).

Knochengewebe bildet ebenfalls über den Horeckercyclus Kohlendioxyd (D. V. COHN, 1962; D. S. BERNSTEIN, 1961). Unter anaeroben Bedingungen entsteht aus Knochenschnitten zugesetzter ^{14}C-Glucose $^{14}CO_2$ mit nur 6% der spezifischen Aktivität wie unter aeroben Bedingungen (G. M. VAES, 1962a). Aerob bildet 1-^{14}C-Glucose mehr $^{14}CO_2$ als 6-^{14}C-Glucose, wenn beide Metaphysenschnitten in vitro zugesetzt werden (D. S. BERNSTEIN, 1961; R. C. GREINLICH, 1965; A. NEUBERGER, 1933). Das markierte CO_2 kann durch decarboxylierende Reaktionen im Horeckercyclus oder durch Oxalacetatdecarboxylierung entstanden sein. Das nicht markierte CO_2 muß aus anderen decarboxylierenden Glucose-unabhängigen Reaktionen stammen.

Zwischenferment und 6-Phosphogluconsäuredehydrogenase, beide NADP-abhängig, sind im Knochengewebe im Verhältnis 1,3 : 1 nachgewiesen worden (J. W. HEKKELMANN, 1964). Beide Enzyme sind in Osteoblasten (K. BALOGH, 1961, 1963; D. G. WALKER, 1961), das Zwischenferment zusätzlich in Osteoclasten, Osteocyten und Odontoblasten lokalisiert worden.

Der Horeckercyclus und der Embden-Meyerhofweg der Glykolyse laufen im Knochengewebe im Verhältnis 1:3—5 ab (R. C. GREINLICH, 1956). Man errechnete, daß normalerweise 85% der Milchsäure im Knochen über den Embden-Meyerhofweg und 15% über den Horeckercyclus gebildet werden (A. NEUBERGER, 1953). Ob das Parathormon, das NADP-abhängige Enzyme hemmt, in den Horeckercyclus eingreift, ist bisher nicht erwiesen.

c) Aminosäurestoffwechsel

Weiteres Kohlendioxyd wird im Knochengewebe durch Decarboxylieren von Glykokoll gebildet (G. M. VAES, 1962a). Diese Reaktion soll im Zusammenhang mit dem Baustoffwechsel besprochen werden.

5. Übersicht der Hormon- und Vitaminwirkungen im Betriebsstoffwechsel

Wir stehen noch in den Anfangsstadien des Verständnisses der Regulation des Betriebsstoffwechsels im Knochen. Wir kennen bisher einige Angriffspunkte am Knochen wirksamer Hormone und Vitamine.

Parathormon	Aktivierung der aeroben Glykolyse, Hemmung der Atmung, Hemmung des Citratabbaus durch Isocitricodehydrogenase- oder Aconitaseinaktivierung, Aktivierung der Brenztraubensäuredecarboxylierung.
Vitamin D	Aktivierung der oxydativen Decarboxylierung von α-Ketosäuren durch Aktivieren der Thiaminkinase.
Oestradiol	Aktivierung der Glykogensynthese, Aktivierung der Citratbildung, Aktivierung des Citratabbaus.

II. Baustoffwechsel des Knochengewebes und seine Regulation

1. Matrixproteine

a) Kollagen

α) Kollagensynthese. Untersuchungen über die Kollagensynthese sind zum großen Teil im permanenten oder embryonalen Knorpel durchgeführt worden (P. EBERT, 1963; D. PROCKOP, 1962, 1963; G. MANNER, 1963; R. KRETSINGER, 1964). Das Charakteristische dieser Synthese ist die Umwandlung von Prolin und Lysin in die für Kollagen typischen Aminosäuren Hydroxyprolin und Hydroxylysin. Diese Umwandlung muß in Knorpel- und Knochenzellen vor sich gehen. Man kann die bisherigen Befunde zu einem Schema der Hydroxyprolin- und Kollagenbildung zusammenfassen (B. PETERKOVSKY, 1963).

Modifiziertes Schema der Kollagenbildung nach PETERKOVSKY (1963):

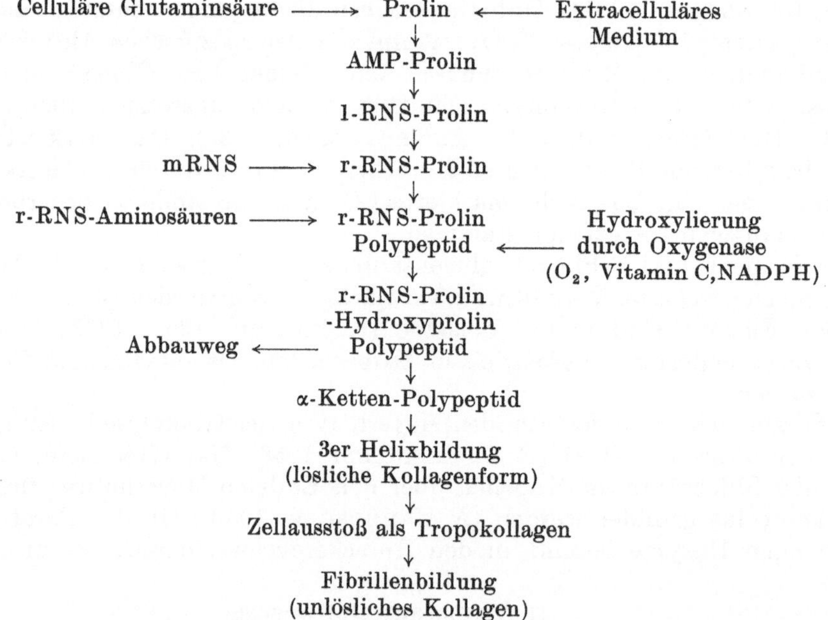

(AMP=Adenosinmonophosphat, RNS=Ribonucleinsäure, NADP=Nicotinsäureamid-adenin-dinucleotid-phosphat.)

Wir müssen annehmen, daß die Hydroxylierung von Prolin nach der Synthese der prolinhaltigen Polypeptidvorstufen am Mikrosom erfolgt. Das nach der Hydroxylierung von den Mikrosomen abgelöste Polypeptid entspricht einer α-Kette des Kollagens mit 110000 Molekulargewicht. Wahrscheinlich unterscheidet sich die Kollagensynthese im verknöcherungsfähigen Knorpel und im Knochen nicht von der im embryonalen und permanenten Knorpel. Sie findet in Osteoblasten statt. Innerhalb von 24 Std. findet man bei

Ratten $H^{14}CO_3$- oder ^{14}C-Glycin bereits in extracellulär strukturierte Matrix des verknöchernden Knorpels und des Knochens eingebaut (R. C. GREINLICH, 1956; A. NEUBERGER, 1953; Q. T. SMITH, 1961, 1963).

Der Einbau ^{14}C-Glycins in die Kollagenmatrix vollzieht sich auch in vitro (G. M. VAES, 1962a) bei Knochenschnitten. Unter anaeroben Bedingungen ist der Einbau um 75% geringer als unter aeroben. Ca. 10% des ^{14}C-Glycins werden zu $^{14}CO_2$ decarboxyliert und der Rest in der Matrix wiedergefunden (G. M. VAES, 1962b). Setzte man ^{14}C-Prolin Metaphysenschnitten junger Ratten zu (B. FLANAGAN, 1962), fand man 70% der Aktivität in der unreifes Kollagen enthaltenden alkalilöslichen Matrixfraktion, 12% im reifen unlöslichen Kollagen und 18% im entstandenen CO_2. Ein Glucosemangel im Inkubationsmedium führte zu um 45% höherer Decarboxylierung und zu um 20% geringerer Aufnahme von ^{14}C-Prolin in Zellfraktionen des Knochens. Weitere Versuche mit ^{14}C-Prolin sprechen dafür (B. FLANAGAN, 1962; W. DEISS, 1962), daß auch im Knochen die Hydroxylierung des Prolins in der Zellfraktion erfolgt.

Für die Kollagensynthese im verknöchernden Gewebe sind Threonin, Arginin, Tryptophan, Methionin, Histidin, Leucin, Isoleucin, Valin, Phenylalanin, Lysin und Tyrosin als essentielle Aminosäuren anzusehen (J. D. BIGGERS, 1957). Hydroxylysin und Hydroxyprolin entstehen aus Lysin bzw. Prolin. Glutaminsäure, Asparaginsäure, Glycin, Prolin, Serin, Alanin können durch Transaminierung aus Abbauprodukten der Glucose gebildet werden (J. D. BIGGERS, 1957; B. FLANAGAN, 1964). Innerhalb von 21 Std haben Metaphysenschnitte von Ratten ^{14}C-Glucose in Aminosäure-^{14}C zu 80% umgesetzt (Tabelle 31).

Tabelle 31. *Prozentuale Verteilung von ^{14}C auf Aminosäuren der Knochenmatrix nach Zusatz von C^{14}-Glucose zu Metaphysenschnitten von Ratten* (B. FLANAGAN, 1964)

	%
Glutaminsäure	29
Alanin	31
Asparaginsäure	13
Prolin	9
Hydroxyprolin	8
Glycin	7
Serin	3

Die Transaminasen, die α-Ketoglutarsäure in Glutaminsäure, Brenztraubensäure in Alanin und Oxalessigsäure in Asparaginsäure überführen, sind im verknöchernden Gewebe nachgewiesen (L. TESSARI, 1959).

Parathormon hemmt die Synthese von Kollagen im Knochen in vitro (G. M. VAES, 1962; C. L. JOHNSTON, 1962) und in vivo (Q. T. SMITH, 1961) bis zu 50% und zwar auf einem der letzten Schritte der Synthese (B. FLANAGAN, 1964a). ^{14}C-Prolin wird in Calvarien bei Parathyreoideaextrakt-vorbehandelten Ratten zu 80% langsamer in Matrix-gebundenes Hydroxyprolin umgewandelt als bei Kontrollen (C. L. JOHNSTON, 1962). Außerdem steigert Parathyreoideaextrakt die Aktivität der Glutamatoxalacetattransaminase in Metaphysen (L. TESSARI, 1960). Es wäre danach vorstellbar, daß Parathormon Aminosäuren verstärkt in den Krebscyclus überführt.

Glucocorticoide, die die Verknöcherung hemmen (Z. LARON, 1963; S. BERNICK, 1963), hemmen ebenfalls die Synthese von Kollagenmatrix im Knochen (Q. T. SMITH, 1963; G. M. VAES, 1962b).

Somatotropes Hormon steigert dagegen die Synthese von Matrixkollagen nach Versuchen an Calvariafragmenten und Metaphysenschnitten (G. M. VAES, 1962b) hypophysektomierter Ratten.

Insulin erhöht in vitro Metaphysenschnitten zugesetzt den ^{14}C-Glycineinbau in die Matrix um 30% (D. M. VAES, 1962).

Thyroxin senkt den ^{14}C-Glycineinbau (D. M. VAES, 1962).

β) Kollagenabbau. Der Abbau des Kollagens im Knochen erfolgt, wie wir heute wissen, wahrscheinlich durch eine Kollagenase, allenfalls noch, wie im Knorpel, nach Denaturieren durch Proteasen. Neutralsalzlösliche Kollagenvorstufen sind leichter denaturierbar als reifes Kollagen (H. HÖRMANN, 1964).

WALKER u. Mitarb. (1964) wiesen in Metaphysenknochen junger Ratten erstmalig ein kollagenolytisches Enzym mit einem pH-Optimum von 8,0 nach, das natives säurelösliches Kollagen in kurzer Zeit abbaute. Diese Kollagenase war ebenso aktiv wie Bakterienkollagenase (J. GROSS, 1962). Die kollagenolytische Aktivität des Knochens ist durch

Parathormonvorbehandlung der Tiere zu verfünffachen (D. G. Walker, 1964). In der Gewebekultur setzt Parathormon zunehmend Hydroxyprolin aus Calvarien frei (B. Stern, 1963). Auf Gelatine oder Sehnenkollagen übt Parathormon in vitro diesen Einfluß nicht aus. Wir haben also in der Kollagenase des Knochens ein typisches, von dem Parathormon abhängiges Enzym vor uns. Kollagen weicher Bindegewebe wird durch Parathormon nicht abgebaut. Bevorzugt in Osteoclasten, aber auch in Osteoblasten, Odontoblasten und Osteocyten kommt Leucinaminopeptidase außerdem vor (M. Tanzer, 1963; M. S. Burstone, 1960; G. M. Jeffree, 1965).

Die Kollagenolyse führt zu einem Matrixumsatz im Knochen. Dieser turnover kann in vivo an Hand der Hydroxyprolinausscheidung im Harn oder direkt durch den Umsatz von ^{14}C-markiertem Knochenkollagen gemessen werden. Gerber (1960) führte Versuche mit ^{14}C-Prolin durch und beobachtete, daß sich Knochenkollagen in einer schnellen und einer langsamen Komponente umsetzt. Die Umsatzzeit der schnellen Komponente — lösliches Kollagen — betrug 4 Tage, die der langsamen Komponente — unlösliches Kollagen — 40 Tage. Knochenkollagen wird also wesentlich schneller als Hautkollagen — 25 und 150 Tage (G. Gerber, 1960) — und Sehnenkollagen — 110 Tage — umgesetzt. Jüngere Individuen setzen im Knochen mehr Kollagen um als ältere (A. Neuberger, 1953; Q. T. Smith, 1963). Durch den Einfluß des Parathormons auf die Kollagenolyse im Knochen ist die Korrelation zwischen Knochenabbau und Hydroxyprolinausscheidung im Harn beim Menschen begründet (T. Dull, 1963; H. Kaiser, 1964; L. Klein, 1964; B. E. C. Nordin, 1964).

b) Kollagenunähnliche Matrixproteine, Synthese und Abbau

Wahrscheinlich bilden sich die kollagenunähnlichen Matrixproteine, die als Kittsubstanzen fungieren, im verknöchernden Knorpel und Knochen ebenso, wie wir es von den Mucoproteiden des permanenten Knorpels her wissen (R. D. Campo, 1962). Der Abbau dieser Matrixproteine könnte sich durch eine saure Protease und durch Kathepsin erklären lassen, die beide im verknöcherungsfähigen Knorpel von Hühnerembryonen (J. T. Dingle, 1961, 1961a, 1965; C. B. Sledge, 1965) und im Knochen von Hühnerembryonen (J. T. Dingle, 1965; L. F. Bélanger, 1965), Mäusen (G. Vaes, 1965) und Ratten (G. Vaes, 1964a) nachgewiesen wurden.

Tabelle 32. *Kathepsinaktivität (Einheiten/g Knochen) in partikelfreier cytoplasmatischer Fraktion des Homogenats* (G. Vaes, 1964a)

Calvaria	Metaphyse Tibia und Femur	Diaphyse Tibia und Femur
0,260	0,346	0,250

Die Protease hat ein pH-Optimum von 3,0 und ist Lysosomen-gebunden (J. T. Dingle, 1961, 1961a). In der Zone hypertropher Knorpelzellen ist sie besonders aktiv (J. T. Dingle, 1965). Auch Osteocyten bilden enzymaktive Lysosomen (L. F. Belanger, 1965). Das Enzym wird durch Vitamin A verstärkt aus den Zellen freigesetzt (H. B. Fell, 1962; J. T. Dingle, 1965). Es spaltet nur kollagenunähnliche Proteine. Glucocorticoide hemmen seine Wirkung (C. B. Sledge, 1965). Parathormon stimuliert die Proteasesekretion der Knochenzellen in Calvariakulturen, die Säuerung des Mediums und gleichzeitig die Knochenresorption (G. Vaes, 1965).

Das Kathepsin spaltet ebenfalls nur kollagenunähnliche Proteine. Die Kathepsinaktivität ist bei Ratten in partikelfreien Metaphysenhomogenaten höher als in Diaphysen und Calvariahomogenaten gefunden worden (G. Vaes, 1964a) (Tabelle 32).

2. Mucopolysaccharide, Synthese und Abbau

Verknöcherungsfähiger Knorpel zeigt in vivo ebenso wie permanenter Knorpel (J. Kawiak, 1963; H. Bostroem, 1952) eine intensive Chondroitinschwefelsäuresynthese (D. D. Dziewiatkowski, 1949, 1951; H. J. Dulce, 1960; J. Weatherell, 1963), die mit Metachromasie einhergeht. Auch in vitro bilden Epiphysenknorpel Chondroitinschwefelsäure A und C (H. GROSSFELD, 1963). Zwischenprodukte des $^{35}SO_4$-Einbaus sind aus Epiphysenknorpeln 9 Tage alter Ratten isoliert worden (J. PICARD, 1964). Man fand Adenosin-5-Phosphosulfat (A-5-PSO_4), 3-Phosphoadenosin-5-Phosphosulfat (3-P-A-5-P-SO_4) Uridindiphosphogalaktosamin-N-Acetylsulfat (UDPGal-N-Acetyl-S) und Chondroitinschwefelsäure. Wir dürfen annehmen, daß der Sulfateinbau, wie bei Knorpelzellen bekannt, in drei Stufen verläuft (F. D'ABRAMO, 1957).

1. $SO_4^{2-} + ATP^{4-} \xrightarrow{Mg}$ A-5-P-$SO_4^{2-} + PP^{4-}$ (ATP-Sulfurylase)
2. A-5-P-$SO_4^{2-} + ATP^{4-} \xrightarrow{Mg}$ 3-P-A-5-P-$SO_4^{4-} + ADP^{3-}$ (Adenosin-5-Phosphosulfokinase)
3. 3-P-A-5-P-SO_4^{4-}+Mucopolysaccharid $\xrightarrow{ATP+Mg}$ Chondroitinsulfat + AMP + P (Mucopolysaccharidsulfotransferase).

Es ist noch nicht erwiesen, ob niedermolekulare Chondroitinschwefelsäure als Primermolekül (J. B. ADAMS, 1961, 1960) für die Chondroitinschwefelsäuresynthese nötig ist, oder polymeres Chondroitin als Vorstufe sulfuriert wird (K. MEYER, 1956a).

Glucose wird von verknöcherungsfähigem Knorpel in Glucosamin und Galaktosamin umgewandelt (W. R. MURPHY, 1956). Die Hexosaminsynthetaseaktivität dieser Knorpel ist hoch (J. D. CIPERA, 1960, 1962; H.-J. DULCE, 1960a, b).

Somatotropes Hormon und Insulin steigern die Mucopolysaccharidsynthese im verknöcherungsfähigen Knorpel (D. S. BERNSTEIN, 1961). Man könnte sich vorstellen, daß durch diese Funktion des somatotropen Hormons in der Epiphysenfuge quellbare Matrix erhalten wird, an deren Rand sich das Längenwachstum elastisch vollzieht. Auch Parathormon (C. D. GURI, 1964) und Vitamin D_3 (J. D. CIPERA, 1960, 1963) erhöhen die Mucopolysaccharidsynthese im verknöcherungsfähigen Knorpel.

Mit zunehmender Verknöcherung bildet Knochengewebe eine Matrix, die weniger saure Mucopolysaccharide enthält (H.-J. DULCE, 1960, 1960b) (Tabelle 33).

Tabelle 33. *Gehalt des verknöchernden Knorpels und Knochens an Mucopolysaccharidbausteinen in % der asche- und fettfreien Trockensubstanz (AFTS)* (H.-J. DULCE, 1960, 1960b)

	Hexosamin % AFTS	Sulfat % AFTS	Uronsäure % AFTS	N % AFTS
Rind, 25—30 cm Scheitelsteißlänge, verknöcherungsfähiger Epiphysenknorpel, Tibia und Femur	6,90	3,58	6,59	10,5
Diaphysenknochen Tibia und Femur	1,52	0,68	0,79	12,2
Ratte, 3 Wochen alt, verknöchernder Epiphysenknorpel, Tibia und Femur	2,20	0,70	1,40	12,1
Diaphysenknochen, Tibia und Femur	0,66	0,28	0,22	12,5

Knochengewebe vermag sulfatierte Mucopolysaccharide nur in geringem Umfang zu synthetisieren. WEATHERELL u. Mitarb. (1963) wiesen nach, daß mit einsetzender Verknöcherung der Sulfatgehalt des Knochens stark abnimmt. $^{35}SO_4$ wird mehr als anorganisches Sulfat und weniger als Estersulfat gebunden (D. HOWELL, 1964; D. D. DZIETWIATKOWSKI, 1951, 1952; AMPRINO, 1955). Auch die Hexosaminsynthetaseaktivität ist im verknöchernden Gewebe niedriger als im verknöcherungsfähigen und im permanenten Knorpel (H. J. DULCE, 1960a, 1960b; A. A. CASTELLANI, 1956; W. DEISS, 1962) (Tabelle 34).

Das Entstehen von Glucuronsäure aus Glucose-1-Phosphat, Uridintriphosphat, Mg^{2+}, und NAD zeigte CASTELLANI (1957) in Epiphysenhomogenaten junger Kaninchen.

Das somatotrope Hormon steigert den Sulfateinbau in verknöchernde Epiphysen (W. R. MURPHY, 1956). Thyreotropes Hormon und Thyroxin unterstützen diese Wirkung noch. Durch Parathormon wird im Knochen, wie JOHNSTON (1965, 1962) in vitro an Calvarien parathyreoideaextraktbehandelter Ratten zeigen konnte, vermehrt Hexosamin synthetisiert. In der weiteren Folge kommt es aber anscheinend doch im Rahmen des Matrixabbaus zur Abnahme des Hexosamingehaltes im Knochen (C. C. JOHNSTON, 1961). Wir wissen, daß gleichzeitig SO_4 vermehrt im Harn und Serum erscheint (F. BRONNER, 1960). Anabole Hormone aktivieren den Sulfateinbau in die Knochenmatrix (K. KOWALEWSKI, 1958, 1958a) (Tabelle 35).

Tabelle 34. *Hexosaminsynthetaseaktivität in Homogenaten von Knochen und Knorpeln beim Rind* (H. J. DULCE, 1960a)

	μg Hexosamin/Std je g AFTS
Rind, 25—30 cm Scheitelsteißlänge, verknöcherungsfähiger Epiphysenknorpel	298
Diaphysenknochen	95
Ratte, 3 Wochen alt, verknöchernder Epiphysenknorpel	101
Diaphysenknochen	99

Ansatz: Enzymnachweis nach dem Verfahren von CASTELLANI (1956).
AFTS = asche- und fettfreie Trockensubstanz

Unter dem Einfluß von Glucocorticoiden (Cortison und Cortisol) wird dagegen die Synthese der sauren Mucopolysaccharide im Knochen, gemessen am $^{35}SO_4$-Einbau und Hexosamingehalt gehemmt (K. KOWALEWSKI, 1958, 1958a; W. H. ROOKS, 1963). Vitamin A und Vitamin D fördern anscheinend die Synthese saurer Mucopolysaccharide im verknöchernden Gewebe über den Sulfateinbau (D. D. DZIEWIATKOWSKI, 1954a, 1954).

Einzelne mucopolysaccharidabbauende Enzyme sind bisher nur im Knochen nachgewiesen worden. Aufgrund histochemischer Beobachtungen müssen wir annehmen, daß in Knochenzellen β-D-Glucuronidase, die Disaccharideinheiten spaltet, und β-D-Glucosidase sowie β-D-Galaktosidase vorkommen (W. GUBISCH, 1961; F. SCHLAGER, 1959, 1960). VAES (1964) wies in Calvarien, Meta- und Diaphysenhomogenaten junger Ratten darüberhinaus durch fraktionierte Zentrifugation im Cytoplasma lokalisierbare Hyaluronidase und partikelgebundene β-N-Acetylaminodesoxyglucosidase nach. Gleichzeitig bestätigte er das Vorkommen von β-Glucuronidase.

Tabelle 35. *Aufnahme von Sulfat in den Femurknochen 3 Wochen alter Hähnchen unter Steroidgaben* (K. KOWALEWSKI, 1958, 1958a)

	^{35}S Imp./min × 1000/100 mg Femurknochen
Kontrolle	6,23
50 mg 17-Äthyl-19-Nortestosteron	15,87
50 mg Methyltestosteron	8,07
50 mg Testosteronpropionat	8,10
50 mg Cortison	1,98
50 mg Cortison + 17-Äthyl-19-Nortestosteron	10,18
50 mg Cortison + 50 mg Methyltestosteron	3,51
50 mg Cortison + 50 mg Testosteronpropionat	3,22

Die Tiere erhielten 24 Std nach der letzten Hormondosis 1 mc ^{35}S/kg subcutan als Na_2SO_4 injiziert. Die gesamten Hormonmengen wurden in 3 Wochen gegeben.

Alle bisherigen chemischen (H.-J. DULCE, 1960), histochemischen (W. EGER, 1963) und autoradiographischen (C. P. LEBLOND, 1950) Untersuchungen von Knochen verschiedener Entwicklungsstadien lassen erkennen, daß im Zuge der Verknöcherung der Gesamtgehalt an Mucopolysacchariden abnimmt, und zusätzlich neutrale sulfatfreie Mucopolysaccharide an die Stelle der sulfathaltigen sauren Mucopolysaccharide treten. Der eigentliche Umsatz der Chondroitinschwefelsäure muß, wie BOWNESS (1963) bei Hunden nachwies, in dem Vorstadium der verknöcherungsfähigen Epiphysenplatte besonders hoch sein, höher noch als im permanenten Knorpel, viel höher aber als in Metaphysenknochen. BOWNESS (1963) schließt aus seinen Beobachtungen, daß die Chondroitinschwefelsäure erst zu niedermolekularen Bruchstücken depolymerisiert und dann desulfuriert wird. Im permanenten Knorpel beträgt die Halbwertszeit von Chondroitinschwefelsäure C anhand der Messungen bei Kaninchen altersabhängig zwischen 3—30 Tagen (Tabelle 36).

Tabelle 36. *Halbwertzeiten der Chondroitinschwefelsäure C und des Keratosulfats in Tagen nach in vivo-Einfluß von Hormonen*

	Junge Tiere Tg.	Erwachsene Tiere Tg.	Erwachsene Tiere/Tg.			
			+ Wachstumshormon	+ Testosteron	+ Oestrogen	+ Cortison
Chondroitinschwefelsäure C .	28—30	3—5	28—30		25	3—4
Keratosulfat . . .		60	8	47	21	5

Präparationen aus dem Nucleus pulposus des Kaninchens, Chondroitinschwefelsäure C anhand von Galaktosamin-^{14}C gemessen, Keratosulfat anhand von Glucosamin-^{14}C gemessen nach ^{14}C-Glucosegabe (E. A. Davidson, 1963).

Bei Ratten errechnet sich die Halbwertzeit aufgrund der ^{35}S-Markierung zu 17 Tagen (H. Bostroem, 1952; Ch. W. Danko, 1961), bei Meerschweinchen zu 87 Tagen (R. Lotmar, 1960).

3. Knochenmineral

Nur im verknöchernden Gewebe und im Knochen tritt das Mineral in einer selbständigen kristallinen Phase auf. Wir finden zwar im permanenten Knorpel Calcium gegenüber der extracellulären Flüssigkeit ca. 30-fach angereichert (H.-J. Dulce, 1960). Es kommt aber nicht zur Ausfällung, weil der hohe Anteil des Knorpels an Chondroitinschwefelsäure das Calcium ebenso wie andere Erdalkalien und Kupfer chelatartig bindet (J. R. Dunstone, 1960).

Das Knochenmineral als kristalline Phase steht im Lösungsgleichgewicht mit der extracellulären Flüssigkeit. Sowohl die Kristallisation als auch die Mineralauflösung sind letztlich physiko-chemische Vorgänge in der extracellulären Flüssigkeit, auf die der Stoffwechsel von Knochenzellen und die Funktion anderer Organe sowie die Mineralzufuhr Einfluß nehmen können. Um einen Einblick in den Baustoffwechsel und den Umsatz des Knochenminerals zu erhalten, muß das Lösungsgleichgewicht zwischen Knochenmineral und extracellulärer Flüssigkeit quantitativ und seiner Art nach untersucht werden. Quantitative Daten gewinnt man in vivo durch Bilanzstudien, die sich auch auf einzelne Verteilungsschritte der im Knochenmineral vertretenen Ionen erstrecken. Die Art des Lösungsgleichgewichtes bestimmt man in Modellversuchen und durch in vivo Beobachtungen.

a) Bilanz- und Umsatzstudien

In erster Linie beschäftigen sich Untersuchungen mit Bilanz und Umsatz von Calcium und Phosphat als den Hauptanteilen des Knochenminerals. Beim Erwachsenen beträgt der im Knochenmineral gebundene Calciumanteil ca. 1,7—2 % des Körpergewichtes. Dieses Calcium ist aufgrund seines Lösungsgleichgewichtes mit der extracellulären Flüssigkeit durch zahlreiche Fließgleichgewichte, die an der extracellulären Flüssigkeit angreifen, beeinflußbar. Man kann die in den Calciumumsatz des Organismus eingehenden Verteilungsschritte zu einem Schema zusammenfassen (Abb. 2).

Zum Prüfen einzelner Verteilungsschritte wird im Tierversuch ^{45}Ca mit einer Halbwertzeit von $1{,}64 \cdot 10^4$ Tagen und beim Menschen zweckmäßig ^{47}Ca mit einer Halbwertzeit von 4,7 Tagen eingesetzt.

Im Schema sind fünf der Messung zugängliche Substrate enthalten.

1. Knochenmineral als schwer austauschbarer Calciumpool (K).
2. Extracelluläre Flüssigkeit (EZF) = Interstitielle Flüssigkeit + Plasma als leicht austauschbarer Calciumpool (P).

3. Harn als Träger ausgeschiedenen Calciums (H_S).
4. Faeces als Träger ausgeschiedenen Calciums (F_S).
5. Ernährung als Träger zugeführten Calciums (Z_N).

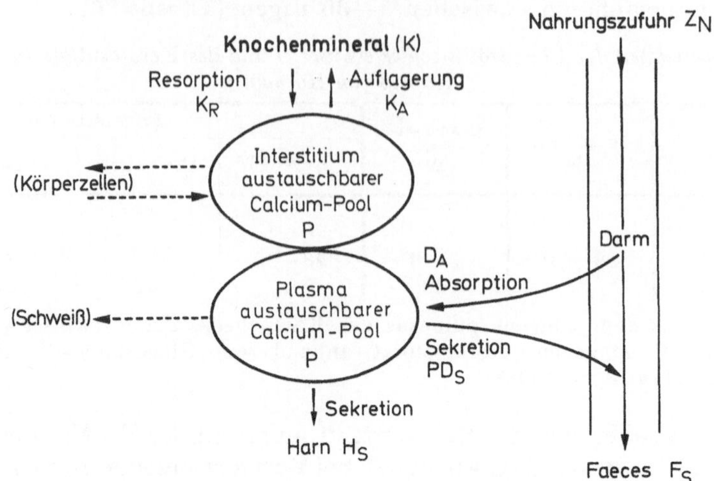

(PD_S = Pool-Darmsekretion, D_A = Darmabsorption)

Abb. 2

Diese Substrate bilden die Grundlage für Berechnungen der Gesamtbilanz und der das Lösungsgleichgewicht des Knochenminerals quantitativq estimmenden Reaktionen. Solange mit der Nahrung nicht ein Calciumüberschuß zugeführt wird, kann man die Calciumsekretion in den Schweiß (0,5—4 m Val/l) (E. EISENBERG, 1961), sowie die Abwanderung von Calcium in Körperzellen (B. MULRYAN, 1964) und schwer austauschbar in den permanenten Knorpel vernachlässigen. Die Gesamtbilanz (Bi in 24 Std) errechnet sich unter diesen Voraussetzungen zu

$$\mathrm{Bi} = Z_N - H_S - F_S \qquad \text{(I)}$$

$$\mathrm{Bi} = K_A - K_R. \qquad \text{(II)}$$

Das bedeutet, Messungen der Calciumzufuhr und -ausfuhr ohne Zuhilfenahme von Isotopen lassen bereits eine orientierende Aussage über Knochen auf- oder abbauende Vorgänge zu, weil $K_A - K_R = Z_N - H_S - F_S$ ist. K_A kann aber exakter mit Hilfe von Calciumisotopen nach

$$K_A = U_P - H_S - PD_S \qquad \text{(III)}$$

innerhalb von 6 Tagen ermittelt werden, weil frischgebildeter Apatit ca. 7 Tage überdauert, ehe er wieder zerfällt.

Die Umsatzrate (U_P) für Calcium im schnell austauschbaren Pool kann man nach einmaliger Injektion von Calciumisotopen aus dem Aktivitätsabfall im Plasma bestimmen (G. BAUER, 1957).

$$U_P = \text{Gesamtcalcium im schnell austauschbaren Pool} \cdot \frac{0{,}693}{T/2}$$

$$T/2 = \text{Halbwertsverweildauer für } {}^{45}\text{Ca im Plasma.}$$

Durch Extrapolieren der spezifischen Aktivität des Calciums im Plasma innerhalb des ersten Tages nach der Injektion einer definierten ^{45}Ca-Menge wird der gesamte schnell austauschbare Calciumpool ermittelt. Zwischen dem 3.—6. Tag ist das Fließgleichgewicht eingetreten. ^{45}Ca wird in dieser Zeit gleichmäßig in den Knochen und Knorpel eingelagert und in Harn, Faeces und Schweiß ausgeschieden. Erst ab 7. Tag ist aufgrund apatitauflösender Vorgänge mit einem rückläufigen Erscheinen von ^{45}Ca aus dem Knochen zu rechnen. Man hat deshalb versucht, aus diesem späten Teil der Kurve K_R abzuleiten. PD_S errechnet man anhand der spezifischen Aktivität der Faeces im Zeitraum des Aktivitätsabfalles im Plasma nach einmaliger Injektion.

Im Tierversuch wird K_A direkt durch Analyse markierten Knochens festgestellt. K_R ergibt sich aus der Differenz von Bi und K_A nach (II) oder der Analyse der Plasmaaktivitätskurve von BAUER (1957). D_A ergibt die Gleichung

$$D_A = Z_N + PD_S - F_S . \qquad \text{(IV)}$$

Die Halbwertsverweilzeit für ^{45}Ca im Organismus des Erwachsenen beträgt ca. 260 Tage (F. BRONNER, 1956). Der schnell austauschbare Calciumpool wurde bei Erwachsenen von mehreren Autoren (G. BAUER, 1957; B. LINDQUIST, 1959; P. DOERING, 1963) zu ca. 5 g entsprechend 70—100 mg/kg Körpergewicht bestimmt (Tabelle 37).

Tabelle 37. *Altersabhängigkeit der Höhe des leicht austauschbaren Calciumpools und des Calciumumsatzes aus dem Pool beim Menschen* (G. BAUER, 1957)

Körpergewicht (kg)	Alter	Leicht austauschbarer Calciumpool (P) g	U_P		K_A		PD_S+H_S	
			mg	%/Tag	mg	% Pool/Tag	mg	% Pool/Tag
4,3	1 Monat	0,78	390	50	281	36	109	14
6,9	5 Monate	1,07	424	39,6	365	34,1	59	5,5
12,9	1,5 Jahre	3,01	605	20,1	543	18,0	62	1,9
32	11 Jahre	5,15	989	19,2	785	15,2	204	4,0
61	22 Jahre	6,96	1071	15,4	788	11,3	283	4,1
70	26 Jahre	5,23	815	15,6	467	8,9	348	6,7
58	43 Jahre	4,61	659	14,3	362	7,8	297	6,5
65	51 Jahre	5,07	643	12,7	363	7,2	280	5,5
70	58 Jahre	4,35	735	16,9	493	11,3	242	5,6
65	60 Jahre	4,3	908	21,1	563	13,1	345	8,0
86	63 Jahre	7,58	1266	16,7	437	5,8	829	10,9

OEFF (1962) fand höhere (7,5—8,8 g), RAGAN (1964) niedrigere Werte (2,9—4,5 g) für P. Die Höhe dieses Calciumpools ist altersabhängig. In der Wachstumsphase beobachteten BAUER u. Mitarb. (G. BAUER, 1957; B. LINDQUIST, 1959; G. D. MCPHERSON, 1965) einen Pool von 150—295 mg/kg Körpergewicht, der deutlich höher als beim Erwachsenen lag. Der Umsatz im schnell austauschbaren Pool beträgt bei Erwachsenen 15 % täglich, bei Kindern 20 % täglich und bei Säuglingen 40—50 % täglich. Die Höhe der täglichen Calciumauflagerung im Knochen wurde von zahlreichen Untersuchern bestätigt (G. BAUER, 1957; B. LINDQUIST, 1959; P. DOERING, 1963; CH. RAGAN, 1964; F. W. LAFFERTY, 1964) (Tabelle 37). DOERING (1963) differenzierte auch noch PD_S und H_S (Tabelle 38).

Tabelle 38. *Erwachsener ca. 60 Jahre* (nach DOERING, 1963)

Ca-Pool	5,2 g	
U_P	. . . .	772 mg = 14,9 %/Tag
K_A	. . . .	516 mg = 9,8 %/Tag
PD_S	. . . .	106 mg = 2 %/Tag
H_S	. . . .	159 mg = 3 %/Tag

OEFF (1962) bestätigte die Höhe der PD_S mit ca. 2 % des Pools täglich. Dagegen fanden er und RAGAN (1964) eine geringere Harnausscheidung von ca. 1,4 % des Pools täglich. Auf Grund langfristiger Versuche (P. DOERING, 1963) ist zu erwarten, daß die Werte für K_A, PD_S und H_S niedriger als in den Tabellen angegeben liegen. Der Anteil des endogenen am fäcalen Calcium kann zufuhrabhängig 20—90 % betragen (P. DOERING, 1963). Im höheren Lebensalter besteht anscheinend eine Neigung zum Calciumverlust, weil K_A konstant bleibt, PD_S und H_S aber zunehmen.

Bei einer Zufuhr von 600—800 mg Calcium täglich werden im Darm des Erwachsenen ca. 37 % Calcium resorbiert (J. L. DEGRAZIA, 1964). Im Alter ist die Resorption geringer (A. CANIGGIA, 1964/65).

Bei Kindern findet sich eine Knochenneubildungsrate von 0,55 % des Skelets/Tag, bei Erwachsenen (30—50 Jahre) von 0,05 %, bei alten Menschen von 0,02 % (B. LINDQUIST, 1959).

Die Calciumresorption (K_R) im Knochen beträgt beim gesunden Erwachsenen 334 bis 515 mg/täglich (F. W. LAFFERTY, 1964), also etwa soviel wie K_A. Damit bleibt die Bilanz des Lösungsgleichgewichtes zwischen Knochenmineral und der extracellulären Flüssigkeit ausgeglichen. Das Gleichgewicht zwischen K_A und K_R ist für die Knochenbildung und das Wachstum — die Massenzunahme — und für die Knochenresorption — die Massenabnahme — bestimmend.

Man kann beim Menschen die K_A auch mit Hilfe des Strontium-Verteilungsraumes bestimmen (E. EISENBERG, 1961). Aus U_P und H_S errechnet man dann K_A. PD_S fällt weg, weil i. v. appliziertes Strontium kaum in den Darm ausgeschieden wird. Bei Knochenkranken verwertet man als weiteres indirektes Maß für K_A die alkalische Phosphatase, für K_R die Hydroxyprolinausscheidung im Harn (F. W. LAFFERTY, 1964). Die Korrelation der Wertepaare betrug 50 %.

Bei Nagetieren verhält sich der Calciumumsatz im Knochen anders als bei Menschen und Affen (G. MILHAUD, 1963). Der leicht austauschbare Pool wird täglich zu ca. 60—70 % umgesetzt. Der größte Teil davon geht in die Größe K_A ein. LINDQUIST (1959) bestimmte die Calciumauflagerung und Resorption an einzelnen Abschnitten der Röhrenknochen von jungen Ratten (Tabelle 39). In der Mandibel der Ratte ist die Calciumresorption besonders stark (H. JEFFAY, 1961).

Tabelle 39. *Calciumumsatz im Tibiaknochen einer 50 g schweren Ratte* (B. LINDQUIST, 1959)

	Epi/Metaphyse	Diaphyse
Calciumgehalt (mg)	36	30
Ca-Auflagerung (mg/Tag)	3,36	0,72
Ca-Resorption (mg/Tag)	2,88	0,24
Nettovermehrung (mg/Tag)	0,48	0,48

Die Knochenneubildungsrate liegt bei der wachsenden Ratte bis zu 10 % des Skelets täglich (W. F. NEUMAN, 1955).

Bei eierlegenden Vögeln ist der Calciumumsatz im Organismus sehr viel rascher als bei Säugetieren und beim Menschen. Mit der Eischale gehen beim Huhn 1,8—2 g Calcium verloren (M. V. L'HEUREUX, 1949; W. MUELLER, 1964; C. TYLER, 1940). In den Reaktionen K_A und K_R werden deshalb im Durchschnitt täglich 1 g Calcium umgesetzt (W. MUELLER, 1964). In der Eischalenbildungsphase beträgt die Entnahme aus dem Knochen ca. 1,5 g Calcium. Man bezeichnet diese Phase als den negativen Bilanztag. In der Ruhephase ist dafür K_R kleiner als K_A, um den Knochen zu regenerieren. Der Ausgleich erfolgt durch den sog. positiven Bilanztag. Durchschnittlich stammen 50 % des Eischalencalciums aus dem Knochen und 50 % unmittelbar aus der Darmresorption (D_A). Der Calciumumsatz im Knochen von Legehühnern ist im wesentlichen auf den spongiösen Knochen begrenzt (W. MUELLER, 1964; S. HURWITZ, 1964, 1965). Der austauschbare Pool beträgt ca. 4,4 g entsprechend 20 % des Körpercalciums (W. MUELLER, 1964). Die Calciumkonzentration in der extracellulären Flüssigkeit liegt bei Legehühnern zwischen 20—30 mg % mit Gipfeln in der Eibildungsphase. Das Calcium ist zum größten Teil proteingebunden.

b) Austauschvorgänge am Knochenmineral und Knochen

Die Art der Austauschvorgänge von Calcium und Phosphor zwischen extracellulärer Flüssigkeit und Knochenmineral wird durch physikalisch-chemische Reaktionen und durch cellulär gesteuerte Reaktionen beschrieben. Schon durch histochemische Markierung, etwa mit Calcium-affinem Alizarin (F. PROELL, 1933; F. HEUCK, 1960, 1960a) oder Tetracyclin (K. H. IBSEN, 1964; J. DELEU, 1964), konnte gezeigt werden, daß im Knochen leichter und schwerer zugängliches Calcium vorkommt (K. H. IBSEN, 1964).

Wir kennen heute drei Stufen, nach denen die rein physiko-chemischen Austausch- und Einbauvorgänge von Calcium und Phosphat am Knochenmineral ablaufen.

I. Eindringen der Ionen in die Hydrathülle der Kristallite und Adsorption an deren Oberfläche.

II. Gleichioniger Austausch an der Oberfläche der Kristalle.

III. Eindringen der Ionen in Fehlordnungsstellen des Kristallgitters, mit Idealisierung des Gitters und eventuelle Umwandlung der Einheitszellen.

Gleichzeitig wird Calcium an noch verbliebene saure Mucopolysaccharide in der Knochenmatrix schwer reversibel chelatartig gebunden (W. EGER, 1963; O. EICHLER, 1962). Bei Dentin und Zahnschmelz nannte EICHLER (1962) den Vorgang den b-Prozeß. Diese sog. Calciumfängereigenschaft ist aber im Knochen vernachlässigbar klein (H.-J. DULCE, 1960; O. EICHLER, 1962) (Tabelle 40).

Tabelle 40. *Calciumgehalt in Knorpel und Knochen bei Rinderfeten* (H.-J. DULCE, 1960)

	Rinderfeten, 3 Monate alt	
	Gesamt-calciumgehalt % FTS	Grundsubstanz gebundenes Ca % FTS[1]
Permanenter Septumknorpel	1,6	1,4
Verknöcherungsfähiger Epiphysen-knorpel, Femur	1,8	1,0
Diaphysenknochen, Femur	22,9	0,0

[1] Errechnet nach Abzug des an anorganisches Phosphat gebundenen Calciums unter Zugrundelegen eines Hydroxylapatits. (FTS = fettfreie Trockensubstanz)

Phosphat wird dagegen in der Knochenmatrix zusätzlich an Orten neutraler Mucopolysaccharide, wahrscheinlich organisch gebunden (W. EGER, 1963; H.-J. DULCE, 1960, 1960b). Man spricht deshalb von der Phosphatfängereigenschaft der Knochenmatrix. Knorpelmatrix nimmt kaum Phosphat auf.

Die cellulär gesteuerten physiko-chemischen Reaktionen zwischen extracellulärer Flüssigkeit und Knochenmineral betreffen die

IV. Kristallgitterneubildung

und die

V. Kristallgitterauflösung.

Die Vorgänge I und II sind konzentrationsabhängig und reversibel. Die daran teilnehmenden Calciumionen werden mit dem leicht austauschbaren Pool (P) erfaßt.

Die Vorgänge III und IV sind teilweise konzentrationsunabhängig und irreversible. Sie werden durch K_A erfaßt. Die Höhe von K_A kann lediglich durch die Calciumaufnahme in die organische Matrix weicher Bindegewebe verfälscht werden.

Der Vorgang V wird in vivo durch K_R gemessen.

In vivo erkennt man, daß ^{45}Ca und ^{32}PO$_4$ im Bereich der Epiphysen und Verknöcherungszonen schneller eingebaut werden als in Diaphysen oder Zahnschmelz (W. D. ARMSTRONG, 1948; G. HEVESY, 1940). Versuche an Hunden beweisen, daß ^{45}Ca und ^{32}P am intensivsten in den Wachstumszonen des Knochens aufgenommen werden (J. STRANDH, 1965).

Aufnahmeraten von ^{45}Ca und ^{32}PO$_4$ bei Hunden (J. STRANDH, 1965) sind:

Periostaler Lamellenknochen 12—13 × 10^{-3} %/Std
Haverssche Systeme Compacta 10—11 × 10^{-3} %/Std
Endostale Spongiosa Lamellen 6,3—7,6 × 10^{-3} %/Std

$$\%/\text{Std} = 100 \frac{a_1 t_2 - a_1 t_1}{\int_{t_1}^{t_2} a_2 t\,(dt) - \int_{t_1}^{t_2} a_1 t\,(dt)}$$

$a_1 t_{1,2}$ = spez. Aktivität im Knochen/Std im Zeitintervall
$a_{1,2} t$ = spez. Aktivität im Plasma/Std.

Periostaler Knochen hat nach mikroradiographischen Messungen tatsächlich einen höheren Kalksalzgehalt als Haverssche Systeme (F. HEUCK, 1963).

An Hand des Aktivitätsabfalls von ^{45}Ca oder ^{47}Ca im Serum von Ratten (G. C. BAUER, 1955) und Menschen (L. LUTWAK, 1964) lassen sich zwei schnelle Phasen des Calciumeinbaus (1 Std und 4—8 Std) ableiten, die den Vorgängen I und II zugeordnet werden können.

Matrixfreies, glykolveraschtes Knochenpulver nimmt ^{45}Ca oder ^{32}P aus Pufferlösung ebenfalls in einer schnellen Phase (2—4 Std) und einer langsamen Phase auf (L. RICHELLE, 1960; M. FALKENHEIM, 1947, 1951; E. E. UNDERWOOD, 1952). Während der ersten Phase kann man die ^{32}P-Aufnahme durch die Freundlichsche Adsorptionsisotherme und später durch zusätzliche Diffusionsvorgänge in Kristalle hinein beschreiben. Der Phosphataustausch hängt von der Größe der Oberfläche der Kristalle des Knochenminerals ab (M. FALKENHEIM, 1947; E. E. UNDERWOOD, 1952), der Calciumaustausch weniger (K. B. DAWSON, 1955; E. E. UNDERWOOD, 1952). An dem Austausch nehmen ca. 12—20% der P-Atome (M. FALKENHEIM, 1947; W. F. NEUMAN, 1950) und 14—32% der Calciumatome (M. FALKENHEIM, 1951; W. F. NEUMAN, 1950; E. E. UNDERWOOD, 1952) des Knochenminerals teil. Nach DALLEMAGNE (1955, 1955a) sind nur ca. 15%, nämlich der sog. Calciumüberschuß, von $1^1/_2$ Calcium/Apatitmolekül austauschbar. Durch Glühen auf 900° nimmt die austauschbare Calciummenge auf 0,5—2% ab (M. FALKENHEIM, 1951). Synthetischer Hydroxylapatit tauscht innerhalb von 24 Std ca. 11% seines Calciums gegen ^{45}Ca aus (W. F. NEUMAN, 1955). In alkoholischer Lösung findet der Austausch in vitro bis zu 10 Std nur in einer Phase statt (L. RICHELLE, 1960), während er in wäßriger Lösung in zwei Phasen, einer schnellen und einer langsamen, bis zu 50 Std verläuft. Die langsame Phase dürfte dem Vorgang II, dem isoionischen Austausch entsprechen, der nach den Befunden von RICHELLE (1960) ca. 20% der Adsorption im Vorgang I beträgt.

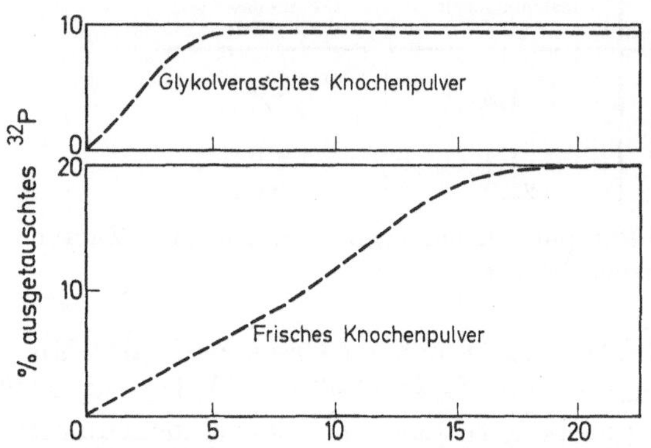

Abb. 3. Aufnahme von ^{32}P in Knochenpulver von Kaninchenfemur (W. F. NEUMAN, 1950a). Austausch in Phosphatpufferlösung von pH 7,2

Die Halbwertszeiten für den ^{45}Calciumaustausch im glykolveraschten Knochenpulver werden mit 1—2 Std (M. J. DALLEMAGNE, 1955; E. E. UNDERWOOD, 1952), im Dentin mit 8 Std genannt (E. E. UNDERWOOD, 1952). In vivo stehen nach Berechnungen von ROBINSON (1952) für den Oberflächenaustausch nach Vorgang I und II nur ca. 2,5% des Knochenminerals zur Verfügung. Auf dieser relativ kleinen Fläche müßte der oben genannte Austausch ca. 15% der Calciumatome erreichen.

Der irreversible Schritt III der Einbauvorgänge am Knochenmineral ist bei in vitro Versuchen nur an unveraschtem Knochenpulver, das von frischgebildetem Knochen stammt (M. FALKENHEIM, 1951; E. E. UNDERWOOD, 1952; W. F. NEUMAN, 1950, 1950a) und an synthetischem Hydroxylapatit (W. F. NEUMAN, 1955) zu erkennen. Die Isotopenaufnahme verläuft kontinuierlich und erreicht schließlich nach Tagen ein höheres Maximum als bei veraschtem Knochenpulver (W. F. NEUMAN, 1950a) (Abb. 3, Tabelle 41).

In vivo ist also die Aufnahmekapazität des Knochens für Ionen größer als bei durch Veraschen erhaltenem Knochenmineral. Das kommt besonders in den frischgebildeten Anteilen des Knochens zum Ausdruck. Gleichzeitig behindert anscheinend die Matrix die Verteilung der Ionen in den Stufen I und II. Von HEVESY (1940) und NEUMAN (1950, 1950a) wird dieser, nur bei unveraschtem Knochenpulver zu beobachtende und im Gegensatz zu I und II über Tage verlaufende Vorgang III als „Rekristallisation" bezeichnet. Die Rekristallisation ist durch Erhöhen der Versuchstemperatur anfänglich zu steigern, nimmt aber bei noch höheren Temperaturen sofort ab. In alkoholischer Lösung tritt keine Rekristallisation auf (L. RICHELLE, 1960).

Unter der Rekristallisation des Knochenminerals stellen wir uns am besten eine Umwandlung der Kristallgitterstruktur vor. Ionen besetzen dabei Fehlstellen im Kristallgitter, oder durch heteroionischen Austausch treten Ca^{++} für H^{+} oder PO_4^{3-} für CO_3^{2-} in das Gitter ein. Auf diese Weise wird das Gitter idealisiert, und einzelne Einheitszellen bilden sich um. Wir sollten deshalb den Ausdruck „Rekristallisation" mit „Umkristallisation" übersetzen. Die physiologische Alterung des Knochenminerals oder das Veraschen führen physiko-chemisch zur Fehlstellenbesetzung und Idealisierung des Gitters, so daß die Ionenaufnahme im Schritt III ausbleibt.

SCHMALZRIED (1963) hat bei Ionenkristallen derartige Fehlordnungstypen nachgewiesen und gezeigt, daß Ionen, dem elektrochemischen Potentialgradienten folgend, in Fehlstellen eines benachbarten, tieferliegenden Kristallgitters einspringen können. Durch die Rekristallisation in der Stufe III könnte hiernach die biologische Evolution der Elementarzellen des Kristallgitters im Knochenmineral während des Lebens beschrieben werden.

Tabelle 41. *^{32}P-Austausch von Knochenpulver des Kaninchenfemur* (W. F. NEUMAN, 1950a)

	% austauschbares P nach 48 Std in $^{32}PO_4$-Puffer, pH 7,2		
	frischer Knochen		glykolveraschter Knochen
	einschließlich organisches Phosphat	ohne organisches Phosphat	
Subperiostaler Knochen	50,4	ca. 35	12,7
Metaphysenknochen	29,3	ca. 21	13
Diaphysenknochen, Compacta	9,2	ca. 9	13,4

Das Knochenpulver war auf 60—100 mesh gemahlen.

Der Calciumaustausch am unveraschten Knochenpulver in den Stufen I—III vollzieht sich mit einer Halbwertzeit zwischen 8—20 Tagen (M. FALKENHEIM, 1951; E. E. UNDERWOOD, 1952). Die Schritte I und II des Ioneneinbaus in das Knochenmineral sind von der Ionenstärke der extracellulären Flüssigkeit abhängig, der Schritt III dagegen nicht (F. BRONNER, 1956; W. F. NEUMAN, 1953). Wahrscheinlich sind diese Schritte Wasserstoffionen-abhängig. Bei Acidose kann Calcium und Natrium aus dem Knochenmineral zur Pufferung herangezogen werden.

Die cellulär gesteuerte Bildung und Umwandlung des Knochenminerals in den Schritten IV und V wird in den Abschnitten Knochenbildung und Knochenauflösung behandelt.

Neben Calcium und Phosphat sind auch alle anderen im Knochenmineral vorkommenden Ionen an seinem Umsatz beteiligt.

Der Natriumumsatz ist im Knochen achtmal schneller als der Calciumumsatz (W. D. ARMSTRONG, 1955). Permanenter Knorpel hat einen noch höheren Natriumumsatz (G. B. FORBES, 1959, 1960). Ca. 30—46% des Körpernatriums liegen im Knochen (M. POST, 1962; M. M. REIDENBERG, 1961; W. H. BERGSTROEM, 1955; G. NICHOLS, 1956). Es beteiligen sich beim Menschen normalerweise nur ca. 10% des Knochennatriums an Austauschvorgängen (G. B. FORBES, 1959; G. NICHOLS, 1956). Im Falle einer Acidose können, ohne daß der Apatit angegriffen wird, beim erwachsenen Organismus ca. 30%, beim wachsenden Organismus ca. 70—80% des Knochennatriums schnell mobilisiert werden (G. B. FORBES, 1959; M. POST, 1962; M. M. REIDENBERG, 1961; D. S. MUNRO, 1959; W. H. BERGSTROEM, 1955, 1956; G. NICHOLS, 1956). STOLL (1956) und NEUMAN (1962) berechneten nach experimentellen Daten, daß in der Hydrathülle des Knochens ca. 0,08 m Mol Na/g und in der Gitteroberfläche ca. 0,12 m Mol Na/g Knochenmineral gebunden werden. Die in der Hydrathülle liegenden Natriumionen sind bei Stoffwechselacidosen offensichtlich leicht mobilisierbar. Mit ihrem Austausch verliert der Knochen gleichzeitig äquimolar Carbonat (W. H. BERGSTROEM, 1954, 1956).

Kalium tritt fast ausschließlich in der Hydrathülle des Knochenminerals auf (W. F. NEUMAN, 1962; W. R. STOLL, 1956) und ist schnell quantitativ austauschbar (Tabelle 42). Ca. 9% des Körperkaliums finden wir im Knochen (M. POST, 1962; M. M. REIDENBERG, 1961; W. H. BERGSTROEM, 1955).

Der Umsatz des Magnesiums ist im Knochen altersabhängig (S. BREIBART, 1960), aber in der Nähe der Verknöcherungszone offensichtlich am stärksten (A. C. FIELD, 1960). Im Magnesiummangelzustand sind ca. 50% des Magnesiums aus dem Knochen mobilisierbar (M. M. REIDENBERG, 1961).

Fluor beeinflußt den Baustoffwechsel des Knochenminerals empfindlich. Mit steigendem Fluorgehalt nimmt die Kristallgröße und -Perfektion des Knochenminerals zu (I. ZIPKIN, 1962; A. S. POSNER, 1964; J. C. MUHLER, 1956) und damit die Löslichkeit und der Ionenabtausch an seinen Oberflächen ab (Abb. 4). Das führt zu geringerem Citrat- und Carbonatgehalt.

Citrat und Carbonat werden von Knochenpulver ebenso wie Calcium und Phosphat in einer schnellen (I) und einer langsamen (II) Phase aufgenommen (W. D. ARMSTRONG, 1956, 1955) Carbonat auch in zwei Phasen abgegeben. Ca. 20—38% des Knochencitrats und 8% des Knochencarbonats sind in vitro leicht austauschbar (W. D. ARMSTRONG, 1965), Veraschen und Phosphationenzusatz verringern die Citrataufnahmefähigkeit. Der Carbonataustausch erfolgt in vivo und in vitro zusammen mit einer äquivalenten Natriummenge (W. D. ARMSTRONG, 1955; W. H. BERGSTROEM, 1954; A. E. SOBEL, 1945).

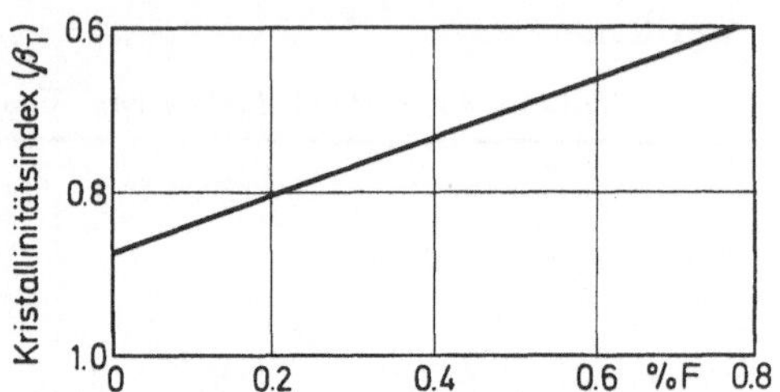

Abb. 4. Abhängigkeit der Kristallinität des Knochenminerals vom Fluorgehalt (A. S. POSNER, 1964). % F in Asche von crista iliaca. Gemessen die Millerindices 211, 112, 300, 302. β_T = Breite bei halbem Maximum für alle Reflektionen in einem Template

Tabelle 42. *Alkalianteile im synthetischen, 7 Tage alten Hydroxylapatit nach 7stündiger Inkubation in ^{22}Na- und ^{42}K-Cl-Lösungen bei pH 7,4 und 25°* (W. F. NEUMAN, 1962)

	K	Na
m Mol/g Knochen, austauschbar .	0,50	0,60
m Mol/g Knochen, nicht austauschbar	0,03	0,27

c) Intestinale Resorption der Bausteine des Knochenminerals

Die Aufnahme von Calcium im Darm (D_A) erfolgt im Duodenum und im Ileum aktiv gegen einen Konzentrationsgradienten und im übrigen Intestinum und Colon passiv durch Diffusion (Y. CHANG, 1964; D. V. KIMBERG, 1961; P. T. CHANDLER, 1962). Im Verlauf des Ileums ist die Calciumaufnahme quantitativ am größten (C. F. CRAMER, 1965). Im Alter wird die aktive Transportleistung geringer (D. V. KIMBERG, 1961). Die Resorption von Calcium im Darm ist innerhalb physiologischer Grenzen pH-unabhängig (R. H. WASSERMAN, 1962; F. R. MICOZ, 1962; J. S. CHARNOCK, 1963). Bei jüngeren Tieren reguliert der Calciumbedarf des Organismus auf einem uns unbekannten Weg die Calciumaufnahme über den Darm (D. V. KIMBERG, 1961). Bei älteren Individuen gibt es diese Regulation nicht.

Die Calciumsekretion erstreckt sich über den ganzen Darm (P. T. CHANDLER, 1962; M. V. L'HEUREUX, 1949). Bei Ratten ist sie im Intestinum aktiv energieabhängig, im Colon passiv.

Im Gegensatz zum Calcium wird anorganisches Phosphat hauptsächlich im Colon und Coecum aufgenommen (P. T. CHANDLER, 1962).

Fluor diffundiert passiv durch die Darmwand (G. STOOKEY, 1964, 1964a).

d) Renale Ausscheidung der Knochenmineralbausteine

Calcium wird in den Harn glomerulär filtriert und tubulär rückresorbiert (W. E. LASSITER, 1962; P. J. HOWARD, 1959). Die Tubuli resorbieren beim Gesunden normalerweise 97—98% der filtrierten Menge von 6,7 mg Calcium/min (D. BERNSTEIN, 1962). Verstärktes Calciumangebot über die extracelluläre Flüssigkeit verringert die Filtrationsrate von Phosphat und steigert die tubuläre Phosphatrückresorption (A. LAVENDER, 1963).

Anorganisches Phosphat wird ebenfalls glomerulär filtriert, aber nur zu ca. 80% im Tubulus rückresorbiert.

4. Regulation des Knochenmineralumsatzes

An der Regulation des Umsatzes der apatitischen Calciumphosphate im Knochen sind Parathormon, Calcitonin, Glucocorticoide, Sexualhormone, Thyroxin, somatotropes Hormon und Vitamin D beteiligt. Angriffspunkte der regulierenden Wirkung sind nicht nur

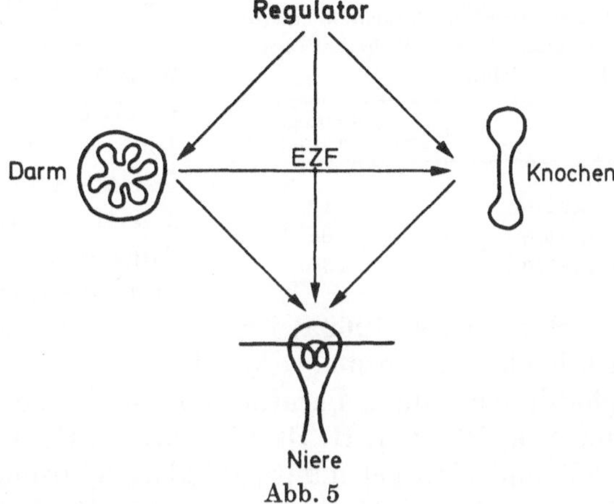

Abb. 5

unmittelbar der Knochen, sondern meist auch Niere und Darm. Auf diese Weise wird durch Vermitteln über die extracelluläre Flüssigkeit (EZF) der Baustoffwechsel des Knochenminerals zusätzlich beeinflußt (Abb. 5).

a) Parathormon

Das Parathormon ist ein aus der Nebenschilddrüse stammendes Polypeptid vom Molekulargewicht 8600, das von RASMUSSEN (1960) und AURBACH (1964) gereinigt dargestellt wurde. Seine quantitative Aminosäurezusammensetzung ist bekannt (H. RASMUSSEN, 1960). In der Regel werden heute aber noch wenig gereinigte Parathyreoideaextrakte klinisch und experimentell angewendet. Nicht alle käuflichen Parathyreoideaextrakte sind biologisch im Calciumhaushalt wirksam (H.-J. DULCE, 1961).

α) Wirkung am Knochen. Wir besitzen heute genügend Beweise dafür, daß Parathormon Knochenmineral mobilisiert. In den Knochen eingebrachtes Nebenschilddrüsengewebe löst Knochenmineral auf (BARNICOT, 1948). Injizierter Parathyreoideaextrakt mobilisiert ^{45}Ca bei Ratten, deren Knochen Wochen vorher markiert waren, in vivo (H. JEFFAY, 1964; K. R. WOODS, 1956) und in vitro (G. M. VAES, 1962; C. COOPER, 1965). Der Aschegehalt von Knochen nimmt dabei ab (A. SCHMID, 1961). Auch die Zahl der calcifizierenden Osteone hängt vom Parathormon ab (J. JOWSEY, 1958). Selbst in vitro Kulturen von Knochenschnitten zugesetztes Parathormon steigert die Knochenmineralauflösung (L. G. RAISZ, 1963, 1965; P. GAILLARD, 1955). Calcium und Phosphat werden gemeinsam mobilisiert (Tabelle 43).

Die Calciummobilisation durch Parathormon ist durch Actinomycin D, einem Hemmstoff der messenger RNS-Synthese, zu hemmen (M. V. HEUREUX, 1949). Man diskutiert deshalb den Wirkungsmechanismus des Parathormons am Knochen cellulär über die Osteoclasten.

β) Intestinale Wirkung. Der Calcium- und Phosphattransport durch die Darmwand in die extracelluläre Flüssigkeit wird durch Parathormon gesteigert (C. F. Cramer, 1963; A. B. Borle, 1963). Diese Wirkung ist eventuell von kleinen Vitamin D-Mengen abhängig. Die bei Hyperparathyreoidismus öfter zu beobachtende Magensaftvermehrung und Hyperacidität ist wahrscheinlich auf die Hypercalcämie zurückzuführen (W. L. Donegan, 1960; R. Ottenjann, 1963).

γ) Renale Wirkung. Parathormon beeinflußt direkt die renalen Ausscheidungsmechanismen für Calcium und Phosphat. Änderungen der Calcium- und Phosphorkonzentration in der extracellulären Flüssigkeit und die Mobilisation des Knochenminerals werden dadurch aber nicht allein erklärt.

Phosphatelimination. Injektionen von Parathyreoideaextrakt führen beim Menschen und beim Tier innerhalb von 3 Std zu einer Phosphatdiurese (gP/Tag) (F. Albright, 1929, 1942; P. L. Munson, 1955; E. Jahan, 1948; P. Chandler, 1951; E. Ellsworth, 1934; H. E. Schaefer, 1962; E. H. Beutner, 1960; H. H. Hiatt, 1957), die durch Actinomycin D-Gaben nicht beeinflußt wird (A. H. Tashjian, 1964). Bei Nebenschilddrüsentumoren ist die Phosphatdiurese typisch (J. J. Canary, 1962; M. Harrison, 1960; D. Bernstein, 1962a). Nach einer Adenomoperation sinkt die Phosphatausscheidung schnell auf Normalwerte ab.

Tabelle 43. *^{45}Ca-Abgabe von markierten Knochenschnitten nach Parathyreoideaextraktzusatz zum Nährmedium* (L. G. Raisz, 1963)

	% ^{45}Ca-Abgabe gegenüber Kontrollen
0,01 IE Parathyreoideaextrakt/ml	12
0,1 IE Parathyreoideaextrakt/ml	66
1,0 IE Parathyreoideaextrakt/ml	136

Ursache der Phosphatdiurese unter Parathormon sind eine gesteigerte glomeruläre P-Filtration (H. E. Schaefer, 1962; H. H. Hiatt, 1957; S. H. Widrow, 1962; W. Eger, 1956; P. Handler, 1952) und eine gehemmte tubuläre Phosphorrückresorption (H. E. Schaefer, 1962; W. Eger, 1956; S. H. Widrow, 1962; H. H. Hiatt, 1957; A. Samiy, 1965; S. Talpers, 1959). Einmalige Injektion von 40 Einheiten Parathyreoideaextrakt Lilly führt beim Menschen zu einer Erhöhung der glomerulären P-Filtration von 2,8 auf 3,8 mg/min und einer Erniedrigung der tubulären P-Rückresorption von 92,8% auf ca. 85,9% (H. E. Schaefer, 1962). Die gesteigerte P-Filtration ist wahrscheinlich auf eine unter Parathormon verstärkte Nierendurchblutung zurückzuführen (H. H. Hiatt, 1957; C. R. Blackburn, 1954). Parathormon hemmt hauptsächlich die Phosphatrückresorption in den proximalen Tubuli, wie tierexperimentell mit der Stop-flow-Methode nachgewiesen werden konnte (A. Samiy, 1965, 1960). Die Phosphatdiurese und Hemmung der Phosphatrückresorption tritt auch nach direkter Infusion des Parathormons in die Nierenarterie auf.

Calciumelimination. Klinisch beobachtete man bei hyperparathyreotischen Patienten eine Zunahme der Calciumausscheidung pro Tag und des Calcium/Kreatinin Quotienten im Harn (B. E. Nordin, 1959), wenn calciumarme Standardkost, die beim Gesunden zu 150 mg Harncalcium/Tag führt, verabreicht wurde. Bei hypoparathyreotischen Patienten bewirkte Parathormoninjektion dagegen eine Abnahme der Calciumclearance (D. Bernstein, 1963). Erklärbar werden diese Befunde durch die Beobachtung, daß Parathormon die tubuläre Calciumrückresoption (H. Rasmussen, 1961; W. Eger, 1956; S. H. Widrow, 1962) wahrscheinlich im distalen Bereich (S. H. Widrow, 1962) aktiviert. Die ausgeschiedene Calciummenge wird dann durch die Differenz zwischen filtriertem und rückresorbiertem Calcium bestimmt. Überwiegt die gesteigerte Filtration bei hohem Plasmacalcium wird mehr, überwiegt die Rückresorption, weniger Calcium ausgeschieden.

Alle weiteren regulativen Einflüsse des Parathormons auf andere Organe sind für den Umsatz des Knochenminerals von untergeordneter Bedeutung. Es ist bekannt, daß Parathormon die Milchsekretion und die Phosphatsekretion in die Milch steigert (A. S Todd,

1962; S. DJOJOSOEBAGIO, 1964). Weiter wissen wir, daß der Calcium-efflux und Phosphat-influx bei Mitochondrien aktiviert wird (J. SALLIS, 1963, 1963a; H. RASMUSSEN, 1964; M. FANG, 1964).

b) Thyreocalcitonin-Calcitonin

Beide Hormone sind Polypeptide vom Molekulargewicht ca. 3000. Sie senken den Plasmacalciumspiegel (D. H. COPP, 1962, 1962a; I. MACINTYRE, 1965; P. HIRSCH, 1964). Thyreocalcitonin wurde aus Schilddrüsen (P. F. HIRSCH, 1963, 1964; I. MACINTYRE, 1966, 1965; G. FOSTER, 1964; R. TALMAGE, 1965), Calcitonin aus Nebenschilddrüsen (D. H. COPP, 1962, 1962a, 1965; A. CARE, 1965) dargestellt. Nach MACINTYRE u. Mitarb. (1965) handelt es sich um die gleiche Substanz. Thyreocalcitonin hemmt die Knochenresorption (I. MACINTYRE, 1966) und verstärkt den Calciumeinbau in den Knochen (P. J. GAILLARD, 1966), wie in vitro Versuche zeigen.

c) Vitamin D

Vitamin D beeinflußt dosisabhängig den Baustoffwechsel des Knochenminerals (B. LINDQUIST, 1952; W. GRAB, 1953). Das mit der Nahrung zugeführte Vitamin D wird nur in Anwesenheit von Galle im oberen Dünndarm resorbiert und in den Knochen transportiert (W. HEYMANN, 1937; D. SCHACHTER, 1964). Mikrosomen und Mitochondrienmembranen der Nieren- und Darmschleimhautzellen binden Vitamin D bevorzugt (A. NORMAN, 1964, 1964a).

Tabelle 44. *Calcium- und P-Bilanz rachitischer Kinder unter Vitamin D-Zufuhr* (F. ALBRIGHT, 1938)

	Ca-Zufuhr g/Tag	Faeces-Ca g/Tag	Harn-Ca g/Tag	Absorbierte Ca-Menge g/Tag	Bilanz-Ca g/Tag
Kontrollperiode über 3 Tage . .	2,4	1,16	0,48	1,24	+0,76
Versuchsperiode mit Vitamin D 3 Tage, 600000 IE/täglich . .	2,4	0,35	0,87	2,05	+1,18
	P-Zufuhr g/Tag	**Faeces-P g/Tag**	**Harn-P g/Tag**	**Absorbierte P-Menge g/Tag**	**Bilanz-P g/Tag**
Kontrollperiode über 3 Tage . .	3,51	0,61	2,25	2,90	+0,65
Versuchsperiode mit Vitamin D 3 Tage, 600000 IE/täglich . .	3,51	0,37	2,14	3,14	+1,0

α) Vitamin D- und *Calcium- und Phosphor-Bilanz.* Bei rachitischen Ratten (B. B. MIGIKOVSKY, 1949) und bei rachitischen Kindern positiviert Vitamin D die Calcium- und P-Bilanz (H. E. HARRISON, 1959; F. ALBRIGHT, 1938; S. H. LIU, 1941) (Tabelle 44). Bei 70—88jährigen Patienten wurde eine negative Ca-Bilanz durch Vitamin D-Gaben ausgeglichen (G. TORO, 1958) (Tabelle 54).

Bei hypoparathyreotischen Patienten verbessert Vitamin D teilweise die Calcium- und P-Bilanz (F. ALBRIGHT, 1937; L. LUTWAK, 1964). Es ist anzunehmen, daß das retinierte Calcium und Phosphat im Knochen als Calciumphosphat verbleiben. Tatsächlich ist der Aschegehalt der Knochen rachitischer Kinder auf 22—32% der Trockensubstanz (normal 56—60%) verringert (L. HARRIS, 1956). Durch Vitamin D-Zufuhr steigt die Mineralisation der Knochen bei rachitischen Ratten an (J.-D. GONIN, 1962).

β) Wirkung am Knochen. Ein Angriffspunkt des Vitamins D am Knochen ist, was die Mineralisation anbelangt, fraglich. Nur aus einzelnen experimentellen Befunden wird ein unmittelbarer Einfluß des Vitamins D hergeleitet. Diese Befunde reichen aber für den endgültigen Beweis nicht aus. Bei Vitamin D-behandelten rachitischen Ratten ist ^{45}Ca gegen Skeletcalcium schneller austauschbar als bei unbehandelten Tieren (H. E. HARRISON, 1950). Der gesamte Calciumumsatz nimmt durch Vitamin D-Therapie zu (Tabelle 45).

Bei gesunden Menschen wurde mit ^{47}Calcium unter Vitamin D-Therapie ein Abfall der Knochenanbaurate gefunden und ein Anstieg nur bei einer pathologischen Osteolyse

(H. Frischauf, 1962). Lindquist (1952) bestimmte bei rachitischen Ratten die für die maximale Calciumresorption im Darm nötige Vitamin D-Menge, steigerte dann die Vitamin D-Dosis und konnte so noch eine Zunahme des ^{45}Calciumeinbaus im Knochen beobachten. Bei diesen Befunden blieben aber die Calcium- und Phosphor-Konzentrationen der extracellulären Flüssigkeit unberücksichtigt. In vitro wurde nämlich bewiesen, daß Schnitte rachitischer Epiphysenknorpel im Serum rachitischer Tiere nicht, im Serum

Tabelle 45. *^{45}Calciumumsatz in Femurknochen rachitischer Ratten* (B. Lindquist, 1959)

	Rachitis	Mit Vitamin D behandelte Rachitis
Calciumgehalt (mg)	12	13
Calciumauflagerung (mg/Std)	0,05	0,11
Calciumresorption (mg/Std)	0,05	0,09
mg austauschbare Calciumfraktion	0,55	1,0

gesunder Tiere gut mineralisieren (S. v. Pfaundler, 1904). Bei rachitischen Ratten stieg linear proportional zum Vitamin D abhängigen P-Anstieg im Serum der ^{45}Calciumeinbau im Knochen an (B. Lindquist, 1952) (Abb. 6).

Da auch bei Kindern die Rachitis durch i. v. Injektionen von anorganischem Phosphat zu heilen ist (D. Fraser, 1957), muß man mit Recht in Frage stellen, ob Vitamin D die

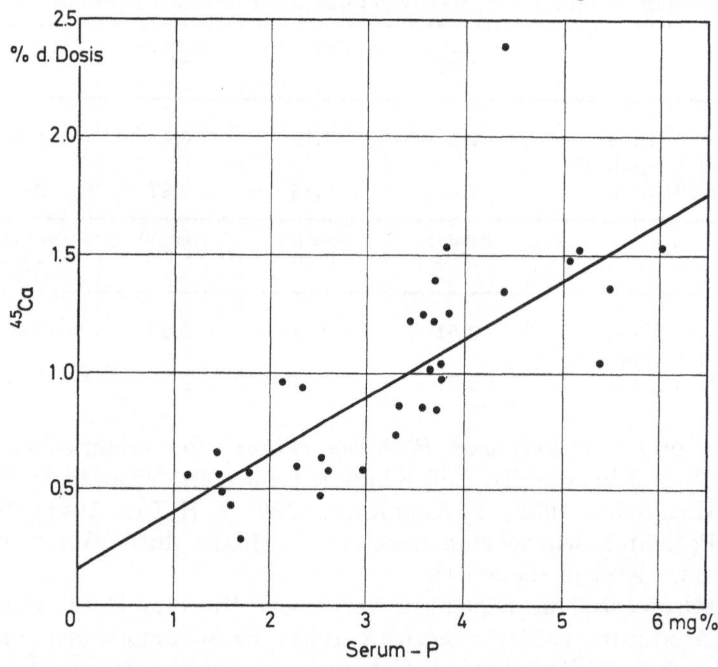

Abb. 6. Beziehung zwischen Serum P und Auflagerungsgeschwindigkeit von ^{45}Calcium im Knochen bei Vitamin D behandelten rachitischen Ratten (B. Lindquist, 1952)

Mineralisation des Knochens unmittelbar reguliert. Es wäre lediglich vorstellbar, daß Vitamin D das örtliche Entstehen von anorganischem aus organischem Phosphat beschleunigt.

Höhere Dosen Vitamin D mobilisieren anscheinend Calcium aus dem Knochen. Nicolaysen (1956) und Bauer (1955a) erhöhten durch Vitamin D-Gaben bei Ratten den Plasmacalciumspiegel selbst dann, wenn keine Calciumresorption über den Darm mehr möglich war.

γ) Intestinale Wirkung. Die Darmschleimhaut ist der Hauptwirkungsort des Vitamins D im Calcium- und Phosphorstoffwechsel. Im Vitamin D-Mangelzustand werden weniger

Calcium und Phosphor im Darm resorbiert (L. J. HARRIS, 1956; R. NICOLAYSEN, 1956; H. E. HARRISON, 1961, 1950; D. GREENBERG, 1945; J. W. MIGICOVSKY, 1955). Bei Tieren und bei Menschen wird bereits innerhalb einer Stunde nach Vitamin D-Gabe die Phosphor- und Calciumresorption im Dünndarm gesteigert (R. NICOLAYSEN, 1943, 1956; D. GREENBERG, 1945; H. E. HARRISON, 1950; B. B. MIGICOVSKY, 1955; A. R. TEREPKA, 1962; H. McKAY, 1943). Das Vitamin wirkt damit bei der Calciumresorption im Darm dem Parathormon synergistisch (Tabelle 46, Tabelle 49).

Tabelle 46. *Calciumresorption bei parathyreoidektomierten Ratten unter 70 E Vitamin D/Woche und 0,041% Ca; 0,4% P in der Kost* (F. C. GRAN, 1960)

	Ca-Zufuhr mg/Tag	Ca-Resorption mg/Tag
Kontrollgruppe	3,9	0,4
Vitamin D-Gruppe	4,4	1,4

Die P-Resorption ist allerdings vom Calciumangebot abhängig (W. GRAB, 1953). Bei gesunden Tieren mit ausreichender Calciumzufuhr kann der Vitamin D-Effekt ausbleiben (R. NICOLAYSEN, 1937). Vitamin D_2, Vitamin D_3 und Ultraviolett-Bestrahlung unterscheiden sich in ihrer qualitativen Wirkung nicht. Im Ileum wird der Calciumeinstrom am stärksten aktiviert (R. H. WASSERMAN, 1962a; J. D. SALLIS, 1962; R. NICOLAYSEN, 1951), am meisten Calcium resorbiert wird aber im Duodenum und Jejunum (Tabelle 47).

Tabelle 47. *^{45}Calciumaufnahme in 2 Std aus in vivo abgebundenen Darmabschnitten bei rachitischen Küken* (R. H. WASSERMAN, 1962a)

	Darmabschnitt	% ^{45}Ca resorbiert	% ^{45}Ca Aufnahme in Tibia
Rachitis	Duodenum	37	1,6
Rachitis + Vitamin D_3 [1]		98	4,7
Rachitis	Jejunum	37	1,6
Rachitis + Vitamin D_3 [1]		87	3,8
Rachitis	Ileum	6	0,18
Rachitis + Vitamin D_3 [1]		22	0,95

[1] 500 IE Vitamin D_3 innerhalb 16 Std vor ^{45}Ca-Gabe.

Anhand der Konzentrationsgradienten für ^{45}Calcium diesseits und jenseits der Darmschleimhaut ist zu beweisen, daß Vitamin D den aktiven, energieabhängigen gegen das Konzentrationsgefälle gerichteten Calcium-Influx beeinflußt und ermöglicht (G. A. WILLIAMS, 1962; D. SCHACHTER, 1960; D. V. KIMBERG, 1961). Bei Nagern findet dieser aktive Calciuminflux hauptsächlich im Duodenum, weniger im Jejunum und Ileum statt (Tabelle 48).

Tabelle 48. *^{45}Calciumkonzentration* Serosaseite: *Mucosaseite nach in vitro-Inkubation isolierter Darmschlingen der Ratte* (G. A. WILLIAMS, 1962)

		^{45}Ca-Konzentration $\frac{\text{Serosaseite}}{\text{Mucosaseite}}$
Kontrolltier	Duodenum	4,8
Vitamin D[1] behandeltes Tier	Duodenum	7,1
Kontrolltier	Jejunum	0,8
Vitamin D[1] behandeltes Tier	Jejunum	1,3
Kontrolltier	Ileum	0,9
Vitamin D[1] behandeltes Tier	Ileum	1,9

[1] 20000 IE Vitamin D/täglich.

Die passive, energieunabhängige, dem Konzentrationsgradienten folgende Diffusion von Calcium durch die Darmschleimhaut, die 0,5—1,6 μ Mol Ca/150 min beträgt und überwiegend im Duodenum und Ileum auftritt (H. HARRISON, 1965), ist ebenfalls durch Vitamin D zu beschleunigen. Fehlt die Darmschleimhaut, wirkt Vitamin D nicht auf die passive Diffusion. Aus der Duodenalmucosa hat man nach Vitamin D-Behandlung rachitischer Küken einen Calcium-bindenden Proteinfaktor isoliert (A. TAYLOR, 1965). Der aktive, durch Vitamin D aktivierbare Calciumtransport in der Darmschleimhaut ist von der Zellatmung abhängig (D. SCHACHTER, 1960a, 1961, 1964a). Hemmstoffe der Atmung senken den Konzentrationsgradienten an der Darmschleimhaut für Calcium gegen 1,0 (D.V. KIMBERG, 1961). Hemmstoffe der Proteinsynthese (Puromycin und Actinomycin D) und Nebennierenrindenblocker hemmen den Vitamin D-induzierten aktiven Calciumtransport ebenfalls (A. TAYLOR, 1965; J. D. SALLIS, 1962). Nach Versuchen an atmenden Darmmitochondrien mit aktivem Calciumaustausch könnte der Angriffspunkt des Vitamins D im subcellulären Bereich liegen (G. ENGSTROM, 1964).

Tabelle 49. *Calcium- und Phosphorausscheidung bei 5 Wochen alten Ratten unter Vitamin D-Behandlung* (R. NICOLAYSEN, 1956)

	Harnausscheidung		Darmresorption	
	mg Ca/Tag	mg P/Tag	mg Ca/Tag	mg P/Tag
Diät 0,25% Ca; 0,35% P				
Kontrolle	0,5	7,9	19	21
Vitamin D-Behandlung	1,2	9,9	24	26
Diät 0,48% Ca; 0,35% P				
Kontrolle	0,7	1,2	19	13
Vitamin D-Behandlung	4,0	2,6	34	20
Diät 0,96% Ca; 0,35% P				
Kontrolle	8,0	0,4	32	8
Vitamin D-Behandlung	19,0	0,3	65	18

Ob Vitamin D unabhängig vom Calciumangebot den Phosphattransport durch die Darmschleimhaut aktivieren kann, ist noch nicht erwiesen. Wir wissen bisher, daß der gegen ein Konzentrationsgefälle serosawärts gerichtete, calciumabhängige Phosphattransport bei Tieren in erster Linie im Jejunum und im kleineren Umfang im Duodenum stattfindet (H. E. HARRISON, 1961; J. D. SALLIS, 1962; W. BAUER, 1932; D. SCHACHTER, 1961). Im Ileum fehlt er. Der Phosphattransport im Jejunum ist durch Atmungsgifte zu hemmen und bei rachitischen Tieren durch Vitamin D_3 zu steigern. Der Phosphattransport im Duodenum wird mehr durch Glykolysehemmstoffe inaktiviert (J. D. SALLIS, 1962).

δ) Renale Wirkung. Die renale Calciumausscheidung wird durch Vitamin D erhöht (Tabelle 49) (R. NICOLAYSEN, 1956; G. FANCONI, 1961; B. FLANAGAN, 1964), ohne daß sich die Calcium-Clearance wesentlich verändert (D. BERNSTEIN, 1963). Demnach muß das Calciumangebot über den Plasmastrom zugenommen haben. Gleichzeitig wird der atmungsabhängige Calcium-efflux der Nierenmitochondrien in Abwesenheit von Parathormon durch Vitamin D aktiviert (G. ENGSTROM, 1964).

Die renale P-Ausscheidung nimmt unter Vitamin D-Behandlung oft zu (A. R. TEREPKA, 1962; G. STALDER, 1957; R. NICOLAYSEN, 1956), teilweise aber auch ab (G. STALDER, 1957). Wahrscheinlich steigert das Vitamin D in höheren Dosen die tubuläre Phosphorrückresorption (H. E. HARRISON, 1954, 1961), die bei rachitischen Kindern erniedrigt ist (G. STALDER, 1957). Es wirkt damit im tubulären P-Transport dem Parathormon antagonistisch. Zur Phosphaturie, die nach Vitamin D-Behandlung viel später als nach Parathormongaben auftritt, kommt es erst, wenn die filtrierte P-Menge mehr als die tubuläre P-Rückresorption zunimmt. Die Vitamin D-Wirkung auf die P-Rückresorption der Niere ist atmungsunabhängig (H. E. HARRISON, 1954), die Parathormon induzierte und O_2 verbrauchende Phosphataufnahme der Nierenmitochondrien benötigt kein Vitamin D (H. RASMUSSEN, 1963).

d) Glucocorticoide

α) Calcium-Bilanz. Cortisol negativiert nach längerer Verabreichung beim Erwachsenen die Calcium-Bilanz (A. LICHTWITZ, 1955). Bei Kindern treten auf diese Weise Wachstumsstörungen auf (G. BOURNE, 1956; Z. LARON, 1962). Erst im höheren Lebensalter können Glucocorticoide negative Calcium-Bilanzen auch positivieren (G. TORO, 1958).

β) Wirkung am Knochen. Cortison verhält sich beim Einbau von Calcium in den Knochen dem Vitamin D antagonistisch (L. F. BÉLANGER, 1960). Seine eigentliche Wirkung auf die Mineralisation ist aber noch nicht klar abgegrenzt. Es liegen Befunde vor, wonach

Tabelle 50. *Transferrate für Calcium (mVal/sec) in der Mineralisierungsreaktion bei Hunden* (E. R. GARRETT, 1964)

	219—260 Tage alt	341—375 Tage alt
Kontrolle	$4{,}1 \cdot 10^{-4}$	$3 \cdot 10^{-4}$
6-Methylprednisolonbehandlung (2 mg/kg/Tag)	$1{,}8 \cdot 10^{-4}$	$1{,}7 \cdot 10^{-4}$

der Calcium- und Phosphoreinbau in das Knochenmineral gehemmt wird (I. CLARK, 1959; J. D. GONIN, 1962; E. KROKOWSKI, 1964; Z. LARON, 1962). Die Transferrate für Calcium in der Reaktion zwischen leicht austauschbarem Pool und Knochenmineral wird durch Glucocorticoide verringert (E. R. GARRETT, 1964) (Tabelle 50).

Man hat aber bei Tieren nach Cortisolbehandlung auch eine Dichtezunahme des Knochens (CH. C. LOBECK, 1960) und eine Steigerung der Calciumaufnahme beobachtet (G. S. GORDAN, 1963; A. B. BORLE, 1960).

γ) Intestinale Wirkung. Versuche nach oraler und parenteraler ^{45}Ca bzw. ^{47}Ca Gabe sprechen dafür, daß Glucocorticoide sowohl die Calciumresorption als auch die Calciumsekretion im Darm steigern (I. CLARK, 1959; E. J. COLLINS, 1962) (Tabelle 51, 52).

Tabelle 51. *Ausscheidung von oral verabfolgtem ^{45}Calcium bei Ratten* (I. CLARK, 1959)

	Kontrolle	Mit Cortisol behandelt
	% ^{45}Ca ausgeschieden	
Harn	0,59	3,6
Faeces	34,5	31,5

Tabelle 52. *Ausscheidung von parenteral verabfolgtem ^{47}Calcium beim Hund* (E. J. COLLINS, 1962)

	Kontrolle	Mit Methylprednisolon[1] behandelt
	% ^{47}Ca ausgeschieden	
Harn	0,81	1,10
Faeces	12,72	36,2

[1] 2 mg 6-Methylprednisolon/kg/täglich über 20 Tage.

Die Transferrate der Sekretion nimmt bei jungen Hunden unter Glucocorticoiden von $0{,}48 \cdot 10^{-4}$ deutlich auf $0{,}78 \cdot 10^{-4}$ mVal Ca/sec zu, bei älteren von $1{,}12 \cdot 10^{-4}$ auf $0{,}97 \cdot 10^{-4}$ mVal Ca/sec etwas ab (E. R. GARRETT, 1964). Für die Bilanz ist ausschlaggebend welcher der beiden Schritte in der Darmschleimhaut überwiegt. Bei in vitro-Versuchen hemmte dagegen Cortison den Calcium-influx im Duodenum (G. A. WILLIAMS, 1961, 1962; J. D. FINKELSTEIN, 1962).

δ) Renale Wirkung. Bilanzversuche mit parenteral appliziertem ^{47}Ca zeigen bereits, daß 6-Methylprednisolon auch die Calciumausscheidung im Harn steigert (E. J. COLLINS, 1962). Es wird die tubuläre Calciumrückresorption gehemmt, wie LAAKE (1960) beim Menschen nachweisen konnte. In ähnlicher Weise wirkt Cortison auf die tubuläre Phosphorrückresorption, so daß eine Phosphaturie unabhängig vom Parathormon auftritt (Z. LARON, 1957; W. R. BOSS, 1952).

e) Mineralocorticoide und Katecholamine

Da das Knochenmineral einen Natriumspeicher des Organismus darstellt, ist zu erwarten, daß Mineralocorticoide auch das Knochennatrium regulieren. Adrenalektomie führt zum Abfall des Knochennatriums (M. M. REIDENBERG, 1961; D. S. MUNRO, 1959), seines austauschbaren Anteiles (D. S. MUNRO, 1959) und seiner spezifischen Aktivität (D. R. ROVNER, 1963). Substitution mit Desoxycorticosteronacetat läßt das Knochennatrium wieder ansteigen (M. M. REIDENBERG, 1961). Aldosterongaben erhöhen bei gesunden Ratten die spezifische ^{22}Natriumaktivität des Knochens (D. R. ROVNER, 1963). Wahrscheinlich ist aber die Wirkung der Mineralocorticoide auf das Knochennatrium indirekt durch ihren Einfluß auf die extracelluläre Natriumkonzentration und die renale Natriumausscheidung bedingt.

Adrenalin führt bei Ratten zu einer von der Kreatininausscheidung unabhängigen Calciurie, die durch Hemmstoffe der Nebennierenmarkfunktion verhindert werden kann (E. MOREY, 1964). Bei gesunden Ratten wird gleichzeitig die Phosphorausscheidung verringert, während sich bei parathyreoidektomierten Ratten die Phosphorausscheidung unter Adrenalingabe dem Calcium synergistisch verhält.

f) Oestrogene und Androgene

Oestrogenbehandlung positiviert die Calciumbilanz (A. LICHTWITZ, 1955; G. TORO, 1958) (Tabelle 54). Die Calciumausscheidung im Harn wird geringer, die Ausscheidung mit den Faeces bleibt teilweise konstant (F. ALBRIGHT, 1948; E. SHORR, 1945; P. H. HENNEMANN, 1957). Oestrogene hemmen die tubuläre renale Phosphatrückresorption und führen damit gleichzeitig zur Phosphaturie (J. R. NASSIM, 1956). Bei Vögeln und Säugetieren wird das retinierte Calcium im Knochen bevorzugt in den spongiösen Bereichen der Röhrenknochen und Wirbelkörper abgelagert (A. J. AHO, 1961; M. SILBERBERG, 1956; C. A. PFEIFFER, 1938; J. GOVAERTS, 1951; G. MANUNTA, 1957). Bruchfestigkeit und Knochendichte nehmen auf diese Weise zu (R. EDGREN, 1956; I. GEDALIA, 1964). Das Ca/P-Verhältnis im Knochen nimmt bei oestrogenisierten Ratten ab (M. SILBERBERG, 1956). Oestradiol und Parathormon wirken unabhängig voneinander am Knochen (G. MANUNTA, 1957a). Nach Untersuchungen bei Ratten und Mäusen hemmen Oestrogene die Calciumresorption in der Reaktion K_R (B. LINDQUIST, 1960) und steigern die Aufnahmerate für Calcium im Knochen (R. E. RANNEY, 1959, 1959a). Der leicht austauschbare Calciumpool vergrößert sich dabei. Der Phosphorumsatz wird in beiden Reaktionen K_A und K_R gesteigert (R. E. RANNEY, 1959a). Die Phosphoreinlagerung überwiegt aber die Phosphorresorption, so daß es parallel zur Calciumeinlagerung zur verstärkten Mineralisation kommt (Tabelle 53).

Tabelle 53. *Calcium- und Phosphoreinlagerung in den Tibiaknochen bei Mäusen nach Oestrogengabe* (R. E. RANNEY, 1959, 1959a)

	Tibia % ^{32}P/g	Anlagerung γ P/g/Std	Leicht austauschbarer P-Pool γ P/g
Kontrolle	9,47	82,5	$2,56 \cdot 10^3$
Oestronbehandlung (0,8—1,2 mg/kg)	12,1	112	$2,96 \cdot 10^3$

	Tibia % ^{45}Ca/g	Anlagerung γ Ca/g/Std	Leicht austauschbarer Ca-Pool γ Ca/g
Kontrolle	39,9	22,3	$1,75 \cdot 10^3$
Oestronbehandlung (0,8—1,2 mg/kg)	43,5	33,4	$2,59 \cdot 10^3$
Parathyreoideaextraktbehandlung (165 E/kg)	35,1	19,4	$1,56 \cdot 10^3$

Messung 24 Std nach Injektion von ^{45}Ca und ^{32}P.

Bei Reptilien wirken Oestrogene dagegen demineralisierend (K. SIMKISS, 1961). Mit physiologischem Rückgang der Oestrogenbildung beim Menschen beobachten wir einen Knochenschwund — die sog. klimakterische Osteoporose (I. A. ANDERSON, 1950; P. H. HENNEMANN, 1957).

Auch Androgene positivieren die Calciumbilanz des Organismus und fördern die Mineralisation (G. TORO, 1958; E. C. REIFENSTEIN, 1947; A. LICHTWITZ, 1955; F. ALBRIGHT, 1948) (Tabelle 54). Beobachtungen von LAFFERTY (1964a) und REIFENSTEIN (1947) sprechen dafür, daß die Knochenresorption gehemmt wird. Gleichzeitig vergrößert sich der austauschbare Calciumpool (G. S. GORDAN, 1963). Bei Frauen ist diese Wirkung der Androgene schwächer (B. E. NORDIN, 1965). 9-Fluor und 11-Hydroxy-substituierte-

Tabelle 54. *Calciumbilanz (mg Ca/kg Körpergewicht/Tag) bei 70—88jährigen Patienten unter Sexualhormoneinflüssen* (G. TORO, 1958)

	Vor Hormongabe				Während Hormongabe			
	Zufuhr	Harnausscheidung	Faecesausscheidung	Bilanz	Zufuhr	Harnausscheidung	Faecesausscheidung	Bilanz
Testosteronproprionat 30 Tage, 30 mg/tgl. . .	16,4	3,0	13,7	−0,3	16,1	1,7	12,3	+2,1
Oestradiol, 60 Tage, 1 mg/2× wöchentlich .	16,5	2,5	14,1	−0,1	16,5	2,0	13,7	+0,8
Vitamin D, 600 IE/tgl., 40 Tage	15,4	1,6	15,3	−1,5	15,2	1,5	13,6	+0,1

Testosterone verlieren sogar den Einfluß auf die Calciumbilanz (M. M. PECHET, 1962). In der Wachstums- und Entwicklungsphase eines Organismus überwiegt die wachstumsbeschleunigende Wirkung des Testosterons seine mineralisierende, so daß der Calciumgehalt der Knochen vorübergehend sogar abnehmen kann (A. J. AHO, 1961).

g) Somatotropes Hormon (STH)

Das somatotrope Hormon begünstigt morphologisch das Skeletwachstum, ohne die Skeletreifung zu beeinflussen (C. W. ASHLING, 1956). Testosteron wirkt in dieser Hinsicht synergistisch, Oestrogene wirken dagegen antagonistisch. Im Wachstumsalter führt somatotropes Hormon zu einer positiven, bei Erwachsenen dagegen zu einer negativen Calciumbilanz (S. HANNA, 1961; G. F. MAZZNOLI, 1965). Die Calciumausscheidung im Harn (H_S) und die Calciumresorption im Darm (D_A) wird regelmäßig gesteigert. Die Calciumsekretion in den Darm (PD_S) ist aber bei Erwachsenen größer und führt zu der negativen Bilanz, wenn die Calciumzufuhr nicht erhöht wird (S. HANNA, 1961; G. F. MAZZNOLI, 1965; D. M. BERGENSTAL, 1960; B. E. NORDIN, 1965a). Bei einer positiven Bilanz mineralisiert der wachsende Knochen, bei einer negativen Bilanz demineralisiert er, und es kann zum Knochenschwund kommen.

Die Phosphorbilanz positiviert das somatotrope Hormon parallel zur Stickstoffbilanz immer (D. M. BERGENSTAL, 1960; B. E. NORDIN, 1965a). Im Harn beobachtet man deshalb eine abnehmende Phosphorausscheidung (P. H. HENNEMANN, 1960). Der retinierte Phosphor wird aber zum Teil in der Nucleinsäure- und Proteinsynthese und weniger in der Mineralisation verwertet.

Bei hypophysektomierten Ratten steigert somatotropes Hormon zwar den ^{45}Calciumeinbau in Epiphysenplatten (F. ULRICH, 1951, 1952). Diese Calciumaufnahme könnte aber auch an die wachsende Knorpelmatrix gebunden und nicht mineralisationsbedingt sein. Bei gesunden Tieren fehlt diese Wirkung des STH. Ein unmittelbarer Angriffspunkt in der Mineralisation des Knochens kann für somatotropes Hormon bisher nicht diskutiert werden. Experimentell begründet ist nur die Steigerung der Calciumresorption (D_A) in der Darmschleimhaut (G. F. MAZZNOLI, 1965a), wodurch der Plasmacalciumspiegel häufig ansteigt (B. E. NORDIN, 1965). Das kann seinerseits zur Hemmung der Parathormonausschüttung und zur Mineralisation führen. In der Duodenalschleimhaut wird der aktive Calcium-influx, der nach Hypophysektomie abnimmt, durch somatotropes Hormon und auch luteotropes Hormon gesteigert (J. D. FINKELSTEIN, 1962) (Abb. 7, Tabelle 55).

In der Niere aktiviert das somatotrope Hormon die tubuläre Phosphatrückresorption, womit die Hyperphosphatämie begründet ist (P. H. HENNEMANN, 1960).

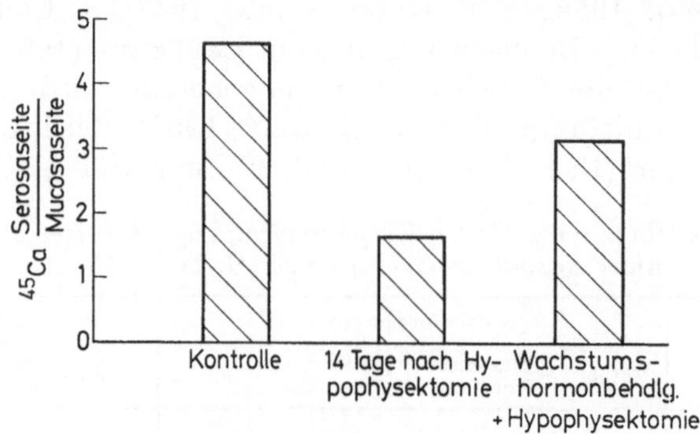

Abb. 7. Einfluß von somatotropem Hormon auf die Calciumaufnahme durch die Duodenalschleimhaut bei der Ratte (J. F. FINKELSTEIN, 1962)

Tabelle 55. *Calciumtransfer (m µMol/min/5 Darmsäcke) in der Duodenalschleimhaut 35 Tage alter Ratten* (J. F. FINKELSTEIN, 1962)

	Hypophysektomierte Tiere 14 Tage nach Operation	Kontrolltiere
Ca-Influx, Medium → Mucosa	85	147
Ca-Efflux, Mucosa → Medium	74	78
Ca-Nettotransfer, Mucosa	+11	+69
Ca-Influx, Serosa → Medium	12	17
Ca-Efflux, Medium → Serosa	25	26
Ca-Nettotransfer, Serosa	−13	−9

h) Schilddrüsenhormon

Im Wachstumsalter fördert Schilddrüsenhormon das Knochenwachstum und die Knochenreifung durch Mineralisation der Epiphysenlinien. Im Erwachsenen-Organismus, ausgenommen im hohen Alter (G. TORO, 1958), negativiert Schilddrüsenhormon die Calciumbilanz. Die renale und faecale Calciumausscheidung nimmt zu (S. M. KRANE, 1956; R. M. FORBES, 1965; P. B. COOK, 1959; J. GREEN, 1951). Knochen von Thyroxin-behandelten Tieren zeigen in vitro einen geringeren Calciumumsatz (E. C. KHOO, 1965) und Aschegehalt (A. E. SOBEL, 1960). Knochenkulturen in vitro zugesetztes Thyroxin senkt ebenfalls den ^{45}Calciumumsatz (F. W. LENGEMAN, 1962).

Bei Thyreotoxikose fand man dagegen einen höheren ^{45}Calciumumsatz im Knochen (S. M. KRANE, 1956), was jedoch nicht gegen eine Demineralisation spricht. In der Duodenalschleimhaut hemmt Thyroxin die aktive Calciumresorption (J. D. FINKELSTEIN, 1962; R. M. FORBES, 1965) und aktiviert die Calciumsekretion im übrigen Darm (P. B. COOK, 1959). In der Niere steigert Schilddrüsenhormon die tubuläre Phosphatrückresorption, wodurch die Phosphat-Clearance abnimmt (V. PARSONS, 1964; R. HARDEN, 1964; O. BIJVOET, 1965).

i) Vitamine

Vitamin B_6 wirkt bei Ratten calciuretisch und hemmt die renale Phosphatausscheidung (A. SCHMID, 1965).

Vitamin C steigert die Calciumresorption im Darm, aber nicht den Mineralisationsgrad des Knochens (G. BOURNE, 1956), obwohl sich mehr Knochengewebe ausbildet. Vitamin C wirkt über die Matrixbildung. Bei Skorbut findet man eine positive Calciumbilanz, weil pathologische Bindegewebsmatrix Calcium aufnimmt (G. BOURNE, 1956). Die Phosphorretention im Knochen nimmt ab.

5. Übersicht der Hormon- und Vitaminwirkungen im Baustoffwechsel des Knochens

Parathormon: Aktivierung der Knochenmineralmobilisation; Aktivierung der Kollagenolyse und Matrix-Proteolyse; Hemmung der Kollagensynthese; Aktivierung der Mucopolysaccharidsynthese; Aktivierung der P- und Ca-Ausscheidung im Harn; Aktivierung der Ca- und P-Resorption im Darm; Negativieren der Ca- und P-Bilanz.

Thyreocalcitonin: Aktivierung der Mineralisation; Positivieren der Ca-Bilanz.

Glucocorticoide: Aktivierung der Ca- und P-Ausscheidung im Harn; Aktivierung der Ca-Resorption und -Sekretion im Darm; Negativieren der Ca- und N-Bilanz; Hemmung der Mucopolysaccharidsynthese; Hemmung der Kollagensynthese.

Oestrogene und Androgene: Aktivierung der Mineralisation; Aktivierung der Synthese von Matrixproteinen; Aktivierung der Phosphatausscheidung im Harn; Positivieren der Ca- und N-Bilanz.

Somatotropes Hormon: Aktivierung der Kollagensynthese; Aktivierung der Mucopolysaccharidsynthese; Aktivierung der Ca-Ausscheidung im Harn; Aktivierung der Ca-Resorption und -Sekretion im Darm; Hemmung der Phosphatausscheidung; Negativieren der Ca-Bilanz (Erwachs.); Positivieren der P + N-Bilanz.

Schilddrüsenhormon: Aktivierung der Ca-Ausscheidung im Harn; Aktivierung der Mucopolysaccharidsynthese; Hemmung der Ca-Resorption im Darm; Hemmung der P-Ausscheidung im Harn; Negativieren der Ca-Bilanz.

Vitamin A: Aktivierung der Matrixproteolyse; Aktivierung der Mucopolysaccharidsynthese.

Vitamin C: Aktivierung der Kollagensynthese.

Vitamin D: Aktivierung der Mucopolysaccharidsynthese; Aktivierung der Ca- und P-Resorption im Darm; Aktivierung der Ca-Ausscheidung im Harn; Hemmung der Phosphatausscheidung im Harn; Positivieren der Ca- und P-Bilanz.

III. Spezielle Enzymaktivitäten im verknöchernden Gewebe

1. Alkalische Phosphatase

Mit der Umwandlung kleinzelligen Knorpels in der enchondralen Verknöcherungszone in hypertrophen, verknöcherungsfähigen Säulenknorpel und in der periostalen Verknöcherungszone tritt cellulär und extracellulär alkalische Phosphatase auf (G. MAJNO, 1951; M. S. BURSTONE, 1960; M. TEAFORD, 1964; R. S. SIFFERT, 1951; A. BOSE, 1960; H. B. FELL, 1929; M. MARTLAND, 1924; H. A. HARRIS, 1932; G. BEVELANDER, 1950; O. HÖVELS, 1959; H. KELLER, 1962; J. VINCENT, 1963; D. B. KROON, 1952). Permanenter Knorpel besitzt nur sehr geringe Aktivität an alkalischer Phosphatase (H.-J. DULCE, 1960a, 1960b). Alle an der Verknöcherung beteiligten Zellen: Osteoblasten, Osteocyten, Odontoblasten sind reich an alkalischer Phosphatase. Osteoclasten enthalten weniger von diesem Enzym (A. BOSE, 1960; J. VINCENT, 1963; D. B. KROON, 1952). In der Gewebekultur entwickeln nur die später mineralisierenden Knochenanlagen und nicht die Knorpelanlagen Phosphataseaktivität (H. B. FELL, 1930, 1931).

Die alkalische Phosphatase ist eine uneinheitliche Phosphomonoesterase. Sie wird in der Regel als β-Glycerophosphatase oder als Paranitrophenylphosphatase gemessen (D. B. KROON, 1952; R. S. SIFFERT, 1951; M. S. BURSTONE, 1960; M. TEAFORD, 1964; J. VINCENT, 1963; I. LORCH, 1946; M. TANZER, 1963; G. M. JEFFREE, 1965; J. S. GREENSPAN, 1965; A. G. PEARSE, 1966; R. SOGGNAES, 1955; G. VAES, 1965).

Ihr pH-Optimum liegt mit β-Glycerophosphat als Substrat zwischen pH 9,5—10,0 (I. Motzok, 1961), mit p-nitrophenylphosphat als Substrat gemessen bei pH 8,7. Das Enzym ist durch 10^{-3}m Magnesium (H. D. Jenner, 1931; R. S. Grier, 1949; O. Bodansky, 1937, 1949), Kobalt (R. Cloetens, 1939), Mangan (R. Cloetens, 1939) und Vitamin D (R. Zetterström, 1951; J. D. Cipera, 1963) aktivierbar und durch 10^{-5} molar Beryllium (R. S. Grier, 1949), Oxalat, Citrat, Calcium (H. D. Jenner, 1931; R. S. Grier, 1949) sowie bei β-Glycerophosphat als Substrat durch Gallensäuren (O. Bodansky, 1937) hemmbar. Damit entspricht das Enzym des Knochens der aus Nierengewebe von Cloetens (1941, 1941 a) dargestellten und in Leber (A. J. Emery, 1955) und Darmschleimhaut (D. Evered, 1964) nachgewiesenen Phosphatase I. Die alkalische Paranitrophenylphosphatase ist durch Gallensäure nicht hemmbar. Die Hauptaktivität der alkalischen Phosphatase ist an die Mikrosomenfraktion des Knochens gebunden (G. Vaes, 1965)a. Die alkalische Phosphatase des Knochens wandert elektrophoretisch wie Nieren- und Serumphosphatase (P. Butterworth, 1965).

Hekkelmann (1966) lenkte kürzlich die Aufmerksamkeit auf eine nur im Knochen und nicht in Leber und Niere vorkommende alkalische Phosphatase, die bei pH 8,8 NADP als Substrat in NAD umwandelt (Tabelle 56).

Tabelle 56. *Abbau von $2\cdot10^{-4}$ molar NADP und NAD-Lösungen durch Extrakte von Kaninchendiaphysen* (J. W. Hekkelmann, 1966) 37°, pH 8,8, Trispuffer, 0,5% Desoxycholsäure.

	m μMol/min/g FG	
	pH 8,8	pH 7,4
NAD-Abbau	13,9 ± 1,5	5,4 ± 0,8
NADP-Abbau	695 ± 85	147 ± 27
NAD-Bildung aus NADP	712 ± 74	139 ± 22

Das zellständige Enzym steht in seinen Eigenschaften der Paranitrophenylphosphatase nahe. Inwieweit NADP als biologisches Substrat der alkalischen Phosphatase bei den örtlichen pH-Verhältnissen auftritt, muß untersucht werden.

Die Funktion der alkalischen Phosphatase im Knochen ist bisher nicht eindeutig geklärt. Früher hat man geglaubt, daß sie unmittelbar mit der Mineralisation zu tun habe, weil sie verstärkt anorganisches Phosphat aus Phosphosäureestern entstehen läßt. Heute bringt man die alkalische Phosphatase vielfach mit der Bildung verknöcherungsfähiger Matrix in Verbindung, ohne ihren Angriffspunkt in der Synthese näher zu kennen. Wie sich ein NADP-Abbau im verknöchernden Gewebe auf die Mineralisation auswirkt, ist zur Zeit noch offen. In Korrelation zur Bildung verknöcherungsfähiger Matrix nimmt die alkalische Plasmaphosphatase zu.

2. Saure Phosphatase

Eine saure Phosphatase ist als typisches Enzym exkretorischer Zellen hauptsächlich in den Osteoclasten des Knochens lokalisiert (M. S. Burstone, 1960; F. Schajowicz, 1958; G. M. Jeffree, 1965; A. G. Pearse, 1966; K. Balogh jr., 1965). Dort ist sie an die Lysosomenfraktion gebunden (A. G. Pearse, 1966; G. Vaes, 1965a). Ihr pH-Optimum liegt bei 5,5. Als Substrat der Messung dient p-nitrophenylphosphat oder Glucose-6-Phosphat. Eine biologische Funktion der sauren Phosphatase bei der Knochenresorption ist noch nicht bekannt. Wir wissen nur, daß nach Parathormoninjektion und während der Eischalenbildung (T. G. Taylor, 1965) ihre Aktivität im Plasma ansteigt (K. M. Morris, 1966).

3. Proteinphosphokinase

Verknöcherungsfähiger Knorpel und Knochen besitzen eine Phosphokinase, die Knochengelatine bei pH 7,4—8,0, Schmelzmatrixprotein und Kollagen mit Adenosintriphosphat (ATP) als Donator phosphoryliert (S. Krane, 1965, 1965a). Die Phosphorylierung findet am Serin des Kollagens statt. Möglicherweise bildet das Enzym die Phosphoproteine des Zahnschmelzes. Über phosphorylierte Matrixproteine des übrigen Knochens und ihre Bedeutung bei der Mineralisation liegen aber keine weiteren Beobachtungen vor.

4. Anorganische Pyrophosphatase

Im verknöchernden Gewebe sind höhere Aktivitäten Magnesium-aktivierbarer anorganischer Pyrophosphatase als im permanenten Knorpel nachgewiesen worden (P. CERLETTI, 1958; H.-J. DULCE, 1960a; H. D. JENNER, 1931) (Tabelle 57).

Das Enzym hat zwei pH-Optima, im verknöcherungsfähigen Knorpel bei pH 5,5 und 7,5 und im Knochen bei pH 5,0 und 8,5 (P. CERLETTI, 1958). Man nimmt aber an, daß

Tabelle 57. *Aktivität der anorganischen Pyrophosphatase bei pH 7,4. Substrat: Pyrophosphat* + $MgCl_2$ (H.-J. DULCE, 1960a, 1960b)

	µMol P/g AFTS/Std					
	Rinderfeten			Kalb	Ratte	
	25—30 cm Scheitel-Steiß-Länge	50—70 cm Scheitel-Steiß-Länge	1 m Scheitel-Steiß-Länge		3 Wochen alt	6—7 Wochen alt
Homogenate						
Permanenter Knorpel	280		121	135	214	485
Verknöchernde Epiphyse	923	820	826	381	1842	2106
Diaphysenknochen	190				632	794

AFTS = asche- und fettfreie Trockensubstanz.

alkalische Phosphatase und anorganische Pyrophosphatase dasselbe Enzymprotein besitzen und die aktiven Zentren pH-abhängig gebildet werden. Als Substrat der Pyrophosphatase ist von FLEISCH (1965) anorganisches Pyrophosphat im nicht mineralisierbaren Sehnenkollagen nachgewiesen worden. WILHELM (1966) zeigte in Zellen des verknöcherungsfähigen Knorpels ebenfalls kondensierte Phosphate, die in anderen Körperzellen fehlten. Da FLEISCH (1965) kondensierte Phosphate als Kristallisationshemmstoff für Calciumphosphate nachwies, sah er die Bedeutung der anorganischen Pyrophosphatase im Zusammenhang mit der Mineralisation.

5. Carboanhydratase

In Knochenzellen von Küken kommt, ebenso wie in Wasserstoffionen-produzierenden Erythrocyten, Nieren- und Magenschleimhautzellen reichlich Carboanhydratase (CAH) vor (H.-J. DULCE, 1960d, 1961; F. KÖRBER, 1964) (Tabelle 58, 59). Als Substrat dieses Enzyms gilt das von Zellen gebildete Kohlendioxyd. Es wird vermutet, daß dieses Enzym am Mechanismus der Knochenauflösung beteiligt ist.

Tabelle 58. *Carboanhydratasegehalt in Organen von Küken* (F. KÖRBER, 1964)

	CAH/E/mg DNS
Epiphyse	866
Niere	1211
Blut	1600

DNS = Desoxyribonucleinsäure.

Tabelle 59. *Carboanhydrataseaktivität im Knochen von Küken* (F. KÖRBER, 1964; H.-J. DULCE, 1961)

Küken 200 g	CAH/E/100 mg FG
Epiphyse	61
Metaphyse	6,3
Diaphyse	2,6
Bandscheibenknorpel . . .	0,2

FG = Frischgewicht.

6. Weitere Enzyme

In der Mineralisationszone sind weiterhin 5-Nucleotidase (J. L. REIS, 1950) und Pyridinnucleotidasen (R. VAN REEN, 1961), in Osteoclasten Phosphoamidase (A. G. PEARSE, 1966; F. SCHAJOWICZ, 1964), β-Hydroxybuttersäuredehydrogenase und Glutaminsäuredehydrogenase (D. G. WALKER, 1961), in lysosomalen Fraktionen von Knochenhomogenaten Desoxyribonuclease und Ribonuclease (G. VAES, 1965a) und im partikelfreien Überstand Katalase (G. VAES, 1965a) nachgewiesen worden. Einer bestimmten Funktion im Stoffwechsel konnte man aber diese Enzyme noch nicht zuordnen.

7. Regulation spezieller Enzymaktivitäten

a) Alkalische Phosphatase

Nach Gaben von Parathyreoideaextrakt in vivo wurde einerseits bei Ratten ein Anstieg der Aktivität der alkalischen Phosphatase in Femurdiaphysen (H. L. Williams, 1941) und bei Mäusen ein Abfall der Enzymaktivität in Calvariakulturen beobachtet (G. Vaes, 1965, 1966).

Vitamin D_2- und D_3-Phosphat aktivieren die alkalische Phosphatase (R. Zetterstroem, 1951; E. Werner, 1958). Bei rachitischen Ratten steigert Vitamin D_3 in vivo die Aktivität des Enzyms in Epiphysen (J. D. Cipera, 1963; H.-J. Dulce, 1959).

Somatotropes Hormon steigert die Aktivität der alkalischen Phosphatase im Knochen nur bei hypophysektomierten Tieren (J. C. Mathies, 1949, 1952), bei gesunden Tieren führt es zu einem Absinken der Enzymaktivität (W. E. Wilkins, 1935).

Thyroxin, thyreotropes Hormon (J. C. Mathies, 1952; H. L. Williams, 1941; C. H. Whicher, 1943), Androgene, Oestrogene (H. L. Williams, 1941; K. W. Buchwald, 1947), Progesteron, und gonadotropes Hormon (C. H. Whicher, 1943) erhöhen bei Ratten die Enzymaktivität.

b) Saure Phosphatase

Parathyreoideaextrakt erhöht nach in vivo Injektionen die Aktivität des Enzyms in Calvariahomogenaten um 46% (G. Vaes, 1965a, 1966), wobei gleichzeitig eine Säuerung des Mediums beobachtet wird.

c) Anorganische Pyrophosphatase

Bei rachitischen Ratten ist die Aktivität des Enzyms verringert und wird durch Vitamin D_3-Behandlung erhöht (J. D. Cipera, 1963; H.-J. Dulce, 1959).

d) Andere Enzyme

Bei Parathyreoideaextrakt-vorbehandelten Mäusen fand Vaes (1965a und 1966), daß Calvarien vermehrt Desoxyribonuclease, β-Glucuronidase und β-Galaktosidase bilden.

Extracelluläre Flüssigkeit und Knochen

I. Knochenmineralbausteine und Knochenenzyme in der extracellulären Flüssigkeit

Die extracelluläre Flüssigkeit besteht aus intravasaler und interstitieller Flüssigkeit. Intravasal besitzt der Erwachsene 5% und interstitiell 15% des Körpergewichtes an extracellulärer Flüssigkeit. Nur die fast proteinfreie, interstitielle Flüssigkeit steht mit dem Knochen in unmittelbarer Verbindung. Die 7% Protein enthaltende, intravasale Plasmaflüssigkeit ist der Analyse gut zugänglich. Wir finden folgende Zusammensetzungen der extracellulären Flüssigkeit:

Tabelle 60

Intravasaler Anteil (Blutplasma, Mensch)

Ca	9,5—10,5 mg %
P anorg.	3—4,5 mg %
Mg	2—2,5 mg %
Na	142 m Mol/l
K	4,5 m Mol/l
Cl	103 m Mol/l
F	0,016 mg %
Standard HCO_3^-	27 mMol/l
Citrat	1—2 mg %
Alkalische Phosphatase	10—40 IE/l (Jung, 1956; Haas, 1966)
Anorganische Pyrophosphatase	positiv (E. Pitkänen, 1960)

Interstitielle Flüssigkeit (Mensch)

Ca	5—6 mg %
P anorg.	3,2—4,7 mg %
Mg	1,5—2,0 mg %
Na	135 m Mol/l
K	4,3 m Mol/l
Cl	108 m Mol/l
F	0,017 mg %
Standard HCO_3^-	28 m Mol/l
Citrat	1—2 mg %
Alkalische Phosphatase	positiv
Anorganische Pyrophosphatase	positiv

1. Calcium- und anorganischer Phosphor-Gehalt

Individuell schwankt der Plasmacalciumspiegel bei Gesunden nur sehr wenig (± 0,2 mg %) (G. Fanconi, 1959; W. Niepmann, 1961; A. M. Feldstein, 1963). Menschen mit normacidem Magensaft haben Werte gegen 9,5 mg %, solche mit hyperacidem Werte gegen 10,5 mg % (W. Niepmann, 1961). Bei Ratten ist der Calciumspiegel ernährungsabhängig (6—12 mg %), beim Menschen nicht (A. E. Sobel, 1945; Munson, 1955). Bei Hühnern beträgt das Serumcalcium im embryonalen Stadium 5,1 mg % (T. Taylor, 1963), später 10,5 mg % und mit Einsetzen der Legeperiode 20—30 mg % (M. R. Urist, 1960). Mit steigendem Lebensalter ändert sich der Plasmacalciumspiegel kaum (G. Fanconi, 1959), der Phosphorspiegel nimmt dagegen von 5,3—8,5 mg % bei Neugeborenen (R. G. Clutre, 1954) auf 3—4 mg % bei 30—70jährigen Erwachsenen (G. Fanconi, 1959) ab. Kinder bis zu 12 Jahren haben 4,4—5,2 mg % anorganisches P im Plasma. Bei Ratten liegt der P-Spiegel mit 8—10 mg % höher (A. E. Sobel, 1945; Munson, 1955), bei Hühnern mit nur 2 mg % (A. Grollman, 1927) niedriger als beim Menschen.

Das Produkt Ca · P (mg %)^2 im Plasma findet man im Erwachsenenalter beim Menschen konstant um 35—40 (mg %)^2.

a) Calcium-Fraktionen in der extracellulären Flüssigkeit

Das Calcium liegt in der intravasalen Flüssigkeit in drei Fraktionen vor:

α) ultrafiltrable Calciumionen,

β) ultrafiltrable undissosiierte Calciumchelate,

γ) nicht ultrafiltrables und adialysables Calcium-Proteinat.

α) Ultrafiltrable Ca-Ionen. In der interstitiellen Flüssigkeit und im Harn finden wir nur Calciumionen und Calciumchelate. Bei pH 7,35 und $\mu = 0{,}15$ sind in der extracellulären Flüssigkeit 45—55 % des Gesamtcalciums = 4,5—5,5 mg % Calciumionen (H. F. Logan, 1960; L. MacLeod, 1964; J. Etori, 1959; F. C. McLean, 1935). Das gesamte ultrafiltrable Calcium beträgt bei pH 7,35 50—60 % = 5—6 mg % des Gesamtcalciums (E. Müller, 1953; R. G. Smith, 1932; A. S. Prasad, 1960; H. F. Logan, 1960; F. C. McLean, 1935; O. Greengard, 1964). Bei pH 5 würden ca. 90 % des Calciums, bei pH 9,0 nur 25 % dialysabel sein (H. F. Logan, 1960). Diese Befunde erklären wahrscheinlich, weshalb klinisch bei pH-Schwankungen des Blutes (pH 7,1—7,6) sich die Menge des ionisierten Calciums ändert (B. v. Schulthess-Sallmann, 1958; A. S. Prasad, 1960). In der extracellulären Flüssigkeit eines Menschen von 70 kg errechnen sich insgesamt ca. 700 mg ultrafiltrables Calcium (= α + β Fraktion). Von 30 mg % Plasmacalcium bei Vögeln in der Legeperiode werden nur ca. 11,5 mg % ultrafiltrabel gefunden (M.-R. Urist, 1960). Während der 17-stündigen Eischalenbildung nimmt das ultrafiltrable Calcium im Serum ab (D. Polin, 1957).

β) Ultrafiltrable Ca-Chelate. Es errechnen sich im Plasma des Menschen maximal nur 5 % des Gesamtcalciums = 0,5 mg % als Calciumchelate (H. F. Logan, 1960). Nur ein sehr kleiner Teil der Calciumchelate in der extracellulären Flüssigkeit ist Calciumcitrat. Nach Messungen von Henning (1951) müssen bei 2 mg % Citrat im Serum weniger als 0,1 mg % Calcium chelatgebunden sein. Nach Citratzusatz hat man im Serum keine niedermolekularen, organischen Calciumkomplexe elektrophoretisch nachweisen können (D. M. Greenberg, 1932). Man vermutet, daß Phosphat und Carbonat anorganische Calciumkomplexe bilden (J. Greenwald, 1945). Wahrscheinlich ist der Anteil des chelatgebundenen Calciums noch geringer als 5% des Gesamtcalciums.

γ) Nicht ultrafiltrable Ca-Proteinate. 45—50% des Plasmacalciums = 4,5—5,0 mg % sind proteingebunden. Im Liquor mit ca. 1% Proteingehalt findet man insgesamt nur 0,28 mg % nicht ionisiertes Calcium (H. F. Logan, 1960). Bei einem 70 kg schweren Erwachsenen würden wir in der gesamten extracellulären Flüssigkeit ca. 150 mg Calcium als Proteinat gebunden vorfinden. Die Bindung des Calciums ist locker und reversibel (E. Müller, 1953; R. Klement, 1953). Physiologisch gebunden sind 0,015 mMol-Ca/g Serumprotein (I. R. Held, 1964). Die maximale Calciumbindungskapazität für Serumproteine beträgt ca. 0,06—0,1 mMol/g (D. M. Greenberg, 1939; H. F. Logan, 1960). Beim Menschen sind demnach die Serumproteine mit Calcium nicht gesättigt. Die Calciumbindung findet in vivo bevorzugt an Albuminen und β-Globulinen statt (A. S. Prasad, 1958, 1960; F. C. McLean, 1935; I. R. Held, 1964). In vitro binden die α-Globuline am meisten Calcium (I. R. Held, 1964; F. C. McLean, 1935; A. S. Prasad, 1958) (Tabelle 61). Die thermodynamischen Daten für die Albumin-Calcium-Bindung beim Rind errechnete Katz (1953):

Tabelle 61. *Calciumbindung an Serumproteinfraktionen in vitro* (I. R. Held, 1964; F. C. McLean, 1935; A. S. Prasad, 1958)

	mg Ca/g Protein	Mol Ca/Mol Protein
Albumin	0,62—0,72	1,08—1,23
α-Globulin	0,64	3,2
β-Globulin	0,57	1,3
γ-Globulin	0,28	1,1

$$\Delta F^0 = 3870 \text{ cal/Mol}$$
$$\Delta S^0 = 14 \text{ cal/Mol}$$
$$\Delta H^0 = 0$$
$$\text{pH} = 8{,}0.$$

Änderungen des Albumin/Globulin-Quotienten von ± 0,6 führen hiernach zu Plasmacalciumveränderungen von ± 0,28 mg % (F. C. McLean, 1935).

Bei Legehühnern mit hohem Plasmacalciumspiegel tritt ein calciumbindendes Phosphorproteid und Lipoproteid in dem β-Globulinbereich auf, das 50 mg Ca/g Protein bindet (M. R. Urist, 1958; D. M. Greenberg, 1939; O. Greengard, 1964).

Zwischen ionisiertem Calcium und dem Calciumproteinat besteht ein Gleichgewichtszustand (F. C. McLean, 1935).

$$\frac{[Ca^{++}] \cdot [Protein^{2-}]}{[Ca\ Protein]} = K' \ (= \text{Dissoziationskonstante})$$

Daraus ist abzuleiten, daß die Proteinkonzentration im Serum die Calciumionenkonzentration beeinflussen muß. Es sind deshalb Nomogramme von McLean und Hastings (1935) entwickelt worden, die es gestatten, aus Serumprotein und Gesamtcalcium bei pH-Konstanz von 7,35 die Calciumionenkonzentration zu errechnen. Bei pH 7,35, 25° und Albumin/Globulin = 1,8 beträgt der negative Logarithmus der Dissoziationskonstanten für Calciumproteinat beim Rind: pK' = 2,22 ± 0,07 (F. C. McLean, 1935). Im Serum des Menschen wurden pK-Werte für Calciumproteinat von 1,97—2,28 nachgewiesen (F. C. McLean, 1935). Der pK für Calciumalbuminat beträgt 2,03 ± 0,11, derjenige für Calciumglobulinat 2,24 ± 0,08 (F. C. McLean, 1935).

b) Anorganische Phosphor-Fraktion in der extracellulären Flüssigkeit

Das anorganische Phosphat ist normalerweise zu ca. 15% proteingebunden (H. F. Logan, 1960; A. Grollman, 1927). Physiologisch sind die Serumproteine im Gegensatz zum Calcium mit anorganischem Phosphat wahrscheinlich fast gesättigt.

2. Magnesium-Gehalt

Bei Hühnern nimmt der Magnesiumspiegel im Serum von 5,5 mg % im frühen Embryonalstadium (T. G. TAYLOR, 1963) auf 2,4 mg % nach dem Schlüpfen ab. Ratten haben normalerweise einen Magnesiumspiegel im Plasma von 3—5 mg % (H. BENJAMIN, 1933). 70—85 % des Gesamtmagnesiums im Plasma sind ionisiert (H. HAAS, 1965; F. C. MCLEAN, 1935; L. MACLEOD, 1964). 15—30 % sind proteingebunden. Die pK-Werte sind den Calciumproteinaten ähnlich. Bei einem 70 kg schweren Menschen errechnen sich von 220 mg Magnesium in der gesamten extracellulären Flüssigkeit 200 mg als Magnesiumionen (H. HAAS, 1965).

3. Enzym-Gehalt

Die alkalische Phosphatase im Plasma nimmt im Laufe des Lebensalters ab (R. G. CLUTRE, 1954). Nur in der Gravidität finden wir einen Anstieg (W. JUNG, 1956). Es ist noch nicht erwiesen, daß derartige Anstiege auf die Ausschüttung von Knochenphosphatase zurückzuführen sind. Im Stadium der Eischalenbildung bei Vögeln nimmt die alkalische Phosphatase zu, im Stadium der Oviposition dagegen die saure Phosphatase (TAYLOR, 1965). Im Serum sind Pyrophosphatasen mit den pH-Optima von 4,7, 8,5 und 11,0 nachgewiesen worden. Die Fraktion mit dem pH-Optimum 8,5 ist an die α_2-Globulin-Fraktion gebunden (E. PITKÄNEN, 1960).

II. Regulation der Zusammensetzung der extracellulären Flüssigkeit

1. Parathormon

a) Calcium-Gehalt

Physiologisch unterliegen von 10 mg % Plasmacalcium ca. 4 mg % der Regulation durch Parathormon. Diese Regulation ist unabhängig von den Nieren nachweisbar (A. GROLLMAN, 1954; R. TALMAGE, 1953; G. S. STEWART, 1951). Nach Entfernen der Nebenschilddrüsen sinkt beim Menschen, bei Säugetieren und Vögeln die Plasmacalciumkonzentration in wenigen Stunden von 9,5—10,5 mg % auf 5,9—7,0 mg % ab (J. J. CANARY, 1962; S. M. KRANE, 1957; J. R. CORTELYOU, 1960; H. MORII, 1963; P. H. HENNEMANN, 1957; R. GOLDSMITH, 1965; R. V. TALMAGE, 1956; H. R. PERKINS, 1953; S. U. TOVERUD, 1964). Bei Legehühnern mit 30 mg % Calcium fällt der Plasmacalciumspiegel auf 8—11 mg % ab (M. R. URIST, 1960). Bei rachitischen, parathyreoidektomierten Ratten können sogar Werte von 3,8 mg % erreicht werden (H. RASMUSSEN, 1963a). Ratten sind gegenüber einem Abfall der Blutcalciumkonzentration nicht allzu empfindlich (A. D. KENNY, 1962a). Bei den übrigen Tieren und beim Menschen beobachtet man bei 7 mg % bereits Tetanien, die mit weiterem Absinken des Calciumspiegels zum Tode führen. Am Abfall der Calciumkonzentration sind beim Menschen und Säuger (D. POLIN, 1958) zu 70 % die Calciumionen und zu 30 % das Calciumproteinat, bei Legehühnern (M. R. URIST, 1960; D. POLIN, 1957) zu 80 % phosphoproteidgebundenes Calcium und nur zu 20 % Calciumionen beteiligt. Nach einer Parathyreoidektomie ist die Erholungsphase im Oxalattoleranztest verlängert (G. S. STEWART, 1951; H. ORIMO, 1964).

Wirksame Parathormonextrakte erhöhen dosisabhängig innerhalb von 3—6 Std das Plasmacalcium bei nebenschilddrüsenlosen Tieren (R. TALMAGE, 1953; E. C. CAMERON, 1963; H. R. PERKINS, 1953; J. R. ELLIOTT, 1956, 1956a; S. U. TOVERUD, 1964) auf ca. 10 mg %, bei gesunden Individuen max. auf ca. 18 mg % (R. TALMAGE, 1953; G. M. VAES, 1962; Z. LARON, 1958; A. GROLLMAN, 1927; P. L. MUNSON, 1955). Bei Legehennen kann der Calciumspiegel durch Parathyreoideaextrakt um 10—30 mg % gesteigert werden (D. POLIN, 1957a; M. R. URIST, 1960). Nur wenige der käuflichen Parathormonpräparate sind allerdings im Calciumhaushalt wirksam (H.-J. DULCE, 1961a). Aufgrund der Plasmacalcium-erhöhenden Wirkung beim Hund hat man die Aktivität des Parathormons in Collipeinheiten und USP-Einheiten definiert. 1 USP-Einheit gleich $^1/_{100}$ der Hormonmenge, die beim Hund 18 Std nach Injektion das Plasmacalcium um 1 mg % erhöht.

Durch Parathormon werden die diffusiblen Calciumionen und das proteingebundene Calcium im Verhältnis 3:2 erhöht (P. H. Hennemann, 1957). Nur bei Legehühnern wird die Fraktion des phosphoproteidgebundenen Calciums bevorzugt vermehrt (M. R. Urist, 1960). Vitamin D begünstigt die Wirkung des Parathormons auf das Plasmacalcium (H. C. Harrison, 1958; H. Rasmussen, 1963a; H. G. Haas, 1966; S. U. Toverud, 1964). Ohne Vitamin D spricht der Organismus auf Parathormon weniger an. Durch Actinomycin D kann der Einfluß des Parathormons auf den Plasmacalciumspiegel fast aufgehoben werden (A. H. Tashjian, 1964; R. Eisenstein, 1964). Damit ist der Beweis erbracht, daß Parathormon im Zellstoffwechsel wahrscheinlich des Knochens innerhalb der Proteinsynthese angreift. Die Calciummobilisation aus den Knochendepots über die extracelluläre Flüssigkeit unter Parathormoneinfluß wird bei einer Peritonealwäsche besonders deutlich (R. V. Talmage, 1956).

b) Anorganischer Phosphor-Gehalt

Im Gegensatz zum Calcium steigt nach Parathyreoidektomie der Gehalt an anorganischem P im Plasma an. Beim Menschen findet man postoperativ Daueranstiege auf 6—10 mg % P (J. J. Canary, 1962; S. M. Krane, 1957), bei Ratten auf 10—18 mg % (R. Talmage, 1953; A. D. Kenny, 1962; P. L. Munson, 1955), die sich in 2—3 Wochen spontan normalisieren (J. R. Cortelyou, 1962). Unter einer P-armen Diät bleibt bei Ratten das Plasma-P trotz Parathyreoidektomie normal (H. Rasmussen, 1963). Parathormoninjektionen senken vornehmlich bei parathyreoidektomierten Tieren das erhöhte Plasma-P (P. L. Munson, 1955; R. Talmage, 1953). Ursache hierfür wird die auftretende Phosphaturie sein. Bei gesunden Tieren ist diese Wirkung unregelmäßiger (P. H. Hennemann, 1957; H. Bengain, 1933; G. M. Vaes, 1962; Z. Laron, 1958; A. Grollmann, 1927). Actinomycin-D beeinflußt die phosphaturische und Plasma-P-senkende Wirkung des Parathormons nicht (A. H. Tashjian, 1964; R. Eisenstein, 1964). Bei nephrektomierten Tieren steigern Parathormoninjektionen den Plasma-P-Spiegel, wodurch ein extrarenaler Angriffspunkt des Parathormons im P-Haushalt erwiesen ist (A. Grollman, 1954; R. V. Talmage, 1956).

c) Magnesium-, Citrat-, Mucoproteid-Gehalt

Das Plasma-Magnesium (A. Grollman, 1954; F. Heaton, 1964; I. McIntyre, 1963), das Plasma-Citrat (J. R. Elliott, 1956, 1956a; P. H. Hennemann, 1957; S. Freeman, 1956) und die Serummucoproteide (M. R. Shetlar, 1956) verhalten sich unter der Regulation durch Parathormon anscheinend wie das Plasmacalcium.

2. Thyreocalcitonin-Calcitonin

Calcium-, anorganischer Phosphor-, Magnesium-Gehalt

Aus Nebenschilddrüse und Schilddrüse stammen Hormone, die den Plasmacalciumspiegel senken. MacIntyre (1965) vertritt die Meinung, daß es sich um ein und dasselbe Hormon handelt. Das von Copp (1961, 1965, 1962, 1962a, 1964) aus tierischen Nebenschilddrüsen dargestellte sog. Calcitonin, ein Polypeptid, führt beim Menschen (H. G. Haas, 1947, 1966), bei Hunden und Schafen innerhalb von 20 min zu einem kurzfristigen Absinken des Plasmacalciumspiegels um 2 mg %, begleitet von einem Abfall des Magnesium- und Phosphorspiegels.

Talmage (1965), P. Hirsch (1964), A. Care (1966), G. Foster (1964a) sowie Gudmunsson (1966) isolierten dagegen aus der tierischen Schilddrüse das sog. Thyreocalcitonin — ein Polypeptid mit dem Molekulargewicht von 3000 (J. MacIntyre, 1965) —, das bei Ziegen, Ratten und Schweinen den Plasmacalciumspiegel innerhalb von 20 min bis 2 Std um 2 mg % langfristig senkt, was COPP (1965) bei Schafen im Umfang von 1 mg % auch bestätigt. Der Plasmamagnesiumspiegel wird durch Thyreocalcitonin nicht beeinflußt (Abb. 8 und 9).

Durch Thyreocalcitonin, dessen Wirksamkeit auf das Plasmacalcium Actinomycin-D und Nebenschilddrüsen unabhängig ist (H. A. SOLIMAN, 1965; I. MACINTYRE, 1966), wird gleichzeitig der Plasmaphosphorspiegel erniedrigt (P. HIRSCH, 1964). Hypercalcämien können mit dem Hormon erfolgreich beeinflußt werden (I. MACINTYRE, 1966; H. A. SOLIMAN, 1965). Nebenschilddrüsen-Extrakte senkten bei GUDMUNSSON (1966) im Gegensatz zu COPP den Plasmacalciumspiegel nicht. Thyroxin hemmt die Thyreocalcitoninwirkung auf das Plasmacalcium (HIRSCH, 1964a).

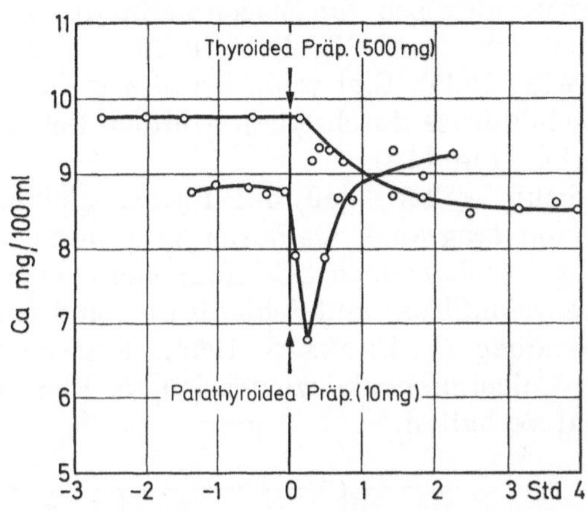

Abb. 8. Vergleich der Wirkung von injizierten Schilddrüsen- und Nebenschilddrüsenpräparationen auf den Plasmacalciumspiegel bei Schafen (D. H. COPP, 1965)

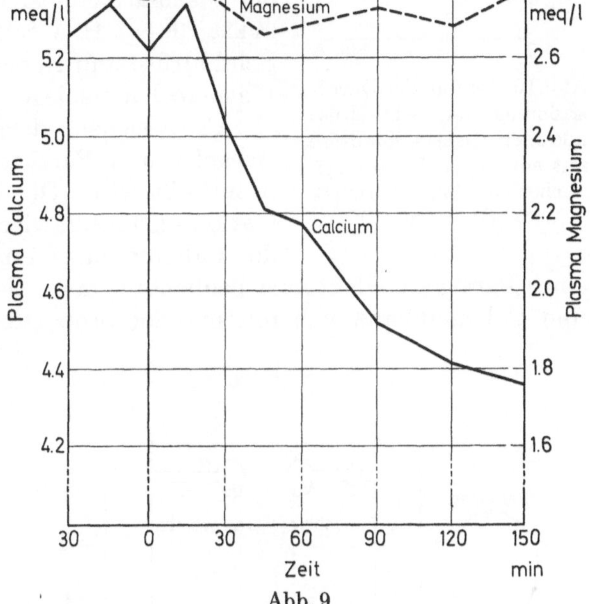

Abb. 9

Abb. 9. Wirkung eines Schilddrüsenextraktes bei der Ziege auf den Plasmamagnesium- und Plasmacalciumspiegel (G. FOSTER, 1964)

3. Das Regelsystem: Calcium- und Magnesiumionenkonzentration im Plasma, Parathormon-, Calcitonin-Thyreocalcitoninausschüttung

a) Reiz für Hormonausschüttung

Adäquater Reiz für die Ausschüttung von Parathormon und der Calcitonine ist der Plasmacalciumspiegel. Ein Senken der Calciumionenkonzentration im Plasma durch Äthylendiamintetraessigsäure-Infusion (D. H. COPP, 1963; KALLIOMÄKI, 1961), sowie ein selektives Durchströmen der Nebenschilddrüse mit Äthylendiamintetraessigsäurelösung (COPP, 1961a) führt innerhalb von wenigen Stunden zu einem Calciumionenanstieg im extracellulären Raum, wie er durch Parathormoninjektionen erreicht werden kann. Parallel mit der calciumionenabhängigen Ausschüttung parathormonwirksamer Substanz geht der Einbau von α-Aminobuttersäure in die Nebenschilddrüsen (L. RAISZ, 1965a). Einen ähnlichen Reiz auf die Parathormonausschüttung scheint auch ein Magnesiummangel auszuüben (I. MACINTYRE, 1963). Infundiert man intravenös Calciumionen, steigt der Calciumspiegel, sofern Nebenschilddrüsen vorhanden sind, nicht proportional an (D. H. COPP, 1963), perfundiert man die isolierte Schilddrüsen-Nebenschilddrüsenregion mit Calciumionen angereicherter Lösung, nimmt der Plasmacalciumspiegel unmittelbar ab (G. FOSTER, 1964a; D. H. COPP, 1962, 1965, 1961a; I. MACINTYRE, 1964). Diese Befunde werden mit einem Rückgang der Parathormon- und dem Auftreten der Thyreocalcitoninausschüttung erklärt.

b) Erfolgsorgane des Reizes

Über das Erfolgsorgan des Reizes für die Ausschüttung eines Calcitonins bestehen aber immer noch Unklarheiten. COPP (1964, 1965) konnte bei Schafen mit dem Durchströmen isolierter Nebenschilddrüsen mit hypercalcämischer Lösung einen schnellen Abfall des Plasmacalciumspiegels erreichen, der beim Durchströmen der isolierten Schilddrüse (D. H. COPP, 1962) ausblieb (Abb. 10).

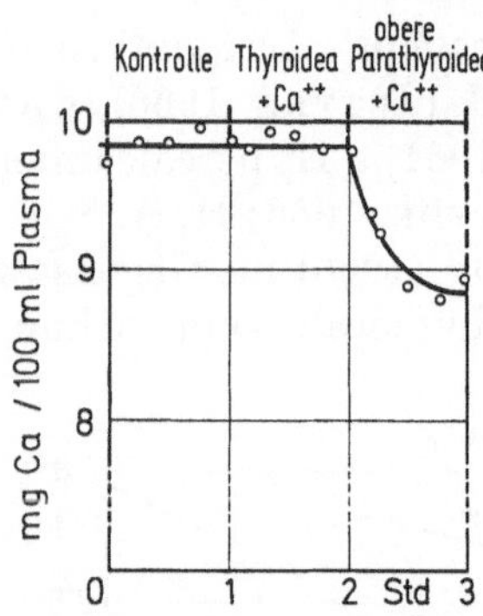

Abb. 10. Einfluß der Durchströmung von Schilddrüse und oberer Nebenschilddrüse mit mit Calciumionen angereichertem Blut (12,8 mg % Ca^{++}) (H. COPP, 1965)

J. MACINTYRE (1965) und G. FOSTER (1964a, 1964b) beobachteten im Gegensatz dazu bei der hypercalcämischen Durchströmung der isolierten Schilddrüse des Hundes einen Abfall des Plasmacalciums um ca. 0,6 mg %. Beim Durchströmen der isolierten Nebenschilddrüsen von Ziegen nahm dagegen der Plasmacalciumspiegel nicht ab (I. MACINTYRE, 1966; G. FOSTER, 1964a; H. A. SOLIMAN, 1965). Erst wenn bei diesen Tieren Schilddrüse und Nebenschilddrüse durchströmt wurden, fiel der Plasmacalciumspiegel (Abb. 11 und 12).

Als gesichert darf heute gelten, daß der Plasmacalciumspiegel durch Parathormon langsamer als durch ein Calcitonin beeinflußt wird. Die Regelmechanismen ,,Calciumionenkonzentration im Plasma: Nebenschilddrüse und Schilddrüse" sind von der Calciumbilanz unabhängig (F. BRONNER, 1966). Erst nach einer Parathyreoidektomie beobachtet man, daß Calciumionenkonzentration im Plasma und Calciumbilanz sich miteinander proportional verhalten.

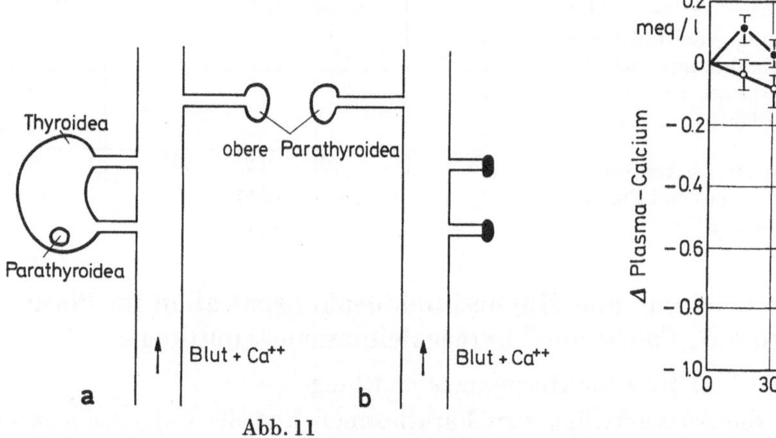

Abb. 11

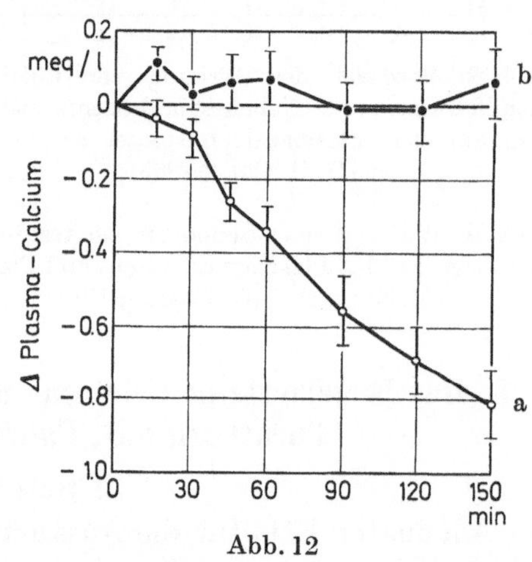

Abb. 12

Abb. 11. Schematische Abbildung der Perfusion von Schilddrüse und Nebenschilddrüse bei Ziegen (G. FOSTER, 1964a)

Abb. 12. Hypercalcämische Durchströmung isolierter äußerer Nebenschildrüsen (b) und des gesamten Nebenschilddrüsenapparates bei der Ziege (a) (G. FOSTER, 1964a)

4. Vitamin D

a) Calcium-Gehalt

Durch Vitamin D kann der Plasmacalciumspiegel bis zur Hypercalcämie gesteigert werden (W. GRAB, 1966; S. U. TOVERUD, 1964; J. R. ELLIOTT, 1956a, 1956; R. EISENSTEIN, 1964; G. GUROFF, 1963). Vitamin D übt diesen Einfluß unabhängig von der Nebenschilddrüse aus (F. C. GRAN, 1960; J. R. ELLIOTT, 1956; S. U. TOVERUD, 1964). Vitamin D_3 ist wirksamer und weniger toxisch als Vitamin D_2 (W. GRAB, 1953; P. CHEN, 1964). Es wird relativ mehr nichtionisiertes Calcium als ionisiertes Calcium erhöht (S. T. ANNING,

1948; F. Albright, 1948). Die Plasmacalciumerhöhung unter Vitamin D kann durch Actinomycin D verhindert werden (R. Eisenstein, 1964). Im schweren Vitamin D-Mangelzustand sinkt der Plasmacalciumspiegel teilweise bis zu 6—7 mg % ab (P. Chen, 1964; F. C. Gran, 1960; H. E. Harrison, 1959). Der Mensch und die Maus reagieren auf Vitamin D empfindlicher als Ratte und Hund (B. Lavrov, 1964). Wir nehmen heute an, daß Vitamin D das Plasma-Calcium erhöht, weil es die Calciumresorption im Darm primär steigert (F. Albright, 1948).

b) Anorganischer Phosphor-Gehalt

Der Plasma-P-Spiegel wird durch Vitamin D ebenfalls erhöht (A. E. Sobel, 1945; P. S. Chen, 1962). Rachitische Kinder hatten vor der Vitamin D-Behandlung ca. 3 mg % $P_{anorg.}$ und nach Therapie ca. 6 mg % $P_{anorg.}$ im Plasma (H. E. Harrison, 1959). Bei Ratten findet man teilweise andere Ergebnisse, weil hier der Einfluß des Vitamins D auf den Plasma-P-Spiegel stark von der oralen P-Zufuhr abhängt (A. E. Sobel, 1945; H. Rasmussen, 1963a). Der dem Calcium parallele P-Anstieg ist wahrscheinlich die Folge einer Depression der Parathormonausschüttung und einer stärkeren renalen Phosphorrückresorption. Der gleichzeitige Calcium- und P-Anstieg im Plasma kann Ursache einer heterotropen Mineralisation bei Erwachsenen unter Vitamin D-Therapie werden.

c) Citrat-, Carbonat-, Phosphatase-Gehalt

Der Citratspiegel im Plasma wird unter Vitamin D-Therapie (G. Fanconi, 1961; R. L. Hartles, 1964; J. R. Elliott, 1956; H. E. Harrison, 1959) erhöht, der Carbonatgehalt des Plasmas gesenkt (A. E. Sobel, 1945). Die Aktivität der alkalischen Phosphatase des Plasmas, die bei der Rachitis bis auf 150 IE/m^2 erhöht sein kann, normalisiert sich während der Vitamin D-Behandlung (H. E. Harrison, 1959; J. R. Campbell, 1965).

5. Glucocorticoide

a) Calcium-Gehalt

Cortison und Cortisol erniedrigen den Plasmacalcium-Gehalt im ionisierten und proteingebundenen Anteil (A. B. Borle, 1960b; B. E. Nordin, 1965a; Z. Laron, 1958; W. C. Thomas, 1958; H. Stoerk, 1963), ausgenommen bei Kaninchen und rachitischen Ratten (Z. Laron, 1956; N. Matsuda, 1956). Bei Menschen mit Morbus Addison beobachtet man Calciumwerte von 11—14 mg % (C. Leeksma, 1957).

b) Anorganischer Phosphor- und Citrat-Gehalt

Der $P_{anorg.}$- und Citratgehalt im Plasma fallen unter Glucocorticoid-Therapie und beim Cushingsyndrom (B. E. Nordin, 1965a) wie der Calciumspiegel ab (Z. Laron, 1957, 1958; B. E. Nordin, 1965a; L. R. Sataline, 1962; A. B. Borle, 1960b; H. C. Harrison, 1959; G. Guroff, 1963). Beim Morbus Addison steigen die Plasma-P-Werte bis zu 7 mg % an (C. Leeksma, 1957). Glucocorticoide verhalten sich demnach in ihrer Wirkung auf die extracelluläre Flüssigkeit dem Vitamin D antagonistisch.

6. Oestrogene — Androgene

Calcium-, anorganischer Phosphor- und Phosphatase-Gehalt

Oestrogengaben können beim Menschen den Plasmacalcium- und Phosphor-Spiegel zeitweilig herabsetzen (B. E. Nordin, 1965a; F. Roth, 1961). Anscheinend wird gleichzeitig die β- und γ-Globulinfraktion des Plasmas erhöht (G. Manunta, 1957b). Bei Vögeln mit intakten Nebenschilddrüsen führen Oestrogengaben dagegen grundsätzlich in wenigen Tagen zu einem dosisabhängigen Anstieg des Calciums und Phosphors im Plasma (D. Polin, 1958; P. Siegmund, 1961; R. H. Hennemann, 1955; M. R. Urist, 1960). Es werden Grenzwerte bis zu 160 mg % Ca erreicht, wovon nur ca. 9 mg % Ca ultrafiltrabel sind (M. R. Urist, 1960). Als Ursache der Calciumerhöhung hat man das Auftreten calciumbindender β-Lipoproteide und Phosphorproteide im Plasma erkannt (M. R. Urist, 1958), die auch physiologisch in der Legeperiode gebildet werden. Actinomycin D vermag die Synthese dieser Proteide und die Calciumerhöhung zu verhindern (O. Greengard, 1964). Nur bei parathyreoidektomierten Hähnchen senken Oestrogene die Calciumionenkonzentration des Plasmas (D. Polin, 1958). Die Phosphatase-Aktivitäten im Plasma von Ratten nehmen nach Oestrogentherapie ab (K. W. Buchwald, 1947). Über Einflüsse von Androgenen auf den Plasma-, Calcium- und P-Spiegel ist wenig bekannt.

7. Peptidhormone der Hypophyse

Calcium-, anorganischer Phosphor- und Magnesium-Gehalt

Bei der Akromegalie wird ein Anstieg des Phosphors und oft auch des Calciums im Plasma bei einem Abfall des Plasmamagnesiums verzeichnet (B. E. Nordin, 1965a; S. Hanna, 1961). Andererseits senken Peptidfraktionen wie Corticotropin und α-β-melanocytenstimulierendes Hormon aus der Hypophyse bei Kaninchen den Plasmacalciumspiegel thyreocalcitoninähnlich (H. Friesen, 1964).

8. Thyroxin

Nach klinischen Beobachtungen erhöht Thyroxin den Plasmacalciumspiegel antagonistisch zum Thyreocalcitonin ohne den Plasma-P-Gehalt zu beeinflussen (B. E. Nordin, 1965a).

III. Das primäre Mineralisationsprodukt und seine Reifung

Man bezeichnet das im Stadium frischer Mineralisation zuerst gebildete Knochenmineral als primäres Mineralisationsprodukt. Lange Jahre glaubte man, sekundäres Calciumphosphat würde als einfacher gebautes Salz zuerst ausfallen und in ein apatitisches Calciumphosphat, das wir heute als Defektapatit oder Hydrogenhydroxylapatit bezeichnen würden, unter Abgabe von Phosphorsäure übergehen (I. Greenwald, 1942; B. Kramer, 1928; J. Raaflaub, 1961a; H. C. Hodge, 1950).

$$9\,CaHPO_4 \times 2\,H_2O \rightarrow Ca_9H_2(PO_4)_6(OH)_2 + 3\,H_3PO_4 + 16\,H_2O.$$

Man fand im jungen Knochen einen Ca/P-Gewichtsquotienten von 1,29 (P. Cartier, 1950; M. Polonowski, 1951) wie bei Ca HPO_4 und erst im älteren Knochen solche von 1,94 wie bei einem apatitischen Calciumphosphat (M. J. Dallemagne, 1948, 1942). Röntgenpulverdiagramme vom geglühten Knochenmineral junger Kaninchen (K. H. Ibsen, 1964) zeigten bis zu 1% Pyrophosphat, das beim Glühen aus Ca H PO_4 entstehen kann. In vivo begann die Mineralisation bei rachitischen Ratten tatsächlich erst, wenn in der extracellulären Flüssigkeit das Löslichkeitsprodukt von Ca HPO_4 mit $3{,}4 \times 10^{-6}$ überschritten wurde (H. C. Hodge, 1950, 1955). Unmittelbar im frischen Knochen oder Zahnschmelz ist aber sekundäres Calciumphosphat niemals röntgenstrukturanalytisch nachgewiesen worden (C. Huggins, 1937; A. Hirschman, 1947, 1953; H. H. Roseberry, 1931; H. C. Hodge, 1955, 1950).

Heute dürfen wir begründet annehmen, daß das primäre Mineralisationsprodukt ein nichtkristallines, mit der heutigen Röntgenbeugungsanalyse nicht differenzierbares Calciumphosphat ist (E. D. Eanes, 1966; Harper, 1966), das erst später kristallin wird und in substituierte Gitterstrukturen von Hydroxylapatit — $Ca_{10}(PO_4)_6\,(OH)_2$, Defektapatit — $Ca_9H_2(PO_4)_6(OH)_2$ [von Dallemagne (1956) unglücklich als α-Tricalciumphosphathydrat bezeichnet], und Octacalciumphosphat — $Ca_8H_2(PO_4)_6 \times 5\,H_2O$ übergeht (R. Quicker, 1967; D. Carlstroem, 1956; M. J. Dallemagne, 1956; J. Macgregor, 1965; O. R. Trautz, 1955; A. S. Posner, 1964). Die nichtkristalline Phase ist mit einem molaren Ca/P-Quotienten von 1,48 dem Octacalciumphosphat sehr ähnlich (E. D. EANES, 1966). Im reifen Knochen des Menschen und des Rindes liegen ca. 55—60 % des Knochenminerals in einer kristallinen Phase vor und 40—45 % in der nicht kristallinen, sog. amorphen Phase (E. D. EANES, 1966; HARPER, 1966), die durch Magnesiumionen und Carbonationen stabilisiert wird. Innerhalb der kristallinen Phase treten wahrscheinlich nur zwei hexagonale Gitter auf (D. TAVES, 1963); hauptsächlich das mit dem Defektapatit isomorphe Apatitgitter

Achslänge a = 9,42—9,44 Å
c = 6,88 Å

(A. S. POSNER, 1964; O. R. TRAUTZ, 1955; D. CARLSTROEM, 1956) und zu ca. 2 % (R. QUIKKER, 1967) das Octacalciumphosphatgitter

Achslänge a = 19,87 Å
b = 9,63 Å
c = 6,88 Å

(W. E. BROWN, 1962).

In beiden Gittern führen Substitutionen mit Carbonat, Fluorid und anderen Ionen zu leichten Veränderungen der Achslängen. Im Laufe der Alterung gehen Defektapatit und Octacalciumphosphat anscheinend auch in vivo in gröber kristallinen und im Gitter idealisierten Hydroxylapatit über (J. MACGREGOR, 1965; W. NEUMAN, 1963).

Diesen neuen Auffassungen über Entstehen und Altern des primären Mineralisationsproduktes widersprechen die meisten früheren Befunde nicht. Defektapatit und Octacalciumphosphat bilden beim Glühen über 300° Pyrophosphat (C. HUGGINS, 1937; W. N. NEBERGALL, 1960). Defektapatit ist in vitro bei Phosphatüberschuß zu synthetisieren (P. LERCH, 1965) und altert unter Wasserstoffionen-Abgabe und Calciumaufnahme. Junge Osteone geben beim Glühen 3 mal mehr Pyrophosphat ab als ältere (K. H. IBSEN, 1964). In vitro im carbonatreichen Medium mineralisierter rachitischer Knorpel hat einen molaren Rest-Calcium/Phosphorquotienten von 1,33 ähnlich wie Octacalciumphosphat (A. HIRSCHMANN, 1965) (Rest-Calcium = Gesamt-Calcium — Carbonatcalcium). Bei einem Ca × P-Produkt von ca. 10^{-6} ist die Kristallisation nicht nur von $Ca\,HPO_4$ sondern auch von Defektapatit, Octacalciumphosphat und Hydroxylapatit zu erwarten. Die sog. Rekristallisation NEUMANs beschreibt wahrscheinlich den Übergang der nichtkristallinen in die kristalline Phase mit Idealisierung des Apatitgitters. In vitro ist es bereits gelungen, durch Mischen von Calciumionenlösung und Phosphationenlösung im alkalischen Bereich bei 25—37° ein dem Knochenmineral ähnliches Mineralisationsprodukt anorganisch zu fällen (H. MOELLER, 1932; P. LERCH, 1965; E. D. EANES, 1966; D. BOULET, 1961). Bei aequimolaren Calcium- und Phosphorkonzentrationen oder einem Calciumüberschuß bildet sich ein gelartiges, nicht kristallines Produkt mit einer Oberfläche von ca. 130 m^2/g, das anscheinend ein Gemisch von Defektapatit und Octacalciumphosphat darstellt und in kristallinen Hydroxylapatit mit einem Ca/P-Gewichtsquotienten von 2,04—2,13 übergeht. Unter derartigen Bedingungen wird die Kristallisation von $Ca\,HPO_4$ nicht mehr beobachtet (H. NEWESELY, 1965). Bei einem Phosphatüberschuß im Medium von 25—200 % bildet sich primär kristalliner Defektapatit mit einem Ca/P-Gewichtsquotienten von 1,82—1,97 (H. MOELLER, 1932; P. LERCH, 1965). Biologisch sind aequimolare Mischungsverhältnisse zu erwarten. Deshalb kann $Ca\,HPO_4$ überhaupt nicht entstehen.

Hydroxylapatit steht mit Defektapatit im Hydrolysegleichgewicht.

$$Ca_{10}(PO_4)_6(OH)_2 + 2H_2O \rightleftharpoons Ca_9H_2(PO_4)_6(OH)_2 + Ca^{++} + 2OH^-,$$

das auch als

$$Ca_{10}(PO_4)_6(OH)_2 + 2H^+ \rightleftharpoons Ca_9H_2(PO_4)_6(OH)_2 + Ca^{++}$$

beschrieben werden kann.

Durch ein OH-Ionenangebot wird das Gleichgewicht zu Gunsten des Hydroxylapatits verschoben (D. TAVES, 1963). Durch ein Wasserstoffionenangebot wird dagegen das Gleichgewicht zu Gunsten des Defektapatits verschoben. Treten an die Stelle des OH-Ionenangebots Bicarbonationen, wird wahrscheinlich ein Carbonat-substituierter, besser löslicher, gegenüber H-Ionen empfindlicher Apatit gebildet. Eine Säuerung wandelt biologisch in Gegenwart von Magnesiumionen ein Carbonatapatitgitter offensichtlich leichter in das Whitlockitgitter um, ohne daß Defektapatit entsteht.

$$Ca_{10}(PO_4)_6CO_3 + 2H^+ + Mg^{++} = 3(Ca, Mg)_3(PO_4)_2 + H_2O + CO_2 + 2Ca^{++}.$$

Bei der Zahnkaries wurden derartige Whitlockitkristalle gefunden (I. GREENWALD, 1942; A. S. POSNER, 1964; H. J. HOEHLING, 1961). MULLER u. Mitarb. (1966) fanden bei Ratten im Vitamin D-Mangelzustand Knochenmineral mit unreiferer Kristall- und Apatitstruktur.

IV. Einflüsse auf die Kristallisation von Calciumphosphaten

Solange keine Hindernisse bestehen, wachsen bei der Kristallisation große Calciumphosphatkristalle auf Kosten der besser löslichen kleinen (A. E. SOBEL, 1960a).

1. Calcium-, Phosphat-, Carbonat-Ionenüberschuß

Ein Phosphationenüberschuß im Lösungsmittel lenkt die Calciumphosphatkristallisation in Richtung eines Defektapatits, ein Calciumionenüberschuß dagegen mehr in Richtung eines reifen Hydroxylapatits (H. MOELLER, 1932). Titrationen von Phosphatpufferlösungen mit Calciumhydroxyd, wobei nacheinander Ca HPO_4, Octacalciumphosphat und Apatite ausfallen, sind für die biologische Anwendung von geringem Interesse (H. C. HODGE, 1955). BACHRA (1963) wies nach, daß Phosphationen bei pH 7,3 gleichzeitig das Entstehen von Calciumcarbonatkristallen verhindern, und umgekehrt Bicarbonationen (22×10^{-3} Mol/l) die Bildung eines einheitlichen Hydroxylapatits so stören, daß ein amorphes carbonatangereichertes, besser lösliches Calciumphosphat mit einem Ca/P-Gewichtsquotienten von 1,4—2,3 entsteht (B. N. BACHRA, 1963, 1963a, 1962, 1965, 1965a). GREENWALD (1945) hatte diese Beziehung voraus berechnet. Eine Kristallisation von Calciumcarbonat, wie sie in Otolithen stattfindet, kann biologisch erst bei einem P/C-Verhältnis von 1:300 stattfinden (B. N. BACHRA, 1963, 1963a).

2. Induktionsstoffe

Modellfällungen von Hydroxylapatit (Mol. Ca/P = 1,62) bei $\mu = 0{,}16$ und 37° werden durch Apatitimpfkristalle oder Kollagenfibrillen bereits bei niederen $Ca^{++} \times P_{anorg.}$-Ionenprodukten von $0{,}4$—$2{,}4 \times 10^{-6}$ (Mol/l)^2 induziert (D. TAVES, 1964; H. FLEISCH, 1964; B. N. BACHRA, 1965). Spontan findet die Kristallisation erst bei einem $Ca^{++} \times P_{anorg.}$-Ionenprodukt von $2{,}4$—$4{,}0 \times 10^{-6}$ (Mol/l)^2 statt (H. FLEISCH, 1961). Bleiionen induzieren in biologischen Konzentrationen von 10^{-6}—10^{-7} molar ebenfalls die Apatitkristallisation beim $Ca^{++} \times P_{anorg.}$-Ionenprodukten von ca. 2×10^{-6} (Mol/l)^2 (H. FLEISCH, 1965a).

3. Fluorid-Ionen

Fluoridionen fördern dagegen in biologischen Konzentrationen von 1—5 γ % entsprechend 0,5—5 μ Mol/l die Keimbildung und Kristallisation von Hydroxylapatit zu Ungunsten von Octacalciumphosphat. Deshalb ist biologisch im schwach basischen Bereich nur ein sehr geringer Anteil von kristallinem Octacalciumphosphat zu erwarten. Die Fluorionen setzen die Austauschfähigkeit des Calciums zwischen dem Knochenmineral und der extracellulären Flüssigkeit herab (C. YATES, 1964) und hemmen die Aufnahme von

Carbonat in die Position von Hydroxyl. Dadurch wird die Bildung eines stabilen unlöslichen Knochenminerals begünstigt (H. NEWESELY, 1960, 1965; W. E. BROWN, 1962; D. TAVES, 1964).

4. Magnesium-Ionen

Magnesiumionen ($0,5 \times 10^{-3}$ Mol/l) verzögern die Kristallisation von Hydroxylapatit und fördern das Entstehen eines nicht kristallinen Calciumphosphatcarbonats (B. N. BACHRA, 1965, 1965a), das EANES u. Mitarb. (1966) im Knochenmineral beschrieben haben. Sie begünstigen zwar in vitro die Whitlockitbildung aus Calciumionen- und Phosphationenlösungen (H. NEWESELY, 1965, 1966; E. HAYEK, 1958). Die biologische Magnesiumkonzentration liegt aber hierzu 3 Zehnerpotenzen zu niedrig.

5. Hemmstoffe

Alle an Calciumphosphatkristalle adsorbierbaren Ionen können Hemmstoffe des Kristallwachstums werden (A. E. SOBEL, 1960a; D. TAVES, 1963). Deshalb ist in der extracellulären Flüssigkeit zur Keimbildung eine gewisse Übersättigung nötig. Weitere Hemmstoffe der Kristallisation sind Calciumchelatbildner, Oberflächengifte und Schwermetalle. Biologische Calciumchelatbildner sind Adenosintriphosphat, Citrat, anorganisches Pyrophosphat (C. NEUBERG, 1949; R. E. GOSSELIN, 1949) und Aminosäuren (W. DIRSCHERL, 1959). Die quantitative Bedeutung der Aminosäuren ist sicher gering (M. HARDEL, 1965). Kondensierte Phosphate und Pyrophosphate können gleichzeitig als Oberflächengift die Kristallisation von Calciumsalzen hemmen (H. FLEISCH, 1966, 1966a, 1964a, 1966b), so daß die Apatitbildungsprodukte $[Ca] \times [P_{ges.}]$ auf $10,8 \times 10^{-6}$ $(Mol/l)^2$ ansteigen (H. FLEISCH, 1964) (Tabelle 62). Beryllium- und Kobaltionen hemmen das Kristallwachstum in Konzentrationen von 10^{-4} molar (H. FLEISCH, 1964b).

Tabelle 62. *Einfluß von Pyrophosphat und Polyphosphat auf die Mineralisation von Hühnerembryonenfemur in der Gewebekultur* (H. FLEISCH, 1966b)

	µg Trockengewicht	µg Hydroxyprolin	% Mineral[1]
Kontrollfemur	1050	20,9	100
Femur + 4 µg P-Grahamsalz/ml Medium .	1077	20,2	53,4
Femur + 16 µg P-Grahamsalz/ml Medium	1004	19,9	17,9
16 µg Pyrophosphat-P/ml Medium . . .	1023	18,7	39

[1] Photometrie der Röntgenbeugungslinien 121, 112.

V. Löslichkeit des Knochenminerals in vitro und in vivo

Für das Beurteilen der biologischen Mineralisation und Demineralisation hat die Löslichkeit des Knochenminerals zentrale Bedeutung. Löslichkeiten werden in der physikalischen Chemie anhand der sog. Löslichkeitsprodukte bestimmt. Unter den Löslichkeitsprodukten (LP) versteht man das molare, auf die Zahl der Kristallgitterteilchen einer Einheitszelle bezogene Ionenprodukt im Lösungsmittel über dem Niederschlag eines Salzes bei konstanter Temperatur und Ionenstärke. Diese Definition setzt allerdings voraus, daß die im Salz vorkommenden Einheitszellen bekannt und einheitlich sind, die Gitterteilchen stöchiometrisch in Lösung gehen, und sich die Gitterstruktur des Salzes beim Auflösen nicht ändert. Beim Knochenmineral treffen diese Voraussetzungen nicht zu, und man darf deshalb nicht von einem Löslichkeitsprodukt im strengen Sinne sprechen. Die Kristallgitterstruktur setzt sich aus nicht stöchiometrisch verteilten, verschiedenen teilweise isomorph substituierten Einheitszellen zusammen, die beim Lösen einer pH-abhängigen Umwandlung unterliegen und deren Ionen ungleichmäßig in Lösung gehen. Man kann die Löslichkeit des Knochenminerals bei konstanter Temperatur und Ionenstärke und konstantem pH deshalb nur aufgrund der molaren Ionenprodukte in einem Lösungsmittel oder der extracellulären Flüssigkeit ermitteln, ohne die Zahlenwerte auf eine bestimmte Einheitszelle zu beziehen. Diese Ionenprodukte sind mit den Ionenprodukten beim Lösen definierter Calciumsalze zu vergleichen. Bei Calciumphosphaten empfehlen sich folgende Produkte zum Beurteilen der Löslichkeit:

$$[Ca^{2+}] \times [P_{anorg}]$$
$$[Ca^{2+}] \times [HPO_4^{2-}]$$
$$[Ca^{2+}] \times [PO_4^{3-}]$$
$$[Ca^{2+}] \times [CO_3^{2-}].$$

Jedes Einrechnen gemessener molarer Ionenkonzentrationen in Formeln von Calciumphosphaten ($Ca_3(PO_4)_2$, $Ca_{10}(PO_4)_6(OH)_2$ u.a.) und Angaben von Löslichkeitsprodukten oder pK-Werten (L. E. HOLT, 1925, 1925a; J. MACGREGOR, 1960) sind fragwürdige Hilfsmaßnahmen, die zu falschen Aussagen über den Sättigungsgrad der extracellulären Flüssigkeit an Knochenmineral führen müssen.

1. Lösungsgleichgewicht: extracelluläre Flüssigkeit/Knochenmineral

a) $Ca^{2+} \times P_{anorg.}$-Ionenprodukt in der extracellulären Flüssigkeit

In der extracellulären Flüssigkeit des Menschen, deren pH mit 7,4, Temperatur 38° und CO_2-Gehalt mit 25 m Mol/l anzusetzen ist, berechnen wir ein $Ca^{2+} \times P_{ges.\,anorg.}$-Ionenprodukt von 15—17 (mg %)^2 oder $1{,}3$—$1{,}5 \times 10^{-6}$ (Mol/l)^2 (H. FLEISCH, 1961). Das $Ca^{++} \times HPO_4^{2-}$-Produkt beträgt $1{,}2$—$1{,}3 \times 10^{-6}$ (Mol/l)^2, das $Ca^{++} \times PO_4^{3-}$-Produkt ca.

Tabelle 63. *Ionenprodukte (Mol/l)² von Calciumphosphaten und Calciumcarbonat in Lösungsmedien in vivo und in vitro bei 38° und pH 7,4*

	$Ca^{++} \times HPO_4^{2-}$	$Ca^{++} \times PO_4^{3-}$	$Ca^{++} \times CO_3^{2-}$
In vivo extracelluläre Flüssigkeit	$1{,}2$—$1{,}3 \times 10^{-6}$	$5{,}2 \times 10^{-11}$	$0{,}13 \times 10^{-6}$
in vitro: Serum-Sättigung			
mit Knochenpulver	$0{,}66$—$0{,}94 \times 10^{-6}$	$2{,}9$—$4{,}1 \times 10^{-11}$	$0{,}11 \times 10^{-6}$
mit Mischapatit	$0{,}2 \times 10^{-6}$	$1{,}7 \times 10^{-11}$	$0{,}05 \times 10^{-6}$
mit Mischapatit und Calciumcarbonat	$0{,}5 \times 10^{-6}$	$2{,}37 \times 10^{-11}$	$0{,}12 \times 10^{-6}$
in vitro: Synthetische carbonathaltige extracelluläre Flüssigkeit, Sättigung			
mit Knochenpulver	$0{,}61 \times 10^{-6}$	$2{,}6 \times 10^{-11}$	$0{,}11 \times 10^{-6}$
mit Mischapatit	$0{,}25 \times 10^{-6}$	$0{,}88 \times 10^{-11}$	$0{,}01 \times 10^{-6}$
mit Mischapatit und Calciumcarbonat	$0{,}08 \times 10^{-6}$	$0{,}26 \times 10^{-12}$	$0{,}03 \times 10^{-6}$

LP in extracellulärer Flüssigkeit $CaHPO_4 = 3{,}2 \times 10^{-6}$ (Mol/l)^2, $CaCO_3 = 0{,}21 \times 10^{-6}$ (Mol/l)^2.

$5{,}2 \times 10^{-11}$ (Mol/l)^2 (vergleiche hierzu Tabelle 63). Der Berechnung liegen Messungen des pH (= 7,4), der Calciumionenkonzentration (= $1{,}3$—$1{,}4 \times 10^{-3}$ Mol/l) und der gesamten anorganischen Phosphorkonzentration (= 10^{-3} Mol/l) sowie die pK'_{1-3}-Werte von SENDROY (1927) zugrunde.

Mit dem $Ca^{++} \times P_{anorg.}$-Ionenprodukt darf nicht verwechselt werden das $Ca \times P_{anorg.}$-Produkt, das sich nur auf intravasale Flüssigkeit, die nicht mit dem Knochenmineral in Kontakt steht, bezieht und weniger aussagt. Es beträgt beim Menschen ca. 30—40 (mg %)^2 = $2{,}6$—$2{,}8 \times 10^{-6}$ (Mol/l)^2 (L. E. HOLT, 1925b; H. C. HODGE, 1955). Bei Nagern und Küken liegen diese Werte mit 95 (mg %)^2 entsprechend $7{,}5 \times 10^{-6}$ (Mol/l)^2 höher (G. M. VAES, 1962; R. V. TALMAGE, 1956; P. S. CHEN, 1964). Nach einer Parathyreoidektomie (A. GROLLMAN, 1954; R. V. TALMAGE, 1956) und bei der menschlichen (L. E. HOLT, 1925b) und experimentellen Rachitis (A. E. SOBEL, 1934; P. S. CHEN, 1964; H. RASMUSSEN, 1963a) nimmt das $Ca \times P$-Produkt auf 15—30 (mg %)^2 ab, was auf eine Abnahme der Löslichkeit des Knochenminerals hindeutet.

b) $Ca^{2+} \times CO_3^{2-}$-Ionenprodukt in der extracellulären Flüssigkeit

Bei 40—60 mm Hg CO_2 und pH 7,4 besteht in der extracellulären Flüssigkeit ein $Ca^{2+} \times CO_3^{2-}$-Ionenprodukt von ca. $0{,}13 \times 10^{-6}$ (Mol/l)^2 (B. HASTINGS, 1927). Das molare CO_3/PO_4-Verhältnis in der extracellulären Flüssigkeit und im Knochenmineral stehen zueinander in fester Beziehung (A. E. SOBEL, 1955).

c) Löslichkeit des Knochenminerals in vitro

Knochenpulver des Menschen löst sich in vitro im Serum bei pH 7,3, 37°, 5,5 % Protein und 17 mMol CO_2/l auf, bis im Überstand bei Sättigung ein $Ca^{2++} \times P_{ges.\,anorg.}$-Ionenprodukt von 0,64—1,24 $\times 10^{-6}$ (Mol/l)^2 erreicht ist (M. A. LOGAN, 1939). Im Plasmaultrafiltrat und im synthetischen Ultrafiltrat als Lösungsmittel wurden ähnliche Werte nämlich 0,8—0,9 $\times 10^{-6}$ (Mol/l)^2 entsprechend $Ca^{2+} \times P_{anorg.}$ ca. 10 (mg %)^2 gemessen (H. FLEISCH, 1961). Ca. 3,3—4,8 mg % Calcium stehen mit Knochenpulver unter biologischen Bedingungen im Lösungsgleichgewicht (C. C. JOHNSTON, 1962a). Errechnet man pH abhängig die Anteile von PO_4^{3-}- und HPO_4^{2-} am gesamten anorganischen P, dann ergibt sich ein $Ca^{2+} \times HPO_4^{2-}$-Produkt von 0,66–0,94 $\times 10^{-6}$ (Mol/l)^2 und ein $Ca^{2+} \times PO_4^{3-}$-Produkt von 2,9–4,1 $\times 10^{-11}$ (Mol/l)^2. MACGREGOR (1962, 1962a) wies nach, daß der CO_2-Gehalt des Lösungsmittels die Löslichkeit des Phosphats im Lösungsgleichgewicht starkt beeinflußt. Im CO_2-freien Medium wird Phosphat des Knochenminerals nur bis zu $0{,}2 \times 10^{-3}$ Mol/l aufgelöst, bei 25 mMol CO_2/l zu $0{,}65 \times 10^{-3}$ Mol/l. Bei pH 7,0 würde das Knochenmineral mit den bei pH 7,4 in der nativen extracellulären Flüssigkeit gemessenen Calcium, HPO_4^{2-} und PO_4^{3-}-Ionenkonzentrationen im Lösungsgleichgewicht stehen (J. MACGREGOR, 1960). Daraus darf man schließen, daß die extracelluläre Flüssigkeit an Knochenmineral übersättigt aber metastabil ist und nur durch eine leichte Säuerung in der unmittelbaren Nähe des Knochenminerals das Lösungsgleichgewicht bestimmt und aufrecht erhalten wird. In der Literatur regelmäßig angegebene Löslichkeitsprodukte für Knochenmineral in der extracellulären Flüssigkeit (pLP $Ca_3(PO_4)_2$ u. a.) (M. A. LOGAN, 1940, 1939; J. MACGREGOR, 1960, 1962) sind praktisch nicht verwertbar. Messungen chemischer Potentiale im Lösungsüberstand von Knochenmineral von Kindern und Erwachsenen sprechen dafür, daß die extracelluläre Flüssigkeit im Kindesalter wahrscheinlich mit einem Octacalciumphosphat-reicheren und im erwachsenen Alter mit einem Hydroxylapatit-reicheren Knochenmineral im Lösungsgleichgewicht steht (MACGREGOR, 1965). Beim Aequilibrieren frischer Knochenschnitte in Serum oder Nährmedium beobachtet man im Lösungsgleichgewicht eine ähnliche Calciumionenkonzentration wie in den Versuchen mit Knochenpulver (G. VAES, 1966, 1962; C. COOPER, 1965). Stammen die Schnitte von parathormonbehandelten Tieren sind die Calciumionenkonzentrationen um $0{,}2 \times 10^{-3}$ Mol/l höher als normal. Knochenschnitte cortisonbehandelter Tiere setzen dagegen im Lösungsgleichgewicht weniger anorganischen Phosphor in das Nährmedium frei (S. SCHARTUM, 1961).

d) Löslichkeit synthetischer Calciumphosphate

Nur das Ca $HPO_4 \times 2\,H_2O$ ist ein um pH 5,0 beständiges einheitlich definiertes Salz, dessen Löslichkeit als regelrechtes Löslichkeitsprodukt zu ermitteln ist. Bei der Ionenstärke der extracellulären Flüssigkeit von $\mu = 0{,}16$ und 38° beträgt im Sättigungszustand das $[Ca^{2+}] \times [HPO_4^{2-}]$ Ionenprodukt $3{,}2 \times 10^{-6}$ (Mol/l)^2 (L. E. HOLT, 1925a; M. A. LOGAN, 1940; M. J. SHEAR, 1928). Dieser Wert entspricht dem stöchiometrischen Löslichkeitsprodukt pLP $= 6{,}4 \times 2{,}3 \times \sqrt{\mu}$. Alle anderen Calciumphosphate sind während eines Löslichkeitsversuches nicht als stöchiometrisch konstant anzusprechen. Es treten beim Lösen Umwandlungen von Tricalciumphosphaten über Defektapatit und Octacalciumphosphat bis zum Hydroxylapatit auf. Die Löslichkeit des Calciumphosphats ist oft geprüft worden. Man glaubte mit einem reinen Tricalciumphosphat ($Ca_3(PO_4)_2$) (L. E. HOLT, 1925, 1925b; M. A. LOGAN, 1940; H. C. HODGE, 1955, 1950; J. SENDROY, 1927a; B. HASTINGS, 1927) zu arbeiten, hatte aber in Wahrheit ein Gemisch von Tricalciumphosphat, Defektapatit, Octacalciumphosphat und Hydroxylapatit eingesetzt. Deshalb sind die Angaben über definierte Löslichkeitsprodukte wiederum nicht zu verwerten. Man muß sich mit einfachen Ionenprodukten im Sättigungszustand begnügen.

Äquilibriert man einen Mischapatit (Gewicht Ca/P = 2,1) bei 38° und pH 7,7 mit Serum (L. E. HOLT, 1925a) wird im Lösungsgleichgewicht ein $Ca^{++} \times P_{ges.\,anorg.}$-Ionenprodukt von $0{,}22 \times 10^{-6}$ $(Mol/l)^2$ im Überstand gemessen. Das $Ca^{++} \times HPO_4^{2-}$-Ionenprodukt beträgt $0{,}2 \times 10^{-6}$ $(Mol/l)^2$, das $Ca^{++} \times PO_4^{3-}$-Ionenprodukt $1{,}7 \times 10^{-11}$ $(Mol/l)^2$. Äquilibriert man Mischapatit bei 38° und pH 7,3 mit einer Carbonat-angereicherten, der extracellulären Flüssigkeit ähnlichen Elektrolytlösung ($\mu = 0{,}13$) findet man ein $Ca^{++} \times P_{ges.\,anorg.}$-Ionenprodukt von $0{,}3 \times 10^{-6}$ $(Mol/l)^2$, ein $Ca^{++} \times HPO_4^{2-}$-Ionenprodukt von $0{,}25 \times 10^{-6}$ $(Mol/l)^2$ und ein $Ca^{++} \times PO_4^{3-}$-Ionenprodukt von $0{,}88 \times 10^{-11}$ $(Mol/l)^2$ (L. E. HOLT, 1925a). Gereinigter Hydroxylapatit ist anscheinend noch etwas unlöslicher (D. BOULET, 1961). Verschiedene Versuche sind auch im carbonatfreien Medium ausgeführt worden (J. SENDROY, 1927a; L. E. HOLT, 1925a). Sie lassen erkennen, daß apatitische Calciumphosphate in Wasser und carbonatfreiem Medium schlechter als in der extracellulären Flüssigkeit löslich sind. Wir errechnen aufgrund der vorstehenden Messungen, daß im Serum bei pH 7,4 ca. $0{,}6$—$0{,}7 \times 10^{-3}$ Mol $Ca^{++}/l = 2{,}4$—$2{,}8$ mg % Calcium mit apatitischem Calciumphosphat im Lösungsgleichgewicht stehen. Auch Mischungen von apatitischem Calciumphosphat und Calciumcarbonat stehen mit nur 4 mg % Calcium im Lösungsgleichgewicht (J. SENDROY, 1926a). Biologisch werden aber 5—5,5 mg % Calciumionen in der extracellulären Flüssigkeit gemessen. Es müssen also im Organismus Calciumionen über die physikalisch-chemische Löslichkeit hinaus in Lösung gebracht werden. Wir wissen, daß hier die celluläre Funktion des Parathormons ursächlich einsetzt.

e) Löslichkeit von synthetischem Calciumcarbonat

Calciumcarbonat kann bei Löslichkeitsversuchen als stöchiometrisch einheitlich definierte Substanz gelten. HASTINGS (1927) leitete für das Löslichkeitsprodukt von Calciumcarbonat die allgemeine Formel $pLP_{CaCO_3} = 8{,}58 - \frac{4{,}94\sqrt{\mu}}{1+1{,}61\sqrt{\mu}}$ ab. Sättigt man Serum bei 38° pH 7,42 und 31×10^{-3} Mol CO_2/l mit Calciumcarbonat, beträgt das $Ca^{++} \times CO_3^{2-}$-Ionenprodukt, das dem Löslichkeitsprodukt entspricht, $0{,}21 \times 10^{-6}$ $(Mol/l)^2$ (B. HASTINGS, 1927). In einer der extracellulären Flüssigkeit ähnlichen Elektrolytlösung ($\mu = 0{,}16$, pH = 7,38, $CO_2 = 25$—30×10^{-3} Mol/l) stellt sich ein $[Ca^{++}] \times [CO_3^{2-}]$-Sättigungsionenprodukt von $0{,}03$—$0{,}05 \times 10^{-6}$ $(Mol/l)^2$ ein (B. HASTINGS, 1927; J. SENDROY, 1927a). Phosphationen steigern die Löslichkeit von Calciumcarbonat (J. GREENWALD, 1945).

f) Löslichkeit eines Gemisches von synthetischem Mischapatit und Calciumcarbonat

Nach Untersuchungen von SENDROY (1927a) lösen sich Apatit-Calciumcarbonat-Gemische im Serum besser als Mischapatit allein. Man findet als Sättigungsionenprodukt für

$$[Ca^{++}] \times [HPO_4^{2-}] = 0{,}5 \times 10^{-6}\ (Mol/l)^2$$
$$[Ca^{++}] \times [PO_4^{3-}] = 2{,}37 \times 10^{-11}\ (Mol/l)^2$$
$$[Ca^{++}] \times [CO_3^{2-}] = 0{,}12 \times 10^{-6}\ (Mol/l)^2.$$

Die gelöste Calciumionenmenge beträgt 10^{-3} Mol/l = 4 mg %. In carbonathaltiger (30 mMol CO_2/l) der extracellulären Flüssigkeit ähnlicher Elektrolytlösung ($\mu = 0{,}16$) werden bei pH 7,4 nach Sättigung mit Apatit-Calciumcarbonat-Gemisch ein

$[Ca^{++}] \times [HPO_4^{2-}]$-Ionenprodukt von $0{,}08 \times 10^{-6}$ $(Mol/l)^2$,

$[Ca^{++}] \times [PO_4^{3-}]$-Ionenprodukt von $0{,}26 \times 10^{-12}$ $(Mol/l)^2$

und ein $[Ca^{++}] \times [CO_3^{2-}]$-Ionenprodukt von $0{,}03 \times 10^{-6}$ $(Mol/l)^2$

bestimmt (J. SENDROY, 1927a; B. HASTINGS, 1927) (Tabelle 63).

2. Sättigungsgrad der extracellulären Flüssigkeit

Ein Vergleich der aktuellen Ionenprodukte für $CaHPO_4$ und $CaCO_3$ in der extracellulären Flüssigkeit mit den unter diesen Bedingungen verwendbaren Löslichkeitsprodukten für $CaHPO_4$ und $CaCO_3$ zeigt, daß die extracelluläre Flüssigkeit biologisch weder an sekundärem Calciumphosphat noch an Calciumcarbonat übersättigt ist. Die Lösungsversuche mit Apatiten und Knochenpulver in Serum oder in Carbonat-angereicherter, synthetischer, extracellulärer Flüssigkeit führen nicht zu Sättigungskonzentrationen, die die Löslichkeitsprodukte des sekundären Calciumphosphats und Calciumcarbonats erreichen.

Ein Vergleich des $Ca^{++} \times PO_4^{3-}$-Ionenproduktes in der extracellulären Flüssigkeit in vivo mit in vitro erhaltenen entsprechenden Sättigungsionenprodukten beweist, daß die extracelluläre Flüssigkeit für Knochenmineral und Mischapatit übersättigt ist. Die Sättigungsgrenzen werden in der extracellulären Flüssigkeit gegenüber den in vitro-Versuchen um ca. das Doppelte überschritten. Ein weiterer Beweis für die physiologische Übersättigung der extracellulären Flüssigkeit an Knochenmineral ist die Abnahme des $Ca^{++} \times P_{ges.\,anorg.}$-Ionenproduktes von 15—18 (mg %)^2 auf ca. 10(mg %)^2 im Plasmaultrafiltrat nach Aequilibrieren mit Knochenpulver (H. Fleisch, 1961). Ähnliche Ergebnisse wurden beim Aequilibrieren von Serum und synthetischer, extracellulärer Flüssigkeit mit Knochenpulver erhalten (D. M. Greenberg, 1932). Die Löslichkeit eines Gemisches von Mischapatit und Calciumcarbonat ist der Löslichkeit von Knochenpulver außerordentlich ähnlich. Derartige Gemische können also zu Vergleichen mit Knochenmineral bei Löslichkeitsbetrachtungen herangezogen werden. Der CO_2-Anteil der extracellulären Flüssigkeit trägt wesentlich zur Löslichkeit des Knochenminerals bei.

Im plasmatischen Raum wird die Übersättigung sicherlich durch die Serumproteine als Kristallisationshemmstoffe stabilisiert. Im interstitiellen Raum könnten kondensierte Phosphate, Magnesiumionen oder niedermolekulare Peptide die Kristallisation und Keimbildung hemmen. In der unmittelbaren Umgebung des Knochens vermutet Macgregor (1960) zusätzlich einen schwachen Säuremantel, der lokal die Übersättigung zur Sättigung herabsetzt und den Lösungsvorgang physiologisch reguliert. Es ist aber auch bekannt, daß Calciumphosphate leicht bei pH 7,4 in vitro stabile, übersättigte Lösungen bilden, die erst bei $Ca^{2+} \times P_{ges.\,anorg.}$-Ionenprodukten von $2{,}4$—$4{,}0 \times 10^{-6}$ (Mol/l)^2, einer stärkeren Übersättigung als im Serum beobachtet wird, Keime bilden und auskristallisieren (H. Fleisch, 1964; A. E. Sobel, 1934, 1955). Wahrscheinlich ist die Kristallisation eines apatitischen Calciumphosphates eine Reaktion zu hoher Ordnung, als daß sie spontan hinreichend schnell verläuft (I. Greenwald, 1942).

Mineralisations- und Verknöcherungsvorgang

Am Lösungsgleichgewicht zwischen extracellulärer Flüssigkeit und Knochen sind physiko-chemische Austauschvorgänge — wie beschrieben — ohne Veränderung der Knochenmasse und zellabhängige Aufbau- und Abbauvorgänge mit Veränderung der Knochenmasse beteiligt. Nur in seltenen Fällen führen Calcium-, Phosphor- und Basenverluste über Darm und Niere physiko-chemisch zu zellunabhängigen Verlusten der Knochenmasse. Solange Nebenschilddrüsen vorhanden sind, kann der Organismus das Lösungsgleichgewicht zellabhängig unter Massenveränderungen des Knochens regulieren. Man spricht von den Phasen der Verknöcherung und Knochenauflösung.

I. Voraussetzungen der Mineralisation und Verknöcherung

Die Übersättigung der extracellulären Flüssigkeit an apatitischen Calciumphosphaten ist eine in vivo regelmäßig erfüllte Voraussetzung der Verknöcherung. Der Verknöcherung und biologischen Mineralisation liegen aber eigentlich zellabhängige Mechanismen im präossealen und knöchernen Gewebe zugrunde, die Keimzentren schaffen, Kristallisationshindernisse beseitigen, die Metastabilität der extracellulären Flüssigkeit herabsetzen und ihre Übersättigung verstärken. Wir gliedern diese Faktoren unter drei funktionellen Gesichtspunkten.

1. Induktion von Kristallkeimen durch
   a) Proteinstrukturen
   b) Abbau von Kristallisationshemmstoffen
      α) Mucopolysacchariden
      β) Pyrophosphat, kondensierte anorganische und organische Phosphate
   c) Metalle und seltene Erden
2. Steigerung der Übersättigung der extracellulären Flüssigkeit durch
   a) Calciumanreicherung
   b) PO_4^{3-}-Anreicherung
3. Herabsetzen der Metastabilität der extracellulären Flüssigkeit durch Carbonatanreicherung.

Diesen Faktoren den ihnen biologisch zukommenden Wert beizumessen, war die Aufgabe experimenteller Verknöcherungs- und Mineralisationsstudien.

II. Experimentelle Studien zur Verknöcherung und Mineralisation

1. Kristallkeimbildung

a) Proteinstrukturen

Bereits BUCHER (1961) beobachtete, daß in übersättigten Calciumchlorid- und Phosphatpufferlösungen Kollagenstrukturen die Kristallisation induzieren. In den letzten Jahren haben mehrere Arbeitsgruppen (B. STRATES, 1958; D. TAVES, 1964; A. E. SOBEL, 1965; H. FLEISCH, 1964b, 1961a, 1966, 1961, 1961b; B. N. BACHRA, 1965, 1966) aus mineralisiertem und nichtmineralisiertem Bindegewebe Kollagenfibrillen hergestellt, die unmittelbar oder nach einer Vorbehandlung bei pH 7,3—8,0, 37° und $\mu = 0{,}16$ als Keimbildner in Mineralisationslösungen wirkten. Entkalkte Dentinmatrix senkte das $Ca^{2+} \times P_{ges.\,anorg.}$-Bildungsprodukt für Knochenmineral in Mineralisationslösungen von 2,3 auf $1{,}7 \times 10^{-6}\,(\mathrm{Mol/l})^2$ (C. C. SOLOMONS, 1960), Sehnenkollagen von 50 auf 16 $(\mathrm{mg}\,\%)^2$ (H. FLEISCH, 1961a, 1964b, 1961b), andere Kollagenpräparationen auf 20—40 $(\mathrm{mg}\,\%)^2$ (A. E. SOBEL, 1965; B. N. BACHRA, 1959). Knochenkollagene induzieren die Mineralisation am regelmäßigsten (B. STRATES, 1958). Unlösliches Kollagen hat sich in vitro als der schlechteste Induktor erwiesen (A. E. SOBEL, 1965), Gelatine induziert überhaupt nicht (R. MARSHALL, 1966). Rekonstituiertes, gereinigtes Kollagen mineralisiert in vivo in der Peritonealhöhle (ST. E. MERGENHAGEN, 1960). Die Fähigkeit zur Kristallkeimbildung und Induktion der Kristallisation hängt anscheinend von der Art der Präparation und der Herkunft des Materials ab. Um korrekte Aussagen zuzulassen, müssen die Kollagenfibrillen frei von jedem anorganischen Kristallkeim gewonnen werden (B. N. BACHRA, 1966).

Kollagenfibrillen präcipitieren an ihrer Oberfläche verschiedene apatitische Calciumphosphate und zwingen den Kristallen die Größe und die Orientierung mit der c-Achse parallel zur Faserachse auf (B. N. BACHRA, 1966). Wahrscheinlich erfolgt die Orientierung der Apatitkristalle mechanisch durch die 640 Å-Periode der Fibrillen (O. R. TRAUTZ, 1963; R. MARSHALL, 1966; A. HALLSWORTH, 1964; A. E. SOBEL, 1960a) und die Größenbegrenzung der Kristalle durch die intermolekularen Bindungen der Tropokollagenmolekeln (H.-J. HÖHLING, 1966). Die Apatitkristallisation findet nach diesen Beobachtungen an isomorphen Proteinstrukturen statt.

Die Keimbildung durch Kollagen ist letztlich ein chemischer Vorgang, bei dem die Überstruktur des Proteins eine Rolle spielt. Nur Fibrillen mit der 640 Å-Periodik und mit freien NH_2-Seitenketten bilden in übersättigten Apatitlösungen Kristallkeime (B. N. BACHRA, 1965, 1966). ε-NH_2-Gruppen, die im Kollagen zu 50% frei vorkommen (R. WUTHIER, 1964; A. HALLSWORTH, 1964), sind an der Tertiärstruktur des Kollagens beteiligt (C. C. SOLOMONS, 1960; H. FLEISCH, 1964; B. N. BACHRA, 1965). Blockieren dieser Gruppen

(M. R. URIST, 1966; R. MARSHALL, 1966), Hitzedenaturierung und Dehydratation heben die Fähigkeit des Kollagens zur Apatitkeimbildung auf. Kupferionen, die Carboxyl-Gruppen blockieren, hemmen die Keimbildung aber nicht das Weiterwachsen von Apatitkristallen auf Keimen (M. R. URIST, 1966; A. E. SOBEL, 1965, 1949). Als weitere Hemmstoffe der Keimbildung sind bekannt Protaminsulfat (M. R. URIST, 1966), Strontiumionen, Alizarin (M. R. URIST, 1966; W. H. HARRIS, 1965), Oxytetracyclin, Jodacetamid, Pyrophosphat (H. FLEISCH, 1961, 1962, 1962a, 1962b, 1966b) und wahrscheinlich auch saure Mucopolysaccharide.

URIST (1966) und BACHRA (1966) vertreten die Meinung, daß die Kollagenmolekel durch günstige räumliche Anordnung polarer Gruppen fähig ist, das Ionenpaar Ca^{2+} und PO_4^{3-} so einzufangen, daß es als Keimzentrum einer Einheitszelle dienen kann. Wahrscheinlich geht das PO_4^{3-} eine festere Bindung mit dem Kollagen ein. Analytische Untersuchungen verknöchernden Knorpels in frühen Verknöcherungsstadien hatten bereits ergeben, daß die Mineralisation mit einer Phosphatanreicherung ohne Calciumanreicherung im Gewebe beginnt (H.-J. DULCE, 1960, 1960b). In Gegenwart von Phosphationen rekonstituiertes Kollagen mineralisiert in vitro besser als in Kochsalzlösung rekonstituiertes Kollagen (ST. E. MERGENHAGEN, 1960). Erst KRANE und GLIMCHER (1964, 1966) wiesen nach, daß Phosphat primär an Kollagen gebunden ist oder sekundär gebunden werden kann. Kristallisierte Kollagenfibrillen nehmen pro Mol 150 Mol anorganisches Phosphat meist in organischer Bindung auf (M. GLIMCHER, 1964). Der größte Teil des organischen Phosphats im Kollagen ist Esterphosphat, als Kohlenhydratphosphat und Serinphosphat (M. GLIMCHER, 1964; KRANE, 1966), der kleinere Teil Aminosäurephosphat in einer N-P-Bindung. Im Dentinkollagen ist Orthophosphoserin nachgewiesen worden (M. J. GLIMCHER, 1964a). An der N-P-Bindung sind 50% der ε-Aminogruppen des Lysins und Hydroxylysins beteiligt (R. WUTHIER, 1964; H. RASMUSSEN, 1962). Es wird vermutet, daß phosphoryliertes Kollagen von den Osteoblasten synthetisiert wird (B. N. BACHRA, 1966; P. CARTIER, 1950; A. POLONOWSKI, 1951). Eine Proteinphosphokinase ist im Knochen nachgewiesen (S. M. KRANE, 1966). Ob alkalische Phosphatase bei dieser Synthese mitwirken kann, ist offen. Wir dürfen heute der Arbeitshypothese folgen, daß Kollagen des künftigen Knochens durch eine günstige Überstruktur und eine Phosphorylierung zur Apatitkeimbildung befähigt ist.

b) Abbau von Kristallisationshemmstoffen

Im verknöcherungsfähigen Knorpel tritt die Mineralisation erst ein, wenn die sauren Mucopolysaccharide, die die Kristallisation von Calciumsalzen hemmen (H.-J. DULCE, 1960, 1960b; N. F. MACLAGAN, 1958), abgebaut werden (Tabelle 64).

Tabelle 64. *Mucopolysaccharid- und Mineralgehalt in Knorpel und Knochen von 3 Monate alten Rinderfeten* (H.-J. DULCE, 1960b)

	Gehalt an sauren Mucopolysacchariden in % organischer Matrix	Calciumgehalt % FTS	$P_{anorg.}$-Gehalt % FTS
Septumknorpel	22,8	1,6	0,1
Verknöchernder Epiphysenknorpel	17,1	1,8	0,41
Diaphysenknochen	3,0	22,9	10,75

Hexosamin, Sulfat, Uronsäuregehalt. FTS = fettfreie Trockensubstanz.

Die Calciumfängereigenschaft von sauren Mucopolysacchariden kann nicht als Ursache, sondern eher als Hindernis der Mineralisation angesehen werden.

Die im knöchernen Gewebe von Osteoblasten gebildeten Phosphatasen betrachtet man als einen der lokalen Faktoren der Mineralisation, weil sie organische Phosphate und anorganische kondensierte Phosphate, die Hemmstoffe der Keimbildung und Calciumchelatbildner sind, abbauen. Plasmaultrafiltrat, das Pyrophosphat enthält, und reines anorganisches Pyrophosphat setzen das $Ca^{2+} \times P_{ges.\,anorg.}$-Bildungsprodukt im Medium bei der Kristallisation von Apatit an Kollagenfibrillen auf ca. $2{,}8 \times 10^{-3}$ (Mol/l)^2 herauf. Erst Pyrophosphatasezugabe senkt das Produkt wieder auf ca. $1{,}8 \times 10^{-3}$ (Mol/l)^2 (H. FLEISCH, 1964b, 1961), wodurch bewiesen ist, daß nach Beseitigen der Hemmstoffe die Kristallisation bei kleinerer Ca^{2+} und P-Konzentration beginnt. Es ist bestätigt, daß verknöchernde Gewebe gegenüber hyalinem Knorpel einen hohen Gehalt an alkalischer Phosphatase und anorganischer Pyrophosphatase aufweisen (H.-J. DULCE, 1960a, 1960b; CERLETTI, 1958).

c) Anreicherung von Metallen und seltenen Erden

Experimentelle in vivo- und in vitro-Untersuchungen von G. GABBIANI (1965, 1965a, 1966), FLEISCH (1965a) und E. SCHIFFMANN (1966) sprechen dafür, daß Blei, Eisen und seltene Erden auf Kollagenmatrix Kristallkeime bilden, an denen sich das Wachstum apatitischer Calciumphosphate in übersättigten Lösungen orientiert. Es ist vorstellbar, daß diese Metalle selbst primär unlösliche Phosphate bilden.

2. Steigerung der Übersättigung

In Mineralisationslösungen treten Calciumphosphatkristallisationen spontan auf, wenn das $Ca^{++} \times P_{ges.\,anorg.}$-Ionenprodukt 35—60 (mg %)^2 erreicht. Es sind deshalb bei der biologischen Mineralisation celluläre Vorgänge zu erwägen, die lokal das $Ca^{++} \times P_{ges.\,anorg.}$-Ionenprodukt über 16—20 (mg %)^2 steigern.

a) Calciumanreicherung

Die von Chondroblasten und Osteoblasten gebildete Chondroitin-Schwefelsäure verknöchernder Gewebe wurde vielfach als Calciumfänger betrachtet, die in der Zone der Verknöcherung die Calciumionenkonzentration so stark erhöht, daß Knochenmineral kristallisiert. Diese Vorstellung wird mit in vitro Versuchen an Knorpelschnitten rachitischer Ratten begründet, bei denen die Mineralisation davon abhängt, ob calciumbindende Chondroitinschwefelsäure vorhanden ist (A. E. SOBEL, 1952, 1955, 1954; P. G. SHIPLEY, 1926; P. G. SHELLING, 1928; C. P. LEBLOND, 1955, 1950; M. LAMM, 1958; P. S. RUBIN, 1949).

Der Theorie steht aber entgegen, daß gerade das chondroitinsulfatreichste Gewebe, der hyaline Knorpel in vivo nicht verkalkt und Chondroitinschwefelsäure als Calciumchelatbildner Kristallisationen hemmt. Permanenter Knorpel und verknöchernder Knorpel hat Calcium gegenüber der extracellulären Flüssigkeit ca. 35fach angereichert, ohne zu mineralisieren (H.-J. DULCE, 1960, 1960b). Diese Calciumanreicherung geschieht ohne äquivalente Phosphoranreicherung (C. P. LEBLOND, 1955; W. EGER, 1964). Es ist zu erwarten, daß Knorpel in vitro erst dann mineralisiert, wenn Chondroitinschwefelsäure mit Calcium abgesättigt ist, wie es FREUDENBERG und SZENT GYÖRGY (1920, 1921, 1921a) nachwiesen. Auch ohne frei verfügbare Chondroitinschwefelsäure ist eine Mineralisation in vitro möglich, wenn statt des anorganischen Phosphates organisches Phosphat in Mineralisationslösungen angeboten wird (Z. B. MILLER, 1952). Aufgrund eigener Untersuchungen (H.-J. DULCE, 1960) und derjenigen von DZIEWIATKOWSKI (1951a, 1952), M. A. LOGAN (1935), EGER (1964), muß man heute annehmen, daß erst mit dem Abbau der Chondroitinschwefelsäure die Mineralisation des Knorpels oder Bindegewebes ermöglicht wird, und nicht die Calciumfängereigenschaft der sauren Mucopolysaccharide unmittelbare Ursache der Mineralisation ist. Bei diesem Abbau könnten gespeicherte Calciumionen frei werden, die die Übersättigung der extracellulären Flüssigkeit lokal steigern. Die in vivo-Mineralisation ist erst dort histochemisch nachweisbar, wo die sauren Mucopolysaccharide fehlen (W. EGER, 1964).

b) Phosphatanreicherung

Bereits in den ersten Stadien der Verknöcherung ist eine Phosphatanreicherung ohne Calciumanreicherung im Vergleich zum permanenten Knorpel nachweisbar (H.-J. DULCE, 1960, 1960b; M. J. DALLEMAGNE, 1948; LEBLOND, 1955; W. EGER, 1964). Das Phosphat reichert sich an Orten neutraler Mucopolysaccharide an (W. EGER, 1964). Man spricht von der Phosphatfängereigenschaft der Knochenmatrix. Vitamin D steigert diese Phosphatanreicherung (J.-G. JOSHI, 1956). Zum großen Teil ist das Phosphat organisch gebunden als Phospholipid (WHITEHEAD, 1959), als Proteinphosphat (KRANE, 1966; A. POLONOWSKI, 1951; M. GLIMCHER, 1964) oder als ester- und energiereiches Anhydridphosphat (H. G. ALBAUM, 1952; P. CARTIER, 1955, 1955a; J. PICARD, 1960). Es entsteht in der Steigerung des Zellstoffwechsels im Knochen unter Glykogenabbau (H. G. ALBAUM, 1952; P. A. MARKS, 1950, 1953, 1950a; A. B. GUTMAN, 1950). In vitro verbessern diese organischen Phosphate die Mineralisation des verknöcherungsfähigen Knorpels (J. S. NIVEN, 1934; R. ROBISON, 1930, 1934; A. LANZETTA, 1963; P. CARTIER, 1955, 1950, 1955a; J. PICARD, 1960). Man sieht ihre Funktion in vivo bei der Matrixsynthese. Die Kristallisation durch Übersättigung begünstigen könnten sie nur, wenn aus ihnen lokal PO_4^{3-} entstünde. Derartige organische Phosphate spaltende Phosphatasen zeichnen zwar knöchernes Gewebe aus, sie treten aber früher als die Mineralisation auf (H. B. TELL, 1934), so daß aus kinetischen Gründen das Entstehen größerer Mengen von Ester- und Pyrophosphaten unwahrscheinlich ist. NEUMAN (1951) glaubt, daß die extracelluläre Phosphatase des Knochens, ohne die in vivo keine Verknöcherung beobachtet wird, adsorbierte organische Phosphate und Pyrophosphate, die Hemmstoffe der Kristallkeimbildung sind, spaltet. Da Inhibitoren der alkalischen Phosphatase, 10^{-2} molar CN^{1-} (H. GOLDENBERG, 1954; R. ROBISON, 1934), 10^{-2} molar Histidin (H. H. HIATT, 1953), 10^{-3} molar Ag^{1+} (J. WALDMANN, 1950, 1948) die in vitro-Mineralisation in anorganischen Mineralisationslösungen nicht hemmen, kann die Phosphatase nicht unmittelbar im Mineralisationsvorgang am Entstehen einer Phosphatübersättigung beteiligt sein. Abgesehen davon, liegt ihr pH-Optimum mit pH 9,8—10,5 weit außerhalb bekannter biologischer Bereiche.

Eine PO_4^{3-}-Anreicherung tritt andererseits am leichtesten auf, wenn der pH-Wert im verknöchernden Gewebe ansteigt. Beim Verschieben des pH-Wertes von 7 auf 8 in der Nähe der Osteoblasten würde sich ohne Verändern des gesamten anorganischen Phosphats die PO_4^{3-}-Konzentration um das 10—15fache erhöhen und eine Kristallisation wäre möglich. In vitro fördern OH-Ionen tatsächlich ein Weiterwachsen des Apatitgitters (D. TAVES, 1963). Diese Arbeitshypothese sollte an Aufmerksamkeit gewinnen, da nachgewiesen werden konnte, daß embryonale Knochen in der Gewebekultur bei pH 8 schneller als bei pH 7 wachsen (H. SCHRYVER, 1964).

3. Herabsetzung der Metastabilität der extracellulären Flüssigkeit

Im sog. Line-Test beschleunigt eine carbonathaltige Mineralisationslösung die Verkalkung von Knorpelschnitten rachitischer Ratten (R. ROBISON, 1930a). Die Metastabilität calcium- und phosphathaltiger Mineralisationslösungen nimmt bereits unabhängig von diesem Versuch mit steigendem Carbonatgehalt ab (B. N. BACHRA, 1965). Lokale CO_2-Produktion der Knochenzellen könnte deshalb die Mineralisation fördern.

III. Biologische Induktoren der Verknöcherung

Man hat im lebenden Organismus mehrfach nach Stoffen gesucht, die den chemischen Reiz für die Entwicklung knöchernen Gewebes darstellen können. Blasenzellaufschwemmungen von Milliporfiltern umhüllt und Tieren implantiert erzeugen in ihrer Umgebung Knochen (A. J. FRIEDENSTEIN, 1962). Zellfreie Extrakte besitzen diese Eigenschaften nicht, wohl aber osteogenetisches Gewebe (P. GOLDHABER, 1961) und Rückenmark (J. LASH, 1957). LEVANDER (1938, 1941, 1946, 1945) stellte aus Periost, Knochenmark und Knochen alkoholische Extrakte her, die bei Kaninchen subcutan oder intramusculär injiziert in einigen Fällen zur Knorpel- und Knochenbildung führten. Wäßrige Extrakte wirkten nicht. ROTH (1950) bestätigte diese Versuche später mit alkoholischen Extrakten aus Knochenpulver. Man nimmt an, daß der osteogenetische Faktor Lipoidcharakter hat, klärt aber nicht, inwieweit bei den Versuchen dystrophische Verkalkungen auszuschließen sind.

Physiko-chemischer Induktor der Kristallorientierung bei der Mineralisation kann der bei jeder Druckbelastung des jungen Knochens auftretende piezoelektrische Effekt sein (M. H. SHAMOS, 1963; I. YASUDA, 1955). Ebenso ist der elektrochemische Potentialgradient in einem fehlgeordneten, stöchiometrisch uneinheitlichen Kristallgitter als die treibende Kraft der Idealisierung und Stabilisierung des Kristallgitters zu betrachten (H. SCHMALZRIED, 1963).

IV. Theorie des Verknöcherungsvorganges

Die derzeitigen Kentnisse über Aufbau und Stoffwechsel des verknöchernden Gewebes und die Beobachtungen an Mineralisationsmodellen lassen folgende Vorstellungen über den Ablauf der Verknöcherung zu.

Morphologische Leistung des Gewebes:

1. Bildung osteogenetischer Zellen → Osteoblasten,
2. Steigerung der Durchblutung.

Chemische Leistung der osteogenetischen Zellen:

1. Bildung einer an sauren Mucopolysacchariden armen phosphorylierten Kollagenmatrix mit Keimzentren.
2. Abbau kristallisationshemmender Phosphate und saurer Mucopolysaccharide (Phosphatasen).
3. Abbau von Glykogen — Auftreten von Atmung und ATP-Bildung.
4. Anreicherung von PO_4^{3-} durch lokale Alkalisierung (Hypothese).

Physikalische Einflüsse bei der Mineralisation:

1. Wachstumsorientierung der Osteone und Trabekel durch piezoelektrische Kräfte.
2. Stabilisierung des Kristallgitters durch elektrochemische Potentiale (Umkristallisation und Reifung).

Die Knorpel- und Bindegewebsbildung, wobei neben Kollagen viel Glykogen und saure Mucopolysaccharide entstehen, sind vorbereitende Leistungen des Organismus für die Verknöcherung.

Der Vorgang der Knochenauflösung

Das Knochengewebe befindet sich physiologisch, ohne daß Massenverluste auftreten, in einem ständigen Umbau. Am Umbau beteiligt ist die physiko-chemische Re- oder Umkristallisation (F. NEUMAN, 1950a) und das Wechselspiel zwischen zellabhängiger Bildung und Auflösung. Die Auflösung ist von den Osteoclasten und Osteocyten sowie vom Parathormon abhängig und umfaßt Knochenmineral und Knochenmatrix. Die um Osteoclasten im Bereich der Trabekel auftretende Auflösung wird als Osteoclasie (G. VAES, 1966), die um Osteocyten an der Peripherie der Osteone auftretende Auflösung als Osteolyse bezeichnet (L. F. BÉLANGER, 1966; P. H. VITTALI, 1966). Auflösung ohne Neubildung, wie auch umgekehrt, führt zu Knochenerkrankungen. Demineralisationen ohne Matrixauflösung können in seltenen Fällen knochenzellunabhängig bei dekompensierten Acidosen vorkommen (C. YATES, 1964; T. H. INGALLS, 1943).

I. Voraussetzung der Knochenauflösung und Demineralisation

Knochenmineral kann im Organismus nur aufgelöst werden, wenn sich seine Löslichkeitsbedingungen verbessern und die Mineralbaustoffe über die extracelluläre Flüssigkeit abfließen. Bessere Löslichkeitsbedingungen entstehen durch Herabsetzen der Ca^{2+} und PO_4^{3-}-Ionenkonzentrationen in der interstitiellen Flüssigkeit oder durch Ansäuern. Ansäuern verändert verschiedene Ionen

$$H^+ + OH^- = H_2O$$
$$H^+ + CO_3^{2-} = HCO_3^{1-} = CO_2 + OH^-$$
$$H^+ + PO_4^{3-} = HPO_4^{2-}$$

und führt beim Carbonatapatit zum Gitterzerfall mit Whitlockitbildung (Karieskristalle), während Hydroxylapatit zunächst in Defektapatit übergeht. Hat die Ca^{2+} und PO_4^{3-}-Ionenkonzentration in der extracellulären Flüssigkeit nur um $^1/_3$ abgenommen, kann sich Knochenmineral bereits auflösen. Die Knochenmatrix kann nur durch proteolytischen Abbau aufgelöst werden. An Zellen gebundene, knochenauflösende Mechanismen müssen deshalb in derartigen chemischen Reaktionsabläufen gesucht werden. Die meisten Studien dieser Art werden unter intensivem Parathormoneinfluß durchgeführt, weil Parathormon die Proteolyse des Bindegewebes und die Stoffwechselacidose fördert und Knochenmineral mobilisiert.

II. Auflösung des Knochenminerals durch Stoffwechselsäuren oder H^+-Ionensekretion

Histochemisch hat man um Osteoclasten eine Säuerung beobachten können. In der Gewebekultur bilden Knochenschnitte unter Parathormoneinfluß mehr Säure als unbehandelte Kontrollen (G. Vaes, 1966). In 2—3 Tagen betragen die Differenzen 0,2—0,5 pH-Einheiten. Diese pH-Differenzen, die einem Verdoppeln bis Vervierfachen der H-Ionenkonzentration entsprechen, müssen zum Absinken der örtlichen PO_4^{3-}-Konzentration auf $^1/_3$—$^1/_5$ und damit zur Knochenmineralauflösung führen. Es können anscheinend bis zu 3 μ Mol Ca/mg Zell-N/Stunde aus Knochen mobilisiert werden (F. Körber, 1964). Quantitative Messungen der auf Zell-N bezogenen H-Ionensekretion im Knochen liegen bisher noch nicht vor. Wir kennen aber quantitativ die Mengen einiger von Metaphysenschnitten gebildeten Säureanionen, die einen gewissen Rückschluß auf die sezernierten H-Ionenaequivalente gestatten (Tabelle 65).

Tabelle 65. *Säureanionenbildung durch Metaphysenschnitte von Nagern in Glucose- und sauerstoffhaltigem Nährmedium*

Lactat: ca. 2,0—2,6 μ Mol/mg Zell-N/Stunde (A. B. Borle, 1960a; G. Vaes, 1961)
Citrat: ca. 0,023—0,035 μ Mol/mg Zell-N/Stunde (A. B. Borle, 1960a; G. Vaes, 1961)
Carbonat: ca. 0,06 μ Mol/mg Zell-N/Stunde

1. Milchsäure

Die aerob gebildete Milchsäure ist etwa der bisher bekannten lösbaren Calciummenge aequivalent. Ihre Produktion ist in der Metaphyse größer als in der Diaphyse (G. Vaes, 1966) und wird durch Parathormon aerob um ca. 30% gesteigert (G. Vaes, 1962; A. B. Borle, 1960a). Parallel zur Milchsäurebildung steigt in Calvariakulturen (pH 7,4) und Metaphysenschnitten das Ca × P-Produkt im Medium an (G. Vaes, 1962; S. Schartum, 1962; C. W. Cooper, 1965; C. Yates, 1965). G. Vaes (1966) errechnete, daß die unter Parathormon vermehrt gebildete Milchsäure (4,4 μ Mol/g Knochen/Stunde) ca. 0,55 mg Knochenmineral mobilisieren könnte. Eine ganze Reihe von Befunden sprechen aber dagegen, daß Milchsäure die unmittelbare knochenmineralauflösende Substanz ist. Das Parathormon erhöht den Plasmacalciumspiegel bedeutend schneller als die aerobe Glykolyse im Knochen (A. D. Kenny, 1962a). Es gibt bei Ratten genetische Knochenresorptionsstörungen mit normaler Lactatbildung im Knochen (G. M. Vaes, 1963). Adrenalin kann die Lactatbildung im Knochen ohne Calciummobilisation steigern (A. D. Kenny, 1962a). Die Calciummobilisation in Calvariakulturen tritt trotz Milchsäureproduktion nicht auf, wenn mit Luft an Stelle von 95% O_2 begast wird (A. D. Kenny, 1959). Wir müssen deshalb weitere Untersuchungen über die Milchsäure als H-Ionendonator bei der Demineralisation abwarten.

2. Citronensäure

Die Theorie, Citronensäure sei Ursache der Resorption des Knochenminerals, ist abzulehnen, weil die im Knochen unter Parathormoneinfluß bildungsfähigen Citratmengen 80—100fach geringer sind (G. Vaes, 1966; A. B. Borle, 1960), als die mobilisierbaren Calciummengen. Knochenmineralauflösende Säuren müssen mindestens im aequivalenten Verhältnis zu den in Lösung gehenden Calciumionen gebildet werden. Die Atmung der Knochenzellen mit 0,5 μ Mol O_2/mg Zell-N/Stunde gestattet nicht die Bildung von 2—3 μ Mol Citrat/mg Zell-N/Stunde (D. M. LASKIN, 1960; G. M. VAES, 1963). Parathormon steigert die Citratbildung im Knochen nur um das 2—3fache (D. M. LASKIN, 1960; A. B. BORLE, 1960). Oestradiol erhöht in vitro die Citratproduktion ohne begleitenden Anstieg des Ca × P-Produktes im Medium (G. M. VAES, 1961). Schon die Korrelation zwischen Citratanstieg im Knochen und Calciummobilisation ist bisher nicht exakt nachgewiesen (A. D. KENNY, 1959). Die Theorie der Knochenauflösung durch Citronensäure kann damit als überholt gelten.

3. Kohlensäure

Die im Knochenstoffwechsel über den Citratcyclus (G. AURBACH, 1964), den Pentosephosphatweg und die Aminosäuredecarboxylierung, auch unter Parathormoneinfluß (D. V. COHN, 1962) gebildete Kohlensäure reicht quantitativ ebenfalls nicht aus, um die Demineralisation zu erklären. Die Säureauflösung des Knochenminerals unter Mitwirken der Kohlensäure muß aber heute deshalb diskutiert werden, weil den Osteoclasten und Osteocyten von der extracellulären Flüssigkeit her genügend CO_2 angeboten werden kann, und man im Knochen hohe Aktivitäten der Kohlensäureanhydratase gefunden hat (H.-J. DULCE, 1960d), die biologisch CO_2 zu H_2CO_3 hydratisiert, aus der wieder H-Ionen dissoziieren

$$CO_2 + H_2O \xrightleftharpoons{CAH} H_2CO_3 \rightleftharpoons H^+ + HCO_3^-.$$

Hauptsächlich H-Ionen produzierende Zellen wie Nieren und Magenschleimhautzellen besitzen dieses Enzym. Hyaliner Knorpel, der nicht verknöchert, besitzt es nicht (H.-J. DULCE, 1960d). Unterstützt wird diese Hypothese durch Befunde bei Hühnern und Hähnchen, die zeigen, daß ein physiologisch oder durch Oestrongaben erhöhter Plasmacalciumspiegel durch den Carboanhydratasehemmstoff Diamox zu senken ist (P. SIEGMUND, 1960; H.-J. DULCE, 1960c; W. BAUDITZ, 1960). Auch in dem Aethylendiamintetraessigsäuretoleranzversuch hemmen Diamox und Thiocyanat die Regeneration des Plasmacalciumspiegels (P. SIEGMUND, 1961).

4. Aktive Wasserstoff-Ionensekretion

Eine aktive H-Ionensekretion finden wir in Tubuluszellen der Niere und Belegzellen der Magenschleimhaut. Bei Lebermitochondrien aktiviert Parathormon in Gegenwart von Magnesiumionen die Calcium- und H-Ionensekretion, die Atmung und die PO_4^{3-}-Aufnahme (H. RASMUSSEN, 1964). Der H^+/PO_4^{3-}-Ionenaustausch der Mitochondrien erfolgt im Verhältnis 1 : 1. Ein derartiger Sekretionsmechanismus wäre auch für die Osteocyten und Osteoclasten anzunehmen. Thiocyanat ist der typische Hemmstoff der aktiven H-Ionensekretion (H. W. DAVENPORT, 1940; W. S. REHM, 1945) und hemmt die calciummobilisierende Wirkung des Parathormons (W. BAUDITZ, 1960), die von der Atmung abhängig ist (A. D. KENNY, 1959). Da auch Carboanhydratase-Hemmstoffe die Calciummobilisation (P. SIEGMUND, 1961) und Säuresekretion (H. D. JANOWITZ, 1952; R. W. BERLINER, 1951) hemmen, muß man bei Knochenzellen eine Verknüpfung der aktiven H-Ionensekretion (H-Flux) mit dem Carboanhydrasegleichgewicht und einem H-Ionendonator diskutieren (Abb. 13).

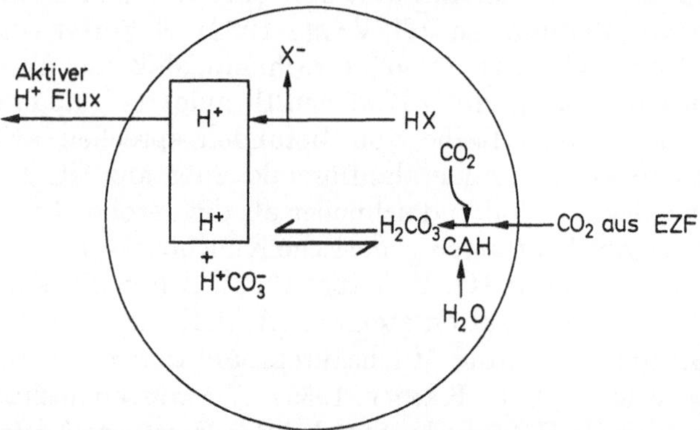

Abb. 13. Schema der H-Ionen-Sekretion der Osteoclasten. CAH = Carboanhydratase, X = organisches Anion

Als Arbeitshypothese nehmen wir an, daß eine hohe Carboanhydratase-Aktivität in Osteoclasten die Pufferwirkung der Kohlensäure schwächt, so daß H-Ionen der stärkeren Stoffwechselsäuren aktiv nach außen abgegeben werden. Ist die Carboanhydratase gehemmt, könnte die Pufferwirkung der Kohlensäure voll wirksam werden und zur Abnahme der H-Ionensekretion führen, so daß weniger Knochenmineral aufgelöst wird. Als H-Ionendonator (HX) wäre Milchsäure vorstellbar. Parathormon greift möglicherweise in den aktiven H-Ionen-Flux an der Zellmembran ein.

III. Auflösung des Knochenminerals durch Calciumchelatbildner

Die Hypothese von der Auflösung des Knochenminerals durch von Knochenzellen gebildete Calciumchelatbildner hat sich bisher nicht als richtig erwiesen. Bei einem O_2-Verbrauch von 0,5µ Mol/mg Zell-N/Stunde können Knochenzellen nicht in der Lage sein, die für die Calciummobilisation von ca. 2µ Mol/mg Zell-N/Stunde nötigen Mengen an Chelatbildnern zu synthetisieren. Citronensäure bindet weniger als $^1/_5$ ihres Molekulargewichts an Calcium (K. Klinke, 1951; W. Henning, 1951a; E. Heinz, 1951). Die Stabilitätskonstante für Calciumcitrat beträgt 10^3. Knochenzellen bilden maximal 0,04µMol Citrat/mg Zell-N/Stunde. Wie aus Studien an der Zahnhartsubstanz hervorgeht, scheiden auch Aminosäuren (Stabilitätskonstanten der Calciumchelate $10^{1,5-2,0}$) als Calciumchelatbildner für die Mineralauflösung aus (Hardel, 1967). Die Vorstellungen von Schatz (1960) sind physiko-chemisch und experimentell unbegründet.

IV. Auflösung der Knochenmatrix

Die Matrixauflösung erfolgt durch die Parathormon-abhängige Kollagenase und lysosomale Protease (G. Vaes, 1966), wobei Kollagen und Mucoproteid gemeinsam parallel zur Demineralisation abgebaut werden. Wir müssen deshalb in der Regel vom Knochenabbau oder Knochenschwund sprechen. Die reine Demineralisation ohne Matrixschwund ist vom biochemischen Standpunkt aus seltener zu erwarten.

V. Theorie der Knochenauflösung

Wir dürfen heute folgende Vorstellungen vom Ablauf der Knochenauflösung haben.

Morphologische Leistung des Gewebes:
1. Bildung der Osteoclasten.
2. Aktivieren des Osteocytenstoffwechsels.

Chemische Leistung knochenauflösender Zellen:
1. Aktive H-Ionensekretion mit H-Ionendonator und Carboanhydratase.
2. Kollagenolyse und Proteolyse der Matrix.
3. Bildung saurer Mucopolysaccharide.

Physikalische Einflüsse:
1. Aufhebung des piezoelektrischen Effekts bei Inaktivität der Knochen.
2. Demineralisation im Lösungsgleichgewicht.

Hormone greifen wahrscheinlich auch in die chemischen Leistungen der Osteoclasten oder Osteocyten ein, z.B. Glucocorticoide in die Mucopolysaccharidbildung, Parathormon in die H^+-ionensekretion und Kollagenolyse.

Schlußbetrachtung

Das Gleichgewicht zwischen Knochenbildung und Knochenauflösung bestimmt den biologischen Bestand des Knochens. Eine positive Ca-Bilanz spricht für eine Mineralisation oder Knochenbildung, eine negative für eine Demineralisation oder einen Knochenschwund. Im Wachstum überwiegt physiologisch die Knochenbildung. Sonst treffen wir in der Regel bei länger bestehendem Ungleichgewicht auf Krankheitserscheinungen.

Literatur

Adams, J. B.: The biosynthesis of chondroitin sulphate. Biochem. J. **76**, 520—533 (1960).

—, and K. G. Rienits: The biosynthesis of chondroitin sulphates influence of nucleotides and hexosamines on sulphate incorporation. Biochim. biophys. Acta (Amst.) **51**, 567—578 (1961).

Aho, A. J., M. Groenroos, E. Raijola, and M. Kajanen: On the prolonged influence of gonadal hormones and of diet with a high Ca/P-ratio on bone in the rat. Acta endocr. (Kbh.) **37**, 63 (1961).

Albaum, H. G., A. Hirshfeld, and A. E. Sobel: Calcification. VI. Adenosine triphosphate content of preosseous cartilage. Proc. Soc. exp. Biol. (N.Y.) **79**, 238 (1952).

— — — Calcification. VIII. Glykolytic enzymes and phosphorylated intermediates in preosseus cartilage. Proc. Soc. exp. Biol. (N.Y.) **79**, 682 (1952a).

Albright, F., C. H. Burnett, P. H. Smith, and W. Parson: Pseudohypoparathyroidism, an example of Seabright-bantam-syndrom. Report of 3 cases. Endocrinology **30**, 922 (1942).

—, and R. Ellsworth: Studies on the physiology of the parathyroid glands: I. Calcium and phosphorus studies in a case of idiopathic hypoparathyreoidism. J. clin. Invest. **7**, 183 (1929).

—, and E. C. Reifenstein: The parathyroid glands and metabolic bone disease. Baltimore: Williams & Wilkins Co. 1948.

—, and H. W. Sulkowitch: Vitamin D-Wirkung auf Ca- und P-Umsatz. J. clin. Invest. **17**, 305 (1938).

Amprino: Ciba Foundation Symposium on bone structure and metabolism, p. 89. J. & A. Churchill, Ltd., 1955.

Anderson, A. J.: Some studies on the relationship between sialic acid and the mucopolysaccharide protein complexes in human cartilage. Biochem. J. **82**, 372 (1962).

Anderson, I. A.: Postmenopausal osteoporosis, clinical manifestations and treatment with oestrogens. Quart. J. Med. **19**, 67 (1950).

Anning, S. T., J. Dawson, D. E. Dolby, and J. T. Ingram: Toxic effects of calciferol. Quart. J. Med. **17**, 203—228 (1948).

Armstrong, W. D.: Radiotracer studies of hard tissues. Ann. N.Y. Acad. Sci. **60**, 670 (1955).

—, and C. P. Barnuni: Concurrent use of radioisotopes of Ca and P in study of metabolism of calcified tissues. J. biol. Chem. **172**, 199 (1948).

—, and L. Singer: Ciba Foundation Symposium on bone structure and Metabolism, p. 103—113. Boston: Little, Brown & Co.

Ashling, C. W., and H. M. Evans: In: G. Bourne, The biochemistry and physiology of bone, p. 671. New York: Academic Press 1956.

Aurbach, G., B. Houston, and J. Potts: Stimulation by parathyroid hormone of the mitochondrial utilization of reduced pyridine nucleotide. Biochem. biophys. Res. Commun. **17**, 464 (1964).

Bachra, B. N.: Precipitation of calcium carbonates and phosphates from metastable solutions. Ann. N.Y. Acad. Sci. **109**, 251 (1963a).

— Proc. of the 12th Congr. of the Eur. organization for research on fluorine and dental caries prevention. Utrecht, June 1965, 95 (1966).

—, and A. E. Sobel: Calcification. XXV. Mineralisation of reconstituted collagen. Arch. Biochem. **85**, 9 (1959).

—, and O. R. Trautz: Carbonic anhydrase and the precipitation of apatite. Science **137**, 337 (1962).

— —, and S. Simon: Precipitation of calcium carbonates and phosphates. I. Spontaneous precipitation of calcium carbonates and phosphates under physiological conditions. Arch. Biochem. **103**, 124 (1963).

— —, and S. L. Simon: Precipitation of calcium carbonates and phosphates. III. A precipitation diagram for the system calcium-carbonate-phosphate and the heterogeneous nucleation of solids in the metastability region. Advanc. Fluor. Sent. Caries Prevention **3**, 101 (1965).

— — — Precipitation of calcium carbonates and phosphates. III. The effect of magnesium and fluoride ions on the spontaneous precipitations of calcium carbonates and phosphates. Arch. oral. Biol. **10**, 731 (1965a).

Bale, W. F., M. L. Lefevre u. H. C. Hodge: Über den anorganischen Aufbau der Zähne. Naturwissenschaften **24**, 636—637 (1936).

Balogh, K.: Histochemical study of oxidative enzyme systems in teeth and peridental tissues. J. dent. Res. **42**, 1457 (1963).

— H. R. Dudley, and R. B. Cohan: Oxidation enzyme activity in skeletal cartilage and bone. Lab. Invest. **10**, 839 (1961).

Balogh jr., K.: Histochemical localization of acid phosphatase activity in teeth after decalcification with EDTA. J. Histochem. Cytochem. **13**, 303 (1965).

Barbieri, E.: Some relationships between the pancreatic β-cells and the metabolism of the epiphyseal cartilage. I. Cartilage ATP concentration of young alloxan diabetic rats. Experientia (Basel) **13**, 370 (1957).

— II. Cartilage cocarboxylase activity of young alloxan diabetic rats. Experientia (Basel) **13**, 371 (1957a).

Barnicot: The local action of the parathyroid and other tissues on bone in intracerebral grafts. J. Anat. (Lond.) **82**, 233—248 (1948).

Baud, C. A., and S. Slatkine: Fluoride metabolism. 2nd Eur. Symp. on calcified tissues. Liège 1964.

Bauditz, W., u. P. Siegmund: Über die Hemmwirkung des Thiocyanats auf den Plasmacalciumanstieg nach Parathormon. Klin. Wschr. **38**, 1220 (1960).

BAUER, G., and B. LINDQUIST: Bone salt metabolism in humans studied by means of radiocalcium. Acta med. scand. **158**, 143 (1957).

BAUER, G. C., A. CARLSSON, and B. LINDQUIST: Some properties of the exchangeable bone calcium. Acta physiol. scand. **35**, 67 (1955).

BAUER, G., A. CARLSON, and B. LINDQUIST: A comparative study on the metabolism of Sr^{90} and Ca^{45}. Acta physiol. scand. **35**, 56 (1955a).

BAUER, W., and A. MARBLE: Studies on the mode of action of irradiated ergosterol. II. Its effect on the calcium and phosphorus metabolism of individuals with calcium deficiency diseases. J. clin. Invest. **11**, 21 (1932).

BEEK, J.: The carbohydrate content of collagen. J. Amer. Leather Chemists' Ass. **36**, 696 (1941).

BÉLANGER, L. F., T. SEMBA, S. TOLNAI, D. H. COPP, L. KROOK, and C. GRIES: The two faces of resorption. 3rd Eur. Symp. on calcified tissues. Davos 1965.

— — — — — — The two faces of resorption. Aus: Calcified tissues 1965. Proceedings of the 3rd Eur. Symp. on calcified tissues held at Davos. Berlin-Heidelberg-New York: Springer 1966.

BELLO, J.: Ester-like groups in different collagens and gelatins. Nature (Lond.) **185**, 241 (1960).

BENGAIN, H., and F. A. HESS: The forms of the calcium and inorganic phosphorus in human and animal sera. III. A comparison of physiological and experimental hypercalcima. J. biol. Chem. **103**, 629 (1933).

BENJAMIN, H., A. F. HESS, and J. GROSS: The forms of magnesium in serum and milk. J. biol. Chem. **103**, 383 (1933).

BERGENSTAL, D. M., and M. B. LIPSETT: Metabolic effects of human growth hormone and growth hormone of other species in man. J. clin. Endocr. **20**, 1427 (1960).

BERGSTROEM, W. H.: The relationship of sodium and potassium to carbonate in bone. J. biol. Chem. **206**, 711 (1954).

— The participation of bone in total body sodium metabolism in the rat. J. clin. Invest. **34**, 997 (1955).

— The sceleton as an electrolyte reservoir. Metabolism **5**, 433 (1956).

BERLINER, R. W., T. J. KENNEDY, and J. ORLOFF: Relationship between acidification of the urine and potassium metabolism. Effect of carbonic anhydrase inhibition on potassium excretion. Amer. J. Med. **11**, 274 (1951).

BERNICK, S., and ·B. ERSHOFF: Histochemical study of bone in cortisone-treated rats. Endocrinology **72**, 231 (1963).

BERNSTEIN, D., C. R. KLEEMAN, and M. H. MAXWELL: The effect of calcium infusions, parathyroid hormone, and vitamin D on renal clearance of calcium. Proc. Soc. exp. Biol. (N.Y.) **112**, 353—354 (1963).

BERNSTEIN, D.: Studies on the renal clearance of phosphate and the role of the parathyroid gland in its regulation. J. clin. Endocr. **22**, 641 (1962a).

— C. R. KLEEMAN, R. E. CUTLER, J. T. DOWLING, and M. H. MAXWELL: Comparison of renal clearance of calcium during infusions of calcium chloride and calcium gluconate. Proc. Soc. exp. Biol. (N.Y.) **110**, 671 (1962).

— B. LEBOEUF, and G. F. CAHILL: Studies on glucose metabolism in cartilage in vitro. Proc. Soc. exp. Biol. (N.Y.) **107**, 458 (1961).

BEUTNER, E. H., and P. L. MUNSON: Time course of urinary excretion of inorganic phosphate by rats after parathyroidectomy and after injection of parathyroid extract. Endocrinology **66**, 610 (1960).

BEVELANDER, G., and P. L. JOHNSON: A histochemical study of the development of membrane bone. Anat. Rec. **108**, 1 (1950).

BIGGERS, J. D., K. A. LAWSON, J. A. LUCY, and M. WEBB: The chemical composition of longbone rudiments from the embryonic chick. Biohim. biophys. Acta (Amst.) **54**, 236—248 (1961).

— M. WEBB, R. C. PARKER, and G. M. HEALY: Cultivation of embryonic chick bones on chemically defined media. Nature (Lond.) **180**, 825 (1957).

BIJVOET, O., and C. MAJOOR: The renal tubular reabsorption of phosphate in thyrotoxicosis. Clin. chim. Acta **11**, 181 (1965).

BLACKBURN, C. R., W. J. HENSEY, K. D. GRANT, and F. B. WRIGHT: Studies on intravascular hemolysis in man. The pathogenesis of the initial stages of acute renal failure. J. clin. Invest. **33**, 825—834 (1954).

BODANSKY, O.: Are phosphatases of bone, kidney, intestine and serum identical? Use of bile acids in their differentiation. J. biol. Chem. **118**, 341 (1937).

— The influence of magnesium and cobalt on the inhibition of phosphatases of bone, intestine and osteogenic sarcoma by amino acids. J. biol. Chem. **179**, 81 (1949).

BOEDTKER, H., and P. DOTY: A native and denaturated state of the soluble collagen. J. Amer. chem. Soc. **78**, 4267 (1956).

BORLE, A. B.: Some effects of adrenalectomy and prednisolone administration on extracellular fluid and bone composition in the rat. Endocrinology **66**, 508 (1960b).

— H. T. KEUTMANN, and W. F. NEUMAN: Role of parathyroid hormone in phosphate transport across rat duodenum. Amer. J. Physiol. **204**, 704 (1963).

— G. NICHOLS, S. M. ZOTTU, and G. LANGE: Metabolic studies of bone in vitro. II. The metabolic patterns of accretion and resorption. J. biol. Chem. **235**, 1211 (1960a).

— N. NICHOLS, and G. NICHOLS: Metabolic studies of bone in vitro. I. Normal bone. J. biol. Chem. **235**, 1206 (1960).

BOSE, A.: Localisation of alkaline phosphatase in the development of the vertebral column in chick. Experientia (Basel) **16**, 144 (1960).

BOSS, W. R., C. M. OSBORN, and A. A. RENZI: Effects of adrenal cortical extract on renal function in hypophysectomized rats. Endocrinology **51**, 66—74 (1952).
BOSTROEM, H.: On the metabolism of the sulfate group of chondroitinsulfuricacid. J. biol. Chem. **196**, 477 (1952).
BOULET, D., and J. R. MARIER: Precipitation of calcium phosphates from solutions at near physiological concentrations. Arch. Biochem. **93**, 157 (1961).
BOURNE, G.: In: G. BOURNE, The biochemistry and physiology of bone, p. 539. New York: Academic Press 1956.
BOWES, J. H., and J. A. MOSS: Free amino of glucose groups of collagen. Nature (Lond.) **168**, 514—515 (1951).
BOWNESS, J. M.: Metabolism of chondroitinsulphate in the epiphyseal plate of puppies. Biochim. biophys. Acta (Amst.) **78**, 295—303 (1963).
BOYD, E. S., and W. F. NEUMAN: Chondroitinsulfate synthesis and respiration in chick embryonic cartilage. Arch. Biochem. **51**, 475 (1954).
BREIBART, S., J. H. LEE, A. MACCOORD, and G. B. FORBES: Relation of age to radiomagnesium exchange in bone. Proc. Soc. exp. Biol. (N.Y.) **105**, 361 (1960).
BRONNER, F.: Effects of parathyroid extract on metabolism of sulfate in immature rats. Amer. J. Physiol. **198**, 605 (1960).
— R. HARRIS, C. MALETSKOS, and C. BENDA: Studies in calcium metabolism. The fate of intravenously injected radiocalcium in human beings. J. clin. Invest. **35**, 78 (1956).
— P. J. SAMMON, and J.-P. AUBERT: Studies in the regulation of the blood calcium level. 4th Eur. Symp. on calcified tissues, Leiden 1966.
BROWN, W. E., J. P. SMITH, J. R. LEHR, and A. W. FRAZIER: Octacalcium phosphate and hydroxyapatite. Nature (Lond.) **196**, 1048 (1962).
BRUBACHER, H.: Über den Gehalt an anorganischen Stoffen, besonders an Kalk, in den Knochen und Organen normaler und rachitischer Kinder. Z. Biol. **27**, 517—549 (1890).
BRUCHMANN, E.: Über die Wirkungen von Ergosterin-Bestrahlungsprodukten auf Aconitat-Hydratase. Hoppe-Seylers Z. physiol. Chem. **327**, 27—34 (1961).
BUCHER, R.: Neue Gesichtspunkte zur Kalkablagerung. Schweiz. med. Wschr. **48**, 91 (1961).
BUCHWALD, K. W., and L. HUDSON: The biochemical effects of injections of sex hormones into hypophysectomized rats. Endocrinology **41**, 111 (1947).
BURSTONE, M. S.: Histochemical observations on enzymatic processes in bones and teeth. Ann. N.Y. Acad. Sci. **85**, 431 (1960).
— Histochemical demonstration of succinic dehydrogenase activity in osteoblasts. Nature (Lond.) **185**, 866 (1960a).
BUTTERWORTH, P., D. MOSS, E. PITKÄNEN, and A. PRINGLE: Some characteristics of alkaline phosphatase in human urine. Clin. chim. Acta **11**, 220 (1965).
BYWATERS, E. G.: Metabolism of cartilage. Nature (Lond.) **138**, 30 (1936).
— Metabolism of cartilage. Nature (Lond.) **138**, 288 (1936a).
— The metabolism of joint tissues. J. Path. Bact. **44**, 247 (1937).
CAMERON, E. C., and D. H. COPP: Parathyroid control of hypercalcemia due to injection of parathyroid extract in the rat. Proc. Soc. exp. Biol. (N.Y.) **114**, 278 (1963).
CAMPBELL, J. R., and T. A. DOUGLAS: The effect of low calcium intake and vitamin D supplements on bone structure in young growing dogs. Brit. J. Nutr. **19**, 339 (1965).
CAMPO, R. D., and D. D. DZIEWIATKOWSKI: Intracellular synthesis of protein-polysaccharides by slices of bovine corbal cartilage. J. biol. Chem. **237**, 2729 (1962).
CANARY, J. J.: Serial changes in serum calcium and phosphorus concentration and in urinary phosphorus excretion after parathyroid surgery: further evidence for a dual effect of parathyroid hormone. J. clin. Endocr. **22**, 229 (1962).
CANIGGIA, A., C. GENNARI, L. CESARI, and S. ROMANO: Intestinal absorption of ^{45}Ca in adult and old human subjects. Gerontologia (Basel) **10**, 193 (1964/65).
CARE, A., and W. KEYNES: The secretion of calcitonin by the parathyroid glands of the sheep. Brit. J. Endocr. **31**, XXXI (1965).
CARE, A. D., D. WEBSTER, and T. DUNCAN: Species variation to thyrocalcitonin. IV. Eur. Symp. on calcified tissues, Leyden 1966, p. 14.
CARLSTROEM, D., and R. ENGSTROEM: Ultrastructure and distribution of mineral salts in bone tissue. In: The biochemistry and physiology of bone, p. 149. New York: Academic Press 1956.
CARTIER, P.: Biochimie de l'ossification, phosphorylation et calcification. C. R. Soc. Biol. (Paris) **144**, 331 (1950).
—, u. J. PICARD: Die Mineralisation von verknöcherungsfähigem Knorpel in vitro. Bull. Soc. Chim. biol. (Paris) **37**, 485, 661 (1955).
— — Mineralisation verknöcherungsfähigen Knorpels. Bull. Soc. Chim. biol. (Paris) **37**, 1159, 1169 (1955a).
CASTELLANI, A. A., B. DE BERNARD, and V. ZAMBOTTI: Glucuronic acid formation in epiphyseal cartilage homogenate. Nature (Lond.) **180**, 859 (1957).
—, and V. ZAMBOTTI: Enzymatic formation of hexosamine in epiphyseal cartilage homogenate. Nature (Lond.) **178**, 313 (1956).
CERLETTI, P., P. IPATA, and G. TANCREDI: Pyrophosphatases of bone. Experientia (Basel) **14**, 440 (1958).
CHANDLER, P. T., and R. G. CRAGLE: Gastrointestinal sites of absorption and endogenous secretion of Calcium and phosphorus in dairy calves. Proc. Soc. exp. Biol. (N.Y.) **111**, 431 (1962).

CHANG, Y., and D. HEGSTEDT: Lactose and calcium transport in gut sacs. J. Nutr. 82, 297 (1964).
CHARNOCK, J. S.: Calcium accumulation and respiratory activity of the small intestine of the rat. Canad. J. Biochem. 41, 1013 (1963).
CHEN jr., P. S., and B. BOSMANN: Effect of vitamins D_2 and D_3 on serum calcium and phosphorus in rachitic chicks. Nutrition (Lond.) 83, 133 (1964).
— A. R. TEREPKA, and C. OVERSLAUGH: Hypercalcemic and hyperphosphatemic actions of dihydrotachysterol, vitamin D_2 and hytakerol (AT-10) in rats and dogs. Endocrinology 70, 815 (1962).
CIPERA, J. D., B. B. MIGIKOVSKY, and L. F. BÉLANGER: Composition of epiphyseal cartilage. I. Canad. J. Biochem. 38, 807 (1960).
—, and J. S. WILLMER: Composition of epiphyseal cartilage. III. Canad. J. Biochem. 40, 419 (1962).
— — Composition of epiphyseal cartilage. IV. Effect of vitamin D_3 on enzymatic activities in epiphyseal and articular cartilage of rachitic chicks. Canad. J. Biochem. 41, 1490 (1963).
CLARK, I., R. F. GEOFFROY, and W. BOWERS: Effects of adrenal cortical steroids on calcium metabolism. Endocrinology 64, 849 (1959).
CLOETENS, R.: Identification de deux phosphatases «alcalines» dans les organes animaux. Enzymologia 6, 46—56 (1939).
— Reversible Abspaltung des zweiten Metalls der alkalischen Phosphatase. II. Biochem. Z. 308, 37 (1941).
— Über den Aktivierungsmechanismus der alkalischen Phosphatase durch Metallionen. II. Biochem. Z. 307, 352 (1941a).
CLUTRE, R. G., P. G. FIKEKAR, M. K. KELKAR, and J. C. PATEL: Calcium, phosphorus and alkaline phosphatase levels in the sera of five hundred and forty five normal indian children. Ind. U. Med. Sci. 8, 214 (1954).
COHN, D. V.: Influence of parathyroid extract on the metabolism of organic acids by bone slices. Endocrinology 74, 133 (1964).
—, and B. K. FORSCHER: Effect of parathyroid extract on the oxidation in vitro of glucose and the production of $^{14}CO_2$ by bone and kidney. Biochim. biophys. Acta (Amst.) 65, 20—26 (1962).
COLLINS, E. J.: Effect of adrenal steroids on radio-calcium metabolism in dogs. Metabolism 11, 716 (1962).
CONSDEN, R., L. E. GLYNN, and W. M. STANIER: A chemical examination of connective tissue in rheumatic fever. Biochem. J. 55, 248 (1953).
COOK, P. B., J. R. NASSIM, and J. COLLINS: The effects of thyreotoxicosis upon the metabolism of calcium, phosphorus and nitrogen. Quart. J. Med. 28, 505 (1959).
COOPER, C.W., C.W. YATES jr., and R.V. TALMAGE: Some endogenous parathyroid hormone effects manifested by bone in vitro. Proc. Soc. exp. Biol. (N.Y.) 119, 81 (1965).
COPP, D. H.: The parathyroid glands and regulation of blood calcium. Oral Surg. 15, 1249 (1963).
— The hormones of the parathyroid and calcium Homeostasis. In: The parathyroid glands (GAILLARD/TALMAGE/BUDY), p. 73. Chicago: Chicago University Press 1965.
—, and E. C. CAMERON: Demonstration of a hypocalcemic factor (calcitonin) in commercial parathyroid extract. Science 134, 2038 (1961).
— —, and B. A. CHENEY: Evidence for calcitonin — a new hormone for parathyroid that lowers blood. Endocrinology 70, 638 (1962).
—, and B. A. CHENEY: Calcitonin — a hormon from the parathyroid which lowers the calcium-level of the blood. Nature (Lond.) 193, 381 (1962a).
—, and A. G. F. DAVIDSON: Direct humoral control of parathyroid function in the dog. Proc. Soc. exp. Biol. (N.Y.) 107, 342 (1961a).
—, and K. HENZE: Parathyroid origin of calcitonin by the parathyroid glands of the sheep. Endocrinology 75, 49 (1964).
CORTELYOU, J. R.: Phosphorus changes in totally parathyroidectomized rana pipiens. Endocrinology 70, 618—621 (1962).
— HIBNER, A. OWERKO, and J. MULROY: Blood and urine calcium changes in totally parathyroidectomized rana pipiens. Endocrinology 66, 441 (1960).
COURTS, A.: Structural changes in collagen. The action of alkalis and acids in the conversion of collagen into eucollagen. Biochem. J. 74, 238—247 (1960).
CRAMER, C. F.: Participation of parathyroid glands in control of Ca absorption in dogs. Endocrinology 72, 192 (1963).
— Sites of calcium absorption and the calcium concentration of gut contents in the dog. Canad. J. Physiol. 43, 75 (1965).
CROWELL, C. D., H. C. HODGE, and W. R. LINE: Chemical analysis of tooth samples composed of enamel, dentine, and cementum. J. dent. Res. 14, 251—268 (1934).
D'ABRAMO, F., and F. LIPMANN: The formation of adenosine 3'-phosphate-5'-phosphosulfate in extracts of chick embryo cartilage and its conversion into chondroitin sulphate. Biochim. biophys. Acta (Amst.) 25, 211—213 (1957).
DALLEMAGNE, M. J.: Le dépot des matières minérales dans l'os en formation. Acta biol. belg. 1, 95 (1942).
— The theory of primary calcification in bone. Nature (Lond.) 161, 115 (1948).
— P. BODSON et CL. FABRY: Le calcium échangeable de la substance minérale de l'os étudié à l'aide de ^{45}Ca. Biochim. biophys. Acta (Amst.) 18, 394—406 (1955).
—, and CL. FABRY: Ciba Symp. Bone Structure and Metabolism, p. 14. London: J. A. Churchill 1956.
— —, and P. BODSON: The exchange of bone calcium with ^{45}Ca. Experientia (Basel) 11, 142 (1955a).

Danko, Ch. W., and P. M. Bergenstal: Effects of growth hormone and corticosteroids in S^{35} fixation in cartilage. Endocrinology **69**, 769 (1961).
Davenport, H. W.: The inhibition of carbonic anhydrase and of gastric acid secretion by thiocyanate. Amer. J. Physiol. **129**, 505 (1940).
Davidson, E. A., and W. Small: Metabolism in vivo of connective-tissue mucopolysaccharides. I. Chondroitin sulfate C and keratosulfate of nucleus pulposus. Biochim. biophys. Acta (Amst.) **69**, 445—452 (1963).
Dawson, K. B.: Calcium exchange in bone. Biochem. J. **60**, 389—391 (1955).
Degrazia, J. A., and C. Rich: Studies of intestinal absorption of $calcium^{45}$ in man. Metabolism **18**, 650 (1964).
Deiss, W., L. Holmes, and C. C. Johnston: Bone matrix biosynthesis in vitro. I. Labeling of hexosamine and collagen of normal bone. J. biol. Chem. **237**, 3555 (1962).
Deleu, J., and H. Bohr: Uptake of tetracycline by human bone in vitro. Nature (Lond.) **204**, 1103 (1964).
Dickens, F., and H. Weil-Malherbe: Metabolism of cartilage. Nature (Lond.) **138**, 125 (1936).
Dickerson, J. W.: The effect of development on the composition of a long bone of the pigiratand fowl. Biochem. J. **82**, 47 (1962).
Dikshit, P. K., and S. Sriramachari: Mode of action of vitamin D. Indian J. med. Res. **49**, 115 (1961).
Dillmann, G., u. H. D. Cremer: Chondroitinschwefelsäure in Knorpel, Knochen und Zähnen. Biochem. Z. **327**, 368—376 (1956).
Dingle, J. T.: 3rd Eur. Symp. on calcified tissues, Davos 1965.
— J. A. Lucy, and H. B. Fell: Studies on the mode of action of excell of vitamin A. 1. Effect of excess of vitamin A on the metabolism and composition of embryonic chick-limb cartilage grown in organ culture. Biochem. J. **79**, 497—500 (1961).
— — — A possible role of intracellular proteases in the degradation of cartilage matrix. Biochem. J. **79**, 500—508 (1961a).
Dirscherl, W., u. A. Glasmacher: Aufnahme und Abgabe von Ca durch anorganische Knochensubstanz und ihre Beeinflussung durch Eiweiß und Eiweißabbauprodukte. Acta biol. med. germ. **3**, 341 (1959).
Dixon, T. F., and H. R. Parkins: Citric acid and bone metabolism. Biochem. J. **52**, 260—265 (1952).
Djojosoebagio, S., and C. W. Turner: Effects of parathyroid extract, dihydrotachysterol (hytakerol) and calciferol on milk secretion in rats. Endocrinology **74**, 554 (1964).
Doering, P.: Untersuchungen des Claciumstoffwechsels mit Ca^{47} beim Menschen. Klin. Wschr. **41**, 681 (1963).
Donegan, W. L., and H. M. Spiro: Parathyroids and gastric secretion. Gastroenterology **38**, 750 (1960).
Drake, M., and A. Veis: Interchain interactions in collagenfold formation. I. The kinetics of renaturation of γ-gelatin. Biochemistry **3**, 135 (1964).
Dulce, H.-J.: Einfluß von Hyaluronsäure auf Calciumoxalatfällungen. Hoppe-Seylers Z. physiol. Chem. **302**, 49—54 (1955).
— Biochemie des Knochens. Habil.-Schr. Berlin 1959.
— Zur Biochemie der Verknöcherung. I. Mineralgehalt und Grundsubstanzzusammensetzung des hyalinen Knorpels, des verknöchernden Knorpels und des Knochens. Hoppe-Seylers Z. physiol. Chem. **319**, 257—271 (1960).
— Zur Biochemie der Verknöcherung. II. Enzymaktivitäten im hyalinen Knorpel, im verknöchernden Knorpel und im Knochen. Hoppe-Seylers Z. physiol. Chem. **319**, 272—278 (1960a).
— Zur Biochemie der Verknöcherung. III. Mineralgehalt, Grundsubstanzzusammensetzung und Enzymaktivitäten im Callusgewebe und im rachitischen Knochen von Ratten. Hoppe-Seylers Z. physiol. Chem. **320**, 1—10 (1960b).
— Der Stoffwechsel des Knochens im Licht neuer physiologisch-chemischer Erkenntnisse. Verh. Dtsch. Orthop. Ges., 48. Kongr. Berlin 1961.
— Chemische Physiologie und chemische Pathologie des Knochens. Stuttgart: Georg Thieme (in Vorbereitung).
— W. Bauditz u. P. Siegmund: Überprüfung der Wirkung von Parathormonpräparaten auf das Plasma-Calcium von jungen Hähnen. Dtsch. med. Wschr. **86**, Nr 5, 210—211 (1961a).
—, u. P. Siegmund: Zur Biochemie der Knochenauflösung. II. Der Einfluß von Diamox auf das Plasma Calcium östron behandelter Hähne. Hoppe-Seylers Z. physiol. Chem. **320**, 160—162 (1960c).
— — F. Körber u. F. Schütte: Zur Biochemie der Knochenauflösung. III. Über das Vorkommen von Carboanhydratase im Knochen. Hoppe-Seylers Z. physiol. Chem. **320**, 163—167 (1960d).
Dull, T., and P. H. Hennemann: Urinary hydroxyproline as an index of collagen turnover in bone. New Engl. J. Med. **268**, 132 (1963).
Dunstone, J. R.: Ion-exchange reactions between cartilage and various cations. Biochem. J. **77**, 164—170 (1960).
Dziewiatkowski, D. D.: Isolation of chondroitin sulfate-S^{35} from articular cartilage of rats. J. biol. Chem. **189**, 187—190 (1951).
— Radioautography visualization of S^{35} deposition in the articular cartilage and bone of suckling rats following injection of labelled sodium sulfate. J. exp. Med. **93**, 451 (1951a).
— Radioautographic studies of sulfate-sulfur S^{35} metabolism in the articular cartilage and bone of suckling rats. J. exp. Med. **95**, 489 (1952).
— Vitamin A and endochondral ossification in the rat as indicated by the use of sulfur-35 and phosphorus-32. J. exp. Med. **100**, 11 (1954).

DZIEWIATKOWSKI, D. D.: Vitamin D endochondral ossification in the rat as indicated by the use of sulfur-35 and phosphorus-32. J. exp. Med. **100**, 25 (1954a).

— R. BENESCH, and R. E. BENESCH: On the possible utilization of sulfate sulfur by the suckling rat for the synthesis of chondroitin sulfate as indicated by the use of radioactive sulfur. J. biol. Chem. **178**, 931 (1949).

EANES, E. D., R. A. HARPER, I. GILLESSEN, and A. S. POSNER: An amorphous component in bone mineral. 4th Eur. Symp. on calcified tissues. Leiden 1966.

EASTOE, J. E.: The amino acid composition of mammalian collagen and gelatin. Biochem. J. **61**, 589—600 (1955).

— The biochemistry and physiology of bone. In: G. H. BOURNE, p. 81. New York: Academic Press Inc. Publ. 1956.

— Organic matrix of tooth enamel. Nature (Lond **187**, 411 (1960).

—, and B. EASTOE: The organic constituents of mammalian compact bone. Biochem. J. **57**, 453 (1954).

EBERT, P., and D. PROCKOP: Effects of hydrocortisone on the synthesis of sulphated mucopolysaccharides and collagen in chick embryos. Biochim. biophys. Acta (Amst.) **78**, 390—392 (1963).

EDGREN, R., and D. W. CALHOUN: Density as an index of the effects of estrogens on bone. Endocrinology **59**, 631 (1956).

EGER, W.: Kongreßthema IV. Nebenschilddrüse, Nieren, Knochen, Nebenschilddrüsen, Nieren und Skelettsystem. Med. Klin. **51**, 822 (1956).

— Morphologie des Knochenstoffwechsels und seiner Störungen. In: Wirkung und Anwendung anaboler Steroide, S. 82. Kolloquium Berlin 1963. Erschienen im Medicus-Verlag 1964.

EGG-LARSEN, N.: An experimental study on growth and glykolysis in epiphyseal cartilage of rats. Acta physiol. scand. **38**, Suppl. 128, 1 (1956).

EICHLER, O., I. APPEL, R. K. WADHWANI u. R. RITTER: Die Aufnahme von ^{45}Ca bei Zahnkeimen von Hunden in vitro. Hoppe-Seylers Z. physiol. Chem. **310**, 8 (1962).

EISENBERG, E., and G. S. GORDAN: Skeletal dynamics in man measured by nonradioactive strontium. J. clin. Invest. **40**, 1809 (1961).

EISENSTEIN, R., and M. PASSAVOY: Actinomycin D inhibits parathyroid hormone and vitamin D activity. Proc. Soc. exp. Biol. (N.Y.) **117**, 77 (1964).

ELLIOTT, J. R., and S. FREEMAN: Relative effect of vitamin D and parathyroid extract on plasma calcium and citric acid of normal and thyroparathyroidectomized dogs. Endocrinology **59**, 196 (1956).

— — Parathyroid function and the plasma citric acid and calcium response to nephrectomy. Endocrinology **59**, 181 (1956a).

ELLSWORTH, E., and J. E. HOWARD: Studies on the physiology of the parathyroid glands. VII. Some responses of the normal human kidney and blood to intravenous parathyroid extract. John Hopk. Hosp. Bull. **55**, 296 (1934).

EMERY, A. J., and A. L. DOUNCE: Intracellular distribution of alkaline phosphatase in rat liver cells. J. biophys. biochem. Cytol. **1**, 315—330 (1955).

ENGEL, J., u. G. BEIER: Vergleich der molekularen Daten von Tryptocollagen verschiedener Kalbshäute in nativem und denaturiertem Zustand. Hoppe-Seylers Z. physiol. Chem. **334**, 201 (1963).

ENGSTROM, G., and H. DELUCA: Vitamin D-stimulated release of calcium from mitochondria. Biochemistry **3**, 203 (1964).

ETORI, J., and S. M. SCOGGAN: Ionized calcium in biological media. Nature (Lond.) **184**, 1315 (1959).

EVERED, D., and T. STEENSON: Citrate inhibition of alkaline phosphatase. Nature (Lond.) **202**, 491 (1964).

FALKENHEIM, M., W. NEUMAN, and H. C. HODGE: Phosphate exchange as the mechanism for adsorption of the radioactive isotope by the calcified tissues. J. biol. Chem. **169**, 713 (1947).

— E. E. UNDERWOOD, and H. C. HODGE: Calcium exchange, the mechanism of adsorption by bone of calcium. J. biol. Chem. **188**, 805 (1951).

FANCONI, G.: Die Wahrung der biologischen Konstante „Plasmacalcium" und ihre Störungen. Schweiz. med. Wschr. **89**, 471 (1959).

— Physiologie und Pathologie des Calcium- und Phosphatstoffwechsels. Helv. paediat. Acta **16**, 293 (1961).

FANG, M., and H. RASMUSSEN: Parathyroid hormone and mitochondrial respiration. Endocrinology **75**, 434 (1964).

FELDSTEIN, A. M., J. SAMACHSON, and H. SPENZER: Levels of calcium, phosphorus, alkaline phosphatase and protein in effusion fluid and serum in man. Amer. J. Med. **35**, 530 (1963).

FELL, H. B.: Phosphataseaktivität in in vitro wachsender Knochen. Arch. exp. Zellforsch. **11**, 245 (1931).

—, and J. T. DINGLE: Studies on the mode of action of excess of vitamin A. 6. Lysosomal protease and the degradation of cartilage matrix. Biochem. J. **87**, 403 (1963).

—, and R. ROBISON: The growth development and phosphatase activity of embryonic avian femora and limbbuds cultivated in vitro. Biochem. J. **23**, 767—784 (1929).

— — The development and phosphatase activity in vivo and in vitro of the mandibular skeletal tissue of the embryonic fowl. Biochem. J. **24**, 1905—1920 (1930).

FIELD, A. C.: Uptake of magnesium^{-28} by the skeleton of a sheep. Nature (Lond.) **188**, 1205 (1960).

FINE, A., and P. PERSON: Terminal respiration of cartilage tissues. Biochim. biophys. Acta (Amst.) **78**, 729—732 (1963).

FINKELSTEIN, J. D., and D. SCHACHTER: Active transport of calcium by intestine: effects of hypophysectomy and growth hormone. Amer. J. Physiol. **203**, 873 (1962).

Flanagan, B., and G. Nichols: Metabolic studies of bone in vitro. IV. Collagen biosynthesis by surviving bone fragments in vitro. J. biol. Chem. **237**, 3686 (1962).
— — Metabolic studies of bone in vitro. V. Glucose metabolism and collagen biosynthesis. J. biol. Chem. **239**, 1261 (1964).
— — Parathyroid inhibition of bone collagen synthesis. Endocrinology **74**, 180 (1964a).
Fleisch, H.: Neue Gesichtspunkte der Kalkablagerung. Schweiz. med. Wschr. **91**, 858 (1961).
— Role of nucleation and inhibition in calcification. Clin. Orthop. **32**, 170 (1964).
— Physiologie und Biochemie der Knochenbildung. Klin. Wschr. **44**, 360 (1966).
—, and S. Bisaz: Mechanism of calcification: Inhibitory role of pyrophosphate. Nature (Lond.) **195**, 911 (1962).
— — Isolement du plasma de pyrophosphate, un inhibiteur de la calcification. Helv. physiol. pharmacol. Acta **20**, C 52—C 53 (1962a).
— — The inhibitory effect of pyrophosphate on calcium oxalate precipitation and its relation to urolithiasis. Experientia (Basel) **20**, 276 (1964a).
— — Proc. of the First Eur. Bone and Tooth Symp. Oxford 1963, 249 (1964b).
— — Further evidence for the inhibitory role of pyrophosphat in calcification. 2nd Eur. Symp. on calcified tissues, Liège 1965.
— —, and R. Russel: The activating effect of lead on the precipitation of calcium phosphate. Proc. Soc. exp. Biol. (N.Y.) **118**, 882 (1965).
— J. Maerki, and R. Russel: Effect of pyrophosphate on dissolution of hydroxyapatite and its possible importance in calcium homeostasis. Proc. Soc. exp. Biol. (N.Y.) **122**, 317 (1966a).
—, and W. F. Neuman: Mechanism of calcification: Role of collagen, polyphosphates and phosphatase. Amer. J. Physiol. **200**, 6 (1961a).
— — Die Rolle der Phosphatase und der Polyphosphate bei der Kalzifikation von Collagen. Helv. physiol. pharmacol. Acta **19**, C 17—C 18 (1961b).
— F. Straumann, R. Schenk, S. Bisaz, and M. Allgower: Effect of condensed phosphates on calcification of chick embryo femurs in tissue culture. Amer. J. Physiol. **211**, 821 (1966b).
Forbes, G. B.: Metabolic role of sodium in bone. Helv. paediat. Acta **14**, 506 (1959).
— Studies on sodium in bone. J. Paediat. **56**, 180 (1960).
Forbes, R. M.: Mineral utilization in the rat. V. Effects of dietary thyroxine on mineral balance and tissue mineral composition with special reference to magnesium nutriture. J. Nutr. **86**, 193 (1965).
Foster, G. V., A. Baghdiantz, M. A. Kumar, E. Slack, H. A. Soliman, and I. MacIntyre: Thyroid origin of calcitonin. Nature (Lond.) **202**, 1303 (1964a).
Foster, G., M. A. Kumar, A. Baghdiantz, H. Soliman, E. Slack, A. Debats, and I. Mac Intyre: 2nd Eur. Symp. on calcified tissues. Liège 1964b, p. 401—407.
— I. MacIntyre, and A. Pearse: Calcitonin production and the mitochondrion-rich cells of the dog thyroid. Nature (Lond.) **203**, 1029 (1964).
Fraser, D., N. T. Jaco, E. R. Yendt, J. D. Mumm, and E. Liu: The induction of in vitro and in vivo calcification in bones of children suffering from vitamin D-resistant rickets without recourse to large doses of vitamin D. Amer. J. Dis. Child. **93**, 84—85 (1957).
Fraser, R. D. B., and T. P. Macrae: Possible role of water in collagen structure. Nature (Lond.) **183**, 179 (1959).
Freeman, S., and J. R. Elliott: The effect of fluoroacetate upon the plasma citrate response in parathyroidectomy and nephrectomy. Endocrinology **59**, 190 (1956).
Freudenberg, E., u. P. György: Über Kalkbindung durch tierische Gewebe. I. Biochem. Z. **110**, 299—305 (1920).
— — Über Kalkbindung durch tierische Gewebe. II. Biochem. Z. **115**, 96—108 (1921).
— — Über Kalkbindung durch tierische Gewebe. III. Biochem. Z. **118**, 50—54 (1921a).
Friedenstein, A. J.: Humoral nature of osteogenic activity of transitional epithelium. Nature (Lond.) **149**, 698 (1962).
Friesen, H.: Hypocalcemic effect of pituitary polypeptides in rabbits. Endocrinology **75**, 692 (1964).
Frischauf, H., u. H. Jesserer: Untersuchungen über die Wirkung von Vitamin D mit Calcium-47. Wien. klin. Wschr. **74**, 801 (1962).
Gabbiani, G., M. L. Jaqcmin, and R. M. Richard: Soft-tissue calcification induced by rare earth metals and its prevention by sodium pyrophosphate. Brit. J. Pharmacol. Chemother. **27**, 1 (1966).
—, and B. Tuchweber: Inhibition of soft-tissue calcification by parathyroid extract and calcium. Acta endocr. (Kbh.) **49**, 603 (1965).
— — Studies on the mechanism of experimental soft-tissue calcification. Canad. J. Physiol. Pharmacol. **43**, 177 (1965a).
Gabriel, S.: Chemische Untersuchungen über die Mineralstoffe der Knochen und Zähne. Z. physiol. Chem. **18**, 257 (1894).
Gade, M., u. H. J. Einbrodt: Ultraspektroskopische Untersuchungen an freigelegten sogenannten Kalkablagerungen aus menschlichen Organen. Naturwissenschaften **50**, 21 (1963).
Gaillard, P.: Bone culture studies with calcitonin. 4th Eur. Symp. on calcified tissues, Leiden 1966.
Gaillard, P. J.: Parathyroid gland tissue and bone in vitro. Exp. Cell Res., Suppl. **3**, 154—169 (1955).
Gallop, P. M., S. Seifter, and C. Franzblau: Occurrence of "ester-like" linkages in collagen. Nature (Lond.) **183**, 1659 (1959).

Garrett, E. R., R. L. Johnston, and E. J. Collins: Quantification of normal and adrenal steroid affected calcium metabolism in the young dog. J. Pharmacol. exp. Ther. **145**, 357 (1964).

Gedalia, I., A. Frumkin, and H. Zukerman: Effects of estrogen on bone composition in rats at low and high fluoride intake. Endocrinology **75**, 201 (1964).

Gerber, G., G. Gerber, and K. Altmann: Studies on the metabolism of tissue proteins. I. Turnover of collagen labelled with proline U-C[14] in young rats. J. biol. Chem. **235**, 2653 (1960).

Glegg, R. E., and D. Eidinger: A method for fractionating the carbohydrate components of bone. Arch. Biochem. **55**, 19 (1955).

— —, and C. P. Leblond: Some carbohydrate components of reticular fibrils. Science **118**, 614—616 (1953).

Glimcher, H. J., G. Mechanic, L. C. Bonar, and E. J. Daniel: The amino acid composition of the organic matrix of decalcified fetal bovine dental enamel. J. biol. Chem. **236**, 3210 (1961).

Glimcher, M. J., and S. M. Krane: The incorporation of radioactive inorganic orthophosphate as organic phosphate by collagen fibrils in vitro. Biochemistry **3**, 195 (1964).

Glimcher, M. J., and S. M. Krane: The identification of serine phosphate in connective tissue. Biochim. biophys. Acta (Amst.) **90**, 477—483 (1964a).

Glynn, L. E., u. C. A. Reading: 7. Colloquium der Gesellschaft für Physiologische Chemie. Chemie und Stoffwechsel des Binde- und Knochengewebes. Berlin-Göttingen-Heidelberg: Springer 1956.

Goldenberg, H., and A. E. Sobel: Calcification. XII. Catio-linked subibition by fluoride and cyanide ions in β-glyzerophosphate medium. Proc. Soc. exp. Biol. (N.Y.) **85**, 275 (1954).

Goldhaber, P.: Osteogenic induction across millipore filters in vivo. Science **133**, 2065—2067 (1961).

Goldsmith, R., J. Wulsin, and M. Wiester: Effect of thyroparathyroidectomy in the clinical course and the serum calcium and phosphorus concentration in dogs. Endocrinology **76**, 9 (1965).

Gonin, J.-D., et H. Fleisch: Mesure de la formation osseuse par l'incorporation des tétracyclines dans l'os. Helv. physiol. pharmacol. Acta **20**, 23 (1962).

Gordan, G. S., and E. Eisenberg: The effect of estrogens, androgens and corticoids on skeletal kinetics in man. Proc. roy. Soc. Med. **56**, 1027 (1963).

Gosselin, R. E., and E. R. Gochlan: The stability of complexes between calcium and orthophosphate polymeric phosphate and phytate. Arch. Biochem. **45**, 301 (1953).

Gossmann, H. H., and S. Heilenz: Zum Bleigehalt menschlichen Knochengewebes. Dtsch. Med. Wschr. **49**, 2267—2269 (1967).

Govaerts, J., M. J. Dallemagne, and J. Melon: Radiocalcium as an indicator in the study of the action of estradiol on calcium metabolism. Endocrinology **48**, 443 (1951).

Grab, W.: Pharmakologie des Vitamin D. Mschr. Kinderheilk. **101**, 163 (1953).

Gran, F. C.: Vitamin D and calcium absorption in parathyreoidectomiced rats. Acta physiol. scand. **49**, 211 (1960).

Grassmann, W.: 7. Kolloquium der Gesellschaft für Physiologische Chemie. Chemie und Stoffwechsel von Binde- und Knochengewebe. Berlin-Göttingen-Heidelberg: Springer 1956.

— Kollagenforschung unter dem Gesichtswinkel der Praxis. Leder **12**, 165 (1961).

— J. Engel, K. Hannig u. K. Kühn: Zur Bildung von Fibrillen und Long-Spacing Segmenten aus renaturierten Tropocollagenlösungen. Hoppe-Seylers Z. physiol. Chem. **329**, 69 (1962).

— K. Hannig u. A. Nordwig: Über die apolaren Bereiche des Collagenmoleküls, Aminosäuresequenzen des Collagen. VI. Hoppe-Seylers Z. physiol. Chem. **333**, 154 (1963).

— — u. M. Schleyer: Zur Aminosäuresequenz des Kollagens. II. Hoppe-Seylers Z. physiol. Chem. **322**, 71 (1960).

— H. Hoermann u. R. Hafter: Eine quantitative Bestimmung von Kohlenhydraten als Osazone. Anwendung der Methode auf Kollagen und Prokollagen. Hoppe-Seylers Z. physiol. Chem. **307**, 87—96 (1957).

— U. Hofmann u. Th. Nemetschek: Die Querstreifung von Kollagenfibrillen. Naturwissenschaften **39**, 215 (1952).

—, u. H. Schleich: Über den Kohlenhydratgehalt des Kollagens. II. Mitt. zur Kenntnis des Kollagens. Biochem. Z. **277**, 320 (1935).

Green, J., and A. Lyall: Calcium metabolism in hypothyreoidism. Lancet **1951 I**, 828.

Greenberg, D. M.: Mineral metabolism calcium, magnesium and phosphorus. Ann. Rev. Biochem. 8, 278 (1939).

— Studies in mineral metabolism with the aid of artificial radioactive isotopes. VIII. Tracer experiments with radioactive calcium and strontium on the mechanism of vitamin D action in rachitic rats. J. biol. Chem. **157**, 99 (1945).

—, and L. D. Greenberg: Is there an unknown compound of the nature of calcium citrate present in the blood. J. biol. Chem. **99**, 1 (1932).

Greengard, O., M. Gordon, M. Smith, and G. Acs: Studies on the mechanism of diethylstilbestrol-induced formation of phosphoprotein in male chickens. J. biol. Chem. **239**, 2079 (1964).

Greenspan, J. S., and H. J. Blackwood: Histochemical studies of chondrocyte function in the cartilage of the mandibular condyle of the rat. 3rd Eur. Symp. on calcified tissues, Davos 1965.

Greenwald, I.: The solubility of calciumphosphate. II. The solubility product. J. biol. Chem. **143**, 711 (1942).

GREENWALD, I.: The effect of phosphate on the solubility of calcium carbonate and of bicarbonate on the solubility of calcium and magnesium phosphate. J. biol. Chem. **161**, 697 (1945).
GREINLICH, R. C.: An autoradiographic study of organically bound carbon-14 in growing epiphyseal cartilage and bone. J. Bone Jt Surg. A **38**, 611 (1956).
GRIER, R. S., M. B. HOOD, and M. B. HOAGLAND: Observations on the effects of beryllium on alkaline phosphatase. J. biol. Chem. **180**, 289 (1949).
GROLLMAN, A.: The condition of the inorganic phosphorus of the blood with special reference to the calcium concentration. J. biol. Chem. **72**, 565 (1927).
— The role of the kidney in the parathyroid control of the blood calcium as determined by studies in the nephrectomized dog. Endocrinology **55**, 166 (1954).
GROSS, J., J. H. HIGHBERGER, and F. O. SCHMITT: Extraction of collagen from connective tissue by neutral salt solutions. Proc. nat. Acad. Sci. (Wash.) **40**, 679 (1954); **41**, 1—7 (1955).
—, and C. M. LAPIERE: Collagenolytic activity in amphibian tissues: A tissue culture essay. Proc. nat. Acad. Sci. (Wash.) **48**, 1014 (1962).
GROSSFELD, H.: Production of chondroitin sulfate in tissue culture of cartilage. Biochim. biophys. Acta (Amst.) **74**, 193—197 (1963).
GUBISCH, W., u. F. SCHLAGER: Fermente im Knochen und Knorpelgewebe. Acta histochem. (Jena) **12**, 69 (1961).
GUDMUNSSON: The isolation of thyrocalcitonin and a study of its effect in the rat. Proc. roy. Soc. B **164**, 460 (1966).
GURI, C. D., and D. S. BERNSTEIN: Effect of parathyroid hormone on mucopolysaccharide synthesis in rachitic rat cartilage in vitro. Proc. Soc. exp. Biol. (N.Y.) **116**, 702 (1964).
GUROFF, G., M. F. DELUCA, and H. STEENBOCK: Citrate and action of vitamin D on calcium and phosphorus metabolism. Amer. J. Physiol. **204**, 833 (1963).
GUSTAVSON, K. H: New York: Academic Press Inc. Publ. 1956. The chemistry and reactivity of collagen, p. 41
GUTMAN, A. B., and E. B. GUTMAN: Phosphorylase in calcifying cartilage. Proc. Soc. exp. Biol. (N.Y.) **48**, 687—691 (1941).
—, and T. F. YÜ: A concept of the role of enzymes in endochondral calcification. Conf. Metab. Interr. Trans. 2. Conf. New York: J. Macy 1950.
HAAS, H.: Tetanie bei Störungen des Calcium- und Magnesiumstoffwechsels. Schweiz. med. Wschr. **95**, 742 (1965).
HAAS, H. G.: In: Knochenstoffwechsel- und Parathyreoideaerkrankungen. Stuttgart: Georg Thieme 1966.
— U. DUBACH u. H. AFFOLTER: Wirkung des zweiten Nebenschilddrüsenhormons Calcitonin beim Menschen. Helv. med. Acta **31**, 442 (1947).
HAFTER, R., u. H. HOERMANN: Der Einfluß von Pepsin auf die Struktur und die faserbildenden Eigenschaften von Collagen. Hoppe-Seylers Z. physiol. Chem. **330**, 169 (1963).
HAGERTY, R. F., TH. B. CALHOON, W. H. LEE, and J. CUTTINO: Characteristics of fresh human cartilage. Surg. Gynaec. Obstet. **110**, 3 (1960).
HALLSWORTH, A.: Aspects of calcification. The availability of α-amino groups in collagen aggregates. Biochem. J. **93**, 255 (1964).
HANDLER, P., and D. V. COHN: Effect of parathyroid extract on renal function. Amer. J. Physiol. **169**, 188 (1952).
— D. V. COHN, and W. J. DE MARIA: Effect of parathyroid extraction on renal excretion of phosphate. Amer. J. Physiol. **168**, 434—441 (1951).
HANNA, S., M. T. HARRISON, J. MACINTYRE, and R. FRASER: Effects of growth hormone on calcium and magnesium metabolism. Brit. med. J. **1961 II**, No 5243, 12.
HARDEL, M., u. H.-J. DULCE: Berechnung der als Aminosäure-Chelate lösbaren Zahnhartsubstanz. Dtsch. zahnärztl. Z. **20**, 694 (1965).
HARDEN, R., M. HARRISON, W. ALEXANDER, and B. NORDIN: Phosphate excretion and parathyroid function in thyrotoxicosis. J. Endocr. **28**, 281 (1964).
HARRINGTON, W. F., and P. H. v. HIPPEL: Formation and stabilization of the collagen-fold. Arch. Biochem. **92**, 100 (1961).
HARRIS, H. A.: Glykogen in cartilage. Nature (Lond.) **130**, 996 (1932).
HARRIS, L. J.: In: The biochemistry and physiology of bone (G. H. BOURNE). New York: Academic Press 1956.
HARRIS, W. H., and CH. NAGANT DE DEUXCHAINES: Controlled in vivo inhibition of bone formation. Second Eur. Symp. on calcified tissues at the Domaine Provincial de Wegimont 1964, 193 (1965).
HARRISON, H. C., and H. E. HARRISON: Cortisol and citrate metabolism. Amer. J. Physiol. **196**, 943 (1959).
— —, and E. A. PARK: Vitamin D and citrate metabolism. Effect of vitamin D in rats fed diets adequate in both calcium and phosphorus. Amer. J. Physiol. **192**, 432—436 (1958).
HARRISON, H. E.: Mechanisms of action of vitamin D. Pediatrics **14**, 285 (1954).
— Physiology of vitamin D. Helv. paediatr Acta **14**, 434 (1959).
—, and H. C. HARRISON: The uptake of radiocalcium by the skeleton: the effect of vitamin D and calcium intake. J. biol. Chem. **185**, 857 (1950).
— — Intestinal transport of phosphate: action of vitamin D, calcium, and potassium. Amer. J. Physiol. **201**, 1007 (1961).
— — Vitamin D and permeability of intestinal mucosa to calcium. Amer. J. Physiol. **208**, 370 (1965).

Harrison, M., and B. E. Nordin: Renal excretion of phosphorus and hypophosphataemia after parathyroidectomy. Brit. med. J. **1960 I**, No 5168, 245.

Hartles, R. L.: Bone remodelling factors. 2nd Symp. on calcified tissues, Liège 1964.

—, and A. G. Leaver: Citrate in mineralized tissues. I. Citrate in human dentine. Arch. oral Biol. **1**, 297—303 (1960).

Hastings, B., C. D. Murray, and J. Sendroy: Studies of the solubility of calcium salts. I. The solubility of calcium carbonate in salt solutions and biological fluids. J. biol. Chem. **71**, 723 (1927).

Hayek, E., u. H. Newesely: Über die Existenz von Tricalciumphosphat in wäßriger Lösung. Mh. Chem. **89**, 88 (1958).

Heaton, F.: The action of the parathyroid glands during magnesium deficiency in the rat. Biochem. J. **92**, 50 (1964).

Heidemann, E., and W. Riess: Über die Dichte von Collagen. Hoppe-Seylers Z. physiol. Chem. **334**, 224 (1963).

Heinz, E.: Untersuchungen über die Komplexverbindungen des Ca. Biochem. Z. **321**, 401 (1951).

Hekkelmann, J. W.: An enzymological study of bone metabolism and its regulation by parathyroid hormone. 2nd Symp. on calcified tissues, Liège 1964.

— Vortrag Leiden, Symposium Calcified tissues 1966.

Held, I. R., and S. Freeman: Binding of calcium by human plasma proteins under simulated physiologic conditions. J. app. Physiol. **19**, 292 (1964).

Hendricks, S. B., and W. L. Hill: The nature of bone and phosphate rock. Proc. nat. Acad. Sci. (Wash.) **36**, 731 (1950).

— — The inorganic constitution of bone. Science **96**, 255 (1942).

Hennemann, P. H., A. P. Forbes, M. Moldawer, E. F. Dempsey, and E. L. Carroll: Effects of human growth hormone in man. J. clin. Invest. **39**, 1223 (1950).

—, and S. Wallach: A review of the prolonged use of estrogens and androgens in postmenopausal and senile osteoporosis. Arch. intern. Med. **100**, 715 (1957).

Hennemann, R. H., G. M. Bourke, and W. P. Jackson: Depression of serum alkaline phosphatase activity by human serum albumin. J. biol. Chem. **213**, 19 (1955).

Henning, W., N. G. Schmal u. W. Theopold: Über Calcium-Citronensäure-Komplexe. Biochem. Z. **321**, 401 (1951a).

— u. W. Theopold: Über Citronensäure-Calcium-Komplexverbindungen. Z. Kinderheilk. **69**, 55 (1951).

Henschen, C., R. Strauman u. R. Bucher: Röntgenspectrographische Untersuchungen des Knochens. Dtsch. Z. Chir. **236**, 485 (1932).

Herring, G. M.: Comparison of bovine bone sialoprotein and serum orosounicoid. Nature (Lond.) **201**, 709 (1964).

Herring, G. M., and P. W. Kent: Some studies on microsubstances of bovine cortical bone. Biochem. J. **89**, 405—414 (1963).

Hess, W. C., and C. Lee: The presence of chondroitin sulfuric acid in dentine. J. dent. Res. **31**, 506 (1952).

Heuck, F.: Röntgenologische, historadiographische und chemischanalytische Untersuchungen der Konzentration und Verteilung im gesunden und kranken Knochen. Radiologia austriaca **14**, 29 (1963).

—, u. E. Schmidt: Die quantitative Bestimmung des Mineralgehaltes der Knochen im Röntgenbild. Die praktische Anwendung einer Methode zur quantitativen Bestimmung des Kalksalzgehaltes gesunder und kranker Knochen. Fortschr. Röntgenstr. **93**, 523 (1960); **93**, 761 (1960a).

Hevesy, G. Ch., H. B. Levi, and O. H. Rebbe: Rate of rejuvenation of the skeleton. Biochem. J. **34**, 532—537 (1940).

Heymann, W.: Metabolism and mode of action of vitamin D. II. Storage of vitamin D in different tissues in vivo. J. biol. Chem. **118**, 371—376 (1937).

Hiatt, H. H., P. A. Marks, and E. Shorr: Inhibitoren für die Ca-Ablagerung im Knorpel in vitro. J. biol. Chem. **204**, 187 (1953).

—, and D. D. Thompson: The effects of parathyroid extract on renal function in man. J. clin. Invest. **36**, 557 (1957).

Hills, G. M.: The metabolism of articular cartilage. Biochem. J. **34**, 1070—1077 (1940).

Hirsch, P. F., E. Voelkel, and P. L. Munson: Thyrocalcitonin: hypocalcemic hypophosphatemic principle of the thyroid gland. Science **146**, 412 (1964).

Hirsch, P. F., G. F. Gauthier, and P. L. Munson: Thyrocalcitonin. Endocrinology **70**, 244 (1963).

— — — Thyroid hypocalcemic principle and recurrent laryngeal nerve injury as factors affecting the response to parathyroidectomy in rats. Endocrinology **73**, 244 (1964a).

Hirschman, A., and A. E. Sobel: Composition of the mineral deposited during in vitro calcification in relation to the fluid phase. Arch. Biochem. **110**, 237 (1965).

— —, and I. Fankuchen: Calcifications Y an x-ray diffraction study of calcification in vitro in relation to composition. J. biol. Chem. **204**, 13 (1953).

— — B. Kramer, and I. Fankuchen: An x-ray diffraction study of high phosphate bones. J. biol. Chem. **171**, 285 (1947).

Hisamura, H.: Glucoproteid des Knochens. J. Biochem. (Tokyo) **28**, 473 (1938).

Hodge, H. C.: Some observations on the dynamics of calcification. (2nd Conf. Macy Foundation New York.) Metab. Interr. Transact. **73** (1950).

— Some achievements and problems in studying the solubility of the mineral of the hard tissues. Ann. N. Y. Acad. Sci. **60**, 661—669 (1955).

Hoehling, H. J., u. H. Newesely: Krystallisationsversuche und Elektronenbeugungsuntersuchungen zur Aufklärung der chemischen

Verbindung der „Carieskrystalle". Dtsch. Zahnärztebl. **15**, 706 (1961).

HOEHLING H. J., and J. VAHL: Organic matrix and crystal formation in different types of mineralization. 4th Eur. Symp. on calcified tissues, Leiden 1955, 56.

HÖRMANN, H.: 2nd Eur. Symp. on calcified tissues, Liège 1964. Diskussion zum Vortrag von Prof. TRISTRAM über: Collagen, an intercellular macromolecule.

HÖVELS, O., u. D. REISS: Physiologie und Stoffwechsel des D-Vitamins. Ergebn. inn. Med. Kinderheilk. **11**, 206—263 (1959).

HOFFMAN, A., G. LEHMANN u. E. WERTHEIMER: Der Glykogenbestand des Knorpels und seine Bedeutung. Pflügers Arch. ges. Physiol. **220**, 183 (1928).

HOLT, L. E.: Studies in calcification. II. Delayed equilibrium between the calcium phosphates and its biological significance. J. biol. Chem. **64**, 579 (1925b).

— V. K. LAMER, and H. B. CHOWN: Studies in calcification. II. Delayed equilibrium between the calcium phosphates and its biological significance. J. biol. Chem. **64**, 567 (1925).

— — — Studies in calcification. I. The solubility product of secondary and tertiary calcium phosphate under various conditions. J. biol. Chem. **64**, 509 (1925a).

HOWARD, P. J., W. S. WILDE, and R. L. MALVIN: Localization of renal calcium transport. Effect of calcium loads and of gluconate anion on water, sodium and potassium. Amer. J. Physiol. **197**, 337—341 (1959).

HOWELL, D., and L. CARSLON: Sulfur metabolism in cartilage. A study of calcifying regions for microscopic distribution of sulfur and relationship to staining by sudan black. Exp. Cell Res. **34**, 568 (1964).

HUGGINS, C.: The composition of bone and the function of the bone cell. Physiol. Rev. **17**, 119 (1937).

HURWITZ, S.: Bone composition and Ca^{45} retention in fowl as influenced by egg formation. Amer. J. Physiol. **206**, 198 (1964).

— Calcium turnover in different bone segments of laying fowl. Amer. J. Physiol. **208**, 203 (1965).

IBSEN, K. H., and M. R. CHRIST: Relationship between pyrophosphate content and oxytetracycline labelling of bone salt. Nature (Lond.) **203**, 761 (1964).

INGALLS, T. H., G. DONALDSON u. F. ALBRIGHT: Nephrektomie macht Knochenläsionen durch Azidose, PTH macht andere Läsionen. J. clin. Invest. **22**, 603 (1943).

ISAAC, S., F. BRUDEVOLD, F. A. SMITH, and D. E. GAIDNER: Solubility rate and natural fluoride content of surface and subsurface enamal. J. Dent. Res. **37**, 254—268 (1958).

JAHAN, E., and R. PITTS: Effect of parathyroid on renal tubular reabsorption of phosphate and calcium. Amer. J. Physiol. **155**, 42—49 (1948).

JANOWITZ, H. D., H. COLCHER, and F. HOLLANDER: Inhibition of gastric secretion of acid in dogs by carbonic anhydrase inhibitor 2-acetylamino-1,3,4-thiodiazol-5-sulfonamid. Amer. J. Physiol. **171**, 325 (1952).

JEFFAY, H., and H. R. BAYNE: Parathyroid hormone and release of calcium 45 from bone. Amer. J. Physiol. **206**, 415 (1964).

—, and H. R. BAYNE: Bone resorption and ^{45}Ca turnover in growing rats. Amer. J. Physiol. **200**, 335 (1961).

JEFFREE, G. M.: Comparative enzymology of osteoclasts and osteoblasts. 3rd Eur. Symp. on calcified tissues, Davos 1965.

JENNER, H. D., and H. D. KAY: The phosphatases of mammalian tissues. III. Magnesium and the phosphatase system. J. biol. Chem. **93**, 733 (1931).

JOHNSTON, C. C., and W. P. DEISS: Some effects of hypophysectomy and parathyroid extract on bone matrix biosynthesis. Endocrinology **76**, 198 (1965).

— —, and L. B. HOLMES: Effect of parathyroid extract on bone matrix hexosamine. Endocrinology **68**, 484 (1961).

— E. B. MUIER, W. M. SMITH, and W. P. DEISS: Influence of parathyroid activity on the chemical equilibrium of bone calcium in vitro. J. Lab. clin. Med. **60**, 689 (1962a).

JOHNSTON, C. C., W. P. DEISS, and E. B. MINER: Bone matrix biosynthesis in vitro. II. Effects of parathyroid hormone. J. biol. Chem. **237**, 3560 (1962).

JOSHI, J. G., and P. K. DIKSHIT: Effect of vitamin D on the phosphorus content of rachitic rat cartilage. Nature (Lond.) **177**, 4509 (1956).

JOWSEY, J.: The effect of parathyreoidectomy on haversian remodeling of bone. Endocrinology **63**, 903 (1958).

JUNG, W., u. G. STARK: Die alkalische Serumphosphatase im mütterlichen und kindlichen Blut nach Vitamin-D-Gaben in der Spätschwangerschaft. Arch. Kinderheilk. **154**, 23 (1956).

KAISER, H., J. GILL, A. SJOERDSMA, and F. BARTTER: Relation between urinary hydroxyproline and parathyroid function. J. clin. Invest. **43**, 1073 (1964).

KALLIOMÄKI, J. L., R. K. MARKKANEN, and V. A. MUSTONEN: Serum calcium and phosphorus homeostasis in man studied by means of the sodium-EDTA test. Acta med. scand. **170**, 211 (1961).

KAO, K.-Y. T., W. E. HITT, R. L. DAWSON, and TH. M. MACGAVACK: Connective tissue. VII. Changes in protein and hexosamine content of bone and cartilage of rats at different ages. Proc. Soc. exp. Biol. (N.Y.) **110**, 538 (1962).

KATZ, S., and I. M. KLOTZ: Interactions of calcium with serum albumin. Arch. Biochem. **44**, 351 (1953).

KAWIAK, J.: Presence of chondroitin sulphate in chondrocytes. Acta histochem. (Jena) **15**, 153 (1963).

KEANE, B. E., G. SPIEGLER. and R. DAVIS: Quantitative evaluation of bone mineral by a radiographic method. Brit. J. Radiol. **32**, 162 (1959).

KELLER, H., u. U. PETERS: Untersuchungen zur Frage der Bedeutung des Zinks für die Carboanhydratase. Hoppe-Seylers Z. physiol. Chem. **317**, 228 (1962).

KENNY, A. D.: Citric acid production by resorbing bone in tissue culture. Amer. J. Physiol. **197**, No 2 (1959).

— Survival and serum Ca-levels of rats after parathyroidectomy. Endocrinology **70**, 715 (1962a).

— Glycogenolytic action of epinephrine on mouse parietal bone. Endocrinology **71**, 901 (1962).

KHOO, E. C., and K. KOWALEWSKI: Effect of thyroid activity on in vitro bone calcium exchange. Endocrinology **77**, 582 (1965).

KIESOW, L.: Über den Stoffwechsel von Kulturhefen beim Wachstum. Z. Naturforsch. **14**b, 224 (1959).

KIMBERG, D. V.: Active transport of calcium by intestine: effects of dietary calcium. Amer. J. Physiol. **200**, 1256 (1961).

KLEIN, L., F. W. LAFFERTY, O. H. PEARSON, and P. H. CURTISS: Correlation of urinary hydroxyproline, serum alkaline phosphatase and skeletal calcium turnover. Metabolism **13**, 272 (1964).

KLEMENT, R.: Die Zusammensetzung der Knochenstützsubstanz. Hoppe-Seylers Z. physiol. Chem. **184**, 132 (1929).

— M. STREHLE u. H. GROSS: Zur Frage der Bindung des Ca an Serumproteine. II. Naturwissenschaften **8**, 246 (1953).

—, u. G. TRÖMEL: Hydroxyapatit, der Hauptbestandteil der anorganischen Knochen und Zahnsubstanz. Hoppe-Seylers Z. physiol. Chem. **213**, 263—269 (1932).

KLINKE, K., u. B. SCHILLERT: Calciumstoffwechsel und Citronensäure. Universitäts-Kinderklinik der Charité Berlin 1951.

KNESE, K. H.: Die Ultrastruktur des Knochengewebes. Dtsch. med. Wschr. **84**, 1640 (1959).

KÖRBER, F.: Der Carboanhydratase-Gehalt der Knochenzellen und seine mögliche physiologische Bedeutung. Inaug.-Diss. Berlin 1964.

KOWALEWSKI, K.: Uptake of radiosulfate in growing bones of cockerels treated with cortisone and certain anabolic-androgenic steroids. Endocrinology **63**, 759 (1958).

— Uptake of radiosulfur in growing bones of cockerels treated with cortisone and 17 ethyl-19 nortestosterone. Proc. Soc. exp. Biol.(N.Y.) **97**, 432 (1958a).

KRAMER, B., and M. J. SHEAR: Composition of bone. IV. Primary calcification. J. biol. Chem. **79**, 147 (1928).

KRANE, S. M.: Parathyroid damage in man: mechanism of effect on serum levels of calcium and phosphorus. J. clin. Endocr. **17**, 386 (1957).

—, and M. J. GLIMCHER: Protein phosphorus and phosphokinases in connective tissues. 3rd Eur. Symp. on calcified tissues, Davos 1965a.

— — Protein phosphorus and phosphokinases in connective tissue. In: Calcified tissues 1965. Proceedings of the third Eur. Symp. on calcified tissues held at Davos. Berlin-Heidelberg-New York: Springer 1966, p. 168—171.

KRANE, S. M., G. L. GORDON, J. B. STEINBERG, and H. CORRIGAN: The effect of thyroid disease on calcium metabolism in man. J. clin. Invest. **35**, 874 (1956).

— STONE, M. J., and M. J. GLIMCHER: The presence of protein phosphokinase ir connective tissues and the phosphorylation of enamel proteins in vitro. Biochim. biophys. Acta (Amst.) **97**, 77—87 (1965).

KREBS, H. A.: Zit. nach E. G. BYWATERS (1937).

KRETSINGER, R., G. MANNER, B. GOULD, and A. RICH: Synthesis of collagen on polyribosomes. Nature (Lond.) **202**, 438 (1964).

KROKOWSKI, E.: Die Absorption von Röntgenstrahlen im Knochen. Fortschr. Röntgenstr. **91**, 76 (1959).

— Quantitative Verlaufbeobachtung der Kalziumveränderung im Knochen mittels röntgenologischer Substanzanalyse. Fortschr. Röntgenstr. **100**, 359 (1964).

KROON, D. B.: Phosphatase and the formation of protein-carbohydrate complexes. Acta anat. (Basel) **15**, 317 (1952).

KÜHN, K., W. GRASSMANN u. U. HOFMANN: Über die Bildung der Collagenfibrillen aus gelöstem Collagen und die Funktion der kohlenhydrathaltigen Begleitkomponenten. Z. Naturforsch. **24**b, 436 (1959).

— — — Über den Aufbau der Collagenfibrille aus Tropocollagenmolekeln. Naturwissenschaften **47**, 258 (1960).

— J. KÜHN u. K. HANNIG: Einwirkung von Trypsin auf gelöstes Collagen. Hoppe-Seylers Z. physiol. Chem. **326**, 50 (1961).

—, u. E. ZIMMER: Eigenschaften des Tropocollagenmoleküls und deren Bedeutung für die Fibrillenbildung. Z. Naturforsch. **16**b, 648 (1961a).

— — P. WAYKOLE u. P. FIETZEK: Die Wirkung von Alkali auf Collagen. Die Änderung des Ladungsmusters der Tryptocollagenmoleküle sowie die Spaltung der intra- und intermolekularen Bindungen. Hoppe-Seylers Z. physiol. Chem. **333**, 209 (1963).

KUYPER, A. C.: The quantitative precipitation of citric acid. J. biol. Chem. **123**, 405 (1938).

LAAKE, H.: The action of corticosteroids on the renal reabsorption of calcium. Acta endocr. (Kbh) **34**, 60 (1960).

LAFFERTY, F. W., O. H. PEARSON, and P. H. CURTISS: Correlation of urinary hydroxyproline serum alkaline phosphatase and skeletal calcium turnover. Metabolism **13**, 272 (1964).

— G. E. SPENCER, and O. H. PEARSON: Effects of androgens, estrogens and high calcium intakes on bone formation and resorption in osteoporosis. Amer. J. Med. **36**, 514 (1964a).

LAMM, M., and W. F. NEUMANN: On the role of vitamin D in calcification. Arch. Path. **66**, 2 (1948).

LANZETTA, A.: Mineralisierung des ossifizierbaren Knorpels in vitro. Arzneimittel-Forsch. **13**, 149 (1963).

LARON, Z.: The action of cortisone on the teeth of rachitic rats. Arch. Path. **61**, 177 (1956).
— B. ARIE, and D. KENDE: Effectioness of growth hormone to prevent the alterations produced by 6-methylprednisolone (medrol) on the growing bone in rats. Endocrinology **72**, 470 (1963).
—, and J. H. BOSS: Comparative effect of corticosterone and cortisone on rat bones. Arch. Path. **73**, 274 (1962).
— J. D. CRAWFORD, and R. KLEIN: Phosphaturic effect of cortisone in normal and parathyroidectomized rats. Proc. Soc. exp. Biol. (N.Y.) **96**, 649 (1957).
— J. P. MUHLETHALER, and R. KLEIN: The interrelationship between cortisone and parathyroid extracts in rat. Arch. Path. **65**, 125 (1958).
LASH, J., S. HOLTZER, and H. HOLTZER: An experimental analysis of the development of the spinal column. Exp. Cell Res. **13**, 292—303 (1957).
LASKIN, D. M., and M. B. ENGEL: Bone metabolism and bone resorption after parathyroid extract. Arch. Path. **62**, 296 (1956).
— — Relations between the metabolism and structure of bone. Ann. N.Y. Acad. Sci. **85**, 421 (1960).
— B. G. SORNAT, and J. A. BAIN: Respiration and anaerobic glycolysis of transplanted cartilage. Proc. Soc. exp. Biol. (N.Y.) **79**, 474 (1952).
LASSITER, W. E., C. W. GOTTSCHALK, and M. MYLLE: Micropuncture study of renal tubular reabsorption of calcium in normal rodents. Fed. Proc. **21**, 435 (1962).
LAVENDER, A., and T. PULLMAN: Changes in inorganic phosphate excretion induced by renal arterial infusion of calcium. Amer. J. Physiol. **205**, 1025 (1963).
LAVROV, B., and E. TERENT'EVA: Reactions to experimental administration of large doses of vitamin D_2. Fed. Proc. **23**, T 908 (1964).
LEAVER, A. G., J. E. EASTOE, and R. L. HARTLES: Citrate in mineralized tissues. II. Arch. oral Biol. **2**, 120 (1960).
LEBLOND, C. P., L. F. BÉLANGER, and R. C. GREINLICH: Formation of bone and teeth as visualized by radioautography. Ann. N.Y. Acad. Sci. **60**, 631—659 (1955).
— G. W. WILKINSON, L. F. BELANGER, and J. ROBICHON: Radioautographic visulaization of bone formation in the rat. Amer. J. Anat. **80**, 289—341 (1950).
LEEKSMA, C., J. DE GRAEFF, and J. DE COCK: Hypercalcaemia in adrenal insufficiency. Acta med. scand. **156**, 455 (1957).
LENGEMAN, F. W.: Effects of thyroxine upon strontium and calcium metabolism of embryonic bone grown in vitro. Endocrinology **70**, 774 (1962).
LERCH, P., and C. VUILLEUMIER: Physico-chemical methods for the identification of microcrystalline basic calcium phosphates prepared in vitro. 3rd Eur. Symp. on calcified tissues, Davos 1965, p. 132.
LEVANDER, G.: A study of bone regeneration. Surg. Gynec. Obstet. **67**, 705 (1938).
— Über Knochenregeneration. Klin. Wschr. **20**, 40 (1941).
—, and N. WILLSTAEDT: Tissue induction. Nature (Lond.) **155**, 148 (1945).
— — Alcohol-soluble osteogenetic substance from bone marrow. Nature (Lond.) **157**, 587 (1946).
L'HEUREUX, M. V., W. R. TWEEDY, and E. M. ZORN: Excretion of radiocalcium by normal rats. Proc. Soc. exp. Biol. (N.Y.) **71**, 729 (1949).
LICHTWITZ, A.: Le metabolisme du calcium et les stéroides. Kalkstoffwechsel und Steroide. Sem. Hop. Paris **31**, 10, 554 (1955).
LIU, S. H., H. J. CHU, H. C. HSU, H. C. CHAO, and S. H. CHEU: Calcium and phosphorus metabolism. Osteomalacia. Pathogenetic role of pregnancy and relative importance of calcium and Vitamin D supply. J. clin. Invest. **20**, 255 (1941).
LINDQUIST, B.: Effect of vitamin D on the metabolism of radiocalcium in rachitic rats. Acta radiatrica, Suppl. **86**, 41 (1952).
— Über die chemische Dynamik des Knochenminerals. Helv. paediat. Acta **14**, 447 (1959).
— M. A. BUDY, F. C. MCLEAN, and J. L. HOWARD: Skeletal metabolism in estrogen-treated rats studied by means of Ca^{45}. Endocrinology **66**, 100—111 (1960).
LOBECK, CH. C., and R. E. STEINKRAUS: Effects of fasting, adrenalectomy and cortisol on bone composition and density. Amer. J. Physiol. **199**, 1087 (1960).
LOGAN, H. F., R. J. HAVEL, G. S. GORDON, and S. L. WHITTINGTON: Ultracentrifugal analysis of protein-bound and free calcium in human serum. J. biol. Chem. **235**, 3654 (1960).
LOGAN, M. A.: Composition of cartilage, bone, dentin and enamel. J. biol. Chem. **110**, 375—389 (1935).
— Recent advances in the chemistry of calcification. Physiol. Rev. **20**, 522 (1940).
—, and L. W. KANE: Solubility of bone salt. IV. Solubility of bone in biological fluids. J. biol. Chem. **127**, 705 (1939).
LORCH, I.: Demonstration of phosphatase in decalcified bone. Nature (Lond.) **158**, 209 (1946).
LOTMAR, R.: Der Einbau von ^{35}S in die Kostalknorpel von Meerschweinchen unter dem Einfluß verschiedener Glucocorticoide. Experientia (Basel) **16**, 303 (1960).
LUTWAK, L., and J. R. SHAPIRO: Calcium absorption in man: based on large volume liquid scintillation counter studies. Science **144**, 1155 (1964).
LUTWAK-MANN, C.: Aminopolysaccharide sulfate-proteincomplexes. Biochem. J. **34**, 517—528 (1940).
MCCONNELL, D.: The application of mineralogical theories to the "mineral" phase of teeth and bones. Biochim. biophys. Acta (Amst.) **17**, 450 (1955).
MACGREGOR, J., and W. BROWN: Blood: bone equilibrium in calcium homoeostasis. Nature (Lond.) **205**, 359 (1965).

MacGregor, J., and B. E. Nordin: Equilibration studies with human bone powder. J. biol. Chem. **235**, 1215 (1960).
— — Equilibration studies with human bone powder. II. The role of the carbonate ion. J. biol. Chem. **237**, 2704 (1962).
— — Effect of bicarbonate on the behaviour of the ions of human bone powder in vitro. Nature (Lond.) **193**, 65 (1962a).
McIntyre, I.: Calcitonin. Melsunger Berichte, Symp. Kassel 1966.
— S. Boss, and V. A. Troughton: Parathyroid hormone and magnesium homoeostasis. Nature (Lond.) **198**, 1058 (1963).
— G. V. Foster, and M. A. Kumar: Calcium metabolism. Proc. roy. Soc. Med. **57**, 865 (1964).
— — — In: The parathyroid gland, p. 89 (Galliard/Talmage/Budy). Chicago: University Press 1965.
McKay, H., M. B. Patton, M. S. Pittman, G. Stearns, and N. Edelbluete: Effect of vitamin D on calcium retentions. J. Nutr. **26**, 153—159 (1943).
MacLagan, N. F., and A. J. Anderson: Colloidal properties of urinary mucopolysaccharides. Ciba-Symp. on the chemistry and biology of mucopolysaccharides. London: J. & A. Churchill 1958.
McLean, F. C., and A. B. Hastings: The state of calcium in the fluids of the body. J. biol. Chem. **108**, 285 (1935).
MacLeod, L.: Ionized calcium and magnesium in serum. Biochem. J. **91**, 29 P—30 P (1964).
McPherson, G. D.: Estimation of the exchangeable pool in children using ^{48}Ca. 3nd Eur. Symp. on calcified tissues, Davos 1965.
Majno, G., u. C. Rouiller: Die alkalische Phosphatase in der Biologie des Knochengewebes. Histochemische Untersuchungen. Virchows Arch. path. Anat. **32**, 1 (1951).
Manner, G., and B. Gould: Collagen biosynthesis. The formation of hydroxyproline and soluble-ribonucleic acid complexes of proline and hydroxyproline by chick embryo in vivo and by a subcellular chick embryo system. Biochim. biophys. Acta (Amst.) **72**, 243—250 (1963).
Manunta, G., J. Saroff, and C. W. Turner: Metabolism of Ca^{45} in blood, bones and young of lactating rats treated with estradiol. Proc. Soc. exp. Biol. (N. Y.) **94**. 788 (1957).
— — — Relationship between estradiol and parathyroid on retention of Ca^{45} in bone and blood serum of rats. Proc. Soc. exp. Biol. (N. Y.) **94**, 785 (1957a).
— — — Paper electrophoretic study of Ca^{45} binding in sera. Proc. Soc. exp. Biol. (N. Y.) **94**, 790 (1957b).
Marks, P. A., and E. Shorr: Factors which regulate the deposition of Ca and S in rachitic cartilage in vitro. Metabol. Interr. Transact. J. M. Fond. **2**, 191 (1950).
— — A method for evaluating the relation of glycogen to unorganic salt deposition in surviving cartilage slices in vitro. Science **112**, 752 (1950a).
Marks, P. A., H. H. Hiatt u. E. Shorr: Faktoren, die die Ca- und Sr-Einlagerung im Knorpel in vitro beeinflussen. J. biol. Chem. **204**, 175 (1953).
Marshall, R., and M. D. Urist: Origins of current ideas about calcification. Clin. Orthop. Rel. Res. **44**, 13—39 (1966).
Martland, M., and R. Robison: The possible significance of hexosephosphoric esters in ossification. V. The enzyme in the early stages of bone development. Biochem. J. **18**, 1354—1357 (1924).
Mathies, J. C., and O. H. Gaebler: The effect of growth hormone preparations on alkaline phosphatase of the tibia. Endocrinology **45**, 129 (1949).
— E. D. Goodman, and L. Palen: Effects of hypophysectomy, growth hormone and thyroxine on phosphatases of tibia, cliver spleen and kidney of rat. Amer. J. Physiol. **168**, 352 (1952).
Matsuda, N.: Effect of cortisone, DOCA and ACTH upon calcification, of rabbit dentine and amount of serum calcium, inorganic phosphate and total protein. Gunma J. med. Sci. **5**, No 4 (1956).
Mayo, K. M.: II. Quantitative measurement of bone mineral content in normal adult bone. Brit. J. Radiol. **34**, 693 (1961).
Mazznoli, G. F., and L. Terrenato: Intestinal absorption and skeletal dynamic of calcium in acromegaly. In: Calcified tissues (Fleisch), p. 254. London: Blackwood 1965.
Mecca, C., G. R. Martin, E. Schiffmann, and P. Goldhaber: Alteration in citrate metabolism in parathyroid extract-treated calvaria. Proc. Soc. exp. Biol. (N. Y.) **117**, 721 (1964).
Menzel, J., A. S. Pomer, H. Schraer, G. Pakis, and R. C. Likens: Comparative fixation of Sr^{89} and Ca^{45} by calcified tissues as related to fluoride induced changes in crystallinity. Proc. Soc. exp. Biol. (N. Y.) **110**, 609 (1962).
Mergenhagen, St. E., G. R. Martin, A. A. Rizzo, S. W. Wright, and D. Scott: Calcification in vivo of implanted collagen. Biochim. biophys. Acta (Amst.) **43**, 562—565 (1965).
Meyer, K : The mucopolysaccharides of bone. In: Bone structure and metabolism (G. E. W. Wolstenholme and C. M. O'Connor). Ciba Foundation Symp. London: J. & A. Churchill Ltd. 1956.
— E. Davidson, A. Linker, and P. Hoffman: The acid mucopolysaccharides of connective tissue. Biochim. biophys. Acta (Amst.) **21**, 506—518 (1956a).
Micoz, F. R.: Intestinal absorption of Ca-45 and Sr-85 as affected by the alkaline earths and pH. Proc. Soc. exp. Biol. (N. Y.) **110**, 273 (1962).
Migicovsky, B. B., and A. R. G. Emslie: Interaction of calcium, phosphorus and vitamin D. III. Study of mode of action of vitamin D using Ca^{45}. Arch. Biochem. **20**, 325 (1949).
—, and S. Jamieson: Calcium resorption and vitamin D. Canad. J. Biochem. **33**, 202 (1955).

Milhaud, G., A. Cherian, and M. Monkhtar: Calcium metabolism in the rat studies with calcium[45]: Effect of age. Proc. Soc. exp. Biol. (N.Y.) **114**, 382 (1963).

Miller, Z. B., J. Waldman, and F. C. Melean: The effect of dyes on the calcification of hypertrophic rachitic cartilage in vitro. J. exp. Med. **95**, 497 (1952).

Mills, B., and L. Bavetta: Effect of parathyroid extract on succinic dehydrogenase activity in young rats bone and kin. Proc. Soc. exp. Biol. (N.Y.) **118**, 273 (1965).

Moeller, H., u. G. Trömel: Bildung schwer löslicher Calciumphosphate aus wäßriger Lösung und die Beziehung dieser Phosphate zur Apatitgruppe. Z. anorg. Chem. **206**, 227 (1932).

Morey, E., and A. D. Kenny: Effects of catecholamines on urinary calcium and phosphorus in intact and parathyroidectomized rats. Endocrinology **75**, 78 (1964).

Morgulis, S.: Studies on the chemical composition of bone ash. J. biol. Chem. **93**, 455 (1931).

Morii, H., Fujita, and S. Okinaka: Effect of vagotomy and atropine on recovery from induced hypocalcemia. Endocrinology **72**, 173 (1963).

Morris, K. M., and T. G. Taylor: The effect of parathyroid extract on the activity of four acid hydrolases in the plasma of the domestic fowl. 4th Eur. Symp. on calcified tissues, Leiden 1966.

Moss, J. A.: The carbohydrate of collagen. Biochem. J. **61**, 151—153 (1955).

Motzok, I., and H. D. Branion: Studies on alkaline phosphatases. Biochem. J. **80**, 5 (1961).

Müller, E.: Zur Frage der Bindung des Ca im Serum. Naturwissenschaften **16**, 442 (1953).

Mueller, W., R. Schraer, and H. Schraer: Calcium metabolism and skeletal dynamics of laying pullets. Nutrition **84**, 20 (1954).

Muendez, J.: Density of fat and bone mineral of the mammalian body. Metabolism **9**, 472 (1960).

Muhler, J. C.: Effect of fluorides and other solutions on solubility of powdered enamel in acid. Proc. Soc. exp. Biol. (N.Y.) **92**, 849 (1956).

Muller, S. A., A. S. Posner, and H. E. Firschhein: Effect of vitamin D deficiency on the crystal chemistry of bone mineral. Proc. Soc. exp. Biol. (N.Y.) **121**, 844—846 (1966).

Mulryan, B. J., M. Neuman, W. Neuman, and T. Y. Toribara: Equilibration between tissue calcium and injected radiocalcium in the rat. Amer. J. Physiol. **207**, 947 (1964).

Munro, D. S.: The effects of sodium depletion on bone sodium. Proc. roy. Soc. Med. **52**, 258 (1959).

Munson, P. L.: Studies on the role of the parathyroids in calcium and phosphorus metabolism. Ann. N.Y. Acad. Sci. **60**, 776 (1955).

Murphy, W. R., W. H. Daughaday, and C. Hartnett: The effect of hypophysectomy and growth hormone on the incorporation of labeled sulfate into tibial epiphyseal and nasal cartilage of the rat. J. Lab. clin. Med. **47**, 715 (1956).

Nassim, J. R., P. S. Saville, and L. Mulligan: The effect of stilbestrol on urinary PO_4 excretion. Clin. Sci. **15**, 367 (1956).

Nebergall, W. N., and G. Kühl: An investigation of the composition and structure of dental enamel using ignition methods. Naturwissenschaften **47**, 254 (1960).

Neuberg, C., and J. Mandl: Functions of ATP and other phosphoric and derivates. Arch. Biochem. **23**, 499 (1949).

Neuberger, A., and H. G. Slack: The metabolism of collagen from liver, bone skin and tendon in the normal rat. Biochem. J. **53**, 47—52 (1953).

Neuman, W. F.: Bone as an problem in surface chemistry. Trans. Macy Conf. on Metabol. Interr. **2**, 33 (1950).

— R. Bjornerstedt, and B. J. Mulryan: Synthetic hydroxyapatite crystals. II. Aging and strontium incorporation. Arch. Biochem. **101**, 215 (1963).

— V. Disbefano u. B. J. Mulryan: J. biol. Chem. **193**, 227 (1951).

—, and B. J. Mulryan: The surface chemistry of bone. I. Recrystallization. J. biol. Chem. **185**, 705 (1950a).

—, and M. W. Neuman: Ion exchange in bone material. Chem. Rev. **53**, 1 (1953).

— T. Y. Toribara, and B. J. Mulryan: Synthetic hydroxyapatite crystals. Sodium and potassium fixation. Arch. Biochem. **98**, 384 (1962).

—, and H. J. Weikel: Recrystallisation in bone mineral. Ann. N.Y. Acad. Sci. **60**, 685 (1955).

Newesely, H.: Darstellung von „Oktacalciumphosphat" (Tetracalciumhydrogentriphosphat) durch homogene Kristallisation. Mh. Chem. **91**, 1020 (1960).

— Umwandlungsvorgänge bei Calciumphosphaten. 3rd Eur. Symp. on calcified tissues, Davos 1965, p. 136.

— Habil.-Schr. Berlin 1966.

Nichols, G., and N. Nichols: The role of bone in sodium metabolism. Metabolism **5**, 438 (1956).

Nicolaysen, R.: Studies upon the mode of action of vitamin D. Biochem. J. **31**, 107—121, 122—129 (1937).

— The absorption of calcium as a function of the body saturation with calcium. Acta physiol. scand. **5**, 200 (1943).

— The influence of vitamin D on the absorption of calcium from the intestine of rats. Acta physiol. scand. **22**, 260 (1951).

—, and N. Eeg-Larsen,: The mode of action of vitamin D. In: Bone structure and metabolism (G. E. Wolstenholme and C. M. O'Connor). London: J. & A. Churchill 1956.

Niepmann, W.: Experimentelle Untersuchungen zur intestinalen Calcium-Resorption in Abhängigkeit von der Magenacidität beim Menschen. Klin. Wschr. **39**, 1064 (1961).

NIVEN, J. S., and R. ROBISON: The development of the calcifying mechanism in the long bones of the rabbit. Biochem. J. **28**, 2237—2242 (1934).

NORDIN, B. E.: Assessment of calcium excretion. Lancet **1959 II**, 368.

— Hormones and calcium metabolism. Symp. on calcified tissues, Davos 1965a.

— H. FLEISCH, H. J. BLACKWOOD, and M. OWEN: Hormones in calcified tissues, p. 226. Berlin-Heidelberg-New York: Springer 1965.

— D. A. SMITH, I. MACFADYEN, and S. JOHNSTON: The relation between urinary hydroxyprolin and calcium balance in osteoporosis. 2nd Eur. Symp. on calcified tissues, Liège 1964.

NORMAN, A. W., and H. F. DELUCA: Vitamin D and the incorporation of (1-^{14}C) acetate into the organic acids of bone. Biochem. J. **91**, 124—130 (1964).

— — The subcellular location of H^3 vitamin D_3 in kidney and intestine. Arch. Biochem. **107**, 69 (1964a).

— J. LUND, and H. DELUCA: Biologically active forms of vitamin D_3 in kidney and intestine. Arch. Biochem. **108**, 12 (1964b).

OEFF, K., W. SCHWARZKOPFF u. J. M. SCHMIDT-RHODE: Untersuchungen zur Dynamik des Calciumstoffwechsels beim Menschen mit Calcium. Klin. Wschr. **40**, 904 (1962).

OESER, H., and E. KROKOWSKI: Quantitative analysis of inorganic substances in the body. Brit. J. Radiol. **36**, 274 (1963).

ONESON, I., and J. ZACHARIAS: The role of the carbohydrate moiety in the structure of the collagen fibril. Arch. Biochem. **89**, 271 (1960).

ORIMO, H., T. FUJITA, H. MORII, and K. NAKAO: Role of the kidney in recovery from induced hypocalcemia. Endocrinology **75**, 857 (1964).

OTTENJANN, R., F. WIDMEIER u. L. DEMLING: Hypercalcämie und Magensekretion. Klin. Wschr. **41**, 717 (1963).

PARSONS, V., and J. ANDERSON: The maximal renal tubular reabsorptive rate for inorganic phosphate in thyreotoxicosis. Clin. Sci. **27**, 313 (1964).

PEARSE, A. G.: Enzyme cytochemistry and elucidation of bone cell structure. 4th Eureopean Symposium on calcified tissues, Leiden (1966).

PAUTARD, F. G.: Mineralization of keratin and its comparison with the enamel matrix. Nature (Lond.) **199**, 531 (1963).

PECHET, M. M., E. L. CARROLL, and L. S. JACOBS: Studies concerning the nature of the adrenal androgen in man: a specific structural requirement for somatotropic and androgenic activity as measured by the effects on the metabolism of nitrogen, calcium, phosphorus, sodium and potassium. Metabolism **11**, 167 (1962).

PERKINS, H. R., and T. F. DIXON: Parathyroid and bone citrogenase. Science **118**, 139 (1953).

PETERKOFSKY, A., and S. UDENFRIEND: Conversion of proline to collagen hydroxyproline in a cell-free system from chick embryo. J. biol. Chem. **238**, 3966—3977 (1963).

PFAUNDLER, S. v.: Über die Elemente der Gewebsverkalkung und ihre Beziehung zur Rachitisfrage. Jb. Kinderheilk. **60**, 123 (1904).

PFEIFFER, C. A., and W. U. GARDNER: Skeletal changes and blood serum calcium level in pigeons receiving estrogens. Endocrinology **23**, 485 (1938).

PICARD, J., et P. CARTIER: La mineralisation du cartilage ossifiable. IX. Fixation de diverses formes de phosphore par le cartilage ossifiable de rat jeune normal et de rat jeune rachitique. Bull. Soc. Chim. biol. (Paris) **42**, 1105 (1960).

— A. GARDAIS, and L. DUBERNARD: Presence of sulphated nucleotides in the epiphyseal growth cartilage of the rat. Nature (Lond.) **202**, 1213 (1964).

PIEZ, K. A.: Amino acid composition of some calcified proteins. Science **134**, 841 (1961).

—, and J. GROSS: The amino acid composition of some fish collagens: the relation between composition and structure. J. biol. Chem. **235**, 995 (1960a).

— E. WEISS, and M. S. LEWIS: The separation and characterization of the α- and β-components of calf skin collagen. J. biol. Chem. **235**, 1987—1991 (1960).

PITKÄNEN, E.: The pyrophosphatase activity in human blood serum. Scand. J. clin. Lab. **12**, 143 (1960).

POLIN, D., and P. D. STURKIE: The influence of the parathyroids on blood calcium levels and shell deposition in laying hens. Endocrinology **60**, 778 (1957).

— — The blood calcium response of the chicken to parathyroid extracts. Endocrinology **60**, 1 (1957a).

— — Parathyroid and gonad relationship in regulating blood calcium fractions in chickens. Endocrinology **63**, 177 (1958).

POLONOWSKI, M., et P. CARTIER: In vitro calcification. Sur le premier stade biochimique de l'ossification. C. R. Acad. Sci. (Paris) **232**, 119 (1951).

POSNER, A. S., E. D. EANES, and I. ZIPKIN: X-ray diffraction. Analysis of the effect of fluoride on bone, p. 79. 2nd Eur. Symp. on calcified tissues, Liège 1964.

POST, M., and W. C. SHOEMAKER: Bone electrolyte response to intravenous acid loads. Surg. Gynec. Obstet. **115**, 749 (1962).

PRASAD, A. S.: Studies on ultrafiltrable calcium. Arch. intern. Med. **105**, 560 (1960).

—, and E. B. FLINK: The base binding property of the serum proteins with respect to calcium. J. Lab. clin. Med. **51**, 345 (1958).

PROCKOP, D., A. KLAPAN, and S. UDENFRIEND: Oxygen-18 studies on the conversion of proline to collagen hydroxyproline. Arch. Biochem. **101**, 499 (1963).

— B. PETERKOFSKI, and S. UDENFRIEND: Studies on the intracellular localization of collagen synthesis in the intact chick embryo. J. biol. Chem. **237**, 1581 (1962).

Proell, F., u. A. Diener: Modell- und Tierversuche zum Problem der Verkalkung von Knochen. Z. Zellforsch. **18**, 244—253 (1933).

Quicker, R.: Unveröffentlichte Untersuchungen (1968).

— u. H.-J. Dulce: Octacalciumphosphat im Zahnschmelz und seine Beziehung zur Karies. Dtsch. zahnärztl. Z. (1967) (im Druck).

Raaflaub, J.: Über die Basisität der Knochenmineralien. Experientia (Basel) **17**, 443 (1961).

— Nebenschilddrüsen, Knochensystem und Säure-Basen-Haushalt. Schweiz. med. Wschr. **91**, 1417 (1961a).

Raeiha, C. E., and O. Forsander: The activation of vitamin D of the phosphorylation of thiamin. Science **115**, 242 (1952).

— — Vitamin D and phosphorylation of thiamin. Acta paediat. scand. **43**, Suppl. 100, 541 (1954).

Ragan, Ch., and A. M. Briscoe: Effect of exercise of the metabolism of ^{40}calcium and of ^{47}calcium in man. J. clin. Endocr. **24**, 385 (1964).

Raisz, L. G.: Inhibition of actinomycin D on bone resorption induced by parathyroid hormone of vitamin A. Proc. Soc. exp. Biol. (N. Y.) **119**, 614 (1965).

— W. Y. Au, and P. Stern: Regulation of parathyroid activity. The parathyroid glands, p. 50. Chicago: Chicago University Press 1965a.

— W. Y. Au, and J. Tepperman: Effect of changes in parathyroid activity on bone metabolism in vitro. Endocrinology **68**, 783—794 (1961).

Raisz, L. G.: Stimulation of bone resorption by parathyroid hormone in tissue culture. Nature (Lond.) **197**, 1015 (1963).

Ranney, R. E.: Antagonism between estrone and parathyroid extract in their effects upon bone accretion. Endocrinology **65**, 595 (1959).

— The effect of estrogens on bone phosphate accretion, resorption, and exchange in mice. Endocrinology **64**, 783 (1959a).

— The effect of estrone and parathyroid extract on bone citrate metabolism. Endocrinology **67**, 166—169 (1960).

Rasmussen, H.: The nature and properties of the parathyroid hormone. First int. Congr. of endocrinology Copenhagen 1960.

— Parathyroid hormone. Nature and mechanism of action. Amer. J. Med. **30**, 112—128 (1961).

— H. DeLuca, Cl. Arnaud, Ch. Hawker, and M. v. Stedingk: The relationship between vitamin D and parathyroid hormone. J. clin. Invest. **42**, 967—968 (1963).

— — — — — The relationship between vitamin D and parathyroid hormone. J. clin. Invest. **42**, 1940 (1963a).

—, and E. Reifenstein jr.: The parathyroid glands. In: Textbook of endocrinology, ed. by R. H. Williams. Philadelphia and London: W. B. Saunders Press 1962.

— J. Fischer, and C. Arnaud: Parathyroid hormone, ion exchange, and mitochondrial swelling. Proc. nat. Acad. Sci. (Wash.) **52**, 1198 (1964).

Reen, R. van: Metabolic activity in calcified tissues activities aconitase and isocitricodehydrogenase activities in rabbit and dog femurs. J. biol. Chem. **234**, 1951 (1959).

— Metabolism in calcified tissues: pyridine nucleotidases of the rabbit femur. Arch. Biochem. **93**, 242 (1961).

Rehm, W. S., and A. J. Enelow: The effect of thiocyanate on gastric potential and secretion. Amer. J. Physiol. **144**, 701 (1945).

Reidenberg, M. M.: The role of sodium depletion on bone sodium. Arch. intern. Med. **107**, 578 (1961).

Reifenstein, E. C., and F. Albright: The metabolic effects of steroid hormones in osteoporosis. J. clin. Invest. **26**, 24 (1947).

Reis, J. L.: Studies on 5-nucleotidase and its distribution in human tissues. Biochem. J. **46**, XXI—XXII (1950).

Rich, A., and F. H. Crick: (a) The structure of collagen. Nature (Lond.) **176**, 915—916 (1955).

— — (b) The molecular structure of collagen. J. molec. Biol. **3**, 483—506 (1961).

Richelle, L.: Le calcium échangeable de la substance minérale de l'os, étudiée à l'aide du ^{45}Ca. VI. Pourcentage d'échange apparent et remaniement en milieux aqueux et alcoolique. Bull. Soc. Chim. biol. (Paris) **42**, 1125 (1960).

Robison, R., M. MacLeod, and A. H. Rosenheim: The possible significance of hexose phosphoric esters in ossification, IX. part. Biochem. J. **24**, 1927 (1930a).

—, and A. H. Rosenheim: Calcification of hypertroph. Knorpel in vitro. Biochem. J. **28**, 684 (1934).

—, and K. M. Soames: The possible significance of hexosephosphoric esters in ossification. Biochem. J. **24**, 1922 (1930).

Robinson, R. A.: An electron-microscopic study of the crystalline inorganic component of bone and its relationship to the organic matrix. J. Bone Jt Surg. A **39**, 389 (1952).

—, and S. R. Elliott: The water content of bone. J. Bone Jt Surg. A **39**, 167 (1957).

—, and M. L. Watson: Crystall-collagen relationship in bone as observed in the electron microscope. Ann. N.Y. Acad. Sci. **60**, 596 (1955).

Rogers, H. J.: Concentration and distribution of polysaccharide in human cortical bone and the dentine of teeth. Nature (Lond.) **164**, 625 (1949).

— The polysaccharide associated with the organic matrix of bone. Biochem. J. **49**, XII—XIII (1951).

— S. M. Weidmann, and A. Parkinson: Studies on the skeletal tissues. The collagen content of bones from rabbits, oxen and humans. Biochem. J. **50**, 537 (1952).

Rooks, W. H., and R. I. Dorfman: The effect of various steroids on the incorporation of radiosulfur by the growing bones of cockerels. Metabolism **12**, 242 (1963).

Roseberry, H. H., A. B. Hastings, and J. K. Morse: X-ray analysis of bone and teeth. J. biol. Chem. **90**, 395 (1931).

Roth, F.: Die Wirkung der Oestrogene auf den Kalziumspiegel. Gynaecologia (Basel) **152**, 312 (1961).

Roth, H.: Extraktversuche mit konserviertem Knochengewebe. Schweiz. med. Wschr. **80**, 1051 (1950).

Rovner, D. R., D. H. Streeten, L. H. Luis, C. T. Stevenson, and J. W. Conn: Content and uptake of sodium and potassium in bone. Influence of adrenalectomy, aldosterone, desoxycorticosterone and spironolactone. J. clin. Endocr. **23**, 938 (1963).

Rubin, P. S., and J. R. Howard: Histochemical studies on the role of acid metabolism in calcifiability and calcification. First conference 1949. Metab. Interrel. New York: J. Macy, Found. p. 155.

Ruiz-Gijon, J.: Über die chemische Zusammensetzung der Knochen bei Hungerzuständen. Biochem. Z. **308**, 59—63 (1941).

Sallis, J. D., H. DeLuca, and H. Rasmussen: Parathyroid hormone-dependent uptake of inorganic phosphate by mitochondria. J. biol. Chem. **238**, 4098 (1963).

— — — Parathyroid hormone stimulation of phosphate uptake by rat liver mitochondria. Res. Commun. **10**, 266 (1963a).

Sallis, J. D., and E. S. Holdsworth: Influence of vitamin D on calcium absorption in the chick. Amer. J. Physiol. **203**, 497 (1962).

— — Calcium metabolism in relation to vitamin D_3 and adrenal function in the chick. Amer. J. Physiol. **203**, 506 (1962a).

Samiy, A. H., P. Hirsch, and A. Ramsay: Localization of phosphaturic effect of parathyroid hormone in nephron of the dog. Amer. J. Physiol. **208**, 73 (1965).

Samiy, A. H.: Localization of the renal tubular action of parathyroid hormone. Endocrinology **67**, 266 (1960).

Sataline, L. R., C. Powell, and G. Hamwi: Suppression of the hypercalcemia of thyrotoxicosis by corticosteroids. New Engl. J. Med. **267**, 646 (1962).

Schachter, D., W. B. Dowdle, and H. Schenker: Active transport of calcium by the small intestine of the rat. Amer. J. Physiol. **198**, 263 (1960).

— — — Accumulation of Ca^{45} by slices of the small intestine. Amer. J. Physiol. **198**, 275 (1960a).

— J. D. Finkelstein, and S. Kowarski: Metabolism of vitamin D. I. Preparation of radioactive vitamin D and its intestinal absorption in the rat. J. clin. Invest. **43**, 787 (1964).

— D. V. Kimberg, and H. Schenker: Active transport of calcium by intestine: action and bio-assay of vitamin D. Amer. J. Physiol. **200**, 1263 (1961).

— S. Kowarski, and J. Finkelstein: Vitamin D_3: direct action on the small intestine of the rat. Science **143**, 143 (1964a).

Schaefer, H. E., u. A. Schaefer: Über die durch Parathormon-Gesamtextrakt bedingte Änderung der Phosphor- und Calciumausscheidung im Urin. Z. klin. Med. **157**, 382 (1962).

Schajowicz, F., and R. Carbrini: Histochemical distribution of succinic dehydrogenase in bone and cartilage. Science **131**, 1043 (1960).

—, and R. Carbrini: Histochemical localization of acid phosphatase in bone tissue. Science **127**, 1447 (1958).

— — Demonstration of a phosphamidasic activity in bone tissue. Acta histochem. (Jena) **17**, 371 (1964).

Schartum, S., and G. Nichols: Influence of adrenal glucocorticoids on distribution of calcium and phosphorus between bone and its surrounding fluids. Proc. Soc. exp. Biol. (N.Y.) **108**, 228 (1961).

— — Concerning pH gradients between the extracellular compartment and fluids bathing the bone cluneral surface and their relation to Ca-ion distribution. J. clin. Invest. **41**, 1163 (1962).

Schatz, A., and J. J. Martin: Destruction of bone and tooth by proteolysis chelation: Its inhibition by fluoride and application to dental caries. N.Y. J. Dent. **30**, 124 (1960).

Schiffmann, E., B. A. Corcoran, and G. R. Martin: The role of complexed heavy metals in initiating the mineralization of "elastin" and the precipitation of mineral from solution. Arch. Biochem. **115**, 87—94 (1966).

Schlager, F.: Vorkommen und Lokalisation der β-D-Galactosidase in Knochen, Knorpel und im benachbarten Gewebe der weißen Maus. Acta histochem. (Jena) **8**, 176—184 (1959).

— β-D-Glucosidaseaktivität in Knochen, Knorpel und skeletalmuskulatur. Acta histochem. **9**, 320—328 (1960).

Schmalzried, H.: Stofftransport in Ionenkristallen und seine Bedeutung für Reaktionen in festem Zustand. Naturwissenschaften **50**, 62 (1963).

Schmid, A.: Beeinflussung der renalen Ausscheidung von Strontium, Calcium und Phosphat durch Pyridoxin, Pyridoxal und Pyridoxinsäure. Arzneimittel-Forsch. **15**, 28 (1965).

—, u. K. Zipf: Wirkung hoher Parathormondosen auf das Verhalten von Strontium und Calcium in Knochen und Blutserum. Ein Beitrag zum Wirkungsmechanismus von Parathormon. Biochem. Z. **333**, 529 (1961).

Schraer, H., A. S. Posner, R. Schraer, and I. Zipkin: Effect of fluoride on bone "crystallinity" in the growing rat. Biochim. biophys. Acta **64**, 565 (1962).

Schryver, H., and R. Gwatkon: Effect of alkaline media on the growth of embryonic tibiotarsi in organ culture. Nature (Lond.) **202**, 822 (1964).

Schulthess-Sallmann, B. v.: Der Einfluß experimenteller Azidose und Alkalose auf die Ultrafiltrierbarkeit des Plasmakalziums und die Kalziumausscheidung im Urin beim Menschen. Helv. med. Acta **25**, 601 (1958).

Sendroy, J., and A. B. Hastings: Studies of the solubility of calcium phosphate in salt solutions and biological fluids. J. biol. Chem. **71**, 783 (1927).

Sendroy, J., and A. B. Hastings: Studies of the solubility of calcium salts. III. The solubility of calcium carbonate and tertiary calcium-phosphate under various conditions. J. biol. Chem. **71**, 797 (1927a).

Shamos, M. H., L. S. Lavine, and M. I. Shamos: Piezoelectric effects in bone. Nature (Lond.) **197**, 81 (1963).

Shear, M. J., and B. Kramer: Composition of bone. J. biol. Chem. **79**, 125 (1928).

Shelling, D., B. Kramer, and E. Orent: Studies upon calcification in vitro. J. biol. Chem. **77**, 157 (1928).

Shetlar, M. R., R. Howard, W. Joel, C. L. Courtright, and E. C. Reifenstein: The effects of parathyroid hormone on serum glycoprotein and seromucoid levels and on the kidney of the rat. Endocrinology **59**, 532 (1956).

Shipley, P. G., B. Kramer, and J. Howland: Studies upon calcification in vitro. Biochem. J. **20**, 379 (1926).

Shorr, E.: The possible usefulness of estrogens and aluminium hydroxide gels in the management of renal stones. J. Urol. (Baltimore) **53**, 507 (1945).

Siegmund, P., u. H.-J. Dulce: Zur Biochemie der Knochenauflösung. I. Einfluß des Carboanhydratase-Inhibitors 2-Acetamino-1.3.4-thiodiazol-sulfonamid-(5) (Diamox) auf den Calciumstoffwechsel von Legehennen. Hoppe-Seylers Z. physiol. Chem. **320**, 149—159 (1960).

— — Zur Biochemie der Knochenauflösung. IV. Einfluß von Thiocyanat auf den Calciumstoffwechsel bei Legehennen. Hoppe-Seylers Z. physiol. Chem. **320**, 212—217 (1960a).

— — F. Körber u. E. Schütte: Über den Einfluß von Carboanhydraseinhibitoren auf erhöhte Plasma-Calcium-Werte und das Vorkommen von Carboanhydrase (CAH) im Epiphysenknorpel und Knochen. Naturwissenschaften **46**, 358 (1959).

— F. Körber u. H.-J. Dulce: Pharmakologische Beeinflussung des durch Oestron erhöhten Calcium-Spiegels von Hähnen. Naunyn-Schmiedebergs Arch. exp. Path. Pharmak. **240**, 327 (1961).

Siffert, R. S.: The role of alkaline phosphatase in osteogenesis. J. exp. Med. **93**, 415 (1951).

Silberberg, M., and R. Silberberg: Steroid hormones and bone. In: The biochemistry and physiology of bone (G. H. Bourne), p. 623. New York: Academic Press 1956.

Simkiss, K.: Influence of large doses of oestrogens on the structure of the bones of some reptiles. Nature (Lond.) **190**, 1217 (1961).

Sledge, C. B.: 3rd Eur. Symp. on calcified tissues, Davos 1965.

Smith, Q. T.: Labeled glycine of collagens of different-aged normal and cortisone-treated rats. Amer. J. Physiol. **205**, 827 (1963).

—, and W. D. Armstrong: Collagen metabolism of rats in various hormonal and dietary conditions. Amer. J. Physiol. **200**, 1330 (1961).

Smith, R. G., and H. R. Sternberger: Diffusible and non-diffusible blood serum calcium following intravenous injections of calcium salts. J. biol. Chem. **96**, 245 (1932).

Sobel, A. E.: Local factors in the mechanism of calcification. Ann. N.Y. Acad. Sci. **60**, 713 (1955).

— Second Eur. Symp. on calcified tissues at the Domaine Provincial de Wegimont 1964, 291 (1965).

— G. Bonorris, and M. Sideman: Effect of cortisone, thyroxine and cold on femurs of guinea pigs. Amer. J. Physiol. **199**, 1087 (1960).

—, and M. Bürger: Calcification. XIV. Investigation of the role of chondroitinsulfate in the calcifying mechanism. Proc. Soc. exp. Biol. (N.Y.) **87**, 7 (1954).

— A. R. Goldfarb, and B. Kramer: Studies of incurable ricketts. I. Respective role of the local factor and vitamin D in healing. Proc. Soc. exp. Biol. (N.Y.) **31**, 869 (1934).

—, and A. Hanok: Calcification. VII. Reversible inactivation of calcification in vitro and related studies. J. biol. Chem. **197**, 669 (1952).

—, and P. A. Laurence: Crystal growth in mineralizing tissues. Biochim. biophys. Acta (Amst.) **41**, 1—8 (1960a).

— S. Nobel, and A. Hanok: The reversible inactivation of calcification in vitro. Proc. Soc. exp. Biol. (N.Y.) **72**, 68 (1949).

— M. Rockenmacher, and B. Kramer: Carbonate content of bone in relation to the composition of blood and diet. J. biol. Chem. **158**, 475—489 (1945).

Soggnaes, R.: Microstructure and histochemical characteristics of the mineralized tissues. Ann. N.Y. Acad. Sci. **60**, 545 (1955).

Soliman, H. A. Robinson, G. V. Foster, and I. MacIntyre: Mode of action of calcitonin. Calcified tissues, Davos, p. 242. Berlin-Heidelberg-New York: Springer 1965.

Solomons, C. C., and W. F. Neuman: On the mechanisms of calcification in the remineralization of dentin. J. biol. Chem. **8**, 235 (1960).

Stack, M. V.: The chemical nature of the organic matrix of bone, dentin and enamel. Ann. N.Y. Acad. Sci. **60**, 585 (1955).

Spratt, J. L., and G. A. R. Boho: Parathyreoid hormone and whole body oxidation of glucose, pyruvate and citrate by the intact rat. Arch. int. Pharmacodyn. **141**, 95 (1963).

Stalder, G.: Endogene Phosphat-Clearance bei Vitamin-D-Mangelrachitis und rachitogener Tetanie, ihre Beeinflussung durch Vitamin D_2. Int. Z. Vitaminforsch. **27**, 382 (1957).

Strandh, J., A. Bengtsson, and H. Jorulf: The rates of uptake of calcium and phosphorus in microscopic bone structure. J. Bone Jt Surg. A **47**, 146 (1965).

Strates, B., and W. F. Neuman: On the mechanisms of calcification. Proc. Soc. exp. Biol. (N.Y.) **97**, 3 (1958).

STEENBOCK, H., and S. A. BELLIN: Vitamin D and tissue citrate. J. biol. Chem. **205**, 985 (1953).

STEGEMANN, H., u. G. F. JUNG: Über die anorganische Trockensubstanz nach Formamidaufschluß. Hoppe-Seylers Z. physiol. Chem. **320**, 272 (1960).

STERN, B., G. MECHANIC, M. J. GLIMCHER, and P. GOLDHABER: The resorption of bone collagen in tissue culture. Biochem. biophys. Res. Commun. **13**, 137 (1963).

STEWART, G. S., and H. F. BOWEN: Funktion der Parathyreoidea nach Nephrektomie. Endocrinology **48**, 568 (1951).

STOERK, H., A. PETERSON, and V. JELINEK: The blood calcium lowering effect of hydrocortisone in parathyroidectomized rats. Proc. Soc. exp. Biol. (N.Y.) **114**, 690 (1963).

STOLL, W. R., and W. F. NEUMAN: The uptake of sodium and potassium ions by hydrated hydroxyapatite. J. Amer. chem. Soc. **78**, 1585 (1956).

STOOKEY, G., D. CRANE, and J. C. MUHLER: Further studies on fluoride absorption. Proc. Soc. exp. Biol. (N.Y.) **115**, 295 (1964a).

— E. DELLINGER, and J. MUHLER: In vitro studies concerning fluoride absorption. Proc. Soc. exp. Biol. (N.Y.) **115**. 298 (1964).

STRUG, P.: Röntgenologische und chemisch-analytische Bestimmung des Ca-Gehaltes im Knochen. Inaug.-Diss. Berlin 1964.

TALMAGE, R. V., and J. R. ELLIOTT: Changes in extracellular fluid levels of calcium phosphate and citrate ions in nephrectomized rats following parathyroidectomy. Endocrinology **59**, 27 (1956).

— F. W. KRAINTZ, R. C. FROST, and L. KRAINTZ: Evidence for a dual action of parathyroid extract in maintaining serum calcium and phosphate levels. Endocrinology **52**, 318 (1953).

— J. NEUENSCHWANDER, and I, KRAINTZ: Evidence for the existence of thyrocalcitonin in the rat. Endocrinology **76**, 103 (1965).

TALPERS, S., and D. STEIN: Tubular reabsorption of P as a measure of parathyroid activity. Metabolism 8, 170 (1959).

TANZER, M., and R. HUNT: Osteoclasts: Organization in chick embryo bone. Science **141**, 1270 (1963).

TASHJIAN, A. H., D. A. ONTJES, and T. L. GOODFRIEND: Mechanism of parathyroid hormone action: effects of actinomycin D on hormone-stimulated ions movements in vivo and in vitro. Biochem. biophys. Res. Commun. **16**, 209—215 (1964).

TAVES, D.: Similarly of octacalcium phosphate and hydroxyapatite structures. Nature (Lond. **200**, 1312 (1963).

—, and W. F. NEUMAN: Factors controlling calcification in vitro: fluoride and magnesium. Arch. Biochem. **108**, 390 (1964).

TAYLOR, A., and R. H. WASSERMAN: A vitamin D_3-dependent factor influencing calcium binding by homogenates of chick intestinal mucosa. Nature (Lond.) **205**, 248 (1965).

TAYLOR, T. G.: The sodium and potassium of bone mineral. Experientia (Basel) **16**, 109 (1960).

— The nature of bone citrate. Biochim. biophys. Acta (Amst.) **39**, 148 (1960a).

— Calcium and magnesium in the blood and bones of chick embryos. Biochem. J. **87**, 7 P (1963).

— A. WILLIAMS, and J. KIRKLEY: Cyclic changes in the activities of plasma acid and alkaline phosphatase during egg-shell calcification in the domestic fowl. 3rd Eur. Symp. on calcified tissues, Davos 1965.

TEAFORD, M., and A. WHITE: Alkaline phosphatase and osteogenesis in vitro. Proc. Soc. exp. Biol. (N.Y.) **117**, 541 (1964).

TELL, H. B., and R. ROBISON: The development of the calcifying mechanism in avian cartilage and ateoid tissue. Biochem. J. **28**, 2243 (1934).

TEREPKA, A. R., and P. S. CHEN jr.: Comparison of the effects of crystalline dihydrotachysterol, vitamin D_2 and parathyroid extract on calcium and phosphorus metabolism in man. J. clin. Endocr. **22**, 1007 (1962).

TORO, G., P. G. ACKERMANN, and W. B. KOUNTZ: Effect of some hormones on calcium balance in elderly subjects. Proc. Soc. exp. Biol. (N.Y.) **97**, 819 (1958).

TESSARI, L.: The effect of parathyroid extract upon transaminase activity in metaphysical bone. Endocrinology **66**, 890 (1960a).

—, and L. PARRINI: Glutamic-pyruvic transaminase in rabbits long bones. Nature (Lond.) **184**, 904 (1959).

—, e D. TAGLIABNE: Sulla specificata dell'azione della vitamina D sulla cartilagine di accrescimento: biosintesi della cocarbossilasi. Acta vitamin. (Milano) **14**, 97 (1960).

THOMAS, W. C., and H. G. MORGAN: The effect of cortisone in experimental hypervitaminosis D. Endocrinology **63**, 57 (1958).

TODD, A. S., O. T. FOSGATE, R. G. CRAGLE, and T. H. KAMAL: Parathyroid action on calcium, phosphorus, magnesium and citric acid in doing cattle. Amer. J. Physiol. **202**, 987 (1962).

TOVERUD, S. U.: The effect of parathyroid hormone and vitamin D on serum calcium in rats. Acta physiol. scand. **62**, 391 (1964).

TRAUTZ, O. R.: X-ray diffraction on biological and synthetic apatites. Ann. N.Y. Acad. Sci. **60**, 696 (1955).

—, and B. N. BACHRA: Oriented precipitation of inorganic crystals in fibrous matrices. Arch. oral Biol. 8, 601—613 (1963).

TRISTRAM, G. R., H. NEURATH, and K. BAILEY: In: The proteins, vol. 1, part A, p. 181. New York: Academic Press 1953.

TROTTER, M., and R. R. PETERSEN: The relationship of ash and organic weight of human skeletons. J. Bone Jt Surg. A **44**, 669 (1962).

TULPULE, P. G., and V. N. PATWARDHAN: Mode of action of vitamin D. The effect of vitamin D deficiency in the rat on anaerobic glycolysis and pyruvate oxidation by epiphyseal cartilage. Biochem. J. **58**, 61—65 (1954).

Tyler, C.: P- und Ca-Stoffwechsel und chemische Knochenstruktur. Biochem. J. **34**, 202 (1940).

Ulrich, F., W. O. Reinhardt, and Choh Hao Li: The effects of hypophyseal growth hormone on the metabolism of Ca^{45} in hypophysectomized rats. Endocrinology **49**, 213—217 (1951).

— — — Some aspects of the role of pituitary hormones in calcium metabolism. II. Growth hormone. Acta endocr. (Kbh.) **10**, 117—127 (1952).

Underwood, E. E., and H. C. Hodge: Calcium exchange in enamel and dentin as shown by calcium. J. dent. Res. **31**, 64 (1952).

Urist, M. R., and J. M. Adams: Effects of various blocking reagents upon local mechanism of calcification. Arch. Path. **81**, 325—342 (1966).

— N. M. Deutsch, G. Pomerantz, and F. C. McLean: Interrelations between actions of parathyroid hormone and estrogens on bone and blood in avian species. Amer. J. Physiol. **119**, 851 (1960).

— O. A. Scheide, and F. C. McLean: The partition and binding of calcium in the serum of the laying hen and of the estrogenized rooster. Endocrinology **63**, 570 (1958).

Vaes, G. M.: Hydrolytic enzymes and lysosomes in bone cells. 2nd Symp. on calcified tissues, Liège 1964, p. 51—62.

— 2nd Eur. Symp. on calcified tissues, Davos 1964a.

— Acid hydrolases, lysosomes and bone resorption induced by parathyroid hormone. 3rd Eur. Symp. on calcified tissues, Davos 1965.

— Hydrolytic enzymes and lysosomes in bone cells. 2nd Eur. Symp. on calcified tissues, Liège 1965a, p. 51—62. Berlin-Heidelberg-New York: Springer 1965a, Calcified tissues, p. 56.

— In: La résorption osseuse et l'hormone parathyroidienne, p. 79. Louvain: Impr. E. Warny 1966.

—, and G. Nichols: Metabolic studies of bone in vitro. III. Citric acid metabolism and bone mineral solubility. Effect of parathyroid hormone and estradiol. J. biol. Chem. **236**, 3323 (1961).

— — Effects of a massive dose of parathyroid extract on bone metabolic pathway. Endocrinology **70**, 546 (1962).

— — Oxygen tension and the control of bone cell metabolism. Nature (Lond.) **193**, 379 (1962a).

— — Metabolism of glycin-1-C^{14} by bone in vitro: effects of hormones and other factors. Endocrinology **70**, 890 (1962b).

— — Bone metabolism in a mutant strain of rats which lack bone resorption. Amer. J. Physiol. **205**, 461 (1963).

Veis, A., J. Anesey, and J. Cohen: The long range reorganization of gelatin to the collagen structure. Arch. Biochem. **94**, 20 (1961).

—, and R. J. Schlueter: Presence of phosphate-mediated cross-linkages in hard tissue collagens. Nature (Lond.) **197**, 1204 (1963).

Verzar, F.: Differenzierung verschiedener Vernetzungen. Hoppe-Seylers Z. physiol. Chem. **335**, 38 (1963).

Vierenstein, K.: Untersuchungen über den Stoffwechsel des normalen Gelenkknorpels. Z. Orthop. **92**, 4 (1959).

Vincent, J.: Microscopic aspects of mineral metabolism in bone tissue with special reference to calcium, lead and zinc. Clin. Orthop. **26**, 2116 (1963).

Virtama, P.: Quantitative determination of bone minerals from roentgenograms. Experientia (Basel) **13**, 236 (1957).

Vittali, P. H.: Osteocyte activity in metabolic bone disease. 4th Eur. Symp. on calcified tissues, Leiden 1966.

Voogd der Straaten, W. A. de: Some data concerning the mode of action of patathyroid hormone on bone tissue. Gen. comp. Endocr. **3**, 737 (1963).

Waldmann, J.: Calcification of hypertrophic epiphyseal cartilage in vitro following in activation of phosphatase and other epiphyseals. Proc. Soc. exp. Biol. (N.Y.) **69**, 262 (1948).

— Effect of inactivation of enzymes on calcification of cartilage in vitro. Metab. Interrel. **2**, 203 (1950).

Walker, D. G.: Citric acid cycle in osteoblasts and osteoclasts. Bull. Johns Hopk. Hosp. **108**, 80 (1961).

— C. M. Zapiere, and J. Gross: A collagenolytic factor in rat bone promoted by parathyroid extract. Biochem. biophys. Res. Commun. **15**, 397 (1964).

Wasserman, R. H.: Studies on vitamin D_3 and the intestinal absorption of calcium and other ions in the rachitic chick. J. Nutr. **77**, 69 (1962a).

—, and A. Taylor: Intestinal pH and absorption and deposition of Ca^{47} in the rachitic chick. Proc. Soc. exp. Biol. (N.Y.) **109**, 633 (1962).

Weatherell, J., and S. M. Weidmann: The distribution of organically bound sulphate in bone and cartilage during calcification. Biochem. J. **89**, 265 (1963).

Werner, E.: Cholesterin-phosphatsäureester und seine Umwandlungsprodukte zu Vitamin D_3-Phosphatsäureester als Substrate alkalischer Phosphatasen. Hoppe-Seylers Z. physiol. Chem. **311**, 178—184 (1958).

Whicher, C. H., and E. M. Watson: Effects of thyrotropic hormone, gonadotropic factor, pituitary growth substance and insulin upon the phosphatase content of rat femur. Endocrinology **33**, 83 (1943).

Whitehead, R. G., and S. M. Weidmann: Trichloracetic acid-insoluble phosphatase compounds. Nature (Lond.) **183**, 4665 (1959).

Widrow, S. H., and N. O. Levinski: The effect of parathyroid extract on renal tubular Ca reabsorption in the dog. J. clin. Invest. **41**, 2151 (1962).

Wilhelm, G.: The problem of calcification of skeletal tissue. 4th Eur. Symp. on calcified tissues. Leiden 1966.

WILKINS, W. E., J. A. CALHOUN, C. PILCHER, and E. M. REGEN: The influence of pituitary growth hormone of bone and kidney. Amer. J. Physiol. **112**, 477 (1935).

WILLIAMS, G. A., E. W. BOWSER, W. J. HENDERSON, and V. UZGIRIS: Ca-absorption in the rat in relation to excessive vitamin D and cortisone. Proc. Soc. exp. Biol. (N.Y.) **110**, 889 (1962).

— N. BOWSER, W. J. HENDERSON, and V. UZGIRIS: Effects of vitamin D and cortisone in intestinal absorption of calcium in the rat. Proc. Soc. exp. Biol. (N.Y.) **106**, 664 (1961).

WILLIAMS, H. L., and E. M. WABON: Influence of hormones upon phosphatase content of rat femur. Endocrinology **29**, 258 (1941).

WILSON, H. R.: The molecular arrangement in α-keratin. J. molec. Biol. **6**, 474 (1960).

WOOD, G. C.: The heterogeneity of collagen solutions and its effect on fibril formation. Biochem. J. **84**, 429 (1962).

WOODARD, H. Q.: The elementary composition of human cortical bone. Hlth Phys. **8**, 513 (1962).

WOODS, K. R., and W. D. ARMSTRONG: Action of parathyroid extracts on stable bone mineral using radiocalcium as tracer. Proc. Soc. exp. Biol. (N.Y.) **9**, 255 (1956).

WUTHIER, R., P. GRON, and J. IRVING: The reaction of 1-fluoro-2,4-dinitrobenzene with bone. Studies on the relationship between bone collagen and apatite. Biochem. J. **92**, 205 (1964).

YATES, C., S. DOTY, and R. V. TALMAGE: Effects of sodium fluoride on calcium homeostasis. Proc. Soc. exp. Biol. (N.Y.) **115**, 1103 (1964).

—, and R. V. TALMAGE: Influence of endogenous parathyroid hormone on citrate and lactate production by bone in vitro. Proc. Soc. exp. Biol. (N.Y.) **119**, 88 (1965).

YASUDA, I., K. NOGUCHI, and T. SATA: Dynamic callus and electric callus. J. Bone Jt Surg. Boston **37**, 1292—1293 (1955).

ZETTERSTRÖM, R., and M. LJUNGGREN: The activation of alkaline phosphatase from different organs by phosphorylated vitamin D_2. Acta chem. scand. **5**, 283 (1951).

ZIPKIN, I., A. S. POSNER, and E. D. EANES: The effect of fluoride on the x-ray diffraction pattern of the apatite of human bone. Biochim. biophys. Acta (Amst.) **59**, 255—258 (1962).

C. Die radiologische Erfassung des Mineralgehaltes des Knochens

Von

F. Heuck

Mit 160 Abbildungen

I. Einleitung

Das Skelet dient dem Organismus nicht nur als Stützapparat, sondern auch als wichtige Mineralreserve. Die Erkennung von Veränderungen des Mineralgehaltes in einem Knochen war bisher nur durch die Röntgenuntersuchung oder die histologische Analyse einer Gewebeprobe leicht zugänglicher Skeletbezirke möglich. Zwar erlaubt die histologische Untersuchung eines Knochenpunktates, die Struktur des gewonnenen Gewebes zu beurteilen, doch ist hierzu stets ein Eingriff erforderlich, der für Kontrolluntersuchungen nach Behandlung einer Knochenerkrankung nicht beliebig oft wiederholt werden kann.

Die Röntgenuntersuchung des Skeletes muß sich auf die Beurteilung der äußeren Form und der Makrostruktur (Strukturen 1. und 2. Ordnung nach Knese 1958) der Knochen beschränken. Eine Abnahme oder Zunahme des Mineralgehaltes der Tela ossea sowie ein Abbau oder Umbau im Bereich der Strukturen 3.—5. Ordnung werden sich dem röntgenologischen Nachweis entziehen müssen, da sie im Grenzgebiet zum mikroskopischen Bereich ablaufen.

Der Knochen nimmt auf Grund seiner ununterbrochenen Stoffwechselaktivität an allen normalen und pathologischen Lebensvorgängen teil. Es ist daher verständlich, daß der Knochenstoffwechsel von allen Änderungen des normalen Stoffwechsels mit beeinflußt wird. Manche Fehlsteuerungen des Stoffwechsels, insbesondere des Mineralhaushaltes, werden zuerst durch Veränderungen des Skeletsystems angezeigt. Der Knochen spielt dadurch in der gesamten klinischen Medizin eine wichtige Rolle. Viele primäre und sekundäre Erkrankungen des Skeletes, die mit Veränderungen des Kalksalzgehaltes der Knochenmatrix einhergehen, lassen sich aber nur bei rechtzeitiger Erkennung mit Erfolg behandeln. Deshalb wurde versucht, mit verschiedensten Methoden bereits frühzeitig Änderungen des Mineralgehaltes der Knochen allein durch radiologische Untersuchungen zu erfassen. Da die Bemühungen der verschiedensten Arbeitsrichtungen und Forschungsvorhaben bisher noch nicht zu einem Abschluß gelangen konnten, ist es schwierig, heute schon eine umfassende und vollständige Übersicht zu geben. Viele Methoden sind noch nicht ausgereift oder für die praktische radiologische Arbeit kaum brauchbar; nur wenige konnten eine breitere klinische Anwendung finden und haben Ergebnisse gebracht.

Es soll dennoch versucht werden, die bisher vorliegenden anatomischen und physikalischen Grundlagen der radiologischen Meßverfahren darzustellen, die methodischen Möglichkeiten und Grenzen aufzuzeigen und bisher erarbeitete Ergebnisse von Kalksalzmessungen des gesunden und kranken Knochens zusammenzustellen. So können die Basis für eine breitere Anwendung der in der klinischen Radiologie bereits brauchbaren Meßmethoden geschaffen und weitere Anregungen zur Mitarbeit auf diesem Forschungsgebiet der Medizin gegeben werden.

II. Anatomische Grundlagen radiologischer Messungen des Mineralgehaltes von Knochen

1. Der Knochen als Organ und Skeletbaustein

Der einzelne Knochen stellt einen *Gewebsverband* dar, so daß er als „*Organ*“ angesehen werden kann. Die lebende Knochensubstanz setzt sich zusammen aus dem eigentlichen Knochengewebe (der Tela ossea), dem Markgewebe (Reticulo-Endothel: blutbildendes Mark, später Fettmark), den Bindegewebselementen der periostalen und endostalen Zonen, den blutführenden Gefäßen und dem Nervengewebe.

Das *Knochengewebe* selbst — die Tela ossea — setzt sich aus zwei verschiedenen, miteinander eng verbundenen Komponenten zusammen, dem organischen und dem anorganischen Teil. Der organische Teil nimmt etwa zwei Drittel des Knochengewebsvolumens ein und besteht aus Zellen, kollagenen Fasern und Kittsubstanz. In die *organische Grundsubstanz* sind die *anorganischen Mineralbestandteile* eingelagert, die als Calciumverbindungen, vorwiegend in Form von Phosphaten, Carbonaten, Citraten und anderen Salzen vorkommen. Der Hauptbestandteil der Kalksalze des Knochengewebes liegt nach unserem heutigen Wissen als *Hydroxylapatit* vor (s. Beitrag DULCE, S. 15).

Eine wesentliche Aufgabe des eigentlichen Knochengewebes besteht in der Depotfunktion für lebensnotwendige Mineralien. Das Knochenmark ist die Bildungsstätte der Blutzellen. Die röntgenologische Darstellung eines Knochens muß als Summationsbild der verschiedenen Gewebselemente, die im „Organ Knochen“ zusammengeschlossen sind, verstanden werden.

Der einzelne Knochen ist in seiner Form, Größe und Struktur auf die spezifisch statische Aufgabe eines Bausteines des Skeletes — das dem Makroorganismus als Stützgerüst dient — ausgerichtet. Die äußere Form und die Grundzüge der Architektur der Bauelemente eines jeden Knochens werden maßgeblich durch genetische Faktoren geprägt. Daneben spielen endogene, insbesondere hormonelle und geschlechtsspezifische sowie exogene Einflüsse (Ernährung, Belastung u.a.) bei der Knochenbildung eine Rolle.

2. Der strukturelle Aufbau der Knochen

Für die radiologische Beurteilung des Knochens ist sowohl die Kenntnis der Makrostruktur als auch der Mikrostruktur des Knochengewebes von Bedeutung, über die in diesem Handbuch KNESE berichtet. Nach den Untersuchungsergebnissen von KNESE (1958) sind die beiden Komponenten des Knochengewebes, die Kollagenfasern und die anorganischen Einlagerungen, im Sinne eines „Verbundbaues“ zusammengefügt. Der Autor unterscheidet in diesem „Verbundbau“ Strukturen verschiedener Ordnungsstufen:

Strukturen 1. Ordnung: Compacta-Spongiosa-Verteilung im Knochen.
Strukturen 2. Ordnung: topographische Verteilung der Lamellensysteme.
Strukturen 3. Ordnung: Lamellensysteme (Osteone).
Strukturen 4. Ordnung: einzelne Lamellen.
Strukturen 5. Ordnung: Kollagenfasern und die sie umgebenden anorganischen und organischen Substanzen.

Im Bereich der *röntgenologisch darstellbaren Strukturen* 1. Ordnung eines Knochens ist neben der *Spongiosa* und der *Compacta* die unterschiedlich dicke *Corticalis* für die *globale Bestimmung der Kalksalzkonzentration* im Knochen von Bedeutung (Abb. 1). Die Corticalis (auch Knochengrenzlamelle genannt) umschließt den spongiösen Knochen und geht im Bereich der Metaphysen der Röhrenknochen in die Compacta der Diaphysen über. Bei Systemerkrankungen des Skeletes (Osteopathien), die mit einer Transformation des Knochens oder einem Abbau (Rarefikation) der Spongiosa einhergehen, bleibt die Corticalis erstaunlich lange erhalten und intakt, sie kann jedoch eine Verschmälerung erfahren.

Meist kommt es erst nach einem Einbruch dieser Knochenlamelle, also einer Kontinuitätstrennung, schließlich auch zum Abbau und zur Auflösung der Corticalis. Im angloamerikanischen Schrifttum wird die Corticalis nicht besonders berücksichtigt, doch spielt sie in der Knochenpathologie und der Radiologie der Systemerkrankungen des Skeletes eine besondere Rolle.

Das „Verbundbausystem" des Knochens ist für die Statik des Skeletes von Bedeutung. Die einzelnen Struktureinheiten weisen einen unterschiedlichen Gehalt an anorganischen Kalksalzen in der organischen Grundsubstanz auf. Der Aufbau der Lamellen aus Kollagenfasern ist wahrscheinlich örtlich verschieden, aber für den Ort wiederum spezifisch (KNESE,

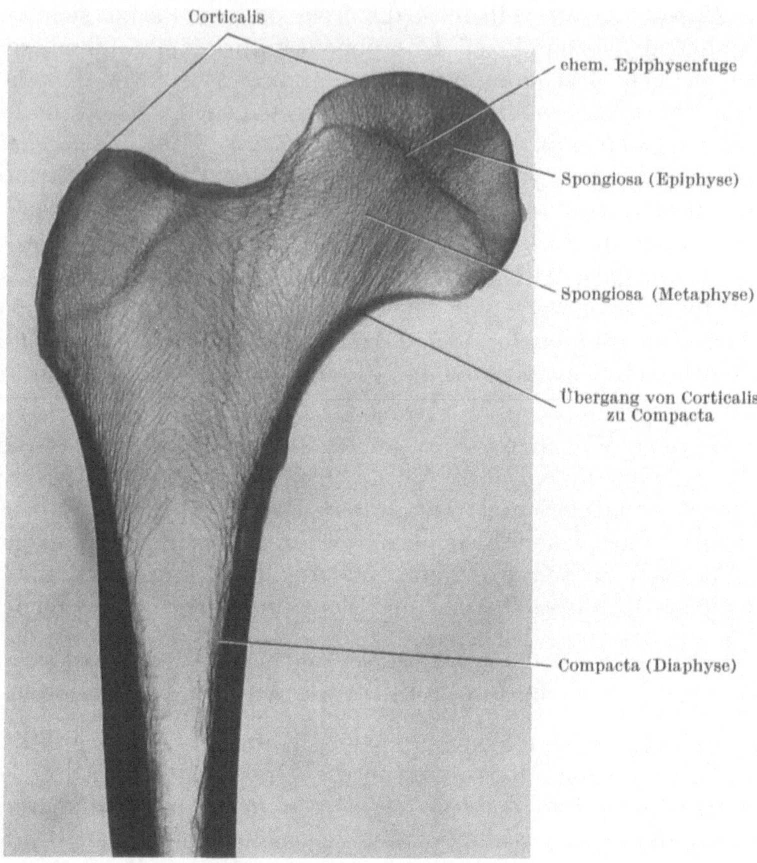

Abb. 1. Die Strukturen 1. Ordnung eines Knochens, dargestellt am proximalen Femur

RITSCHL und VOGES 1954). Mit Hilfe *mikroradiographischer Untersuchungen* der Tela ossea können die im mikroskopischen Bereich liegenden *erheblichen Unterschiede* der Kalksalzkonzentration in den Lamellensystemen (Osteonen) dargestellt werden (s. Beitrag von ENGSTRÖM, S. 296). Die interessanten Ergebnisse biophysikalischer Untersuchungen des Knochengewebes waren Anlaß, die unterschiedliche Verteilung der Kalksalze in der Tela ossea des *kranken Knochens* zu untersuchen. Mit Hilfe mikroradiographischer und chemisch-analytischer Methoden konnte eine *eindeutige Abnahme des Kalksalzgehaltes im eigentlichen Knochengewebe* bei Osteopathien (hepatogene und diabetische Osteopathie, primärer und sekundärer Hyperparathyreoidismus u.a.) gefunden werden (HEUCK 1962). Im kranken Knochen fanden sich Zonen eines stark verminderten Kalksalzgehaltes, die ein ganzes Osteon (Strukturen 3. Ordnung) einnehmen können. Größere Unterschiede in der Kalksalzkonzentration fanden sich im Bereich osteoider Säume (HEUCK 1963). Vergleichende histologische und mikroradiographische Untersuchungen des Osteopathieknochens, insbesondere des primären und sekundären Hyperparathyreoidismus, konnten den Beweis einer osteolytischen Aktivität der Osteocyten erbringen (HEUCK 1966, 1968). Die Osteolyse wird durch eine periosteocytäre Entkalkung der Tela ossea eingeleitet. Der Knochenabbau oder -umbau folgen nach. Aus den Zonen besonderer Stoffwechselaktivität konnten die Knochenkalksalze mit Hilfe von Calciumkomplexbildnern (EDTA) relativ rasch aus dem Knochengewebe herausgelöst werden (HEUCK 1963). Es handelt sich um Zonen der sog. ,,mobilen Calciumfraktion" des Knochens. Im kranken Knochengewebe ist also nicht nur ein Abbau durch die Tätigkeit der Osteoklasten zu finden oder ein gestörter Aufbau durch mangelhafte Osteoblastentätigkeit festzustellen, sondern es kann eine *echte Entkalkung* der Tela ossea nachgewiesen werden.

Das bisher vorliegende gesicherte Wissen über die Lebensvorgänge im Knochengewebe ist noch sehr lückenhaft und unvollkommen. Die Forschungsergebnisse der letzten Jahre haben Zweifel an der Gültigkeit unserer bisherigen Vorstellungen über die Biodynamik des Knochens geweckt.

3. Die wechselseitigen Beziehungen zwischen Struktur und Mineralkonzentration (Hydroxylapatit-Konzentration, Apatitwert) in Knochen

Die Bestimmung des Anteiles der anorganischen Fraktion — vorwiegend der Kalksalze — am Gesamtvolumen eines Knochens kann mit sehr verschiedenen Methoden vorgenommen werden. Die größte Genauigkeit wird die chemische Analyse des Knochens erbringen (s. bei DULCE, S. 12). Dabei kann von der *Frischsubstanz des Gesamtknochens* (Tela ossea + Knochenmark + Blut- oder Gewebsflüssigkeit + Fett + übrige Gewebe), von der Trockensubstanz des Gesamtknochens (entwässerter Knochen), von der fettfreien Frischsubstanz oder der fettfreien Trockensubstanz eines Knochens oder einer Knochenprobe ausgegangen werden. Die gefundenen Werte können in Gewichtsprozenten (mg %), Volumenprozenten (mg/ml) oder als spezifisches Gewicht angegeben werden.

Am lebenden Menschen können Rückschlüsse auf den Mineralgehalt im Skelet (halbquantitative oder quantitative Messungen der Kalksalzkonzentration eines Knochens) nur mit Hilfe physikalischer Methoden ermöglicht werden. Die einzelnen Elemente, aus denen der Gewebsverband Knochen zusammengesetzt ist, absorbieren Röntgenstrahlen oder Gammastrahlen (eines Isotops) unterschiedlich. Die Größenordnung der Absorption (oder Schwächung) ist von der Ordnungszahl der Elemente, der Dicke und der Dichte der durchstrahlten Medien abhängig. Einen zusätzlichen Einfluß haben die Qualität der verwendeten Strahlung und die Makrostruktur des Knochens (s. auch S. 126). So ist das Röntgenbild kein ,,Schattenbild", sondern seine Transparenz ist abhängig von materiellen und räumlichen Gegebenheiten des untersuchten Knochens.

Von WEECH und SMITH wurde bereits 1923 im Experiment bewiesen, daß die Strahlenabsorption im Knochen ausschließlich durch die Anwesenheit von Calcium bedingt ist. Neben einem in Formalin fixierten Humerus wurde ein zweiter, in 5%iger Salpetersäure entkalkter Humerus geröntgt und gezeigt, daß nur der normale Humerus einen guten Kontrast gibt. Als Gegenkontrolle wurden ein von der organischen Grundsubstanz befreiter Humerus und ein normaler, unbehandelter Humerus nebeneinander aufgenommen. Der Kontrastschatten beider Knochen war gleich und somit der Gegenbeweis schlüssig geführt.

Die radiologische Messung der Kalksalzkonzentration eines Knochens am Lebenden kann im allgemeinen nur auf den *Gesamtknochen* (also die ,,Frischsubstanz") bezogen werden. Ein Vergleich der mit unterschiedlicher Methodik (chemisch-analytisch, radiologisch u.a.) gewonnenen Werte der Kalksalzkonzentration eines Knochens oder Knochenbezirkes ist nur dann möglich, *wenn alle Werte auf die Frischsubstanz des Gesamtknochens* berechnet werden. Der erhaltene Globalwert wird im allgemeinen in mg *Knochenmineral (oder Hydroxylapatit)* pro ml Gesamtknochen (mg/ml) angegeben. Aus der bekannten Zusammensetzung des Hydroxylapatit kann *der Calciumgehalt* in dem untersuchten (also durchstrahlten) Knochen berechnet werden.

Die Werte der globalen Kalksalzkonzentration (oder Hydroxylapatitkonzentration) in einem Knochenabschnitt sind einmal von dem *Verhältnis Knochengewebe/Markgewebe*, zum anderen von dem *Mineralisationsgrad* der Tela ossea, also der Kalksalzkonzentration im eigentlichen Knochengewebe, abhängig. Bei gesunden Menschen behält der Knochen bis in das Greisenalter die Grundzüge der äußeren Form und der Architektur bei. Lediglich die inneren Strukturen der Bälkchen, Lamellen und Röhrensysteme der Spongiosa, der Osteone und Schaltlamellen der Compacta der Diaphysen erfahren im Laufe des Alterungsprozesses eine Transformation, die mit einem *Verlust an Knochengewebssubstanz* einhergeht. Diese *Strukturauflockerung* der Bauelemente des Knochens muß zwangsläufig zu einer Abnahme der *globalen Kalksalzkonzentration* im Gesamtknochen führen und zwar auch dann, wenn der Kalksalzgehalt der Tela ossea selbst *unverändert* bleibt oder sogar *zunimmt*.

Chemische Analysen von Knochen oder Knochenproben aus verschiedenen Skeletpartien haben gezeigt, daß die Zusammensetzung der Knochen während des Alterungsprozesses Änderungen erfährt (Heuck und Schmidt 1960; Frercks und Heuck 1969; Dulce in diesem Handbuch, S. 12). In der *Spongiosa* ist eine Verminderung des Knochengewebes zugunsten des Markgewebes, und hier besonders des Fettmarkes festzustellen. Der *Wassergehalt* nimmt in allen Knochen ab, während der *Fettgehalt* zunimmt. Die *Tela ossea* weist nur eine geringfügige Abnahme des Kalksalzgehaltes im Laufe des Alterungsprozesses auf, im 9. Dezennium konnte sogar eine Zunahme der Kalksalzkonzentration festgestellt werden. Die *Diaphysencompacta* erfährt eine *Volumenabnahme*, also eine Verschmälerung durch „endostalen Abbau", die eine Verbreiterung des Markraumes zur Folge hat. Der von K. Weiss (1957) geprägte Begriff der „Entknochung" konnte inzwischen durch die chemische Analyse bestätigt werden. Die *Grundtendenz der Alterungsvorgänge* im Knochen, die zur Altersosteoporose führen, ist monoton und sowohl im spongiösen als auch im kompakten Knochen gleichermaßen zu beobachten. Das Mikroradiogramm des Knochengewebes von gesunden Greisen ergibt keine eindeutigen Abweichungen in der Verteilung und Konzentration der Kalksalze gegenüber dem Kalksalzmosaik im mittleren Lebensalter.

Bei *Systemerkrankungen* des Skeletes (Osteopathien) weist der pathologisch veränderte Knochen Störungen des Umbaues auf, die mit einer Volumenabnahme (Osteoporose) oder Volumenzunahme (Osteosklerose) des Knochengewebes in den spongiösen Partien und mit einer Verschmälerung oder Verdickung der Compacta der Diaphysen der Extremitätenknochen einhergehen. Die Verschiebung der Relation Knochengewebe/Markgewebe wird eine Abnahme bzw. Zunahme der *globalen Kalksalzkonzentration* in den untersuchten *spongiösen* Knochen ergeben. Die *Abbau- oder Anbauprozesse der Compacta* werden sich in gleicher Weise in einer Zunahme oder Abnahme der globalen Kalksalzkonzentration im Gesamtvolumen des Knochens (unter Einschluß des Knochenmarks!) ausdrücken. Neben einer Bestimmung der globalen Kalksalzkonzentration werden *Messungen der Compactadicke der Diaphysen* wichtige Informationen über die gestörten Lebensvorgänge des „Organs Knochen" vermitteln können. Die Methoden der radiologischen Morphometrie, ihre Möglichkeiten und Grenzen, die bisher erhobenen Befunde an gesunden Menschen und die Ergebnisse einer klinischen Anwendung von Compacta-Messungen bei Systemerkrankungen des Skeletes sollen daher in den nachfolgenden Kapiteln mit berücksichtigt werden.

Eine Zunahme oder Abnahme des Knochengewebsvolumens im Gesamtknochen (oder der Frischsubstanz) infolge krankhaft gestörter Transformationsvorgänge kann — insbesondere bei solchen Systemerkrankungen, die durch eine Störung im Mineralhaushalt des Makroorganismus induziert worden sind — von einer *stärkeren Entkalkung* des bereits vorhandenen Knochengewebes oder einer *mangelhaften Verkalkung* der neu angebauten Tela ossea begleitet werden. Die krankhafte Steigerung des Mineralisationsgrades der Tela ossea über das normale Maß hinaus kommt seltener vor. Solche Vorgänge werden sowohl die globale Kalksalzkonzentration in den spongiösen als auch in den kompakten Knochenbezirken beeinflussen. Da eine Bestimmung des *Knochengewebsvolumens* am Lebenden in der Spongiosa nicht möglich ist, kommt der Compacta-Messung, also der Bestimmung des Verhältnisses Knochengewebe/Markgewebe im Bereich der Diaphysen große Bedeutung für die Skeletanalyse zu. Die Kombination von Compacta-Messungen und radiologischer Bestimmung der Kalksalzkonzentration im Diaphysenbereich wird Hinweise auf den Mineralisationsgrad des Knochengewebes selbst geben können. Bei den meisten Systemerkrankungen des Skeletes sind die Transformationsvorgänge und die zur Entkalkung führenden Prozesse nicht unabhängig voneinander, sondern meist nebeneinander zu finden.

Für die richtige Beurteilung der radiologischen Meßwerte einer globalen Kalksalzkonzentration in spongiösen Knochen (z.B. in den Wirbelkörpern, den Epiphysen und Metaphysen der Extremitätenknochen usw.) ist *die Kenntnis der Corticalisdicke* des untersuchten Knochenbezirkes von Bedeutung. Die Dicke der Corticalis ist *sehr unterschiedlich*, insbesondere dort, wo spongiöse Knochenpartien in die Compacta der Diaphysen übergehen, wie in den metaphysären Abschnitten der Röhrenknochen. Das Verhältnis *der Corticalis zu dem Volumen der spongiösen Partie* eines Knochens ist bei kleinen Knochen nicht ohne Einfluß auf die globale Kalksalzkonzentration des Gesamtknochens. Eine dicke Corticalis wird die Relation Knochengewebe/Markgewebe zugunsten des Knochengewebes verschieben und einen höheren Normalwert ergeben. In den Halswirbelkörpern ist die Relation Corticalis/Spongiosa eine andere als z.B. in den Lendenwirbelkörpern, so daß die Unterschiede der globalen Kalksalzkonzentration in diesen Knochen zwanglos zu verstehen sind (s. S. 283).

Das Verhältnis von Corticalis/Spongiosa ist neben der Architektur der Bauelemente eines Knochens und dem Mineralisationsgrad der Tela ossea für die *Belastungsfähigkeit* des einzelnen Skeletbausteines und damit die *Statik des Stützgerüstes* überhaupt von entscheidender Bedeutung. Die äußere Form eines Knochens bleibt solange erhalten, bis die Abbauvorgänge und/oder der Kalksalzverlust der Tela ossea zur *statischen Insuffizienz*, zur „Umbauzone" oder pathologischen Fraktur führen (s. S. 269).

Die Beurteilung der oben geschilderten krankhaften Vorgänge in einem Knochen mit Hilfe des Röntgenbildes oder spezieller Untersuchungsverfahren (Vergrößerungstechnik, Tomographie usw.) gehört zu den schwierigsten Aufgaben der klinischen Radiologie. Gröbere Struktur- und Formänderungen eines Knochens wie Osteolysen oder Osteosklerosen können wesentlich leichter erkannt werden. *Eine diskrete Abnahme oder Zunahme der globalen Kalksalzkonzentration im Knochen kann nur mit Hilfe radiologischer Meßverfahren frühzeitig und für eine Therapie rechtzeitig erfaßt werden.* Da alle Meßwerte auf das Gesamtvolumen eines Knochens bezogen werden müssen, gehört zur kritischen Beurteilung die *gleichzeitige Beachtung* von Form, Größe, Struktur oder Architektur der Bauelemente des untersuchten Knochens, um Fehlschlüsse zu vermeiden. Nur dann wird diese neue radiologische Information von den verschiedenen Fachgebieten der klinischen Medizin richtig gewertet und verwendet werden!

III. Grenzen und Möglichkeiten einer subjektiven Beurteilung des Knochen-Mineralgehaltes aus dem Röntgenbild

1. Der Informationswert der einfachen Röntgenaufnahme

Der Gehalt des Knochengewebes an Elementen mit einer höheren Ordnungszahl wie Calcium (20) und Phosphor (15) hat eine stärkere Absorption von *energiearmen Röntgenstrahlen* zur Folge, wie sie bei 30—60 kV Anodenspannung erzeugt werden. So stellt sich das Knochengewebe gegenüber den Weichteilen mit Elementen niedrigerer Ordnungszahl (etwa 7,5) auf der photographischen Schicht eines Röntgenfilmes relativ gut dar. Mit zunehmender Anodenspannung werden die Absorptionsunterschiede zwischen Knochen und Weichteilen geringer, um schließlich — z.B. bei 300—500 kV — kaum mehr erkennbar zu sein. Die Strahlenabsorption durch den Knochen wird ferner von der *Konzentration* der Kalksalze bestimmt. So ist es möglich, zu Lebzeiten einen Einblick in den

Ablauf krankhafter Prozesse im Skelet zu gewinnen. *Umschriebene*, pathologisch gesteigerte *Abbauvorgänge* sowie ein *verstärkter Anbau* oder eine Sklerose des Knochens können ohne Schwierigkeiten röntgenologisch erkannt und analysiert werden. Dagegen fallen *diffuse*, pathologische Prozesse, selbst wenn sie mit erheblichen Veränderungen des Mineralgehaltes einhergehen, sehr spät im Röntgenbild auf. Die Frage, *wann* eine Atrophie oder Entkalkung des Knochens *röntgenologisch erkannt werden kann*, ist Gegenstand umfangreicher klinisch-röntgenologischer und experimenteller Untersuchungen gewesen.

Tabelle 1. *Änderungen der Filmschwärzung in Abhängigkeit von unterschiedlichen Knochenmineralmengen sowie ihrer Verteilung im Modellversuch*

Relativer Anteil von Mineral im Phantom (in % des Gewichtes)	Änderung der Schichtdicke des Mineralgehaltes in %	Ausmaß der Mineraländerung im Gesamtvolumen in %	Änderung der Filmschwärzung in %	
			Verteilung	
			gleichmäßig	ungleichmäßig
5	5	0,25	0,8	—
10	5	0,50	1,6	—
15	5	0,75	2,4	—
20	5	1,00	*3,0*	—
30	5	1,50	*4,0*	—
40	5	2,00	*5,9*	—
5	10	0,50	1,6	1,0
10	10	1,00	*3,2*	2,6
15	10	1,50	*4,8*	4,1
20	10	2,00	*6,4*	5,8
30	10	3,00	*7,9*	6,8
40	10	4,00	*10,4*	9,2
5	15	0,75	2,5	2,1
10	15	1,50	*4,8*	4,6
15	15	2,25	*6,9*	6,2
20	15	3,00	*8,2*	7,1
30	15	4,50	*11,6*	10,2
40	15	6,00	*15,4*	*13,9*
5	20	1,00	*3,4*	3,0
10	20	2,00	*6,6*	6,1
15	20	3,00	*9,2*	8,7
20	20	4,00	*11,2*	10,0
30	20	6,00	*15,6*	*14,1*
40	20	8,00	*20,5*	*17,6*
5	30	1,50	*5,2*	5,1
10	30	3,00	*9,8*	8,6
15	30	4,50	*14,0*	*13,4*
20	30	6,00	*16,9*	*15,3*
30	30	9,00	*25,1*	*19,0*
40	30	12,00	*32,2*	*23,1*

Die in Kursivdruck gesetzten Änderungen der Filmschwärzung waren mit dem Auge festzustellen.

[Virtama, P.: Ann. Med. intern. Fenn. **49**, 57 (1960), Tab. 1]

Baastrup (1923), Rieder (1937) und Sudeck (1938) bezeichneten die Röntgenuntersuchung des Skeletes als eine sehr grobe Methode, da man mit dieser beim Menschen erst eine Knochenatrophie von 10—13 Gewichtsprozenten feststellen könne. Nach Coryn (1937) tritt ein Kalkverlust von mindestens 10% röntgenologisch in Erscheinung.

Lachmann und Whelan (1935) haben die Möglichkeiten und Grenzen röntgenologischer Untersuchungsmethoden des Knochens hinsichtlich der Erkennung von Entkalkungsosteopathien, insbesondere der Osteoporose aufgezeigt. Im Experiment wurden durch Maceration und Entkalkung menschlicher Knochen konzentrische und exzentrische Atrophien nachgeahmt, wie sie auch beim Lebenden gefunden werden. Es kann röntgenologisch nicht festgestellt werden, ob eine Knochenatrophie durch Halisterese (also Entkalkung) oder durch celluläre Resorption des Knochengewebes zustande kommt. Die Annahme, eine Entkalkung von 10—15% könne noch erkannt werden, wird als falsch bezeichnet, da sie auf Tierversuchen basiere. Nur unter sehr günstigen Umständen können in einigen Knochen Entkalkungen unter 20% noch visuell diagnostiziert werden. Im allgemeinen sind erst Calciumverluste von 20—40% erkennbar. Der Grad der eben noch nachweisbaren Verkalkung variiert sehr in den verschiedenen Knochen des Skeletes aber auch in einzelnen Bezirken desselben Knochens. Die Makrostruktur der Knochen wird in diesem Zusammenhang als ein wichtigerer Faktor betrachtet als das Volumen des Knochens. Ein „negatives" Röntgenbild erlaubt also nicht, eine Osteoporose auszuschließen.

Experimentelle Untersuchungen über *die Bedeutung einer gleichmäßigen oder ungleichmäßigen Verteilung* des voll mineralisierten Knochengewebes (Spongiosabälkchen) und den Einfluß der überlagernden Weichteile auf die *visuelle Beurteilung des Knochenmineralgehaltes* aus dem Röntgenbild hat Virtama (1960) durchgeführt (Tabelle 1). Mit Phantomversuchen konnte er nachweisen, daß Dichteänderungen von 3—4% durch das Auge *dann erfaßt werden können*, wenn das stärker absorbierende Material *gleichmäßig* verteilt ist (Abb. 2a—c). Bei einer *ungleichmäßigen* Verteilung des stärker absorbierenden Materials (also der Kalksalze), konnten erst Unterschiede von 13—14% erkannt werden (Abb. 3a, b). Diese Versuche beweisen, daß *die ungleichmäßige Verteilung der Kalksalze innerhalb des Knochens die bedeutsamste Ursache für die schlechte Erkennbarkeit* einer Verminderung oder

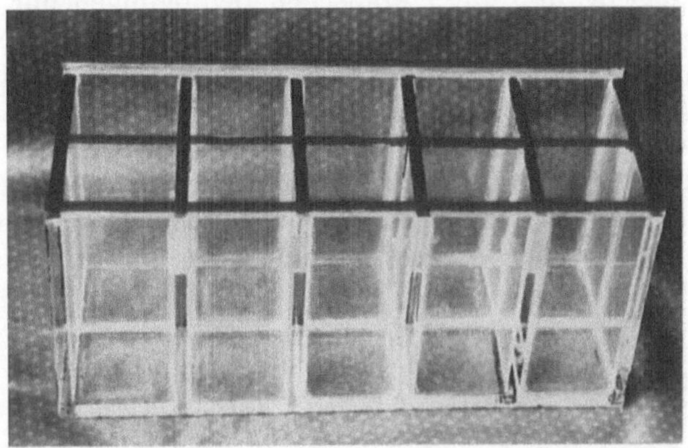

Ab. 2a. Ansicht des Plexiglas-Kastens mit 10 Fächern (2×2×5 cm), die mit unterschiedlichen Mengen von Knochenmehl und Wasser gefüllt wurden. (Nach Virtama, 1960; Abb. 1)

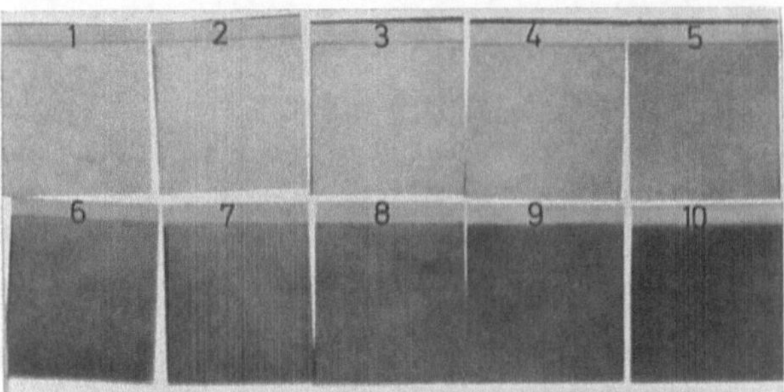

Abb. 2b. Röntgenbild der mit Knochenmehl gefüllten Fächer. Der durchschnittliche Mineralgehalt im Phantom betrug 30%. (Nach Virtama, 1960; Abb. 2a)

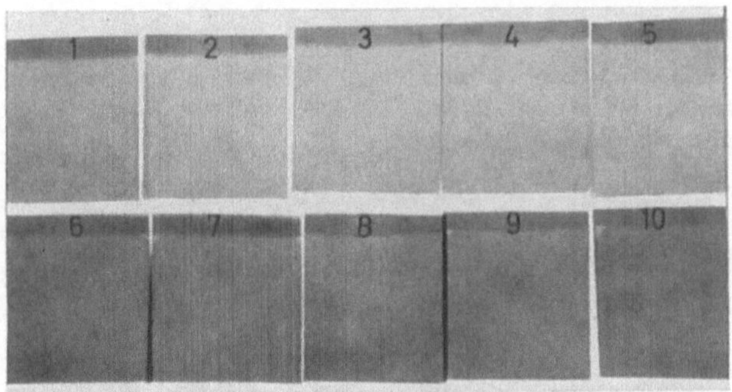

Abb. 2c. Röntgenaufnahme des gleichen Phantoms zusätzlich mit Wasser gefüllt. (Nach Virtama, 1960; Abb. 2b)

Zunahme des Knochenmineralgehaltes ist. Unter günstigsten Bedingungen können Unterschiede von 2% erkannt werden, doch sind gewöhnlich sehr viel größere Unterschiede erforderlich, um sie *deutlich sichtbar* werden zu lassen. Die Angaben von Neeff (1925) und Jacobson (1957), Differenzen von 0,5% seien noch zu erkennen, liegen sicher zu niedrig, während die von Ebert (1957) gefundenen Unterschiede von 5—15% bei einer gleichmäßigen Verteilung des Knochenminerals von Virtama (1960) als zu hoch angesehen werden. Bei normaler Knochenstruktur kann das unbewaffnete Auge höchstens Differenzen von 30% sicher erfassen. So muß z.B. in einem Wirbelkörper der Mineralgehalt um 30—40% erniedrigt sein, um auf dem Röntgenbild erkennbar zu werden.

Baker, Butterworth und Langley (1946) kommen auf Grund von Serienröntgenaufnahmen zu der Ansicht, daß unter klinischen Bedingungen nur etwa 50% mehr oder weniger Calcium im Knochen festgestellt werden könne. Babaiantz (1947) weist darauf hin, daß eine Osteoporose im Röntgenbild wohl erkannt, jedoch nicht klassifiziert werden kann. Untersuchungen am menschlichen *Wirbelkörper* ergaben, daß Entkalkungen von 30% *gerade noch*, von 50—70% *gut* im Röntgenbild sichtbar sind.

Die Schwierigkeit der röntgenologischen Erkennung selbst *umschriebener Entkalkungen* des Knochens geht aus den Untersuchungen von Ardran (1951) hervor. Bohrungen von 3 mm Durchmesser waren in der Wirbelkörperspongiosa nur dann zu erkennen, wenn der

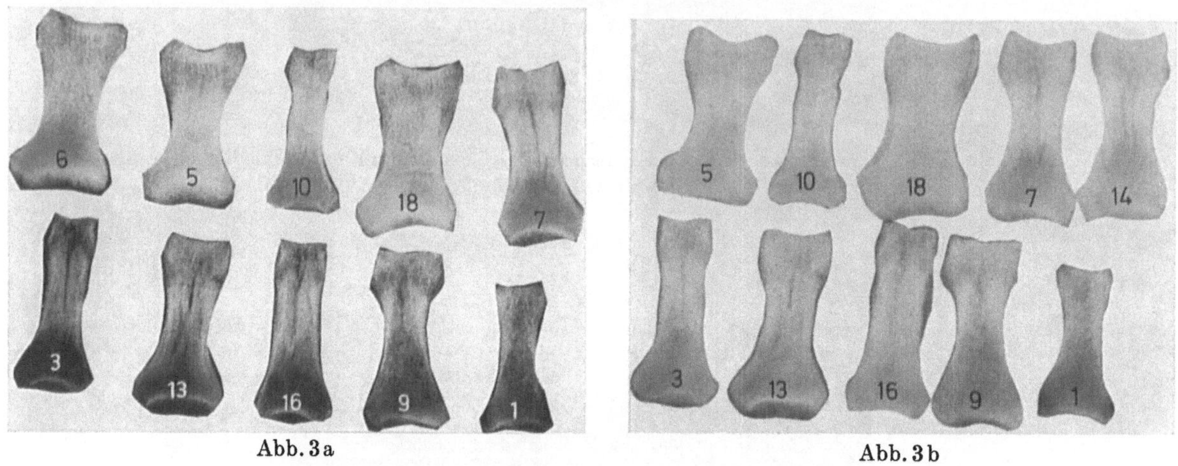

Abb. 3a Abb. 3b

Abb. 3a. Zusammenstellung der Röntgenbilder einer Knochengruppe ohne Wasser. (Nach Virtama, 1960; Abb. 3a)

Abb. 3b. Die Röntgenaufnahmen der gleichen Knochengruppe im Wasserbad in etwas veränderter Zusammenstellung. (Nach Virtama, 1960; Abb. 3b)

Wirbel nicht im Wasserphantom, sondern frei in Luft geröntgt wurde. Ein Defekt von 14 mm Durchmesser war im Wasserphantom nur schwach als „porotische Fläche" sichtbar. In einer experimentellen Studie hat Knutsson (1953) an Knochenpräparaten die Probleme der röntgenologischen Darstellbarkeit von Defekten, strukturellen Veränderungen und Frakturen in der Spongiosa aufgezeigt. Von großem Einfluß auf die Erkennbarkeit eines pathologischen Knochenprozesses sei die *Weichteilüberlagerung* der Knochen, besonders der Wirbelkörper. Der Wert der *Tomographie* zur Verbesserung der röntgenologischen Darstellung und damit Erkennbarkeit von Spongiosadefekten wird besonders hervorgehoben.

Fusi (1953) hat Modelluntersuchungen an Präparaten gesunder Lendenwirbelkörper durchgeführt, um die Möglichkeiten der röntgenologischen Erfassung einer Osteoporose zu bestimmen. Knochenscheiben aus den Lendenwirbelkörpern wurden in 5%iger Salpetersäure entkalkt und dann röntgenologisch untersucht. Am *isolierten Wirbelknochen* konnte eine Abnahme des Kalkgehaltes von ca. 3% erkannt werden, doch gilt dies nur für das Präparat! Am Patienten kann dagegen röntgenologisch erst eine Verminderung des Kalkgehaltes der Wirbelkörper um mindestens 60% des normalen Wertes erfaßt werden.

Vergleichende röntgenologische und chemisch-analytische Untersuchungen zur Frage der Darstellbarkeit von *Entkalkungen der Fingerknochen* hat Cobb (1951) angestellt. Einer röntgenologisch eben noch erkennbaren Veränderung in einem Knochenpräparat lag ein chemisch-analytisch ermittelter Unterschied des Kalksalzgehaltes von 9% zu Grunde, während bei einem ganzen Finger erst ein Unterschied von etwa 25% auffiel. Da die Vergleiche an einem relativ leicht zu untersuchenden, d.h. nur durch wenig Weichteile bedeckten Knochen des Körpers durchgeführt worden sind, dürfte eine Entkalkung der Wirbelsäule sehr viel schwerer zu entdecken sein.

KELLGREN und BIER (1956) haben die Röntgenbilder von 259 Fällen einer *rheumatischen Arthritis* verschiedenen Untersuchern (vier Klinikern und zwei Radiologen) zur Beurteilung vorgelegt. Die gefundenen *Unterschiede in der Beurteilung* waren besonders groß hinsichtlich einer reinen *Entkalkung des Knochens. Destruktionen* konnten sehr viel *deutlicher erkannt werden,* doch wurde ihre Ausdehnung von den verschiedenen Untersuchern unterschiedlich beurteilt. Nach einem Jahr wurden dieselben Röntgenfilme erneut zur Auswertung vorgelegt. Bei dem gleichen Untersucher fanden sich auch nach einem Jahr keine Differenzen in der Beurteilung der Filme.

Untersuchungen zur Detailerkennbarkeit im Röntgenbild hat RÖHLER (1957) durchgeführt. Er kommt zu dem Ergebnis, daß *kleine und kontrastarme Details* sowohl subjektiv als auch objektiv nur begrenzt auf dem Röntgenfilm erfaßt werden können, da die Filmschwärzung gewissen Schwankungen unterliegt. Die Möglichkeiten einer Erfassung werden bestimmt durch das Verhältnis der Gradation des Filmes zur mittleren Schwärzungsschwankung der Emulsion. Hieraus kann gefolgert werden, daß feinere Änderungen der Spongiosastruktur *nicht erkannt* werden können, jedoch *in der Gesamtabsorption erscheinen müssen.* Das Auge kann Leucht-Dichteunterschiede am Lichtkasten zwar wahrnehmen, aber nicht unterscheiden, ob sie echt sind oder nicht, d.h., ob sie durch Details hervorgerufen werden, die tatsächlich vorhanden sind. Derartige Differenzen lassen sich *nur durch photometrische Messungen* erfassen.

Im *Tierversuch* hat LANDOFF (1942) die Nachweisbarkeit einer *Knochenatrophie* infolge Immobilisation, nach einer akuten Arthritis und bei dem sog. Sudeck-Syndrom studiert. Röntgenologisch war eine Differenz des Kalkgehaltes nur dann mit einiger Sicherheit feststellbar, wenn Unterschiede von 10—15% vorlagen. Unterschiede der Projektion des Knochens im Röntgenbild machen die Feststellung eines atrophischen Prozesses schwierig. Das Röntgenbild allein kann nicht als Indikator für eine zunehmende Atrophie oder eine Ausheilung derselben angesehen werden. Ferner können atrophische Prozesse unterschiedlicher Genese nicht miteinander verglichen werden.

Ein großer praktischer Wert kommt allen Feststellungen experimenteller Art nicht zu. *Die Schwierigkeiten der Beurteilung des Kalkgehaltes der Knochen* aus dem Röntgenbild sind in *verschiedenen Faktoren* begründet. Nicht nur die unterschiedliche Projektion des gleichen Knochens bei verschiedenen Aufnahmen und die ungleichmäßige Verteilung der Knochenmineralien im Knochen selbst, sondern auch photographische Fehler spielen eine Rolle. Von besonderer Bedeutung sind die Dauer der Strahlenexposition des Filmes und der Entwicklungsprozeß. Eine Über- oder Unterbelichtung sowie eine Fehlentwicklung des Röntgenfilmes können sowohl eine Verminderung als auch eine Vermehrung des Kalksalzgehaltes vortäuschen.

Die Beurteilung des Kalksalzgehaltes der Knochen aus dem Röntgenbild ist also einerseits von *dem subjektiven Eindruck* des Beobachters, andererseits von *zahlreichen physikalischen Faktoren* abhängig, die bei dem Zustandekommen des Röntgenbildes eine Rolle spielen. Nur eine größere Erfahrung wird es erlauben, Vermutungen über Veränderungen des Kalksalzgehaltes auf Grund einer erhöhten Strahlendurchlässigkeit des Knochens, also einer verminderten Dichte desselben, zu äußern (Tabelle 2). Angaben über einen Kalksalzverlust des Skeletes sollten bei der Beurteilung von Systemerkrankungen zurückhaltend bewertet werden, während röntgenologische Hinweise auf *Struktur- und Konturveränderungen,* auf Deformitäten, Umbauzonen oder pathologische Frakturen eine größere Beweiskraft für das Vorhandensein einer primären oder sekundären Knochenerkrankung besitzen. In dem von MAASS (1951/52) bearbeiteten Krankengut der Kieler Medizinischen Universitätsklinik war das Symptom des „Glockenthorax" in 25%, das Vorkommen multipler pathologischer Frakturen in 10 % und eine Wirbelsäulenverbiegung (Kyphose, Kyphoskoliose) in etwa 20 % der Fälle festzustellen (Tabelle 3). Das Zusammentreffen von *mehreren Symptomen* besitzt im Hinblick auf die Sicherheit der Diagnose „Entkalkungsosteopathie" entscheidende Bedeutung.

Tabelle 2. *Ergebnis eines Vergleiches zwischen subjektiver Beurteilung von Röntgenbildern und radiologischer Messung des Knochenmineralgehaltes am Beispiel der Lendenwirbelsäule*

Anzahl der Patienten	Objektive Bewertung des Hydroxylapatitgehaltes der Lendenwirbelsäule	Subjektive Deutung des Röntgenbildes			
		∅	+	++	+++
40	∅	70 %	28 %	2 %	—
24	+	33,5 %	66,5 %	—	—
56	++	9 %	23 %	62,5 %	5,5 %
54	+++	—	7 %	39 %	54 %

[KROKOWSKI, E.; Dtsch. med. Wschr. **91**, 60 (1966), Tab. 1]

Tabelle 3. *Zusammenstellung der Kombination von röntgenologisch nachweisbaren Skeletveränderungen bei Osteopathien*

	Glockenthorax	Kyphosen, Skoliosen	Wirbeldeformierungen	Frakturen Loosersche Umbauzonen	Rippentiefstand
Unkombiniert	9	2	5	6	
Rippentiefstand	3	4	3		4 / 1
Frakturen, Loosersche Umbauzonen	1	3	3	12 / 2	
Wirbeldeformierungen	6	7	18 / 17		1
Kyphosen, Skoliosen	2	12 / 15	5		1
Glockenthorax	17 / 19	7	1		
Unkombiniert	12	4	11	2	

Teil a: Linke, obere Hälfte; ausgeprägte Fälle von Systemerkrankungen.
Teil b: Rechte, untere Hälfte; weniger ausgeprägte Fälle von Systemerkrankungen.
Die Häufigkeit der Zuordnung ergibt sich im jeweiligen Schnittfeld der waagerechten und senkrechten Reihen. Die unterteilten Diagonalfelder enthalten die Anzahl der Fälle, die das betreffende Symptom überhaupt aufweisen. (MAASS, K.: Diss. Kiel 1951, Abb. 3).

2. Die Beurteilung des Knochenmineralgehaltes durch visuellen Vergleich mit einem Referenzsystem

Bei den ersten Versuchen, die subjektive Beurteilung des Knochenkalksalzgehaltes aus dem Röntgenbild zu *objektivieren*, wurde der visuelle Vergleich zwischen der Filmschwärzung *durch den Knochen* und der Filmschwärzung durch *ein bekanntes Referenzsystem* angestrebt. Die einfachste Form eines Referenzsystems oder „Standardwertes" zur Beurteilung der röntgenologischen Dichte von Knochen bestand in einem normal kalkhaltigen, präparierten Leichenknochen.

Untersuchungen mit einem solchen *„Standardknochen"* sind von STEVEN (1947) am Handskelet durchgeführt worden. Als Referenzsystem wurde ein Metacarpale II des Erwachsenenskeletes empfohlen (Abb. 4). Zur Nachahmung der Weichteile wurde der entfettete Knochen zunächst in Paraffin eingebettet. Da dieses Einbettungsmaterial weniger absorbierte — also nicht den Weichteilen entsprach —, wurde der Knochen in eine Mischung aus 5 Gewichtsteilen Paraffin und 5 Gewichtsteilen Bienenwachs mit

1 Gewichtsteil Sägemehl eingelegt. Dieses Gemisch ergab zufriedenstellende Befunde (Abb. 5). Mit Hilfe des „Phantomknochens" sollte *die Beurteilung der Knochendichte* bei Rheumatikern von Aufnahme- und Entwicklungsbedingungen unabhängig gemacht werden. Die ersten Untersuchungen wurden bei rheumatischer Arthritis (Abb. 6), Spondylitis ankylopoetica und Gicht (Abb. 7) durchgeführt. Es sei möglich, rheumatische Erkrankungen von der Gicht zu differenzieren, da das Auftreten einer generalisierten Osteoporose beim Rheumatismus ein entscheidend wichtiger Faktor sei.

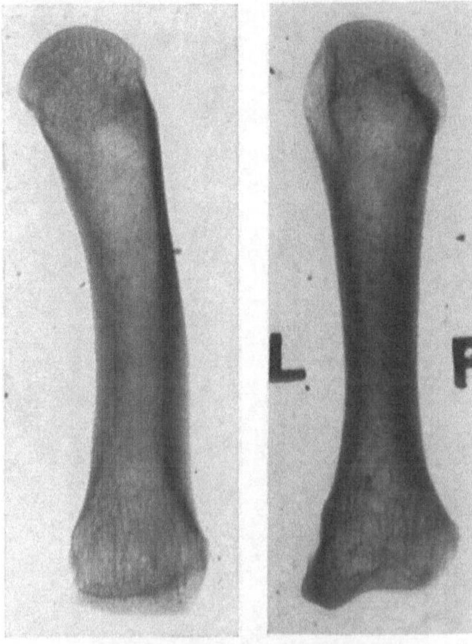

Abb. 4. Röntgenaufnahme des „Standardknochens" von STEVEN (1947) in 2 Ebenen. Die Seitenaufnahme zeigt eine Dicke von 3 cm distal und von 4 cm proximal (zum Handgelenk hin)

Die Möglichkeiten und Grenzen der einfachen *visuellen Abschätzung* des Mineralgehaltes der Knochen der Hand beim Verwenden eines Satzes von *Standardknochen* (Fingerknochen) haben LAITINEN, VIRKKUNEN und VIRTAMA (1958) aufgezeigt. Das Ergebnis der visuellen Beurteilung durch verschiedene Untersucher wurde mit den Knochendichtewerten, bestimmt nach der Methode der Silberanalyse von VIRTAMA (1957), verglichen. Die Abweichungen waren gering, so daß die Methode für den klinischen Gebrauch gut geeignet erscheint.

Von NACHLASS und PARKE (zit. nach STEIN, 1937) wurde der visuelle Vergleich zwischen der Knochendichte und einem *treppenförmigen Vergleichskörper* empfohlen.

Den *visuellen Schwärzungsvergleich* zwischen einem Aluminiumphantom und dem Daumenknochen hat BALZ (1968) empfohlen. Der Vergleichskörper besteht aus zwei Plexiglasplatten von 5 mm Dicke (als Weichteilersatz, dem Durchmesser der Weichteile

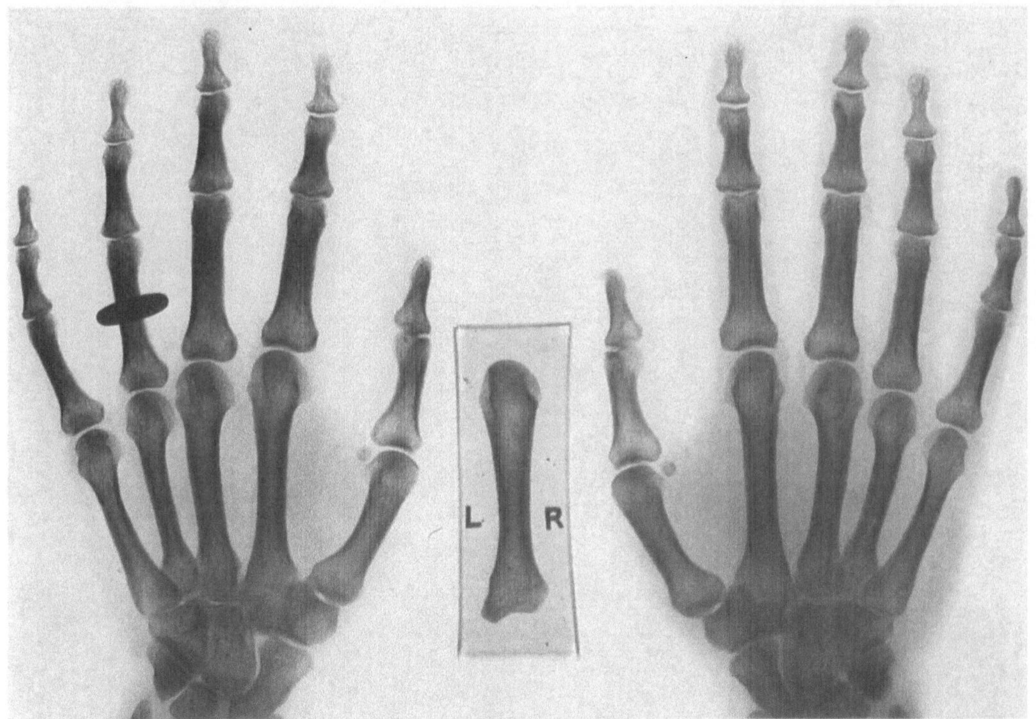

Abb. 5. Röntgenaufnahme der Hände eines gesunden Erwachsenen mit dem „Standardknochen". (Nach STEVEN, 1947)

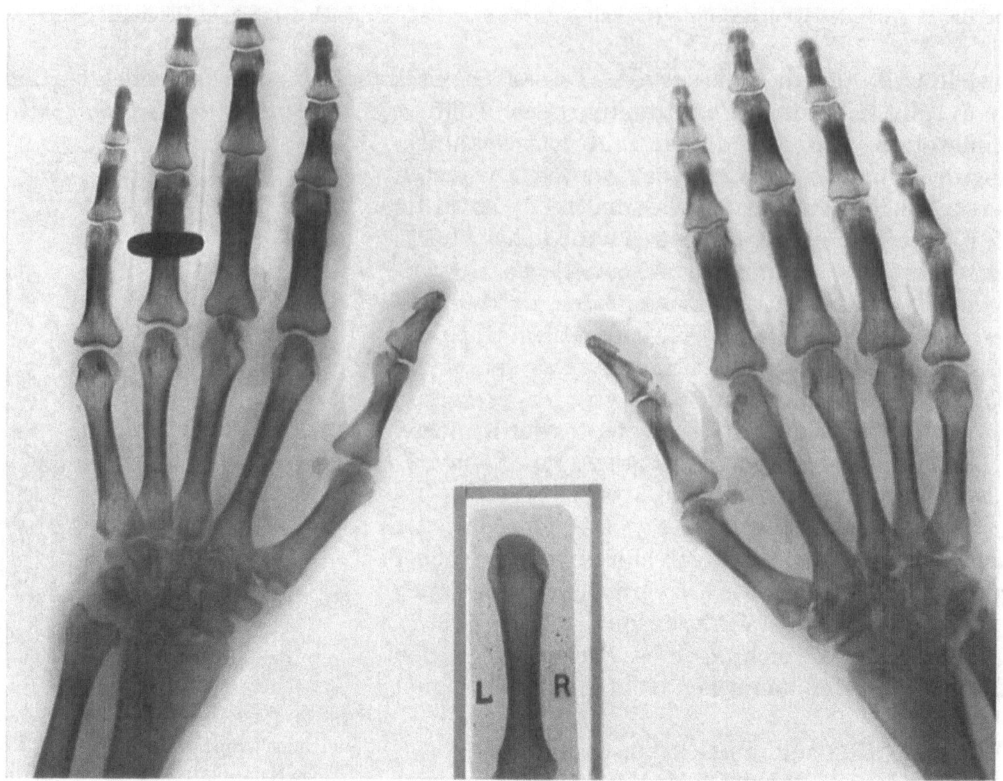

Abb. 6. Röntgenaufnahme der Hände bei rheumatischer Arthritis mit dem „Standardknochen" (die Aufnahme wurde freundlicherweise von STEVEN zur Verfügung gestellt)

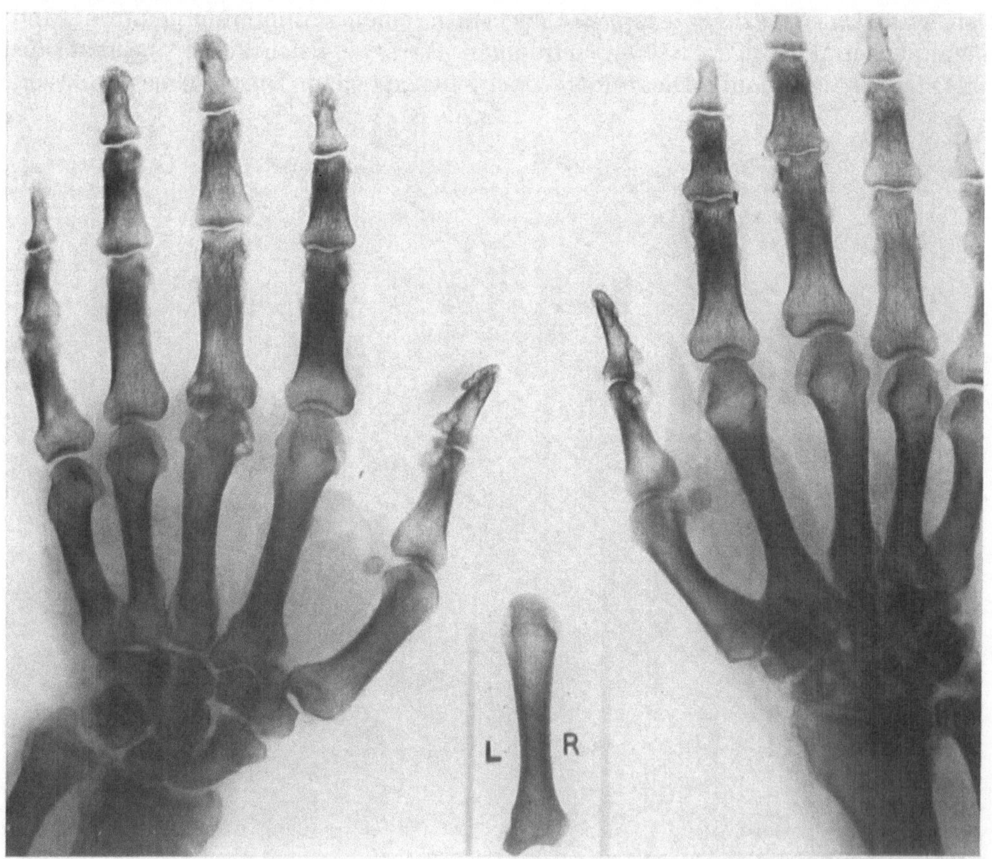

Abb. 7. Röntgenaufnahme der Hände bei Gicht zusammen mit dem „Standardknochen" (die Aufnahme wurde freundlicherweise von STEVEN zur Verfügung gestellt)

entsprechend), zwischen die ein Aluminiumblech von 4,0 und 4,6 mm Dicke (als Referenzsubstanz für den Knochen) eingefügt wird. Die Kontrolle der richtigen Lage von Daumen und Referenzsystem erfolgt durch einen folienlosen Film. Der zur Auswertung verwendete Film wird in eine 9×12 Folienkassette zwischen hochverstärkende Folien eingelegt. Der Röntgenfilm liegt der Folie jedoch nicht an, sondern es wird eine 1 mm dicke Plexiglasscheibe auf beiden Seiten dazwischen gelegt. Hierdurch wird die Aufnahme unscharf, die Spongiosazeichnung verwaschen und die Schwärzung des Filmes praktisch homogen (Abb. 8). Die Aufnahmeexposition wird mit einem Fokus-Objektabstand von 100 cm und einem Objekt-Filmabstand von 50 cm durchgeführt. Bei dieser Vergrößerungstechnik wird die Streustrahlung unwirksam und die Meßstelle des Daumenknochens für den visuellen Vergleich erheblich vergrößert. Ferner sollen Film- und Folienfehler weitgehend ausgeschaltet

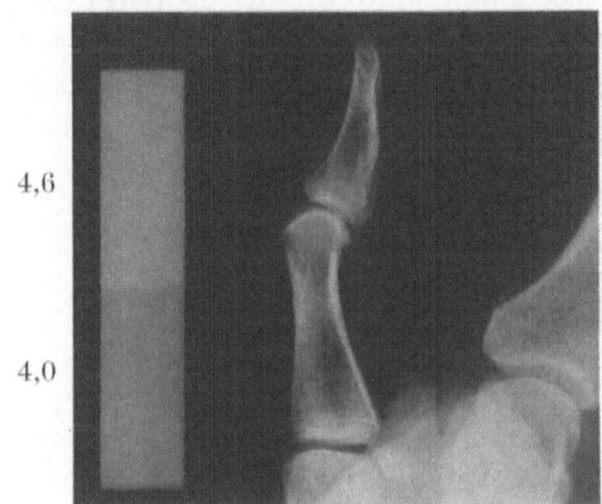

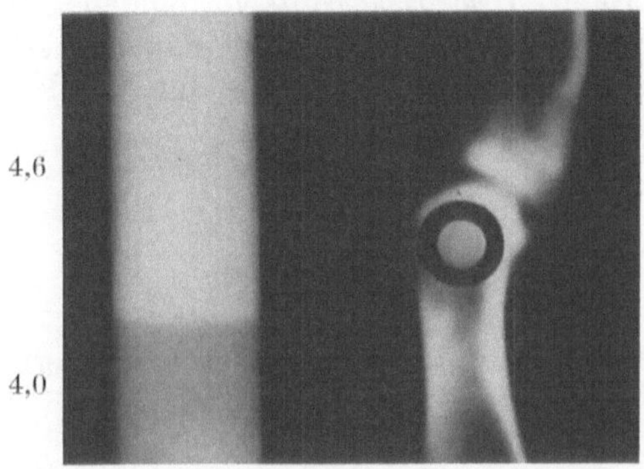

Abb. 8. Standardaufnahme (links) und Vergrößerungsaufnahme des Daumens und des Referenz-Systems bei einem Objekt-Filmabstand von 50 cm (rechts) zur visuellen Schätzung des Knochenmineralgehaltes. (Nach BALZ, 1968)

werden. Der visuelle Vergleich der Filmschwärzung in der Knochenregion und der Region des Aluminiumreferenzsystems erfolgt nach Zerschneiden der Filme vor einem Schaukasten. Mit Hilfe eines Schwärzungsmessers und einer weiteren Aluminiumstufe können jedoch genauere Meßwerte ermittelt werden.

IV. Theoretische Grundlagen radiologischer Messungen des Knochenmineralgehaltes

1. Die physikalischen Grundlagen

Der Knochen kann als *ein Gemisch aufgefaßt werden*, das sich aus zwei die Röntgenstrahlen oder Gammastrahlen *unterschiedlich absorbierenden Elementgruppen* zusammensetzt:

1. der organischen Grundsubstanz (vorwiegend Wasserstoff, Kohlenstoff, Sauerstoff und Stickstoff);

2. den anorganischen Kalksalzen.

Die Frage, in welcher Form der Mineralanteil im Knochen vorliegt, scheint noch nicht endgültig geklärt zu sein. Die Ergebnisse der meisten röntgenspektrographischen Untersuchungen sprechen dafür, daß die Calcium- und Magnesiumsalze des Knochens *in der Hauptsache einen Hydroxylapatit mit Beimengungen von Carbonatapatit bilden*. Die Entstehung des Hydroxylapatits im Knochengewebe ist noch nicht geklärt. Es wird angenommen, daß die Bildung aus dem sekundären Calciumphosphat oder dem Pyrophosphat erfolge. Der Nachweis dieser Vorstufen ist schwierig, da sie meist bei der Zerstörung der organischen Matrix mit entfernt werden und nur dann gefunden werden können, wenn der Knochen mehr als 25% des sekundären Phosphats enthält.

Bisher wurde die Bestimmung der absoluten Menge der Knochenmineralien aus dem Röntgenbild für nicht möglich gehalten, weil die Konstanz der Zusammensetzung der Kalksalze nicht allgemein anerkannt wurde. Nach den Untersuchungen von GABRIEL (1894), KLEMENT (1929/38) und HEUCK und SCHMIDT (1954/60) weist die anorganische Knochensubstanz des normalen Skeletes unabhängig von Alterungsvorgängen ein weitgehend konstantes Verhältnis von $CaO:P_2O_5$ auf. Geringfügige Abweichungen in dem Quotienten $CaO:P_2O_5$ kommen dadurch zustande, daß *neben dem Hydroxylapatit* noch Phosphate, Carbonate, Citrate und andere Calciumverbindungen im Knochen vorliegen (NETTER 1959). Diese Abweichungen sind allein für die Biochemie des Knochens von Interesse und wegen ihrer Geringfügigkeit bei der radiologischen Messung des Mineralgehaltes im Knochen ohne Belang (s. hierzu DULCE, S. 15).

Bedeutungsvoll *für die Absorption der Röntgenstrahlen* sind die in größerer Menge *in Form des Hydroxylapatits* vorhandenen schweren Elemente *Calcium* und *Phosphor*. In welcher Weise die Stoffe miteinander verbunden sind, ist für die Strahlenabsorption bedeutungslos. Die Absorption läßt sich durch folgende Exponentialgleichung darstellen:

$$I = I_0\, e^{-\mu d}$$

I_0 = eingestrahlte Intensität
I = geschwächte Intensität
μ = Schwächungskoeffizient
d = Schichtdicke.

Diese Gleichung kann man auch folgendermaßen schreiben:

$$I = I_0 e^{-\frac{\mu}{\varrho} w}$$

$\frac{\mu}{\varrho}$ = Massenschwächungskoeffizient
w = Flächengewicht ($w = \varrho \cdot d$)
ϱ = spezifisches Gewicht.

Die Schwächungskoeffizienten setzen sich aus Einzelkomponenten zusammen. Für den Massenschwächungskoeffizienten μ/ϱ kann unterschieden werden:

$$\frac{\mu_K}{\varrho_K} = \frac{\mu_1}{\varrho_1} \cdot \frac{m_1}{100} + \cdots \quad \cdots + \frac{\mu_n}{\varrho_n} \cdot \frac{m_n}{100}$$

$\frac{\mu_K}{\varrho_K}$ = Massenschwächungskoeffizient des Knochens;

$\frac{\mu_1}{\varrho_1}, \cdots, \frac{\mu_n}{\varrho_n}$ = Massenschwächungskoeffizienten der Komponenten des Knochens;

$m_1, \cdots, m_n$ = Gewichtsprozente der Komponenten des Knochens.

Der Massenphotoabsorptionskoeffizient r/ϱ ist von der Wellenlänge λ der verwendeten Röntgenstrahlung und von der Kernladungszahl Z des absorbierenden Stoffes abhängig (Abb. 9).

$$\frac{r}{\varrho} = 4{,}86 \cdot 10^{-3} \cdot Z^{3,12} \cdot \lambda^3 - 1{,}37 \cdot 10^{-6}\, Z^{5,18} \cdot \lambda^4$$

für $\lambda < \lambda K$ und $Z \geqq 3$, mit λ_K = Fluoreszenzwellenlänge.

In durchstrahlten Medien entsteht die Intensitätsschwächung durch photoelektrische Absorption (r/ϱ), durch Streuprozesse (σ/ϱ = Massenstreukoeffizient klassische Streuung, Compton-Streuung) und bei Energien über 1,02 MeV (ultraharte Röntgenstrahlen) zunehmend durch Paarbildung (π/ϱ = Massenpaarbildungskoeffizient), indem aus einem Strahlenquant ein Elektron und ein Positron entsteht.

$$\frac{\mu}{\varrho} = \frac{r}{\varrho} + \frac{\sigma}{\varrho} + \frac{\pi}{\varrho}.$$

Bei zunehmender Spannung, also kürzerer Wellenlänge, tritt der Photoeffekt gegenüber dem Compton-Effekt zurück (Abb. 10, Tabelle 4), wodurch die Ordnungszahl der einzelnen

Substanzen an Bedeutung verliert, so daß die Absorptionsdifferenz und damit der Kontrast zwischen den Weichteilen und dem Knochengewebe gering wird. Es sollte nach Möglichkeit mit einer weichen Strahlung gearbeitet werden, um einen guten Kontrast zu erzielen.

Die Strahlenabsorption in einem Stoffgemisch (z. B. dem Knochen) setzt sich additiv *aus den einzelnen Koeffizienten* der Bestandteile zusammen.

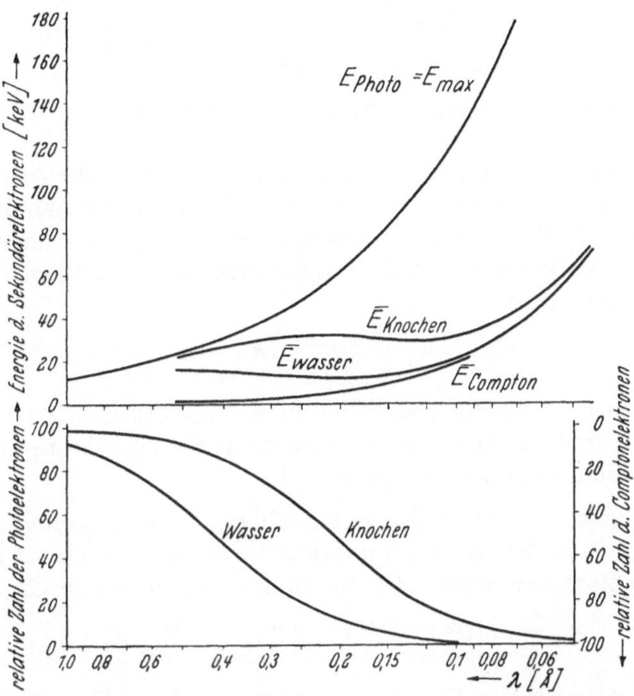

Abb. 9. *Oben:* Energie der Sekundärelektronen in Abhängigkeit von der Strahlenqualität (E_{photo} = Energie der ausgelösten Photoelektronen, E_{compton} = mittlere Energie der Comptonelektronen, E_{knochen} = mittlere Energie sämtlicher im Knochen ausgelösten Elektronen, E_{wasser} = mittlere Energie sämtlicher im Wasser ausgelösten Elektronen). *Unten:* Prozentualer Anteil der Photo- und Comptonelektronen. (Nach KROKOWSKI, 1959; Abb. 4)

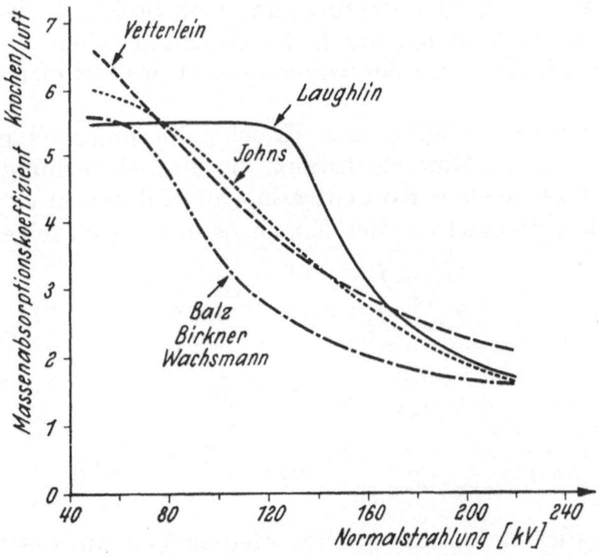

Abb. 10. Der Massenabsorptionskoeffizient von Knochen relativ zu Luft in Abhängigkeit von der Strahlenqualität (gemessen von verschiedenen Autoren). (Nach KROKOWSKI, 1959; Abb. 3)

Tabelle 4. *Zusammenstellung der charakteristischen röntgenphysikalischen Daten für den Knochen*

Photoeffekt	Comptoneffekt	Paarbildung	Dichte (g/cm³)	Beobachter
$Z_{eff} = 15,4$				VETTERLEIN
$Z_{eff} = 13,8$	$N_{eff} = 3,00 \cdot 10^{23}$	$Z_{eff} = 10,0$	1,85	JOHNS
$Z_{eff} = 13,8$—14				SPIERS
	$N_{eff} = 3,16 \cdot 10^{23}$	$Z_{eff} = 6,21$	1,85	JOYET u.a.
$Z_{eff} = 15$			1,9	GRASHEY, BIRKNER
			1,470	HELLRIEGEL
$Z_{eff} = 14,0$	$N_{eff} = 3,1 \cdot 10^{23}$	$NZ = 31 \cdot 10^{23}$	1,5	KROKOWSKI

[KROKOWSKI, E.: Fortschr. Röntgenstr. **91**, 76 (1959), Tab. 1]

In dieser Gleichung müssen alle im Knochen analytisch nachweisbaren Atome berücksichtigt werden. Die Elemente der organischen Grundsubstanzen mit kleinem Schwächungskoeffizienten (O, N, C, H u.a.) können gegenüber den Elementen der Knochenkalksalze Ca und P mit großem Schwächungskoeffizienten vernachlässigt werden. So ist folgende Gleichung möglich:

$$\frac{\mu_k}{\varrho_k} = \left(\frac{\mu}{\varrho}\right)_{org} \cdot \frac{m_{org}}{100} + \left(\frac{\mu}{\varrho}\right)_{Ca,P} \cdot \frac{m_{Ca,P}}{100}$$

$\left(\frac{\mu}{\varrho}\right)_{org}, \left(\frac{\mu}{\varrho}\right)_{anorg}$ = Massenschwächungskoeffizient der organischen Knochenbestandteile (Mittelwert) und der anorganischen Knochenbestandteile (Mittelwert),

m_{org}, m_{anorg} = Gewichtsprozente entsprechend.

Da das Calcium-Phosphor-Verhältnis im Knochen nur sehr geringfügige Abweichungen erkennen läßt, kann aus den Schwächungskoeffizienten von Ca und P auf den Gehalt an Kalksalzen geschlossen werden. Hieraus ergibt sich folgende Gleichung:

$$\ln \frac{I_o}{I} = \left[\left(\frac{\mu}{\varrho}\right)_{org} \cdot \frac{m_{org}}{100} + \left(\frac{\mu}{\varrho}\right)_{anorg} \cdot \frac{m_{Ca,P}}{100}\right] \cdot d \cdot \varrho_k$$

Diese Beziehung gilt exakt nur für eine monochromatische Strahlung, doch ist sie auch noch anwendbar, wenn die Untersuchungen mit einer polychromatischen Strahlung durchgeführt werden, deren Strahlenhärte gleich der der monochromatischen ist, da dann von Aufnahme zu Aufnahme eine gleichbleibende Intensitätsverteilung der ausgestrahlten Wellenlängen gewährleistet ist.

Zur *Messung der Konzentration* der Knochenkalksalze ist die Kenntnis der Schwächungskoeffizienten der organischen und anorganischen Stoffe, die Ermittlung der Intensitätsabnahme der Röntgenstrahlung durch die Weichteile allein I_w und die Weichteile mit Knochen I_{wk} sowie die Kenntnis des Durchmessers des untersuchten Knochens notwendig (Abb. 11).

Messungen ohne Berücksichtigung des Knochendurchmessers geben lediglich eine Information über die gesamte Mineralsubstanz, die die Schwächung der Strahlung verursachte. Über die interessierende Konzentration an Kalksalzen sind daher keine Aussagen möglich. Für die Untersuchung des Knochens ergibt sich folgende Gleichung:

$$I_w = I_0 \, e^{-\mu_{org} D}$$

$$I_{wk} = I_0 \, e^{-\mu_{org}(D-\Delta) - \mu_{org} \Delta},$$

Daraus folgt:

$$\frac{I_w}{I_{wk}} = e^{+(\mu_{anorg} - \mu_{org}) \Delta},$$

$$\mu_{anorg} - \mu_{org} = \frac{\ln \frac{I_w}{I_{wk}}}{\Delta}.$$

Die Meßergebnisse werden dann eine größere Genauigkeit aufweisen, wenn die Unterschiede der Schwächung der Strahlung durch die organische und die anorganische Fraktion des Knochens möglichst groß sind. Diese Voraussetzungen sind bei niedrigen Spannungen von 50—60 kV am günstigsten. Bei ansteigender Anodenspannung werden die Unterschiede schließlich so gering, daß auch die Schwärzung auf dem Röntgenfilm fast die gleiche ist. Eine photometrische Auswertung der Filme birgt dann eine hohe Fehlerquote (s. S. 26).

Zur Bestimmung der Kalksalzkonzentration im Knochen ist es bei allen Meßverfahren erforderlich, die Intensität sowohl innerhalb wie außerhalb des „Knochenschattens" zu messen. Die gemessenen Intensitäten können dann mit denen hinter einem Referenzsystem (knochenähnliches Material, Aluminium, Metall-Legierungen usw.) verglichen werden und Schwächungsgleichwerte angegeben oder die Kalksalzkonzentration unmittelbar berechnet werden. Zur Bestimmung der Intensitätsverhältnisse I_w/I_{wk}, I_w/I_{anorg} und I_w/I_{org} bzw. der Schwächungsgleichwerte können verschiedene Meßgeräte Verwendung finden.

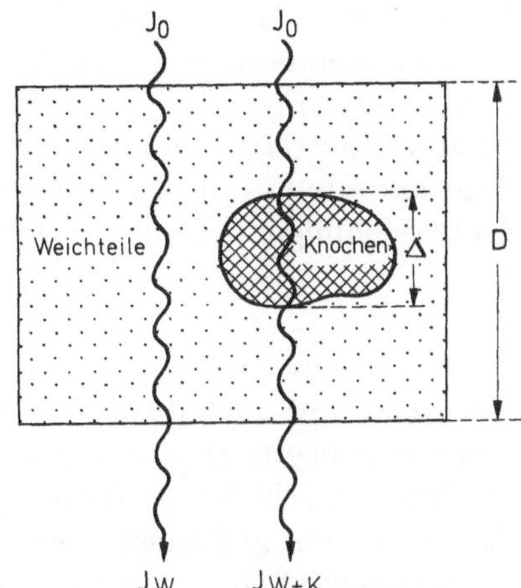

Abb. 11. Schematische Darstellung der Schwächung einer Röntgenstrahlung durch Knochen und Weichteile

2. Die direkten Messungen der Strahlenabsorption (praktische Dosimetrie)

a) Die Ionisationskammer

Die Ionisationskammer erlaubt bei geringstem apparativem Aufwand genaue Intensitätsmessungen. Der gemessene Knochenquerschnitt muß jedoch wegen der niedrigen Empfindlichkeit und wegen der kleinen verfügbaren Intensitäten in der Größenordnung von cm² liegen. Es sind daher Aussagen über den strukturellen Aufbau des Knochens nicht möglich.

Die Meßwerte sind als Mittelwerte über einen größeren Querschnitt des Knochens anzusehen. Es ergeben sich hierdurch stärkere Einschränkungen in der Auswahl des zu untersuchenden Skeletabschnitte. Der Knochendurchmesser sollte zur Vereinfachung der Auswertung der Messungen über den Querschnitt des zu untersuchenden Areals konstant sein. Für diese Messungen gut geeignet ist die Gegend der Femurcondylen (Vose 1958; Györgyi und Bozóky 1961), da in dieser Skeletregion sowohl das Strahlenbündel gut eingeblendet als auch die zur Messung benutzte Ionisationskammer fest und in ihrer Lage zur Strahlenquelle konstant angebracht werden kann. Die Meßkammer hat also stets denselben Abstand vom Brennfleck der Strahlenquelle.

b) Das Geiger-Müller-Zählrohr

Die Empfindlichkeit des Geiger-Müller-Zählrohres ist sehr groß. Hierdurch wird eine Ausblendung des Strahlenbündels ermöglicht, so daß lokale Intensitätsmessungen durchgeführt werden können. Als Strahlenquelle ist *ein Gamma-Strahler* geeignet, der eine konstante Intensität besitzt. Zur Messung ist eine *präzise Verschiebung* des Strahlenbündels oder des zu untersuchenden Objektes erforderlich. Werden diese Voraussetzungen erfüllt, so sind Messungen auch in umschriebenen Arealen oder Aussagen über Strukturen des untersuchten Objektes möglich.

c) Das Proportional-Zählrohr

Die Empfindlichkeit des Proportional-Zählrohres ist zwar geringer als die des Geiger-Müller-Zählrohres, doch sind auch Messungen mit fein ausgeblendetem Strahlenbündel möglich. Hierdurch können Untersuchungen des strukturellen Aufbaues von Knochen vorgenommen werden. Darüber hinaus erlaubt die Proportionalität von Impulshöhe und Energie des absorbierten Strahlungsquants beim Proportional-Zählrohr die Gewinnung eng begrenzter Spektralbereiche. Die Ermittlung einer Schwächung bei bestimmten

Wellenlängen durch den Knochen bedeutet eine wesentliche Verbesserung der Untersuchungsbedingungen. Für die Aussiebung der Spektralbereiche der Strahlung ist ein Linearverstärker und ein Ein- oder Mehrkanalanalysator erforderlich. FROMMHOLD und SCHOKNECHT (1959/60) haben über eine solche Meßapparatur berichtet, die mit Molybdän-Eigenstrahlung unter Verwendung eines Proportional-Zählrohres arbeitet. Für derartige Untersuchungen ist ein beträchtlicher apparativer Aufwand erforderlich.

d) Der Szintillationszähler

Der Szintillationszähler besitzt in dem interessierenden Wellenlängenbereich die höchste Empfindlichkeit. Er erlaubt ebenso wie das Proportionalzählrohr die Aussiebung eines eng begrenzten Spektralbereiches. Durch eine starke Ausblendung des Röntgenstrahlenbündels ist es daher ebenfalls möglich, Informationen über die Struktur des Knochens zu gewinnen. Der Szintillationszähler erfordert ein leistungsfähiges Hochspannungsgerät höchster Konstanz und für die spektralen Messungen wie das Proportionalzählrohr einen Linearverstärker mit Ein- oder Mehrkanalanalysator. Derartige Einrichtungen sind sehr umfangreich und kostspielig.

3. Die Messung der Filmschwärzung

Seit Entdeckung der Röntgenstrahlen sind die photographischen Effekte dieser Strahlen sehr genau studiert worden. Die Brom-Silber-Emulsion eines Filmes wird durch Röntgenstrahlen geschwärzt. Die Untersuchungen dieses Phänomens basieren auf dem Gesetz von BUNSEN und ROSCOE ($E = I \times t$) und auf der charakteristischen Kurve von HURTER und DRIFFIELD, die das Verhältnis von Dichte zum Logarithmus der Exposition darstellt. Da die Schwärzung des Filmes bei konstanter Wellenlänge und Belichtungsdauer sowie gleichbleibenden Entwicklungsbedingungen nur von der Strahlungsintensität abhängt, können den festgestellten Schwärzungen Intensitäten zugeordnet werden.

Das *Filmverfahren* zeigt zwar gegenüber den oben beschriebenen Methoden eine *geringere Empfindlichkeit und Genauigkeit*, doch ermöglicht es *eine gute Orientierung* über die zu untersuchenden Knochenbezirke. Es sind somit wiederholte Untersuchungen an einem *bestimmten Knochenareal* möglich. Weiterhin besitzt der Film ein extrem hohes räumliches Auflösungsvermögen und ermöglicht *genaue Aussagen über die Knochenstruktur*.

Bei konstanter Belichtungszeit ist der Zusammenhang zwischen Schwärzung und Intensität durch die Schwärzungskurve gegeben. Diese Schwärzungskurve verläuft bei Verwendung einer Röntgenstrahlung anfangs gradlinig, weist später eine Krümmung auf und strebt einem Maximum zu. Bei extrem hohen Intensitäten ist eine Verminderung der Schwärzung festzustellen. BARKLA und MARTYN fanden 1913, daß sich der durch Röntgenstrahlen erzeugte photographische Effekt bei einer bestimmten Intensität mit der Wellenlänge veränderte, d.h. je härter die Strahlung, um so geringer der photographische Effekt. Diese Beobachtung ist später bestätigt worden. KIEFFER und SEIDEMANN (1946) konnten feststellen, daß eine charakteristische Kurve für Filmmaterial, Entwicklung und eine bestimmte Strahlenqualität dazu benutzt werden können, um genaue Messungen relativer Intensitäten aus der Schwärzung eines Filmes durchzuführen. Im Anfangsbereich ist die Schwärzung der Intensität proportional. Bei allen densitometrischen Meßmethoden zur Bestimmung der Kalksalzkonzentration im Knochen wird nach Möglichkeit in diesem linearen Bereich gearbeitet, da hier die Auswertung besonders einfach ist.

Die *Filmschwärzungen* können auf verschiedene Weise gemessen werden. Das *Silber kann* in der entwickelten Filmschicht direkt *durch eine chemische Analyse*, *Neutronenaktivierung* oder eine *Röntgenfluoreszenzanalyse* bestimmt werden. Diese Untersuchungsmethoden sind sehr genau, jedoch für die klinische Praxis aufwendig und umständlich. Ihre Anwendung erstreckt sich vorwiegend auf optisch nicht mehr faßbare Schwärzungen des Filmes. Eine weitere Methode zur Analyse der Filmschwärzung besteht in der *Transparenzmessung*. Sie ist die in der Praxis übliche Methode. Die Durchlässigkeit eines Filmes für sichtbares Licht ist von dem Schwärzungsgrad der Filmemulsion abhängig. Die Schwärzung S (im englischen Schrifttum density $= D$) ist definiert als dekadischer Logarithmus des Verhältnisses der Lichtintensitäten L_0 und L_1 mit schwächendem Film ($S = \log L_0/L_1$). Eine quantitative Aussage über die Lichtintensitäten L_0 und L_1 und damit über die Schwärzung ist durch photometrische Messung möglich.

Faktoren, welche die Photometrie beeinflussen, hat WILSEY (1934) studiert. Er kommt zu dem Ergebnis, daß es kaum einen Weg geben wird, um die Photometrie mit Methoden durchzuführen, die die photographischen Eigenschaften des Filmes ganz ausschließen, so daß bleibende und absolute Werte erzielt werden können. Die numerischen Werte werden immer abhängig sein von den speziellen Eigenschaften des benutzten photographischen Materials. Im allgemeinen jedoch zeigt das photographische Phänomen durch Röntgenstrahlenbelichtung weniger Variationen als bei Belichtung mit normalem, sichtbarem Licht. Die besonderen Probleme der Photometrie bei Verwendung der Hartstrahltechnik hat MATTSON (1955) untersucht. Der Einfluß von Streustrahlen auf die photometrische Auswertung der Röntgenfilme muß besonders beachtet werden. Auf die Photometrie sind weiterhin folgende Faktoren von Einfluß: Veränderungen der Empfindlichkeit der Emulsion, Veränderungen des Entwicklungsgrades, der Zeit-Intensitätsfaktor, der Unterbrechungsfaktor, die spektrale Empfindlichkeit des photographischen Materials und der Kontrast. Zur Vermeidung von Fehlern durch diese Faktoren sollte insbesondere eine *Standardisierung* der Belichtung und der Behandlung der Filme angestrebt werden.

Die Probleme und Fehler der Densitometrie des Knochens haben BISMUTH (1959) beschäftigt. Als wichtigste Schwierigkeit sind die Streustrahlung durch Weichteilüberlagerung zu nennen. Die von VOSE (1959) vorgeschlagenen *direkten* Absorptionsmessungen seien weniger geeignet als die Verfahren der Densitometrie von Röntgenfilmen. Die Densitometrie sei einfach, leicht reproduzierbar, durch den Film zu belegen und für Verlaufskontrollen gut geeignet.

a) Der Einfluß von Filmmaterial, Entwicklung und Verarbeitung

Es ist oft versucht worden, *unmittelbar* aus den Schwärzungswerten eines Filmes auf die Dichte der geröntgten Gegenstände zu schließen, ohne daß es bisher gelang, ein Verfahren zu entwickeln, das für die klinische Radiologie brauchbar wäre. Die größten Schwierigkeiten bereiten die unterschiedlichen photographischen Eigenschaften der verschiedenen Filmemulsionen und die Qualität der Verstärkerfolien. Untersuchungen über die Bedeutung dieser Faktoren für eine densitometrische Auswertung von Röntgenfilmen haben MORGAN und VAN ALLEN (1949) durchgeführt. Von HEUCK und SCHMIDT (1960) wurde die Brauchbarkeit verschiedener Filmqualitäten (folienlose Filme, Folienfilme, Materialuntersuchungsfilme) für eine photometrische Auswertung der Filme zur Messung der Mineralkonzentration im Knochen geprüft. Der Einfluß der Eigenschaften und Qualität verschiedener *Folien* auf die Filmschwärzung wurde in zahlreichen Untersuchungen eingehend studiert (s. bei FROMMHOLD 1956; WIDENMANN 1957; HEUCK und SCHMIDT 1960; SCHOBER, dieses Handbuch Bd. III, S. 10—42). Die Ergebnisse waren unterschiedlich. Einerseits wurde ein deutlicher Einfluß handelsüblicher Folien auf photometrische Messungen von Röntgenfilmen festgestellt (BALZ und BIRKNER 1956), andererseits konnten nur geringe Schwärzungsdifferenzen eines Röntgenfilmes gefunden werden, die durch das verwendete Folienmaterial induziert worden sind (HEUCK und SCHMIDT 1960). Die mit Verstärkungsfolien verarbeiteten Filme haben durch einen hohen Gammawert eine relativ große Empfindlichkeit, was bei geringen Schwärzungsunterschieden durch die dargestellten Gegenstände von Nutzen ist.

Von großem Einfluß auf photometrische Messungen ist die *Gleichmäßigkeit des Filmgusses*, da Guß-Schlieren erhebliche Fehler hervorrufen können (VIRTAMA 1957). Prüfungen der Homogenität des Filmmaterials wurden von HINESS (1968) mit einer Gammastrahlung vorgenommen und bei einer mittleren Schwärzung von $S = 1$ Schwankungen von 2,2% gefunden.

Eine Unter- oder Überbelichtung der Filme sollte vermieden werden, da die Auswertung von Schwärzungsdifferenzen nur im gradlinigen Teil der Gradationskurve sinnvoll ist. Die Prüfung der Filme auf Reproduzierbarkeit eines Intensitätsverhältnisses ergab einen mittleren Fehler von $\pm 1{,}4\,\%$ (HINESS 1968).

Die große Bedeutung der *Entwicklung und Verarbeitung* der Röntgenfilme für eine photometrische Auswertung, insbesondere zur quantitativen Messung des Knochenmineralgehaltes ist von allen Arbeitsgruppen hervorgehoben worden. Sehr eingehend wurden diese Fragen, Probleme und Zusammenhänge von VIRTAMA (1957) bearbeitet.

Die zur Entwicklung und Verarbeitung der Röntgenfilme von den einzelnen Untersuchern verwendeten Chemikalien sind sehr unterschiedlich, so daß kein Fabrikat besonders empfohlen werden kann. Das Verhalten verschiedener handelsüblicher Filme bei der Entwicklung in verschiedenen Entwicklerlösungen ist von FREY (1957) untersucht worden. Die Zahl der Fehler, welche durch die *Filmbearbeitung* zustande kommen können, ist groß. Die *Entwicklungszeit* eines Filmes ist für photometrische Messungen von Bedeutung (VIRTAMA 1957; HEUCK und SCHMIDT 1960).

Von den Hersteller-Firmen wird im allgemeinen eine Entwicklungszeit von 3—5 min empfohlen. HENNY (1934) hat gezeigt, daß Filme mit derselben Emulsionsnummer, die nicht 5 min, sondern 6 min entwickelt worden sind, Fehler bis zu 100 % aufweisen können. Eine zu lange Entwicklung des Filmes verursacht eine deutliche Erhöhung des Grauschleiers (auch „Schleierschwärzung" genannt, die ihre Ursache in einer Reduzierung des unbelichteten Bromsilbers zu Silber während des Entwicklungsprozesses hat). Bei einer photometrischen Messung von Schwärzungswerten ist die *Schleierschwärzung* zu berücksichtigen. Der Einfluß der *Entwicklertemperatur* und der *Bewegung der Entwicklerflüssigkeit* während des Entwicklungsprozesses auf die Gleichmäßigkeit des Entwicklungsvorganges und damit auf die Filmschwärzung ist verschiedentlich untersucht worden (MERGLER 1957; VIRTAMA 1957). Unter den bekannten Entwicklungsmethoden sind die Pinselentwicklung und die Sprudelentwicklung am genauesten, jedoch sehr umständlich. Nach den Untersuchungen von HEUCK und SCHMIDT (1960) sind eine Umlaufpumpe oder Sprudelentwicklung nicht unbedingt erforderlich. Es genügt eine sorgfältige und *ausgiebige Bewegung* der Filme bei der Handentwicklung (VIRTAMA 1957; HEUCK und SCHMIDT 1960; HINESS 1968). Bei der Entwicklung der Filme mit einer *Entwicklungsmaschine* treten Unterschiede in der Filmschwärzung (Flecke, Streifen und Schlieren) auf, die bei der photometrischen Auswertung erheblich stören. Der gegenwärtige Stand der Maschinenentwicklung läßt die auf diesem Wege bearbeiteten Filme für densitometrische Analysen ungeeignet erscheinen.

Bei der Handentwicklung der Röntgenfilme sollte vor dem *Fixierprozeß* eine *Zwischenwässerung* von etwa 1 min eingeschaltet werden. Die *Nachwässerung* der Filme ist mit 30—40 min ausreichend. Eine besondere Behandlung der Filme erübrigt sich, wenn sie stets mit der notwendigen Sorgfalt fixiert, gewässert und getrocknet werden.

Vor jeder photometrischen Auswertung sollte in den Bereichen eines Filmes, die von der ungeschwächten Primärstrahlung geschwärzt worden sind, eine *Kontrolle des „Leerwertes"* vorgenommen werden (HEUCK und SCHMIDT 1960). Bei genügend großem Fokus-Film-Abstand ist an diesen Stellen die Strahlungsintensität etwa gleich, so daß die Schwärzungswerte übereinstimmen müssen. Unterschiede können nur durch ungleichmäßigen Guß der Filmemulsion oder schlechte Verarbeitung der Filme zustande kommen, so daß derartige Aufnahmen für quantitative densitometrische Analysen nicht geeignet sind.

b) Der Einfluß der Strahlenqualität

Für die Untersuchung der Kalksalzkonzentration im Knochen wäre eine *monochromatische Röntgenstrahlung* am besten geeignet (OMNELL 1957; ROCKOFF 1965). Ein solches Verfahren erfordert jedoch sehr lange Belichtungszeiten, so daß für Untersuchungen an Mensch und Tier nur die *polychromatische Strahlung Verwendung gefunden hat.*

Der Kontrast der Röntgenaufnahme eines Knochens hängt maßgeblich von der Strahlenqualität ab. Eine harte Strahlung ergibt geringe Kontraste, während eine weiche Strahlung große Bildkontraste erzeugt. Bei voluminösen Objekten ist die Schwächung der weichen Röntgenstrahlung so erheblich, daß lange Belichtungszeiten erforderlich werden und eine hohe Strahlenbelastung auftritt. Es muß daher in solchen Fällen durch Erhöhung der Röhrenspannung ein Kompromiß zwischen der Belichtungszeit und dem Bildkontrast gesucht werden. Die spektrale Verteilung der *bildgebenden Austrittsstrahlung* hängt von der Objektdicke ab, da die langwellige Strahlung stärker absorbiert wird als die kurzwellige, wodurch mit zunehmender Eindringtiefe eine Aufhärtung der Strahlung erfolgt. Hierdurch wird das Röntgenbild zunehmend kontrastärmer. Mit zunehmender Spannung und Eindringtiefe werden dem aufgehärteten Röntgenstrahlenbündel durch den Compton-Effekt weichere Strahlen als Streustrahlung beigemischt. Von einer bestimmten Eindringtiefe ab führt die Überlagerung dieser beiden Effekte zu einem Gleichgewicht in der spektralen Verteilung. Dieses Gleichgewicht wird um so früher eintreten, je begrenzter der Wellenlängenbereich der einfallenden Röntgenstrahlung und je höher die Erzeugungsspannung an der Röntgenröhre ist. Eine Röntgenstrahlung erfährt bei dem Durchtritt durch das Objekt nicht nur eine Qualitätsänderung, sondern induziert auch die störende Streustrahlung (s. S. 128).

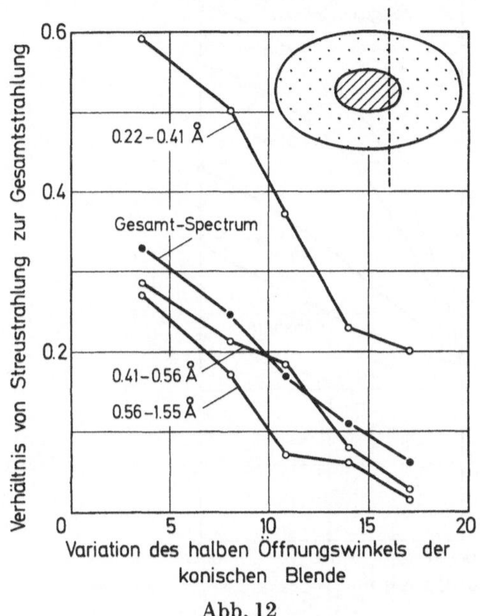

Abb. 12

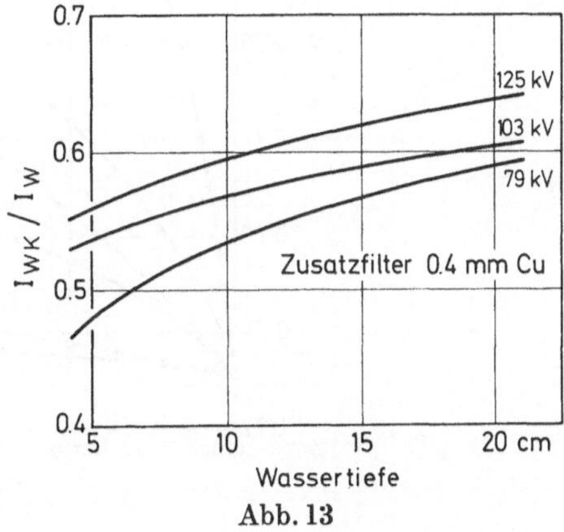

Abb. 13

Abb. 12. Verhältnis der Streustrahlung zur Gesamtstrahlung aufgetragen gegen den halben Öffnungswinkel einer konischen Bleiblende. Als Streukörper wurde ein Phantom benutzt, das aus einem Femurpräparat eingebettet in Fleisch bestand. (Nach Mayer, Trostle, Ackerman, Schraer und Sittler, 1960; Abb. 7)

Abb. 13. Abhängigkeit des Kontrastes von der Wassertiefe bei verschiedenen Röhrenspannungen. (Nach Hiness, 1968; Abb. 7)

Die Intensität der Streustrahlung in Abhängigkeit vom Winkel zum Primärstrahl für verschiedene Wellenlängenbereiche untersuchten Mayer, Trostle, Ackerman, Schraer und Sittler (1960). Sie erhielten die in Abb. 12 wiedergegebenen Kurven an einem Femurpräparat eingebettet in Weichteile. Ähnliche Ergebnisse wurden für andere Knochen und Weichteilpräparate in verschiedenen Lagen zum Primärstrahl ermittelt.

In Modellversuchen an einem Knochenphantom konnte Hiness (1968) feststellen, daß die Verwendung einer härteren Strahlung (Erhöhung der Röhrenspannung und Zunahme der Strahlenfilterung) die Untersuchungen des Knochenkalksalzgehaltes von der Schichtdicke der Weichteile und der Lokalisation des Knochens in den Weichteilen weitgehend unabhängig macht (Abb. 13). Diese Beobachtung ist für radiologisch-densitometrische Messungen des Knochenmineralgehaltes von Bedeutung.

c) Der Einfluß der Streustrahlung

Der Kontrast der Filmschwärzungen wird maßgeblich durch die Streustrahlung beeinflußt. Die klassische Streuung von Elementen mittlerer Ordnungszahl ist in dem interessierenden Energiebereich gering. Die störende Streustrahlung stammt überwiegend von Compton-Prozessen und ruft auf dem Röntgenfilm einen gleichmäßigen Untergrund zusätzlicher Schwärzung hervor. Der Kontrast ist also von dem Ausmaß der überlagerten Streustrahlung abhängig. Die Intensität der Streustrahlung kann herabgesetzt werden durch die Verwendung einer Streustrahlenblende, durch die Anwendung der Abstandstechnik *(„Grödel-Technik")* und durch die Einblendung des Primärstrahlenbündels.

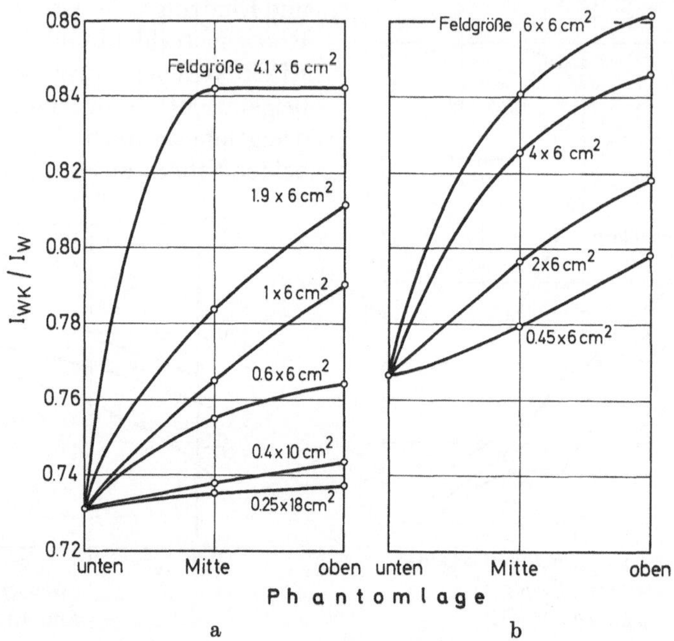

Abb. 14. a Abhängigkeit des Intensitätsverhältnisses I_{wk}/I_w von der Tiefenlage des kontrastierenden Körpers bei verschiedenen Feldgrößen. Röhrenspannung 79 kV. (Nach HINESS, 1968; Abb. 9). b Abhängigkeit des Intensitätsverhältnisses I_{wk}/I_w von der Tiefenlage des kontrastierenden Körpers bei verschiedenen Feldgrößen. Röhrenspannung 93 kV. (Nach HINESS, 1968; Abb. 10)

Eine *Streustrahlenblende* besteht aus parallel liegenden Bleilamellen, so daß nur die geschwächte Primärstrahlung und die parallel dazu verlaufende Streustrahlung den Film erreichen können. Bei stehender Blende werden sich die Bleilamellen auf dem Film abzeichnen und die photometrische Auswertung beeinträchtigen. Durch eine Bewegung der Blende kann die Streifenzeichnung der Bleilamellen zwar beseitigt werden, doch tritt wegen des Betriebes mit fallender Last eine ungleichmäßige Belichtung der verschiedenen Filmbezirke auf. Die Bewegung der Blende kann unregelmäßig sein, wodurch ebenfalls unterschiedliche Schwärzungen der nebeneinander belichteten Filmpartien zustande kommen.

Durch eine Vergrößerung des Film-Objekt-Abstandes kann mit Hilfe der sog. *Abstandstechnik („Grödel-Technik")* die Streustrahlung weitgehend von dem Röntgenfilm ferngehalten werden (SPIEGLER 1957; ZIELER 1966). Bei einem Objekt-Film-Abstand von 10—20 cm (im Mittel 15 cm nach SPIEGLER 1957) kann der Streustrahlenanteil so erheblich vermindert werden, daß die aus dem Objekt austretende Streustrahlung wegen der diffusen Richtungsverteilung den Film nur noch zu einem geringen Teil trifft. Von SPIEGLER (1959) ist der Einfluß der Streustrahlen auf die Filmschwärzung bei filmnaher und filmferner Lage eines Phantoms in einem aus Wasser bestehenden Streukörper untersucht worden. Er fand Unterschiede der Filmschwärzung, die sich mit zunehmendem

Abstand des Filmes vom Streukörper (Wasserbad) verringerten. HEUCK und SCHMIDT (1960) haben mit zwei gleich dicken Knochenscheiben aus der Mitte der Tibia ähnliche Untersuchungen durchgeführt und festgestellt, daß die durch Streustrahlen bedingte störende Schwärzung im Spannungsbereich von 50—80 kV bei Verwendung eines Folienfilmes und einer Rasterblende (Objekt-Film-Abstand wenigstens 10 cm, an manchen Flachblendentischen mehr) keine bedeutende Rolle spielt. Betont sei jedoch, daß HEUCK und SCHMIDT (1960) zur Bestimmung der Kalksalzkonzentration ein Referenzsystem verwendeten, so daß der zu untersuchende Knochen und das Referenzsystem von der Streustrahlung *in gleicher Weise* beeinflußt wurden.

Ferner kann durch *enge Einblendung* des Primärstrahlenbündels der Anteil der Streustrahlung an der Gesamtstrahlung vermindert werden. Über den Wert der Einblendung des Strahlenbündels liegen Untersuchungen von KEANE (1959), KEANE, SPIEGLER, DAVIS (1959), DOYLE (1961), OKUYAMA (1965) und HINESS (1968) vor. Ein langes, schmales Strahlenbündel bietet die günstigsten Bedingungen zur Berücksichtigung der Weichteile (Abb. 14a und b nach HINESS 1968). Die enge Einblendung des Primärstrahlenbündels ergibt gegenüber der Verwendung einer Streustrahlenblende und der Abstandstechnik zusätzlich den Vorteil einer geringeren Strahlenbelastung für den Patienten. Allerdings ist die Festlegung der zu messenden Knochenregion, insbesondere die Zuordnung zu der durchstrahlten Schichtdicke des Knochens mit Hilfe einer Aufnahme in der 2. Ebene schwierig. Für die Untersuchungen sollte daher ein Bereich gewählt werden, in dem die Schichtdicke des untersuchten Knochens konstant ist oder die zur Messung verwendete Region festgelegt werden kann.

d) Die Messung der Schichtdicke des Knochens

Zur Bestimmung der in der klinischen Medizin interessierenden *Konzentration der Kalksalze* in der Volumeneinheit eines Knochenabschnittes (Gesamtvolumen oder Frischsubstanz des Knochens, s. S. 109) aus der Schwächung einer Strahlung ist die Kenntnis der *Schichtdicke* des untersuchten Knochens erforderlich. Die durchstrahlte Dicke der Knochenregion kann am einfachsten durch eine Aufnahme in der zur Meßrichtung senkrechten Ebene bestimmt werden.

Von verschiedenen Arbeitsgruppen wurde die Frage einer möglichst genauen Messung des Knochendurchmessers am Ort der Untersuchung geprüft. Kompliziert geformte Knochen wie Darmbein, Sitzbein, Schulterblatt, Wirbelkörper u.a. sind in ihren geometrischen Dimensionen schwer zu erfassen und lassen daher nur ungenaue Angaben über die durchstrahlte Dicke zu. Günstige Voraussetzungen für die Dickenmessung liegen bei Fersenbein, Radius, Ulna, Femur und anderen Extremitätenknochen vor, die deshalb für die radiologische Messung der Mineralkonzentration bevorzugt worden sind.

Besonders einfach ist die Messung des Durchmessers in der Mitte der Röhrenknochen (Diaphysen), wo die Compactastärke kontrastreich zur Darstellung kommt, da hier nur wenig Spongiosa ausgebildet ist. Die Meßgenauigkeit im Bereich der Diaphysen wurde von HINESS (1968) an einem Knochenphantom (Plexiglas und Tricalciumphosphatpulver) unter verschiedenen Bedingungen der Feldgröße und des Objekt-Film-Abstandes geprüft. Weder die Feldgröße noch der Objekt-Film-Abstand zeigten einen nennenswerten Einfluß auf die Meßwerte.

Bei niedrigerer Röhrenspannung war die Streuung der Meßwerte geringer als bei Verwendung hoher Spannung, was auf den größeren Kontrast der mit weicher Strahlung angefertigten Aufnahmen zurückzuführen ist. Die *direkte Ausmessung* der Schichtdicke war genauer als die *photometrische Dickenmessung*, da das Auge für die Festlegung der Grenzen einen größeren Bereich heranzieht, während die Körnigkeit der Filmemulsion zu Fehlern bei der photometrischen Messung führen kann. Durch die direkte Messung kommt ein geringer positiver Fehler von 1—3%, durch die photometrische Messung ein geringer negativer Fehler von 1—2% zustande. Diese Fehler können bei Extrapolation auf den Objekt-Film-Abstand von 0 noch verringert werden. Da neben der Mineralkonzentration des Knochens im Bereich der Diaphysen auch die Dicke der Compacta der Diaphysen für die Beurteilung von Systemerkrankungen des Skeletes wichtig ist, kommt dem Ergebnis dieser Untersuchungen besondere Bedeutung zu (s. S. 223).

e) Die zur Messung verwendeten Photometer (Densitometer)

In den bisher vorliegenden Mitteilungen haben die photometrischen (oder densitometrischen) Meßverfahren zwar Erwähnung gefunden, doch sind solche Methoden in der Praxis der klinischen Radiologie noch weitgehend unbekannt. Die Bemühungen einzelner Arbeitskreise, neue Informationen mit Hilfe densitometrischer Untersuchungsmethoden zu erhalten und damit weitere Teilgebiete der klinischen Medizin auf eine exakte, naturwissenschaftliche Basis zu stellen, sind für zukünftige Entwicklungen von großem Wert.

Unter der Vielzahl vorhandener Photometer sind nur wenige für die routinemäßige Auswertung von Röntgenfilmen geeignet. Die Densitometrie *verschiedener Filmformate* ohne *Zerstückelung der Röntgenfilme* erlauben nur einzelne Meßgeräte. Es erscheint daher sinnvoll, einige Hinweise auf geeignete Untersuchungsgeräte aus dem Schrifttum besonders zusammenzufassen, um auch der Technik die Wünsche und Forderungen der klinischen Radiologie deutlich zu machen.

Die physikalischen Voraussetzungen für die Brauchbarkeit von Densitometern zur Auswertung von Röntgenfilmen hat WEBBER (1941) untersucht. Er empfiehlt Glasfilter, die die Hitze der Strahlung absorbieren und *vorwiegend grünes Licht* hindurchlassen, welches den größten Effekt auf die Photozelle hat.

Von ENGSTRÖM, WEGSTEDT und WELIN (1948) wurde ein Densitometer entwickelt, mit dem unter *gleichzeitiger visueller Beobachtung* des Filmes die Schwärzung an einem bestimmten Punkt gemessen werden kann. Das Gerät ist daher besonders geeignet für die Auswertung von Röntgenaufnahmen. Bei relativen Messungen wurde eine Fehlerbreite von 0,5% festgestellt.

Die Arbeitsgruppe von P. B. MACK hat seit 1927 eine Reihe von Meßinstrumenten entwickelt, die zur Bestimmung der Knochenmasse und der Knochendichte geeignet sind.

Eine besondere Apparatur zur röntgenologischen Bestimmung der Knochendichte haben MACK, VOSE und NELSON (1959) zusammengestellt. Das Gerät erlaubt eine Korrektur der Meßlinie des Vergleichskörpers aus einer Aluminiumlegierung. Diese Möglichkeit bringt eine Erleichterung in der Handhabung und einen *hohen Grad der Reproduzierbarkeit* der Messungen mit sich. Die sehr aufwendige Meßapparatur besteht aus vier Teilen:

1. Einer Knorr-Albers-Meßeinrichtung, die in ihren Dimensionen so modifiziert wurde, daß die Röntgenaufnahmen im rechten Winkel zum durchfallenden Lichtstrahl befestigt werden können.
2. Einem Aufzeichnungsgerät zur Registrierung der Filmdichtekurven (Modell Edomax E).
3. Einem zweiten Edomax E, der die nicht linearen Dichtekurven korrigiert.
4. Einer Instron-Ergänzungseinrichtung.

Das Besondere dieses Instrumentariums zur Bestimmung der Knochendichte besteht darin, daß alle *Unregelmäßigkeiten* in der Meßkurve des Knochens sofort *zu einer linearen Kurve korrigiert werden* und die Strahlenabsorption direkt angezeigt wird. Für die Messung wird zuerst die Dichtekurve des Referenzsystems aufgeschrieben, dann werden die Werte der korrigierten Knochenmeßlinie mit Hilfe einer besonderen Formel in äquivalente Volumina umgerechnet. Die Apparatur korrigiert automatisch eine Über- oder Unterbelichtung des Filmes, so daß auch innerhalb großer Belichtungsunterschiede noch richtige Werte ermittelt werden können. Die günstigsten Meßbedingungen wurden bei 40 mAs und 50 kV Anodenspannung gefunden. Es sind Untersuchungen an Knochenpräparaten durchgeführt worden. Der photometrisch ermittelte Wert wurde bei 50 Knochenproben durch nachfolgende Veraschung der Knochen kontrolliert. Die Untersuchungen ergaben, daß die benutzte Aluminiumlegierung die Röntgenstrahlen sehr ähnlich absorbiert wie der Knochen. Zur Korrektur der geringen Unterschiede muß die Strahlenabsorption durch die Aluminiumlegierung mit dem Faktor 1,0075 multipliziert werden, um der Absorption durch das Knochenkalksalz gleichzukommen.

Die photometrische Auswertung von Röntgenfilmen kann mit Hilfe des „Eppendorf-Photometers" unter Verwendung des Spezialaufsatzes für Elektrophoreseuntersuchungen durchgeführt werden, wenn der Röntgenfilm in entsprechend schmale Streifen *zerschnitten* wird (Heuck und Schmidt 1960). Neben dem Röntgenbild zur Beurteilung von Form und Struktur des Knochens ist dann jedoch noch eine weitere Aufnahme für die photometrische Bestimmung des Mineralgehaltes im Knochen erforderlich.

Von der Firma Dr. B. Lange (Berlin) wurde nach Angaben von Heuck und Schmidt (1954/59/60) ein Spezialphotometer konstruiert, bei dem die *Zerstückelung* der zur Photometrie benutzten Röntgenaufnahmen *nicht erforderlich* ist. Mit diesem Photometer können Röntgenaufnahmen bis zu einem Format von 35×35 cm ausgewertet werden. Zu dem Lange-Photometer wird das Multiflex-Galvanometer (MGF 2) der gleichen Firma verwendet.

Von Rockoff (1965) wurde ein vollautomatisch arbeitendes Mikrodensitometer mit Registriersystem beschrieben, das die quantitative radiologische Analyse verschiedener Untersuchungsmethoden erlaubt. Die Knochenspongiosa kann hinsichtlich der Bälkchendichte und -dicke untersucht werden. Die Leistungsfähigkeit des Gerätes wird am Beispiel eines Calcaneuspräparates demonstriert.

Eine Methode zur densitometrischen Auswertung von Röntgenfilmen, die auf dem Prinzip des „räumlichen Differenzmeßverfahrens" beruht, wurde von Vanselow, Heuck und Piepgras (1968) entwickelt. Bei gleichzeitiger Subtraktion störender Überlagerungen (z.B. durch Weichteilschatten oder Luft) können die Schwärzungswerte eines Referenzsystems und des Knochens zueinander in Beziehung gesetzt werden. Es ist nicht erforderlich, den Röntgenfilm zu zerschneiden. Die Apparatur wurde zu densitometrischen Messungen für die Kreislaufanalyse am Menschen entwickelt. Die Vorteile der Meßeinrichtung für densitometrische Bestimmungen der Kalksalzkonzentration im Knochen wurden erprobt.

V. Methoden zur Bestimmung des Knochenmineralgehaltes durch direkte Messung der Strahlenabsorption

Die Bestimmung von „*Schwächungsgleichwerten*" des Knochens, sowie halbquantitative und quantitative Messungen der globalen Mineralkonzentration im Gesamtvolumen Knochen auf *röntgenologisch-photometrischem Wege* machen die Elimination oder Standardisierung zahlreicher Störfaktoren erforderlich (s. S. 124—130). Es ist daher versucht worden, einen Teil der Schwierigkeiten und Probleme dieser Methoden dadurch zu umgehen, daß die *Strahlenabsorption durch den Knochen* mit Hilfe geeigneter Dosimeter (Ionisationskammern, Szintillationszähler u.a.) *direkt gemessen* und aus dem Meßergebnis auf den Mineralgehalt des Gesamtknochens rückgeschlossen wird. Die physikalischen Grundlagen dieser Meßverfahren wurden von Spiers (1946) ausführlich bearbeitet.

1. Die Absorptionsmessungen mit einer normalen polychromatischen Röntgenstrahlung

Über eine Methode zur Bestimmung *der Knochendichte* durch Messungen der Röntgenstrahlenabsorption im Knochengewebe hat Vose (1958) berichtet. Das *Prinzip der Methode* beruht darauf, das Verhältnis der *eintretenden Intensität* zur *austretenden Intensität* einer Röntgenstrahlung in Beziehung zu setzen *zum Durchmesser des durchstrahlten Knochens* (Abb. 15). Die theoretischen Grundlagen der Methode wurden eingehend dargelegt. Da das Verhältnis der Strahlenabsorption durch den Knochen einerseits und die Weichteile andererseits bei Änderung der Wellenlänge einer Strahlung ebenfalls verändert wird, ist es für Kontrollmessungen mit der beschriebenen Methode erforderlich, die *Anodenspannung konstant* zu halten. Zur Bestimmung der *Qualität der benutzten Röntgenstrahlung* wurde eine besondere Meßmethode angegeben, bei der mit Hilfe einer 6 mm dicken Aluminiumschicht in einem Abstand von 50 cm das Verhältnis zwischen der Durchdringungsfähigkeit der Strahlung und der effektiven Spannung ermittelt wird. Die zu Meßzwecken verwendete Strahlung wurde bei einer Anodenspannung von 68 kV erzeugt und mit 0,5 mm Aluminium gefiltert. Das Strahlenbündel sollte möglichst stark eingeblendet werden. Die Untersuchungen können praktisch mit jeder Diagnostikröhre durchgeführt werden (Abb. 16). Als Dosis-Meßgerät diente ein Victoreen-Minometer (Modell 287), das bei konstanter Wellenlänge der Röntgenstrahlung nur einen kleinen Meßfehler besitzt.

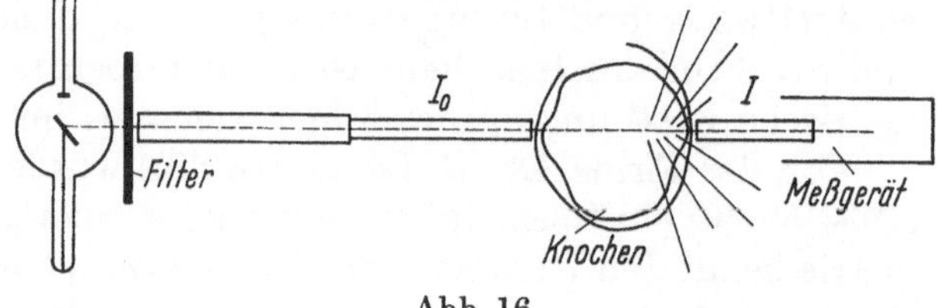

Abb. 16

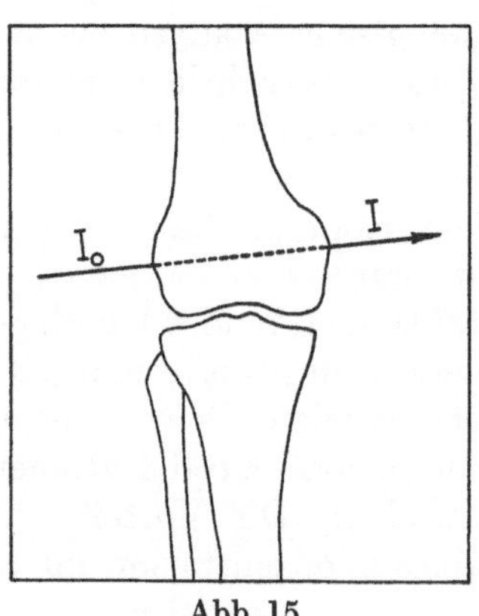

Abb. 15

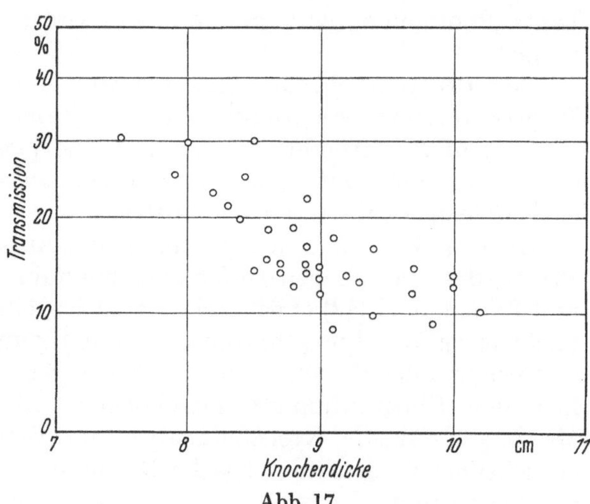

Abb. 17

Abb. 15. Schematische Darstellung der Meßanordnung. (Nach VOSE, 1958; Abb. 6)

Abb. 16. Die schematische Darstellung des Prinzips zur Messung des „Transmissionsfaktors“. (Nach VOSE, 1958; Abb. 1)

Abb. 17. Ergebnisse von Messungen des „Transmissionsfaktors“ der Femurcondylen verschiedener Versuchspersonen. (Nach VOSE, 1958; Abb. 8)

Die Messungen wurden am *distalen Femurende im Bereich der Condylen* durchgeführt, da hier die den Knochen bedeckenden Weichteile sehr dünn sind. Nach Messung des Femurdurchmessers im Bereich der Femurcondylen wird die vom Knochen absorbierte Röntgenstrahlung ermittelt. Bei dieser Messung wird der Mineralanteil des Knochengewebes am stärksten absorbieren. Der organische Anteil des Gesamtknochens, bestehend aus Grundsubstanz und dem Fettgewebe, beträgt im Meßbezirk etwa 35 % des gesamten Knochengewichtes. Da die Weichteile ein kleineres effektives Atomgewicht besitzen als Calcium und Phosphor des Knochenminerals, sind ihre Absorptionskoeffizienten relativ klein. Die genaue Zusammensetzung des Gesamtknochens kann nicht ermittelt werden, so daß sich VOSE mit einem Wert begnügt, der als „*Transmissionsfaktor*“ (Verhältnis zwischen Knochendicke und Transmission in Prozent ausgedrückt) ein Maß für die Strahlenabsorption ist (Abb. 17). Zehn Messungen an ein und demselben Knochen ergaben eine mittlere Abweichung des Meßergebnisses vom arithmetischen Mittel um 2 %. Der durch das Meßinstrument verursachte Fehler ist sehr klein, so daß die Abweichungen durch Änderungen der Meßposition am Knochen bedingt sein dürften.

In einer späteren Arbeit hat VOSE (1959) die *Fehlerbreite* der Meßmethode an *frischen Tierknochen* geprüft, die nach der röntgenologischen Untersuchung verascht wurden. Diese Kontrolle ergab eine durchschnittliche Abweichung von 0,7 % bei einer *maximalen Schwankung von 3,4 %*. An einer Untersuchungsreihe von 76 knochengesunden Personen

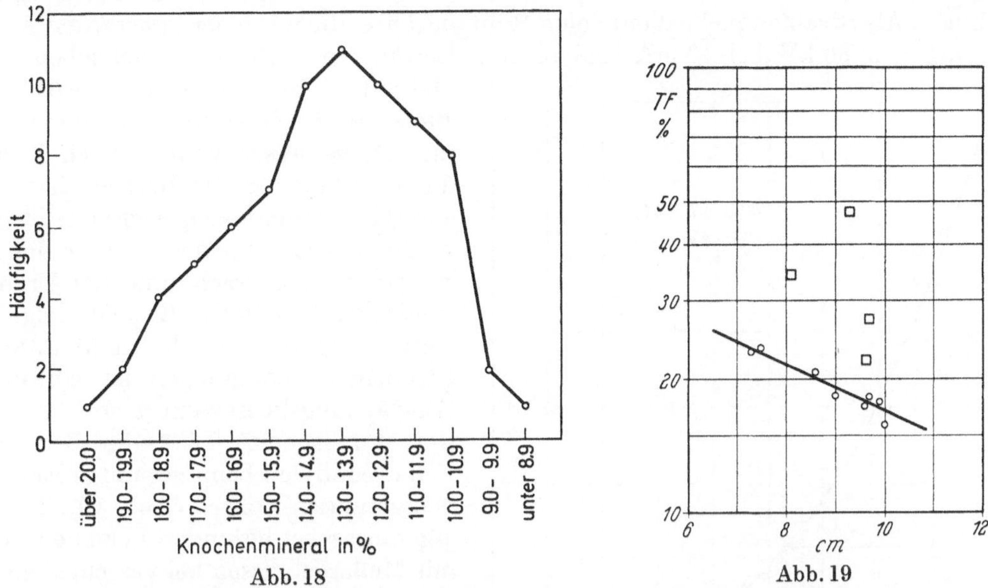

Abb. 18. Häufigkeitsverteilung der Meßwerte des Knochenmineralgehaltes der Spongiosa der Femurcondylen von 76 Erwachsenen beiderlei Geschlechtes. (Nach VOSE, 1959; Abb. 5)

Abb. 19. Darstellung der Meßergebnisse des „Transmissionsfaktors" bei gesunden und kranken Menschen. ○ = Normalwerte, □ = pathologische Werte. (Nach GYÖRGYI und BOZOKY, 1961; Abb. 5)

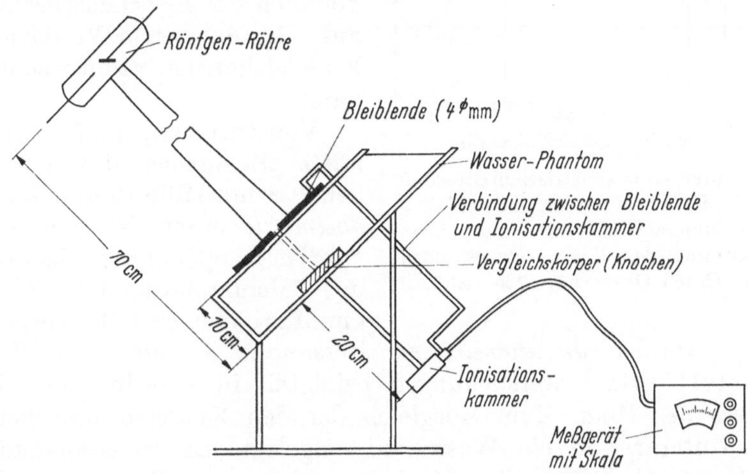

Abb. 20. Schematische Darstellung der Anordnung zur direkten Messung der Strahlenabsorption durch die Ulna. (Nach OKUYAMA, 1965; Abb. 4)

beiderlei Geschlechts und verschiedenen Alters konnte VOSE (1959) feststellen, daß der Mineralgehalt in der Femurspongiosa *außerordentlich variiert* (Abb. 18). Bei etwa 25 % der untersuchten Personen war eine Schwankungsbreite des Knochenmineralgehaltes der Femurcondylenspongiosa zwischen 12 und 14,9 % nachweisbar. Nach Zusammenstellung der Meßergebnisse wird vorgeschlagen, die Knochen auf Grund ihrer Dichte in verschiedene Klassen einzuteilen.

Auch von EDHOLM und JACOBSON (1959) wurde eine polychromatische Röntgenstrahlung zu direkten Absorptionsmessungen benutzt.

Das Prinzip der Untersuchungsmethode von VOSE (1958) haben GYÖRGYI und BOZÓKY (1961) angewandt, um Messungen des Transmissionsfaktors bzw. des linearen Schwächungskoeffizienten im Bereich der Femurcondylen mit einem Ionisationsmeßgerät vorzunehmen. Als Strahlenquelle diente eine Röntgenröhre, die mit einer konstanten Anodenspannung von 80 kV bei 10 mA und einer Filterung von 2,5 mm Al betrieben wurde. Methodisch ist so vorgegangen worden, daß zuerst die Dosisleistung ($I = 0$) in mR/min in Luft gemessen wurde. Nach Kenntnis des Durchmessers im Bereich der Femurcondylen wurde das eng begrenzte Strahlenbündel in die Achse des zu untersuchenden Körperteiles gebracht und der Transmissionsfaktor ermittelt. Es sind einige Meßwerte mitgeteilt worden, und unter den gegebenen Bedingungen ist ein linearer Schwächungskoeffizient μ von 0,17—0,19 (im Durchschnitt 0,177) im Bereich der Femurcondylen beim gesunden Erwachsenen gefunden worden (Abb. 19). Die Meßergebnisse bei gesunden Personen können mit Meßergebnissen bei verschiedenen Erkrankungen verglichen werden (Tabelle 5). In dem Diagramm sind einige Beispiele zusammengestellt. Der lineare Schwächungskoeffizient bzw. der Transmissionsfaktor wird durch den Mineralgehalt im Gesamtvolumen des Knochens beeinflußt, so daß aus den gemessenen Werten auf die globale Kalksalzkonzentration geschlossen werden kann.

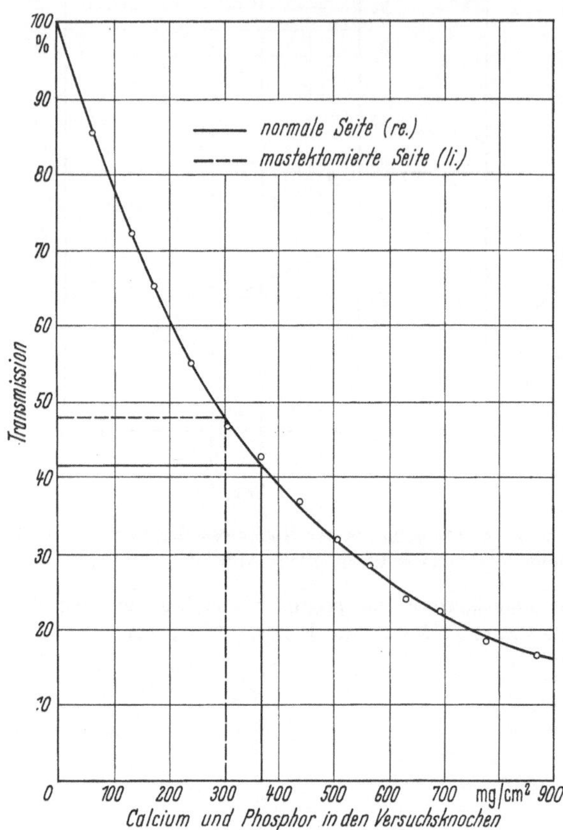

Abb. 21. Beispiel der direkten dosimetrischen Messung des Calciumgehaltes der Ulna beider Arme einer 50jährigen Frau. Niedriger Mineralgehalt der linken Ulna als Folge der Inaktivität des linken Armes nach Mamma-Amputation. (Nach OKUYAMA, 1965; Abb. 8)

Von OKUYAMA (1965) wurden *quantitative Messungen* des Knochenmineralgehaltes mit Hilfe *direkter Röntgenstrahlendosimetrie* unter Verwendung eines *Standardknochenphantoms* [zusammengesetzt aus Calciumphosphat $Ca_3(PO_4)_2$ und Calciumkarbonat $CaCO_3$] vorgenommen. Zu Vergleichszwecken wurden *densitometrische Messungen* an derselben Knochenregion ausgeführt (s. S. 191). Die Untersuchungen erfolgten in verschiedenen Punkten des *distalen Abschnittes der Ulna*. Zum Ausgleich der den Knochen umgebenden Weichteile wurde der Unterarm in ein Wasserbad eingelegt. Es ist besonders bemerkenswert, daß die *Streustrahlung* bei *allen Messungen* eine große Rolle spielte. Aus diesem Grunde wurde der Streuanteil für den Knochen und das Referenzsystem — auch im Wasserphantom — mit Hilfe einer besonderen Bleiblende vermindert (Abb. 20). Durch diese Maßnahme konnten genauere Meßwerte erzielt werden. Das Prinzip der von OKUYAMA (1965) beschriebenen Untersuchungsmethode entspricht dem von HEUCK und SCHMIDT (1954/59/60) angegebenen Verfahren der vergleichenden Absorptionsmessung von Knochen und einem Referenzsystem aus *knochenäquivalentem Material (Hydroxylapatit)*. Ergebnisse größerer Reihenuntersuchungen an *gesunden Versuchspersonen* wurden bisher nicht vorgelegt. Als Beispiel der Anwendung des Meßverfahrens sind in Abb. 21 und Tabelle 6 die Mineralwerte (Calcium-Phosphor-Werte) der Ulna beider Arme einer 50jährigen Frau

Tabelle 5. *Ergebnisse der Messungen des „Transmissionsfaktors" bei einigen Skeleterkrankungen*

		TF %	lg TF	× cm	μ
1. H. J. St. p. contus. gen. sin. Pellegrini-Stiedascher Kalkschatten am li. Femur	rechter Femur	17,4	—1,75	9,6	0,182
	linker Femur	27,4	—1,29	9,7	0,133
2. H. E. St. post osteotomiam fem. d.	rechter Femur	22,2	—1,50	9,6	0,157
	linker Femur	18,7	—1,68	9,9	0,186
3. G. J. Exostosis tibiae utr.	rechter Femur	17,7	—1,73	9,9	0,175
	linker Femur	15,8	—1,85	10,0	0,185
4. Si. An. Sarcoma tibiae sin.	rechter Femur	23,5	—1,45	8,4	0,173
	linker Femur	34,6	—1,06	8,1	0,131
	rechter Knöchel	17,5	—1,74	6,3	0,275
	linker Knöchel	25,0	—1,39	6,5	0,214
5. Sü. Ar. St. p. arthroplast. gen. d.	rechter Femur	47,0	—0,76	9,3	0,082
	linker Femur	20,8	—1,45	8,6	0,168
6. C. J. M. Perthes + subluxatio coxae d.	rechter Femur	55,5	—0,59	6,0	0,098
	linker Femur	44,4	—0,81	6,6	0,123
7. S. M. Synovitis gen. sin.	rechter Femur	34,8	—1,05	7,8	0,135
	linker Femur	64,2	—0,44	8,1	0,054
8. B. A. Myelodysplasia	rechter Femur	32,6	—1,12	8,4	0,133
	linker Femur	33,0	—1,11	8,9	0,125
9. T. J. St. p. poliomyelitid. et osteotom. fem. d.	rechter Femur	12,1	—2,11	12,1	0,175
	linker Femur	9,3	—2,38	9,3	0,256

[GYÖRGYI, G., u. I. BOZÓKY: Fortsch. Röntgenstr. **94**, 667 (1961), Tab. 1]

Tabelle 6. *Beispiel der Anwendung eines kombinierten Meßverfahrens.*
50jähr. ♀ mit Mamma-Carcinom li., Messung 17 Monate nach Mastektomie

	Reihe der Meßpunkte 4,5 cm prox. vom Proc. styl.	Photometerwerte	Transmission in %	Äquivalenter Mineralgehalt in mg/cm² E.M.C.	Dicke der Ulna in cm	Mineralgehalt in mg/cm²
	Wasserphantom PMMA*	0,127	100	0		
rechte Ulna (gesunde Seite)	A	0,101				
	B	0,067				
	C	0,056				
	D	0,053	41,7	371	1,10	337
	E	0,062				
	F	0,063				
	G	0,071				
linke Ulna (mastektom. Seite)	A	0,086				
	B	0,071				
	C	0,073				
	D	0,061	48,0	305	1,07	285
	E	0,061				
	F	0,064				
	G	0,083				

* PMMA = Polymethylmetacrylat. [OKUYAMA, T.: Nippon Acta radiol. **25**, 775 (1965), Tab. 3]

dargestellt. Nach Mamma-Amputation links fand sich ein niedrigerer Mineralgehalt (höherer „Transmissionswert") verglichen mit der gesunden Seite.

Mit einem besonderen *Szintillationszählrohr* haben MASON und RUTHVEN (1965) im Laboratorium Messungen am Knochen unter Verwendung eines schmalen Röntgenstrahlenbündels niedriger Energie vorgenommen. Das Ergebnis wurde direkt in eine Kurve transformiert. Zur Untersuchung wurde die *Mittelphalanx des 5. Fingers links* herangezogen. Die Brauchbarkeit des Verfahrens wurde an einem Phantomfinger geprüft. Es fand sich eine Reproduzierbarkeit des Meßverfahrens von 3—6%. Größere Meßreihen sind bisher nicht vorgelegt worden.

2. Die Absorptionsmessungen mit monochromatischer Röntgenstrahlung

Die Verwendung einer monochromatischen Röntgenstrahlung zur Untersuchung des Knochenmineralgehaltes haben FROMMHOLD und SCHOKNECHT (1959/60) vorgeschlagen. Als Strahlenquelle diente eine Feinstrukturröhre mit Molybdän-Anode und Punktfokus (MC 50, C.H.F. Müller, Hamburg). Die Apparatur wurde mit einer elektronisch stabilisierten Spannung betrieben (Abb. 22a und b). Die erzeugte Strahlung fällt auf einen Kalkspatkristall, nachdem sie zuvor durch eine Spaltblende eingeengt worden ist. Durch Reflexion

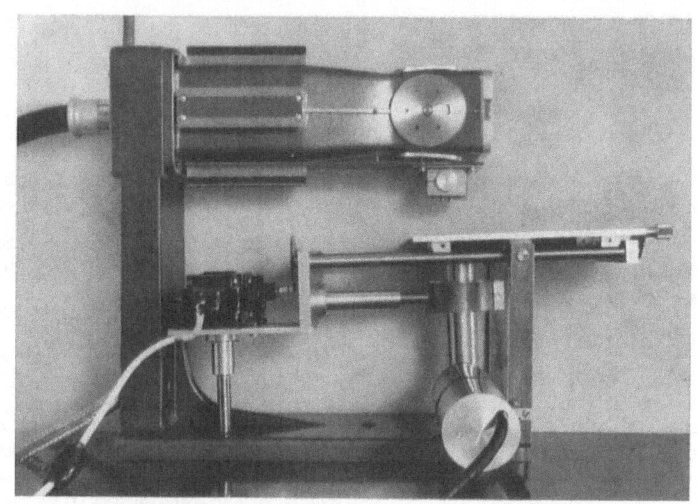

a

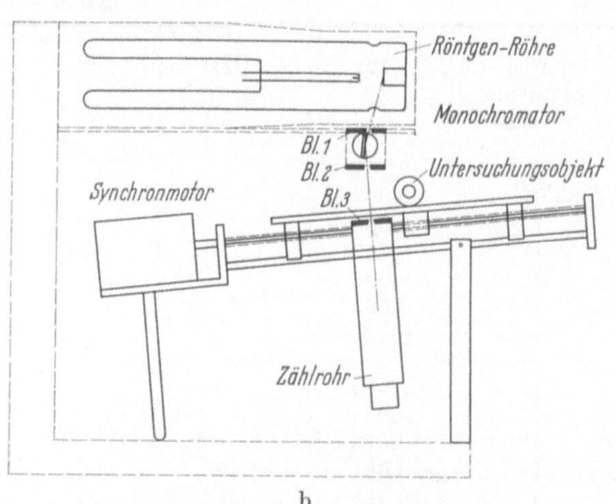

b

Abb. 22. Spezialröntgenapparat (C. H. F. Müller) MC 50 in Verbindung mit dem Feinstrukturuntersuchungsapparat Mikro. 111 zur Untersuchung der Absorption und Feinstruktur von Knochen (a) und schematische Darstellung der Meßapparatur (b). (Nach FROMMHOLD und SCHOKNECHT, 1960; Abb. 3 und 1)

an dem Kalkspatkristall entsteht die monochromatische Strahlung. Mit Hilfe einer zweiten Spaltblende werden aus der reflektierten Strahlung die Mo $K\alpha_1$- und die $K\alpha_2$-Linie ausgeblendet und die Strahlenbündel auf eine Strichlänge von 3 mm begrenzt (Abb. 23). Die Wellenlänge dieser Strahlung beträgt 0,71 Å. Die Intensität der Strahlung wird durch eine unmittelbar hinter der zweiten Blende befindliche Metallfolie herabgesetzt. Die gefilterte monochromatische Röntgenstrahlung trifft auf das Untersuchungsobjekt. Die aus dem Objekt austretende geschwächte Strahlung passiert eine weitere, dritte Blende zur Beseitigung der Streustrahlung und wird von einem Glockenzählrohr mit Krypton-Füllung gemessen, das im Proportionalbereich betrieben wird. Die Zählrohrimpulse werden über einen Vorverstärker dem Verstärker und Ratemeter eines Strah-

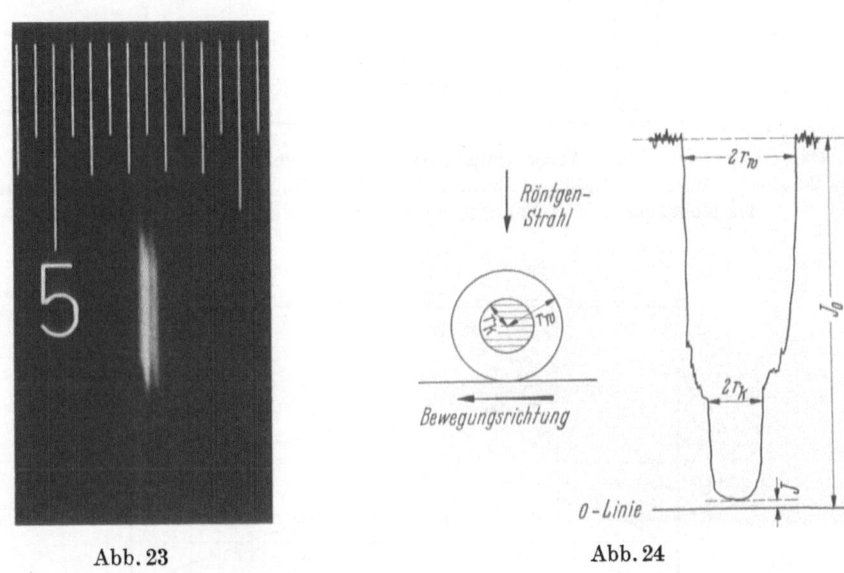

Abb. 23. Aufnahme des Röntgenstrahles ($K\alpha_1$, $K\alpha_2$) nach der Kristallreflexion mit Vergleichsmaßstab (ein Skalenteil = 0,5 mm). (Nach FROMMHOLD und SCHOKNECHT, 1960; Abb. 2)

Abb. 24. Idealisierter Querschnitt durch einen Finger und Beispiel für eine Absorptionskurve bei Durchlaufen des Röntgenstrahles in der angegebenen Bewegungsrichtung. (Nach FROMMHOLD und SCHOKNECHT, 1960; Abb. 4)

lungsmeßgerätes mit angeschlossenem Tintenschreiber zugeführt. Zur Messung kann auch ein Szintillationsmeßkopf [NaJ(T_1)-Kristall von 25 mm Durchmesser und 5 mm Dicke] in Verbindung mit einem Photomultiplier verwendet werden.

Die physikalisch-technischen Bedingungen des Meßverfahrens begrenzen die Anwendung der Methode zunächst auf dünne Skeletabschnitte, z.B. Fingerknochen. So sind die ersten Messungen am *Mittelglied des 5. Fingers* durchgeführt worden. Als *Kenngröße für den Kalkgehalt des Knochens* dient der lineare Absorptionskoeffizient für Mo K-Strahlung. Durchläuft der zu untersuchende Finger des Patienten den ausgeblendeten Röntgenstrahl, so zeichnet die Apparatur automatisch die Absorptionskurve der Strahlung durch den Knochen auf (Abb. 24). In der Möglichkeit, neben *der Gesamtabsorption* in Abhängigkeit vom Kalkgehalt des Knochens auch Unterschiede der Absorption durch Corticalis und Spongiosa, also *die Knochenstruktur* und damit die Art des Knochenabbaues erfassen zu können, sehen die Autoren einen erheblichen Vorteil ihrer Methode. Die ersten Untersuchungsergebnisse an gesunden Personen verschiedenen Alters und Geschlechtes lassen mit zunehmendem Alter ein *Absinken des Kalkgehaltes* im Mittelglied des 5. Fingers erkennen (Abb. 25). Eindeutige Unterschiede des Knochenkalkgehaltes zwischen den beiden Geschlechtern fanden sich in den untersuchten Knochenbezirken nicht (Abb. 26a und b). Die praktische Anwendungsmöglichkeit der Methode bei Knochenerkrankungen wird an

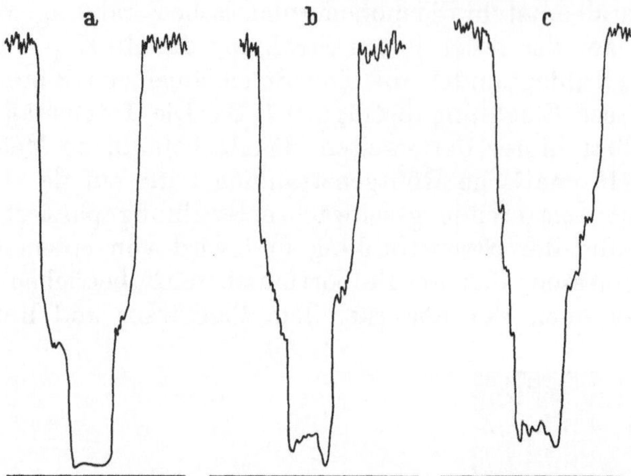

Abb. 25a—c. Die charakteristischen Absorptionskurven der Fingerknochen von Patienten verschiedener Altersstufen (a 20jähriger Mann, b 44jähriger Mann, c 78jähriger Mann) geben auch Hinweise auf die Struktur des Knochens. (Nach FROMMHOLD und SCHOKNECHT, 1960; Abb. 7)

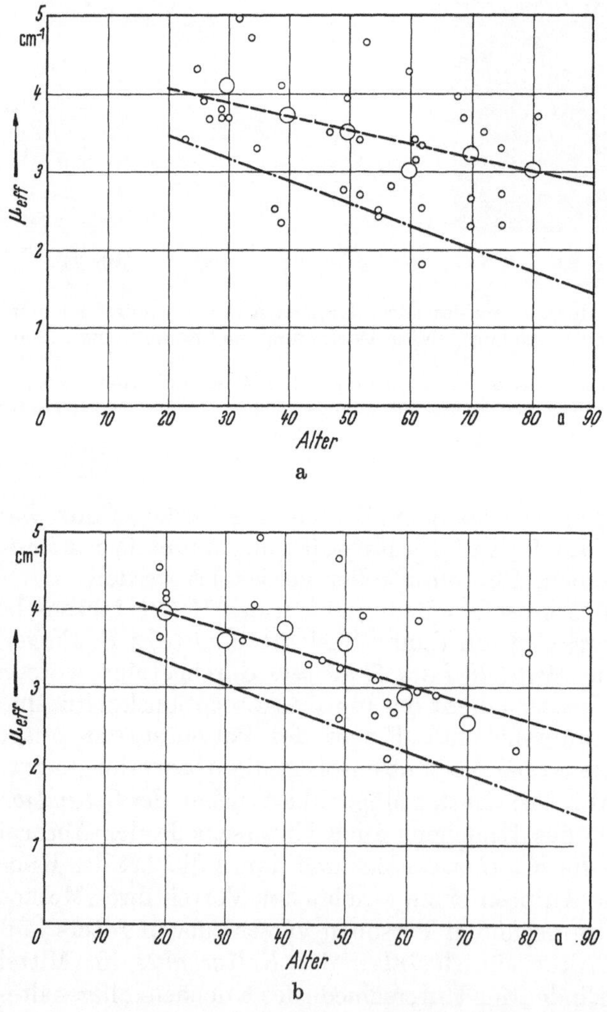

Abb. 26a u. b. Darstellung der Meßergebnisse (effektive Absorptionskoeffizienten) in den verschiedenen Altersgruppen (a Männer, b Frauen). (Nach FROMMHOLD und SCHOKNECHT, 1960; Abb. 5 und 6)

einigen Absorptionskurven gezeigt, die von solchen Patienten gewonnen wurden, bei denen eine Demineralisation des Fingerskeletes (z.B. nach Ruhigstellung eines Armes wegen einer Oberarmhalsfraktur) eingetreten war (Abb. 27).

Von Jacobson und Lindberg (1964) ist ein Röntgenspektrophotometer entwickelt worden, das eine mit Hilfe einer Spezialröhre erzeugte *monochromatische Strahlung* verwendet. Die Referenzsysteme aus verschiedenen Substanzen (Wasser, Jodverbindungen, Hydroxylapatit) werden zur Analyse der Zusammensetzung von Körpergeweben oder anderen Stoffen so im Strahlenkegel plaziert, daß die Photomultiplier-Meßeinheit mit Hilfe eines komplizierten elektronischen Systems das Meßergebnis in kurzer Zeit ermitteln kann.

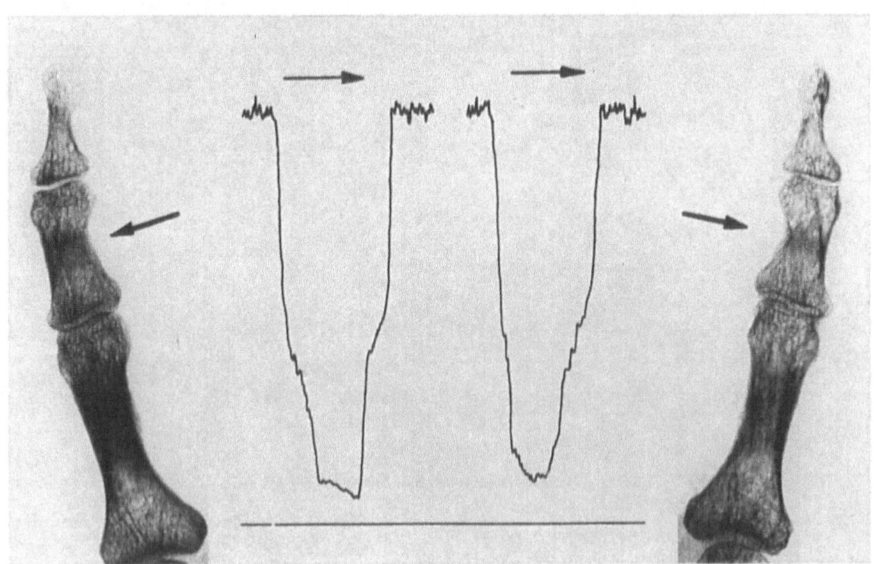

Abb. 27. Absorptionskurven durch die Mitte des Mittelgliedes vom 5. Finger beider Hände geschrieben. 64jährige Frau mit Pseudarthrose nach Oberarmhalsfraktur rechts. Deutliche Unterschiede des Kalkgehaltes und der Struktur der beiden Knochen. (Nach Frommhold und Schoknecht, 1960; Abb. 9)

3. Die Absorptionsmessungen mit der γ-Strahlung von Isotopen

Mit einer γ-Strahlung von ^{192}*Iridium* untersuchten Gershon-Cohen, Cherry und Boehnke (1958) die Knochendichte. Es können auch *andere Isotope* (z.B. ^{170}Thulium) verwendet werden, doch sollte die Ermittlung der Absorptionskoeffizienten für die im Knochen vorkommenden Stoffe möglich sein. Die durch Weichteile einerseits und Knochen andererseits absorbierte Strahlung wurde mit einem Hochleistungszählrohr erfaßt und auf ein elektronisches System übertragen. Praktisch wurden die Untersuchungen so durchgeführt, daß zuerst die Absorption durch die Weichteile, dann die Absorption durch Weichteile und Knochen festgestellt wurde. Als *Vergleichsphantom* für die Weichteile diente eine *Wasserschicht*. Mit Hilfe des elektronischen Systems der Meßapparatur können die Absorptionswerte für Weichteile und Knochen (γ-Massenabsorptionskoeffizient) zueinander in Beziehung gesetzt werden und dann *rechnerisch direkt der Wert für die Knochendichte* (und damit den Kalkgehalt) abgelesen werden. Die Reproduzierbarkeit einer Messung mit normaler Röntgenaufnahme-Einrichtung liegt bei etwa 2—5%, während die Abweichung bei Verwendung einer γ-Strahlung nur 1% betragen soll. Durch *Vergleichsmessungen* an einem Ochsenschwanz und nachfolgender *chemischer Analyse* der untersuchten Knochen konnte ein Fehler der Meßmethode *von etwa 10%* ermittelt werden.

Mit Hilfe eines besonderen Markierungssystems (Bleigitter mit bekannten Abständen) wurden Untersuchungen *am 3. und 4. Lendenwirbelkörper* durchgeführt. Das Strahlenbündel wurde auf 1,25 cm eingeblendet, so daß die Messungen repräsentativ für den

Mittelwert der Knochendichte sind (Abb. 28). Die Ergebnisse der Messungen an der Wirbelsäule eines 96 Jahre alten Mannes, eines 28 Jahre alten Mannes und einer 77 Jahre alten Frau wurden gegenübergestellt. Bei der 77jährigen Frau konnte eine fortgeschrittene Osteoporose der gesamten Wirbelsäule festgestellt werden. Diese Meßmethode ist genauer als die subjektive Beurteilung von Röntgenaufnahmen. Die applizierte Strahlendosis betrug maximal 10 mR. Die Lendenwirbelsäule dürfte jedoch als Meßregion nicht optimal

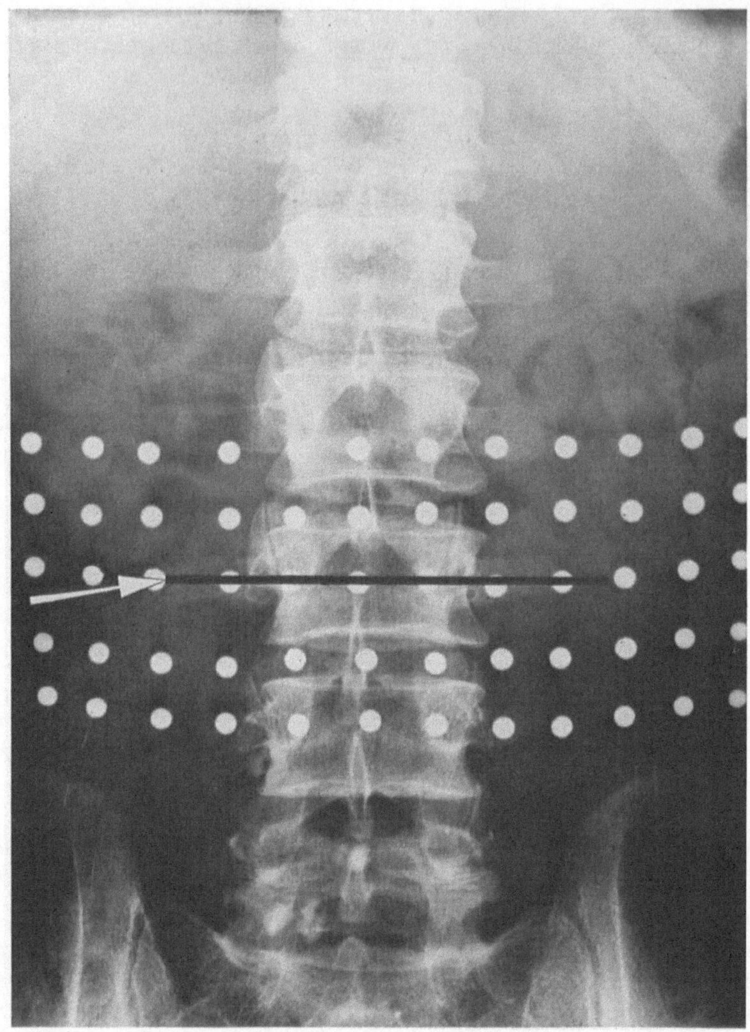

Abb. 28. Röntgenbild der Wirbelsäule eines 28jährigen gesunden Mannes mit dem Markierungssystem nach GERSHON-COHEN, CHERRY und BOEHNKE (1958) zur Messung der Knochendichte mit einer Gammastrahlung. Der Meßweg durch den 3. Lendenwirbel ist eingezeichnet

geeignet sein. Von den Autoren wird *der Beckenknochen 5 cm lateral vom Sacroiliacalgelenk* empfohlen, da dieser Knochenbezirk wohl immer frei von anderen Einflüssen, wie sekundären Veränderungen bei einer Arthritis, sein dürfte.

Ein Meßverfahren zur Bestimmung des Knochenmineralgehaltes mit Hilfe der *direkten Photon-Absorption durch den Knochen* haben CAMERON, GRANT und MCGREGOR (1962), CAMERON und SORENSON (1965) entwickelt und geprüft. Als *Strahlenquelle* wurde eine Probe von 35 mC ^{125}J mit einer Strahlungsenergie von 28,5 keV verwendet. Die Größe des Strahlenaustrittsfensters wird mit 3 mm im Durchmesser, später mit 1×5 mm angegeben. Die ganz weiche Strahlung wurde durch eine 0,06 mm dicke Zinnfolie absorbiert.

Zinn hat eine K-Absorptionskante von 29 keV und eliminiert die 31 und 35 keV-Komponenten des ^{125}J. Die Strahlenquelle wurde dem Meßgerät genau gegenüber angeordnet und besaß eine wirksame Fläche von 0,7 mm^2. Der Natriumjodidkristall hat einen Durchmesser von 1 cm bei einer Dicke von 2 mm und sitzt einem Photomultiplier auf. Der Photomultiplier ist mit einem Impulshöhenanalysator verbunden, dessen Informationen durch verschiedene Registriergeräte aufgezeichnet werden. In späteren Mitteilungen empfehlen die Autoren die Verwendung eines Computers, um eine noch schnellere Auswertung zu erreichen.

MAZESS, CAMERON, O'CONNOR und KNUTZEN (1964) untersuchten *den Einfluß der umgebenden Weichteile* an Leichenknochen und fanden einen Korrelationsquotienten von 0,96 zwischen dem gemessenen Mineralgehalt und den danach ermittelten Knochen- und Aschegewichten. Sie folgerten daraus, daß diese Meßtechnik die bisher genaueste sei, um den Knochenmineralgehalt auch bei einer Überlagerung durch Weichteile zu bestimmen. Die Methode wurde ferner dazu verwendet, um Einflüsse der Ernährung auf den Knochenmineralgehalt von Hühnerküken zu untersuchen. Bei diesen Messungen fand sich ein Korrelationsquotient von 0,95 in vivo und 0,99 in vitro.

Eine weiterentwickelte Technik wurde von CAMERON und SORENSON (1965) auf ihre Zuverlässigkeit geprüft. Ferner wurde untersucht, inwieweit die Werte der Absorptionsmessung reproduzierbar sind und als *Indikator für den wirklichen Mineralgehalt* verwendet werden können. Nach zufriedenstellenden Ergebnissen wurde eine Einrichtung zu Messungen am lebenden Menschen konstruiert. Bei Messungen des *Radius*, der *Metacarpalia* und der *Phalangen* wird der Unterarm in einer Holzhalterung fixiert und hierdurch während des Meßvorganges absolut ruhig gestellt. Von oben wird der Meßbezirk des Armes mit einem Gummischlauch fixiert, der eine 2%ige Kochsalzlösung enthält und von einem Plexiglasfenster komprimiert wird, um die Weichteildicke des Armes anzugleichen. Die Strahlenquelle kann mit unterschiedlicher Geschwindigkeit (0,54; 0,79 und 1,58 mm/s) über den Knochen bewegt werden. Im allgemeinen wurde die mittlere Geschwindigkeit benutzt. In Modellversuchen mit Glasplatten und Kunststoff ist der Einfluß der Weichteile, der Qualität der verwendeten Strahlung und der Meßinstrumente auf das Meßergebnis überprüft worden.

Neben ^{125}J sind *die Isotope* ^{241}Am *und* ^{210}Pb auf ihre Eignung für Messungen des Knochenmineralgehaltes geprüft worden (CAMERON und SORENSON 1968). Die besten Ergebnisse wurden mit der γ-Strahlung des ^{125}J erzielt.

Mit einem weiterentwickelten Meßsystem wurden über einige Wochen *Verlaufsmessungen des Knochenmineralgehaltes vom linken Radius* bei einem gesunden, 26 Jahre alten Mann durchgeführt. Die Ergebnisse von 3—6 an *demselben Tage* vorgenommenen Messungen zeigen gewisse Abweichungen nach oben und unten, also eine deutliche Streuung, doch war die Standardabweichung von 1,3% gering und beweist die Reproduzierbarkeit der Methode.

Als Meßpunkte wurden *am Radius die Epiphyse, Metaphyse und Diaphysen-Mitte* empfohlen. Ferner erscheint *die Spongiosa des posterioren Anteiles vom Calcaneus* und *die Compacta der Humerusdiaphyse* zu Meßzwecken geeignet. Von SORENSON, CAMERON und MAZESS (1968) wurden Reihenuntersuchungen an *der Compacta der Diaphysen von Radius und Humerus* bei Kindern und Erwachsenen begonnen, um den Einfluß von Alter, Geschlecht und Besonderheiten der einzelnen Knochen erfassen zu können. Bei wiederholten Messungen an demselben Patienten waren nur geringe Abweichungen des Meßergebnisses von ungefähr 1% festzustellen. Die Meßwerte verschiedener Personen ergaben Unterschiede von 20—22% im kompakten Knochen. Die Gegenüberstellung der durch Absorptionsmessungen erhaltenen Mineralwerte (angegeben in g/cm^2) und der Aschewerte zeigt eine Standardabweichung von 2%, so daß bei Verlaufskontrollen Änderungen des Mineralgehaltes um 5% erfaßt werden können.

Eine Verschiebung des Verhältnisses von Ca:P im Knochenmineral (z.B. durch das Vorkommen anderer Kalksalze neben dem Hydroxylapatit) wird größere Unterschiede des Meßergebnisses zur Folge haben. Die *Zusammensetzung der Kalksalze* ist also nicht ohne Bedeutung für radiologische Absorptionsmessungen von Knochen.

Angeregt durch das Prinzip der Meßmethode von CAMERON und SORENSON (1962/65) haben LANZL und STRANDJORD (1964) eine Meßeinrichtung entwickelt, die mit Hilfe von ^{125}J die Transmission der γ-Strahlung durch einen *Fingerknochen* zu untersuchen erlaubt. Die ersten Vorversuche wurden an Kaninchenknochen durchgeführt. Zur Messung der Tiere mußte eine besondere Halterung konstruiert werden. Als Meßobjekt am Menschen erschien der Knochen *des Mittelgliedes vom 2. Finger der linken Hand* besonders geeignet, da die Weichteile hier nur sehr gering entwickelt sind. Die spongiösen Knochen der Wirbelsäule, des Beckenskeletes und des Calcaneus werden zwar eine stärkere Demineralisation aufweisen als die gemischten, vorwiegend kompakten kleinen Handknochen, doch macht die Korrektur der Weichteile, welche die größeren spongiösen Knochen bedecken, Schwierigkeiten. Von STRANDJORD und LANZL (1965) wurde eine U-förmige Halterung für den zu untersuchenden Finger konstruiert, die an den Seiten eine Skala besitzt, um den Meßpunkt bei späteren Kontrollen wieder genau reproduzieren zu können (Abb. 29a und b). Die Messung wird einmal durch Weichteile + Knochen + Weichteile und einmal nur seitlich am Knochen vorbei durch die reinen Weichteile vorgenommen (Abb. 30). Dann wird der Knochen um 90° gedreht und noch einmal durch die Weichteile gemessen. Die Dicke des Knochens wird mit Hilfe von Röntgenaufnahmen in 2 Ebenen direkt bestimmt. Da die *γ-Strahlung des ^{125}J relativ hart ist*, müssen die umliegenden Weichteile des Fingers nach Ansicht der Autoren *nicht unbedingt berücksichtigt* werden.

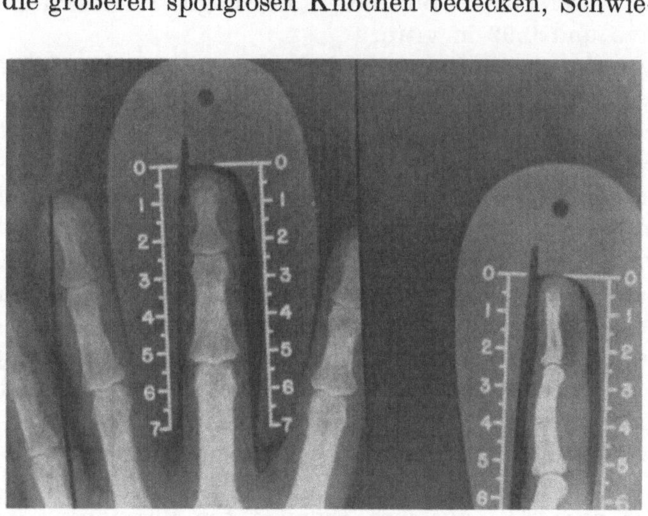

Abb. 29a

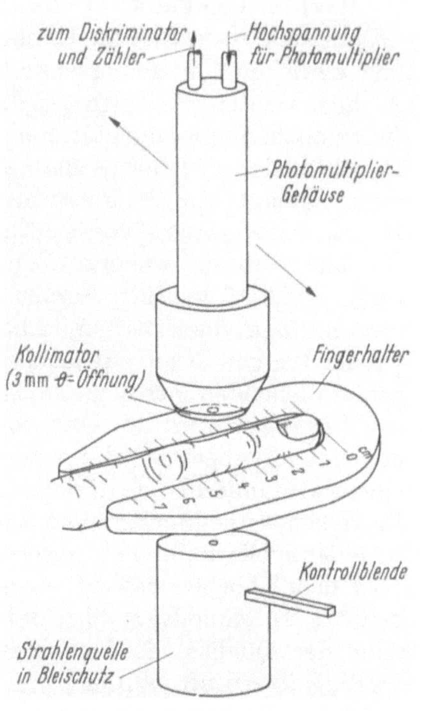

Ab. 29b

Abb. 29a. Spezialhalterung für einen Finger zur Messung des Knochenmineralgehaltes mit einer Gammastrahlung. (Nach STRANDJORD und LANZL, 1965; Abb. 3)

Abb. 29b. Schema der Meßanordnung zur Bestimmung des Knochenmineralgehaltes mit der Gammastrahlung des ^{125}J. (Nach STRANDJORD und LANZL, 1965; Abb. 4)

Die *Meßeinrichtung* (Abb. 29) besteht aus einer zylindrischen Plastikkapsel mit dem Isotop und einem Messingbehälter, der zur Strahlenabsorption oder als Strahlenschutz dient. Der Strahlenaustritt wird durch eine verschiebbare Blende gewährleistet. Das Austrittsfenster hat das Format $0{,}3 \times 2{,}0$ mm. Die durchfallende γ-Strahlung wird von einem Thallium-aktivierten, 2 mm dicken Natrium-Jodid-Kristall registriert. Um diesen Kristall vor einfallendem Licht und vor Feuchtigkeit zu schützen, liegt eine 0,13 mm dicke Beryllium-Folie darüber. Diese Folie absorbiert nur 1% der Strahlung, da die Dicke sehr gering und die Atomzahl sehr niedrig sind. Der Kristall wird von einem Metallmantel umschlossen, um noch Streustrahlung zu absorbieren. Die Kollimatoröffnung des Meßkopfes hat einen Durchmesser von 3 mm. Die durch einfallende Strahlung in dem Kristall induzierten Lichtimpulse werden von einem Photomultiplier aufgenommen. Über einen Impulshöhenanalysator werden die Signale an ein Meßgerät weitergegeben und registriert. Die Meßeinrichtung ist so konstruiert, daß sie Transmissionsmessungen über die ganze Breite des Meßfeldes automatisch durchführt. Der Finger wird dabei stillgehalten, während Strahlenquelle und Strahlungsempfänger in einer Halterung fixiert sind und motorisch bewegt werden, um den Finger langsam abzutasten. Die Einzelmessungen werden mit 1 mm Abstand durchgeführt. Ist der Finger einmal überfahren, so bleibt der Motor stehen und die ganze Meßeinrichtung wird 1 mm zur Seite verschoben. Dann geht die Messung in der anderen Richtung weiter. Die Untergrundstrahlung muß von den Meßwerten abgezogen werden (Differentialmeßverfahren).

Die Meßwerte werden ausgedrückt als lineare Koeffizienten der Absorption des ganzen Knochens. Der Durchmesser der Phalanx kann auf dem Röntgenbild ermittelt werden. Ein Knochen gleichen Durchmessers, der eine dünnere Compacta besitzt, wird niedrigere lineare Koeffizienten der Absorption ergeben. Dieser Fall wäre bei einer Osteomalacie gegeben. STRANDJORD und LANZL (1965) haben Untersuchungen an gesunden Frauen und Frauen nach der Menopause durchgeführt (s. auch S. 251). Ferner wurden Patienten mit einer Osteoporose nach Hormonbehandlung kontrolliert. Reihenuntersuchungen nach Cortison-Therapie wurden begonnen.

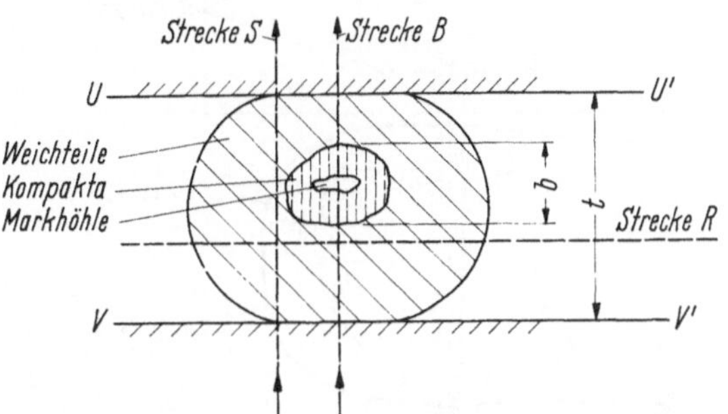

Abb. 30. Schema zur Durchführung der Messung des Knochenmineralgehaltes mit Gammastrahlen unter Berücksichtigung der Weichteilabsorption. (Nach DAVIS, STRANDJORD und LANZL, 1966; Abb. 3)

STRANDJORD, FORLAND, LANZL und COX (1968) fanden neben einem *Absinken der Knochendichte* bei gesunden Männern und Frauen *mit fortschreitendem Alter* erheblich *verminderte Dichtewerte* der Fingerknochen von 20 Patienten mit chirurgisch bestätigtem *Hyperparathyreoidismus* (s. S. 262). Durch postoperative *Kontrollmessungen konnte eine langsame Zunahme der Knochendichte objektiv nachgewiesen werden.* Die Autoren halten mit CAMERON und SORENSON (1965) vier Punkte ihres Meßverfahrens für bedeutsam:

1. Die durch das Objekt hindurchgeschickte Strahlung wird *direkt* von einem Szintillationsmeßgerät registriert.
2. Die benutzte Strahlung ist monochromatisch.
3. Die γ-Strahlung und der Detektor sind sehr gut fokussiert.
4. Der Einfluß der umgebenden Weichteile wird mit berücksichtigt.

Von JOHNSTON (1968) wurde die Methode nach CAMERON und SORENSON (1965) zur *Messung der Knochenmasse im Radius* verwendet. Eine Meßlinie wurde 3 cm distal vom Radiusende in den vorwiegend spongiösen Knochen und eine zweite Meßlinie 8 cm distal vom Radiusende, also in dem kompakten Knochen gewählt. Die mittlere Abweichung bei wiederholten Messungen an demselben Patienten betrug 2,5% (2,4—3,9%), wobei der Fehler durch die Meßeinrichtung kleiner ist als der durch den Meßvorgang bedingte individuelle Fehler. Die Messungen ergaben bei Männern größere Knochenmasse als bei Frauen. Neger besaßen mehr Knochenmasse als Weiße. In einer Gruppe von 157 weißen Frauen verschiedenen Alters wurde eine signifikante Verminderung der Knochenmasse nach dem 50. Lebensjahr gefunden. In einer kleineren Gruppe von 66 Männern war ein deutlicher Abfall des Knochengewebsvolumens nach dem 60. Lebensjahr festzustellen. Solche Frauen, die eine Zusammensinterung der Wirbelkörper erkennen ließen, hatten eine geringere Knochenmasse 3 cm distal vom Radiusende, also im spongiösen Knochen, während die Messung 8 cm vom distalen Ende entfernt keinen krankhaften Befund ergab. Der Vergleich einer kleineren Gruppe von Frauen nach der Menopause zeigte infolge Oestrogen-Behandlung (bei 15 Frauen) eine deutlich größere Knochenmasse im spongiösen Radiusbezirk (3 cm oberhalb des distalen Radiusendes) als bei einer Vergleichsgruppe (insgesamt 57 Frauen).

Über eine weitere klinische Anwendung der Methode von CAMERON und SORENSON (1965) zur Bestimmung des Knochenmineralgehaltes und erste Meßergebnisse bei Gesunden und Kranken haben EVENS, PAK, BARTTER und ASHBURN (1968) berichtet. Die Messungen wurden am *linken Radius* und der *linken Ulna* in einem Areal $11{,}2\times 5$ cm ($4^1/_2$ inch) proximal vom Metacarpal-Phalangealgelenk durchgeführt. Der Unterarm lag im Wasserbad. Die Reproduzierbarkeit der Messungen wurde an 50 Patienten geprüft und eine Abweichung von $0{,}2\pm 0{,}1$ % gefunden. Wiederholte Messungen an einem Standardknochen (Hundeknochen und Kunststoff) im Laufe von 3 Monaten (insgesamt 11 Messungen) ergaben eine Standardabweichung von 2 %. Bei 8 gesunden Menschen und 2 Patienten ohne eine aktive Knochenerkrankung ergaben *Kontrollmessungen* in Abständen von 1 und 10 Wochen eine durchschnittliche Abweichung von ± 1 %. Neben Untersuchungen an knochengesunden Menschen sind bei verschiedenen Systemerkrankungen Einzelmessungen und Kontrollmessungen durchgeführt worden. Die Meßmethode ist geeignet, Veränderungen des Knochenmineralgehaltes durch therapeutische Maßnahmen zu erfassen.

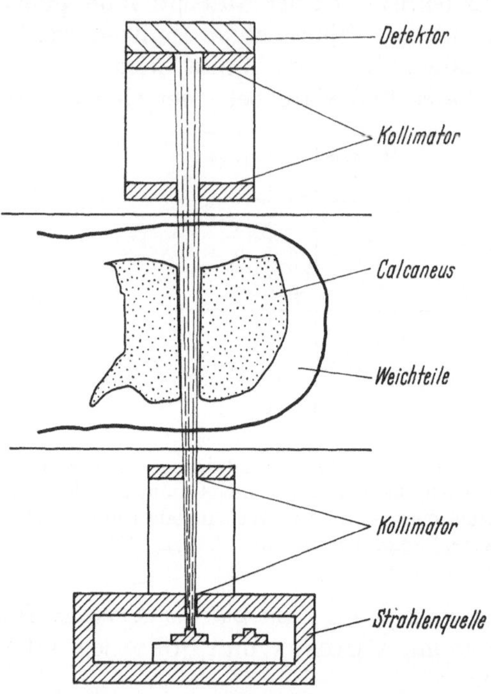

Abb. 31. Schema der Meßanordnung zur Bestimmung des Knochenmineralgehaltes (im Calcaneus) mit Gammastrahlen unterschiedlicher Energie der Isotope ^{125}J und ^{241}Am. (Nach COHEN und GILSON, 1965; Abb. 1)

Die Verwendung von *zwei unterschiedlichen γ-Strahlen* der Isotope ^{125}J (100 mC) und ^{241}Am (1 mC) zu Absorptionsmessungen im Bereich der Spongiosa des Calcaneus haben COHEN und GILSON (1965) empfohlen (Abb. 31). Die Strahlenbündel werden auf 2 mm im Durchmesser eingeblendet. Als Strahlenempfänger diente ein Natriumjodid-Kristall mit einer Meßapparatur, die auch die Streustrahlung registrierte. Die theoretisch-physikalischen Grundlagen dieser gemischten Meßmethode sind eingehend dargelegt worden. Der Meßfehler beträgt ± 1 %, bei Verwendung von 10 mC ^{241}Am kann der Fehler auf $\pm 0{,}8$ %, bei einer Mischung von 400 mC ^{125}J und 40 mC ^{241}Am auf weniger als $\pm 0{,}5$ % herabgesetzt werden. Bei diesem Prinzip könnte die Meßeinrichtung sehr klein und dadurch transportabel sein.

Von NILSSON (1968) wurde als *Strahlenquelle* ^{241}*Am* und als Meßgerät ein Szintillationsdetektor benutzt, um die *posttraumatisch auftretende Entkalkung* in der *Spongiosa der Femurcondylen* nach Tibiaschaftfrakturen zu erfassen. Ferner wurden die *posttraumatische Osteopenie* und Veränderungen *im Humerus* bei *Erfrierungen* untersucht. Die Beeinflussung des Knochens durch einen hohen oder niedrigen *Fluorgehalt des Wassers* wurde an der Spongiosa des *distalen Femurendes* bei einer größeren Bevölkerungsgruppe studiert. Vergleichsmessungen gesunder und *diabetischer Frauen* wurden begonnen.

Von SHIMMINS, GILLESPIE, HAMILTON und SMITH (1968) wurde ein Gerät konstruiert, um den Knochenmineralgehalt mit drei verschiedenen Isotopen (^{137}Cs, ^{241}Am, ^{170}Th) messen zu können. Wenn die Absorptionskoeffizienten für die benutzten Energien bekannt sind, so ist es möglich, Knochen und Weichteile getrennt zu erfassen. Die Isotope ^{137}Cs und ^{241}Am wurden für Messungen der Ulna (Mitte und distal) und des Radius (Mitte und distal) benutzt. Messungen mit einer einzigen Strahlung nach Einlegen des zu untersuchenden Knochens in ein Wasserbad ergaben die genauesten und am besten zu reproduzierenden Werte. Mit ^{241}Am wurde der Femur im mittleren Drittel nach Kompression der Weichteile untersucht. Die zur Messung des Mineralgehaltes erforderliche Bestimmung der Dicke der Knochen erfolgte mit einer Röntgenaufnahme.

VI. Methoden zur radiologisch-densitometrischen Bestimmung des Knochenmineralgehaltes

1. Die direkte photometrische (oder densitometrische) Bestimmung von Dichte oder Mineralkonzentration der Knochen

Die Möglichkeiten der Filmschwärzungsmessung zur Bestimmung der „Knochendichte" wurden bereits wenige Jahre nach der Entdeckung W. C. Röntgens erkannt. Als erster beschrieb 1897 DENNIS ein Verfahren zur Densitometrie der Knochen. PRICE (1901) berichtete über die Verwendung einer Treppe zur Bestimmung der Dichte von Knochen und Zähnen. Zunächst wurden diese Mitteilungen nicht beachtet. Erst nach 1930 waren die Probleme einer *direkten densitometrischen Untersuchung des Knochenmineralgehaltes* und des photometrischen Vergleichs von „Röntgenschatten" der Knochen mit der Filmschwärzung durch einen Vergleichskörper bestimmter Schichtdicke Gegenstand intensiver Forschungen (WILSEY 1934; KIEFFER und SEIDEMANN 1946; MORGAN und VAN ALLEN 1949; MATTSON 1951; MEES 1954 u.a.). Die ersten *experimentellen Untersuchungen* im Laboratorium wurden an *Zahnschliffen* vorgenommen (HODGE, BALE, WARREN und VAN HUYSEN 1935; HODGE, VAN HUYSEN und WARREN 1935/37/38; HODGE, VAN HUYSEN, WILSEY und WARREN 1936; HODGE und WARREN 1936; HODGE, WILSEY, VAN HUYSEN und WARREN 1937 u.a.). Die Ergebnisse dieser Untersuchungen sind von *grundlegendem Wert*, doch lassen sie sich nicht ohne weiteres auf solche Bedingungen übertragen, wie sie für Untersuchungen an *Leichenknochen* oder am *Knochen des lebenden Menschen* vorliegen.

Zur Bestimmung des Kalkgehaltes von Knochen am Lebenden konstruierte SANDERS (1935, 1937) ein Photometer, bei dem die Photozelle an ein Voltmeter angeschlossen war, so daß der während der Messung auftretende Ausschlag des Voltmeters abgelesen werden konnte. Zur exakten Messung wird jedoch die Verwendung eines *Referenzsystems* empfohlen (s. S. 152).

Eine Verbesserung der photometrischen Auswertung von Röntgenfilmen haben MACK, O'BRIEN, SMITH und BAUMAN (1939) versucht, indem sie ein *Mikrophotometer* konstruierten, das kontinuierlich die Lichtabsorption durch die photographische Schicht des Filmes registrieren kann. Mit einer besonderen Halterung wird das Röntgenbild über einen feststehenden Lichtstrahl motorisch bewegt und gleichzeitig der photometrisch ermittelte Wert über ein Spiegelgalvanometer auf einer Trommel mit Photopapier festgehalten. Dieses Instrument kann Meßlinien der Röntgenaufnahmen von Knochen oder Zähnen registrieren. Durch Bezug der Meßkurve auf eine Nullinie können die Dichtewerte ähnlicher Abschnitte des Knochens oder der Zähne bestimmt und die ermittelten Werte verschiedener Individuen miteinander verglichen werden. Es ist ferner möglich, die Dichtewerte von Knochen oder Zähnen mit den Dichtewerten bekannter Mineralzusammensetzungen in Beziehung zu setzen.

Von WEBBER (1941) ist ein Densitometer konstruiert worden, mit dem die „röntgenologische Dichte" von Knochen *direkt* ermittelt werden kann. In den Bezirken erhöhter Gewebsdichte (also geringerer Schwärzung) wird automatisch eine höhere Empfindlichkeit der Meßeinrichtung eingestellt. Mit dieser Methode wurde die relative Gewebsdichte/mm^2 auf dem Röntgenfilm an Tierknochen bestimmt. Durch Kontrolle der gefundenen Densitometerwerte mit dem Mineralgehalt der veraschten Knochen wurde versucht, eine *charakteristische Gewebsdichte* für den Knochen herauszufinden. Auf diesem Wege wurde eine halbquantitative oder quantitative Bestimmung des Knochenmineralgehalts angestrebt.

BROWN und BIRTLEY (1951) haben eine Methode zur Ermittlung der *direkten Dichteeinheiten* auf Grund der Exposition einer Filmemulsion ausgearbeitet. Das konstruierte Gerät erlaubt, die Expositionskurve neben der Densitometerkurve aufzutragen und kann für jeden Film und jedes Plattenmaterial verwendet werden, wenn die charakteristische Filmschwärzungskurve bekannt ist.

Pais und Forni (1951) haben Modelluntersuchungen über die Möglichkeit der *photometrischen Erkennung einer Entkalkung des Knochens* vorgenommen. Als Knochenprobe diente ein Stück Calcaneusspongiosa, das in Abschnitten entkalkt wurde, um dann den photometrischen Wert und seine Veränderungen zu ermitteln. Diese Untersuchungen stellen Vorversuche zur Messung des Mineralgehaltes im Knochen dar. Später hat Forni (1951) weiter an einer Methode gearbeitet, um die radiologische Untersuchung des Skeletes im Hinblick auf die Dichte der Knochen auszubauen.

Virtama, Kajanoja, Hopsu und Telkkä (1960) haben Untersuchungen über die Dichte einer größeren Zahl menschlicher *Finger- und Handknochen* durchgeführt. Die Untersuchungen wurden an den Carpalia, Metacarpalia und Fingerknochen von 5 Männern und 5 Frauen vorgenommen. Die Knochen der *Männer* waren *dichter* als die der *Frauen*. Der *dichteste Handwurzelknochen* war das *Os lunatum*. Die proximalen Phalangen waren weniger dicht als die übrigen Fingerknochen. Bei Kenntnis der Dichte eines *Handwurzelknochens*, eines *Metacarpale* und *einer Phalanx* kann der Mineralisationsgrad der Handknochen mit ziemlicher Genauigkeit bestimmt werden. Die Dichtewerte der beiden Hände können sehr unterschiedlich sein, so daß auch empfohlen wird, beide Hände zu untersuchen.

Virtama und Telkkä (1961) führten Untersuchungen über die *Spongiosastruktur und die Trabekel des Knochens menschlicher Finger* durch. Von 40 Fingerknochen aus 10 Skeleten sind densitometrische Kurven in drei Bereichen gewonnen worden. Die Unterschiede der Kurven des gesunden Knochens, verglichen mit denen des osteoporotischen Fingerknochens, werden erläutert. Die Ergebnisse der Gegenüberstellung der Knochendichte und der Trabekelzahl stimmen gut überein (s. auch Rockoff, 1968). Es wird jedoch ausdrücklich betont, daß auf Grund von Dichtemessungen im Bereich der Extremitäten nicht auf die Dichte anderer Knochen des Skeletes, insbesondere der Wirbelkörper geschlossen werden kann.

Von Hiness (1968) wurden Modelluntersuchungen an einem Knochenphantom aus Plexiglas in Wasser durchgeführt, um festzustellen, wie genau der Mineralgehalt von Knochen *mit Hilfe der Schwächungskoeffizienten allein aus Röntgenaufnahmen* bestimmt werden kann. Der Knochen wurde durch eine Mischung aus Plexiglas (Plexiglaspulver) und Tricalciumphosphat bei unterschiedlichen Mengen des Calciumphosphates repräsentiert. Die densitometrisch ermittelten Werte des Kalksalzgehaltes lagen sowohl bei einer Konzentration des Tricalciumphosphats von 75% wie bei einer Konzentration von 50% *über den tatsächlichen Werten*. Bei der 50%igen Mischung war eine höhere Abweichung von +3,8 bis +17,6% (Mittelwert +10,4%) festzustellen. Es ist bemerkenswert, daß die Röntgen-Kontrollaufnahmen eine *deutliche Inhomogenität der Mischungen* aufdeckten. Diese Abweichungen zeigen Parallelen zu den Beobachtungen von Heuck und Schmidt (1960) über den Einfluß eines „Teilchenfaktors" auf das Ergebnis densitometrischer Messungen eines Stoffgemisches aus einem stärker und einem schwächer absorbierenden Stoff, wie ihn der Knochen darstellt (s. S. 149). Auf Grund dieses Fehlers studierte Hiness (1968) in weiteren Versuchen die Abweichung der densitometrischen Messung einer vorgegebenen Lösung von Calciumchlorid ($Ca\,Cl_2$) unterschiedlicher Konzentration in einem Plexiglasrohr als Knochenmodell, das in einem Wasserbad dem Film nahe (unten liegend) oder fern (in der Mitte oder am oberen Wasserspiegel liegend) angeordnet war. Auch bei diesem Modellversuch zeigten die densitometrischen Messungen eine Abweichung nach oben, also *einen etwas höheren Wert der Kalksalzkonzentration*. Dabei waren die Abweichungen dann besonders groß, wenn das *Strahlenbündel breiter* und die vorgegebene Konzentration des Kalksalzes niedriger waren (25%ige Lösung). Bei Verwendung eines *eng eingeblendeten Strahlenbündels* waren die Abweichungen von den Sollwerten wesentlich geringer. Noch genauer waren die densitometrischen Werte bei einer mit 0,4 mm Cu gefilterten Strahlung, die mit 103 kV Anodenspannung erzeugt und eng eingeblendet worden war. Diese Bedingungen lieferten trotz des verringerten Kontrastes gute Meßwerte bei prozentualen Abweichungen vom Sollwert von +4,5 bis −0,65%. Aus diesen Beobachtungen spricht der *große Einfluß der Streustrahlung* auf das Meßergebnis (s. S. 128).

2. Die Bestimmung des Knochenmineralgehaltes durch vergleichende Schwärzungsmessungen

Am lebenden Menschen ist es außerordentlich schwierig und praktisch nicht möglich, aus den Schwärzungswerten eines Filmes *unmittelbar* auf den Kalksalzgehalt des zu untersuchenden Knochens zu schließen. Die Filmschwärzung ist nicht nur von der Zusammensetzung der durchstrahlten Gewebe und der Knochensubstanz abhängig, sondern wird von zahlreichen weiteren Faktoren beeinflußt, die eingehend erörtert worden sind (s. S. 124—130). Diese Störfaktoren lassen sich dadurch weitgehend ausschalten, daß die Schwächung der Strahlung durch das Knochengewebe mit der Schwächung durch ein *Referenzsystem* bekannter Zusammensetzung verglichen wird.

a) Die geeigneten Vergleichskörper oder Referenzsysteme

Die Objektivierung der „röntgenologischen Dichte" eines Knochens ist mit verschiedenen Referenzsystemen angestrebt worden. Die chemische Zusammensetzung der Vergleichskörper war zunächst bedeutungslos. Es wurden jedoch vorwiegend solche Substanzen empfohlen, die in ihrer chemischen Zusammensetzung dem Knochen ähnlich sind, deren physikalisches Verhalten im Hinblick auf die Schwächung der Röntgenstrahlen also nur geringfügige Abweichungen erwarten ließ. Mit Hilfe der *gleichzeitigen Darstellung eines Referenzsystems neben dem zu untersuchenden Knochen auf demselben Film* ist es möglich, einen jederzeit *reproduzierbaren Meßwert* zu erhalten, wenn die Strahlenexposition Filmschwärzungswerte ergibt, die auf dem *linearen Teil der Gradationskurve* des Filmes liegen. Die photometrisch ermittelte Filmschwärzung des Vergleichskörpers wird zu der Filmschwärzung des zu untersuchenden Knochens in Beziehung gesetzt und diejenige Schichtdicke des Vergleichskörpers bestimmt, die denselben Schwärzungswert wie der zu untersuchende Skeletbezirk aufweist. An und für sich wird bei diesem Verfahren die Schwärzung nur als Indikator benutzt, um festzustellen, ob Schwärzungsgleichheit zwischen dem zu untersuchenden Bezirk und einer entsprechenden Schichtdicke des Referenzsystems besteht. Sind die Schwärzungsunterschiede des Referenzsystems fein genug, so braucht nicht interpoliert zu werden und das Meßverfahren ist unabhängig von der Gradationskurve des Filmes.

Die bisher verwendeten *Vergleichskörper* waren aus Aluminium, Aluminiumlegierungen oder anderen Metallen hergestellt und besaßen Keilform oder Treppenform. Ferner sind Referenzsysteme aus knochenähnlichem Material wie Elfenbein, Rinderknochen, Knochenpulver und Calciumverbindungen benutzt worden. Das Ergebnis des Vergleiches der Schwächung der Röntgenstrahlung durch den Knochenbezirk einerseits und das Referenzsystem andererseits wird als „Schwächungsgleichwert" angegeben. Die Bestimmung des sog. Schwächungsgleichwertes auf der Aluminiumbasis erlaubt, den Calciumgehalt des Knochens auf *rechnerischem Wege* zu ermitteln. Es muß jedoch betont werden, daß die so errechneten Werte der Kalksalzkonzentration im allgemeinen nicht durch eine chemische Analyse des interessierenden Knochenbezirkes kontrolliert worden sind. Diese Methoden stellen dennoch gegenüber der einfachen Betrachtung des Röntgenbildes einen wesentlichen Fortschritt dar.

Der Bezugswert („Schwächungsgleichwert") des jeweils verwendeten Referenzsystems ist jedoch *abhängig* von der zur Untersuchung benutzten *Qualität der Strahlung*, so daß Vergleiche der mit unterschiedlichen Methoden gewonnenen Meßwerte nicht möglich sind. Eine Röntgenstrahlung, die z.B. bei 40 bzw. 100 kV Anodenspannung entsteht, wird durch *Aluminium* einerseits, Phosphor und Calcium andererseits unterschiedlich geschwächt (Abb. 32). Die polychromatische Röntgenstrahlung wird nur dann von zwei Objekten *in gleicher Weise* geschwächt, wenn sie auch die gleiche Zusammensetzung und die gleiche Masse besitzen. Die Referenzsysteme aus Aluminium und Aluminiumlegierungen erschweren daher einen Vergleich der verschiedenen Untersuchungsergebnisse.

Die *knochenähnlichen Referenzsysteme* (Elfenbein, Rinderknochen, Knochenpulver u.a.) sind nicht jederzeit reproduzierbar, da Unterschiede in der Zusammensetzung des Materials bestehen.

Dies ist nur ein Teil der Problematik, die es bisher unmöglich machte, von verschiedenen Untersuchern erarbeitete Werte miteinander zu vergleichen oder einen Absolutwert der Mineralkonzentration von Knochen zu bestimmen. In einer grundlegenden Arbeit hat OMNELL (1957) daher empfohlen, die Referenzsysteme aus einem Material herzustellen, das ungefähr die gleichen Atomgewichte besitzt wie der zu untersuchende Knochen. SPIEGLER (1959) hat sich mit den physikalischen Grundlagen von Messungen zur quantitativen Auswertung von „Röntgenschatten" beschäftigt. Über die physikalischen Eigenschaften verschiedener Referenzsysteme (Treppen aus Aluminium, Alu-

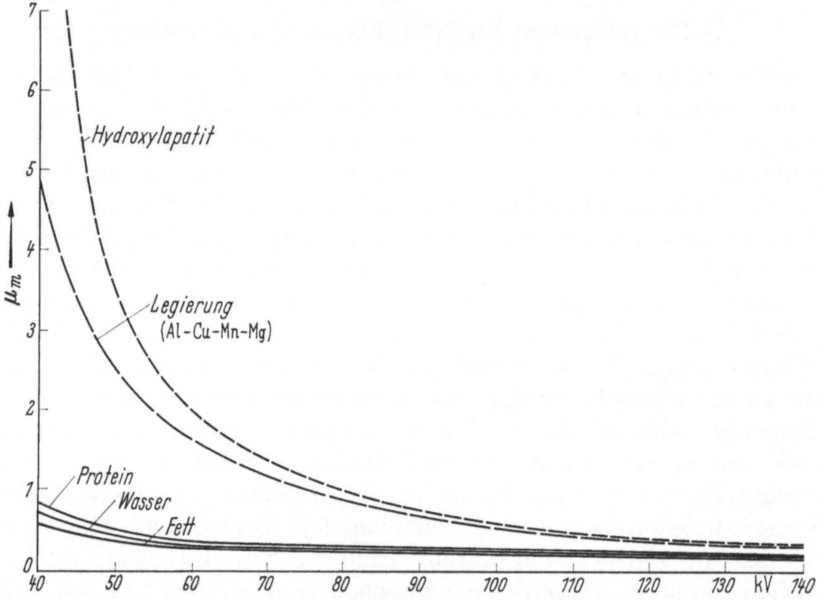

Abb. 32. Unterschiede der Massenschwächungskoeffizienten der verschiedenen Körpergewebe, einer Aluminiumlegierung und von Hydroxylapatit in Abhängigkeit von der Röhrenspannung. (Nach VOSE, 1965; Abb. 2)

miniumlegierungen, Plexiglas u.a.), welche zu photometrischen Untersuchungen geeignet sind, haben SEEMANN und ROTH (1960) berichtet. Eine photometrische (oder densitometrische) Analyse ist *dann von der Strahlenqualität und anderen Faktoren unabhängig*, wenn die Vergleichsmessungen an dem *gleichen* Stoff oder sehr ähnlichen Stoffmischungen vorgenommen werden. Die Entwicklung von solchen Referenzsystemen, deren chemische Zusammensetzung reproduzierbar und deren physikalische Eigenschaften dem Knochen gleich sind, brachte einen bedeutsamen Fortschritt (HEUCK und SCHMIDT 1954/59/60; OKUYAMA 1965; PRIBOTH, BÖRNERT und FRITZSCHE 1966; MEEMA 1963/64).

Einige wichtige Fragen zur Bestimmung des Mineralgehaltes im Knochen mit verschiedenen Methoden haben SPIEGLER und KEANE (1961) bearbeitet. Für das richtige Verständnis der Meßergebnisse ist es bedeutsam, die *Grundbegriffe „Flächendichte" und „Konzentration"* klar zu erfassen. Die *Flächendichte* des Knochenminerals (hauptsächlich Calciumphosphate in Form des Hydroxylapatit) ist die Gesamtmasse des Minerals, die über der Flächeneinheit liegt und in mg/cm^2 angegeben wird. So definiert ist die Flächendichte unabhängig von der Packungsdichte (Auflockerung) der aufgeschichteten Substanz. Da die Flächendichte auch ein Maß der effektiven Gesamtschicht an Mineral ist, die der Röntgenstrahl bei der Durchdringung des Knochens vorfindet, kann demnach von „effektiver Gesamtdicke" an Stelle der „Flächendichte" gesprochen werden. Bei gegebener Strahlenqualität und streufreier Abbildung hängt die Absorption im Mineral des Knochens lediglich von der Flächendichte ab. Wenn jedoch Streustrahlung den Film erreicht, so ist die Annahme, daß die Gesamtabsorption nur von der Flächendichte abhängig sei, nicht mehr richtig.

Bei *gleicher Flächendichte* des Minerals könnte ein osteoporotischer Femur eines Riesen die gleiche Strahlenabsorption erreichen wie ein Femur von durchschnittlichen Dimensionen. Es ist daher *nicht* die „effektive Gesamtdicke" des Minerals ein Maß für die Mineralisation, sondern die *Konzentration*, also die *Masse Mineral* in der *Volumeneinheit Gesamtknochen* (mg/ml) für die Beurteilung der Lebensvorgänge im Knochen bedeutsam (KEANE, SPIEGLER und DAVIS 1959; HEUCK und SCHMIDT 1954/60).

Die *Abweichungen der Meßergebnisse densitometrischer Bestimmungen* der Kalksalzkonzentration gegenüber *chemisch-analytischen Befunden* oder vorgegebenen Werten führten zu der Vermutung, daß die Absorption der Röntgenstrahlung in Stoffmischungen von der Art der Verteilung der Stoffe und dem Grad der Homogenität des dichteren Mediums abhängt (HEUCK und SCHMIDT 1960; HINESS 1968; s. S. 146). Die Röntgenstrahlenabsorption in Stoffmischungen verdient daher besondere Beachtung.

b) Die Strahlenabsorption in Stoffmischungen („Teilchenfaktor")

Der Vergleich von Röntgenaufnahmen des proximalen Femurabschnittes läßt bei annähernd *gleicher* Kalksalzkonzentration in der Volumeneinheit der Schenkelhalsspongiosa deutliche *Strukturunterschiede* grober oder feiner Spongiosabälkchen und Lamellen erkennen. Bei Untersuchungen an spongiösen Knochen muß also geprüft werden,

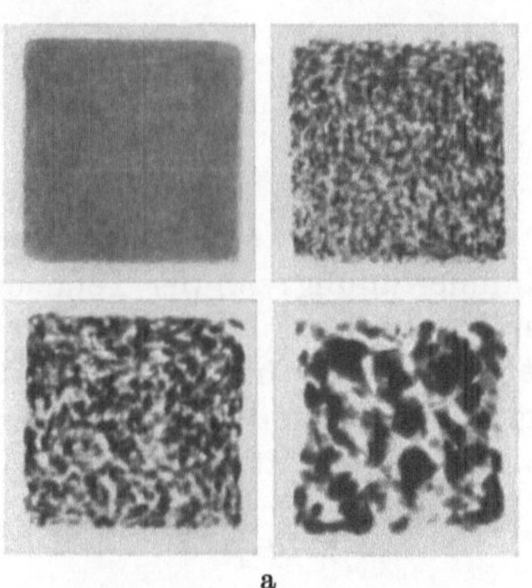

a

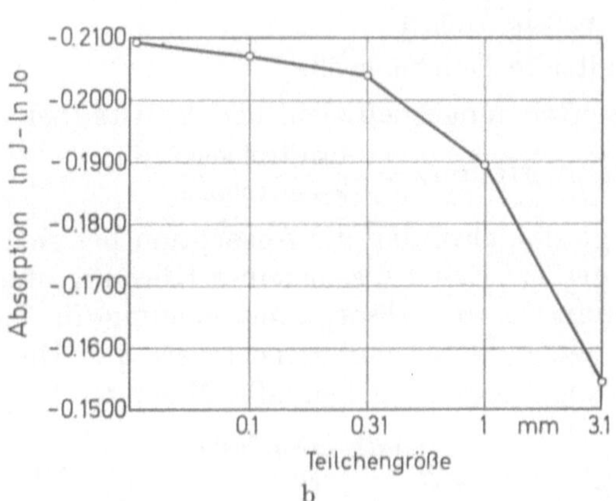

b

Abb. 33. a Röntgenbild vier gleich großer Würfel mit einer Kantenlänge von 2 cm aus einem Gemisch von Paraffin und Marmor mit gleicher Konzentration, aber verschiedener Teilchengröße des Marmors. (Nach HEUCK und SCHMIDT, 1960; Abb. 7). b Graphische Darstellung der Röntgenstrahlenabsorption in Abhängigkeit von der Teilchengröße des Hydroxylapatits in einer Mischung. (Nach HEUCK und SCHMIDT, 1960; Abb. 6)

in welchem Ausmaß die Verteilung der anorganischen Substanz im Gesamtknochen die Röntgenstrahlenabsorption beeinflußt, inwieweit also die Absorption von der Struktur und Größe der Spongiosabälkchen abhängt. Von HEUCK und SCHMIDT (1960) wurde geprüft, ob bei der Mischung einer molekular-dispersen, geringe Absorption aufweisenden Komponente mit einer solchen, die durch eine große Absorption charakterisiert ist, Differenzen im Gesamtabsorptionswert der Mischung auftreten, je nachdem, ob die stark absorbierende Komponente fein- oder grobkörnig ist (Abb. 33a).

Aus der folgenden Überlegung ergibt sich *die Bedeutung der Korngröße für die Absorption:*

Betrachtet man ein Pulver aus Teilchen mittleren Durchmessers x, die über das durchstrahlte Volumen vom Querschnitt l und der Höhe d regellos so verteilt sind, daß sie vom Gesamtvolumen V den Anteil $v = q \cdot V$ mit kompakter Materie erfüllen, so ergibt sich $q = v/V$ als die Raumerfüllung, also den Bruchteil, den das Volumen aller Teilchen pro Gesamtvolumen ausmacht.

Für den Fall $q = 1$ würde nach der obigen Überlegung von einer einfallenden Lichtenergie I_0 nur der Anteil $I = I_0 \cdot e^{-\mu \cdot d}$ wieder austreten, wenn μ der totale Schwächungskoeffizient der Materie ist.

Für den Fall $q < 1$ betrachten wir zunächst eine Schicht der Dicke x. Da in dieser die Teilchen der Dicke x nur nebeneinander liegen können, ist der Bruchteil q dieser Schicht mit absorbierender Materie erfüllt, während der Bruchteil $1-q$ nicht absorbierende Materie enthält. Von der auf diese Schicht fallenden Lichtenergie I_0 geht der Anteil $(1-q)\, I_0$ ungeschwächt hindurch, während der Rest durch Absorption geschwächt wird. Insgesamt erhält man für die durch diese Schicht hindurchgegangene Energie den Wert

$$I_1 = (1-q)\, I_0 + q I_0 e^{-\mu x} = I_0 (1-q+q e^{-\mu x}).$$

In der zweiten Schicht der Dicke x geschieht mit der Energie I_1 das gleiche, so daß nach Durchlaufen der beiden Schichten nur noch die Energie

$$I_2 = (1-q)\, I_1 + q I_1 e^{-\mu x} = I_1 (1-q+q e^{-\mu x}) = I_0 (1-q+q e^{-\mu x})^2$$

vorhanden ist.

Nach Durchlaufen von $n = d/x$ Schichten ist dann nur noch die Energie

$$I = I_0 (1-q+q e^{-\mu x})^n = I_0 (1-q+q e^{-\mu x})\, d/x$$

vorhanden. Daraus ergibt sich

$$\ln \frac{I}{I_0} = \frac{d}{x} \ln (1-q+q e^{-\mu x}),$$

worin also bedeuten

x = mittlere Teilchengröße;

μ = Schwächungskoeffizient des Apatits (bei 40 kV 2,23);

q = Raumerfüllung = $\frac{\text{Apatitvolumen}}{\text{Gesamtvolumen}}$.

Es zeigt sich also, daß die Absorption bei gleicher Raumerfüllung von der Teilchengröße abhängig ist. Erst bei sehr feiner Körnung und dadurch homogener Verteilung geht diese Gleichung in die Absorptionsgleichung für homogenes Material über und man erhält einen neuen Schwächungsgleichwert $q\mu$. Dieses ergibt sich, wenn man in der letzten Gleichung x gegen 0 gehen läßt. Nach der Regel von de l'Hopital ist

$$\lim_{x \to 0} \frac{\ln (1-q+q e^{-\mu x})}{x/d} = -q \cdot \mu \cdot d \quad \text{bzw.} \qquad \ln \frac{I}{I_0} = -q \cdot \mu \cdot d$$

Berechnet man die Abhängigkeit der Absorption von der Teilchengröße im Bereich zwischen 0 (ideale Lösung) und den Teilchengrößen, in denen der Hydroxylapatit im Knochengewebe vorkommt, so ergibt sich für eine Mischung, die 300 mg Apatit pro cm^3 Substanz enthält die graphische Darstellung der Abb. 33b.

In diesem Zusammenhang interessiert ferner die Frage, ob die Stärke der Streuung in einer Stoffmischung inhomogener Zusammensetzung auch von der Teilchengröße des stärker absorbierenden Stoffes der Mischung beeinflußt wird. Es fand sich, daß der Einfluß der Streustrahlung auf die Filmschwärzung bei einer kurzwelligen Primärstrahlung (erzeugt bei 100 kV Anodenspannung) unabhängig von der Teilchengröße ähnlich ist. Bei einer weicheren Strahlung (erzeugt bei 80 und 60 kV Anodenspannung) fand sich, daß der Phantomkörper mit den kleinsten Teilchen das größte Streuvolumen entwickelte.

Diesen Überlegungen und Befunden kommt zunächst nur geringe praktische Bedeutung zu, doch sollten sie bei Meßungenauigkeiten insbesondere in spongiösen Knochen beachtet werden. Die von VIRTAMA (1957/60) gefundenen Absorptionsunterschiede bei gleichem Aschegehalt und gleicher Schichtdicke des Knochens, die als Folge einer ungleichmäßigen Verteilung der Knochensalze angesehen wurden, könnten ebenso wie die Meßungenauigkeiten in den Versuchen von HINESS (1968) durch den Einfluß der Teilchengröße (Teilchenfaktor) der stärker absorbierenden Kalksalze erklärt werden.

c) Die Berücksichtigung der Weichteile

Der Einfluß der jeden Knochen umgebenden mehr oder weniger voluminösen Weichteile auf die Meßgenauigkeit bereitete bei allen bisher ausgearbeiteten Methoden besondere Schwierigkeiten. Die Verschleierung eines vorhandenen Kalksalzverlustes durch *überlagernde Weichteile* ist nicht unbekannt und wiederholt untersucht worden (Lachmann und Whelan 1935; Shackman und Harrison 1948; Ardran 1951 u.a.). Ein *direkter Vergleich* der Dichte des zu untersuchenden Knochens mit einem gleichzeitig auf demselben Film *neben dem Knochen dargestellten Referenzsystem* ist nicht möglich, da die umgebenden Weichteile das Meßergebnis erheblich beeinträchtigen können.

Die *Eliminierung* des Weichteilfaktors ist folgendermaßen möglich:

1. durch rechnerische Berücksichtigung der Strahlenabsorption durch die Weichteile (Morgan 1946; Engström und Welin 1949; Mack, Brown und Trapp 1949) und

2. dadurch, daß der zu untersuchende Knochen und die ihn umgebenden Weichteile zusammen mit dem Referenzsystem in einem *Wasserbad* geröntgt werden, das sowohl die Extremität als auch den Vergleichskörper umhüllt und somit eine gleichmäßige Strahlenabsorption sowie Streuung gewährleistet (Jackson 1951; Keane, Spiegler und Davis 1959).

Lefebvre, Bismuth und Chaumont (1964) haben sich mit dem Einfluß der Absorptionsunterschiede, die durch das Fettgewebe in den Weichteilen und im Knochen selbst bedingt sind, auf die densitometrischen Messungen mit einer Aluminium-Treppe als Referenzsystem beschäftigt. Die in den Weichteilen vorhandenen *Fettgewebsanteile* ergeben Absorptionsdifferenzen, die sich auch durch eine Aufnahme im Wasserbad nicht vollständig ausgleichen lassen. Eine bessere Angleichung an die inhomogene Zusammensetzung der Weichteile kann durch ein *Alkoholbad* (50—70%iger Äthylalkohol) erreicht werden (Heuck 1968). Mit diesem Verfahren ist die Untersuchung kleiner Extremitätenknochen (Hand, Unterarm oder Fuß) möglich, ein Grund, weshalb meist das Handskelet herangezogen wurde (Keane, Spiegler und Davis 1959). Ein besonderer Vorteil der Ausschaltung der Weichteile durch ein ,,Standardvolumen" liegt darin, daß *die Belichtungs- und Entwicklungsbedingungen* bei diesen Methoden *konstant gehalten werden können*, so daß die *praktische* Durchführung der Kalksalzmessung erleichtert wird.

Von Spiegler und Keane (1961) ist besonders darauf hingewiesen worden, daß nicht nur die den Knochen umgebenden Weichteile berücksichtigt werden müssen, sondern auch die Anteile der organischen Substanz in einem Knochen selbst. Bei entsprechender Schichtdicke dieses Knochens können sie fast die Hälfte der von den Knochenkalksalzen hervorgerufenen Schwächung der Primärstrahlung ausmachen.

Von Rethmeier (1955), Heuck und Schmidt (1954/60) wurde versucht, den Einfluß der Weichteile dadurch auszuschalten, daß z.B. bei der Untersuchung zur Bestimmung des Kalksalzgehaltes der Handknochen oder der Femurhalsspongiosa der Vergleichskörper unmittelbar neben den Knochen *unter die umgebenden Weichteile* gelegt wurde. Zum Ausgleich der Rundung des Oberschenkels wurde die Hydroxylapatittreppe in einen stumpfen Keil aus Paraffin oder Columbian-Paste (Paraffin, Bienenwachs und Sägemehl) eingebettet, deren Strahlenabsorption der der Weichteile ähnlich ist. Diese Referenzsysteme sollten so lokalisiert werden, daß die Weichteile fest auf den Phantomkörper gepreßt werden und eine glatte, parallele Begrenzung der durchstrahlten Schicht resultiert (ähnliche Anordnung wie Henny 1950). Der Weichteilschatten überlagert somit in gleicher Weise den Knochen und das Referenzsystem.

Die Lage von Femurknochen und Referenzsystem innerhalb der Weichteile ist allerdings unterschiedlich. Nach den Ergebnissen der Untersuchungen von Hiness (1968) kann bei Verwendung einer härteren Strahlung (103 kV Anodenspannung und 0,4 mm Cu-Filterung) und einer engen Einblendung des Strahlenbündels eine Lageabweichung zwischen Knochen und Vergleichskörper zugelassen werden, und zwar sowohl hinsichtlich der Dicke und Tiefenlage des Knochens bzw. des Referenzsystems in den Weichteilen als auch hinsichtlich der Dicke des Gesamtkörpers, ohne daß sich nennenswerte Fehler ergeben.

Dieser Sachverhalt erlaubt eine Vereinfachung der radiologischen Methode der Mineralgehaltsbestimmung im Knochen. So ist es wegen der verringerten Dickenabhängigkeit der Schwächungskoeffizienten möglich, unabhängig von der Dicke des zu untersuchenden Knochens einen zylindrischen Vergleichskörper von konstantem, genau auszumessendem Durchmesser und genau einstellbarer Konzentration zur Bestimmung der Schwächungskoeffizienten (μ anorganisch — μ organisch) zu verwenden. Da die Schwächungskoeffizienten jeweils durch Messung von Intensitätsverhältnissen, also aus Relativwerten einer Aufnahme gewonnen werden, können die Aufnahmen des zu untersuchenden Knochens und des Vergleichskörpers *getrennt hergestellt* werden, sofern die Röhrenspannung hinreichend konstant ist. Dadurch ist es möglich, Knochen und Vergleichskörper bei den Schwächungsmessungen an der gleichen Stelle des Strahlungsfeldes senkrecht zur Strahlrichtung anzuordnen, so daß Feldinhomogenitäten keine Rolle spielen und Änderungen der Weglänge im Absorber vermieden werden. Ferner erübrigt sich in einem solchen Falle die gemeinsame Einbettung von Untersuchungsobjekt und Vergleichskörper in gewebsäquivalentes Material, was die technische Durchführung der Mineralgehaltsbestimmung erheblich vereinfacht.

Auf Grund der Ergebnisse von Phantommessungen ist der Fehler in der Mineralgehaltsbestimmung nach dem angegebenen Verfahren bei Knochen, die eine präzise Dickenbestimmung erlauben, mit $\pm 5\%$ anzusetzen (Hiness 1968). Bei kompliziert geformten Knochen macht die Dickenmessung Schwierigkeiten, so daß mit größeren Fehlern zu rechnen ist. Diese werden von der Genauigkeit der Dickenmessung bestimmt. Wie auf S. 129 erörtert, ist die direkte Ausmessung der Dicke auf dem Röntgenfilm der photometrischen Bestimmung überlegen.

3. Die klinische Anwendung von Methoden der vergleichenden Schwärzungsmessung

a) Die Bestimmung eines „Schwächungsgleichwertes" mit Referenzsystemen aus Aluminium oder anderen Metallen

Vergleichskörper aus Aluminium oder Aluminiumlegierungen wurden von verschiedenen Arbeitsgruppen verwendet, da die Strahlenabsorption durch Aluminium der durch Calcium ähnlich ist. Voraussetzung für vergleichende Untersuchungen ist jedoch, daß die Qualität der Strahlung von Aufnahme zu Aufnahme konstant gehalten wird, da die Messungen von der Wellenlänge abhängig sind. Die Angabe der „Schwächungsgleichwerte" in Schichtdicke Aluminium kann bei Kenntnis der entsprechenden Schichtdicke Knochen in die Mineralkonzentration des untersuchten Knochens umgerechnet werden. Bei 50 kV Anodenspannung entspricht die Dicke von *1 mm Aluminium einer Flächendichte von 130 mg/cm² Calciumphosphat.* Mit Hilfe dieser Beziehung und einer Korrektur für die Verdrängung von organischer Substanz durch die effektive Mineralschicht können Mineralkonzentrationen geschätzt werden (Spiegler 1959).

Die ersten Versuche zur Objektivierung der Knochendichte mit Hilfe eines Aluminium- und Elfenbeinkeiles sind nach Stein (1937) von Sanders (1937), Nachlass und Parke (1937) durchgeführt worden. Die densitometrisch gemessenen Schwärzungswerte des Knochens wurden zu den äquivalenten Schwärzungsintensitäten des Vergleichskörpers auf dem Röntgenfilm in Beziehung gesetzt und die entsprechende Schichtdicke des Vergleichsmaterials ermittelt. Mit Hilfe dieser Methode war es möglich, die röntgenologische Dichte des normalen Knochens mit den Werten kranker Knochen zu vergleichen.

Von dem Gedanken ausgehend, Knochenentkalkungen bei einer Polyarthritis bereits im Anfangsstadium der Krankheit erfassen zu können, haben Engström und Welin (1949) eine Methode zur quantitativen Bestimmung des Kalkgehaltes in der Volumeneinheit Knochen entwickelt. Dieser Meßwert sei treffender als die Angabe des Calciumgehaltes in der Gewichtseinheit, da die Menge Calcium in der Volumeneinheit den Kontrast im Röntgenbild bestimme. Als Referenzsystem wurden *drei Aluminiumtreppen* verschiedener Dicke benutzt (Abb. 34). Die Aufnahmen sind auf folienlosen Feinkornfilmen unter konstanten Belichtungsbedingungen bei 44 kV Anodenspannung und gleichmäßiger Verteilung der Strahlung über die Filmfläche angefertigt worden. Die photometrische Auswertung der Filme wurde mit einem besonders konstruierten Densitometer vorgenommen (s. auch S. 130). Die Meßfläche wurde mit 2 mm² angegeben. Die Strahlenabsorption durch die Weichteile wurde aus der Schwächung von Knochen und Weichteilen einerseits und der alleinigen Weichteilschwächung andererseits rechnerisch berücksichtigt. Die Messungen sind im distalen und proximalen Bereich der Basalphalanx des Daumens und an der Grund- und Mittelphalanx des Zeigefingers durchgeführt worden. Auf die verschiedenen Fehlerquellen des Untersuchungsverfahrens wird eingegangen und besonders betont, daß unterschiedliche Anodenspannungen, also verschiedene Strahlenqualitäten, Meßfehler ergeben, da der Massenschwächungskoeffizient für Aluminium und Kalksalze bei verschiedenen Spannungen nicht gleich ist. Zur Beseitigung dieses Fehlers sind die Aufnahmen mit weitgehend gleicher Spannung und gleicher Belichtungszeit angefertigt worden. Ferner können Fehler durch die Korrektur der Weichteilabsorption zustande kommen.

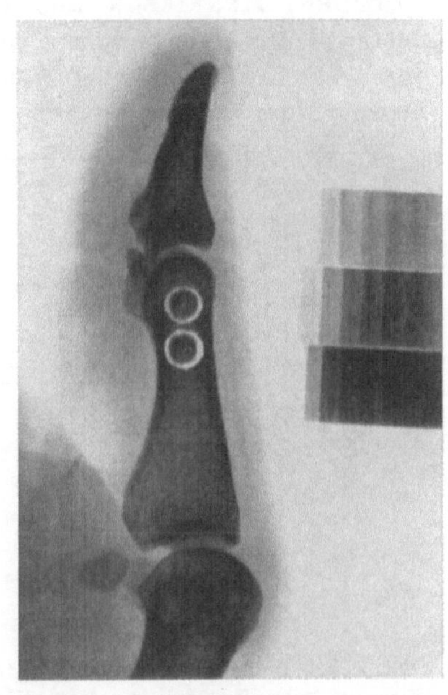

Abb. 34. Darstellung von Daumenknochen mit dreiteiligem Aluminium-Referenzsystem. Die Meßzonen sind eingezeichnet. (Nach ENGSTRÖM und WELIN, 1949; Abb. 1)

Nach Klassifizierung der Patienten vom klinischen Standpunkt aus (Ödeme, Funktionsstörungen und andere klinische Symptome, Muskelatrophie usw.) sind die Meßergebnisse von 160 Röntgenaufnahmen bei 10 Frauen und 10 Männern, welche an rheumatischen Erkrankungen litten, ausgewertet worden. Im Vergleich zu einem Kollektiv von jeweils 10 knochengesunden Männern und Frauen fand sich eine *deutliche Verminderung des Knochenkalkgehaltes bei Polyarthritis*. In fast 50 % der Fälle lag der Calciumgehalt unterhalb der Fehlergrenze des Normalkollektivs, wodurch die Abnahme gesichert erscheint. Bei schweren klinischen Veränderungen fanden sich häufiger pathologische Werte, so daß eine gute Übereinstimmung der klinischen Klassifikation mit dem Calciumgehalt des Knochens gefunden werden konnte. Die Abnahme des Calciumgehaltes fand sich nicht nur in den gelenkbildenden Knochenpartien der Epiphysen und Metaphysen, sondern auch im Bereich der Compacta der Diaphysen. Die Entkalkung muß also diffus erfolgen. Einmal wurde bei schwerer Verminderung des Kalkgehaltes durch *therapeutische Maßnahmen eine gute Besserung festgestellt*.

Neben einer *Aluminiumtreppe* oder einem *Aluminiumkeil* wurde von BARTELHEIMER (1951) und MAASS (1951) ein in Paraffin eingebetteter *Mittelhandknochen* eines gesunden Menschen als Referenzsystem verwendet. Das erste, von EPPINGER benutzte Referenzsystem soll nach MAASS ein *Glasphantom* aus treppenweise übereinander gekitteten Objektträgern gewesen sein. Das von MAASS zur Auswertung benutzte Meßgerät erlaubt mit Hilfe eines *Graukeiles* den Schwärzungswert des Aluminiumphantoms für den zu untersuchenden Knochen direkt mit dem Auge abzulesen. Die Messungen wurden am *Radius* (1 cm proximal vom Radiocarpalgelenk), *Os capitatum* und in der *Mitte der distalen Metaphyse des Os metacarpale secundum* vorgenommen. Die Aluminiumschwächungsgleichwerte von 18 normalen und 21 kalkarmen Handskeleten sind gemessen worden. Bei kalkarmen Knochen liegen diese Werte erheblich unter den Normalwerten. Da Differenzen des *normalen Kalkgehaltes* zwischen der *rechten* und der *linken* Seite gefunden werden konnten, wird empfohlen, beide Seiten zu untersuchen oder der *rechten Seite* den Vorzug zu geben. Neben den Aluminiumwerten des Knochens muß ferner die *Dicke des Knochens* — also das durchstrahlte Volumen — berücksichtigt werden, um zu brauchbaren Ergebnissen zu kommen. Da zwischen Breite und Dicke des Knochens eine weitgehend konstante Relation besteht, läßt sich der eine Wert aus dem anderen ermitteln. Durch wiederholte Auswertung einer Aufnahme sind Streuungen von $\pm 0{,}1$ bis $\pm 0{,}2$ mm Aluminium beobachtet worden, woraus ein praktischer Fehler von etwa 2,5% und ein maximaler Fehler von 5% resultiert. Der Wert einer objektiven Beurteilung der Knochen wird vor allem in der Kontrolle *therapeutischer Maßnahmen* während des Krankheitsablaufes einer *Entkalkungsosteopathie* gesehen.

Björn, Henrikson und Omnell (1951) haben über eine röntgenologisch-photometrische Methode berichtet, *periapikale* Läsionen im Bereich des Unterkiefers mit Hilfe eines Aluminiumreferenzsystems quantitativ zu kontrollieren. Die Röntgenaufnahmen müssen unter absolut gleichen Bedingungen an *derselben Stelle* angefertigt werden.

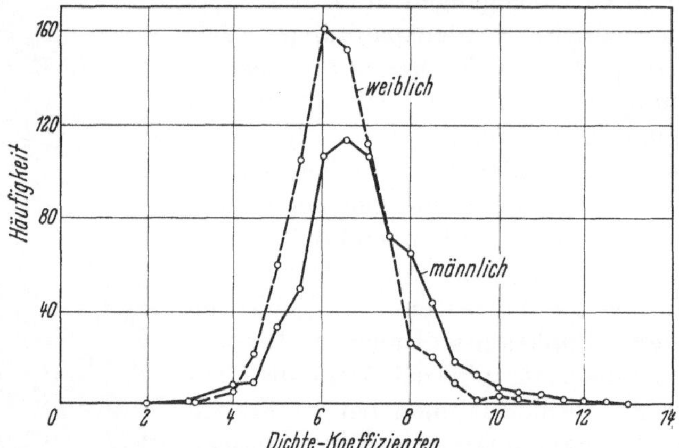

Abb. 35. Die Knochendichtekoeffizienten des Calcaneus (etwa 1200 Versuchspersonen). Die Zahlen der Ordinate geben an, wie oft ein bestimmter Wert erscheint. Durchgezogene Linie = männlich, gestrichelte Linie = weiblich. (Nach McFarland, 1954; Abb. 2)

Fusi (1952) hat versucht, die „Knochendichte" des *2. und 3. Lendenwirbelkörpers* zu bestimmen. Als Referenzsystem dienten *Treppen aus reinem Aluminium* von 2 cm Breite und 8 cm Länge mit einer Stufenhöhe von 1—8 mm. Das Volumen der Lendenwirbelkörper wurde durch Aufnahmen in 2 Ebenen ermittelt. Die photometrische Auswertung erfolgte mit einem Mikrophotometer von Hartmann und einem Zusatzprisma nach Lummer-Brodhun. Besondere Beachtung wurde dem Problem der unterschiedlichen Weichteilüberlagerung infolge Luftfüllung des Darmes geschenkt. Es wird empfohlen, die Messungen in einem Bereich durchzuführen, der frei von Darmluft ist. Aus den Meßergebnissen kann der Calcium- und Phosphorgehalt berechnet und das Verhältnis Ca:P bestimmt werden. Es sind Untersuchungen an *Normalpersonen* durchgeführt worden. Der methodische Fehler wurde nicht bestimmt, z.B. durch Vergleich der Meßwerte mit den tatsächlichen chemisch-analytisch gefundenen Werten von Calcium und Phosphor im Knochen. Nach Angaben des Autors sollen sich Abweichungen von der Norm bei einer Osteoporose oder Sklerose erfassen lassen.

Richards (1953) hat die Strahlendurchlässigkeit des Unterkieferknochens untersucht und in mm-Aluminiumäquivalent angegeben. Er fand große individuelle Unterschiede, die jedoch nicht auf Weichteilüberlagerungen zurückgeführt werden können.

Einen standardisierten *Keil aus einer Aluminiumlegierung* verwendete McFarland (1954) als Vergleichskörper. Basierend auf den Untersuchungen von Brown und Birtley (1951) ermittelte der Autor an 1200 Fällen den „Knochendichtekoeffizienten" des *Calcaneus* und teilte die Ergebnisse der Messungen an gesunden Erwachsenen nach der

„Knochendichte" in 10 „Klassen" ein. Ferner fanden sich Altersunterschiede und geschlechtsgebundene Verschiedenheiten des Knochendichtekoeffizienten (Abb. 35). Mit Hilfe eines konstanten Faktors wurde versucht, die photometrisch erhaltene „Knochendichte" in g Knochenasche/cm³ Knochen umzurechnen. Da die Elimination des durch die Weichteilüberlagerung bedingten Fehlers schwierig ist, sollten die Untersuchungen auf den Calcaneus und die Knochen von Hand und Unterarm beschränkt werden. In diesen Skeletabschnitten kann eine Weichteilkorrektur vorgenommen werden. Die Reproduzierbarkeit des Meßverfahrens wurde mit 30 Bestimmungen an derselben Person und 30 Messungen auf demselben Film geprüft und ein Fehler von 5% gefunden. Eine Überprüfung der densitometrisch ermittelten Werte des Aschegehaltes von Knochen durch die chemische Analyse wurde nicht vorgenommen.

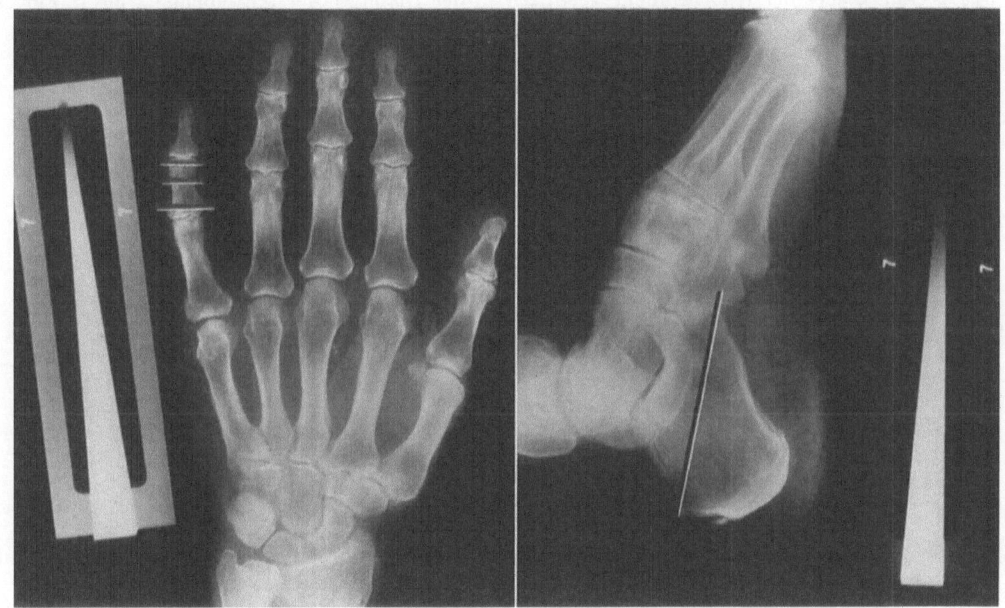

Abb. 36. Darstellung der Meßwege durch das Mittelglied des 5. Fingers und den Calcaneus. (Nach Gershon-Cohen, Schraer und Blumberg, 1955; Abb. 1)

Einen Vergleichskörper aus einer *Aluminium-Zink-Legierung* verwendeten Gershon-Cohen, Schraer und Blumberg (1955) zu Untersuchungen der Knochendichte des *Handskeletes* und des *Calcaneus* älterer Menschen, um die sog. *Altersosteoporose* zu erforschen (Abb. 36). Mit Hilfe eines besonderen Faktors (0,32) konnte der Knochenaschegehalt pro cm³ Gewebe berechnet werden. Es wird jedoch betont, daß dieser Faktor noch durch weitere, experimentelle Untersuchungen genauer zu bestimmen wäre. Die Knochendichte alter Frauen war größer als diejenige alter Männer (Abb. 37a—c).

Eine weitere praktische Anwendung dieser Untersuchungsmethode erfolgte durch Schraer (1958), der die Knochendichte von *Calcaneus und Phalangen* bei Kindern beiderlei Geschlechts untersuchte. Als Referenzsystem diente eine „Standardtreppe" aus einer Legierung von Aluminium (92,8%) und Zink (7,2%) mit 14 cm Länge und 1,4 cm Breite. Am breitesten Teil hat die Treppe einen Abfall von 0,1. Die Absorptionseigenschaften dieses Materials sind denen der Knochenasche sehr ähnlich. Als Strahlenquelle kann jeder Röntgenapparat benutzt werden. Der Fokus der Röhre sollte möglichst klein sein, die Anodenspannung zwischen 50 und 60 kV gewählt werden. Folienlose Filme sind besser geeignet als anderes Filmmaterial. Zur Densitometrie wird ein Mikrophotometer mit elektronischem Komputer verwendet (Schraer 1965). Die Messungen wurden so durchgeführt, daß zuerst eine Dichtekurve des Referenzsystems und dann die Dichtekurve

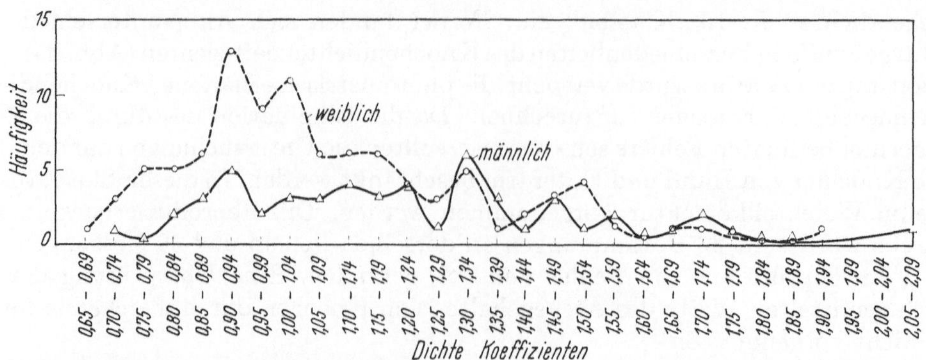

Abb. 37a. Verlaufskurve der Knochendichtekoeffizienten der Diaphyse der Mittelphalanx des 5. Fingers der linken Hand. (Nach GERSHON-COHEN, SCHRAER und BLUMBERG, 1965; Abb. 3)

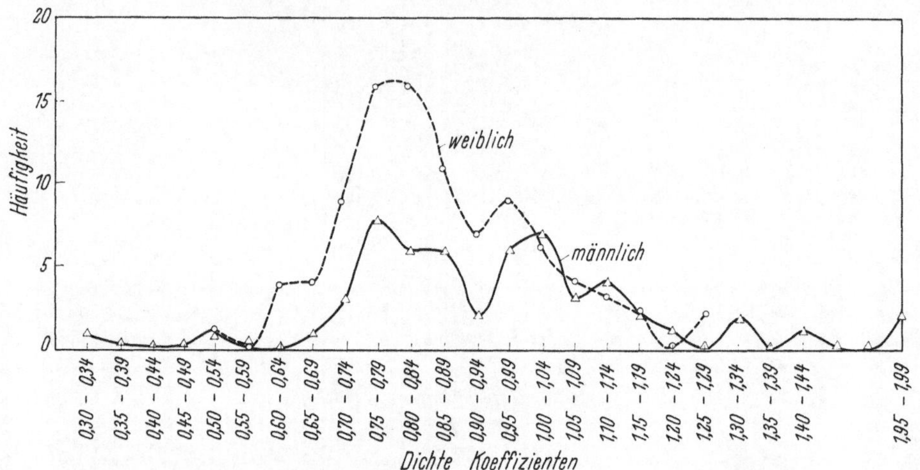

Abb. 37b. Verlaufskurve von Knochendichtekoeffizienten (Mittelwerte) der Metaphyse der Mittelphalanx des 5. Fingers der linken Hand. (Nach GERSHON-COHEN, SCHRAER und BLUMBERG, 1955; Abb. 4)

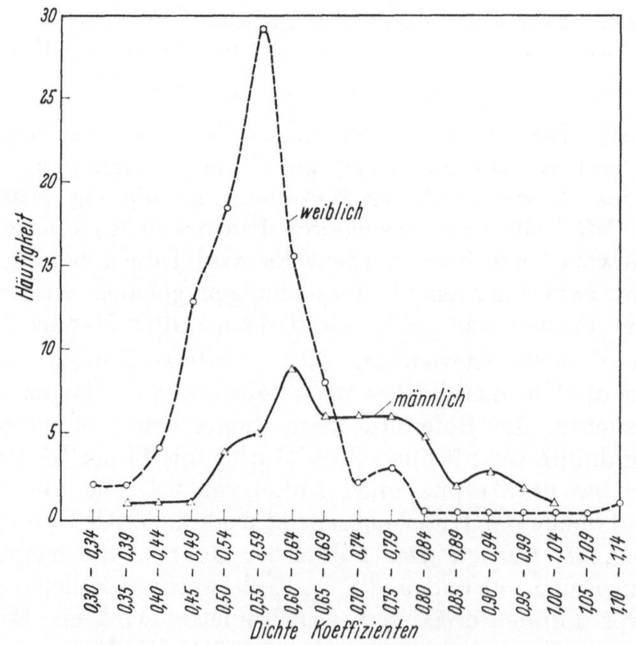

Abb. 37c. Verlaufskurve der Knochendichtekoeffizienten des Calcaneus. (Nach GERSHON-COHEN, SCHRAER und BLUMBERG, 1955; Abb. 2)

des Knochens aufgenommen wurden (Abb. 38a und b). Die Genauigkeit der verwendeten Meßgeräte und die Reproduzierbarkeit des Ergebnisses wurde sehr eingehend und an verschiedenen Tagen von mehreren Arbeitsgruppen geprüft. Es konnte eine durchschnittliche Differenz zwischen den Messungen von 2,66%, das ist ein Fehler von 0,4, gefunden werden (SCHRAER 1965).

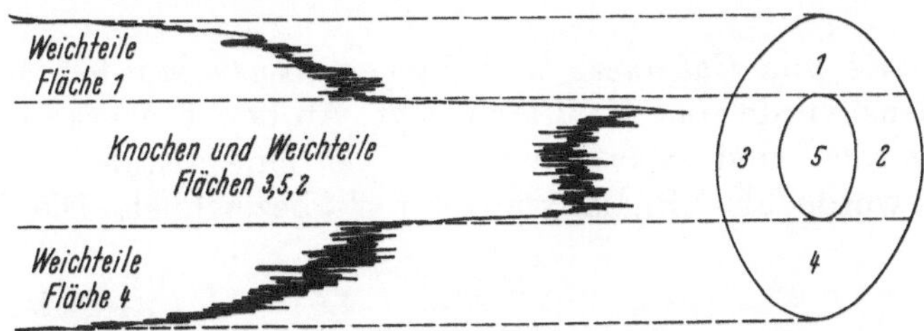

Abb. 38a. Schematische Darstellung eines Fingers mit der gemessenen Densitometerkurve. (Nach SCHRAER, 1958; Abb. 1)

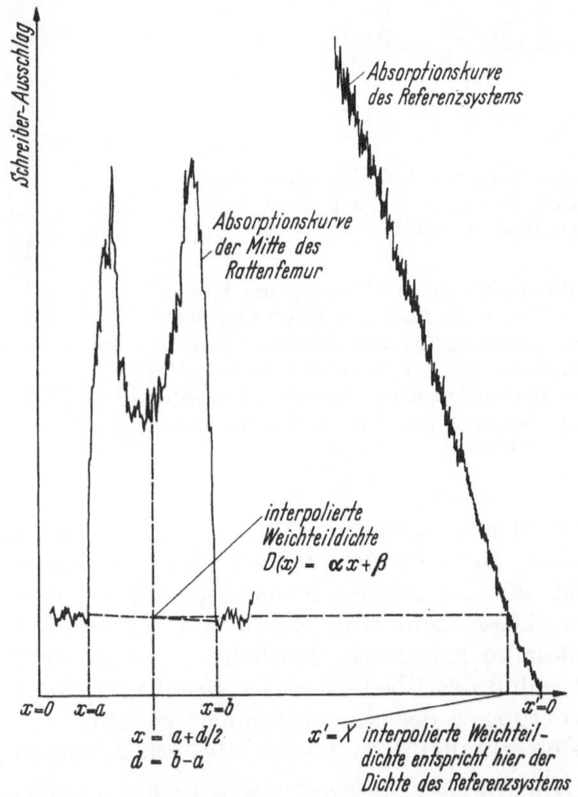

Abb. 38b. Darstellung der Densitometerkurven durch Knochen und Referenzsystem. (Nach SCHRAER, 1965; Abb. 3)

Von BAKER und SCHRAER (1958) wurden mit dieser Methode radiologische Bestimmungen des Trockengewichtes von Knochenpräparaten vorgenommen. An 11 Präparaten des menschlichen Femur wurde die Methode zunächst erprobt und festgestellt, daß eine densitometrische Messung bei Auswertung vieler Meßwege durch den Knochen (21) die größte Genauigkeit besitzt, doch sind noch 4 Meßwege brauchbar. Bei nur einem mittleren Meßweg können bereits Informationen gewonnen werden, die für Routinereihenuntersuchungen verwertbar sind. Weitere Untersuchungen wurden am Humerus und Femur der Skelete von 61 Weißen und 17 Negern durchgeführt. Das Trockengewicht von Humerus und Femur kann als repräsentativ für das gesamte Skelet angesehen werden.

Die Ergebnisse können nicht ohne weiteres auf die Verhältnisse beim lebenden Menschen übertragen werden, da die Weichteile unberücksichtigt geblieben sind. Mit diesen Meßmethoden sei jedoch die Analyse des Skeletes bei kranken Menschen möglich. Der Weichteileffekt fand in den Untersuchungsreihen am Menschen dadurch Berücksichtigung, daß der Dichtekoeffizient der Weichteile von der Gesamtabsorption subtrahiert wurde (SCHRAER 1958).

Zur Densitometrie von *Calcaneus* und *Fingerknochen* wurden Meßlinien festgelegt. Durch den Calcaneus wurde *eine Meßlinie* gelegt. An den Fingerknochen sind *drei Querlinien* gemessen worden, und zwar eine proximale, eine distale und eine zentrale. Die mittlere Meßlinie wurde als „Phalanxmittellinie" bezeichnet. Die Werte dieser Meß-

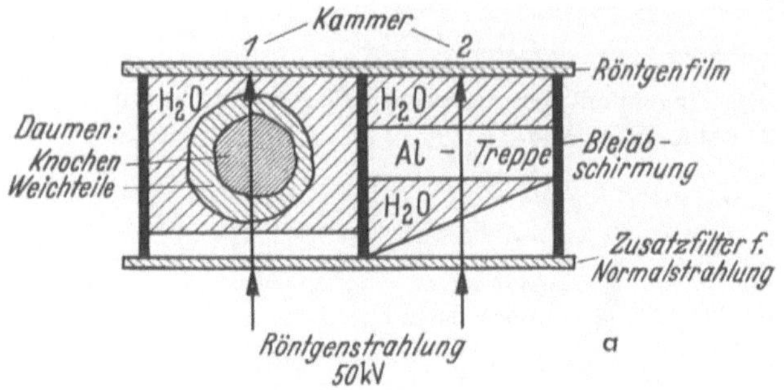

Abb. 39. Schematische Darstellung der Aufnahmeanordnung des Daumens und der Aluminiumtreppe. (Nach BALZ und BIRKNER, 1956; Abb. 1)

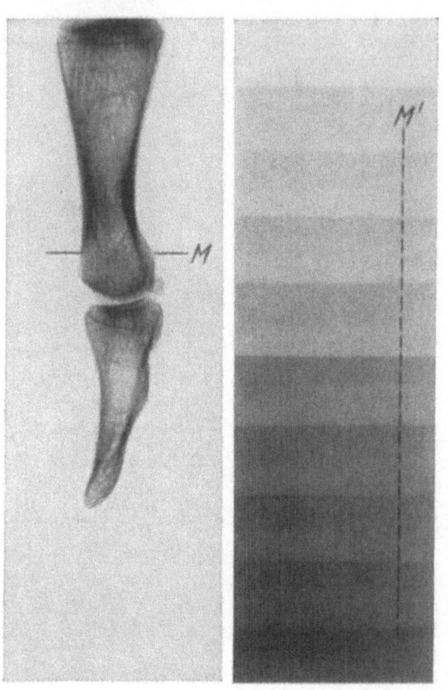

Abb. 40. Beispiel eines Röntgenfilmes zur Messung des Schwächungsgleichwertes (AL—SGW) nach BALZ und BIRKNER (1956). *M* Meßstelle: $^1/_8$ der Grundphalanxlänge vom distalen Phalanxende aus gemessen. *M'* Meßlinie der der Knochenmeßstelle (*M*) zugehörigen Weichteildicke (Daumenkammerbreite minus Knochendurchmesser). (Nach BALZ, BIRKNER und SCHMITT-ROHDE, 1957; Abb. 2)

ergebnisse wurden addiert und das Resultat als *Mittelwert* des *Knochendichtekoeffizienten* der Meßlinien angegeben. Der „*Dichtekoeffizient*" wird in Gramm der Aluminium-Zink-Legierung ausgedrückt, die in ähnlicher geometrischer Form dieselbe Strahlung wie das Meßobjekt absorbiert. Diese Zahl wird durch das Volumen des Knochens dividiert (Tabelle 18). Im Kindesalter konnte ein deutlicher Anstieg der Dichtekoeffizienten aller Knochen bis zum Abschluß des Wachstums festgestellt werden (Abb. 94). Mit der Meßmethode können Änderungen des Knochenmineralgehaltes bei osteoporotischen und osteomalacischen Systemerkrankungen des Skeletes erfaßt werden (SCHRAER 1965).

Die Messung des *Aluminium-Schwächungsgleichwertes* von Knochen haben BALZ und BIRKNER (1956) mit einer besonders modifizierten Untersuchungsmethode vorgenommen, die es erlaubt, ein bestimmtes Knochenvolumen unabhängig von seinen umgebenden Weichteilen zu einem Vergleichskörper in Beziehung zu setzen. Zur Untersuchung wurden *die Knochen des Daumens* oder *der Fingerglieder* gewählt. Die Aufnahmevorrichtung besteht aus zwei gleich großen Kammern aus Plexiglas (Abb. 39). In die erste Kammer, die mit Wasser gefüllt ist, wird der Daumen eingetaucht. Hierdurch soll erreicht werden, daß jeweils eine *definierte Weichteilschicht* durchstrahlt wird. In der zweiten Kammer wird der Knochen durch eine *Aluminiumtreppe*, die den Knochen umgebenden Weichteile durch eine Wasserschicht vor und hinter der Treppe ersetzt (Abb. 40). Die Keilform der ersten Wasserschicht dient hierbei zur Nachbildung der jeweiligen Weichteildicke. Die Aluminiumtreppe befindet sich frei in der Luft. Die seitliche und die untere Begrenzung der Kammern erfolgt durch Bleiabschirmungen, um möglichst gleichmäßige Streuverhältnisse innerhalb der Kammern zu erzielen. Zur Gewinnung einer definierten, praktisch homogenen Strahlung wurde mit 50 kV Anodenspannung und einer Gesamtfilterung von 3 mm Al eine Normalstrahlung nach WACHSMANN (1950) hergestellt. Die Entfernung vom Fokus zur Aufnahmeanordnung betrug 250 cm, um eine parallele Strahlung zu erhalten. Zur Erzielung eines möglichst hohen Gammawertes wurden anfangs Filme mit Verstärkungsfolien verwendet, später jedoch folienlose Filme benutzt. Die photometrische Auswertung erfolgte durch ein Selen-Photoelement mit angeschlossenem Galvanometer (Dr. B. LANGE, Berlin-Zehlendorf). Die Messung ermittelt diejenige Aluminiumschichtdicke, die bei konstantem Weichteilvolumen die gleiche Schwärzung aufweist wie die zu untersuchende Knochenregion. Das Ergebnis wird als *Aluminiumschwächungsgleichwert (Al-SGW)* angegeben. Eine Berechnung des Kalkgehaltes ist nicht vorgenommen worden.

Tabelle 7

Aufnahmen	Osteoporosegrad							Gesamt
	0	0—1	1	1—2	2	2—3	3	
Thorax	139	9	55	4	3	—	—	210
Lendenwirbelsäule 2 E.	65	9	57	6	27	1	7	172
Lendenwirbelsäule ap.	9	2	7	2	3	1	3	27
Lendenwirbelsäule seitl.	7	1	11	—	2	—	2	23
Brustwirbelsäule 2 E.	17	—	25	3	12	1	2	60
Halswirbelsäule	16	6	11	—	3	1	—	37
Becken	20	2	10	2	4	—	2	40
Schädel	16	3	3	1	1	—	—	24
Pyelogramm . . .	26	3	13	—	2	—	—	44
Sonstiges	20	5	8	2	8	—	2	45
	335	40	200	20	65	4	18	682

[WAGNER, A., u. J. SCHAAF: Dtsch. Arch. klin. Med. **207**, 364 (1961), Tab. 1]

WAGNER und SCHAAF (1961) haben einen Vergleich zwischen der *visuellen Beurteilung* des Entkalkungsgrades in verschiedenen Skeletabschnitten und den Befunden photometrischer Messungen von „Aluminiumschwächungsgleichwerten" (Al-SGW) des Daumenknochens (ermittelt nach der Methode von BALZ und BIRKNER 1956; s. S. 158) angestellt. In der Untersuchungsreihe wurden 682 Röntgenaufnahmen des Stammskeletes (Wirbelsäule, Becken, Schädel, Thorax) und der Extremitäten von 360 Patienten 3 Ärzten in Abständen von mindestens 1 Woche jeweils zweimal zur *Beurteilung* vorgelegt. Die Angaben über den Patienten wurden auf den Röntgenbildern abgedeckt. Das Ausmaß der osteoporotischen Veränderungen wurde in 3 Stufen klassifiziert: I. beginnende bzw. leichtgradige Osteoporose; II. deutliche mittelgradige Osteoporose; III. schwere Osteoporose, oft mit Deformierungen der entsprechenden Skeletabschnitte. Das Fehlen osteoporotischer Veränderungen wurde mit 0 bezeichnet. Zur Orientierung für nachfolgende Berechnungen zeigt Tabelle 7 an, wie die 682 Aufnahmen insgesamt von den 3 Untersuchern beurteilt worden sind. Die in der Tabelle 7 aufgeführten Spalten 0—1, 1—2 und 1—3 sind so zu verstehen, daß die Beurteiler bei den 6 Untersuchungen dreimal den niedrigeren und dreimal den höheren Osteoporosegrad angegeben hatten. Wie groß die Unterschiede sind, wenn der *gleiche Untersucher* die *gleichen Bilder* zu *verschiedenen Zeiten* zur Beurteilung vorgelegt bekommt, zeigt Tabelle 8. In den einzelnen Spalten der Tabelle ist dabei verzeichnet, zwischen welchen Graden die Beurteilung schwankte, wenn die Bilder bei beiden Untersuchungen verschieden klassifiziert wurden. Es zeigt sich, daß der Untersucher I bei 20%, der Untersucher II bei 21% und der Untersucher III bei 19% aller Bilder, die ihm zur 2. Beurteilung vorgelegt wurden, zu einer anderen Entscheidung kam als bei der vorausgegangenen Untersuchung. In den weitaus meisten Fällen handelte es sich um kleine Differenzen, also Unstimmigkeiten in der Beurteilung einer leichten oder deutlichen Osteoporose. Die Aufgliederung in die verschiedenen Skeletabschnitte

Tabelle 8

Aufnahme	Untersucher I Differenz der Beurteilung								Untersucher II Differenz der Beurteilung								Untersucher III Differenz der Beurteilung							
	Gesamt	0:1	1:2	2:3	0:2	1:3	Summe	%	Gesamt	0:1	1:2	2:3	0:2	1:3	Summe	%	Gesamt	0:1	1:2	2:3	0:2	1:3	Summe	%
Thorax	210	27	10	—	—	—	37	19	210	29	7	—	—	—	36	17	210	19	6	—	—	—	25	12
LWS 2 E.	172	12	19	3	—	—	34	20	172	18	15	3	—	—	36	21	172	17	16	5	—	—	38	22
LWS ap.	27	2	6	2	—	—	10	36	27	4	3	5	—	—	12	44	27	7	—	2	—	—	9	33
LWS seitlich	23	3	—	—	—	—	3	13	23	2	4	—	—	—	6	26	23	2	3	1	—	—	6	26
BWS 2 E.	60	2	8	5	—	—	15	25	60	6	7	2	2	—	17	28	60	6	4	—	—	—	10	17
HWS 2 E.	37	5	2	1	—	—	8	22	37	6	5	—	1	—	12	32	37	7	1	—	1	—	9	24
Becken	40	5	3	2	—	—	10	23	40	6	4	—	—	—	10	25	40	5	2	2	—	—	9	22
Schädel	24	2	—	1	—	—	3	14	24	2	1	—	—	—	3	12	24	4	1	—	—	—	5	20
Pyelogramm	44	8	—	—	—	—	8	19	44	6	—	—	—	—	6	14	44	5	1	1	—	—	7	16
Sonstiges	45	8	4	—	—	—	12	27	45	1	4	2	—	—	7	16	45	8	2	—	—	—	10	22
	682	74	52	14	—	—	140	20	682	80	50	12	3	—	145	21	682	80	36	12	1	—	129	19

[WAGNER, A., u. J. SCHAAF: Dtsch. Arch. klin. Med. **207**, 364 (1961), Tab. 2]

zeigt, daß die Aufnahmen des Thoraxskeletes, des Schädels, die Ausscheidungsurogramme und andere verhältnismäßig gut übereinstimmen. Dabei muß aber berücksichtigt werden, daß bei den letztgenannten Aufnahmen durchweg seltener eine Osteoporose angenommen worden ist. Wenn man die Anzahl der nicht übereinstimmenden Urteile nur auf die Zahl der Aufnahmen bezieht, bei denen mindestens einmal eine Osteoporose angenommen wurde, so findet man bei der Lendenwirbelsäule mit 70—85% (Beurteilung der seitlichen Aufnahmen) die größte Übereinstimmung. Auch die Brustwirbelsäule schneidet mit 69% recht gut ab, während bei den Beckenaufnahmen nur in 50%, den Rippenaufnahmen in 58%, den Extremitätenaufnahmen in 61%, den Pyelogrammen in 64% der gleiche Osteoporosegrad angenommen wurde wie bei der Voruntersuchung. Ein Vergleich der Urteile verschiedener Untersucher ergibt an der Wirbelsäule die beste Übereinstimmung, während im Bereich der übrigen Skeletregionen nur eine geringe Übereinstimmung in der visuellen Beurteilung festzustellen ist.

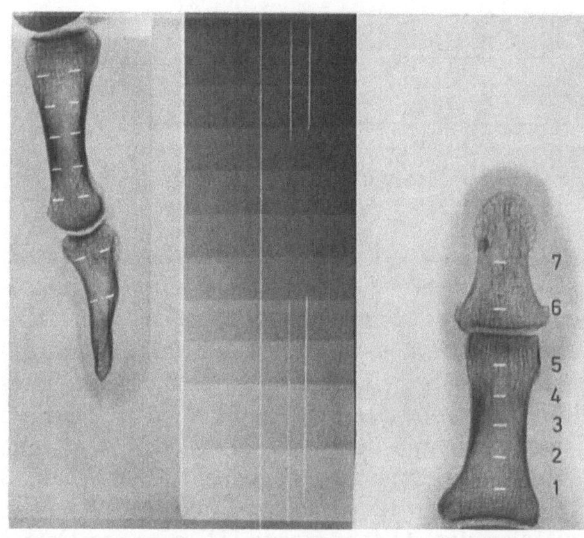

Abb. 41. Darstellung des Daumens mit eingezeichneten Meßbezirken und Aluminium-Treppe zur Bestimmung des Aluminium-Schwächungsgleichwertes (AL-SGW). (Nach WAGNER und SCHAAF, 1961; Abb. 8)

Von den 360 Patienten wurden gleichzeitig Röntgenaufnahmen eines oder beider Daumen im Wasserbad mit einem Aluminiumreferenzsystem angefertigt und an insgesamt 7 Meßpunkten der Grund- und Endphalanx des Daumens (Abb. 41) der Aluminium-Schwächungsgleichwert (Al-SGW) nach der Methode von BALZ und BIRKNER (1956) gemessen. Von diesen 7 Punkten liegen 1, 5 und 6 in einem compactafreien, rein spongiösen Knochenabschnitt. In den Punkten 2 und 4 wird die Compactamanschette in wechselndem Ausmaß durchstrahlt. Diese zeigt erhebliche Unterschiede in der Dicke. Meist ist sie in der Mitte, in manchen Fällen aber auch im Bereich des Meßpunktes 4 am dicksten, so daß beträchtliche Differenzen zustande kommen. Dies gilt auch für Punkt 7, da sich eine von der Spitze ausgehende Sklerosierungszone häufig bis zur Mitte erstreckt und somit einen Vergleich der verschiedenen Fälle unmöglich macht. Für die Auswertung wurden daher nur folgende Meßstellen herangezogen: 1. Köpfchen des Daumengrundgliedes (Punkt 5); 2. Basis des Daumengrundgliedes (Punkt 6); 3. Mittelwert der Meßstellen 3, 4 und 5 (gemäß dem 1. Vorschlag von BALZ und BIRKNER); 5. Mittelwert der Meß-Stellen des Daumengrundgliedes und 6. Mittelwert aller 7 Meßstellen. Die Meßergebnisse wurden nach dem Lebensalter der Patienten geordnet und von jeweils 5 Jahren ein Mittelwert errechnet. Die Kurven der Aluminiumschwächungsgleichwerte zeigen im Laufe des Alterns alle einen ähnlichen Verlauf — der Aluminiumschwächungsgleichwert sinkt ab (s. auch S. 205). Die getrennte Darstellung der Al-SGW von Männern und Frauen läßt erkennen, daß beim weiblichen Geschlecht der höchste Al-SGW *früher* erreicht wird als beim männlichen Geschlecht, allerdings auch bereits früher (nach dem 35. Lebensjahr) und *deutlicher* (nach dem 50. Lebensjahr) ein Abfall des Al-SGW eintritt (Abb. 42).

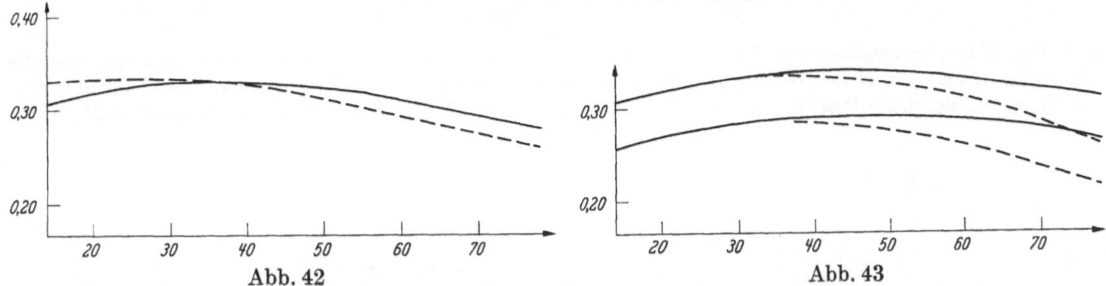

Abb. 42. Der Aluminiumschwächungsgleichwert vom Köpfchen des Daumengrundgliedes (Meßstelle 5) in den verschiedenen Lebensjahrzehnten bei beiden Geschlechtern (männlich = ausgezogene Linie, weiblich = gestrichelte Linie). (Nach WAGNER und SCHAAF, 1961; Abb. 4)

Abb. 43. Mittlerer Aluminiumschwächungsgleichwert sämtlicher Untersuchungen (mit und ohne Osteoporose = gestrichelte Linie) und der Fälle, bei denen auf Grund der Beurteilung des Röntgenbildes keine Osteoporose angenommen wurde (ausgezogene Linie). Die obere Kurve zeigt Meßstelle 5, die untere Kurve Durchschnittswerte der Meßstellen 1, 5 und 6. (Nach WAGNER und SCHAAF, 1961; Abb. 5)

Mit den Ergebnissen dieser Untersuchung wurden die Befunde der visuellen Beurteilung von Brust- und Lendenwirbelsäule verglichen. Der Berechnung der Durchschnittskurven wurden aber nur solche Fälle zugrunde gelegt, die nach der visuellen Beurteilung keine Osteoporose aufwiesen. Die auf diese Weise ermittelten Kurven waren daher besonders in den höheren Altersklassen deutlich flacher. Die Abb. 43 läßt dies am Beispiel der Mittelwerte der Meßstellen 1, 5 und 6 erkennen. Um neben dieser Durchschnittskurve noch weitere Bezugslinien zu erhalten, wurde von jedem Jahrgang der höchste und niedrigste Al-SGW derjenigen Patienten ausgesucht, die keine Osteoporose aufwiesen und auch hier von jeweils 5 Jahren ein Mittelwert berechnet. Da durch diese Rechenoperationen notgedrungen auch Al-SGW von Patienten ohne Osteoporose ober- und unterhalb dieser Bezugslinie liegen müssen, fällt eine genauere Beschreibung der so gewonnenen Schleife — etwa als Normbereich — schwer. Es wurden daher ganz unverbindlich die beiden Zonen oberhalb der Durchschnittskurve A und B, die beiden unteren C und D genannt (Abb. 44a). Werden die durchschnittlichen Al-SGW für alle Personen, bei denen nach dem Röntgenbild keine Osteoporose anzunehmen war, berechnet und mit denjenigen der Osteoporosegruppe I, II und III verglichen, so finden sich an allen Meßstellen jeweils sichere Unterschiede in dem Sinne, daß die Patienten ohne Osteoporose einen höheren Al-SGW als die der Gruppe I und diese wiederum einen höheren als die der Gruppen II und III haben (Tabelle 9). Die Analyse im einzelnen ergibt, daß sich im Bereich der spongiösen Knochen die beste Übereinstimmung zwischen den Aluminiumschwächungsgleichwerten und dem Ergebnis der visuellen Beurteilung fand (Abb. 44b). Auch an den übrigen Meßstellen war eine gute Übereinstimmung zwischen dem Al-SGW

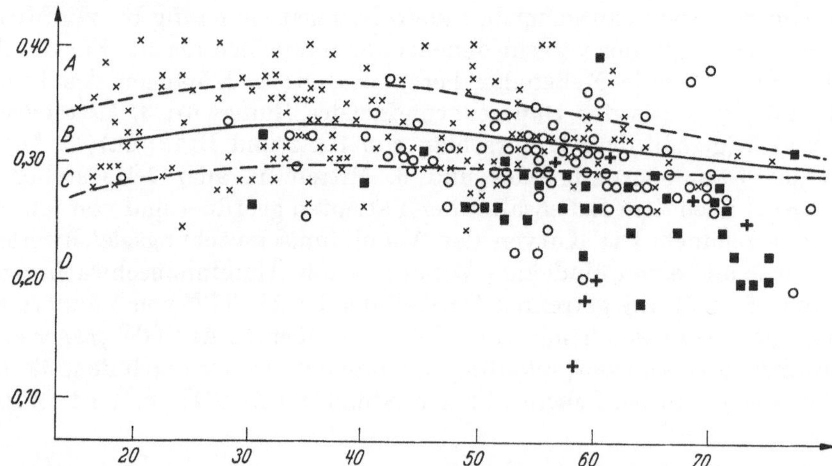

Abb. 44a. Zusammenstellung des Aluminiumschwächungsgleichwertes des Köpfchens vom Daumengrundglied (Meßstelle 5) und des visuell bestimmten Osteoporosegrades (× = 0 keine Osteoporose, ○ = 1 leichte Osteoporose, ■ = 2 deutliche Osteoporose, + = 3 schwere Osteoporose). (Nach WAGNER und SCHAAF, 1961; Abb. 7)

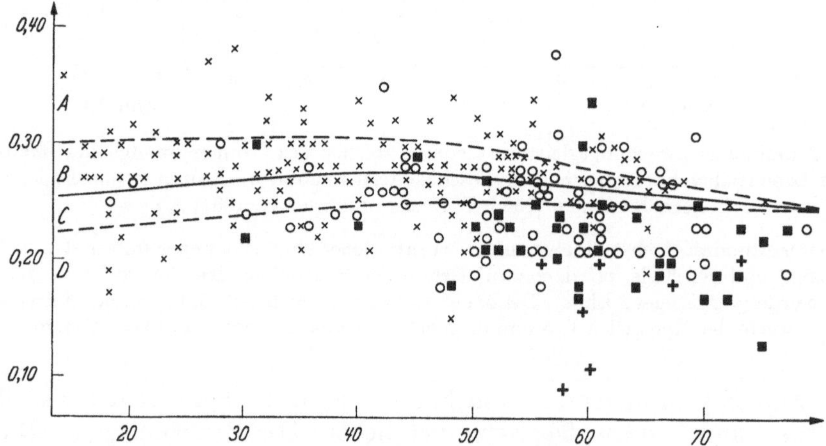

Abb. 44b. Zusammenstellung der Aluminiumschwächungsgleichwerte der Basis des Daumenendgliedes (Meßstelle 6) mit dem visuell bestimmten Osteoporosegrad. (Nach WAGNER und SCHAAF, 1961; Abb. 8)

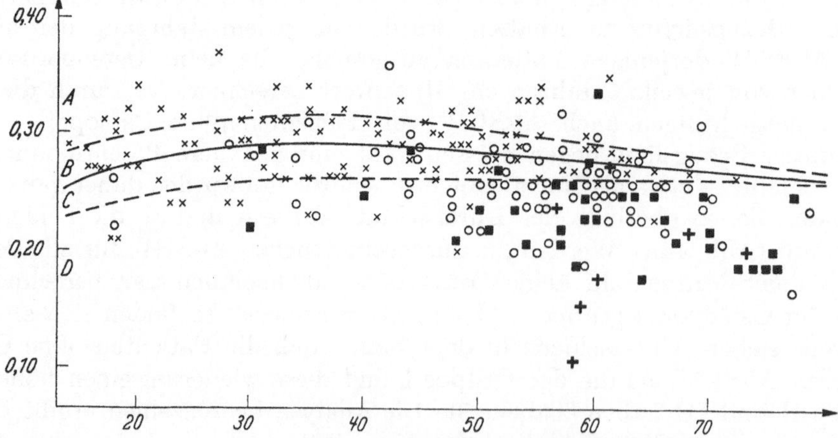

Abb. 44c. Zusammenstellung der Durchschnittswerte der Aluminiumschwächungsgleichwerte von drei Meßstellen der Daumenknochen (Meßstelle 1, 5 und 6 nach Abb. 41) mit dem visuell bestimmten Osteoporosegrad. (Nach WAGNER und SCHAAF, 1961; Abb. 6)

Tabelle 9

Photometrische Meßstellen (vgl. Abb. 41)	Mittlerer Al-SGW bei Patienten mit Osteoporosegrad			
	0	I	II	III
5. (3 Meßstellen am Köpfchen des Daumengrundgliedes)	0,34	0,30	0,28	0,24
6. (spongiöser Knochen am Daumendglied)	0,30	0,25	0,23	0,16
Mittelwert aus 1, 5 und 6 (spongiöser Knochen)	0,28	0,25	0,23	0,20
Mittelwert aus 3, 4 und 5 (mit Compacta)	0,40	0,35	0,33	0,27
Mittelwert der Meßstellen am Daumengrundglied	0,35	0,31	0,30	0,25
Mittelwert von allen 7 Meßstellen	0,34	0,30	0,29	0,23

[WAGNER, A., u. J. SCHAAF: Dtsch. Arch. klin. Med. **207**, 364 (1961), Tab. 4]

und dem visuell bestimmten Osteoporosegrad festzustellen (Abb. 44c). Trotz dieser recht günstigen Ergebnisse der Auswertung bleiben WAGNER und SCHAAF (1961) skeptisch. Es fanden sich bei gleichem Al-SGW ganz verschiedene Osteoporosegrade und umgekehrt Fälle, bei denen der gleiche Grad einer Osteoporose angenommen wurde und stark differierende Al-SGW nachweisbar waren. Die Untersuchungen zeigten, daß in gewissem Umfang doch eine Übereinstimmung zwischen beiden Methoden besteht. Bei Messung an spongiösen Knochen ließen sämtliche Patienten mit schwerer, 97% der Patienten mit deutlicher und 81% der Patienten mit leichter Osteoporose einen Al-SGW erkennen, der unter dem Durchschnitt für das entsprechende Lebensalter lag. Die Streubreite des Al-SGW ist aber bereits bei den als normal befundenen Fällen so groß, daß sich zwangsläufig auch in späteren Jahren die Al-SGW verschiedener Osteoporosegrade infolge individueller Variationen überschneiden müssen. Die Messung des Al-SGW kann die visuelle Osteoporose-Diagnostik nicht ohne weiteres ersetzen. Die großen Nachteile, die bei einer vom subjektiven Urteil abhängigen Untersuchung immer wieder gegeben sind, können zwar durch die objektive Photometrie ausgeschaltet werden, doch erfaßt die Meßmethode nur *einen* Skeletbezirk. Besondere Bedeutung kommt der objektiven Knochendichtemessung bei Verlaufsbeobachtungen zur Beurteilung des Knochenmineralgehaltes nach der Behandlung einer Osteopathie oder bei länger dauernder Corticosteroidbehandlung zu.

MAINLAND (1956) setzt sich mit den *Schwierigkeiten* und der *klinischen Bedeutung* der verschiedenen Knochendichtemessungen kritisch auseinander. Er geht vor allem auf die Beseitigung der störenden Strahlenabsorption durch die Weichteile und die Brauchbarkeit der einzelnen Methoden ein. Insbesondere zeigt er Probleme auf, die der Einführung solcher Methoden in der Praxis entgegenstehen und eine Anerkennung der Methoden bisher verzögert haben. Die Fehlermöglichkeiten der Verfahren und die Faktoren, die ein objektives Ergebnis verschleiern können, werden im einzelnen aufgezählt. Für eigene Untersuchungen benutzte der Autor *Referenzsysteme aus Aluminium oder Elfenbein* und drückte die Knochendichte in der *äquivalenten Schichtdicke von Aluminium* aus. Nach seinen Forschungen eignen sich für die densitometrische Untersuchung des Knochenkalkgehaltes am lebenden Menschen vor allem der *Calcaneus*, die *Fingerknochen* und das *distale Ende von Radius und Tibia.* In umfangreichen Untersuchungsreihen wurde die Änderung der Knochendichte in den *verschiedenen Lebensaltern* bei gesunden Menschen untersucht (s. S. 204). Später sind vergleichende Dichtemessungen bei *rheumatischen Erkrankungen* vorgenommen worden. Hierbei ist besonders auf die Unterschiede der Knochendichte nach *Cortisonbehandlung* und nach anderen Behandlungsmethoden geachtet worden (s. S. 205).

Bestimmungen der Knochendichte am *Alveolarfortsatz des Unterkiefers von Hunden* hat OMNELL (1957) durchgeführt. Auf Grund *theoretischer Überlegungen* wird die Frage geprüft, ob sich bei Verwendung monochromatischer Röntgenstrahlung der Absolutgehalt des Knochens an Knochenasche bestimmen ließe. Für Untersuchungen an Mensch und Tier muß eine polychromatische Strahlung Verwendung finden, da eine monochromatische

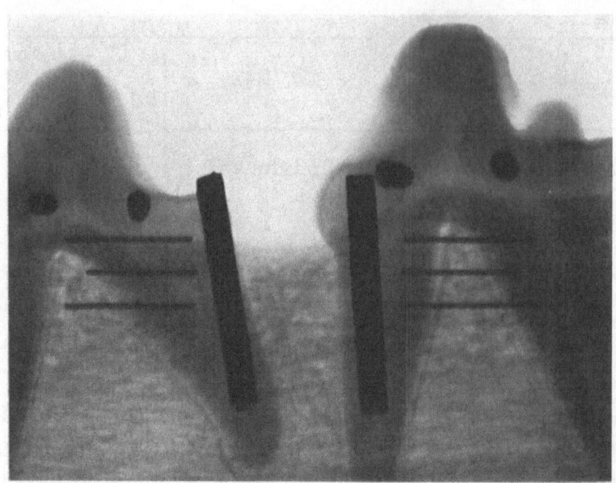

Abb. 45a. Vergrößerte Röntgenaufnahme des Unterkieferknochens von Hunden zur densitometrischen Messung der Knochendichte. (Nach OMNELL, 1957; Abb. 7)

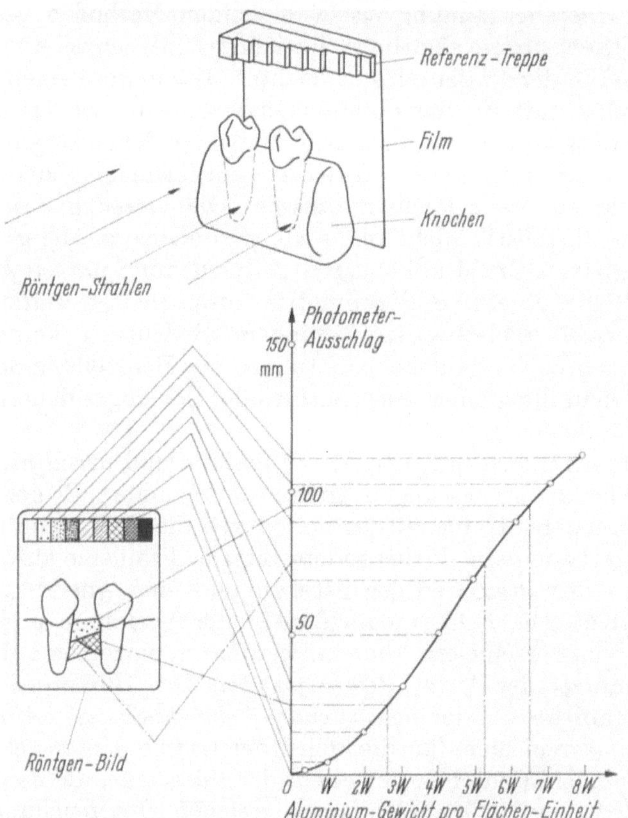

Abb. 45b. Schematische Darstellung der Auswertung der Röntgenaufnahmen des Unterkieferknochens mit Aluminiumtreppe. (Nach OMNELL, 1957; Abb. 3)

Strahlung extrem lange Belichtungszeiten erfordert. Zur quantitativen Analyse wird eine *Treppe aus Aluminium* benutzt (Abb. 45a und b). Die ermittelten Werte werden in Gewichtseinheiten Al angegeben. Die Probleme der Absorption der Röntgenstrahlung durch unterschiedlich zusammengesetzte Stoffe sowie andere Fehlerquellen werden eingehend besprochen und ihr Einfluß auf die Messungen geprüft. Die Meßfehler werden mit 1,6—3,9 bzw. 2,2—5,5% angegeben. Entkalkung und Kalkeinlagerung im spongiösen Knochen des Alveolarfortsatzes am Unterkiefer von Hunden wurden unter experimentell erzeugten krankhaften Bedingungen *fortlaufend untersucht.* Für Vergleichszwecke wurde eine Apparatur konstruiert, die es erlaubt, die Position von Röhre, Objekt und Film immer *exakt zu reproduzieren.* Die Untersuchungen beschäftigten sich vorwiegend mit der Demineralisation des Unterkieferknochens.

Grundlegende Arbeiten über die physikalischen Gesetzmäßigkeiten der radiologischen Messung des Mineralgehalts in Knochen *mit Hilfe einer Aluminiumtreppe* hat SPIEGLER (1959) veröffentlicht. Es wird empfohlen, den Knochenmineralgehalt als „Flächengewicht“ in mg/cm^2 (Masse/Flächeneinheit) oder als „effektive Schichtdicke“ anzugeben. Die Strahlenabsorption einer weichen Röntgenstrahlung (bei 50 kV Anodenspannung erzeugt) durch 1 mm Aluminium entspricht einem Flächengewicht von 130 mg/cm^2 des Knochenminerals (Calciumphosphat in Form des *Hydroxylapatit*). Bei Kenntnis der Schichtdicke des durchstrahlten Knochens kann die Mineralkonzentration in mg/cm^3 (ml) berechnet werden. Später haben SPIEGLER und KEANE (1961) vorgeschlagen, die Mineralwerte in Bruchteilen des *voll mineralisierten Knochens* auszudrücken. Die Dichte des Knochenminerals liegt bei 3, so daß ein Knochen die Mineralkonzentration von 3000 mg/cm^3 aufweisen müßte, wenn er *voll mineralisiert* wäre. Der Knochen der Femurdiaphysencompacta (HEUCK und SCHMIDT 1960) ist also nur zu 45 Gewichtsprozenten mineralisiert, die Diaphysencompacta des Ochsenfemur zu 55 Gewichtsprozenten.

KEANE, SPIEGLER und DAVIS (1959) untersuchten mit Hilfe einer *Aluminiumtreppe* (14 Stufen von 5 mm Breite und 0,5 mm Höhe) den Mineralgehalt des Knochens der *Ulna in verschiedenen Bezirken* bei Hand- und Geistesarbeitern. Handarbeiter bzw. Menschen, die ihre Hand stark gebrauchten (Sportler, Busfahrer) zeigten einen höheren Mineralgehalt des Ulnaknochens als Geistesarbeiter. Der störende Einfluß der umgebenden Weichteile wurde durch Einlegen des Unterarms in ein Wasserbad eliminiert (Abb. 46a und b). Zur Bestimmung des Mineralgehaltes der Ulna müssen *zwei Aufnahmen* des Unterarmes in *zueinander senkrecht stehenden Ebenen* hergestellt werden. Für spätere Kontrollmessungen an demselben Patienten ist nur noch eine Aufnahme erforderlich, da sich der Durchmesser des Knochens nicht wesentlich ändert. Die Exposition erfolgte bei 80 kV Anodenspannung, 4 mA und einem Fokus-Film-Abstand von 90 cm auf Ilfex-Film. Da bei der relativ harten Strahlung der Streueffekt groß ist, wurde die Filmkassette zur Beseitigung der Streustrahlung in *einem Abstand von 20 cm vom Objekt* placiert. Die photometrische Auswertung der Filme wurde an verschiedenen Meßpunkten der Ulna vorgenommen. Der *Mineralgehalt (g/cm^3)* kann bei Kenntnis der Schichtdicke des Knochens *berechnet* werden. Bei 38 Kontrollmessungen wurde ein Meßfehler von nur 8% gefunden, so daß man erwarten darf, Änderungen des Mineralgehaltes von 15—20% erfassen zu können. Der Mineralgehalt der Ulna schwankt erheblich zwischen 200 mg und 400 mg/cm^3. Die höheren Werte wurden dort gefunden, wo der Knochen röhrenförmig wird, d.h. wo die Compacta beginnt. Kontrollen der röntgenologisch ermittelten Werte mit chemischen Analysen sind nicht durchgeführt worden.

Mit der Untersuchungsmethode von KEANE, SPIEGLER und DAVIS (1959) hat MAYO (1961) Messungen im Bereich des *unteren Ulnaendes* und des *Processus posterior des Calcaneus* vorgenommen. Für die Messungen an der Ulna wird die Methode nicht abgewandelt. Zur Messung des Calcaneus wird die Ferse in eine Plexiglasbox mit Wasser eingelegt und auf eine 6 cm vom Boden des Gefäßes erhöhte Brücke gestützt. Der Fuß muß knapp in die Plexiglasbox hineinpassen. Das *Referenzsystem (Aluminiumtreppe)* wird hinter dem Calcaneus aufgestellt (Abb. 47a und b). Der Film wird in einem Abstand von 20 cm von der Wasserbox entfernt aufgestellt. Das Strahlenbündel sollte möglichst genau in einem Winkel von 90° auf die Plexiglasbox einfallen. Die *Schichtdicke der Knochen* wird aus einer Aufnahme in der *2. Ebene* ermittelt. Der Vergrößerungsfaktor sollte berücksichtigt werden. Die Meßfläche des verwendeten Densitometers betrug 8×4 mm, so daß individuelle Unterschiede der Spongiosatrabekel nicht ins Gewicht fielen. Für Auswertungen an der Ulna wurde das Meßfeld in Längsrichtung zum Schaft angeordnet. Die *Meßpunkte der Ulna* wurden *2, 4* und *6 cm* proximalwärts von der Gelenkfläche ausgewählt. Der

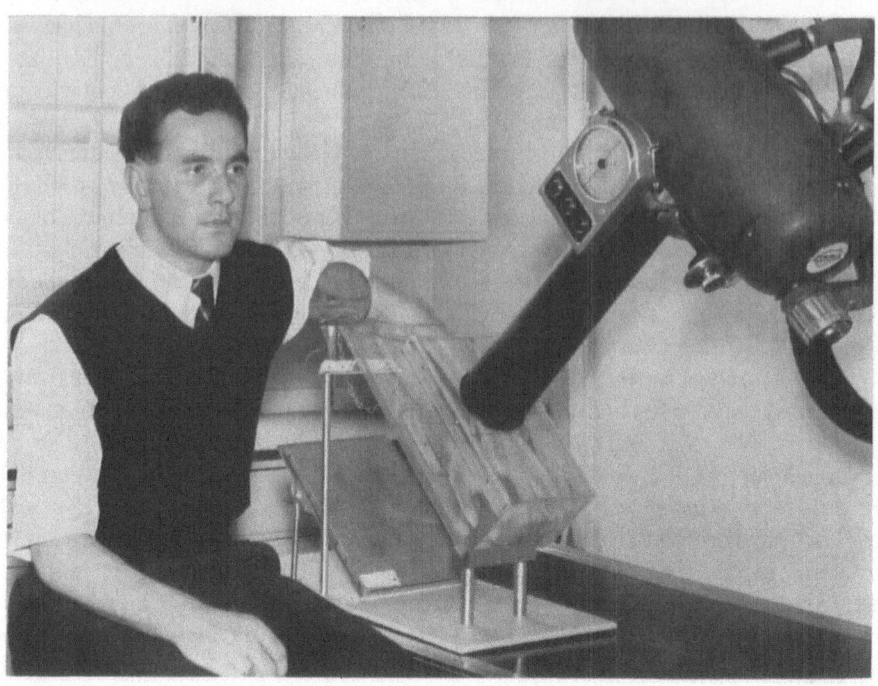

Abb. 46a. Aufnahmeanordnung von Unterarm und Referenzsystem im Wasserbad zur Untersuchung der Ulna. (Nach KEANE, SPIEGLER und DAVIS, 1959; Abb. 4)

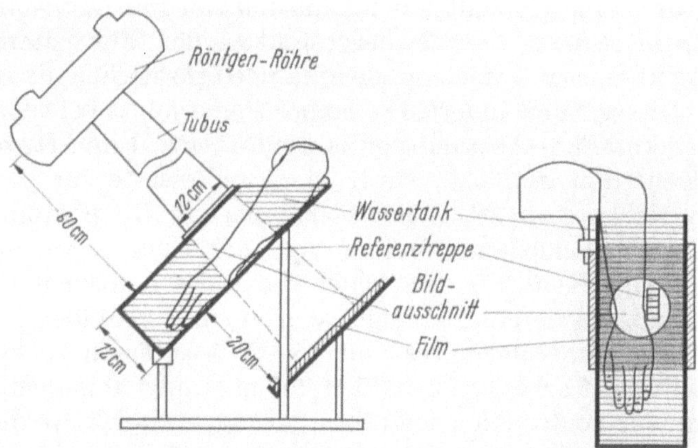

Abb. 46b. Schematische Zeichnung einer Aufnahmeanordnung zur Messung des Mineralgehaltes der Ulna. (Nach KEANE, SPIEGLER und DAVIS, 1959; Abb. 3). Der Objekt-Filmabstand beträgt 20 cm, um den Streuanteil zu verringern (Groedelsche Abstandstechnik)

Meßpunkt des Calcaneus wurde in der *Mitte der beiden engsten Stellen des Processus posterior calcanei* gewählt. Es wurde festgestellt, daß um diesen Meßpunkt herum ein Bezirk von 3—4 cm^2 vorhanden ist, in dem nur geringe Variationen der radiologischen Dichte zu finden sind. Dies erleichtert die Messung (s. auch HEUCK und SCHMIDT 1960). Da die Knochen nicht homogen sind, insbesondere im Bereich des Schaftes der langen Röhrenknochen wie z.B. der Ulna, ist es besser, vom *durchschnittlichen Mineralgehalt* als von der „Knochendichte“ zu sprechen. Der Mineralgehalt in der Diaphysencompacta ist sehr hoch. In *spongiösen Knochen* wie dem Calcaneus sind die Kalksalze gleichmäßiger verteilt und der durchschnittliche Mineralgehalt nähert sich der wirklichen Dichte.

Von DOYLE (1961) wurde in Anlehnung an die Methode von KEANE, SPIEGLER und DAVIS (1959) ein Meßverfahren zur Bestimmung des Mineralgehaltes im distalen Ab-

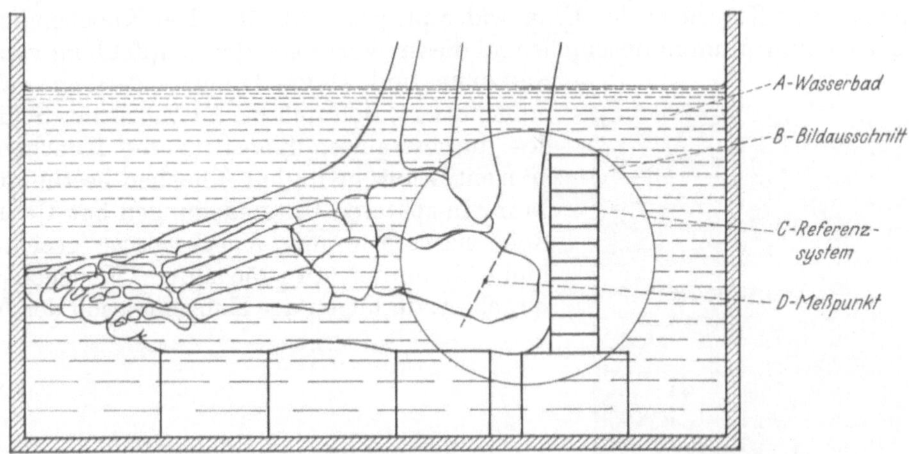

Abb. 47a. Aufnahmeanordnung des Calcaneus und der Aluminiumtreppe im Wasserbad zur quantitativen Messung des Knochenmineralgehaltes. (Nach MAYO, 1961; Abb. 1)

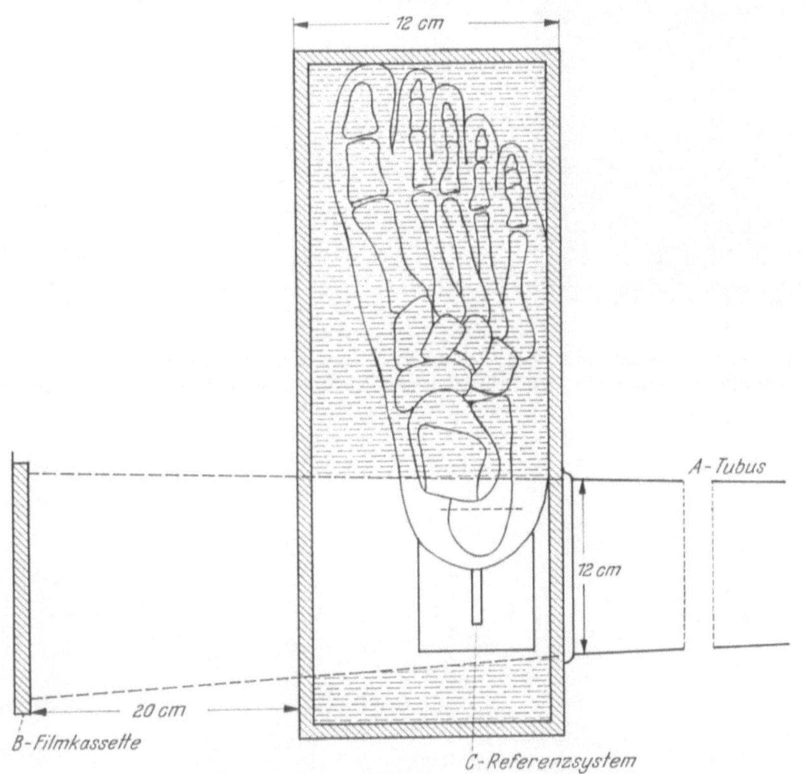

Abb. 47b. Darstellung der Aufnahmeanordnung von Abb. 47a in anderer Ebene. (Nach MAYO, 1961; Abb. 2)

schnitt der Ulna entwickelt. Als Referenzsystem wird eine Aluminiumtreppe benutzt. Der Unterarm und das Referenzsystem werden zusammen in eine Plexiglasbox, die mit Wasser gefüllt ist, eingelegt (Abb. 46). Das Referenzsystem besitzt 8 Treppen mit 0,5 mm Treppenabstand und einer Länge von 9 cm. Mit einem Mikrodensitometer wird der Röntgenfilm ausgewertet, wobei das Referenzsystem und der zu untersuchende Ulnabezirk zueinander in Beziehung gesetzt werden (Abb. 48a und b). Die punktförmigen Messungen erfolgten in der Mitte des Ulnaschaftes entlang der Längsachse in einer Zone 1—8 cm proximal von der distalen Grenze der Ulna in Abständen von 0,5 cm (Abb. 49). Die Meßwerte jedes einzelnen Punktes auf dieser Meßstrecke wurden in eine Kurve eingetragen, die den

Mineralgehalt des Knochens der Ulna widerspiegelt (Abb. 50). Die Knochendichte wird ausgedrückt in mm Aluminiumschicht und dieser Wert nach der Empfehlung von KEANE, SPIEGLER und DAVIS (1959) mit dem Faktor 130 multipliziert, wodurch bei Kenntnis der Schichtdicke des durchstrahlten Knochens die Knochenmineralkonzentration in mg/ml Knochen bestimmt werden kann. In späteren Untersuchungen hat DOYLE (1965) Referenzsysteme mit *Knochenasche* geeicht, wobei 1 mm Aluminium etwa 155 mg/cm² Knochenasche entsprach. Änderungen der Konzentration der Knochen-

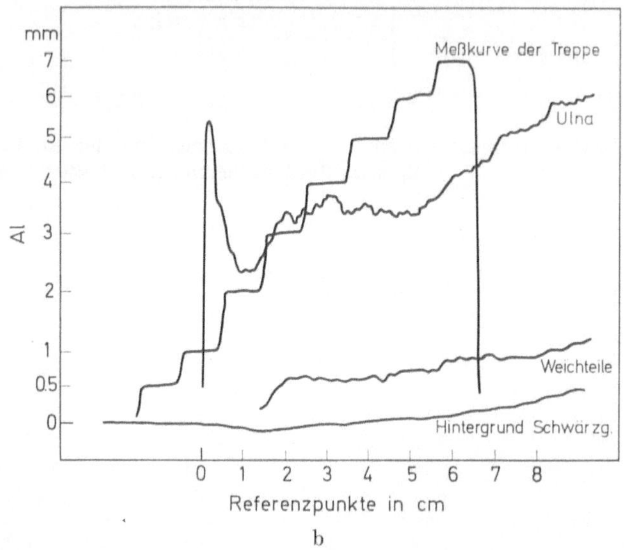

a b

Abb. 48. Beispiel einer Röntgenaufnahme im Wasserbad (a) und der Densitometerkurven durch Ulna, Referenzsystem und Weichteile zur Messung der Mineralkonzentration in Knochen (b). (Nach DOYLE, 1961; Abb. 4)

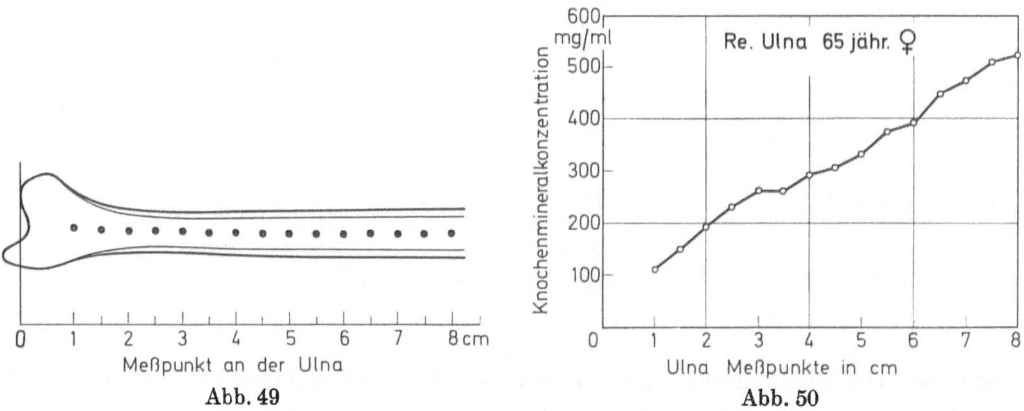

Abb. 49 Abb. 50

Abb. 49. Schematische Darstellung der Meßpunkte im Bereich des distalen Ulnadrittels zur Bestimmung der Mineralkonzentration. (Nach DOYLE, 1961; Abb. 3)

Abb. 50. Darstellung des Kurvenverlaufes einer normalen Ulna (65jährige Frau) in den einzelnen Meßpunkten. Der Wert von etwa 100 mg/ml Knochenmineral im Knochenmeßpunkt 1 liegt an der unteren Grenze der Norm. (Nach DOYLE, 1961; Abb. 5)

asche sowie der Aluminiumdicke einerseits und der Strahlenqualität andererseits konnten keine wesentlichen Verschiebungen im Meßergebnis bringen, so daß auch Aluminiumreferenzsysteme geeignet erscheinen. Allerdings dürfte ein Referenzsystem aus reinem *Hydroxylapatit* überlegen sein (HEUCK und SCHMIDT 1954/59/60). In solchen Abschnitten, in denen die Compacta dünn ist, wie am distalen Ende, war ein niedriger Knochenmineralgehalt von 100 mg/ml zu finden, der bis zum Meßpunkt 8 cm proximal vom distalen Ulnaende an steigt und Werte von 500—600 mg/ml erreicht. Die dickere Compacta des Knochens ist sicher von Einfluß auf das Meßergebnis.

Als *Index* für den gesamten Mineralisationsgrad eines Knochens hat DOYLE (1965) für die Ulna das Verhältnis der Mineralkonzentration in einem Bezirk 1 cm proximal der distalen Grenzlamelle zu der Mineralkonzentration in dem Bezirk 8 cm proximal empfohlen. Es wurden Normalwerte dieses „Index" bei 75 Männern und 78 Frauen ermittelt (s. S. 214).

Die Meßmethode von KEANE, SPIEGLER und DAVIS (1959) wurde in geringer Abwandlung von BJÖRK (1965) angewendet. Die Aluminiumtreppe aus *reinem Aluminium* besitzt 8 Stufen (0,5—7 mm dick), die auf 0,005 mm genau gearbeitet sind. Zur Ver-

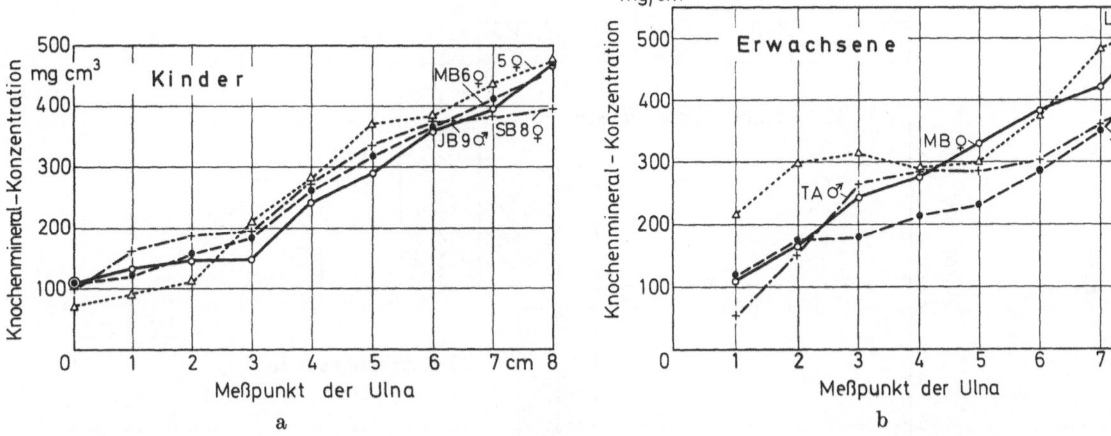

Abb. 51. Darstellung der Ergebnisse der radiologischen Messung des Knochenmineralgehaltes der Ulna gesunder Kinder (a) und gesunder Erwachsener (b). Die relativ große Streubreite bei Kindern ist deutlich erkennbar. (Nach BJÖRK, 1965; Abb. 2)

meidung von Luftblasen im Wassertank wurde ein Netzmittel hinzugefügt. Die Aufnahmebedingungen für die Ulna betrugen 80 kV bei 80 mAs. Auf konstante, sorgfältige Entwicklung und Bearbeitung der Filme muß Wert gelegt werden. Die photometrische Auswertung der Filme erfolgte nach der Methode von DOYLE (1961), die mehrere Meßzonen an der Ulna berücksichtigt. Die Meßwerte wurden in einem Diagramm dargestellt. Es wurden 200 Messungen an 10 Normalpersonen (Abb. 51a und b) und 50 Patienten durchgeführt (s. S. 258). Das Verfahren ist in der klinischen Radiologie insbesondere für Verlaufskontrollen von Systemerkrankungen des Skeletes brauchbar und hat sich bewährt.

HODGKINSON, EXTON-SMITH und CROWLEY (1963) haben Ergebnisse von Dichtemessungen des Knochens der Grundphalanx vom 3. Finger der linken Hand (bei Erkrankungen auf der linken Seite der rechten Hand) mitgeteilt. Als Referenzsystem diente eine Aluminiumtreppe. Unter standardisierten Aufnahmebedingungen (55 kV, 100 mA, 0,3 sec, Fokus-Film-Abstand 1 m) wurden Röntgenaufnahmen des 3. Fingers angefertigt. Zur Auswertung des Röntgenbildes wird nach Abdecken eines Meßbezirkes die Dichte des Knochens mit der Dichte der Aluminiumtreppe photometrisch verglichen. Nach der Formel:

$$\text{Knochendichte} = \frac{\text{Transmission des Knochens} \times 1000}{\text{Transmission der Treppe} \times \text{Knochendiameter}^2}$$

werden die Ergebnisse in ganzen Zahlen ausgedrückt. Die Prüfung der Genauigkeit ergab eine Schwankung der Meßwerte um 2 Einheiten. Daneben sind Röntgenaufnahmen der Wirbelsäule angefertigt worden, um pathologische Frakturen erkennen zu können. Die

Dichtewerte der Fingerknochen von 25 Patienten mit Wirbelveränderungen verschiedenster Genese variierten zwischen 4 und 11 bei einem Mittelwert von 7, während sich bei 19 gesunden, gut ernährten Frauen Werte zwischen 9 und 16 bei einem Mittelwert von 12 fanden. Bei 36 Patienten ohne nachweisbare Wirbelveränderungen wurden Dichtewerte von 6—13 bei einem Mittelwert von 10 gefunden (Abb. 52). Die Übereinstimmung der Meßergebnisse mit dem klinischen Krankheitsbild war gut.

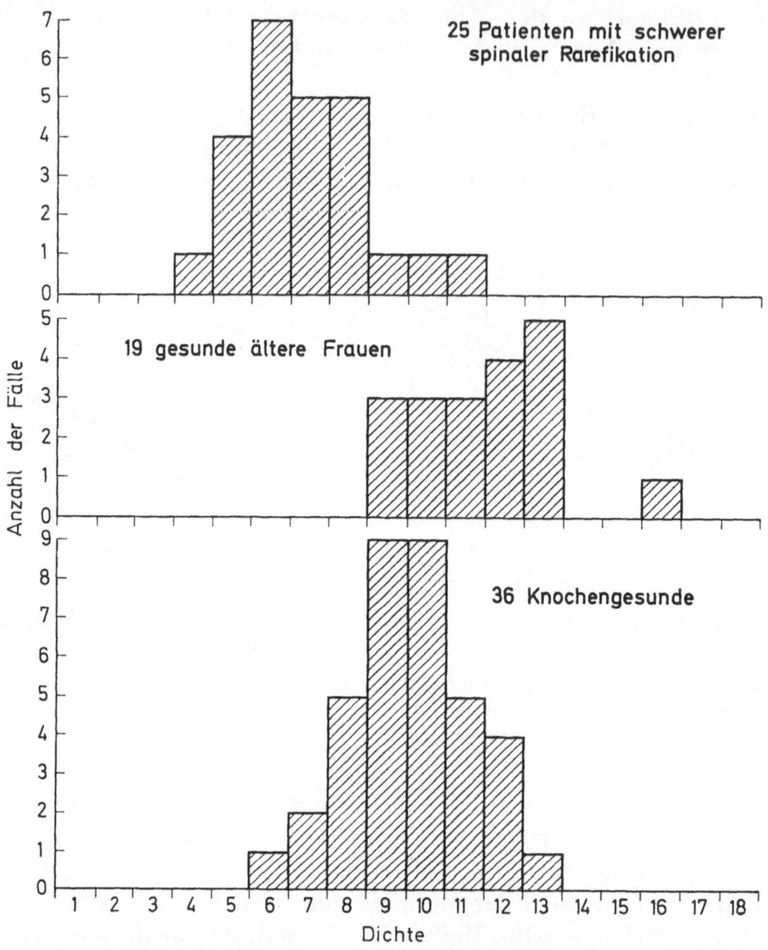

Abb. 52. Graphische Darstellung der Ergebnisse von Dichtemessungen des Knochens der Grundphalanx vom 3. Finger der linken Hand. (Nach Hodgkinson, Exton-Smith und Crowley, 1963; Abb. 1, 2 und 3). *Unten:* Knochendichte bei 36 Patienten ohne Wirbelveränderungen (Normalfälle). *Mitte:* Knochendichte bei 19 aktiven älteren Frauen (Altersosteoporose, sonst normal). *Oben:* Knochenwerte von 25 Patienten mit schweren osteoporotischen Wirbelveränderungen

Von Fanucci und Loasses (1962) wurde, basierend auf den Untersuchungen von Turano (1952/53) eine Methode zur Objektivierung der Dichte des Wirbelknochens entwickelt, bei der als Vergleichskörper Aluminium verwendet wird. Die Meßwerte wurden in äquivalenter Schichtdicke Aluminium angegeben. Zunächst wurde die Brauchbarkeit der Methode an 28 Lendenwirbelpräparaten erprobt, deren Dichte-Index angegeben wird. Bei gesunder Wirbelsäule fand sich eine Differenz der Indexwerte zwischen 0,8—1,65, während die osteoporotischen Veränderungen der Wirbelkörper eine Schwankung des densitometrischen Dichte-Index zwischen 0,256 und 0,723 ergaben.

Mouvet (1964) beschäftigte sich mit den Möglichkeiten, die Absorptionskurve von Referenzsystemen aus Aluminium zu verbessern. Ferner wird eine Bleiblende mit quadratischem oder rechteckigem Ausschnitt verwendet, um die Schwierigkeiten, die durch die polychromatische Strahlung und die Streustrahlung auftreten, zu vermindern.

Lefebvre, Bismuth und Chaumont (1964) haben mikro-densitometrische Vergleichsmessungen mit einer Aluminiumtreppe als Referenzsystem durchgeführt. Bei 30 bis 60 mg Ca/cm² konnten noch Unterschiede von 2,6 mg Ca/cm² festgestellt werden.

Von der Überlegung ausgehend, daß die meisten Knochen mehr oder weniger stark durch Weichteile überlagert werden, haben Mäntyla, Telkkä, Wegelius und Virtama (1964) densitometrische Untersuchungen über die Brauchbarkeit der Mineralkonzentration der Zähne als Indikator für die Knochendichte und damit den Knochenkalksalzgehalt angestellt, um die Schwierigkeiten der Weichteilabsorption und Streuung zu umgehen. Als Referenzsystem fand eine Aluminiumtreppe Verwendung. Die Untersuchungen wurden an 38 Schneidezähnen des Oberkiefers und 24 Schneidezähnen des Unterkiefers durchgeführt. Zum Vergleich wurde ferner die Knochendichte des *Unterkiefers* herangezogen. Durch die densitometrische Auswertung der folienlosen Spezial-Kodakfilme wurden die Dichtewerte von Zähnen und Knochen in *Aluminium-Schichtdicke* angegeben.

Der kritische *Vergleich* der Dichtewerte *der Zähne* mit den Meßwerten des *Unterkieferknochens* ergab keine Abhängigkeit voneinander. *Der Zahn ist an einem raschen Austausch von Calciumsalzen nicht beteiligt* und muß als Gebilde mit eigenen Stoffwechselgesetzen betrachtet werden. Die Untersuchungsreihe ergab keine Korrelation der Dichte der Zähne und der Dichte des Unterkieferknochens. Die Dichte der Zähne kann daher *nicht als ein Indikator* für die Kalksalzkonzentration des Knochengewebes des Unterkiefers oder anderer Knochen des Skeletes angesehen werden.

Die Anwendung einer Computer-Meßeinrichtung zur Bestimmung des Knochenmineralgehaltes hat Mack (1965) erprobt. In ihrer Arbeitsgruppe wurden seit 1927 verschiedene Methoden entwickelt und neben Referenzsystemen aus Elfenbein (s. S. 174) solche aus Aluminium oder Aluminiumlegierungen (93,4% Aluminium, 0,6% Mangan, 1,5% Magnesium, 4,5% Kupfer) verwendet. Das komplizierte Meß-System erlaubt die Durchführung verschiedener Untersuchungsmethoden. Die Ergebnisse können entweder direkt abgelesen werden, oder mit Hilfe einer mathematischen Formel in das äquivalente Referenzvolumen und in die äquivalente Referenzmasse umgewandelt werden, da die Dichte der Aluminiumverbindung bekannt ist. Ein Referenzsystem aus einer Aluminiumlegierung kann nach einer Eichung zur Bestimmung des Knochenkalksalzgehaltes Verwendung finden. Die Eichungen wurden so durchgeführt, daß chemisch reine Calciumverbindungen oder Mischungen von Verbindungen bekannten Gewichtes in Plastik eingebettet und auf demselben Film mit dem Referenzsystem dargestellt wurden. Durch diese Eichung können die Meßwerte in Hydroxylapatit-Einheiten angegeben werden. Am Lebenden müssen bei einer Knochenuntersuchung immer die Weichteile mitberücksichtigt werden, so daß im Gesamtbild neben dem Knochenmineral auch Protein, Wasser und Fett erscheinen. Die Massenabsorptionskoeffizienten dieser Substanzen sind abhängig von der für die Anfertigung des Bildes benutzten Strahlenenergie. Vergleichsuntersuchungen zwischen den gemessenen Werten und den chemisch-analytischen Werten von Knochenproben verschiedener Herkunft (Tierknochen und Menschenknochen) ergaben eine gute Übereinstimmung. Die Reproduzierbarkeit der Methode wurde an 8 Calcaneusaufnahmen getestet, die innerhalb einer $^1/_2$ Std angefertigt worden sind. Es konnte eine Genauigkeit von 99% gefunden werden.

Ein Referenzsystem, bestehend aus einem Keil (Neigung 5:1) einer *Aluminium-Legierung (93,4% Al, 4,5% Cu, 1,5% Mg, 0,6% Mn)* mit einem *in Plexiglas eingebetteten Zylinder aus 40% menschlicher Knochenasche* (bei 575°C verascht) und 60% Kasein hat Vose (1965) entwickelt, um Untersuchungen des Mineralgehaltes *im Femurhals* und in *der Wirbelsäule* durchführen zu können. Die Weichteilüberlagerung wird bei Untersuchungen am Femur dadurch korrigiert, daß das Phantom unter die Weichteile des Oberschenkels geschoben wird, so daß die Weichteildicke für Knochen und Phantom gleich ist. Bei Untersuchungen der Wirbelsäule wird die Weichteil- und Muskelschicht des Patienten durch Plexiglasplatten ersetzt, die zur gleichen Dicke übereinander geschichtet werden können. Die Strahlenabsorption durch Plexiglas entspricht zwar nicht der Strahlenabsorption durch die Weichteile des Patienten, doch kann der geringe Fehler bei der Densitometrie ausgeglichen werden. Wichtig ist es, bei Verlaufskontrollen immer die gleiche Schichtdicke des Plexiglases zu verwenden. Das gesamte Referenzsystem wird zur Vermeidung eines unnötigen Streustrahleneinflusses in Blei eingeschlossen, zumal die Aufnahme des Phantoms und die Aufnahme der Wirbelsäule *auf demselben Film, aber getrennt exponiert werden.* Bei Verwendung einer Strahlung von 60 kV Anodenspannung und einer Filterung von 3 mm Aluminium wurde die beste Reproduzierbarkeit der Meßergebnisse festgestellt. Die Filme sollten sofort entwickelt und verarbeitet werden, da *nach 24 Std entwickelte Filme Unterschiede der Schwärzung bis zu 15%* zeigten. Die Ursache dieser Unterschiede ist bisher ungeklärt. Zur Auswertung der Filme wird ein Spezial-Mikrophotometer mit einem Kurvenschreiber benutzt, das für densitometrische Messungen geeignet ist. Die Fehlerbreite des Photometers wird mit 2% angegeben. Eine Verringerung der Fehler ist durch doppelte Auswertung jedes Filmes möglich. Es können jedoch nicht alle Fehler densitometrischer Messungen völlig beseitigt werden. Es soll versucht werden, die Technik des Meßverfahrens zu verbessern und die Genauigkeit weiter zu erhöhen.

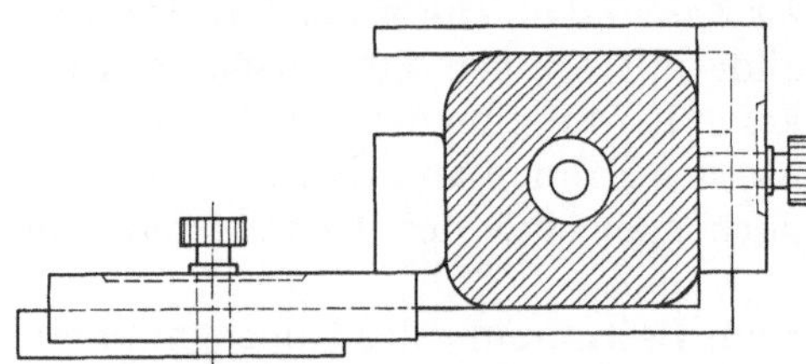

Abb. 53. Schematische Darstellung der Plexiglas-Halterung zur Kompression der Weichteile des Oberarmes. (Nach MAROTTA, 1955; Abb. 8)

Von VOSE und PYKE (1966) wurden Untersuchungen über den Einfluß der Zusammensetzung des Wirbelkörpers auf die Röntgenstrahlen-Absorption durchgeführt. In 105 Fällen sind Aufnahmen der Wirbelsäule in 2 Ebenen mit einem Aluminiumreferenzsystem angefertigt worden, um den Mineralgehalt bestimmen zu können. Später wurde der 3. Lendenwirbelkörper herauspräpariert, getrocknet, entfettet und gewogen. Der Calciumgehalt wurde durch Veraschung der Knochen bestimmt. Die Strahlenabsorptions-Messung (ausgedrückt in Aluminium-Gleichwerten) stellt ein sehr genaues Maß für den Aschegehalt eines Knochens dar.

Neben Aluminium und Aluminium-Legierungen wurden auch andere *Metalle oder Metall-Legierungen* als Referenzsystem verwendet. MAROTTA (1955) wählte eine Reihe von Metallstäben (deren Zusammensetzung nicht genauer definiert wird) in einem Plexiglasphantom als Referenzsystem. Jeder Metallstab repräsentiert eine bestimmte Menge an Calcium/cm^2. Die *Eichung* dieser Metallstäbe erfolgte zuvor mit einer *bekannten Calciumphosphatlösung.* Das erste Metallphantom entsprach 0,67 g Calcium/cm^2, das zweite 1,6 g Calcium/cm^2, das dritte 1,74 g Calcium/cm^2. Die Kalksalzbestimmung wurde in der *Diaphyse des Humerus* durchgeführt. Zur Standardisierung der Weichteile wurde der Oberarm durch eine Plexiglaseinrichtung komprimiert (Abb. 53). Die Filmschwärzungswerte der Phantome wurden photometrisch ermittelt und zu den Schwärzungswerten des Knochens in Beziehung gesetzt. Die densitometrischen Messungen am Knochen erfolgten im Gebiet der Markhöhle. Der Durchmesser wurde durch eine *Aufnahme in der 2. Ebene ermittelt.* Eine Tabelle, die durch besondere Berechnungen zusammengestellt wurde, gestattet es, aus den Photometerwerten (Ca/cm^2) direkt die Menge des Calcium/cm^3 Knochengewebe abzulesen. Es werden einige Beispiele gegeben.

Die Methode von MISASI, SAVOIA und SORRENTINO (1957) basiert auf den Voruntersuchungen von MAROTTA (1955). Die Röntgenstrahlenabsorption durch drei *unterschiedlich dicke Kupferbänder*, die auf zwei Schlitten aus Kunststoff angebracht worden sind und zusammen mit dem planparallel komprimierten Extremitätenabschnitt geröntgt wurden, kann zu der Strahlenabsorption des Knochens in Beziehung gesetzt werden. Aus den photometrisch ermittelten Schwärzungswerten kann mit Hilfe einer Tabelle der Calciumgehalt/cm^2 gefunden werden. Chemisch-analytische Kontrolluntersuchungen der photometrisch ermittelten Werte zur exakten Bestimmung des methodischen Gesamtfehlers sind von den genannten Autoren nicht vorgelegt worden.

b) Die Messungen mit Referenzsystemen aus Elfenbein

Elfenbein ist eine Substanz, die *in ihrer chemischen Zusammensetzung dem Knochengewebe sehr ähnlich ist* und daher in Form von Keilen, Treppen oder Zylindern oft als Referenzsystem Verwendung gefunden hat. Eine chemisch-analytische Bestimmung des Calciumgehaltes der verwendeten Elfenbeinphantome erlaubt *die Umrechnung* der miteinander vergleichbaren photometrischen Werte *in Werte des Calciumgehaltes vom Knochen.*

Umfangreiche Untersuchungen aller Faktoren und Probleme, die bei einer objektiven Bestimmung des Kalkgehaltes des Skeletes am Patienten beachtet werden müssen, sind von De Does, Gorter und Seeder (1933) und Endtz (1934) vorgelegt worden. Das Prinzip der von De Does, Gorter und Seeder (1933) benutzten Meßmethode besteht darin, zusammen mit dem zu untersuchenden Knochen einen Vergleichskörper zu röntgen, *dessen Calciumgehalt bekannt ist.* Der Kalkgehalt der Radiusknochen wurde gemessen, indem die Strahlenabsorption des Knochens mit der Absorption durch einen *Elfenbeinkeil* (1 cm breit, 2 cm lang, 0,5 cm hoch) verglichen wurde. Zur Röntgenaufnahme wird der Elfenbein-Vergleichskörper so neben den Knochen gelegt, daß *er von den Weichteilen überlagert* wird, um die Weichteilabsorption direkt zu kompensieren. Durch chemische Analyse wurde der Calciumgehalt des Elfenbeinphantoms festgestellt, so daß auf photometrischem Wege bestimmt werden konnte, wieviel mg Ca/cm^3 des untersuchten Knochens vorlagen. Durch Verwendung eines Phantoms aus Elfenbein können Änderungen der Belichtungszeit, der Qualität der Röntgenstrahlen und Variationen der Entwicklungszeit vernachlässigt werden. Bei Benutzung desselben Phantoms ergab die Methode eine gute Reproduzierbarkeit.

Endtz (1934) hat fortlaufende Bestimmungen des Knochenkalkgehaltes bei der *Rachitis* und der *kindlichen Osteoporose* durchgeführt und fand Unterschiede des Kalkgehaltes zwischen der Verkalkungszone und dem Schaft, die nach Behandlung besonders deutlich waren.

Später verwendete Stein (1937) ebenfalls *Elfenbein* als Vergleichskörper, da die Strahlenabsorption dieser Substanz ähnlich der von Calcium und Phosphor ist. Ein kleineres Treppenphantom (Nachlass und Parke 1937) hat den Nachteil, daß infolge des schrägen Verlaufs der Röntgenstrahlen nur ein geringer Teil des Treppenschattens ausgewertet werden kann. Das von Stein benutzte treppenförmige Referenzsystem aus Elfenbein besaß daher Stufen von 2 mm Höhe, die auf 0,05 mm genau angefertigt worden sind. Die untere Stufe wurde bei 3 mm, die obere bei 30 mm gewählt. Für die Untersuchungen von *Beckenknochen, Femur* und *Wirbelknochen* muß das Referenzsystem eine Stufenhöhe 18 und 45 mm besitzen. Als Photometer wurde ein Universal-Weston-Photometer mit einer Lichtquelle von 100 W/115 V und einem Kondensor benutzt, um einen Lichtstrahl großer Intensität und nahezu gleichmäßiger Zusammensetzung zu erzeugen. Die Wärmeenergie wurde durch ein Filter vermindert, um Verbrennungen des Filmes zu vermeiden. Die Meßeinrichtung besitzt einen hohen Grad an Genauigkeit. Selbst bei unterschiedlicher Belichtung der Filme (Überbelichtung oder Unterbelichtung) sind die Werte noch brauchbar. Die Röntgenfilme müssen zur Photometrie nicht zerschnitten oder beschädigt werden. Durch Eintragen des Photometerwertes der Knochen in ein besonders *geeichtes Diagramm* kann der Dichtewert des Knochens in mm Elfenbein *direkt* abgelesen werden. Es wird empfohlen, immer zwei Aufnahmen anzufertigen, wobei einmal die Elfenbeintreppe und einmal der darzustellende Knochen im Zentralstrahl liegen sollten. Das Referenzsystem soll möglichst *in der Nähe des zu untersuchenden Objektes* placiert werden. Die Genauigkeit der beschriebenen Methode wird mit 10% angegeben. In einer Anmerkung wird darauf hingewiesen, daß gemeinsam mit Warren ein Wasserphantom entwickelt worden sei, das zusammen mit dem Elfenbeinphantom die durch die Weichteile bedingten Fehler ausschließen soll. Dies sei besonders wichtig für Untersuchungen am Becken, am proximalen Femur und an der Wirbelsäule.

Eine *Anzahl von Elfenbeinzylindern* mit einem Durchmesser von 12 mm und einer Höhe zwischen 1 und 18 mm sowie einer Höhendifferenz von 1 mm verwendete Bywaters

(1948) als Vergleichskörper. Die Meßeinrichtung zur Photometrie bestand aus einer Selen-Photozelle mit einem Spiegelgalvanometer. Vor Bestimmung der Dichte des Knochens wird *eine Eichkurve in mm Elfenbein* ermittelt. Die Fehlermöglichkeiten (unterschiedliche Leistung der Röntgenröhre, Unterschiede in der Zusammensetzung des Entwicklers, Einfluß der Entwicklungszeit und -temperatur u.a.) werden ausführlich diskutiert und festgestellt, daß bei Verwendung eines Elfenbein-Vergleichskörpers die meisten Fehler unberücksichtigt gelassen werden können. Die Beseitigung des Fehlers, der durch die Weichteile bedingt ist, bereitet Schwierigkeiten, da bei größeren Weichteilmassen exakte Untersuchungen unmöglich werden. Das mit einer inhomogenen Röntgenstrahlung hergestellte Bild gemischter Gewebe könne theoretisch nicht unmittelbar mit dem Bild der Elfenbeinzylinder verglichen werden, so daß unter solchen Bedingungen die Verwendung einer Aluminiumtreppe angeraten wird. Wichtig ist es daher, eine möglichst große Homogenität der Röntgenstrahlung anzustreben. Bei Serienuntersuchungen und Verlaufskontrollen ist es schwierig, exakt denselben Meßbezirk des Knochens wiederzufinden. Die gefundenen Abweichungen lagen jedoch unter $\pm 5\%$. Der Autor empfiehlt die Methode auch für den klinischen Routinebetrieb und zur *Beobachtung des Krankheitsverlaufes von Knochenveränderungen.* Es wurden Untersuchungen am *Handskelet bei rheumatischen Erkrankungen* durchgeführt und *Änderungen des Kalkgehaltes nach einer Fraktur* und deren Behandlung im Gipsverband studiert.

Marchal (1948) hat eine Methode angegeben, mit der es *gleichzeitig* möglich ist, *kontinuierliche Spannungsänderungen* abzulesen. Als Schwärzungsgradmesser diente deshalb *ein Aluminiumkeil,* an dem ein Streifen aus *reinem Silber* befestigt wurde. Die Untersuchungen können nun mit einer polychromatischen Strahlung, die im Spannungsbereich von 50—65 kV ansteigend erzeugt werden kann, durchgeführt werden. Als Referenzsystem für den Knochen wird *ein Keil aus Elfenbein* oder *kompaktem Knochen* verwendet, der *direkt auf die Weichteile* der zu untersuchenden Region gelegt wird. Die Methode kann bei einem Gewebsödem ungenau werden, da die Strahlendurchlässigkeit um 50% schwanken kann. Die photometrische Auswertung der Röntgenfilme erfolgte mit einem Vassy-Mikrodensimeter. Zunächst werden die Schwärzungsbezirke von Aluminium und Silber ausgemessen und auf diese Weise die mittlere benutzte Spannung festgelegt. Dann werden die Schwärzungswerte des Referenzsystems und des Knochens ermittelt. Die praktische Anwendung der Methode wird an *dem Fingerknochen* eines 11jährigen Kindes erprobt. Da die Dichte des Knochens im Röntgenbild allein durch die eingelagerten Kalksalze des Knochens bedingt ist, erlaubt die Bestimmung der Dichtekurve des Referenzsystems *eine Berechnung der Calciumsalze* im ausgewerteten Knochenbezirk. Eine Kontrolle der berechneten Calciumwerte des Knochens durch chemische Analyse wurde nicht durchgeführt.

Eingehende Untersuchungen unter Berücksichtigung aller *theoretischen Voraussetzungen* zur Bestimmung der Knochendichte aus dem Röntgenbild sind von Mack, Brown jr. und Trapp (1949) vorgelegt worden. Als Vergleichskörper diente eine *Elfenbeintreppe* (Abb. 54). Durch die Streustrahlung entstand eine relativ gleichmäßige, zusätzliche Schwärzung des Filmes. Ihre Beseitigung gelang durch Filter oder Schlitzblenden. Sie konnte ferner dadurch reduziert werden, daß eine langwellige Strahlung benutzt wurde, doch waren bei größeren Objekten wegen der erforderlichen sehr langen Belichtungszeiten Grenzen gesetzt. Die benutzte Anodenspannung lag zwischen 45 und 55 kV. Der zu untersuchende Knochenabschnitt wurde in *2 Ebenen* geröntgt und die Elfenbeintreppe in einer bestimmten Standardposition mit aufgenommen. Von größter Bedeutung war die Festlegung einer *exakten Meßlinie durch den Knochen,* um eine möglichst große Reproduzierbarkeit des Verfahrens zu erreichen (Abb. 55). Die photometrischen Messungen erfolgten mit einem Mikrophotometer besonderer Bauart (s. S. 130). Die Meßlinie durch den Knochen wurde in eine bestimmte Anzahl von Segmenten eingeteilt. Die unter jedem Segment gemessene Fläche wurde ermittelt (Abb. 56). Mit Hilfe einer Formel wurde aus den Segmentwerten ein Mittelwert für die gesamte Meßlinie berechnet und in Einheiten der Elfenbeinschichtdicke ausgedrückt. Dieser korrigierte Wert der „*äquivalenten Elfen-*

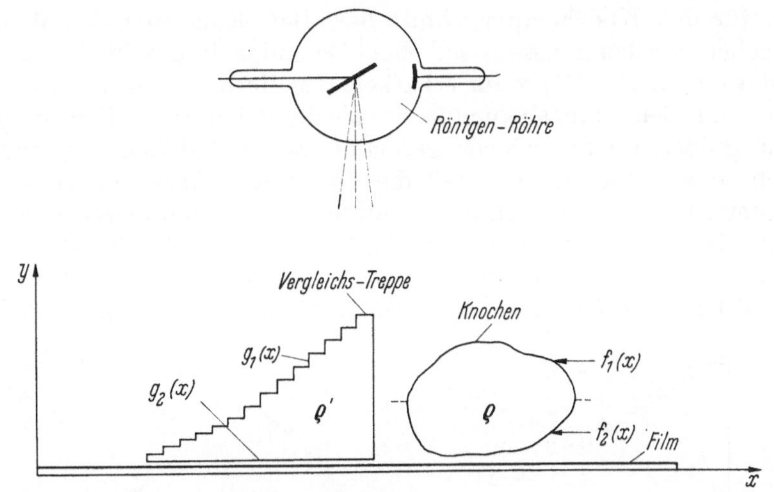

Abb. 54. Schematische Darstellung der Aufnahmeanordnung mit Elfenbeintreppe. (Nach MACK, BROWN und TRAPP, 1949; Abb. 3)

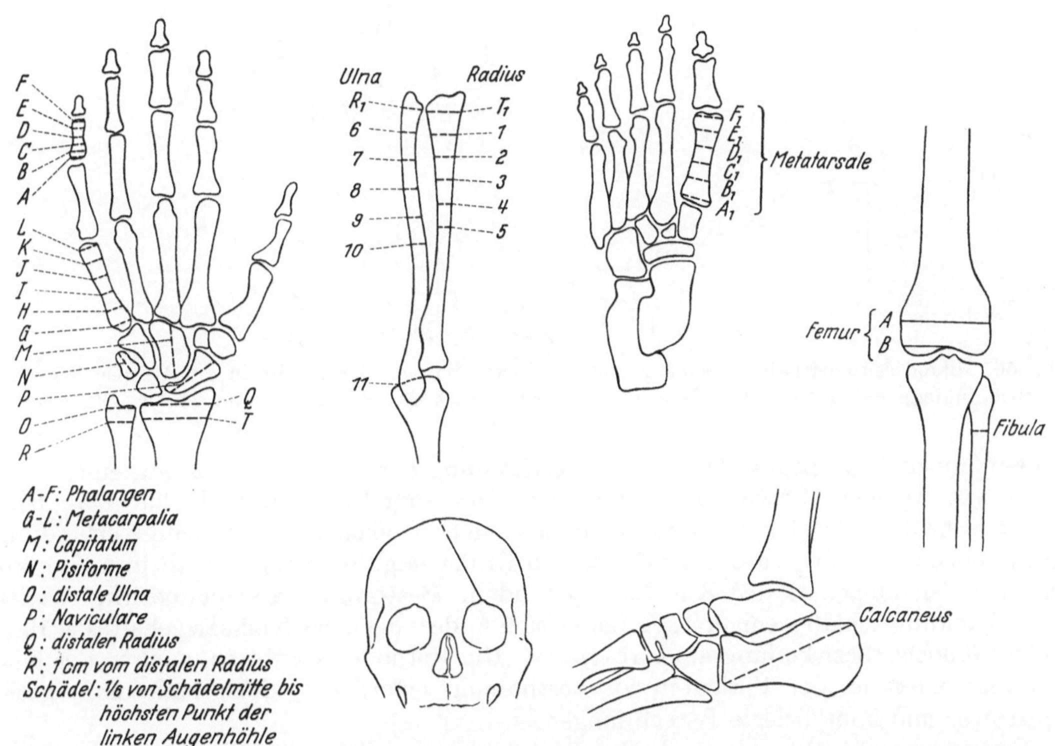

Abb. 55. Schematische Darstellung der Meßlinien an den verschiedenen Knochenpartien. Die Meßlinie des Schädels reicht von der Medianlinie zum höchsten Punkt der linken Orbita. Vom Metacarpale V und dem Mittelglied des 5. Fingers sind mehrere Meßlinien gewählt worden. Von Radius, Ulna und Metatarsale I wurden in einigen Messungen ebenfalls mehrere Linien berücksichtigt. (Nach MACK, BROWN und TRAPP, 1949; Abb. 7 und 8)

beinschichtdicke" jeder Meßlinie wurde durch den *Mittelwert der Dichte des Knochens* dividiert und dann mit dem Wert der *Elfenbeindichte in g/cm³* multipliziert. Das Ergebnis ist die „*Elfenbeindichte*" *des Knochens in g Elfenbeinäquivalent/cm³ Knochen.* Dies ist ein Faktor, der das Verhältnis von Knochendichte zur spezifischen Dichte des Elfenbeinkeiles darstellt. Er kann *in g Knochenasche/Volumeneinheit umgerechnet* werden. Eine Vereinfachung der Methode stellt die Angabe des mittleren Elfenbeindickeäquivalentes in Zentimeter für den Knochenquerschnitt dar. Bei Beachtung der Meßlinien, die besonders angegeben werden müssen, soll eine Genauigkeit des Meßverfahrens von fast 100% erreicht werden. Die Reproduzierbarkeit der Methode wurde unter verschiedenen Entwicklungs- und Belichtungsbedingungen an der Ulna eines Kindes geprüft und es konnten keine größeren Unterschiede gefunden werden. Belichtung und Entwicklung müssen jedoch so gewählt werden, daß die Gradationskurve des verwendeten Filmes Berücksichtigung findet. Es wurden quantitative Messungen an *einigen tausend* Röntgenaufnahmen der Knochen von *Calcaneus*, *Fuß* (Metatarsale I), *Hand* (Mittelglied des li. Kleinfingers, Metacarpale V li., Os capitatum, Os pisiforme, Os naviculare, distale Enden von Radius und Ulna), *Ellenbogen*, *Kniegelenk*, *Hüftgelenk*, *Femur*, *Patella* und *Schädel*

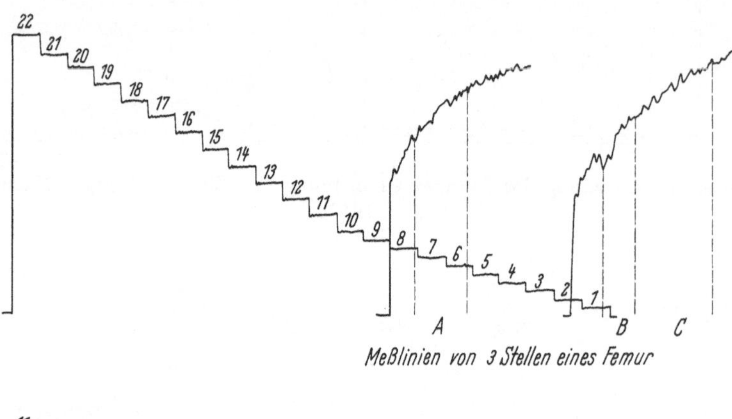

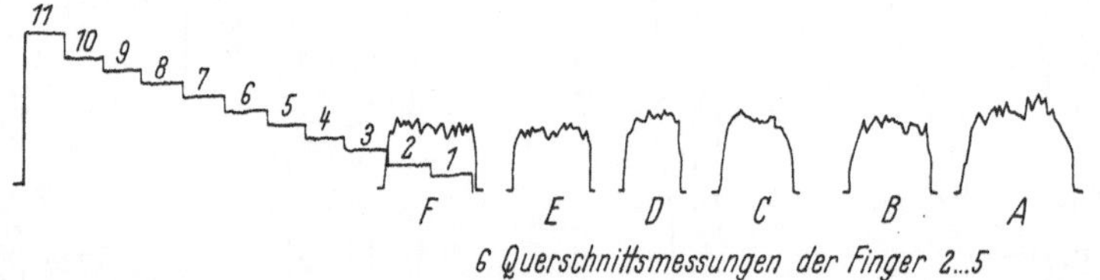

Abb. 56. Mikrodensitometrisch gewonnene und korrigierte Kurven der Meßlinien am Beispiel der Fingerknochen (unten) und des distalen Femurendes (oben). (Nach Mack, Brown und Trapp, 1949; Abb. 10)

vorgenommen und festgestellt, daß die Bestimmung der Knochendichte mit einer Fehlerbreite von wenigen Prozenten möglich ist. Die vorgelegte Methode hat eine betont theoretische Basis. Da der lebende Knochen als Calciumspeicher dient, Calciumverbindungen aufnimmt oder abgibt, wurden Einflüsse von Ernährung, Schwangerschaft und Krankheit auf den Calciumgehalt des Knochens gefunden. Bestimmte Knochenbezirke reagieren schnell, und innerhalb weniger Tage finden sich Änderungen des Kalksalzgehaltes, während andere Knochenbezirke langsamer reagieren. Die Methode erlaubt es, auch in der Klinik den Calciumstatus der Patienten zu bestimmen, erfordert jedoch eine umfangreiche Apparatur und komplizierte Berechnungen.

Rethmeier (1955) benutzte als Vergleichskörper ein *Elfenbeinphantom in einer Metallhalterung*, das *unter die Weichteile* placiert und zusammen mit dem zu untersuchenden Knochen geröntgt wurde (Abb. 57). Die Untersuchungen sind am *Handskelet von Kindern* durchgeführt worden. Zur photometrischen Auswertung der Filme wurde ein besonders konstruiertes Densitometer verwendet, das mit Hilfe eines mikroskopischen Systems die Schwärzung kleinster Felder im Knochen sowie im Elfenbeinkeil zu messen erlaubt. Die Beseitigung des Einflusses der durch die Weichteile bedingten Strahlenabsorption konnte dadurch erreicht werden, daß das Elfenbeinphantom zwischen Zeigefinger und Daumen unter die Weichteile placiert wurde. Da die Maße und die Zusammensetzung des Elfenbeinkeiles bekannt sind, ist es möglich, einen *Schätzwert der Menge des Calciumphosphates/ Volumeneinheit des Knochens* zu gewinnen. Größere Untersuchungsreihen mit diesem Verfahren sind nicht durchgeführt worden.

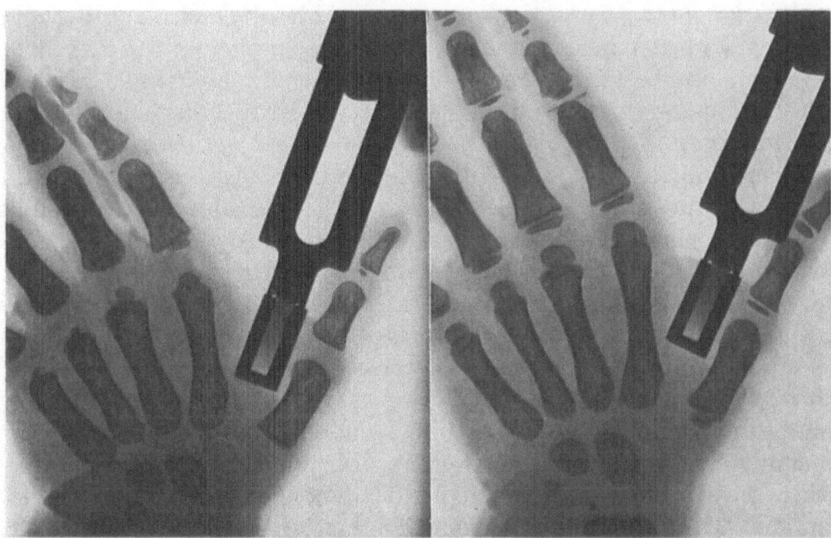

Abb. 57. Röntgenaufnahmen der rechten Hand zusammen mit der Elfenbeintreppe in einer Metallhalterung zur Kontrolle der Kalksalzkonzentration bei einem Kind. (Nach RETHMEIER, 1955; Abb. 3)

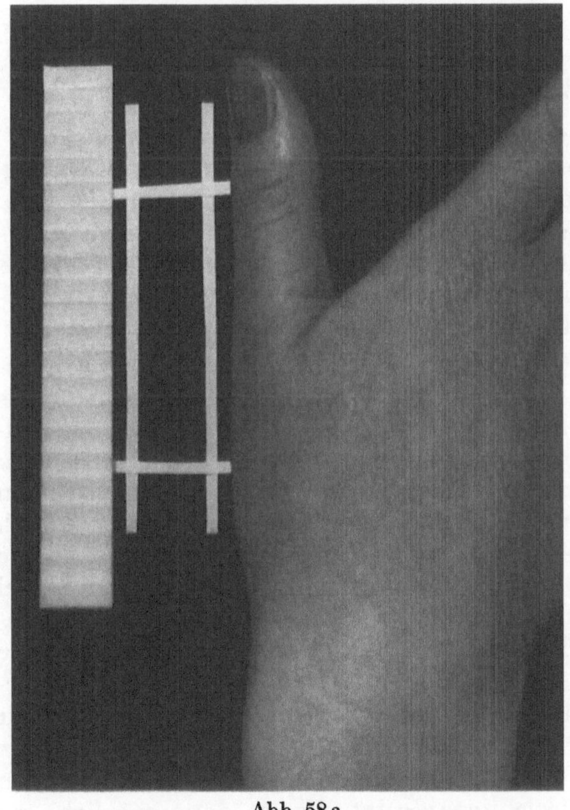

Abb. 58a

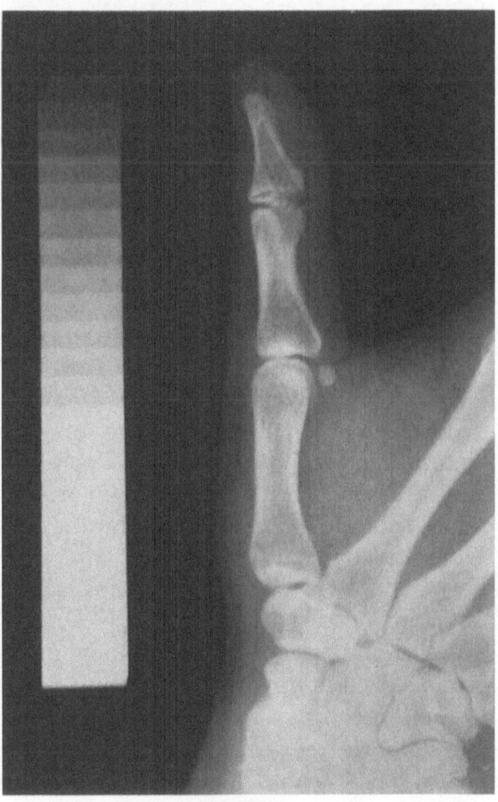

Abb. 58b

Abb. 58a. Aufnahmeanordnung des rechten Daumens zusammen mit der Elfenbeintreppe

Abb. 58b. Röntgenaufnahme von Daumenknochen und Elfenbeintreppe entsprechend 58a. (Nach SCHMID, 1960; Abb. 1)

SCHMID (1960) verwendete als Referenzsystem ebenfalls eine *Elfenbeintreppe* folgender Abmessungen: 11 cm lang, 1 cm breit, die ersten 10 Stufen 1 mm hoch, die nächsten 12 Stufen 2 mm hoch, alle Stufen 5 mm lang (Abb. 58a und b). Zu Messungen wurde *die*

Diaphyse der Mittelphalanx des rechten Daumens gewählt, obgleich Veränderungen des Kalkgehaltes an diesem Knochen nicht so rasch erkennbar sein dürften wie an Knochen, die vorwiegend aus Spongiosa bestehen. Die Compacta der Mittelphalanx reagiert wesentlich träger. Die Bestimmung der Dichte der Mittelphalanx ist technisch einfach durchzuführen und mit den wenigsten Fehlerquellen behaftet. Deshalb eignet sich diese Skeletregion für Serienuntersuchungen besonders gut. Die Auswertung des Röntgenfilmes erfolgte mit einem Apparat für die Papierelektrophorese (Integraph Firma Bender & Hobein, München), der durch einen Linsenvorsatz modifiziert wurde. Neben der Elfenbeintreppe wird das Röntgenbild des Daumens ausgeschnitten und photometriert. Der zur Messung verwendete Lichtpunkt wandert von der markierten *Mitte der distalen Diaphyse zur Mitte der proximalen Diaphyse* der Mittelphalanx des rechten Daumens. Die Knochendichte wird mit der äquivalenten Dichte des Referenzsystems verglichen und *in Stufenwerten der Elfenbeintreppe* ausgedrückt. In einem zweiten Arbeitsgang kann das Verhältnis von Knochendichte zur Elfenbeintreppe bestimmt und die prozentuale Knochendichte von 1 cm^2 Daumenmittelphalanx ermittelt werden. Die Methode soll eine Genauigkeit von ± 5% erreichen. Es wurden Untersuchungen der Knochendichte von 1 cm^2 der Daumenmittelphalanx bei 325 Patienten mit einer Polyarthritis oder Arthrosis deformans im Alter von 5—85 Jahren durchgeführt (s. S. 269). Vom 5.—25. Lebensjahr kommt es zu einer Zunahme des Mineralgehaltes im Knochen, der dann zunächst ziemlich konstant bleibt, um vom 60. Lebensjahr an langsam abzunehmen. Die *individuelle Streubreite* war bei Berechnung auf 1 cm^2 Phalangenfläche *relativ groß*.

c) Die Messungen mit Referenzsystemen aus Knochenmaterial

Der erste Versuch, als *Referenzsystem Knochen* zu verwenden, geht auf STEVEN (1947) zurück. Er verglich die entkalkten Knochen der Hand von Rheumatikern mit einem sog. „Standardknochen" (s. S. 117). Es handelte sich um einen normalen Mittelhandknochen, der zur Reproduktion der Weichteilabsorption in ein Gemisch von Paraffin, Bienenwachs und Sägespäne eingebettet wurde. Auf diese Weise konnte frühzeitig eine generalisierte Osteoporose festgestellt werden. Einen solchen „Standardknochen" haben auch BARTHELHEIMER (1951) und MAASS (1951) zusätzlich neben einem Al-Referenzsystem verwendet.

Zu dem von HENNY (1950) vorgelegten Untersuchungsverfahren werden *als Phantomkörper dünne, planparallel geschliffene Tafeln aus Rinderknochen* benutzt. Der Knochen ist als Vergleichskörper deshalb besonders geeignet, weil *unbeabsichtigte Differenzen* der Anodenspannung von zwei aufeinanderfolgenden Röntgenaufnahmen das Meßergebnis *nicht* beeinflussen. HENNY hebt hervor, daß die Anwendung langwelliger Röntgenstrahlen (etwa bei 50 kV Anodenspannung erzeugt) die günstigsten Ergebnisse liefere. Durch Übereinanderschichten verschieden dicker Scheiben läßt sich eine beliebige Knochendicke herstellen. Mit Hilfe einer Apparatur aus Plexiglas können die Weichteile planparallel zusammengedrückt werden. Die Untersuchungen sind an der Diaphyse des Femur durchgeführt worden. Zur Verminderung der Streustrahlung wurde eingeblendet und eine Bucky-Blende benutzt. Die Phantome sind während der Aufnahme senkrecht zur Femurachse angeordnet und überragen den Femurknochen nach beiden Seiten (Abb. 59). Zur Bestimmung *des Durchmessers* der Femurknochen ist eine Aufnahme *in der 2. Ebene* erforderlich. Die Dichtewerte *des Femur* werden photometrisch ermittelt und zu den Dichtewerten des Knochenphantoms in Beziehung gesetzt. Es ist dann möglich, die Dichte des Femur in mm Knochenphantomdicke anzugeben. Dividiert man die äquivalenten mm des Knochenphantoms durch die Dicke der Corticalis, so erhält man eine äquivalente Dicke eines mm der Femurcorticalis in Phantomeinheiten. Wird eine quantitative *chemische* Calcium- und Phosphorbestimmung des Phantommaterials durchgeführt, so kann der Mineralgehalt des Femur *in mg Ca und P/mm³ Femurcorticalis* errechnet werden. In einer 1934 veröffentlichten Arbeit hat HENNY die Faktoren, die für die Dichtemessung eines Filmes von Bedeutung sind, beschrieben. Es wurde ein Densitometer konstruiert, das einen Meßfehler von 2% aufweist. Die Meßfehler werden sorgfältig besprochen. Nach Ermittlung des Kalkgehaltes der Femurdiaphyse gesunder Personen können pathologische Veränderungen schon bei der ersten Untersuchung erkannt werden. Rapide Änderungen des Calciumgehaltes des Skeletes lassen sich wahrscheinlich in den spongiösen Anteilen der Knochen besser erfassen, wofür der proximale Femurabschnitt besonders geeignet erscheint.

Ein Referenzsystem aus *kompaktem Knochen* oder Elfenbein benutzte auch MARCHAL (1948), dessen Methode auf S. 174 beschrieben wurde.

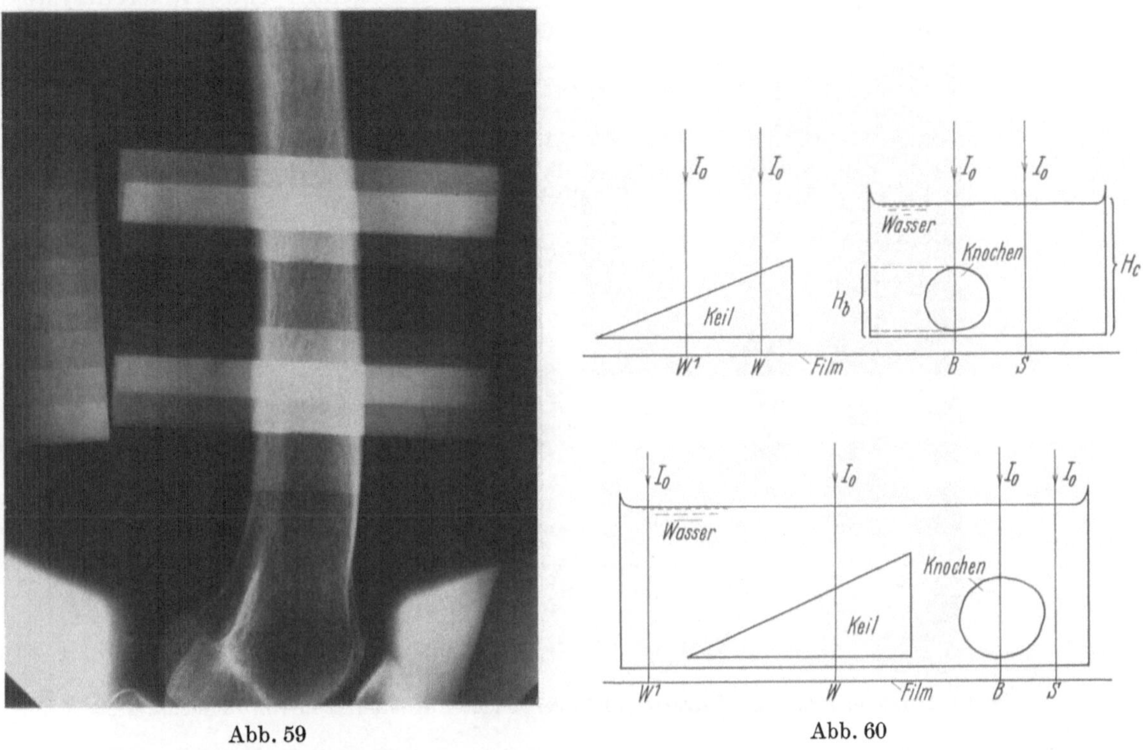

Abb. 59 Abb. 60

Abb. 59. Röntgenaufnahme des Femur zusammen mit den beiden Tafeln aus Rinderknochen, die im rechten Winkel zur Femurlängsachse angeordnet sind. (Nach HENNY, 1948; Abb. 3)

Abb. 60. Schematische Darstellung der Versuchsanordnung des Referenzsystems *außerhalb und innerhalb* eines Wasserbades zur Bestimmung des Streueffektes der Weichteile auf die photometrische Messung des Knochenmineralgehaltes. (Nach JACKSON, 1951; Abb. 3 und 4)

Mit den Problemen der Weichteilabsorption und der Streuung durch die Weichteile bei Knochendichtemessungen hat sich JACKSON (1951) beschäftigt (Abb. 60). Als Vergleichskörper wurde ein *Knochenkeil* aus dem Schaft des Femur eines Ochsen benutzt.

Bei bekannten Dimensionen des Keiles kann aus der Länge die Dichte berechnet werden. Zur Standardisierung der durch die Weichteile bedingten Fehler wurde der Knochenkeil zusammen mit dem zu untersuchenden Skeletabschnitt oder einem Phantom in einem *Wasserbad* geröntgt. Die photometrische Auswertung der Röntgenfilme erfolgte mit einem Weston-Photographic-Photometer, Modell 877. Die Dichte eines bestimmten Knochenbezirkes wurde zu der entsprechenden Dichte des Vergleichskeils in Beziehung gesetzt und die „*äquivalente Keildicke*" (EWT) für den zu untersuchenden Knochen ermittelt. Besondere Untersuchungen sind durchgeführt worden um festzustellen, welchen Einfluß die Anodenspannung und Stromstärke, die Belichtungszeit und Filmemulsion auf die Messungen ausüben können. Ferner ist geprüft worden, welchen Einfluß die Entwicklung der Filme besitzt. Es sind verschiedene Versuche zur Erfassung der durch die Weichteile bedingten Absorption und Streuung angestellt worden, deren Ergebnisse zu einer Ablehnung der „Subtraktionsmethode" der Weichteile, wie sie von BYWATERS (1948) sowie ENGSTRÖM und WELIN (1949) angewendet wurde, führten. Das Absorptionsphänomen durch die Weichteile kann nicht als eine einfache Proportion angesehen werden, da auch der Streueffekt der Weichteile berücksichtigt werden muß. Auch von MACK u. Mitarb. (1949) sind die „Weichteileffekte" beachtet worden, die nur dann vernachlässigt werden können, wenn die Weichteile sehr dünn sind wie z.B. über den Phalangen und dem Calcaneus. Der von HENNY (1950) beschrittene Weg einer Berücksichtigung der Weichteilabsorption vernachlässigt den Streueffekt. Die einfache *Subtraktionsmethode* kann nur begrenzt verwendet werden, so daß die Darstellung eines Referenzsystems zusammen mit dem zu untersuchenden Knochenbezirk im Wasserphantom empfohlen

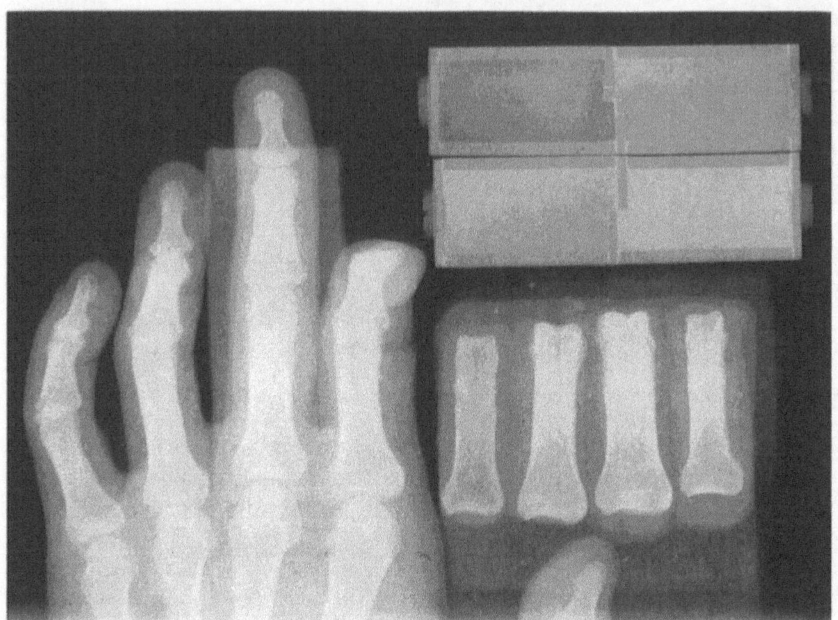

Abb. 61. Darstellung der von VIRTAMA (1957) verwendeten Kombination von Referenzsystemen

wird. Wenn subcutan größere Fettmengen vorhanden sind, so können selbst dadurch Unterschiede auftreten, die beachtet werden sollten.

Versuche zur Bestimmung des Mineralgehaltes im Knochen am lebenden Menschen und Tier haben TARJÀN, SÁNDI und DEÁK (1954) durchgeführt und als Referenzsystem eine *Knochentreppe* oder einen *Knochenkeil* verwendet. Mit Hilfe der vergleichenden Densitometrie von Referenzsystem und interessierendem Knochenareal kann der Mineralgehalt von Knochen *in vivo* gemessen und fortlaufend kontrolliert werden. Die Methode wurde zu Reihenuntersuchungen im Tierexperiment benutzt, um den Mineralgehalt und die Knochenfestigkeit nach Gabe von Citronensäure oder Vitamin D bei unterschiedlicher Calciumdiät an Ratten zu prüfen. Das Verfahren wurde auch zu diagnostischen Zwecken und Kontrolluntersuchungen am Menschen empfohlen.

VIRTAMA (1957) hat Methodik und Ergebnisse seiner Untersuchungen zur Ermittlung des Mineralgehaltes der Knochen aus dem Röntgenbild in einer Monographie zusammengefaßt. Als Vergleichskörper benutzte er *normale Knochen* verschiedener Dicke sowie durch krankhafte Vorgänge *entkalkte Knochen* und ein *Treppenphantom aus Knochenpuder von Rinderknochen* (Abb. 61). Die Phantomknochen wurden in einem besonderen Gemisch aus Paraffin und Bienenwachs zusammen mit Sägespänen (Columbienpaste) eingebettet, um den „Weichteileffekt" zu standardisieren. Unter Umgehung der Photometrie wurde mit Hilfe einer titrimetrischen Methode nach VOLHARD *der Silbergehalt der Emulsion* der Röntgenfilme ermittelt. Der Vorteil der Methode liegt darin, daß die Dichtebestimmung an einer *biologischen Einheit*, nämlich *dem ganzen Knochen* durchgeführt werden kann.

Die Röntgenbilder der zu untersuchenden Fingerphalangen wurden aus dem Film herausgeschnitten. Vor der Silberbestimmung wurde *die Fläche* des Filmes mit Hilfe einer Glasplatte bestimmt, die in 2,5 mm²-Quadrate eingeteilt war. Um die Meßgenauigkeit zu erhöhen, wurden die Aufnahmen zuvor vergrößert. Für die Untersuchungen wurden folienlose Filme benutzt, die einen hohen Silbergehalt besitzen. Zur chemischen Analyse des Silbergehaltes wurde die Emulsion mit 5%iger Salpetersäure vom Filmschichtträger abgelöst und eine Titration gegen 0,05—0,02 n NH_4SCN-Lösung oder KSCN-Lösung durchgeführt. Als Indikator diente $Fe(III)NH_4(SO_4)_2$-Lösung. Bei Zimmertemperatur lag der Fehler der Methode bei 1,5—3,5 mg Ag um 6,7 µg Ag oder wenigstens 0,3%. Die Untersuchungen folienloser Filme ergaben Schwankungen von ± 2 mg/cm². Mit zunehmender Größe der untersuchten Fläche wird die Differenz kleiner. Änderungen der Filmdichte, die nicht durch die Strahlenabsorption zustande kommen, werden auf Änderungen der Spannung, der Entwicklung und der Emulsion des Filmes zurückgeführt. Zur Ausschaltung dieser Fehler wurde ein Referenzsystem verwendet, das aus *Ochsenknochenpulver (in Plexiglasgefäße eingepreßt)* und aus einem *menschlichen Fingerknochen (der in ein Columbien-Paste-Paraffin-Wachs-Sägespäne-Gemisch eingebettet war*, das ähnlich wie die Weichteile absorbiert*)* zusammengesetzt war. Die Anodenspannung während der Aufnahme lag zwischen 40 und 60 kV. Um eine möglichst gleichmäßige Filmschwärzung zu erreichen, wurde eine Entwicklungsmaschine konstruiert und die Herstellungsbedingungen der Filme standardisiert. Mit dieser Methode wurden die *Basalphalangen* von 86 Leichen untersucht. Für jeden Fall sind vier Filme hergestellt worden. In 46 Fällen, in denen wenigstens zwei Filme zuverlässige Werte ergaben, wurde die *dritte Basalphalanx der linken Hand* herausgelöst, von Weichteilen befreit und ihr Volumen mit der spezifischen Gewichtsmethode bestimmt. Durch Veraschen der Knochen bei 850° in 8 Std wurde der Mineralgehalt festgestellt. Diese Werte sind mit den ermittelten Silberwerten verglichen worden. Mit Hilfe einer Formel kann die Knochenasche/cm³ berechnet werden. Der Vergleich der Silberanalysen mit den chemisch-analytisch gefundenen Mineralwerten des Knochens ergab Standardabweichungen von $\pm 3{,}6$%. Als besonderer Vorteil der Bestimmung des Silbergehaltes der Emulsion wird die einfache Ausführbarkeit der Methode genannt. Durch eine *einzige Silberanalyse* kann der Mineralgehalt des *gesamten Knochens* bestimmt werden. Die Ergebnisse der Bestimmung *des Aschegehaltes in g/cm³* sind in Tabellen zusammengestellt. VIRTAMA beobachtete erstmals gewisse Absorptionsunterschiede zwischen den Phantomen und dem Knochen gleichen Aschegehaltes und gleicher Schichtdicke. Er führte diese Unterschiede auf eine *ungleichmäßige Verteilung* des die Röntgenstrahlen am stärksten absorbierenden Stoffes, nämlich des Calciumphosphates zurück. Später hat VIRTAMA (1959) über seine Untersuchungsergebnisse an der *Spongiosa* und der *Compacta von Fingerknochen* berichtet.

Die beschriebenen Untersuchungsmethoden erlauben, die Dichte eines Knochens zu der Dichte des jeweils verwendeten Referenzsystems in Beziehung zu setzen und normale mit krankhaft veränderten Knochen zu vergleichen. Es wurde versucht, die in der praktischen Röntgenologie bisher übliche, unzuverlässige und von subjektiven Faktoren bestimmte Beurteilung des Kalkgehaltes der Knochen auf Grund einer einfachen Betrachtung von Röntgenaufnahmen durch eine objektive Bestimmung der Dichte des Knochens abzulösen. Aus den Werten der vergleichenden Dichtemessungen kann dann auf rechnerischem Wege oder durch chemisch-analytische Vergleichsuntersuchungen der Aschegehalt, der Calciumgehalt oder die Gesamtmenge der anorganischen Kalksalze des Knochens ermittelt werden.

d) Die Messungen mit Referenzsystemen aus definierten, reproduzierbaren Calciumverbindungen

Die *Inkonstanz* der zum Vergleich verwendeten Elfenbeinphantome oder Referenzsysteme aus Knochen bzw. knochenähnlichem Material führte zu der Überlegung, *klar definierte und reproduzierbare Calciumverbindungen* als Vergleichskörper heranzuziehen.

So hat BAUD (1957) ein Verfahren zur Bestimmung des Kalksalzgehaltes der Knochen im makroskopischen und mikroskopischen Bereich beschrieben, bei dem je ein Vergleichskörper aus *Tricalciumphosphat* und Elfenbein Verwendung fand (Abb. 62). Mit Hilfe von $Ca_3(PO_4)_2$-Tabletten wurden sehr gute Resultate erzielt. Es konnte festgestellt werden, daß die Unterschiede des Mineralgehaltes bei pathologischen Veränderungen in den verschiedenen Skeletabschnitten unterschiedlich sind, verglichen mit dem normalen Knochen.

Die Methode von REICH, LEVITIN und FELTON (1958) benutzt als Referenzsystem ein *Calcium-Chlorid-Phantom* mit einer Aluminiumtreppe. Dieses Referenzsystem wird zusammen mit der zu untersuchenden Hand in einem mit Wasser gefüllten Aluminiumgefäß geröntgt (Abb. 63). So konnten Fehler, die durch die Belichtung, die Entwicklung, die Filmemulsion usw. zustande kommen können, weitgehend ausgeschaltet werden. Der

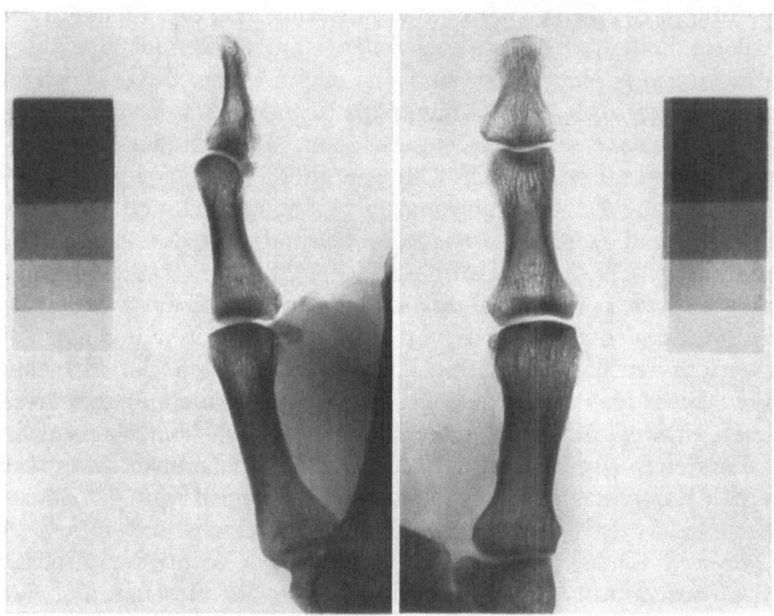

Abb. 62. Röntgenaufnahme des Daumens mit dem Referenzsystem von BAUD (1957, Abb. 2)

Vergleichskörper aus $CaCl_2$ bestand aus einem Kunststoffblock, in den runde Löcher von 1 cm Durchmesser und 1 cm Tiefe gebohrt wurden, die mit $CaCl_2$-Pulver ausgefüllt und mit einer Glasplatte verschlossen wurden. Geringe Absorptionsdifferenzen bestehen lediglich zwischen dem Fettgewebe und den umgebenden Weichteilen. Die Strahlenabsorption durch die Weichteile des Fingers beträgt bei dieser Versuchsanordnung etwa 2% weniger als im freipräparierten Knochen. Die Auswertung der folienlosen Röntgenfilme erfolgte mit einem Kodak-Color-Densitometer vom Diffusionstyp bei einer Meßfläche von 1,25 mm im Durchmesser. Es wurden die *lateralen, proximalen Abschnitte der zweiten Phalanx des Zeigefingers* untersucht. Dieser Knochen besitzt dünne Corticalisschichten und kann gut in einer zweiten Ebene dargestellt werden. Zur Ermittlung des Calciumgehaltes wurden die Knochendichte gegen die Dichtewerte des Calcium-Vergleichskörpers und der Aluminiumtreppe dargestellt und in *mg Ca/mm³ des geprüften Knochens umgerechnet* (Abb. 64a—c). Der durch die Belichtung auftretende Fehler lag unter 2%. Eine Prüfung der Methode durch ein anderes Röntgeninstitut zeigte Schwankungen von annähernd 14%. Die chemisch-analytische Kontrolluntersuchung der geröntgten Knochen ergab Unterschiede zwischen Dichtemessung und chemisch-analytisch ermitteltem Calciumwert von annähernd 15%. Dieser Fehler sei gegenüber dem sonst auftretenden Fehler von etwa 50% gering, so daß die Methode insbesondere für Verlaufskontrollen bei Systemerkrankungen des Knochens empfohlen wird.

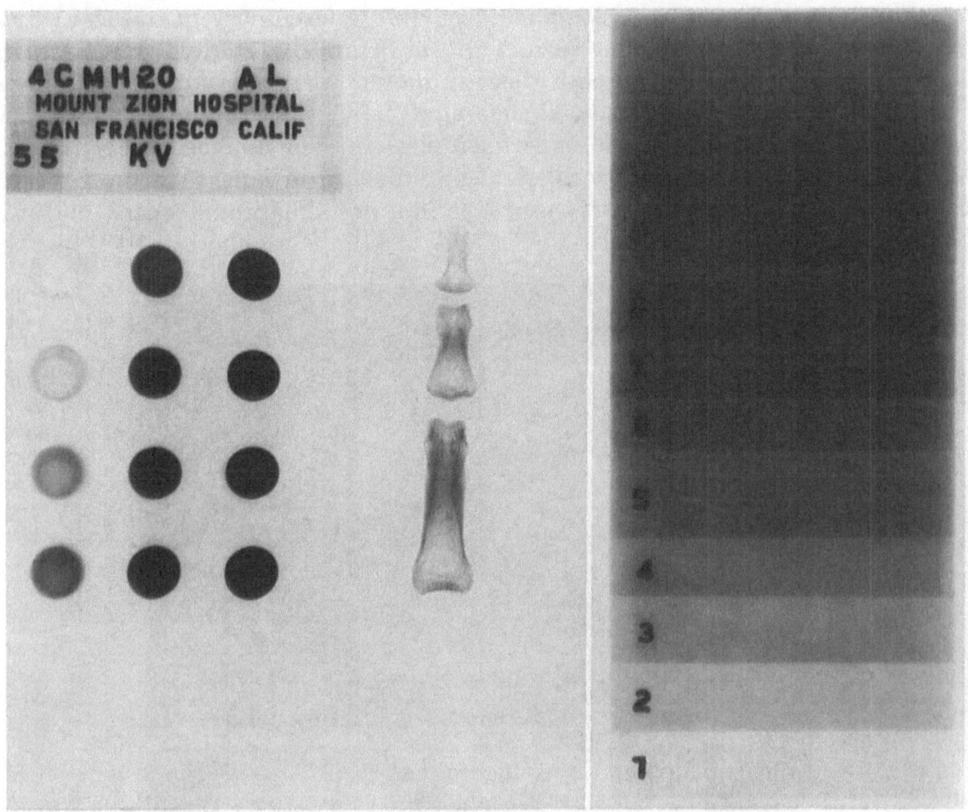

Abb. 63. Beispiel einer Röntgenaufnahme des Referenzsystems von REICH, LEVITIN und FELTON (1958, Abb. 1), bestehend aus einer Aluminiumtreppe und verschiedenen Konzentrationen von Calciumchlorid in einer Kunststoffplatte

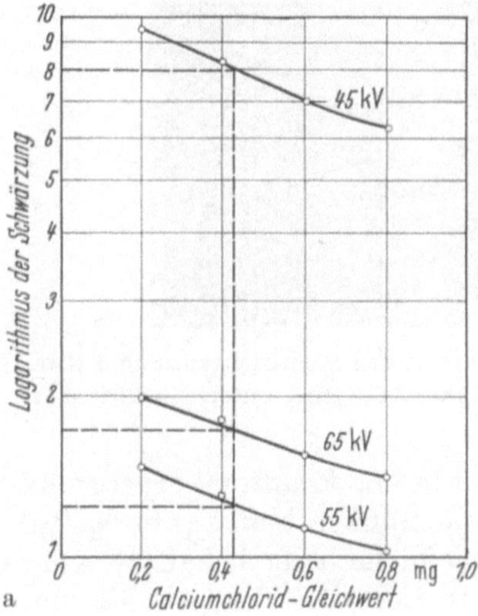

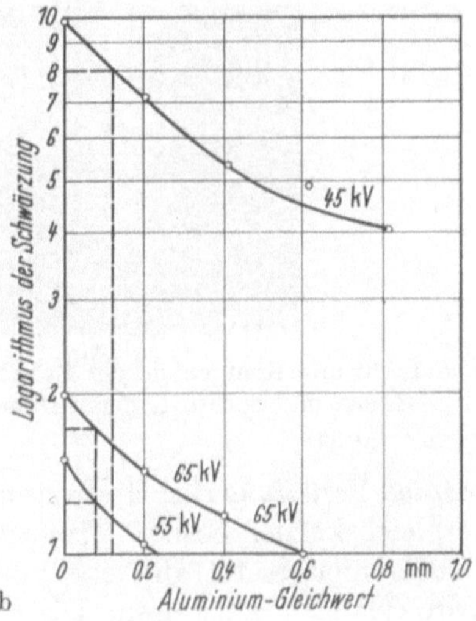

Abb. 64. Darstellung des Einflusses der Strahlenqualität auf die Schwärzungskurve des Calciumchlorid-Referenzsystems (a) und einer Aluminiumtreppe (b). (Nach REICH, LEVITIN und FELTON, 1958; Abb. 2 und 3). c Die zweifache Auswertung eines Röntgenfilmes ergibt nur einen geringen Fehler. (Nach REICH, LEVITIN und FELTON, 1958; Abb. 5 und 6)

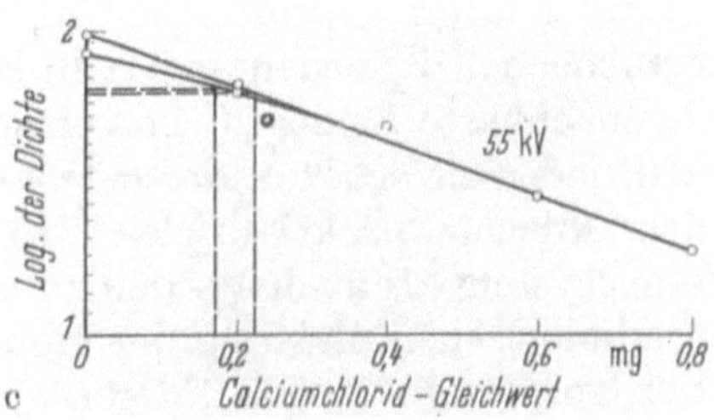

Von HEUCK und SCHMIDT (1954/59/60) ist ein Referenzsystem aus *Hydroxylapatit und Kunstharz* hergestellt worden (Abb. 65). Der Hauptbestandteil der anorganischen Knochensubstanz, der Hydroxylapatit, liegt in diesem Vergleichskörper in Teilchen von der Größenordnung der Spongiosabälkchen und Lamellen vor, da theoretische Überlegungen und Berechnungen sowie experimentelle Untersuchungen ergeben haben, daß die Teilchengröße der stärker absorbierenden Substanz in einer Mischung verschieden absorbierender Stoffe für die Gesamtabsorption des Phantomkörpers und die vergleichenden Messungen nicht belanglos ist (s. S. 149). Besondere Bedeutung hat die

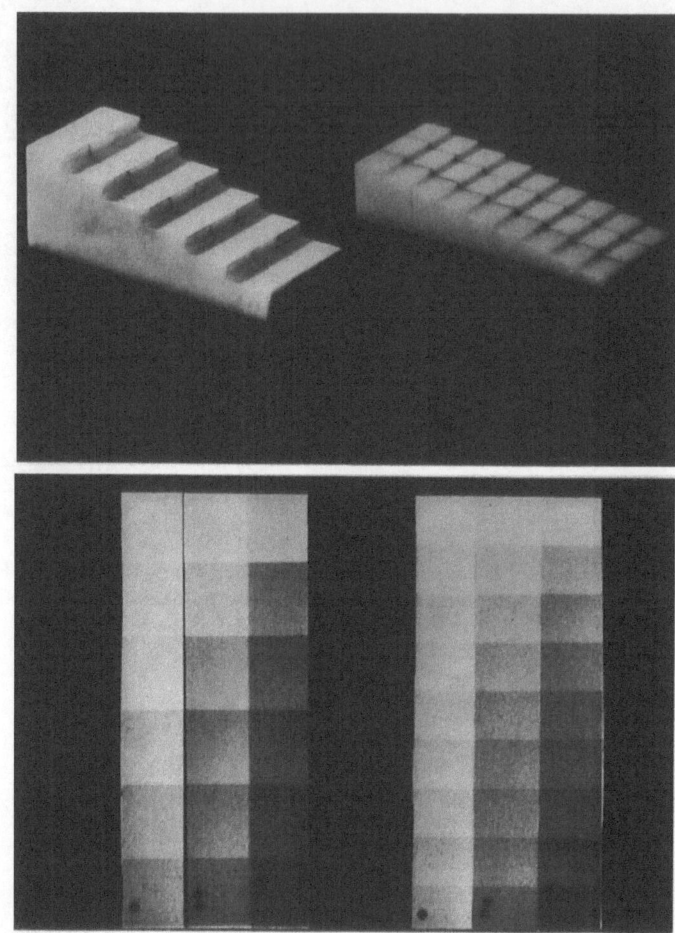

Abb. 65. Aufsicht und Röntgenbild der Referenzsysteme (Treppen aus Hydroxylapatit und Kunstharz) nach HEUCK und SCHMIDT, deren Dimensionen und Konzentrationen unterschiedlich sind

gleichmäßige Verteilung der Hydroxylapatitteilchen in der Phantomkörpergrundsubstanz. Der Vergleichskörper besitzt *Treppenform* und war zunächst aus zwei, später aus drei Teilen zusammengesetzt, die eine jeweils unterschiedliche, aber bekannte Konzentration an Hydroxylapatit aufweisen. Die Apatitkonzentration der Treppenteile wurde durch *chemische Analyse* geprüft. Die *Größe* des Referenzsystems sollte den Dimensionen der zu untersuchenden Knochen angepaßt sein, um den unbekannten Knochen jeweils zwischen zwei benachbarte Schichtdicken einschachteln zu können. Das Referenzsystem besitzt den Vorteil, jederzeit *exakt reproduzierbar* zu sein. In seinen physikalischen Eigenschaften ist es dem Knochen praktisch gleich, so daß sich alle Fehler (s. S. 124—130) sowohl auf das Referenzsystem als auch auf den zu untersuchenden Knochen in gleicher Weise auswirken. Zur radiologischen Messung der globalen Kalksalzkonzentration sollten solche Knochenpartien ausgewählt werden, deren gegenüberliegende Flächen planparallel begrenzt sind.

Von Heuck und Schmidt wurden die spongiösen Partien des Femurhalses und des Calcaneus, später auch des Radius (Quintar 1962) untersucht (Abb. 66, 67, 68).

Zur Berücksichtigung der Weichteilüberlagerung erfolgte die Untersuchung des Calcaneus zunächst in einem Wasserbad. Die in den Weichteilen vorhandenen Fettgewebsanteile ergeben geringe Absorptionsdifferenzen (s. S. 151), spielen jedoch im Gesamtfehler keine entscheidende Rolle. Eine bessere Angleichung der Absorptionsunterschiede durch Fett und Muskulatur kann mit 70%igem Alkohol erreicht werden. Die Untersuchung des Radius erfolgte ebenfalls im Wasserbad oder Alkoholbad. Für die

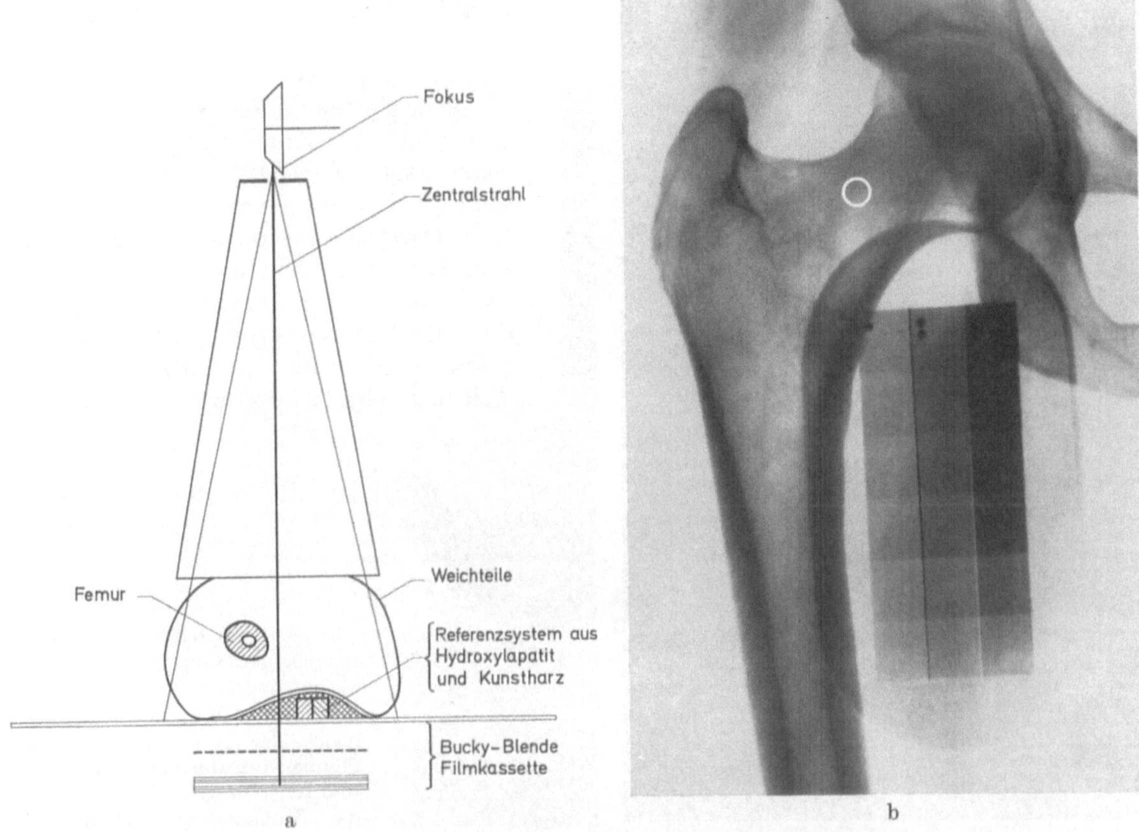

Abb. 66. Schematische Darstellung der Aufnahmeanordnung von (a) Oberschenkel und Referenzsystem und (b) Röntgenaufnahme des proximalen Femurabschnittes mit Apatittreppe. (Nach Heuck und Schmidt, 1960; Abb. 5 und 12)

Untersuchung des Femurhalses wurde die Hydroxylapatittreppe zum Ausgleich der Rundung des Oberschenkels in einen stumpfen Keil aus Paraffin oder Columbienpaste (Paraffin, Bienenwachs und Sägespäne), deren Strahlenabsorption der der Weichteile ähnlich ist, eingebettet und dieses Phantom unter die Weichteile des Oberschenkels gelegt. Auf diese Weise drücken die Weichteile des Oberschenkels fest auf das Phantom, so daß die aufliegenden Bezirke glatt begrenzt sind. Zur Erzielung einer gleichmäßigen Dicke des Oberschenkels wurde von der Röhrenseite her mit einem Spezialtubus komprimiert (Abb. 66a). Der Oberschenkelweichteilschatten überlagert somit gleichzeitig auch das Referenzsystem.

Die Röntgenaufnahmen können mit *jeder in der Medizin gebräuchlichen Röntgenapparatur* hergestellt werden. Die Röhre sollte einen möglichst kleinen Fokus besitzen. Die verwendete Strahlenqualität sollte so beschaffen sein, daß *möglichst große Absorptionsdifferenzen* erhalten werden. Eine Filterung der erzeugten Strahlung durch ein mindestens 2 mm dickes Aluminiumfilter ist erforderlich. Die Aufnahmen des Calcaneus und Radius wurden mit einer Anodenspannung von 50—60 kV hergestellt. Für die Untersuchung des Femurhalses ist eine höhere Spannung erforderlich. Der Objekt-Film-Abstand betrug bei Verwendung eines handelsüblichen Buckytisches etwa 10—20 cm und Verwendung eines Vertigraphen (stehendes Buckyblenden-Stativ) etwa 10—15 cm, so daß diese Aufnahmeanordnung bereits ausreichend den von Spiegler (1959) geforderten Bedingungen eines größeren Objekt-Film-Abstandes zur Verminderung des weichen, langwelligen Streustrahlenanteiles Rechnung trägt (s. S. 165).

Die Bedeutung der verschiedenen Filmmaterialien, der Entwicklungszeit, der verwendeten Folien sowie der Änderung der Strahlenqualität und der Einfluß der Streustrahlenblende auf das Meßergebnis wurden sorgfältig untersucht. Alle Störfaktoren lassen sich ausschalten, da sie in gleicher Weise auf den Schwärzungswert des Knochens wie auf den Schwärzungswert des Referenzsystemes Einfluß haben. Durch die gleichzeitige Darstellung von Referenzsystem und Knochen können jederzeit *reproduzierbare Werte* gewonnen werden, wenn die Strahlenexposition Schwärzungswerte ergibt, die auf dem linearen Teil der Gradationskurve des Filmes liegen. Diese Forderung muß bei dem Verfahren zur Bestimmung des „Apatitwertes" unbedingt eingehalten werden.

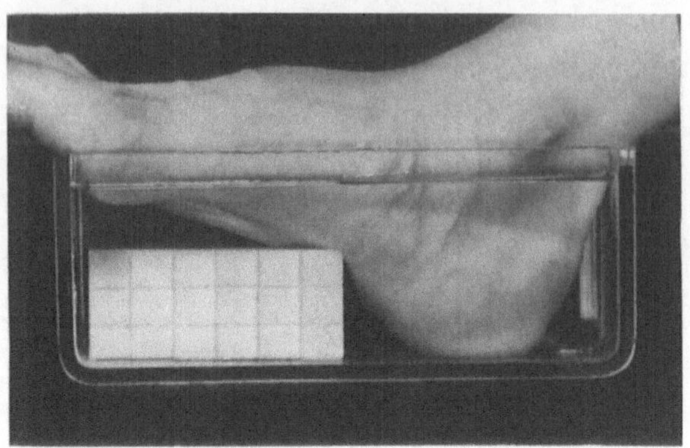

a

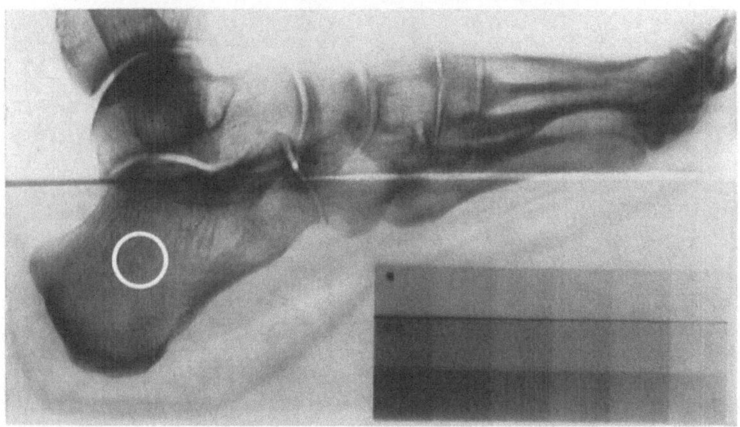

b

Abb. 67. Darstellung der Aufnahmeanordnung von Referenzsystem und Calcaneus im Wasserbad (oder Alkoholbad) zum Ausgleich der Weichteile (a) und Röntgenaufnahme von Calcaneus und Referenzsystem zur Messung der Kalksalzkonzentration (b). (Nach Heuck und Schmidt, 1960; Abb. 7 und 8)

Die Auswertung der Röntgenfilme wurde mit einem Spezialphotometer der Firma Lange vorgenommen. Der Verlauf der Schwärzungskurven der Apatittreppen hängt von der Konzentration des Hydroxylapatit in der organischen Substanz ab. Die photometrisch erhaltenen Schwärzungswerte werden in ein Koordinatensystem eingetragen, und zwar die Schwärzungswerte auf der Ordinate und Schichtdicke der Treppen auf der Abszisse (Abb. 69). So erhält man die Schwärzungskurven der Treppenteile unterschiedlichen Apatitgehaltes. Der Abstand von benachbarten Schwärzungskurven ist gegeben durch die Differenz der Treppen an Hydroxylapatit in der Volumeneinheit. Dann wird die durch eine Aufnahme in der zweiten Ebene gewonnene Schichtdicke des Knochens gegen den Schwärzungswert der zu untersuchenden Knochenregion ebenfalls in das Koordinatensystem eingetragen. Der Abstand von zwei Schwärzungskurven der Hydroxylapatittreppen voneinander entspricht der bekannten Differenz dieser beiden Treppen an Hydroxylapatit. Liegt der Schwärzungswert des Knochens zwischen diesen beiden Werten,

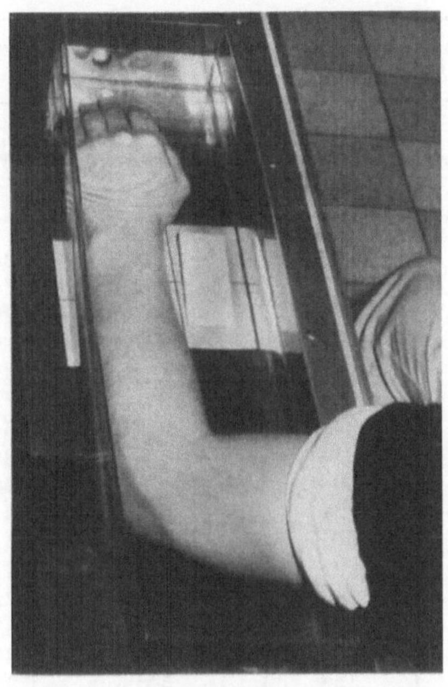

a

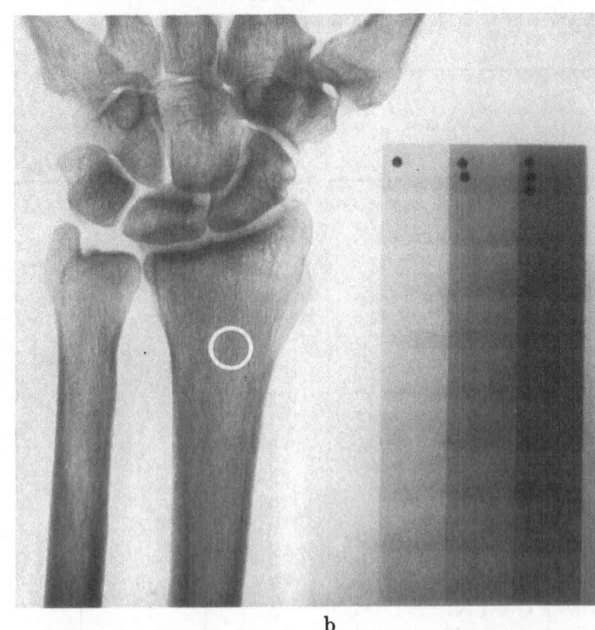

b

Abb. 68. Aufnahmeanordnung von Unterarm und Referenzsystem im Wasserbad (oder Alkoholbad) (a) und Darstellung von Radius und Referenzsystem auf einem Röntgenfilm (b). (Nach QUINTAR, 1962; Abb. 4 und 5)

so muß auch sein Gehalt an Hydroxylapatit zwischen den Werten der beiden Treppen liegen. Da sich *alle möglichen Fehler* während des Untersuchungsganges *sowohl auf das Referenzsystem* als auch auf den zu *untersuchenden Knochen* auswirken, können sie weitgehend vernachlässigt werden. Der durch den photometrischen Meßvorgang selbst bedingte Fehler kann durch wiederholte Messungen und *Bestimmung des Mittelwertes* im Endergebnis klein gehalten werden. Eine größere Fehlerquelle kann in einer *ungenauen Messung* des zu untersuchenden Knochendurchmessers liegen. Die Aufnahme in der zweiten Ebene muß *exakt* eingestellt werden und der Vergrößerungsfaktor ist bei jeder Messung zu berücksichtigen! Die zur Untersuchung verwendeten Knochenzonen von Femurhals, Calcaneus und Radius sind in den Abb. 66, 67, 68 markiert. Mit dieser Methode kann *jeder Skeletabschnitt* auf seinen Mineralgehalt untersucht werden.

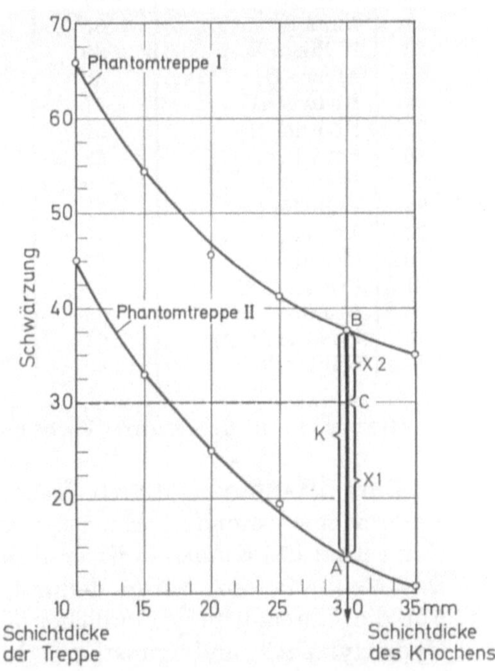

Abb. 69. Schematische Darstellung zur Auswertung der Röntgenaufnahmen und Berechnung der Kalksalzkonzentration im untersuchten Knochenbezirk. (Nach HEUCK und SCHMIDT, 1960; Abb. 13)

Die *Fehlerbreite* der Methode von HEUCK und SCHMIDT (1954/59/60) wurde an 34 Patienten ermittelt, bei denen der Mineralgehalt des Knochens intravitam mit dem später *post-mortal* aus dem Knochenpräparat chemisch-analytisch ermittelten Mineralgehalt verglichen wurde (Tabelle 10). Die Abweichung der chemisch-analytischen Kontrolluntersuchung von den photometrisch ermittelten Werten betrug max. $\pm 10\%$ (Abb. 70), die Standardabweichung war noch geringer. Diese Kontrolle erlaubt Aussagen über die Gesamtfehlerbreite der Methode und gibt somit ein Urteil über ihre Brauchbarkeit in der klinischen Radiologie.

Tabelle 10. *Kontrolle des radiologisch gemessenen Mineralgehaltes im Gesamtvolumen des spongiösen Knochenanteils von Femurhals und Calcaneus durch die chemische Analyse von Autopsiematerial in 34 Fällen („knochengesunde" und „knochenkranke" Personen)*

Nr.	Name	Alter	Geschlecht	Chemisch ermittelter Wert in mg/ml	Photometrisch ermittelter Wert in mg/ml	Abweichung des photometrischen Wertes vom chemisch ermittelten Wert	
						in mg/ml	in %
1.	Erika P.	7	f	253	232	−21	−8,25
2.	Renate S. . . .	13	f	224	210	−14	−6,25
3.	Paul S.	23	m	376	360	−16	−4,25
4.	Lisa P.	24	f	343	339	− 4	−1,16
5.	Karl J.	26	m	420	419	− 1	−0,25
6.	Arno K.	32	m	276	274	− 2	−0,73
7.	Gerd H.	34	m	368	370	+ 2	+0,56
8.	Frieda S. . . .	39	f	208	214	+ 6	+2,88
9.	Gerda V.	43	f	297	280	−17	−5,75
10.	Paul H.	46	m	247	222	−25	−5,6
11.	Rudolf W. . . .	49	m	297	305	+ 8	+2,7
12.	Hermann P. . .	51	m	280	292	+12	+4,3
13.	Dora B.	54	f	296	285	−11	−3,72
14.	Kurt K.	55	m	317	311	− 6	−1,88
15.	Hermann M. . .	57	m	303	304	+ 1	+0,36
16.	Gerd K.	57	m	327	322	− 5	−1,36
17.	Erich W. . . .	61	m	368	365	− 3	−0,82
18.	Karl C.	62	m	260	251	− 9	−3,46
19.	Marie R.	62	f	226	247	+21	+9,3
20.	Otto C.	64	m	207	219	+12	+5,8
21.	Anna S.	65	f	431	438	+ 7	+1,64
22.	Wilhelm B. . . .	65	m	355	328	−27	−7,6
23.	Albert G. . . .	66	m	292	280	−12	−4,1
24.	Hedwig H. . . .	67	f	375	370	− 5	−1,36
25.	Heinrich D. . .	67	m	363	343	−20	−5,5
26.	Paul R.	68	m	397	402	+ 5	+1,26
27.	Heinz M.	70	m	252	259	+ 7	+2,8
28.	Wilhelm C. . . .	71	m	393	409	+16	+4,08
29.	August H. . . .	75	m	223	204	−19	−8,5
30.	Hermann S. . .	77	m	300	304	+ 4	+1,36
31.	Friedrich C. . .	85	m	242	226	−16	−6,6
32.	Bruno W.*) . .	55	m	251	243	− 8	−3,4
33.	Friedrich C.*) . .	64	m	246	258	+12	+8,2
34.	Günter R. . . .	60	m	390	352	−38	−9,75

*) Calcaneus

[HEUCK, F., u. E. SCHMIDT: Fortschr. Röntgenstr. **93**, 761 (1960), Tab. 8]

Durch HANSEN u. Mitarb. (1961) ist für die Untersuchung von Säuglingen und Kleinkindern eine besondere Einrichtung entwickelt worden, die es erlaubt, gleichzeitig die Extremität des Kindes zu fixieren und den Calcaneus im Wasserbad zu röntgen (Abb. 71). Das Meßverfahren wurde dadurch auch in der Pädiatrischen Radiologie anwendbar. Für die Untersuchung kindlicher Knochen war es erforderlich, das Referenzsystem aus Hydroxylapatit und Kunstharz durch eine dritte Treppe zu erweitern, deren Apatitkonzentration niedriger war. Dem Volumen des kindlichen Knochens entsprechend mußten auch kleinere Treppen hergestellt werden.

Nach vorangegangenem gründlichem Studium der Chemie der Knochencalciumphosphate sind HEUCK und SCHMIDT (1960) zu der Überzeugung gelangt, daß die Bestimmung der Konzentration des Hydroxylapatit in der Volumeneinheit Knochengewebe eine *Verständigung verschiedener Untersucher* auf einheitlicher Basis erlaubt. Wenn die Konzentration des Hydroxylapatit pro ml Knochensubstanz bei Patienten mit Knochenerkrankungen bestimmt werden kann, so ist es möglich, aus diesem Wert den *Calciumgehalt*, den *Aschegehalt* oder auch das *spezifische Gewicht* der Knochen zu berechnen, da die

Zusammensetzung der organischen Knochengrundsubstanz und des Knochenmarkes annähernd konstant sind und das Volumen des organischen Teiles im Knochengewebe aus dem Gesamtvolumen und dem Apatitvolumen berechnet werden kann. Es wird daher empfohlen, den „*Apatitwert*“ des Knochens als *neuen* Begriff in die klinische Radiologie einzuführen. Die *praktische Anwendung* der Meßmethode in der klinischen Radiologie und die bisher am menschlichen Skelet ermittelten „Apatitwerte“ des gesunden und kranken Knochens werden später ausführlicher beschrieben (s. S. 218).

Das Prinzip der radiologischen Meßmethode des Knochenkalksalzgehaltes von Heuck und Schmidt (1954/59/60) wurde in der *Veterinärmedizin* durch Priboth, Börnert und Fritzsche (1966) praktisch angewendet. Die Untersuchungen wurden am *7. Schwanz-*

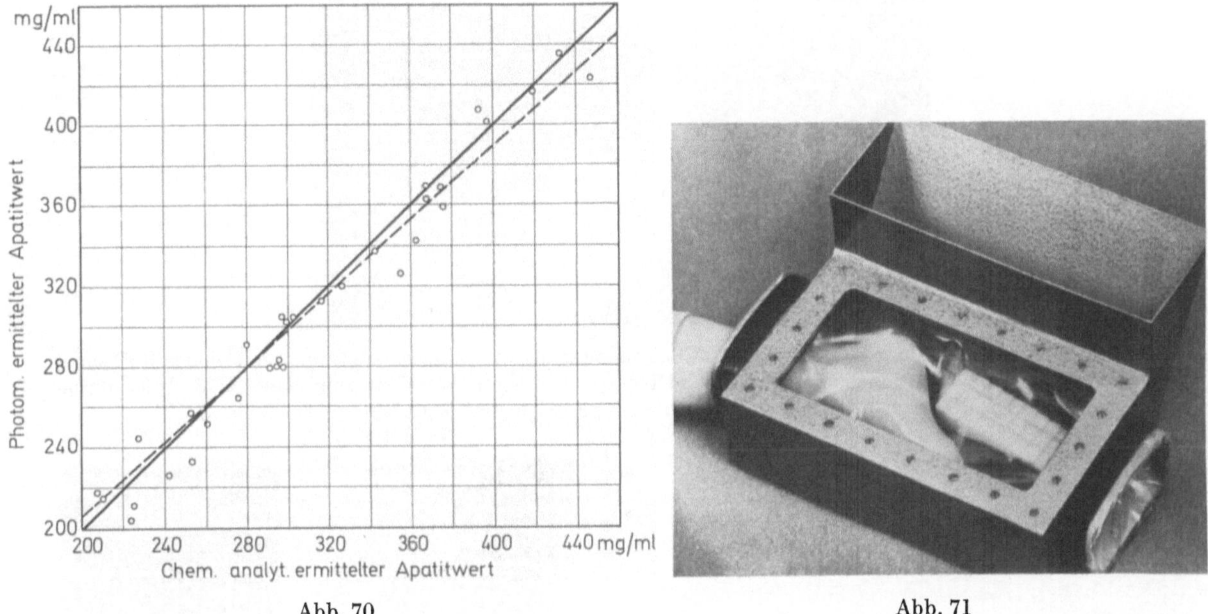

Abb. 70 Abb. 71

Abb. 70. Vergleich der photometrisch bestimmten Mineralkonzentration im Knochen mit der postmortal im entsprechenden Bezirk durchgeführten chemisch-analytischen Bestimmung des Kalksalzgehaltes. (Nach Heuck und Schmidt, 1960; Abb. 24). Die gestrichelte Linie stellt die Regressionsgrade nach statistischer Auswertung dar

Abb. 71. Aufnahmeanordnung des kindlichen Fußes in einer besonderen Halterung (Plexiglaskasten mit Wasser) zusammen mit dem Referenzsystem zur Darstellung des Calcaneus. (Die Aufnahme wurde freundlicherweise von Hansen zur Verfügung gestellt)

wirbel junger Rinder durchgeführt. Die proximale Diaphyse dieses Wirbels erwies sich wegen der parallel zueinander verlaufenden seitlichen Begrenzungen als günstiges Untersuchungsobjekt. Der Vergleichskörper wurde aus drei fest miteinander verbundenen treppenförmigen Teilen zusammengesetzt. Er bestand aus Knochenasche der Rinderknochenspongiosa die in ein Kunstharz (Piacryl) einpolymerisiert wurde. Die Konzentration an Knochenasche in jedem der 3 Teile des Vergleichskörpers ist unterschiedlich. (Teil I enthält 325 mg/ml, Teil II enthält 227 mg/ml, Teil III enthält 86 mg/ml Knochenasche.) Der Vergleichskörper war 9,5 cm lang und 3,2 cm breit. Die oberste Stufe war 2 cm hoch. Die einzelnen Treppenstufen des Vergleichskörpers haben eine Höhe von 2 mm, die unterste Stufe beginnt mit einer Höhe von 4 mm. Die erforderliche Eichung des Vergleichskörpers wurde auf chemisch-analytischem Wege exakt durchgeführt.

Zur Berücksichtigung der den Knochen umgebenden Weichteile wurde der Schwanz in einem mit Wasser gefüllten Plexiglasgefäß mit einer Strahlung von 60 kV Anodenspannung und einer Stromstärke von 12 mA bei einem Fokus-Filmabstand von 1,5 m geröntgt (Abb. 72). Zuvor wurde der 7. Schwanzwirbel durch Abzählen mit einem Bleidraht markiert. Die Schichtdicke des Wirbels wurde durch eine Aufnahme in der 2. Ebene ermittelt, die exakt durchgeführt werden muß. Bei Messung der Schichtdicke ist der Vergrößerungsfaktor zu berücksichtigen, der etwa 6% betrug. Die photometrische Aus-

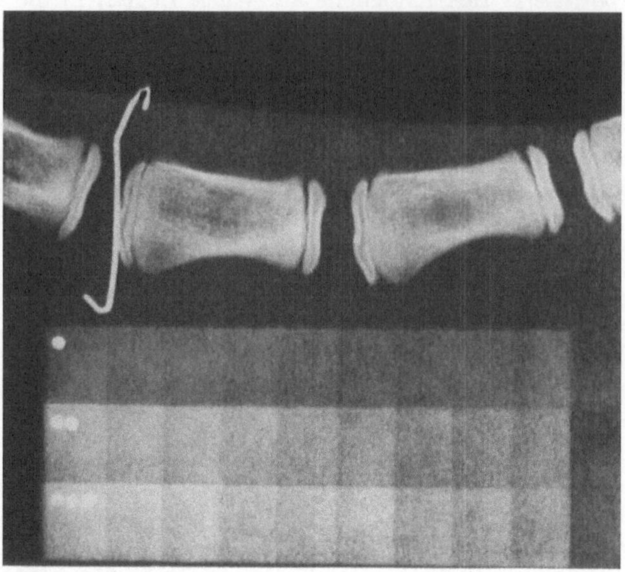

Abb. 72. Beispiel einer Röntgenaufnahme des 7. Schwanzwirbels von Rindern zusammen mit einem Referenzsystem aus Knochenasche und einem Kunststoff. Die proximale Epiphyse (Meßregion) des 7. Wirbels ist durch einen Bleidraht markiert. (Nach PRIBOTH, BÖRNERT und FRITZSCHE, 1966; Abb. 3)

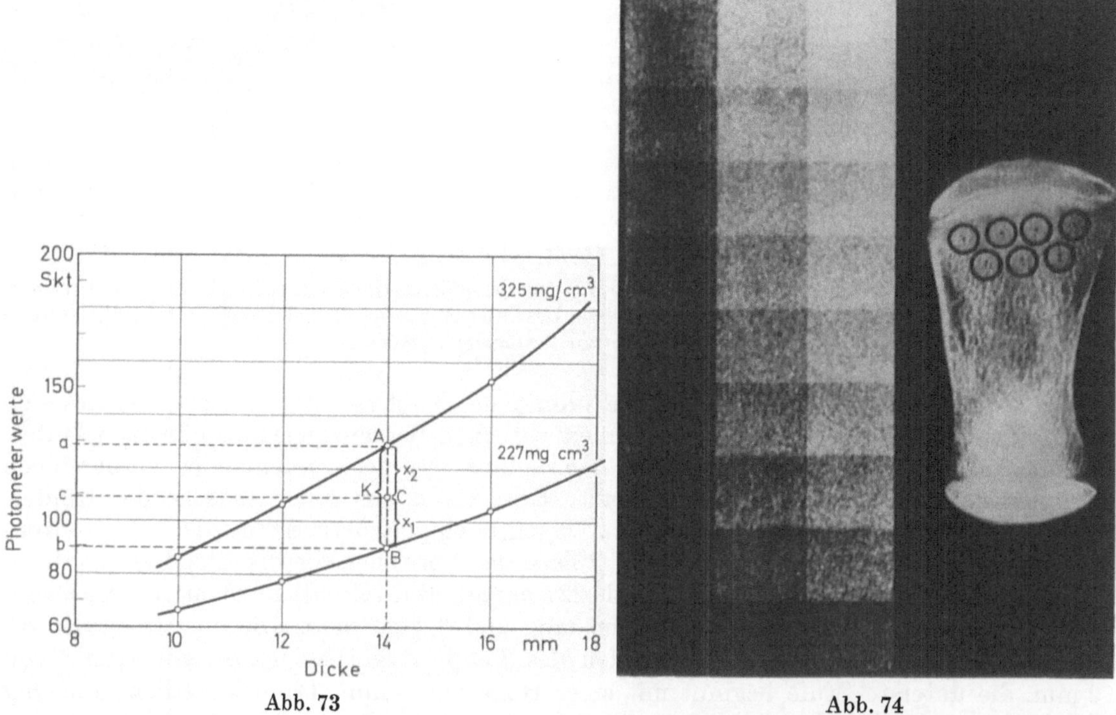

Abb. 73 Abb. 74

Abb. 73. Eichkurven zur Berechnung des Aschegehaltes im Knochen des 7. Schwanzwirbels von Rindern. (Nach PRIBOTH, BÖRNERT und FRITZSCHE, 1966; Abb. 7)

Abb. 74. Röntgenbild eines isolierten 7. Schwanzwirbelknochens mit dem verwendeten Referenzsystems aus Rinderknochenasche. Die hier zur Photometrie verwendeten Knochenbezirke sind durch Kreise markiert. (Nach PRIBOTH, BÖRNERT und FRITZSCHE, 1966; Abb. 8)

wertung erfolgt in ähnlicher Weise wie es HEUCK und SCHMIDT (1960) angeben. Zunächst werden die zwei oder drei Teile des Referenzsystems stufenweise photometriert und die Meßwerte graphisch dargestellt. Es entstehen dabei zwei Kurven (Abb. 73). Auf der Abszisse ist die Dicke (Höhe) der Stufen des Referenzsystems in Millimeter angegeben, auf der Ordinate der zur jeweiligen Stufe gehörende Photometermeßwert in Skaleneinheiten. Dann wird der interessierende Knochenabschnitt an mehreren Punkten photometriert (Abb. 74). Aus den erhaltenen Skalenteilenwerten errechnet man den Mittelwert. Dieser wird an dem Abszissenwert ins Koordinatensystem eingetragen, der der Dicke des untersuchten Knochens an der Untersuchungsstelle entspricht. Die Mineralkonzentration wird dann berechnet.

Zur Kontrolle der röntgenologisch-photometrisch ermittelten Werte wurden die entsprechenden Knochenproben aus der proximalen Diaphyse des 7. Schwanzwirbels entnommen und chemisch analysiert. Die Volumenbestimmung der Knochenprobe erfolgte auf pyknometrischem Wege. In Tabelle 11 sind die röntgenologisch-photometrischen und die chemisch-analytisch bestimmten Werte der Mineralkonzentration (Aschegehalt) in der proximalen Diaphyse des 7. Schwanzwirbels vom Rind dargestellt. Bei Verwendung folienloser Filme fanden sich Differenzen zwischen den Werten von maximal 8,5%, während bei Verwendung von Folienfilmen Abweichungen bis zu 10,4% festgestellt werden konnten. Den Fehlermöglichkeiten wurde im einzelnen nachgegangen. Die von 29 gesunden Jungrindern röntgenologisch-photometrisch ermittelten Aschenwerte der proximalen Diaphyse des 7. Schwanzwirbels lagen zwischen 222 und 385 mg/ml. Untersuchungen von kranken Tieren ergaben eine Verminderung der Kalksalzkonzentration (oder Aschewerte) im Knochen.

Tabelle 11. *Kontrolle des röntgenologisch-photometrisch „in vivo" ermittelten quantitativen Aschegehaltes der proximalen Diaphyse des 7. Schwanzwirbels durch die chemische Analyse bei 29 klinisch gesunden, 8-12 Monate alten Jungmastbullen*

Lfd. Nr.	Chemisch ermittelter Wert mg/cm³	Photometrisch ermittelter Wert mg/cm³	Abweichung der photometrisch ermittelten Werte vom chemischen Wert	
			mg/cm³	%
1	335	340	+ 5	+ 1,5
2	224	240	+16	+ 7,1
3	342	385	+43	+12,6
4	365	375	+10	+ 2,7
5	309	283	−26	− 8,4
6	238	222	−16	− 6,7
7	229	222	− 7	− 3,1
8	273	243	−30	−11,0
9	257	264	+ 7	+ 2,7
10	246	230	−16	− 6,5
11	280	291	+11	+ 3,9
12	271	300	+29	+10,7
13	279	268	−11	− 3,9
14	261	255	− 6	− 2,3
15	280	283	+ 3	+ 1,1
16	325	285	−40	−12,3
17	322	315	− 7	− 2,2
18	311	340	+29	+ 9,3
19	305	291	−14	− 4,6
20	287	281	− 6	− 2,1
21	285	319	+34	+11,9
22	292	301	+ 9	+ 3,1
23	343	372	+29	+ 8,5
24	368	380	+12	+ 3,3
25	381	371	−10	− 2,6
26	386	375	−11	− 2,9
27	375	381	+ 6	+ 1,6
28	313	351	+38	+12,1
29	354	342	−12	− 3,4

[PRIBOTH, W., D. BÖRNERT u. H. FRITZSCHE: Zbl. Vet.-Med. **13** A, 628 (1966), Tab. 5]

Von OKUYAMA (1965) wurden radiologische Messungen des Knochenmineralgehaltes unter Verwendung eines reproduzierbaren, knochengleichen Referenzsystems nach dem Prinzip der Methode von HEUCK und SCHMIDT (1954/59/60) bestehend aus einer Mischung von *Calciumphosphat und Calciumkarbonat* in Kunststoff (Methylmetacrylat) eingebettet (Abb. 75) — mit Hilfe direkter Strahlenmessungen (s. S. 134) und photometrischer Messungen von Röntgenfilmen durchgeführt. Als Meßort wurden zwei Knochenzonen der *distalen Ulna*, etwa 3 und 4 cm proximal vom Handgelenk gewählt (Abb. 76). Die Aufnahmeanordnung von Strahlenquelle, Unterarm und Referenzsystem in einem Wasserbad (zum Ausgleich der Weichteilabsorption) war für die Röntgenaufnahmen die

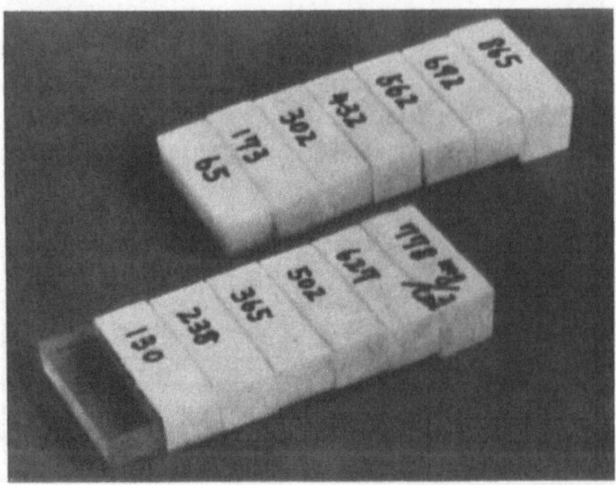

Abb. 75. Die Referenzsysteme aus Calciumphosphat und Calciumcarbonat in einem Kunststoff, wie sie von Okuyama (1965, Abb. 12) entwickelt worden sind

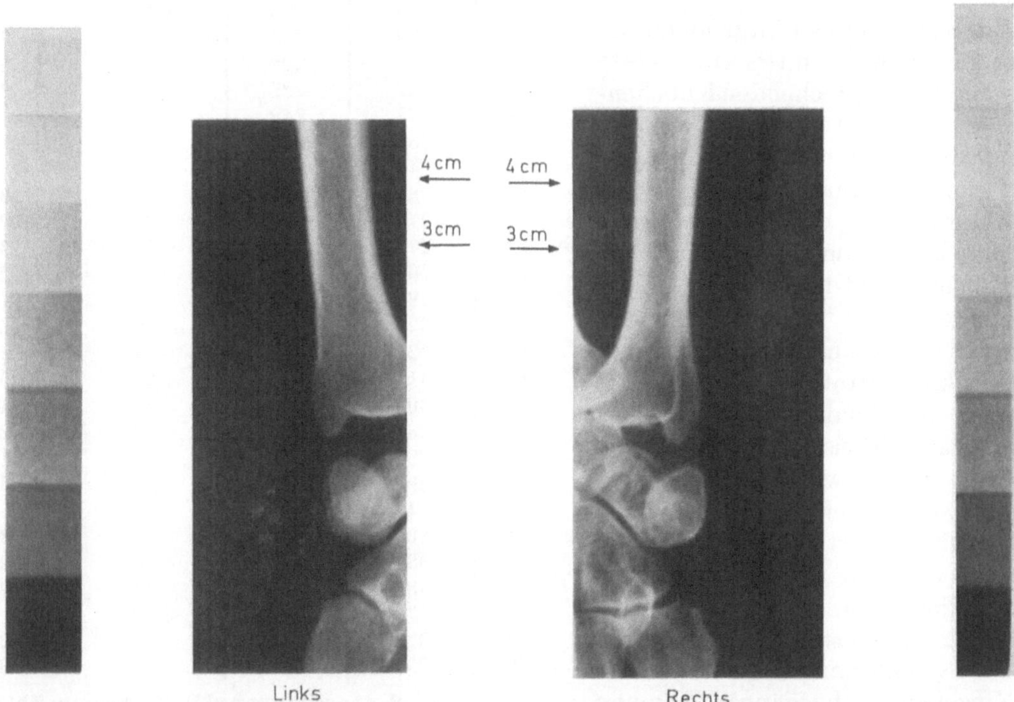

Abb. 76. Röntgenaufnahme der distalen Ulnaregion zusammen mit dem Referenzsystem zur Messung des Knochenkalksalzgehaltes. (Nach Okuyama, 1965; Abb. 17)

gleiche wie für die Strahlenabsorptionsmessungen (s. S. 133, Abb. 20). Mit Hilfe einer besonderen objektnahen Bleiblende wurde versucht, die störende Streustrahlung zu vermindern (Abb. 77a und b). Aus dem gleichen Grunde wurde nach der Groedelschen Abstandstechnik zwischen Filmkassette und Wasserphantom ein Abstand von 20 cm gewählt. Jeder einzelne Meßwert der Zone 3 und 4 cm proximal vom Processus styloideus ulnae wurde aus mehreren Photometerwerten im Bereich der Meßzone als *Mittelwert* errechnet. Die Photometerwerte werden gegen den Calcium- und Phosphorgehalt des Referenzsystems (in mg/ml bekannt als E.M.C. = „Equivalent Mineral Contents") zusammen mit den Meßwerten der Ulna in ein Koordinatensystem eingetragen. Aus diesem Schema kann dann die Mineralkonzentration der zu untersuchenden Knochen direkt abgelesen werden (Abb. 78). Die densitometrisch gefundene Kalksalzkonzentration der Ulna bei

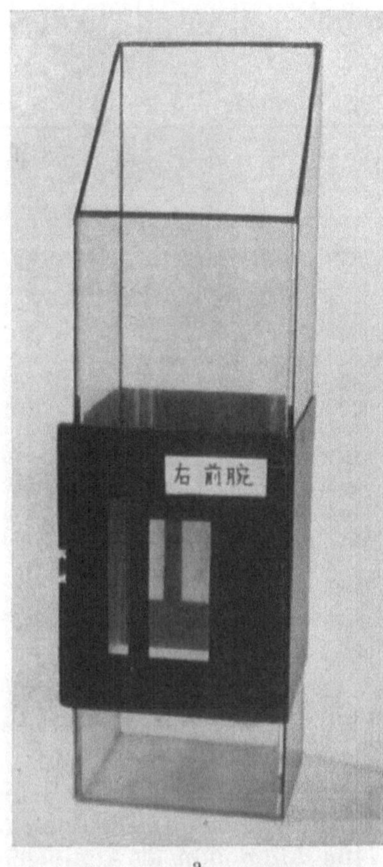

a

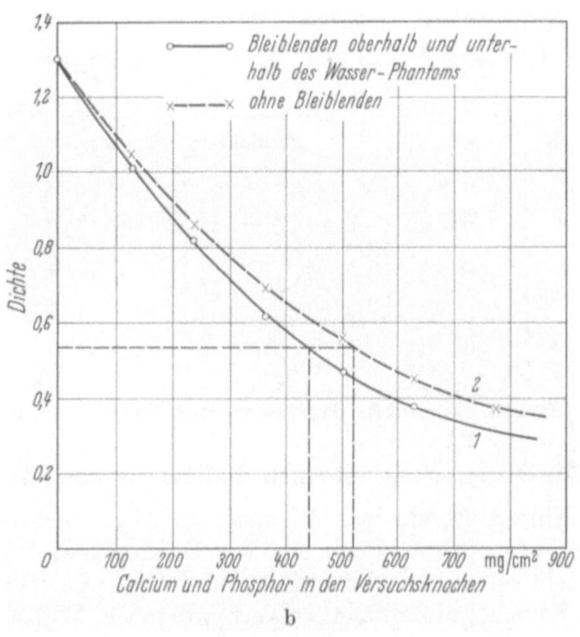

b

Abb. 77. Plexiglaskasten mit objektnaher Bleiblende zur Verminderung der Streustrahlung. (Nach OKUYAMA, 1960; Abb. 15.) Der Einfluß der Bleiblende auf das Meßergebnis ist in Abb. 77b dargestellt. (Nach OKUYAMA, 1965; Abb. 13)

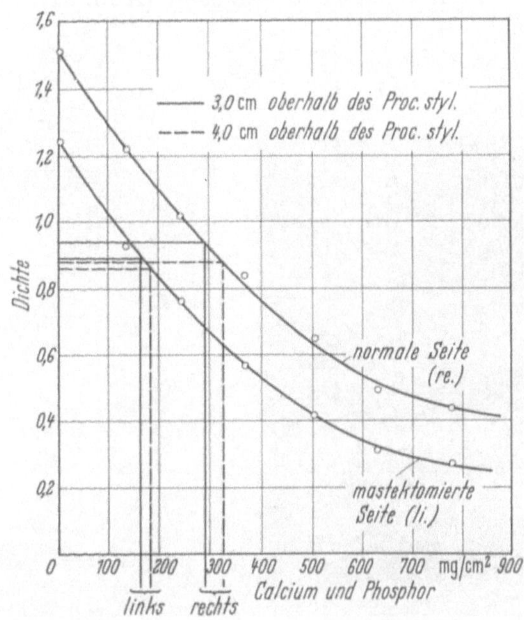

Abb. 78. Schematische Darstellung der Eichkurven des Referenzsystems zusammen mit den Meßwerten 3 und 4 cm oberhalb des Processus styloideus ulnae am Beispiel einer diffusen Atrophie der Knochen des linken Armes nach Mamma-Amputation. (Nach OKUYAMA, 1965; Abb. 18)

Gesunden schwankt zwischen 260 und 400 mg/ml. Von ADACHI und OKUYAMA (1966) werden einige Meßergebnisse vorgelegt (Tabelle 12).

Tabelle 12. *Einige Ergebnisse der Messungen des Mineralgehaltes der Ulna bei Gesunden*

Fall	Alter und Geschlecht	Beruf	Meßpunkt proximal vom Proc. styloid. in cm	Äquivalenter Mineralgehalt in mg/cm² E.M.C.	Dicke der Ulna in cm	Mineralgehalt in mg/cm³
W. K.	31, ♂	med.-techn. Ass.	re. 3	360	1,23	293
			4	380	1,23	310
			li. 3	333	1,19	281
			4	363	1,21	300
A. N.	17, ♂	Student	re. 3	346	1,20	288
			4	360	1,12	321
S. T.	32, ♂	Arzt	re. 3	394	1,16	339
			4	424	1,14	372
			li. 3	357	1,16	308
			4	417	1,15	363
T. O.	32, ♂	Arzt	re. 3	395	1,20	330
			4	433	1,21	358

[ADACHI, T., and T. OKUYAMA: Bull. Tokyo med. dent. Univ. **13**, 349 (1966), Tab. 6]

e) Die Messung mit einem Referenzsystem aus Kaliumhydrogenphosphat (K_2HPO_4)

Eine Methode zur *Messung der Hydroxylapatitkonzentration* im Knochen der Diaphysencompacta haben MEEMA, HARRIS und PORRETT (1964) entwickelt. Als Referenzsystem wurde zunächst eine Aluminiumtreppe verwendet (Abb. 79a und b). Die Berechnung des Knochenmineralgehaltes erfolgte in der Weise, daß 1 mm Aluminium als Äquivalent für 150 mg Mineralsubstanz angesehen wurde. Als Meßort wurde das proximale Ende des Radius etwa 1—2 cm distalwärts von der Tuberositas radii gewählt (Abb. 80). In diesem Bereich ist die Compacta relativ gleichmäßig dick. Zur Aufnahme werden der Unterarm und der Vergleichskörper in ein Wasserbad eingelegt (Abb. 81). Da bei dem Spannungs-

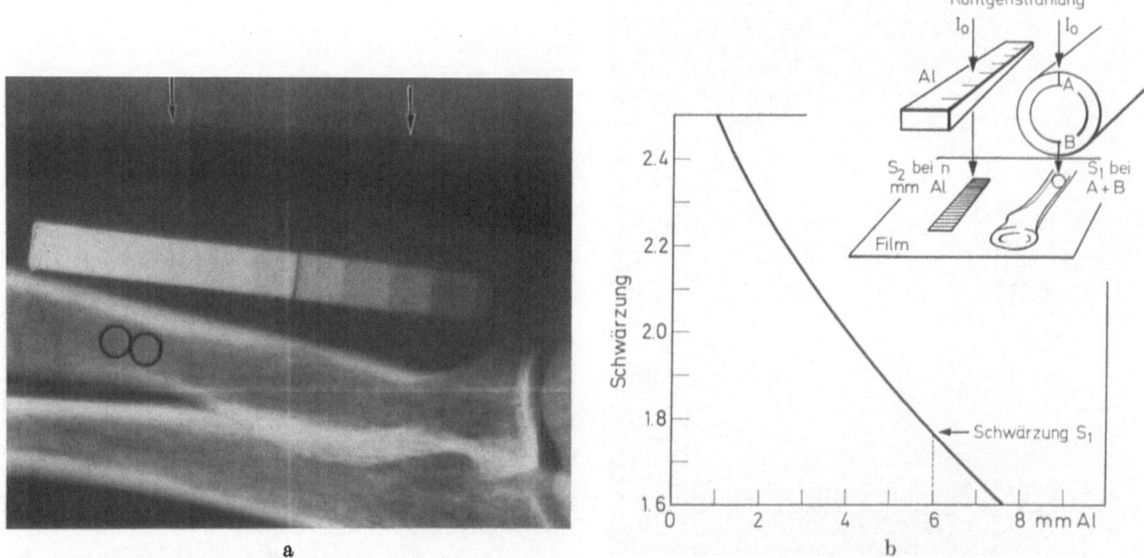

Abb. 79. Darstellung des Radius mit Markierung des Meßbezirkes und einer Aluminiumtreppe (a) und schematische Darstellung des Prinzips zur radiologischen Messung des Knochenmineralgehaltes (b). (Nach MEEMA, HARRIS und PORRETT, 1964; Abb. 1, 2, 15)

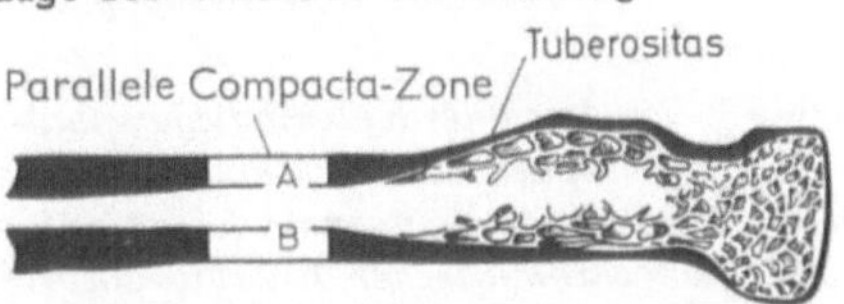

Abb. 80. Meßbezirk im Bereich des Radius 1—2 cm distal der Tuberositas radii. (Schematische Darstellung nach MEEMA, HARRIS und PORRETT, 1964; Abb. 5)

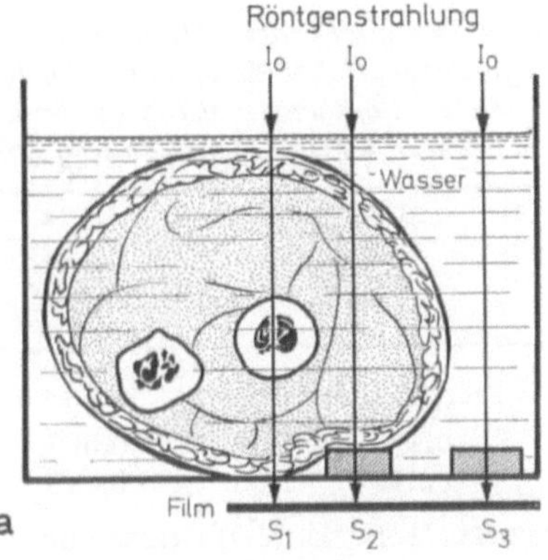

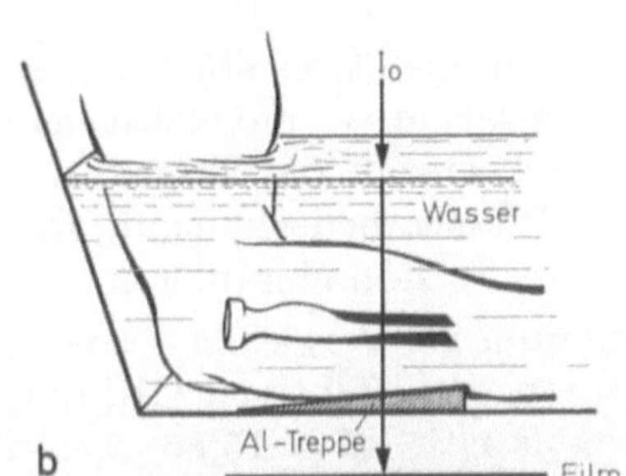

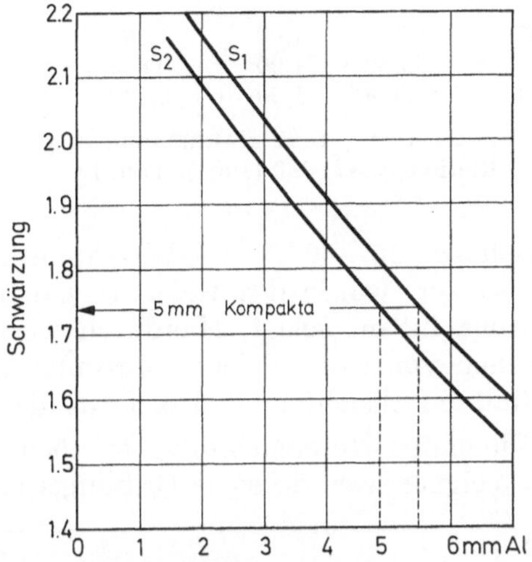

Abb. 81. Schematische Darstellung der Aufnahmeanordnung von Unterarm und Referenzsystem im Wasserbad (a und b) und der densitometrischen Auswertung des Röntgenfilmes (rechts). (Nach MEEMA, HARRIS und PORRETT, 1964; Abb. 6)

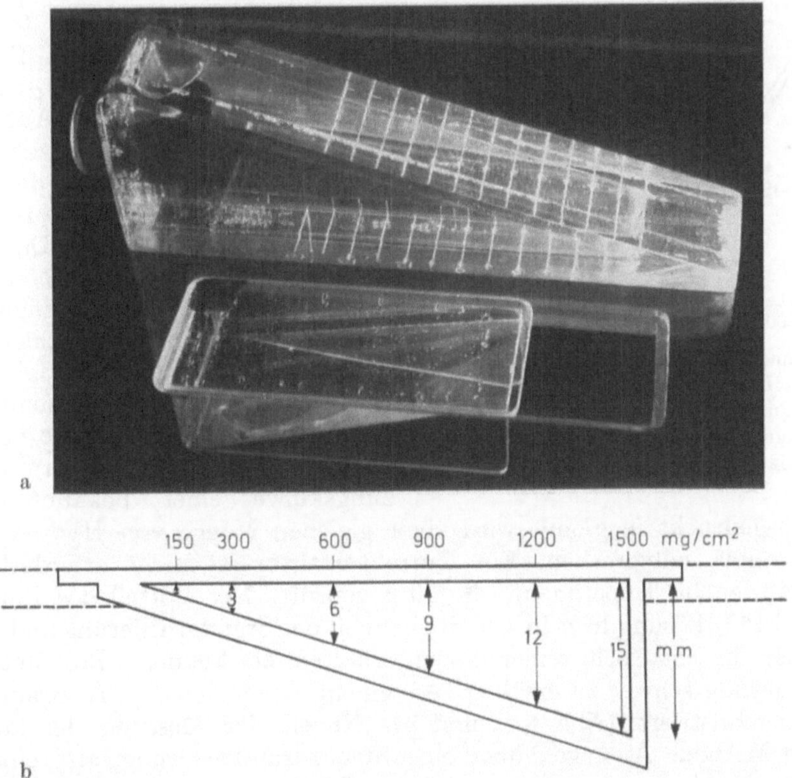

Abb. 82. Das K_2HPO_4-Referenzsystem (nach MEEMA, HARRIS und PORRETT, 1964; Abb. 3) in Aufsicht (oben) und Aufnahmeanordnung (unten) (a). Skizze des keilförmigen Referenzsystems (Plexiglasgefäß mit K_2HPO_4) mit Angaben der Eichwerte in mg/cm² (b). (Nach MEEMA, HARRIS und PORRETT, 1964; Abb. 10)

Tabelle 13. *Vergleich der Kaliumdiphosphat-(KP-) und Hydroxylapatit-(HA-) Mengen, welche den gleichen Anteil einer Röntgenstrahlung unterschiedlicher monochromatischer Energie absorbieren*

Kev	KP ($\bar{Z}$ = 15.59) μ/ϱ	KP m	HA ($\bar{Z}$ = 15.86) μ/ϱ	HA m
35	1,32	1,00	1,39	0,95
50	0,582	1,00	0,607	0,96
70	0,338	1,00	0,348	0,97

[MEEMA, H. E., C. K. HARRIS, and R. E. PORRETT: Radiology 82, 986 (1964), Tab. 1]

Tabelle 14. *Vergleich der Aluminium-(Al-) und Hydroxylapatit-(HA-) Mengen, welche den gleichen Anteil einer Röntgenstrahlung unterschiedlicher monochromatischer Röntgenstrahlung absorbieren*

Kev	Al ($\bar{Z}$ = 13) μ/ϱ	Al m	HA ($\bar{Z}$ = 15.86) μ/ϱ	HA m
35	0,834	1,00	1,39	0,60
50	0,413	1,00	0,607	0,68
70	0,273	1,00	0,348	0,78

[MEEMA, H. E., C. K. HARRIS, and R. E. PORRETT: Radiology 82, 986 (1964), Tab. 2]

bereich von 45—60 kV Anodenspannung das Muskelgewebe etwas stärker absorbiert als das Wasser, wurde das Referenzsystem *unter die Muskulatur*, möglichst nahe an den Knochen heran, gelegt. Hierdurch wird erreicht, daß sowohl die Treppe als auch der Knochen von etwa gleicher Muskulatur, Fett und Wasser bedeckt sind. Der störende Einfluß der Weichteile ließ sich auf diese Weise am sichersten eliminieren.

Die ersten Untersuchungen ergaben, daß Aluminium als Vergleichskörper nicht optimal geeignet war, da seine Ordnungszahl $Z = 13$ von der effektiven Ordnungszahl des Hydroxylapatit $Z = 15{,}86$ wesentlich abweicht (Tabelle 14). Die Schwärzungskurven eines Referenzsystems aus Aluminium und Hydroxylapatit sind daher nicht gleich und bei unterschiedlicher Anodenspannung treten größere Unterschiede auf (s. S. 148). Aus diesem Grunde wurde ein Referenzsystem aus einer 100%igen *K_2H PO_4-Lösung* in einem Plastikgefäß entwickelt (Abb. 82a und b). Diese Substanz hat die effektive Ordnungszahl $Z = 15{,}59$, so daß der Unterschied zum Hydroxylapatit ($Z = 15{,}86$) nur sehr gering ist (Tabelle 13). Da die Massenabsorptionskoeffizienten dieser beiden Substanzen unter gleichen Bedingungen nur auf den effektiven Ordnungszahlen beruhen, ist ein direkter Vergleich möglich (Abb. 83). So kann die Filmschwärzung im Bereich der interessierenden Bezirke verglichen werden und die photometrisch ermittelte Schwärzungskurve einer bekannten Menge an K_2H PO_4, ausgedrückt in g/cm², wird einer gleichen Menge von Hydroxylapatit, ausgedrückt in g/cm², entsprechen. Ein Korrekturfaktor ist nicht erforderlich. Die Bedingungen wurden im Experiment sorgfältig geprüft. Der Vorteil des Referenzsystems aus einer K_2H PO_4-Lösung liegt in der Möglichkeit der Standardisierung und das Referenzsystem immer in chemisch reiner Form erhalten zu können. Bei Metallegierungen ist diese Forderung schwer zu erfüllen. An einem Beispiel wird die Brauchbarkeit des Verfahrens demonstriert (Abb. 84a und b). Neben der Messung der Compactadicke erlaubt diese Methode Aussagen über eine Strukturauflockerung, also einen Knochenabbau oder -umbau in der Compacta (s. S. 237). Die Strukturauflockerung der Diaphysencompacta wird als „corticale Osteoporose" bezeichnet. Derartige Veränderungen sind im allgemeinen nicht mit Hilfe des Röntgenbildes am Lebenden zu erkennen. Ein Meß-

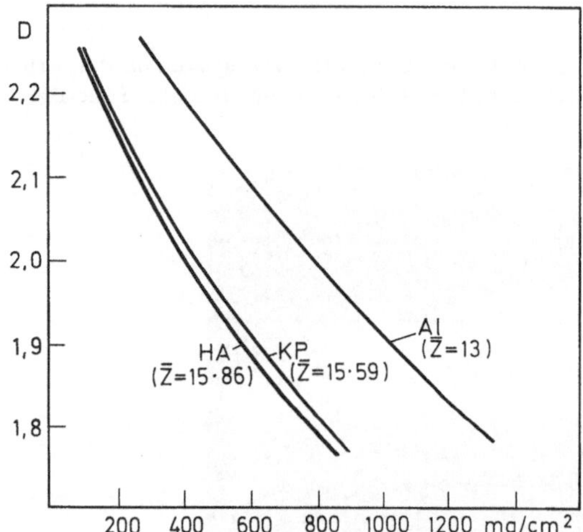

Abb. 83. Zusammenstellung der Schwärzungskurven einer Röntgenaufnahme von K_2HPO_4, Hydroxylapatit und Aluminium angefertigt bei 50 kV Anodenspannung. (Nach MEEMA, HARRIS und PORRETT, 1964; Abb. 4)

verfahren zur Bestimmung der Kalksalzkonzentration im kompakten Knochen erlaubt zwar den Nachweis einer „corticalen Osteoporose", doch kann es nicht unterscheiden zwischen einer *Strukturauflockerung* der Compacta, also einem *Knochenabbau im Sinne der Spongiosierung* oder einer *Entkalkung des Knochengewebes.* Mit dem Meßverfahren sind Untersuchungsergebnisse bei gesunden und kranken Menschen gewonnen worden (s. S. 237).

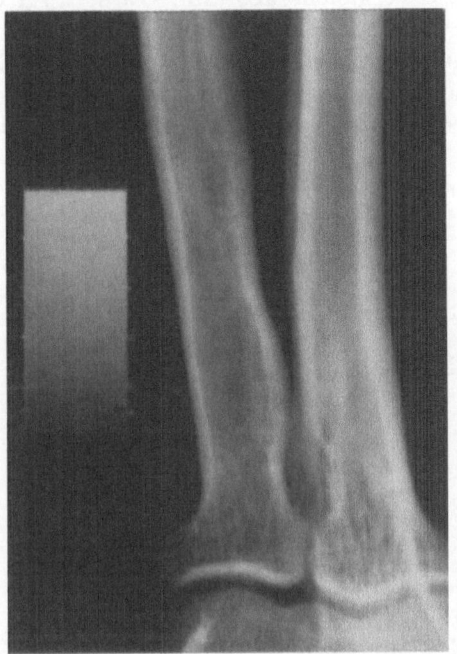

a

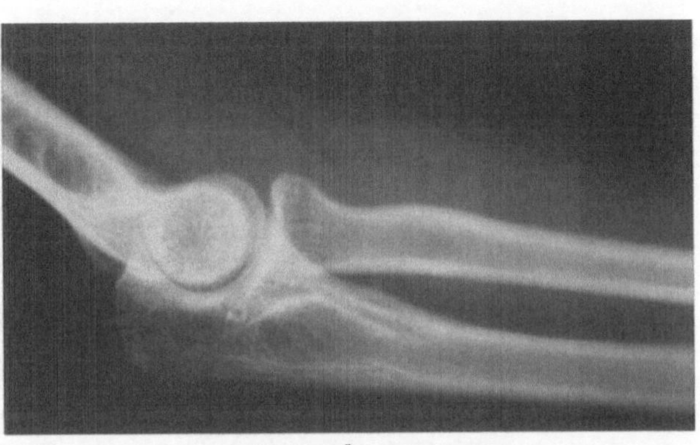

b

Abb. 84. Röntgenaufnahme der Meßregion des Radius mit dem K_2HPO_4-Referenzsystem im Wasserbad (Nach MEEMA, HARRIS und PORRETT, 1964; Abb. 15) (a). Darstellung des Radius in der 2. Ebene zu Abb. 84a (b)

f) Vergleichende photometrische Messungen bei Verwendung verschiedener Strahlenqualitäten

Die Möglichkeit, den Kalksalzgehalt durch vergleichende photometrische Messungen unter Verwendung differenter Strahlenqualitäten bei Herstellung von zwei verschiedenen Röntgenaufnahmen zu ermitteln, ist sowohl theoretisch (OMNELL 1957) als auch praktisch (KROKOWSKI u. Mitarb. 1959/68) untersucht worden. Durch die Anwendung *verschiedener Strahlenqualitäten* ist allein die *Ordnungszahl* der durchstrahlten Stoffe für das Meßergebnis von Bedeutung, so daß diese bei Untersuchungen des Knochens ein *Maß für den Calciumgehalt* ist. Der Flächenwert (SPIEGLER 1959) kann auch *ohne* Kenntnis der Dicke des durchstrahlten Knochens bestimmt werden, wenn zwei unterschiedliche Röntgenstrahlenqualitäten benutzt werden. Dagegen ist zu einer Aussage über die *Mineralkonzentration* im Gesamtvolumen Knochen *die Kenntnis der Dicke* des durchstrahlten Volumens notwendig. Diese Methoden müssen sich also mit den gleichen Schwierigkeiten der Messung des Durchmessers unregelmäßig geformter Knochen auseinandersetzen, wie sie für die anderen radiologischen Untersuchungsmethoden aufgezeigt worden sind (s. S. 129).

Auf der Basis vergleichender Schwärzungsmessungen bei Anwendung differenter Strahlenqualitäten haben KROKOWSKI u. Mitarb. (1959/61/68) eine Methode zur Bestimmung des Mineralgehaltes im Knochen entwickelt (Abb. 85). Die erforderlichen Anodenspannungen werden mit 50—250 kV angegeben. Als *Vergleichskörper* zur Eliminierung der Weichteilabsorption und Bestimmung des „Wasser-Schwächungsgleichwertes" *(H_2O — SWG)* wurde *ein mit Wasser gefülltes Plexiglasphantom* benutzt (Abb. 86a—c).

Die theoretische Ableitung der Methode stützt sich auf folgende Überlegungen (Abb. 87):

Der Schwächungsgleichwert einer bestimmten Schicht Weichteilgewebe (SGW_w) ergibt sich aus dem Schwächungskoeffizienten für Weichteil (μ_w), der Dicke der Gewebsschicht (d) und dem Schwächungskoeffizienten für die Vergleichssubstanz: Wasser (μH_2O) bzw. Plexiglas (Abb. 87, Gl. 1). Dementsprechend müssen bei Errechnung des Schwächungsgleichwertes für eine Schicht, in der Knochen in Weichteilgewebe eingebettet ist (wk), die Dicke des Knochens (Δ) und des Weichteilgewebes (d) sowie die entsprechenden Schwächungskoeffizienten (μ_k und μ_w) berücksichtigt werden (Abb. 87, Gl. 2). Der

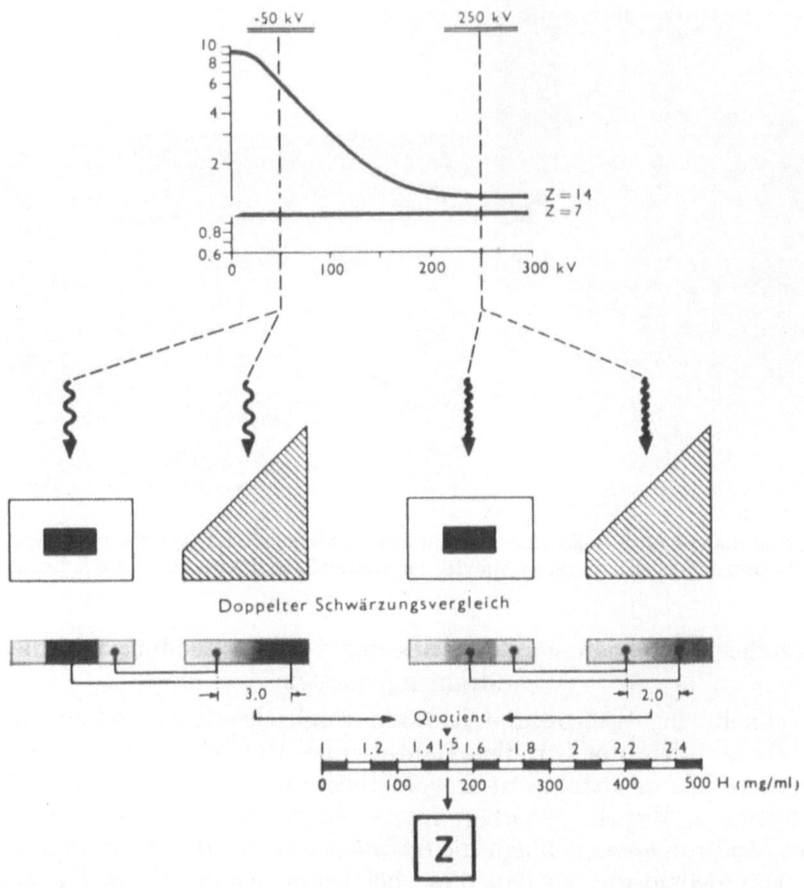

Abb. 85. Schematische Übersicht des Untersuchungsganges zur „radiologischen Substanzanalyse". (Nach Krokowski, 1959)

Schwächungsgleichwert für Knochen allein entspricht der Differenz nach Gl. 3a. Rechnerisch ergibt sich Gl. 3b als *Schwächungsgleichwert des Knochens*

$$SGW_k = \frac{\mu K \Delta}{\mu H_2O}.$$

Bildet man aus den Schwächungsgleichwerten des Knochens bei verschiedener Spannung (Abb. 88) den Quotienten, so hebt sich die Dicke (Δ) durch Kürzung auf. — Der gewonnene Zahlenwert kann als *relatives Maß für den Gehalt an anorganischer Knochensubstanz* angesehen werden Gl. 4.

$$\frac{(SGW_K)\ 62\,kV}{(SGW_K)\ 250\,kV} = K.$$

Die ersten Untersuchungen sind an der *Wirbelsäule* durchgeführt worden (Krokowski und Schlungbaum 1959), da diese Knochen bei Osteopathien bevorzugt und am stärksten verändert sein sollen. Für Untersuchungen an der *Lendenwirbelsäule* hat sich eine Wasserschicht von 18 cm als zweckmäßig herausgestellt.

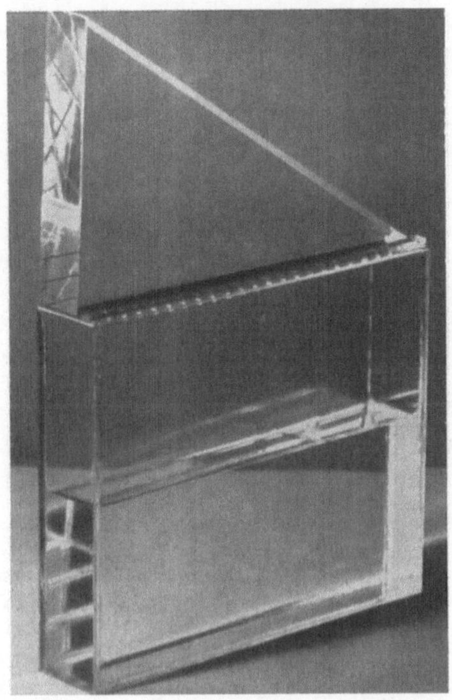

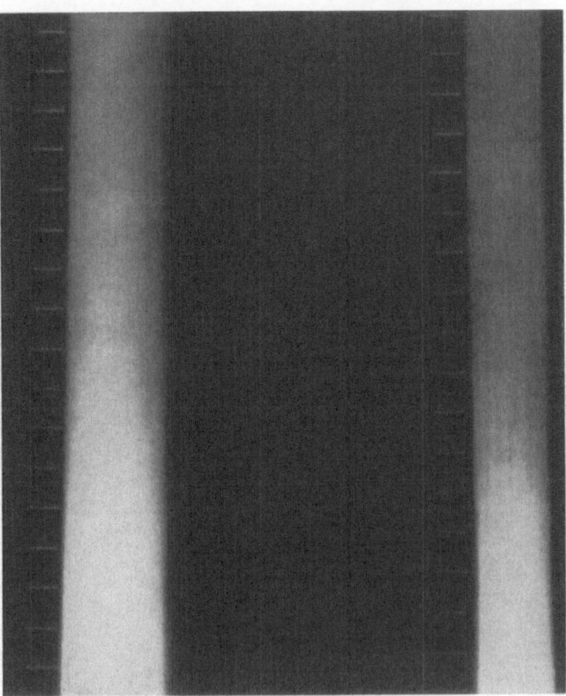

Abb. 86a Abb. 86b

Abb. 86a. Das Referenzsystem (Plexiglaskeil und Wassergefäß)

Abb. 86b. Röntgenaufnahme des Phantoms (mit 250 kV links und 62 kV rechts). (Nach KROKOWSKI und SCHLUNGBAUM, 1959; Abb. 2 und 3)

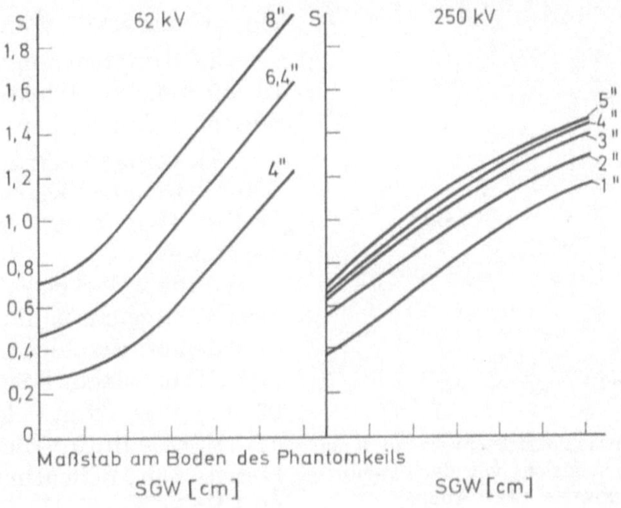

Abb. 86c. Ergebnis der Schwärzungsmessungen von Phantomaufnahmen bei verschiedenen Belichtungszeiten und Röhrenspannungen. (Nach KROKOWSKI und SCHLUNGBAUM, 1959; Abb. 4)

Die Schwächung der Röntgenstrahlen durch die Weichteile wird von der Schwächung durch Weichteile + Knochen subtrahiert, um den *reinen Schwächungsgleichwert* des Knochens für eine entsprechende Wasserschichtdicke zu erhalten. Die Neigung des Plexiglaskeiles von 45° hat zur Folge, daß der abgelesene Wert genau der Differenz $SGW_{wk} - SGW_{w}$, also dem Schwächungsgleichwert des Knochens (SGW_{k}) entspricht. Der Quotient der SGW bei 62 und 250 kV Anodenspannung ist der gesuchte *Faktor K*. Die Meßergebnisse von 24 Untersuchungen (Tabelle 15) ergaben bei *knochengesunden Personen* einen Wert

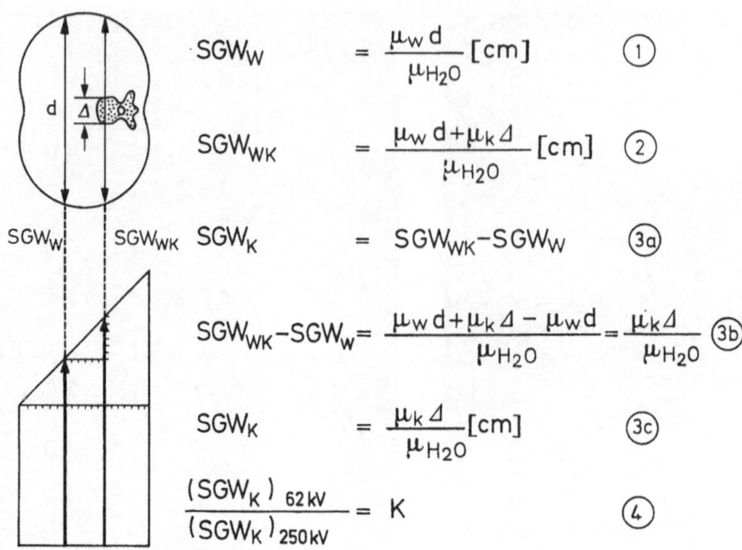

Abb. 87. Zusammenstellung der theoretischen Ableitung der Formeln zur Methode der „vergleichenden Schwächungsmessung“ oder „Substanzanalyse“. (Nach Krokowski und Schlungbaum, 1959; Abb. 5)

für den *Faktor K* von 1,90 ($\pm$0,12). Alle störenden Einflüsse von seiten des Röntgenfilmes, der Filmbearbeitung, der umgebenden Weichteile und anderer technischer Fehlermöglichkeiten werden nach Ansicht der Autoren durch die Methode eliminiert. Die „*vergleichende Schwächungsmessung*“ erlaubt eine Objektivierung der Diagnose „Osteoporose“. Die Methode soll nach später durchgeführten Vergleichen der Meßwerte mit den Ergebnissen chemischer Analysen (Strug 1964; Imig 1966) die Bestimmung des Mineralgehaltes in allen Skeletabschnitten mit einer Genauigkeit von $\pm$4 % erlauben.

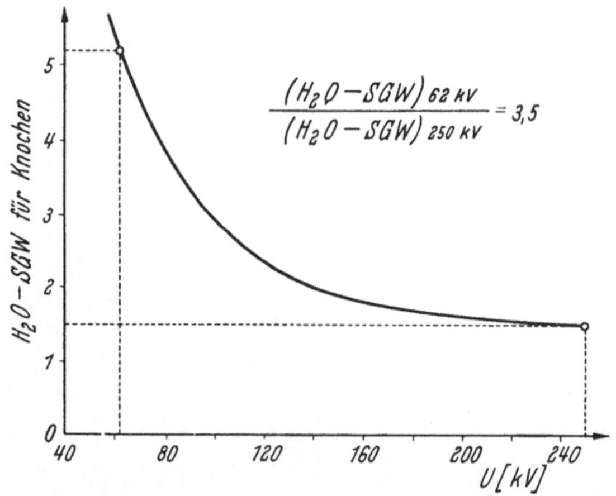

Abb. 88. Der Wasser-Schwächungsgleichwert für Knochen (H_2O-SGW) in Abhängigkeit von der Strahlenhärte. (Nach Krokowski, 1959; Abb. 5)

Die Untersuchungstechnik wurde in nachfolgenden Arbeiten modifiziert und wie folgt beschrieben:

Als Aufnahmegerät dient ein spezielles 200 kV-Diagnostikgerät der Firma C. H. F. Müller (Hamburg) mit einem Zusatzgenerator.

Von dem Wirbelsäulenabschnitt werden zwei Röntgenaufnahmen mit jeweils verschiedenen Strahlenqualitäten (60 und 200 kV) bei einem Fokus-Filmabstand von 90 cm angefertigt. Der Aufnahmetisch enthält eine Bucky-Blende mit Hartstrahlraster. Die Belichtungszeiten liegen bei 60 kV je nach Umfang des Patienten zwischen 1 und 5 sec, bei der 200 kV-Aufnahme zwischen 0,12 und 0,32 sec. Bei der 200 kV-Röhre ist zusätzlich ein 6 mm starkes Kupferfilter eingesetzt, so daß eine Halbwertschicht von 3,7 mm Kupfer resultiert.

Die Strahlenabsorption ist bei der 60 kV-Röntgenstrahlung von Ordnungszahl, Dicke und Dichte des absorbierenden Mediums abhängig (Abb. 89).

Die photometrische Messung wird auf den beiden Aufnahmen (mit 60 und 200 kV Anodenspannung angefertigt) jeweils an identischen Stellen (Durchmesser 6 mm) im Zwischenwirbelloch (Weichteil) und im angrenzenden Teil des Wirbelkörpers (im allgemeinen am 4. Lendenwirbelkörper) vorgenommen.

Tabelle 15. *Zusammenstellung der Ergebnisse der Bestimmungen des „Faktors K" bei 24 Untersuchungen*

Nr.	Name	Geschlecht	Alter	62 kV			250 kV			K = (SGW$_k$) 62 kV / (SGW$_k$) 250 kV	Diagnose	
				S$_w$	S$_{wk}$	SGW$_k$ (cm)	S$_w$	S$_{wk}$	SGW$_k$ (cm)		röntgenologisch	klinisch
1	K. M.	w.	69	0,53	0,36	4,6	0,77	0,76	3,0	1,53	Osteoporose II	Osteoporose
2	E. St.	m.	66	0,94	0,59	6,2	0,70	0,69	3,2	1,94	o. B.	o. B.
3	M. G.	w.	62	0,82	0,50	5,7	0,69	0,68	3,0	1,90	o. B.	o. B.
4	K. Sch.	m.	62	0,84	0,59	5,4	1,13	1,12	3,0	1,80	o. B.	o. B.
5	E. Th.	m.	61	0,95	0,70	5,1	0,80	0,74	3,8	1,34	Osteoporose III	Osteoporose
6	A. M.	w.	59	1,18	0,33	11,5	1,09	0,80	6,8	1,69	Osteoporose II	Osteoporose
7	J. G.	m.	59	0,90	0,37	8,2	1,23	1,14	4,4	1,86	o. B.	o. B.
8	R. L.	m.	58	0,39	0,26	5,9	1,03	1,02	3,0	1,97	o. B.	o. B.
9	G. F.	w.	58	0,78	0,50	5,0	0,97	0,96	3,0	1,67	Osteoporose II	Osteoporose
10	P. R.	m.	58	0,51	0,28	7,3	0,94	0,89	3,6	2,02	o. B.	o. B.
11	A. K.	m.	55	0,98	0,68	5,5	1,34	1,33	3,0	1,83	o. B.	o. B.
12	W. Sch.	m.	55	0,38	0,165	8,8	1,01	0,90	4,4	2,00	o. B.	o. B.
13	W. W.	m.	53	0,23	0,20	5,0	0,48	0,40	4,3	1,16	Osteoporose IV	Osteoporose
14	A. B.	m.	51	0,54	0,36	5,6	0,99	0,97	3,3	1,70	Osteoporose I	o. B.
15	M. G.	w.	49	0,93	0,67	5,3	0,88	0,87	3,1	1,71	Osteoporose I	o. B.
16	E. A.	w.	48	1,28	0,92	5,9	1,35	1,34	3,0	1,97	o. B.	o. B.
17	A. G.	w.	48	0,64	0,39	5,7	0,91	0,90	3,0	1,90	o. B.	o. B.
18	H. H.	w.	47	0,36	0,325	4,0	0,72	0,70	3,2	1,25	Osteoporose IV	Osteoporose
19	H. S.	w.	46	0,69	0,50	4,6	1,10	1,05	3,8	1,21	Osteoporose IV	Osteoporose
20	H. St.	w.	45	1,70	1,50	4,7	1,61	1,59	3,2	1,47	Osteoporose III	Osteoporose
21	L. P.	w.	43	0,65	0,46	6,4	1,05	1,03	3,3	1,94	o. B.	o. B.
22	H. L.	m.	42	0,48	0,38	4,4	0,55	0,54	3,1	1,42	Osteoporose III	?
23	Ch. B.	w.	39	0,46	0,31	5,7	0,66	0,65	3,0	1,90	o. B.	o. B.
24	K. L.	m.	34	0,94	0,50	7,8	1,10	0,97	5,0	1,56	Osteoporose II	Osteoporose

[KROKOWSKI, E., u. W. SCHLUNGBAUM: Fortschr. Röntgenstr. **91**, 740 (1959), Tab. 1]

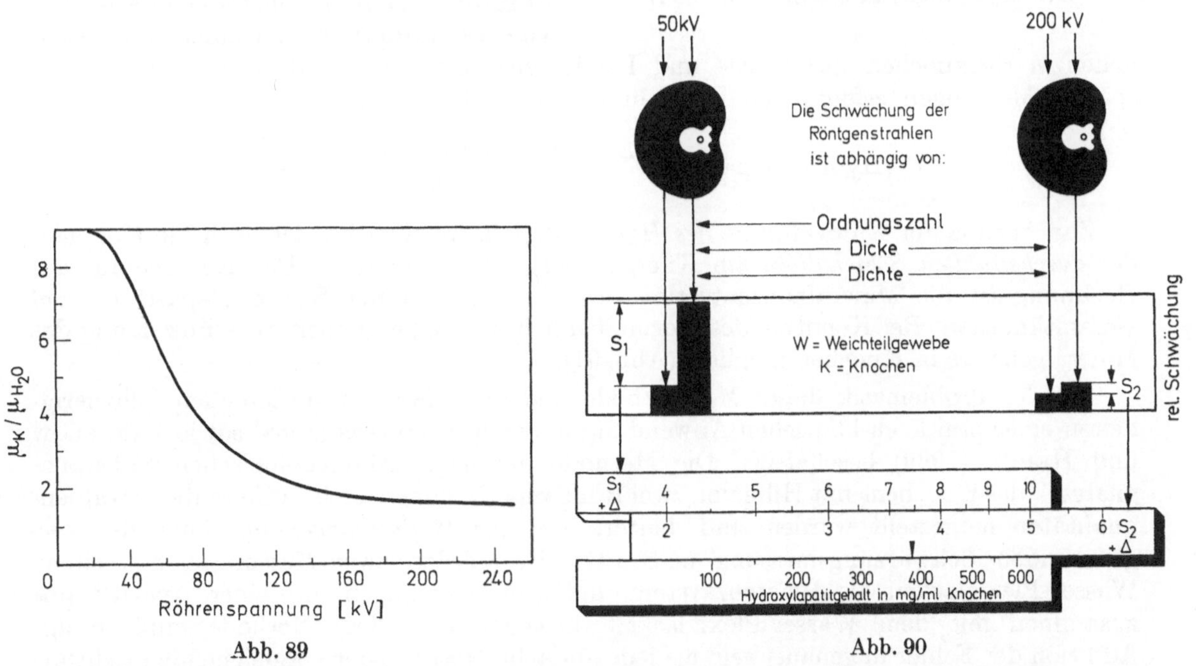

Abb. 89

Abb. 90

Abb. 89. Das Verhältnis der Schwächung im Knochen zur Schwächung in Wasser in Abhängigkeit von der Röhrenspannung (für den Fall $\mu d \ll 1$). (Nach KROKOWSKI und SCHLUNGBAUM, 1959; Abb. 1)

Abb. 90. Schematische Darstellung der röntgenologischen Bestimmung des Hydroxylapatitgehaltes im Knochen nach KROKOWSKI mit Hilfe eines speziellen Rechenschiebers. (Nach KROKOWSKI, 1965; Abb. 1)

Bei einer Röntgenstrahlung von 200 kV dagegen sind für die Absorption im wesentlichen Dichte und Dicke des Mediums bestimmend; die relativ hohe Ordnungszahl von Calcium hat auf die Absorption keinen Einfluß. Bei 60 kV ist die Schwächungsdifferenz (S 1) zwischen durchstrahltem Weichteilgewebe und Knochen erheblich, bei 200 kV nur sehr gering (S 2). Der Quotient S 1/S 2 stellt somit ein Maß für die Calciumkonzentration im Knochen dar.

Es wird ein Kodak-Film mit einer Auer HV-Folie verwendet und maschinell entwickelt. Zur Photometrie wird ein Photometer der Firma B. Lange, Berlin, benutzt. Die Filmschwärzung wird photometrisch bestimmt und auf eine Standardschwärzung bezogen. Diese Standardschwärzung wird durch Aufnahme eines Plexiglaskeiles mit Wasser gewonnen und als Schwächungsgleichwert ausgedrückt, um von den Eigenschaften des verwendeten Filmmaterials (Gradation, Schleier, Verstärkerfolie usw.) und der Filmverarbeitung unabhängig zu sein. Mit den gemessenen Werten kann auf einem Spezial-Rechenschieber (Abb. 90) direkt der Hydroxylapatitgehalt in mg pro ml Knochen abgelesen werden (KROKOWSKI 1963).

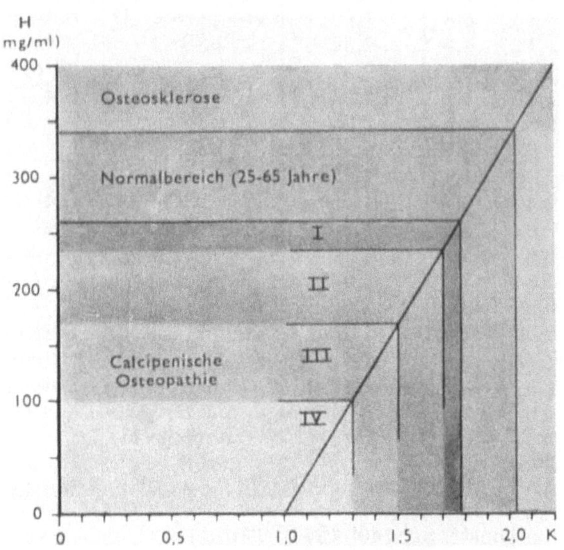

Abb. 91. Schematische Darstellung von *K*-Wert und Hydroxylapatitgehalt. (Nach KROKOWSKI)

Die *Umrechnung des K-Faktors* in die äquivalente Mineralkonzentration wurde durch vergleichende Untersuchungen mit Hilfe des Referenzsystems aus Hydroxylapatit und Kunststoff von HEUCK und SCHMIDT (1960) und chemischen Analysen von 18 autoptisch gewonnenen menschlichen Wirbelknochen der Brust- und Lendenwirbelsäule versucht (STRUG 1964). Für spätere Messungen erfolgte die Umrechnung nach der Formel:

$$\text{H (Hydroxylapatit)} = \frac{K \text{ (ermittelter Knochenwert)} - 1}{0{,}003}.$$

Zur Angabe der *Konzentration des Hydroxylapatit* im Knochen ist noch die Kenntnis der *durchstrahlten Schichtdicke* am Knochenmeßareal erforderlich. Das Endergebnis der Rechnung ist die Mineralkonzentration des Knochens in mg Hydroxylapatit pro ml Gesamtknochen. Bei Kenntnis des Normalbereiches ist eine quantitative Bewertung des Mineralgehaltes in Knochen möglich (Abb. 91).

Mit der Problematik dieser Meßmethode und den hieraus resultierenden Schwierigkeiten einer praktisch-klinischen Anwendung haben sich HINESS (1968) sowie VANSELOW und HEUCK (1969) beschäftigt. Die Methode der sog. „röntgenologischen Substanzanalyse" des Knochens mit Hilfe von zwei Röntgenaufnahmen die bei differenten Strahlenqualitäten hergestellt worden sind, basiert auf *vier Meßvorgängen* im Sinne der vergleichenden Schwärzungsmessung (s. S. 197). Es werden zwei Messungen mit einem Wasser-Plexiglaskeil als Referenzsystem und zwei Messungen mit einer Apatittreppe zusammen mit dem Wasser-Plexiglaskeil durchgeführt. Diese Methode muß infolge Addition der Fehler ungenauer sein als jede einfache Methode der vergleichenden Schwärzungsmessung. Unter Beachtung der Fehlermöglichkeiten des Meßvorganges sind die bisher erarbeiteten Ergebnisse (s. S. 214) über „Normalwerte" und Änderungen der Mineralkonzentration bei Systemerkrankungen des Skeletes dennoch für die weitere wissenschaftliche und klinische Arbeit bedeutungsvoll.

VII. Ergebnisse radiologischer Messungen der Knochendichte und Mineralkonzentration bei Gesunden

Mit den zusammengestellten, auf unterschiedlichen physikalischen und technischen Prinzipien entwickelten Untersuchungsmethoden zur Bestimmung des Knochenmineralgehaltes und der Knochenmasse sind bisher nur wenige Ergebnisse ermittelt worden. Für weitere Forschungen und die Einführung praktisch brauchbarer Meßmethoden in die Routinearbeit der klinischen Radiologie sind alle bereits vorliegenden Meßergebnisse als Grundlage von großem Wert. Nur dann, wenn über den Knochenmineralgehalt des *gesunden Menschen* ausreichende Kenntnisse vorliegen, können krankhafte Abweichungen erfaßt werden. In den nachfolgenden Kapiteln sollen alle umfangreicheren Untersuchungsergebnisse zusammengestellt werden. Es sind nur einzelne Mosaiksteine zu dem noch fehlenden Fundament eines Wissens über den „Normbereich" der Verteilung und Konzentration der Knochenkalksalze, der Knochenmasse und Knochenstrukturen bei Mensch und Tier. Zur Festlegung von „Normalwerten" des Mineralgehaltes der verschiedenen Knochen des Skeletes in den einzelnen Altersgruppen beider Geschlechter bei verschiedenen Rassen und Umweltseinflüssen bedarf es noch umfangreicher Forschungsarbeit!

1. Der Knochenmineralgehalt — ausgedrückt in „Schwächungsgleichwerten"

Es liegen von den verschiedensten Arbeitsgruppen Untersuchungsergebnisse vor, die den Knochenkalksalzgehalt einiger Knochenregionen in der Schichtdicke von Aluminium oder Aluminiumlegierungen, Elfenbein oder anderem Material, das als Referenzsystem Verwendung gefunden hat, ausdrücken.

Die ersten, vergleichbaren Meßergebnisse des Knochenkalkgehaltes *verschiedener Zonen vom Daumengrundglied, der Mittel- und Grundphalanx des Zeigefingers* haben ENGSTRÖM und WELIN (1949) erarbeitet (s. S. 152). Mit Hilfe einer Aluminiumtreppe als Referenzsystem wurde unter Berücksichtigung der Weichteilabsorption die erhaltene Knochenabsorption durch eine Formel so ausgedrückt, daß eine direkte Beziehung zum Calciumgehalt des Knochengewebes besteht. Der erhaltene Wert für die Calciumsalze pro mm Knochenschichtdicke ist also ein Globalwert für den Gesamtknochen, so daß bei einem Knochen mit dicker Corticalis dieser Wert größer sein muß als bei einem Knochen mit dünner Corticalis oder mit einem verminderten Kalksalzgehalt. Die Normalwerte wurden an den *Fingerknochen von 10 Männern und 10 Frauen ermittelt* und jeweils in zwei gleich große Gruppen unterteilt. Die Untersuchungsbedingungen waren so einheitlich wie möglich, um verwertbare und vergleichbare Ergebnisse zu erhalten. Die Meßpunkte lagen im Bereich der distalen Spongiosapartie und der etwas weiter proximal gelegenen Partie des Überganges zur Compacta vom Daumengrundglied. Am Zeigefinger wurde im Mittelglied in ähnlicher Weise gemessen, im Grundglied erfolgte die Messung proximal im Bereich der Epiphyse und etwas weiter distal von diesem Meßpunkt. Die gewonnenen Ergebnisse sind in Tabelle 16 zusammengestellt, aus denen die Absorptionswerte für die

Tabelle 16. *Mittelwerte und Standardabweichung der Al-Schichtdicken, die in den untersuchten Zonen von Daumen- und Fingerknochen die gleiche Strahlenabsorption aufweisen*

Meßpunkt	Männlich		Weiblich	
	Serie 1	Serie 2	Serie 1	Serie 2
Daumen dist.	2,47 ± 0,38	2,88 ± 0,25	3,14 ± 0,39	2,76 ± 0,51
Daumen prox.	3,15 ± 0,36	3,58 ± 0,56	4,21 ± 0,41	4,12 ± 0,50
Zeigefinger ganz dist.	2,45 ± 0,37	2,71 ± 0,26	2,98 ± 0,40	3,06 ± 0,63
Zeigefinger dist.	2,10 ± 0,31	2,19 ± 0,26	2,52 ± 0,30	2,39 ± 0,29
Zeigefinger prox.	3,10 ± 0,53	3,19 ± 0,13	3,72 ± 0,63	3,49 ± 0,72
Zeigefinger ganz prox.	3,87 ± 0,41	3,90 ± 0,45	4,56 ± 0,44	4,20 ± 0,47

[ENGSTRÖM, A., and S. WELIN: Acta radiol. (Stockh.) **31**, 483 (1949), Tab. 10]

untersuchte Knochenregion zusammen mit den Absorptionswerten der Weichteile hervorgehen. Der Kalksalzgehalt des Knochens kann aus den gefundenen Werten berechnet werden. Da die Schwächung der Röntgenstrahlen und damit der Kontrast der Röntgenaufnahmen durch die stärker absorbierenden Kalksalze *pro Volumeneinheit* zustande kommt, halten es ENGSTRÖM und WELIN für sinnvoller, die *Kalksalzkonzentration in Volumeneinheiten Gesamtknochen anzugeben* und nicht, wie in den ersten methodischen Arbeiten empfohlen, in Gewichtseinheiten.

Von MAASS (1951) sind im Bereich der *distalen Radiusmetaphyse*, der *Mitte des Os capitatum* und der *Mitte der distalen Metaphyse des Metacarpale II* von 18 gesunden Händen die „*Aluminiumwerte*" ermittelt worden (Tabelle 17). Es fällt auf, daß die Knochen der

Tabelle 17. *Die „Aluminium-Werte" einiger normaler und pathologisch veränderter Knochen des Handskelets (distale Radiusmetaphyse, Mitte Os capitatum, Mitte distale Metaphyse des Metacarpale II)*

Normal von 18 Händen			Entkalkt von 21 Händen			
Radius	Capitatum	Metacarpale II	Radius	Os capitatum	Metacarpale II	
8,1	7,3	5,0	6,9	6,4	4,2	Durchschnitt links
8,8	8,0	5,8	7,2	6,4	4,8	Durchschnitt rechts
7,4—8,7	6,4—8,1	4,4—5,5	5,2—7,5	5,1—7,6	2,4—5,4	Extremwerte links
8,0—9,5	7,3—9,2	5,0—6,8	6,2—8,6	4,6—7,7	3,6—5,3	Extremwerte rechts

[MAASS, K.: Diss. Kiel 1951, Abb. 9]

rechten Hand, verglichen mit der linken Seite, eine höhere Strahlenabsorption aufweisen, also auch einen höheren Kalkgehalt besitzen müssen. Dieser Unterschied wird auf eine gewisse Inaktivität der linken Extremität gegenüber rechts zurückgeführt. Ähnliche Befunde haben auch QUINTAR (1962), KROKOWSKI und STEINER (1961) erhoben. Bei Untersuchungen des globalen Kalksalzgehaltes in der Radiusspongiosa oder in der Spongiosa der Knochen des Handskeletes sollte entweder der rechten Hand der Vorzug gegeben werden oder *beide Hände* untersucht werden. Die Schwankungsbreite zwischen den höchsten und den niedrigsten „Aluminiumwerten" war in den drei Knochen der untersuchten Hände groß. Zur richtigen Beurteilung ist die Kenntnis der *Knochendicke* im Bereich der gemessenen Knochenpartie wertvoll, da feingliedrige Hände manchmal einen niedrigeren Schwächungswert aufweisen als plumpe, große und grobe Hände. Da zwischen der Knochenbreite und der Knochendicke von Radius und Metacarpale II eine konstante Relation gefunden wurde, konnte bei diesen Knochen auch die Knochenschichtdicke bei der Beurteilung berücksichtigt werden. Der Vergleich von „Aluminiumwerten" der Knochen in 21 kranken Händen von *Patienten mit Osteoporose oder Entkalkungsosteopathien* zeigte deutlich eine Überlappung der niedrigsten „Aluminiumwerte" der gesunden Handknochen mit den höchsten „Aluminiumwerten" bei Systemerkrankungen des Skeletes. Bemerkenswert ist, daß die Schwankungsbreite der „Aluminiumwerte" von gesunden Knochen wesentlich geringer war als die Schwankungsbreite der kranken Knochen.

In größeren Untersuchungsreihen hat MAINLAND (1956) Schwächungsgleichwerte für verschiedene Knochenregionen, ausgedrückt in der „*äquivalenten Aluminiumdicke*", bei Gesunden und Kranken ermittelt (Methode s. S. 163). Die densitometrischen Untersuchungen wurden in folgenden Knochenpartien von 5 Knochen des Handskeletes durchgeführt: *distales Radiusende, Mitte des Os lunatum, Mitte des Os capitatum, Mitte der Diaphyse des Metacarpale V* und *Mitte der Diaphyse der Mittelphalanx des 5. Fingers*. Es sind insgesamt 50 gesunde männliche Versuchspersonen im Alter von 20—84 Jahren und 12 gesunde weibliche Versuchspersonen im Alter von 19—30 Jahren zur Untersuchung herangezogen und mehrfach kontrolliert worden. An den 5 verschiedenen Knochen des Handgelenkes und der Hand sind Altersunterschiede bestimmt worden. Bei 32 Männern ist sowohl die rechte als auch die linke Hand gemessen worden. Die Knochen der rechten Hand besitzen eine deutlich höhere Dichte als die der linken Hand, mit Ausnahme des Os lunatum. Beziehungen zwischen Knochendichte und Körpergewicht fanden sich nicht. Die Dichtewerte der weiblichen Handknochen lagen eindeutig niedriger als die der männlichen Handknochen mit Ausnahme der Phalanx des 5. Fingers. Der linear ansteigende Verlust der mittleren Dichte wird mit 5% im Laufe von 20 Jahren angenommen. Die Dimensionen der Knochen scheinen von geringerer Bedeutung zu sein. Die an den Knochen des Handskeletes erhobenen Befunde können jedoch nicht als repräsentativ für alle übrigen Knochen des Skeletes betrachtet werden.

Aus diesem Grunde hat MAINLAND (1957) die Altersunterschiede der *„röntgenologischen Dichte“* des *Calcaneus* an 42 Männern und 12 Frauen studiert. Von 31 Männern sind sowohl der *linke* als auch der *rechte Calcaneus* densitometrisch untersucht worden. Durch mehrfache Messungen und Kontrollmessungen sowie durch wiederholte Anfertigung von Röntgenaufnahmen desselben Knochens konnte eine Standardabweichung von

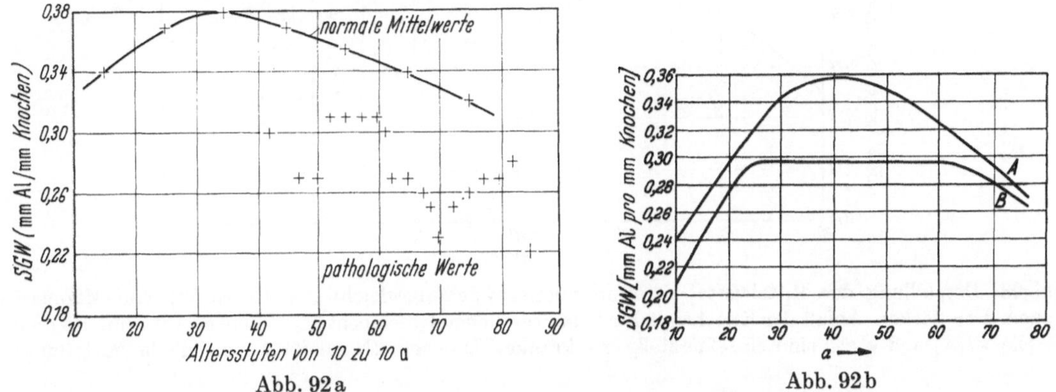

Abb. 92a

Abb. 92b

Abb. 92a. Mittelwert von je 3 Meßstellen der rechten und linken Grundphalanx des Daumens in Aluminium-Schwächungsgleichwerten (Al-SGW) pro mm Knochen bei gesunden und einigen Patienten mit Osteopathien dargestellt. (Nach BALZ und BIRKNER, 1956; Abb. 4)

Abb. 92b. Darstellung der Mittelwerte der Al-SWG von Corticalis und Spongiosa der Phalangen in den einzelnen Lebensjahrzehnten A; in B sind zum Vergleich die Mittelwerte der Al-SWG des Phalanx-Köpfchens dargestellt, das fast nur aus Spongiosa besteht. Der Einfluß auf das Meßergebnis der Compacta wird deutlich. (Nach BALZ, BIRKNER und SCHMITT-ROHDE, 1957; Abb. 4b)

$\pm 6,2$% gefunden werden. Die im Gesamtkollektiv erkennbaren Unterschiede der Knochendichte des Calcaneus, ausgedrückt in *Aluminiumschichtdicke*, sind mit 0,55 mm oder — berechnet auf die Gesamtdichte — mit 7,1% angegeben worden. Ein Zusammenhang zwischen der Knochendichte und dem Konstitutionstyp oder dem Körpergewicht fand sich nicht. Die Mittelwerte der Knochendichte zeigten keine deutlichen Unterschiede zwischen den beiden Geschlechtern, doch ist für eine bindende Aussage die Zahl der durchgeführten Untersuchungen wohl noch zu gering. Über Veränderungen der Knochendichte im Laufe des Alterungsprozesses sind auf Grund der kleinen Zahl ebenfalls noch keine Aussagen möglich gewesen.

Bei Untersuchungen über die *calcipenischen Osteopathien* und ihre frühzeitige Erkennung haben BALZ, BIRKNER und SCHMITT-ROHDE (1957) die praktische Anwendung des von BALZ und BIRKNER entwickelten Untersuchungsverfahrens in der Klinik dargelegt. Sie fanden bei 103 *gesunden Menschen* einen Anstieg der Durchschnittswerte des *„Aluminiumschwächungsgleichwertes“* bis zum 30. Lebensjahr (Abb. 92a und b). Dies entspricht dem bis zu diesem Lebensalter stetig zunehmenden Mineralgehalt der Knochen. Im 5. Lebensjahrzehnt beginnt ein *Abfall des globalen Mineralgehaltes*, der sich in einer Verminderung des Schwächungsgleichwertes ausdrückt und bei *Frauen weitaus deutlicher ist als bei Männern* (Abb. 93). Der Abfall des „Aluminiumschwächungsgleichwertes“ drückt die Abnahme des Gesamtmineralgehaltes in der durchstrahlten Knochenpartie aus, ist also unabhängig von dem Kalksalzgehalt des einzelnen Struktur- und Bauelementes der Knochen. Es waren deutliche Unterschiede des Alterungsprozesses im Kurvenverlauf von reiner Spongiosa und solchen Knochenpartien, die von einer dickeren Corticalis umgeben waren, festzustellen.

Knochendichtemessungen zur *Bestimmung der physiologischen Altersosteoporose* sind von Gershon-Cohen, Schraer und Blumberg (1955) durchgeführt worden. Von 149 gesunden Patienten (52 männlichen und 97 weiblichen) im Alter von 63—98 Jahren wurden Skeletaufnahmen der *linken Hand* und des *linken Fußes* angefertigt. Der „*Dichtekoeffizient*" (s. S. 156) des *Calcaneus* betrug beim weiblichen Geschlecht 0,55—0,59, beim männlichen Geschlecht 0,60—0,64. Es fand sich also eine geringere Dichte des Calcaneus

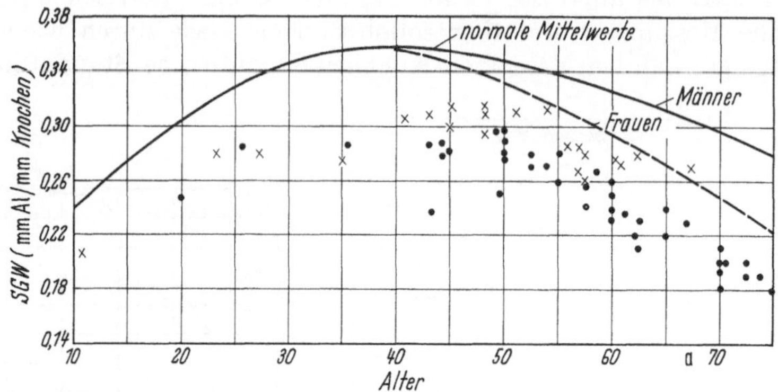

Abb. 93. Darstellung der Mittelwerte der Aluminiumschwächungsgleichwerte (Al-SGW) von Männern und Frauen. Der stärkere Abfall der Knochendichte beim weiblichen Geschlecht im 5. Lebensjahrzehnt ist deutlich. Die × (♂) und ● (♀) sind einzelne Meßwerte kranker Knochen. (Nach Balz, persönliche Mitteilung)

beim weiblichen Geschlecht. Die „Dichtekoeffizienten" im Bereich der *Diaphysen der Mittelphalangen des 5. Fingers der linken Hand* zeigten bei Frauen größere Schwankungen als bei Männern, während im *Metaphysengebiet* die Dichtekoeffizienten denen des Calcaneus ähnlich waren. Der Dichtekoeffizient der Diaphysen der Mittelphalanx des 5. Fingers war bei beiden Geschlechtern größer als der des Calcaneus. Vergleiche zwischen dem Osteoporosegrad verschiedener Knochenbezirke ergaben keine Übereinstimmung. Die individuellen Differenzen der Knochendichtewerte waren groß. Bedeutungsvoller als der Mittelwert zahlreicher Untersuchungen ist die *Kontrolle der Meßwerte einer einzelnen Person über einen längeren Zeitraum*, um z.B. krankhafte Veränderungen frühzeitig erkennen zu können.

Eine Reihe von Untersuchungen über die normale röntgenologische Knochendichte des *Calcaneus* und der *Phalangen* von beiden Geschlechtern innerhalb verschiedener *jugendlicher Altersgruppen* hat Schraer (1958) vorgelegt. Es wurden der „*mittlere Knochendichtekoeffizient*" (s. S. 156) und die Standardabweichungen im Bereich der Spongiosa des *linken Calcaneus* von 738 Jungen und 746 Mädchen, ferner der *Diaphysenmitte und der Metaphyse der II. Phalanx (Mittelglied) des 5. Fingers der linken Hand* bei 395 Mädchen und 624 Jungen — alle im Wachstumsalter von 7—20 Jahren — untersucht und ausgewertet (Tabelle 18). Der „Mittelwert des Knochendichtekoeffizienten" beider Knochen steigt bei beiden Geschlechtern mit fortschreitendem Alter an (Abb. 94). Die Dichtewerte des Calcaneus bei Mädchen in den Altersgruppen 13—15 und 16—20 Jahre und der Diaphysenmeßlinie des Fingerknochens bei Jungen in den Altersgruppen 7—9 und 10 bis 12 Jahre fielen aus dem Rahmen und wurden als eine Ausnahme angesehen. Der „Knochendichtekoeffizient" der Phalanx ist bei Mädchen deutlich größer als bei Jungen im gleichen Alter. Eine Ausnahme scheint hier die Altersgruppe von 7—9 Jahren zu machen, in der auch die Calcaneuswerte der Jungen deutlich höher lagen als die der Mädchen. Für alle Altersgruppen und beide Geschlechter trifft zu, daß sich die *Knochendichtekoeffizienten mit dem Alter der Kinder beträchtlich erhöhen.* Die Unterschiede zwischen den

Tabelle 18. *Mittelwerte der Dichtekoeffizienten des Calcaneus und der Fingerknochen bei Kindern zwischen 7 und 20 Jahren (s. Abb. 94)*

Alter	Männlich			Weiblich		
	Mittelwert	St.-A.	Anzahl	Mittelwert	St.-A.	Anzahl
			Calcaneus			
7—9	0,60	0,09	138	0,60	0,09	139
10—12	0,67	0,10	183	0,63	0,08	138
13—15	0,74	0,10	254	0,68	0,10	296
16—20	0,82	0,05	163	0,68	0,09	173
			Phalanx-Ende			
7—9	0,64	0,11	77	0,71	0,16	97
10—12	0,66	0,16	101	0,80	0,18	56
13—15	0,89	0,21	225	1,02	0,18	135
16—20	1,03	0,19	221	1,11	0,18	107
			Phalanx-Mitte			
7—9	1,02	0,23	77	1,10	0,21	97
10—12	1,03	0,28	101	1,25	0,30	56
13—15	1,32	0,30	225	1,64	0,22	135
16—20	1,43	0,24	221	1,74	0,31	107

St.-A. = Standardabweichung.
[SCHRAER, H.: J. Pediat. 52, 416 (1958), Tab. 2]

untersuchten Knochenpartien können zwanglos mit der anatomischen Struktur und dem Aufbau der untersuchten Knochen verstanden werden. Die Fingerknochen haben eine sehr viel dickere Corticalis oder Compacta von wesentlich höherem globalen Mineralgehalt als eine spongiöse Knochenpartie. Die Unterschiede zwischen den Geschlechtern können durch die im Wachstumsalter auftretende frühere Reife und den früheren Epi-

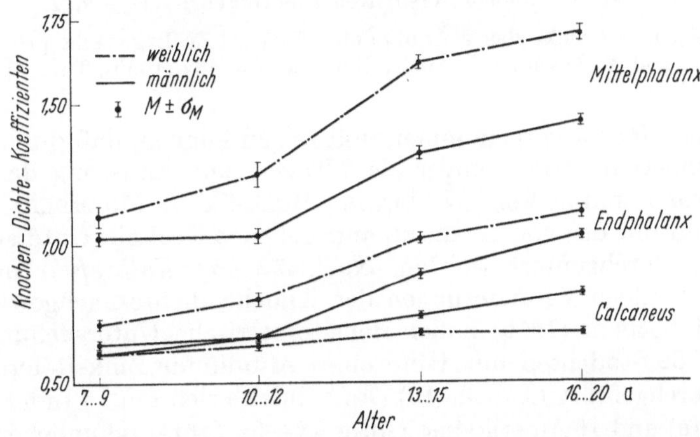

Abb. 94. Die Änderung des Knochendichtekoeffizienten von Calcaneus und Fingerknochen bei Kindern in Abhängigkeit von Alter und Geschlecht. (Nach SCHRAER, 1958; Abb. 2)

physenschluß des weiblichen Geschlechtes erklärt werden. Das *wachsende Skelet* verhält sich also anders wie das Skelet des Erwachsenen. Die vermehrte Knochendichte des Calcaneus beim männlichen Geschlecht kann auf den *Einfluß hormoneller Faktoren* zurückgeführt werden. Ein zunehmender Anstieg des Knochendichtekoeffizienten bei beiden Geschlechtern mit zunehmendem Alter konnte auch in anderen Knochen festgestellt werden.

Am Menschen wurden bisher noch keine *Verlaufskontrollen* durchgeführt, um geringe Veränderungen der Knochendichte zu erfassen. SCHRAER (1958) hat Kontrollunter-

Tabelle 19. *Ergebnisse densitometrischer Untersuchungen von Fingerknochen bei Indern und Amerikanern*

Inder (Männer)					Inder (Frauen)				
Lfd. Nr.	Alter	Gewicht	Größe	Dichte-Koeffizient *	Lfd. Nr.	Alter	Gewicht	Größe	Dichte-Koeffizient *
1	25	106	162,5	0,69	9	28	114	155,0	0,96
2	25	128	170,0	0,81	10	23	161	172,5	1,05
3	44	116	170,0	0,94	11	25	142	165,0	1,13
4	47	142	170,0	0,97	12	33	119	155,0	1,20
5	25	146	167,5	0,97	13	36	93	160,0	1,23
6	28	149	172,5	1,03	14	25	120	160,0	1,25
7	40	174	170,0	1,25	15	36	120	152,5	1,26
8	25	126	160,0	1,31	16	26	88	152,5	1,27
Mittelwerte	32 ± 10	136 ± 21	167,5 ± 5	1,00 ± 0,2		29 ± 5	120 ± 24	160 ± 7,5	1,17 ± 0,11

Mittelwert der Dichtekoeffizienten aller untersuchten Inder: *1,08 ± 0,16*

Amerikaner (Männer)					Amerikaner (Frauen)				
Lfd. Nr.	Alter	Gewicht	Größe	Dichte-Koeffizient *	Lfd. Nr.	Alter	Gewicht	Größe	Dichte-Koeffizient *
17	26	141	170,0	0,69	25	21	111	162,5	0,88
18	25	173	175,0	0,89	26	27	144	165,0	0,93
19	23	172	172,5	0,95	27	20	117	162,5	1,07
20	27	218	187,5	1,10	28	22	130	160,0	1,11
21	21	160	170,0	1,29	29	24	104	152,5	1,18
22	18	170	177,5	1,31	30	32	151	170,0	1,25
23	25	142	175,0	1,39	31	31	150	170,0	1,26
24	26	151	170,0	1,43	32	22	112	155,0	1,30
Mittelwerte	23 ± 3	166 ± 25	175 ± 5	1,13 ± 0,27		24 ± 5	127 ± 19	162,5 ± 7,5	1,12 ± 0,15

Mittelwert der Dichtekoeffizienten aller untersuchten Amerikaner: *1,12 ± 0,21*

* Der Dichtekoeffizient drückt das g-Äquivalent einer Al-Zn-Legierung pro cm³ Knochen aus. [WILLIAMS, D. E., and A. SAMSON: J. Amer. diet. Ass. **36**, 462 (1960), Tab. 1]

suchungen an *jungen Ratten* vorgenommen und zeigen können, daß durch eine *kalkhaltige Nahrung* bereits innerhalb von weniger als 7 Tagen eine Änderung der Knochendichte nachgewiesen werden kann. Von WILLIAMS, MCDONALD, MORRELL, SCHOFIELD und MCLEOD (1957) sind mit der von SCHRAER angegebenen Technik Untersuchungen an der *Calcaneusspongiosa* durchgeführt worden. Nach *längerer Kalkzufuhr* mit der Nahrung konnten keine eindeutigen Veränderungen der Knochendichte nachgewiesen werden.

WILLIAMS und SAMSON (1960) haben densitometrische Untersuchungen der Fingerknochen 2—5 bei 32 Studenten mit Hilfe eines Aluminium-Zink-Referenzsystems nach SCHRAER (1958) durchgeführt (Tabelle 19). Es handelte sich um 16 Inder oder Pakistaner (Alter 22—47 Jahre) und 16 Amerikaner (Alter 18—32 Jahre) männlichen und weiblichen Geschlechts. Die Meßwerte wurden nach SCHRAER als „Dichtekoeffizient" angegeben, die das Gewicht in Gramm der Aluminium-Zinkverbindung repräsentieren, welche die Röntgenstrahlung in gleicher Weise absorbiert wie 1 cm³ des durchstrahlten Knochens. Es fanden sich Werte von 1,10 g Aluminiumäquivalent/cm³ mit einer Standardabweichung von 0,19 und einem mittleren Fehler von 0,03. Die Beurteilung der Meßergebnisse aller Versuchspersonen ergab keinerlei Hinweise auf Zusammenhänge zwischen den Dichtekoeffizienten des Knochens und rassischen Unterschieden, dem Geschlecht, dem Alter, dem Gewicht oder der Größe der Versuchspersonen.

Zur Bestimmung der normalen Dichte von Knochen wurde nicht nur Aluminium, sondern auch Elfenbein als Standard- oder Referenzsystem verwendet. SCHMID (1960) untersuchte 325 Patienten im Alter von 5—85 Jahren, die entweder *knochengesund* waren oder an einer *chronischen Polyarthritis* bzw. *Arthrose* erkrankt waren (Methode s. S. 177). Er fand eine beträchtliche Zunahme der Knochendichte der *Diaphyse des Daumengrundgliedes* vom 5.—25. Lebensjahr. Danach war bis zum 60. Lebensjahr eine relative Konstanz der Knochendichte festzustellen, während nach dem 60. Lebensjahr ein deutliches Absinken der Knochendichtewerte gefunden wurde (Abb. 150). Die Knochendichte wurde bei diesen Messungen als Vergleichswert in Prozent angegeben, der sich auf eine Elfenbeintreppe als Referenzsystem bezieht. Eine Umrechnung in Aschewerte oder vergleichbare Werte einer Calciumverbindung (z.B. Hydroxylapatit) erfolgte nicht. Die gefundenen „*Normalwerte*" *für die Diaphyse der Daumengrundphalanx* können daher nur zu Meßwerten kranker Knochen in Beziehung gesetzt werden, die mit demselben Meßverfahren, also auf derselben Basis gewonnen worden sind (s. S. 269).

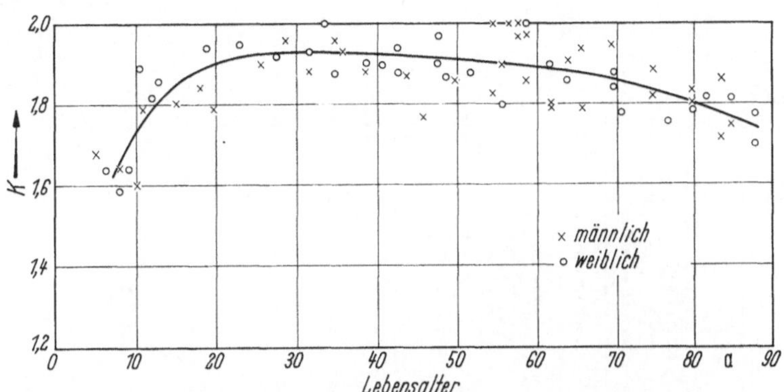

Abb. 95. Verteilung der K-Werte der Wirbelknochen von Gesunden in Abhängigkeit von Alter und Geschlecht. (Nach KROKOWSKI, persönliche Mitteilung)

Mit der von KROKOWSKI (1959) entwickelten Untersuchungsmethode (s. S. 200) haben KROKOWSKI und SCHLUNGBAUM (1959) an einer größeren Zahl gesunder und kranker Menschen Untersuchungen des „Schwächungsgleichwertes" *der Wirbelspongiosa* (sog. „K-Wert") vorgenommen. Der Vergleich gefundener K-Werte mit 100 klinischen, z.T. durch eine Knochenpunktion auch autoptisch bestätigten Befunden führte zur Festlegung des Normalbereiches in Abhängigkeit von Lebensalter und Geschlecht (Abb. 95). Bis zum 3. Lebensjahrzehnt ist ein Ansteigen des K-Wertes der Wirbelspongiosa festzustellen. Danach bleiben die K-Werte zunächst konstant, um im 5. oder 6. Lebensjahrzehnt wieder abzusinken. In späteren Mitteilungen dieser Arbeitsgruppe wurde der K-Wert in Hydroxylapatitwerte umgerechnet (s. S. 202 und Abb. 96).

Radiologische, chemische und histologische Untersuchungen über die Wirbelosteoporose an Knochenpräparaten der *Lendenwirbelsäule* von 100 Sektionen haben CALDWELL und COLLINS (1961) durchgeführt. Eine Aluminiumtreppe diente als Referenzsystem für die radiologische Dichtemessung. Der Calciumgehalt wurde durch chemische Analyse ermittelt und in mg/cm³ Gesamtknochen angegeben. Er schwankt zwischen 38 und 102 mg Ca pro cm³ Knochen. In 75% der Fälle fanden sich Werte zwischen 50—84 mg/cm³ (Tabelle 20). Die hohen Calciumwerte wurden bei jungen Menschen gefunden, während im Laufe des Alterungsprozesses ein Absinken der Calciumkonzentration festzustellen war. Sowohl der Calciumgehalt wie die radiologische Dichte waren beim männlichen Geschlecht höher als beim weiblichen Geschlecht, und zwar in jedem Lebensalter (Tabelle 21). Die vom Calciumgehalt abhängige Verminderung der Knochendichte mit dem Alter war statistisch signifikant. Eine Abgrenzung des „osteoporotischen" Knochens gegen den normalen Knochen war weder radiologisch noch chemisch-analytisch oder histologisch möglich. Die Ergebnisse zeigen die Problematik der Osteoporose-Diagnostik auf.

Mit Hilfe von Schwächungsgleichwerten sind zwar gewisse Informationen über den Mineralgehalt des Knochengewebes zu gewinnen, doch wurde immer wieder angestrebt,

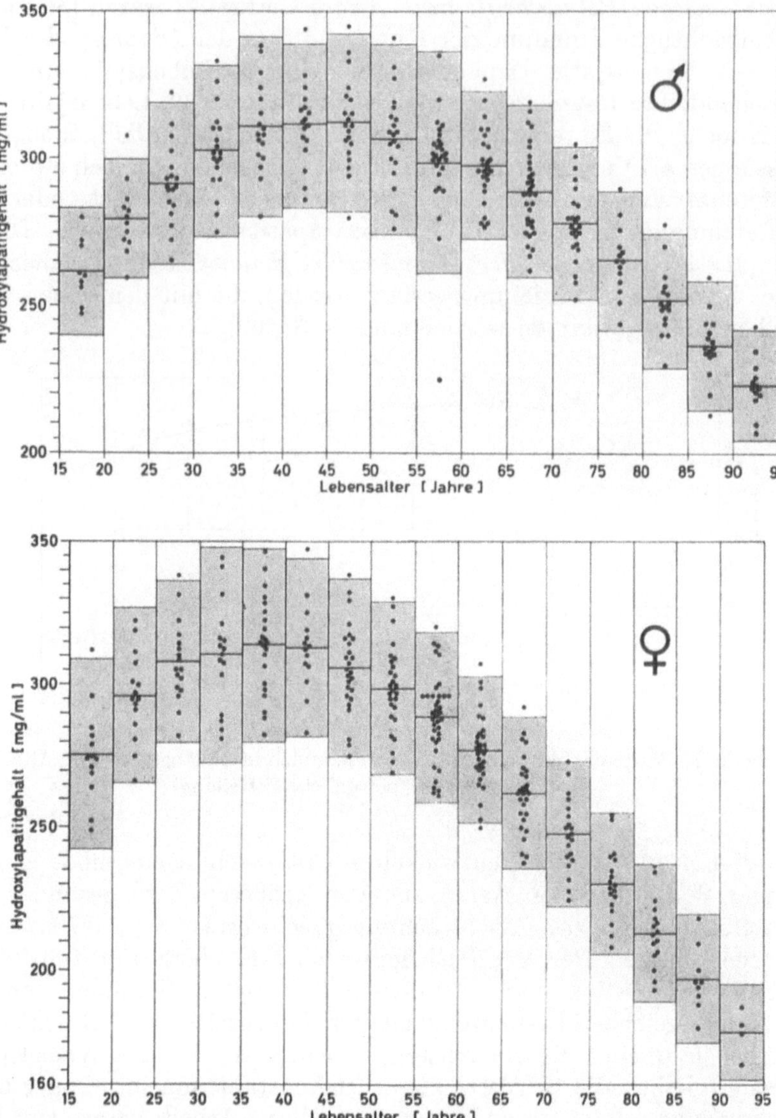

Abb. 96. Verteilung und Streuung der Normalwerte des Hydroxyl-Apatitgehaltes der Lendenwirbelkörper in Abhängigkeit von Lebensalter und Geschlecht. (Nach KROKOWSKI und HAASNER, 1968; Abb. 1)

Tabelle 20. *Calciumgehalt in mg/cm³ der Lendenwirbelkörper, geordnet nach der radiologischen Dichte (ausgedrückt in Einheiten des Vergleichskörpers aus Aluminium)*

Radiologische Dichte in Einheiten des Referenzsystems	Calcium in mg/cm³		Gesamtzahl der Fälle	Männlich		Weiblich	
	Mittelwerte	Bereich		Anzahl der Fälle	Durchschnittsalter in Jahren	Anzahl der Fälle	Durchschnittsalter in Jahren
4	48	—	1	0	—	1	88
5	53	38— 67	18	8	70,1	10	66,9
6	62	47— 76	32	19	60,5	13	68,8
7	75	60— 94	31	18	53	13	58,2
8	84	69—101	12	9	37	3	52,3
9	89	71—102	4	2	54,5	2	35,5
10	95	92— 97	2	2	29,5	0	—
			100	58		42	

[Caldwell, R. A., and D. H. Collins: J. Bone Jt. Surg. B **43**, 346 (1961), Tab. 2]

Tabelle 21. *Durchschnittswerte der radiologisch bestimmten Dichte von Lendenwirbelkörpern von Personen beiderlei Geschlechts geordnet nach Dezennien*

Altersgruppen	Männlich		Weiblich	
	Zahl der Fälle	Durchschnitts-Dichtewerte	Zahl der Fälle	Durchschnitts-Dichtewerte
0—10	—	—	—	—
11—20	5	8	—	—
21—30	3	7,3	2	8,5
31—40	4	7,25	2	7,0
41—50	6	7,5	2	8,0
51—60	10	6,9	8	6,6
61—70	20	6,2	14	5,8
71—80	8	6,5	12	5,75
81—90	2	5	2	5

[Caldwell, R. A., and D. H. Collins: J. Bone J. Surg. B **43**, 346 (1961), Tab. 3]

aus den verschiedensten Schwächungsgleichwerten entweder den tatsächlichen Calciumgehalt, den Aschegehalt oder den Hydroxylapatitgehalt der untersuchten Knochenregion zu ermitteln.

2. Die Berechnung der Mineralkonzentration (Hydroxylapatitgehalt) aus Schwächungsgleichwerten

Unter Berücksichtigung der physikalischen und biologischen Gegebenheiten ist die Berechnung des Hydroxylapatitgehaltes (oder Calciumgehaltes bzw. Aschegehaltes) aus verschiedenen Schwächungsgleichwerten durchaus möglich. Die Bedeutung eines solchen methodischen Vorgehens für die klinische Radiologie kann nur dann beurteilt werden, wenn die Fehlerbreite der Untersuchungsverfahren bekannt ist. Die rechnerisch gefundenen Meßergebnisse müssen auf ihre Übereinstimmung mit den chemisch-analytisch kontrollierten Werten der Kalksalzkonzentration im *gleichen Knochenareal* überprüft werden. Auf diesem Wege kann der Gesamtfehler einer Methode bestimmt werden. Solche Vergleichsuntersuchungen sind jedoch nur selten durchgeführt worden. An dem Knochenforschungszentrum der Pennsylvania-Universität in den Vereinigten Staaten erkannten Mack u. Mitarb. (1959) die Notwendigkeit einer chemisch-analytischen Kontrolle der errechneten Werte des Kalkgehaltes. So wurden die in vorangegangenen Untersuchungsreihen (Mack 1949) errechneten Werte des Knochenmineralgehaltes und dadurch das Berechnungsverfahren selbst kontrolliert. An 50 Knochenstücken menschlichen und tierischen Materials durchgeführte Vergleichsuntersuchungen ergaben nur geringe Abweichungen des *errechneten Mineralwertes* von den chemisch-analytisch gefundenen Werten des Kalksalzgehaltes.

Die praktische Durchführung eines solchen Untersuchungsverfahrens in der klinischen Radiologie haben Keane, Spiegler und Davis (1959) versucht (s. S. 165). Der Berechnung des Kalksalzgehaltes liegt die „effektive Mineraldicke“ zugrunde, wobei 1 mm Al-Äquivalent = 130 mm/cm^2 Knochenmineral gesetzt wird. Aus diesem „Flächenwert“ kann die *Konzentration der Kalksalze im Volumen Knochen* (g/cm^3) errechnet werden, wenn die durchstrahlte *Schichtdicke des Knochens* bekannt ist (Tabelle 22). Es wurde der Kalksalzgehalt der Ulna *in Nähe des Handgelenkes* bei solchen Menschen, die einer stärkeren Belastung des Handgelenkes (z.B. Busfahrer und Feuerwehrmänner) und solchen, die einer geringeren Belastung des Handgelenkes während des Lebens ausgesetzt waren, untersucht (Tabelle 23). Die gefundenen Werte schwanken zwischen 200 und 400 mg/cm^3 im Meßbereich der Ulna. Der niedrige Kalksalzgehalt wird als überraschender Befund registriert. Für die große Härte und Stabilität des Knochens dürfte jedoch auch die Makrostruktur von Bedeutung sein.

Tabelle 22. *Gegenüberstellung der verschiedenen Ergebnisse der quantitativen Bestimmung des Mineralgehaltes mit einer radiologischen Methode*

Meßstelle oberhalb des Proc. styloid.	1 Dem Aluminium entsprechende Dicke (t)	2 Effektive Mineraldicke (trn)	3 Dicke der Ulna lateral gem. (l)	4 Mineral-Konzentration (tm/l)
2 cm	2,0 mm	0,26 g/cm²	1,30 cm	0,20 g/cm³
4 cm	3,0 mm	0,39 g/cm²	1,35 cm	0,29 g/cm³
6 cm	3,7 mm	0,48 g/cm²	1,35 cm	0,36 g/cm³

[KEANE, B. E., G. SPIEGLER, and R. DAVIS: Brit. J. Radiol. 32, 162, (1959), Tab. 1]

Tabelle 23. *Resultate der Messungen des Mineralgehaltes der Ulna*

Personen	Beruf	Alter	Meßpunkt über dem Proc. styl. cm	Effektive Mineraldicke g/cm²	Lateraler ⌀ der Ulna cm	Mineralgehalt g/cm³
1	Keine körperliche Arbeit	32	2	0,37	1,3	0,28
			4	0,42	1,2	0,35
			6	0,58	1,25	0,46
2	Keine körperliche Arbeit	66	2	0,17	1,1	0,15
			4	0,33	1,05	0,32
			6	0,54	1,2	0,45
3	Feuerwehrmann	65	2	0,52	1,55	0,33
			4	0,65	1,3	0,50
			6	—	—	—
4	Autobusfahrer	57	2	0,49	1,15	0,42
			4	0,56	1,1	0,51
			6	0,62	1,2	0,52
5	Student (Rugbyspieler)	22	2	0,43	1,2	0,37
			4	0,57	1,2	0,47
			6	0,70	1,2	0,58

[KEANE, B. E., G. SPIEGLER, and R. DAVIS: Brit. J. Radiol. 32, 162 (1959), Tab. 2]

Normalwerte des Mineralgehaltes von *Ulna* (2 cm proximal von der distalen Gelenkfläche) und *Calcaneus* hat MAYO (1961) mit einer modifizierten Methode nach SPIEGLER u. Mitarb. (s. S. 165) bei 103 gesunden Personen ermittelt (Abb. 97). Die Meßwerte der Ulna lagen alle über 200 mg/ml (bis auf einen Wert, der wohl aus der Reihe fällt). Der Mittelwert der Ulna betrug beim *männlichen Geschlecht 370 mg/ml*, beim *weiblichen Geschlecht 325 mg/ml* mit einer Standardabweichung von 84,5 bzw. 87 mg/ml. Es wurden geringe Unterschiede zwischen rechter und linker Ulna gefunden, jedoch keine Konstanz in Abhängigkeit von Rechts- oder Linkshändern. Die Mineralkonzentration im *rechten Calcaneus* betrug durchschnittlich *bei Männern 180 mg/ml*, bei *Frauen 175 mg/ml* mit einer Standardabweichung von 38 bzw. 37 mg/ml bei größeren Einzelabweichungen. Zunächst sind beide Calcanei untersucht worden, doch fanden sich keine wesentlichen Unterschiede, so daß die Messungen der normalen Mineralkonzentration allein am rechten Calcaneus fortgesetzt wurden. Zwischen dem *Mineralgehalt* des Knochens und der *Dichte der Spongiosaarchitektur* war eine gute Übereinstimmung festzustellen. Die Meßergebnisse

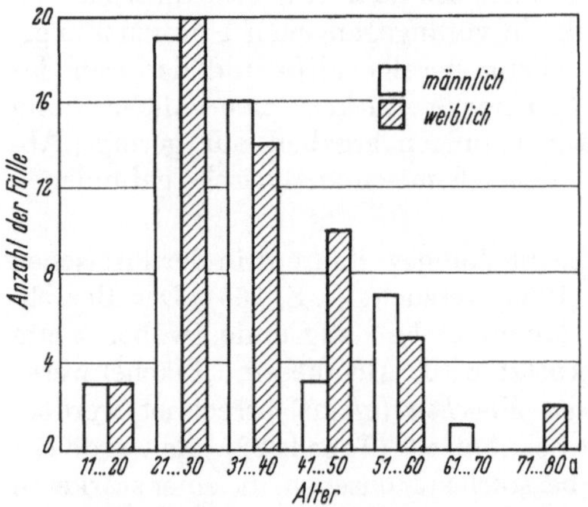

Abb. 97. Die Alters- und Geschlechtsverteilung der Normalfälle. (Nach MAYO, 1961; Abb. 3)

der einzelnen Altersgruppen lassen beim weiblichen Geschlecht einen *geringen Abfall* der Mineralkonzentration mit dem Alter erkennen, während diese Tendenz beim männlichen Geschlecht nicht so deutlich ist (Abb. 98a und b). Eine Abhängigkeit des Knochenmineralgehaltes von *Größe* und *Gewicht* war nicht festzustellen. Hervorzuheben sind *die großen*

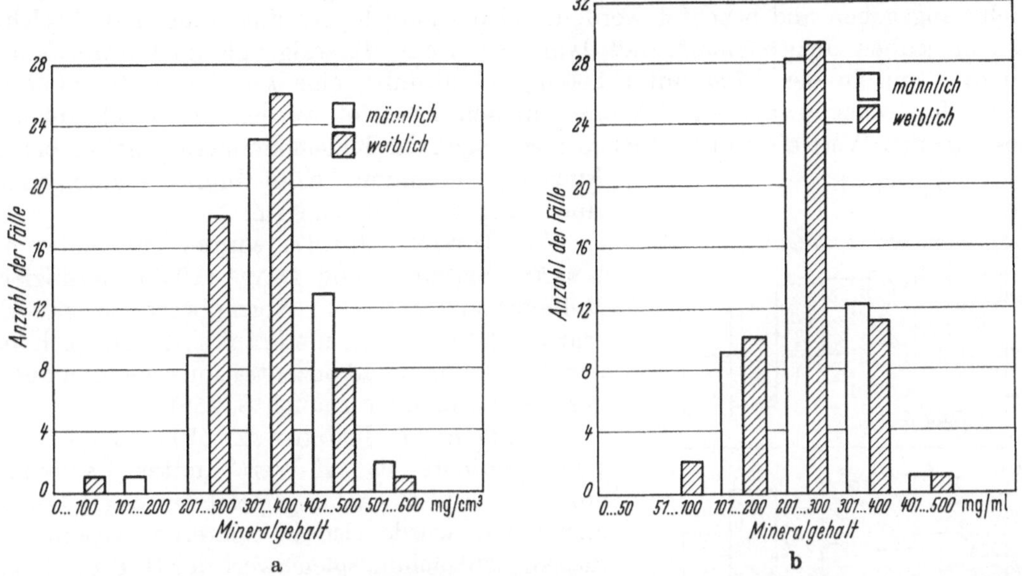

Abb. 98a. Häufigkeitsverteilung der Mineralkonzentration in der Ulna 2 cm proximal vom Handgelenk. (Nach MAYO, 1961; Abb. 4)

Abb. 98b. Häufigkeitsverteilung der Mineralkonzentration im Calcaneus. (Nach MAYO, 1961; Abb. 6)

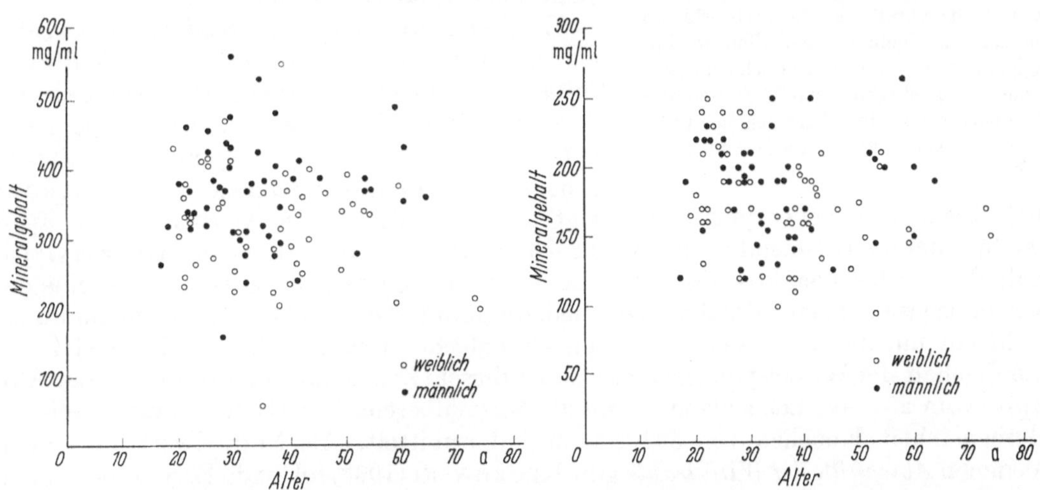

Abb. 99. Verteilung der Meßwerte des Knochenmineralgehaltes von Ulna (links) und Calcaneus (rechts) beim männlichen und weiblichen Geschlecht. (Nach MAYO, 1961; Abb. 8 und 9)

individuellen Unterschiede der globalen Kalksalzkonzentration von Knochen (Abb. 99). Diese Faktoren sollten beachtet werden und sind nicht nur für die untersuchten Knochenregionen von Interesse, sondern auch von Einfluß auf die Meßergebnisse des „Compactaindex" der Diaphysen (BARNETT und NORDIN 1960; s. S. 225). Eine besondere Bedeutung für die Größenordnung der globalen Kalksalzkonzentration eines Knochenbezirkes wird *der spezifischen Spongiosaarchitektur des Einzelindividuum* zugeschrieben. So ist es nicht möglich, den „Normalwert" des Mineralgehaltes von Knochen festzustellen, ohne *individuelle Besonderheiten* zu berücksichtigen. Bei einem Einzelindividuum mit hohem

Mineralgehalt im Knochengesamtvolumen kann — wenn eine krankhafte Verminderung der globalen Kalksalzkonzentration eintritt — auch dann noch ein Wert gemessen werden, der in den „Normbereich" fällt, wenn bereits ein relativ hoher Mineralverlust eingetreten ist. So kann der Wert von Messungen des Mineralgehaltes durch diese Probleme begrenzt sein. Aus den genannten Gründen sollte daher immer die Lage des Meßwertes zum „Normbereich" angegeben und beachtet werden. Wiederholte Kontrollmessungen sind wichtig! Es bleibt jedoch unzweifelhaft, daß dann, wenn der Mineralgehalt im *Calcaneus* unter 110 mg/ml und in der *Ulna* unter 200 mg/ml absinkt, eine *krankhafte Verminderung* vorliegt. Die oben genannten Faktoren müssen beachtet werden, doch schränken sie keineswegs den Wert der radiologischen Messungen des Knochenmineralgehaltes bei dem Einzelindividuum und Kontrolluntersuchungen über einen längeren Zeitraum ein.

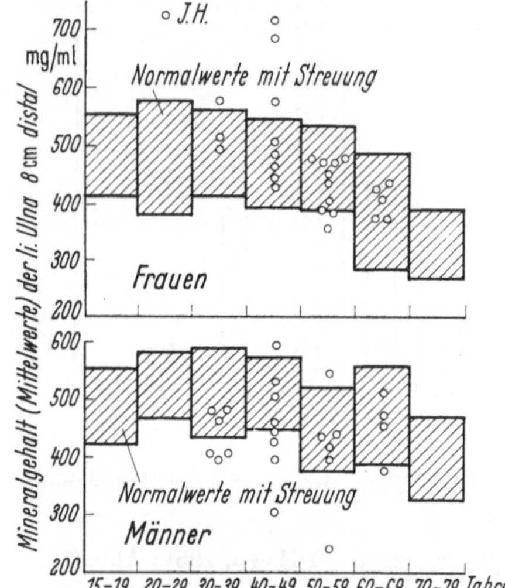

Abb. 100. Streubreite der Normalwerte des Knochenmineralgehaltes der Ulna in Abhängigkeit von Alter und Geschlecht (zusammen mit Meßwerten von 27 Frauen und 24 Männern sowie einer Akromegalie aufgetragen). (Nach DOYLE, 1967; Abb. 1)

Von DOYLE (1961/67) wurden mit einer nach KEANE, SPIEGLER und DAVIS (1959) modifizierten Meßmethode (s. S. 166) Normalwerte an der Ulna erarbeitet (Abb. 100), um krankhafte Abweichungen der Knochenmineralkonzentration erkennen und abgrenzen zu können (s. auch S. 258).

Nachdem von KROKOWSKI (1959) zunächst die Knochendichte als „K-Wert" unter Verwendung eines Wasser-Schwächungsgleichwertes (H_2O-SGW) angegeben wurde, ist in späteren Arbeiten aus diesem Schwächungsgleichwert der Hydroxylapatitgehalt berechnet worden. Die Berechnung basiert auf dem Vergleich des radiologisch-photometrisch ermittelten Meßwertes (Methode s. S. 200) mit chemischen Analysen desselben.

Es sind *Normalwerte des Hydroxylapatitgehaltes* in der Spongiosa von *Wirbelkörper*, *Radius* und *Calcaneus* mitgeteilt worden. Die Ergebnisse der Untersuchungen des 3. Lendenwirbelkörpers lassen eine Abhängigkeit des Hydroxylapatitgehaltes vom Lebensalter erkennen (OESER und KROKOWSKI 1961). Bis zum 4. Lebensjahrzehnt steigt der Mineralgehalt im Wirbelknochen an und sinkt bis zum 90. Lebensjahr um etwa 20—40% ab (Abb. 101). Wird der Hydroxylapatitgehalt der Wirbelspongiosa gegen das Lebensalter aufgetragen, so ergibt sich eine gegen die Altersachse geneigte Parabel. Der Scheitelpunkt der Parabel liegt beim männlichen Geschlecht um das 45., beim weiblichen Geschlecht etwa um das 38. Lebensjahr. Der Mineralgehalt der Wirbelspongiosa ist also zu diesem Zeitpunkt am größten. In der Altersgruppe vom 25.—65. Lebensjahr wurde als Normalbereich ein Hydroxylapatitgehalt pro Volumeneinheit Knochen von 307 ± 33 mg/ml ermittelt. Als Normalwerte für die verschiedenen *Abschnitte der Wirbelsäule* gibt KROKOWSKI (1963) folgende Ergebnisse bekannt:

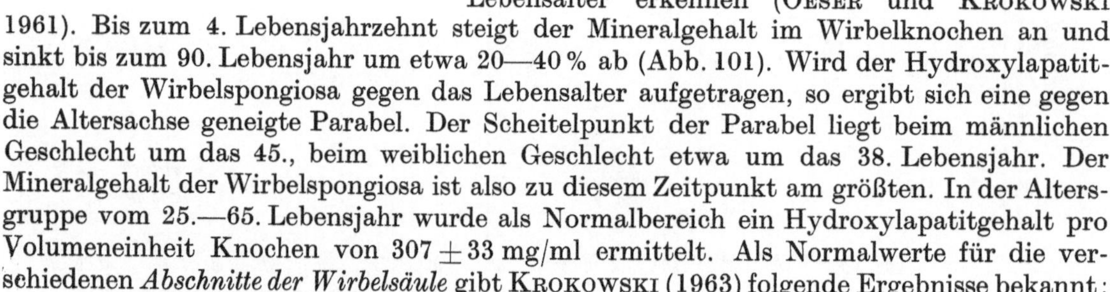

In der Halswirbelsäule 300—350 mg/ml,
in der Brustwirbelsäule 250—275 mg/ml und
in der Lendenwirbelsäule 275—300 mg/ml.

In einer späteren Untersuchungsreihe haben KROKOWSKI u. Mitarb. (1967) über die Altersabhängigkeit des Hydroxylapatitgehaltes in der Wirbelspongiosa des 4. LWK auf Grund von 615 Untersuchungen (297 ♂ und 318 ♀) an knochengesunden Personen berichtet (Tabelle 24). Die an der Wirbelsäule erhobenen Befunde werden als Grundlage einer genauen Definition der Knochenentkalkung verwendet. Für eine Osteoporose war bisher die Einteilung in juvenile, präsenile und senile Osteoporose gebräuchlich. Von KROKOWSKI wird diese Einteilung derart ergänzt, daß durch Vergleich mit der *physiologischen Alterskurve* eine *Involutionsosteoporose* und eine *präsenile Osteoporose* von der *pathologischen Osteoporose* abgegrenzt werden. KROKOWSKI meint, daß bei der sog. „physiologischen Osteoporose" die mit steigendem Lebensalter zunehmende Demineralisation in allen Skeletabschnitten synchron verlaufe, während bei der generalisierten „pathologischen Osteoporose" zuerst das Stammskelet, dann das Beckenskelet, der Femurkopf

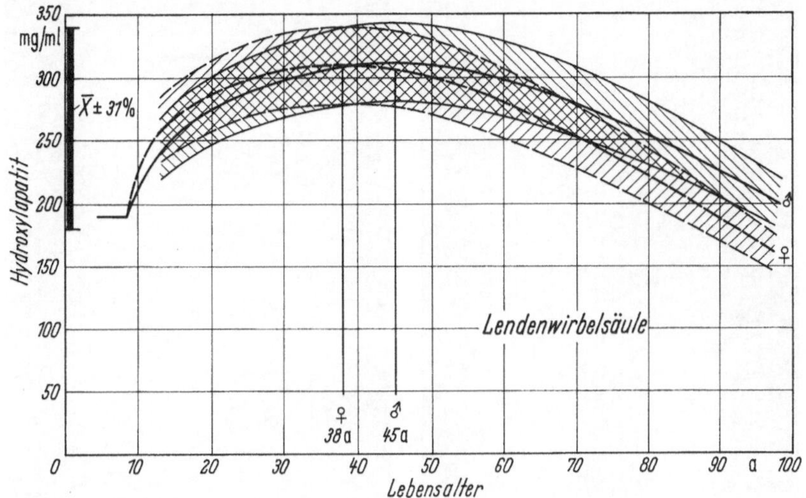

Abb. 101. Hydroxylapatitgehalt in der Wirbelspongiosa (3. und 4. Lendenwirbelkörper) in Abhängigkeit von Alter und Geschlecht. (Nach KROKOWSKI, 1965/67)

Tabelle 24. *Ergebnisse der Messungen des Hydroxylapatitgehaltes vom 4. Lendenwirbelkörper, angegeben in mg/ml Gesamtknochen*

Altersgruppen (Jahre)	♂				♀			
	Anzahl n	Mittelwert $\bar{x}$	2σ	Normbereich $\bar{x} \pm 2\sigma$	Anzahl n	Mittelwert $\bar{x}$	2σ	Normbereich $\bar{x} \pm 2\sigma$
15—19	9	261,44	21,6	239,84—283,04	13	275,54	33,4	242,14—308,94
20—24	12	279,50	20,4	259,10—299,90	15	295,93	30,6	265,33—326,53
25—29	18	291,17	27,4	263,77—318,57	17	307,76	28,2	279,56—335,96
30—34	19	302,53	29,0	273,53—331,53	16	310,13	37,6	272,53—347,73
35—39	17	310,65	30,6	280,05—341,25	22	313,55	33,6	279,95—347,15
40—44	17	311,12	27,8	283,32—338,92	14	312,71	31,2	281,51—343,91
45—49	20	312,20	30,2	282,00—342,40	26	305,42	30,8	247,62—336,22
50—54	21	306,52	32,4	274,12—338,92	27	298,48	30,2	268,28—328,68
55—59	27	298,56	37,6	260,96—336,16	38	288,39	29,6	258,79—317,99
60—64	26	297,69	25,2	272,49—322,89	31	277,00	25,6	251,40—302,60
65—69	32	288,84	29,2	259,64—318,04	28	261,96	26,4	235,56—288,36
70—74	24	278,04	26,0	252,04—304,04	20	247,65	25,4	222,25—273,05
75—79	14	265,29	23,8	241,49—289,09	18	230,33	24,8	205,53—255,13
80—84	16	251,50	23,0	228,50—274,50	16	213,00	24,2	188,80—237,20
85—89	16	236,50	22,0	214,50—258,50	9	196,89	22,4	174,49—219,29
90—94	13	222,92	18,8	204,12—241,72	4	178,25	16,8	161,45—195,05

[STRESEMANN, E., u. E. KROKOWSKI: Klin. Wschr. **45**, 564 (1967), Tab. 1]

und Schenkelhals und schließlich die peripheren Skeletabschnitte betroffen seien. Der Bestimmung des Hydroxylapatitgehaltes in der Wirbelsäule komme daher die größere Bedeutung zu gegenüber Messungen der Kalksalzkonzentration von Knochen in peripheren Skeletabschnitten.

In der *distalen Metaphyse des Radius* (Abb. 102a und b) wurde, verglichen mit den in der Wirbelsäule gefundenen Werten des Knochenmineralgehaltes, ein analoger Kurvenverlauf der Hydroxylapatitkonzentration während des Alterungsprozesses gefunden (Abb. 101), doch ist die Abnahme des Mineralgehaltes in diesem Knochen mit zunehmendem Lebensalter größer (OESER und KROKOWSKI 1961; KROKOWSKI und

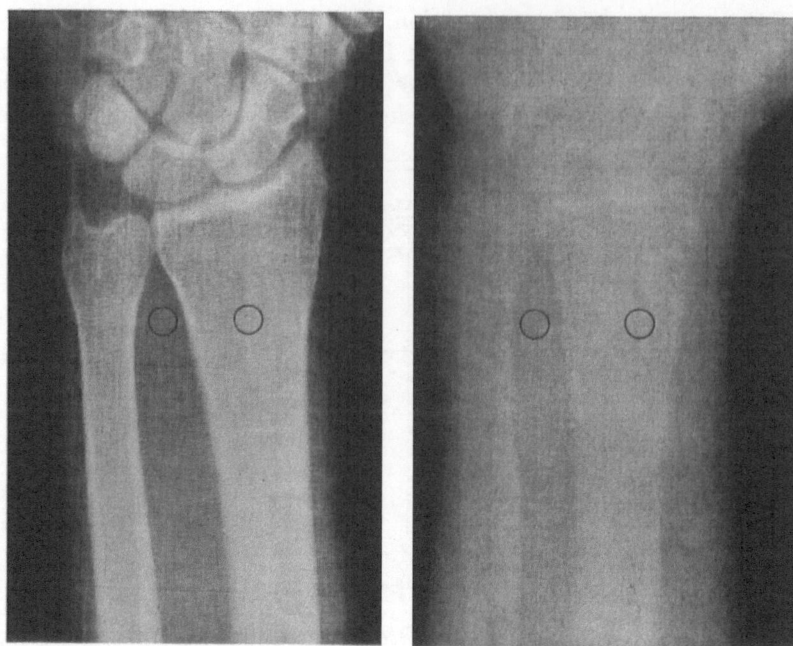

Abb. 102a. Röntgenaufnahme des Radius mit Meßzonen (○) bei 45 und 250 kV Anodenspannung hergestellt. (Nach KROKOWSKI und STEINER, 1961; Abb. 2a und b)

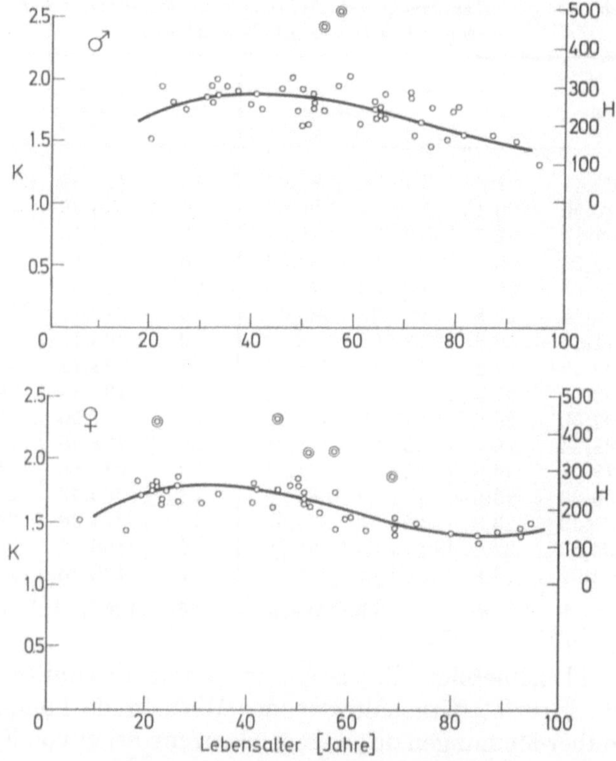

Abb. 102b. Meßwerte der Radiusspongiosa in Abhängigkeit vom Lebensalter beim männlichen (oben) und weiblichen (unten) Geschlecht. (Nach KROKOWSKI und STEINER, 1961; Abb. 4)

STEINER 1961). Vom 40.—80. Lebensjahr soll nach den Ergebnissen von KROKOWSKI (1962) der Hydroxylapatitgehalt der Radiusmetaphyse um fast 40% absinken. Als Normalbereich für das 25.—65. Lebensjahr wird ein Hydroxylapatitgehalt von 267 ±

66 mg/ml Knochen bei männlichen und von 233 ± 53 mg/ml Knochen bei weiblichen Personen angegeben. Die *normale Variationsbreite des Apatitgehaltes* soll in der Wirbelspongiosa ± 11 %, in der Radiusspongiosa ± 25 % betragen. Die größere Schwankungsbreite des Kalksalzgehaltes im peripheren Knochen wird mit individuell unterschiedlicher Belastung erklärt. Körperlich arbeitende Menschen weisen einen höheren Hydroxylapatitgehalt in der Radiusspongiosa auf. Der Hydroxylapatitgehalt in den Wirbelkörpern ließ keine beruflich bedingten Unterschiede erkennen. Aus diesen Befunden wird geschlossen, daß bereits die aufrechte Haltung und der aufrechte Gang des Menschen einen genügenden Reiz zur maximalen Kalksalzeinlagerung in die Wirbelkörper darstellen.

In weiteren Untersuchungen wurde der Hydroxylapatitgehalt der *Calcaneusspongiosa* ermittelt (Abb. 103). Auch hier fand sich eine altersabhängige Verminderung des Knochen-

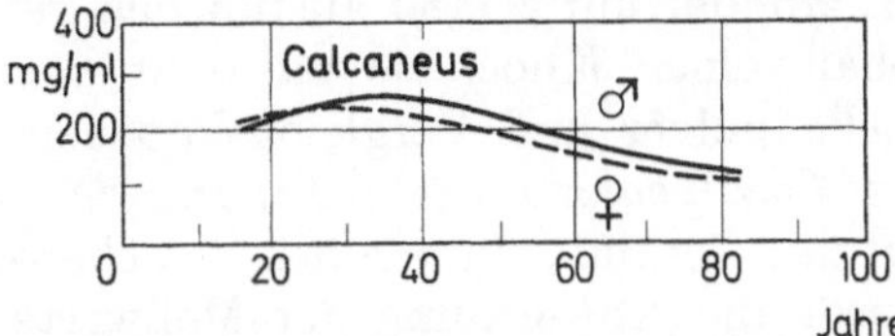

Abb. 103. Ergebnisse der Messung der Hydroxylapatitkonzentration im Calcaneus in Abhängigkeit von Alter und Geschlecht. (Nach KROKOWSKI, 1965; Abb. 2)

mineralgehaltes. In allen untersuchten Knochenpartien war mit der Methode von KROKOWSKI eine Abnahme der Hydroxylapatitkonzentration im Laufe des Alterungsprozesses festzustellen. Dieser Befund spricht für die Existenz einer *Altersosteoporose*, die in allen Abschnitten des Skeletes auftritt. Der Kurvenverlauf der Hydroxylapatitkonzentration in den untersuchten Skeletregionen zeigt gleiche Unterschiede bei den Geschlechtern.

Tabelle 25. *Ergebnisse von Untersuchungen des Knochenmineralgehaltes im Grundglied des 3. Fingers der linken Hand*

Männer					Frauen				
Lfd. Nr. nach VIRTAMA	Alter	wirklicher Knochen-mineralgehalt in mg/ml	photometrisch ermittelter Knochen-mineralgehalt in mg/ml	Fehler	Lfd. Nr. nach VIRTAMA	Alter	wirklicher Knochen-mineralgehalt in mg/ml	photometrisch ermittelter Knochen-mineralgehalt in mg/ml	Fehler
2	39	497	432	065	20	33	540	525	015
34	42	485	483	002	33	41	464	457	007
25	46	449	459	010	22	43	532	556	024
31	47	490	499	009	18	50	455	463	008
32	49	373	388	015	46	53	387	395	008
45	52	465	468	003	9	55	533	554	021
1	58	387	378	009	12	56	523	539	016
5	58	490	480	010	13	57	499	496	003
26	58	472	463	009	14	59	492	488	004
10	60	470	468	002	3	60	482	473	007
4	62	408	415	069	15	61	499	493	006
8	62	464	467	003	28	64	429	426	003
6	63	518	533	015	30	64	295	350	055
37	65	388	393	005	7	65	422	428	006
40	65	505	509	004	17	69	528	529	001
27	66	406	415	009	42	70	481	468	013
23	68	507	495	012	44	70	470	466	004
24	69	515	504	011	39	71	525	523	002
21	71	358	377	019	11	74	366	342	024
19	74	523	525	001	36	76	484	478	006
41	77	541	558	017	38	78	469	468	001
16	80	493	479	014	29	80	541	557	016
					43	82	521	517	004
					35	85	352	355	003

[VIRTAMA, P.: Acta anat. (Basel) **31**, Suppl. 29 (1957), Tab. 18 und 19]

Der Altersknick liegt beim männlichen Geschlecht im 40. Lebensjahr, beim weiblichen Geschlecht etwas früher, im 35. Lebensjahr. Während der Pubertät sei ein plötzlicher Anstieg des Hydroxylapatitgehaltes im Knochen festzustellen.

Von Oeser und Krokowski (1963) wird auf einen *Anstieg des Mineralgehaltes der Zähne* im Wachstumsalter zwischen 6 und 18 Jahren aufmerksam gemacht. Danach sei ein konstanter Abfall festzustellen. Diese Beobachtung stimmt jedoch nicht mit den Untersuchungsergebnissen anderer Autoren überein (Mäntylä, Telkkä, Wegelius und Virtama 1964). Bei einer Caries sei eine Verminderung des Kalksalzgehaltes in den Zähnen festzustellen. Dieser Befund entspricht der lokalen Demineralisation, wie sie für eine Caries charakteristisch ist.

Ein anderer Weg zur *Berechnung* des Aschegehaltes der Knochen ist von Virtama (1957) beschritten worden. Mit der auf S. 180 ausführlich geschilderten Methode wurde der unbekannte Aschegehalt eines Knochens zu dem bekannten Aschegehalt eines Referenzsystems aus Knochenpulver und Vergleichsknochen in Beziehung gesetzt. Die Messungen wurden an der *Basalphalanx des 3. Fingers der linken Hand* durchgeführt. Der Aschegehalt wurde auf das Gesamtvolumen des Knochens bezogen. Durch chemisch-analytische Kontrollen wurde die Abweichung der Meßwerte ermittelt. An einem Sektionsmaterial von 46 männlichen und weiblichen Präparaten konnte der Aschegehalt pro Volumeneinheit Knochen in der Basalphalanx des 3. Fingers der linken Hand gemessen werden. Zur Erleichterung eines Vergleiches mit den Ergebnissen anderer Untersuchungen und zur Darstellung der Alters- und Geschlechtsunterschiede wurde das Untersuchungsmaterial von Virtama nach Alter und Geschlecht der Probanden neu geordnet (Tabelle 25).

3. Die Ergebnisse der direkten Messung der Hydroxylapatitkonzentration („Apatitwert“)

Durch methodische Unterschiede der bisher erarbeiteten Meßverfahren war eine *Verständigung* verschiedener Untersucher über den Knochenmineralgehalt von gesunden und kranken Menschen erschwert. Es war unmöglich, die mit unterschiedlichen Methoden erarbeiteten Normalwerte miteinander zu vergleichen. Die Referenzsysteme aus Rinderknochen, Elfenbein und Knochenpulver bestehen aus einem Material, dessen Zusammensetzung Schwankungen unterworfen ist, so daß die gemessenen Werte nicht exakt reproduziert werden können. Die Verwendung von Vergleichskörpern aus Aluminium, Aluminiumlegierungen und anderen Metallen erfordert konstante Untersuchungsbedingungen, da die Meßergebnisse nicht unabhängig von der verwendeten Strahlenqualität sind.

Zur quantitativen Bestimmung der Kalksalzkonzentration im Gesamtvolumen eines Knochenbezirkes wurde daher von Heuck und Schmidt (1954/59/60) die Verwendung eines reproduzierbaren und knochengleichen Referenzsystems empfohlen (Methode s. S. 184). Diese radiologische Methode vergleicht die Strahlenabsorption eines umschriebenen Knochenareals unbekannten Kalksalzgehaltes mit der Strahlenabsorption derselben Schichtdicke eines Referenzsystems, das zusammengesetzt ist aus dem im Knochen vorwiegend vorhandenen Kalksalz — dem Hydroxylapatit — und einem Kunststoff (Polyacrylharz). Das Meßergebnis wurde als *„Apatitwert“* in die klinische Radiologie eingeführt. Aus den Apatitwerten kann der Calciumgehalt in mg/ml Knochensubstanz errechnet werden (1 mg Hydroxylapatit enthält 0,3989 mg Calcium). Die Bestimmung der Hydroxylapatitkonzentration erfolgte bevorzugt in spongiösen Knochenpartien, da hier bereits frühzeitig krankhafte Abweichungen, insbesondere bei Systemerkrankungen des Skeletes auftreten. Von Heuck und Schmidt (1960) wurden Messungen in der Mitte der Spongiosa des Femurhalses (225 Probanden) und der Spongiosa des Calcaneus (120 Probanden) bei erwachsenen, knochengesunden Menschen durchgeführt.

Mit der Methode von Heuck und Schmidt (1960) hat Hansen (1964) Untersuchungen der Kalksalzkonzentration in der *Calcaneusspongiosa bei 370 knochengesunden Säuglingen und Kindern* im Alter von 2 Tagen bis zu 16 Jahren vorgenommen. Trotz eines erstaunlich großen Normalbereiches fand sich ein statistisch signifikanter Anstieg des Hydroxylapatitgehaltes im Gesamtvolumen des Calcaneus während der Kindheit von 110 auf fast 200 mg/ml (Abb. 104). Bei allen Versuchen zur Analysierung und Objektivierung der ver-

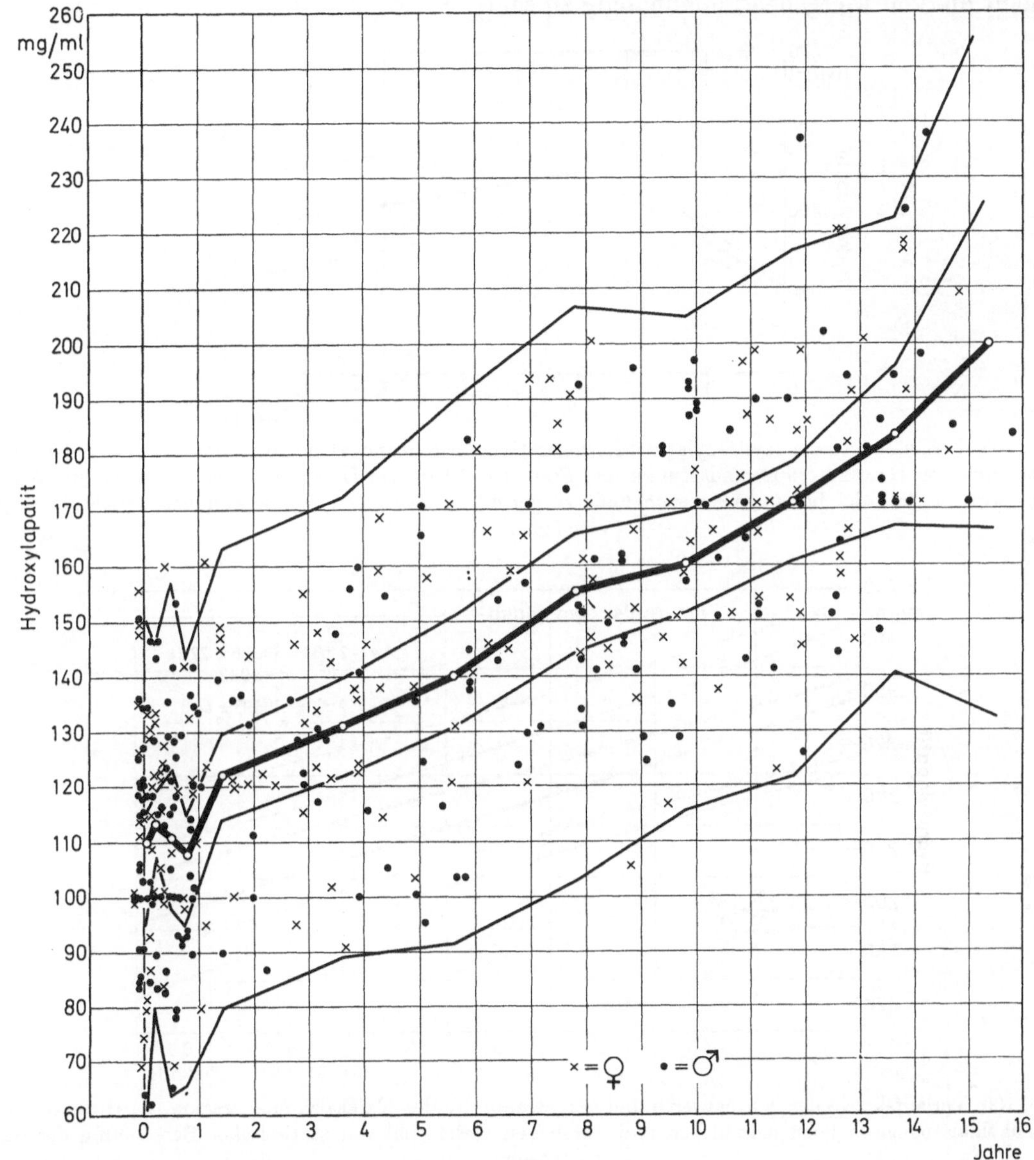

Abb. 104. Mittlere Kalksalzkonzentration im Calcaneus während der Kindheit mit Streubereich der Mittelwerte und Normalbereich, $N = 370$. (Nach HANSEN, 1962/64; Abb. 2)

schiedenen Entwicklungspotenzen des Kindes in Messung der Körperhöhe, des Körpergewichtes und des Knochenalters ist eine regelmäßig wiederkehrende erhebliche Streubreite des „Normalen“ festzustellen, die durch eine Vielzahl nicht immer analysierbarer Faktoren bedingt ist unter denen die Konstitution, die Ernährung und der phasenhafte Ablauf der Entwicklung sicher eine wesentliche Rolle spielen. Da jedes Kind in diesem Sinne sich nach einem individuellen Gesetz entwickelt, erfahren alle Vergleiche mit Durchschnittswerten eine wesentliche Einschränkung besonders im Hinblick auf die exakte Abgrenzung gegenüber krankhaften Werten. HANSEN (1964) nimmt an, daß unter physiologischen Bedingungen die Belastung einen maßgeblichen Reiz für die Mineralisation darstellt. Diese Ansicht wird dadurch gestützt, daß die Korrelation zwischen Mineralgehalt und Körpergewicht viel enger ist als diejenige zwischen Mineralgehalt und Längenwachstum bzw. Knochenreife. Die Wirkung androgener Hormone während der puberalen Entwicklung sowie diejenige therapeutisch zugeführter anaboler Steroide scheint hiervon weitgehend unabhängig zu sein.

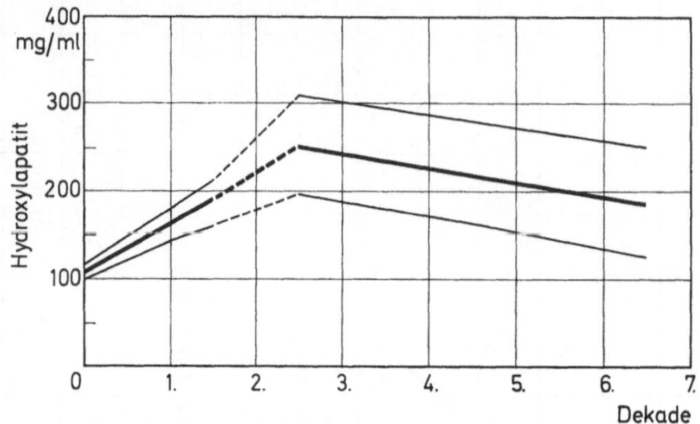

Abb. 105. Verlaufskurve der Hydroxylapatitkonzentration der Calcaneusspongiosa zusammengestellt nach den Meßwerten von Hansen (1962) und Heuck und Schmidt (1960). Im Übergangsbereich vom 2. zum 3. Jahrzehnt war die Zahl der bisher gemessenen Fälle zu gering, so daß hier nur eine annähernd richtige Angabe möglich war

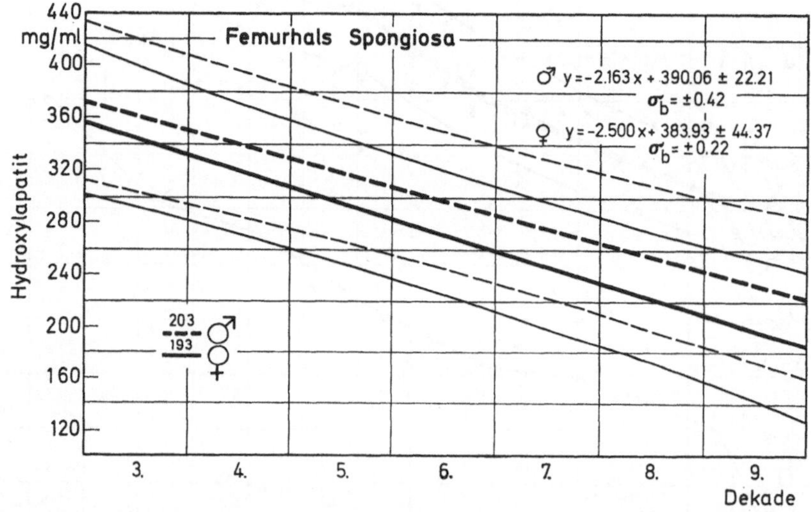

Abb. 106. Verlaufskurve der Normalwerte und der Streubreite der Kalksalzkonzentration (Apatitwert) in der Schenkelhalsspongiosa beim männlichen und weiblichen Geschlecht mit statistischer Berechnung der Streubreite

Die „Normalwerte" in den nachfolgenden Lebensjahrzehnten haben Heuck und Schmidt (1959/60) ermittelt (Abb. 105). Die Meßergebnisse der globalen Kalksalzkonzentration der Schenkelhalsspongiosa und der Calcaneusspongiosa in den einzelnen Dezennien lassen erkennen, daß vom 4. oder 5. Lebensjahrzehnt an ein Abfall des „Apatitwertes" eintritt (Abb. 106 und 107). Der Gipfel der Kurve der Hydroxylapatitkonzentration liegt also im 3. Lebensjahrzehnt. Danach ist ein *kontinuierliches Absinken* des Knochenmineralgehaltes als Ausdruck des *normalen Alterungsprozesses* zu beobachten. Diese altersabhängigen Veränderungen der Konzentration der Kalksalze im Gesamtvolumen eines Knochens stimmen in der Grundtendenz mit den Untersuchungsergebnissen anderer Autoren überein, die „Schwächungsgleichwerte" oder „Dichtekoeffizienten" des Knochengewebes ermittelt haben. Bemerkenswert ist die *erhebliche Streubreite der Normalwerte* der Kalksalzkonzentration bei beiden Geschlechtern. Beim männlichen Geschlecht war im allgemeinen eine etwas höhere Kalksalzkonzentration in den untersuchten Knochenregionen festzustellen. Die statistische Auswertung einer größeren Untersuchungsreihe ergibt signifikante Differenzen der Kalksalzkonzentration bei den Geschlechtern lediglich im Bereich der Femurhalsspongiosa, während die Calcaneusspongiosa und die Spongiosa der Radiusmetaphyse (QUINTAR 1962) keine statistisch signifikanten Geschlechtsunterschiede aufweisen (HEUCK und KÖHLER 1969). Der Normbereich dieser drei Spongiosapartien streut relativ breit (Abb. 106—108).

Wie bereits das einfache Röntgenbild des Skeletes erkennen läßt, ist die Dichte verschiedener Bezirke des gleichen Knochens sowie verschiedener Knochen des gleichen

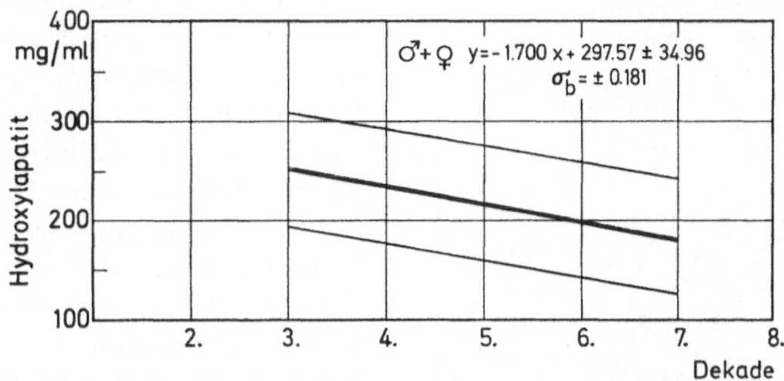

Abb. 107. Knochenmineralgehalt im Calcaneus bei Erwachsenen beiderlei Geschlechts und Streubreite der Norm. In der Calcaneusspongiosa fanden sich keine signifikanten Unterschiede der Hydroxylapatitkonzentration zwischen dem männlichen und weiblichen Geschlecht. (Nach HEUCK, 1968)

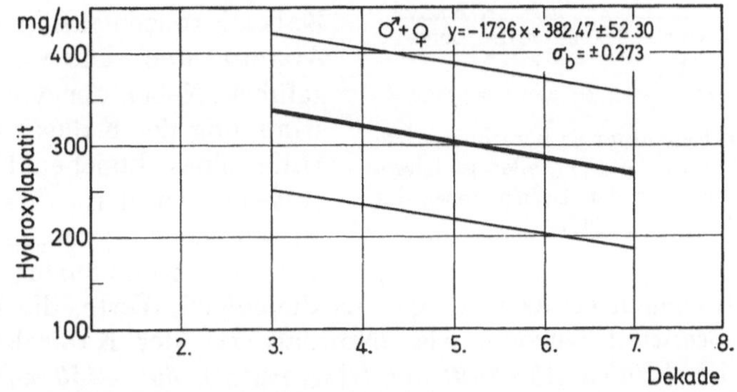

Abb. 108. Knochenmineralgehalt in der Metaphyse des Radius (Apatitwerte nach HEUCK und SCHMIDT, 1960) bei beiden Geschlechtern. Es war kein signifikanter Unterschied zwischen den Geschlechtern nachweisbar. Statistische Berechnung der Regressionslinie und Streubreite

Skeletes sehr unterschiedlich. Es kann also erwartet werden, daß auch die Hydroxylapatitkonzentration in der Knochenfrischsubstanz an verschiedenen Punkten ein und desselben Knochens außerordentlich differieren muß, da sich die Meßwerte auf das durchstrahlte Gesamtvolumen eines Knochenbezirkes beziehen. Unterschiede der Struktur und Architektur eines Knochens sind für den Apatitwert nicht ohne Bedeutung (s. S. 149). Der *Globalwert* der Hydroxylapatitkonzentration in *reiner Spongiosa* schwankt zwischen 180 und 400 mg/ml. In solchen Knochenbezirken, in denen die Spongiosa von einer dickeren *Corticalis* oder bereits von der Compacta umschlossen wird, müssen die Werte höher liegen. Die Unterschiede in der Hydroxylapatitkonzentration verschiedener Knochen und Knochenabschnitte des Skeletes werden von Morphologie und Makrostruktur der untersuchten Knochen abhängig sein. Diese Tatsache sollte bei der klinischen Anwendung und Wertung dieser radiologischen Meßverfahren zur Skeletanalyse beachtet werden.

Eine nähere Analyse der Meßergebnisse des „Apatitwertes" in den verschiedenen Lebensaltern bei gesunden Menschen erlaubt gewisse Aussagen. Die im Säuglings- und Kleinkindesalter beobachtete „physiologische Osteoporose" kann nur dadurch erklärt werden, daß nach der Geburt eine Transformation des geflechtartigen Knochens in den *spongiösen* Knochen erfolgt. Nach dem 1. Lebensjahr ist keine eindeutige Verminderung der Knochenkalksalzkonzentration zu beobachten. Zwischen dem 11. und 15. Lebensjahr ist ein steilerer Anstieg der Apatitkurve erkennbar, der mit dem *Wachstumsschub in der Pubertät* parallel geht und offenbar in Beziehung zur Gonadenreifung steht. Die Zunahme der Kalksalzkonzentration bis in das 3. Lebensjahrzehnt spricht dafür, daß *Mineralisation und Wachstum nicht parallel gehen* und mit dem Epiphysenfugenschluß Knochenbildung und Knochentransformation noch nicht abgeschlossen sind. Ein Vergleich der Globalwerte der Kalksalzkonzentration beider Geschlechter in der Schenkelhalsspongiosa (Abb. 109) zeigt keine Unterschiede im 3. Lebensjahrzehnt, danach ein stärkeres Absinken des Apatitwertes beim weiblichen Geschlecht und im hohen Greisenalter wiederum keine statistisch zu sichernden Unterschiede zwischen den Geschlechtern (HEUCK und KÖHLER 1969).

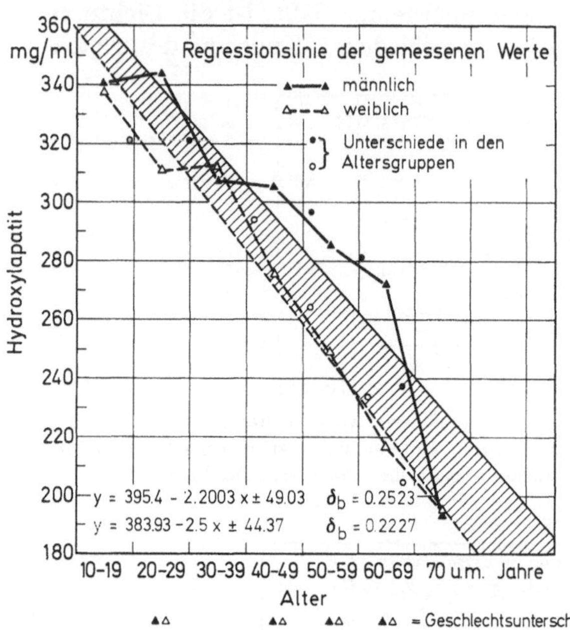

Abb. 109. Die aus den Originalwerten berechneten Regressionsgeraden. ○ (♂) und • (♀) stellen gesicherte Unterschiede (T-Test) zwischen den Altersgruppen dar. (Nach HEUCK, 1968)

Vergleichende Untersuchungen der Kalksalzkonzentration in *der Ulna* haben ADACHI und OKUYAMA (1966) durchgeführt. Neben der densitometrischen Bestimmung der Kalksalzkonzentration mit Hilfe eines knochenähnlichen Referenzsystems wurden direkte Absorptionsmessungen vorgenommen. Die densitometrisch gefundenen Werte des Knochenkalksalzgehaltes lagen etwas niedriger als diejenigen Werte, die mit Hilfe der Absorptionsmessung ermittelt wurden. Als „Normalwert" der Kalksalzkonzentration gesunder Menschen im *distalen Abschnitt der Ulna wurden 300—450 mg/ml* (mit Hilfe der Absorptionsmessung) bzw. *260—400 mg/ml* (mit Hilfe densitometrischer Messungen) angegeben. Bei Rechtshändern wurde eine etwas höhere Mineralkonzentration des Knochens in der rechten Ulna festgestellt.

Die *Kombination* von Messungen der Compactadicke zur *Bestimmung der Knochenmasse* und densitometrischer Messungen zur *Bestimmung der Kalksalzkonzentration* in dem gleichen durchstrahlten Knochenbezirk sind geeignet, gewisse Aussagen über die *Kalksalzkonzentration im Knochengewebe selbst* zu geben (s. S. 237). Mit der Methode von MEEMA, HARRIS und PORRETT (1964), die als Referenzsystem eine gesättigte Kaliumhydrogenphosphatlösung verwendeten (Methode s. S. 194), wurden in der *Compacta* der proximalen *Radiusdiaphyse* bei gesunden Männern und Frauen Kalksalzkonzentrationen von 1000—1400 mg/ml gefunden (Tabelle 26). Die Untersuchungsbefunde stimmen mit den Resultaten von ARNOLD (1968) gut überein, der mit Hilfe der chemischen Analyse Werte von 1191—1212 mg/ml Knochenmineral in der Diaphysencompacta des Femur feststellte. Von HINESS (1968) wurde nach der Methode von MEEMA, HARRIS und PORRETT (1964) die Mineralkonzentration von Knochenpräparaten aus der Mitte der Femurdiaphyse gemessen. Die Kalksalzkonzentration variierte zwischen 940 und 1430 mg/ml bei einem Mittelwert von 1150 mg/ml. Die Untersuchungen von FRERCKS (1968) ergaben

Tabelle 26. *Hydroxylapatitgehalt der Compacta der proximalen Radiusdiaphyse bei Normalpersonen*

Männer			Frauen		
Alter	Hydroxylapatit-Werte in mg/ml	kombinierte Compactadicke in mm	Alter	Hydroxylapatit-Werte in mg/ml	kombinierte Compactadicke in mm
19	1060—1080	7,8—7,9	19	1230—1330	6,0—7,0
19	1100	7,0	20	1230—1250	6,0—6,5
21	1060—1100	6,9—7,0	21	1120—1200	6,0—6,3
22	1130—1180	7,4—7,8	21	1150—1200	6,0
28	1200—1260	8,6—9,0	25	1360	5,5
31	1180	7,2	25	1220	6,0
33	1150—1190	6,4	26	1230	5,3
38	1140—1170	7,0	30	1330—1410	5,3—6,0
39	1120—1140	7,0—7,4	30	1120—1140	6,3—6,7
40	1000—1100	6,0	31	1150—1190	5,2
40	1180	8,5	31	1120—1150	6,3—6,7
40	1140	5,6	32	1200—1380	5,8—6,1
40	1330—1340	8,0	38	1140	5,8
43	1070—1140	7,0—7,2	39	1360—1370	5,5—6,0
47	1170—1190	6,3—7,0	41	1270—1290	6,0—6,2
49	1130	7,0	42	1240	5,5
54	1100—1120	8,0	43	1160—1290	5,0—5.8
60	1200	7,0	44	1080	5,0
			46	1140—1180	6,0—6,4
			62	1250—1370	6,2—6,8

[MEEMA, H, E., C. K. HARRIS, and R. E. PORRETT: Radiology 82, 986 (1964), Tab. 4]

eine Apatitkonzentration in der Compacta der Femurdiaphyse von 1150—1200 mg/ml im 3. Dezennium, die auch im Laufe des Alterungsprozesses kaum eine Änderung erkennen ließ.

Eine möglichst genaue Kenntnis der Globalwerte der Knochenkalksalzkonzentration in verschiedenen Knochen des Skeletes ist wünschenswert, um in der klinischen Radiologie schon frühzeitig krankhafte Veränderungen des „Apatitwertes" erkennen zu können, die Ausdruck einer Entkalkungsosteopathie oder einer pathologischen Osteosklerose sind. Dadurch wird eine *rechtzeitige* Therapie ermöglicht, so daß die gefürchteten pathologischen Frakturen und Umbauzonen mit all ihren sekundären Folgeerscheinungen wie irreversiblen Skeletdeformitäten, Bewegungsstörungen u.a. verhütet werden können.

VIII. Die radiologische Morphometrie von Knochen

Die Bestimmung des Knochengewebsvolumens im „*Organ Knochen*" mit Hilfe der radiologischen Morphometrie der einzelnen Knochen, also der Bausteine des gesamten Skeletes, vermittelt wichtige Befunde, die zum besseren Verständnis der *Biomorphose* dieses Gewebsverbandes während des Alterungsprozesses beitragen können.

Die in allen Lebensphasen von Mensch und Tier ununterbrochen ablaufenden *Austausch- und Umbauvorgänge* in jedem Knochen führen während der Wachstumsperiode zu einer *Größenzunahme* des Gesamtknochens bei *gleichzeitiger Transformation* der inneren Bauelemente und Strukturen (Spongiosa, Corticalis, Compacta, Osteone, Lamellen). Das erwachsene Individuum läßt im Laufe des Alterungsprozesses bei weitgehend konstanter äußerer Form und Größe jedes Knochens charakteristische art- und geschlechtsspezifische Transformationsprozesse erkennen, die mit einer Verminderung des ursprünglichen Knochengewebsvolumens innerhalb des Gesamtvolumens eines Knochens einhergehen. Es handelt sich hierbei um einen normalen, physiologischen Vorgang im *Organ Knochen*, dessen biochemische Zusammenhänge noch weitgehend ungeklärt sind.

In der *Spongiosa* kommt es zur Abnahme von Zahl und Größe der Bälkchen und Lamellen, die *Corticalis* und die *Compacta* erfahren eine von der endostalen Zone des

Markraumes aus fortschreitende Volumenabnahme. Während dieser *Reduktion der Masse des Knochengewebes* innerhalb des Organes Knochen bleibt die *Kalksalzkonzentration* in der Tela ossea des gesunden Individuum *weitgehend normal* (s. S. 233). Unter krankhaften Bedingungen (z.B. bei Störungen im Mineralhaushalt, Resorptionsstörungen des Darmkanals u.a.) kann eine Abnahme, seltener eine Zunahme der Kalksalzkonzentration im Knochengewebe auftreten. Bereits Cooke (1955) war der Ansicht, daß eine *gleichmäßige* Resorption der Knochensalze von der Knochenoberfläche her erfolge. Der Entkalkungsvorgang in der Compacta ist daher schwerer zu erfassen als in der Spongiosa, da die Knochenlamellen und Osteone im Vergleich zu den Trabekeln des spongiösen Knochens sehr viel zahlreicher und dichter gepackt angeordnet sind. Der spongiöse Knochen ist zur *Früherfassung* von Entkalkungsosteopathien besser geeignet.

Bei jeder krankhaften Störung, die sich auf die Lebensvorgänge des gesamten Skeletsystems auswirkt, sind zwei, *im Endergebnis verschiedene pathologische Prozesse* zu erfassen:

1. Die Abnahme oder Zunahme des Knochengewebsvolumens (der Knochenmasse).
2. Die Verminderung oder Erhöhung der Konzentration der Kalksalze im Knochengewebe (der Tela ossae).

Da beide Prozesse bei *Systemerkrankungen* des Knochens häufig *gleichzeitig nebeneinander ablaufen*, wobei der eine oder andere Vorgang überwiegen kann, sind *radiologische Messungen der Dicke von Compacta oder Corticalis* von großem Wert. Die radiologischen Messungen der *globalen Mineralkonzentration* im Gesamtvolumen von spongiösen Knochen können *nicht differenzieren* zwischen Verlust an Knochengewebssubstanz oder Verlust an Kalksalzen in der Tela ossea. So bringt die *kombinierte Anwendung* mehrerer radiologischer Meßmethoden eine für die Klinik sehr nützliche Erweiterung der Information über den Zustand des Skeletes.

1. Die Messungen der Compacta und Corticalis

Die Messung der Compactadicke (im englischen Schrifttum Corticalisdicke) wird an Röntgenaufnahmen vorgenommen. Für Absolutmessungen müssen daher der Vergrößerungsfaktor bei kleinem Fokus-Objekt-Abstand und großem Objekt-Film-Abstand, die geometrische Unschärfe durch die Projektionsbedingungen, die Konturunschärfe infolge Überbelichtung oder zu harter Strahlung und die unregelmäßige Begrenzung der Compactainnenkontur zum Markraum hin, besonders in der Übergangszone der Metaphyse zu spongiösen Knochenpartien, beachtet werden, um gröbere Fehler zu vermeiden (Virtama u. Mitarb. 1960; Barnett und Nordin 1960; Meema u. Mitarb. 1962; Garn u. Mitarb. 1964; Hiness 1968 u.a.).

Einige dieser *Fehlerquellen* werden dann unbedeutend, wenn ein *Index* ermittelt wird (Barnett und Nordin 1960), also die Compactadicke (oder der Markraum) zum Gesamtdurchmesser des interessierenden Knochenbezirkes in Beziehung gesetzt wird. Die Meßgenauigkeit hängt ferner von dem verwendeten *Meßinstrument* ab, und es sind von einem einfachen Längenmaß oder einem Meßzirkel bis zu komplizierten Meßgeräten verschiedenste Methoden auf ihre Genauigkeit geprüft worden (Meema u. Mitarb. 1962; Garn u. Mitarb. 1962, 1968).

Untersuchungen von Merz, Trotter und Peterson (1956) haben gezeigt, daß gewisse *Beziehungen der Knochenmasse des Femurschaftes zum Gesamtskelet* bestehen müssen. *Planimetrische Untersuchungen* der Compacta ergaben eine große Streubreite, so daß es besser sei, solche Messungen von Untersuchungen an der Spongiosa getrennt vorzunehmen. Die Diaphysencompacta kann z.B. im Bereich des *Femurschaftes* und der *Metacarpalia* gut gemessen werden. Es wurden bereits Standardwerte für beide Knochen ermittelt.

Die Dicke der Diaphysencompacta von *Fingerknochen* als Maß für das *Knochengewebsvolumen* und damit den *Mineralgehalt* zu betrachten, veranlaßten Virtama und Mähönen (1960) an 26 Präparaten von Basalphalangen Vergleichsuntersuchungen durchzuführen.

Die Knochenpräparate sind in jeweils fünf verschiedenen Projektionen geröntgt worden. Von allen Röntgenaufnahmen wurden Vergrößerungen hergestellt (Abb. 110). Mit Hilfe dieser vergrößerten Röntgenbilder konnte der *prozentuale Anteil des Flächengewichtes* der Diaphysencompacta zum Flächengewicht des übrigen Knochens in Beziehung gesetzt werden und als „*Corticalisrelation*“ oder „*Corticalisverhältnis*“ angegeben werden. Danach wurde das Volumen der geröntgten Knochen pyknometrisch bestimmt und innerhalb

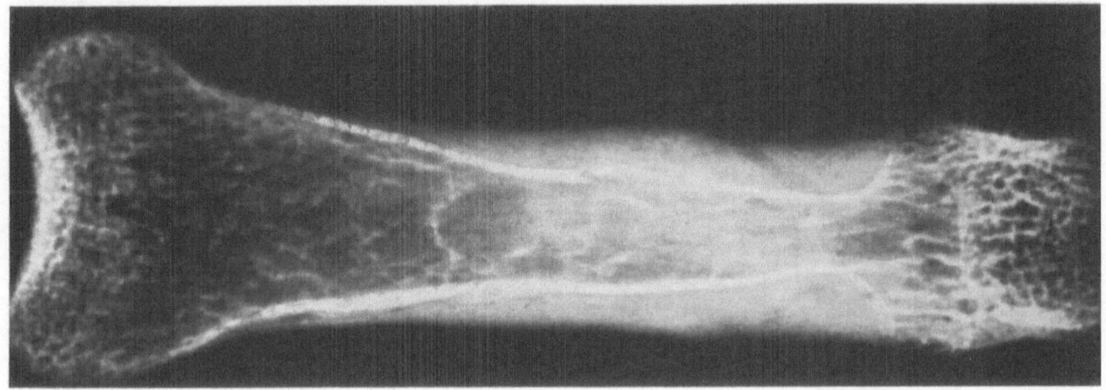

Abb. 110. Vergrößerte Aufnahme von einem der Fingerknochen, die als Ausgangsmaterial der Methode zur Bestimmung der „Corticalisrelation“ dienten. (Nach VIRTAMA und MÄHÖNEN, 1960; Abb. 1)

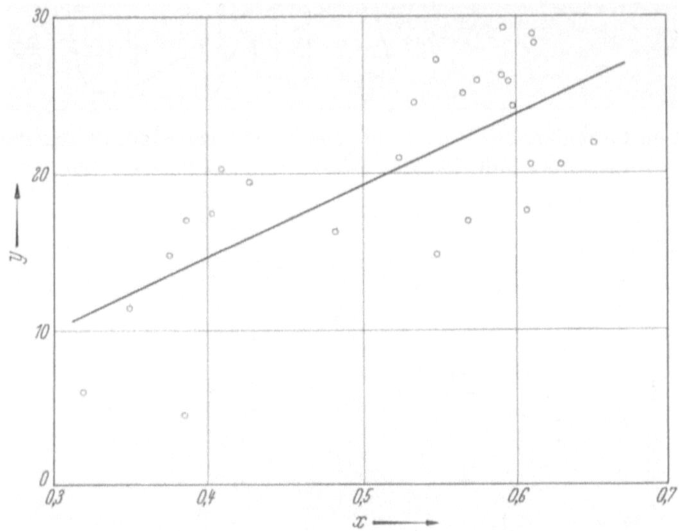

Abb. 111. Darstellung der Streuung des Mineralgehaltes (x) im Verhältnis zum Corticalisanteil in Prozent (y). (Nach VIRTAMA und MÄHÖNEN, 1960; Abb. 2)

von 24 Std eine Veraschung bei 800°C vorgenommen. So konnte der Mineralgehalt des Knochens in g Asche/cm^3 Gesamtknochen ermittelt werden. Diese Werte wurden mit dem arithmetischen Mittel der entsprechenden prozentualen Anteile der Compacta am Gesamtknochen verglichen (Abb. 111). Die Fehlerbreite der Bestimmung des Compacta-anteiles wird mit 1,6% angegeben. Der arithmetische Mittelwert des Verhältnisses der Compacta zum Gesamtknochen betrug 20,2%, der arithmetische Mittelwert des Mineralgehaltes der Knochen betrug 0,520 g/cm^3. Die Meßergebnisse der „Corticalisrelation“ zeigten eine erstaunlich gute Übereinstimmung mit den Bestimmungen des Mineralgehaltes im Knochen. Die Methode wird zur Erfassung einer *Osteoporose* im Fingerknochen empfohlen.

Aus Ergebnissen der Compactamessung (oder Corticalismessung) haben BARNETT und NORDIN (1960) einen *Index* berechnet, der die Relation der alleinigen Compactadicke zum Gesamtdurchmesser der Diaphyse im Meßareal erfaßt (Abb. 112a—d). Der „Barnett-

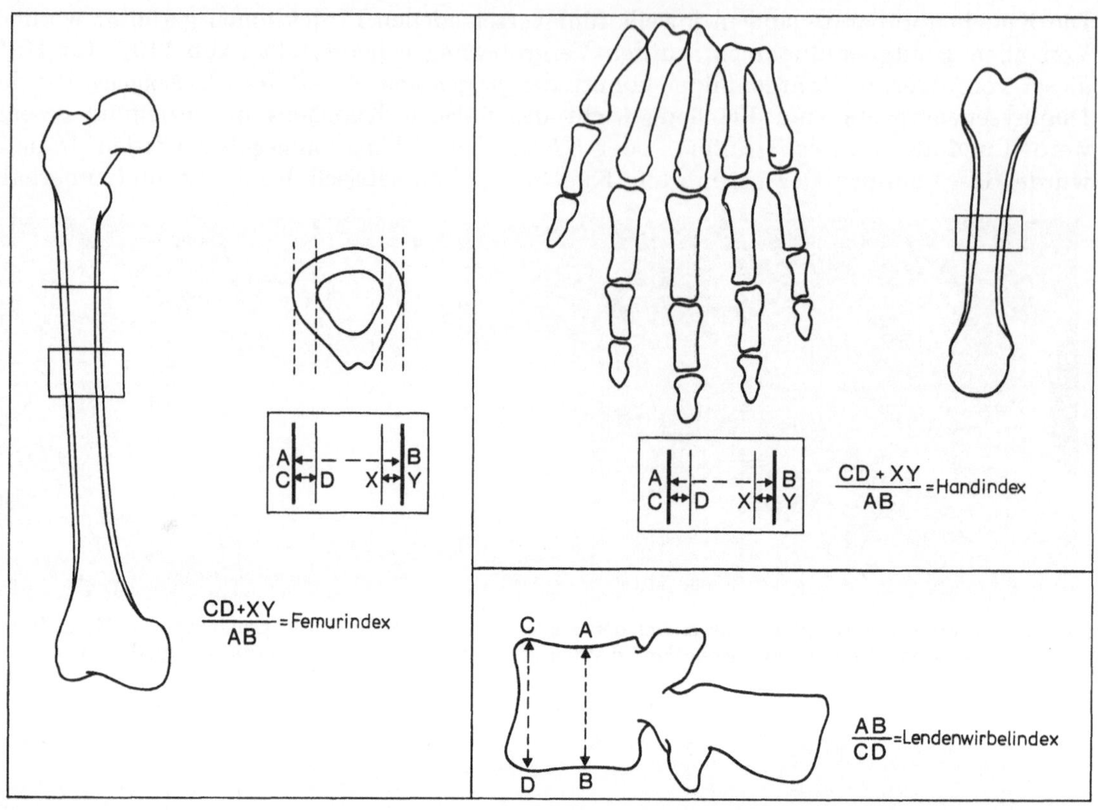

Abb. 112a. Meßschema zur Bestimmung des Compacta-Index („peripherer Index") und des Wirbelkörper-Index („zentraler Index"). (Nach BARNETT und NORDIN, 1960)

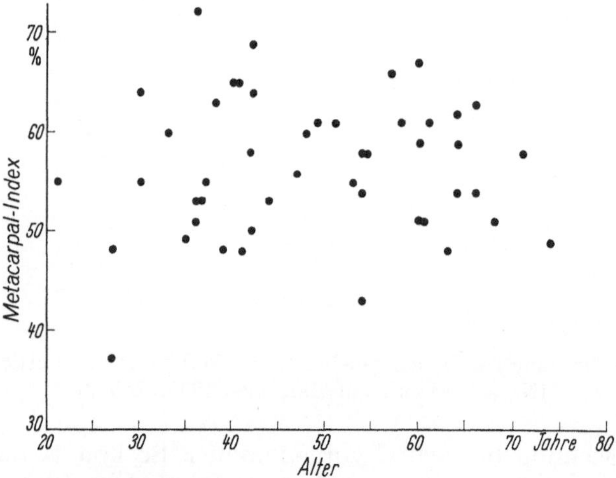

Abb. 112b. Verteilung des Metacarpalindex bei gesunden Männern in den einzelnen Altersgruppen. (Nach NORDIN, BARNETT, SMITH und ANDERSON, 1965; Abb. 9)

Nordin-Index" gibt die Corticalisdicke in Prozent des Gesamtdurchmessers an. Er wurde bestimmt für die Femurdiaphyse, die Diaphyse des Metacarapale II (BARNETT und NORDIN 1960; NORDIN, BARNETT, SMITH und ANDERSON 1965) und für die Mitte der Diaphyse der Tibia (BERNARD und LAVAL-JEANTET 1962). Die Compacta des Femur wird in der Übergangszone zwischen mittlerem und cranialem Drittel ausgemessen, da dort die größte Dicke festzustellen ist. Der II. Mittelhandknochen weist die größte Compactadicke im mittleren Schaftanteil auf (Abb. 112e). Bei *gesunden Menschen* liegt die untere Grenze des Corticalisindex für das Metacarpale II bei 43—44%, für den Femur bei 45%.

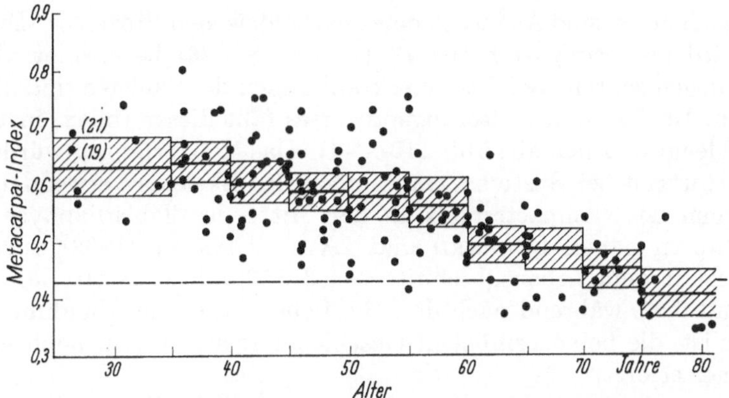

Abb. 112c. Metacarpalindex mit Standardabweichung bei gesunden Frauen in den einzelnen Dezennien. (Nach NORDIN, BARNETT, SMITH und ANDERSON, 1965; Abb. 6)

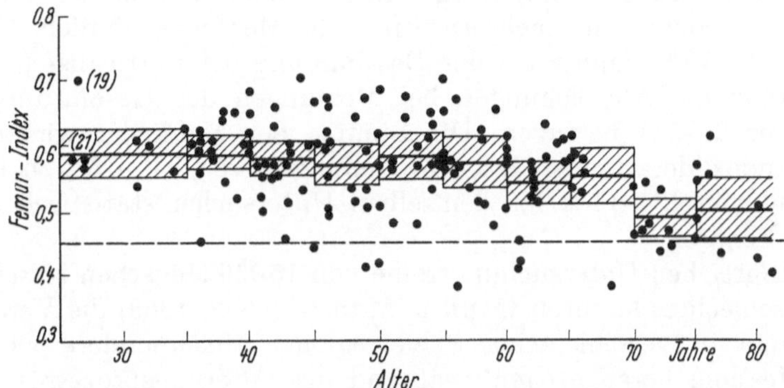

Abb. 112d. Femurindex mit Standardabweichung bei gesunden Frauen in den einzelnen Dezennien. (Nach NORDIN, BARNETT, SMITH und ANDERSON, 1965; Abb. 7)

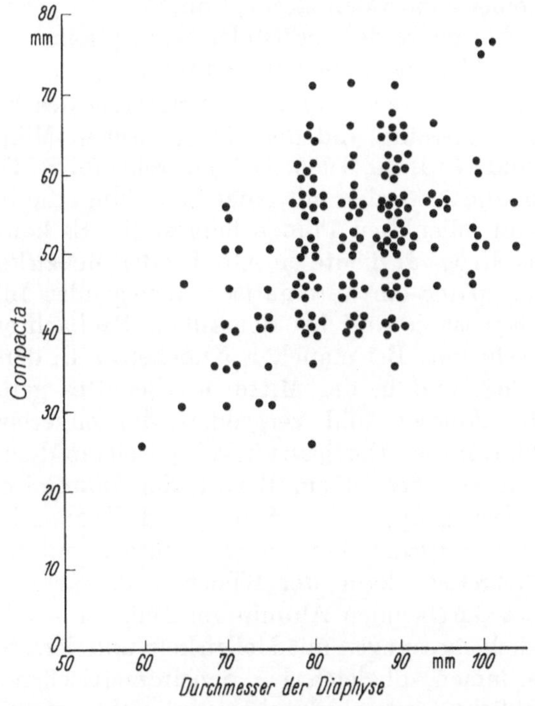

Abb. 112e. Gegenüberstellung von Gesamtdurchmesser des Metacarpalschaftes und der Compactadicke bei 151 Männern aller Altersgruppen, die eine Abhängigkeit dieser Meßgröße voneinander zeigt. (Nach NORDIN, BARNETT, SMITH und ANDERSON, 1965; Abb. 5)

Abweichungen nach unten sind Ausdruck eines pathologischen Prozesses. Die *Summe* dieser beiden Werte wird als „*peripherer Index*" (s. auch S. 226) bezeichnet, dessen Normalwerte über 88 % liegen sollten. Bei Systemerkrankungen des Skeletes sind niedrigere Werte gefunden worden. Im Laufe des Alterungsprozesses fällt dieser Index, insbesondere beim weiblichen Geschlecht deutlich ab (Abb. 112c—d). Das Meßverfahren wurde verschiedentlich zu Untersuchungen bei Systemerkrankungen des Skeletes verwendet (s. S. 243).

Untersuchungen des Compactaindex in der Mitte der Tibiadiaphyse im Alter von 3 bis über 60 Jahren haben BERNARD und LAVAL-JEANTET (1962) durchgeführt. Der Compactaindex ist in dem Lebensabschnitt von 3—50 Jahren relativ konstant und liegt zwischen 0,39 und 0,57, während nach dem 50. Lebensjahr eine Abnahme des Compactaindex erkennbar ist, die beim weiblichen Geschlecht relativ rasch, beim männlichen Geschlecht langsamer erfolgt.

Die *Fehler dieser Meßmethoden,* die auf unterschiedliche Durchführung der Messung, also den untersuchenden Arzt zurückgeführt werden können, sind von ADAMS, DAVIES, KILPATRICK und SWEETMAN (1968) festgestellt worden. Sowohl bei demselben Untersucher als bei verschiedenen Beobachtern waren die Meßfehler ähnlich. Die größten Abweichungen von 11—15 % kamen bei der Bestimmung der Corticalis- (oder Compacta-) Dicke vor, während die Abweichungen bei Messungen des Gesamtdurchmessers vom Metacarpale II nur 2—5 % betrugen. Die Summe der Meßfehler wirkte sich auf den Barnett-Nordin-Index derart aus, daß Abweichungen von 11—15 % bei verschiedenen Untersuchern und von 12—14 % bei demselben Untersucher statistisch gesichert nachgewiesen werden konnten.

In einer umfangreichen Untersuchungsreihe von 15036 Menschen *verschiedener Rassen* und beiderlei Geschlechtes konnten GARN u. Mitarb. (1962, 1968) die Veränderungen der Diaphysencompacta in verschiedenen Skeletregionen (insbesondere wurde das Metacarpale II zur Messung herangezogen) während des Alterungsprozesses feststellen. Die endostale Zone der Compacta zeigt die stärksten Umbauvorgänge bei gesunden und kranken Menschen. Es können drei verschiedene Phasen unterschieden werden:

1. die juvenile Phase einer endostalen Resorption,
2. die hormonelle Reifungsphase der endostalen Apposition,
3. die Erwachsenenphase der endostalen Resorption.

Vergleichende methodische Untersuchungen zur Erfassung des Knochenschwundes mit Hilfe einer Compactadickenmessung und der radiologischen Mikrodensitometrie haben GARN, FEUTZ, COLBERT und WAGNER (1963, 1965) durchgeführt. Die Röntgenaufnahmen zur Messung der Compactadicke werden mit einer Strahlung, die bei 30—50 kV Anodenspannung erzeugt wird, auf folienlosen Filmen hergestellt. Es können aber auch Folienfilme benutzt werden. Als *Meßgerät* diente ein Greif- oder Meßzirkel mit einer ablesbaren Genauigkeit von 0,1 mm, später ein automatisch anzeigendes Instrument. Die *Reproduzierbarkeit der Messungen* ist sowohl bei demselben Beobachter als auch unter verschiedenen Beobachtern sehr gut. Bei manchen Knochen, z.B. den Metacarpalia, sollten einige Hilfspunkte festgelegt und in der Mitte des Schaftes gemessen werden. Dieses Vorgehen vereinfacht das Ablesen und vergrößert die Zuverlässigkeit der Messung. SMITH u. Mitarb. (1964) haben die „Corticalisdicke" jeweils in dem Bereich ermittelt, wo die Markhöhle am engsten ist. Dies ist ein Bezirk, der anatomisch von Bedeutung ist. Die Meßergebnisse der Arbeitsgruppen von SMITH und GARN zeigen gute Übereinstimmung. Die radiologischen *Compactadickemessungen* wurden mit mikrodensitometrischen Verfahren verglichen. Theoretisch kann der Knochen als *einfacher Zylinder* angesehen werden und die Compacta durch einen Aluminium-Zylinder als Modell ersetzt werden. Vergleichende Compactadickemessungen mit Meßzirkeln und densitometrischen Methoden scheinen gut übereinzustimmen, obgleich bei densitometrischen Messungen über den ganzen Knochen der wirkliche Corticalisdurchmesser nicht erfaßt wird. Bei Messungen mit Meßzirkeln wird die Markhöhle vom Gesamtdurchmesser des Knochens subtrahiert. Die Autoren haben an einer großen Anzahl von Röntgenaufnahmen des *Metacarpale II*

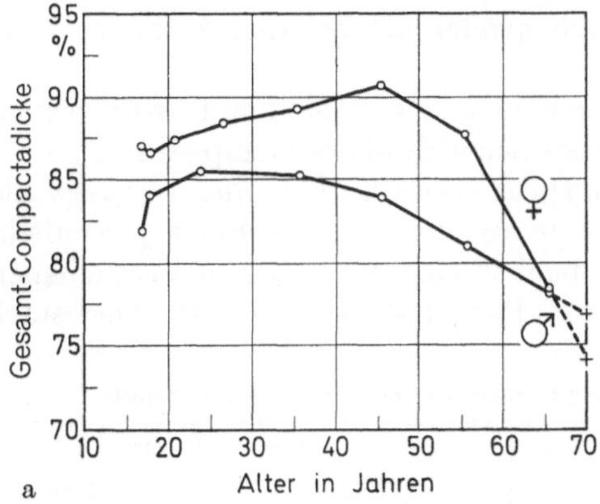

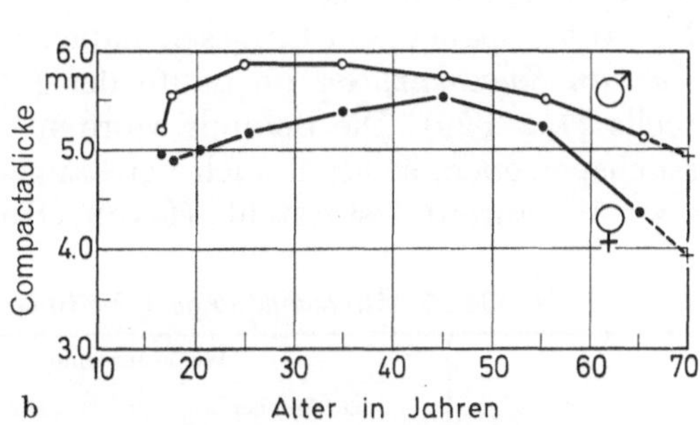

Abb. 113a. Veränderungen des kompakten Knochens in der Mitte des Metacarpale II bei Männern und Frauen im Laufe des Alterungsprozesses ausgedrückt in Prozent zum Gesamtdurchmesser der Diaphyse. (Nach GARN, ROHMAN und NOLAN, 1964; Abb. 4)

Abb. 113b. Darstellung der Alterskurve der Compactadicke (Absolutwerte) in der Mitte des Metacarpale II bei beiden Geschlechtern. (Nach GARN, ROHMAN und NOLAN, 1964; Abb. 3)

Dickenmessungen mit einem Zirkel und densitometrische Messungen mit einem Aluminiumvergleichskörper durchgeführt. Beide Meßergebnisse stimmen gut überein. Die Methode sei ausreichend reproduzierbar und für klinische Untersuchungen wertvoll.

Nach Untersuchungen von GARN, ROHMANN und NOLAN (1964) mit dieser Methode am Metacarpale II (462 Normalpersonen im Alter von 16—75 Jahren) ist die Compactadicke bei Männern größer als bei Frauen (Abb. 113a). Nach dem 5. Lebensjahr fand sich eine Abnahme der Compactadicke bei beiden Geschlechtern, doch war die Verschmälerung bei Frauen wesentlich größer als bei Männern, was mit der Menopause in Zusammenhang stehen dürfte (Abb. 113b). Bei 575 Familienuntersuchungen (Vergleich Vater—Tochter, Vater—Sohn, Mutter—Tochter, Mutter—Sohn) fanden sich Anzeichen für eine x-gebundene Erblichkeit des kompakten Knochens. Solche Männer, die ein großes Compactavolumen besitzen, lassen einen größeren Compactaverlust erkennen, als Männer mit primär geringem Compactavolumen. Bei Frauen mit sehr geringer Compactadicke wird oft eine pathologische Osteoporose angenommen. Wahrscheinlich handelt es sich jedoch auch um Fälle von idiopathischer Osteoporose oder Abortivformen der Osteogenesis imperfecta. Zur Feststellung von Unterschieden im Alterungsprozeß des Skeletes bei *verschiedenen Rassen* sind sowohl Weiße als auch Neger, Japaner und Chinesen untersucht worden. Nach dem 5. Lebensjahrzehnt konnte bei beiden Geschlechtern, sowohl bei Weißen als auch bei Schwarzen, eine Verminderung der Compactadicke gefunden werden. Der Verlust an Knochensubstanz betrug beim *männlichen Geschlecht* maximal 20%, beim *weiblichen Geschlecht* bis zu 31%. Die Japaner und Chinesen ließen die gleiche Tendenz des Alterungsgeschehens an der Diaphysencompacta erkennen (Abb. 114), doch waren die

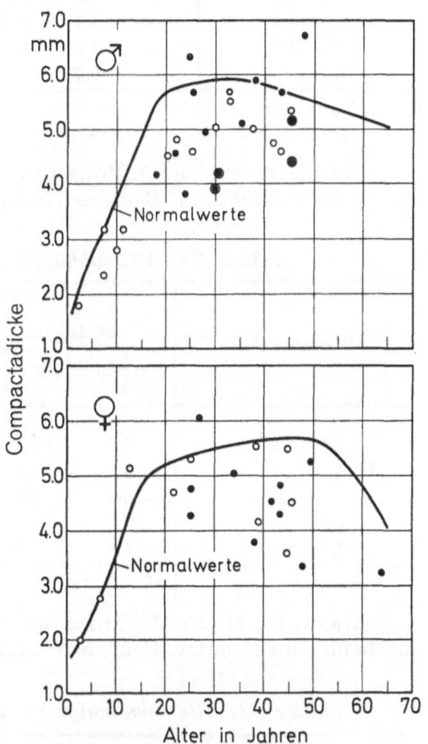

Abb. 114. Zusammenstellung der Compactadicke des Metacarpale II beim männlichen und weiblichen Geschlecht in Abhängigkeit vom Lebensalter und rassischen Einflüssen (Chinesen und Japaner in Amerika geboren ○, vergleichbare Gruppe in Asien geboren ● und amerikanische weiße Bevölkerung ——). (Nach GARN, PAO und RIHL, 1964; Abb. 1)

Verluste an Knochenmasse bei den Frauen noch größer als bei den Männern (GARN, PAO und RIHL 1964).

Obwohl die Compactadicke erhebliche Unterschiede der einzelnen Rassen erkennen ließ — die Japaner und Chinesen haben eine wesentlich dünnere Compacta —, war *der Verlust an Knochenmasse* im Laufe des Alterungsprozesses *bei allen Rassegruppen* gleich (Tabelle 27, 28, 29). Die Befunde wurden nicht nur an einem Querschnitt verschiedener Versuchspersonen, sondern auch bei Langzeitbeobachtungen der gleichen Versuchsperson (bis zu 35 Jahren) festgestellt (GARN, ROHMANN, PAO und HULL 1965). Der stärkste

Tabelle 27. *Altersabhängige Verminderung der Compactadicke des 2. Metacarpale*

Altersgruppen	Weiße aus Ohio						Neger aus Missouri					
	267 Männer			352 Frauen			111 Männer			117 Frauen		
	Zahl der Fälle	Mittelwerte mm	Standardabweichung	Zahl der Fälle	Mittelwerte mm	Standardabweichung	Zahl der Fälle	Mittelwerte mm	Standardabweichung	Zahl der Fälle	Mittelwerte mm	Standardabweichung
25—34	62	5,9	0,6	153	5,4	0,8	24	5,3	0,7	24	4,8	0,7
35—44	92	5,8	0,7	85	5,5	0,7	24	5,2	0,6	25	4,6	0,5
45—54	60	5,7	0,7	61	5,2	0,7	22	4,6	0,6	22	4,0	0,6
55—64	34	5,3	0,6	31	4,6	0,6	20	4,7	0,6	20	3,9	0,8
65—..	19	4,7	0,4	22	3,7	0,7	21	4,3	1,0	26	3,3	0,7
Abnahme der Dicke	20%			31%			19%			31%		

(GARN, ST. M., CH. G. ROHMANN, E. M. PAO, and E. I. HULL: Progress in development of methods on bone densitometry. Conf. in Washington D. C., 1965, Tab. 1a)

Tabelle 28. *Altersabhängige Verminderung der Compactafläche des 2. Metacarpale*

Altersgruppen	Weiße aus Ohio				Neger aus Missouri			
	267 Männer		352 Frauen		111 Männer		117 Frauen	
	Anzahl der Fälle	Mittelwerte mm^2	Anzahl der Fälle	Mittelwerte mm^2	Anzahl der Fälle	Mittelwerte mm^2	Anzahl der Fälle	Mittelwerte mm^2
25—34	62	59,6	153	44,7	24	57,1	24	43,6
35—44	92	58,5	85	45,7	24	53,3	25	45,1
45—54	60	59,7	61	43,8	22	50,7	22	39,0
55—64	34	58,5	31	42,2	20	53,1	20	38,5
65—..	19	50,6	22	36,6	21	48,8	26	34,1
Verminderung	15%		18%		15%		22%	

(GARN, ST. M., CH. B. ROHMANN, E. M. PAO, and E. I. HULL: Progress in development of methods on bone densitometry. Conf. in Washington D. C., 1965, Tab. 1b)

Tabelle 29. *Altersabhängige Verminderung des Compactaindex* (NORDIN) *des 2. Metacarpale*

Altersgruppen	Weiße aus Ohio				Neger aus Missouri			
	267 Männer		352 Frauen		111 Männer		117 Frauen	
	Anzahl der Fälle	Mittelwerte *	Anzahl der Fälle	Mittelwerte *	Anzahl der Fälle	Mittelwerte *	Anzahl der Fälle	Mittelwerte *
25—34	62	63	153	67	24	56	24	59
35—44	92	62	85	68	24	56	25	54
45—54	60	60	61	66	22	49	22	49
55—64	34	54	31	57	20	50	20	47
65—..	19	50	22	46	21	46	26	39

(GARN, ST. M., CH. G. ROHMANN, E. M. PAO, and E. I. HULL: Progress in development of methods on bone densitometry. Conf. in Washington D. C., 1965, Tab. 1c)

* Gemessen nach dem Nordin-Index. Bemerkenswert ist es, daß der Index bei den Frauen zu Beginn höher ist.

Verlust an Knochensubstanz fand sich bei beiden Geschlechtern zwischen dem 4. und 5. sowie dem 6. und 7. Lebensjahrzehnt. Bemerkenswert ist die Beobachtung einer *Zunahme der Knochenmasse* bei 49 Frauen und einigen Männern. In *einem* Fall war über drei aufeinanderfolgende Jahrzehnte ein *Knochenanbau* festzustellen. Bei der Mehrzahl der untersuchten Personen konnte jedoch ein Verlust an Knochensubstanz im Bereich der Diaphyse nachgewiesen werden.

Messungen des *endostalen* und *periostalen* Durchmessers vom Metacarpale II bei drei verschiedenen Bevölkerungsgruppen wurden von SPENCER, SAGEL und GARN (1968) durchgeführt. Alle drei Bevölkerungsgruppen zeigen ähnliche Werte. Zunächst war bei beiden Geschlechtern bis zum 11. Lebensjahr kein Unterschied festzustellen, dann stiegen die Werte beim männlichen Geschlecht bis zum 20. Lebensjahr etwas an. Vom 40. Lebensjahr an konnte ein Absinken des Parameters besonders deutlich beim weiblichen Geschlecht gefunden werden (GARN, ROHMANN und WAGNER 1968).

Das *endostale Wachstum* des Knochens hält bei beiden Geschlechtern bis zur *4. Dekade* an und ist während der Schwangerschaft beim weiblichen Geschlecht besonders eindrucksvoll. Zu Anfang der *5. Dekade* beginnt ein *endostaler Knochenabbau*, der in der 6. und 7. Dekade ständig fortschreitet und ansteigt. Beim *weiblichen Geschlecht* kann in der 5. Dekade bereits ein Verlust der Compactadicke von 40% eintreten (Tabelle 30). Im Bereich der endostalen Zone ist der Knochen beim weiblichen Geschlecht sehr viel empfindlicher als beim männlichen Geschlecht und ist wesentlich größeren Umbau- und Abbauprozessen unterworfen.

Im Gegensatz zu früheren Ansichten liegt der Beginn der Phase einer endostalen Resorption des Erwachsenenalters um das 40. Lebensjahr bei beiden Geschlechtern und allen Rassen. Die *geschlechtsspezifischen Unterschiede* der endostalen Resorption sind in allen Skeletbezirken beträchtlich. In der juvenilen Phase ist eine hohe endostale Resorptionsrate beim männlichen Geschlecht charakteristisch. Der Zeitpunkt des Beginns der

Tabelle 30. *Vergleich der Knochenverminderung in 3 Ländern bei beiden Geschlechtern*

Altersgruppen	Männer				Frauen			
	Anzahl der Fälle	Compactadicke in mm	Compactafläche in %	Nordin-Index	Anzahl der Fälle	Compactadicke in mm	Compactafläche in %	Nordin-Index
				Vereinigte Staaten, Ohio				
30	62	5,9	86,1	62,8	153	5,4	89,1	68,4
40	92	5,8	85,0	62,4	85	5,5	89,6	67,9
50	60	5,7	84,0	60,0	61	5,2	88,3	65,8
60	35	5,3	79,4	54,6	40	4,6	81,3	56,8
70	23	5,0	78,0	53,2	32	3,9	71,8	47,0
80	12	4,9	78,6	53,8	22	3,3	63,7	39,8
				Guatemala				
30	89	5,45	87,3	64,3	159	5,03	90,3	68,9
40	92	5,19	85,5	61,9	137	4,77	87,5	64,7
50	62	5,38	85,8	62,3	101	4,73	85,9	62,6
60	42	5,12	83,5	59,5	51	3,91	76,8	51,9
70	24	4,72	79,0	54,3	38	3,73	72,9	47,9
80	11	4,80	80,3	55,6	17	3,22	66,9	42,5
				El Salvador				
30	57	5,34	85,5	61,9	101	5,19	91,0	70,1
40	46	5,40	85,9	62,6	80	5,05	89,4	67,5
50	22	5,51	86,4	63,2	71	4,87	87,3	64,4
60	29	5,11	83,4	59,3	48	4,02	78,4	53,6
70	14	4,80	77,7	52,9	29	3,74	73,4	48,6
80	11	4,44	76,4	51,4	8	3,11	62,9	39,0

(GARN, ST. M., CH. G. ROHMANN, and B. WAGNER: Fed. Proc. **26**, 1729 (1967), Tab. 1)

endostalen Apposition liegt beim weiblichen Geschlecht früher als beim männlichen Geschlecht. Die endostale Apposition ist in der Reifungsphase beim weiblichen Geschlecht größer. Während des Alterungsprozesses ist die endostale Resorption beim weiblichen Geschlecht 2,5—3mal größer als beim männlichen Geschlecht. Bemerkenswert ist, daß diese Gesetzmäßigkeit für verschiedene Rassen in gleicher Weise Gültigkeit hat. Mit dem endostalen Abbau während des Alterns ist ein oft nur diskreter subperiostaler Anbau im Diaphysenbereich festzustellen, der bereits im 4. Jahrzehnt beginnen kann.

Der *Compactaindex* des II. Metacarpale wurde auch von BUGYI (1965) an 200 Röntgenaufnahmen der Hand bestimmt. Im Laufe des Wachstums ist nicht nur eine Zunahme der *Länge* der Röhrenknochen festzustellen, sondern auch ein *Breitenwachstum* der Diaphysen,

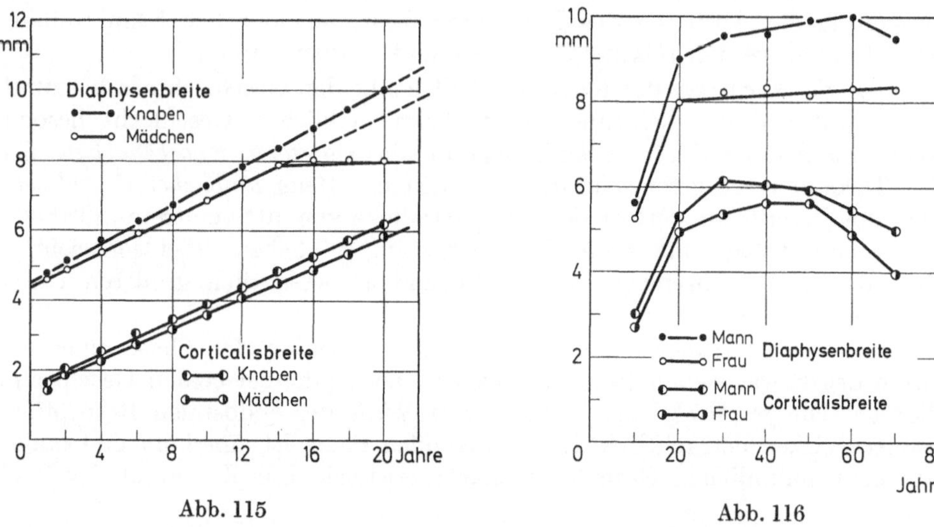

Abb. 115

Abb. 116

Abb. 115. Darstellung der Meßwerte des Breitenwachstums der Compacta der Diaphyse des 2. Metacarpalknochens im mittleren Abschnitt (unten) und der Diaphysenbreite allein (oben). (Nach BUGYI, 1965, Abb. 1)

Abb. 116. Darstellung der Meßwerte von Corticalisbreite und Diaphysendurchmesser des Metacarpale II im Erwachsenenalter. (Nach BUGYI, 1965; Abb. 2)

das zwischen dem 11.—18. Lebensjahr zum Abschluß kommen soll (Abb. 115). Der Gesamtdurchmesser der Diaphyse bleibt beim weiblichen Geschlecht vom 20. Lebensjahr an konstant, während er beim männlichen Geschlecht noch bis zum 60. Lebensjahr zunehmen kann und erst im 7. Jahrzehnt eine Verschmälerung aufweist. Die Compactadicke nimmt bei Männern noch bis zum 30. Lebensjahr zu, bei Frauen konnte eine geringe Zunahme noch bis zum 50. Lebensjahr gefunden werden. Vom 40. Lebensjahr ab ist eine geringe, aber stetige Verminderung der Compactadicke (Compactaindex) beim männlichen Geschlecht festzustellen, während bei Frauen erst später, aber dann wesentlich schneller, eine Verschmälerung der Compacta erfolgt (Abb. 116).

Von MEEMA (1962) wurden Messungen der „*kombinierten Corticalisdicke*" am *proximalen Radius* durchgeführt. In einem Bezirk des Radius 1—2 cm distal der Tuberositas radii sind die glatten Konturen der Diaphysencompacta zur Messung gut geeignet. Auf einer seitlichen Aufnahme, die in Supinationsstellung des Unterarmes gewonnen wurde, können die Meßpunkte bestimmt werden (Abb. 80 und 84b). Die Summe der beiden gemessenen Compactadicken (A + B) ergibt den von MEEMA (1962) zugrunde gelegten Wert (C) der „*kombinierten Corticalisdicke*". Mit dieser Methode wurden Untersuchungen an Gesunden und Kranken durchgeführt (s. S. 223 und 237).

Die Untersuchungsergebnisse des Radius basieren auf Messungen an Röntgenaufnahmen von 356 Männern und 295 Frauen der Altersgruppen von 20 über 70 Jahre. Der *untere Grenzwert* der normalen „kombinierten Corticalisdicke" beträgt 5 mm. Das weibliche Geschlecht läßt im Alter von etwa 50—70 Jahren in der Hälfte des Kollektivs ein Absinken dieses Wertes auf 4 mm, seltener noch weniger, erkennen. Die entsprechende männliche Altersgruppe zeigte nur in 2% des Kollektivs Werte unter 4 mm. Eine Verminderung der „kombinierten Corticalisdicke" auf etwa 4 mm kann also noch nicht als eindeutig pathologisch betrachtet werden, da die *individuelle Schwankungsbreite der Compacta* (bzw. Corticalis) recht groß ist.

In einer weiteren Untersuchungsreihe von insgesamt 1214 Patienten mit *klinisch normalem Skelet* konnten MEEMA und MEEMA (1963) die Resultate der Messungen einer „kombinierten Corticalisdicke" bestätigen. In der Altersgruppe von 21—45 Jahren betrugen die Normalwerte des *Radius* bei Männern 5—10 mm, bei Frauen 5—8 mm. Die Meßergebnisse der „kombinierten Corticalisdicke" des *Humerus* betrugen bei Männern 7—15 mm, bei Frauen 7—12 mm. Nach dem 45. Lebensjahr war sowohl beim männlichen als auch beim weiblichen Geschlecht ein geringfügiges Absinken der „kombinierten Corticalisdicke" festzustellen. Die Zusammenstellung der Mittelwerte der „kombinierten Corticalisdicke" von Humerus und Radius zeigt bei beiden Geschlechtern sowohl für den Humerus als auch für den Radius eine Abnahme der Meßwerte, doch liegen die Radiuswerte niedriger als die Werte des Humerus. Beim weiblichen Geschlecht sind beide Werte niedriger. Da der Gesamtdurchmesser von Humerus und Radius bei beiden Geschlechtern in den Altersgruppen von 21 bis über 70 Jahren konstant bleibt, liegt der Abnahme der „kombinierten Corticalisdicke" ein echter endostaler *Knochenabbau* zugrunde. Der Verlust der Corticalisdicke nach dem 45. Lebensjahr wird für den *Humerus mit 7%*, für den *Radius mit 8%* angegeben. Beim weiblichen Geschlecht ist der Radius der empfindlichere Indicator für eine Abnahme der „Corticalisdicke". Eine gleichzeitige Messung des Humerus vermag den diagnostischen Wert dieser Methode nur wenig zu erhöhen. Beim männlichen Geschlecht dagegen scheint der Humerus ein sicherer Indikator zum Nachweis einer Osteoporose zu sein, doch müssen die Untersuchungsergebnisse noch weiterhin bestätigt werden. Nach dem 70. Lebensjahr ist eine deutliche Atrophie der Compacta bei beiden Geschlechtern zu erkennen. Das weibliche Geschlecht zeigt schon nach der Menopause ein Absinken der „kombinierten Corticalisdicke", so daß im Bereich des Radius 73% der untersuchten Frauen Werte von 4 mm und weniger aufwiesen. Das männliche Kollektiv zeigte nach dem 70. Lebensjahr nur in 10% Werte, die unter 4 mm liegen. Da die Untersuchungen an klinisch völlig gesunden Personen durchgeführt worden sind, können die erhobenen Befunde einer *Verminderung* der „kombinierten Corticalisdicke" während des Alterungsprozesses als Ausdruck der sog. *„physiologischen Altersosteoporose"* betrachtet werden. Bei Kenntnis der Normalbefunde sind die Messungen der Corticalis- oder Compactadicke gut geeignet, einen Verlust an Knochenmasse (Osteoporose oder Osteopenie) anzuzeigen. Die Meßmethoden sind der einfachen Röntgenaufnahme überlegen, da sie unabhängig von der Schwärzung des Filmes durchgeführt werden können.

Der Corticalisverlust eines Knochens bei Erkrankungen wird zu der gesunden Corticalis in Relation gebracht und in Prozent ausgedrückt. Zur Sicherung des Informationswertes werden Messungen an *beiden* Extremitäten empfohlen.

Von VIRTAMA, KAJANOJA und TELKKÄ (1963) wurde die „Corticalisrelation" oder das „Corticalisverhältnis" des menschlichen *Femur* im Hinblick auf die klinische Brauchbarkeit als Maß für den Mineralgehalt untersucht. Die Verschmälerung der Diaphysencompacta der Röhrenknochen sei ein wichtiges Zeichen der Osteoporose. Vergleichende Untersuchungen wurden an 53 *Femurknochenpräparaten* von 18 Männern und 9 Frauen im Alter zwischen 25 und 82 Jahren durchgeführt, die aus der Sammlung des Anatomischen Institutes der Universität Helsinki stammten. Von den Knochen wurden Röntgenaufnahmen in verschiedenen Projektionen angefertigt, um die Gesamtfläche des Knochens zur Fläche der Diaphysencompacta (oder Corticalis) planimetrisch in Beziehung setzen zu können (s. VIRTAMA und MAHÖNEN 1960). Das „Corticalisverhältnis" wurde gewonnen, indem die Corticalisfläche durch die Fläche des Gesamtknochens dividiert und mit 10 multipliziert wurde. Das Trockengewicht wurde durch das Knochenvolumen dividiert, um die „Knochendichte" zu ermitteln. Es fand sich eine gute Relation zwischen dem „Corticalisverhältnis" und dem Mineralgehalt, ausgedrückt in der „Knochendichte" (Abb. 117).

BARNETT und NORDIN (1960) bestimmten den „*Corticalisindex*" durch Messung der medialen und lateralen Compactadicke in der Mitte des Femurschaftes (s. S. 225). Die Summe dieser Werte wird durch den Schaftdurchmesser (Diaphysendurchmesser) geteilt und dieser Wert mit 100 multipliziert *(Barnett-Nordin-Index)*. Die Korrelation zwischen dem Barnett-Nordin-Index des menschlichen Femur und dem Mineralgehalt war weniger deutlich als zwischen dem „Corticalisverhältnis" und dem Mineralgehalt. Funktionelle Momente können dem Femur eine sehr unregelmäßige äußere Form geben, durch die es schwierig wird, das „Corticalisverhältnis" durch den „Corticalisindex" (BARNETT u. NORDIN 1960) zu ersetzen. Dennoch kann auch diese Methode als Indikator für den Knochenabbau Verwendung finden, insbesondere zu wiederholten Vergleichsuntersuchungen bei Knochenkrankheiten. Der „Corticalisindex" gibt jedoch keine Auskunft über eine *Entkalkung* des Knochens. Es wird betont, daß die Messung des „Corticalisverhältnisses" (also die planimetrische Untersuchung) eine wesentlich genauere Aussage erlaubt als die Bestimmung des „Corticalisindex" (Messung der Compacta nur an *einer* Stelle).

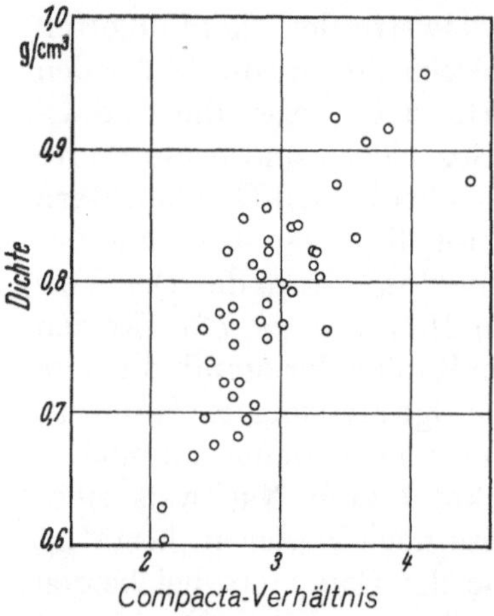

Abb. 117. Abhängigkeit des Compactaverhältnisses von der Dichte am Beispiel des Femur. (Nach VIRTAMA, KAJANOJA und TELKKÄ, 1963; Abb. 1)

SMITH und WALKER (1964) fanden bei 2030 *morphometrischen* Messungen der Compacta der Femurdiaphyse von älteren Frauen eine Verminderung der Compactadicke mit gleichzeitiger Zunahme des Markvolumens. Da der Durchmesser der Diaphyse breiter wurde, muß der subperiostale Knochenanbau größer sein als die endostale Resorption.

Messungen der Dicke der Diaphysencompacta können leicht an *verschiedenen Knochen* des Skeletes durchgeführt werden, wodurch ein besserer Überblick über das Gesamtskelet gewonnen werden kann (VIRTAMA 1965). Die Ergebnisse umfangreicher Messungen an der Diaphysencompacta verschiedener Extremitätenknochen haben HELELÄ und VIRTAMA (1968) vorgelegt, um herauszufinden, welche Knochen am besten geeignet sind. An über 10000 Fällen wurde das Ausmaß der Abweichungen der Corticalisdicke in verschiedenen Altersgruppen, die Beziehungen zum Mineralgehalt, zu Größe und Gewicht, Alter und Beruf untersucht.

Gewisse *Zusammenhänge* zwischen der *Abnahme der Dicke der Femurcompacta* und dem *Aschegehalt der Wirbelspongiosa* fanden ARNOLD und BARTLEY (1965) bei Untersuchungen von Autopsiematerial (Abb. 118a, b, c). Eine Atrophie der Femurcompacta ist stets zusammen mit einer Wirbelatrophie festzustellen, d.h. sie kommt niemals bei normalen Wirbeln vor. Beim weiblichen Geschlecht ist eine erhebliche Reduktion der Compactadicke im Verhältnis zur Wirbelkörpermineralisation festzustellen. Die *progressive Atrophie* der Compacta ist bei Frauen sehr viel deutlicher als bei Männern. Nur ein kleiner Teil der Männer zeigt einen ähnlichen Altersgang der Diaphysencompacta wie die weiblichen Patienten. Die Wirbelatrophie beginnt mit dem 30. Lebensjahr und hat mit 90 Jahren den Tiefpunkt erreicht. Sie findet sich bei beiden Geschlechtern, doch sind die Werte bei den Frauen während des ganzen Lebens etwas niedriger als bei den Männern. Die Femurcompacta wird bei Frauen während des ganzen Lebens dünner, während sie bei Männern konstant zu sein scheint. Hierin kann ein Grund dafür gesehen werden, daß Wirbelfrakturen und Schenkelhalsfrakturen bei Frauen häufiger auftreten als bei Männern.

Messungen der Compactadicke der *Rippen* und des *Schlüsselbeines* haben FISCHER und HAUSSER (1968) bei Personen vom 15. Lebensjahr an und in allen Decennien durchgeführt. Für jede Altersgruppe wurden 100 Röntgenaufnahmen des Thoraxskeletes ausgewertet. Die Messungen der Compacta- (oder Corticalis-) dicke sind im Bereich der cranialen Compacta

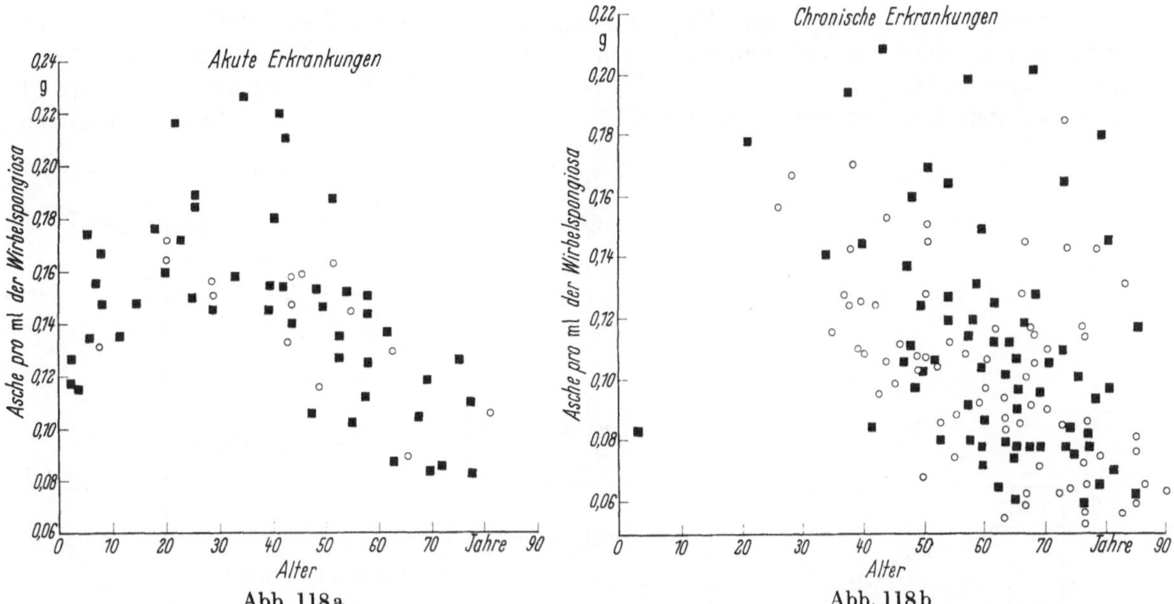

Abb. 118a

Abb. 118b

Abb. 118a. Ergebnisse der Bestimmung des Aschegehaltes in der Wirbelsäule (Mitte des Wirbelkörpers) aufgetragen gegen das Lebensalter (Patienten waren an akuten Erkrankungen gestorben!) bei Männern (■) und Frauen (○). Eine Altersregression ist deutlich erkennbar. (Nach ARNOLD und BARTLEY, 1965; Abb. 1)

Abb. 118b. Bei chronischen Erkrankungen ist der *Abfall* des Aschegehaltes der Wirbelkörper ähnlich. Die etwas höheren Werte entsprechen einer Sklerose bei chronisch Nierenkranken (sklerotische Form des sekundären Hyperparathyreoidismus ?). (Nach ARNOLD und BARTLEY, 1965; Abb. 2)

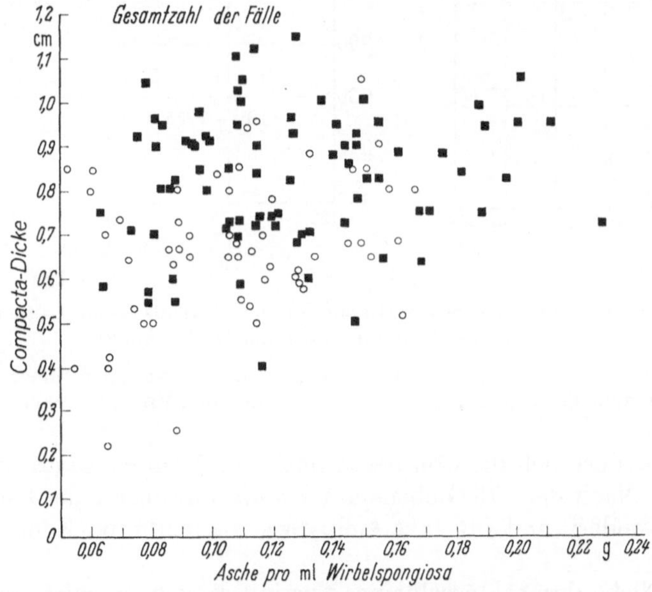

Abb. 118c. Gegenüberstellung von Aschegehalt der Wirbelkörper und Compactadicke des Femur. (Nach ARNOLD und BARTLEY, 1965; Abb. 3)

der 4. oder 5. Rippe in Höhe der Scapularlinie und der cranialen Compacta des Schlüsselbeines im Bereich des mittleren Schaftdrittels ausgeführt worden. Es wurden jeweils zwei Messungen in einem Abstand von 1 cm vorgenommen und hieraus der Mittelwert bestimmt. Als Meßinstrument diente eine Schublehre mit einer Meßgenauigkeit von 0,1 mm. Es sind Messungen bei gesunden Personen und bei Patienten mit Systemerkrankungen des Skeletes oder einer generalisierten Mitbeteiligung des Skeletes bei verschiedenen Erkrankungen durchgeführt worden.

Nachdem die Compacta der Rippe zu Beginn des 3. Decenniums ihre normale Dicke erreicht hat, wird sie mit zunehmendem Alter dünner (Abb. 119a). Der Mittelwert nimmt gleichmäßig von 1,63 ± 0,27 auf 0,54 ± 0,25 mm ab. Der Compactaabbau beträgt also, auf den Ausgangswert bezogen, 67% bei beiden Geschlechtern. Beim weiblichen

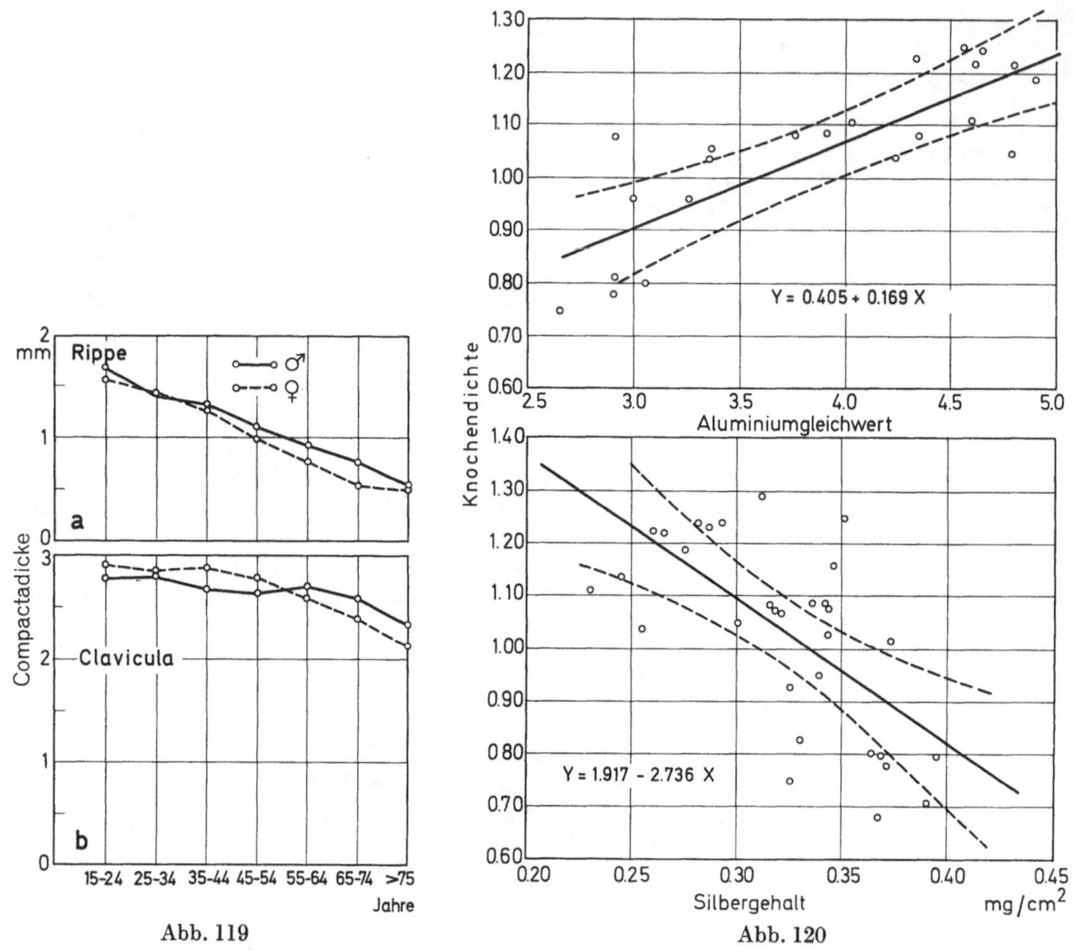

Abb. 119. Normalwerte der Compactadicke von Rippen (a) und Clavicula (b) im Laufe des Alterungsprozesses. (Nach Fischer und Hausser, 1969; Abb. 2)

Abb. 120. Gegenüberstellung der Aluminiumwerte und der Ergebnisse einer Silberanalyse des Filmes zur Bestimmung der Knochendichte. (Nach Helelä und Virtama, 1968; Abb. 2)

Geschlecht verschmälert sich die Compacta nach der Menopause stärker als beim männlichen Geschlecht. Nach dem 75. Lebensjahr ist die Compacta bei beiden Geschlechtern hochgradig verschmälert und oft läßt sich diese hauchdünne Zone nicht mehr genau messen.

Die Compactadicke des Schlüsselbeines verringert sich im mittleren Drittel während des Alterungsprozesses von 2,84 ± 0,45 auf 2,21 ± 0,58 mm. Auf den Ausgangswert bezogen beträgt der Compactaabbau 22% bei beiden Geschlechtern (Abb. 119b). Die Veränderungen sind also weniger deutlich als die der Rippencompacta. Beim weiblichen Geschlecht ist die Schlüsselbeincompacta in den ersten vier Altersgruppen auffallend dicker als beim männlichen Geschlecht. Der Abbau der Schlüsselbeincompacta beginnt bei Frauen zwei Decennien früher als bei Männern und erreicht auch stärkere Grade. Die Meßergebnisse wurden statistisch gesichert.

Der Informationswert *verschiedener radiologischer Meßmethoden* zur Bestimmung der Knochendichte der Ulna wurde von Helelä und Virtama (1968) an 32 Präparaten dieses Knochens untersucht. Im distalen, spongiösen Teil der Ulna wurde das spezifische Gewicht mit den Ergebnissen densitometrischer Untersuchungen und einer Silberanalyse der Filmemulsion verglichen (Abb. 120). Die besten Ergebnisse wurden durch die Densitometrie des Filmes erzielt, doch waren die Befunde einer Messung der Compactadicke ähnlich. Es wird daher empfohlen, die einfache Compactamessung den komplizierteren Meßmethoden vorzuziehen.

Aus allen bisher vorliegenden Mitteilungen über den Wert von Corticalis- oder Compactamessungen geht hervor, daß *möglichst vielseitige und kombinierte Untersuchungen* des Skeletes durchgeführt werden sollten, um den Informationswert radiologischer Meßmethoden zur Bestimmung des Mineralgehaltes und der Knochenmasse zu verbessern.

2. Kombinierte morphometrische und densitometrische Untersuchungen der Compacta

Von H. E. Meema und S. Meema (1968) sind kombinierte Messungen der Compactadicke (oder Corticalisdicke) und der Dichte des Knochens nach der von Meema, Harris und Porrett (1964) entwickelten Methode (s. S. 194) durchgeführt worden.

Meema, Harris und Porrett (1964) haben Normalwerte des Hydroxylapatitgehaltes im proximalen Drittel der Diaphyse des Radius beim männlichen und weiblichen Geschlecht ermittelt (Tabelle 26). Verglichen mit diesen Normalwerten kann eine *Strukturauflockerung* der Diaphysencompacta (auch „corticale Osteoporose" genannt) eindeutig festgestellt werden (Abb. 121a und b). Es muß jedoch beachtet werden, daß auch eine Demineralisation des nicht abgebauten oder aufgelockerten kompakten Knochens gleiche Meßwerte ergeben kann. Diese Methode erlaubt also nicht nur, die „corticale Osteoporose" festzustellen, sondern auch eine *echte Demineralisation der Tela ossea* nachzuweisen (s. S. 238), wie sie bei verschiedenen Stoffwechselerkrankungen vorkommt (Tabelle 31). Die kombinierte Meßmethode gibt Informationen über 1. die Knochenmasse, 2. den Knochenmineralgehalt im untersuchten Skeletbezirk.

Von Meema und Meema (1968) sind der Einfluß einer frühzeitigen Kastration auf den Knochen und Veränderungen nach der Menopause untersucht worden.

Tabelle 31. *Einige Fälle mit niedrigem Hydroxylapatitgehalt der proximalen Diaphysencompacta des Radius. Die Werte wurden photometrisch ermittelt*

Fall	Alter und Geschlecht	Klinische Angaben	Hydroxylapatitgehalt in mg/ml	Kombinierte Compactadicke
1. M. W.	27 ♀	Rheumatische Arthritis (?) Gynäkologische Totalexstirpation	830—920	6,0—6,5 mm
2. E. L.	72 ♂	Senile Osteoporose mit multiplen Wirbelfrakturen	800—870	4,6—5,4 mm
3 C. B.	18 ♀	Sekundärer Hyperparathyreoidismus (chronische Pyelonephritis, autoptisch gesichert)	in vivo: 830—960 autoptisch: 800—900	6,0 mm
4. M. M.	60 ♀	Fraglicher Hyperparathyreoidismus, Operation ergab kein Adenom	830—910	3,2—4,0 mm
5. H. E.	46 ♂	sekundärer Hyperparathyreoidismus (chronische Pyelonephritis, autoptisch gesichert)	840—960	5,0—5,5 mm
6. F. L.	44 ♂	Cortison-Cushing	870—970	7,0 mm
7. E. C.	72 ♀	Morbus Cushing bei Nebennieren-Carcinom	860—980	4,3—4,5 mm
8. C. C.	31 ♀	Malabsorptions-Osteopathie	860—890	3,6—4,2 mm

[Meema, H. E., C. K. Harris, and R. E. Porrett: Radiology 82, 986 (1964), Tab. 5]

Die Beziehungen zwischen der Compactadicke und der Dichte des mittleren Abschnittes vom *Metacarpale II* haben WOLANSKI und EAGEN (1965) untersucht. Die Messungen der Compactadicke wurden mit einem Zirkel auf folienlosen Filmen durchgeführt. Die Dichtemessungen erfolgten in der Mitte zwischen den lateralen Begrenzungen des Knochens. Bei den Messungen sind die verschiedenen Faktoren wie Entwicklungstechnik, Belichtung, Schleierschwärzung und Einfluß der Strahlenfilterung berücksichtigt worden. Zur Untersuchung sind 176 Männer und 153 Frauen im Alter zwischen 2 und

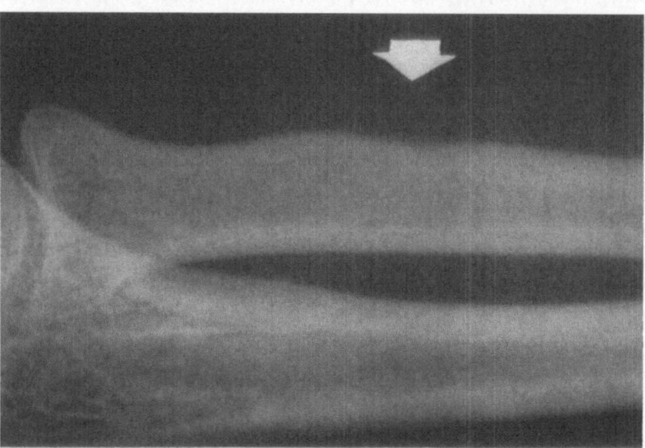

Abb. 121a. Subperiostale Resorption und Strukturauflockerung an der Tuberositas radii bei sekundärem Hyperparathyreoidismus. (Nach MEEMA, HARRIS und PORRETT, 1964; Abb. 16)

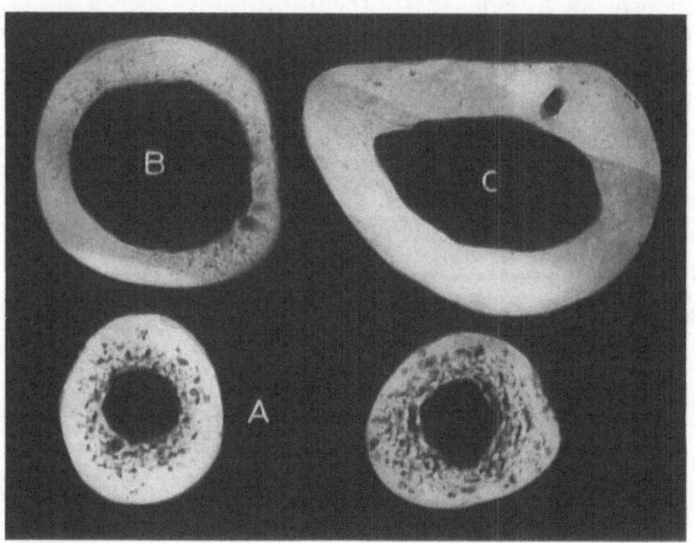

Abb. 121b. Röntgenaufnahmen von Radiusquerschnitten in verschiedenen Bezirken mit teilweise deutlicher Strukturauflockerung im Sinne der beginnenden Spongiosierung. (Nach MEEMA, persönlich zur Verfügung gestellt)

74 Jahren herangezogen worden, die alle Einwohner der gleichen Stadt waren. Die Weichteilabsorption wurde rechnerisch berücksichtigt. Die Compactadicke steigt zwischen dem 3. und 20. Lebensjahr steil an und erreicht bei Frauen im 24. Lebensjahr, bei Männern im 28. Lebensjahr den höchsten Wert. Dann kommt es zu einer Verminderung der Compactadicke. Von der Pubertät an ist die Compacta bei den Jungen dicker als bei den Mädchen.

Interessant ist die Feststellung einer Änderung der *Weichteildichte*. Sie fällt bis zum 10. Lebensjahr leicht ab und steigt dann rapide bis zum 20. und 23. Lebensjahr wieder an, um schließlich langsam erneut bis zum 28. Lebensjahr bei den Männern und bis zum 35. Lebensjahr bei den Frauen abzufallen. Danach bleibt sie mehr oder weniger konstant. Während Frauen zwischen 15 und 27 Jahren einen höheren Wert für die Weichteildichte zeigen als Männer, ist es im späteren Lebensalter umgekehrt.

Die *Knochendichte* steigt zwischen dem 3. und 22. Lebensjahr sehr deutlich an, um bis zum 30. Lebensjahr nur noch langsam zuzunehmen. Danach fällt sie allmählich ab, und zwar bei den Männern etwas langsamer als bei den Frauen. Etwas steiler ist der Abfall nach der Menopause, also vom 50. Lebensjahr ab. Bis zum 20. Lebensjahr ist die Knochendichte bei Jungen höher als bei Mädchen, während vom 20.—55. Lebensjahr die Dichte im Metacarpale II bei den Frauen größer ist als bei den Männern. Später kehrt sich das Verhältnis wieder um.

Es wurde ferner das Verhältnis von Knochendichte zu Compactadicke untersucht. Bis zum 25. Lebensjahr steigt bei beiden Geschlechtern die Knochendichte im Verhältnis zur Compactadicke sehr rasch an und fällt vom 25.—37. Lebensjahr ab. In den Altersgruppen zwischen dem 37. und 50. Lebensjahr kann ein weiterer Anstieg der Knochendichte bei Männern beobachtet werden. In den später folgenden Jahren bleibt die Dichte gleichmäßig. Bei den Frauen ist ein weiterer Anstieg vom 37.—48. Lebensjahr festzustellen. Vom 50. Lebensjahr an fällt die Knochendichte relativ rasch ab. Ein Vergleich der beiden Geschlechter zeigt, daß die Veränderungen bis zum 50. Lebensjahr sehr ähnlich sind, obwohl die relative Dichte bei den Männern etwas höher liegt. Etwa vom 57. Lebensjahr an ist die relative Knochendichte bei den Frauen niedriger als bei den Männern. Es ist ein fast regelmäßiges Nebeneinander und Parallellaufen der Compactadicke und der Knochendichte im Alter zwischen 2 und 27 bzw. 34 Jahren bei Männern und von 2—28 bzw. 31 Jahren bei Frauen zu beobachten. Die parallel verlaufenden Linien zeigen eine größere Dicke bei den Männern und eine etwas höhere Dichte bei den Frauen. Nach diesem Zeitpunkt sind die Veränderungen bei den Geschlechtern sehr verschieden. Während man beim weiblichen Geschlecht eine starke Verminderung der Knochendichte und eine langsame Abnahme der Compactadicke feststellen kann, bleibt bei den Männern die Compactadicke auch dann unverändert, wenn die Knochendichte abzufallen beginnt. Erst später kommt es zu einer Verminderung der Compactadicke bei etwa gleichbleibender Knochendichte.

Diese Methoden erlauben eine genaue Analyse des Knochens in vivo. Der kombinierten Messung von Compactadicke und Knochendichte kommt große Bedeutung bei der Differenzierung von Osteoporose und Osteomalacie zu.

3. Spezielle radiologische Untersuchungen an der Wirbelsäule

Bei klinisch-radiologischer Beurteilung von Systemerkrankungen des Skeletes wurde der sog. „Stammosteoporose" eine besondere Bedeutung zugemessen. Hierbei sollte die Wirbelsäule frühzeitig und zuerst Knochenabbau und Entkalkungsvorgänge erkennen lassen. So ist es verständlich, daß eine Reihe spezieller densitometrischer Untersuchungsmethoden und andere Meßverfahren zur radiologischen Beurteilung der Wirbelsäule entwickelt worden sind. Einige dieser Methoden haben bereits praktische Anwendung gefunden, andere sind von theoretischem Interesse und sollen zusammengefaßt dargelegt werden.

a) Untersuchungen von Dichte oder Struktur der Wirbelkörper

Neben solchen radiologischen Methoden, die zur Dichtemessung von Wirbelkörpern ein Referenzsystem verwenden und auf S. 199 abgehandelt worden sind, ist die Methode der Bestimmung der „relativen Wirbeldichte" zu nennen (Nordin 1960).

Die stärkere Entkalkung der Wirbelsäule als rein spongiöser Knochen und die deutlich erkennbaren Transformationsvorgänge mit Verlust der horizontalen Bälkchenstrukturen bei Betonung der vertikalen Strukturen haben Nordin (1960) veranlaßt, eine Methode

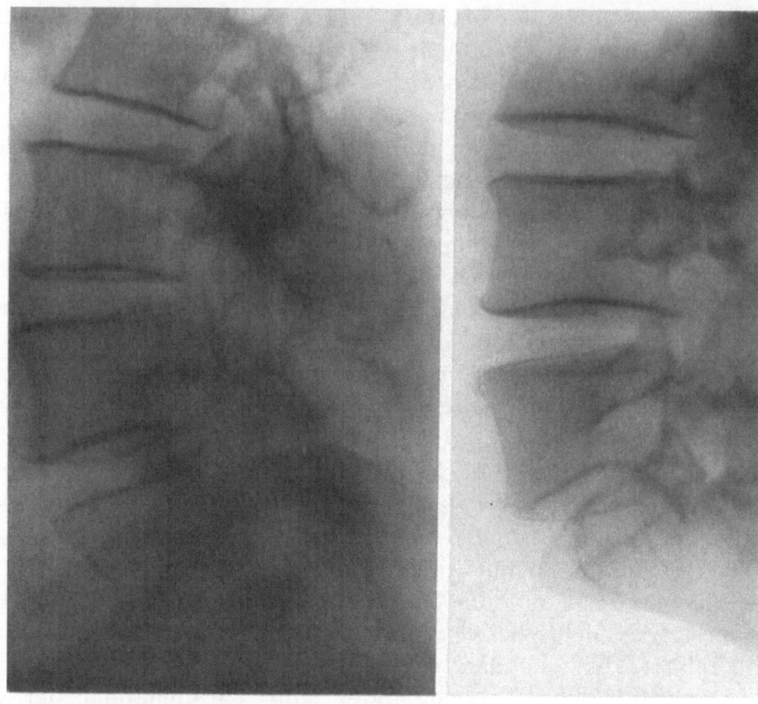

Abb. 122a. Beispiel einer seitlichen Röntgenaufnahme der unteren Lendenwirbelsäule mit der „Standardwirbelsäule" als Vergleichsphantom. (Nach NORDIN)

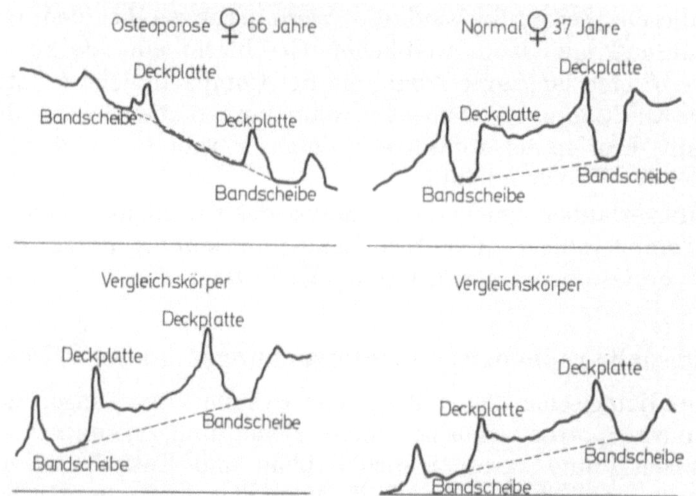

Abb. 122b. Gegenüberstellung der Densitometerkurven des Vergleichskörpers („Standardwirbelsäule") und der Densitometerkurven einer osteoporotischen Wirbelsäule (li.) sowie einer normalen Wirbelsäule (re.) (von NORDIN persönlich zur Verfügung gestellt)

zu entwickeln, die die Dichte des Wirbelknochens zu der Dichte des Bandscheibenraumes in Beziehung setzt. Die Dichteunterschiede werden mit den Dichteunterschieden einer normalen Lendenwirbelsäule verglichen, die unmittelbar neben dem Patienten auf demselben Film aufgenommen wird (Abb. 122a und b). Die „Standardwirbelsäule" wird in einer Plexiglasbox in Formalin aufbewahrt und in streng seitlicher Lage, analog der Position des zu untersuchenden Patienten auf einer Übersichtsaufnahme oder einem Tomogramm dargestellt. Die photometrische Auswertung erfolgte mit einem Laurence-Locarte oder Joyce-Loebel-Densitometer, das einen 1 mm breiten Schlitz zur kontinuierlichen Messung der Dichte besitzt. Die Dichteunterschiede zwischen der Bandscheibenzone und dem Wirbelkörper des Patienten werden dividiert durch die entsprechenden Unterschiede der „Standardwirbelsäule" und hierdurch die „relative Wirbelkörperdichte" erhalten (Abb. 123a und b). Liegt die relative Wirbelkörperdichte bei 1,0, so sagt dies aus, daß zwischen dem

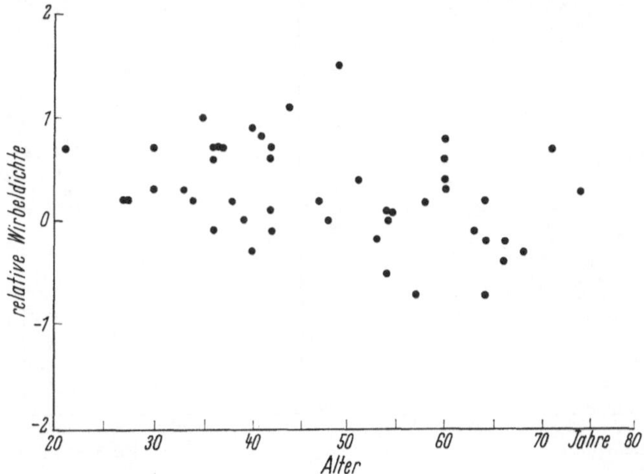

Abb. 123a. Die „relative Wirbeldichte" bei 47 gesunden Männern in den verschiedenen Dezennien. (Nach NORDIN, BARNETT, SMITH und ANDERSON, 1965; Abb. 16)

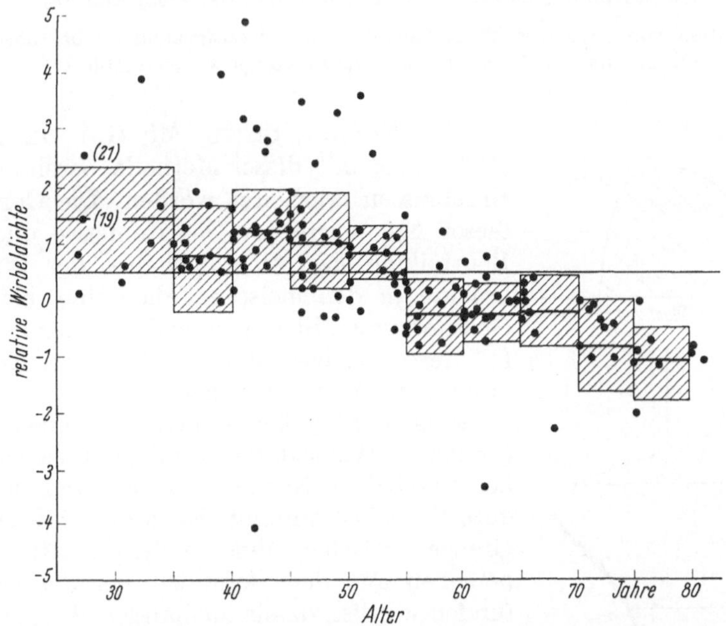

Abb. 123b. Die „relative Wirbeldichte" mit Standardabweichung bei 152 gesunden Frauen in den verschiedenen Dezennien. (Nach NORDIN, BARNETT, SMITH und ANDERSON, 1965; Abb. 15)

Patienten und dem Standard kein Unterschied besteht. Die relative Wirbelkörperdichte 0 gibt an, daß zwischen dem Bandscheibenraum und dem Wirbelkörper selbst keine Dichteunterschiede bestehen, so daß angenommen werden kann, der Knochen ist völlig demineralisiert. Bei dieser Interpretation müßte jedoch die unterschiedliche Strahlenabsorption durch Fett und Weichteile berücksichtigt werden! Durch diese physikalische Tatsache sind wahrscheinlich auch die hin und wieder mitgeteilten negativen Werte der relativen Wirbelkörperdichte zu verstehen. Der Fehler der Methode wird mit $\pm 0{,}15$ bei wiederholten Messungen des gleichen Filmes und mit $\pm 0{,}30$ bei Auswertung verschiedener Filme desselben Patienten angegeben.

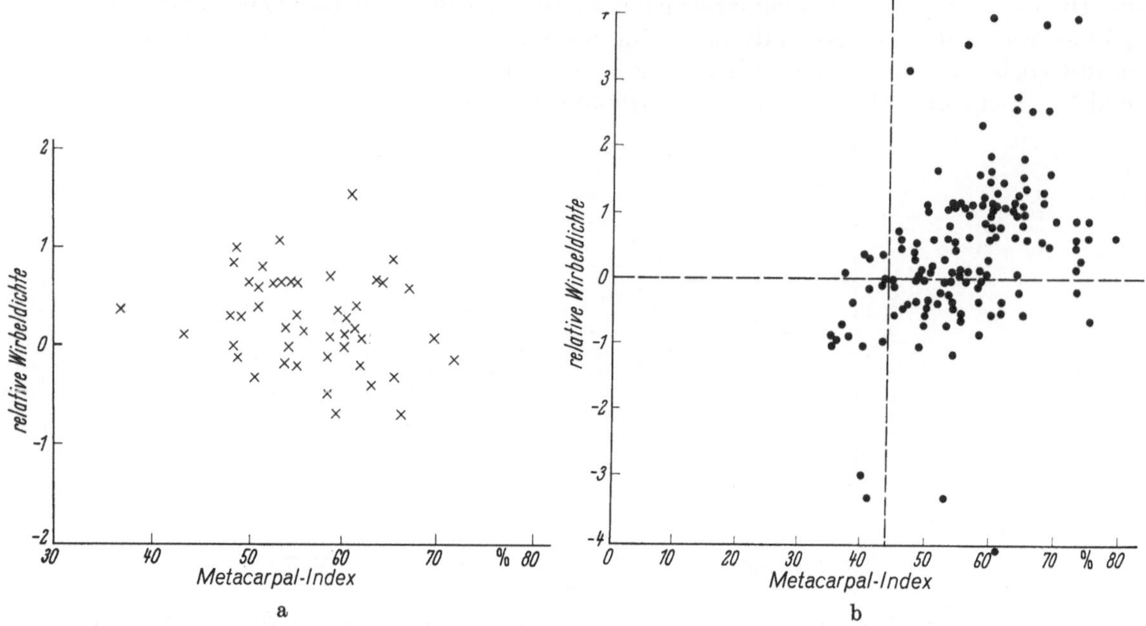

Abb. 124a. Relation von „relativer Wirbeldichte" zum „Metacarpalindex" bei 47 normalen Männern. (Nach Nordin, Barnett, Smith und Anderson, 1965; Abb. 18)

Abb. 124b. Relation von „relativer Wirbeldichte" zum „Metacarpalindex" bei normalen Frauen. (Nach Nordin, Barnett, Smith und Anderson, 1965; Abb. 17)

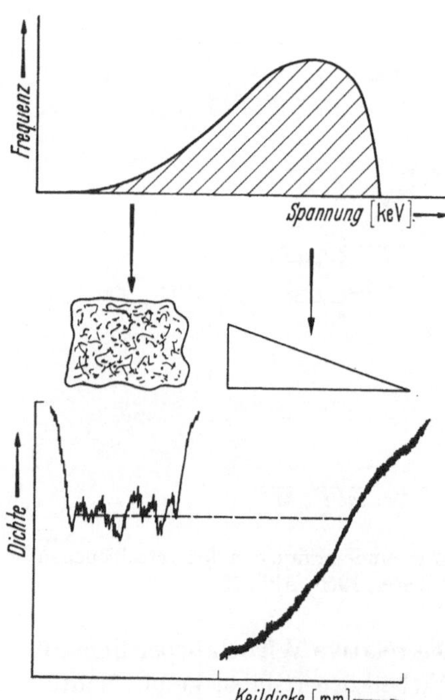

Abb. 125. Schematische Darstellung der Methode der Mikrodensitometrie von Wirbelspongiosa (mit Referenzsystem). (Nach Rockoff, 1965; Abb. 1)

Von Nordin, Smith, Mc. Gregor und Anderson (1965) sind mit dieser Methode bereits eine Reihe von Ergebnissen erarbeitet worden. Die Gegenüberstellung dieser Ergebnisse der Densitometrie und der visuellen Beurteilung des Mineralgehaltes der Wirbelkörper erbrachte in den meisten Fällen eine relativ gute Übereinstimmung. Mit zunehmendem Alter fand sich ein Abfall der „relativen Wirbeldichte" bei Normalpersonen, besonders bei Frauen nach der Menopause. Die Auswertung der Meßergebnisse verschiedener Methoden („relativer Wirbeldichte" und „Metacarpalindex") ergab bei weiblichen Normalpersonen und bei Osteoporose gute Übereinstimmung. Es konnte jedoch keine scharfe Grenze zwischen den Meßergebnissen von Normalpersonen und den Befunden bei der Osteoporose gefunden werden, da sie ineinander übergehen (Abb. 124a und b).

Vergleichsuntersuchungen von Messungen der Wirbeldichte („relative Wirbeldichte" nach Nordin, 1960) mit den Ergebnissen der Messungen des „Bikonkavitätsindex" der Wirbelkörper ergaben dann krankhafte Veränderungen des Index, wenn sich die Wirbeldichte der Dichte des Bandscheibenraumes anzugleichen begann. Bei einer Osteoporose kann die Wirbeldichte auch geringer sein als die Bandscheibendichte (Nordin, Barnett, Mc Gregor und Nisbet 1962).

Eine mikrodensitometrische Methode, kombiniert mit einem Analog-Rechner zur Bestimmung der Breite und Zahl der Spongiosabälkchen auf Röntgenaufnahmen menschlicher

Wirbelkörper ist von ROCKOFF (1968) entwickelt worden (Abb. 125). In einer vorläufigen Studie konnten die Knochenmasse, die Kompressionsfähigkeit des Knochens, der Calcium-Phosphor- und Magnesiumgehalt von Lendenwirbelkörpern mit Hilfe der neuen Methode bestimmt werden. Es fand sich eine gute Korrelation zwischen der am Lebenden in situ bestimmten Breite der vertikal und horizontal orientierten Spongiosabälkchen-Schatten und der Knochenmasse, der Kompressionsfähigkeit und dem Mineralgehalt der Wirbelspongiosa.

b) Untersuchungen der Wirbelkörperdeckplatten

Neben der densitometrischen Messung der „relativen Wirbeldichte" (s. S. 240) wurde von BARNETT und NORDIN (1960) ein besonderes Meßverfahren zur Erkennung osteoporotischer Veränderungen im Bereich der Wirbelsäule, insbesondere zum Nachweis pathologischer Frakturen und Zusammensinterung von Wirbeln angegeben. Der sog. „Bikonkavitäts-Index" stellt den Quotienten aus der geringsten meßbaren Wirbelhöhe und der höchsten meßbaren Wirbelhöhe multipliziert mit dem Faktor 100 dar. Größere Sicherheit als die seitliche Übersichtsaufnahme bietet die Messung an Tomogrammen der Wirbelsäule, die 1—1,5 cm neben der Mittellinie gewonnen werden sollten.

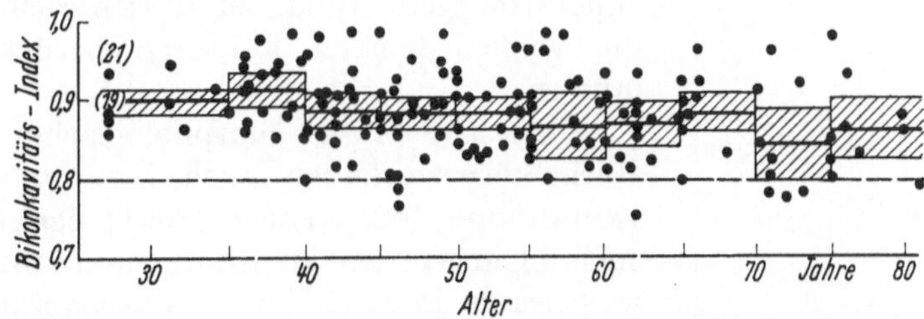

Abb. 126. Bikonkavitätsindex und Standardabweichungen in den einzelnen Dezennien (Normalwerte von 152 Frauen). (Nach NORDIN, BARNETT, SMITH und ANDERSON, 1965; Abb. 8)

Die Messungen wurden am 3. und 4. Lendenwirbelkörper bei seitlicher Projektion vorgenommen. Der normale Meßwert des „Bikonkavitäts-Index" sollte mindestens 80% ergeben und im Laufe des Alterungsprozesses nicht abfallen; es sei denn, es liegt eine Entkalkung oder ein stärkerer Knochenabbau vor (Abb. 126). Der „Bikonkavitäts-Index" wurde von KUHLENCORDT, KRUSE, LOZANO-TONKIN, WIENERS und BARTELHEIMER (1967) an Schichtaufnahmen des 3. und 4. Lendenwirbelkörpers bei Systemerkrankungen des Knochens ermittelt. Dieser „zentrale Index" wird einem „peripheren Index" (Summe des Compacta-Index von Femur und Metacarpale) an die Seite gestellt (s. auch S. 226).

VIRTAMA, GÄSTRIN und TELKKÄ (1962) haben Untersuchungen zur Brauchbarkeit des „Bikonkavitätsindex" der Wirbelkörper als Maß für die Knochendichte durchgeführt. Ferner wurde die Ansicht von BARNETT und NORDIN (1960) überprüft, nach der die *Bikonkavität der Lendenwirbelsäule* von besonderem Interesse sei. Das Untersuchungsmaterial aus der Sammlung des Anatomischen Institutes Helsinki bestand aus drei Wirbelsäulen von Männern im Alter zwischen 36 und 62 Jahren, einer Wirbelsäule einer Frau von 45 Jahren und 28 einzelnen Brust- und Lendenwirbelkörpern — insgesamt also 99 Wirbelkörpern. Der „Bikonkavitätsindex" der Wirbelkörper wurde röntgenologisch nach der Methode von BARNETT und NORDIN (1960) ermittelt (s. S. 226). Die Dichte der Wirbelkörper wurde durch Trockengewichtsbestimmung und Volumenbestimmung mit einem Pyknometer gefunden. Die Knochendichte wurde ausgedrückt in Gewicht der fettfreien Knochensubstanz (g)/Volumeneinheit (cm³). Die durchschnittliche Knochendichte aller untersuchten Wirbelkörper betrug 0,427 g/cm³. An der *Halswirbelsäule* fanden sich die höchsten Dichtewerte, im Bereich der Brustwirbelsäule nur wenig höhere Werte als im Bereich der Lendenwirbelsäule. Die relativ hohe Dichte der Halswirbelkörper kann durch ihr kleineres Volumen und die andere Relation von Corticalis zu Spongiosa zustande kommen. Die Ermittlung der Bikonkavitätswerte ergab, daß die Brustwirbelkörper weniger bikonkav sind als die Halswirbelkörper und die Lendenwirbelkörper. In der Mitte der Brustwirbelsäule sind auch die normalen Wirbelkörper häufig keilförmig deformiert, und zwar nicht nur bei Fällen von Osteoporose. Die Bikonkavität der Lendenwirbelkörper ist deutlicher als die der Halswirbelkörper (Tabelle 32). Besonders abweichend waren die Befunde am 5. Lendenwirbelkörper. Die Gegenüberstellung des „Bikonkavitätsindex" und der Knochendichte ergab keine eindeutigen Zusammenhänge (Abb. 127). Es trifft wohl zu, daß der Anteil bikonkaver Wirbel bei einer Osteoporose höher ist als bei gesunden Wirbelsäulen, doch spielen das Gewicht des Menschen, traumatische Faktoren oder Mikrotraumen eine Rolle. Ferner dürfte die Form der Zwischenwirbelscheiben einen Einfluß auf die Deckplatten der Lendenwirbelkörper haben. Wahrscheinlich spielen auch embryologische Störungen eine Rolle. Der „Bikonkavitätsindex" stellt zwar eine relativ einfache morphologische Methode zur Beurteilung der Wirbelsäule dar, doch handelt es sich hierbei um einen Röntgenbefund, zu dessen richtiger Beurteilung die verschiedensten Faktoren berücksichtigt werden müssen.

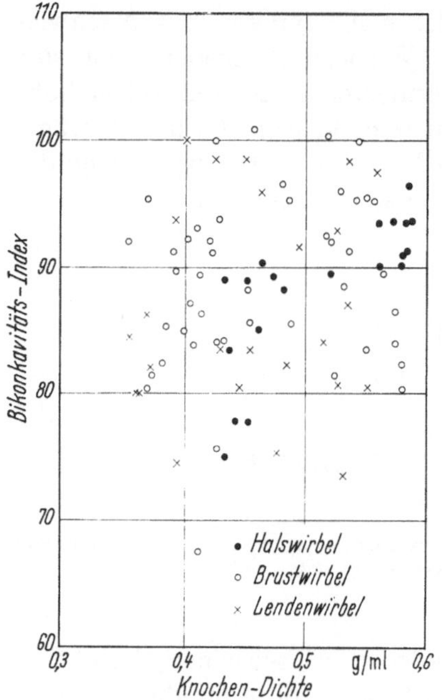

Abb. 127. Gegenüberstellung von Bikonkavitätsindex und Knochendichte in den verschiedenen Abschnitten der Wirbelsäule. (Nach Virtama, Gästrin und Telkkä, 1962; Abb. 4)

Über Ergebnisse morphologischer Messungen von Wirbelkörpern haben auch Dubouloz, Legré, Merjanian und Serratrice (1961) berichtet. Die Untersuchungen wurden an Röntgenaufnahmen der Lendenwirbelsäule in zwei Ebenen durchgeführt. Bei anterior-posteriorer Projektion kann eine Abweichung der Wirbelkörperhöhe bis zu 2 mm zwischen rechts und links noch als normal angesehen werden. Die noch normalen Höhenunterschiede der Lendenwirbelkörper bei seitlicher Projektion wurden mit 3 mm bei L 1 und mit 2 mm bei den übrigen Lendenwirbelkörpern angegeben. Von 93 Normalpersonen aus sitzenden und manuell arbeitenden Berufen wiesen signifikant mehr Frauen als Männer vornehmlich im Alter von 20—29 Jahren eine Tendenz zur Keilform des Wirbels auf. Unter den Patienten, die wegen posttraumatischer Beschwerden untersucht worden sind, waren 90% Männer im Alter zwischen 30—39 Jahren. Eine Differenz zwischen der hinteren und vorderen Höhe des Wirbelkörpers um mehr als 3 mm war meist traumatisch bedingt.

Experimentelle Untersuchungen über die *Dichte der Wirbeldeckplatten* als Maß für eine Osteoporose haben Virtama, Telkkä und Helelä (1965) durchgeführt. Eine krankhafte Störung drückt sich in einem Wirbelkörper zuerst in der Verminderung der *Anzahl der Trabekel*, insbesondere der horizontal verlaufenden aus (Rockoff 1968). Diese Veränderungen sind jedoch am lebenden Menschen wegen der überlagernden Weichteile äußerst schwer erkennbar. Der Wirbelkörper wird im Röntgenbild durch die *Corticalisschale* abgrenzbar, welche das Spongiosanetz umschließt. Ein Verlust der Spongiosa bis zu einem Viertel des Ausgangswertes beeinflußt das Röntgenbild nicht, wenn die Corticalis unverändert bleibt (Knutsson 1953). Die Corticalis der Deckplatten der Wirbelkörper reagiert bei einer Störung offenbar relativ langsam. Selbst bei einer Osteoporose bleiben die Deckplatten besonders betont. Diese Tatsache wurde von Murray (1961) und Julkunen (1962) als bedeutsam für die Diagnose einer Osteoporose angesehen, da die Deckplatten in solchen Fällen stärker in Erscheinung treten. Die „radiologische

Dichte" der Deckplatten hängt jedoch auch von aufnahmetechnischen und physikalischen Faktoren ab. So wurde die Brauchbarkeit der radiologischen Messung der Dichte der Wirbeldeckplatten durch vergleichende chemische Untersuchungen geprüft. In einer Serie von 28 Brust- und Lendenwirbelkörperpräparaten von Leichen im Alter von 30 Jahren wurde das Trockengewicht bestimmt. Die Dichte wurde aus Trockengewicht

Tabelle 32. *Knochendichte- und Bikonkavitäts-Indexwerte von 3 Wirbelsäulen*

	Wirbelsäule I		Wirbelsäule II		Wirbelsäule III	
	Knochendichte	Bikonkavitäts-index	Knochendichte	Bikonkavitäts-index	Knochendichte	Bikonkavitäts-index
Hals-Wirbelsäule	0,601	—	0,461	—	0,501	—
	0,596	—	0,450	89,0	0,491	—
	0,582	93,7	0,452	77,8	0,459	—
	0,587	93,7	0,432	89,0	0,480	88,2
	0,572	93,7	0,441	77,8	0,472	89,3
	0,579	82,4	0,432	75,0	0,463	90,4
	0,560	93,6	0,437	83,5	0,460	85,1
Mittelwerte:	0,582	90,9	0,444	82,1	0,475	88,3
Brust-Wirbelsäule	0,563	89,6	0,431	84,2	0,451	88,3
	0,556	92,5	0,425	84,1	0,421	91,2
	0,550	95,6	0,413	86,3	0,409	93,2
	0,541	95,4	0,419	92,1	0,406	83,9
	0,543	100,0	0,424	100,0	0,411	89,4
	0,536	91,3	0,427	93,8	0,390	91,3
	0,528	96,0	0,411	67,6	0,399	85,0
	0,520	92,0	0,426	75,7	0,392	89,7
	0,531	88,5	0,486	85,5	0,384	85,3
	0,523	81,5	0,404	87,2	0,381	82,4
	0,516	92,5	0,402	92,3	0,369	80,4
	0,518	100,4	0,452	85,6	0,373	81,5
Mittelwerte:	0,533	84,6	0,425	86,2	0,399	86,8
Lenden-Wirbelsäule	0,526	93,0	0,429	83,5	0,368	86,2
	0,514	84,2	0,462	96,0	0,361	80,1
	0,534	87,0	0,401	100,0	0,354	84,5
	0,526	80,7	0,493	91,7	0,372	82,1
	0,531	73,5	0,392	93,7	0,363	80,1
Mittelwerte:	0,526	83,7	0,435	93,0	0,363	82,6

[Virtama, P., G. Gästrin, and A. Telkkä: Clin. Radiol. **13**, 128 (1962), Tab. 1]

und Volumen ermittelt. Der Aschegehalt betrug 57% der Trockendichte, der Calciumgehalt 39% des Aschegehaltes. Vor der chemischen Analyse wurden diese Wirbelkörper unter verschiedenen Bedingungen zusammen mit einer Aluminiumtreppe als Referenzsystem im Wasserphantom geröntgt (Tabelle 33). Die Röntgenfilme wurden densitometrisch ausgewertet unter besonderer Berücksichtigung der Deckplatten. Die *„relative Dichte"* (Virtama, Telkkä und Helelä 1965) der Deckplatten wurde dadurch ermittelt, daß ihre durchschnittliche Dichte von der durchschnittlichen Dichte der Wirbelspongiosa subtrahiert wurde. Die Brustwirbelsäule ist für Untersuchungen der „relativen Dichte" der Wirbeldeckplatten am besten geeignet. Im Bereich der Lendenwirbelsäule stören die Weichteilüberlagerungen erheblich und bringen ungünstige Bedingungen. Die „relative Dichte" der Wirbelendplatten ist offenbar ein geeigneteres Maß zur Erfassung einer Osteoporose als der Nachweis von Wirbeldeformitäten.

Tabelle 33. *Gegenüberstellung der Ergebnisse von Messungen der „relativen Dichte" der Wirbeldeckplatten* und des Mineralgehaltes der Wirbel bei unterschiedlichem Weichteilmantel und verschiedener Strahlenqualitäten

Mineralgehalt in mg/ml	Relative Dichte der Deckplatten								
	10 cm Wasser			20 cm Wasser			30 cm Wasser		
	60 kV	80 kV	100 kV	60 kV	80 kV	100 kV	60 kV	80 kV	100 kV
322	11,2	10,6	7,1	6,0	3,4	3,2	3,2	2,7	0,5
470	7,9	6,0	3,2	4,0	3,1	3,0	1,1	0,9	0,1
411	6,5	4,2	2,2	3,1	3,8	2,5	0,8	0,1	0,1
413	9,4	8,0	6,8	5,4	3,8	2,1	1,1	0,6	0,0
469	5,1	4,0	2,0	3,8	2,4	1,2	1,3	0,6	0,5
397	9,1	8,1	5,6	5,1	6,1	2,1	2,1	1,0	0,6
512	7,2	6,3	3,3	5,8	3,4	1,5	0,9	0,9	0,9
496	3,4	3,1	1,8	2,4	2,0	0,9	1,6	0,2	0,1
326	8,1	7,0	4,8	6,2	5,2	2,6	1,4	0,6	0,2
492	8,0	6,2	4,1	7,1	4,8	2,5	1,7	0,5	0,2
464	8,8	6,9	3,2	4,8	5,7	3,1	2,1	0,4	0,1
399	5,4	4,7	3,3	4,1	4,0	3,1	2,3	0,1	0,0
412	10,6	7,9	5,2	6,0	5,8	2,1	2,8	0,1	0,8
478	5,4	4,8	2,3	3,8	2,9	1,1	0,9	0,1	0,2
492	4,9	4,2	2,1	3,6	3,2	0,8	1,3	0,1	0,0
394	7,6	6,2	4,1	5,1	5,0	0,8	0,9	0,2	0,4
427	7,5	7,0	5,6	5,0	4,1	3,1	2,0	1,2	0,4
502	6,9	5,6	4,1	6,1	2,6	0,6	0,4	0,4	0,3
443	6,2	5,0	3,2	5,4	2,0	0,2	0,6	0,5	0,3
472	9,6	8,0	5,1	6,3	3,2	0,9	0,9	0,6	0,4
451	6,7	6,0	4,3	5,8	4,1	2,2	3,1	0,9	0,6
486	6,6	6,1	3,8	3,9	3,0	2,1	0,7	0,6	0,4
363	9,5	8,1	6,1	5,8	3,0	1,7	1,0	0,7	0,4
424	4,5	4,2	2,7	2,6	2,0	1,8	1,9	0,6	0,4
516	6,2	5,1	3,3	3,1	2,7	0,6	0,8	0,6	0,0
479	4,5	4,1	3,7	2,1	2,5	0,7	0,6	0,3	0,0
420	5,0	3,8	3,0	2,8	2,0	0,9	0,4	0,2	0,0
401	8,5	8,5	5,8	3,6	2,1	1,0	0,6	0,4	0,0

[VIRTAMA, P., A. TELKKÄ, and T. HELELÄ: Brit. J. Radiol. 38, 360 (1965), Tab, 1]

IX. Die praktische Anwendung radiologischer Messungen in der klinischen Medizin

Die bisher mit verschiedenen Untersuchungsmethoden erarbeiteten „Normwerte" einiger Knochen oder Knochenbezirke des menschlichen Skeletes können als Grundlage angesehen werden, um krankhafte Abweichungen festzustellen. Neben der Messung von *Einzelwerten* sind *Verlaufskontrollen* während eines Krankheitsablaufes von Bedeutung. Der Erfolg oder Mißerfolg einer therapeutischen Maßnahme kann objektiviert werden. Nachfolgend sollen Untersuchungsergebnisse des Knochenmineralgehaltes und der Compactadicke bei verschiedenen Erkrankungen nach klinischen Gesichtspunkten zusammengestellt werden, um die Möglichkeiten dieser neuen radiologischen Meßmethoden für die einzelnen Fachgebiete der Medizin darzulegen.

1. Der Einfluß körperlicher Belastung oder Ruhigstellung (Immobilisation) auf den Knochenmineralgehalt

Es ist bekannt, daß nach *längerer Ruhigstellung* einer Extremität eine Abnahme der Knochendichte röntgenologisch nachgewiesen werden kann. Umgekehrt wurden bisher keinerlei Zusammenhänge zwischen *stärkerer körperlicher Belastung* und dem globalen Knochenmineralgehalt gefunden. So hat MAYO (1961) *Langzeituntersuchungen am Calcaneus* durchgeführt, um den Einfluß der statischen Belastung auf den Kalksalzgehalt des

Knochens zu prüfen. Als Versuchspersonen wurde eine größere Gruppe von Soldaten, die einem intensiven Übungsdrill unterzogen worden waren, und eine Kontrollgruppe aus dem Krankenhauspersonal ausgewählt. Es fanden sich *keine eindeutigen Unterschiede des Knochenmineralgehaltes vom Calcaneus bei den beiden Gruppen.* Die Kalksalzkonzentration des Calcaneus war bei den Soldaten vielleicht etwas höher, doch handelte es sich bei diesen ausschließlich um junge Menschen.

Eine Objektivierung der *nach Ruhigstellung eines Gliedes* oder *Bettruhe* auftretenden Veränderungen im Knochen hat die Arbeitsgruppe von Mack versucht. Mit einer mikrodensitometrischen Meßmethode konnte die Demineralisation von Knochen nicht nur nach Ruhigstellung eines Gliedes sondern auch während einer Schwangerschaft (Mack, Brown und Trapp 1949) gefunden werden. Systematische Untersuchungen an einem Kollektiv ausgewählter junger Männer, die während der *Versuchsdauer von einigen Wochen* einer strengen Bettruhe unterzogen wurden, hat Mack (1965) durchgeführt. Die Zusammensetzung und die Menge der diätetischen Nahrung wurde im Hinblick auf den Calcium- und Phosphorgehalt genau bestimmt. Die Ausscheidung von Calcium und Phosphor in Stuhl und Urin wurden fortlaufend kontrolliert. Im Stuhl fand sich eine höhere Calciumausscheidung als im Urin, während die Phosphorausscheidung im Urin höher war. Bei den verschiedenen Versuchspersonen war die Calciumausscheidung im Stuhl und Urin unterschiedlich, jedoch abhängig von der aufgenommenen Calciummenge. Bei geringem Nahrungscalcium war die Calciumausscheidung im Urin am höchsten, bei Aufnahme einer mittleren Calciummenge war die Ausscheidung ebenfalls mittelmäßig und bei der Aufnahme einer hohen Calciummenge war die Ausscheidung sehr gering. Diese Befunde konnten sowohl bei den Versuchspersonen während der Bettruhe als auch bei ambulanten nicht bettlägerigen Patienten gefunden werden. Die densitometrische Messung der Kalksalzkonzentration in der *Mitte des Calcaneus* ergab *nach 14tägiger Bettruhe die höchsten Werte bei der Gruppe mit einer negativen Calciumbilanz.* In den untersuchten Knochen der *Phalangen des 2.—5. Fingers* waren die Veränderungen nach 14tägiger Bettruhe geringer. Nach 30 Tagen Bettruhe fand sich eine *deutliche Verminderung der Knochendichte in den Fingerknochen.* Dieser Befund läßt darauf schließen, daß der Knochenabbau erst nach 14 Tagen beginnt oder deutlich wird.

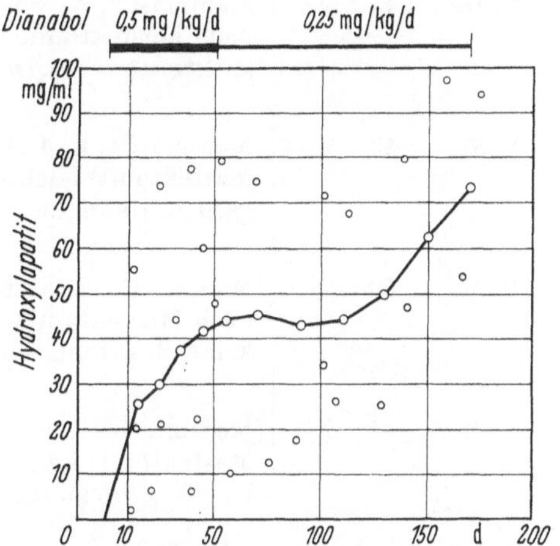

Abb. 128. Anstieg der Hydroxylapatitkonzentration im Calcaneus nach Behandlung mit anabolen Steroiden bei Inaktivitätsosteoporose im Kindesalter (Durchschnittswerte von 5 Kindern). (Nach Hansen, 1962; Abb. 6)

Den Anstieg der Hydroxylapatitkonzentration in der Calcaneusspongiosa konnte Hansen (1962) bei Inaktivitätsosteoporose im Kindesalter nach Behandlung mit anabolen Steroiden durch quantitative radiologische Messungen objektivieren (Abb. 128).

Ergebnisse densitometrischer Kontrolluntersuchungen der *Spongiosa des Calcaneus bei 140 dauernd bettlägerigen Kindern* hat Vose (1968) vorgelegt. Die Untersuchungen wurden zur Objektivierung eines Therapieerfolges durchgeführt. Bei allen Kindern konnte vor der einzuleitenden Behandlung *eindeutig eine Inaktivitätsosteoporose* festgestellt werden. Nach Behandlung mit *Fluor-Präparaten* und *Hormonen* fand sich eine *deutliche Zunahme der Knochendichte* (Knochenmasse) im untersuchten Knochenareal. Die Behandlung mit *Phosphorpräparaten* (0,18 mg/kg/Tag) ergab nach 18 Monaten *keine deutlichen Unterschiede* der Calcaneusdichte verglichen mit unbehandelten Kindern.

Die Inaktivitätsatrophie des Knochens nach *Mammaamputation* haben Adachi und Okuyama (1966) an der *Ulna* (3 und 4 cm proximal des Processus styloideus ulnae) gemessen (Methode s. S. 133 und 191). Gegenüber der gesunden Seite war ein deutlich erniedrigter

Tabelle 34. *Ergebnisse der Mineralgehaltsmessungen bei einigen Krankheiten*

Fall	Alter und Geschlecht	Klinische Diagnose	Meßpunkt proximal vom Proc. styloid. in cm	Äquivalenter Mineral-Gehalt in mg/cm² E.M.C.	Dicke der Ulna in cm	Mineralgehalt in mg/cm³
A. T.	53 ♀	Mamma-Ca. li. 33 Monate nach	3	290	1,08	269
		Mastektomie schweres Ödem und	re. 4	326	1,08	302
		schwere Bewegungseinschränkung	3	165	0,97	170
			li. 4	180	1,00	180
T. A.	71 ♀	Senile Osteoporose	3	100	0,95	105
			li. 4	115	0,97	109
Y. H.	53 ♀	Mamma-Ca. re. 3 Monate	3	322	1,32	244
		nach Mastektomie Ödem (—),	re. 4	338	1,28	264
		leichte Bewegungseinschränkung	3	302	1,28	236
			li. 4	347	1,20	289
N. M.	48 ♀	Mamma-Ca. li. 4 Monate nach	3	334	1,16	288
		Mastektomie leichtes Ödem,	re. 4	346	1,15	300
		geringe Bewegungseinschränkung	3	262	1,15	228
			li. 4	282	1,10	257
S. M.	50 ♀	Mamma-Ca. bilateral 18 Mon.	3	271	0,93	291
		nach Mastektomie, kein Ödem	re. 4	310	0,95	326
		keine Bewegungseinschränkung	3	248	0,91	272
			li. 4	283	0,96	295
K. M.	44 ♀	Mamma-Ca. li. 6 Monate nach	3	376	1,11	338
		Mastektomie kein Ödem,	re. 4	400	1,12	357
		leichte Bewegungseinschränkung	3	260	1,11	234
			li. 4	285	1,12	254

[ADACHI, T., and T. OKUYAMA: Bull. Tokyo dent. Univ. **13**, 349 (1966), Tab. 6]

Tabelle 35. *Ergebnisse der densitometrischen Messung des Mineralgehaltes der Ulna nach Mamma-Amputation*

Fall	Alter und Geschlecht	Mastektomierte Seite	Monate nach Operation	Ödem	Bewegungseinschränkung	Transmission %	Äquivalenter Mineralgehalt mg/cm² E.M.C.	Dicke der Ulna cm	Mineralgehalt mg/cm³
M. S.	24 ♀	rechts	8	wenig	gering	re. 38,4	407	1,00	407
						li. 42,7	363	0,96	379
U. Y.	32 ♀	rechts	4	(—)	gering	re. 38,6	410	1,15	357
						li. 41,6	372	1,05	356
T. N.	36 ♀	rechts	2	(—)	schwer	re. 42,8	357	0,98	364
						li. 45,7	325	0,90	361
S. M.	49 ♀	bilateral	3	(—)	(—)	re. 49,0	294	0,98	300
						li. 48,0	305	0,98	311
Y. K.	34 ♀	rechts	5	(—)	(—)	re. 43,0	328	1,20	273
						li. 41,0	347	1,24	280

[OKUYAMA, T.: Nippon Acta Radiol. **25**, 775 (1965), Tab. 4]

Mineralgehalt der Ulna besonders dann zu finden, wenn auf der operierten Seite ein Oedem des Armes vorlag (Tabelle 34 und 35).

Von BJÖRK und LEMPERG (1967) wurden Vergleichsuntersuchungen des Knochenmineralgehaltes in der *Tibia* nach *Unterschenkelamputationen* durchgeführt (Methode s. S. 169). Alle Patienten hatten im Knochen des Amputationsstumpfes einen deutlich verminderten Kalksalzgehalt (Tabelle 36).

Über eine *Abnahme des Knochenkalksalzgehaltes nach Lähmungen* haben KROKOWSKI, KROKOWSKI und SCHLIACK (1963) berichtet. Der Knochenkalksalzgehalt nimmt zwar

Tabelle 36. *Ergebnisse von Messungen des Knochenmineralgehaltes der Tibia nach Amputation*

Alter in Jahren	Grund der Amputation	Muskelfunktion	Maximale Laufstrecke	Knochenmineralgehalt der Tibia in mg/cm³		Quotient der Werte des normalen zum amputierten Bein
				amputiertes Bein	normales Bein	
69	chron. Inf.	gut	200 m	60	180	0,33
52	congenitale Mißbildung	schlecht	100 m	36	85	0,42
62	Trauma	mäßig	1000 m	30	62	0,49
33	Trauma	sehr gut	unbegrenzt	104	182	0,57
49	Trauma	sehr gut	unbegrenzt	58	94	0,62
46	Trauma	mäßig	unbegrenzt	220	300	0,72
35	Trauma	schlecht	unbegrenzt	200	265	0,76
50	Trauma	gut	unbegrenzt	92	112	0,82

[Björk, L., u. R. Lemperg: Acta radiol. (Stockh.) 6, 575 (1967), Tab. 1]

während der Immobilisation einer Extremität nach einem Trauma sehr rasch ab, doch erfolgt die Verminderung der globalen Kalksalzkonzentration bei Lähmungen wesentlich langsamer. Nach etwa $2^1/_2$—3 Jahren ist die maximale Calciumabnahme erreicht (Abb. 129). Ein Minimalgehalt an Hydroxylapatit bleibt im Knochen erhalten. Bei jungen Menschen ist die Abnahme der globalen Kalksalzkonzentration in einem Knochen größer als bei alten Menschen. Verglichen mit dem Ausgangswert war in den mittleren Altersklassen (25 bis 65 Jahre) ein Absinken des Apatitwertes um 40—50%, im höheren Lebensalter nur um 20—30% unter dem Normwert festzustellen. Das Ausmaß der *relativen* Hydroxylapatitverminderung nach einer Extremitätenlähmung ist also vom Lebensalter abhängig, während der absolute Endwert vom Alter unabhängig ist. Ein bestimmter Minimalgehalt an Hydroxylapatit bleibt auch in der gelähmten Extremität erhalten. Aus dem Seitenvergleich der gesunden Extremität mit der gelähmten Extremität soll annähernd auf die *Dauer der Parese* geschlossen werden können. Simulierte Lähmungen lassen sich von echten Lähmungen unterscheiden, ein Befund der auch bei *gutachterlichen Fragen* von Bedeutung sein kann.

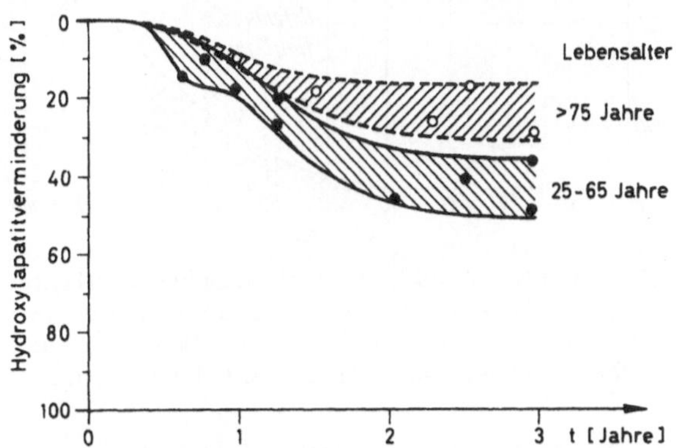

Abb. 129. Abnahme der Hydroxylapatitkonzentration in der Radiusspongiosa einer gelähmten Extremität in Abhängigkeit von der Dauer der Parese. (Nach Krokowski, Krokowski und Schliack, 1963)

2. Meßergebnisse bei der „präsenilen" oder „postmenopausischen" Osteoporose (sog. „pathologische Osteoporose")

Der normale Alterungsprozeß des gesunden Menschen führt zu einer Abnahme des Knochengewebsvolumens im Gesamtvolumen eines Knochens, ohne daß das Knochengewebe selbst krankhafte Veränderungen aufweist. Diese „physiologische Altersosteoporose" wird gegen die „pathologische Osteoporose" abgegrenzt. Da unser Wissen über die normalen und pathologischen Lebensvorgänge des Knochengewebes noch sehr lückenhaft ist, sollen die bei der „pathologischen Osteoporose" gefundenen Untersuchungsergebnisse gesondert zusammengestellt werden.

Nach der Theorie von Albright und Reifenstein (1948) soll bei einer pathologischen Osteoporose vor allem die Wirbelsäule, das Beckenskelet und eventuell der Schädelknochen betroffen sein. Diese Theorie widerspricht der von Albright selbst geäußerten Vorstellung, daß es sich bei der Osteoporose um eine Störung der Knochenbildung handeln soll. Eine hormonelle Dysregulation dürfte sowohl beim weiblichen als auch beim männlichen Geschlecht das gesamte Skeletsystem betreffen, so daß die Knochenveränderungen auch im Bereich der Extremitäten auftreten müssen. Die Vorstellung, daß bei einer „pathologischen Osteoporose" ebenso wie bei der „physiologischen Osteoporose" alle Knochen des Skeletes betroffen sind, ist nicht neu (COOKE 1955).

KROKOWSKI (1966) meint dagegen, daß die „physiologische Involutionsosteoporose" in *allen Skeletabschnitten* mit steigendem Lebensalter synchron zunimmt, während die „pathologische Osteoporose" im Stammskelet beginnt und erst in späteren Stadien die peripheren Skeletpartien erfaßt (Abb. 130). Durch die „zentrifugale" Ausbreitung der pathologischen Osteoporose vermögen Bestimmungen des Kalksalzgehaltes an peripheren Knochen eine beginnende oder leichte Osteoporose nicht zu erfassen. Diese Vorstellungen einer besonderen Rolle des Stammskeletes wurden durch biochemische und radiologische Befunde an verschiedenen Skeletpartien sowohl während des normalen Alterungsprozesses, als auch bei Systemerkrankungen des Skeletes widerlegt (DOYLE 1967; MEEMA u. Mitarb. 1964, 1968; HEUCK 1968).

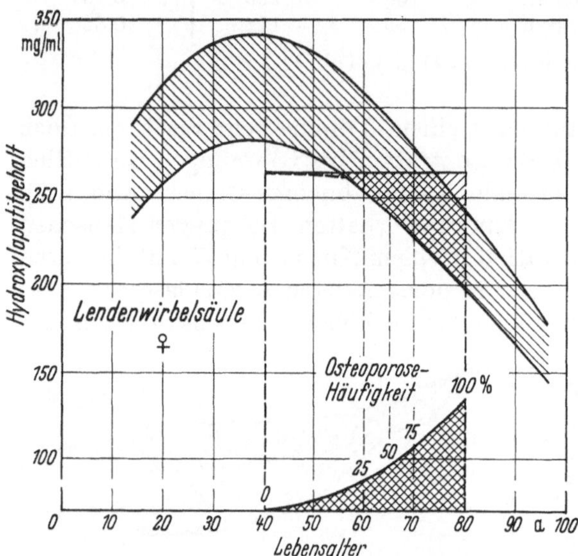

Abb. 130. Physiologische Altersabhängigkeit des Hydroxylapatitgehaltes der Wirbelspongiosa und prozentuale Osteoporosehäufigkeit nach visueller Beurteilung des Röntgenbildes. (Nach KROKOWSKI, 1966; Abb. 2)

Eine Störung des Knochenumbaues konnte bei der Osteoporose nicht nachgewiesen werden, ebenso wie der Eiweißmangel keine Osteoporose hervorrufen kann. Nach den heute gültigen Vorstellungen spielt der *Calciummangel* eine bedeutende Rolle, der alimentär, durch gestörte intestinale Resorption oder vermehrte Ausscheidung hervorgerufen sein kann.

Auf Grund von Calcium-Bilanz-Untersuchungen konnte NORDIN (1962) bei 29 Patientinnen mit einer Osteoporose (bestimmt an der Wirbelsäule mit Hilfe des Barnett-Nordin-Index) feststellen, daß in der Mehrzahl der Fälle ein Calciummangel vorliegt. Dieser Befund spricht gegen die Vorstellungen von ALBRIGHT (1948), nach denen die Osteoporose die Folge einer Störung der Matrixbildung im Knochen ist.

Wahrscheinlich spielen auch die im Knochen selbst ablaufenden Regulationsvorgänge, die von dem Parathormon und seinem Antagonisten, dem Thyreocalcitonin, gesteuert werden, eine bedeutende Rolle.

Zum Verständnis der im höheren Lebensalter häufiger nachweisbaren Osteoporose des Skeletes wurde in erster Linie die hormonelle Umstellung während des Klimakteriums der Frau und im Greisenalter des Mannes angeschuldigt. So spielte *der Begriff der „präsenilen Osteoporose"* eine große Rolle. Das weibliche Geschlecht soll von einer Osteoporose doppelt so häufig betroffen sein wie das männliche Geschlecht und es ist ein Verhältnis von 1:2 bis 1:4 genannt worden (ANDERSON 1939; KESSON, MORRIS und MCCUTCHEON 1947 u.a.).

Nach den bisher vorliegenden Untersuchungsergebnissen ist ein *plötzlicher rascher Abfall der globalen Kalksalzkonzentration* in den untersuchten Knochenpartien während und unmittelbar nach der Menopause, der auf eine krankhafte Störung hinweisen könnte, nicht festzustellen gewesen. Der Begriff der „postmenopausischen Osteoporose" wurde zweifelhaft. Von einigen Autoren wurde die Existenz dieser Sonderform der Osteoporose abgelehnt (HEUCK 1965; KROKOWSKI 1967).

Zu diesem Fragenkomplex wurden Kontrolluntersuchungen der Knochendichte bei 25 Frauen, die *während der Menopause* in einem Fall mit Hyperthyreose *eine Hormontherapie* erhielten, von BALZ, BIRKNER und SCHMITT-ROHDE (1957) vorgelegt. Nach einer Behandlungsdauer von 6—8 Wochen konnte ein *Anstieg* des „Aluminiumschwächungsgleichwertes“ (Methode s. S. 158) gefunden werden (Abb. 131a und b). Auch SCHMID (1963) konnte einen *Anstieg* der niedrigen Knochendichtewerte nach abwechselnder Behandlung mit *Anabolica oder Calciumpräparaten* bei der *senilen* Osteoporose und der *Involutionsosteoporose* feststellen (Abb. 150). Der Aufenthalt in sonnigem Höhenklima hatte die gleiche Wirkung auf den Knochen und eine Zunahme der Knochendichte zur Folge. Alleinige Klimakammerbehandlung war dagegen ohne Einfluß auf die Knochendichte. Bei einigen Patienten konnte weder die Sonnenbehandlung noch die Klimatherapie die Knochendichte verändern. Die Wirkung regelmäßig durchgeführter *Gymnastik* oder *Durchwärmungstherapie* wurde von SCHMID (1963) an 27 Patienten untersucht. Im Kontrollzeitraum von 3 Monaten

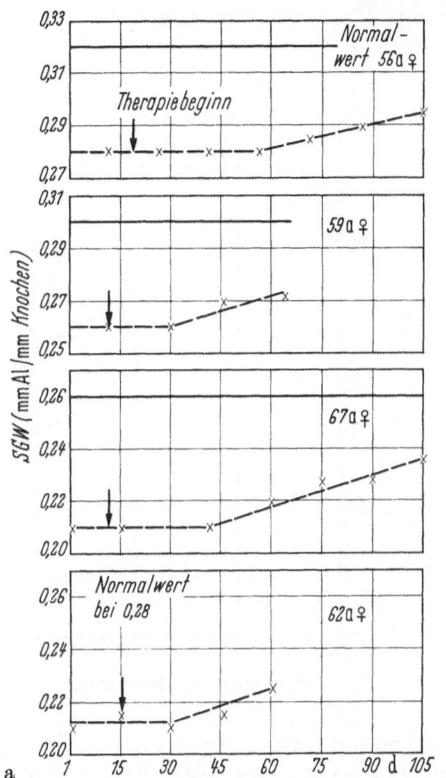

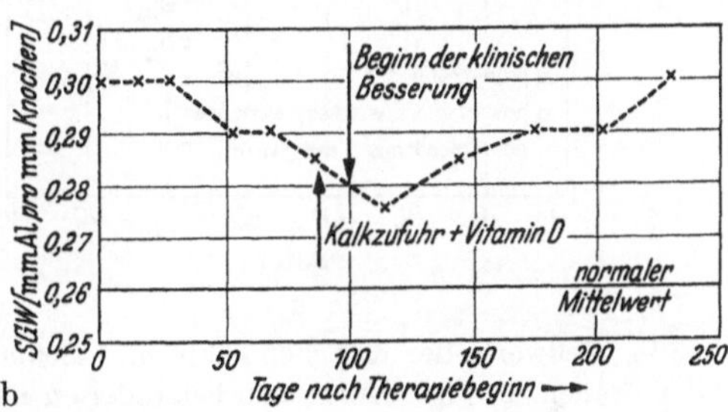

Abb. 131a. Zunahme der Knochendichte nach Hormonbehandlung der postmenopausischen Osteoporose. (Nach BALZ, persönliche Mitteilung)

Abb. 131b. Eigenartiger Kurvenverlauf des Aluminiumschwächungsgleichwertes bei Hyperthyreose einer 68jährigen Frau unter Sexualhormontherapie und späterer Kalk- und Vitamin D-Zufuhr. Thyreostatica wurden nicht gegeben. (Nach BALZ, BIRKNER und SCHMITT-ROHDE, 1957; Abb. 10)

fand sich *keine signifikante Beeinflussung der Knochendichte* solcher Patienten, die eine Osteoporose aufwiesen.

Von KROKOWSKI (1965) wurden an 416 Patienten beiderlei Geschlechts, die das 45. Lebensjahr überschritten hatten, geprüft, welche Zusammenhänge zwischen den subjektiven „Osteoporoseschmerzen“ als erstem klinischen Symptom der Osteoporose und den objektiven Meßwerten der Mineralkonzentration in den Wirbelkörpern bestehen. Es zeigte sich weder hinsichtlich der Altersverteilung, noch bezüglich der Lokalisation und des Schweregrades eine Korrelation zwischen subjektivem und objektivem Befund. Selbst zu osteoporotischen Wirbelkörperzusammenbrüchen bestand keine vollkommene und direkte Korrelation. Etwa 20% der Patienten mit Skeletschmerzen wiesen einen normalen, altersentsprechenden Hydroxylapatitgehalt der Wirbelsäule auf. Eine direkte kausale Bindung zwischen Osteoporose und Skeletschmerz sei daher abzulehnen.

Die Wirkung einer Hormontherapie auf die sog. „postmenopausische Osteoporose“ haben STRANDJORD und LANZL (1965) studiert (Methode s. S. 142). Es wurden 25 junge Frauen vor der Menopause, 69 Patientinnen nach der Menopause ohne Hormontherapie, 71 Patientinnen mit Hormontherapie und 30 Patientinnen mit unregelmäßiger Hormontherapie im Hinblick auf den Knochenkalksalzgehalt kontrolliert.

Unabhängig von der Hormontherapie konnte ein Absinken der globalen Kalksalzwerte im Knochen mit zunehmendem Alter gefunden werden. Die einer Hormontherapie unterzogenen Patientinnen (alle drei Behandlungsgruppen) zeigten eine gewisse Verminderung oder Herabsetzung der Knochenveränderungen im Sinne der Altersosteoporose. Der osteoporotische Knochen zeigte jedoch die gleiche Zusammensetzung wie normaler Knochen. In einer späteren Mitteilung haben DAVIS, STRANDJORD und LANZL (1966) sowie STRANDJORD, FORLAND, LANZL und COX (1968) über das Ergebnis einer langjährigen Oestrogenbehandlung während der Menopause berichtet und — verglichen mit

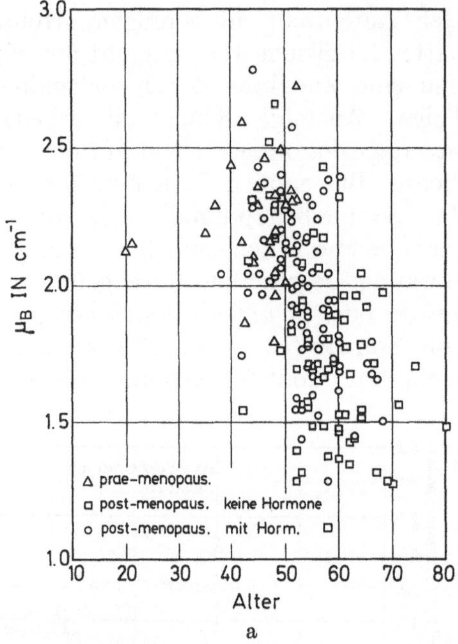

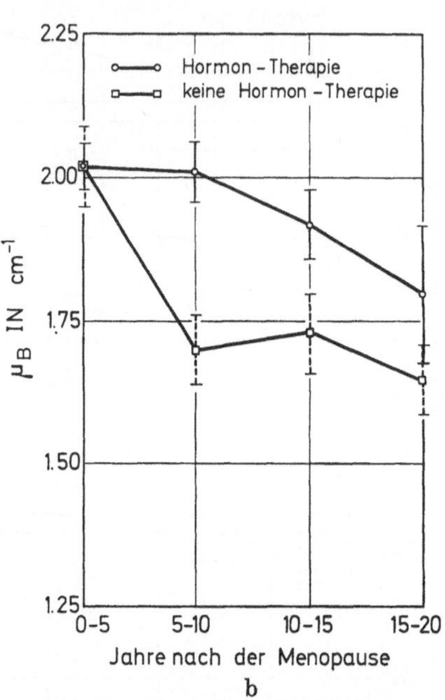

Abb. 132a. Meßwerte der Knochendichte im Calcaneus vor und nach der Menopause bezogen auf das Lebensalter der Frauen. Die mit Hormonen behandelten Patientinnen zeigen nur gering höhere Werte verglichen mit dem unbehandelten Kollektiv. (Nach DAVIS, STRANDJORD und LANZL, 1966; Abb. 4)

Abb. 132b. Vergleich der Knochendichte im Calcaneus von Patientinnen, die mit Hormonen behandelt worden sind und Patientinnen, die ohne eine Hormonbehandlung geblieben sind, bezogen auf die Jahre nach der Menopause. (Nach DAVIS, STRANDJORD und LANZL, 1966; Abb. 5)

unbehandelten Frauen — einen etwas geringeren globalen Kalksalzwert des Knochens gefunden (Abb. 132a und b).

Demgegenüber sprechen die Ergebnisse von KROKOWSKI (1967), HEUCK (1965) u. a. gegen einen kausalen Zusammenhang zwischen Oestrogenmangel in der Menopause und einer Osteoporose. Mit zunehmendem Alter sinkt der Hydroxylapatitgehalt im Skelet *kontinuierlich* um 20—40% ab. Diese physiologische Altersregression ist zwar bei Frauen deutlicher als bei Männern, doch konnte keine Stufen- oder Knickbildung im Verlauf der Regressionskurve nachgewiesen werden. Es ist verständlich, daß dieser Befund mit dem Hormonausfall nach der Menopause in Zusammenhang gebracht wird, doch konnte ein frühzeitiges Einsetzen der Verminderung des Hydroxylapatitgehaltes im Sinne der „postklimakterischen Osteoporose" nach aus therapeutischen Gründen vorzeitig eingeleiteter Menopause nicht festgestellt werden. Umgekehrt konnte durch Substitution mit weiblichen Hormonen eine Rückbildung dieser Osteoporoseform nicht erreicht werden.

Aus den verschiedenartigen Untersuchungsergebnissen geht hervor, daß der hormonelle Einfluß auf den Knochen nicht allein für die Altersosteoporose verantwortlich sein kann. Es spielen noch andere, bisher unbekannte Faktoren eine Rolle. Nach der Menopause ist ein krankhaftes stärkeres Absinken der globalen Kalksalzkonzentration oder eine rapide

Abnahme der Knochenmasse nicht festzustellen. Die Feststellung einer über das physiologische Maß hinausgehenden Veränderung des Knochens sollte immer den Verdacht auf eine andersartige Störung im Mineralhaushalt des Organismus wecken.

3. Meßergebnisse bei generalisierten Osteopathien

a) Allgemeine Befunde

Die radiologische Messung des Knochenmineralgehaltes ist nicht nur für die frühzeitige Erkennung von Systemerkrankungen des Skeletes, sondern auch für die Kontrolle des Behandlungsergebnisses von Bedeutung. Eine erfolgreiche Behandlung kann nur dann durchgeführt werden, wenn noch keine irreversiblen Schäden am Skelet aufgetreten sind. Die radiologischen Messungen können sowohl eine Verminderung als auch eine Zunahme der Knochenkalksalzkonzentration objektivieren.

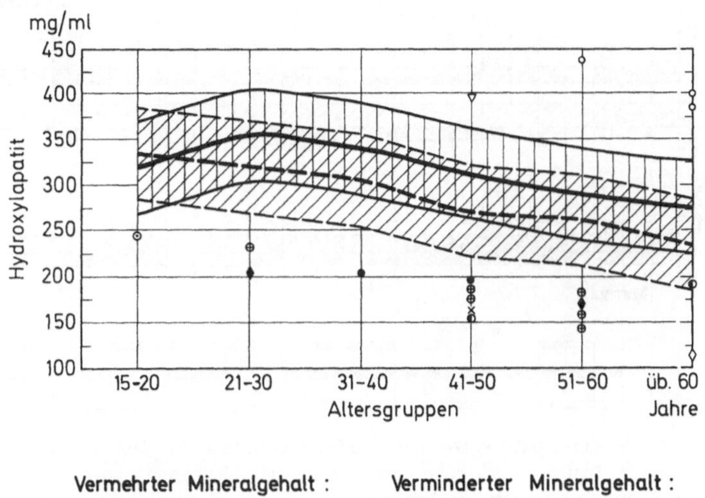

Abb. 133. Einzelmeßwerte der Apatitkonzentration in der Schenkelhalsspongiosa bei Osteopathien zusammen mit dem Streubereich der Normalwerte. (Nach Heuck, 1963; Abb. 1)

Eine größere Anzahl von Untersuchungsergebnissen der Kalksalzkonzentration in der Schenkelhalsspongiosa und Calcaneusspongiosa bei *verschiedenen Systemerkrankungen* des Skeletes haben Heuck und Schmidt (1960) mitgeteilt (Abb. 133). Mit der gleichen Methode (s. S. 219) konnte Hansen (1962) bei Kindern eine Änderung der Kalksalzkonzentration in der Calcaneusspongiosa bei verschiedenen Osteopathien und Bluterkrankungen vorlegen. Die *Wirkung von Hormonpräparaten* (Testosteronderivaten) auf den kranken Knochen konnte objektiviert werden. Die Behandlung der Osteogenesis imperfecta mit anabolen Steroiden ergab bei 2 Kindern keine nachweisbare Wirkung, während bei einer 17jährigen Patientin der Kalksalzgehalt des Knochens im Laufe von 7 Monaten bis zur Norm anstieg. Dieser Befund veranlaßte Hansen (1962) zu der Annahme, daß pathogenetische Unterschiede der einzelnen Osteogenesis-Formen bestehen könnten. Sehr eindrucksvoll war die Wirkung anaboler Steroide auf die sekundären Knochenveränderungen bei akuten Hämoblastosen. Durch eine relativ hohe Dosierung konnten die generalisierte Osteoporose und die zum Teil beträchtlichen statischen Beschwerden sowie die subepiphysäre Spongiosaatrophie und die osteolytischen Prozesse günstig beeinflußt werden.

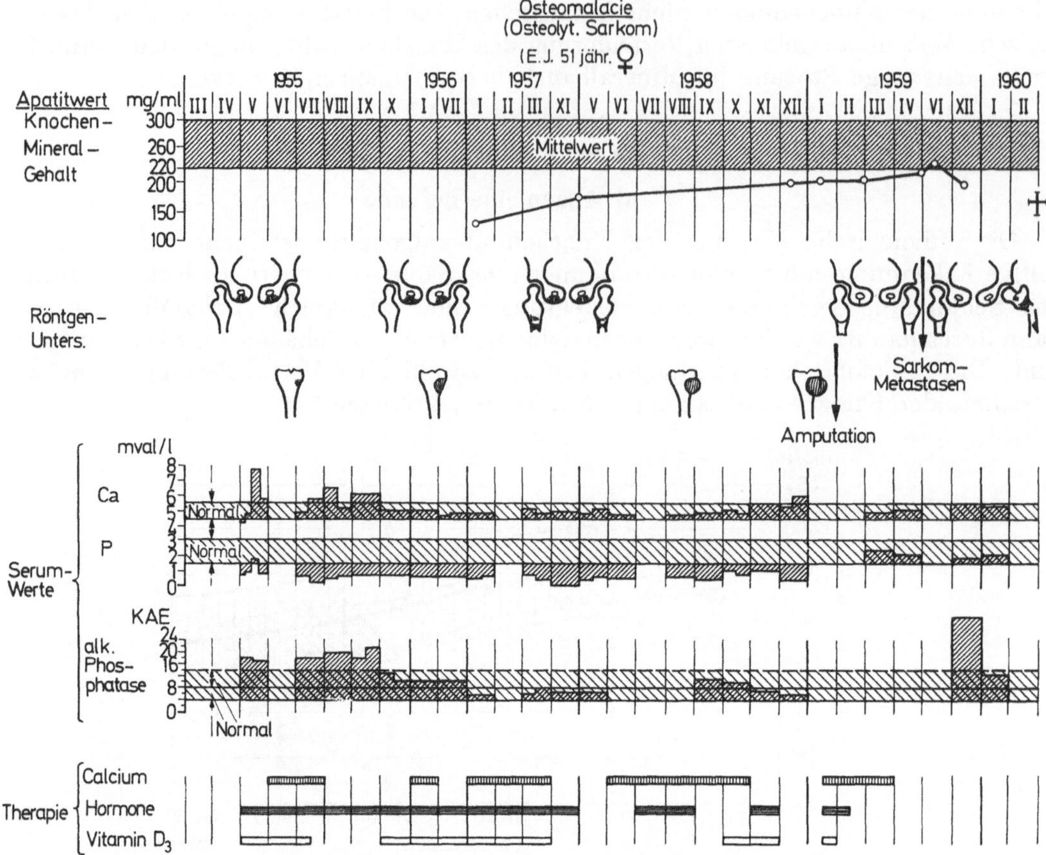

Abb. 134. Verlaufskontrolle des Apatitwertes bei einer Osteomalacie (53jähr. ♀) über mehrere Jahre (oben). Im Beobachtungszeitraum traten zahlreiche Loosersche Umbauzonen auf, die unter therapeutischen Maßnahmen abheilten. Gleichzeitig stieg der Apatitwert in den Normbereich an. Die Patientin starb an einem metastasierenden osteolytischen Sarkom des Tibiakopfes. (HEUCK, 1962; Abb. 6)

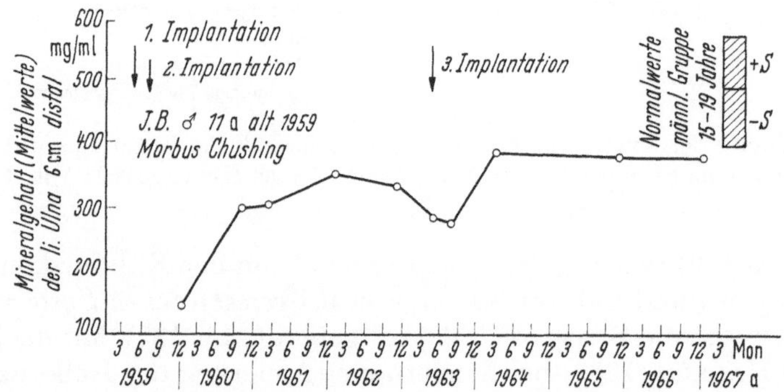

Abb. 135. Verlaufsbeobachtung des Knochenmineralgehaltes der Ulna bei hypophysärem Cushing nach Behandlung mit zweimaliger Implantation von 198 Au und einer dritten Implantation von 90 Y in die Hypophyse. (Nach DOYLE, 1967; Abb. 6)

In einer umfangreichen Untersuchungsreihe *älterer Menschen* haben MORGAN, GILUM, GIFFORD und WILCOX (1962) den Einfluß der Ernährung auf den Knochenmineralgehalt (ausgedrückt in der Knochendichte) studiert. Die Gegenüberstellung der Meßergebnisse von solchen alten Menschen, die zu Hause leben und solchen die in einem Altersheim untergebracht sind, ergab einen niedrigeren Knochenmineralgehalt bei den Altersheiminsassen. Die Untersuchungen weisen auf den Wert der radiologischen Messung des Knochenmineralgehaltes in der *geriatrischen Forschung* hin.

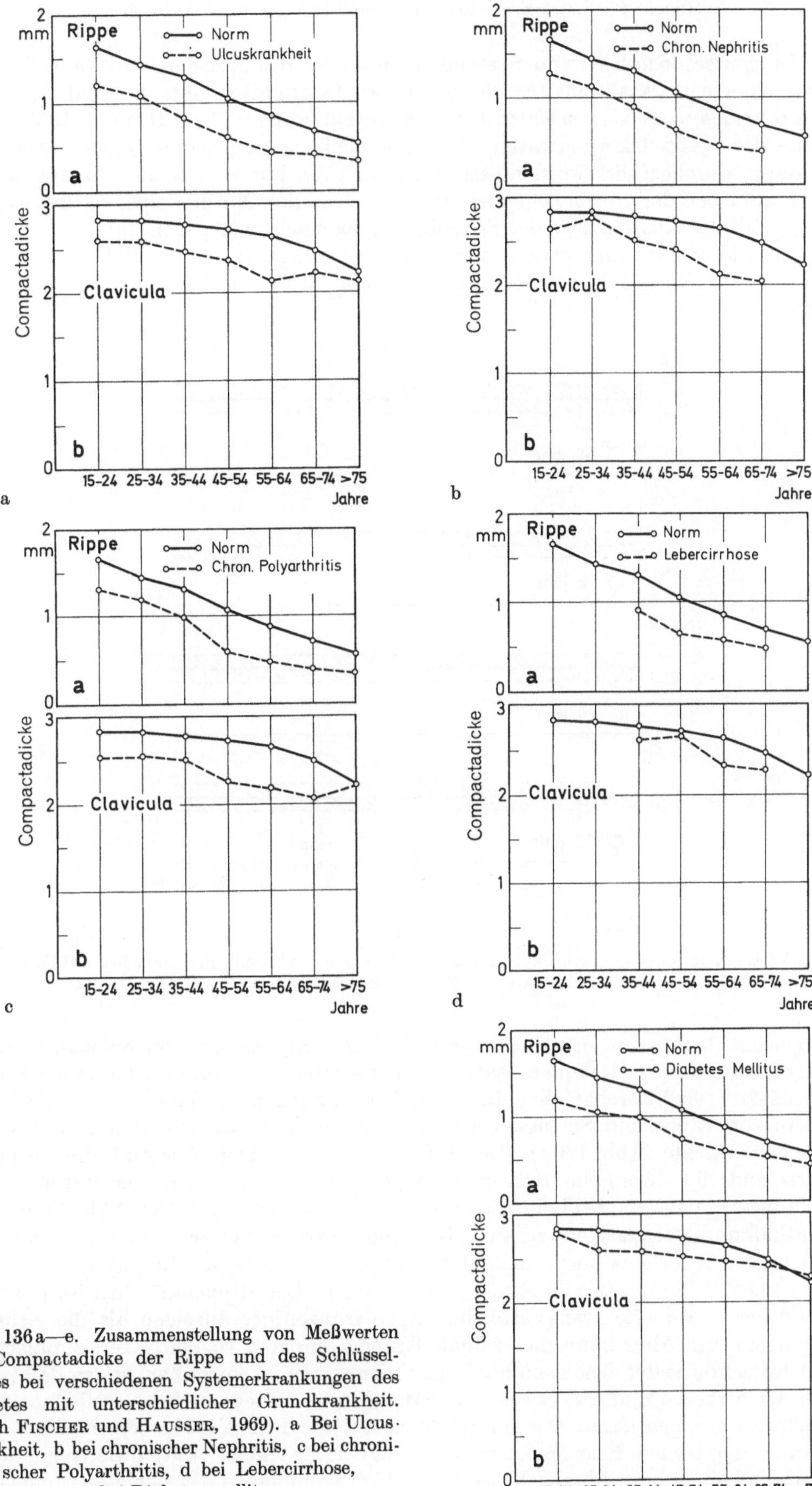

Abb. 136a—e. Zusammenstellung von Meßwerten der Compactadicke der Rippe und des Schlüsselbeines bei verschiedenen Systemerkrankungen des Skeletes mit unterschiedlicher Grundkrankheit. (Nach FISCHER und HAUSSER, 1969). a Bei Ulcuskrankheit, b bei chronischer Nephritis, c bei chronischer Polyarthritis, d bei Lebercirrhose, e bei Diabetes mellitus

Bei *Langzeitbehandlungen* von Systemerkrankungen des Skeletes wird die Objektivierung des Knochenkalksalzgehaltes die wichtigste Information sein. Es sind nur *wenige Kontrolluntersuchungen über mehrere Jahre* mitgeteilt worden. Von HEUCK (1962) ist die Kontrolle der Kalksalzkonzentration der Schenkelhalsspongiosa bei einer *Osteomalacie* über 3 Jahre durchgeführt worden. Es zeigte sich ein kontinuierlicher Anstieg der zunächst weit unter der Norm liegenden Werte bis in den Normbereich (Abb. 134). Der erneute Abfall des Apatitwertes der Schenkelhalsspongiosa war durch die hier lokalisierte osteolytische Metastase eines osteogenen Sarkoms bedingt, an der die Patientin verstarb. Über eine Verlaufsbeobachtung bei hypophysärem Cushing hat DOYLE (1967) berichtet (Abb. 135).

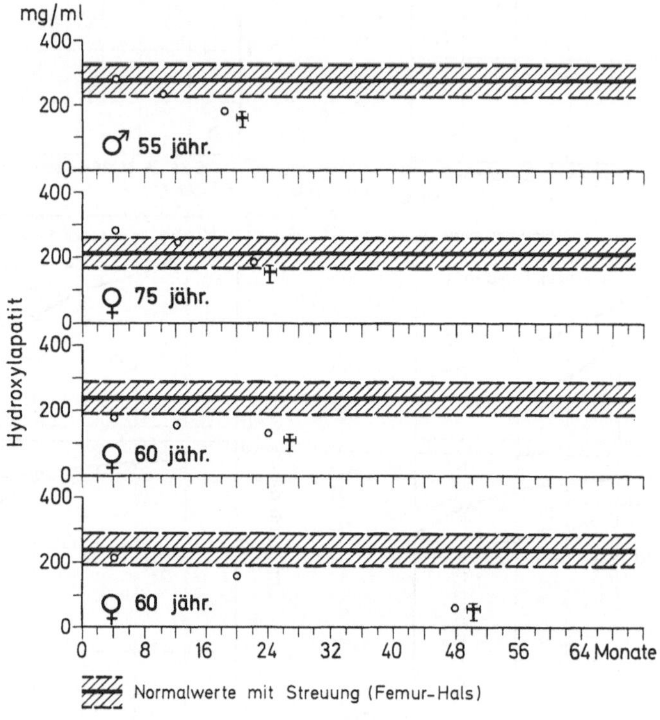

Abb. 137. Verlaufskontrollen der Hydroxylapatitkonzentration in der Schenkelhalsspongiosa bei Patienten mit diffusen Knochenveränderungen als Folge eines Plasmocytom. (Nach HEUCK, 1968)

Vergleichende Messungen der *Compactadicke der Rippen und des Schlüsselbeines* bei verschiedenen mit einer Demineralisation einhergehenden Erkrankungen haben FISCHER und HAUSSER (1958) durchgeführt. Bei allen Erkrankungen war eine *Verschmälerung* der Compacta von Rippe und Schlüsselbein festzustellen. Der stärkste Abbau fand sich bei der Ulcuskrankheit (Abb. 136a). Dann folgen mit geringem Abstand die chronische Nephritis und die chronische Polyarthritis (Abb. 136b und c). Am geringsten war die Compactaverschmälerung bei Lebercirrhose und beim Diabetes mellitus (Abb. 136d und e). Die Entkalkungsosteopathien zeigen also einen Compactaabbau von der endostalen Oberfläche des Knochens ausgehend, der deutlich stärker ist als die physiologische Verschmälerung der Compacta von Rippe und Clavicula. Der Rippenknochen ist wesentlich empfindlicher und dürfte krankhafte Störungen frühzeitiger anzeigen als die Schlüsselbeincompacta. Im Alter kann die craniale Rippencompacta so stark verschmälert sein, daß ein fortschreitender Knochenabbau hier nicht mehr nachweisbar ist, so daß nun im Bereich der dickeren und erst etwas später deutlich reagierenden Schlüsselbeincompacta der Nachweis erfolgen kann. Der im Hinblick auf die Intensität unterschiedliche Compactaabbau der beiden Knochen macht es möglich, in einem weiten Bereich auch für den Einzelfall einen brauchbaren Hinweis auf Umbauvorgänge des Skeletes zu gewinnen.

An einigen Beispielen hat KROKOWSKI (1964) Veränderungen der Hydroxylapatitkonzentration in Wirbelkörpern bei einer *diffusen Metastasierung* vor und nach Strahlenbehandlung tumoröser Knochendestruktionen, während einer Corticosteroidmedikation (Abb. 144) und nach Anabolica-Behandlung gemessen. Besonders eindrucksvoll konnte das Absinken der Hydroxylapatit-Konzentration in der Wirbelspongiosa bei der Corticosteroid-Osteoporose und im Zusammenhang mit dem Auftreten pathologischer Frakturen gezeigt werden.

Fortschreitende Zerstörungen des Knochens, die in den makroskopischen Dimensionen erkennbar sind, werden dann, wenn sie im mikroskopischen Bereich ablaufen, nur mit

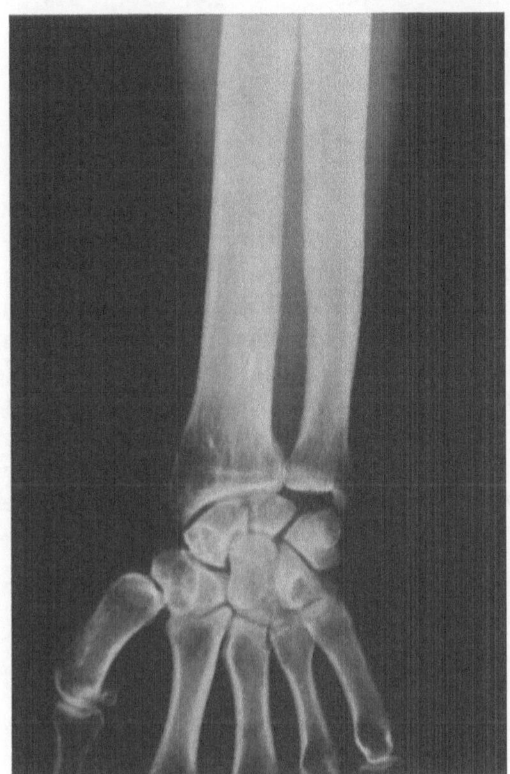

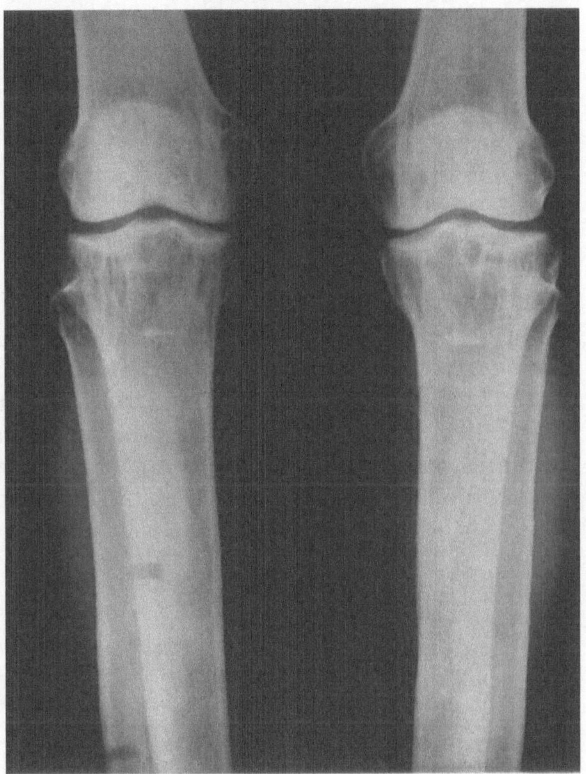

Abb. 138. Hyperostosis generalisata, Röntgenbild zu dem Meßwert 3 in Tabelle 37. (Nach ADACHI und OKUYAMA 1966; Abb. 15 und Tabelle 5)

Hilfe der radiologischen Messung der Kalksalzkonzentration im Gesamtvolumen des Knochens frühzeitig erfaßt werden können. Hier ist vor allem an das *diffuse Plasmocytom* zu denken. Von HEUCK (1968) wurde über Verlaufsbeobachtungen der Kalksalzkonzentration in der Femurhalsspongiosa beim Plasmocytom berichtet (Abb. 137).

Einige Meßergebnisse der Mineralkonzentration der Ulna (3 und 4 cm proximal des Processus styloideus ulnae) bei *generalisierten Skeleterkrankungen* haben ADACHI und OKUYAMA (1966) vorgelegt (Methode s. S. 133 und 191). Neben Osteoporosen wurde eine *Hyperostosis generalisata* (Abb. 138) untersucht und hierbei an beiden Armen eine *hohe* Mineralkonzentration gefunden (Tabelle 37).

Nach der Methode von CAMERON und SORENSON (s. S. 140) haben EVENS, ASHBURN, PACK und BARTTER (1968) Untersuchungen bei verschiedenen Systemerkrankungen des Skeletes (Osteoporose, Osteogenesis imperfecta, Osteomalacie, Hyper- und Hypoparathyreoidismus, Marmorknochenkrankheit) durchgeführt und eine gute Übereinstimmung der klinischen Befunde mit den gemessenen Dichtewerten gefunden.

Tabelle 37. *Ergebnisse der densitometrischen Mineralgehaltsbestimmung in der Ulna bei einigen Erkrankungen*

Fall	Alter und Geschlecht	Diagnose	Transmission %	Äquivalenter Mineralgehalt mg/cm² E.M.C.	Dicke der Ulna in cm	Mineralgehalt in mg/cm³
T. N.	66 ♂	Senile Osteoporose	re. 45,6	327	1,68	195
			li. 49,5	292	1,60	183
T. A.	70 ♀	Senile Osteoporose	re. 80,4	73	1,00	73
		Rhabdomyo-Sarkom linker Ellenbogen	li. 74,2	107	0,95	113
M. I.	26 ♂	Hyperostosis	re. 31,9	511	1,47	348
		generalisata	li. 35,6	450	1,38	326
S. Y.	15 ♂	Blutergelenk	re. 35,7	450	1,15	391
		linker Ellenbogen	li. 53,5	253	0,92	278

[OKUYAMA, T.: Nippon Acta radiol. **25**, 775 (1965), Tab. 5]

b) Der Knochenkalksalzgehalt bei hormonellen Störungen

Bei 15 Patienten mit zum Teil *schwerer Thyreotoxikose* (10 Frauen und 5 Männer) fand DOYLE (1967) im Bereich der Ulna eine niedrige Mineralkonzentration bei Frauen, während nur 3 der 5 Männer eine eindeutige Verminderung des Kalksalzgehaltes erkennen ließen (Abb. 139). Über Veränderungen der Compactadicke und der Knochendichte in Abhängigkeit voneinander haben MEEMA und MEEMA (1968) berichtet und *hormonelle Einflüsse* (insbesondere nach einer frühzeitigen Kastration) auf den Knochen untersucht. Von DOYLE (1967) wird empfohlen, die Untersuchungen an den spongiösen Knochen getrennt von Messungen der Compactadicke zu betrachten. Mit der von ihm modifizierten Methode (s. S. 168) sind verschiedene *hormonelle Störungen* untersucht worden. Bei

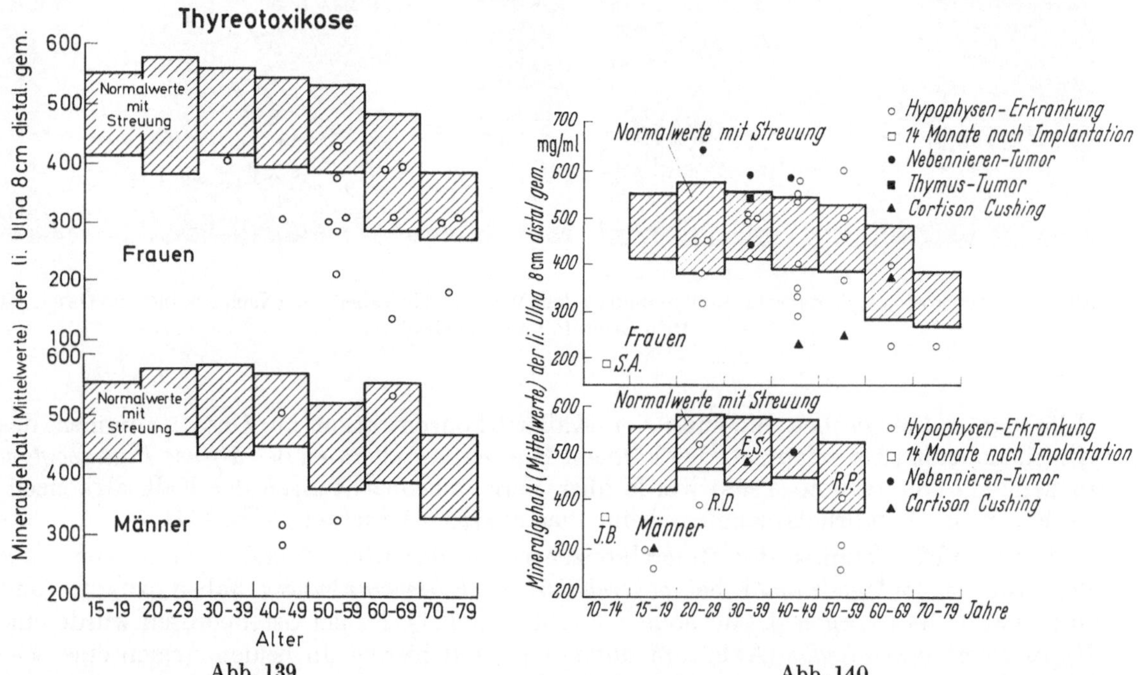

Abb. 139 Abb. 140

Abb. 139. Zusammenstellung von Einzelmeßwerten des Knochenmineralgehaltes in der Ulna bei Thyreotoxikose-Patienten. Die Streubreite der Normalwerte von Männern (unten) und Frauen (oben) ist eingetragen. (Nach DOYLE, 1967; Abb. 7)

Abb. 140. Darstellung mehrerer Meßwerte des Knochenmineralgehaltes in der Ulna bei verschiedenen hormonellen Erkrankungen. Die Werte sind zusammen mit der Streubreite der Normalwerte von Männern (unten) und Frauen (oben) eingetragen. (Nach DOYLE, 1967; Abb. 2)

51 Patienten mit einer *Akromegalie* fand sich kein Anhalt für eine Verminderung des globalen Mineralgehaltes im Knochen, also eine Osteoporose (Abb. 100).

Beim *Morbus Cushing* (insgesamt 42 Patienten mit *hypophysärem Cushing, Nebennieren-Cushing* und *medikamentösem Cushing*) wurde nur bei einem Drittel der unter-

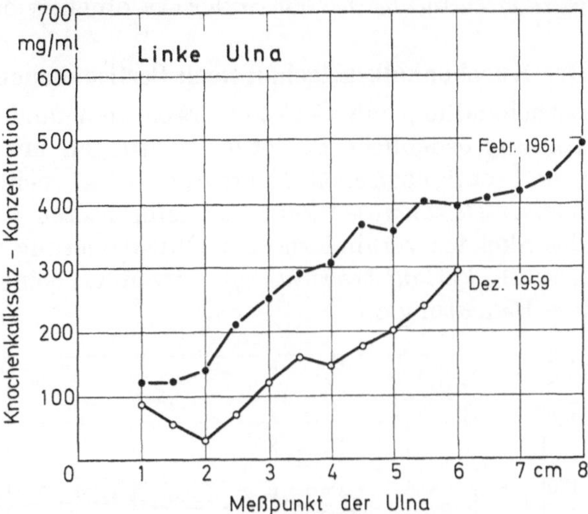

Abb. 141. Verlaufskontrolle des Knochenmineralgehaltes im Bereich der verschiedenen Meßzonen der Ulna (gemessen nach der Methode von Doyle, 1961) bei einem Morbus Cushing, der durch Hypophysenimplantation behandelt wurde. (Nach Fraser, 1962; Abb. 4)

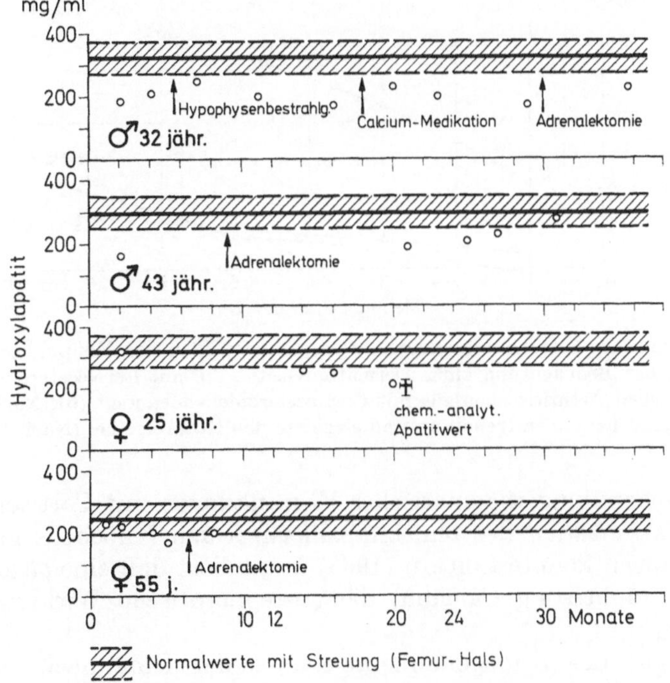

Abb. 142. Verlaufskontrolle der Apatitwerte in der Schenkelhalsspongiosa bei einigen Fällen von Morbus Cushing. (Nach Heuck, 1968)

suchten Kranken eine Verminderung des Knochenmineralgehaltes der Ulna festgestellt (Abb. 140). Einige Kranke mit normalem Mineralgehalt der Ulna zeigten dennoch pathologische Frakturen an den Rippen und den Wirbelkörpern. Mit der Meßmethode von Doyle (1961) hat Fraser (1962) Kontrolluntersuchungen beim Cushing-Syndrom nach therapeutischer Hypophysenimplantation vorgenommen (Abb. 141).

Die von HEUCK (1965/68) gemessenen Werte der Kalksalzkonzentration in spongiösen Knochen beim *Morbus Cushing* zeigten gegenüber der Norm eine deutliche Verminderung. In einigen Fällen wurden *Verlaufskontrollen des „Apatitwertes"* in der Schenkelhalsspongiosa vorgenommen und nach operativer Entfernung z.B. eines Nebennierentumors der *Anstieg der Kalksalzkonzentration im Gesamtknochen* objektiviert (Abb. 142).

c) Der Knochenkalksalzgehalt nach Cortisonbehandlung

Nach einer Langzeitbehandlung mit Cortison-Präparaten fanden sich unter dem Bild des *medikamentösen Cushing* erhebliche Skeletveränderungen mit *Abnahme der globalen Kalksalzkonzentration* und pathologischen Frakturen. Eine rechtzeitige therapeutische Beeinflussung der *„Cortison-Osteoporose"* kann die gefürchteten *pathologischen Frakturen und Deformierungen* des Skeletes verhindern. Der Objektivierung der globalen Knochenkalksalzkonzentration und *Verlaufsbeobachtungen* während einer Cortisonbehandlung kommt daher besondere Bedeutung zu.

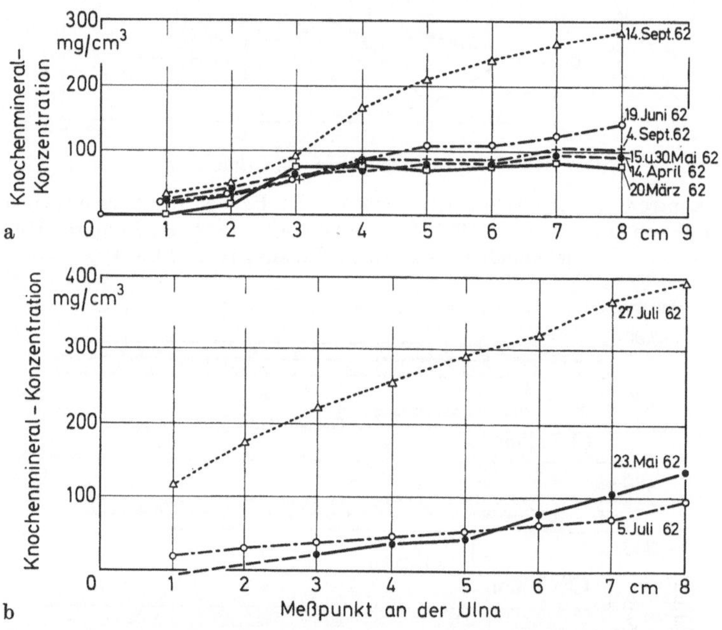

Abb. 143. Verlaufskontrolle des Knochenmineralgehaltes in den verschiedenen Meßpunkten der Ulna (Methode nach DOYLE, 1961) bei der Beobachtung einer Dermatomyositis, die mit Corticosteroiden behandelt wurde (a) und einer rheumatischen Arthritis ebenfalls mit Corticosteroiden behandelt (b). Nach Verminderung der Cortisondosis stieg der Knochenmineralgehalt an und erreichte den Normbereich. (Nach BJÖRK, 1965; Abb. 3)

Während der Behandlung rheumatischer Erkrankungen mit Cortison ist eine *zusätzliche stärkere Demineralisation* des ohnehin kalksalzarmen Knochens gefürchtet. Durch Kontrolluntersuchungen konnte SCHMID (1963) feststellen, daß eine *gleichzeitige Gabe von Calciumpräparaten* (täglich 4 g Calcium) die „osteoporotische Wirkung" der Cortisonderivate verhindert.

Kontrollmessungen des Knochenmineralgehaltes der Ulna nach Behandlung einer Dermatomyositis mit Corticosteroiden hat BJÖRK (1965) vorgelegt. Durch Verminderung der Cortison-Medikation konnte ein gewisser Anstieg der Mineralkonzentration festgestellt werden (Abb. 143a und b). Die gleiche Tendenz fand sich auch im Laufe der Behandlung des Rheumatismus.

Den Einfluß einer Corticoid-Behandlung auf den *globalen Mineralgehalt der Wirbelkörper* haben STRESEMANN und KROKOWSKI (1967) untersucht. Bei 101 Patienten mit chronischem Bronchialasthma, die einer Corticosteroidbehandlung unterzogen wurden, fand sich in 26% nach mehrmonatiger bis mehrjähriger Therapie eine Osteoporose

(Abb. 144). Im Laufe von weiteren 1—2 Jahren nahm diese Osteoporose noch zu. Da bereits vor Beginn der Corticoidtherapie ein ähnlicher Häufigkeitsgrad der Osteoporose gefunden werden konnte, soll die Corticoidbehandlung lediglich eine *bereits vorhandene* Osteoporosebereitschaft fördern.

Bei solchen Patienten, die längere Zeit mit *Cortison* behandelt wurden, ist die Messung der „relativen Wirbeldichte" nach Meinung von NORDIN, SMITH, MC GREGOR und ANDERSON (1965) sehr kompliziert und schwierig, da Alter und Geschlecht des Patienten, die Grundkrankheit, der Typ des verabfolgten Cortison-Präparates und die Dauer der Medikation von Einfluß sind. Die Untersuchungen wurden so durchgeführt, daß die „relative Wirbeldichte" zur verabreichten Gesamtdosis Cortison in Beziehung gesetzt wurde. Es konnte deutlich eine Abhängigkeit der „relativen Wirbeldichte" von der verabreichten Cortisondosis festgestellt werden.

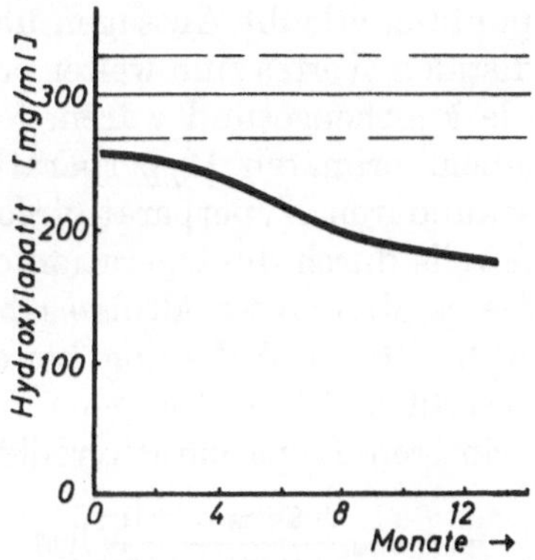

Abb. 144. Verlaufsbeobachtung des Apatitwertes der Wirbelspongiosa (3. Lendenwirbelkörper) nach $1^1/_2$jähriger Corticosteroidbehandlung wegen Asthma bronchiale (43jähriger Mann). (Nach KROKOWSKI, 1964; Abb. 9c)

d) Der Knochenkalksalzgehalt beim Hyperparathyreoidismus

Beim *Hyperparathyreoidismus* kann sowohl eine deutliche Abnahme der Knochenkalksalzkonzentration als auch eine Zunahme festgestellt werden. Die Zunahme ist vor allem bei der *sekundären Form des Hyperparathyreoidismus* nicht selten (DOYLE 1966). Nach operativer Entfernung des Nebenschilddrüsentumors kann eine *Rückkehr* der erniedrigten Kalksalzwerte *zur Norm* (Abb. 145) objektiviert werden (HEUCK 1968).

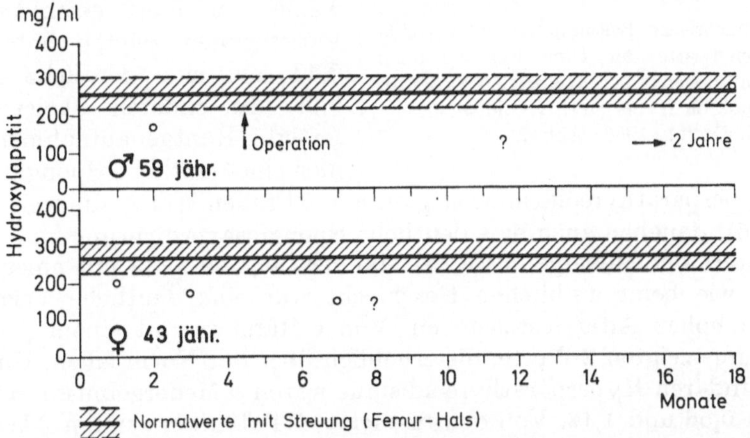

Abb. 145. Kontrollmessungen der Hydroxylapatitkonzentration in der Schenkelhalsspongiosa bei 2 Patienten mit einem primären Hyperparathyreoidismus. Nach operativer Entfernung eines großen Nebenschilddrüsenadenoms stieg bei dem 59 Jahre alten Mann im Laufe von über 2 Jahren der zunächst verminderte Apatitwert zur Norm an (oberes Diagramm). (Nach HEUCK, 1968)

Ergebnisse von Messungen des Knochenmineralgehaltes beim *primären und sekundären Hyperparathyreoidismus* hat DOYLE (1961, 1966) vorgelegt. Die ersten auffallenden Werte von Messungen des Mineralgehaltes im distalen Drittel der Ulna nach der Methode von KEANE, SPIEGLER und DAVIS (1959) konnten bei einer 31 Jahre alten Frau mit einem Nebenschilddrüsenadenom gefunden werden. Der Mineralgehalt lag ungewöhnlich hoch und die Spongiosastruktur zeigte eine deutliche Verdichtung. In einer Reihe weiterer Untersuchungen von primärem und sekundärem Hyperparathyreoidismus hat DOYLE (1966) die ursprüngliche Untersuchungsmethodik derart variiert, daß er das Meßergebnis in der Mitte der Ulna 1 cm proximal vom distalen Ende mit dem Meßergebnis 8 cm proximal in Beziehung setzte. Das Verhältnis der Aluminiumäquivalente an beiden Meßpunkten erlaubt Aussagen über den spongiösen Anteil des Knochens. Das Verhältnis des distalen Wertes zum weiter proximal gelegenen Wert wurde bei 75 Männern und 78 Frauen, die knochengesund waren, festgestellt. Ferner wurde bei 18 Frauen und 6 Männern mit einem primären Hyperparathyreoidismus und bei 5 Frauen und 9 Männern mit einem sekundären Hyperparathyreoidismus dieser Mineralindex bestimmt. Die Diagnose wurde jeweils durch die Operation oder die Obduktion gesichert. Als Beispiel für die Ableitung dieses Mineralverhältnisses beim Gesunden sei auf Abb. 48—50 verwiesen, während in Abb. 146 die Ableitung bei einer Patientin mit primärem Hyperparathyreoidismus dargestellt ist. Die Röntgenaufnahmen des Skeletes zeigten bei allen Patienten mit einem primären Hyperparathyreoidismus nur sehr spärliche subperiostale Resorption im Bereich der Fingerknochen, während die Patientin mit einem sekundären Hyperparathyreoidismus deutliche Symptome der subperiostalen Compactaresorption erkennen ließ. Beim weiblichen Geschlecht fanden sich Normalwerte bei 0,32 des genannten Mineralisationsverhältnisses der beiden Meßpunkte der Ulna mit einer Streuung von 0,084. Erst in höherem Alter war ein geringer Abfall der Normalwerte beim weiblichen Geschlecht festzustellen. Die 18 erkrankten Frauen mit primärem Hyperparathyreoidismus zeigten 14mal Werte, die unter den Normalwerten lagen, während zwei Werte nur wenig verändert erschienen. Nur zwei Patientinnen zeigten höhere Werte von 0,43 und eine deutliche Erhöhung von 0,88. In anderen Skeletregionen angefertigte Röntgenaufnahmen zeigten auch hier eine deutliche Spongiosklerose. Beim sekundären Hyperparathyreoidismus zeigten alle 5 Frauen Werte, die weit über der Norm lagen (Abb. 146), daneben auch eine deutliche Spongiosaverdichtung.

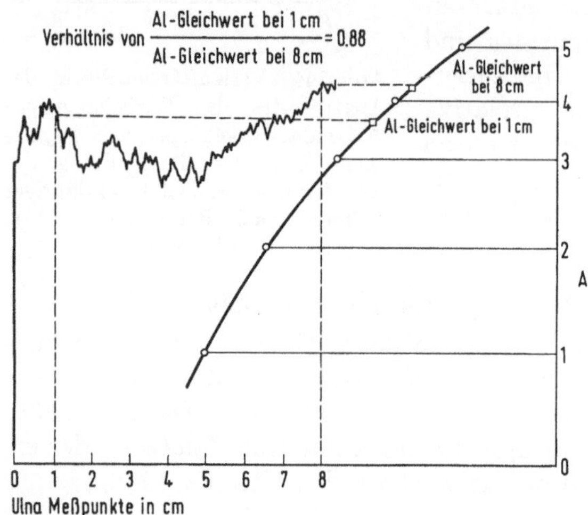

Abb. 146. Densitometrische Bestimmung des Verhältnisses der Al-Gleichwerte der Ulna 1 cm zu 8 cm proximal vom Handgelenk bei 31jähriger Patientin mit einem primären Hyperparathyreoidismus. (Nach DOYLE, 1966; Abb. 2)

Der Mittelwert der Meßergebnisse bei Männern lag bei 0,39 mit einer Streuung von 0,076. Ebenso wie beim weiblichen Geschlecht war eine deutliche Verminderung des Wertes erst im hohen Alter festzustellen. Von 6 Männern mit einem primären Hyperparathyreoidismus zeigten 2 Werte, die erheblich über der Norm lagen. Unter 9 Männern mit einem sekundären Hyperparathyreoidismus waren 6 Meßergebnisse extrem hoch und lagen zwischen 0,56 und 1,12. Von den restlichen 3 Patienten zeigten 2 Werte, die etwas über den Normalwerten, jedoch noch innerhalb der Streubreite lagen. Nur 1 Patient ergab Werte unterhalb der Normbreite, doch handelte es sich bei ihm um eine in diesem Zusammenhang bedeutsame Zweiterkrankung an Hypogonadismus.

Es konnte also festgestellt werden, daß bei einem primären Hyperparathyreoidismus nur selten ein erhöhter Mineralgehalt vorkommt, während beim sekundären Hyperparathyreoidismus häufig eine Verdichtung der Spongiosa im distalen Ulnaabschnitt mit Zunahme des globalen Mineralgehaltes auftritt. Die Geschlechtsunterschiede der Mineralkonzentration der Ulna, die beim primären Hyperparathyreoidismus zu beobachten waren, sind bemerkenswert.

Eine Verminderung der Knochendichte der Fingerknochen bei operativ bestätigtem *Hyperparathyreoidismus* konnten STRANDJORD, FORLAND, LANZL und COX (1968) bei 17 von 20 Kranken nachweisen (Methode s. S. 142). Bei einigen Patienten wurde durch *postoperative Kontrollmessungen* ein langsamer Anstieg der Knochendichte als Ausdruck einer Heilung festgestellt.

e) Der Knochenkalksalzgehalt bei gastrointestinalen Erkrankungen

Die Ergebnisse radiologischer Messungen der globalen Kalksalzkonzentration bei 24 gastrointestinalen Osteopathien verschiedener Genese hat HEUCK (1968) mitgeteilt (Tabelle 38). Bei 17 Kranken war der Knochenkalksalzgehalt in der Femurhalsspongiosa gegenüber der Norm deutlich vermindert. Verlaufskontrollen der Apatitwerte während der Behandlung einer Resorptionsstörung können den Anstieg der Mineralkonzentration

Tabelle 38. *Ergebnisse der Messung der Kalksalzkonzentration in der Femurhalsspongiosa bei verschiedenen gastrointestinalen Osteopathien*

Erkrankung	Alter (in Jahren)	Apatitwert (mg/ml)	Mittlerer Normalwert Apatit in mg/ml
Malabsorptions-Syndrom			
Loni O.	32	230	300
Elsbeth B.	37	160	280
Elfriede J.	48	140	270
Mary M.	50	200	260
Irma N.	50	170	260
Grete H.	52	190	250
Lilly F.	55	270	240
Heinrich M.	55	190	275
Hildegard B.	56	240	240
Herta G.	56	240	240
Ernst G.	57	180	270
Anna L.	61	240	230
Pauline M.	62	190	230
Frieda H.	65	170	220
Martha K.	65	200	220
Hepatogene Osteopathie			
Peter M.	51	220	280
Wilhelm L.	56	230	275
August H.	70	190	250
Frieda E.	71	195	220
Prankreatogene Osteopathie			
Inge E.	30	280	300
Kurt K.	58	200	270
Wilhelm G.	76	150	230
Sprue			
Christa H.	35	280	275
Waldemar L.	67	210	250

[HEUCK, F., in: Aktuelle Gastoenterologie (Bartelheimer und Heisig), S. 174, Tab. 1. Stuttgart: Thieme 1968.]

oder ein weiteres Absinken über einen längeren Beobachtungszeitraum von Monaten oder Jahren registrieren (Abb. 147). Bei einer stärkeren Abnahme der Kalksalzkonzentration im Gesamtknochen nimmt die Frakturneigung erheblich zu, bis schließlich der „kritische Apatitwert" (s. S. 269) erreicht ist und die Zerrüttung der Spongiosa mit pathologischer Fraktur, Umbauzone oder Spontanfraktur auftreten. Die radiologisch-densitometrischen Kontrolluntersuchungen der Kalksalzkonzentration in verschiedenen Knochen des Skeletes sind auch bei Bilanzuntersuchungen von Bedeutung, da sie das Depotorgan für Calcium und andere Mineralien kontrollieren und den Einbau oder das Herauslösen der Knochenkalksalze anzeigen können.

Von NORDIN, SMITH, MC GREGOR und ANDERSON (1965) wurden Veränderungen der „*relativen Wirbeldichte*" (Methode s. S. 239) bei 30 Männern und 39 Frauen, die an einer *Steatorrhoe* erkrankt waren, ermittelt. Bei solchen Patienten, die zusätzlich an einer

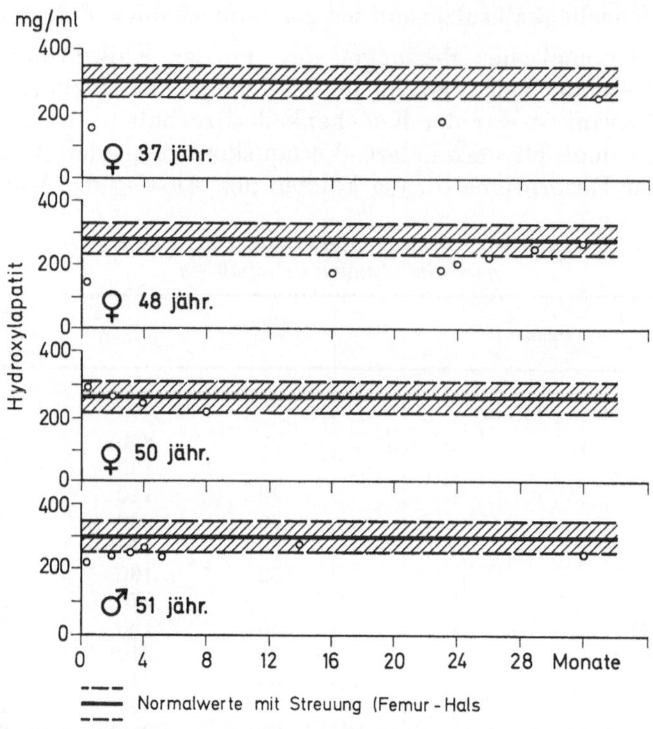

Abb. 147. Verlaufskontrollen der Hydroxylapatitkonzentration bei 4 Patienten mit einer gastro-intestinalen Osteopathie. Nicht in allen Fällen fand sich ein deutlich verminderter Apatitwert der Schenkelhalsspongiosa. Eine Objektivierung des Kalksalzgehaltes ist insbesondere im Hinblick auf die Behandlung von Interesse. (Nach HEUCK, 1968)

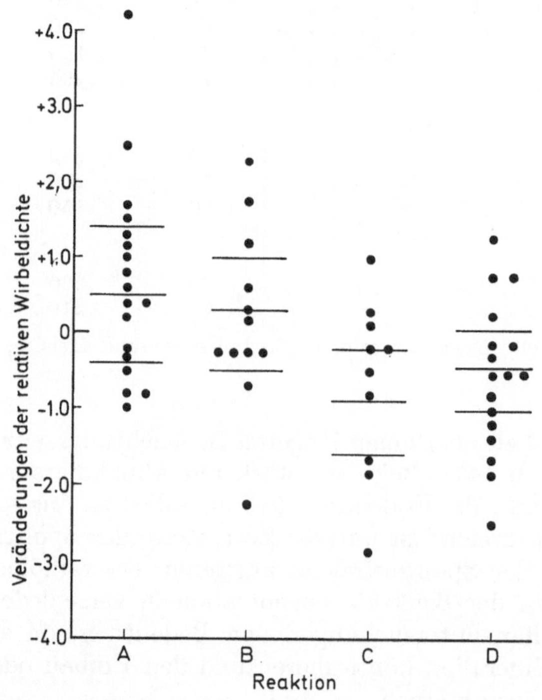

Abb. 148. Veränderungen der relativen Wirbeldichte (RWD) nach Calciumtherapie der Osteoporose im Laufe eines Jahres nach klinischen Symptomen, insbesondere Rückenschmerzen, geordnet. A Schmerzfrei, B eindeutige Besserung, C zweifelhafte Besserung, D unverändert oder verschlimmert. Die horizontalen Striche bedeuten Mittelwerte ± 2 Standardfehler. (Nach NORDIN und SMITH, 1964; Abb. 5)

Osteomalacie erkrankt waren, fand sich eine erhöhte „relative Wirbeldichte“ bei meist niedrigem Metacarpalindex (s. S. 242). Diese Befunde scheinen dafür zu sprechen, daß sich *das Verhältnis von Spongiosa zu Compacta* bei *gastro-intestinalen Osteopathien*, insbesondere der Steatorrhoe *umgekehrt* proportional verhält, also eine Zunahme der Spongiosadichte mit einer Verminderung der Compactadicke einhergeht.

Der Einfluß einer *Calciumtherapie* auf Knochenveränderungen wurde bei 66 Patienten untersucht. Ein Jahr lang sind 6 g Calciumglycerophosphat (entsprechend 1 g Calcium) täglich verabreicht worden. Die Abb. 148 zeigt die „relative Wirbeldichte“ aufgetragen gegen die subjektiven Beschwerden der Patienten, wobei eingeteilt wurde in: A schmerzfrei, B sehr gute Besserung, C zweifelhafte Besserung, D keine Änderung des Zustandes. Als gebessert angesehen werden solche Patienten, bei denen eine Zunahme der „relativen Wirbeldichte“ um mehr als den Faktor 0,2 festzustellen ist. Als stationär angesehen werden Veränderungen der „relativen Wirbelsäule“um + 0,2 und als verschlechtert eine Abnahme der „relativen Wirbeldichte“ um mehr als 0,2. Es sollten wiederholt Kontrollmessungen durchgeführt werden. Die Verfasser sind der Ansicht, daß aus den Ergebnissen der Untersuchungen eine deutliche Veränderung der Wirbeldichte nicht festzustellen ist.

f) Der Knochenkalksalzgehalt bei Osteosklerosen

Eine *Zunahme der globalen Kalksalzkonzentration* von Knochen fand sich bei der Osteomyelosklerose (Heuck 1965), bei der Marmorknochenkrankheit (Doyle 1967), bei

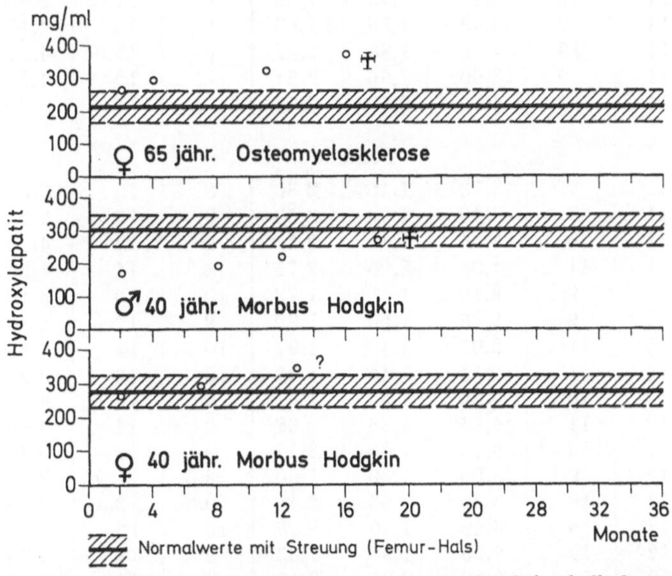

Abb. 149. Verlaufskontrollen der Hydroxylapatitkonzentration in der Schenkelhalsspongiosa bei verschiedenen sklerosierenden Erkrankungen des Knochens. (Nach Heuck, 1968)

Leukämien und der Lymphogranulomatose mit osteosklerotischen Reaktionen (Heuck 1968) und in einigen Fällen von sekundärem Hyperparathyreoidismus (Doyle 1966). In *Verlaufskontrollen* konnte die stetige Zunahme des Knochenkalksalzgehaltes beobachtet werden (Abb. 149; Heuck 1968).

Bugyi (1964/65) benutzte den Compacta-Index der proximalen Humerusdiaphyse zur Beurteilung einer Hyperostose als Frühzeichen der verstärkten *Fluoreinwirkung* auf das Skelet.

4. Der Knochenkalksalzgehalt bei Polyarthritis

Die Polyarthritis geht mit einer *Abnahme des Kalksalzgehaltes* in den gelenkbildenden Knochenpartien einher. Bei uncharakteristischen klinischen Symptomen kann die Objektivierung des Entkalkungsgrades ein wichtiger Befund der chronischen Polyarthritis sein.

Tabelle 39. *Absorptionsmessungen an Daumen mit rheumatischen Knochenveränderungen*

Fall und Seite	Klinische Gruppe	Breite des Knochens (mm)	Breite der Weichteile (mm)	Referenz-Gleichwert			Breite des Knochens (mm)	Breite der Weichteile (mm)	Referenz-Gleichwert		
				Knochen und Weichteile	Weichteile	pro mm Knochen			Knochen und Weichteile	Weichteile	pro mm Knochen
		Basalphalanx distal gemessen					Basalphalanx proximal gemessen				
					Männer						
21 L	II	14	12	4,00	2,40	2,06	12	13	3,50	2,20	1,97
R		14	13	4,10	2,25	2,17	12	14	4,20	2,25	2,49
22 L	III	13	14	3,80	2,35	1,97	12	14,5	3,45	1,70	2,10
R		15	16	3,55	2,20	1,61	13	16	3,25	2,00	1,65
23 L	III	14	11	3,75	2,05	2,04	11	14	4,45	2,15	2,95
R		15	11	4,35	1,95	2,35	11	14	4,75	2,10	3,25
24 L	II	14	10	3,85	1,70	2,24	11	12	3,90	1,60	2,78
R		15	8	4,15	0,85	2,57	11	11	3,80	1,10	2,95
25 L	II	14	11	4,25	1,80	2,46	12	13	4,60	1,90	3,01
R		14	11	4,45	2,20	2,48	12	12	4,60	2,10	2,96
26 L	III	13	13	2,90	1,90	1,50	10	15	3,05	1,80	1,97
R		13	13	3,40	2,15	1,79	11	15	3,80	2,20	2,30
27 L	II	12	12	3,50	1,30	2,38	9	16	4,10	1,35	3,62
R		11	14	4,35	2,00	2,94	9	16	5,55	2,10	4,70
28 L	II	14	8	2,75	1,60	1,55	11	9	2,35	1,70	1,44
R		14	10	3,15	1,45	1,82	12	11	2,80	1,60	1,69
29 L	I	14	12	3,45	1,85	1,85	10	16	4,15	1,80	3,04
R		14	13	4,25	1,80	2,42	10	15,5	4,75	1,80	3,72
30 L	II	14	10	3,90	1,95	2,21	11	12	4,10	1,80	2,87
R		14	12	4,55	2,40	2,32	11	14	5,00	2,45	3,29
					Frauen						
31 L	I	11	7	3,10	1,45	2,30	8	10	3,50	1,35	3,45
R		11	8	3,40	1,30	2,53	9	10	3,75	1,35	3,42
32 L	II	11	10	3,45	1,40	2,52	9	12	4,50	1,60	3,97
R		11	11	4,05	2,05	2,75	8	14	4,85	2,05	4,43
33 L	III	11	9	2,40	1,10	1,73	10	10	3,10	1,35	2,43
R		12	9	2,25	1,50	1,39	9	12	2,80	1,55	2,61
34 L	III	11	11	2,95	1,40	1,97	10	12	3,35	1,40	2,58
R		12	11	2,75	1,45	1,67	10	12	3,20	1,55	2,35
35 L	I	12	13	3,20	1,95	1,84	9	16	4,15	1,65	3,44
R		13	11	4,25	1,85	2,62	9	14	4,90	2,00	4,19
36 L	III	12	10	3,25	1,60	2,12	9	12	3,80	1,70	3,29
R		12	9	3,05	1,80	1,90	9,5	11	3,55	1,60	2,84
37 L	III	12	10	3,30	1,65	2,12	9,5	13,5	3,60	1,85	2,65
R		12	10	3,40	1,80	2,15	10	12	3,55	1,80	2,57
38 L	II	12	12	2,95	1,50	1,83	9	14	3,20	1,60	2,48
R		12	11,5	3,50	2,00	2,10	9	14	3,75	2,00	2,81
39 L	III	12	10	3,20	1,35	2,16	9	13	4,30	1,35	3,89
R		12	10	3,75	1,85	2,38	9	13	4,50	1,95	3,72
40 L	II	12	9	2,60	1,30	1,71	10	12	3,50	1,30	2,79
R		12	10	3,50	1,70	2,27	11	12	3,60	1,60	2,51

[ENGSTRÖM, A., and S. WELIN: Acta radiol. (Stockh.) **31**, 483 (1949), Tab. 11 u. 12]

ENGSTRÖM und WELIN (1949) haben mit der von ihnen angegebenen Methode (s. S. 152) eine Verminderung des Knochenkalkgehaltes in der *Grundphalanx des Daumens* und der Mittelphalanx des Zeigefingers bei 10 Frauen und 10 Männern, die an *rheumatischen Erkrankungen* litten, festgestellt (Tabelle 39—41). Die Kranken wurden in *drei Gruppen* eingeteilt. In den Gruppen 1 und 2 waren die Ergebnisse der Messungen nur zum Teil krankhaft, während in der Gruppe 3 häufiger eine Verminderung des Kalksalzgehaltes festgestellt wurde. Die Verminderung des Kalkgehaltes fand sich nicht nur in den Metaphysen und Epiphysen, sondern auch in den Diaphysen. Dieser Befund spricht dafür,

Tabelle 40. *Absorptionsmessungen der Zeigefinger von Männern mit rheumatischen Knochenveränderungen*

Fall und Seite	Klinische Gruppe	Breite des Knochens (mm)	Breite der Weichteile (mm)	Referenz-Gleichwert			Breite des Knochens (mm)	Breite der Weichteile (mm)	Referenz-Gleichwert		
				Knochen und Muskeln	Weichteile	pro mm Knochen			Knochen und Muskeln	Weichteile	pro mm Knochen
		Mittalphalanx weit distal					Mittelphalanx distal				
21 L	II	11	11	3,05	1,40	2,14	16	8	3,60	1,45	1,95
R		11	10	2,40	1,45	1,56	15	8	3,20	1,45	1,66
22 L	III	11	10	2,30	1,65	1,37	15	7	2,75	1,85	1,44
R		10	12	2,45	1,55	1,60	14	12	2,95	1,75	1,53
23 L	III	11	10	2,65	1,35	1,82	15	7	2,90	1,55	1,61
R		10	10	3,35	1,60	2,55	13	8	3,55	1,70	2,23
24 L	II	10	9	2,85	1,50	2,14	14,5	8,5	2,90	1,50	1,54
R		12	8	2,70	1,70	1,67	15	7	3,45	1,85	1,94
25 L	II	11	10	3,15	1,40	2,26	15	7	3,40	1,55	1,94
R		11	11	3,40	1,75	2,29	15	8	3,70	1,85	2,03
26 L	III	10	11	2,30	1,30	1,62	13	9	2,05	1,35	1,15
R		10	12	2,50	1,85	1,49	14	9	2,50	1,95	1,45
27 L	II	9	11	3,20	1,45	2,67	14	7	3,55	1,45	2,18
R		9	11	3,15	1,50	2,59	14	7	3,60	1,75	2,14
28 L	II	11	11	2,20	1,25	1,43	16	6	2,65	1,25	1,44
R		11	10	2,65	1,65	1,69	16	6	3,15	1,65	1,79
29 L	I	10	10	2,55	1,65	1,73	14	8	2,95	1,80	1,63
R		11	10	2,85	1,80	1,82	14	8	3,40	1,80	1,97
30 L	II	11	8,5	2,50	1,25	1,78	15	6	3,20	1,50	1,84
R		10,5	9	2,60	1,60	1,77	15	6	2,80	1,75	1,53
		Basalphalanx proximal					Basalphalanx weit proximal				
21 L	II	14	11	5,15	2,10	3,01	12	13	4,95	2,10	3,52
R		13	11	4,50	1,95	2,78	11	13	4,45	2,05	3,04
22 L	I	15	10	3,25	2,15	1,53	11,5	14,5	3,05	1,90	1,73
R		13	11	3,60	1,75	2,00	11	13	3,20	1,90	2,19
23 L	II	13	11	3,90	1,85	2,32	11	14	4,45	2,00	3,02
R		14	10	4,30	2,05	2,46	12	13	5,30	2,15	3,48
24 L	II	15	8	4,40	1,65	2,55	12	11	4,75	1,75	3,26
R		12	12	4,55	2,30	2,82	12	13	4,55	2,30	2,80
25 L	III	15	9	4,75	1,80	2,72	11	13	5,80	1,95	4,30
R		14	11	4,65	1,95	2,71	11	13	5,20	2,00	3,74
26 L	II	12	14	3,00	1,60	1,79	10	16	3,70	1,70	2,65
R		12	13	3,70	2,20	2,13	10	16	5,30	2,30	3,88
27 L	II	11	13	5,15	1,90	3,75	11	12	5,60	2,00	4,15
R		13,5	10,5	4,30	2,10	2,50	10	15	5,60	1,65	4,61
28 L	III	14	9	3,55	2,05	1,96	13	10	3,90	2,05	2,32
R		13	10	3,25	1,80	1,90	13	10	3,90	1,80	2,40
29 L	III	13	11	4,20	1,75	2,62	9	15	5,30	1,75	4,75
R		12,5	10	4,95	2,00	3,21	12	12	5,00	2,00	3,33
30 L	II	13,5	8,5	3,95	1,60	2,46	11	12	4,15	1,70	2,96
R		14	9	4,40	2,10	2,55	11	12	4,65	2,10	3,23

[ENGSTRÖM, A., and S. WELIN: Acta radiol. (Stockh.) **31**, 483 (1949), Tab. 13]

daß die Reduktion des Kalkgehaltes bis zu einem gewissen Grad *diffus* sein kann. In einem Falle wurde die *Zunahme* des Kalkgehaltes im Knochen nach Therapie *objektiviert*.

Durch einen Vergleich der Knochendichtewerte von gesunden Menschen mit den Dichtewerten bei der *chronischen Polyarthritis* fand SCHMID (1960/63) ein deutliches Absinken unter die Norm. Bei einfachen *Arthrosen* war die Verminderung der Dichte nicht so deutlich (Abb. 150). Nach Behandlung der chronischen Polyarthritis mit Glucocorticoiden kam es in einer Anzahl von Fällen zur weiteren Abnahme des Knochenmineralgehaltes um 20—30%, obgleich die Gelenkschmerzen verschwanden. Durch gleich-

Tabelle 41. *Absorptionsmessungen der Zeigefinger von Frauen mit rheumatischen Knochenveränderungen*

Fall und Seite	Klinische Gruppe	Breite des Knochens (mm)	Breite der Weichteile (mm)	Referenz-Gleichwert Knochen und Muskeln	Referenz-Gleichwert Weichteile	Referenz-Gleichwert pro mm Knochen	Breite des Knochens (mm)	Breite der Weichteile (mm)	Referenz-Gleichwert Knochen und Muskeln	Referenz-Gleichwert Weichteile	Referenz-Gleichwert pro mm Knochen
		Mittelphalanx weit distal					Mittelphalanx distal				
31 L	I	9	7	2,45	1,15	2,80	11	6	2,80	1,15	2,29
R		8	9,5	3,15	1,55	2,88	11	7	3,00	1,55	2,18
32 L	II	9	9	3,65	1,65	2,56	12	7	3,05	1,65	2,04
R		9	9	3,45	1,40	2,47	12	7	2,75	1,40	1,86
33 L	III	8	10	2,50	1,40	2,15	12	7	2,45	1,45	1,59
R		9	9	1,80	1,30	1,28	12	7	2,15	1,50	1,33
34 L	III	8	10	2,40	1,45	2,00	12	9	3,05	1,65	1,95
R		8,5	10	2,00	1,15	1,62	13	7	2,40	1,20	1,53
35 L	I	9	11	2,60	1,10	2,21	13	8	3,00	1,35	1,92
R		9	11	2,50	1,40	1,93	13	8	2,50	1,50	1,48
36 L	III	10	9	2,60	1,15	2,05	13	7	2,15	1,40	1,28
R		9	9	2,70	1,30	2,28	12	6	2,75	1,50	1,87
37 L	III	10	9	2,35	1,30	1,73	13	7	2,90	1,50	1,82
R		9	9	2,40	1,40	1,88	13	7	2,70	1,45	1,68
38 L	II	8	11	2,10	1,10	1,85	11	9	2,55	1,20	1,83
R		8	12	2,15	1,35	1,68	13	8	2,80	1,50	1,72
39 L	III	8	10	2,15	1,20	1,48	12	8	2,65	1,35	1,73
R		8,5	10	2,30	1,70	1,63	13,5	6,5	3,00	1,70	1,82
40 L	II	9	10	2,25	1,25	1,76	11	8	2,80	1,35	1,82
R		9	10	2,50	1,30	2,03	12	8	2,85	1,50	1,88
		Basalphalanx proximal					Basalphalanx weit proximal				
31 L	I	10	8	3,80	1,35	3,20	9	10	3,45	1,30	3,08
R		11	8	4,30	1,65	3,12	9	10	5,00	1,90	4,45
32 L	II	10	11	5,50	1,85	4,43	10	12	7,60	1,85	6,59
R		10	11	4,30	1,70	3,41	9	13	5,10	1,90	4,42
33 L	III	12	9	3,05	1,60	1,96	10	12	4,30	1,55	3,45
R		11	9	3,30	1,90	2,23	10	12	4,40	2,00	3,31
34 L	III	11	12	3,70	1,95	2,44	10	13	4,60	1,95	3,50
R		9	14	3,15	1,60	2,42	9	14	3,50	1,60	2,80
35 L	I	11	11	3,85	1,40	2,86	10	12	4,80	1,45	4,01
R		10	12	4,10	1,60	3,23	10	13	4,65	1,50	3,80
36 L	III	11	10	2,90	1,30	2,03	11	10	3,75	1,35	2,84
R		13	7	3,20	1,55	2,04	11	10	4,20	1,75	3,05
37 L	III	12	10	3,85	2,10	2,40	10	13	4,85	2,50	3,49
R		13	10	3,60	1,75	2,18	11	13	3,80	1,85	2,54
38 L	II	10	12	3,15	1,40	2,38	10	12	3,95	1,45	3,16
R		11	10	3,35	1,50	2,39	10	11	3,95	1,75	3,03
39 L	III	11	11	3,30	1,50	2,32	9	13	3,85	1,50	3,29
R		12	10	3,70	2,10	2,29	9	13,5	4,45	2,15	3,52
40 L	II	12	9	3,15	1,40	2,13	11	12	4,10	1,60	2,83
R		11	11	3,40	1,60	2,36	11	11	4,70	1,70	3,50

[Engström, A., and S. Welin: Acta radiol. (Stockh.) **31**, 483 (1949), Tab. 14]

zeitige Gabe von Androgenen konnte diese Nebenwirkung der Glucocorticoide beseitigt werden, ohne daß der therapeutische Effekt ausblieb.

Der Einfluß einer Cortison-Calcium-Medikation wurde von Schmid (1963) bei 12 Patienten mit einer *primär-chronischen Polyarthritis* während mehrerer Monate untersucht. Bei der Verabreichung von Cortisonpräparaten vermag *allein die medikamentöse Zufuhr von Calcium* im Alter zwischen 18 und 47 Jahren das Auftreten einer schweren Osteoporose zu hemmen.

Über Untersuchungsergebnisse der globalen Knochenkalksalzkonzentration in drei verschiedenen und entfernt voneinander lokalisierten spongiösen Knochenpartien des

Skeletes von Rheumakranken hat HEUCK (1968) berichtet. In der Radiusmetaphyse fanden sich zum Teil erhebliche Verminderungen des Knochenkalksalzgehaltes, insbesondere bei Lokalisation der rheumatischen Erkrankung im Handgelenk und den Fingergelenken. Die Calcaneusspongiosa zeigte ein ähnliches Verhalten bei Lokalisation der Erkrankung im Bereich des Fußgelenkes. Bemerkenswert ist die nicht selten zu findende gleichzeitige Verminderung der globalen Kalksalzkonzentration in der Schenkelhalsspongiosa. Die Beobachtung einer Abnahme der Knochenkalksalzkonzentration *in allen untersuchten Spongiosapartien* berechtigt zu der Vermutung, daß nicht nur lokale Faktoren, sondern auch solche Veränderungen, die das gesamte Skeletsystem betreffen, bei der Polyarthritis eine Rolle spielen.

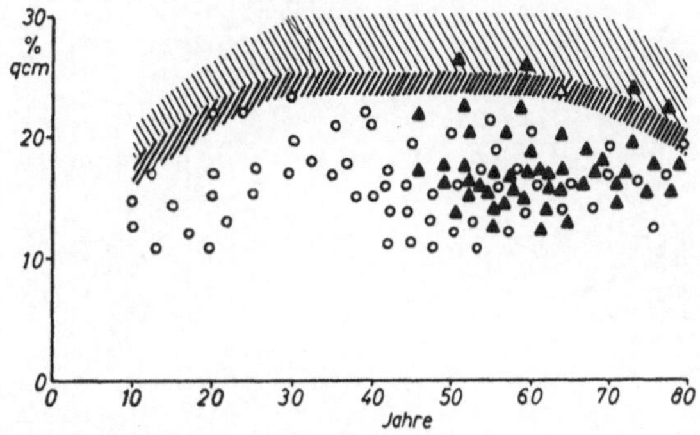

Abb. 150. Zusammenstellung der Meßwerte des Daumenknochens bei chronischer Polyarthritis ○ und bei Arthrosen ▲ mit dem normalen Streubereich. (Nach SCHMID, 1960/63; Abb. 4)

5. Knochenmineralgehalt und Frakturrisiko

Die Belastungsfähigkeit oder die statische Insuffizienz eines Knochens als Baustein des Skeletes ist nicht nur von der Form und Struktur des Knochens, sondern auch von der Relation des Knochengewebes zum Knochenmark und von der Kalksalzkonzentration im Knochengewebe selbst (Tela ossea) abhängig. Die Knochenmasse und die Knochenkalksalzkonzentration sowohl global gemessen als auch im Knochengewebe selbst ermittelt, sind daher wichtige Informationen zur Abschätzung des *Frakturrisikos* in einzelnen Knochen.

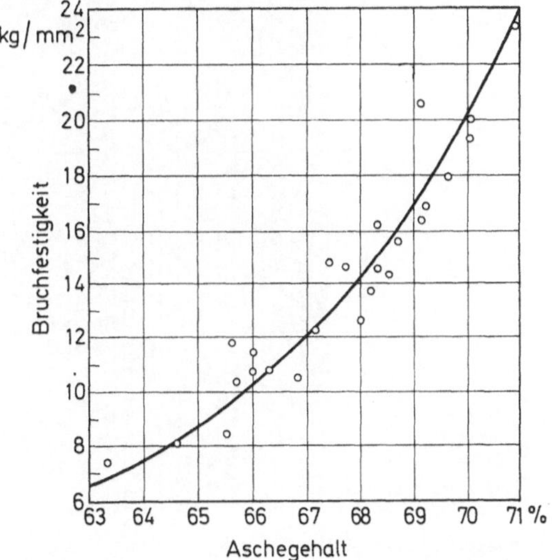

Abb. 151. Abhängigkeit der Bruchfestigkeit des Knochens vom Aschegehalt dargestellt am Beispiel der Diaphysencompacta des Femur. (Nach VOSE und KUBALA, 1958; Abb. 3)

Die *Bruchfestigkeit* bei Biegungsbelastung wurde von VOSE und KUBALA (1959) an 25 fixierten und getrockneten Femurpräparaten geprüft. Mit einer radiologischen Meßmethode (s. S. 131) wurde der Aschegehalt an verschiedenen Stellen der Femurdiaphyse bestimmt und eine exponentielle Abhängigkeit der zur Kontinuitätstrennung erforderlichen „Bruchkräfte" vom Aschegehalt festgestellt (Abb. 151).

Von HEUCK (1963) wurde durch langzeitige Kontrolluntersuchungen des Kalksalzgehaltes von Knochen bei Osteopathien der „kritische Apatitwert" bestimmt. Dieser Wert gibt die untere Grenze der globalen Hydroxylapatitkonzentration im spongiösen Knochen an, bei der eine Zusammensinterung der Spongiosa im Sinne der pathologischen Fraktur einsetzen kann (Abb. 152). Der „kritische Apatitwert" der Schenkelhalsspongiosa wurde bei 80—120 mg/ml gefunden.

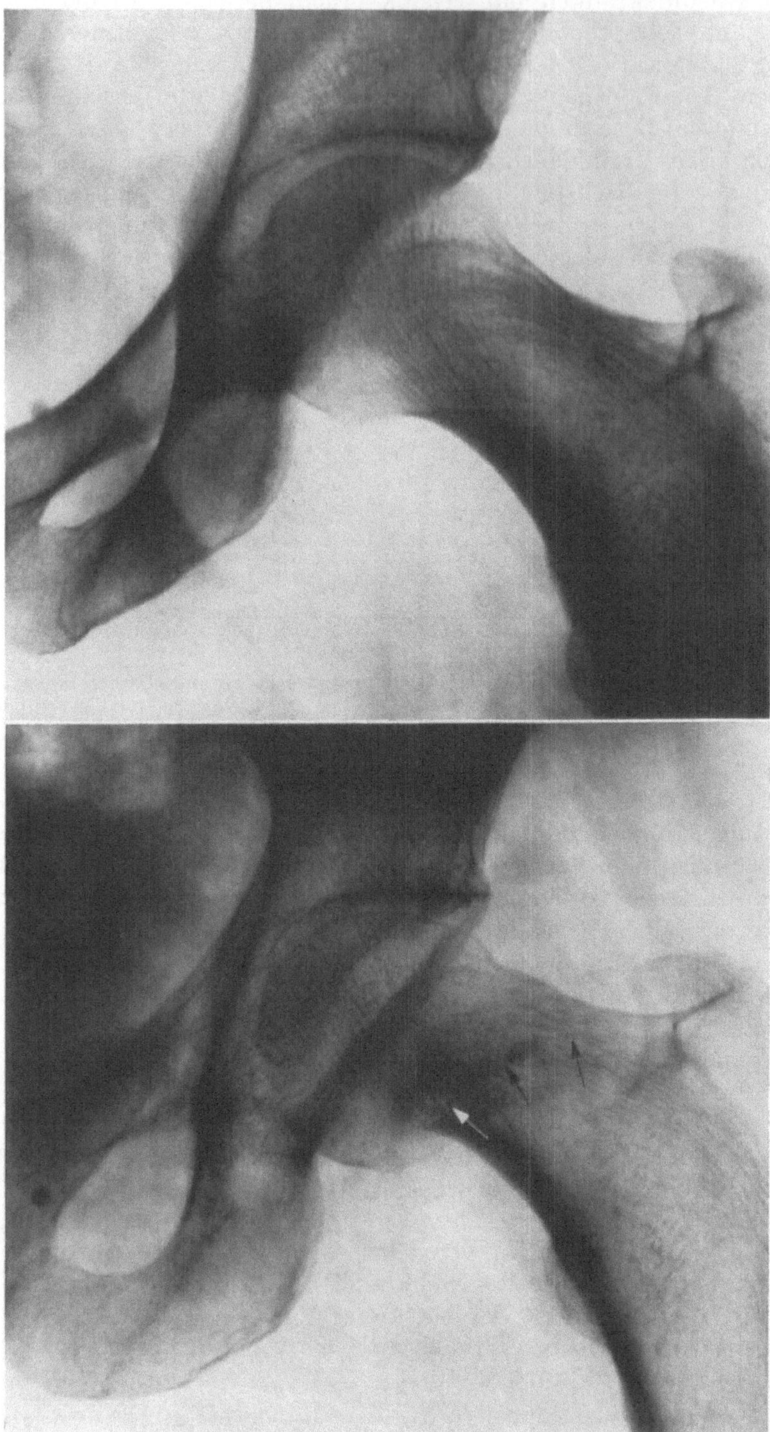

Abb. 152. Frühbefund einer Umbauzone im Schenkelhalsbereich bei Osteopathie infolge chronischer Lebercirrhose. Der postmortal chemisch-analytisch bestimmte Apatitwert betrug 120 mg/ml. (Nach HEUCK, 1968; Abb. 5)

Die Zusammenhänge zwischen dem *Mineralgehalt des Knochens und der Bruchfestigkeit* untersuchten VOSE und MACK (1963) an 10 Präparaten des proximalen Femurabschnittes. Als Maß für den Mineralgehalt wurden die radiologisch-densitometrisch gefundenen Mineralwerte im Bereich der Mitte des Femurhalses (Wardsches Dreieck) herangezogen

(Methode s. bei MACK, VOSE und NELSON 1959, S. 131). Die am Präparat gemessenen Werte lagen zwischen 260 mg und 510 mg/cm³ Knochen, während in den mehr lateral oder medial gelegenen wesentlich dichteren Zonen Werte von 740—1000 mg oder 1350 bis 1830 mg in cm³ Knochen gemessen wurden. Zwischen der höchst zulässigen Belastung sowie der Art der Fraktur (insbesondere der Biegung des Knochens!) und der radiologischen Dichte des Knochens, welche den Mineralgehalt repräsentiert, fand sich ein enger Zusammenhang.

KROKOWSKI (1963) hat Kontrolluntersuchungen an der Wirbelsäule durchgeführt und festgestellt, daß eine Wirbelfraktur dann droht, wenn der globale Hydroxylapatitgehalt des Wirbelknochens den Wert von 175 mg/ml unterschreitet (s. auch HAASNER, KROKOWSKI und RACH, 1967). Dieser Wert wird als „Bruchgrenze" bezeichnet und soll vom Lebensalter, Geschlecht und der Lokalisation innerhalb der Wirbelsäule unabhängig sein (Abb. 153).

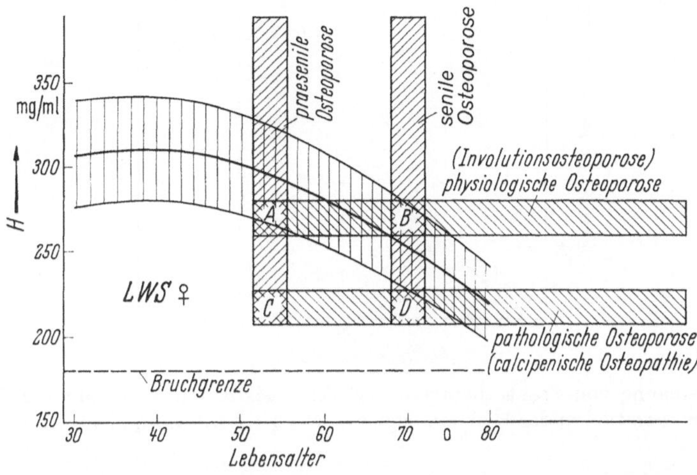

Abb. 153. Schematische Darstellung der Beziehung der „Bruchgrenze" des Wirbelkörpers zu der Mineralkonzentration im Gesamtknochen. (Nach KROKOWSKI, 1967; Abb. 2)

In den einzelnen Abschnitten der Wirbelsäule fand sich ein unterschiedlicher Hydroxylapatitgehalt im Gesamtvolumen der Wirbelkörper. Als Meßwerte werden angegeben: für die Halswirbelsäule 300—350 mg/ml, für die Brustwirbelsäule 250—275 mg/ml und für die Lendenwirbelsäule 275—300 mg/ml. Bei einer generalisierten Osteoporose soll die „Bruchgrenze" in den einzelnen Abschnitten unterschiedlich rasch erreicht werden. Hierdurch wird die Bevorzugung der Brustwirbelsäule bei osteoporotischen Wirbelfrakturen erklärt. In der Halswirbelsäule sollen osteoporotische Wirbelfrakturen, also Zusammensinterungen infolge einer starken Verminderung der globalen Kalksalzkonzentration nicht vorkommen. Bei der Beurteilung dieser Fragen sollte jedoch die Relation der Corticalis des Wirbels zum Gesamtvolumen nicht unbeachtet bleiben (s. S. 283). Jede Formänderung eines Halswirbelkörpers sei immer durch ein Trauma oder eine Knochenzerstörung bedingt. In diesem Zusammenhang weist KROKOWSKI (1963) besonders auf die Unterschiede der Häufigkeit und Lokalisation *osteoporotischer* und *traumatisch bedingter* Wirbelfrakturen hin. Ferner hat KROKOWSKI (1962) auf die Zusammenhänge zwischen Altersosteoporose und Frakturrisiko aufmerksam gemacht, indem er die Häufigkeit von Radiusfrakturen mit zunehmendem Alter der Abnahme des Globalwertes der Hydroxylapatitkonzentration im Radius gegenüberstellte (Abb. 154 und 156).

Die stärkere Verminderung der Compactadicke im Bereich der Diaphysen hat MEEMA (1962) veranlaßt, Untersuchungen der „kombinierten Corticaliswerte" der proximalen Radiusdiaphyse (Methode s. S. 237) bei 50 Frauen mit *Schenkelhalsfrakturen* und 20 Frauen mit *Wirbelkompressionsfrakturen* im Alter von über 70 Jahren durchzuführen. Es fanden sich Werte von 2 oder 3 mm, also eine *deutliche Verschmälerung* der Diaphysencompacta. Ein

Vergleichskollektiv von über 70 Jahre alten Frauen *ohne irgendeine Frakturneigung* ließen diese erhebliche *Verminderung* des Knochengewebsvolumens in der Radiusdiaphyse *vermissen*. Auch bei Männern mit Wirbelfrakturen fanden MEEMA und MEEMA (1963) eine *geringere* kombinierte Corticalisdicke des Radius. Verglichen mit einer gleichaltrigen gesunden Gruppe von Männern lagen die Werte um etwa 2 mm niedriger. Diese Beobachtungen veranlaßten MEEMA und MEEMA (1963), das Auftreten von Kompressionsfrakturen im Bereich der Wirbelsäule als sicheres Zeichen für eine pathologische Osteoporose anzusehen. Schenkelhalsfrakturen und Radiusfrakturen waren im Greisenalter beim weiblichen Geschlecht wesentlich häufiger zu finden als beim männlichen Geschlecht.

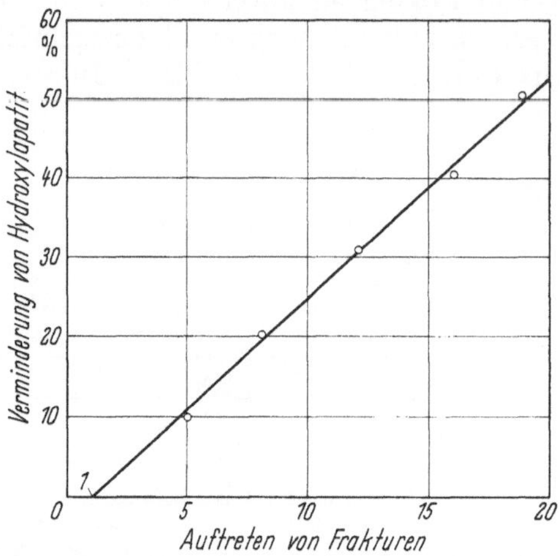

Abb. 154. Gegenüberstellung von Frakturhäufigkeit (Frakturrisiko) und Verminderung der Hydroxylapatitkonzentration in der Radiusspongiosa. (Nach KROKOWSKI, 1962; Abb. 4)

6. Der Knochenmineralgehalt nach Frakturen und beim „Sudeck-Syndrom"

Auf die Bedeutung der Objektivierung der Knochenkalksalzkonzentration während der Frakturheilung, bei einer *Atrophie* des Knochens und bei dem sog. „Sudeck-Syndrom" wurde hingewiesen. Ergebnisse von Kontrolluntersuchungen der „Aluminiumschwächungsgleichwerte" des Daumenknochens nach Unterarmfrakturen, vorwiegend Radiusfrakturen, hat BALZ (1968) vorgelegt. Bei solchen Frakturen, die *ohne* ein Sudeck-Syndrom heilten, konnte nur eine kurzfristige, vorübergehende Verminderung der Knochendichte im Daumengrundglied festgestellt werden. Die Radiusfrakturen *mit* einem Sudeck-Syndrom zeigten eine nachhaltige und meist *sehr lang dauernde* Verminderung der Knochendichte des Daumengrundgliedes. Die Messungen wurden mit Kontrollen auf der gesunden Seite verglichen und die Ergebnisse gemeinsam dargestellt (Abb. 155a und b). Von MAZZA und VACCHERI (1957) wurde die Entkalkung des Knochens nach Frakturen und bei der sog. Sudeckschen Knochenatrophie untersucht. Neben einer rein visuellen Auswertung der Röntgenaufnahmen sind photometrische Messungen der Schwärzung des Filmes mit Hilfe eines Apparates nach VIALLI-ROMANINI vorgenommen worden. Die Knochendichte wird nach diesem Verfahren zu verschiedenen Zeiten bestimmt und zum Alter des Patienten und zum Ort der Fraktur in Beziehung gesetzt. Angaben über den Kalkgehalt des Knochengewebes werden nicht vorgelegt. In den distal von der Fraktur liegenden Knochenbezirken ist die Demineralisation ausgeprägter als proximal. Ein Unterschied zwischen chirurgischer und konservativer Behandlung ergab sich hinsichtlich des Mineralverlustes der Knochen nicht. Densitometrische Kontrollen der *Frakturheilung* haben VOSE, MACK, BROWN und MEDLEN (1961) an der Tibia von Albinoratten durchgeführt (Methode s. S. 131). Eine vollständige Frakturheilung konnte nach etwa 77 Tagen festgestellt werden. Das Ergebnis wurde durch histologische Kontrolluntersuchungen ergänzt.

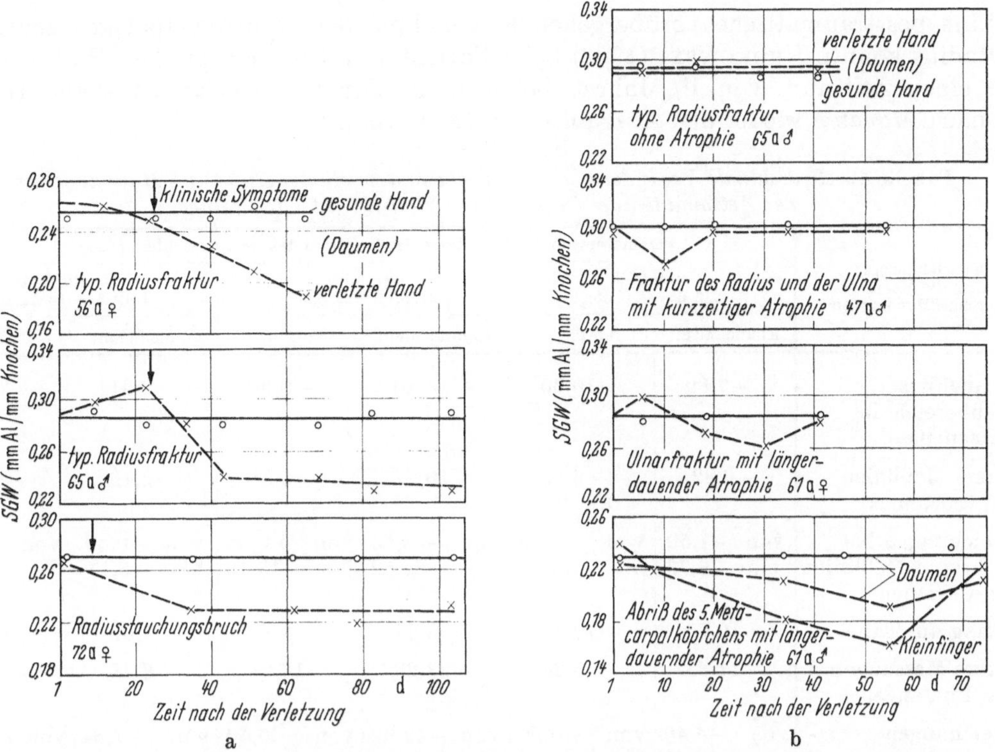

Abb. 155a. Ergebnis von Messungen der Aluminiumschwächungsgleichwerte im Daumenknochen (nach BALZ und BIRKNER, 1956) in Abhängigkeit von der Frakturheilung. (BALZ, persönliche Mitteilung)

Abb. 155b. Die Meßwerte des Aluminiumschwächungsgleichwertes in dem Daumenknochen stimmen mit dem klinischen Befund einer Sudeckschen Atrophie während der Frakturheilung gut überein. (BALZ, persönliche Mitteilung)

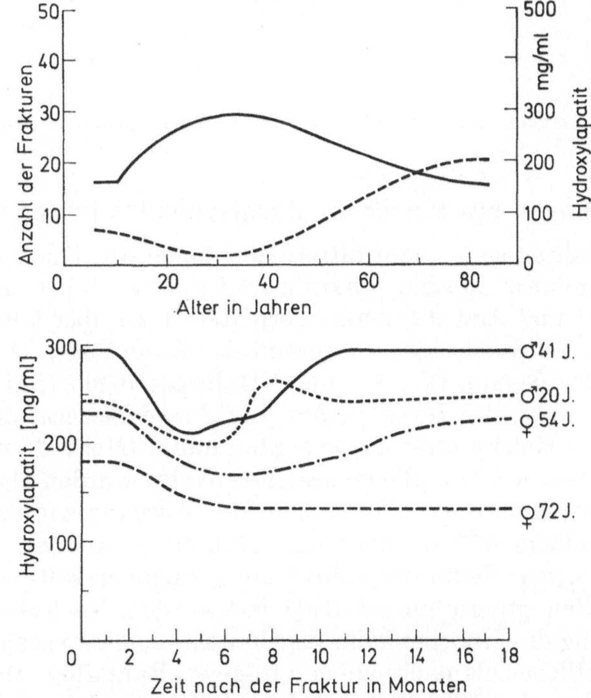

Abb. 156. Gegenüberstellung von Frakturrisiko und Hydroxylapatitgehalt in der Radiusspongiosa (oben) und der Verlaufskontrollen des Apatitwertes in der Radiusspongiosa bei einigen Frakturen über mehrere Monate. (Nach KROKOWSKI, 1962; Abb. 3 und 5)

Eine posttraumatische vorübergehende Abnahme der Hydroxylapatitkonzentration im Radius konnte KROKOWSKI (1962) bei 4 Patienten mit einer typischen Radiusfraktur über einen Zeitraum von $1^1/_2$ Jahren beobachten. Der Hydroxylapatitgehalt erreichte erst nach *Monaten* wieder den Ausgangswert (Abb. 156).

Tabelle 42. *Prozentuale Veränderung der Knochenmasse einiger Fuß- und Handknochen der Astronauten der Gemini IV-, V- und VII- Raumflüge*

Knochenbezirk, an dem die Messungen durchgeführt wurden	Veränderungen der Knochenmasse in % (auf das Referenzsystem bezogen)					
	Gemini IV 3. 6. 65—7. 6. 65		Gemini V 21. 8. 65—29. 8. 65		Gemini VII 4. 12. 65—18. 12. 65	
	Kommandant	Co-Pilot	Kommandant	Co-Pilot	Kommandant	Co-Pilot
Gebräuchlicher Meßbereich des Calcaneus	−7,80	−10,30	−15,10	−8,90	−2,91	−2,84
Mehrere Meßlinien am Calcaneus	−6,82	−9,25	−10,27	−8,88	−2,46	−2,54
Abweichungen bei mehreren Meßlinien am Calcaneus	von −1,50 bis −9,73	von −2,08 bis −13,42	von +3,55 bis −29,52	von +0,55 bis −13,76	von −0,49 bis −5,17	von +1,39 bis −7,66
Messung am Talus	−10,69	−12,61	−13,24	−9,87	−7,06	−4,00
Mehrere Messungen der Phalangen 5—2	−11,85	−6,24	−23,20	−16,98	−6,78	−7,83
Abweichungen der Meßwerte der Phalangen 5—2	von −4,40 bis −12,20	von −0,50 bis −14,30	von −19,60 bis −26,10	von −0,40 bis −22,10	von −1,84 bis −12,07	von −2,19 bis −14,86
Mehrere Messungen der Phalangen 4—2	−4,19	−8,65	−9,86	−11,80	−6,55	−3,82
Abweichungen der Meßwerte der Phalangen 4—2	von −1,28 bis −11,27	von +0,49 bis −15,28	von −6,00 bis −13,10	von − 5,30 bis −16,90	von −2,88 bis −9,11	von −1,66 bis −8,54
Messungen am Capitatum	−4,48	−17,64	−17,10	−16,80	−4,31	−9,30

[MACK, P. B., P. A. LACHANCE, G. P. VOSE, and F. B. VOGT: Amer. J. Roentgenol. **100**, 503 (1967), Tab. 1]

7. Kontrollmessungen des Knochenkalksalzgehaltes in der Raumfahrtmedizin

In den letzten Jahren sind quantitative Messungen des Knochenkalksalzgehaltes bei Astronauten durchgeführt worden (MACK, LA CHANGE, VOSE und VOGT 1967). Der russische Kosmonaut und Arzt JEGEROFF berichtete 1964 über hohe Calciumverluste des Knochens durch die Schwerelosigkeit während des Raumfluges (KROKOWSKI 1966). Bei den Raumfahrern der Gemini IV-, V- und VII-Besatzungen sind radiologische Dichtemessungen des *Calcaneus*, der *Handknochen*, der *Fingerknochen*, des *Capitatum* und des *Talus* mit Hilfe eines Referenzsystems aus Aluminium (Methode nach MACK u. Mitarb., s. S. 174) vorgenommen worden. Die gemessenen Werte wurden als ,,Schwächungsgleichwerte“ des Referenzsystems angegeben und zu den Ausgangswerten in Beziehung gesetzt (Tabelle 42). Nach einem 8 Tage dauernden Raumflug fanden sich die stärksten Entkalkungen. Ein 14tägiger Raumflug führte zu geringeren Entkalkungen, insbesondere dann, wenn täglich Bewegungsübungen absolviert wurden. Nach einem 4tägigen Raumflug war die Verminderung des Knochenkalksalzgehaltes weniger ausgeprägt als nach 8tägigem Raumflug, aber deutlicher als nach einem 14tägigen Raumflug. Die Befunde lassen vermuten, daß die Dauer des Raumfluges keinen Einfluß auf die Knochenentkalkung hat. Im Bereich der untersuchten Knochen fanden sich Unterschiede. Die Calcaneusspongiosa und die Talusspongiosa zeigten deutlichere Kalksalzverluste als die Fingerknochen

Tabelle 43. *Dichtevergleich der Calcanei von drei Raumschiffbesatzungen*

Verlauf der Meßlinien	Gemini IV Veränderung in 4 Tagen in %		Gemini V Veränderung in 8 Tagen in %		Gemini VII Veränderung in 14 Tagen in %	
	Kommandant	Co-Pilot	Kommandant	Co-Pilot	Kommandant	Co-Pilot
1 mm höher	−7,09	−9,80	−14,10	−8,70	−3,99	−3,13
Normal	−7,80	−10,27	−15,10	−8,78	−2,91	−2,84
1 mm tiefer	−7,26	−10,30	−11,04	−7,00	−3,00	−2,81
2 mm tiefer	−5,47	−9,04	−10,05	−7,97	−3,50	−2,08
3 mm tiefer	−6,91	−10,27	−11,10	−8,17	−3,09	−2,43
4 mm tiefer	−7,91	−10,95	−11,49	−8,66	−2,99	−3,88
5 mm tiefer	−6,42	−12,29	−13,81	−8,51	−2,87	−2,64
6 mm tiefer	−7,05	−10,98	−14,68	−7,90	−3,04	−1,13
7 mm tiefer	−8,14	−10,54	−13,94	−8,53	−3,85	−1,79
8 mm tiefer	−7,84	−10,43	−29,52	−10,48	−5,17	−2,01
9 mm tiefer	−7,72	−8,99	−17,45	−8,49	−3,82	−1,93
10 mm tiefer	−9,18	−13,12	−21,64	−9,69	−2,84	−3,34
11 mm tiefer	−7,09	−11,92	−20,84	−9,03	−3,97	−3,35
12 mm tiefer	−7,93	−9,36	−12,77	−8,62	−3,55	−2,33
13 mm tiefer	−8,35	−8,52	−12,26	−9,26	−3,10	−2,33
14 mm tiefer	−8,27	−10,29	−8,13	−9,21	−1,45	−2,73
15 mm tiefer	−3,04	−11,18	−4,83	−8,65	−2,06	−1,01
16 mm tiefer	−5,19	−11,82	−4,34	−9,99	−1,53	−2,10
17 mm tiefer	−6,69	−13,42	−7,94	−8,03	−2,78	−4,38
18 mm tiefer	−7,21	−11,65	−7,63	−9,96	−1,57	−7,66
19 mm tiefer	−6,48	−9,56	−9,86	−9,81	−1,90	−4,01
20 mm tiefer	−8,98	−9,65	−8,20	−13,76	−1,82	−0,27
21 mm tiefer	−7,67	−9,80	−8,42	−12,47	−1,18	−0,56
22 mm tiefer	−9,73	−8,45	−9,03	−13,27	−0,51	−1,01
23 mm tiefer	−6,78	−8,08	−9,21	−13,42	−0,49	+1,39
24 mm tiefer	−9,04	−10,33	−3,85	−12,36	−0,86	−0,68
25 mm tiefer	−6,74	−8,31	+2,16	−10,80	−0,96	−2,05
26 mm tiefer	−4,75	−7,18	+3,09	−10,03	−1,34	−4,77
27 mm tiefer	−4,34	−4,26	+3,55	−8,07	−1,10	−3,69
28 mm tiefer	−2,84	−6,16	+2,65	−8,98	−1,53	−3,23
29 mm tiefer	−3,06	−3,03	−1,05	+0,55	−1,72	−2,09
30 mm tiefer	−1,50	−2,08	−3,25	−6,44	−1,72	−1,45
31 mm tiefer	−3,87	−2,96	−5,43	−7,54	−0,95	−2,95
32 mm tiefer	−4,42	−3,41	−2,66	−10,15	−1,51	−4,72
33 mm tiefer	−5,15	−4,55	−12,56	−8,21	−0,54	−2,30
34 mm tiefer	−6,24	−2,63	−10,69	−6,21	−1,48	−3,81
35 mm tiefer	−8,81	−2,80		−12,69	−1,97	−2,44
36 mm tiefer		−7,57			−2,76	−5,63
37 mm tiefer		−10,82				−3,96
38 mm tiefer		−10,18				−2,51
39 mm tiefer						−2,06
40 mm tiefer						+8,22
Mittelwerte	−6,82	−9,25	−10,23	−9,10	−2,46	−2,54

[Mack, P. B., P. LaChance, G. P. Vose, and F. B. Vogt: Amer. J. Roentgenol. **100**, 503 (1967), Tab. 2]

(Tabelle 43 und 44). Der *spongiöse Knochen* erwies sich auch bei diesen Kontrolluntersuchungen als *empfindlicher*. Ein Vergleich der gefundenen Skeletveränderungen mit der gemessenen Aufnahme und Ausscheidung von Calcium ergab keine Zusammenhänge zwischen Demineralisation und Calciumaufnahme. Dagegen wird dem Einfluß von Bewegungsübungen auf den Knochenmineralgehalt eine große Bedeutung zugeschrieben.

Später hat Vose (1968) über einen Knochensubstanzverlust bei *Hunden* nach kurzdauerndem Zustand der *Schwerelosigkeit* berichtet. Die Regeneration dieses relativ raschen Knochenverlustes erfolgt sehr viel langsamer als der Verlust selbst. Es ist bemerkenswert, daß *die Erholungszeit des Knochens* gegenüber der Geschwindigkeit des Knochenabbaues oder Kalksalzverlustes *sehr viel länger dauert*.

Tabelle 44. *Dichtevergleich der 2.—5. Phalangen von 3 Raumschiffbesatzungen*

Lage der Meßpunkte	Veränderungen der Knochenmasse in % (gemessen als g-Äquivalent des Referenzsystemes)					
	Gemini IV-Flug 3. 6. 65—7. 6. 65		Gemini V-Flug 21. 8. 65—29. 8 65		Gemini VII-Flug 4. 12. 65—18. 12. 65	
	Kommandant	Co-Pilot	Kommandant	Co-Pilot	Kommandant	Co-Pilot
distales Phalanx-Ende	−9,7	−4,9	−22,2	−18,3	−4,6	−10,9
1 mm höher	−9,6	−14,3	−22,3	−19,0	−9,3	−3,3
2 mm höher	−9,5	−8,3	−21,5	−17,7	−8,3	−10,5
3 mm höher	−10,3	−2,4	−22,9	−22,1	−10,4	−10,5
4 mm höher	−10,1	−0,5	−20,6	−20,2	−12,1	−12,2
5 mm höher	−10,2	−1,9	−19,6	−20,9	−6,8	−6,5
6 mm höher	−9,8	−3,8	−21,3	−18,3	−3,5	−14,9
7 mm höher	−6,2	−3,5	−21,9	−19,6	−1,8	−7,8
8 mm höher	−4,4	−3,4	−23,3	−17,9	−3,3	−6,3
9 mm höher	−3,5	−5,1	−23,1	−22,0	−4,7	−5,0
10 mm höher	−7,6	−3,3	−23,5	−17,3	−4,3	−4,2
11 mm höher	−7,8	−4,6	−23,5	−15,8	−3,8	−3,5
12 mm höher	−10,7	−7,1	−24,2	−14,2	−4,9	−2,2
13 mm höher	−12,2	−5,5	−26,1	−15,5	−6,2	−2,3
14 mm höher	−10,6	−5,4	−24,3	−0,4	−10,7	−4,2
15 mm höher	−11,7	−5,1	−24,3	−14,7	−8,9	−2,5
16 mm höher		−7,5	−23,8	−16,5	−8,4	−7,9
17 mm höher		−8,4	−25,9		−7,1	

[MACK, P. B., P. LACHANCE, G. P. VOSE, and F. B. VOGT: Amer. J. Roentgenol. **100**, 503 (1967), Tab. 3]

X. Die Anwendung radiologischer Meßmethoden in der experimentellen Medizin und der Veterinärmedizin

Die radiologische Messung des Knochenmineralgehaltes und die Möglichkeit, Verlaufskontrollen über einen längeren Zeitraum durchzuführen, ist auch für die Veterinärmedizin von Interesse und besitzt große Bedeutung für die experimentelle Medizin und Biologie. In den letzten Jahren wurde eine Reihe interessanter Befunde mitgeteilt.

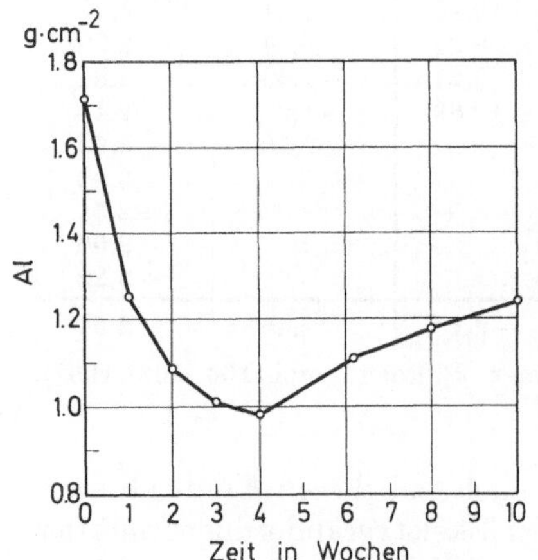

Abb. 157. Verlaufskurve des Aluminiumwertes der Spongiosa des Unterkiefers von Hunden als Folge einer Fremdkörperwirkung. (Nach OMNELL, 1957; Abb. 12)

Langdauernde Kontrolluntersuchungen des Unterkieferknochens von Hunden hat OMNELL (1957) mit Hilfe eines Referenzsystems aus Aluminium durchgeführt (Methode s. S. 163). Es wurde der Einfluß von Amalgan-Fremdkörpern und Knochenbohrungen auf die Kalksalzkonzentration der Unterkieferspongiosa studiert. Die Meßwerte der Knochendichte, ausgedrückt in Aluminiumäquivalenten, sind ein Maß für die Änderung der Kalksalzkonzentration des Knochens (Abb. 157).

Knochendichtemessungen an Rattenknochen haben SCHRAER, SCHRAER, TROSTLE und D'ALFONSO (1959) durchgeführt. Als Referenzsystem diente die von SCHRAER (s. S. 155) verwendete Aluminium-Zink-Legierung in Keilform. Als Meßort diente der Femur der Ratten, durch den drei Meßlinien gezogen wurden (Abb. 158, Tabelle 45 und 46). Die Gegenüberstellung der röntgenologisch ermittelten Knochendichtekoeffizienten (Massenschwächungskoeffizient) der Knochenasche und der Calciumwerte zeigte die beste Übereinstimmung im Bereich der proximalen Meßlinie des Femur (Tabelle 47).

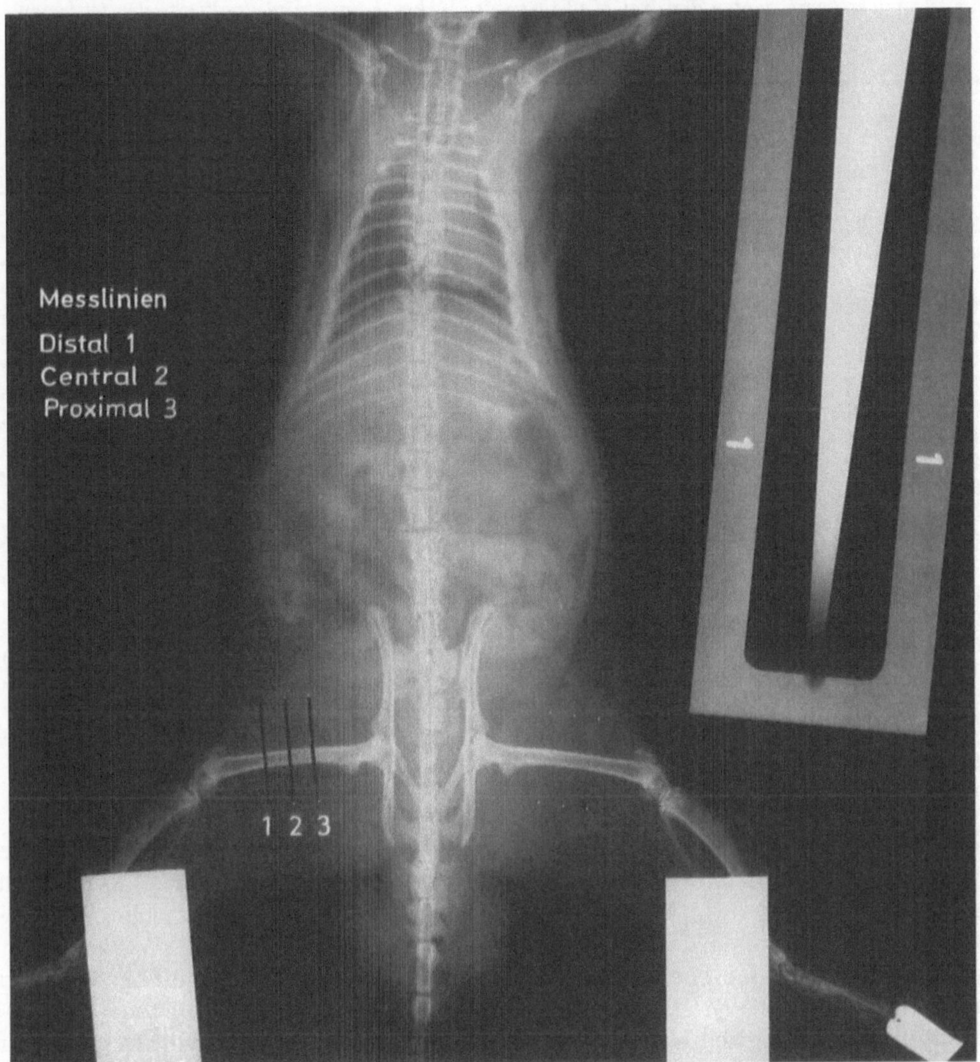

Abb. 158. Röntgenbild einer Ratte mit dem Referenzsystem aus einer Aluminiumlegierung und den drei Meßlinien durch den Femurknochen (s. Tabelle 45 und 46). (Nach SCHRAER, SCHRAER, TROSTLE und D'ALFONSO, 1959; Abb. 3)

Tabelle 45. *Beziehungen der Röntgen-Dichtekoeffizienten von distaler, zentraler und proximaler Meßlinie zueinander*

	r
Distale zur zentralen Meßlinie	0,93
Distale zur proximalen Meßlinie	0,83
Proximale zur zentralen Meßlinie	0,90

[SCHRAER, H., R. SCHRAER, H. G. TROSTLE, and A. D'ALFONSO: Arch. Biochem. **83**, 486 (1959), Tab. 2]

Tabelle 46. *Durchschnittswerte der Dichtekoeffizienten der drei Meßlinien*

Meßlinie	Mittelwert	Standard-Abweichung
Distal	0,37	0,13
Zentral	0,50	0,10
Proximal	0,66	0,21
Durchschnitt	0,51	0,17

[SCHRAER, H., R. SCHRAER, H. G. TROSTLE, and A. D'ALFONSO: Arch. Biochem. **83**, 486 (1959), Tab. 3]

Eine Einheit des Röntgenmassenkoeffizienten entspricht 9,8 mg Calcium oder 29,5 mg Knochenasche. Durch die relativ hohe Ordnungszahl des Calcium gegenüber andereren Stoffen im Knochen wird schon eine geringe Verminderung des Calciumgehaltes eine relativ große Änderung der Strahlenabsorption im Knochen zur Folge haben. Bei mono-

Tabelle 47. *Dichtekoeffizienten der drei Meßlinien des linken Femur und die Werte der fettfreien Trockensubstanz, der Knochenasche sowie des Calcium der entsprechenden proximalen und distalen Knochensegmente*

Nummer der Tiere	Röntgen-Dichtekoeffizienten				Dichtewerte		
	Meßlinien			Mittelwerte	getrocknete Knochen	Knochenasche	Calcium
	distal	zentral	proximal		g/cm³	g/cm³	g/cm³
13	0,375	0,485	0,615	0,492	0,671	0,372	0,138
14	0,479	0,689	0,794	0,654	0,838	0,508	0,191
15	0,299	0,442	0,632	0,458	0,666	0,361	0,140
16	0,326	0,437	0,625	0,463	0,667	0,371	0,136
17	0,273	0,417	0,566	0,419	0,571	0,285	0,108
18	0,430	0,488	0,653	0,524	0,790	0,499	0,169
19A	0,382	0,515	0,706	0,534	0,794	0,474	0,177
20A	0,279	0,467	0,568	0,438	0,588	0,296	0,111
21	0,480	0,745	0,861	0,695	0,862	0,529	0,202
22	0,237	0,320	0,531	0,363	0,588	0,263	0,098
23	0,262	0,302	0,466	0,343	0,526	0,235	0,089
24	0,351	0,466	0,580	0,466	0,536	0,273	0,104
26	0,495	0,609	0,768	0,624	0,902	0,537	0,197
27A	0,214	0,252	0,427	0,298	0,532	0,261	0,098
28	0,428	0,586	0,910	0,641	0,812	0,474	0,177
29	0,506	0,699	0,757	0,654	0,824	0,492	0,189
30	0,370	0,440	0,477	0,416	0,511	0,227	0,084
31	0,346	0,492	0,768	0,535	0,773	0,456	0,171
32	0,368	0,465	0,639	0,491	0,746	0,434	0,169
45	0,543	0,737	0,929	0,736	0,892	0,556	0,210

[SCHRAER, H., R. SCHRAER, H. G. TOSTLE, and A. D'ALFONSO: Arch. Biochem. **83**, 486 (1959), Tab. 6]

chromatischer Strahlung ist dieser Effekt noch deutlicher als bei einem breiteren Strahlenspektrum. Durch schrittweise Entkalkung der Rattenknochen wurde festgestellt, daß schon Veränderungen des Calciumgehaltes von 4—7% photometrisch erfaßt werden können. Diese Ergebnisse decken sich mit den Befunden von FUSI (1953), der durch Entkalkungsversuche an Rippenknochen Calciumverluste von ungefähr 3% feststellen konnte. Die Meßwerte von spezifischem Gewicht der Knochen, Knochenasche, Calciumgehalt und röntgenologisch ermittelter Dichte der Rattenknochen wurden zueinander in Beziehung gesetzt und festgestellt, daß der Mineralgehalt des Rattenknochens mit Hilfe photometrischer Meßverfahren genau bestimmt werden kann.

Eine experimentelle Osteoporose konnten VIRTAMA und KALLIO (1961) im Tierversuch an Ratten *nach Calciummangeldiät* erzeugen und durch radiologische Untersuchungen objektivieren. Die Dicke der Diaphysencompacta von Femur, Humerus und Tibia (Abb. 159a und b) und die Dichte der Wirbelknochen (Abb. 160a und b) der Ratten wurden untersucht. Nach 6 Monaten einer calciumarmen Diät war der Verlust des Knochenminerals etwa 10% und vom 7. Monat an stieg die Demineralisationsrate erheblich an.

Den Einfluß des Calciumgehaltes der Nahrung auf Volumen und Dichte des Knochens haben SCHRAER, SIAR und SCHRAER (1963) an 28 Ratten untersucht (Methode s. S. 155). Die radiologischen Kontrollmessungen wurden am Femur und dem 7. Schwanzwirbel vorgenommen und bis zu 59 Tagen fortgesetzt. Geringe Änderungen der Kalksalzkonzentration konnten erfaßt werden.

Von SPENCER, GARN und COULOMBE (1966) wurden quantitative Untersuchungen der Altersabhängigkeit der Diaphysencompacta bei Ratten durchgeführt.

Mit Hilfe densitometrischer Methoden hat TARJÁN (1963) im Tierexperiment *Zusammenhänge zwischen der Ernährung und der Knochenbildung* studiert. Als Referenzsystem wurde eine Aluminiumtreppe oder ein Aluminiumkeil verwendet. Die Meßmethode wurde auf der Basis der Arbeiten von ENGSTRÖM und WELIN (1949), MACK, BROWN und TRAPP (1949) sowie OMNELL (1957) entwickelt. In größeren Versuchsreihen an Ratten ist neben der densitometrischen Bestimmung der Knochendichte gleichzeitig die Elastizität und die Festigkeit der Röhrenknochen gemessen worden. Es konnte festgestellt werden, daß Oxalsäure in der Nahrung die Knochenbildung bei Ratten nur vorübergehend störend beeinflussen kann. Nach regelmäßiger Zufuhr von Oxalsäure mit der Nahrung gewöhnen sich die Tiere an diesen Stoff, so daß schließlich keine deutlichen Ossifikationsstörungen mehr festzustellen sind. Untersuchungen der Einwirkung von Citronensäure auf die Knochenbildung ergaben auch bei solchen Tieren, die mit einer Vitamin D-freien Diät ernährt worden waren, ein einwandfreies Knochenwachstum. Es wurde im Gegenteil

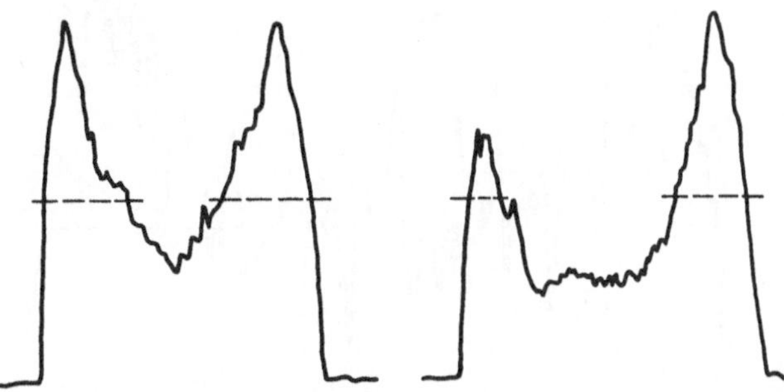

Abb. 159a. Beispiel einer Densitometerkurve durch den gesunden (links) und den osteoporotischen (rechts) Femur einer Ratte nach Calciummangeldiät. (Nach VIRTAMA und KALLIO, 1961; Abb. 3 und 4)

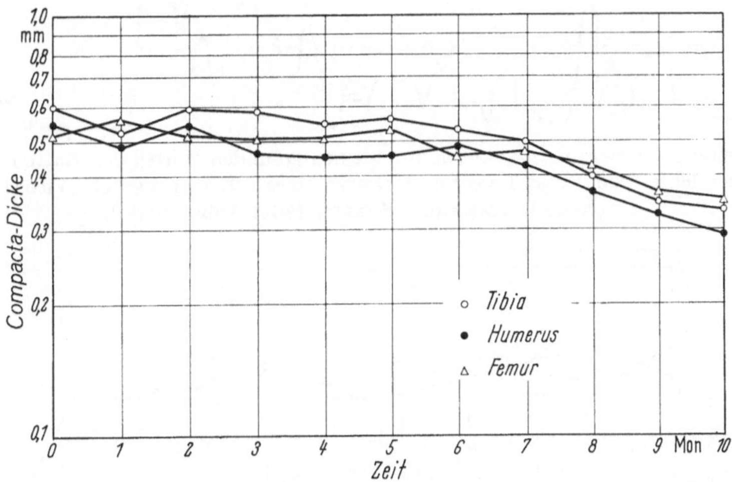

Abb. 159b. Abnahme der Compactadicke von Tibia (○), Femur (●) und Humerus (△) bei Ratten nach Calciummangeldiät. (Nach VIRTAMA und KALLIO, 1961; Abb. 10)

festgestellt, daß die mit Citronensäure, aber ohne Vitamin D ernährten Tiere einen hochwertigeren Knochen entwickeln als die mit Vitamin D ernährten Tiere. Ferner wurde der Einfluß einer proteinarmen und proteinreichen Diät auf die Knochenbildung studiert. Eine Diät, die weniger als 12% Eiweiß enthält, wirkt sich ungünstig aus. Ebenso beeinflußt eine Diät mit mehr als 20% Eiweiß die Knochenbildung negativ. Ein mittlerer Eiweißgehalt der Nahrung ist für die Ossifikation am günstigsten.

KALLAI und TARJÁN (1963) untersuchten den Zusammenhang zwischen der *Knochenfestigkeit* und dem *Mineralgehalt*, der als *Aluminiumäquivalent* mit Hilfe der Röntgendensitometrie bestimmt wurde. Die Meßergebnisse wurden durch chemische Analysen kontrolliert. Der mittlere Meßfehler betrug 3,53%, er konnte durch doppelte Auswertung von 2 Röntgenaufnahmen auf 2,01% reduziert werden. Der Aschegehalt, die Bruchfestigkeit, der Elastizitätsmodul und der densitometrisch gemessene Aluminiumäquivalentwert des *Femur von weißen Ratten* wurden zueinander in Beziehung gesetzt. Auf Grund der berechneten Regressionsgleichungen kann der in vivo bestimmte Aluminiumäquivalentwert Informationen über die beiden wichtigsten biologischen Aufgaben des Knochengewebes liefern — über den Mineralgehalt und die statische Belastbarkeit, charakterisiert durch die Bruchfestigkeit des Knochens.

Die *Knochenheilungsrate bei Ratten* haben VOSE, MACK, BROWN und MEDLEN (1961) mit Hilfe densitometrischer Methoden untersucht. Als Referenzsystem diente eine Alu-

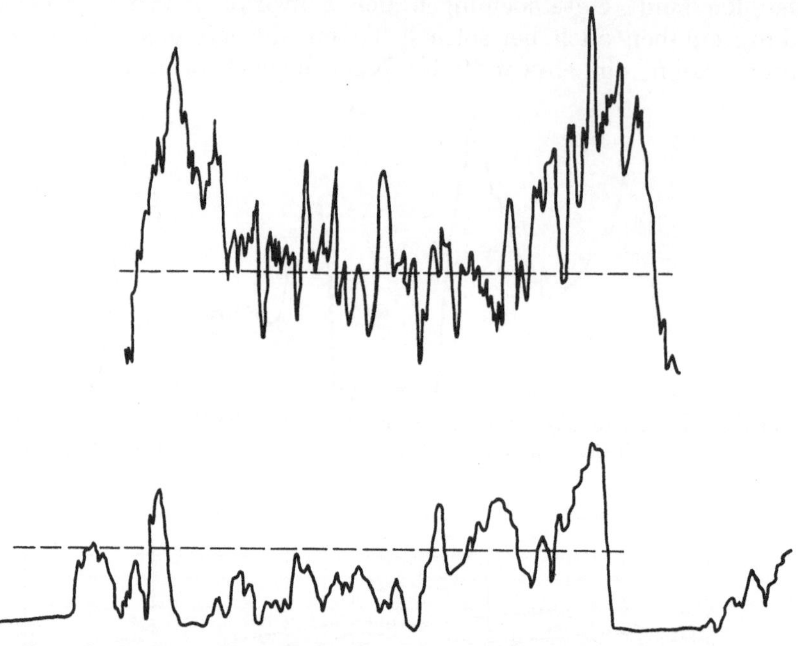

Abb. 160a. Darstellung der Densitometerkurve durch einen gesunden Wirbel der Ratten mit der berechneten normalen Bälkchendichte (oben) und Densitometerkurve eines osteoporotischen Wirbels der Ratte (unten). (Nach VIRTAMA und KALLIO, 1961; Abb. 7 und 8)

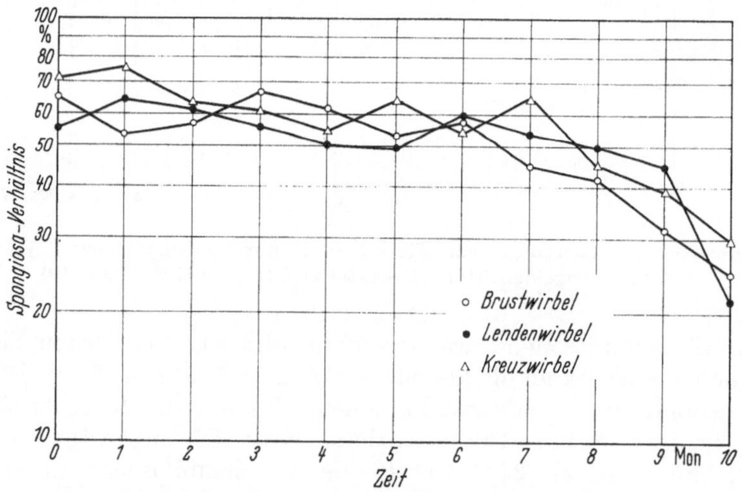

Abb. 160b. Abnahme der Trabekeldichte in den Brustwirbeln (○), Lendenwirbeln (•) und Kreuzwirbeln (△) der Ratte nach Calciummangeldiät. (Nach VIRTAMA und KALLIO, 1961; Abb. 11)

miniumtreppe. Die Ablagerung von neuem Knochen wurde durch tägliche Messungen kontrolliert und nach 77 Tagen eine vollständige Regeneration festgestellt. Gleichzeitig durchgeführte histologische Untersuchungen des Knochengewebes ergaben eine gute Übereinstimmung mit den Ergebnissen der radiologischen Messungen.

Messungen der Knochenkalksalzkonzentration *beim Rind* haben PRIBOTH, BÖRNERT und FRITZSCHE (1966) durchgeführt. Die ersten Ergebnisse wurden am 7. Schwanzwirbel

Tabelle 48. *Gegenüberstellung des röntgenologisch-photometrisch und chemisch-analytisch „in vitro" ermittelten Aschegehaltes der proximalen Diaphyse des 7. fleischfreien Schwanzwirbelknochens von klinisch gesunden sowie osteopathiekranken etwa 9—12 Monate alten Jungbullen*

Nummer des Tieres	1	2	3	4	5	6	7	8	9	10
Alter (Monate)	10	9	12	9	11	10	10	12	11	12
Klinische Diagnose	gesund	Osteopathie	gesund	Osteopathie	Osteopathie	Osteopathie	gesund	gesund	gesund	Osteopathie
chemisch-analytischer Wert mg/cm³	246	173	223	211	211	221	286	292	253	217
Diasinex ohne Folie										
Photometrie	248	175	235	205	194	236	276	308	253	208
Abweichung (mg/cm²)	+2	+2	+12	−6	−17	+15	−10	+16	±0	−9
Abweichung (%)	+0,8	+1,2	+5,4	−2,8	−8,1	+6,8	−3,5	+5,5	±0,0	−4,2
Orwo RF 4 ohne Folie										
Photometrie	230	167	242	198	194	214	304	300	242	202
Abweichung (mg/cm²)	−16	−6	+19	−13	−17	−7	+18	+8	−11	−15
Abweichung (%)	−6,5	−3,5	+8,5	−6,5	−8,1	−3,2	+6,3	+2,7	−4,4	−6,9
Orwo Rapid RF 2 mit Folie										
Photometrie	266	160	246	191	194	214	263	279	278	203
Abweichung (mg/cm²)	+20	−13	+23	−20	−17	−7	−20	−13	+25	−14
Abweichung (%)	+8,1	−7,5	+10,3	−9,5	−8,1	−3,2	−7,0	−4,5	+9,9	−6,5
Supervidox mit Folie										
Photometrie	259	158	229	189	193	243	262	310	250	197
Abweichung (mg/cm²)	+13	−15	+6	−22	−18	+22	−24	+18	−3	−20
Abweichung (%)	+5,3	−8,7	+2,7	−10,4	−8,5	+10,0	−8,4	+6,2	−1,2	−9,2

[Priboth, W., D. Börnert u. H. Fritzsche: Zbl. Vet.-Med. **13 A**, 628 (1966), Tab. 1, 2, 3 u. 4]

von Jungmastbullen ermittelt. Bei *kranken Tieren* konnte eine deutliche Verminderung des Apatitwertes der Wirbelspongiosa gefunden werden (Tabelle 48).

Vergleichsuntersuchungen der *Knochendichte* oder des Knochenmineralgehaltes von *Wirbelkörpern* bei Mensch und Tier haben Hoffmann und Fabian (1966) durchgeführt. Bei *Katzen* im Alter von 1—16 Jahren zeigte die Wirbelspongiosa eine strähnige Transformation und erhöhte Transparenz im Alter. Während beim Menschen in der mittleren Brustwirbelsäule und der mittleren Lendenwirbelsäule die niedrigsten Hydroxylapatitwerte gefunden wurden (Krokowski, 1965), ist bei Katzen im thorako-lumbalen Übergangsbereich der Wirbelsäule der niedrigste Hydroxylapatitgehalt festgestellt worden. Die gefundenen Werte der Hydroxylapatitkonzentration in Wirbelkörpern waren bei der *Katze* durchschnittlich höher als beim Menschen, und dies dürfte auf die andere Relation von Corticalis zu Spongiosa und Unterschiede in der Makrostruktur des Knochens zurückzuführen sein.

In einer späteren Untersuchungsreihe fand Hoffmann (1967) neben einer deutlichen Abnahme des Kalkgehaltes der Wirbelkörper bei Katzen während des Alterungsprozesses eine stärker ausgeprägte Osteoporose bei alten kastrierten Tieren. Untersuchungen des Kalkgehaltes im Skelet von Hunden zeigten ebenfalls die bekannten Veränderungen im Laufe des Alterungsprozesses. Parallel mit einer Verminderung des Kalksalzgehaltes ist eine strähnige Transformation der Knochenstruktur der Wirbelkörper als Ausdruck der Altersosteoporose festzustellen. Die Altersosteoporose wird also nicht nur beim Menschen, sondern auch beim Wirbeltier beobachtet. Die globale Kalksalzkonzentration eines Knochens ist sowohl beim Menschen als auch Tier von der Funktion des einzelnen Knochens und statischen Faktoren abhängig.

Strandjord und Lanzl (1965) haben mit der Methode von Cameron und Sorenson (1965, s. S. 142) Untersuchungen an den Femurknochen von *Kaninchen* durchgeführt. Von Babcock und Montilla (1965) wurden mit der gleichen Methode quantitative

Messungen des Knochenmineralgehaltes an der Tibia *des Haushuhnes* durchgeführt, das einen sehr labilen Calciumstoffwechsel aufweist. Die Standardabweichung der Messung (Methode s. S. 143) wird mit 3% angegeben. Es ist 3 und 5 cm proximal vom Tibiotarsalgelenk gemessen worden. Die Meßergebnisse des linken und rechten Beines zeigten gute Übereinstimmung. Nach einer Calciummangelernährung wurde ein erhebliches Absinken des Kalksalzgehaltes festgestellt. Gleichzeitig setzte die Eierproduktion aus. Die Untersuchungsergebnisse lassen erkennen, daß der Knochen der Tibia den Calciumverlust im gesamten Körper reflektiert. Ferner sind Vergleichsuntersuchungen zwischen Hühnern, die einer energischen Bewegung unterzogen worden sind, und solchen, die sich kaum bewegt haben, vorgenommen worden. Die Ernährung ist in beiden Kollektiven gleich gewesen. Es fanden sich keine Veränderungen des Knochenkalksalzgehaltes innerhalb einer Untersuchungsdauer von 14 Tagen. Untersuchungen des Tibiaknochens bei jungen Hennen ergaben einige Zeit vor dem ersten Eierlegen einen rapiden Anstieg der Knochendichte und des Knochengewichtes. Unmittelbar vor dem Eierlegen fand sich ein rapider Abfall der Knochenkalksalzkonzentration und danach eine Normalisierung. In weiteren Untersuchungsreihen wurde nachgewiesen, daß eine ausreichende tägliche Calciumzufuhr mit der Nahrung für die Eierproduktion und die Resistenz der Tiere gegenüber Erkrankungen eine entscheidende Rolle spielt.

XI. Schlußbetrachtungen

Die vorliegende Zusammenstellung zeigt, daß verschiedene Wege beschritten werden können, um den Mineralgehalt eines Knochens und das Knochengewebsvolumen zu messen. Für die klinische Radiologie sind nur solche Untersuchungsverfahren geeignet, die leicht durchgeführt werden können und einen relativ geringen Fehler aufweisen. Eine Verständigung verschiedener Arbeitsgruppen über die Kalksalzkonzentration der Knochen des Skeletes ist nur auf einer einheitlichen Basis möglich. Die Einführung des „Apatitwertes" von Knochen, also die Bestimmung der Konzentration der Knochenkalksalze (repräsentiert durch den Hydroxylapatit) in der Volumeneinheit Gesamtknochen, der in mg/ml angegeben werden sollte, erscheint zweckmäßig.

Die bisher vorliegenden Untersuchungsergebnisse lassen erkennen, daß sowohl die einzelnen Knochen des Skeletes als auch verschiedene Bezirke innerhalb eines Knochens Unterschiede der Kalksalzkonzentration aufweisen. Besonders groß sind die Differenzen des Kalksalzgehaltes im Gesamtvolumen zwischen spongiösen Knochenpartien der Epiphysen- und Metaphysenregion und den kompakten Zonen der Diaphysen der Röhrenknochen (Tabelle 49). Ferner sind Unterschiede der globalen Kalksalzkonzentration im Organ „Knochen" zwischen dem weiblichen und männlichen Geschlecht gefunden worden, wobei die Knochen des männlichen Geschlechtes im allgemeinen einen etwas höheren Mineralgehalt aufweisen als die des weiblichen Geschlechtes. Im Laufe des Alterungsprozesses ist zunächst vom Säuglingsalter bis zur Pubertät ein stetiges Ansteigen der globalen Kalksalzkonzentration in den Knochen der verschiedensten Skeletregionen festzustellen, dem dann eine gewisse Konstanz folgt. Vom 4.—5. Lebensjahrzehnt an ist ein kontinuierliches Absinken der globalen Kalksalzkonzentration nachweisbar. Die altersabhängigen Veränderungen der Mineralkonzentration gehen mit Strukturänderungen des Knochens einher, die in den makroskopischen Dimensionen auch im Röntgenbild deutlich erkennbar werden. Morphometrische Untersuchungen haben eine Abnahme des Knochengewebsvolumens (der Knochenmasse) in allen Abschnitten der bisher untersuchten Diaphysen ergeben. Auffallend ist die recht große Schwankungsbreite der Normalwerte verschiedener Individuen im gleichen Altersbereich, die allein durch konstitutionelle Faktoren, Umwelteinflüsse, genetische und rassische Komponenten erklärt werden kann.

Die Möglichkeiten radiologisch-densitometrischer Untersuchungsverfahren zur Bestimmung der Hydroxylapatitkonzentration im Knochen und morphologischer Untersuchungen

Tabelle 49. *Zusammenstellung der bisher ermittelten globalen Mineralkonzentrationen*

Skelet-Bereich	Meßergebnisse	Art der Bestimmung	Autoren
Wirbelsäule	♂ und ♀ 270—340 mg/ml	Photometrie, differente Strahlenqualitäten	OESER und KROKOWSKI (1961)
Halswirbelsäule	♂ und ♀ 300—350 mg/ml	Photometrie, differente Strahlenqualitäten	KROKOWSKI (1963)
Brustwirbelsäule	♂ und ♀ 250—375 mg/ml	Photometrie, differente Strahlenqualitäten	KROKOWSKI (1963)
Lendenwirbelsäule	♂ und ♀ 275—300 mg/ml	Photometrie, differente Strahlenqualitäten	KROKOWSKI (1963)
4. Lendenwirbel	♂ und ♀ 310 mg/ml	Photometrie, differente Strahlenqualitäten	KROKOWSKI u. Mitarb. (1965/67)
Radius, distale Metaphyse	♂ 200—320 mg/ml ♀ 180—280 mg/ml	Photometrie, differente Strahlenqualitäten	KROKOWSKI und STEINER (1961)
Radius, distale Metaphyse	♂ 200—380 mg/ml ♀ 180—350 mg/ml	Photometrie, Apatit-Referenzsystem	QUINTAR (1962)
Radius, proximale Diaphyse	♂ und ♀ 1000—1400 mg/ml	Photometrie, K_2HPO_4-Referenzsystem	MEEMA, HARRIS und PORRETT (1964)
Ulna distal 2 cm prox. Proc. styl. 4 cm prox. Proc. styl. 6 cm prox. Proc. styl.	 ♂ und ♀ 200 mg/ml ♂ und ♀ 290 mg/ml ♂ und ♀ 360 mg/ml	Photometrie, Al-Referenzsystem	KEANE, SPIEGLER und DAVIS (1959)
Ulna, 2 cm prox. des dist. Gelenkes	♂ 370 mg/ml (± 84,5 mg/ml) ♀ 325 mg/ml (± 87,0 mg/ml)	Photometrie, Al-Referenzsystem	MAYO (1961)
Ulna, 8 cm prox. des dist. Gelenkes	♂ 420—580 mg/ml ♀ 420—550 mg/ml	Photometrie, Al-Referenzsystem	DOYLE (1967)
Ulna	♂ 260—400 mg/ml ♀ 300—450 mg/ml	Photometrie, Ca-Referenzsystem	OKUYAMA (1965)
Fingerknochen, Basalphalanx des 3. Fingers	♂ 360—540 mg/ml ♀ 350—450 mg/ml	Silber-Analyse, Knochen-Referenzsystem	VIRTAMA (1957)
Femurhals-Mitte	♂ 280—380 mg/ml ♀ 250—350 mg/ml	Photometrie, Apatit-Referenzsystem	HEUCK und SCHMIDT (1959/60)
Femur-Diaphysen-Mitte	♂ und ♀ 1150 mg/ml	Photometrie, K_2HPO_4-Referenzsystem	HINESS (1968)
Tibia	♂ und ♀ 200—300 mg/ml	Photometrie, Al-Referenzsystem	BJÖRK und LEMPERG (1967)
Calcaneus-Mitte	♂ 220—280 mg/ml ♀ 200—265 mg/ml	Photometrie, Apatit-Referenzsystem	HEUCK und SCHMIDT (1959/60)
Calcaneus	♂ 180 mg/ml (± 38,0 mg/ml) ♀ 175 mg/ml (± 37,0 mg/ml)	Photometrie, Al-Referenzsystem	MAYO (1961)
Calcaneus	♂ 250 mg/ml ♀ 220 mg/ml	Photometrie, differente Strahlenqualitäten	KROKOWSKI (1965)

zur Objektivierung des Knochenschwundes als Ausdruck physiologischer oder pathologischer Prozesse sind bisher noch nicht allgemein erkannt und genutzt worden. Die Erfassung des Apatitgehaltes bei der normalen Altersosteoporose, der Inaktivitätsatrophie des Knochens, einer Osteopathie, einem Sudeck nach Frakturen und bei der Begutachtung kann von großem Wert sein, da es bisher unmöglich war, den Grad einer Änderung der Mineralkonzentration des Knochens objektiv zu bestimmen.

Ein weiteres Anwendungsgebiet der radiologischen Bestimmung der Kalksalzkonzentration von Knochen liegt in der Möglichkeit Untersuchungen durchführen zu können, ohne den Knochen selbst zerstören zu müssen wie es für jede chemisch-analytische Methode Voraussetzung ist. Über den Rahmen der klinischen Radiologie hinaus dürften derartige Untersuchungen auch in der theoretischen und experimentellen Medizin, der Anatomie, der Pathologie, der Gerichtsmedizin, der Anthroprologie und der Veterinärmedizin von Interesse sein.

Literatur

Adachi, T., and T. Okuyama: A study of the quantitative analysis on the mineral contents of the bone by X-rays. Bull. Tokyo med. dent. Univ. **13**, 349—367 (1966).

Adams, P. H., G. T. Davies, J. Kilpatrick, and P. Sweetman: Barnett-Nordin-index: Observer error study. Symposium Ossium, London 1968 (im Druck).

Albright, F., and E. C. Reifenstein: The parathyroid glands and metabolic bone diseases. Baltimore: Williams & Wilkins Co. 1948.

Anderson, J. B., J. Shimmins, and D. A. Smith: A new technique for the measurement of metacarpal density. Brit. J. Radiol. **39**, 443—450 (1966).

Anderson, W. D. A.: Renal lesion in hyperparathyroidism. Endocrinology **24**, 272—378 (1939).

Ardran, G. M.: Bone destruction non demonstrable by radiography. Brit. J. Radiol. **24**, 107—109 (1951).

Arnold, J. S.: External and trabecular morphologic changes in lumbar vertebrae in aging. Conference on Progress in Methods of Bone Mineral Measurements, Bethesda, Maryland 1968 (im Druck).

—, and M. H. Bartley: Rates of involution of vertebrae and femur in aging. In: Progress in development of methods in bone densitometry. Conference in Washington D.C. 1965, p. 149. NASA, Sci. Techn. Inf. Div. Washington D.C. 1966.

Atkinson, P. J., J. A. Weatherell, and S. M. Weidmann: Changes in density of the human femoral cortex with age. J. Bone Jt Surg. B **44**, 496—502 (1962).

Baastrup, C. I.: The acute bone atrophy and its roentgen picture. Acta radiol. (Stockh.) 364 (1923).

Babaiantz, L.: Les ostèoporoses. Radiol. clin. (Basel) **16**, 291—322 (1947).

Babcock, S. W., and J. Montilla: Quantitation of bone mineral measurement in the domestic hen. In: Progress in development of methods on bone densitometry. Washington D.C. 1965, p. 95—102. NASA, Sci. Techn. Inf. Div. Washington D.C. 1966.

Baker, P. T., J. L. Angel, M. A. Little, and R. B. Mazess: Studies on bone density: Age, sex, race, altitude and nutritional factors. Department of Sociology and Anthroprology, The Pennsylvania State University, University Park, Pa. Privately printed 1964.

—, and H. Schraer: The estimation of dry skeletal weight by photometry of roentgenograms. Hum. Biol. **30**, 171—184 (1958).

Baker, S. L., E. C. Butterworth, and F. A. Langley: The calcium- and nitrogen-content of human bone tissue. Cleaned by Microdissection. Biochem. J. **40**, 391—396 (1946).

Balz, G.: Beurteilung des Mineralgehaltes im Knochen ohne photometrische Messung. Symposium Ossium, London 1968 (im Druck).

—, u. R. Birkner: Die Bestimmung des Aluminiumschwächungsgleichwertes von Knochengewebe am Lebenden. Strahlentherapie **99**, 221—227 (1956).

— — u. J. M. Schmitt-Rohde: Über die calcipenischen Osteopathien und ihre Diagnostik mit Hilfe eines besonderen Röntgenverfahrens. Ärztl. Wschr. **12**, 209—213, 233—237 (1957).

— — u. F. Wachsmann: Experimentelle Untersuchungen über die Absorption von Röntgenstrahlen in verschiedenen Geweben. Strahlentherapie **97**, 382—388 (1959).

Barkla, C. G., and G. H. Martyn: The photographic effects of X-rays and X-ray-spectra. Phil. Mag. **25**, 296—300 (1913).

Barnett, E., and B. E. C. Nordin: The radiological diagnosis of osteoporosis: A new approach. Clin. Radiol. **11**, 166—174 (1960).

— — Radiological assessment of bone density. Brit. J. Radiol. **34**, 683—692 (1961).

Bartelheimer, H.: Formen und Entstehungsbedingungen der Entkalkungsosteopathien. Ärztl. Wschr. **6**, 606—614 (1951).

— Mineralhaushalt und Knochen, Klinik. Fortschr. Röntgenstr. **86**, Beih. 39, 59—66 (1957).

Baud, Ch.-A.: Radiographies et microradiographies osseuses quantitatives. Rev. suisse Méd. **46**, 329—331 (1957).

Beaulieu, M., H. Brasseur, M. J. Dallemagne et J. Melon: Critique des methodes de mineralisation de l'os. Arch. int. Physiol. **57**, 411—418 (1949/50).

Béhar, M., Ch. Rohmann, D. Wilson, F. Viteri, and St. M. Garn: Osseous development in children with kwashiorkor. Fed. Proc. **24**, 338 (1964).

Bernard, J., et M. Laval-Jeantet: L'épaisseur relative de la corticale du tibia, application à l'évaluation des ostéoporoses et des ostéoscleroses. Presse méd. **68**, 889—892 (1960).

Bismuth, V.: La densimétrie de l'os par les rayons x. Presse méd. **67**, 1933—1936 (1959).

Björk, L.: Radiographic determination of the bone mineral content in osteoporosis. Acta radiol. (Stockh.) **3**, 218—224 (1965).

—, and R. Lemperg: Radiographic determination of the bone mineral content in amputation stumps. Acta radiol. (Stockh.) **6**, 575—578 (1967).

Björn, H., C.-O. Henrikson u. K.-A. Omnell: Registrering av Röntgentäthen hod det periapikala Benet. Svensk tandläk.-T. **2**, 115—118 (1951).

Breitling, G., u. K.-H. Vogel: Dosisverteilung bei der Bestrahlung inhomogener Medien mit schnellen Elektronen. Strahlentherapie **122**, 321—340 (1963).

Brown, W. N.: Bone density computing machine. Proc. Electronics Conf. **5**, 64 (1949).

—, and W. B. Birtley: A densitometer which records directly in units of emulsion exposure. Rev. Sci. Instr. **22**, 67—72 (1951).

Bunsen, R., and H. E. Roscoe: Photo-chemical researches. V. On the direct measurement of the chemical action of sunlight. Phil. Trans. B **153**, 139—160 (1863).

Bugyi, B.: Über Altersabhängigkeit des kortikalen Index des 2. Metakarpalknochens. Anat. Anz. **116**, 378—383 (1965).

Bywaters, E. G. L.: The measurement of bone opacity. Clin. Sci. **6**, 281—287 (1948).

Caldwell, R. A., and D. H. Collins: Assessment of vertebral osteoporosis by radiographic and chemical methods post-mortem. J. Bone Jt Surg. B **43**, 346—361 (1961).

Cameron, J., and J. A. Sorenson: Measurement of bone mineral by the direct photon absorption method: Principles and instrumentation. Conference on Progress in Methods of Bone Mineral Measurements, Bethesda, Maryland 1968 (im Druck).

Cameron, J. R., R. Grant, and R. MacGregor: An improved technic for the measurement of bone mineral content in vivo. Radiology **78**, 117 (1962).

— R. B. Mazess, and J. A. Sorenson: Precision and accuracy of bone mineral determination by direct photon absorptiometry. Invest. Radiol. **3**, 141—150 (1968).

—, and J. A. Sorenson: Bone mineral measurement by improved photon absorption technique. In: Progress in development of methods on bone densitometry, Washington D.C. 1965, p. 87—92. NASA, Sci. Techn. Inf. Div. Washington D.C. 1966.

Chaumont, P., M. Laval-Jeantet, J. Lefebvre et N. Balmain: A propos des causes d'erreur en densitometrie osseuse. Symposium Ossium, London 1968 (im Druck).

Cignolini, P.: Nuova tecnica per la radiodensimetria dello scheletro. Radiol. pract. **10**, 3—8 (1960).

Cobb, S.: Zit. nach Virtama 1951.

Cohen, M. J., and A. J. Gilson: Precision methods using soft penetration radiation for bone densitometry. In: Progress in development of methods on bone densitometry, Washington D.C. 1965, p. 103—112. NASA, Sci. Techn. Inf. Div. Washington D.C. 1966.

Colbert, Ch.: Bone mineral measurement from X-ray images. Conference on Progress in Methods of Bone Mineral Measurements, Bethesda, Maryland 1968 (im Druck).

Cooke, A. M.: Osteoporosis. Lancet **1955 I**, 877, 929.

Coryn, G.: Introduction. A l'étude des affections endocriniennes du squelette. Presse méd. **1937**, 90, 93, 103, 611.

Davis, M. E., N. M. Strandjord, and L. H. Lanzl: Estrogens and the aging process. J. Amer. med. Ass. **196**, 219—224 (1966).

Deák, P., R. Tarján u. E. Sándi: Über die röntgenphotometrische Registrierung von Veränderungen der Knochenstruktur. Magy. Radiol. **5**, 97—101 (1953).

Deitrick, J. E., G. D. Whedon, and E. Shorr: The effects of immobilization upon various metabolic and physiologic functions of normal man. Amer. J. Med. **4**, 3—36 (1948).

Dennis: Zit. nach Mack, zit. nach Vose. 1897.

Does, J. J. de, E. Gorter u. W. A. Seeder: Een objektieve methode om in vivo het kalkgehalte van het beenstelsel te bepalen in het bijzonder bij rachitis. Ned. T. Geneesk. **77**, 25—31 (1933).

Doyle, F. H.: Ulnar mineral concentration in metabolic bone diseases. Brit. J. Radiol. **34**, 698—712 (1961).

— The measurement of the mineral content of living bones. Proc. roy. Soc. Med. **58**, 165—166 (1965).

— Quantitative bone changes in hyperparathyroidism. J. Physiol. (Lond.) **184**, 61—64 (1966).

— Radiological findings in hyperparathyroidism. Some quantitative observations. In: Progress in radiology. XI. Int. Congr. Radiol. 1965, vol. I, p. 492—497 Amsterdam, Excerpta Med., Int. Congr. Ser. No 105, 1967.

— Some quantitative radiological observations in primary and secondary hyperparathyroidism. Brit. J. Radiol. **39**, 161—167 (1966).

— Radiological assessment of endocrine effects on bone. Radiol. Clin. N. Amer. **5**, 289—302 (1967).

— Age-related bone changes in women. Conference on Progress in Methods of Bone Mineral Measurement, Bethesda, Maryland 1968 (im Druck).

DUBOULOZ, P., J. LEGRÉ, R. MERJANIAN et G. SERRATRICE: Étude radiologique et valeur statistique des corps vertébraux lombaires à tendance cunéiforme. J. Radiol. Électrol. **42**, 629—641 (1961).

EBERT, H. G.: Bringt die Kontrastverstärkung von Röntgenfilmen praktischen Nutzen? Fortschr. Röntgenstr. **87**, 530—536 (1957).

EDHOLM, P., and B. JACOBSON: Quantitative determination of iodine in vivo. Acta radiol. (Stockh.) **52**, 337—346 (1959).

ENDTZ, A. W.: Een Methode om in vivo het kalkgehalte van het Beenstelsel te Bepalen. Leiden, Holland: N. V. Boek — en Steendrukkerij Eduard Ijdo 1934.

ENGSTRÖM, A.: Quantitative micro- and histological elementary analysis by roentgen absorption spectrography. Acta radiol. (Stockh.), Suppl. **63**, (1946).

— L. WEGSTEDT, and S. WELIN: A simple portable densitometer. Acta radiol. (Stockh.) **30**, 440—442 (1948).

—, and S. WELIN: A method for the quantitative roentgenological determination of the amount of calcium salts in bone tissue. Acta radiol. (Stockh.) **31**, 483—502 (1949).

EVANS, F. G., C. C. COOLBAUGH, and M. LEBOW: An apparatus for determining bone density by means of S^{90}. Science **114**, 182—185 (1951).

EVENS, R. G., CH. Y. C. PAK, F. C. BARTTER, and W. ASHBURN: Clinical application of in vivo measurement of bone mineral content by a photon absorption method. Conference on Progress in Methods of Bone Mineral Measurements, Bethesda, Maryland 1968 (im Druck).

EZOP, J. J., and T. G. STINCHCOMB: Design and applications of β-excited X-ray sources. In: Progress in development of methods on bone densitometry. Washington D.C. 1965, p. 127—136. NASA, Sci. Techn. Inf. Div. Washington D.C. 1966.

FANUCCI, A., e A. LOASSES: Le alterazoini fondamentali dello scheletro nella moderna radiologia clinica. Nunt. radiol. (Roma) **24**, 753—800 (1958).

— — Metodo per l'obiettivazione radiologica dell'osteoporosi. Nunt. radiol. (Firenze) **28**, 439—449 (1962).

FISCHER, E., u. D. HAUSSER: Die Kompaktadicke der Rippe und des Schlüsselbeines bei Erwachsenen und der Einfluß demineralisierender Erkrankungen (1969, im Druck).

FORNI, I.: Presentazione di un fotometro a cellula fotoelettrica per diafanometria radiografica. Atti 35. Congr. S.I.O.T. 1951, p. 278.

FOURMAN, P.: Calcium metabolism and bone. Oxford: Blackwell 1960.

FOWLER, J. F.: Absorbed dose near bone: A conductivity method of measurement. Brit. J. Radiol. **30**, 361—366 (1957).

FRASER R., The problem of osteoporosis. Critical review. J. Bone Jt Surg. B **44**, 485—495 (1962).

FRERCKS, J.: Vergleichende chemisch-analytische Untersuchungen des spongiösen und kompakten Knochens aus fünf verschiedenen Skeletbezirken. Diss. Kiel 1968.

FRERCKS, J., u. F. HEUCK: (In Vorbereitung.)

FREY, K. W.: Untersuchungen über das Verhalten von Röntgenfilmen in mehreren handelsüblichen Röntgenentwicklern. Fortschr. Röntgenstr. **87**, 378—383 (1957).

FREYBURG, G.: Die radiologische Bestimmung der Knochendichte bei Frakturen und Distorsionen des Unterarmgebietes zwecks frühzeitiger Erfassung von Knochenatrophien. Diss. Freie Universität Berlin 1958.

FROMMHOLD, W.: Verstärkerfolie und Bildgüte. Untersuchungen an deutschen Folienfabrikaten. Fortschr. Röntgenstr. **84**, 719—740 (1956).

—, u. G. SCHOKNECHT: Untersuchungen über die Absorption und Feinstruktur von Knochen mittels monochromatischer Röntgenstrahlung. Fortschr. Röntgenstr. **93**, 358—366 (1960).

FUSI, G.: Tentativi di fotometria della densita radiografica scheletrica. Radiol. med. (Torino) **38**, 261—272 (1952).

— Saggio sperimentale sulle prime manifestazioni radiologiche di osteoporosi. Radiol. clin. (Basel) **22**, 123—129 (1953).

GABRIEL, S.: Chemische Untersuchungen über die Mineralstoffe der Knochen und Zähne. Hoppe-Seylers Z. physiol. Chem. **18**, 257—303 (1894).

GARN, ST. M.: An annotated bibliography on bone densitometry. Amer. J. clin. Nutr. **10**, 59—67 (1962).

— Dynamics of change at the enosteal surface of tubular bones. Conference on Progress in Methods of Bone Mineral Measurements, Bethesda, Maryland 1958 (im Druck).

— CH. ROHMANN, and P. NOLAN JR.: Studies on the development of compact bone in normal individuals and in endocrine and nutritional abnormalities. Department of Growth and Genetics, Fels Research Institute, Yellow Springs, Ohio. Privately printed 1963.

— M. BÉHAR, CH. ROHMANN, F. VITERI, and D. WILSON: Catch-up bone development during treatment of kwashiorkor. Fed. Proc. **24**, 1424 (1964).

— E. FEUTZ, C. COLBERT, and B. WAGNER: Comparison of cortical thickness and radiographic microdensitometry in the measurement of bone loss. In: Progress in development of methods on bone densitometry. Washington D.C. 1965, p. 65—75. NASA, Sci. Techn. Inf. Div. Washington D.C. 1966.

— E. N. PAO, and M. E. RIHL: Compact bone in Chinese and Japanese. Science **143**, 1439—1440 (1964).

—, and CH. ROHMANN: Interaction of nutrition and genetics in the timing of growth and development. Pediat. Clin. N. Amer. **13**, 353—379 (1966).

— — M. BÉHAR, F. VITERI, and M. A. GUZMÁN: Compact bone deficiency in protein-calorie malnutrition. Science **145**, 1444—1445 (1964).

GARN, ST. M., CH. ROHMANN, and M. A. GUZMÁN: Malnutrition and skeletal development in the pre-school child. Pre-school child malnutrition. National Academy of Sciences Washington D.C. 1968, p. 43—62.

— —, and P. NOLAN: The development nature of bone changes during aging. In: Relations of development and aging (ed. JAMES E. BIRREN), p. 41—61. Springfield (Ill.): Ch. C. Thomas 1964.

— — E. M. PAO, and E. I. HULL: Normal "osteoporotic" bone loss. In: Progress in development of methods in bone densitometry. Conference in Washington D. C. 1965, p. 187. NASA, Sci. Tech. Inf. Div. Washington D. C. 1966.

— —, and B. WAGNER: Bone loss as a general phenomenon in man. Fed. Proc. **26**, 1729—1736 (1967).

— — —, and W. ASCOLI: Continuing bone growth throughout life: A general phenomenon. Amer. J. Phys. Anthrop. **26**, 313—317 (1967).

GERSHON-COHEN, J., N. H. CHERRY, and M. BOEHNKE: Bone density studies with a gamma gage. Radiat. Res. **8**, 509—515 (1958).

—, and J. F. MCCLENDON: Roentgenographic studies of osteoporosis. I. Replacement of common salt by a balanced salt diet of rats. Radiology **61**, 261—265 (1953).

— A. M. RECHTMAN, H. SCHRAER, and N. BLUMBERG: Asymptomatic fractures in osteoporotic spines of the aged. J. Amer. med. Ass. **153**, 625—627 (1953).

— H. SCHRAER, and N. BLUMBERG: Bone density measurements of osteoporosis in the aged. Radiology **65**, 416—419 (1955).

GLOCKER, R., u. E. MACHERAUCH: Röntgen- und Kernphysik für Mediziner und Biophysiker. Stuttgart: Georg Thieme 1965.

GOLL, K. H., u. W. DÖPKE: Über den Kalziumgehalt des Knochens. Z. ges. inn. Med. **16**, 1019—1023 (1961).

GOODMAN, L. S., and B. LEVIN: In vivo measurement of the mineral content of a section of the radius. Conference on Progress in Methods of Bone Mineral Measurements, Bethesda, Maryland 1968 (im Druck).

GOULD, D. M.: Generalized decreased bone density. Amer. J. med. Sci. **223**, 569—580 (1952).

GUZMÁN, M. A., CH. ROHMANN, M. FLORES, ST. M. GARN, and N. S. SHRIMSHAW: Osseous growth of Guatemalan children fed a protein-calorie supplement. Fed. Proc. **24**, 338 (1964).

GYÖRGYI, G., u. L. BOZÓKY: Der lineare Schwächungskoeffizient als ein Maßstab des Mineralgehaltes der Knochen. Fortschr. Röntgenstr. **94**, 667—672 (1961).

HAAS, H. G.: Die Abklärung von Knochenkrankheiten. Internist (Berl.) **7**, 558—564 (1966).

HAASNER, E., E. KROKOWSKI u. K. RACH: Normalwerte des Hydroxylapatitgehaltes im Skelet in Abhängigkeit von Lokalisation, Lebensalter und Geschlecht. Klin. Wschr. **45**, 575—578 (1967).

HALL, M. C.: The trabecular pattern of the neck of the femur with particular reference to changes in osteoporosis. Canad. med. Ass. J. **85**, 1141—1144 (1961).

—, and M. ROSSER: The structure of the upper end of the humerus with reference to osteoporotic changes in senescence leading to fractures. Canad. med. Ass. J. **88**, 290—294 (1963).

HANSEN, H. G.: Zur Anwendung anabol wirksamer Steroide bei Kindern. Mschr. Kinderheilk. **110**, 236—240 (1962).

— Zur Wirkung anaboler Steroide auf das Skeletsystem mit besonderer Berücksichtigung der Mineralisation. Kolloquium „Wirkung und Anwendung anaboler Steroide", Schering AG Berlin 1963. Berlin: Medicus-Verlag 1964, S. 277—281.

—, u. R. v. PATAY: Persönliche Mitteilung 1961.

HAUSSER, D.: Die Kompaktadicke der Rippe und des Schlüsselbeines als Index für den Mineralgehalt des Skelets (röntgenologische Untersuchungen am Lebenden). Diss. Tübingen 1967.

HELELÄ, T., and P. VIRTAMA: Cortical thickness of long bones as an estimate of mineral content. Symposium Ossium, London 1968 (im Druck).

— — Bone density of the ulna. Invest. Radiol. **3**, 103—107 (1968).

HENNY, G. C.: An instrument for measuring the density of roentgen films. Amer. J. Roentgenol. **31**, 550—554 (1934).

— Roentgenographic estimation of the mineral content of bone. Radiology **54**, 202—210 (1950).

HEUCK, F.: Der röntgenologische Nachweis generalisierter Osteopathien. Internist (Berl.) **3**, 252—267 (1962).

— Röntgenologische, historadiographische und chemisch-analytische Untersuchungen der Konzentration und Verteilung der Kalksalze im gesunden und kranken Knochen. Radiol. Austr. **14**, 29—56 (1963).

— Beurteilung des Kalksalzgehaltes der Knochen bei Osteopathien, Schering-Koll. Berlin 1963. Berlin: Medicus-Verlag 1964, S. 113—119.

— Ergebnisse chemisch-analytischer und historadiographischer Untersuchungen der Knochenkalksalze bei Osteopathien. Verh. Dtsch. Path. 47. Tgg 1963. Stuttgart: Gustav Fischer 1963, S. 182—186.

— Die Messung des Kalksalzgehaltes im Knochen bei Osteopathien. Med. Klin. **60**, 954—959 (1965).

— Radiologische Aspekte der Osteoporose. Dtsch. med. Wschr. **92**, 2272—2277 (1967).

— Der Knochen bei gastrointestinalen Erkrankungen. In: BARTELHEIMER u. HEISIG, Aktuelle Gastroenterologie, S. 174—190. Stuttgart: Georg Thieme 1968.

— Quantitative measurement of bone mineral content with densitometric methods. 2. Conference on Progress in Methods of Bone Mineral Measurement Febr. 1968 in Bethesda, Maryland USA (im Druck).

Heuck, F.: Results of quantitative measurements of bone mineral in general osteopathies. Symposium Ossium London 1968 (im Druck).

—, u. Ch. Lauritzen: Veränderungen von Mineralgehalt und Struktur des Femur nach gynäkologischer Strahlentherapie. Strahlentherapie **66**, 87—92 (1967).

—, u. E. Schmidt: Röntgenologische und chemisch-analytische Untersuchungen des pathologisch veränderten Knochens. Fortschr. Röntgenstr. **81**, Verhandl.-Bd. 37, 27(1954).

— — Zur Osteoporose bei Diabetes mellitus. Verh. dtsch. Ges. inn. Med. **62**, 464—467 (1956).

— — Mikroradiographische und chemische Untersuchungen des Knochens bei chronischen Lebererkrankungen. Fortschr. Röntgenstr. **90**, Verhandl.-Bd. 41, 87 (1959).

— — Neue Erkenntnisse über die Zusammensetzung der Knochensalze und ihre direkte Bestimmung in der Volumeneinheit Knochengewebe. IX. Int. Congr. Radiol. 1959 München, Vortrag 306.

— — Die quantitative Bestimmung des Mineralgehaltes der Knochen aus dem Röntgenbild. Fortschr. Röntgenstr. **93**, 523—554 (1960).

— — Die praktische Anwendung einer Methode zur quantitativen Bestimmung des Kalksalzgehaltes gesunder und kranker Knochen. Fortschr. Röntgenstr. **93**, 761—783 (1960).

Hiness, R.: Untersuchungen zur Mineralgehaltsbestimmung von Knochen. Diss. Tübingen 1968.

Hioco, D.: Physiopathologie und Therapie der Osteoporose. Dtsch. med. Wschr. **91**, 1079—1083 (1966).

Hodge, H. C., W. F. Bale, S. L. Warren, and G. van Huysen: Factors influencing the quantitative measurement of the roentgenray absorption of tooth slabs. IV. Absorption coefficient factors. Amer. J. Roentgenol. **34**, 817—838 (1935).

— G. van Huysen, and S. L. Warren: Factors influencing the quantitative measurement of the roentgenray absorption of tooth slabs. I. Radiation factors. Amer. J. Roentgenol. **34**, 523—528 (1935).

— — — Factors influencing the quantitative measurement of the roentgenray absorption of tooth slabs. II. Filter factors. Amer. J. Roentgenol. **34**, 529—538 (1935).

— — — Factors influencing the quantitative measurement of the roentgenray absorption of tooth slabs. X. Tissue factors. Amer. J. Roentgenol. **40**, 269—282 (1938).

—, and S. L. Warren: Factors influencing the quantitative measurement of the roentgenray absorption of tooth slabs. V. Theory of the step tablet. Amer. J. Roentgenol. **36**, 391—407 (1936).

— R. B. Wilsey, G. van Huysen, and S. L. Warren: Factors influencing the quantitative measurement of the roentgenray absorption of tooth slabs. VII. Densitometric factors. Amer. J. Roentgenol. **37**, 385—403 (1937).

Hodkinson, H. M., A. N. Exton-Smith, and M. F. Crowley: Diagnosis and assessment of osteoporosis. Postgrad. med. J. **39**, 433—437 (1963).

Hölscher, W.: Die radiologische Bestimmung der Knochendichte zwecks Kontrolle therapeutischer Maßnahmen bei internistischen Erkrankungen des Knochensystems. Diss. Freie Universität Berlin 1958.

Hoffmann, G.: Alters- und physiologische Schwankungen des Mineralgehaltes im Knochen. Berl. Med. **13**, 366—367 (1962).

— Deutung der Kalziumverteilung im Skelet aus Statik und Abstammung. Z. ärztl. Fortbild. **56** (1967).

—, u. G. Fabian: Der Mineralgehalt des Skelets beim Menschen und bei der Katze, eine vergleichende röntgenologische Betrachtung. Forsch. Praxis, Fortbild. (Berl.) **17**, 351—353 (1966).

Hopsu, V. K., P. Kajanoja, A. Telkkä, and P. Virtama: The density of some small bones of human extremities with special reference to the reliability of volume measurement methods. Anat. Anz. **109**, 247—254 (1961).

Hurter, F., and V. C. Driffield: J. Soc. chem. Ind. **9**, 455 (1890).

Imig, H.: Vereinfachung der quantitativen Absorptionsmessung zur Calciumbestimmung im menschlichen Skeletsystem. Diss. Freie Universität Berlin 1966.

Ingalls, N. W.: Observations on bone weights. Amer. J. Anat. **48**, 45—98 (1931).

Jackson, H.: Problems in the measurement of bone density. Brit. J. Radiol. **24**, 613—616 (1951).

Jacobson, B.: An image transforming scanning photometer for displaying small density gradients. Acta radiol. (Stockh.) **48**, 376—384 (1957).

— X-ray spectrophotometry in vivo. Amer. J. Roentgenol. **91**, 202—210 (1964).

—, and B. Lindberg: X-ray spectrophotometer for simultaneous analysis of several elements. Rev. Sci. Instr. **35**, 1316—1319 (1964).

Jaeger, R. G.: Dosimetrie und Strahlenschutz, physikalische und technische Daten. Stuttgart: Georg Thieme 1959.

Johns, H. E.: The physics of radiation therapy. Canada 1953 (zit. nach Krokowski).

Johnston, C. C.: Measurement of bone mass in the radius. Conference on Progress in Methods of Bone Mineral Measurements, Bethesda, Maryland 1968 (im Druck).

Jowsey, J.: Mineral density in normal and osteoporotic bone. Conference on Progress in Methods of Bone Mineral Measurements, Bethesda, Maryland 1968 (im Druck).

Joyet, G., C. Trümpy-Eggenberger u. W. Mauderli: Das Brown-Boveri-Betatron 1953, S. 36. Zit. nach Krokowski 1959.

Julkunen, H.: Rheumatoid spondylitis. Acta rheum. scand., Suppl. **4**, (1962).

JURIST, J. M.: Ulnar vibrating properties. Conference on Progress in Methods of Bone Mineral Measurements, Bethesda, Maryland 1968 (im Druck).
KÁLLAI, L., u. R. TARJÁN: Zusammenhang der Knochenfestigkeit mit dem in vivo gemessenen röntgendensitometrischen Äquivalent. Kisérl. Orvostud. **15**, 25—28 (1963).
— — The in vivo determination of bone apatite and bone density by X-ray densitometry. Acta vet. Acad. Sci. hung. **13**, 311—322 (1963).
KEANE, B. E., G. SPIEGLER, and R. DAVIS: Quantitative evaluation of bone mineral by a radiographic method. Brit. J. Radiol. **32**, 162—167 (1959).
KELLGREN, J. H., and F. BIER: Radiological signs of rheumatoid arthritis. Ann. rheum. Dis. **15**, 55—60 (1956).
KESSON, C. M., N. MORRIS, and N. MCCUTCHEON: Generalized osteoporosis in old age. Ann. rheum. Dis. **6**, 146—161 (1947).
KIEFFER, J., and R. M. SEIDEMAN: Photographic measurement of radiation quality and quantity. Science **104**, 596—600 (1946).
KIVILAAKSO, E., and E. PALOLAMPI: On the density of the ulna and on the relationship between density and cortical thickness. Acta anat. (Basel) **60**, 325—331 (1965).
KLAPPER, E. A., and P. B. MACK: Regression curves for representative urinary calcium and bone mass values. In: Progress in development of methods in bone densitometry. Conf. in Washington D.C. 1965, p. 179. NASA, Sci. Tech. Inf. Div. Washington D.C. 1966.
KLEMENT, R.: Die Zusammensetzung der Knochenstützsubstanz. Hoppe-Seylers Z. physiol. Chem. **184**, 131—142 (1929).
— Die anorganische Skeletsubstanz. Ihre Zusammensetzung, natürliche und künstliche Bildung. Naturwissenschaften **26**, 145—152 (1938).
KNESE, K.-H.: Knochenstruktur als Verbundbau. In: Zwanglose Abhandlungen auf dem Gebiet der normalen und pathologischen Anatomie, H. 4. Stuttgart: Georg Thieme 1958.
— Eine Erörterung neuerer Untersuchungen über die Bedeutung der Spongiosaarchitektur. Homo, Suppl. **2**, 172—178 (1959).
— Die Ultrastruktur des Knochengewebes. Dtsch. med. Wschr. **84**, 1640—1644 (1959).
— Neuere Untersuchungen über die Knochenbildung und ihre Beeinflussungsmöglichkeiten. Dtsch. zahnärztl. Z. **14**, 925—932 (1959).
— I. RITSCHL u. D. VOGES: Quantitative Untersuchungen der Osteonverteilung im Extremitätenskelet eines 43jährigen Mannes. Z. Zellforsch. **40**, 519—570 (1954).
KNUTSSON, F.: A qualitative comparison between the standard type of examination and tomography for certain intraosseous structural changes. Brit. J. Radiol. **26**, 113—121 (1953).
KROKOWSKI, E.: Die Absorption von Röntgenstrahlen im Knochen. Fortschr. Röntgenstr. **91**, 76—84 (1959).
KROKOWSKI, E.: Die typische Radiusfraktur. Schweiz. med. Wschr. **92**, 1120—1122 (1962).
— Die Substanzanalyse in der Röntgendiagnostik. Röntgenhinweise **9**, 16—19 (1963).
— Zur quantitativen Beurteilung von osteoporotischen und traumatischen Wirbelfrakturen. Z. ärztl. Fortbild. **52**, 413—415 (1963).
— Quantitative Verlaufsbeobachtung der Kalziumveränderung im Knochen mittels röntgenologischer Substanzanalyse. Fortschr. Röntgenstr. **100**, 359—366 (1964).
— Osteoporoseschmerz und Röntgenbefund. Dtsch. med. J. **16**, 393—395 (1965).
— Quantitative röntgenologische Bestimmung des Skelet-Calciumgehaltes. Verh. dtsch. Ges. inn. Med. **71**, 607—613 (1965).
— Röntgenologische Analysetechnik zur Bestimmung des Calciumgehaltes im Knochen. Medizinalmarkt **9**, 424—429 (1965).
— Die quantitative Bewertung der Osteoporose. Z. Orthop. **101**, 269—273 (1966).
— Möglichkeiten zur Bestimmung des Skelet-Calciumgehaltes in der Klinik. Dtsch. med. Wschr. **91**, 60—66 (1966).
— Kritische Bemerkungen zum Begriff der postmenopausischen Osteoporose. Geburtsh. u. Frauenheilk. **26**, 968—972 (1966).
— Physiopathologie und Therapie der Osteoporose. Dtsch. med. Wschr. **91**, 2230—2231 (1966).
— Die röntgenologische Bestimmung des Knochencalciums und Mikroradiographie. Med. Mitt. Melsungen **40**, 69—78 (1966).
— Definition und Bestimmung der Osteoporose. Münch. med. Wschr. **108**, 1288—1290 (1966).
— Moderne Fragen der röntgenologischen Skeletdiagnostik. Röntgenstrahlen **15**, 46—49 (1966).
— Frühdiagnose und Verlauf der Osteoporose. Münch. med. Wschr. **109**, 1981—1984 (1967).
—, u. E. HAASNER: Die Osteoporose in heutiger Sicht. Kurz und Gut **1**, 2—4 (1967).
— — Aktuelle Bedeutung der quantitativen Bestimmung des Skelet-Calciumgehaltes. Wehrmed. Mschr. **12**, 229—232 (1968).
— — Analyse und Auswertung der Osteoporosetherapie. Med. Klin. **63**, 1097—1101 (1968).
— P. SCHAEFER, I. FALCK u. P. KOEPPE: Quantitative Untersuchungen zur Calciumtherapie der Osteoporose. Med. Klin. **36**, 1394—1396 (1967).
—, u. W. SCHLUNGBAUM: Die Objektivierung der röntgenologischen Diagnose „Osteoporose“. Fortschr. Röntgenstr. **91**, 740—746 (1959).
—, u. D. STEINER: Röntgenologische Bestimmung des Kalziumgehaltes im menschlichen Skelet. Med. Klin. **56**, 2073—2076 (1961).
—, u. E. STRESEMANN: Röntgenologische Bestimmung des Mineralisationsgrades der Wirbelsäule von Kranken mit chronischem Bronchialasthma. Klin. Wschr. **45**, 370—373 (1967).
KUHLENCORDT, F., H.-P. KRUSE, C. LOZANO-TONKIN, H. WIENERS u. H. BARTELHEIMER: Vergleichende röntgenologische und morphometrische Untersuchungen bei der Osteoporose. Klin. Wschr. **45**, 1020—1023 (1967).

LACHMAN, E.: Osteoporosis: The potentialities and limitations of its roentgenologic diagnosis. Amer. J. Roentgenol. **74**, 712—715 (1955).
—, and M. WHELAN: The roentgen diagnosis of osteoporosis and its limitations. Radiology **25**, 165 (1935).
LAITINEN, H., M. VIRKKUNEN, and P. VIRTAMA: Demineralization of the finger bones in rheumatoid arthritis. Acta rheum. scand. **4**, 266—275 (1958).
LANDOFF, G. A.: Experimentelle Untersuchungen über die Knochenatrophie infolge einer Immobilisation und einer akuten Arthritis. Acta chir. scand., Suppl. **71** (1942).
LANZL, L. H., and N. STRANDJORD: Radioisotopic device for measuring bone mineral. Proceedings of Symposium on Low-Energy-X- and Gamma-Sources and Applications held at Illinois Institute of Technology Research Institute Chicago (Ill.) 1964, p. 257—276.
LAUGHLIN, J. S.: X-ray energy measurements. Atomics **3**, 54 (1952).
LEFEBVRE, J., V. BISMUTH et P. CHAUMONT: La densitométrie de l'os chez l'enfant. J. Radiol. Électrol. **45**, 11—16 (1964).
LOBODZIEC, W., and B. LUBAS: Influence of transverse dimensions of bone on roentgen dose distribution for different qualities of primary radiation. Acta radiol. (Stockh.) **4**, 471—480 (1966).
MAASS, K.: Untersuchungen zur röntgenologischen Diagnose der osteogenen Systemerkrankungen und Beschreibung einer Methode zur feineren Beurteilung des Kalkgehaltes der Knochen im Röntgenbild. Diss. Kiel 1951.
MACK, P. B.: Results from study of bone density in appraisal of calcium status. Milbank Memorial Fund 1950, p. 30—63.
— Electronic densitometer as a means of assessing bone density. Yearbook Physiol. Anthrop. **8**, 315 (1952).
— Radiographic bone densitometry. In: Progress in development of methods on bone densitometry, Washington D.C. 1965, p. 31—46. NASA, Sci. Techn. Inf. Div. Washington D.C. 1966.
— Calcium loss studies during human bed rest: A preliminary report. Progress in development of methods in bone densitometry. Conference in Washington D.C. 1965, p. 169. NASA Sci. Techn. Inf. Div. Washington D.C. 1966.
— W. N. BROWN, and H. D. TRAPP: The quantitative evaluation of bone density. Amer. J. Roentgenol. **61**, 808—825 (1949).
— P. A. LA CHANCE, G. P. VOSE, and F. B. VOGT: Bone demineralization of foot and hand of gemini-titan IV, V and VII astronauts during orbital flight. Amer. J. Roentgenol. **100**, 503—511 (1967).
— A. T. O'BRIEN, J. M. SMITH, and A. W. BAUMAN: A method for estimating the degree of mineralization of bones from tracings of roentgenograms. Science **89**, 467 (1939).
MACK, P. B., and F. B. VOGT: Assessment of bone mass by roentgenographic density techniques. Conference on Progress in Methods of Bone Mineral Measurement Bethesda, Maryland 1968 (im Druck).
— G. P. VOSE, and J. D. NELSON: New development in equipment for the roentgenographic measurement of bone density. Amer. J. Roentgenol. **82**, 303—310 (1959).
MÄNTYLÄ, M., A. TELKKÄ, C. WEGELIUS, and P. VIRTAMA: Teeth as indicators of bone density. Acta odont. scand. **22**, 365—371 (1964).
MAINLAND, D.: Elementary medical statics. The principles of quantitative medicine. Philadelphia: W. B. Saunders Co. 1952.
— Measurement of bone density. Ann. rheu. Dis. **15**, 115—118 (1956).
— A study of age differences in the X-ray density of the adult human calcaneus. J. Geront. **12**, 53—61 (1957).
— A study of age differences in the X-ray density of five bones in the adult human wrist and hand. J. Geront. **12**, 284—291 (1957).
—, and L. HERRERA: Clinical surveys. In: J. M. STEELE (ed.), Methods in medical research, vol. 6, p. 159—171. Chicago: Year Book Publ. 1954.
MARCHAL, M.: Le microdensigramme osseux chez l'homme et l'évaluation pondérale du calcium osseux par les rayons x. C. R. Acad. Sci. (Paris) **226**, 526—528 (1948).
MAROTTA, U.: Metodo roentgenografico per il dosaggio del calcio nell'osso. R. C. Ist. sup. Sanità **18**, 463—487 (1955).
MASON, R. L., and C. RUTHVEN: Bone density measurements in vivo: Improvement of X-ray densitometry. Science **150**, 221—222 (1965).
MATTSSON, O.: Practical photographic problems in radiography. Acta radiol. (Stockh.), Suppl., 120 (1955).
MAYER, E. H., H. G. TROSTLE, E. ACKERMAN, H. SCHRAER, and O. D. SITTLER: A scintillation technique for the X-ray determination of bone mineral content. Radiat. Res. **13**, 156—167 (1960).
MAYO, K. M.: Quantitative measurement of bone mineral content in normal adult bone. Brit. J. Radiol. **34**, 693—698 (1961).
MAZESS, R., J. R. CAMERON, R. O'CONNOR, and D. KNUTZEN: Accuracy of bone mineral measurement. Science **145**, 388—389 (1964).
MAZESS, R. B., J. CAMERON, and J. A. SORENSON: A comparison of radiologic methods for determining bone mineral content. Conference on Progress in Methods of Bone Mineral Measurements, Bethesda, Maryland 1968 (im Druck).
MAZZA, A., e M. VACCHERI: Determinazioni fotometriche della demineralizzazione dei monconi di frattura delle ossa lunghe. Radiother. Radiobiol. Fis. med. **12**, 463—468 (1957).
MCCLENDON, J. F., and J. GERSHON-COHEN: Experimental "senile" osteoporosis. Amer. J. Roentgenol. **82**, 300—306 (1959).

McFarland, W.: Evaluation of bone density from roentgenograms. Science **119**, 810—811 (1954).

Meema, H. E.: The occurence of cortical bone atrophy in old age and osteoporosis. J. Canad. Ass. Radiol. **13**, 27—32 (1962).

— Cortical bone atrophy and osteoporosis as a manifestation of aging. Amer. J. Roentgenol. **89**, 1287—1295 (1963).

— C. K. Harris, and R. E. Porrett: A method for determination of bone-salt content of cortical bone. Radiology **82**, 986—997 (1964).

—, and S. Meema: Measurable roentgenologic changes in some peripheral bones in senile osteoporosis. J. Amer. Geriat. Soc. **11**, 1170—1182 (1963).

— — The interrelationships between cortical bone thickness, mineral mass and mineral density in human radius: A roentgenologic-densitometric study. Conference on Progress in Methods of Bone Mineral Measurements, Bethesda, Maryland 1968 (im Druck).

Mees, C. E. K.: The theory of the photographic process. New York: MacMillan Co. 1954.

Mergler, H.: Über die Beeinflussung der Schwärzung medizinischer Röntgenfilme durch Verarbeitungsbedingungen. Röntgen-Bl. **10**, 170—173 (1957).

Merz, A. L., M. Trotter, and R. R. Peterson: Estimation of skeletal weight in the living. Amer. J. phys. Anthrop. **14**, 589—610 (1956).

Misasi, N., A. Savoia e L. Sorrentino: L'utilizzazione di un metodo roentgen-fotometrico per il dosaggio del calcio nello ossa, nella pratica ortopedica. Clin. ortop. **9**, 113—117 (1957).

Morgan, A. F., H. L. Gilum, E. D. Gifford, and E. B. Wilcox: Bone density of an aging population. Amer. J. clin. Nutr. **10**, 337—346 (1962).

Morgan, R. H.: An analysis of the physical factors controlling the diagnostic quality of roentgen images. Amer. J. Roentgenol. **55**, 67—89 (1946).

—, and W. W. van Allen: The densitometry of roentgenographic films and screens. Radiology **52**, 832—845 (1949).

Mouvet, W.: Dosage non destructif de la composante minérale du tissu osseux par densitomètrie radiographique. C. R. Acad. Sci. (Paris) **259**, 2309—2311 (1964).

Mueller, W. J., R. Schraer, and H. Schraer: Calcium metabolism and skeletal dynamics of laying pullets. J. Nutr. **84**, 20—26 (1964).

Murray, P. D. F.: The physiology of supporting tissue. Ann. Rev. Physiol. **9**, 103—118 (1947).

Nachlass, I. W., and E. A. Parke: Zit. nach Stein 1937.

Neef, Th.: Beiträge zur Metalluntersuchung mittels Röntgenstrahlen. Z. techn. Physik **6**, 208—215 (1925).

Nelson, J. D., P. B. Mack, and G. P. Vose: New design of a linearizing recording densitometer. Rev. Sci. Instr. **29**, 316 (1958).

Netter, H.: Physikalisch-chemische Grundlagen der Lebensvorgänge. Theoretische Biochemie. Berlin-Göttingen-Heidelberg: Springer 1959.

Nilsson, B.: Clinical studies with measurement of bone mineral content with a single photon beam. Conference on Progress in Methods of Bone Mineral Measurements, Bethesda, Maryland 1968 (im Druck).

Nordin, B. E. C.: The pathogenesis of osteoporosis. Lancet **1961I**, 1011—1015.

— Calcium balance and calcium requirement in spinal osteoporosis. Amer. J. clin. Nutr. **10**, 384—390 (1962).

— The application of basic science to osteoporosis. In: Bone Biodynamics by H. M. Frost. Boston (Mass.): Little, Brown & Co. 1964.

— Bone density patterns in osteoporosis. Conference on Progress in Methods of Bone Mineral Measurements, Bethesda, Maryland 1968 (im Druck).

— E. Barnett, J. MacGregor, and J. Nisbet: Lumbar spine densitometry. Brit. med. J. **1962I**, 1793—1796.

— — D. A. Smith, and J. Anderson: Measurement of cortical bone volume and lumbar spine density. In: Progress in development of methods on bone densitometry. Washington D.C. 1965, p. 21—30. NASA, Sci. Techn. Inf. Div. Washington D.C. 1966.

— J. McGregor, and D. A. Smith: The incidence of osteoporosis in normal women: its relation to age and the menopause. Quart. J. Med., N. S. **35**, 25—38 (1966).

—, and D. A. Smith: Die Behandlung der Osteoporose. Triangel **6**, 273—277 (1964).

— — J. MacGregor, and J. Anderson: The application of measurements of bone volume and spinal density. Progress in Development of Methods in Bone Densitometry. Conference in Washington D.C. 1965, p. 155. NASA, Sci. Techn. Inf. Div. Washington D.C. 1966.

Odland, L. M., K. P. Warrick, and N. C. Esselbaugh: Cooperative nutritional status studies in the western region. II. Bone Density, Montana Agr. Expt. Station Bull. No 534, Jan. 1958.

Oeser, H., u. E. Krokowski: Röntgenstrahlen zur visuellen Knochenbiopsie zwecks Bestimmung des Mineralgehaltes. Dtsch. med. Wschr. **86**, 2431—2434 (1961).

— — Quantitative analysis of inorganic substances in the body. Brit. J. Radiol. **36**, 274—279 (1963).

Okuyama, T.: A study of quantitative analysis on the mineral contents of the bone by X-rays. Nippon Acta radiologica **25**, 775—790 (1965).

Omnell, K.-A.: Quantitative roentgenologic studies on changes in mineral content in vivo. Acta radiol. (Stockh.), Suppl. 148 (1957).

— B. Lindström, F. C. Hoh, and E. Hammerlund-Essler: Method for non-destructive determination of inorganic and organic material in mineralized tissues. Acta radiol. (Stockh.) **54**, 209—219 (1960).

OWEN, M.: Measurement of the variations in calcification in normal rabbit bone. J. Bone Jt Surg. B **38**, 762—768 (1956).

PAIS, C., e I. FORNI: Rapporto fra demineralizzazione sperimentale dell'osso a la sua valuttazione diafanometrica. Atti 35. Congr. S. I. O.T. 1951, p. 281.

PALMER, H. E., W. B. NELP, R. MURANO, C. RICH, and K. G. PAILTHORP: In vivo neutron activation analysis of total body bone mass. Conference on Progress in Methods of Bone Mineral Measurements, Bethesda, Maryland 1968 (im Druck).

PAPWORTH, M. P.: Quantitative assessment of the mineral content of bone: Preliminary investigation. J. Coll. Radiol. Aust. **8**, 78—83 (1964).

PARISH, J. G.: Radiographic measurements of the skeletal structure of the normal hand. Brit. J. Radiol. **39**, 52—62 (1966).

POSNER, A. S.: The chemical and physical nature of bone mineral. Conference on Progress in Methods of Bone Mineral Measurement, Bethesda, Maryland 1968 (im Druck).

PRIBOTH, W., D. BÖRNERT u. H. FRITZSCHE: Zur Methode der röntgenologisch-photometrischen Bestimmung des Aschegehaltes im Knochen beim Rind. Zbl. Vet.-Med. A **13**, 628—644 (1966).

PRICE: Zit. nach MACK, zit. nach VOSE. 1901.

QUINTAR, H.: Quantitative Bestimmung des Kalksalzgehaltes am Radius. Diss. Kiel 1962.

RAKOVSKAJA, M., and M. KOSSAKOVSKAJA: Investigations of the mineralization degree of rat's bones in densimetric evaluation of roentgenograms. Vop. Pitan. **18**, 42—47 (1959).

RAKOWSKA, M., and M. KOSSAKOWSKA: Bone density as a measure of calcium availability in rats. Rocz. Pánstwowego Zakladu Higieny **9**, 345—357 (1959).

REICH, ST. B., J. LEVITIN, and L. R. FELTON: A roentgen method of evaluating density of bone. Amer. J. Roentgenol. **79**, 705—708 (1958).

REID, A. F., and A. H. HALFF: Direct determination of density of solids. Science **135**, 319—320 (1961).

RETHMEIER, B. J.: Densitometrie. De bepaling van het calciumgehalte der beenderen. J. belge Radiol. **38**, 487—500 (1955).

RICH, C., E. KLINK, R. SMITH, B. GRAHAM, and P. IVANOVICH: Sonic measurement of bone mass. In: Progress in development of methods on bone densitometry. Washington D.C. 1965, p. 137—144. NASA, Sci. Techn. Inf. Div. Washington D.C. 1966.

RICH, C., E. J. KLINK, G. L. MULLINS, and C. B. GRAHAM: Sonic measurement of bone mass. J. clin. Invest. **42**, 970 (1963).

RICHARDS, A. G.: Measuring the radiopacity of the lip and mandible. J. dent. Res. **32**, 193—201 (1953).

RIEDER, W.: Die akute Knochenatrophie. Dtsch. Z. Chir. **248**, 269—331 (1936).

ROCKOFF, S. D.: A new versatile microdensitometric system for quantitative radiographic analysis. Radiology **85**, 731—735 (1965).

— Theoretical aspects of radiographic densitometry. In: Progress in development of methods in bone densitometry. Washington D.C. 1965, p. 7—10. NASA, Sci. Techn. Inf. Div. Washington D.C. 1966.

— Radiographic trabecular quantitation of human lumbar vertebrae in situ: method and relation to bone mass, strength, and calcium, phosphorus and magnesium content. Symposium Ossium, London 1968 (im Druck).

—, and R. SELZER: Radiographic trabecular quantitation of human lumbar vertebrae in situ: Theory, relation to bone composition and strength, and progress in digital computer analysis. Conference on Progress in Methods of Bone Mineral Measurements, Bethesda, Maryland 1968 (im Druck).

RÖCKERT, H.: A quantitative X-ray microscopical study of calcium in the cementum of teeth. Acta odont. scand. **16**, Suppl., 25 (1958).

RÖHLER, R.: Untersuchungen zur Detailerkennung im Röntgenbild. Fortschr. Röntgenstr. **86**, 376—378 (1957).

ROHMANN, CH., ST. M. GARN, H. A. GUZMÁN, M. FLORES, M. BÉHAR, and E. PAO: Osseous development of Guatemalan children on low protein diets. Fed. Proc. **24**, 338 (1964).

RUMP, W.: Elektromedizin und Strahlenkunde. München u. Berlin: Urban & Schwarzenberg 1954.

SANDERS, A. P.: Diss. Pennsylvania State College 1937. Zit. nach MACK, BROWN und TRAPP.

SARABRIN, I. G.: Trudy Soveščanija po biologičeskim, Moskva 1952, p. 164.

SAVILLE, P. D.: Predictability of bone ash in the beagle. Conference on Progress in Methods of Bone Mineral Measurements, Bethesda, Maryland 1968 (im Druck).

SCHLUNGBAUM, W., u. E. KROKOWSKI: Absorptionsmessungen zur Objektivierung der radiologischen Diagnose Osteoporose. IX. Int. Congr. Radiol. München 1959, Vortrag 298.

SCHMID, J.: Photometrische Bestimmung der Knochendichte. Z. Rheumaforsch. **19**, 186—197 (1960).

— Kalktherapie bei Osteoporose. Schweiz. med. Wschr. **93**, 1815—1820 (1963).

SCHRAER, H.: Variation in the roentgenographic density of the os calcis and phalanx with sex and age. J. Pediat. **52**, 416—423 (1958).

— Quantitative radiography of the skeleton in living systems. In: Progress in development of methods on bone densitometry. Washington D.C. 1965, p. 11—20. NASA, Sci. Techn. Inf. Div. Washington D.C. 1966.

—, and M. T. NEWMAN: Quantitative roentgenography of skeletal mineralization in malnourished Quechua Indian boys. Science **128**, 476—477 (1958).

—, and R. SCHRAER: Quantitative measurements of bone density changes in rats fed with diets

of different calcium content. Fed. Proc. **15**, 571—572 (1956).
SCHRAER, H., and R. SCHRAER: Quantitative measurement of bone mineral content from roentgenograms. (Abstr.) National Biophysics Conferences, Columbus, Ohio 1957.
— — Bone mass changes in hens observed in vivo during the egg laying cycle. Experientia (Basel) **17**, 255—256 (1961).
— — H. G. TROSTLE, and A. D'ALFONSO: The validity of measuring bone density from roentgenograms by means of bone density computing apperatus. Arch. Biochem. Biophys. **83**, 486—500 (1959).
—, and W. J. SIAR: Bone density and calcium ingestion. Fed. Proc. **19**, 370 (1960).
— —, and R. SCHRAER: Changes in bone mass and density in living rats during the manipulation of calcium intake. Arch. Biochem. Biophys. **100**, 393—398 (1963).
SEDLIN, E. D.: The ratio of cortical area to total cross-section area in rib diaphysis: A quantitative index of osteoporosis. Clin. Orthop. **36**, 161—168 (1964).
SEEMANN, H. E., and B. ROTH: New stepped wedges for radiography. Acta radiol. (Stockh.) **53**, 215—256 (1960).
SHACKMAN, R., and C. V. HARRISON: Occult bone metastases. Brit. J. Surg. **35**, 385—389 (1948).
SHIMMINS, J., F. C. GILLESPIE, M. D. HAMILTON, and D. A. SMITH: The measurement of bone mineral in vivo by photon absorption. Calc. Tissue Res. **2**, Suppl., 40 (1968).
—, and D. A. SMITH: Estimation of bone mineral transfer rate by the measurement of longterm retension of SR^{85}. Metabolism **15**, 436—443 (1966).
SMITH, D. A., J. B. ANDERSON, J. SHIMMINS, J. F. SPIERS, and E. BARNETT: Mineral and density changes in bone with age in normal and pathological states. Conference on Progress in Methods of Bone Mineral Measurements, Bethesda, Maryland 1968 (im Druck).
SMITH, R. W., JR.: Osteoporotic changes in bone mass with age. 92nd Annual Meeting Amer. Publ. Health Ass. Inc. New York 1964.
— Comments on cortical thickness measurements. In: Progress in development of methods in bone densitometry. Conference in Washington D.C. 1965, p. 195. NASA, Sci. Techn. Inf. Div. Washington D.C. 1966.
—, and R. R. WALKER: Femoral expansion in aging women: Implications for osteoporosis and fractures. Science **145**, 156—157 (1964).
SORENSON, J. A., and J. R. CAMERON: Body composition determination by differential absorption of monochromatic X-rays. Symposium of Low-Energy X- and Gamma Source, Chicago, Ill. 1964.
— —, and R. B. MAZESS: Measurement of bone mineral by the direct photon absorption method: Experimental results. Conference on Progress in Methods of Bone Mineral Measurements, Bethesda, Maryland 1968 (im Druck).
SPENCER, R. P., and M. J. COULOMBE: Quantitation of the radiographically determined age dependence of bone thickness. Invest. Radiol. **1**, 144—147 (1966).
— ST. M. GARN, and M. J. COULOMBE: Agedependent changes in metacarpal cortical thickness in two populations. Invest. Radiol. **1**, 394—397 (1966).
— S. S. SAGEL, and ST. M. GARN: Age changes in five parameters of metacarpal growth. Invest. Radiol. **3**, 27—34 (1968).
SPIEGLER, G.: Quantitative Bedeutung des Röntgenschattens. Z. angew. Physik **11**, 65—68 (1959).
—, u. B. E. KEANE: Hart- und Weichsubstanz im Knochen und die Absorption in beiden. Fortschr. Röntgenstr. **94**, 662—666 (1961).
SPIERS, F. W.: Effective atomic number and energy absorption in tissues. Brit. J. Radiol. **19**, 52—63 (1946).
STEIN, I.: The evaluation of bone density in the roentgenogram by the use of ivory wedges. Amer. J. Roentgenol. **37**, 678—682 (1937).
STEVEN, G. D.: X-ray appearences in chronic rheumatism. Ann. rheum. Dis. **6**, 1—14 (1947).
— "Standard bone". A description of radiographic technique. Ann. rheum. Dis. **6**, 184—185 (1947).
STEVENS, J., P. A. FREEMAN, B. E. C. NORDIN, and E. BARNETT: The incidence of osteoporosis in patients with femoral neck fracture. J. Bone Jt Surg., B **44**, 520—527 (1962).
STRANDJORD, N. M., M. FORLAND, L. LANZL, and A. COX: Bone densitometry: Clinical applications. Conference on Progress in Methods of Bone Mineral Measurements, Bethesda, Maryland 1968 (im Druck).
—, and L. H. LANZL: Iodine-125 bone densitometry. In: Progress in development of methods on bone densitometry. Washington D.C. 1965, p. 115—124. NASA, Sci. Techn. Inf. Div. Washington 1966.
— — Estrogens and postmenopausal osteoporosis. In: Progress in development of methods in bone densitometry. Conference in Washinton D.C. 1965, p. 163. NASA Scient. Techn. Inf. Div. Washington D.C. 1966.
STRESEMANN, E., u. E. KROKOWSKI: Der Mineralisationsgrad der Wirbelsäule nach langfristiger Corticosteroidbehandlung des chronischen Bronchialasthmas. Klin. Wschr. **45**, 564—569 (1967).
STRUG, P.: Röntgenologische und chemisch-analytische Bestimmung des Mineral- und Calciumgehaltes im Knochen. Diss. Freie Universität Berlin 1964.
STÜHLER, R.: Über den Feinbau des Knochens. Fortschr. Röntgenstr. **57**, 231—264 (1938).
SUDECK, P.: Kollaterale Entzündungszustände „sog. akute Knochenatrophie" und Dystrophie der Gliedmaßen in der Unfallheilkunde. Berlin 1938.
TARJÁN, R.: Einfluß der Ernährung auf das Knochensystem. IV. Die Rolle des Nahrungseiweißes in der Ossifikation. Acta physiol. Acad. Sci. hung. **8**, 127 (1955).

Tarján, R.: Diet and bones. Nutr. et Dieta (Basel) **3**, 32—51 (1963).
— E. Sándi u. P. Deák: Versuche zur in-vivo-Bestimmung des Mineralstoffgehaltes im Knochensystem. Acta physiol. hung. **5**, Suppl. 38 (1954).
—, u. K. Szóke: Veränderungen der organischen und anorganischen Knochensubstanz sowie der Knochenfestigkeit bei Ratten mit zunehmendem Alter. Hoppe-Seylers Z. physiol. Chem. **308**, 1—4 (1957).
Telkkä, A., H. Kauppinen, and P. Virtama: Correlation of dry weight of human carpal, metacarpal and finger bones to their actual mineral contents. Amer. J. Phys. Anthrop. **20**, 17—19 (1962).
Tettoni, E., E. Comino e S. Perazzo: Intorno alla valutazione radiologica de osteoporosi. Minerva radiol. **9**, 169—175 (1964).
Trotter, M., G. E. Broman, and R. R. Peterson: Densities of bones of white and negro skeletons. J. Bone Jt Surg. A **42**, 50—58 (1960).
Trotter, N.: A preliminary study of estimation of weight of the skeleton. Amer. J. Phys. Anthrop. **12**, 537—552 (1954).
Turano, L.: Studio radiologico dello scheletro senile. Relaz. Congr. Soc. It. Gerontol. Geriatr., Milano 1952.
— Osservazioni radiologiche sul metabolismo dell'osso senile. G. Geront. **1**, 1—11 (1953).
Urist, M. R.: The problem of osteoporosis. Clin. Res. **6**, 377—385 (1958).
— The etiology of osteoporosis. J. Amer. med. Ass. **169**, 710—712 (1959).
— P. S. Zaccalini, N. S. MacDonald, and W. A. Skoog: New approaches to the problem of osteoporosis. J. Bone Jt Surg. B **44**, 464—484 (1962).
Vanselow, K., F. Heuck u. U. Piepgras: Theoretische Grundlagen einer Methode zur Messung der Gewebsdurchblutung am nicht narkotisierten Menschen. Fortschr. Röntgenstr. **108**, 529—536 (1968).
Vanselow, K., u. F. Heuck: (In Vorbereitung.)
Vetterlein, K.-Th.: Über die Ionisation von Röntgenstrahlungen in verschiedenen Geweben. Diss. Erlangen 1949/50.
Vignon, G., et V. Calvel: Une technique de densimétrie osseuse. Rev. lyonn. Méd. **8**, 979—982 (1959).
Virtama, P.: Determination of the mineral content of human finger bones by silver analysis of roentgenograms. Acta anat. (Basel) **31**, Suppl. 29 (1957).
— Quantitative determination of bone minerals from roentgenograms. Experientia (Basel) **13**, 236—237 (1957).
— Assessment of the mineral content of bones from roentgenograms. IX. Int. Congr. Radiol. 1959 München, Vortrag 313.
— Uneven distribution of bone minerals and covering effect of non-mineralized tissue as reasons for impaired detectability of bone density from roentgenograms. Ann. Med. intern. Fenn. **49**, 57—65 (1960).
Virtama, P.: Variations in the ash contents of bones of the extremities. Ann. Med. exp. Fenn. **38**, 127—132 (1960).
— Radiological determination of bone density. Duodecim (Helsinki) **81**, 816—824 (1965).
— G. Gästrin, and A. Telkkä: Biconcavity of the vertebrae as an estimate of their bone density. Clin. Radiol. **13**, 128—131 (1962).
— P. Kajanoja, V. K. Hopsu, and A. Telkkä: Density of human carpal, metacarpal, and digital bones. Ann. Med. exp. Fenn. **38**, 467—471 (1960).
— —, and A. Telkkä: Cortical ratio as an estimate of the mineral content of the human femur. Ann. Med. exp. Fenn. **41**, 3—6 (1963).
—, and E. Kallio: Bone pattern in experimental osteoporosis of the rat. Ann. Med. exp. Fenn. **39**, 154—164 (1961).
—, and H. Mähönen: Thickness of the cortical layer as an estimate of mineral content of human finger bones. Brit. J. Radiol. **33**, 60—62 (1960).
—, and A. Telkkä: Trabecular pattern of the cancellous bone as an estimate of mineral content of human finger bones. Acta anat. (Basel) **46**, 47—52 (1961).
— — Cortical thickness as an estimate of mineral content of human humerus and femur. Brit. J. Radiol. **35**, 632—633 (1962).
— —, and T. Helelä: Relative density of the vertebral end-plates as an estimate of osteoporosis. Brit. J. Radiol. **38**, 360—364 (1965).
Vogt, F. B., L. S. Meharg, and P. B. Mack: Use of a digital computer in the measurement of roentgenographic bone density. Persönliche Mitteilung 1968.
Vose, G. P.: Determination of the organic-inorganic ratio in osseous tissue by X-ray absorption. Analyt. Chem. **30**, 1819—1821 (1958).
— X-ray transmission factor in estimating bone density. Radiology **71**, 96—101 (1958).
— Quantitative determination of osseous and soft fractions of bone by X-ray absorption. Lab. Invest. **8**, 1540—1546 (1959).
— Factors affecting the precision of radiographic densitometry of the lumbar spine and femoral neck. In: Progress in development of methods on bone densitometry. Washington D.C. 1965, p. 47—63. NASA, Sci. Techn. Inf. Div. Washington D.C. 1966.
— X-ray bone densitometry in short and long duration studies. Conference on Progress in Methods of Bone Mineral Measurement, Bethesda, Maryland 1968 (im Druck).
—, and A. L. Kubala: Bone strength — its relationship to X-ray-determined ash content. Human. Biol. **31**, 261—270 (1959).
—, and P. B. Mack: Roentgenologic assessment of femoral neck density as related to fracturing. Amer. J. Roentgenol. **89**, 1296—1301 (1963).
— — S. O. Brown, and A. B. Medlen: Radiographic determination of the rate of bone healing. Radiology **76**, 770—776 (1961).

VOSE, G. P., and R. E. PYKE: Compositional factors affecting vertebral X-ray absorption. Invest. Radiol. **1**, 371—378 (1966).

WACHSMANN, F.: Vorschläge zur Standardisierung der Bestrahlungsbedingungen in der Röntgentherapie. Strahlentherapie **83**, 41—50 (1950).

— H. TIEFEL u. E. BERGER: Messung der Quantität und Qualität gestreuter Röntgenstrahlen. Fortschr. Röntgenstr. **101**, 308—317 (1964).

WAGNER, A., u. J. SCHAAF: Vergleichende Untersuchungen mit und ohne photometrisches Meßverfahren über den Grad osteoporotischer Veränderungen im Röntgenbild. Dtsch. Arch. Klin. Med. **207**, 364—385 (1961).

WEBBER, H. E.: A practical roentgenographic densitometer. Amer. J. Roentgenol. **46**, 104—108 (1941).

WEECH, A. A., and M. S. SMITH: The anatomic base for interpreting roentgenograms in rickets. Amer. J. Dis. Child. **26**, 117—131 (1923).

WEISS, K.: Über das Röntgenbild der Knochenatrophie. Radiol. Austr. **9**, 227—237 (1957).

WHEDON, G. D., J. E. DEITRICK, and E. SHORR: Modification of the effects of immobilization upon metabolic and physiologic functions of normal man by the use of an oscillating bed. Amer. J. Med. **6**, 684—711 (1949).

—, and E. SHORR: Metabolic studies in paralytic acute anterior poliomyelitis II. Alterations in calcium and phosphorus metabolism. J. clin. Invest. **36**, 966—1033 (1957).

WIDENMANN, L.: Untersuchungen über die Abhängigkeit der Filmschwärzung mit handelsüblichen Verstärkerfolien von der Strahlenqualität. Fortschr. Röntgenstr. **87**, 386—397 (1957).

WILLIAMS, D. E., and R. L. MASON: Bone density measurement in vivo. Science **138**, 39—40 (1962).

— B. B. McDONALD, E. MORRELL, F. A. SCHOFIELD, and F. L. MACLEOD: Influence of mineral intake on bone density in humans and in rats. J. Nutr. **61**, 489—505 (1957).

—, and A. SAMSON: Bone density of East Indian and American students. J. Amer. diet. Ass. **36**, 462—466 (1960).

WILSEY, R. B.: The photographic photometry of roentgen rays. Amer. J. Roentgenol. **32**, 789—804 (1934).

WOLANSKI, N., and J. EAGEN: The interrelationship between bone density and cortical thickness in the second metacarpal as a function of age. In: Progress in development of methods on bone densitometry, Washington D.C. 1965, p. 79—84. NASA, Sci. Techn. Inf. Div. Washington D.C. 1966.

YUAN, CHAO-YING: A development of an improved calibration wedge material for the quantitative evaluation of bone density. Masters Thesis, The Pennsylvania State University 1950.

ZIELER, E.: Bildgüte in der Radiologie. Stuttgart: Gustav Fischer 1966.

D. Microradiography of normal bone

By

A. Engström

With 23 figures

1. Introduction

The development of roentgen microscopic procedures has produced new and powerful tools for the study of the structure and composition of osseous tissues. The simple and predictable laws, which govern the interaction between roentgen rays and the material they pass through, make it possible to draw chemical conclusions from roentgen ray absorption data. Thus, it is possible to measure the distribution of mineral salts in a histological section of bone, and by a differential roentgen absorption technique it is also possible to determine the quantity of the inorganic and organic phases simultaneously.

There are several techniques of roentgen microscopy, among which the simplest is "direct contact microradiography". Other techniques such as projection roentgen microscopy or reflection roentgen microscopy can also be used to study the mineralization of bone at the microscopic level, but as these latter much more complicated techniques do not yield a linear resolution better than the direct contact microradiographic procedure only the microradiographic techniques will be described in this survey. The general principles for microradiography have been given elsewhere in this handbook, where also references can be found.

2. Chemical composition of bone and other mineralized tissues

Chemically bone can be divided into an inorganic and an organic fraction. Usually the organic fraction (including water) represents at least half of the weight of the fresh bone. The volume occupied by this fractions is about 70 %. The content of water varies with age of bone and state of growth. Thus the water content may be as high as 70 % in newly forming bone and as small as 10 % in senile, compact bone.

The main portion of the organic fraction of bone contains the fibrous protein collagen. Almost $^9/_{10}$ of the organic fraction consists of this protein which has its characteristic macromolecular organization. In the organic fraction one also finds a few per cent hyaluronic acid and chondroitin sulfate.

The inorganic substance of bone consists mainly of hydroxyapatite $Ca_{10}(PO_4)_6(OH)_2$, carbon dioxide, citrate and water with other ions such as Na, K, Mg, Cl, and F in small amounts. The inorganic fraction is obtained as the bone ash after ignition.

3. The molecular structure of the bone salt

Since the first roentgen crystallographic studies of bone were made, many molecular models of the bone salt have been proposed. Now it is generally agreed (with few exceptions) that the hydrated calcium phosphate has the crystallographic form of hydroxyapatite. A schematic drawing of the molecular arrangement is shown in Fig. 1. The crystallographic unit cell has the dimensions $a = 9.42$ and $c = 6.88$ Å. These values correspond closely to those of hydroxyapatite in mineral form, where $a = 9.421$ and $c = 6.881$ Å. The roentgen diffraction lines of a bone specimen are broadened and the measurements of the profiles of the lines permit the determination of the size of the crystallites.

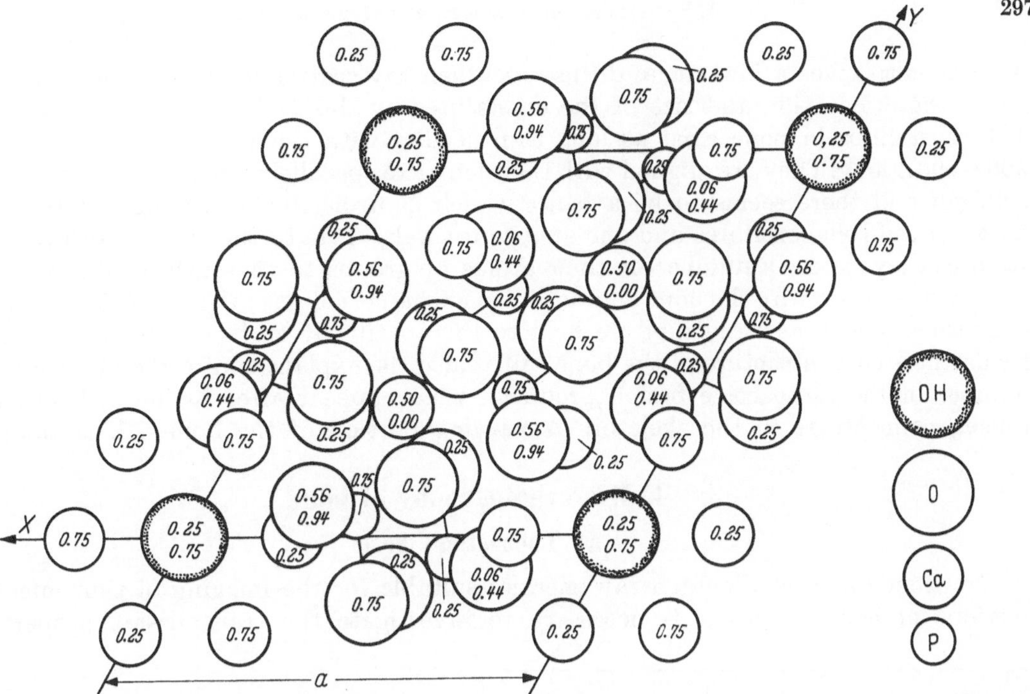

Fig. 1. Molecular arrangement in hydroxyapatite. The figures give fractional height above the basal plane

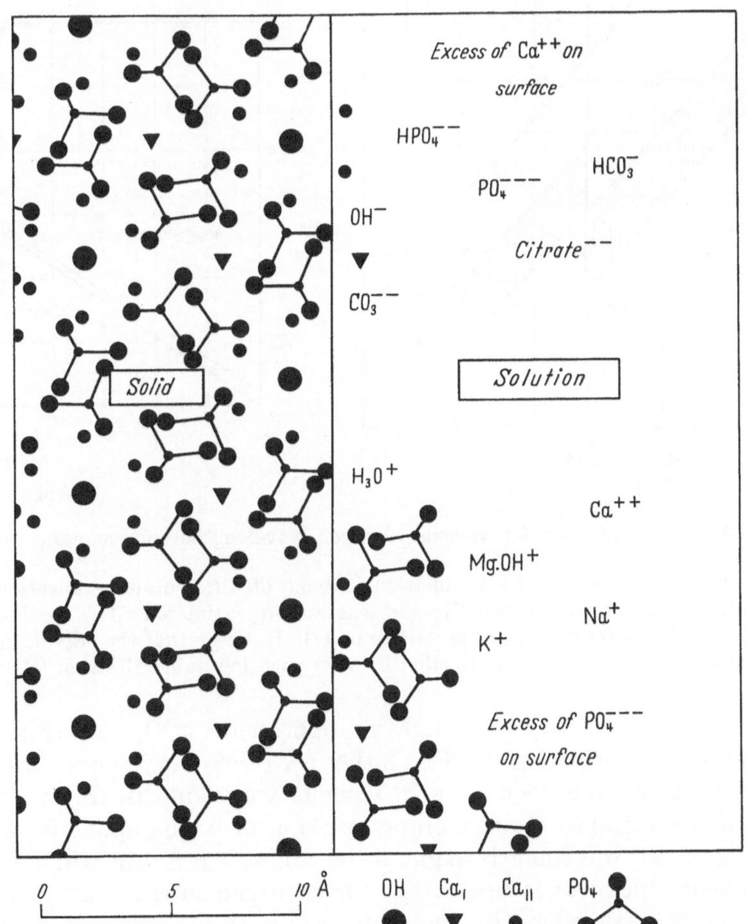

Fig. 2. The surface and part of the core of a hydroxyapatite crystal. It is seen that the crystal can end with either negatively or positively charged groups which can attract other ions of opposite charge (CARLSTRÖM 1955)

As bone also gives a low angle, diffuse roentgen ray scatter it has also been possible to study the orientation and size of the crystallites by this technique to a certain extent. The crystallites in bone exist as long thin needles with the width 30—50 Å and about 300—600 Å long. They are aligned with their long axes parallel to the fiber directions of the collagen and there seems to be a factor which controls the molecular interrelationship between the collagen fibres and the apatite crystals. Due to the small width of the crystallites they expose a number of their atoms or groups to the surface, Fig. 2, and this is the explanation why the bone acts as an ion exchange column. Thus carbonate and other constituents such as strontium are held to the apatite by surface adsorption. The particular molecular structure of the bone salt is also the explanation to the fact that a great number of the radioactive fission products, which appear after fission of heavy atomic nuclei, concentrate in the skeleton. A varying portion of the bone salt is amorphous.

4. Microradiography of bone

a) Theoretical basis

In order to select roentgen ray energies suitable for the imaging of thin microscopic sections of bone tissues it is necessary to investigate the transmission properties for

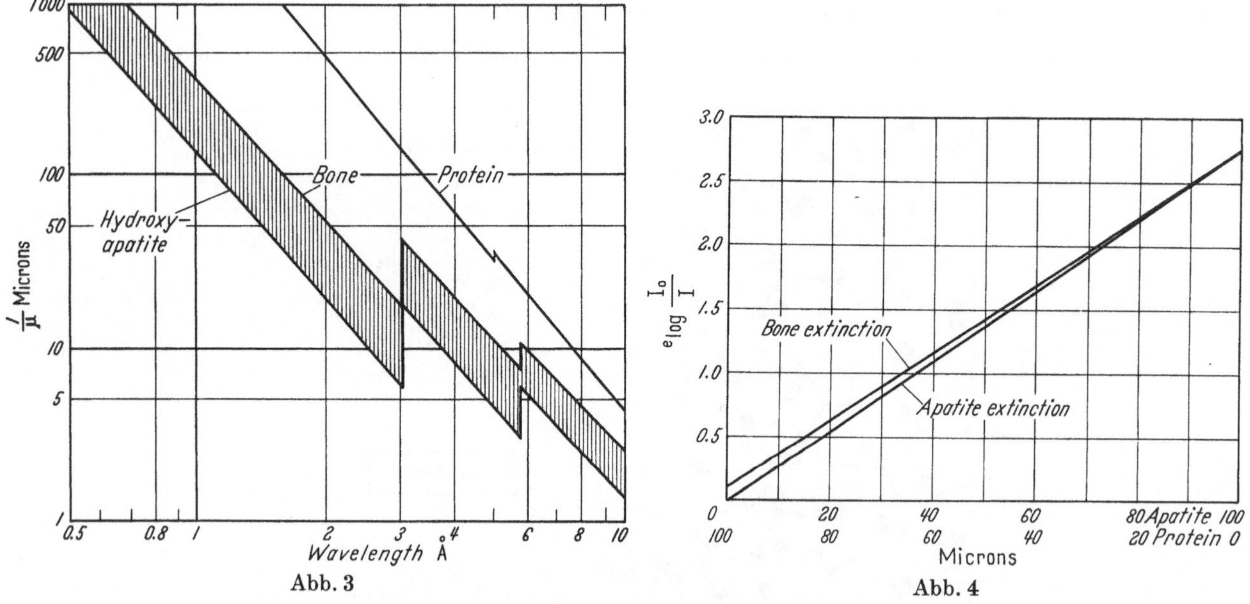

Fig. 3. Layers of bone for various roentgen wavelengths corresponding to $\frac{1}{\mu}$.

Fig. 4. Roentgen ray extinction of 1.54 Å radiation in bone of different mineralization (expressed as the volume ratio, apatite: protein), as compared to the true apatite extinction. The specific gravity of apatite is assumed to be 3.1, and that for dried bone protein to be 1.3. It is seen that the organic material is relatively more responsible for the observed extinction of bone with low mineralization (Wallgren 1957)

roentgen rays of varying energy. A suitable expression is the $1/\mu$-thickness where μ is the linear absorption coefficient. In Fig. 3 the $1/\mu$-thicknesses have been calculated for bone and protein using roentgen rays of various wavelengths. From the diagram it is apparent that, if one wants to study a ground section of bone about 100 microns in thickness, the roentgen ray wavelength ought to be about 1.5 Å. As will be seen from later considerations that thickness is best fitted for roentgen microscopy of bone and a most suitable roentgen ray wavelength, the CuK α-radiation, is easily available. When a microradiogram is recorded with, for example, 1.54 Å roentgen rays the resulting absorption image is due to absorption both of the organic and inorganic fractions. The chemical composition of these fractions and their relative concentrations make it obvious, however, as is illustrated in Fig. 4, that the major part of the absorption takes part in the inorganic fraction, hence a microradiogram recorded under such circumstances will indicate the distribution of mineral salts. More quantitatively, the roentgen ray absorption for any wavelength in bone can be represented by the following equation:

$$I = I_0 \cdot e^{-\left(\frac{\mu}{\varrho} o \cdot m_o + \frac{\mu}{\varrho} i m_i\right)}.$$

In this equation I_0 and I are incident, and transmitted roentgen ray intensities respectively μ/ϱ, indicate the mass absorption coefficient and m the fractional mass. Index o and i stand for organic and inorganic fraction respectively. In order to illustrate the magnitude of the various mass absorption coefficients the following Table 1 gives the actual values

Table 1. *Mass absorption coefficients for various substances*

Wavelength Å	1.0	1.54 (CuKα)	1.93	2.29 (CrKα)	3.0
Hydroxyapatite . . .	25.2	84	148	249	509
Protein	2.2	7.2	13.9	23.8	53
Water	2.8	9.9	19.4	32.4	75
Plastic	1.9	6.3	12.2	20.7	47

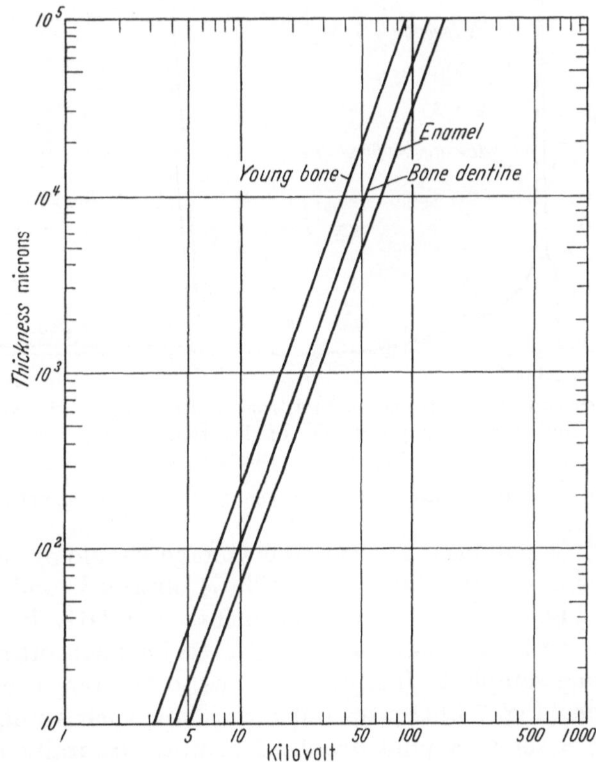

Fig. 5. Suitable energies of the roentgen rays used for radiography of bone

of the mass absorption coefficients for apatite and organic matrix for a series of roentgen wavelengths. It should be noted that the mass absorption coefficient for the plastic material usually employed to embed the bone specimens to facilitate the grinding is similar to that of the organic fraction. In Fig. 5 proper energies of the roentgen rays are given in order to obtain good radiograms of bone specimens of varying thicknesses.

b) Equipment

It is possible to use any type of roentgen ray generator which can be energized with voltages in the range 5—25 kV to obtain good microradiograms of thin bone sections. Thus roentgen tubes with thin beryllium windows are suitable, and grenz ray tubes are of good use. As mentioned above it is feasible to use as pure radiation as possible, and such can be obtained by having a roentgen tube with a copper target. Such tubes are commonly used for roentgen diffraction studies. If the radiation is filtered in a nickel

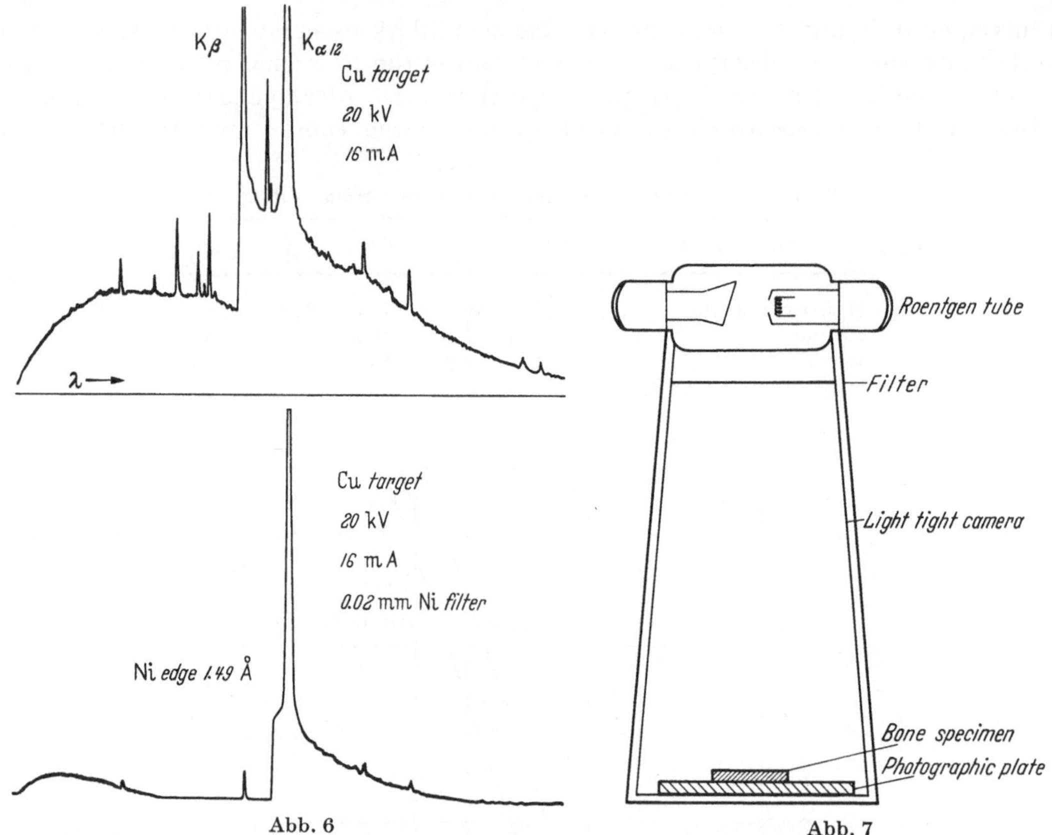

Abb. 6 Abb. 7

Fig. 6. Upper figure: Geiger counter spectrometric registration of the total radiation at 20 kV from a copper target tube. Lower figure: Monochromatizing influence of filtration through a 20 micron nickel filter on the copper line radiation

Fig. 7. Schematic representation of equipment of microradiography of bone

filter and not too high a potential is used (the voltage should not exceed 1.9 times the excitation potential) almost pure CuK α-radiation is obtained, and this is illustrated by the spectral curve in Fig. 6. As the bone specimens are relatively thick in comparison to the thin microtome sections of soft tissues and used for ultrasoft roentgen microradiography, a relatively long sample to film distance has to be used in order to diminish the penumbra in the image. Fig. 7 illustrates a drawing how such an equipment may easily be assembled and Fig. 8 shows a photograph of a unit. Naturally many variations are possible, and descriptions of various types of equipment are found in i.a. the proceedings of the first and second International Symposia on Roentgen Ray Microscopy.

The microradiograms are recorded on fine grained photographic emulsions such as Eastman Kodak Spectroscopic plates 548 or 649, or Kodak Maximum Resolution. Also Lipman Emulsion manufactured by Gevaert in Belgium can be used with great advantage. The film emulsions are developed in fine grained developer and, after processing in the usual way, the emulsion is protected with a thin cover glass mounted with Canada balsam. Photomicrographs of the microradiograms are obtained by usual photomicrography. As the black and white microradiogram has a high contrast, measures have to be taken to prevent glare when photographed through the microscope.

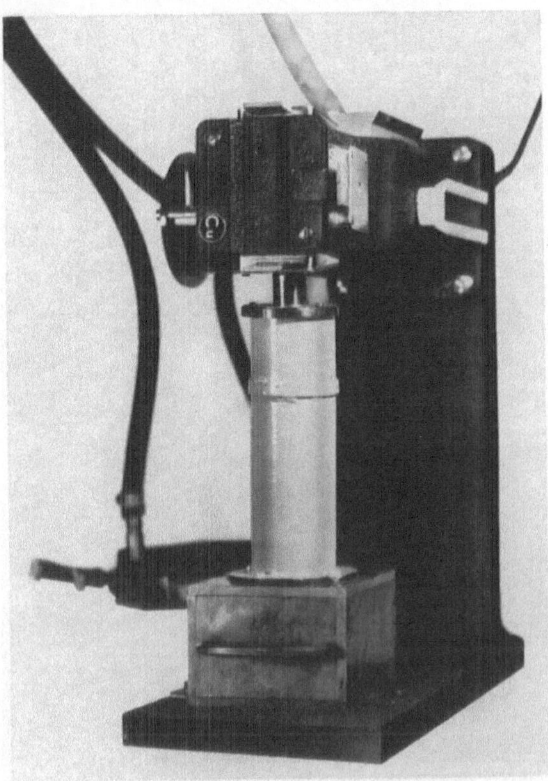

Fig. 8. Photograph of an equipment used for microradiography of bone

c) Preparation of bone specimens

Pieces of compact bone can be ground directly without embedding in a plastic material. Thin slices of bone are cut either by a hand-saw or better in a special cutting machine. Several types of sawing machines (many of them utilizing a milling machine) have been developed, which permit direct cutting of a 100 micron thick sections with plane parallel surfaces. In the best cases microradiograms can be recorded directly of these slices without any special treatment. However, in order to secure good microradiograms the bone sections must be ground and polished. This is done on fine grained emery papers with absolute alcohol used as wetting agent. When extremely thin and clean sections are needed, the grinding has to be done on special plane glass plates with coarse to extremely fine surfaces. Absolute alcohol is used as wetting agent.

Spongious bone or small pieces of bone surrounded by another matrix have to be embedded in a plastic before cutting and grinding. After removal from the organism the bone specimens are dehydrated in alcohol and then transferred to a dilute dilution of methyl methacrylate, which is allowed to penetrate the specimen. After this process the specimens are transferred to a polymerizing solution of methyl methacrylate, and the polymerization is either done by heat or by ultra violet light. Also embedding materials such as araldite may be used with advantage.

5. Microradiographic appearance of normal bone

a) Compact bone

Figs. 9 and 10 show some microradiograms of normal compact bone. It is clearly seen that the Haversian systems have a varying degree of roentgen absorption indicating a

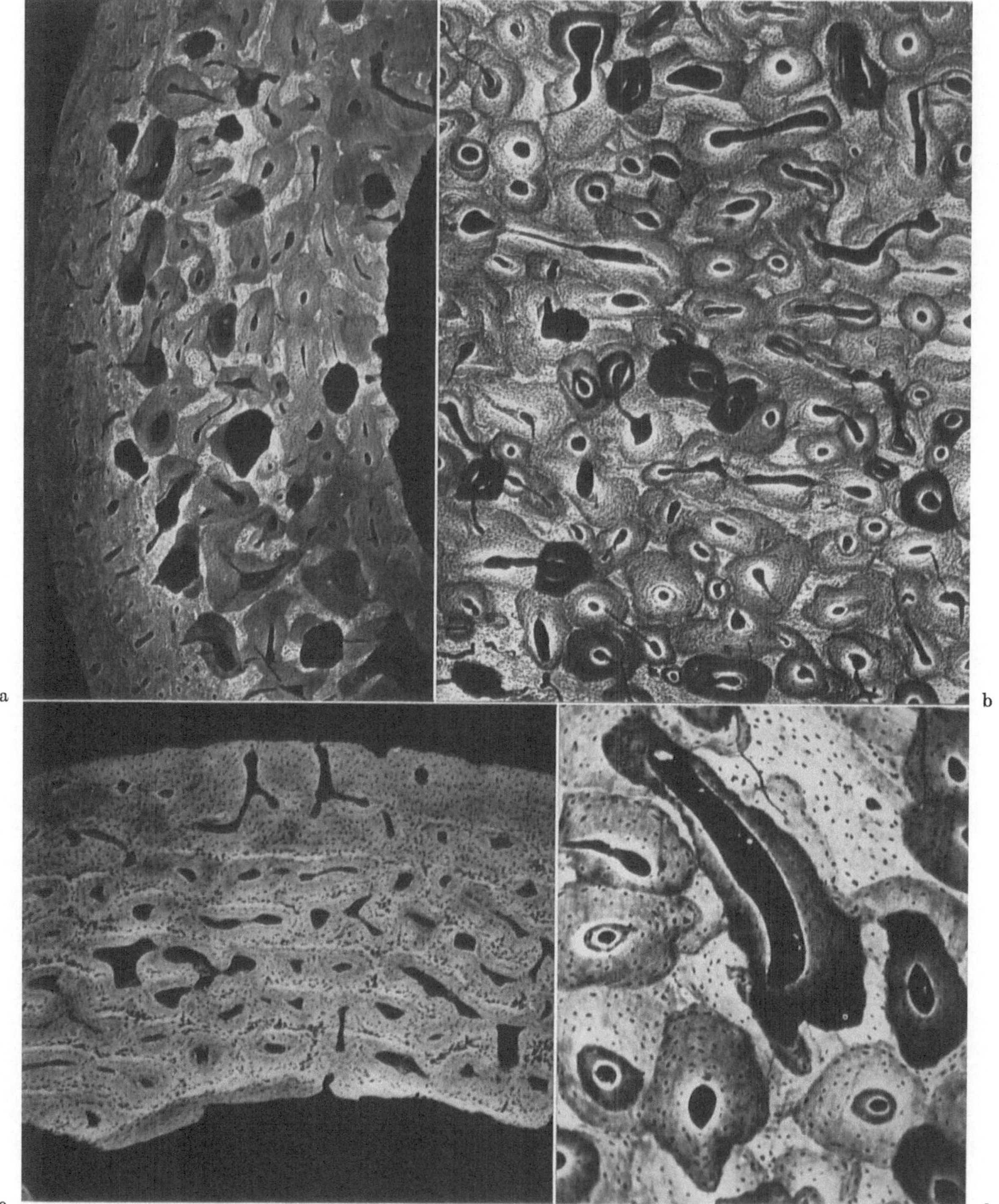

Fig. 9a—d. Microradiograms of normal bone. a Cortical bone from dog. b Cortical bone from a 7 years old human. c Embryonic human bone. d Human adult bone

varying degree of mineralization. From the general topology of growth one can conclude that the young Haversian systems have the smaller content of mineral salts. The osteocytes appear as black holes, indicating no roentgen absorption and therefore there is no apatite present. The Haversian systems can in many places be seen limited by cementing lines having a higher roentgen absorption than the surrounding bone tissue, which indicates higher content of mineral salts than in the osteon itself. The Haversian canals and the Volkmann's canals, which contain organic material, appear as black structures having no roentgen absorption. This observation is one of the experimental proofs for the theoretical deduction shortly mentioned above, and stating that with properly chosen quality of the roentgen beam, the image is given by the inorganic fraction.

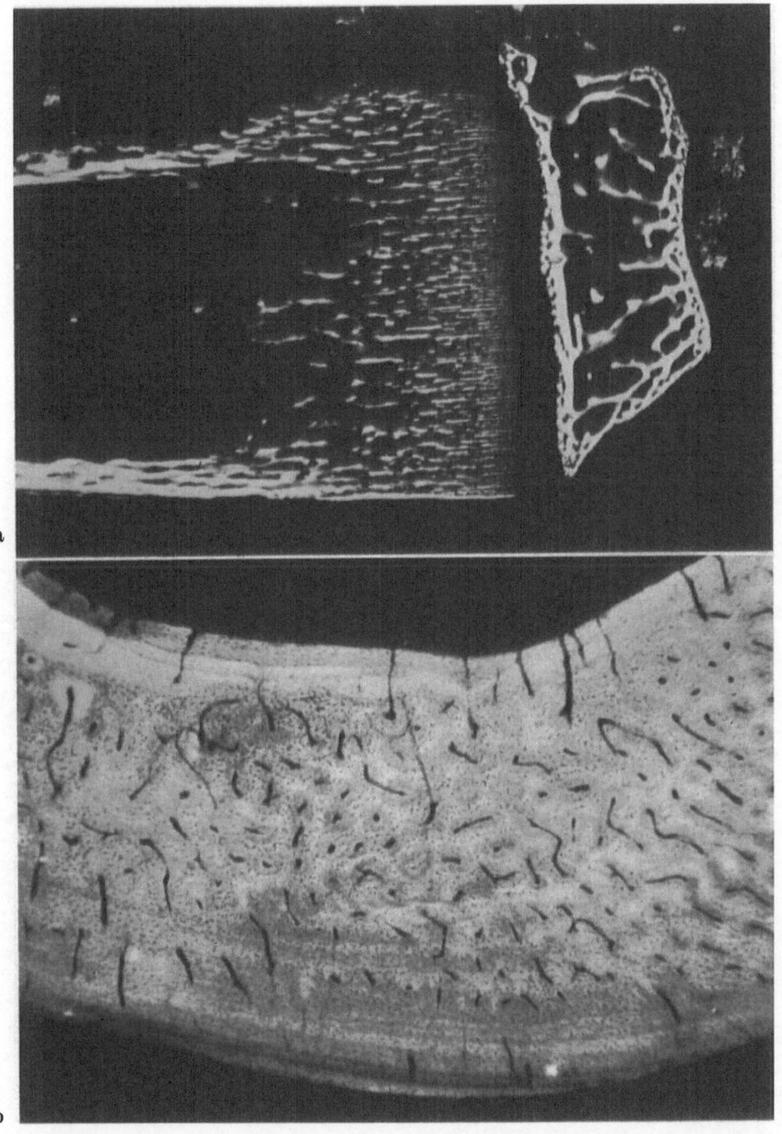

Fig. 10a and b. Microradiograms of rabbit bone. a Epiphyseal region. b Compacta of femur

When examining a microradiogram it must be born in mind that the fine grained emulsions are extremely steep, that is, they have a high γ-value which means that the film emulsion in itself is an amplifyer for small differences in roentgen absorption. It is for this reason that two structures in a microradiograph recorded under the conditions specified above, that is with 1.5 Å roentgen rays, and appearing as black and white, might not differ more than ca. 5—10% in mineral content. Therefore, when 1.5 Å roentgen rays are used, only structures which are at least mineralized to $^3/_4$ of their full physiological mineralization, appear in the microradiogram. Thus, if the lifespan of the Haversian system with regards to its mineral content, is represented by Fig. 11, it is only the latter part which is recorded with such an experimental technique.

In order to record the lowly mineralized parts of e.g. developing bone, roentgen rays of longer wavelengths have to be used and the whole investigation has to be performed in vacuum. As an intermediate between these two experimental approaches, the use of CrK α-radiation, that is the output from a chromium target which is filtered in vanadium,

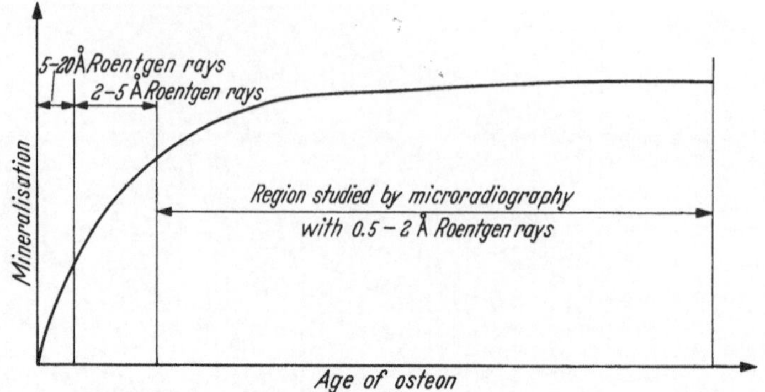

Fig. 11. Schematic drawing of the life span of an osteon

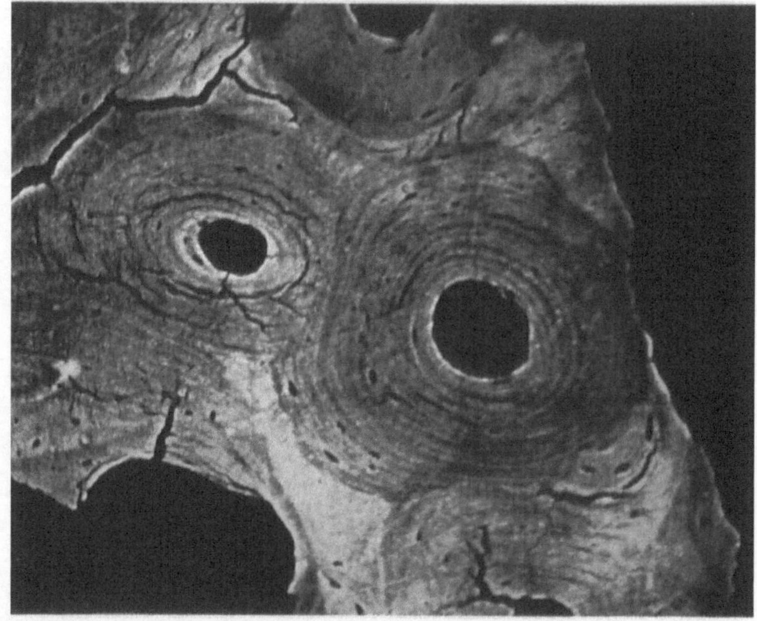

Fig. 12. Microradiographic demonstration of the lamellar structure of Haversian systems, indicating a varying mineral content of the different layers

can be used. The use of CrK α-radiation often gives a much more detailed picture but the fully mineralized structures do not appear so differentiated as with CuK α-radiation.

In conclusion therefore it can be said that in order to study all the ranges of mineralization and to obtain maximum possible differentiation at each step one must employ several roentgen ray wavelengths. It must be noted, however, that when using roentgen rays softer than 1.5 Å the section thickness has to be smaller according to Fig. 5, which might present difficulties in preparing plano-parallel specimens with no cracks. It has been possible to demonstrate the lamellar appearance of the Haversian systems in thin sections using soft roentgen rays as illustrated by Fig. 12.

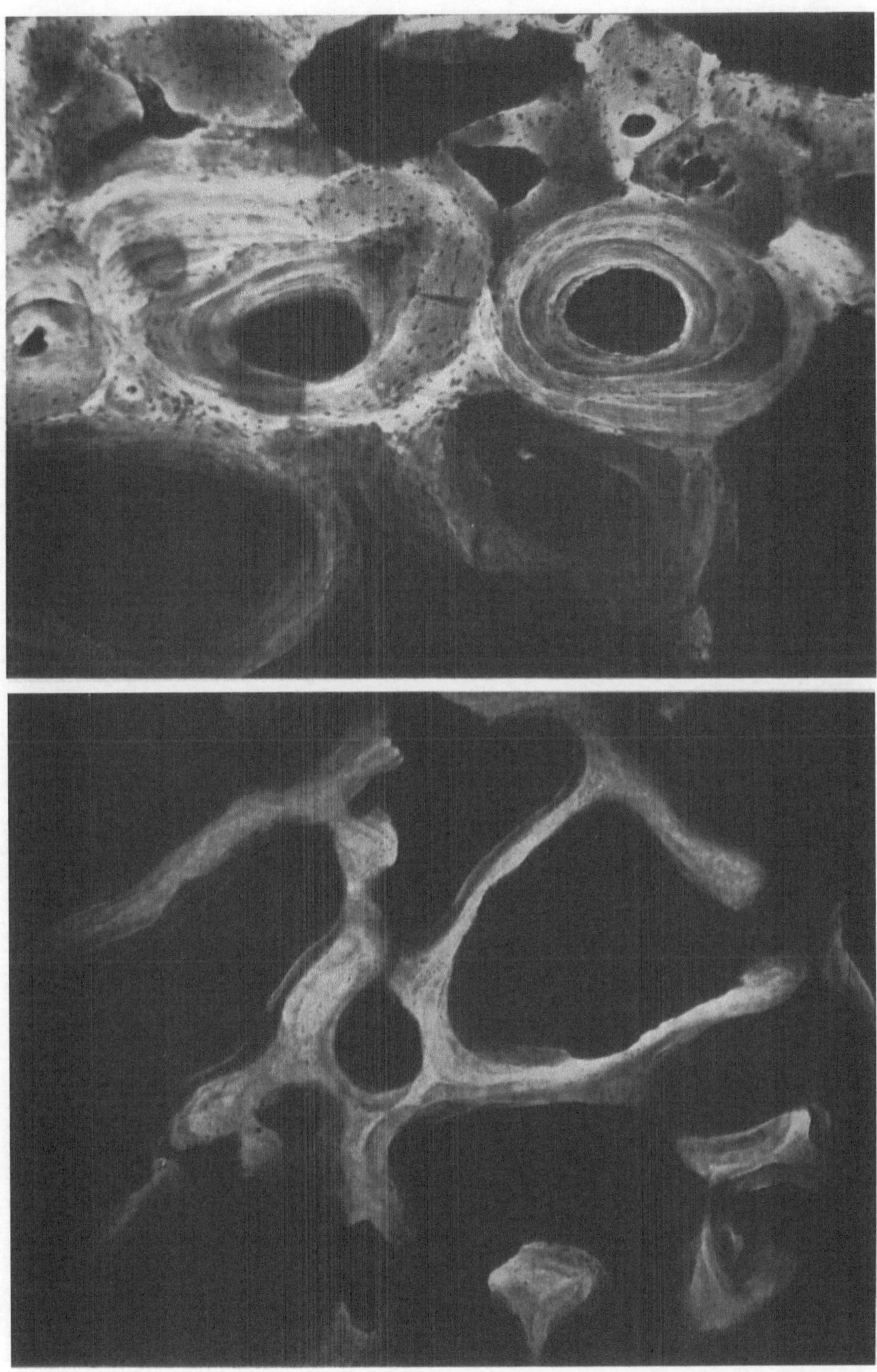

Fig. 13. Microradiograms of spongious bone indicating a rebuilding as judged from the number of lowly mineralized areas. Above bone from a vertebra, below from a rib (animal with hyperparathyroidism)

b) Spongious bone

Also in spongious bone the differences in mineralization are shown by microradiography. Areas of low and high mineralisation vary in a more irregular way than in

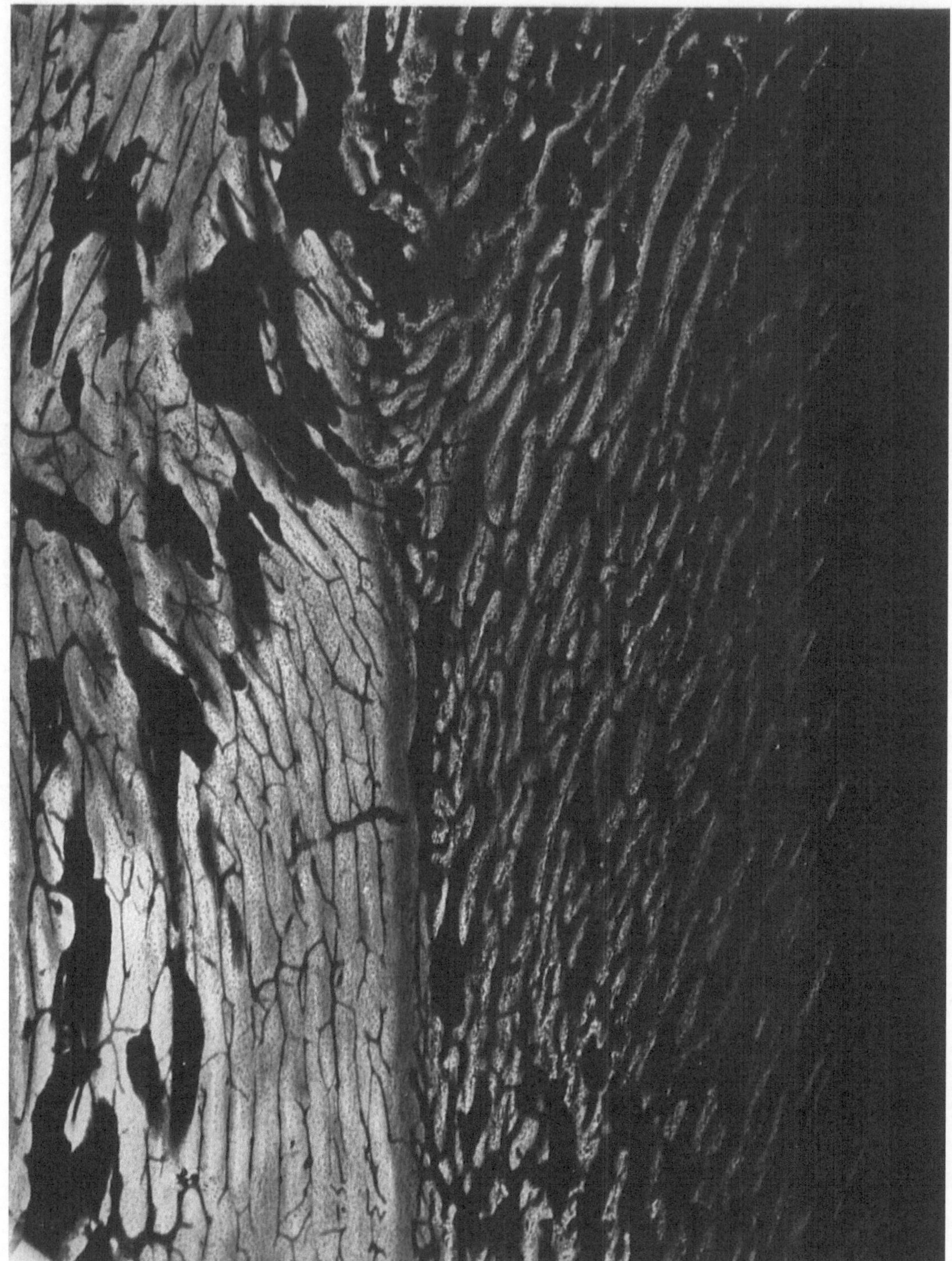

Fig. 14. Microradiogram of a healing fracture (Nilsonne, 1959)

compact bone. In spongious bone it can be shown that the less mineralized areas are the younger ones and this finding has been confirmed in experiments with radioactive isotopes. In Fig. 13 microradiograms of spongious bone are shown. The bone tissue formed around a callus is shown in Fig. 14 where the compact bone can be seen as well as the thin spicules originating in the periosteum.

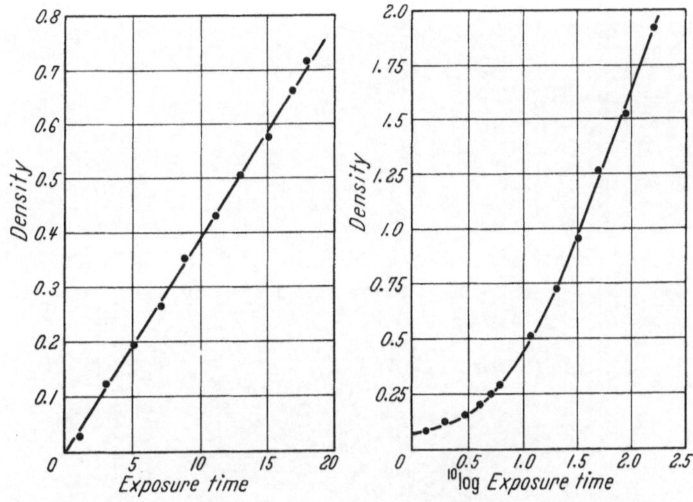

Fig. 15. Density versus incident roentgen intensity for a film emulsion used for microradiography

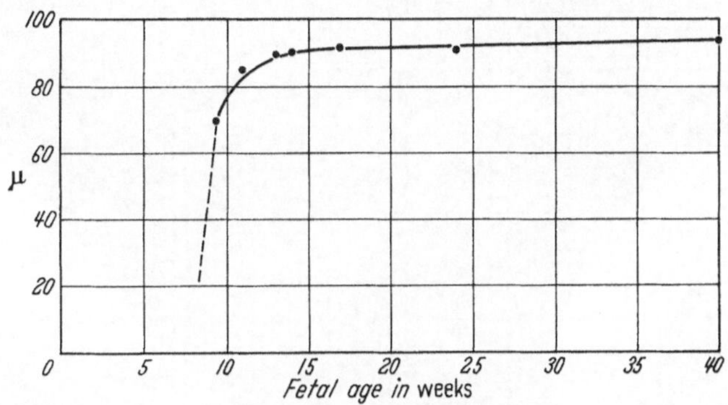

Fig. 16. Rate of mineralization expressed as the linear absorption coefficient in human fetal bone (WALLGREN 1957)

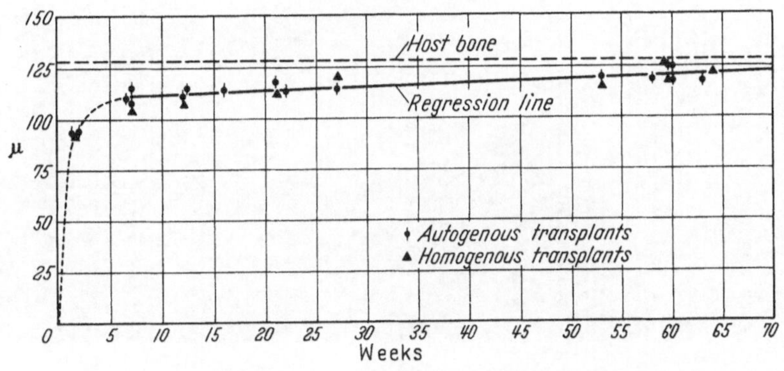

Fig. 17. Rate of mineralization in a healing bone transplant (HOLMSTRAND, 1957)

6. Quantitative microradiography

If the microradiogram is recorded under special conditions, the attenuation of roentgen rays can be quantitatively measured by microphotometry. Two procedures are possible. As the density of the microradiogram, properly developed, is linear with the incident roentgen intensity up to a value of about 0.5 (Fig. 15), microradiograms exposed in this range can be measured in the photometer directly. The incident roentgen intensity is proportional to the photographic density of the microradiogram not covered by the

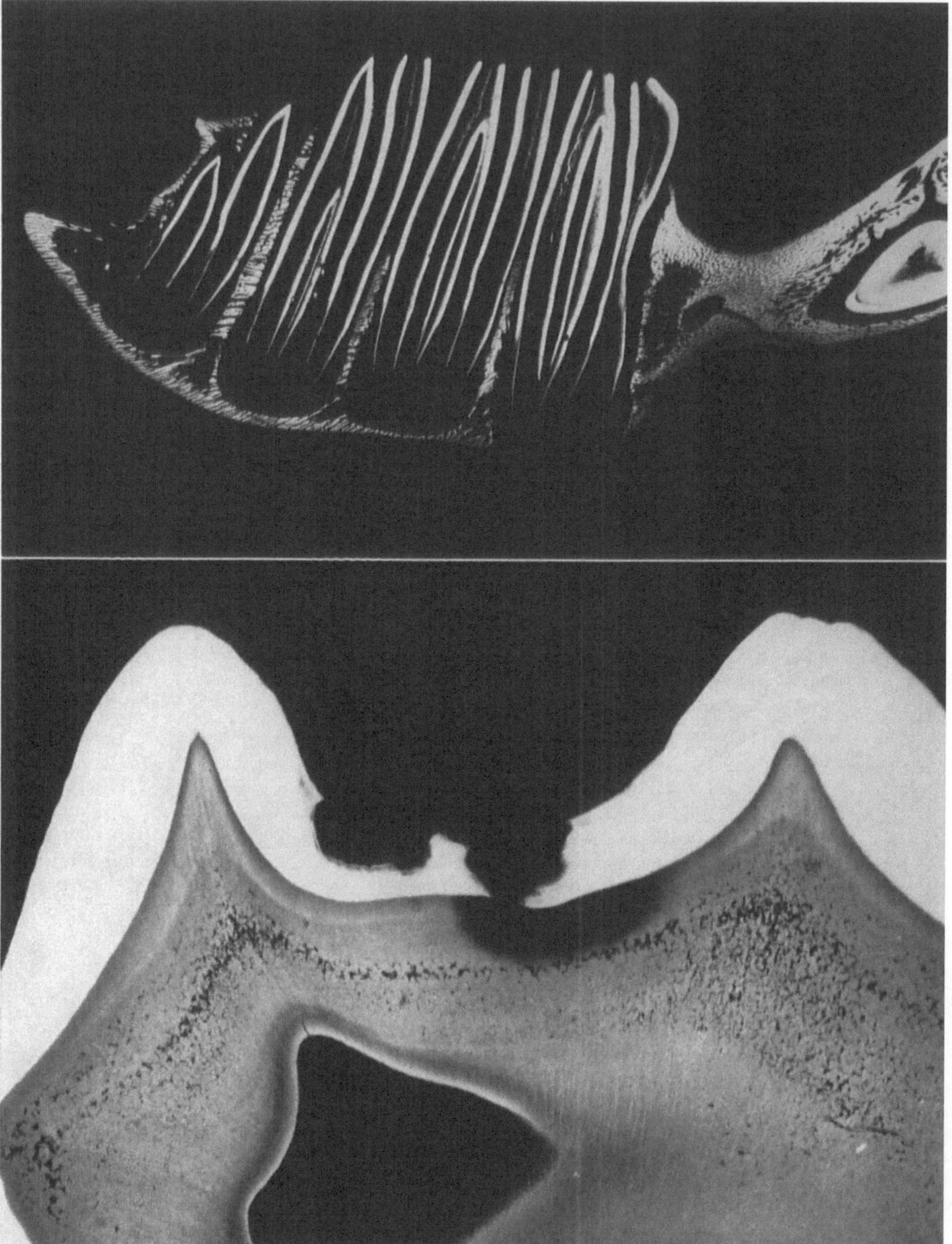

Fig. 18. Top: microradiogram of section through a jaw. Below: microradiogram of a carious tooth

specimen, thus $I_0 = \text{const} \cdot \log \frac{P_0}{P}$ where P_0 is the photometer reading on a non-exposed area of the microradiogram and P the reading of the exposed area where no specimen is present. Correspondingly $I = \text{const} \frac{P_0}{P_s}$ where P_s is the photometer reading in the particular structure to be measured. When monochromatic roentgen radiation, e.g. CuK α-radiation, is used, the amount of mineral salts is computed from the equation

$$I = I_0 \cdot e^{-\mu \cdot d}$$

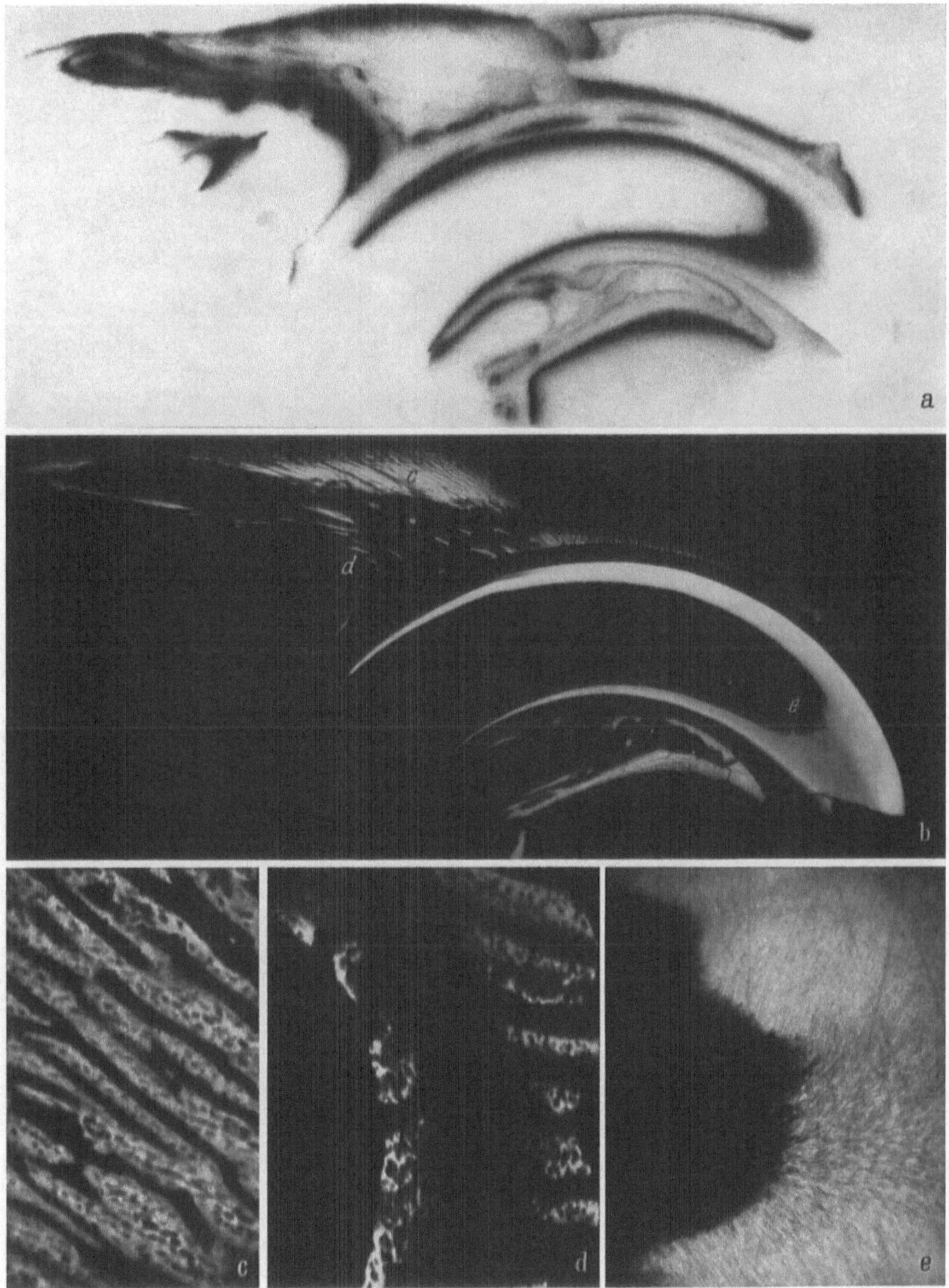

Fig. 19. Radioautogram (a) and microradiograms (b, c, d and e) of the incisor from a rat which had received ^{90}Sr by peritoneal injection (ENGSTRÖM, et al., 1958)

where μ is the linear absorption coeffizient (dimension cm^{-1}) and d the thickness of specimen in cm. If d is measured separately, the equation can be solved for μ. The value of μ for monochromatic radiation and hydroxyapatite can be computed from standard tables, and knowing the density of apatite (3), the theoretical value for hydroxyapatite can be computed. The actual μ measured is lower than the absolute value and the ratio

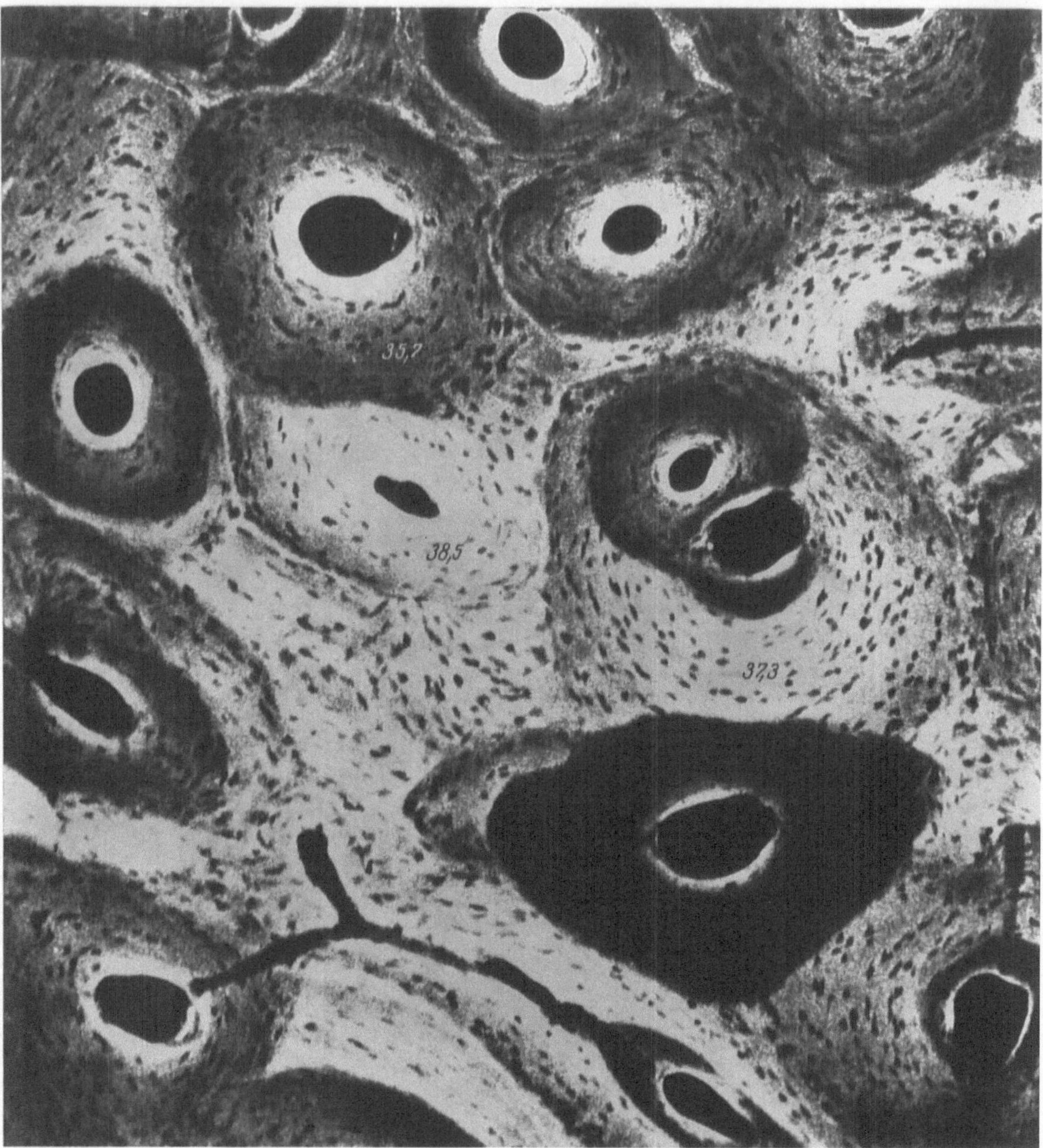

Fig. 20. Hardness of Haversian systems correlate well with the degree of mineralization demonstrated with microradiography (CARLSTRÖM, 1954)

of the two gives the percentage mineralization in a particular structure. The amount of mineral salts can also be expressed in $g \cdot cm^{-2}$ if the equation on page 299 is used.

The disadvantage of the above mentioned method is that the microradiogram must be relatively lightly exposed which presents difficulties in identifying a particular structure in the microphotometer. In order to be able to measure also heavily exposed microradiograms, a reference system in the form of a step wedge is microradiographed simultaneously with the specimen. Thus the photometry of such a recording permits the evaluation of the mineral content of a particular structure in terms of units of step wedge. If the properties of this wedge are known (thickness of steps and material) the absolute amount of mineral salts can be determined. Figs. 16 and 17 show some applications of quantitative microradiography.

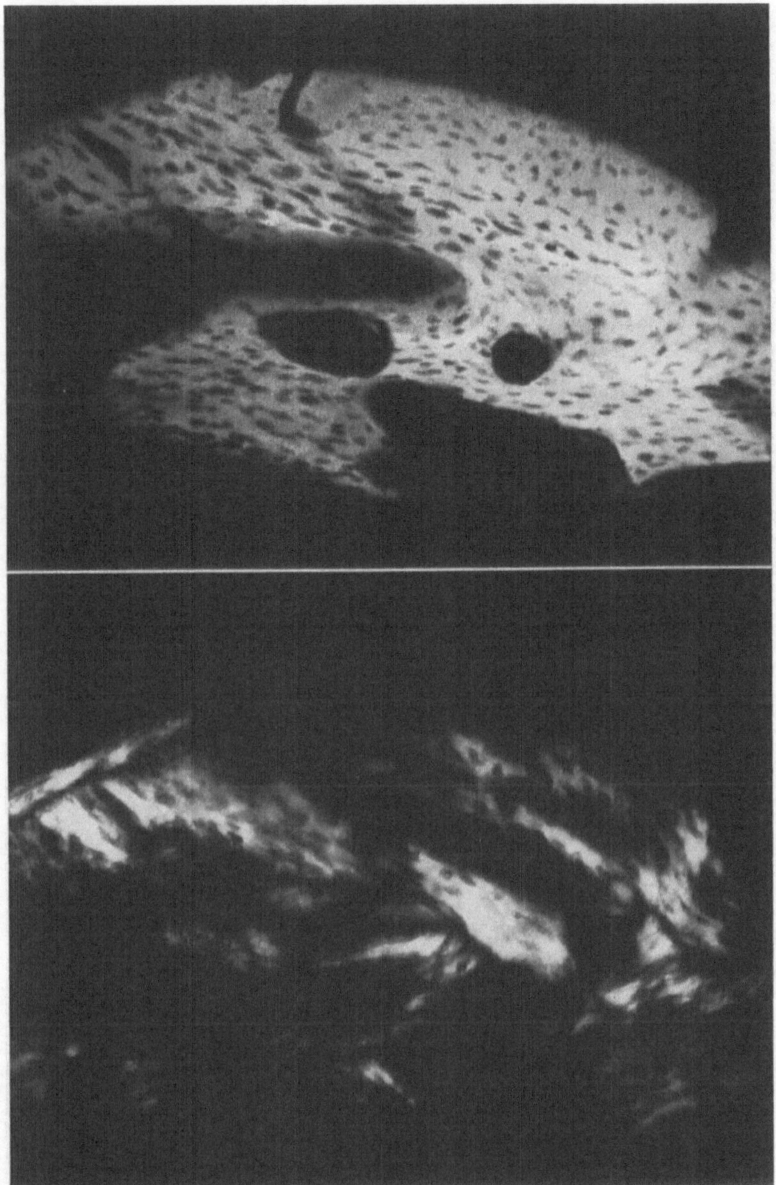

Fig. 21. Microradiogram of ectopic bone and, below, the birefringence of the organic fraction as seen in the polarizing microscope of the same section after decalcification

7. Teeth

Microradiography has been extensively applied to dental problems both what regards the normal development as several pathological conditions. Fig. 18 (top) shows a section through a jaw of a young animal, the high mineral content of the enamel is well seen. In Fig. 18, below, the carious zone in human enamel and the lesions in the dentine are demonstrated well.

In connection with work on the incorporation of radioactive strontium in the organism, rats were injected with ^{20}Sr and sacrificed at various intervals after receiving the dose. Bone specimens were prepared for microradiography, and radioautograms were also prepared of the same sections. Fig. 19a is the radioautogram showing the distribution of ^{20}Sr, 19b the corresponding microradiogram, and enlargements in 19c, e and f. One can see that it is the lowly mineralized tissue that accumulates the radioactivity.

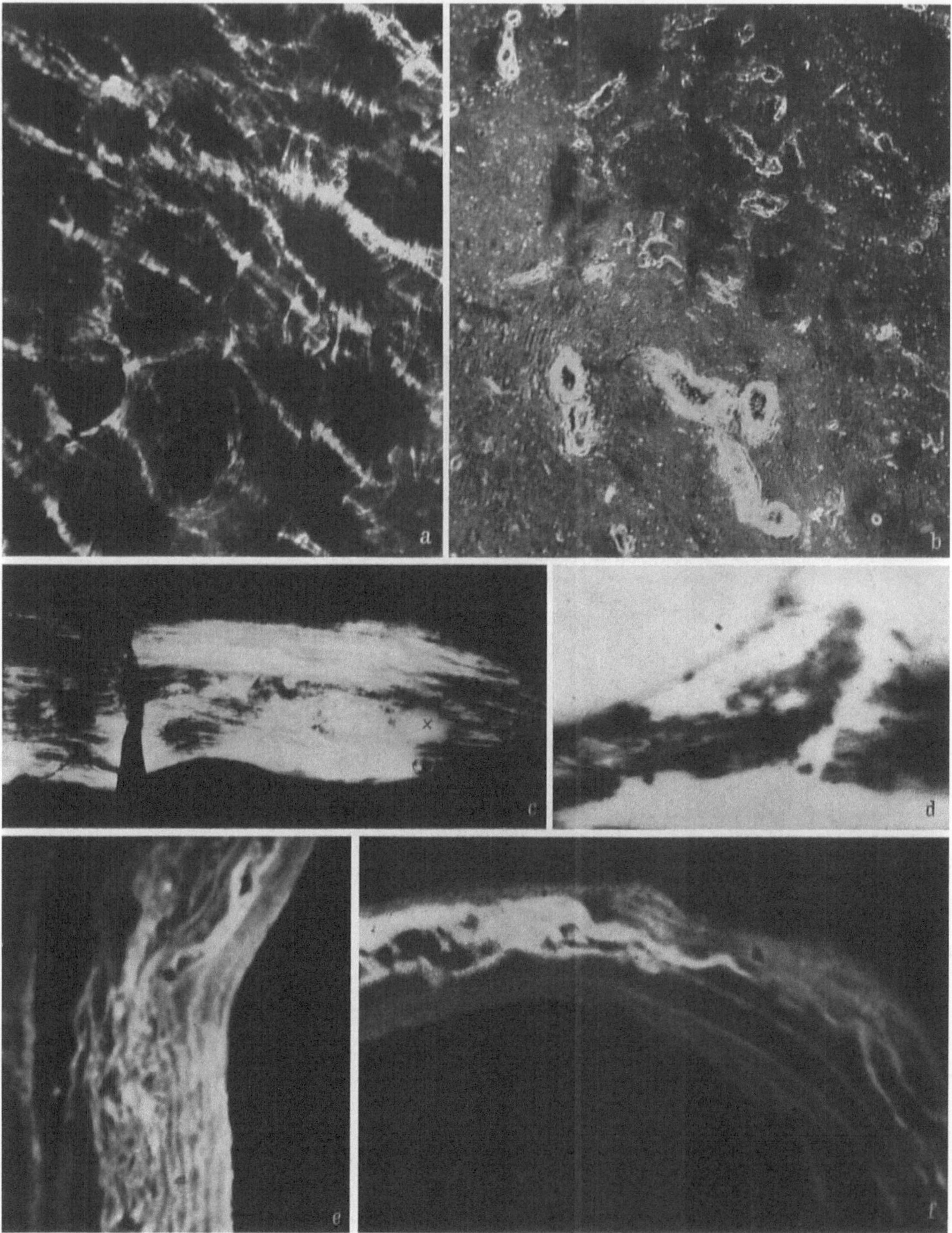

Fig. 22 a—f. Microradiograms of pathological calcifications. a, c, e and f aorta, b Sturge-Weber's disease, and d radioautogram of an aortic calcification after labelling in ^{45}Ca

8. Miscellaneous applications

The results obtained by microradiography and shown in the distribution of mineral salts were checked by microhardness determination. Fig. 20 gives the hardness values for some Haversian systems.

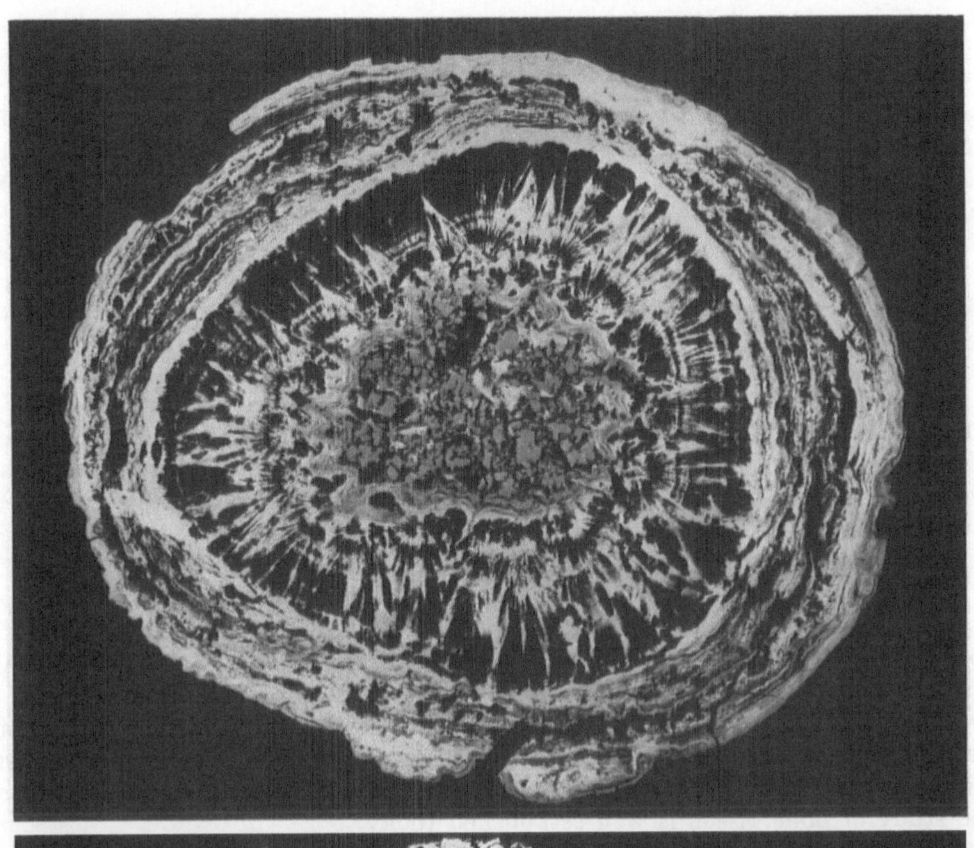

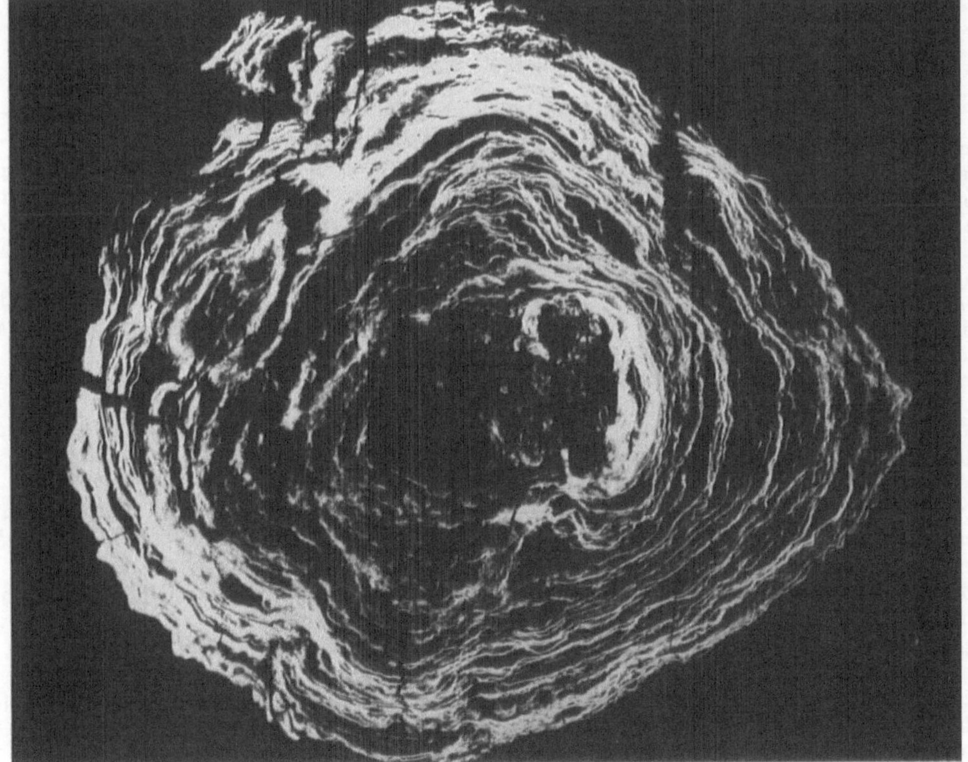

Fig. 23. Microradiograms of sections of urinary concrements

Ectopic bone formed after the injection of alcohol into a muscle of a rabbit is shown in Fig. 21 top, below the appearance in the polarizing microscope after decalcification.

Pathological calcification in blood vessels were microradiographed and the results shown in Fig. 22; a, c, e and f are sections from an arteriosclerotic aorta showing heavily absorbing calcium deposits; d is a labelling in vitro with ^{45}Ca of such a deposit, and the radioautogram shows the ready uptake; b is a section from brain in Sturge-Weber's disease showing the calcification of the small blood vessels.

Finally, in Fig. 23 two microradiograms of urinary calculi are shown. The concrements were embedded in plastic and thin sections cut. The results of the microradiographic investigation were correlated with roentgen diffraction studies.

9. Conclusions

Microradiography has cast considerable light on the amount and the distribution of apatites in mineralized tissues. By microradiography it was for the first time possible to show the differences in mineralization between different Haversian systems. The application of microradiographic techniques to the study of bone has found use in the study of various types of pathological tissues, and in the reference list some publications dealing with such problems are found. The microradiographic appearance of bone, and especially in its quantitative modification, gives us an excellent basis to judge the general structure of bone; it has been suggested that the microradiogram should be used in bone pathology to give the diagnosis of various bone diseases. More important for basic research is that the results given by microradiography are a firm basis upon which the results of other types of investigations, such as staining reactions, enzymatic reactions, the results of radioautography, etc., could be related. That microradiography is an important tool in the study of bone tissue is well established today.

References

Microradiographic technique

Bergman, G.: Studies on mineralized dental tissues. XI. Microradiography as a method for studying dental tissues. Odontologisk Revy **8**, 143 (1957).

—, and B. Engfeldt: Studies on mineralized dental tissues. II. Microradiography as a method for studying dental tissues and its application to the study of caries. Acta odont. scand. **12**, 99 (1954).

Combée, B., and A. Engström: A new device for microradiography and a simplified technique for the determination of the mass of cytological structures. Biochim. biophys. Acta **14**, 432 (1954).

Cosslett, V. E., A. Engström and H. H. Pattee: X-ray Microscopy and Microradiography. New York: Academic Press 1957.

Engström, A.: Quantitative micro- and histochemical elementary analysis by roentgen absorption spectrography. Acta radiol. (Stockh.) Suppl. **63** (1946).

— Historadiography, chapt. 10, p. 489. Physical techniques in biological research, III. edit., G. Oster and A. W. Pollister. New York: Academic Press 1956.

— X-ray micrography. Analysis of elements by microtechniques utilizing absorption emission and scattering of x-rays. Trace Analysis. Edit. Yoe and Koch, p. 493. New York: John Wiley & Sons 1957a.

Engström, A.: Contact microradiography: A general survey. X-ray microscopy and microradiography. Edit. V. E. Cosslett, A. Engström and H. H. Pattee, p. 24. New York: Academic Press 1957b.

— X-ray microscopy, chapt. V, p. 343. Analytical cytology. Edit. R. C. Mellors. New York: McGraw-Hill 1959.

— X-ray microanalysis in biology and medicine. Amsterdam: Elsevier Publ. Co. 1961.

— S. Bellman and B. Engfeldt: Microradiography. A review. Brit. J. Radiol. **28**, 517 (1955).

— V. E. Cosslett, and H. H. Pattee: X-ray microscopy and X-ray microanalysis. Amsterdam: Elsevier Publ. Co. 1961.

—, and R. C. Greulich: High-resolution microradiography using low-voltage x-rays. J. appl. Physics **27**, 758 (1956).

— C. Lagergren and B. Lundberg: Determination of strontium and calcium in bone by x-ray absorptiometry. Exp. Cell Res. **12**, 592 (1957).

—, and B. Lindström: The weighing of cellular structure by ultrasoft x-rays. General cytochemical methods, vol. 1, p. 1. Edit. J. F. Danielli. New York: Academic Press 1958.

ENGSTRÖM A., and B. LUNDBERG: A simple midget x-ray tube for high-resolution microradiography. Exp. Cell Res. **12**, 198 (1957).

— — and G. BERGENDAHL: High resolution microradiography with ultrasoft x-rays. J. ultrastruct. Res. **1**, 147 (1957).

—, and L. WEGSTEDT: Equipment for microradiography with soft roentgen. Acta radiol. (Stockh.) **35**, 345 (1951).

FITZGERALD, P. J., and A. ENGSTRÖM: The use of ultraviolet-microscopy, roentgen-ray-absorption, and radioautographic techniques in the study of neoplastic disease: A discussion of these cytophysical techniques. Cancer (Philad.) **5**, 643 (1952).

HAMMARLUND-ESSLER, E.: A method of preparing ground sections for microradiography and autoradiography with a description of a grinding apparatus. Acta odont. scand. **13**, 167 (1955).

HOH, F. C., and B. LINDSTRÖM: On the theory of quantitative microradiography in biology. J. ultrastruct. Res. **2**, 512 (1959).

WALLGREN, G., and K. HOLMSTRAND: Technical considerations on quantitative microradiography on bone. Exp. Cell. Res. **12**, 188 (1957).

Microradiography of bone and structure of bone

AMPRINO, R., and A. ENGSTRÖM: Studies on x-ray absorption and diffraction of bone tissue. Acta anat. (Basel) **15**, 1 (1952).

CARLSTRÖM, D.: X-ray crystallographic studies on apatites and calcified structures. Acta radiol. (Stockh.) Suppl. **121** (1955).

—, and A. ENGSTRÖM: Ultrastructure and distribution of mineral salts in bone tissue. Chapt. 6, p. 149. The biochemistry and physiology of bone. Edit. G. H. BOURNE. New York: Academic Press 1956.

DAVIES, H. G., and A. ENGSTRÖM: Interferometric and x-ray absorption studies of bone tissue. Exp. Cell Res. **7**, 243 (1954).

ENGFELDT, B., and S.-O. HJERTQUIST: Biophysical studies on bone tissue. XV. A histochemical and microradiographic study on normal bone tissue. Acta path. microbiol. scand. **36**, 385 (1955).

ENGSTRÖM, A.: Structure of bone from the anatomical to the molecular level. Ciba foundation symposium on bone structure and metabolism, p. 3. Edit. G. E. W. WOLSTENHOLME and C. M. O'CONNOR. London: J. & A. Churchill 1956.

— R. BJÖRNERSTEDT, C. J. CLEMEDSON and A. NELSON: Bone and radiostrontium. New York: John Wiley & Sons, and Stockholm: Almqvist & Wiksell 1958.

—, and B. ENGFELDT: Lamellar structure of osteons demonstrated by microradiography. Experientia (Basel) **9**, 19 (1953).

HOLMSTRAND, K.: Biophysical investigations of bone transplants and bone implants. An experimental study. Acta orthop. scand. Suppl. **26** (1957).

HOLMSTRAND, K.: Biophysical investigations of bone transplants. Plast. reconstr. Surg. **19**, 265 (1957).

KARLSSON, K., A. ENGSTRÖM and H. ENGSTRÖM: Microradiographic studies of the auditory ossicles (malleus and incus) and of the osseous labyrinth. Acta radiol. (Stockh.) **42**, 381 (1954).

NILSONNE, U.: Biological investigations of the mineral phase in healing fractures. Acta orthop. scand. Suppl. **37** (1959).

OMNELL, K.-Å.: Quantitative roentgenologic studies on changes in mineral content of bone in vivo. Acta radiol. (Stockh.) Suppl. **148** (1957).

WALLGREN, G.: Biophysical analyses of the formation and structure of human fetal bone. A microradiographic and x-ray crystallographic study. Acta paediat. (Uppsala) Suppl. **113** (1957).

Microradiography of dental tissues

BERGMAN, G.: Studies on mineralized dental tissues. XIII. Combined microradiographic and autoradiographic investigations on carious teeth. J. dent. belge **50**, 75 (1959).

—, and B. ENGFELDT: Studies on mineralized dental tissues. IV. Biophysical studies on teeth and tooth-germs in osteogenesis imperfecta. Acta path. microbiol. scand. **35**, 537 (1954).

— — Studies on mineralized dental tissues. V. Microradiographic investigation of experimentally produced caries and attrition in white rats. Acta odont. scand. **12**, 193 (1954).

— — Studies on mineralized dental tissues. VI. The distribution of mineral salts in the dentine with special reference to the dentinal tubules. Acta odont. scand. **13**, 1 (1955).

ENGFELDT, B., G. BERGMAN and E. HAMMARLUND-ESSLER: Studies on mineralized dental tissues. I. A microradiographic and autoradiographic investigation of teeth and tooth-germs of normal dogs. Exp. Cell. Res. **7**, 381 (1954).

—, and E. HAMMARLUND-ESSLER: Studies on mineralized dental tissues. X. A microradiographic, autoradiographic, and histochemical investigation on dental hard tissues in dogs with experimentally produced vitamin D deficiency. Acta odont. scand. **14**, 293 (1956a).

— — Studies on mineralized dental tissues. IX. A microradiographic study of the mineralization of developing enamel. Acta odont. scand. **14**, 273 (1956b).

HAMMARLUND-ESSLER, E.: Studies on the mineral component of dental enamel by means of microradiography, autoradiography and x-ray diffraction. Trans. roy. Schools of Dentistry Stockholm and Umeå No 5, 1958.

—, and G. BERGMAN: A diamond saw apparatus for cutting hard tissues. Trans. roy. Schools of Dentistry Stockholm and Umeå No **4**, 1 (1958).

OMNELL, K.-Å.: Electrolytic precipitation of zinc carbonate in the jaw. O.S., O. M. & O. P. **12**, 846 (1959).

Other applications of microradiography to hard tissues

CARLSTRÖM, D.: Micro-hardness measurements on single Haversian systems in bone. Experientia (Basel) **10**, 171 (1954).

— B. ENGFELDT, A. ENGSTRÖM and N. RINGERTZ: Studies on the chemical composition of normal and abnormal blood vessel walls. I. Chemical nature of vascular calcified deposits. Lab. Invest. **2**, 325 (1953).

ENGFELDT, B.: Biophysical studies on bone tissue. VI. Biophysical studies on bone tissue from osteogenic sarcoma. Cancer (Philad.) **7**, 815 (1954).

— R. BJÖRNERSTEDT, C.-J. CLEMEDSON and A. ENGSTRÖM: A preliminary study of the in vivo and in vitro uptake of Sr^{90} in bone tissue and the osseous localization of radioactive fission products from atomic explosions. Acta orthop. scand. **24**, 101 (1954).

ENGFELDT, B., and A. ENGSTRÖM: Biophysical studies on bone tissue. XII. Experimentally produced ectopic bone tissue. Acta orthop. scand. **24**, 85 (1954).

HEDENBERG, I.: Macroscopic and microscopic changes and stone formation in the urinary tract in experimentally produced vitamin A deficiency in rats and some notes on the effect of large doses of vitamin A on the uterine, vaginal and vesical epithelium. Acta chir. scand. Suppl. **192** (1954).

LAGERGREN, C.: Biophysical investigations of urinary calculi. An x-ray crystallographic and microradiographic study. Acta radiol. (Stockh.) **133** (1956).

Note added in proof: Since the submission of this manuscript in 1958 considerable improvements in techniques and new results have been obtained. A review is given in the proceedings of 42nd meeting of the Japanese Orthopaedie Association, Tokyo 1969.

E. Struktur und Ultrastruktur des Knochengewebes

Von

K.-H. Knese

Mit 55 Abbildungen

1. Einleitung: Struktur und Ultrastruktur

Der vorliegende Artikel beschäftigt sich mit einigen Fragen der Struktur des Knochengewebes. Zu dieser Erörterung muß zunächst die Morphologie der Gewebekomponenten, der Kollagenfibrillen, der Interfibrillärsubstanz und der Kristalle dargestellt werden. Schließlich sind die Fragen der Knochenbildung und der Strukturentstehung zu diskutieren.

Das Knochengewebe hat eine sehr verwickelte Struktur. Als Struktur eines Stoffes bezeichnen wir das innere Gefüge eines Materials nach Art, Form und Ordnung der Teile. Im Vergleich mit einem Bauwerk hat PETERSEN (1927, 1930) das Gefüge eines Skeletstückes in mehrere übereinander liegende Stufen oder Ordnungen gegliedert. KNESE et al. (1954) und KNESE (1958b, 1959b, c) erweitern die Gliederung von PETERSEN durch Beschreibung einer Struktur zweiter Ordnung. Damit sind im Knochengewebe Strukturen folgender Ordnung zu unterscheiden:

1. Ordnung: Die Compacta-Spongiosa-Verteilung.

2. Ordnung: Die topographisch spezifische Zusammenlagerung von Lamellensystemen als Ausdruck des verschiedenartigen Feinbaues der Skeletelemente.

3. Ordnung: Die Lamellensysteme, Osteone (Haverssche Systeme) und Tangentiallamellen (Schalt- und sog. Generallamellen).

4. Ordnung: Die Lamellen.

5. Ordnung: Die Fasern mit dem sie umgebenden Mantel organischer und anorganischer (kristalliner) Substanzen.

6. Ordnung: Die Molekular-(Ultra-)Struktur der Fasern, der organischen und anorganischen Substanzen.

Im Knochengewebe liegt demgemäß eine Strukturhierarchie vor. „Auf Grund solcher Strukturhierarchie vollbringen die höheren Stufen neuartige, d.h. den tieferen nicht mögliche Leistungen" (W. J. SCHMIDT, 1957). KNESE (1958b) hat die mechanischen Leistungen der Strukturen verschiedener Ordnung des Knochengewebes diskutiert (s. S. 449).

Die Strukturen 6. und z.T. 5. Ordnung können mit dem Lichtmikroskop (Hellfeld) nicht mehr oder nur begrenzt untersucht werden (s. unten). Diese Dimension umfaßt die submikroskopische Morphologie (FREY-WYSSLING, 1953) oder die molekulare und kolloidale Organisation des biologischen Materials (GROSS, 1950). Heute wird häufig von der Ultrastruktur der Gewebe gesprochen.

Die Ordnungsstufen des Knochengewebes mit Ausnahme derjenigen 1. Ordnung wurden an Hand der Lagerung der Kollagenfibrillen (KNESE et al., 1954) aufgestellt; so kamen auch KNESE und TITSCHAK (1962) und KNESE und KNOOP (1961c) zu der Auffassung, das Knochengewebe sei ein Fasergewebe, wobei die Faserordnung auch für die Ordnung aller restlichen Komponenten, unter anderem der Mineralien (s. S. 351), maßgebend ist.

Zur Untersuchung der Struktur in ihren Ordnungsstufen muß jeweils eine bestimmte „Auflösung" gegeben sein, wobei etwa folgende Bereiche angegeben werden können: Röntgen-Brechung

10^{-8}—10^{-5} cm = 6. und 5. Ordnung; Elektronenmikroskop 10^{-6}—10^{-5} cm = 5. und 4. (3.) Ordnung; Lichtmikroskop 10^{-4}—10^{-1} cm = 4. bis 2. Ordnung; Untersuchungen im polarisierten Licht umspannenden großen Bereich von der 2.—6. Ordnung: In der Dimension der 2. bis 4. (5.) Ordnung wird z.B. die Anisotropie der Kollagenfasern dazu benutzt, um Lage und Verlaufsweise der Fasern festzustellen; in der Dimension 5. und 6. Ordnung wird die Ursache der Doppelbrechung und damit die Molekularstruktur der Fasern untersucht.

Die Ultrastruktur kann z.T. aus Untersuchungen mit indirekten Methoden, Doppelbrechung und Röntgenbrechung, erschlossen werden. Jede indirekte Methode birgt aber die Gefahr von Fehldeutungen in sich und kann nur ein gewisses Mittel der Strukturordnung erfassen (Robinson und Watson, 1952; Knese, 1959b), worüber noch zu berichten ist. Es ist daher wünschenswert, das gleiche Material mit verschiedenen Methoden zu untersuchen (Knese, 1959b). Durch das Elektronenmikroskop mit einem Auflösungsvermögen für biologische Objekte von mindestens 20—40 Å gegenüber 5000 Å des Lichtmikroskopes ist ein beachtlicher Teil der submikroskopischen Morphologie „sichtbar" geworden.

2. Die Komponenten des Knochengewebes

a) Die sog. Grundsubstanz

Als Bestandteile des Knochengewebes und z.T. auch der übrigen Stützgewebe sind unter Angabe ihrer „Gewebetopographie" (in Anlehnung an Eastoe, 1956; Gersh und Catchpole, 1960) folgende Stoffe zu nennen:

Osteocyten		Zellproteine Kohlenhydrate Fette lösliche anorganische Salze Wasser
Intercellularsubstanzen	Fibrillen	Kollagen Kohlenhydrate
	Organische Inter- und Perifibrillärsubstanzen	Glykosaminoglycane Saure MPS (Hyaluronsäure)[a] Chondroitin-4-sulfat (A) Chondroitin-6-sulfat (C) Keratansulfat Glykoproteine Proteine (widerstandsfähige ?) Lösliches Kollagen (Tropokollagen)
	Abkömmlinge des Blutplasmas	Wasser Enzyme Immunkörper Stoffwechselprodukte Albumin Globulin Vitamine Hormone Ionen
	Anorganische Kristallite	Hydroxylapatit $+Ca^{++}$, MgH^{+}, Citrat$^{=}$, HCO_3^-, $HPO_4^{=}$, Na^+, K^+
Dazu: Blutgefäße		Kollagen Elastin
Restblut		Wasser Zellproteine Plasmaproteine Salze

[a] Im Knochengewebe nicht (oder vermutlich nicht) vorhanden.

Diese Aufstellung zeigt, daß im Knochengewebe eine Durchdringungsstruktur von Materialien verschiedener Eigenschaften (Knese, 1956a, 1958b) vorliegt; dabei bestehen zwischen diesen Teilen sehr enge, leider nur z. T. aufgeklärte Beziehungen. Weiterhin ist zu unterscheiden zwischen jenen Stoffen, die dem Gewebe eigen sind und jenen, die das Gewebe durchwandern und dem Blut angehören.

Für die verschiedenartigen Aufgaben des Knochengewebes sind wie für die anderen Stützgewebe die Intercellularsubstanzen bestimmend. Robb-Smith (1954) und Gibian (1954) haben das mangelnde Interesse an den Intercellularsubstanzen der Auswirkung der Virchowschen Zellenlehre zugeschrieben. Robb-Smith meint allerdings, es liegt weniger ein Mangel an Kenntnissen als ein wissenschaftlicher Isolationismus vor und setzt sich mit den Gründen einer „connective tissue renaissance" auseinander. Für den Organismus entscheidende Stoffwechselvorgänge sind nicht an Zellen, sondern an die Zwischensubstanzen gebunden, ob mit oder ohne Mitwirkung von Zellen, ist gleichgültig, da ohne die Struktur der Zwischensubstanzen das Substrat für diese Prozesse fehlt. Nach Gibian (1959) tritt neben die „atomistische Cellularität" das Continuum der Bindegewebe. Gibian, als Chemiker weniger durch Lehrtradition gehemmt als ein Biologe oder Mediziner, stellt fest, daß die Zellen der Bindegewebe nicht wie die in drüsigen Organen Träger der Tätigkeit sind (s. unten, Knese und Knoop, 1961c); die Zellen sind nur Aufbauelemente für eine hoch differenzierte Struktur, welche ihrerseits die vornehmlich „mechanische" (nicht im engeren Sinne) Leistung übernimmt. Den Zellen bleiben die ursprünglichen Aufgaben der nutritiven, fermentativen und reparatorischen Leistungen vorbehalten. Der Biologe wird in der Beurteilung der Zelleistung sog. ausdifferenzierter Stützgewebe vorsichtiger sein, kann aber an der zentralen Stellung der Intercellularsubstanz in der sog. Funktion dieser Gewebe nicht vorbeigehen. Dieser Wandel in der Auffassung gilt auch für das Knochengewebe, das nicht mehr nur als ein „Hartgewebe" mit rein mechanischen Aufgaben angesehen werden kann.

Die verschiedenartigen Bauelemente werden als die sog. Komponenten des Stützgewebes, auch des Knochengewebes, zusammengefaßt (unter anderem Robinson, 1952; Knese, 1956a; Sognnaes, 1955). Die Gesamtheit oder ein Teil der Intercellularsubstanzen wird mitunter noch Matrix oder Grundsubstanz benannt. Diese Bezeichnung wurde zuerst von Meckauer (1836) für den Knorpel und von Henle (1841, beide Angaben nach Wassermann, 1956) auch für den Knochen gebraucht; Henle sprach vikariierend und indifferent von Intercellularsubstanz. Bei Erörterung dieses Terminus darf nicht vergessen werden, daß zur damaligen Zeit die Intercellularsubstanz als ein homogenes Material (unter anderem Tomes und de Morgan, 1853) erschien, in das die Zellen eingebettet sind. In den folgenden 100 Jahren war man bemüht, mit den verschiedensten Methoden die Struktur dieser Intercellularsubstanz aufzuklären; die entsprechenden Untersuchungen sind noch nicht abgeschlossen. Der weitere Gebrauch des Ausdruckes Grundsubstanz ist aber nicht mehr gerechtfertigt und nicht nur für Follis (bei Meyer, 1952) zu einem roten Tuch geworden (zur Geschichte siehe Wassermann, 1929, 1956).

Der Terminus Grundsubstanz wird heute für sehr verschiedene Teile gebraucht, für die gesamte Intercellularsubstanz oder nur jene Komponenten, die nach Ausschluß der Fasern verbleiben. Nach Dorfman (1954, 1955) erfolgt die Anwendung des Wortes leichtfertig und führt zu einer Verwirrung der Begriffe, da mit einer unzureichenden Definition umfangreiche und unbewiesene Theorien verbunden werden. Viele der vorliegenden Untersuchungsergebnisse verlieren an Klarheit durch die von dem jeweiligen Autor untergelegte Bedeutung (Semantik, Hall, 1959) der verwandten Termini. Dorfman (1953) beschränkt den Ausdruck auf das amorphe Kontinuum, das sich zwischen den Zellen, Fasern und Gefäßen befindet; das Material besteht aus dem Gewebe eigenen Stoffen und den durchwandernden; diese Grundsubstanz fungiert wegen der hohen elektrischen Ladung als auswählende und kontrollierende Schranke zwischen Kreislauf und Stützgewebe (s. S. 334).

Mit dieser Beschreibung von Dorfman (1953) ist für den Augenblick wohl der altgewohnte Terminus Grundsubstanz gerettet. Schwierig zu entscheiden ist, ob die durchwandernden Stoffe als Bestandteil des Gewebes anzusehen sind. Weiterhin ist zu bedenken, daß eine Reihe von Stoffen, MPS, KH, Proteine, unter anderem lösliches Kollagen, eine differenzierte Molekularstruktur aufweisen und enge Beziehungen zu morphologisch darstellbaren Strukturen, z.B. den Fasern, besitzen. So ist nach Wassermann (1956) eine Unterscheidung zwischen einem amorphen und strukturierten Zustand in der Dimension der submikroskopischen Organisation nicht mehr gerechtfertigt; Fasern und Grundsubstanz erscheinen nur bei lichtmikroskopischen Beobachtungen als klar voneinander zu unterscheidende Elemente. Duran-Reynals (1950) führt aus, daß sich unsere Kenntnisse von der Grundsubstanz aus dem Zustand einer Art Abstraktion in den einer Realität verwandelt haben. Ein wesentlicher Schritt wurde mit der Erkenntnis getan, daß es sich bei dem sog. „spreading factor" um Hyaluronidase handelt; weiterhin gelang die Isolierung verschiedener Polysaccharide und z.T. ihr Nachweis im Schnitt (PAS-Reaktion, Metachromasie).

Unsere Methoden zur Untersuchung morphologischer Elemente haben sich durch Verwendung des Elektronenmikroskops dem makromolekularen Bereich angenähert. Der Schritt von der Stuktur 6. Ordnung, der molekularen, zur Struktur 5, die im Elektronenmikroskop untersucht werden kann, bereitet uns aber noch große Schwierigkeiten. Wir „sehen" z.B. bei Untersuchung der Fibrillogenese und Osteogenese plötzlich strukturierte Elemente, die Fibrillen, ohne angeben zu können, welche Vorgänge im molekularen Bereich zu „sichtbaren" Gebilden führen. Der Schritt zwischen der Struktur 5. und 6. Ordnung erscheint methodisch, aber kaum sachlich bedingt. Es ist zu empfehlen, wie sich das bei vielen Autoren anbahnt, die einzelnen Komponenten der Stützgewebe rein topographisch und materiell zu beschreiben, wie das in der oben wiedergegebenen Aufstellung durchgeführt wurde.

b) Die Osteocyten

Die Zellen des Knochengewebes liegen in mandelkernförmig gestalteten Knochenhöhlchen, von denen Knochenkanälchen ausgehen. In diese Kanälchen entsenden die Osteocyten Cytoplasmafortsätze und stehen mittels dieser Fortsätze untereinander in Verbindung. Auf diesem Wege sollte der Stofftransport innerhalb des Knochengewebes erfolgen. Das Hohlraumsystem ist von einer Art Kapsel ausgekleidet (Rouget, 1858; Neumann, 1863), die von Broesicke (1882) als Grenzscheide bezeichnet wurde (vgl. Weidenreich, 1930; Lipp, 1954).

Die Osteocyten stammen von Osteoblasten ab. Im Verlaufe dieser Umwandlung soll sich der Osteoblast selbst mit Knochensubstanz, dem Knochenhöhlchen, umgeben und damit zum Osteocyten werden. Für diesen Vorgang ist aber Voraussetzung, daß der Osteoblast seine polare Differenzierung aufgibt und auch nach der Periostseite hin Knochensubstanz bildet. Elektronenmikroskopische Beobachtungen (Knese und Knoop, 1958, 1961c) lassen dagegen vermuten, daß der Osteoblast zunächst seine osteogene Tätigkeit einstellt (Abb. 1). Die Zelle wird lang, spindelförmig, das endoplasmatische Reticulum (s. unten) verschwindet zu einem größeren Teil, die Mitochondrien bleiben erhalten. Durch die benachbarten Osteoblasten wird die Zelle von einem präossalen Gewebe umgeben, in dem dann Minerale abgelagert werden (Knese und v. Harnack, 1962; Knese, 1966b). Mit Erreichen der vollen Mineralisation ist morphologisch die Umwandlung zum Osteocyten vollendet (Abb. 2). In die vom Knochenhöhlchen ausgehenden Kanälchen reichen Cytoplasmafortsätze hinein. Nach polarisationsoptischen Untersuchungen von W. J. Schmidt (1959) verlaufen die Kollagenfibrillen in der Grenzscheide der Lacunen in allen Richtungen tangential zur Oberfläche, in den Kanälchen aber in deren Längsrichtung. Nach elektronenmikroskopischen Untersuchungen von Knese und v. Harnack (1962) haben nicht alle Osteocyten eine Wand mit einer „Eigenfaserung". Bei Vorliegen einer eigenen Wand ist die Richtung der sie aufbauenden Fasern z.T. sehr

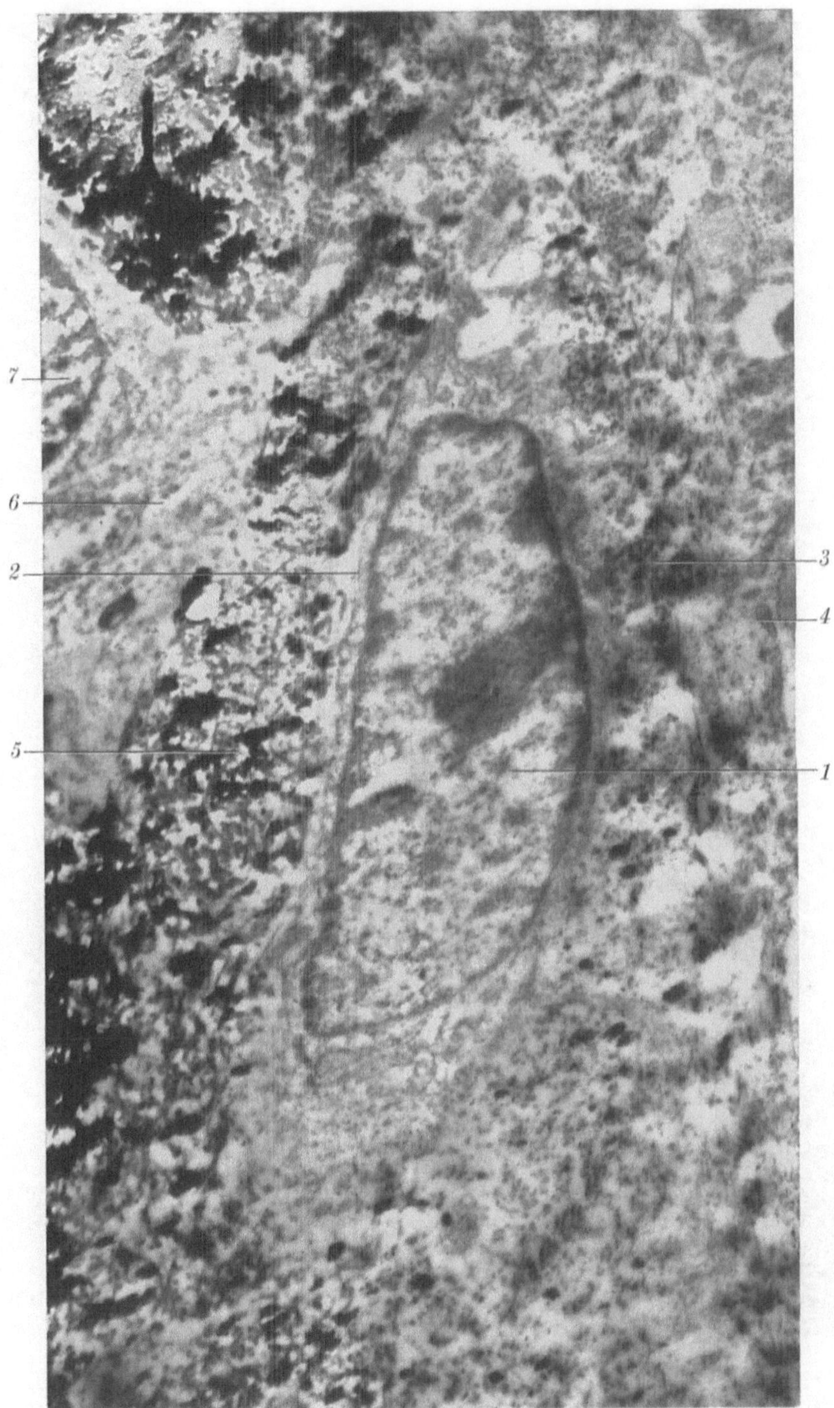

Abb. 1. Einmauerung eines Osteocyten. *1* Kern des Osteocyten; *2* Zellmembran; *3* Periostseite des Knochenhöhlchens noch aus präossalem Gewebe mit geringer Kalkeinlagerung aufgebaut; *4* Cytoplasma des Osteoblasten; *5* Markseite des Knochenhöhlchens mit stärkerer Kalkeinlagerung im präossalen Gewebe; *6* Osteoblast; *7* Osteoblastenkern. Vergr. 15500fach. (Aus: KNESE und KNOOP, 1958)

wechselnd. WASSERMANN und YAEGER (1965) beschrieben weiterhin eine dünne osmiophile Schicht als Lacunenbegrenzung. BOYDE und HOBDELL (1968) sprechen an Hand von Untersuchungen mit Hilfe der Rasterelektronenmikroskopie (scanning electron microscopy) von einer Zufallsorientierung der Fasern in der Lacunenwand im Gegensatz

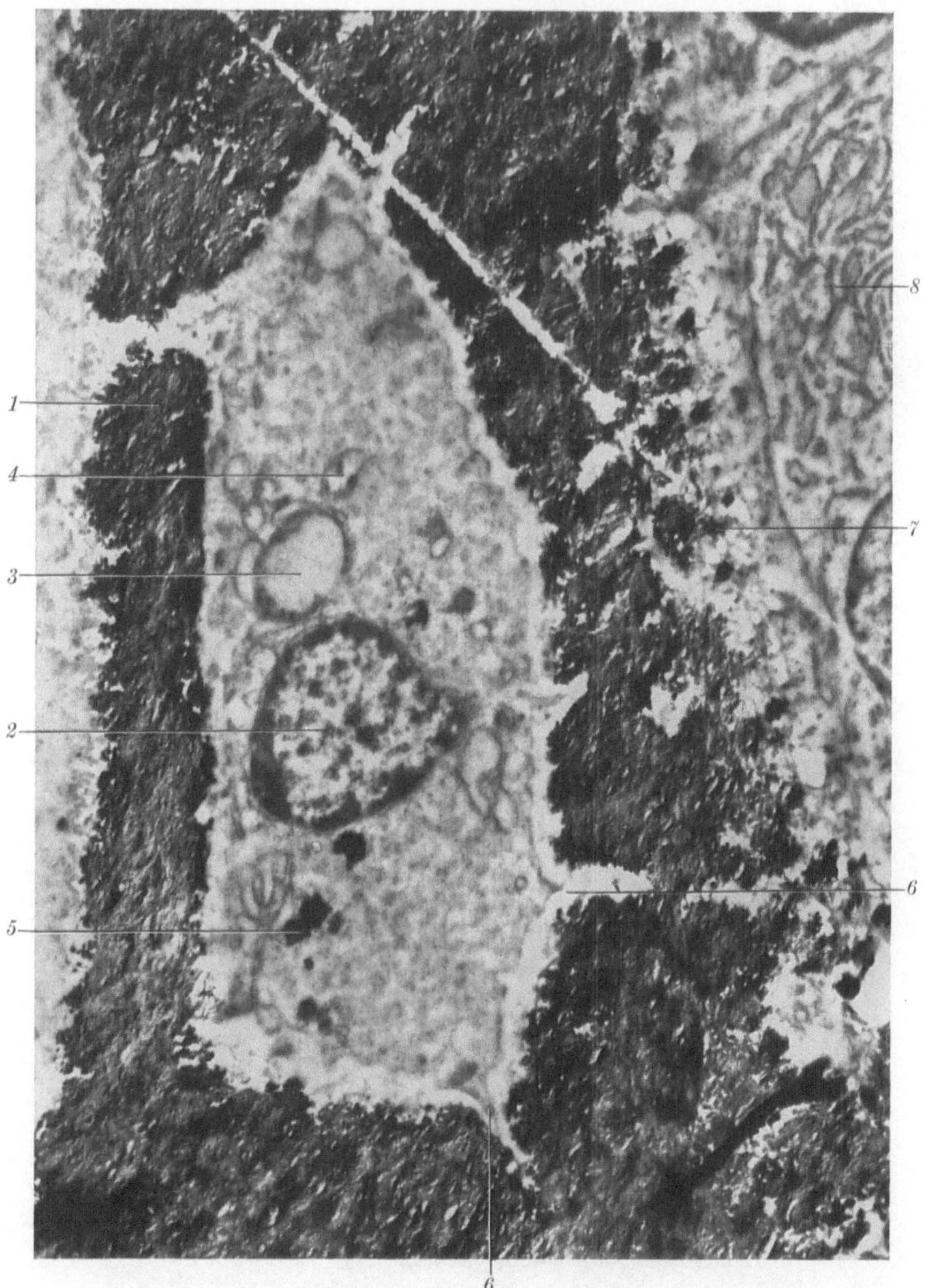

Abb. 2. Osteocyt. *1* Markseite des Knochenbälkchens; *2* Kern des Osteocyten; *3* sog. juxtanucleäre Vacuole; *4* Mitochondrien; *5* osmiophile Granula; *6* Osteocytenfortsätze; *7* präossales Gewebe mit Kalkdrüsen; *8* Cytoplasma des Osteoblasten. Vergr. 11000fach. (Aus: Knese und Knoop, 1958)

zu den orientierten Fasern in Osteoblastennähe. Damit liegt in der Grenzscheide eine „Eigenfaserung" vor, die von der Faserordnung in der restlichen Intercellularsubstanz abweicht und die Möglichkeit gibt, die Grenzscheiden aus ihrer Umgebung zu isolieren. Robinson und Watson (1952) messen elektronenmikroskopisch in Rippe und Femur des Menschen einen Durchmesser der Kanälchen von 1000—2500 Å. Knese und v. Harnack

(1962) 4000—5500 (2800—7600) Å. Die Zellfortsätze haben eine Dicke von 800—1500 Å (vgl. ROBINSON 1964); in dem frei bleibenden Spalt zwischen Fortsatz und Kanälchenwand liegen dann MPS (s. u.). Elektronenmikroskopisch konnten KNESE und v. HARNACK (1962) nur bei einigen Knochenkanälchen eine Wand mit einer Eigenfaserung beobachten. Bei anderen Kanälchen liegen dichte Packungen der Fibrillen mit gleicher Verlaufsweise wie im benachbarten Knochengewebe vor.

Der Osteocyt und seine Umgebung sind als eine Einheit anzusehen (RUTISHAUSER und MAJNO, 1951). Bereits ACHARD (1936) hatte die Basophilie (vgl. LIPP, 1954, s. unten) von Osteocyten und eine Diffusionszone um sie herum aufgezeigt. Die Basophilie beruht bekanntlich, wenn saure Mucopolysaccharide (MPS) auszuschließen sind, auf dem Vorhandensein von Ribonucleinsäuren (RNS); das elektronenmikroskopische Äquivalent der RNS sind die Membranen des endoplasmatischen Reticulum, besetzt mit den sog. Palade-Granula oder Ribosomen. Nach RUTISHAUSER und MAJNO (1951) sind bereits in normalem Knochen auch nekrotische oder sterbende Osteocyten (langsame Nekrose oder Onkose), und zwar in den zentralen Teilen der Spongiosa und an der Peripherie der Haversschen Systeme, zu finden. Die starke Phosphataseaktivität der Osteoblasten ist noch bei jungen Osteocyten erhalten und verschwindet erst bei älteren Zellen (MAJNO und ROUILLER, 1951); die Aktivität tritt bei der Onkose erneut auf. In Osteocyten sind auch PAS-positive Granula, d. h. Polysaccharide, vorhanden (HELLER-STEINBERG, 1951; KNESE und KNOOP, 1961c).

Elektronenmikroskopisch (KNESE und KNOOP, 1958; DUDLEY und SPIRO, 1961) wurden in frisch eingeschlossenen Osteocyten zunächst nur wenig Zellorganellen beobachtet, späterhin (KNESE und v. HARNACK, 1962; KNESE, 1963c, 1966b; BAUD, 1962, 1966; ROBINSON, 1964; BÉLANGER et al., 1965) wurden ein endoplasmatisches Reticulum verschiedenartiger Gestaltung, Mitochondrien, Golgi-Apparat und andere Einlagerungen beschrieben. Während u. a. BAUD (1962) die Aufgabe der Osteocyten in der Aufrechterhaltung des Stoffwechsels und der Kontrolle der MPS sieht, haben KNESE und v. HARNACK (1962) Zeichen für eine Neubildung von Kollagenfibrillen (intraossale Osteogenese) beschrieben. BÉLANGER et al. (1965) beschäftigen sich mit osteolytischen Phänomenen. KNESE (1963c) hat auf die unterschiedliche Gestalt der Osteocyten aufmerksam gemacht (junge, polyedrische im nicht lamellären Zwischengewebe und die flachen im lamellären Knochengewebe) sowie auf die nach Lebensalter wechselnde Zahl der Osteocyten je Flächeneinheit des Schnittes (Abb. 9).

LIPP (1954) kommt auf Grund umfangreicher histochemischer Untersuchungen an Osteocyten zu Vorstellungen über den zelligen Bauplan des Knochengewebes, der dem Organisationsschema anderer Bindegewebe gleicht. Fibrocyten und Knochenzellen stehen nur selten in einem reticulären Zusammenhang; beide sind von einer homogenen, chemisch inaktiven Substanz, der Kittsubstanz im Bindegewebe, den Grenzscheiden im Knochen, umgeben. Die Grenzscheidensubstanz ist auf das netzförmige Kanalsystem beschränkt, an dessen Kreuzungsstellen die Osteocyten liegen. Sie besteht aus einem verschieden stark PAS-positiven KH-Proteinkomplex, der vielleicht neben Lipoiden auch Mucopolysaccharide enthält (vgl. ROBINSON, 1964; JOWSEY, RIGGS und KELLY, 1964; WASSERMANN und YAEGER, 1965).

c) Die Kollagenfibrillen und das Kollagen

α) Morphologie der Kollagenfibrillen

Die Strukturhierarchie des Knochengewebes ergibt sich aus der Lagerungsform der Kollagenfasern. Somit ist dem Kollagen eine etwas umfangreichere Erörterung zu widmen, obwohl ein größerer Teil dieser Untersuchungen nicht am Knochenkollagen durchgeführt wurde.

v. EBNER (1874, 1875) hat durch Untersuchungen im Hellfeld nach Verhinderung der Säurequellung vermittels einer Salzlösung und im polarisierten Licht nachgewiesen, daß im Knochengewebe Kollagenfasern vorhanden sind. Die lamelläre Struktur des Knochengewebes war seit langem bekannt. Nun gab Sharpey (in Quains Anatomy 1856) Fasern an, die diese Lamellen durchdringen. v. Ebner (1875) meint, es könne sich wegen der bei Sharpeys Untersuchungen vorliegenden Säurequellung nicht um Kollagenfasern handeln. Kölliker (1860) führte den Begriff „Sharpeysche Fasern" ein, mit dem bis heute sehr verschiedenartige Fasern bezeichnet werden, die den Knochen mit der Umgebung verbinden. In der 8. Auflage von Quains Anatomy beschreibt Sharpey (1876 nach v. Eggeling, 1911) aber eindeutig den Aufbau der Knochenlamellen aus netzförmig verbundenen Fasern, d.h. die von v. Ebner aufgefundenen Kollagenfasern des Knochengewebes.

Es ist bis heute nicht klar, welche Strukturen in den sog. „perforating fibers" vorliegen, die mitunter die peripheren Knochenschichten durchdringen, und auf die v. Eggeling (1911) den Terminus beschränkt wissen will. Es scheint jedoch auf keinen Fall angebracht, alle Faserverbindungen zwischen dem Knochen und seiner Umgebung als Sharpeysche Fasern zu bezeichnen, wie z.B. die Verbindungen zum Periost oder die im Bereich von Sehnen- und Bandansätzen (Knese, 1956a). Fasern der Sehnen werden als sog. Einstrahlungsknochen (Petersen, 1930) Bestandteil des Knochengewebes (Biermann, 1957; Knese und Biermann, 1958; vgl. Abb. 51). Kollagenfasern verlaufen bekanntlich in Bündeln in leichter haarlockenartiger Wellung, auch in Sehnen (Lerch, 1951). In Sehnen zeigt sich aber bei Annäherung an den Knochen ein gestreckter Verlauf der Fasern (Biermann, 1957), sie erscheinen wie vorgespannt (Knese, 1958b). Einen gestreckten Verlauf zeigen Kollagenfasern stets innerhalb des Knochengewebes und unterscheiden sich damit von Fasern in anderen Stützgeweben.

Die Faserkomponente des Knochengewebes kann an ungefärbten Präparaten nach Entkalkung und Entquellung mit 5% Natriumsulfat im Hellfeld bei starker Abblendung erkannt werden; es tritt das Phänomen der gestreiften und gepunkteten Lamellen auf (s. unten). Die Fasern können versilbert (zuerst Studnička, 1906; vgl. Knese, 1956a) oder mit der Gram-Weigertschen Fibrinfärbung gefärbt werden (Weidenreich, 1923), die neuerlich Smith (1960a, b) wieder angewandt hat. Die Methode der Wahl ist aber die Untersuchung ungefärbter Schnitte im polarisierten Licht, die leider viel zu wenig, vor allem bei jungen Knochen geübt wird (Knese, 1959a). Die sog. Routine-Methoden (z.B. Hämatoxylin-Eosin) sind in keiner Weise dazu geeignet, die Struktur des Knochens aufzuzeigen. Der Gebrauch des Phasenkontrastverfahrens, auch an zuvor gefärbten Präparaten, ist besonders bei Untersuchung von Sehnen- und Bandansatzzonen zu empfehlen und hierbei häufig der Untersuchung im polarisierten Licht überlegen (Biermann, 1957; Knese und Biermann, 1958).

Die Definition des Kollagens ist z.Z. nach Untersuchungsmethode verschieden. Gross (und die folgenden bei Meyer, 1952) bezeichnet als Kollagen eine Klasse von Faserproteinen mit einem bestimmten Weitwinkel-Brechungsmuster, häufig einer Periode von 640 Å, mit einem geringen Gehalt an aromatischen Aminosäuren, aber einem hohen an Pyrolidin-Aminosäuren und Glycin; Hamilton gibt zur Definition sogar den Prozentsatz der einzelnen Aminosäuren an, da Kollagene aller Quellen praktisch gleich aufgebaut sind; nach Meyer (1952) ist der Ausdruck mehrdeutig; er kann histologisch für das sichtbare Licht oder das Elektronenmikroskop bzw. chemisch definiert werden.

Wir folgen dem weit verbreiteten Sprachgebrauch und bezeichnen als „Kollagen" ein Skleroprotein mit bestimmter Aminosäurezusammensetzung, als „Kollagenfibrillen bzw. -fasern" ein faseriges Gebilde von periodischem Aufbau.

Schwierig ist die Abgrenzung gegenüber den Retikulin-, Gitter- oder argyrophilen Fasern (Eastoe, 1967). Bei Anwendung von Silbermethoden zeigen bekanntlich Kollagenfasern eine kolloidale Bräunung, die Gitterfasern aber infolge eines Silberniederschlages eine Schwärzung. Die Arbeitsgruppe Schwarz (1955, 1957) hat versucht, diese Unterscheidung auch bei Untersuchungen im elektronenmikroskopischen Bereich durch Beschreibung einer Innen- und Außenversilberung aufrechtzuerhalten. Die noch immer umstrittene Bedeutung der Argyrophilie (vgl. KRAMER et al., 1953; BAIRATI, 1958) wird unter anderem auf den KH-Anteil der Fasern zurückgeführt (vgl. SCHWARZ et al., 1959).

Argyrophile Fasern wurden als sog. präkollagene Fasern für Vorgänger der Kollagenfasern angesehen (vgl. WASSERMANN, 1929; GUSTAVSON, 1956; GILLMAN, 1968; RAMACHANDRAN, 1967). Im Hinblick auf das Knochengewebe ist von Interesse, daß bei menschlichen Feten von etwa 170 mm SSL ab im Periost argyrophile Fasern (Abb. 6) auftreten (KNESE, 1956a), die mitunter als v. Korffsche (1906, 1907) Fasern bezeichnet werden. Wir kommen auf die sog. präkollagenen Fasern zurück und fassen vorläufig mit WASSERMANN (1956-zusammen: 1. Die sog. Reticulumfasern sind die embryonale Form der Bindegewebs) fasern, 2. die Reticulumfasern gehen kontinuierlich in Kollagenfasern über, 3. die Reticulumfasern sind durch einen geringen Durchmesser und die Neigung Gitter zu bilden ausgezeichnet (s. S. 329).

Die Struktur des Kollagens verschiedenster Herkunft ist in der fibrillären Struktur (RANDALL et al., 1952) und Aminosäurenzusammensetzung (NEUMAN, 1949) gleich, nur das Fischkollagen weist eine andere Zusammensetzung auf (NEUMAN, 1949; EASTOE, 1954, 1967). Aus der kaum zu übersehenden Literatur (BORASKY, 1950; BEAR, 1952; RAMACHANDRAN, 1967, 1968) sollen hier nur jene Tatsachen herausgegriffen werden, die für die Struktur und Biologie des Knochenkollagens von Bedeutung sind.

Im Hinblick auf die Nomenklatur des Kollagens sind die verschiedenen Bereiche des Auflösungsvermögens der Untersuchungsmethoden zu beachten (vgl. KÜNTZEL und PRAKKE, 1941; BEAR, 1952; WASSERMANN, 1956). Die lichtmikroskopisch sichtbare Faser von 20—200 μ Durchmesser besteht aus Fibrillen von 2—10 μ Durchmesser. Elektronenmikroskopisch sehen wir Mikrofibrillen, die häufig nur Fibrillen genannt werden. Diese Mikrofibrillen haben eine Dicke von 200—2000 Å und kommen mit dem letzteren Wert in den Bereich der lichtmikroskopischen Sichtbarkeit. Die Mikrofibrille ist aus Filamenten aufgebaut (SCHMITT et al., 1942; GROSS, 1951), die mitunter auch Primärfibrillen genannt werden. Darüber hinaus wird auf Grund der Untersuchung von Weitwinkel-Röntgen-Diagrammen das Vorhandensein von Protofibrillen angenommen (BEAR, 1952).

Fast zur gleichen Zeit wurde vermittels der Röntgenbrechung (BEAR, 1944; KRATKY und SEKORA, 1943) und des Elektronenmikroskopes (WOLPERS, 1943, 1944; SCHMITT et al., 1942, 1945) eine periodische Struktur der Mikrofibrille von der Länge 640 Å (400—1000) aufgedeckt (Abb. 3). Die gleiche Periode besitzt die Kollagenfibrille des reifen Knochengewebes (WOLPERS, 1949; HUBER und ROUILLER, 1951; ROBINSON, 1951; SCHWARZ und PAHLKE, 1953; ROBINSON und WATSON, 1952, 1955; ASCENZI, 1955).

WYCKHOFF (1952) fand außer Fibrillen mit einer Periode von 650 Å solche mit 210 Å. PORTER (1951, Gewebekultur), RANDALL et al. (1952, embryonale Gewebe), MARTIN (1953, Tibia des Hühnchens) und JACKSON (1955) fanden bei jungen Fibrillen und in frühen Entwicklungsstadien Perioden, die unter 640 Å liegen. KNESE und KNOOP (1958) haben im präossalen Gewebe der Tibia von Rattenfeten die Periode statistisch zu 290 Å $\pm$ 78 bestimmt. In entkalktem jungen periostalen Knochen der Ratte beträgt die Periode etwa 500 Å, im chondralen etwa 400 Å (KNESE und KNOOP, 1961c). ASCENZI und BENEDETTI (1955) haben für den 5. und 6. Fetalmonat die Periode an Schädelknochen menschlicher Feten zu 520—540 Å (Mittel Parietale $5^1/_2$ FM. 534 Å, Grenzwerte 491/581: KNESE 1959b) gemessen. SCHWARZ und PAHLKE (1953) geben vom Fetalleben zum postfetalen ein Anwachsen der Periode von 450 auf 640 Å an.

KNESE und KNOOP (1958) haben auch die Dicke der Fibrillen in verschiedenem Abstand vom Osteoblasten untersucht und finden in drei einander folgenden (Abb. 12) Streifen von jeweils 0,75 μ Breite die Zunahme der Dicke von 300 auf 356 und schließlich auf 430 Å. In entkalktem periostalen Knochen lag die Dicke ebenfalls noch über 400 Å, in enchondralem dagegen bei 800 Å. Aus den Werten von HUBER und ROUILLER (1951) errechnet (KNESE, 1959b) beträgt die Fibrillendicke bei einem 3 Monate alten Kinde 704, beim Erwachsenen 975 Å. Nach SCHWARZ und PAHLKE (1953, umgerechnet von KNESE,

1959b) betragen die Fibrillendurchmesser im Parietale bei Feten von 17 cm: 288; 35 cm: 414; 52 cm: 403 Å, im Femur bei einem Individuum von $1^1/_2$ J.: 422; 4 J.: 601; $7^3/_4$ J.: 497; 67 J.: 615 Å, im Petrosum mit 64 J.: 569; 74 J.: 577 Å. ROBINSON und WATSON (1955) geben die Fibrillendicke für das Kind mit 180—350—530 Å, für Individuen im mittleren Lebensalter mit 800 und für das Greisenalter mit 1000—1500 Å an.

Die beschriebene Änderung der Periode und der Dicke der Kollagenfibrillen wird als Wachstum oder Reifung bezeichnet, ein Vorgang, der von der Fibrillenbildung verschieden ist und in der Aufnahme von in Neutralsalzen löslichem, monomerem (Tropo-) Kollagen (s. S. 329) bestehen soll (PORTER und PAPPAS, 1959; WASSERMANN, 1956; über

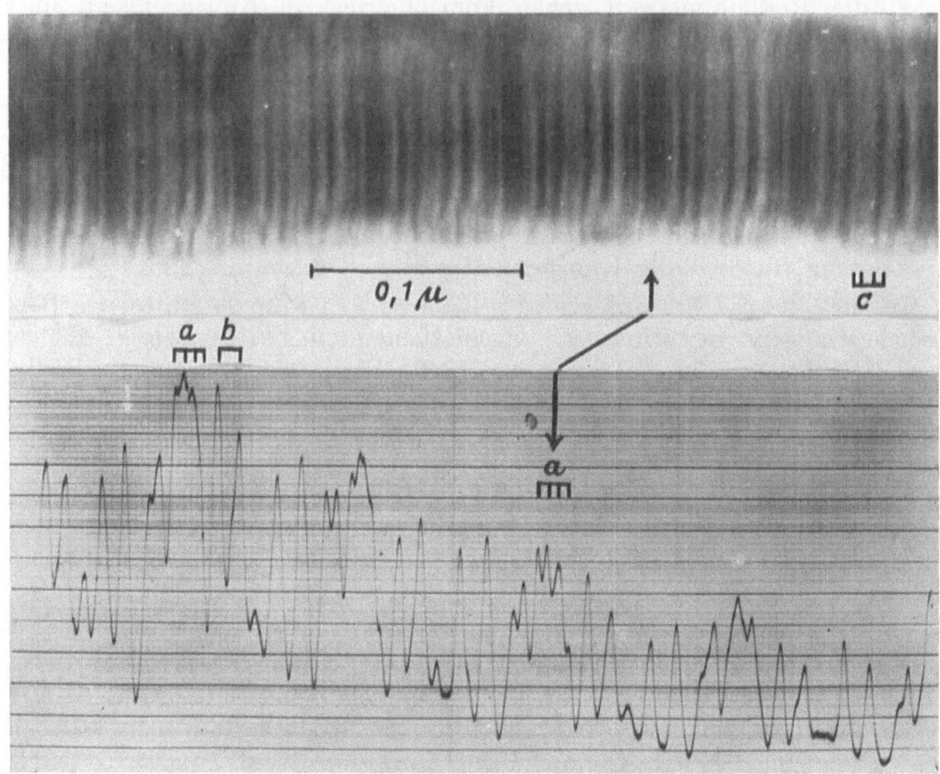

Abb. 3. Mikrofibrille aus dem Lig. nuchae des Menschen mit einer Unterteilung der Periode von 670 Å in 11—13 Unterbanden; Vergr. 26900. Darunter die Photometerkurve. (NEMETSCHEK et al., 1955, aus WASSERMANN, 1956)

Alterung: VERZÁR, 1964; SINEX, 1968). KNESE und TITSCHAK (1962), die diesen Vorgang auch als Zuwachs bezeichnet haben, vermuten auf Grund elektronenmikroskopischer Untersuchungen am Perichondrium und Epiphysenknorpel (KNESE und KNOOP, 1961a), daß die Neubildung von Fibrillen mit einer massiven Ausschüttung von relativ großen Makromolekülen verbunden ist, der Zuwachs aber nicht. WASSERMANN (1956) hat für die Dickenzunahme von Sehnenfibrillen von 500 auf 2000 Å eine Vergrößerung des Querschnittes auf das 16fache und eine Vermehrung der Polypeptidketten von 2000 auf 30000 errechnet. KNESE und TITSCHAK (1962) bestimmten die Volumenzunahme einer Fibrillenperiode von 640 Å und der Faserdicke von 800 Å im mittleren Lebensalter zu 15,7 gegenüber der Fibrille in Osteoblastennähe und zu 7,7 im Vergleich mit einer Fibrille des präossalen Gewebes. Für Fibrillen im Greisenalter mit einer Dicke von 1000 Å lauten die entsprechenden Werte 24,5 bzw. 11,9. Der Zuwachs, d.h. der Anteil des von der Fibrille nach ihrer Bildung durch Materialaufnahme vermehrten Volumens beträgt für eine Fibrillendicke von 800 Å 93,6 % und bei 1000 Å Dicke 95,9 % des endgültigen Volumens einer Periodenlänge.

In etwa 2 μ Abstand vom Osteoblastenrand legen sich die Fibrillen zu Bündeln, d.h. Fasern zusammen (KNESE und KNOOP, 1958). Die Zusammenlagerung erfolgt, wie es von der quergestreiften Muskulatur her bekannt ist, derart, daß die einander entsprechenden Periodenabschnitte auf gleicher Höhe liegen (ROBINSON, 1951; KNESE, 1959b); dabei treten auch Verschiebungen der Fasern gegeneinander auf, die ähnlich wie bei quergestreiften Muskelfasern zu Noniusperioden führen. Durch den Zuwachs der Fibrillen an Dicke wird deren Anzahl je Flächeneinheit des Schnittes herabgesetzt. Diese Flächendichte beträgt bei der Ratte (KNESE und KNOOP, 1961c; KNESE und v. HARNACK, 1962; KNESE, 1963) in Osteoblastennähe 340 Fibrillen je 1 μ^2, im Abstand von 1,5—2,25 μ 300, in noch nicht mineralisiertem präossalem Gewebe 220/μ^2, in entkalktem periostalem Knochen 90/μ^2; Werte für den Menschen liegen nicht vor.

Der geschilderte periodische Aufbau der Kollagenfibrille erscheint elektronenmikroskopisch als eine Folge dunkler und heller Teile, der Makroperiode, die von SCHMITT et al. (1943) als A- und B-, von WOLPERS (1943) als D- und H-Streifen bezeichnet wurden. Der A (H)-Teil mißt etwa 400 Å. Nach Färbung mit Osmiumsäure fanden WOLPERS (1944, 1948), mit Phosphorwolframsäure SCHMITT et al. (1945), mit Uranylacetat NUTTING et al. (1948) 5 intraperiodische Streifen (A: a, b, c, d; B: e). Schließlich wurden 3—7 (GROSS und SCHMITT, 1948) bzw. 8—13 (HOFMANN et al., 1952) solcher Streifen angegeben (Abb. 4). Die Kollagenfibrillen des Knochens zeigen 5 Streifen (ROBINSON und WATSON, 1955; SHELDON und ROBINSON, 1961). GLIMCHER (1960) hat schematisch dargestellt (Abb. 4), daß ursprünglich für jede Periode nur eine Bande und Interbande angenommen wurde. Mit fortschreitender Technik erkannte man eine größere Zahl von Banden, wobei einzelne von ihnen nur eine Breite von 8—10 Å besitzen.

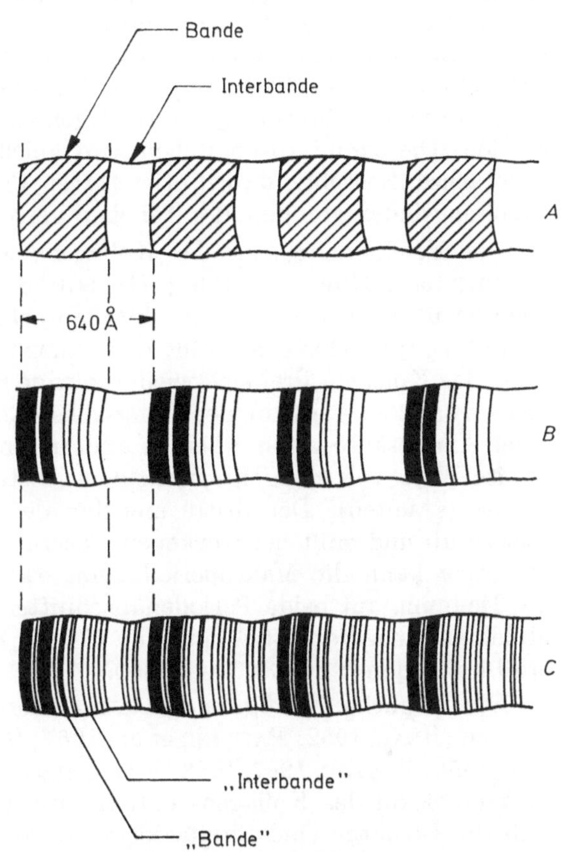

Abb. 4. Schematische Darstellung zur Bezeichnung „Bande und Interbande" des Kollagens. *A* Ursprüngliche Unterscheidung von Bande und Interbande. *B* und *C* Weitere Aufteilung der Periode mit entsprechendem Fortschritt der elektronenmikroskopischen Technik. (Umzeichnung nach GLIMCHER, 1969)

Das Fehlen einer solchen Querstruktur im Elektronenmikroskop beruht nicht auf einer Eigenheit der Fibrille, sondern hängt von präparatorischen und aufnahmetechnischen Bedingungen ab. Die einzelnen Querstreifen verhalten sich gegenüber verschiedenartigen Färbungen (s. oben, vgl. unter anderem KÜHN et al., 1960) unterschiedlich.

NEMETSCHEK (1958) hat die elektronenmikroskopisch sichtbare einfache oder hoch unterteilte Querstreifung in der Abhängigkeit von der Vorbehandlung erörtert und ein Modell entworfen, das diesen Befunden Rechnung trägt. Auf die Abhängigkeit der Fibrillenstruktur von der Vorbehandlung beim Knorpel haben KNESE und KNOOP (1961a) hingewiesen.

Diese Befunde haben die Erörterungen über die Molekularstruktur der Kollagenfibrille stark beeinflußt. Die Kollagenfibrille ist bekanntlich positiv einachsig doppelbrechend, d.h. sie zeigt eine Doppelbrechung nur in Längsachse der Faser, aber nicht senkrecht dazu. Diese Qualität der Kollagenfaser wird bei der Untersuchung des Knochens in der Struktur 2.—4. Ordnung dazu verwandt, um Verlaufsweise und Ordnung der Kollagenfasern zu bestimmen. Kollagenfasern, die mit ihrer Längsachse mehr oder minder in der Präparatebene liegen, erscheinen bei entsprechender Einstellung zwischen gekreuzten Nikols hell, senkrecht zur Schnittebene verlaufende Fasern aber dunkel. Zur Aufklärung der Struktur sind demgemäß mindestens zwei aufeinander senkrecht stehende Schnittebenen zu untersuchen (KNESE, VOGES und RITSCHL, 1954; KNESE und KNOOP, 1961c).

Aus der Erscheinung der Doppelbrechung kann aber auch auf die Molekularstruktur der Kollagenfaser geschlossen werden. Die vorliegenden Beobachtungen (unter anderem PFEIFFER, 1943; ROLLHÄUSER, 1952) sprechen nach den optischen Theorien (W. J. SCHMIDT, 1934, 1957; FREY-WYSSLING 1953) für das Vorliegen einer Eigendoppelbrechung und einer Formdoppelbrechung; die Kollagenfaser kann als ein organischer Kristall angesehen werden. Die submikroskopischen Partikelchen liegen mit ihrer Längsachse parallel zur Faserachse. Zwischen diesen orientierten Partikelchen befindet sich ein Medium, dessen Brechungsindex von dem der Teilchen verschieden ist.

Die Molekularstruktur des Kollagens wurde mit Hilfe chemischer Methoden (u.a. HANNIG und NORDWIG, 1967; GALLOP, BLUMENFELD und SEIFTER, 1967; VEIS, 1967; CARVER und BLOUT, 1967) und Röntgenbrechungsdiagrammen untersucht (ASTBURY, 1950; BEAR, 1952; GUSTAVSON, 1956; RAMACHANDRAN, 1967). Im Röntgenbrechungsdiagramm zeigt das Kollagen drei sich wiederholende Einheiten (ASTBURY, 1950; BEAR, 1952): Die erste von 2,86 Å ist in der Längsachse der Fasern ausgerichtet und gibt die Länge einer Aminosäure an, die beiden andern sind senkrecht zu dieser Achse orientiert. Der zweite Wert von 4,4 Å entspricht dem Abstand der Wasserstoffbrücken in der backbone-Ebene (s. unten). Der dritte meridionale Abstand hängt von dem Quellungsgrad der Fasern ab und mißt bei trockenen Fasern 10,4 Å, bei starker Quellung 15—17 Å. Durch Dehnung kann die Makroperiode von 640 auf 1000—6000 Å verlängert werden, wobei die Dehnung auf beide Periodenabschnitte entfällt, aber im H-Teil stärker ist. Auf die Molekularlänge von 640 Å entfallen 670 bis 700 Aminosäurenreste. Das Molekulargewicht ergibt sich damit zu 63000—65000.

Die mögliche Konfiguration der Aminosäuren im Kollagen ist vielfältig diskutiert worden (BEAR, 1952; PAULING et al., 1951; BEAR et al., 1957; NEMETSCHEK, 1958; GUSTAVSON, 1956; EASTOE, 1967, 1968; RAMACHANDRAN, 1967; HANNIG und NORDWIG, 1967). Das Makromolekül des Kollagens enthält drei umeinander gewundene Polypeptidketten, so daß die Struktur eines dreifaserigen Seiles vorliegt. Diese Tripelhelix ist etwa 3000 Å lang und 13,5 Å dick. Die drei Ketten werden durch Wasserstoffbindungen zwischen den Amid- und Carbonylgruppen gehalten.

β) Chemie des Kollagens

Kollagen gehört zu den Skleroproteinen, die sich abgesehen von der Faserbildung (kristalline Ordnung) durch Schwer- bzw. Unlöslichkeit in Wasser, Salzlösungen usw., sowie der Beständigkeit gegen proteolytische Fermente auszeichnen. 24—35% des gesamten Körpereiweiß wird vom Kollagen gestellt (NEUBERGER, 1955). Nach ROGERS et al. (1952) sind 90—95% des organischen Knochenanteils Kollagen; etwa 15—24% des Knochengewichtes entfallen auf Kollagen (NEUBERGER, 1955); nach Untersuchungen von EASTOE und EASTOE (1954) am Rinderfemur stehen 18,64% Kollagen 1,02% widerstandsfähige Proteine, 0,24% MPS, 69,66% unlösliche und 1,25% lösliche anorganische Anteile sowie 8,18% Wasser gegenüber.

Die Aminosäurenzusammensetzung des Kollagens ist recht gleichartig (unter anderem NEUMAN, 1949; EASTOE, 1955, 1967, 1968): Glycin 23—29%, Prolin 15—16%, Hydroxyprolin 14%, Alanin 11%, Glutaminsäure 12%, Arginin 9%, Leucin 3—4%, Phenylalanin 2,5%, Tyrosin 1%. 70% des gesamten Körper-Glycins und Prolins sowie fast das gesamte Hydroxyprolin sind im Kollagen enthalten (NEUBERGER, 1955); eine geringe Menge Hydroxyprolin (1—2%) enthält Elastin.

Mit markiertem Glycin wurde die Kollagenbildung von HARKNESS et al. (1954), OREKHOVITCH (1952), JACKSON (1957), die durch Osteoblasten von CARNEIRO und LEBLOND (1959) verfolgt. Glycin wurde auch zur Bestimmung des geringen Stoffwechsels des Kollagens angewandt (PERONNE und SLACK, 1951; NEUBERGER und SLACK, 1953; SLACK, 1953; ROBERTSON, 1952; THOMPSON und BALLON, 1956).

Unsere Kenntnisse vom Kollagen wurden durch umfangreiche experimentelle Studien über die Rekonstitution von Fibrillen aus Kollagenlösungen in verdünnten Säuren erheblich erweitert. Bisher gelang diese Rekonstitution von Fibrillen aber nicht mit Knochenkollagen (GLIMCHER, 1959, 1960; GLIMCHER und KRANE, 1968). Diese Untersuchungen basieren auf den Arbeiten von NAGEOTTE (1927). Sie führten zur Unterscheidung mehrerer Kollagene (unter anderem SCHMITT et al., 1942; VANAMEE und PORTER, 1951; NODA und WYCKHOFF, 1951; BAHR, 1950, 1951; JACKSON und RANDALL, 1953). HIGHBERGER, GROSS und SCHMITT (1951) erhielten in Gegenwart von MPS neben Fibrillen mit einer Periode von 640 Å solche mit einer Periode von 2000—2400 Å. Das Material dieser „fibrous long-spacing" (FLS) wurde als Tropokollagen bezeichnet (vgl. GROSS 1952; GROSS et al. 1955; über die verschiedenartigen Aggregationen s. SCHMITT et al. 1955). Im übrigen konnten HIGHBERGER et al. (1951) Kristallite herstellen, die nur aus einer Periode von etwa 2600 Å bestehen. Es ist die „segment long-spacing" (SLS) Form.

Diese Beobachtungen und die Untersuchungen der Fibrillogenese führten schließlich zur Unterscheidung von drei Kollagenen (NEUBERGER, 1955; GRASSMANN, 1955; OREKHOVITCH et al., 1957). PIEZ (1967) schlägt allerdings vor, nur zwischen „löslichem Kollagen" und „Faserkollagen" zu unterscheiden.

1. Tropokollagen. Extrahierbar durch Salzlösungen, Periode 2000 Å. Stoffwechsel hoch aktiv. Tritt in der Interfibrillärsubstanz auf.

2. Prokollagen. Extrahierbar durch Säuren (citratlösliches Kollagen, JACKSON 1957). Ausgefällt durch neutrale und alkalische Lösungen. Periode 640 Å. Stoffwechsel weniger aktiv. Nach OREKHOVITSCH et al. (1948) und BOWES et al. (1953, 1957) enthält dieses Kollagen weniger Hydroxyprolin, aber mehr Tyrosin und Kohlenhydrate. Tritt in neugebildeten Fasern auf.

3. Kollagen. Unlöslich in schwach alkalischen und sauren Lösungen. Periode 650 Å. Stoffwechsel inaktiv. Tritt in ausgebildeten Fasern auf.

Diese Ergebnisse verhalfen dem aus der Lichtmikroskopie stammenden, mitunter heftig kritisierten Begriff des Prokollagens in besser definierter Form zu einer Wiedergeburt. Die summarische Aufstellung soll noch durch folgende Angaben ergänzt werden. Wenn neutralsalzlösliches Kollagen vorhanden ist, fehlen sichtbare Fibrillen; dieses (Tropo)-Kollagen liegt demgemäß nicht in den Fasern, sondern in der nicht fibrillären Intercellularsubstanz (JACKSON, 1957). Das citratlösliche (Pro)-Kollagen erscheint in neugebildeten Fibrillen und in der Außenschicht größerer Fasern (HARKNESS et al., 1954; JACKSON, 1957) bzw. in dünnen argyrophilen Fasern des sich entwickelnden Bindegewebes (GROSS, 1950). EASTOE (1968) weist darauf hin, daß nach SCHMITT (1956) die Aggregation der benachbarten Kollagenmakromoleküle durch elektrostatische Kräfte erfolgt. Da nun keine covalente Bindungen vorhanden sind, ist dieses Fasersystem unstabil. Eine Neutralsalzlösung kann die elektrostatischen Kräfte zwischen den Seitenketten reduzieren und es entsteht eine Lösung von Makromolekülen. Mit „Reifung" der Kollagenfibrillen bilden sich intramolekulare oder intermolekulare kovalente Bindungen (vgl. RAMACHANDRAN, 1967).

In diesem Zusammenhange wollen wir erwähnen, daß die Stellung des Reticulins noch sehr umstritten ist (KRAMER und LITTLE, 1953; ROBB-SMITH, 1957). Nach WINDRUM et al. (1955) besteht Reticulin zu 85% aus Kollagen mit etwas geringerem Prolin- und größerem Hydroxyprolin- und Hydrolysingehalt, 4% Kohlenhydraten und 10—12% fest gebundenen Lipiden. Elektronenmikroskopisch gleicht die Reticulumfaser bekanntlich den Kollagenfibrillen; sie haben nach MELCHER (1966) die Periode von 640 Å.

Die verschiedenen Formen des Kollagens lassen sich nun auf eine Makromolekülform des Tropokollagens in verschiedener sterischer Form polymerisiert zurückführen (SCHMITT,

1956; Glimcher, 1959, 1960; Hodge, 1967). Parallel angeordnete Makromoleküle ohne Verschiebung gegeneinander geben als Einzelsegment die SLS-Form, als Fibrille die FLS-Form. Sind die Makromoleküle gegeneinander verschoben, entsteht, und zwar bei einer Versetzung um ein Viertel ihrer Länge, die Fibrille mit der Periode 640 Å und bei $^1/_{12}$ der Länge jene mit 210 Å. Dabei ergeben sich Überlappungen und Mikrolücken (hole zones), denen eine Bedeutung für die Mineralisation zugesprochen wird (Glimcher 1959, 1960). Mit der Struktur des Knochenkollagens, vor allem in bezug auf die Mineralisation, haben sich Glimcher und Krane (1968) auseinandergesetzt.

Als Endprodukt jeder Faserbildung erscheint das unlösliche Kollagen. Für die Unlöslichkeit wurden unter anderem Bindungen zwischen der Hydroxylgruppe des Hydroxyprolin und einer Keto-imid-Gruppe anliegender Peptidketten verantwortlich gemacht (Gustavson, 1955). Nach Jackson (1954) liegen im Kollagen 60% Wasserstoffbrücken und 40% salzartige Bindungen vor. Jackson (1953) glaubte zunächst an Chondroitinsulfat als stabilisierenden Faktor, kam dann aber (1954) zu der Auffassung, es handelte sich um ein Mucoprotein, daß vom Chondroitinsulfat verschieden ist (s.u.).

Für die Struktur der Kollagenfasern sind KH von großer Bedeutung, wenn auch ihr prozentualer Anteil relativ gering ist (1%, Grassmann und Schleich, 1935; Beck, 1941; Moss 1955). Das Prokollagen enthält etwa 6—8% KH (Banga und Balo, 1957; Eastoe, 1967). Nachgewiesen wurden Glucose, Galaktose (Grassmann und Schleich, 1935; Gallop et al., 1967), beide nach Beck (1941) in äquimolaren Mengen, Mannose (Gross et al., 1952), Fucose (Glegg et al., 1953), Glucosamin (Schneider, 1948). Da Glucuronsäure fehlt, soll kein saures MPS vorliegen (Glegg et al., 1954), wie verschiedentlich vermutet wurde (Mercer, 1952). Bango und Balo (1957) nehmen ein Mucoprotein an, das durch ein entsprechendes Pankreasenzym aufgelöst wird. Einen regelmäßigen Einbau der KH in die Polypeptidketten vermuten Grassmann und Schleich (1935). Meyer (1954) und Schneider (1948, 1949) nehmen eine Verknüpfung der Peptidketten durch eine KH enthaltende Zwischensubstanz an. Im übrigen ist der KH-Gehalt und die Art der Kohlenhydratbindung bei den Kollagenfasern nicht einheitlich (Gross 1950a, b). Die Hexosen sind voraussichtlich in Pyranoseform an die Hydroxylgruppe des Hydroxylysin gebunden (Gallop et al., 1967).

In dem Zusammenhang muß darauf hingewiesen werden, daß Kollagen bei morphologischen Untersuchungen immer mit einer Reihe von Begleitsubstanzen, den Perifibrillärsubstanzen (Knese, 1963a) erscheint. Deswegen wird derzeit häufig vielen speziellen Untersuchungen rekonstituiertes Kollagen zugrundegelegt. Für die Biologie des Kollagens dürften diese Perifibrillärsubstanzen aber von erheblicher Bedeutung sein. Weiterhin möge auf die verschiedenen Kollagenformen hingewiesen werden, die Veis (1967) aufführt: Er unterscheidet das „native Kollagen", das nur von anhängendem Gewebe befreit ist, das „intakte Kollagen", entstanden durch Extraktion der Polysaccharide und der Nichtkollagen-Komponenten, und das „Matrixkollagen", dem alle nicht gebundenen Kollagenkomponenten entzogen wurden, das aber die covalent gebundenen Nichtkollagen-Komponenten enthält.

Elektronenmikroskopische Aufnahmen von Kollagenfibrillen zeigen häufig eine gegen die Umgebung schlecht abgrenzbare Hülle um die Fasern, auch im präossalen Gewebe (Knese und Knoop, 1958). Kuhnke (1958a, b) zeigte, daß eine Destruktion der Fibrillen im Dünnschnitt durch Trypsin und Papain von den Schnittenden her erfolgt, durch Hyaluronidase aber von der Oberfläche ausgeht; der Autor nimmt infolgedessen an, daß eine MPS-haltige Kittsubstanz (vgl. Schwarz, 1955, 1957) nicht nur die einzelnen Fibrillen verbindet, sondern auch deren Oberfläche überzieht. Die Querstreifung geht bei dieser Behandlung verloren. Knese und Knoop (1961a) konnten an den Fibrillen der Fibroelastica des Perichondriums nach Hyaluronidasevorbehandlung undeutlich begrenzte Fibrillen beobachten, deren Querstreifung nur schwach oder überhaupt nicht mehr zu erkennen ist. Im Lichtmikroskop wird nach Hyaluronidasewirkung die Faserstruktur des Periostes und Perichondriums, des Appositionsknorpels und der präossalen Ränder

der Knochenbälkchen deutlich, vermutlich infolge der Auflösung der Inter- bzw. Perifibrillärsubstanz (KNESE und KNOOP, 1961c).

Auf den Kohlenhydratgehalt wird die beim Kollagen wechselnde, beim Reticulin regelmäßig vorhandene PAS-positive Reaktion zurückgeführt (Überblick: McMANUS, 1954; GRAUMANN, 1957). Eine PAS-positive Reaktion kann auch beim Knochen auftreten (WISLOCKI et al., 1947; VINCENT, 1954). Der sog. nicht lamelläre Knochen färbt sich stärker an als der lamelläre; Lamellenknochen zeigt dagegen eine kräftige Ninhydrin-Reaktion auf Proteine (KNESE, 1959b).

γ) *Die Fibrillogenese*

Die Untersuchungen der Fibrillogenese haben große Fortschritte gemacht, da häufig mit biochemischen Untersuchungen morphologische, besonders elektronenmikroskopische, gekoppelt werden. Diskussionspunkt bleibt aber immer noch der Ort der Fibrillogenese oder, etwas anders formuliert, die Beziehung zwischen den Zellen und den intercellulären Fibrillen.

Auf Grund der Untersuchungen über die Rekonstitution von Fibrillen können die Bedingungen der Fibrillogenese in großen Zügen in Anlehnung an JACKSON (1957) charakterisiert werden: Bevor sichtbare Fibrillen auftreten, sind größere Mengen von Sulfo-MPS nachweisbar. Die Fibroblasten, ebenso die Chondroblasten, Osteoblasten und Odontoblasten produzieren einen Kollagenvorläufer, ein Tropokollagen (LOWTHER, 1963) GOULD, 1968). Mit dem Auftreten von sichtbaren Fibrillen ist ein citratlösliches (Pro-; Kollagen nachweisbar. Dieser morphologisch orientierten Beschreibung soll hinzugefügt werden, daß für die Kollagenbiosynthese eine Hydroxylation von Prolin und Lysin zu Hydroxyprolin und Hydroxylysin erforderlich ist. Auch zu den weiteren Fragen der Bildung der Polypeptidketten verweisen wir auf GOULD (1968). Durch weitere Aufnahme von neutralsalzlöslichem Kollagen werden die Fasern dicker, die Fibrillen reifen, die Seitenbindungen nehmen an Stärke zu und damit nimmt die Löslichkeit des Kollagens ab.

Allerdings besteht keine Einigkeit darüber, wie die einzelnen Schritte dieser Kollagenentwicklung ausgelöst werden, noch viel weniger, wodurch sie gesteuert werden; im letzteren Zusammenhange dachte man an eine Reihe von Hormonen und Vitaminen. Es ist noch unklar, ob die Befunde über die Fibrillogenese in vitro auf die Verhältnisse in vivo übertragen werden können (MEYER, 1954). Eine Rolle bei der Fibrillogenese spielen KH, vielleicht MPS, wie seit langem vermutet wird (MEYER, 1946, 1950b; COHN, 1942; PARTRIDGE, 1948; JACKSON und RANDALL, 1953; JACKSON, 1957; GRASSMANN et al., 1957). Eine metachromatische Farbreaktion, die für das Vorhandensein von MPS spricht, ist in Geweben mit einer Fibrillogenese seit langem bekannt. Mit fortschreitender Faserbildung nimmt diese Reaktion an Stärke ab (unter anderem BALASCZ und HOLMGREN, 1949, 1950). MEYER (1954) hat daher an einen Einbau der MPS in die Fibrillen gedacht, den jedoch SYLVÉN (1941) wegen des Fehlens entsprechender Farbreaktionen bestreitet. Allerdings ist auch mit einer Änderung der Eigenschaften der MPS mit der Bindung an Fibrillen zu rechnen (WASSERMANN, 1956). Trotz mancher Widersprüche scheint es JACKSON und BENTLEY (1968) wahrscheinlich, das Glykosaminoglycane, besonders Chondrotinsulfat, mit Kollagen zusammenwirken, um Fibrillen zu bilden. Weiterhin sind sie für die Bildung von Kollagenstrukturen in höheren Ordnungsstufen notwendig, ebenso für strukturelle Stabilität der Bindegewebe. KNESE und v. HARNACK (1926) diskutieren ausführlich an Hand ihrer Untersuchungen der Faserstruktur des Knochengewebes über die Entstehung der Ordnung der Kollagenfibrillen, d.h. über die Prinzipien der Strukturbildung.

Bekannt ist die metachromatische Reaktion der Ränder von Knochenbälkchen, des sog. präossalen Gewebes, die dem ausgebildeten Knochen fehlt (s. unter Osteogenese).

Sehr verschiedenartige Zellen sind, wie nun endgültig anerkannt, zur Faserbildung fähig, nicht nur Fibroblasten, sondern auch die Chondroblasten, Osteoblasten, Odontoblasten, d.h. Bindegewebszellen gleichgültig, ob mesodermaler, ektodermaler oder entodermaler Herkunft. Bekanntlich entstammt das Mesenchym des Kopfgebietes nicht nur dem Mesoderm, sondern auch der ektodermalen Kopfganglienleiste (HARRISON, 1935; VEIT, 1939; DAMAS, 1942, 1944; STARCK, 1944). Diese Beobachtungen haben dazu geführt, die Lehre von der Spezifität der Keimblätter aufzugeben.

Die Fähigkeit der Osteoblasten, Fibrillen zu bilden, wurde auch in Gewebekulturen nachgewiesen (unter anderem WJERESZINSKI, 1924; FELL, 1928/29, 1956; STUDITSKY, 1936; ROULET, 1935).

Vor Erörterung der „Morphologie“ der Fibrillogenese ist noch einmal zu betonen, daß alle morphologischen Methoden nur über ein begrenztes Auflösungsvermögen verfügen. Bei Beachtung dieser methodischen Beschränkung erscheinen viele in der Literatur zu Tage tretende Gegensätze von geringerer Bedeutung, als die Schärfe der Diskussion mitunter vermuten läßt. Eine weitere Entwicklung der Methode wird vermutlich manche der Streitpunkte als gegenstandslos aufzeigen.

Durch das Elektronenmikroskop sind die Untersuchungsmöglichkeiten gegenüber dem Lichtmikroskop um eine Ordnungsstufe verschoben, aber die Situation hat sich für den Beurteiler nicht grundsätzlich geändert. Es liegt ein Sprung vor von Strukturen 6. Ordnung, den nicht unmittelbar „sichtbaren“ (s. S. 318) zu Strukturen 5. Ordnung, den sichtbaren. Dies zeigen die Untersuchungen von JACKSON und SMITH (1957) und SMITH und JACKSON (1957; vgl. HARKNESS et al., 1954) an Gewebekulturen von Osteoblasten. Zunächst ist ein an Hydroxyprolinen reiches Protein nachzuweisen, aber keine Fibrillen; die Umbildung zu sichtbaren Fibrillen ist auf der anderen Seite mit keinem signifikanten Anstieg des Hydroxyprolingehaltes verbunden.

Die Bildung extracellulärer Substanzen ändert das Gefüge der Bildungszonen im elektronenmikroskopischen Bilde derart, daß die Entscheidung, ob in bestimmten Befunden ein präparatives Artefact oder das Äquivalentbild einer Strukturänderung in vivo vorliegt, mitunter nicht leicht ist (KNESE und KNOOP, 1961c; KNESE, 1963a, b). Enge nachbarschaftliche Beziehungen zwischen Zellen und Fibrillen als Zustandbild sprechen nicht ohne weiteres für einen Bildungsvorgang. Aus diesem Grunde wurde der Bildungsprozeß häufig nach einer Verletzung bei der Wundheilung untersucht (z.B. WASSERMANN, 1953). Relativ günstig liegen die Verhältnisse bei der Osteogenese, da die Fibrillenbildung hier an bestimmte Orte gebunden ist (KNESE und KNOOP, 1961c, s. unten).

Die Auffassungen über Ort und Ablauf der Fibrillogenese sind jenen über die Bildung der Intercellularsubstanzen im allgemeinen und die der Knochensubstanz (s. S. 340) sehr ähnlich. Die Deutung gleichartiger Befunde durch verschiedene Untersucher hängt von den allgemeinen Vorstellungen über die Beziehungen zwischen Zellen und Intercellularsubstanzen ab. Folgende Ansichten wurden vertreten:

1. Fibrillen werden intracellulär gebildet (FLEMMING, 1897; MALL, 1902; STUDNIČKA, 1907; LEWIS, 1917; WASSERMANN, 1956; HOWATSON und HAM, 1955).
2. Fibrillen entstehen epicellulär (PORTER und PAPPAS, 1959).
3. Fibrillen entstehen extracellulär (NAGEOTTE, 1916; GROSS, 1956; KAJIKAWA et al., 1959; SCHMITT et al., 1958).

Die unter 1. und 2. genannten Auffassungen sind nicht grundsätzlich voneinander verschieden. Die Synthese von Kollagenvorstufen in Zellen wird heute von keiner Seite bestritten. Sie ist durch Untersuchungen mit markiertem Glycin erwiesen, für die Osteoblasten durch CARNEIRO und LEBLOND (1960); über die verschiedenen Untersuchungen mit markiertem Prolin und Lysin vgl. GOULD (1968). Es ist nur die Frage, wo die Fibrillen zuerst sichtbar werden. Die unter 1. genannten Autoren sprechen von Außenschichten der Zellen, die unter 2. aufgeführten von einer Art Ektoplasma. Noch nicht geklärt erscheint die Frage, wie groß die Makromoleküle sind, die aus der Zelle ausgeschleust werden. Die Annahme einer rein extracellulären Fibrillenbildung hat durch die Untersuchungen über die Fibrillen-Rekonstitution eine wesentliche Stütze erhalten. In Gebieten einer umfangreichen Fibrillenbildung mit überblickbarer Ordnung der Fibrillen, wie bei der Knochenbildung, fällt aber auf, daß Fibrillen mit allen Kennzeichen der Jugendlichkeit nur in Zellnähe liegen.

Während die Vorgänge der Dickenzunahme von Fibrillen verschiedentlich diskutiert wurden, bedarf das Auftreten von Fibrillen mit geringer Periode und deren Anwachsen auf den Wert 640 Å noch weiterer Untersuchungen. PORTER (1951) hat die Vermutung ausgesprochen, daß die Periode von 210 Å eine fundamentale Einheit für biologische Fasern darstellt, da ein gleicher Wert beim Fibrin und Myosin gefunden wurde.

Über die elastischen Gewebe, Morphologie, Histogenese, Biochemie und Pathologie, berichtet ausführlich AYER (1964). Im Hinblick auf die Entstehung von elastischen Fasern wird eine Abkunft von Kollagenfibrillen angenommen. KNESE (unveröffentlicht) beobachtete im Periost von Rinderfeten ab 130 mm SSL die Aufspaltung von Kollagenfibrillen in eine Art Primärfibrillen. Gegenüber dem bisher haarlockenförmigen Verlauf der Kollagenfibrille nehmen diese Primärfibrillen eine gestreckte, drahtige Verlaufsform an. Auf Querschnitten durch die entstehenden elastischen Fasern ist ein Perlkranz von Kollagenfasern an der Oberfläche zu erkennen, ein dichter peripherer und ein weniger dichter zentraler Anteil. In welcher Form und unter welchen Bedingungen diese Umwandlung von Kollagen zu Elastin vor sich geht, ist unbekannt.

d) Die Peri- und Interfibrillärsubstanzen

Nach den Ausführungen in der Einleitung ist in diesem Abschnitt die Struktur der sog. „amorphen" Grundsubstanz, d.h. der morphologisch nicht direkt darstellbaren Komponenten, zu erörtern. Die Einschränkung „nicht direkt" ist erforderlich, weil auf der Gegenwart dieser Stoffe bestimmte Farbreaktionen beruhen, wie die PAS-Reaktion oder die Metachromasie. Es wurde vorgeschlagen, den Terminus Grundsubstanz fallen zu lassen, und die Benennung nach dem topographischen Auftreten der Stoffe und ihrer Konstitution durchzuführen.

Ein Teil der Stoffe hat topographisch enge Beziehungen zu den Fibrillen und ist demgemäß als Perifibrillärsubstanz zu beschreiben, andere liegen als Interfibrillärsubstanzen zwischen den Fibrillen (KNESE, 1963a). Der Konstitution nach sind saure Mucopolysaccharide (MPS), neutrale Heteropolysaccharide (Glykoproteide und -proteine), lösliche Kollagene (GROSS 1958) und weitere Proteine, zu unterscheiden.

Die technisch ungewöhnlich schwierige Bearbeitung des Knochengewebes hat dazu geführt, daß die grundsätzlichen Vorstellungen über den Aufbau der Intercellularsubstanzen fast ausschließlich an anderen Stützgeweben, unter anderem dem Knorpel, gewonnen wurden. Die allgemeinen Fragen der Organisation der Intercellularsubstanz werden daher erst beim Knorpelgewebe erörtert (s. dort). Hier werden nur die am Knochen gewonnenen Ergebnisse aufgeführt.

α) Die sauren Mucopolysaccharide

Das Vorhandensein von mucoiden Stoffen in der Intercellularsubstanz des Knochens wurde bereits von SPULER (1899) vermutet. HAWK und GIES (1901) und SEIFERT und GIES (1904) isolierten durch Extraktion ein Osseomucoid (0,4%), das sich als ein sehr komplexer Stoff erwies, so daß heute kaum noch von „einem" Osseomucoid gesprochen wird. HISAMURA (1938b) trennte das Osseomucoid in zwei Fraktionen, die eine enthält Chondroitinsulfat, die zweite ist durch eine hohe N-Rate ausgezeichnet. Das Vorliegen von Chondroitinsulfat wurde von ROGERS et al. (1951; 0,3—0,4%), MASCHUNE et al. (1951), EASTOE und EASTOE (1954; 0,24%) und GLEGG und EIDINGER (1955) bestätigt (vgl. BALAZS und ROGERS 1965). Letztere Autoren konnten nachweisen, daß das Protein vom Kollagen verschieden ist, da es kein Hydroxylprolin, kleinere Mengen von Glycin, Alanin und Prolin, aber größere von Tyrosin und Leucin enthält.

Die bisher als Mucopolysaccharide bezeichneten Stoffe gehören zu jenen Substanzen, die Aminozucker enthalten. Die Nomenklatur für diese Stoffgruppe ist recht unbefriedigend. Die große Zahl unterschiedlicher Benennungen beruhte zum Teil auf der Unkenntnis des Aufbaues dieser Stoffe. Vor allen Dingen wird der Gebrauch der Vorsilbe „Muco-“ als uncharakteristisch und unzutreffend kritisiert. Es besteht Hoffnung, daß sich die Vorschläge der Nomenklaturkommission der American Chemical Society (Jeanloz, 1960; Balazs und Jeanloz, 1965, 1966) weitgehend durchsetzen werden. Danach werden allgemein Polysaccharide mit Aminozuckern Glykosaminoglycane genannt. Die bisher als Mucopolysaccharide bezeichneten Substanzen mit einer Uronsäure sollen dann Glykosaminoglykurane heißen. Chondrotin-4-Sulfat ersetzt Chondrotinsulfat A, Chondrotin-6-Sulfat Chondrotinsulfat C, Dermatansulfat das Chondrotin-Sulfat B; weitere Bezeichnungen werden mit geringen Abänderungen übernommen, z.B. heißt es nun statt Keratosulfat Keratansulfat. Glykoproteine bzw. Glykopeptide sind Proteine bzw. Peptide mit Kohlenhydraten. Schließlich stellte sich heraus, daß diese Kohlenhydrate häufig nicht nur Polysaccharide, sondern auch Oligosaccharide enthalten und im allgemeinen an Nicht-Kollagenproteine gebunden sind. So wurden auch Bezeichnungen wie Polysaccharidproteinkomplex, Chondrotinsulfat-Proteinkomplex (u.a. Jeanloz, 1960) bzw. komplexe Kohlenhydrate (u.a. Dorfman, 1963) vorgeschlagen.

Von diesen sauren MPS konnten im kompakten Knochen Chondroitin-4-sulfat (0,24% des Trockengewichtes) nachgewiesen werden (Meyer et al., 1956; Meyer, 1956). In Kälberknochen ist vermutlich Chondroitin-6-sulfat vorhanden. Ein phosphoryliertes Polysaccharid, wie es Di Stefano et al. (1953) angeben, konnte Meyer (1956) nicht auffinden. Weiterhin enthält der Knochen ein Keratansulfat (Meyer et al., 1953; Glegg et al., 1953, 1954), das einzige saure Polysaccharid ohne Uronsäure. Keratansulfat hat nichts mit Keratin zu tun, der Name wurde gegeben, weil es zuerst in der Cornea aufgefunden wurde. Schließlich sind noch Hyaluronate und unvollständig sulfurierte Fraktionen vorhanden; diese letzteren Fraktionen sind in ihrer Struktur unbekannt.

Während der Entwicklung ändert sich nicht nur der Gehalt, sondern auch die Konstitution der MPS. Nach Sobel et al. (1953, 1954) erfolgt im Rattenfemur eine Abnahme des Verhältnisses von Hexosamin zu Kollagen. Von den in der Literatur vorliegenden Angaben (Zusammenstellung bei Balazs und Rogers, 1965) können nur jene herangezogen werden, die sich eindeutig auf das Knochengewebe beziehen. Bei Untersuchungen des Callus und der Epiphyse ist stets eine Beimengung von knorpeligen Anteilen möglich und zu berücksichtigen. Nach Rogers (1949) nimmt im menschlichen Femur der Hexosamingehalt (g/100 g Trockengewebe) von 0,2 (9—22 Monate) auf 0,11 (47—61 Jahre) ab.

Die biochemischen Erhebungen werden durch topochemische ergänzt. Mit verschiedenartigen Färbemethoden ist außer dem Vorhandensein bestimmter reagierender Gruppen auch deren topographische Verteilung zu untersuchen. Die Farbreaktionen der Bildungszellen, aber auch der Osteocyten wurden in recht ausführlichen Studien beschrieben (s. S. 348). Unsere Kenntnisse über das färberische Verhalten der Intercellularsubstanz des Knochens sind weniger umfassend. Der Nachweis saurer MPS im Schnitt erfolgt unter anderem durch die metachromatische Farbreaktion (Toluidinblau) und die Anfärbung mit basischen Stoffen. Einen metachromatischen Farbton nimmt häufig, aber nicht immer, das präossale Gewebe an, das in der Form von Rändern Knochenbälkchen umgibt (Follis, 1949; Bevelander und Johnson, 1950; Pritchard, 1952; Knese und Knoop, 1961c; Knese, 1963c). Auf die Bedeutung der metachromatischen Reaktion kommen wir beim Knorpel zurück, wollen hier aber darauf hinweisen, daß diese Reaktion durch sehr viele Faktoren beeinflußt wird. Auch die mit Methylenblau nachgewiesene Basophilie bedarf einer Reihe von Kontrolluntersuchungen. Die Färbung ist in verschiedenem pH zum Nachweis des isoelektrischen Punktes durchzuführen. Für das Knochengewebe liegen entsprechende Untersuchungen von Achard (1936) und Vincent (1954) vor. Zur Entscheidung, ob MPS oder andere saure Substanzen vorliegen, ist eine Kontrolle durch Vorbehandlung mit Hyaluronidase erforderlich.

Häufig wird die PAS-Reaktion (McManus, 1954) zum Nachweis von Polysacchariden angewandt; hierbei werden durch Perjodsäure gebildete Aldehydgruppen durch Schiffsches Reagens (Leukofuchsin) sichtbar gemacht. Stark PAS-positiv sind wiederum die präossalen Säume (Bevelander und Johnson, 1950; Pritchard, 1952; Vincent, 1954; Lacroix, 1960, 1961).

Die Färbungsdifferenzen bei Anwendung der Schmorlschen Färbung zwischen gelb und mehr braun sind ungeklärt. Auffällig ist, daß sich die innerste Lamelle um einen Haversschen Kanal im allgemeinen gelb anfärbt (Knese, 1958b); für diese Lamelle ist eine von den anderen Lamellen abweichende Struktur anzunehmen (Knese, 1956a, 1957; s. S. 377). Der Mechanismus der Eisenhämatoxylin-Färbung (Heidenhain) bedarf ebenfalls einer weiteren Untersuchung, da Teile des Knochengewebes ungefärbt bleiben, andere aber eine starke Schwärzung aufweisen. Für die Unterschiede bei der Azan-Färbung wurde bisher angenommen, daß sich unverkalktes Gewebe (Osteoid) blau, „verkalktes" aber rot anfärbt; eine so einfache Deutung der Farbreaktion ist aber anzuzweifeln (Knese, 1959b, 1963c). Lorentz (1960) hat auf den entscheidenden Einfluß der Vorbehandlung bei Ausfall der Azanfärbung hingewiesen; für die Aufnahme von Azocarmin sollen Amino- und Imino-Gruppen von Bedeutung sein.

β) Die Glykoproteine

Unsere Kenntnisse von der Struktur und Verteilung der Glykoproteine Polysaccharide, die keine Hexuronsäure enthalten, sind sehr gering; diese Stoffe werden heute als Glykoproteine bezeichnet. Hisamura (1938) erhielt aus Knochen eine Fraktion mit Galaktose und Galaktosamin ohne Hexuronsäure. Dische und Osnos (1950) isolierten aus verschiedenen Organen ein Fuco-Mucopolysaccharid, das wahrscheinlich eine Mischung mehrerer Heteropolysaccharide darstellt (s. unten). In der von Glegg, Eidinger und Leblond (1954) aus kompaktem Knochen gewonnenen proteinhaltigen Fraktion konnten Galaktose, Mannose und Fucose nachgewiesen werden. Die neutralen Mucopolysaccharide sind der sog. Serummucoid-Fraktion des Blutplasmas sehr ähnlich. Die genauere Lokalisation der an Extrakten untersuchten Stoffe ist nicht möglich. Balazs und Rogers (1965) meinen, es handle sich (1.) um Plasmaproteine, (2.) Material der Intercellularsubstanz und (3.) Glykopeptide der Erythrocyten. Ob es für den Knochen spezifische Glykoproteine gäbe, kann z.Z. nicht gesagt werden. Bei scorbutischen Tieren wurde im Granulationsgewebe, in dem typische Kollagene nicht entstehen, ein PAS-positives Material aufgefunden, das nach Bradfield und Kodicek (1951) durch Hyaluronidase nicht angegriffen wird.

Die Vermutung einer Verbindung von neutralen Polysacchariden mit Faserelementen legen die Untersuchungen des Reticulins und des kohlenhydratreichen säurelöslichen Kollagens nahe. Dische et al. (1958) fanden im Femurschaft und in Rippen von Kälbern und jungen Rindern zwei neutrale Polysaccharide. Die eine Fraktion ist in Äthanol löslich und enthält 40% KH (Galaktose, Mannose, ein Hexosamin und einen gewissen Betrag Fucose). Die zweite in Äthanol unlösliche Fraktion ist in einem Teil praktisch frei von Hexosamin, enthält Galaktose, Glucose, wenig Fucose und ist mit einem Protein verbunden. Der andere Teil dieser Fraktion weist neben den drei Hexosen einen geringen Betrag Fucose und eine beachtliche Menge Hexosamin auf. Die in Äthanol lösliche Fraktion ist als eine Mischung von Polysacchariden anzusehen. Für das Heteropolysaccharid aus Glucose und Galaktose wird in Anlehnung an Untersuchungen am Glaskörper (Dische und Zelmanes, 1955) angenommen, daß es eine Hülle um die jungen Kollagenfasern bildet; diese Hülle wird während der Faserreifung reduziert oder verschwindet. Der zweite Teil der Fraktion mit dem Hexosamin ist wohl dem in Äthanol löslichen MPS ähnlich. Herring und Kent (1963) haben ein Sialoprotein, ein Glykoprotein mit Sialinsäure aus der Corticalis erwachsener Rinder isoliert.

Untersuchungen mit sehr verschiedenartigen Methoden, biochemischen, topochemischen und elektronenmikroskopischen, legen die Vermutung nahe, daß für die Topographie der organischen Intercellularsubstanzen einmal unmittelbare Beziehungen zu den Fibrillen, zum anderen eine Lagerung zwischen den Fibrillen zu unterscheiden sind. Man muß aber wohl auch damit rechnen, daß gleichartige Stoffe an verschiedenen Orten vorkommen; so hat z.B. RANDALL (bei RANDALL et al., 1953) darauf hingewiesen, daß man Kollagen aus der Umgebung der Fibrillen und aus ihnen selbst gewinnen kann.

Nach GROSS (1958) sind extracellulär die verschiedensten Aggregate von monomerem Tropokollagen zu finden. Die in der Intercellularsubstanz liegenden Proteine, die nicht Kollagen sind, konnten in ihrer Struktur bisher nicht näher untersucht werden. Schwer ist z.Z. auch das sog. widerstandsfähige (resistant) Protein einzuordnen, das in heißem Wasser schwerer löslich ist als Kollagen (STACK, 1951; ROGERS et al., 1952; EASTOE und EASTOE, 1954). Nach den letztgenannten Autoren enthält es kein Hydroxyprolin, der Gehalt an Prolin und Glycin ist geringer als im Kollagen, der Tyrosin-Anteil dagegen sehr hoch.

γ) Die Beziehungen zwischen den Intercellularsubstanzen

Verschiedentlich wurde betont, daß Knochengewebe jeder Untersuchung einen großen Widerstand entgegensetzt. Die Trennung der Komponenten oder die Herauslösung einer von ihnen aus der Durchdringungsstruktur (KNESE, 1956a, 1958b) gelingt nur mit mehr oder minder großen Zerstörungen. Erhebungen aber an den restlichen Stütz- und Bindegeweben haben gezeigt, daß die Struktur der Intercellularsubstanz bei allen im Prinzip gleich oder doch sehr ähnlich ist. Zu einer Gleichstellung des Knochengewebes in seiner Organisation mit den anderen Stützgeweben kam auch LIPP (1954) und zwar bei Untersuchungen, die von den Osteocyten ausgingen. Die Organisation des Knochengewebes und die damit erst möglichen Stoffwechselwege werden u.a. von ROBINSON (1952, 1964), LIPP (1954) und WASSERMANN und YAEGER (1965) dargestellt.

Man kann folgendes Strukturbild des Knochengewebes entwerfen: Das Grundgerüst der Intercellularsubstanz bilden die Kollagenfibrillen, deren Flächendichte sehr hoch liegt, d.h. deren Abstand von einander relativ gering ist. Die Fibrillen verlaufen gestreckt und nicht gewellt, wie das in den anderen Stützgeweben fast durchweg der Fall ist. Die Ordnung der Fibrillen ist für den Knochen spezifisch, sie treten in Schichten, den sog. Lamellen, auf. Durch Bildung von Lamellensystemen und deren verschiedenartige Zusammenlagerung in den Skeletstücken entsteht eine Strukturhierarchie, die unter anderem die mechanische Leistung des Skeletes gewährleistet.

Das Knochengewebe ist ein Fasergewebe, in dem die Ordnung der anderen Komponenten (s. unter Kristallite) von den Fibrillen abhängig ist. Die einzelne Fibrille ist von einem Mantel sog. organischer und anorganischer Perifibrillärsubstanz (KNESE, 1963a) umgeben, zu der auch Wasser gehört (s. S. 337). Die organische Perifibrillärsubstanz besteht aus vermutlich fester gebundenen neutralen Heteropolysacchariden und locker gebundenen sauren MPS. Die anorganischen Substanzen in enger Nachbarschaft mit den organischen überziehen die Fibrille in der Form einer Hülle aus einzelnen Kristalliten.

Zwischen den Fibrillen und ihren Mänteln befindet sich die Interfibrillärsubstanz, deren Grundgerüst vermutlich die sauren MPS, vor allem Chondroitinsulfat A, bilden. Diese MPS sind polymere, aus sich wiederholenden Grundeinheiten aufgebaute Stoffe; sie sind polydispers, d.h. nebeneinander treten Moleküle verschiedener Kettenlänge auf. Viele Befunde sprechen dafür, daß am gleichen Ort entweder mehr nieder- oder hochpolymere MPS überwiegen. GERSH und CATCHPOLE (1949) sprachen früher an Hand verschiedener Farbreaktionen von einem wechselnden „Polymerisationsgrad"; an diesem Terminus wurde heftig Kritik geübt (DORFMAN, 1955). GERSH und CATCHPOLE (1960) finden den Ausdruck heute selbst mißverständlich und haben ihn durch „Aggregation" ersetzt. Die MPS haben Austauschereigenschaften und können erhebliche Mengen Kationen, Na, K, Ca und andere binden (ENGEL et al., 1954; JOSEPH et al., 1954; DORFMAN und MATHEWS, 1956). Weiterhin sind die MPS Träger des extracellulären und extravasalen Wassers (s. unten); im Stützgewebe wird etwa die Hälfte des gesamten Wassers, das $^1/_5$ des Körpergewichtes ausmacht, festgehalten. Der Stofftransport durch das Stützgewebe erfolgt entlang den Kollagenfibrillen (MCMASTER et al., 1950). Für das Knochengewebe hat LIPP (1954) den Stofftransport vermittels der Grenzscheidensubstanz angenommen, die der Perifibrillärsubstanz stofflich vermutlich sehr ähnlich ist.

δ) *Das Wasser und die Komponenten in bezug auf das Volumen*

Den Ausführungen über die „Organisation" der organischen Inter- und Perifibrillärsubstanz ist noch eine kurze Erörterung über die Beziehung zu den anorganischen Kristalliten und der Wasserverteilung anzuschließen. Welche Rolle hierbei die Mucopolysaccharide spielen, konnte noch nicht befriedigend geklärt werden (s. unten). Die anorganische Substanz des Knochens erscheint im Knochen in der Form von Kristalliten (s. S. 351). In einer wäßrigen Suspension bildet der einzelne Kristall mit Umgebung ein Vierzellen-System (NEUMAN und NEUMAN, 1958). Der Kristall besitzt eine Wasserhülle (hydration shell), die polarisierbare Ionen enthält. Diese Hülle schließt sich der Kristalloberfläche an. Zum Schluß folgt das Innere des Kristallgitters. Außerhalb der Wasserhülle liegt eine schwach gebundene weitere Hülle, die von gleicher Zusammensetzung wie die Umgebung ist (Schema bei KNESE, 1963a). Der Ionenaustausch zwischen der umgebenden Lösung und der Hülle geht sehr schnell vor sich, der zwischen Wasserhülle und Kristalloberfläche noch relativ rasch, der mit dem Kristall aber wesentlich langsamer. Die Diffusionsrate in noch nicht mineralisiertem Gewebe ist groß und damit der Ionenaustausch umfangreich. Die Mineralisation geht demgemäß bis zu einem kritischen Wassergehalt mit erheblicher Geschwindigkeit vor sich. Dieser kritische Wassergehalt entspricht etwa 90% der vollen Mineralisation des präossalen Gewebes.

Die Aufklärung der Beziehungen zwischen der Wasserverteilung und dem Mineralanteil geht auf ältere, lange nicht beachtete Untersuchungen von DEAKINS (1942) und DEAKINS und BURT (1944) am Schmelz noch nicht durchgebrochener Zähne des Schweines zurück. Diese Autoren haben die Dichte, das Naß-, Trocken- und Aschegewicht berücksichtigt und eine Beziehung der Komponenten auf das Volumen durchgeführt. Sie kommen zu der Feststellung, daß eine Zunahme des Aschevolumens auf Kosten des Wasservolumens erfolgt. Ein Kristall bildet sich und wächst in einem durch das Wasser vorbestimmten Volumen. Das Wasservolumen zwischen den Kristallen und den Fibrillen wird damit schrittweise kleiner und kleiner. Die organische Phase, das Kollagen bleibt gleich; der maximale Mineralisationsgrad hängt eindeutig von der Menge des organischen Materials ab (ROBINSON und ELLIOT, 1957).

ROBINSON (1960, 1964) hat die Menge der einzelnen Komponenten des Knochengewebes in bezug auf das Volumen näher dargestellt. Die von ROBINSON leider gebrauchte, mißverständliche Bezeichnung Osteoid für die Intercellularsubstanz übernehmen wir im folgenden nicht. Dieser Intercellularsubstanz stellt der Verfasser das Mark-Gefäß-Osteocyten-Volumen gegenüber. Im Hinblick auf die Wasserverteilung in der Intercellularsubstanz unterscheidet ROBINSON zwischen dem Konstitutionswasser und dem „gebundenen" Wasser. Das Konstitutionswasser hat vermutlich mehrere Anteile. Es kann an die Kollagenfibrillen gebunden sein und zwar an die Wasserstoffbindung einer Hydroxylgruppe der einen Protofibrille mit der Imid-Gruppe einer zweiten Protofibrille. Weiterhin besteht eine Verbindung mit den MPS. Das Kristallwasser des Apatites macht nur einen sehr geringen Anteil aus. Das „gebundene Wasser" bleibt als die Wasserhülle der Kristalle von NEUMAN und NEUMAN (1958) als Teil des „freien" Wassers übrig, das vor Einsetzen der Mineralisation im präossalen Gewebe vorhanden war.

Das Verhältnis von Massen- und Volumen-% zueinander gibt die folgende Tabelle (auszugsweise) von ROBINSON (1960) wieder:

Komponenten	Massen-%	Volumen-%	Komponenten	Massen-%	Volumen-%
Mark-Gefäß-Osteocyten-Raum			Intercellularsubstanz		
Wasser	6,70	13,74	Wasser	3,40	6,97
anorganischer Teil	0,05	0,03	anorganischer Teil	66,67	45,56
organischer Teil	0,87	1,26	organischer Teil	22,31	32,44
Summe	7,62	15,03	Summe	92,38	84,97

Der Bezug auf das Volumen ist bei Untersuchungen der Struktur und der Strukturbildung ohne Zweifel wünschenswert, läßt sich aber bei rein morphologischen Untersuchungen kaum erreichen. Ein Schritt auf dieses Ziel hin ist der Bezug auf die Schnittfläche, wie das für die Flächendichte der Fibrillen (KNESE und KNOOP, 1961c) und der Osteone (KNESE et al., 1954; AUERBACH, 1957; KNESE und TITSCHAK, 1962) durchgeführt wurde.

Aus Durchschnittswerten haben FROST (1961, 1962) und ROBINSON (1964) den Volum- und Oberflächenanteil des Hohlraumsystems kalkuliert. Danach ergibt sich für einen sog. typischen Mann von 70 kg Gewicht eine Oberfläche der Knochenhöhlchen und -kanälchen von 700—1100 m^2, die Haversschen Kanälchen machen nur 2—3 m^2 aus (vgl. Poren-Volumen S. 457).

3. Bemerkungen zum Ablauf der Osteogenese

Der Ausspruch C. E. v. BAERS, die Entwicklungsgeschichte sei der Lichtträger der Anatomie, gilt auch für alle Untersuchungen des Knochengewebes. Es liegt daher eine sehr umfangreiche Literatur über die Knochenbildung vor. Die im vorigen Jahrhundert begonnenen morphologischen Untersuchungen an z.T. sehr differentem Material führten zu so verschiedenartigen Vorstellungen, daß eine Klärung, was nun Knochenbildung ist, kaum möglich war (HINTZSCHE, 1927). Eine systematische Nachuntersuchung an menschlichen Feten von 34—421 mm SSL (3 Monate-Kind) zeigte, daß die Beobachtungen der älteren Autoren jeweils nur für einen bestimmten Entwicklungszeitraum gelten (KNESE 1956a). Der Vorgang der Knochenbildung spielt sich in einer Zone von weniger als 1 μ Breite ab, so daß der Ablauf des Bildungsprozesses lichtmikroskopisch nicht zu beobachten war (KNESE und KNOOP, 1958, 1961c). Elektronenmikroskopische Untersuchungen konnten manche strittigen Fragen klären.

Die geschilderten Unklarheiten über das Wesen der Knochenbildung führten zu einer Reihe von Untersuchungen sehr verschiedener Natur. Einmal wurde die Frage der Spezifität der Osteoblasten diskutiert (LACROIX, 1949, 1951a, b; MCLEAN und URIST, 1955). Weiterhin bemühte man sich, einen „Modellfall" der Knochenbildung zu finden, und hat in diesem Zusammenhang dem sog. Follikulin- oder Markknochen der Vögel eine besondere Aufmerksamkeit gewidmet (BLOOM et al., 1941; HELLER et al., 1950; CLAVERT, 1948, 1950). Unter dem Einfluß von Follikelhormon wird eine Art Spongiosa als Ca-Speicher im Markraum aufgebaut, die zur Zeit des Aufenthaltes des Eies in der Schalendrüse wieder abgebaut wird. Sehr umfangreiche Untersuchungen auch unter dem Gesichtspunkt des Ersatzes von Knochen wurden der Transplantation gewidmet (LACROIX, 1951, 1961; MCLEAN und URIST, 1955; LENTZ, 1955). Zum Teil wurde in diesem Zusammenhang das Vorhandensein sog. osteogener Substanzen erörtert (BERTELSEN, 1944; LEVANDER, 1945; LACROIX, 1951). Die alte Frage, inwieweit mechanische Faktoren für die Knochenbildung verantwortlich sind, wurde verschiedentlich aufgegriffen (vgl. MURRAY, 1936; GLÜCKSMANN, 1938, 1942; TISCHENDORF, 1952/54) und in ihren Grundvorstellungen kritisiert (KNESE, 1959a). Bedeutsame Fortschritte wurden in der Kultur von Knochengewebe und ganzer Extremitäten erzielt (FELL, 1928/29, 1956; ROULET, 1935; MURRAY, 1936; BASSETT, 1962). Eine unübersehbare Fülle von Untersuchungen liegt über hormonelle (WILKINS, 1955) und nutritive (SHAW, 1955) Einflüsse auf Knochenbildung und -wachstum vor.

Die Darstellung der bedeutsamen Untersuchungen mittels Radioisotopen, die auf die Arbeiten über ^{32}P (CHIEVITZ und HEVESY, 1935) folgten, ist einem eigenen Kapitel vorbehalten (AMPRINO).

Obwohl seit langem bekannt ist, daß Verkalkung nicht gleich Knochenbildung ist, wurde häufig die Mineralablagerung als der entscheidende Vorgang der Osteogenese angesehen. Der Morphologie der Mineralisation ist ein eigenes Kapitel gewidmet. Der organische Knochenanteil erschien in diesem Zusammenhang nur als ein Kalkfänger, als die „verkalkungsfähige" Grundsubstanz. Die Untersuchungen über diesen Mechanismus sind noch zu keinem endgültigen Ergebnis gekommen (vgl. SCHÜTTE, 1956; GLIMCHER, 1959; URIST, 1964, 1966; GLIMCHER und KRANE, 1968). In diesem Zusammenhang wurde der Verteilung der alkalischen Phosphatase große Aufmerksamkeit gewidmet mit dem Endergebnis, daß über die Aufgaben der Phosphatase bei der Mineralablagerung nichts bekannt ist (MAJNO und ROUILLER, 1951; BOURNE, 1956). Über den Ca- und P-Stoffwechsel liegen ausführliche Darstellungen vor (MORSE, 1956; IRVING, 1957; NEUMAN und NEUMAN, 1958; COMAR und BRONNER, 1960, 1961; LICHTWITZ und PARLIER, 1964).

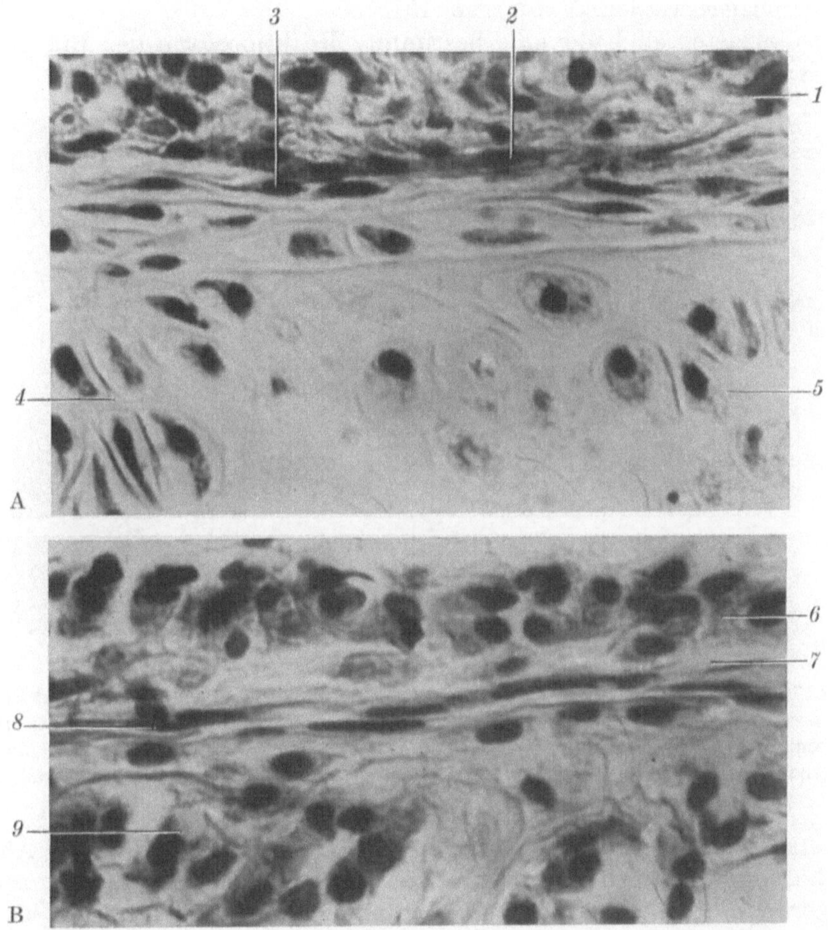

Abb. 5. Rinderfetus 126 mm SSL. Flache Knochenbildungszellen und polare Osteoblasten. A Höhe Proliferations- und Säulenknorpel. *1* Perichondrium; *2* flache Bildungszellen mit geringer Anfärbung des Cytoplasmas; *3* flache Zellen des Appositionsknorpels; *4* Säulenknorpel; *5* Proliferationsknorpel. B Höhe Eröffnungszone. *6* Schicht der polaren Osteoblasten; *7* dünne Knochenlamelle; *8* Schicht der flachen Zellen; *9* Markräume mit Markosteoblasten. Gallocyanin. Objektiv 40. Ok 12,5

Für die vorliegende Erörterung der Knochenstruktur ergibt sich aus diesen Untersuchungen, daß Kristalle mit dem Gitter des Hydroxylapatites in enger Beziehung zu den Kollagenfasern abgelagert werden (s. S. 352). Trotz der polarisationsoptischen Untersuchungen von v. EBNER (1887), der bereits von Mikrokristallen sprach, wurde häufig der Ausdruck „Verkalkung“ im Sinne einer Art kolloidaler Durchtränkung des Gewebes gebraucht. Der Terminus Verkalkung (calcification) ist demgemäß endgültig durch Mineralisation zu ersetzen.

a) Die Osteogenese zu verschiedenen Lebenszeiten

Nach einer ausführlichen Diskussion der sog. Osteoblastenlehre an Hand der älteren Literatur stellte HINTZSCHE (1927) die Ansichten über den Ablauf der Knochenbildung zusammen:

1. Sekretionstheorie (GEGENBAUR, 1864).
2. Umwandlungstheorie, d.h. es wurde die Umwandlung eines Teils des Cytoplasmas in Knochensubstanz angenommen (WALDEYER, 1865).
3. Knochenbildung durch cuticulare Abscheidung (v. EBNER, 1906).
4. Bildung der Kittsubstanz durch Osteoblasten, der Fasern aber durch andere Zellen (Fibroblasten) (v. KORFF, 1906).
5. Abscheidung eines Sekretes, aus dem in der Gewebsflüssigkeit Fibrillen und Kittsubstanz differenziert werden (NAGEOTTE, 1918).
6. Die Osteoblasten sind nur eine bestimmte Reaktionsform der Bindegewebszellen, die bei der Knochenbildung auftritt (LERICHE und POLICARD, 1926).

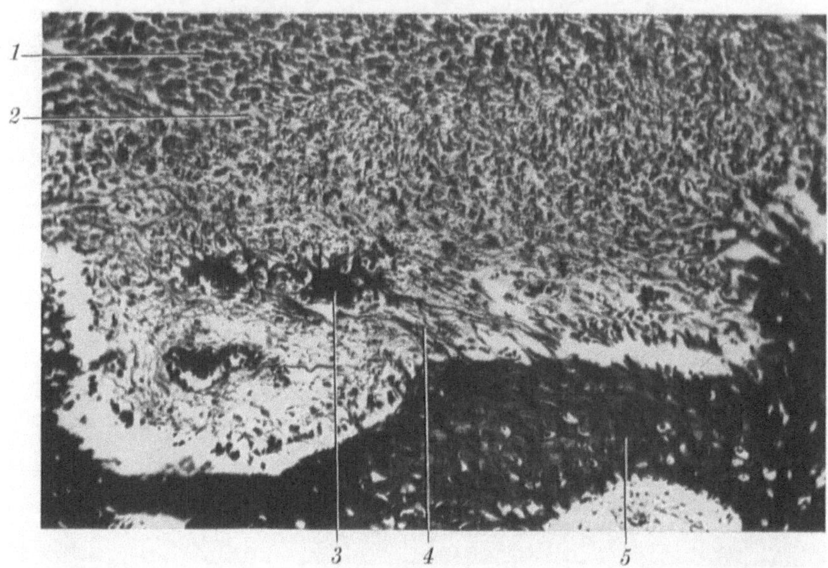

Abb. 6. Fetus 172 mm. Humerus, Mitte. Beginnende Vorbildung präkollagener Fasern und Bälkchenbildung. *1* Fibroelastica mit quer getroffenen dicken Kollagenfaserbündeln; *2* Grenzschicht, in der die Bildung der Fasern der Cambiumschicht stattfindet; *3* Bälkchenanlage; *4* intertrabeculäre Fasern; *5* älteres Bälkchen, das präkollagene Faserwerk ist teilweise kenntlich. Versilberung Bodian. Obj. 20, Ok. 9. (Aus: KNESE, 1956a)

Diese verschiedenen Auffassungen entsprechen fast vollständig den Ansichten, die über die Bildung der Fibrillen und der restlichen organischen Substanzen (s. S. 332) geäußert wurden. Eine endgültige Stellungnahme zu diesen Theorien ist noch nicht möglich. Durch histochemische und elektronenmikroskopische Untersuchungen konnte aber festgestellt werden, daß Cytoplasma nicht in „Knochensubstanz" umgewandelt wird; es liegt stets eine Stoffproduktion vor, die an Zellen und bestimmte Zellorganellen gebunden ist (KNESE und KNOOP, 1961c). Für die Faserbildung wurde von manchen Verfassern (s. S. 332) angenommen, daß Zellen ein Sekret abgeben, aus dem sich intercellulär Fasern bilden. Wir haben für die Fibrillogenese auseinandergesetzt, daß neben der Neubildung von Fibrillen unter unmittelbarer Beteiligung von Zellen stets intercelluläre „Bildungsvorgänge" ablaufen, die als Fibrillenwachstum oder -reifung genauer untersucht wurden (WASSERMANN, 1956; PORTER und PAPPAS, 1959; KNESE und TITSCHAK, 1962). Ähnliche Reifungsvorgänge sind für die übrigen Komponenten des Knochengewebes anzunehmen.

In der älteren Literatur finden sich eine ganze Reihe von Angaben, die für Unterschiede im Ablauf der Osteogenese zu verschiedenen Lebenszeiten sprechen. Knochenbildung ist nicht stets gleichartig, wie v. EBNER (1875) annahm. GEGENBAUR (1864) hatte bereits festgestellt, daß die Entwicklung eines anscheinend gleichen Gewebes sich nach „sehr verschiedenen Normen" vollzieht. Über die lebenszeitlichen Differenzen der Knochenbildung ist heute kaum etwas bekannt, da sich alle neueren Arbeiten auf die

Untersuchung kleiner Laboratoriumstiere beschränken, bei denen nur eine Knochenbildung durch polar gestaltete Osteoblasten auftritt. Erst autoradiographische Untersuchungen haben auch andere Bildungsformen erneut entdeckt (s. unten).

Zur Aufklärung der voneinander abweichenden Angaben älterer Autoren hat KNESE (1956a) eine systematische lichtmikroskopische Nachuntersuchung der Knochenbildung am Menschen über den gesamten Fetalbereich vorgenommen. Alle älteren Beobachtungen konnten als zutreffend bestätigt werden. Demgemäß ist eine Reihe verschiedenartiger Bildungsformen zu beschreiben. BAHLING (1958) hat für das örtliche und zeitliche Auftreten der einzelnen Formen tabellarische Angaben gemacht. KNESE (1956a) unterscheidet folgende Modi:

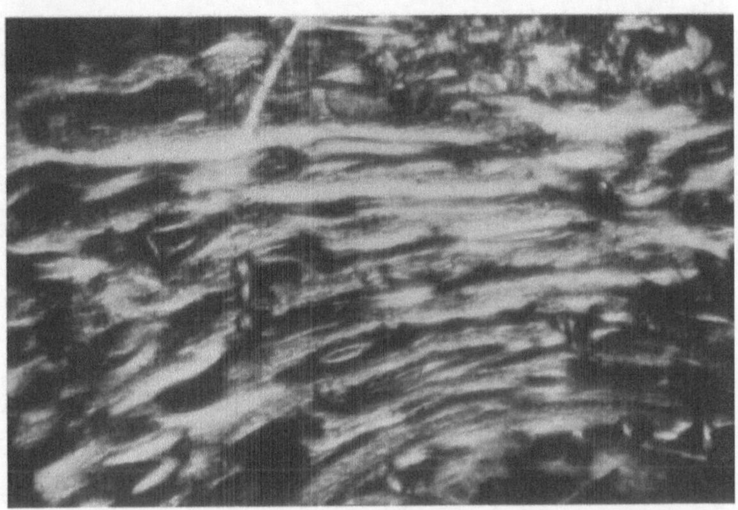

Abb. 7. Fetus 247 mm SSL. Femur, Mitte. Kollagenfaserlagerung in der Form tangentialer Streifen mit lamellenartiger Anordnung. Dazwischen vereinzelt (Faserfilz-)Osteone. Ungefärbt, polarisiertes Licht, Obj. 10, Ok. 8. (Aus: KNESE, 1956a)

A. Knochenbildung durch Umwandlung; sie erwies sich elektronenmikroskopisch ebenfalls als „Sekretion", bei der aber die Bildungszellen verlorengehen oder verdämmern. SCHAFFER (1930) hat das „Verdämmern" von Zellen bei der Knorpelbildung beschrieben (Abb. 5A).

B. Knochenbildung durch polar gestaltete Osteoblasten (Abb. 5B).

C. Knochenbildung unter Vorbildung von Fasern (Modus v. KORFF) (Abb. 6).

D. Bildung periostaler Tangentiallamellen (Abb. 7).

E. Bildung periostaler Kleinstosteone (vgl. KNESE und TITSCHAK, 1962, Abb. 8, s. S. 378).

Weitere topochemische Untersuchungen an Rinderfeten (KNESE, 1963c, 1964a, 1966a) führten zur Unterscheidung mehrerer Osteoblastenformen und zur Aufstellung einer Systematik der Skeletzellen (Abb. 9), für die deutsche und englische (KNESE, 1964a) Termini vorgeschlagen wurden. Die Untersuchungen wurden an Rinderfeten durchgeführt, da bei ihnen ähnliche Formen der Knochenbildung vorliegen wie sie zuvor beim Menschen beobachtet wurden (KNESE, 1956a). Die häufig zur Untersuchung gewählten kleineren Laboratoriumstiere, Ratte und Maus, lassen eine Reihe von Bildungsformen dagegen vermissen (KNESE, 1966a). Sehr viele topochemische und enzymhistochemische Angaben der Literatur beziehen sich demzufolge auf die „frühen" epitheloiden Osteoblasten. Bei der Systematik der Skeletzellen werden zunächst in der Unterscheidung früher, mittlerer und später Bildungsformen zeitliche Faktoren berücksichtigt. Ein weiteres Kriterium ist die topographische Position der Osteoblasten, wobei u.a. zwischen periostalen, metaphysären (enchondralen) und Markosteoblasten zu unterscheiden ist. Der oben genannten Knochenbildung durch Umwandlung ganzer Zellen (A) entsprechen die spindelförmigen

Osteoblasten, die frühen epitheloiden den unter B genannten polaren, die kubischen Osteoblasten dem Modus von KORFF (C) und darauf erscheinen dann die späten epitheloiden Osteoblasten, die z.T. dem Modus D und E zuzuordnen sind. Am Diaphysenende treten im Zusammenhang mit der Ausbildung der encoche d'ossification cytoplasma-

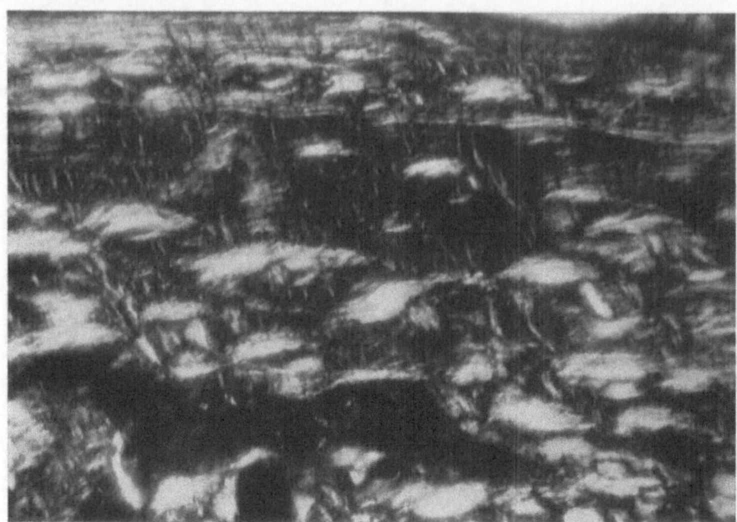

Abb. 8. Neugeborener = 335 mm SSL. Tibia, Mitte. Zirkuläre Kollagenfaseranordnungen mit Differenzierungsgefälle von zentral nach peripher. Links oben Auflagerung periostaler Tangentiallamellen und reihenweise angeordneter Kleinstosteone. Ungefärbt, polarisiertes Licht, Obj. 10, Ok. 8. (Aus: KNESE, 1956a)

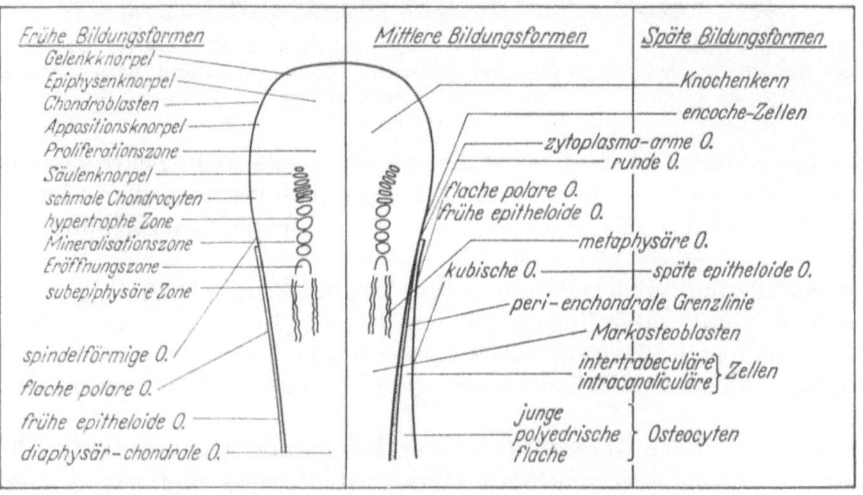

Abb. 9. Diagramm der Verteilung der Skeletzellen, aufgeteilt nach frühen, mittleren und späten Bildungsformen (aus KNESE 1966a). Englische Termini vgl. KNESE (1964a). Wir schlagen nunmehr vor, die Proliferationszone im Epiphysenknorpel als „Transformationszone" zu bezeichnen, da von einem Teil der Autoren die Proliferation auf den Säulenknorpel bezogen wird

arme sowie runde Osteoblasten und encoche-Zellen auf (KNESE, 1968). Manche widersprüchlichen Angaben der Literatur über die Reaktionsformen von Osteoblasten mögen darauf beruhen, daß Osteoblastenformen zu verschiedenen Zeiten an verschiedenen Orten und bei verschiedenen Species untersucht wurden.

Der „Modus v. KORFF" (1906, PETERSEN, 1919) ist dadurch ausgezeichnet, daß im Periost argyrophile Fasern erscheinen, die vermutlich durch Fibroblasten gebildet werden (Abb. 6, vgl. SOGNNAES, 1955; KNESE, 1956a). Weitere mehr rundliche Zellen in Knochennähe „mauern" diese Fasern in die Knochensubstanz ein. Gegenüber histochemischen Färbemethoden verhalten sich beide Zellformen abweichend von den Osteoblasten (KNESE, 1964a). Es handelt sich hierbei um einen Bildungsmodus, der bei menschlichen Feten von etwa 170 mm SSL erscheint und etwa bis zum Ende der Schwangerschaft zu beobachten ist (KNESE, 1956a; BAHLING, 1958).

Die Bildung periostaler Kleinstosteone und Tangentiallamellen (Abb. 8) beginnt in den letzten Fetalmonaten. Sie ist während der gesamten postnatalen Osteogenese zu beobachten (KNESE, 1956b). An Hand von autoradiographischen Untersuchungen über die Ablagerung von ^{45}Ca beim Hunde haben LEA und PONLOT (1958) und PONLOT (1960) diese Bildungsformen erneut beschrieben. Es ist zu hoffen, daß weitere autoradiographische Untersuchungen den postnatalen Bildungsformen ein größeres Interesse entgegenbringen.

b) Die Osteoblasten

Die folgende Zusammenfassung soll einige der für die Strukturbildung bedeutsamen Vorgänge bei der Knochenbildung herausgreifen. Histochemische (FOLLIS und BERTHRONG, 1948, 1949; BEVELANDER und JOHNSON, 1950; PRITCHARD, 1952; MONESI und BETTINI, 1958; KNESE und KNOOP, 1961c; CABRINI, 1961; KNESE, 1966a; FULLMER, 1965) und elektronenmikroskopische Untersuchungen (WILHELM, 1955; SCOTT und PEASE, 1956; ROBINSON und CAMERON, 1956; SHELDON und ROBINSON, 1957; S. F. JACKSON, 1956; KNESE und KNOOP, 1958, 1961a, b, c; ASCENZI und BENEDETTI, 1959; DUDLEY und SPIRO, 1961; SCOTT, 1967) konnten eine Reihe von Vorgängen bei der Knochenbildung klären.

Die seit langem bekannte Basophilie (Abb. 13a) der Osteoblasten (ASKANAZY, 1902) tritt bei der Entwicklung der Osteoblasten aus spindelförmigen Stammzellen über sog. Präosteoblasten auf (HELLER et al., 1950; PRITCHARD, 1952). Die Basophilie schwindet während der Knochenbildung (CAPPELLIN, 1948; CLAVERT, 1950) und beruht auf dem Vorhandensein von Ribonucleinsäuren (RNS), wie die Digestion mit Ribonuclease zeigt (FOLLIS, 1951). Die Basophilie der Osteoblasten nimmt im Lauf der Entwicklung von den spindelförmigen zu den späten Osteoblasten zu (KNESE, 1964a, 1966a). Die basophile Substanz des Cytoplasmas wird als Ergastoplasma (vgl. HAGUENAU, 1958) bezeichnet (Abb. 10). Elektronenmikroskopisch stellt sich dieses Ergastoplasma als ein System von Doppelmembranen dar, zwischen denen Hohlräume, die Zisternen, liegen (Abb. 11). Zum Grundplasma oder Hyaloplasma hin tragen die Membranen (Palade-)Granula die sog. Ribosomen von etwa 150 Å Durchmesser, die als Träger der RNS erkannt wurden (PORTER, 1953; SJÖSTRAND, 1956; PALADE, 1956; HAGUENAU, 1958, 1959). Dieses System stellt das endoplasmatische Reticulum (α-Cytomembranen) dar. Das endoplasmatische Reticulum ist in Osteoblasten stark ausgebildet und entspricht dem Umfange nach etwa dem der Pankreaszellen (Abb. 14).

Ribonucleinsäuren und endoplasmatisches Reticulum stehen mit der Proteinsynthese in engem Zusammenhang (BRACHET, 1950; CASPERSSON, 1950). Bei den Osteoblasten überwiegt die Synthese von Skleroproteinen, die in der Verknöcherungsfront von den Zellen abgegeben werden und dann als Fibrillen des präossalen Gewebes erscheinen (KNESE und KNOOP, 1958, 1961c). Die Tätigkeit der Osteoblasten wurde wegen der Bildung von Stoffen und deren Abgabe an die Intercellularsubstanz von sehr vielen Untersuchern, die verschiedenartige Methoden angewandt haben, mit der von Drüsenzellen verglichen und als eine Art Sekretion beschrieben (Lit. bei KNESE, 1956a; KNESE und KNOOP, 1961a, c). Die Struktur der stoffproduzierenden Drüsenzellen und der skeletogenen Zellen ist sehr ähnlich. Die sekretorische Tätigkeit der Drüsenzellen findet aber in einem ausdifferenzierten Organverband statt und das Zellprodukt wird als Sekret abgeführt. Bei den Stützgeweben werden die von den Zellen abgegebenen Stoffe zu extracellulären Komponenten des Gewebes, die Stoffabgabe ist der entscheidende Anteil der Strukturbildung und der Gewebsdifferenzierung (KNESE und KNOOP, 1961c; KNESE, 1967a, b).

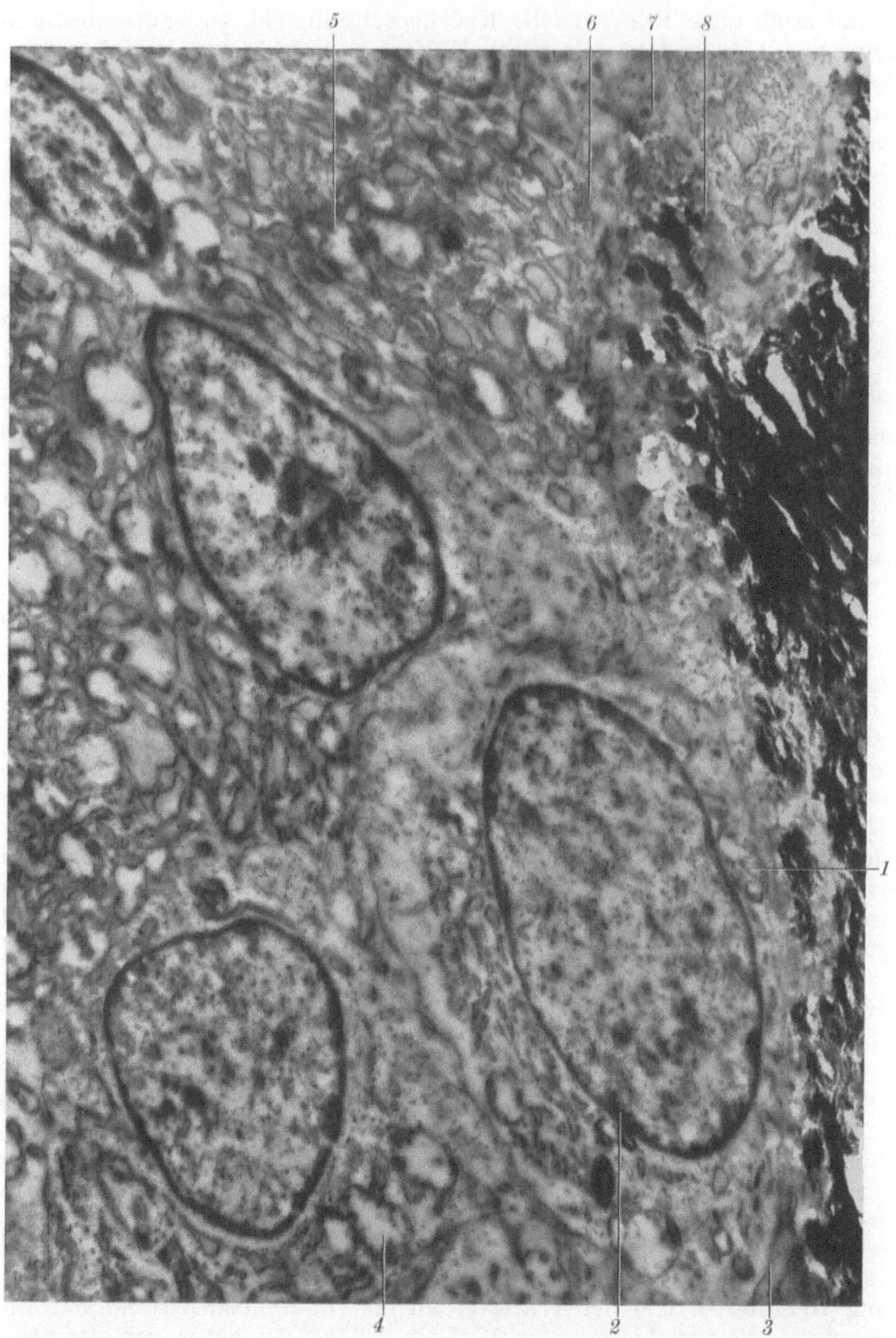

Abb. 10. Osteoblastenlager. *1* Ruhende Osteoblasten mit gering entwickeltem endoplasmatischen Reticulum sowie (*2*) geringer Dichte und feiner Verteilung des Chromatins; *3* Zellmembran; *4* tätige Osteoblasten mit stark entwickeltem endoplasmatischen Reticulum und dichtem verklumpten Chromatin; *5* Mitochondrien; *6* Verbindung zwischen Zelleib des Osteoblasten und präossalem Streifen; *7* überwiegend quergeschnittene Fasern und *8* Kalkablagerungen. Vergr. 16000fach. (Aus: KNESE und KNOOP, 1958)

c) Bildung der Gewebekomponenten

Knochenbildung ist ein Vorgang, der aus mehreren Einzelprozessen zur Bildung der jeweiligen Gewebekomponenten besteht. Eine mehrzeitige Entstehung des Knochen-

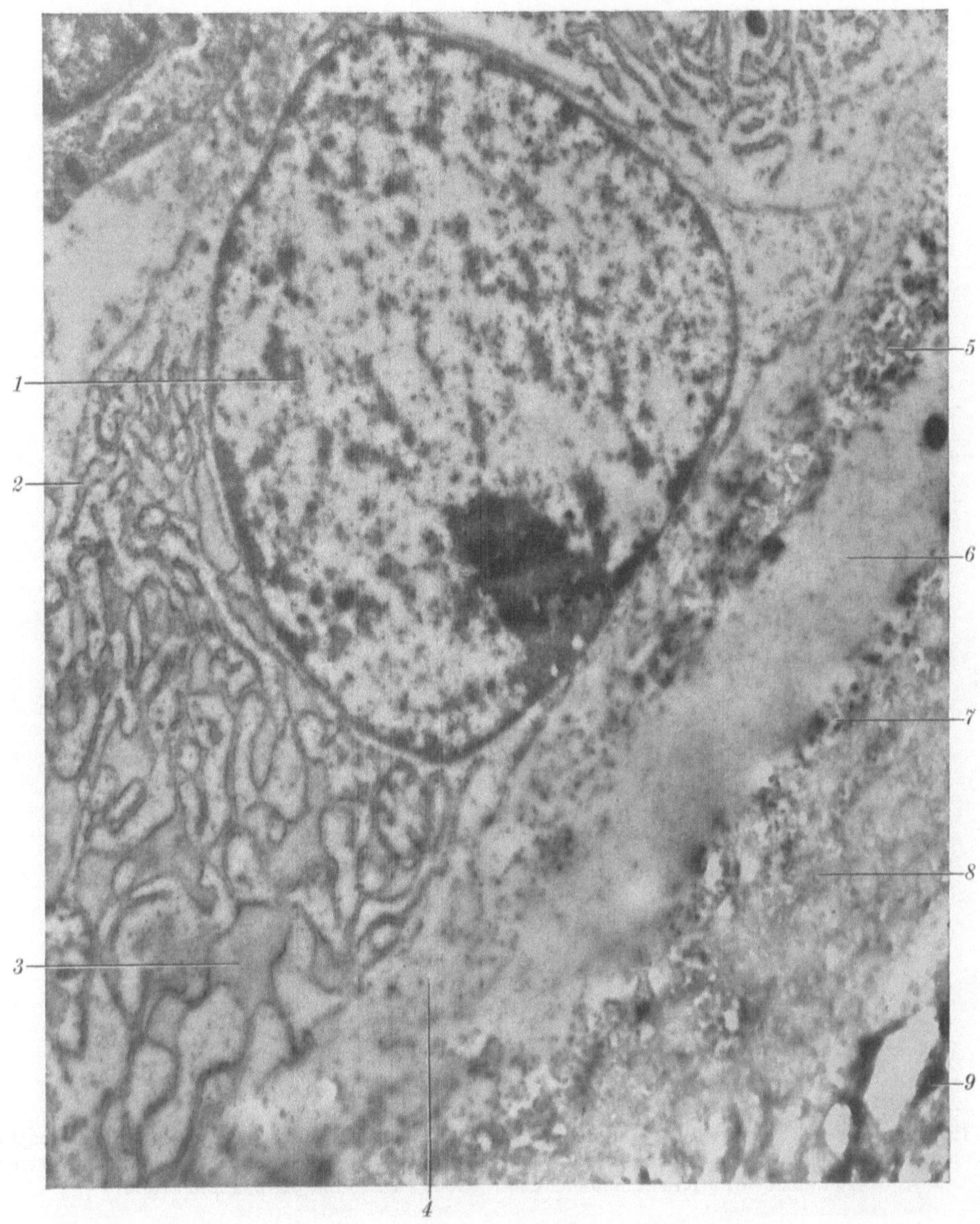

Abb. 11. Zwischenschaltung eines hyalinen bzw. opaken Streifens zwischen Osteoblast und Knochen. *1* Kern mit randständigem Nucleolus; *2* endoplasmatisches Reticulum mit gering entwickelter Zwischensubstanz; *3* endoplasmatisches Reticulum mit stark erweiterten Zisternen; *4* hyaliner Streifen mit wenigen verquollenen Fasern; *5* Faserquer- und Längsschnitte, geringe Menge Zwischensubstanz; *6* strukturloser hyaliner Streifen; *7* Faserquerschnitte auf der Knochenseite des hyalinen Streifens; *8* verquollenes präossales Gewebe; *9* mit Kalkmantel versehene Fasern. Vergr. 15500fach. (Aus: KNESE und KNOOP, 1958)

gewebes wurde verschiedentlich vermutet (SPULER, 1899; v. EBNER, 1906; PETERSEN, 1919; ROBINSON, 1952; KNESE, 1956a). Elektronenmikroskopische Untersuchungen brachten hierfür die endgültige Bestätigung. Sie erlaubten auch Aussagen über den jeweiligen Ort der Bildung der Gewebekomponenten (KNESE und KNOOP, 1961c, KNESE, 1967b). Im übrigen ist seit langem bekannt (unter anderem PARK, 1954), daß z.B. bei Mangelzuständen (Rachitis) zunächst nur die Bildung einer Gewebekomponente gestört ist, sekundär aber weitere Bildungsvorgänge in Mitleidenschaft gezogen werden. Unsere

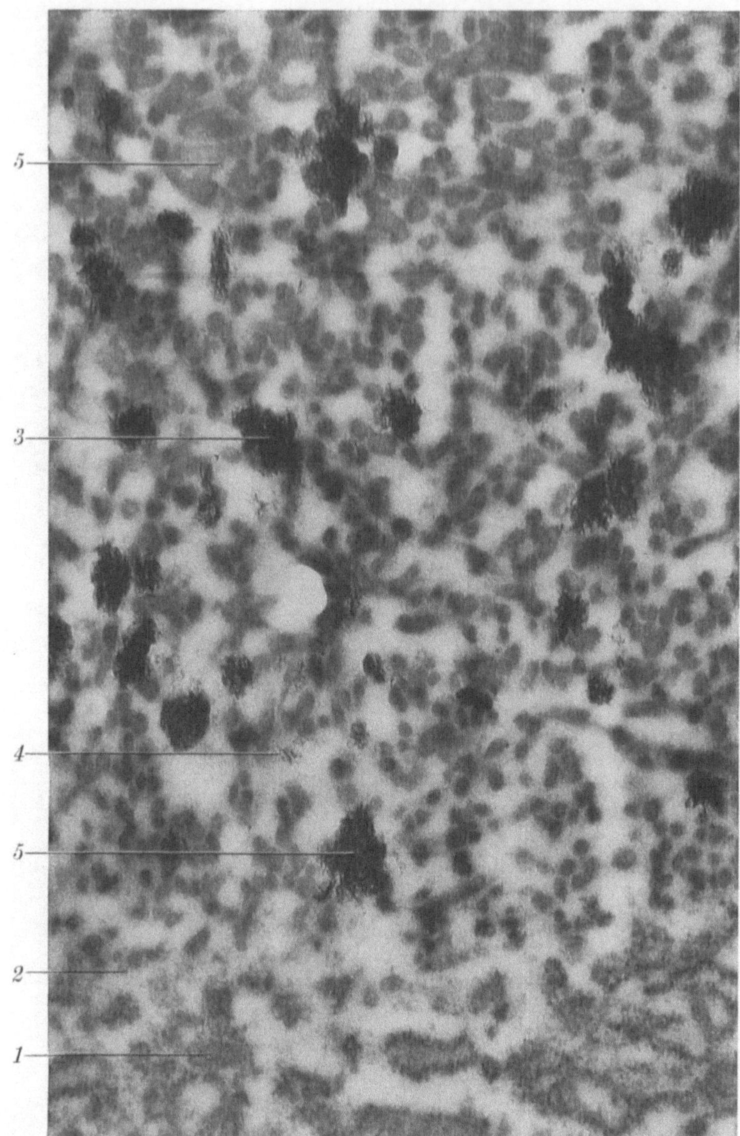

Abb. 12. Tibia eines Rattenfeten, präossales Gewebe. *1* Rand des Osteoblasten mit dem endoplasmatischen Reticulum; *2* dünne Kollagenfibrillen; *3* dicke Kollagenfibrillen, z.T. in Bündeln angeordnet; *4* einzelne Kristallnadeln; *5* Kristallhaufen. Vergr. 65000 (Aufnahme KNESE und KNOOP)

fortschreitende Kenntnis über die Zellstruktur und Zelleistung machen eine detaillierte Diskussion der cytologischen Gestaltung der Osteoblasten im Hinblick auf ihre Tätigkeit möglich (KNESE, 1966b).

Für die Fibrillogenese bei der Knochenbildung gelten die oben genannten Ausführungen, besonders über die Beziehungen zwischen Zellen und Fibrillen. Die Knochenfibrillen treten in der sog. Verknöcherungsfront auf, d.h. die Bildung des präossalen Gewebes, des physiologischen Osteoids, ist durch die Entstehung von Fibrillen morphologisch gekennzeichnet (Abb. 12). Elektronenmikroskopische Untersuchungen haben gezeigt, daß nicht ein präexistierendes Fibrillenwerk „verknöchert", sondern die Fibrillen von den Osteoblasten erst gebildet werden. Bereits GEGENBAUR (1864) hatte auf die Bildung der Fasern ad hoc hingewiesen. Knochengewebe ist demgemäß kein erstarrtes Bindegewebe; dies gilt auch für die desmale Osteogenese (vgl. ASCENZI und BENEDETTI, 1959). Der Ausdruck „Verknöcherung (ossification)" ist demzufolge zu vermeiden und durch Knochenbildung bzw. Osteogenese zu ersetzen. Ob mit dieser Bildung von Fasern ad hoc die Eigenschaft, „Kalkfänger“ zu sein, verbunden ist, kann z. Z. nicht entschieden werden (s. S. 355). Die Ergebnisse der bisherigen Untersuchungen lassen keine Unterschiede zwischen den Knochenfibrillen und denen von anderen Orten erkennen. Allerdings ist eine Rekonstitution von Knochenfibrillen bisher nicht gelungen (s. S. 331).

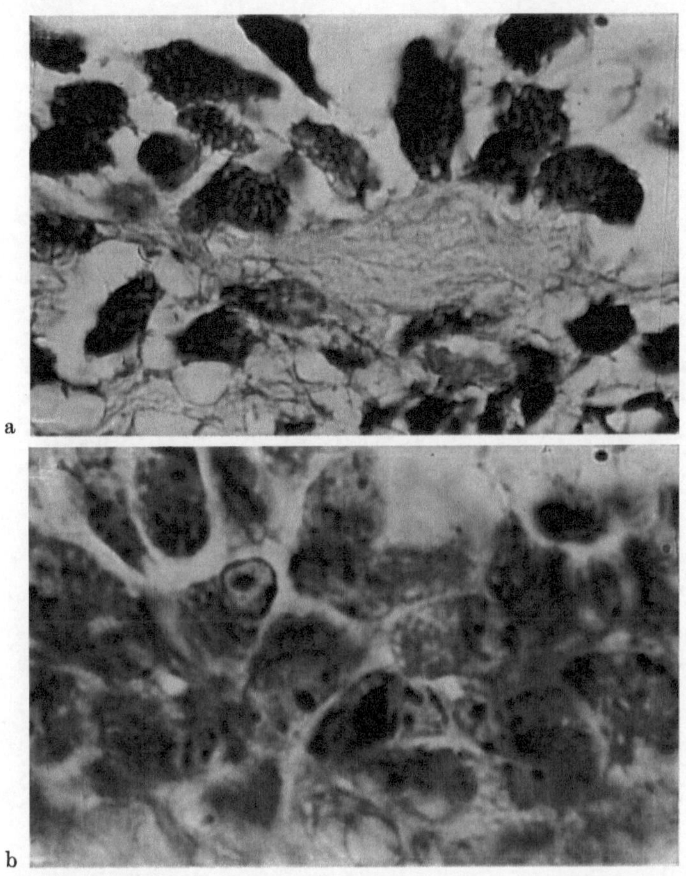

Abb. 13a u. b. Rinderfetus 126 mm SSL, Metacarpus. Osteoblasten. a Färbung mit Methylenblau pH 4,1. Schwache metachromatische Reaktion des Knochenbälkchens. Das Cytoplasma der Osteoblasten zeigt ein kräftig tingiertes Netzwerk. b Färbung mit Toluidinblau pH 4,1. Kern und Nucleolus reagieren orthochromatisch. Das Cytoplasmanetz zeigt eine dunkel violette metachromatische Reaktion, die Netzlücken eine hell violette. Ölimmersion 100, Ok 12,5

Das Cytoplasma der Osteoblasten läßt sich auch mit Methoden zur Darstellung von Kohlenhydraten anfärben; das Ergebnis ist allerdings sehr wechselnd (Knese und Knoop, 1961c). Topochemische Untersuchungen (Knese, 1964a, 1966a) ergaben bei frühen Osteoblastenformen eine schwächere Kohlenhydratreaktion als bei den späteren. Heller-Steinberg (1951) hatte zuerst auf Cytoplasmagranula hingewiesen. Bei Methylenblaufärbung (Abb. 13a) ist eine leichte metachromatische Tönung des Cytoplasma zu beobachten, mitunter in der Form einer Netzstruktur, wie sie auch bei Färbung mit Toluidinblau (Abb. 13b) auftritt (Knese und Knoop, 1961a, c; Tonna und Cronkite, 1959). Diese Farbreaktionen weisen auf Mucopolysaccharide in Osteoblasten hin. Knese und Knoop (1958, 1959, 1961a, c) haben auf Erweiterungen der Zisternen des endoplasmatischen Reticulums hingewiesen (Abb. 11), deren Zusammenhang mit der Bildung des MPS-Proteinkomplexes wahrscheinlich gemacht werden konnte. Bei topochemischen Studien des Periostes kam Knese (1966a) zu der Auffassung, daß besondere Zellen des Periostes, die Cambiumzellen (s. u.), die MPS produzieren. Diese MPS sind extracellulär teilweise von Lipoproteinmembranen umhüllt und werden voraussichtlich in Präosteoblasten wieder

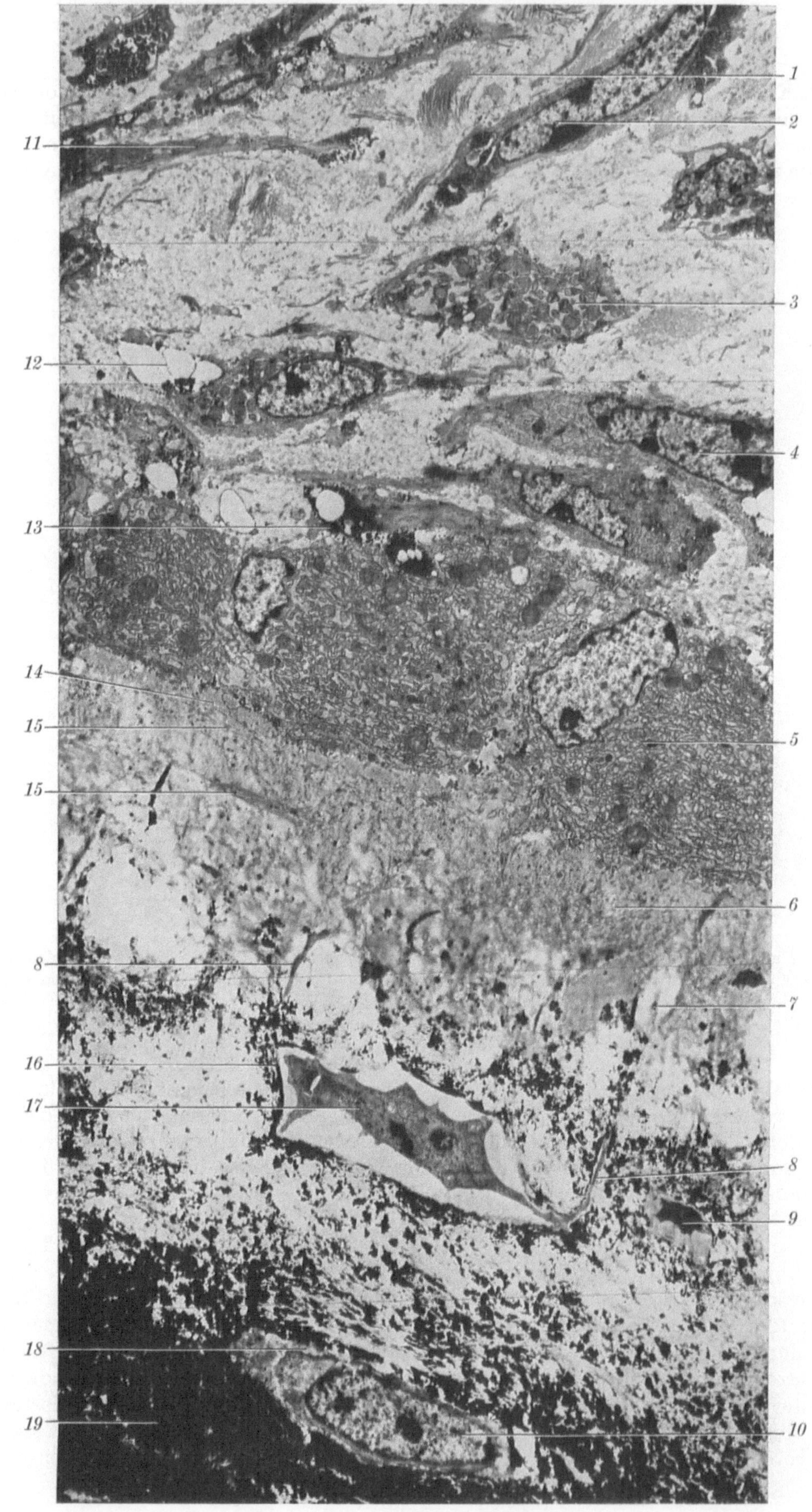

Abb. 14. (Legende s. S. 349)

aufgenommen (Abb. 14). Diese Auffassung konnte elektronenmikroskopisch bestätigt werden (KNESE, 1967a, b).

Die Mineralisation, die Ablagerung von anorganischen Kristalliten, erfolgt erst in dem präossalen Gewebe und zwar in verschieden weiter Entfernung vom Osteoblasten (s. S. 352).

Zur Enzymhistochemie der Osteoblasten weisen wir u.a. auf FULLMER (1965) und CABRINI (1961) hin. Osteoblasten zeigen eine positive alkalische Phosphatase-Reaktion (unter anderem PRITCHARD, 1952; BOURNE, 1956). Die Angaben über saure Phosphatase sind widersprüchlich (FULLMER, 1965). Über Oxydasen berichten FOLLIS und BERTHRONG (1948), BALOGH, DUDLEY und COHEN (1961), über Hydrolasen VAES (1965), über Dehydrogenasen unter anderem FULLMER (1965) sowie TAKADA (1966) und schließlich über Esterasen FULLMER (1965).

Auch die Frage der Entwicklung, Differenzierung oder Zellmetamorphose (KNESE 1956, 1967a) der periostalen Osteoblasten wurde näher untersucht. Einmal wurde eine Markierung der Zellen während der Mitose durch Thymidin durchgeführt (unter anderem TONNA, 1961; YOUNG, 1962; OWEN, 1965). Hierbei ergibt sich, daß nur 4—8% der Osteoblasten markiert werden. Von KNESE (1966a) wurden dann im Periost folgende Zellformen unterschieden: In der Fibroelastica die Fibroblasten und in der Cambiumschicht die sog. Stammzellen, dann Cambiumzellen und Präosteoblasten und schließlich die sog. reifen Osteoblasten (Abb. 14).

d) Das Skeletorgan

Verschiedentlich wurde auf die notwendige Unterscheidung zwischen dem Knochen als Organ und als Gewebe hingewiesen (HINTZSCHE, 1927; WEINMANN und SICHER, 1955; SOGNNAES, 1955; KNESE, 1959a). Außer der Bildung des Knochengewebes ist die des Skeletorgans zu untersuchen. Im allgemeinen begnügt man sich mit der Schilderung, wie aus dem knorpeligen Skeletstück durch Ablagerung einer periostalen Manschette, durch die Markraumbildung und enchondrale Osteogenese sowie das Auftreten von Knochenkernen ein knöchernes Skeletelement wird. An Hand von Untersuchungen der Verteilung von ^{32}P konnten LEBLOND et al. (1950) zeigen, daß ein Teil der enchondralen Bälkchen als sog. Trichter (funnel) in die Diaphyse einbezogen wird. Das zeitliche Auftreten der Knochenkerne, der Schluß der Epiphysen usw. sind vor allem von klinischer Seite her gut untersucht.

Bisher liegt nur eine geringe Anzahl von Studien darüber vor, wie der Ablauf der Knochenbildung zu einem charakteristisch geformten Skeletstück führt. STREETER (1949) hat die Entwicklung des knorpeligen Humerus untersucht, ZAWISCH-OSSENITZ des Femur (1929), der Clavicula (1953), des Occipitale (1957), PRATT (1957, 1959) des Femur der Ratte.

Der periostale Knochen wird in der Fetalzeit in der Form von Trabekeln abgelagert (Abb. 15). PINARD (1952) konnte durch Rekonstruktionen zeigen, daß die im Querschnitt durch ein Skeletstück erscheinenden Trabekel ein Plattensystem bilden. BAHLING (1958) hat die Ordnung und Verteilung der Bälkchen in verschiedenen Querschnitten der großen Extremitätenknochen beim Menschen in der Fetalzeit beschrieben; sie konnte zeigen, wie durch eine wechselnde Apposition an verschiedenen Orten des Knochenumfanges

Abb. 14. Rinderfet 104 mm SSL. Periost, präossales Gewebe und Knochengewebe. *1* Intercelluläre Spalten mit wenigen Kollagenfibrillen; *2* Stammzelle; *3* Cambiumzelle mit erweiterten Zisternen und Mitochondrien; *4* Präosteoblast; *5* reife Osteoblasten; *6* präossales Gewebe; *7* Schrumpfspalten; *8* Osteocytenfortsatz; *9* Osteocytenanschnitt; *10* Osteocyt in fast vollständig mineralisiertem Gewebe; *11* Zellausläufer; *12* osmiophile Membranen; *13* K-H-Einlagerung; *14* hyaliner Streifen; *15* Fibrillenbündel; *16* Mineraleinlagerung in der Wand des Knochenhöhlchens; *17* Osteocyt, etwas geschrumpft; *18* homogene Substanz um einen Osteocyten (Rouget-Neumannsche Scheide?); *19* weitgehend mineralisiertes Knochengewebe; elektronenmikroskopische Vergrößerung 1775. (Aus: KNESE, 1966b)

die bekannte Querschnittsform eines Knochenelementes entsteht. Besonders eindrucksvoll ist dieser Vorgang an der dreikantigen Tibia zu beobachten (Abb. 16).

Auf die enchondrale Osteogenese kommen wir beim Knorpelgewebe zurück.

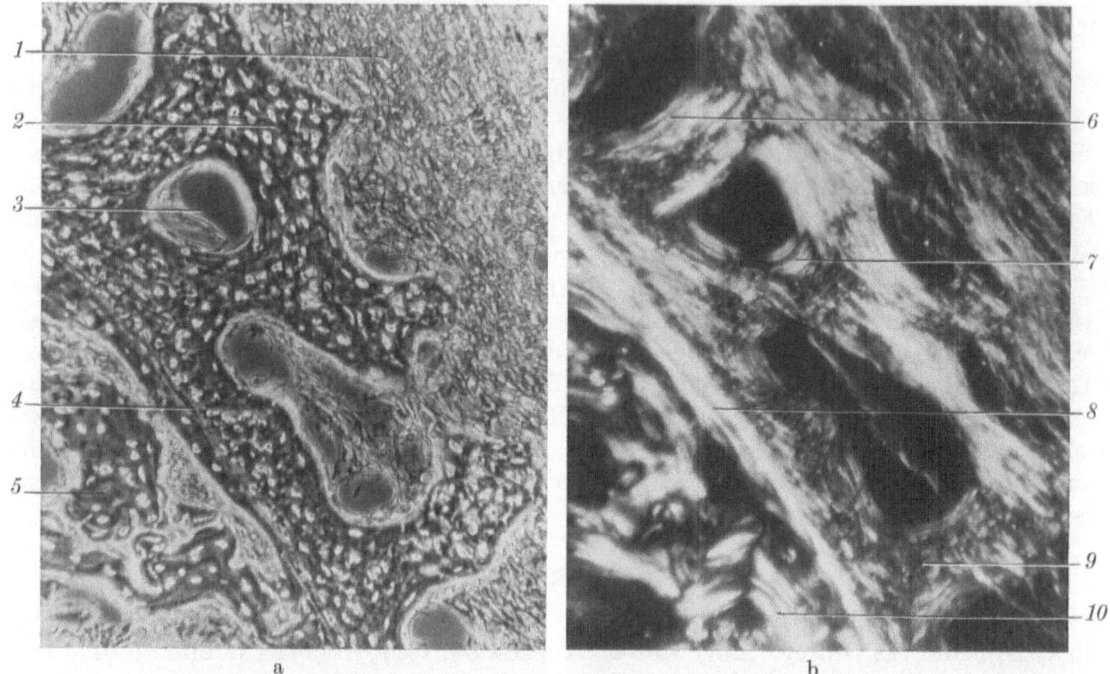

Abb. 15a u. b. Rinderfetus 105 mm SSL, Querschnitt. a Mit Phasenkontrastverfahren, b in polarisiertem Licht. *1* Periost; *2* zirkuläre Bälkchen mit Anlage von radiären Bälkchen; *3* abgeschlossener Gefäßraum; *4* perienchondrale Grenzlinie; *5* enchondraler Knochen; *6* etwas dickere Lamellen um einen Gefäßkanal; *7* dünne Lamellen; *8* chondraler Knochen mit Lamellen auf der Markseite der perienchondralen Grenzlinie; *9* sog. Zwischengewebe; *10* dickere chondrale Knochenlamellen. Obj. 10, Ok. 12,5

4. Die Struktur 5. Ordnung: Kollagenfibrillen und Kristallite

Die Struktur 5. Ordnung des Knochengewebes bilden die Kollagenfibrillen mit ihrem Mantel organischer und anorganischer Substanzen. Die Beziehungen zur organischen Peri- bzw. Interfibrillärsubstanz wurden oben dargestellt. Die anorganischen Einlagerungen treten in der Form des Hydroxylapatites auf, der durch ein bestimmtes Kristallgitter gekennzeichnet ist. Es handelt sich um Kristallite von submikroskopischer Größe. Ihre Gestalt und ihre Beziehungen zu den Kollagenfibrillen sind nunmehr zu erörtern. Einige Bemerkungen über den morphologisch kenntlichen Ablauf der Mineralisation werden angeschlossen.

a) Die Gestalt der Kristalle

Von den Ergebnissen röntgenographischer Untersuchungen (vgl. BRANDENBERGER und SCHINZ, 1945; CARLSTRÖM, 1955; CARLSTRÖM und ENGSTRÖM, 1956; ENGSTRÖM und

Abb. 16. Darstellung der Bälkchenverteilung in einem mittleren Tibia-Querschnitt während der Fetalentwicklung. Die einzelnen Schnitte sind in verschiedenem Maßstab wiedergegeben. Die weiße Linie innerhalb der Bälkchen ist die perienchondrale Grenzlinie; innerhalb der Grenzlinie liegt chondraler Knochen mit Resten von Intercellularsubstanz des Knorpels. Die Ziffern um den einzelnen Querschnitt geben die Körperrichtungen an: *1* posterior; *3* medial; *5* anterior; *7* lateral. Durch Apposition von Bälkchen an verschiedenen Punkten des Querschnittsumfanges entsteht die dreieckige Form des Tibiaquerschnittes. Die intertrabeculären Spalten werden in den marknahen Teilen des Schnittes zur Geburt hin enger. (Aus: BAHLING, 1958; mit Erlaubnis des Verfassers und der Akademischen Verlagsgesellschaft Leipzig)

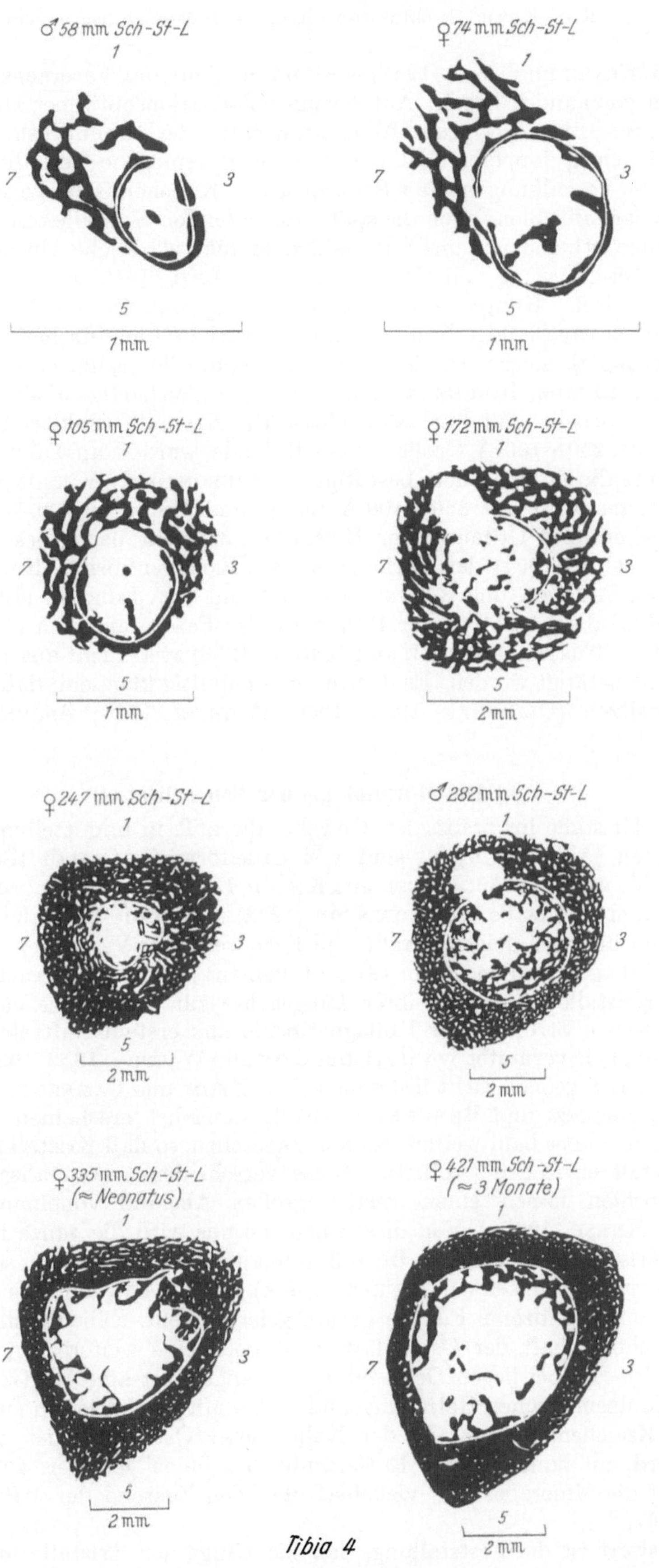

Abb. 16. (Legende s. S. 350)

FINEAN, 1958; CLARK und IBALL, 1957) wird nur erwähnt, daß Faserachse und (c-) Kristallachse parallel zueinander liegen. Auf Grund polarisationsoptischer Untersuchungen beschrieb W. J. SCHMIDT (1947) die Ablagerungsform der submikroskopischen Kristalle, die negativ einachsig doppelbrechend sind, als sog. homogene Verkalkung und stellt ihr die sphäritische Verkalkung in den Schuppen der Knochenfische gegenüber. Die zuerst gebildeten Kollagenfibrillen sollen die später ausfallenden Kristalle orientiert absorbieren.

Im folgenden stützen wir uns auf elektronenmikroskopische Untersuchungen. Nach mechanischer Dissoziierung von Knochen kam ASCENZI (1949, 1955) zu der Auffassung, daß die anorganische Komponente eine netz- oder wabenartige Struktur bildet. Die anorganischen Einlagerungen bestehen aus Körnchen und erscheinen auch bei ihrer ersten Ablagerung als solche. Die isolierte Knochenfibrille besitzt eine vollständige Hülle anorganischer Substanz. ROBINSON (1951) hat eine gleichartige Hülle an Knochen, der im Autoclaven vorbehandelt war, beobachtet. Die Kristalle schildert ROBINSON aber als Tafeln von 500×250×100 Å Größe. Diese Befunde wurden an Dünnschnitten von unvollständig entkalktem Knochen bestätigt (ROBINSON und WATSON, 1952, 1953). Die Größe der Platten wird mit 350—400 Å Länge und Breite und 25—50 Å Dicke etwas kleiner angegeben. Die Ordnung der Kristalle entspricht nach diesen Verfassern und nach BECHER et al. (1954) der Periodizität der Kollagenfibrille. Nach ROBINSON und WATSON (1955), SHELDON und ROBINSON (1957) und S. F. JACKSON (1957) sollen die anorganischen Kristalle sowohl an der Peripherie der Fasern als auch in ihnen liegen. Die letztere Möglichkeit ist nach KNESE und KNOOP (1958) zwar nicht auszuschließen, konnte aber auch nicht betätigt werden. Es dürfte nun endgültig klar sein, daß die Kristalle eine Nadelform besitzen (GLIMCHER, 1959, 1966; ASCENZI, 1964; ASCENZI, BONUCCI und BOCCIARELLI, 1965).

b) Die Morphologie der Mineralisation

Die ersten Kristalle im präossalen Gewebe, die z.T. in unmittelbarer Nachbarschaft der Osteoblasten (Abb. 17) liegen, sind von nadelförmiger Gestalt (SCOTT et al., 1956; ROBINSON und CAMERON, 1956; KNESE und KNOOP, 1958; über das Knorpelmineral s. dort). Nach einer früheren Angabe von ROBINSON (1952) sollten die Kristalle in neugebildetem und reifem Knochen von gleicher Größe und Form sein. Die Verteilung der Kristallnadeln entlang der Kollagenfibrillen (Abb. 18) läßt keinen bevorzugten Anlagerungspunkt erkennen. Die Kristalle liegen mit ihrer Längsachse zur Faserachse etwa parallel. Eine Beziehung zwischen Struktur der Kollagenfibrille und erstem Auftreten von Kristallen, wie sie ursprünglich vermutet wurde (ROBINSON und WATSON, 1952, 1955; S. F. JACKSON, 1957), läßt sich demgemäß nicht feststellen (ROBINSON und CAMERON, 1956; KNESE und KNOOP, 1958; ASCENZI und BENEDETTI, 1959). Zunächst erscheinen einzelne Kristallnadeln, denen sich aber bald weitere Nadeln zugesellen, so daß Kristallnester von drusenähnlicher Gestalt entstehen (Abb. 19). Diese verschiedenen Mineralisationszentren entlang der Fibrillen haben einen relativ großen Abstand voneinander (KNESE und KNOOP, 1958; KNESE, 1963a). Von diesen Zentren aus wird die ganze Fibrille mit einem Mantel von Kristallen überzogen. In voll mineralisiertem Knochen sind die Kollagenfibrillen nicht mehr zu erkennen. KNESE (1963a) gibt an, daß die Kristalle etwa in 5 bis 10 Schichten um die einzelne Fibrille herum gelagert sind. Neben ersten Mineralablagerungen in Nachbarschaft der Osteoblasten ist noch eine weitere Form zu beobachten (KNESE, 1966b). Hierbei liegen Osteocyten, die lange Fortsätze besitzen, mit stark entwickelten endoplasmatischen Reticulum und vielen Mitochondrien in einem von Fibrillen aufgebauten Knochenhöhlchen. In der Nähe dieser Osteocyten ist die Mineralisation stark und wird mit zunehmender Entfernung von ihnen geringer, so daß ein Einfluß der Zellen auf die Mineralisation, vielleicht über den Zustand der MPS, zu erwägen ist (s.u. LIPP, 1967).

Bemerkenswert ist die Feststellung, daß die Länge der Kristalle im reifen Knochen nicht die Länge einer Kollagenperiode überschreitet. Ein ähnlicher Befund konnte für

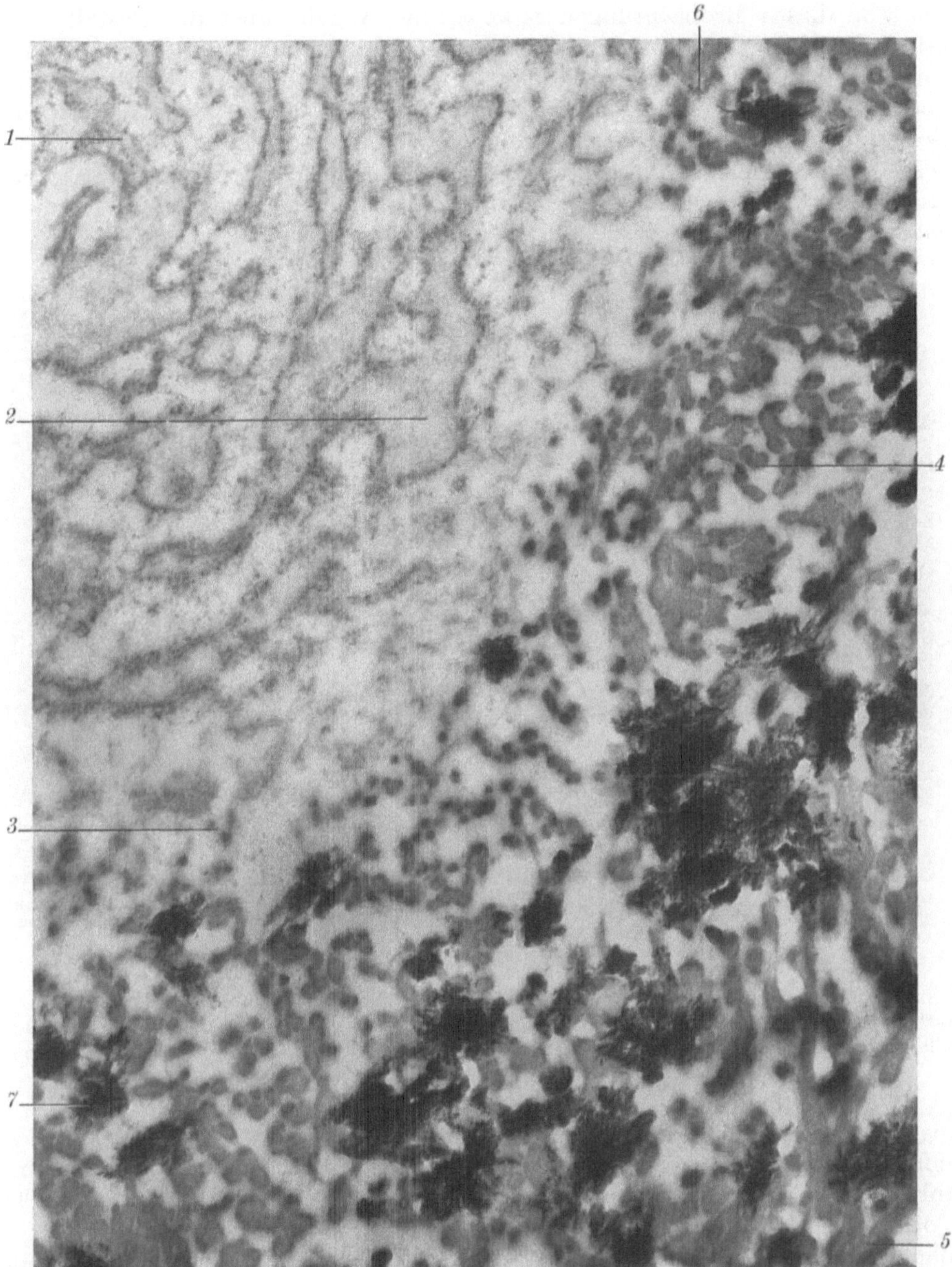

Abb. 17. Übergang von einem Osteoblasten zum präossalen Gewebe. *1* Endoplasmatisches Reticulum mit wenig erweiterten Zisternen zwischen den Membranen; *2* endoplasmatisches Reticulum mit stärker erweiterten Zisternen; *3* dünne Fasern in Osteoblastennähe; *4* dickere Fasern in der Mineralisationszone; *5* Faserlängsschnitte mit Querstreifen; *6* Einzelkristalle; *7* Kristalldrüsen. Vergr. 43000fach. (Aus: KNESE und KNOOP, 1958)

die Kristallnadeln des präossalen Gewebes erhoben werden (KNESE und KNOOP, 1958). Der Zentral-(Mittel-)wert für die Kollagenperiode war 290 Å, für die Kristalle 184,5 Å, der obere Grenzwert ist jedoch für beide mit 368 Å gleich. So liegt die Vermutung einer engen Beziehung zwischen Periode und Kristallgröße nahe, wenn auch hieraus nicht direkt auf den Mechanismus der Kristallablagerung zu schließen ist (s. S. 356). Die Dicke der Kristallnadeln beträgt 54 Å (39—77). Die Kristalle des präossalen Gewebes sind dicker und kürzer als die des Knorpels (KNESE und KNOOP, 1961b).

Eine von diesen Beobachtungen abweichende Angabe über die Gestalt der ersten Kristallpartikelchen machte S. F. Jackson (1957); sie findet granuläre Körper nicht nur an Fibrillen, sondern auch in nicht strukturierten opaken Teilen des präossalen Gewebes. Im Bereich der Fibrillen erfolgt die Anlagerung zwischen den d- und ab-Banden. Die Granula in den unstrukturierten Teilen sollen auf eine noch nicht sichtbare Periodizität hinweisen. Eine entfernte Ähnlichkeit mit den Befunden von S. F. Jackson zeigen die von Glimcher (1959) abgebildeten Mineralablagerungen bei Versuchen in vitro; allerdings besteht bei diesen keinerlei Beziehung zur Kollagenperiode.

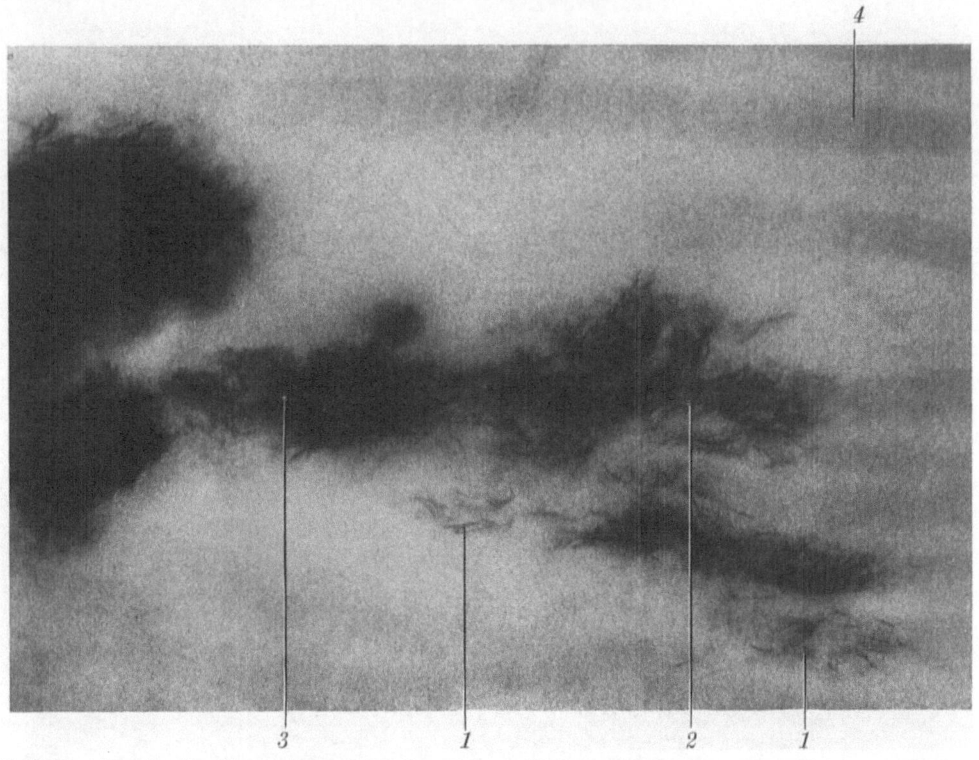

Abb. 18. Tibia einer fetalen Ratte. Präossales Gewebe mit Kollagenfibrillen im Längsschnitt. *1* Einzelkristalle (vermutlich tangentialer Anschnitt des Kristallmantels); *2* Fibrille mit Kristallmantel, Ausrichtung der Kristalle annähernd, aber nicht streng parallel zur Faserachse; *3* dichter Kristallhaufen; *4* Kollagenfibrillen. Vergr. 200000fach (Aufnahme Knese und Knoop)

Die sog. „verkalkungsfähige Grundsubstanz" der älteren Autoren stellt sich elektronenmikroskopisch als das Fibrillenwerk des präossalen Gewebes dar, zu dem wahrscheinlich eine bestimmte Peri- und Interfibrillärsubstanz hinzutritt. An diese Elemente sind offensichtlich die sog. „lokalen Faktoren" der Mineralisation gebunden. Unter morphologischen Aspekten fällt auf, daß im Knochen die Mineralien enge topographische Beziehungen zu den Kollagenfibrillen haben, die Mineraldepots im Knorpel dagegen praktisch frei von Kollagenfibrillen sind (Knese, 1963a). Viele topochemische und biochemische Angaben über die Mineralisation beziehen sich aber auf Befunde am Knorpel; diese Tatsache wird in den Arbeiten nicht immer deutlich, so daß eine kritische Klärung der Befunde z.T. unmöglich ist. Die Verhältnisse am Epiphysenknorpel sind besonders verwickelt, da einmal eine Mineralisation des Knorpels, zum andern dicht darunter in der Metaphyse eine echte Knochenbildung, nämlich die der primären Spongiosa vorliegt. Die beiden Vorgänge, Mineralisation des Knorpels und metaphysäre Osteogenese sind nicht miteinander vergleichbar. Manche Verwirrung mag durch die mangelnde Berücksichtigung dieser diffizilen morphologischen Verhältnisse entstanden sein.

Wegen der vielfältigen und sehr differenten Hypothesen über den Mineralisationsvorgang sei auf Armstrong (1952), Irving (1957), Neuman und Neuman (1958), Glim-

CHER (1959), URIRST, (1964, 1966) sowie GLIMCHER und KRANE (1968) verwiesen. Die vorliegenden Schwierigkeiten haben NEUMAN und NEUMAN (1958) in folgenden Punkten zusammengefaßt:

1. Können Zellen ein Kollagen abgeben, das sich spontan zu Fibrillen aggregiert, die ihrerseits aktiv zum Auffangen von Hydroxylapatit fähig sind?
2. Wirken die Kollagenfibrillen auf die Ordnung der MPS, so daß hierdurch das Auffangen ermöglicht wird?
3. Verlangen die Fibrillen einen Aktivierungsmechanismus, wie z.B. die Phosphorylation?
4. Ist die „epitaxis" nur ein zufälliges Ereignis, dem die Präcipitation folgt?

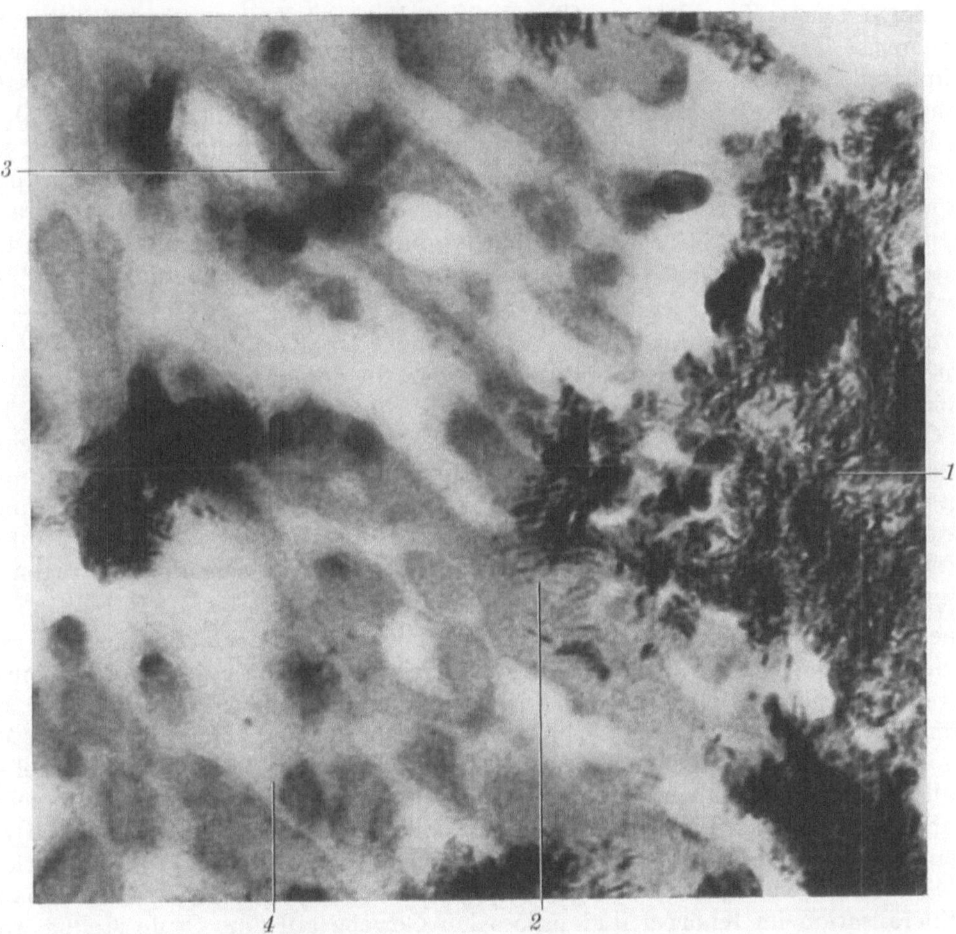

Abb. 19. Faserquerschnitte mit Einzelkristallen (*1*) bzw. Bildung von kleinen Kristalldrusen (*2*); *3* Mantel der Kollagenfaser, wahrscheinlich durch organische Interfibrillärsubstanz gebildet. Vergr. 105000fach. (Aus: KNESE und KNOOP, 1958)

URIST (1966) formuliert sieben Bedingungen bzw. Schritte des Mineralisationsvorganges, von denen wir als morphologisch interessant hier nur die Abgabe von Proteinen und Wasser zur Bildung submikroskopischer Räume nennen (vgl. auch ROBINSON und ELLIOT, 1957; NEUMAN und NEUMAN, 1958). Unter mineralogischen Gesichtspunkten ist wie bei anderen Kristallbildungen auch zwischen der Kern- oder Keimbildung und dem Kristallwachstum zu unterscheiden (GLIMCHER und KRANE, 1968; KNESE, 1963a). URIST (1964, 1966) gibt eine kurze historische Darstellung über die verschiedenen Theorien der Mineralisation und weist auf die Fülle der vorliegenden Befunde hin, GLIMCHER und KRANE (1968) haben die verschiedenartigen Ansichten ausgiebig diskutiert. Ein persönliches Engagement vieler Autoren hat die Diskussion wohl wesentlich erschwert.

In vitro-Versuche sprechen dafür, daß nur native Fibrillen mit der Periode von 640 Å zu einer Kristallkernbildung führen (GLIMCHER, 1959). Elektronenmikroskopische Beobachtungen am präossalen Gewebe lassen aber Kristallablagerungen an Fibrillen einer geringeren Periode und von verschiedener Dicke und dem entsprechend auch in verschieden weitem Abstand von Osteoblasten erkennen (KNESE und KNOOP, 1958).

Im Hinblick auf die Eigenschaften der Kollagenfibrillen, als Kristallfänger zu fungieren, wurde an reaktive polare Seitengruppen (Lysin) des Kollagens gedacht. Es wurde z.T. ein Mechanismus angenommen, der dem der Färbung mit Osmiumsäure und Wolframsäure (BEAR, 1952) bzw. der Versilberung sehr ähnlich ist (WASSERMANN und KUBOTA, 1956; KNESE und KNOOP, 1958). Nach SOBEL (1950, 1955) muß ein lokaler Faktor vorliegen, der in einem Komplex von Chondroitinsulfat und Kollagen in kritischer Stellung zu suchen ist. GLIMCHER (1959) und HODGE (1960) kommen bei Zusammenfassung der experimentellen Ergebnisse zu der Auffassung, daß die Induktion der Kristallisation auf einer heterogenen Kernbildung von Apatit aus einer niederschlagbaren Ca-PO_4-Lösung durch Kollagenfibrillen beruht. Sie hängt nicht von den Makromolekülen „per se“ oder einer bestimmten linearen Ordnung der Makromoleküle ab, sondern von Gruppen von Makromolekülen und Protofibrillen, die sich in seitlicher und Längsrichtung als natives Kollagen polymerisieren. Die Modellversuche von THIELE und KRÖNKE (1955) über das Eindiffundieren von Salzlösungen in ionotrope Gele sprechen ebenfalls dafür, daß die Mineralablagerung von der Faserstruktur abhängt.

SOBEL et al. (1960) haben den Mechanismus der Kernbildung und des Kristallwachstums diskutiert. Die Kernbildung erfordert in der gelösten Phase ein chemisches Potential, das größer als das der Kerne ist. Die Bildung der Gittereinheit von 18 Ionen $Ca_{10}(PO_4)_6(OH)_2$ erfolgt nicht in einem Schritt. Der gesamte Vorgang entspricht einem Schlüssel-Schlüsselloch-Mechanismus. Das Katalysatorsystem ist an Kollagen gebunden und besteht aus einem Mucoprotein, dem glykolytischen Cyclus, ATP und UTP und einem Ca-Ionen konzentrierenden Mechanismus. Es liegt eine selektive Einstellung auf Ca vor, der Vorgang läuft z.B. nicht mit Strontium ab. Einige entscheidende Fragen bleiben aber immer noch ungeklärt.

Recht umstritten ist die Mitwirkung der Mucopolysaccharide bei der Mineralisation (u.a. SOBEL, 1955, vgl. KNESE, 1963a), vor allem da der Gehalt des Knochengewebes an MPS relativ gering ist. Eine erneute Diskussion der möglichen Bedeutung der MPS für die Mineralisation ergibt sich vielleicht bei einem näheren Vergleich zwischen der Mineralisation im Knorpel und jener im präossalen Gewebe (KNESE, 1963a). Im Knorpel sind die Kristalle nicht mit Kollagenfibrillen vergesellschaftet. Ihnen fehlt dementsprechend die Ausrichtung, wie sie im Knochengewebe zu beobachten ist, sie bilden ziemlich regellose Haufen. Die Befunde am Knorpelmineral sprechen dafür, daß die Mineralisation nicht grundsätzlich an Kollagenfibrillen gebunden ist. KNESE (1963a) meint nun, man könne die Mineralisation im Knorpel und präossalen Gewebe auf eine Stufe stellen, wenn die Kristallbildung in einem ionotropen Gel von Chondroitinsulfat angenommen würde.

Bei den lokalen Mechanismen wurde auch an verschiedene Proteine gedacht. So spricht, der Terminus ist sicher nicht glücklich gewählt, URIST (1964, 1966) von einem Elastoid. LIPP (1967) kommt auf Grund fluorescenzmikroskopischer Untersuchung zu der Auffassung, daß ein Calcium tragendes Serumprotein mit Produkten der Osteoblasten Komplexe bildet und damit die Mineralisation einleitet. Diese Angabe würde sich in Übereinstimmung mit der elektronenmikroskopischen Beobachtung von KNESE (1966b) über die starke Mineralisation in der Nähe von Osteocyten befinden.

WALLGREN (1957) hat angegeben, daß das Kristallwachstum von 160 auf 220 Å in kurzer Zeit vor sich geht. Dieses Wachstum läuft der Zunahme der Mineralisation parallel, die vom ersten Erscheinen an in 3 Wochen 85% erreicht und diesen Wert bis zur Geburt beibehält. Die ersten Kristalle zeigen im Hinblick auf das Kollagen keine bestimmte Orientierung, die erst in 1—2 Wochen auftritt.

Das Kristallwachstum erfordert nach SOBEL et al. (1960) eine geringere Energie als die Kernbildung. Die Größe der Hydroxylapatitkristalle liegt in der kolloidalen Dimension, deren Wachstumsgesetze von denen größerer Kristalle abweichen: Je größer ein Partikelchen ist, um so schneller wächst es heran. Spurenkomponenten wie Citrat ändern Größe und Gestalt des Kristalles. Wegen der Vergesellschaftung mit den Faser-Makromolekülen und den MPS erfolgt das Kristallwachstum mehr in der einen als in den beiden anderen Dimensionen, so daß nadelförmige Gebilde von bestimmter Länge entstehen. Das Kristallwachstum beruht vielleicht auch nur auf einer Aggregation von Mikrokristallen. Die Beschränkung des Kristallwachstums durch Anlagerung weiterer Ionen an dessen Oberfläche kann durch verschiedene Ionen, Carbonate, Citrate, auch Phosphate und organische Kationen, bewirkt werden. Vermutlich wird auch der Kontakt mit der extracellulären Flüssigkeit bei der Kristallreifung herabgesetzt, so daß die zum Wachstum erforderlichen Ionen nicht mehr zur Verfügung stehen.

Die hier in Kürze vorgetragenen Theorien über die Mineralisation unter Betonung morphologischer Fakten zeigen, daß es sich bei der Mineralablagerung um einen sehr komplexen Vorgang handelt. Eine befriedigende Hypothese muß das Zusammenspiel sehr verschiedenartiger Phänomene aus verschiedenen Bereichen berücksichtigen, nämlich mineralogischer, biochemischer und morphologischer Phänomene. Obwohl der Vorgang der Mineralablagerung noch weiterer Aufklärung bedarf, ergibt sich aus den bisherigen Untersuchungen, daß im Knochen dem Kollagen eine zentrale Stellung zuerkannt werden muß. Der Knochen ist als ein Fasergewebe aufzufassen, in dem die Ordnung aller übrigen Komponenten vom Kollagen abhängt (KNESE und TITSCHAK, 1962). Damit gewinnen die rein morphologischen Untersuchungen über die Fibrillenordnung im Knochen ein erhöhtes Interesse.

5. Die Formen des Knochengewebes

a) Die Struktur des neu gebildeten Knochengewebes

Nach vollständiger Mineralisation liegt ein junges Knochengewebe vor. Untersuchungen im polarisierten Licht (W. J. SCHMIDT, 1933) und Mikroradiographien (COHEN und LACROIX, 1953; ENGSTRÖM und ENGFELDT, 1953; VINCENT, 1954; AMPRINO, 1952; CARLSTRÖM und ENGSTRÖM, 1956; WALLGREN, 1957) haben gezeigt, daß die Menge der Mineralien in einzelnen Teilen des Knochengewebes verschieden groß ist. Der Grad der Mineralisation wechselt von Lamelle zu Lamelle. Der sog. primäre Knochen enthält mehr Mineralien als der sekundäre. Leider liegen bisher keine elektronenmikroskopischen Untersuchungen (s. unter Lamellen) über die Morphologie von Gebieten unterschiedlichen Mineralgehaltes vor. Da die Mineralkomponente nach dem Mechanismus der Einlagerung und ihrer Ordnung als von den Fibrillen abhängiges Element anzusehen ist, wurde bei der Einteilung der Knochengewebe nur die jeweilige Faserstruktur, aber nicht der Umfang der Mineralisation berücksichtigt. Dieses Vorgehen ist vermutlich nicht ganz korrekt (KNESE und TITSCHAK, 1962).

Die Systematik der Gewebeformen beruht demgemäß auf Angabe der Ordnung der Kollagenfibrillen; die Aufklärung des räumlichen Verlaufes der Fasern ist recht schwierig und hat z. B. für das reife lamelläre Knochengewebe eine Jahrzehnte währende Diskussion hervorgerufen (s. S. 361). Die bisher vorliegenden Einteilungen wurden an Hand lichtmikroskopischer Beobachtungen durchgeführt. Dabei wurde angenommen, daß jeder besonderen Verlaufsform von Fasern eine spezielle Gewebeform entspricht. Weiterhin wurde vorausgesetzt, daß keine Änderungen des Faserverlaufes in einem einmal gebildeten Gewebe stattfinden (v. EBNER, 1875; GEBHARDT, 1901). Zwischen Geweben unterschiedlicher Faserordnung soll schließlich keinerlei genetische Beziehung bestehen. Diese Gewebeformen treten aber in enger Vergesellschaftung im gleichen Schnitt auf (KNESE und TITSCHAK, 1962) und sind einander koordinierte Varietäten des Knochengewebes (v. EBNER, 1875).

Die erste periostale Knochenschicht um das Knorpelmodell (periostale Grundschicht, STRELZOFF 1873) und im weiteren Verlaufe der Entwicklung das Ende der Diaphysenschale erscheinen im Lichtmikroskop als ein homogener Streifen. Im polarisierten Licht ist eine schwache Doppelbrechung zu erkennen, bei älteren Feten mitunter auch eine Unterteilung in Schichten (KNESE, 1956a; KNESE und KNOOP, 1961c). Elektronenmikroskopisch läßt sich ein Fibrillenwerk mit verschiedener Verlaufsweise der Fibrillen nachweisen, d.h. es liegen Lamellen von geringer Dicke vor (KNESE und KNOOP, 1961c).

Abb. 20. Periostales Knochengewebe mit Titriplex (Versen) entkalkt. *1* Lamelle mit Fibrillenlängsschnitten, die Fibrillen lassen die Querstreifung erkennen; *2* Fibrillen, die in die Nachbarlamelle ausscheren; *3* Fibrillenbündel, die die übernächste Lamelle mit längsgeschnittenen Fibrillen erreichen; *4* Lamellen mit Fibrillenquerschnitten. Vergr. 12500fach. (Aus: KNESE und KNOOP, 1961c)

Von diesem ersten periostalen Gewebe abgesehen wird lehrbuchmäßig zwischen einem grobgebündelten, geflechtartigen und einem feingebündelten, lamellären Knochengewebe unterschieden. Der geflechtartige Knochen wird als neugebildetes primäres Knochengewebe angesehen, das bei kleineren Lebewesen wie der Ratte zeitlebens vorliegt (u.a. ERTELT, 1955), bei größeren, auch dem Menschen, durch sekundäres lamelläres ersetzt wird. Die Faserordnung des Knochengewebes ist in gefärbten Präparaten nur ungenügend oder überhaupt nicht, aber im polarisierten Licht recht gut zu erkennen (Abb. 15). Das geflechtartige Gewebe ist dann durch grobe Faserbündel, die scheinbar regellos verlaufen, ausgezeichnet. Nun zeigt aber bereits das präossale Gewebe elektronenmikroskopisch (Abb. 20) vor Einsetzen der Mineralisation eine lamelläre Schichtung, wobei die einzelnen Schichten eine Dicke von 0,7—1,3 μ haben (KNESE und KNOOP, 1961c). Diese Lamellen erscheinen im Lichtmikroskop als eine Art Faserbündel. Bei Bildung des trabeculären Knochens läßt sich weiterhin im polarisierten Licht eine Ordnung erkennen, die der Verlaufsweise nach der späteren lamellären Hülle von Gefäßräumen sehr ähnlich ist (KNESE und KNOOP, 1961c). Es wurde daraufhin vermutet, daß grob gebündeltes geflechtartiges und lamelläres Gewebe nicht grundsätzlich voneinander verschieden sind.

In den letzten Fetalmonaten und in der postnatalen Lebenszeit wird periostal ein Knochengewebe abgelagert, das eindeutig eine Struktur aufweist, nämlich die periostalen Kleinstosteone und sog. periostale Tangentiallamellen (KNESE, 1956a). Ihre Bildung wurde durch autoradiographische Untersuchungen mittels ^{45}Ca von LEA und PONLOT (1958) und PONLOT (1960) beim Hunde bestätigt.

b) Das reife Knochengewebe

Das reife Knochengewebe des Menschen wird als lamelläres bezeichnet. Die Kollagenfasern sind in Schichten zusammengefügt, den Lamellen. Lamellen umgeben als Spezial- oder Haverssche Lamellen Gefäßkanäle, wodurch Haverssche Systeme oder Osteone entstehen. Zwischen diesen Haversschen Systemen liegen weitere Lamellen, deren Ordnung keine Beziehungen zu Gefäßen erkennen läßt; diese Lamellen werden als Schalt- oder Interstitiallamellen bezeichnet. An bestimmten Stellen des äußeren Umfanges des Knochens unter dem Periost treten äußere und zur Markhöhle hin innere Generallamellen hinzu.

α) Die Lamelle (Struktur 4. Ordnung)

Die Lamellenstruktur wurde mit den verschiedensten Methoden untersucht, im Lichtmikroskop an gefärbten oder ungefärbten Schnitten, im polarisierten Licht, an Hand von Mikroradiogrammen, mit Hilfe der Röntgenbeugung und schließlich im Elektronenmikroskop und zwar an Dünnschnitten und Abdrücken. Die Ansichten über den Lamellenaufbau weichen nicht unerheblich voneinander ab. Zunächst war zu klären, ob eine Lamelle ein wohl abgegrenztes individuelles Gebilde ist (unter anderem FILOGAMO, 1946) oder ob ihr eine scharfe Begrenzung fehlt (BURKHARDT, 1929). Zwischen benachbarten Lamellen findet ein umfangreicher Faseraustausch statt (v. EBNER, 1875; PETERSEN, 1935; ROUILLER et al., 1952; TISCHENDORF, 1952/54; KNESE et al., 1954; FRANK et al., 1955). v. EBNER (1875) beschrieb die Lamellenränder als gesägt und BURKHARDT (1929) hat sich mit der Art dieser Zähnelung näher beschäftigt. KNESE et al. (1954) nehmen auf Grund von Untersuchungen im polarisierten Licht an, daß die Lamelle aus einem zentralen Faserkern besteht, der Einzelheiten des Faserverlaufs nicht erkennen läßt (Abb. 21). Beiderseits dieses Kernes schließen sich Faserkämme an, die beim Übergang in den Lamellenkern einen unterschiedlichen „Einsteigwinkel“ aufweisen. Dieser Winkel kann ein rechter oder spitzer sein. Die Verfasser nehmen an, daß der weitere Faserverlauf innerhalb des Lamellenkernes je nach Einstiegwinkel einer rechts- oder linksgängigen Schraubenlinie entspricht. Diese Faserkämme zeigen von Lamelle zu Lamelle große Unterschiede, woraus auch auf einen entsprechend unterschiedlichen Faseraufbau der Lamellen zu schließen ist. Einzelne Faserbündel ziehen durch die Nachbarlamelle hindurch und erreichen die übernächste Lamelle. FRANK et al. (1955) haben den Faserverlauf an Längs- (Abb. 24), Quer- (Abb. 23) und Schrägschnitten (Abb. 22) elektronenmikroskopisch untersucht und kommen in der Unterscheidung zwischen gefiederten und intermediären Lamellen mit bogenförmigem Faserverlauf zu ähnlichen Ergebnissen. KNESE und v. HARNACK (1962) haben die Fibrillenstruktur des Knochengewebes an entmineralisierten Tibien von Jungratten untersucht. Sie fanden eine spitzwinkelige Verflechtung der Fibrillen. Zu längs verlaufenden Fibrillen treten stets quer verlaufende im Sinne einer Bewehrung hinzu. An den Rändern einer Lamelle wird der Verflechtungswinkel größer; Fibrillen und Fibrillenbündel treten in eine Zwischenschicht ein, die zu gleichen Teilen aus quer- und schräggeschnittenen Fibrillen aufgebaut ist. Lamellen können größere Fasermassen austauschen oder sich ohne einen eigentlichen Fibrillenaustausch miteinander verbinden.

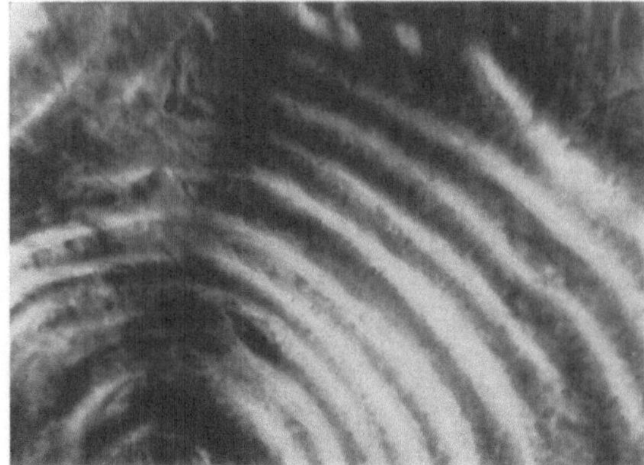

Abb. 21

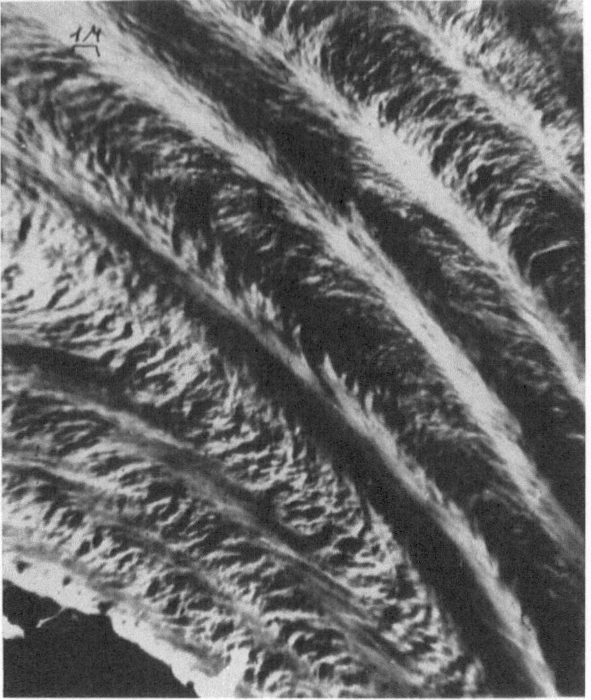

Abb. 22

Abb. 21. Ausschnitt aus einem Osteon mit Faserübertritten. Einstiegwinkel wechselnd. (Polarisiertes Licht, Ölimmersion, Ok. 8, Sammlungsfemur. Aus: Knese, Voges und Ritschl, 1954)

Abb. 22. Tibia des Menschen. Gegen die Querschnittsebene geneigter Schnitt durch ein Osteon in Nähe des Haversschen Kanals (li. unten). An den Kanal schließt sich die abweichend strukturierte innere Lamelle an. Es folgen Lamellen, deren Faserkern durch bogenförmige Fasern verbunden sind, die von einem Lamellenkern zum nächsten ziehen. In der äußeren Lamellengruppe (re. oben) sitzen den Lamellenkernen Faserkämme auf. (Aus: Frank et al., 1955; mit Erlaubnis von Autor und Verlag Masson und Cie. Paris)

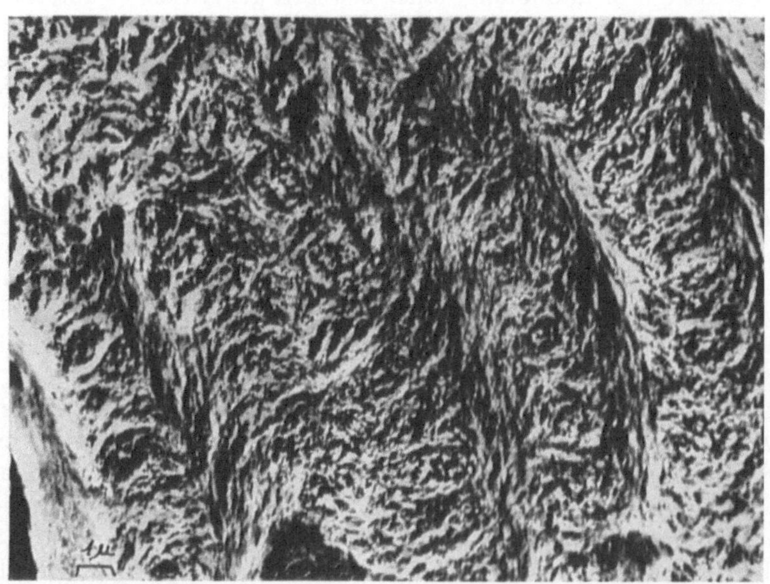

Abb. 23. Femur des Menschen, reiner Osteonquerschnitt: Auf den Haversschen Kanal folgt die innere Lamelle. Die Faserkerne der folgenden Lamellen sind z. T. durch bogenförmig verlaufende Fasern verbunden, z. T. sind Faserkämme vorhanden. (Aus: Frank et al., 1955; mit Erlaubnis von Autor und Verlag Masson und Cie. Paris)

Die Lamelle ist demgemäß kein individuelles Gebilde, sondern eine bestimmte Lagerungsform der Kollagenfbrillen, die in der Strukturhierarchie des Knochens die 4. Ordnung bildet. Die Lamellen stellen weiterhin keine geschlossenen Schichten um den Haversschen Kanal dar, sondern sind vielfältig durchbrochen, sie keilen aus (Petersen 1930), d.h. enden spitzwinklig, verschmelzen mit anderen oder teilen sich zu mehreren Lamellen auf. Es liegt eine ungewöhnliche Vielfalt der „Faserordnung" vor.

Im Lichtmikroskop erscheinen Lamellen gestreift oder gepunktet (v. Ebner, 1887; Ranvier, 1875; Weidenreich, 1930). Aus diesem Erscheinungsbild wurde geschlossen, daß in den gestreiften Lamellen die Fasern in der Schnittebene zirkulär um den Haversschen Kanal herumziehen, in den gepunkteten aber in Richtung des Kanals und senkrecht zum Schnitt angeordnet sind. Diese beiden Faserverlaufsformen wurden als flache und steile Wicklung unterschieden. An den gepunkteten Lamellen ist das Phänomen der Punktwanderung zu beobachten. Bei Einstellung der optischen Ebene auf die untere Schnittfläche und Durchwandern des Schnittes mittels Drehen der Mikrometerschraube bis zur Scharfeinstellung der oberen Schnittfläche „wandern" die Punkte zur Seite. Diese Erscheinung der Punktwanderung spricht dafür, daß die steilen Fasern nicht genau parallel zum Haversschen Kanal, sondern etwas schräg dazu verlaufen. Damit ist ein annähernd schraubiger Verlauf der Fasern in einer Lamelle anzunehmen, allerdings läßt sich der Steigungswinkel dieser Schrauben nicht messen (Kölliker, 1886; Gebhardt, 1906; Petersen, 1930).

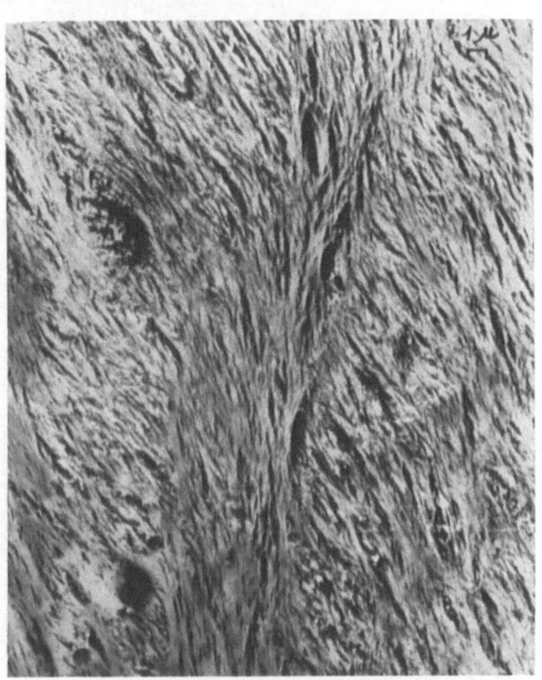

Abb. 24. Tibia des Menschen. Längsschnitt durch ein Osteon. In der Mitte ein Lamellenkern mit Bündelung und Verflechtung der Fibrillen. Nach beiden Seiten zu benachbarten Lamellenkernen scheren Fasern aus, die Faserkämme mit wechselndem Einstiegswinkel bilden. (Aus: Frank et al., 1955; mit Erlaubnis des Autors und Verlages Masson und Cie. Paris)

Auf Grund der optischen Eigenschaften der Kollagenfibrille — sie ist positiv einachsig doppelbrechend — erscheinen im Knochenquerschnitt die flach gewickelten Lamellen im polarisierten Licht hell, die steil gewickelten dunkel. Der Wechsel von Lamellen verschiedener optischer Qualität wurde von Ziegler (1906) auf Lamellen unterschiedlicher Bauart zurückgeführt, nämlich Faserlamellen und solchen aus „Zwischensubstanz". Ruth (1947) unterschied Kollagenfaserlamellen und granuläre Lamellen. Rutishauser et al. (1950) und Rouiller et al. (1952) nahmen anisotrope Faser- und isotrope Zementlamellen an. Die letztgenannten Autoren haben Abdrücke von Knochenschnitten elektronenmikroskopisch untersucht, die, wie die Untersuchungen von Frank et al. (1955) zeigen, für vorliegende Untersuchungen weniger geeignet sind. Ascenzi, Bonucci und Bocciarelli (1965) fanden elektronenmikroskopisch im Femur des Rindes keine sog. Zementlamellen. Dagegen sprechen die Autoren von einer interlamellären Zementzone, die sich durch die Zufallsorientierung der Elemente im polarisierten Licht isotrop verhält. Hierbei handelt es sich offensichtlich um die Zwischenschicht von Knese und v. Harnack (1962) mit dem Faseraustausch zwischen den Lamellen.

Nach Knese et al. (1954) ist der regelmäßige Wechsel von steil und flach gewickelten Lamellen in Osteonen selten (Abb. 25), aber in Tangentiallamellen sehr häufig. In manchen Knochengebieten sind im polarisierten Licht fast nur dunkle Lamellen aufzufinden. Nach

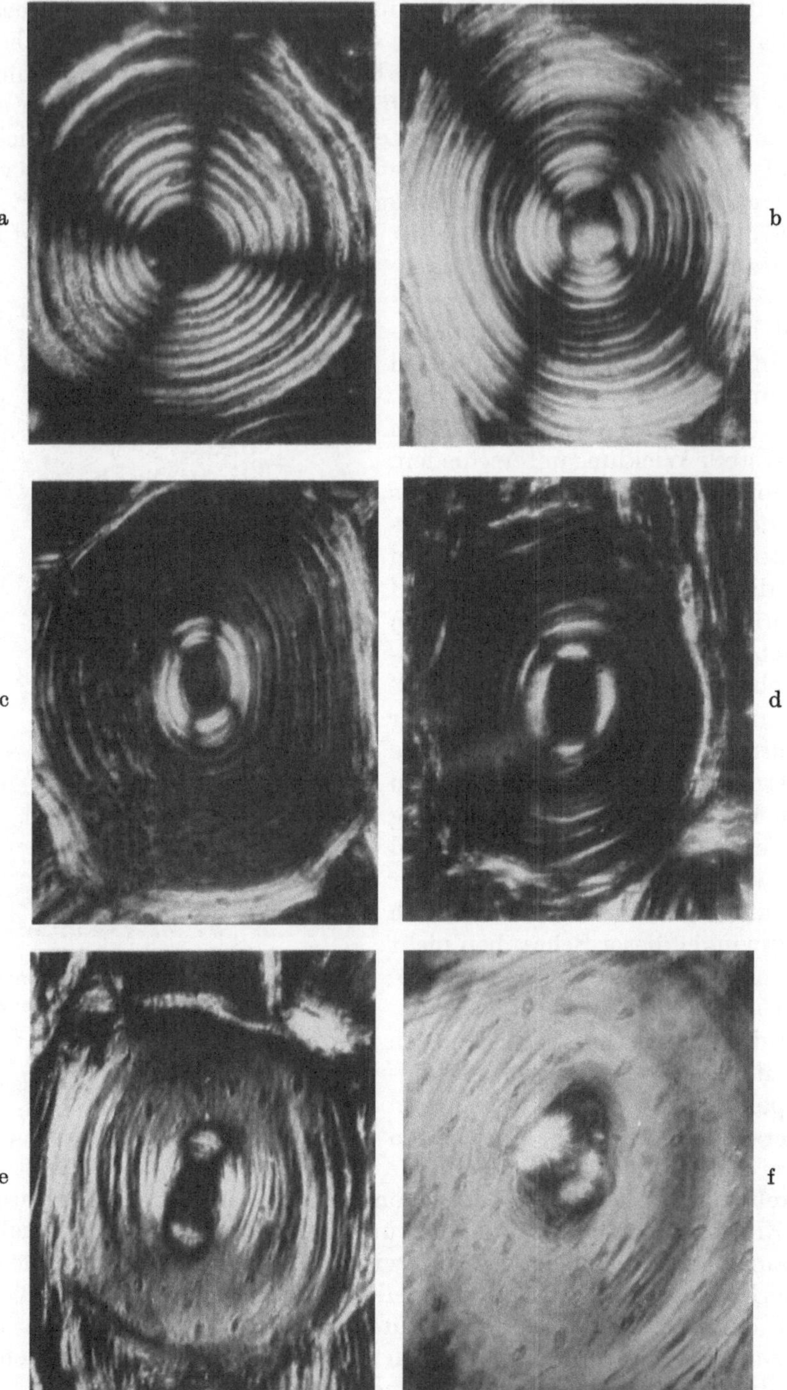

Abb. 25a—f. Steigungsfolgen. a Regelmäßig (Tibia); b überwiegend flach (Humerus); c überwiegend steil (Humerus); d fast nur steil (Tibia); e Faserfilz mit Lamellen (Humerus); f fast reiner Faserfilz (Femur). a 7 Jahre, b—f 43 Jahre. (Polarisiertes Licht, Obj. 40, Ok. 6. Aus: KNESE, VOGES und RITSCHL, 1954)

den bisherigen Ausführungen müßte die Osteonwand dann aus sog. Zementlamellen aufgebaut sein. Ein Längsschnitt durch ein solches Knochengebiet läßt aber im polarisierten Licht dicht nebeneinander liegende, hell aufleuchtende Lamellen erkennen. Damit liegen, wie die älteren Autoren schon angegeben haben, in den dunklen Lamellen steil gewickelte Lamellen vor.

DAVIES und ENGSTRÖM (1954) haben festgestellt, daß die Menge der organischen Substanz über alle Lamellen eines Osteones hin gleichbleibt. Da innerhalb der organischen Substanz das Kollagen an Menge vorherrscht, ist das Vorliegen von Lamellen verschiedener Zusammensetzung recht unwahrscheinlich. Im übrigen haben die Untersuchungen der Osteogenese gezeigt, daß Knochengewebe ohne Kollagen nicht zu einer dem Knochen spezifischen Mineralisation führt. Gegenüber der annähernd gleichbleibenden Menge organischer Substanz der Lamellen wechselt allerdings der Mineralgehalt von Lamelle zu Lamelle erheblich (W. J. SCHMIDT, 1933; AMPRINO und ENGSTRÖM, 1952; AMPRINO, 1952a, b, 1955; COHEN und LACROIX, 1953; ENGSTRÖM und ENGFELDT, 1953; DAVIES und ENGSTRÖM, 1954; VINCENT, 1954; FRANK et al., 1955).

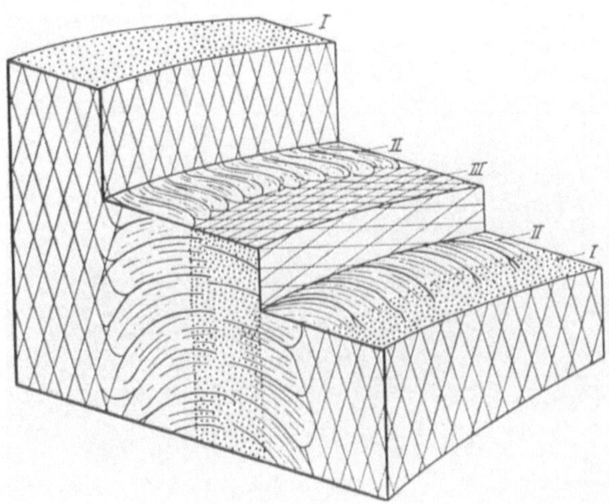

Abb. 26. Schema des Faserverlaufes in benachbarten Lamellen eines regelmäßig gewickelten Osteons. *I* Fasernetze in steilgewickelten Lamellen: Im Längsschnitt sind die Fasern annähernd längs getroffen, im Querschnitt erscheinen die Lamellen als gepunktete Lamellen älterer Autoren. *II* Bogenförmiges Ausscheren von Fasern aus dem Lamellenkern mit Übertritt und Umbiegen in die Nachbarlamellen. *III* Flachgewickelte Lamelle: Im Querschnitt Fasern annähernd längs getroffen und zirkulär um den Haversschen Kanal verlaufend, im Längsschnitt als gepunktete Lamellen. (Schema KNESE, aus BARGMANN, 1959; vgl. KNESE, 1959b, c; mit Erlaubnis des Thieme-Verlages Stuttgart)

Bei jüngeren Individuen finden sich häufiger als bei älteren in der Osteonwand neben Lamellen Bezirke ohne diese Gliederung bzw. kann die gesamte Osteonwand Lamellen vermissen lassen. Diese Bezirke erscheinen im polarisierten Licht hell; sie wurden als Faserfilze (KNESE et al. 1954) bezeichnet. Eine Untersuchung im polarisierten Licht kombiniert mit dem Phasenkontrastverfahren läßt jedoch eine undeutliche lamelläre Gliederung erkennen, so daß eine mangelhafte Ausreifung der Fibrillen angenommen wurde (KNESE 1957). Der Faseraufbau der einzelnen Lamellen ist vermutlich sehr unterschiedlich (KNESE, VOGES und RITSCHL, 1954). Ein paralleler Verlauf der Kollagenfibrillen innerhalb einer Lamelle (GEBHARDT, 1906; FURUTA, 1949) ist wohl recht selten. Im allgemeinen liegt ein matten- oder gitterartiges Geflecht der Kollagenfibrillen vor (v. EBNER 1875; KÖLLIKER 1886; WEIDENREICH 1923; HUBER et al. 1951; ROUILLER et al. 1952; ROBINSON und WATSON 1952; TISCHENDORFF 1952/54). Aus den elektronenmikroskopischen Aufnahmen von ROBINSON und WATSON (1952) ist zu schließen, daß die Netzbildung innerhalb der Lamellen im Femur eine stärkere Durchflechtung als in der Corticalis der Rippe aufweist (Abb. 27). In der Tibia von Jungratten beobachteten KNESE und v. HARNACK (1962) elektronenmikroskopisch überwiegend steil orientierte Lamellensysteme, die in sich ein sehr unterschiedliches Verflechtungssystem zeigen. Im Hinblick auf die „Materialstruktur" (KNESE 1958b) sind zu der Hauptfibrillenrichttung quer verlaufende „Bewehrungsbündel" mitunter in der Form von Arcaden besonders beachtenswert.

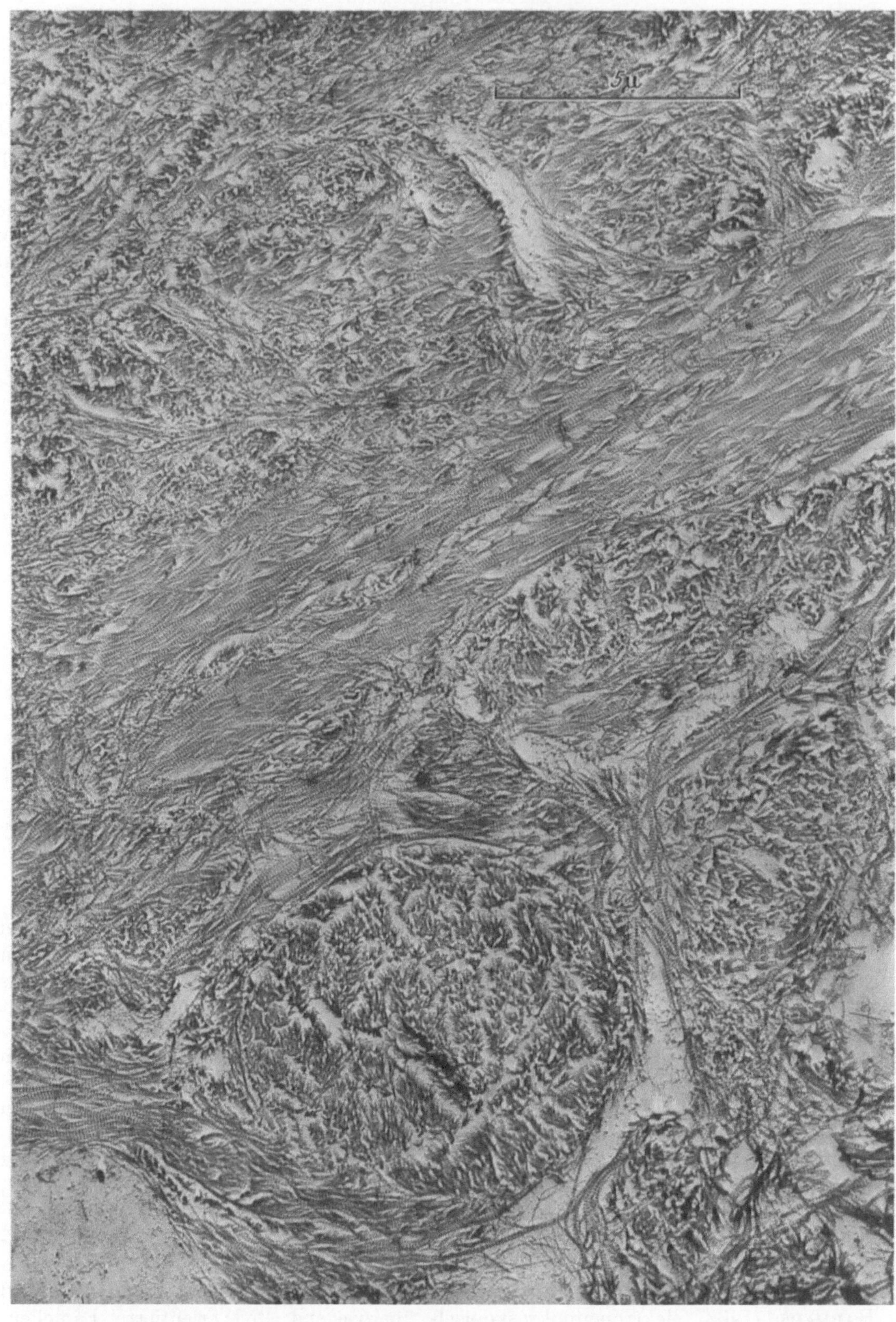

Abb. 27. Entmineralisierter menschlicher Knochen: Laterale Femurwand, Schnitt parallel zur Oberfläche und zur langen Achse des Knochens. In der Mitte längsgeschnittene Kollagenfibrillen, unten ein rundes Bündel, dessen Fibrillen etwa senkrecht dazu verlaufen. (Aus: ROBINSON und WATSON 1952; mit Erlaubnis der Autoren und des Verlegers)

ROUILLER et al. (1952) sowie FRANK et al. (1955) haben die bisherigen Auffassungen über den Lamellen- und Osteonaufbau in Schemata wiedergegeben. KNESE (bei BARGMANN, 1959; KNESE, 1959b, c) hat ein weiteres Schema (Abb. 26) hinzugefügt, das alle bisherigen Beobachtungen berücksichtigt, nämlich den Unterschied von gepunkteten und gestreiften, damit steil und flachgewickelten Lamellen, sowie die Faserverbindungen zwischen den Lamellen. Die Kollagenfibrillen bilden im Lamellenkern ein spitzwinkliges Raumgitter (s. S. 363). Durch die lange Achse des Maschenrhombus ist bestimmt, ob eine flache oder steile Lamelle vorliegt; entsprechend erscheinen dann im Längs- oder Querschnitt Punkte oder Streifen. Aus dem Lamellenkern treten Fasern in die Nachbarlamelle oder in die übernächste ein.

β) Die Lamellensysteme (Struktur 3. Ordnung)

1. Das Osteon. Die Osteonquerschnitte bieten in ihrer Form und in ihrem Wechsel von steil und flach gewickelten Lamellen oder dem Auftreten von Faserfilzen eine ungewöhnlich große Vielfalt. GEBHARDT (1906) unterschied fünf Osteonformen: 1. Osteone ohne Lamellierung, 2. Osteone mit steiler Wicklung, 3. Osteone mit flacher Wicklung, 4. Osteone mit regelmäßigem Wechsel zwischen flach und steil, 5. kombinierte Typen. Diese Einteilung wurde bald als nicht ausreichend erkannt.

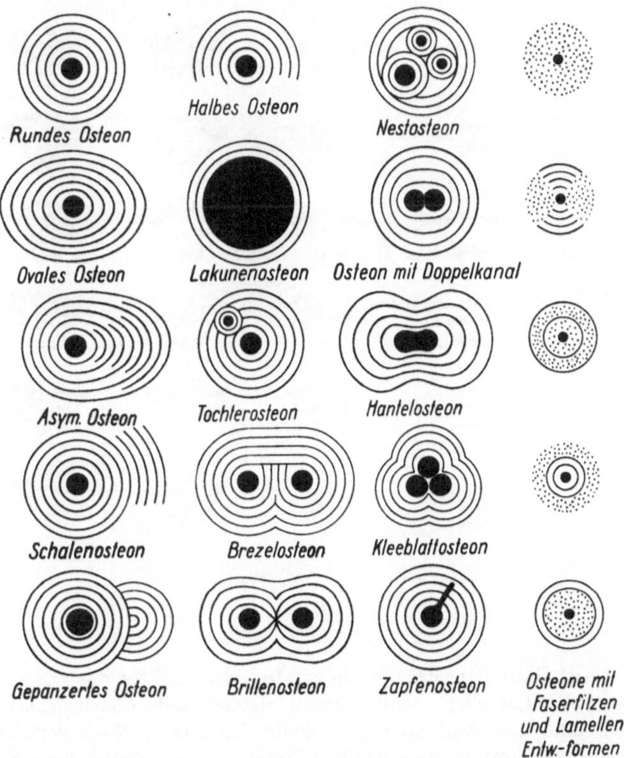

Abb. 28. Schematische Darstellung der Form von Osteonquerschnitten. Beim asymmetrischen Osteon liegt auf einer Seite des Haversschen Kanals eine größere Anzahl von Lamellen als auf der gegenüberliegenden. Dem Schalenosteon und dem gepanzerten Osteon sind in unterschiedlicher Form bogenförmige Lamellen angeschlossen. Tochterosteon, Brezelosteon usw. geben die unterschiedliche Lamellenordnung im Bereich von Gefäßverbindungen wieder. Das Zapfenosteon zeigt ein senkrecht vom Haversschen Kanal abgehendes Gefäß ohne Lamellenumhüllung. In der 4. letzten senkrechten Reihe die Kleinstosteone mit einem Wechsel von Lamellen und Faserfilzen (gepunktet). (KNESE und TITSCHAK, 1962; mit Erlaubnis der Akademischen Verlagsgesellschaft Leipzig)

Eine Systematik der Osteonquerschnittsbilder nach ihrer Form, Größe und nach Art der Steigungsfolge wurde von KNESE et al. (1954), AUERBACH (1957) und KNESE und TITSCHAK (1962) entwickelt. Diese Systematik stellt die Grundlage eines Schlüssels dar, der die Übernahme der Kennzeichen eines Osteons auf eine Lochkarte (Hollerith) und deren maschinelle Bearbeitung zuläßt. Auf diesem Wege konnten 47690 Osteonquerschnitte untersucht werden, die aus den großen Extremitätenknochen eines 43jährigen Mannes, 34 mittleren Tibiaschnitten von 22 Individuen und schließlich dem Metacarpus von je 13 Haus- und Wildschweinen stammen.

Der Form des Osteonquerschnittes nach wurde zwischen Runden, Ovalen, Asymmetrischen, Schalenosteonen usw. unterschieden (Abb. 28). Die Größe des Osteons wird

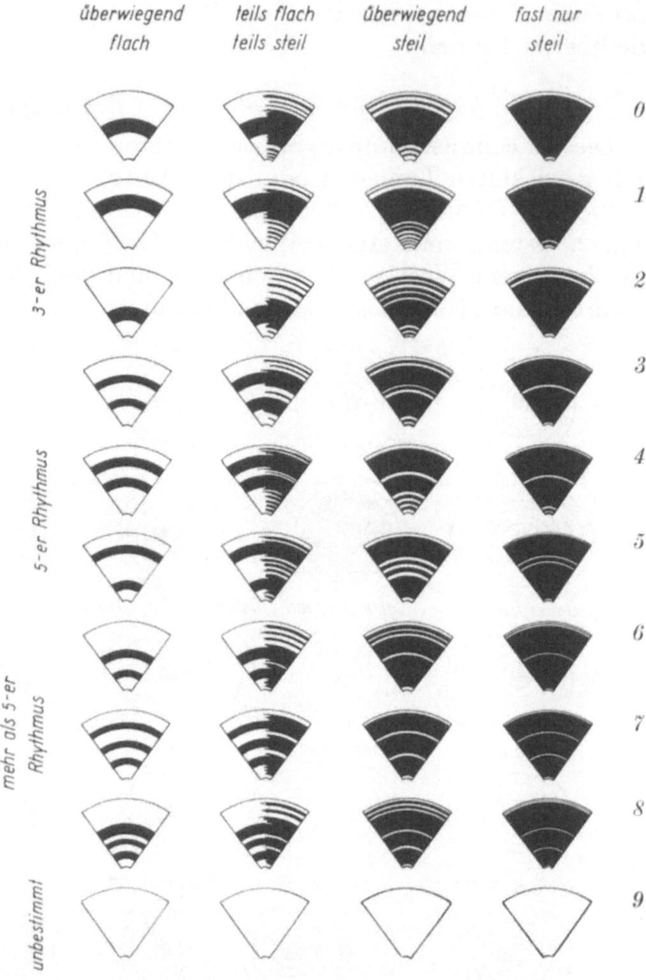

Abb. 29. Schematische Darstellung der Steigungsfolgen in einem Sektor des Osteonquerschnittes. Hell: flach und dunkel: steil gewickelte Lamellen. Überwiegend flache; teils überwiegend flach, teils überwiegend steil; überwiegend steil und fast nur steil gewickelte Lamellen; *0—2* verschiedene Formen des 3er-Rhythmus; *3—6* verschiedene Formen des 5er-Rhythmus; *7—8* verschiedene Formen des mehr als 5er-Rhythmus; *9* davon abweichende seltene Steigungsfolgen. (Die Ziffern geben die Schlüsselzahlen der Lochkarte an.) (KNESE und TITSCHAK, 1962; mit Erlaubnis der Akademischen Verlagsgesellschaft Leipzig)

nach der Lamellenzahl angegeben. Die Systematik der Steigungsfolge, des Wechsels von Lamellen mit verschiedenem Kollagenfaserverlauf bietet wegen der Vielfalt große Schwierigkeiten, da auch die Osteonwand in einander gegenüberliegenden Schnitten unterschiedlich gebaut sein kann (Abb. 29). Schließlich fällt auf, daß steil oder flach gewickelte Lamellen in Gruppen auftreten, so daß eine rhythmische Gliederung der Wand zustandekommt.

Für den seit langem gebrauchten Terminus „Haverssches System" hat BIEDERMANN (1914) das Wort Osteon eingeführt. Diese Bezeichnung wurde verschiedentlich kritisiert, da sie die Vorstellung von einer Baueinheit hervorruft. Das Wort steht seiner Bildung nach neben den rein oder überwiegend cellulär bestimmten Begriffen Neuron und Chondron sowie der Entwicklungs- und Funktionseinheit Nephron (KNESE et al., 1954). Osteone erscheinen als wohl abgrenzbare „individuelle" Einheiten nur in Querschnitten durch Skeletstücke, in Längsschnitten sind sie dagegen überhaupt nicht oder nur mit größter Schwierigkeit und vermutungsweise zu begrenzen. Zur Aufklärung des Osteonaufbaues wurden Osteone rekonstruiert (FILOGAMO, 1944/45; AMPRINO, 1948, Knochen der Hühnersehnen; BLECHSCHMIDT, 1948; KOLTZE, 1951; COHEN et al., 1958). Alle diese Rekonstruk-

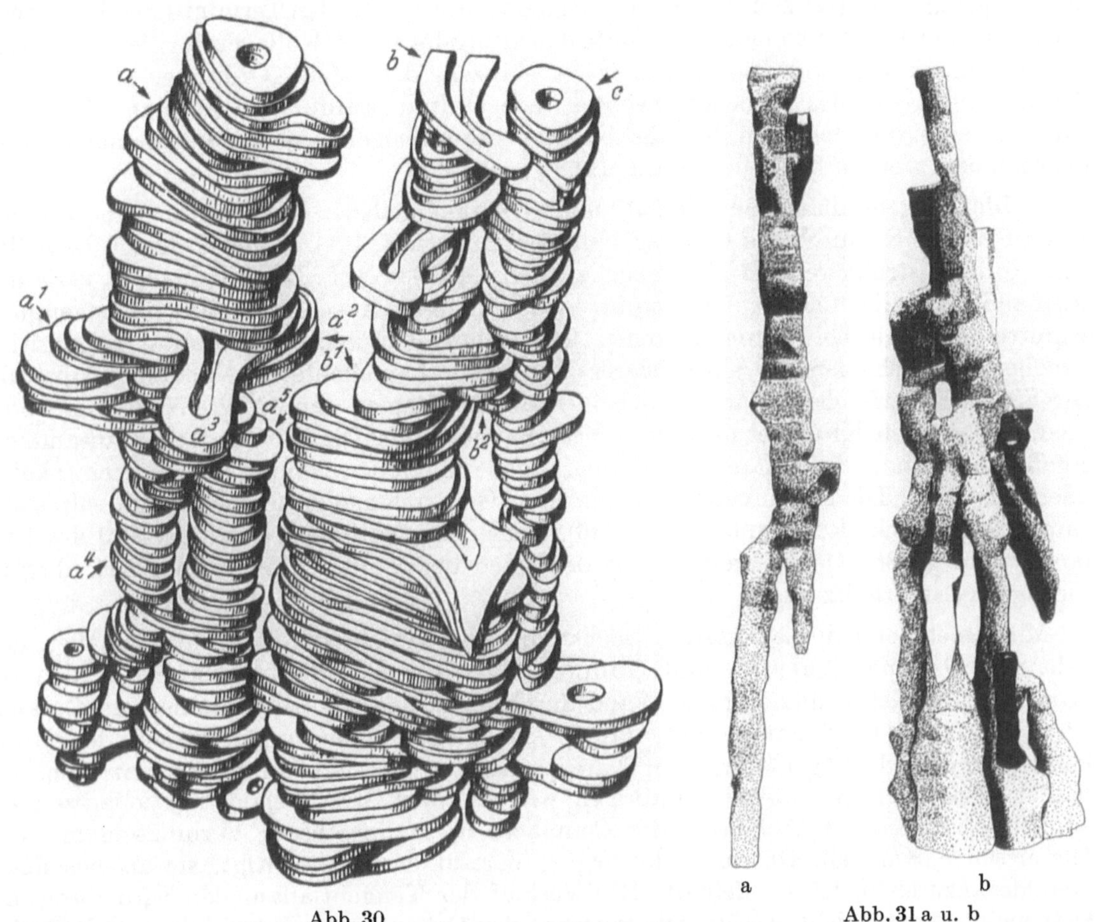

Abb. 30 Abb. 31 a u. b

Abb. 30. Mensch, 65 Jahre. Humerus Höhe der Tub. deltoidea. Graphische Rekonstruktion einer stark verflochtenen Osteongruppe. Das Osteon a zeigt bei a_1, a_2 und a_5 balkonartige Auskragungen bei a_3 eine Gefäßverbindung. Bei a_4 liegt eine Aufteilung in zwei getrennte Osteone vor. Die Osteone b und c sind in Höhe b_2 miteinander verbunden und dann wieder auf eine Strecke voneinander getrennt. Im unteren Teil stoßen die Osteongruppen aneinander. (FILOGAMO 1944/45; mit Erlaubnis des Verfassers und des Verlages Ulrico Hoepli, Milano)

Abb. 31 a u. b. Rekonstruktionen von Osteonen aus der Mitte des Femurschaftes vom Hunde. a Einfache Osteonenform mit spiraligem Verlauf (zwei Windungen auf 1,5 mm). Ein blind endendes Osteon in der Mitte des Modells. b Ein komplexes Osteon, dessen Querschnitte eine stark voneinander abweichende Gestalt aufweisen. Die horizontalen Flächen stellen Anastomosen mit anderen, nicht dargestellten Haversschen Systemen dar. Auf der rechten Seite ein blind endendes Osteon. (Umzeichnung nach COHEN und HARRIS, 1958)

tionen (Abb. 30) ergeben, daß ein Osteon als abgrenzbare Einheit nur von einer zu nächsten Gefäßverzweigung reicht. Im Bereich der Gefäßverbindungen ergeben sich sehr verwickelte Bilder. Die Stärke der Verzweigung wechselt, wobei die Abgänge der sog. Volkmannschen Kanäle (s. S. 368) unbeachtet bleiben können. Nach COHEN et al. (1958) durchziehen die Osteone beim Hunde die Compacta vom Periost zur Markhöhle hin in spiraligem Verlauf (Abb. 31). Die Außenform der Osteone kann stark wechseln und Absätze sowie Verbindungen zu den Schaltlamellen zeigen. Nach FILOGAMO (1946) bleibt der Faserverlauf in verschiedenen Strecken des Osteons gleich; nur bei 20% der untersuchten 200 Osteone wechselt die Fibrillenrichtung in benachbarten Schnitten stärker, aber nicht für alle Lamellen gleichartig.

Das Haverssche System oder Osteon ist demgemäß keine „individuelle" Baueinheit in der Form eines gleichmäßig gestalteten Zylinders; auch die Lamellen stellen keine begrenzten Hohlröhren dar, die wie Sperrholzplatten zum Haversschen System zusammengefügt sind (KNESE, VOGES und RITSCHL, 1954). Mit den Termini Lamelle, Osteon usw. beschreiben wir nur eine bestimmte Lagerungsform der Kollagenfibrillen mit ihrem Mantel organischer und anorganischer Substanzen, d.h. eine „Ordnungs"stufe in der Strukturhierarchie des Knochengewebes. Jede Ordnungsstufe wird mechanischen Aufgaben gerecht, die nicht von den darüber oder darunter gelegenen Ordnungsdimensionen übernommen werden können (KNESE, 1958b; s. S. 453).

2. Die Tangentiallamellen (Schalt- und Generallamellen). Die Ordnung der Haversschen Systeme ist durch das Gefäßsystem bestimmt (s. S. 401). Daneben treten Lamellen ohne direkte strukturelle Beziehungen zu den Gefäßen auf. Diese Lamellen verlaufen zueinander parallel und nehmen größere oder kleinere Abschnitte eines Knochenquerschnittes ein. Hierbei wurde zwischen Generallamellen und Schalt- oder Interstitiallamellen unterschieden. Da ein größerer Teil beider Lamellenformen annähernd parallel zur Knochenoberfläche verläuft und beide Lamellenformen ohne Abgrenzung ineinander übergehen, haben KNESE et al. (1954) diese Lamellen als Tangentiallamellen zusammengefaßt. Am Ende der Diaphyse nehmen solche Lamellen häufig den ganzen Skeletquerschnitt ein. Die sog. inneren oder äußeren Generallamellen umziehen nur selten das ganze Skeletstück (PETERSEN, 1930, 1935). Beide Formen haben an einem Teil des Umfanges ihre größte Mächtigkeit und laufen nach den Seiten hin in einer Art uhrglasförmiger Gestalt spitz aus.

Mit zunehmendem Lebensalter wächst die Zahl der in die Tangentiallamellen eingebauten Osteone (AMPRINO und GODINA, 1954; KNESE, 1958b). Häufig werden die Lamellen von Gefäßkanälen ohne Wand durchzogen, den sog. Volkmannschen Kanälen. W. J. SCHMIDT (1950) hat gezeigt, daß es sich hierbei nicht um perforierende Kanäle handelt, da die Kollagenfasern den Kanälen ausweichen und um sie herumziehen. Die Kanäle ohne eigene Wand sind im übrigen, wie vor allem Osteonrekonstruktionen zeigten, ein Bestandteil des Gefäßnetzes der Compacta in unmittelbarer Verbindung mit den Haversschen Kanälen. Ob ihr mehr querer Verlauf dazu berechtigt, sie als besondere Gebilde anzusehen, ist zweifelhaft. Der Verlauf der Tangentiallamellen wird durch die Osteoneinlagerung nicht gestört. Die zwischen den Osteonen liegenden Tangentiallamellen wurden als Schaltlamellen bezeichnet. Neben dieser Form von Schaltlamellen, die auf die Generallamellen zurückzuführen ist, wurden noch die Osteonfragmente als eine zweite Art beschrieben (KÖLLIKER, 1889).

γ) Die Struktur der Skeletelemente (Struktur 2. Ordnung)

Die Struktur der Skeletelemente des Menschen und der Wirbeltiere war Gegenstand z.T. sehr umfangreicher Untersuchungen (GEBHARDT, 1906; FOOTE, 1913; PETERSEN, 1927; DEMETER und MÁTYÁS, 1928; BOGDASCHEW, 1935; AMPRINO und GODINA, 1947; ERTELT, 1955). Diese Arbeiten haben trotz bedeutender Erweiterung unserer Kenntnisse verschiedene Fragen nicht eindeutig beantworten können, nämlich, ob es einen artspezifischen Aufbau der Skeletelemente gibt, ob die einzelnen Knochen eine typische Struktur aufweisen und in welcher Form die verschiedenen Strukturelemente verteilt sind. In allen untersuchten Skeletelementen waren Osteone unterschiedlicher Bauform und Tangentiallamellen vorhanden.

Der Untersucher steht bei Betrachtung eines Knochenschnittes, wobei nur ganze Querschnitte und nie Bruchteile gewählt werden sollten, vor einer Fülle von Bauelementen, die durch eine reine Betrachtung nicht in allen ihren Eigenheiten erfaßt werden können. KNESE et al. (1954) haben die Untersuchung infolge dessen „mechanisiert", indem sie jedes Osteon nach den oben gegebenen Merkmalen — Form und Steigungsfolge — in einem bestimmten Gebiet (einer Region) mit allen Eigenheiten registrierten und das Ergebnis der Erhebung auf Lochkarten (Hollerith) übernahmen. So wurde eine Art Bevölkerungsstatistik der Osteone ermöglicht. An der Sortiermaschine konnten Anzahl und Verteilung einer bestimmten Osteonquerschnittsform festgestellt werden. Da das Lochkartenverfahren die Prüfung einer unbegrenzten Anzahl von Kombinationen zuläßt, konnte das vorliegende Material von 47 690 Osteonquerschnitten unter sehr verschiedenartigen Gesichtspunkten untersucht werden. Das Ergebnis war, daß die Osteonverteilung die Funktion (im mathematischen Sinne) sehr verschiedenartiger Faktoren ist.

KNESE et al. (1954) kamen nach Untersuchung von Femur, Tibia, Fibula, Humerus, Radius und Ulna eines durch Unfall verstorbenen 43jährigen Mannes zunächst zum Schluß, daß eine bestimmte topographische Verteilung der Osteonsysteme vorliegt, die das einzelne Skeletstück kennzeichnet. Diese topographisch unterschiedliche Zusammenlagerung von Osteonen bezeichnen die Autoren als Struktur 2. Ordnung. Die Einteilung von PETERSEN (1927, 1930) wurde um diese Stufe erweitert; die übrigen Ordnungsstufen von PETERSEN mußten demzufolge um eine Stelle verrückt werden. Die Frage, ob die Osteonverteilung über das Skelet eine zufällige ist oder nicht, haben dann AUERBACH (1957) und KNESE und TITSCHAK (1962) aufgegriffen. Diese Autoren konnten nach Untersuchung einer Reihe von Individuen zeigen, daß ein Strukturmerkmal, z.B. die Osteonform, in einer bestimmten, statistisch formulierbaren Zahl vorliegt. Die Struktur 2. Ordnung ist keine zufällige, sondern eine ortsgemäße. Die Feststellung von VIRCHOW (1875): „Varium et mutabile semper femina, aber es könnte noch besser auf die Knochen angewendet werden", ist damit unzutreffend.

Die Anzahl der Osteonquerschnitte je Flächeneinheit des Knochenquerschnittes wechselt in den einzelnen Skeletstücken. Sie beträgt in einem proximalen Femurschnitt 1030 je cm^2, in einem mittleren 1120, im distalen 1020, im Humerus proximal 1120, in der Mitte 970, distal 1285, in Tibia, Fibula, Radius und Ulna etwas über 800 Osteone je cm^2 (KNESE et al., 1954). AUERBACH (1957) hat für die Tibia die Variation der Flächendichte untersucht und erhält für den gesamten Querschnitt 810 ± 240 Osteone je cm^2, das periphere subperiostale Drittel des Schnittes 950 ± 275, das mittlere 850 ± 315 und das zentrale marknahe Drittel 675 ± 285. Die Flächendichte der Osteonquerschnitte nimmt demgemäß vom Markraum zum Periost hin zu und zwar bei allen untersuchten Schnitten. Die Flächendichte der Osteone ist beim Wildschwein mit 3180 und beim Hausschwein mit 2430 wesentlich höher als beim Menschen. Die Gesamtzahl der Osteone beträgt in einem Schnitt durch die Mitte des Femur 5780, der Tibia 2381 und des Metacarpus beim Wildschwein 2784 und Hausschwein 2062.

Entsprechend der Änderung der Flächendichte der Osteone liegen kleinere Osteone mehr zum Periost hin, größere mehr marknahe, wenn auch nicht ausschließlich, da sich beachtliche Unterschiede zwischen den einzelnen Skeletstücken ergeben. In bestimmten Gebieten (Regionen; KNESE, RITSCHL und VOGES, 1954) sind annähernd gleich große Querschnitte anzutreffen, die fast nur aus Faserfilzen aufgebaut sind (Abb. 32). In anderen Regionen überwiegen Osteone mit steiler Wicklung (Abb. 33), wiederum in anderen in der äußeren Schnitthälfte steile, in der inneren flachgewickelte (Abb. 34). Mitunter ist der mittlere Teil eines Schnittes aus Osteonquerschnitten, der subperiostale und marknahe aus Tangentiallamellen (Generallamellen, s. S. 368) aufgebaut (Abb. 36 und 37). Besonders bei jüngeren Individuen kann die äußere Schnitthälfte nur periostale Kleinstosteone enthalten (Abb. 35). Vergleicht man das gleiche Skeletgebiet (Region) von Menschen verschiedenen Alters, so ergeben sich erhebliche Strukturdifferenzen. Als Beispiel wurde ein Femurschnitt herangezogen, der beim 18- und 25jährigen (Abb. 38) eine große Zahl von Tangentiallamellen, beim 43jährigen aber fast nur Osteone enthält (Abb. 39).

Die Steigungsfolge innerhalb eines Osteonquerschnittes hat Beziehungen zur Osteongröße (KNESE et al., 1954), aber auch zur Lage des Osteons im Skeletquerschnitt (KNESE und TITSCHAK, 1962). Bei kleineren Osteonen überwiegen flache, bei größeren steile Wicklungen. Daneben besteht eine Altersabhängigkeit. In höherem Alter nimmt der prozentuale Anteil der Osteone mit flacher Wicklung auf das Dreifache, solcher mit steiler etwa um ein Drittel zu. Die Faserfilze sinken auf ein Drittel ab. Schließlich ergeben sich, wie oben erwähnt, erhebliche topographische Differenzen in der Steigungsfolge.

KNESE, RITSCHL und VOGES (1954) und KNESE und TITSCHAK (1962) haben in Schemata

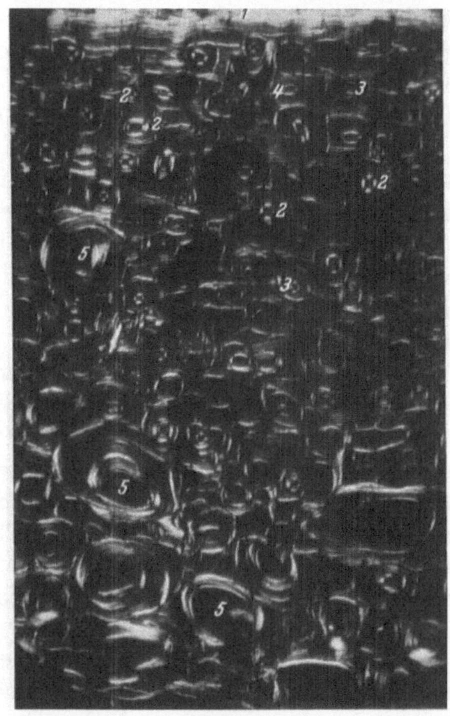

Abb. 32 Abb. 33

Abb. 32. Mann, 43 Jahre. Femur, proximales Viertel. Die ganze Querschnittsbreite besteht aus Osteonen, die von dem Zwischengewebe zum Teil sehr schlecht abgegrenzt sind. Das Zwischengewebe hat überwiegend strähnenartigen Charakter mit radiär und tangential verlaufenden Zügen. *1* Periphere Schicht mit Osteonen, die zum Teil eine undeutliche Lamellierung erkennen lassen; *2* Osteone mit wenig fortgeschrittener Lamellierung; *3* quere Gefäßverbindung zwischen weiteren und engeren längsverlaufenden Kanälen; *4* Osteon mit zentraler Lamellierung und peripherem Faserfilz; *5* Ansammlungen kleinster Faserfilzosteone; *6* ovales Osteon mit Faserfilzen und undeutlich abgegrenzten Lamellen; *7* reines Faserfilzosteon. (KNESE, RITSCHL und VOGES, 1954)

Abb. 33. Mann, 43 Jahre. Tibia proximales Drittel. *1* Periostale Tangentiallamellen, zum Teil mit wenig ausdifferenzierter Lamellierung. Vereinzelte tangentiale Streifen sind im peripheren Schnittdrittel zu erkennen. Hier liegen Osteone verschiedener Größe und mit verschiedener Lamellendifferenzierung. *2* Kleinstosteone mit angedeuteter Lamellierung; *3* ovales Osteon; *4* asymmetrisches Osteon. Die Osteone zeigen überwiegend steile Wicklung. *5* Lacunenosteone mit zum Teil sehr dicker Lamellenwand (KNESE, RITSCHL und VOGES, 1954)

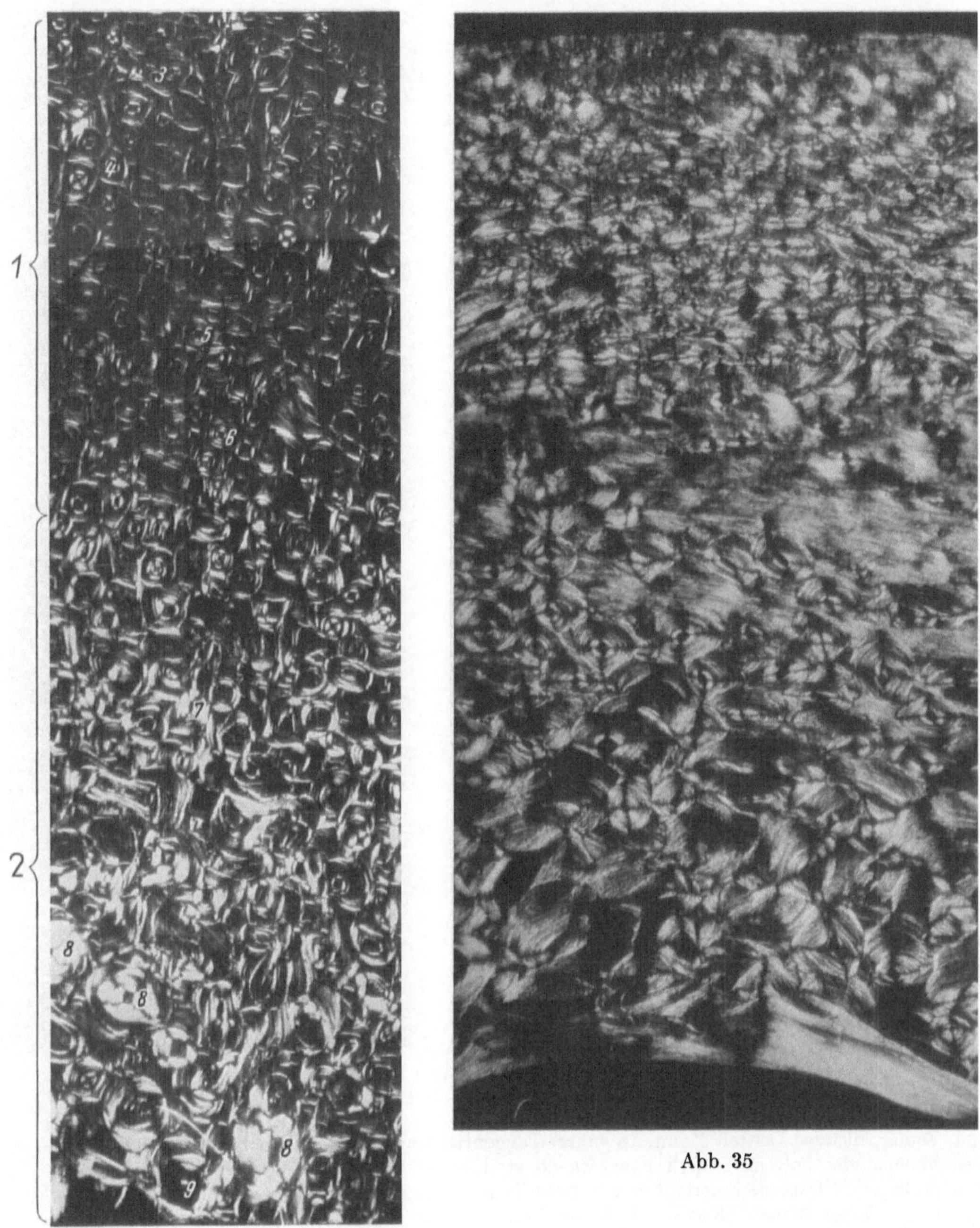

Abb. 34

Abb. 35

Abb. 34. Mann, 43 Jahre. Tibia distales Drittel. Der Schnitt zeigt eine Zweiteilung. Zone *1* Osteone mit ausdifferenzierten Lamellen und überwiegend steiler Wicklung. Zone *2* unregelmäßig geformte Osteone zentral von besonderer Größe mit überwiegend flacher Wicklung und eingestreuten Faserfilzen. Zwischen diesen Osteonen liegen recht kurze Streifen, die zum Teil strähnenartigen Charakter haben. *3* Querverbindung; *4* ovales Osteon; *5* rundes Osteon ohne Lamellierung; *6* rundes Osteon mit annähernd regelmäßiger Wicklung; *7* gepanzertes Osteon; *8* große Faserfilzosteone; *9* lacunärer Raum. (Knese, Ritschl und Voges, 1954)

Abb. 35. Mann, 25 Jahre. Femur, Grenze zwischen distalem und mittlerem Viertel, Vorderseite. Die inneren zwei Drittel des Schnittes sind aus Tangentiallamellen (teils als innere Generallamellen, teils als Schaltlamellen) aufgebaut. Das äußere Drittel enthält periostal aufgelagerte, in Reihen angeordnete Kleinstosteone. Polarisiertes Licht. Vergr. 35fach. (Knese, 1956b; mit Erlaubnis des Verlages F. K. Schattauer, Stuttgart)

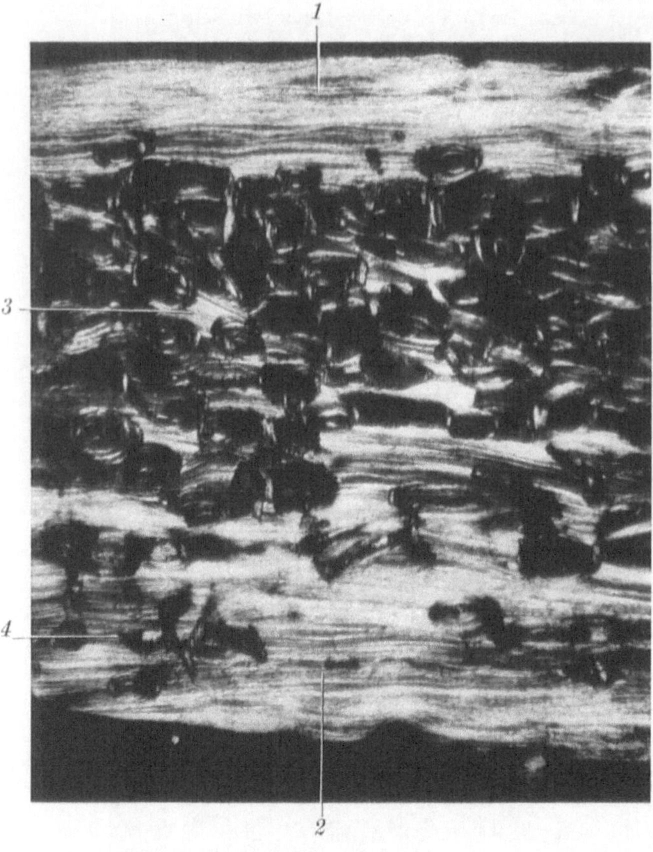

Abb. 36

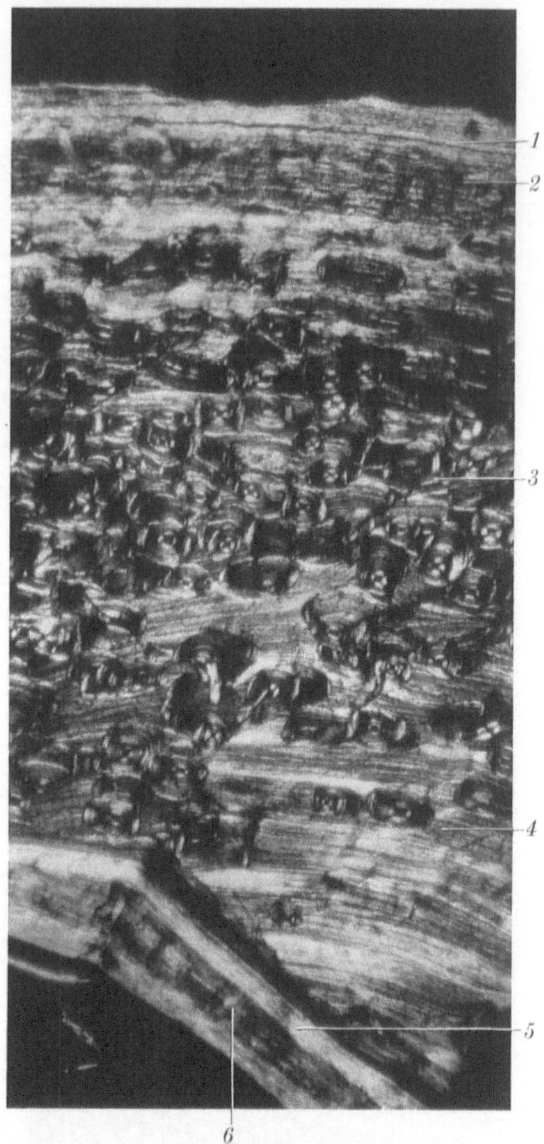

Abb. 37

Abb. 36. Femur, distales Drittel. Mann, 18 Jahre. Tangentiallamellen als äußere (*1*) und innere (*2*) Generallamellen voneinander getrennt durch überwiegend steil gewickelte Osteone, zwischen denen sog. Schaltlamellen (*3*) liegen. *4* Osteone innerhalb der inneren Tangentiallamellen mit zum Teil unvollständiger Wand. Vergr. 35fach. (KNESE, 1958; mit Erlaubnis des Thieme-Verlages, Stuttgart)

Abb. 37. Tibia distales Viertel, Faceis lateralis. Mann, 25 Jahre. In die äußeren Tangentiallamellen (*1*) ist eine Schicht längs verlaufender Gefäßkanäle (*2*) eingebaut, die fast durchweg bereits eine eigene Wand besitzen. Die Mitte des Schnittes (*3*) wird von annähernd gleich großen Osteonen mit dem Steigungswechsel flach-steil-flach eingenommen; *4* Packung von Tangentiallamellen mit wechselnd großen Osteonen, die zum Teil nur eine unvollständige Wand besitzen; *5* innerste Schicht von Tangentiallamellen mit Versetzung gegenüber der vorigen Schicht; *6* Schicht mit längs verlaufenden Gefäßen, die nur eine unvollständige eigene Wand aufweisen. Vergr. 35fach. (KNESE, 1958; mit Erlaubnis des Thieme-Verlages, Stuttgart)

Abb. 38. Femur, Mitte. Vorderwand. Mann, 18 Jahre. Die ganze Querschnittsbreite besteht aus Tangentiallamellen, in die gleichmäßig verteilt Osteone eingelassen sind. *1* Längs verlaufende Gefäßkanäle, die noch keine eigene Wand oder nur Wandteile besitzen; *2* Osteon mit flach gewickelter Wand; *3* überwiegend steil gewickeltes Osteon; *4* unregelmäßig geformtes Osteon; *5* Osteon mit unvollständiger Wand; *6* Schrägschnitte durch Gefäßkanäle; *7* gepanzertes Osteon; *8* Osteone verschiedener Größe, die zum Teil unmittelbar aneinanderstoßen. Vergr. 35fach. (KNESE, 1958; mit Erlaubnis des Thieme-Verlages, Stuttgart)

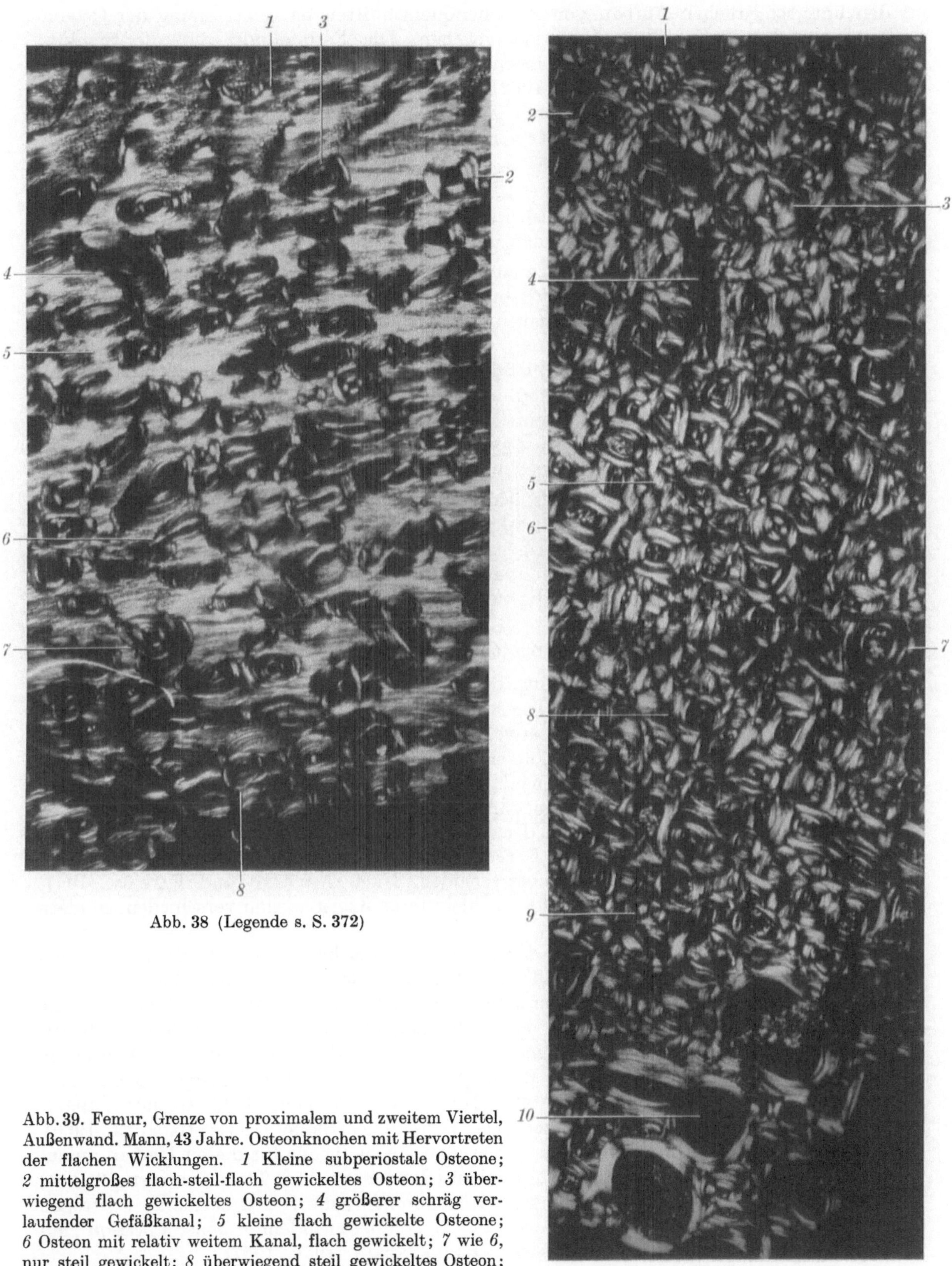

Abb. 38 (Legende s. S. 372)

Abb. 39. Femur, Grenze von proximalem und zweitem Viertel, Außenwand. Mann, 43 Jahre. Osteonknochen mit Hervortreten der flachen Wicklungen. *1* Kleine subperiostale Osteone; *2* mittelgroßes flach-steil-flach gewickeltes Osteon; *3* überwiegend flach gewickeltes Osteon; *4* größerer schräg verlaufender Gefäßkanal; *5* kleine flach gewickelte Osteone; *6* Osteon mit relativ weitem Kanal, flach gewickelt; *7* wie *6*, nur steil gewickelt; *8* überwiegend steil gewickeltes Osteon; *9* regelmäßiges Osteon; *10* Spongiosamaschen. Vergr. 35fach. (KNESE, 1958; mit Erlaubnis des Thieme-Verlages, Stuttgart)

Abb. 39

den unterschiedlichen Aufbau von Knochenquerschnitten nach Verteilung der Osteonformen und des Faserverlaufes wiedergegeben. Die Feststellung, daß die Struktur 2. Ordnung an den Kanten und Flächen eines Skeletstückes unterschiedlich ist (Auerbach, 1957; Knese und Titschka, 1962), läßt einen Zusammenhang zwischen Feinbau und Leistung vermuten; die letzteren Autoren haben Bruchspannung und Steigungsfolge der gleichen Region miteinander verglichen (vgl. Knese, 1958b, s. S. 463).

Durch die Verwendung der Loch-(Hollerith)karte war es möglich, ein „Urmaterial“ zu schaffen, das alle Merkmale eines Osteonquerschnittes enthält. Die Auswertung dieses Urmaterials unter verschiedenen Gesichtspunkten ergab, daß folgende Faktoren für die Struktur der Skeletelemente von Bedeutung sind:

1. Artspezifische Merkmale liegen in der Flächendichte und der Osteongröße vor.
2. Altersspezifische Merkmale spiegeln sich in Osteongröße und Steigungsfolge wider.
3. Skeletspezifische Merkmale ergeben sich aus der örtlich unterschiedlichen Strukturverteilung und der Steigungsfolge.
4. Die Osteonverteilung ist schließlich ein Abbild der Baugeschichte (s. S. 375); dieser Schluß wurde durch die Feststellung nahegelegt, daß eine Reihe von Verteilungsprinzipien der Strukturen sowohl beim Menschen als auch bei den Schweinen auftritt.

Die Struktur 2. Ordnung des Skeletes ist ungewöhnlich verwickelt und hängt von einer ganzen Reihe von Faktoren ab. Die wiedergegebenen Erhebungen haben nur die Ordnung der Kollagenfibrillen berücksichtigt. Bei Untersuchung anderer Gewebekomponenten, die vom Kollagen abhängig sind, treten weitere die Ordnung bestimmende Faktoren hinzu, z.B. bei der Mineralablagerung. Es ist daher nicht verwunderlich, daß für viele Erscheinungen der Mineralverteilung, aber auch für manche Erhebungen über die ^{45}Ca-Ablagerung bisher keine befriedigende Deutung gefunden wurde.

c) Die Baugeschichte des Knochens

Im Hinblick auf die Entwicklung der reifen Knochenstruktur, den sog. Osteonknochen, wird die Auffassung von Tomes und de Morgan (1853) als über jede Kritik erhabener Bestand unseres Wissens angesehen. Der primäre Knochen wird durch einen sekundären ersetzt; durch Resorption entstehen Lacunen, die zu Osteonen aufgefüllt werden. Da aber unter dem Periost ebenfalls Osteone gebildet werden, die sog. periostalen Kleinstosteone, unterschieden einige Autoren (Gross, 1934; Lacroix, 1960) zwischen primären und sekundären Osteonen. Die sekundären Osteone setzen einen Resorptionsprozeß voraus. Beide Osteonformen lassen sich bei manchen Species, z.B. dem Schwein (Gross 1934), nicht voneinander unterscheiden. Nach Amprino und Bairati (1947) sind primärer und sekundärer Knochen nicht in ihrer Konstruktion verschieden, sondern nur nach dem Ort der Bildung.

Die im Lichtmikroskop während der Entwicklung zu beobachtenden Strukturformen erscheinen so verschiedenartig, daß zunächst an einen genetischen Zusammenhang zwischen ihnen nicht gedacht werden kann (v. Ebner, 1875; Gebhardt, 1901). Das reife Knochengewebe ist aber nicht nur aus vollständigen „Osteonen“, sondern auch aus „Bruchstücken“ aufgebaut, so daß eine sog. Breccie vorliegt. Resorption und Apposition als gekoppelte Vorgänge sollen die Mosaikstruktur des Knochens erzeugen (Kölliker, 1889; Gebhardt, 1902; Petersen, 1930; Benoit und Clavert, 1943; Lacroix, 1951); beide Vorgänge zeigen eine gesetzmäßige Verteilung (Brash, 1934; Lacroix, 1960). Bisher gelang es allerdings nicht, den steuernden Mechanismus für diesen Umbau aufzudecken. Neben dem sog. funktionellen Umbau (Petersen, 1930; Tischendorff, 1952/54) wird neuerlich eine hormonelle Kontrolle angenommen; die Sexualhormone, Oestrogen und Androgen, werden als aufbauende, die Nebennierenrindenhormone, Cortison und Hydrocortison, als abbauende angesehen (Reifenstein, 1956, 1957).

v. Ebner (1875) hatte die Forderung erhoben, die Baugeschichte des Knochens aus dem geweblichen Endzustand abzulesen und zwar an Hand der Kittlinien, die als

Resorptions- und Appositionslinien auftreten. Das Musterbeispiel für Anwendung dieser Methode haben PETERSEN und BURKHARDT (1928) bei Untersuchung eines 6jährigen Kindes gegeben.

Die Art des Einbaues von Radioisotopen, vor allem ^{45}Ca, wurde als Bestätigung des Aufbaues von sekundären Osteonen aufgefaßt (LACROIX, 1960; VINCENT 1954; PONLOT, 1960; MARSHALL et al., 1959; MARSHALL, 1960). Diese Untersuchungen führten aber auch zur Neubeschreibung der periostalen Appositionsformen, nämlich der Kleinstosteone und Tangentiallamellen (LEA und PONLOT, 1958; PONLOT, 1960). Ein Teil der Beobachtungen über die Ablagerung von ^{45}Ca ist schwer zu deuten. Es wurden daher sehr verschiedenartige Vorgänge angenommen, die zu einem Einbau von ^{45}Ca führen, nämlich eine Neue ablagerung von Kristallen, ein Kristallwachstum, kurz- oder langfristiger Austausch, ein-Rekristallisation und eine sog. Neuverteilung (redistribution). Gute Kenner der Materie (NEUMAN, BRONNER, COMAR alle bei MARSHALL, 1960) halten die zur Beschreibung der beobachteten Phänomene entwickelte Terminologie für verwirrend, meinen aber, diese Verwirrung sei besser als ein Nichtwissen. Befunde über ^{45}Ca-Ablagerung bedürfen im Hinblick auf begleitende histologische Vorgänge entsprechender ergänzender Untersuchungen. So wurden einige Untersucher durch ihre Befunde über ^{45}Ca-Ablagerungen zu rein morphologischen Untersuchungen veranlaßt (COHEN et al., 1958; JEE und ARNOLD, 1960).

Bedenken gegen die Lehre einer fortlaufenden Resorption und Apposition wurden seit langem geäußert (Literatur bei KNESE und TITSCHAK, 1962). Vor allem fielen verschiedentlich Reste älteren geflechtartigen Knochens zwischen Osteonen auf (TOMES und DE MORGAN, 1853; KÖLLIKER, 1898; GEBHARDT, 1902; WEIDENREICH, 1923, 1930; DEMETER und MÁTYÁS, 1928; SCHAFFER, 1933; AMPRINO, 1937). Es wurde angenommen, daß diese Reste geflechtartigen Knochens erst bei einem erneuten Resorptionsvorgang, der das soeben neugebildete Osteon und nun auch den geflechtartigen Knochen umfaßt, abgebaut werden (GEGENBAUR, 1864, 1867; KÖLLIKER, 1889; AMPRINO, 1937; AMPRINO und GODINA, 1947; LACROIX, 1949).

Die Ausbildung der Lamellen, d.h. die Schärfe ihrer Abgrenzung, ist im gleichen Schnitt und innerhalb eines Osteones sehr unterschiedlich (v. EBNER, 1875; KASSOWITZ, 1879; KÖLLIKER, 1899; MEYBURG, 1901). KAPSAMER (1897) meinte, die Lamellierung beruhe auf einer Differenzierung des Knochengewebes, die mit der Knochenbildung nicht gleichzeitig erfolgt, sondern erst später einsetzt. Weiterhin wurde ein Differenzierungsgefälle vom Markraum zum Periost hin beobachtet (GEBHARDT, 1902; MEYBURG, 1904; DEMETER und MÁTYÁS, 1928; JAFFÉ, 1929; AMPRINO, 1937; KOLTZE, 1951; COHEN et al., 1958). Eine Untersuchung der Verteilung der Osteone nach Größe und Wicklungsform hat diese Beobachtungen bestätigt (KNESE et al., 1954; AUERBACH, 1957; KNESE und TITSCHAK, 1962): Kleinere Osteone liegen mehr zum Periost, größere mehr zum Markraum hin; die Lamellendifferenzierung ist in Nähe der Markhöhle weiter vorangeschritten als subperiostal, die inneren Lamellen eines Osteons jenseits der ersten flachen (s. S. 378) sind besser differenziert als die äußeren. Damit liegt eine Fülle von Befunden vor, die sich schwer mit der Lehre von einer wechselweisen Resorption und Apposition vereinen läßt.

Für eine gerechte Würdigung der Auffassung von TOMES und DE MORGAN (1853) ist zu berücksichtigen, daß den Autoren der Aufbau des Knochengewebes aus Kollagenfasern, Kristallen und weiteren Substanzen unbekannt war. Den Verfassern erschien das Knochengewebe als eine homogene oder granuläre Substanz. Sie sahen Veränderungen der Struktur, die sie nur als Neubildung nach Verschwinden der alten Strukturen erklären konnten. Sie haben demgemäß die Baugeschichte des Knochens aus der Dimension der 2. oder 3. Ordnung beurteilt.

Die oben referierten Befunde über die Komponenten des Knochengewebes zeigen, daß am Ende der Faserentwicklung ein schwerlösliches oder unlösliches Kollagen steht. Der Stoffwechsel des ausgereiften Kollagens ist gering oder gleich Null (PERRONE und SLACK, 1951; NEUBERGER und SLACK, 1953; SLACK, 1953; NEUBERGER, 1955; ROBERTSON, 1952;

Thompson und Ballon 1956). Diese mit Hilfe von Radioisotopen erhobenen Befunde stimmen gut mit den elektronenmikroskopischen Beobachtungen über die Entwicklung der Kollagenfibrille überein. Dem Kollagen kommt eine zentrale Stellung bei der Mineralisation zu. Hierbei erweist es sich als ein „bleibendes" Element. Die angenommene Resorption würde aber einen fortlaufenden Abbau und Neuaufbau des Kollagens erfordern, für den bisher keine Anhaltspunkte vorliegen.

Diese Feststellungen gelten für die regelrechte, sog. normale Entwicklung. Im Gefolge von Traumen einschließlich experimentell gesetzter Läsionen tritt ein Umbau auf, der auch in der histologisch faßbaren Struktur zum Ausdruck kommt (Knese, 1956b). Bei der Heilung von derartigen Defekten treten Vorgänge auf, die nicht mit der regelrechten Entwicklung gleichzusetzen sind (Murray, 1936; Knese, 1959a, 1960). Beobachtungen beim Defektschluß können daher nur mit Vorsicht oder überhaupt nicht auf die regelrechte Entwicklung übertragen werden.

Die vorliegenden Beobachtungen über die „Molekularbiologie" der Komponenten des Knochengewebes und das Verteilungsprinzip der Strukturen innerhalb des Skeletstückes veranlaßten Knese und Titschak (1962), die entscheidenden Vorgänge der Histogenese des Knochengewebes in der Dimension der Ultrastruktur (5. und 6. Ordnung) zu suchen. Der Anschein eines grundsätzlichen Strukturwandels entsteht dann als Äquivalent in den Strukturen 4.—1. Ordnung.

Die Baugeschichte des Knochens wurde bisher von den Beobachtungen im lichtmikroskopischen Bereiche her erörtert. Knese und Titschak (1962) und Knese und v. Harnack (1962) haben demgegenüber den Versuch unternommen, auch die Ultrastruktur zu berücksichtigen. Auf diesem unterschiedlichen Ansatzpunkt beruht im wesentlichen die Diskussion zwischen Amprino (1963) und Knese (1963b). Amprino (1963) sieht weiterhin den Umbau als einzigen Weg zur Entstehung der Knochenstrukturen, voran der Osteone, an. Knese (1963b) weist einmal darauf hin, daß eine größere Zahl von älteren Befunden (vgl. Knese und Titschak, 1962) mit diesen Vorstellungen nicht vereinbar ist. Zum anderen sei der Versuch unternommen worden, die neueren Kenntnisse von der Ultrastruktur und Molekularbiologie der Komponenten des Knochengewebes im Hinblick auf die Baugeschichte des Knochens auszuwerten. Den bisher angenommenen Formen der Entstehung von Osteonen (s.u.) wird ein weiterer Bildungsmechanismus hinzugefügt. Leider fehlt noch eine Diskussion, die neben der Ultrastruktur auch die Befunde mit den Tetracyclinmarkierungen (s.u.) berücksichtigt.

Eine Diskussion aller Vorgänge, die zur Bildung des Skeletstückes führen, steht noch aus, wie die Untersuchungen von Zawisch (1929) über die Entwicklung des Femur, von Leblond et al. (1950) über Einverleibung enchondralen Knochens als Trichter in die Diaphyse, von Pratt (1959) über die Strukturentwicklung im Rattenfemur und die mannigfachen Untersuchungen über das Längenwachstum zeigen. Untersuchungen über die Strukturentwicklung, voran der Osteonbildung, haben sich bisher auf Knochenquerschnitte beschränkt, da nur hier die Osteonstruktur deutlich erkennbar ist.

Eine ausführliche Untersuchung der Querschnittsentwicklung der großen Knochen in der Fetalzeit liegt von Bahling (1958) vor, die den Ort der Apposition, die Verteilung der Knochenbälkchen und die Entstehung der Querschnittsform beschrieb. Bahling hat die Knochenbildung auch quantitativ verfolgt und in Wachstumskurven dargestellt.

Knese und Titschak (1962) haben, gestützt auf eigenes Material und dasjenige von Demeter und Mátyás (1928), die postnatale Zunahme der Osteone in einem mittleren Femurschnitt verfolgt (Abb. 40). Die Anzahl der Osteone beträgt beim Neugeborenen 465, im 5. Jahr 927, im 10. Jahr 1840, im 15. Jahr 2820, im 20. Jahr 3750, im 30. Jahr 5200 und im 40. Jahr 5780, d.h. von der Geburt bis zum 40. Jahr hat sich die Osteonzahl um das 12,5fache vermehrt. Die Querschnittsfläche ist im gleichen Zeitraum von 0,23 auf 5,0 cm^2 angewachsen. Die Autoren haben nun an Hand der bisher bekannten Tatsachen über die Reifung der Gewebekomponenten, besonders des Kollagens, errechnet, daß 43% der Querschnittsfläche des Femur eines 40jährigen auf Apposition und 57% auf die Reifung der Komponenten, den Zuwachs, zurückzuführen sind.

Die postnatale Apposition von Knochengewebe erfolgt in der Form der periostalen Kleinstosteone und Tangentiallamellen. Diese Kleinstosteone sind seit langem bekannt

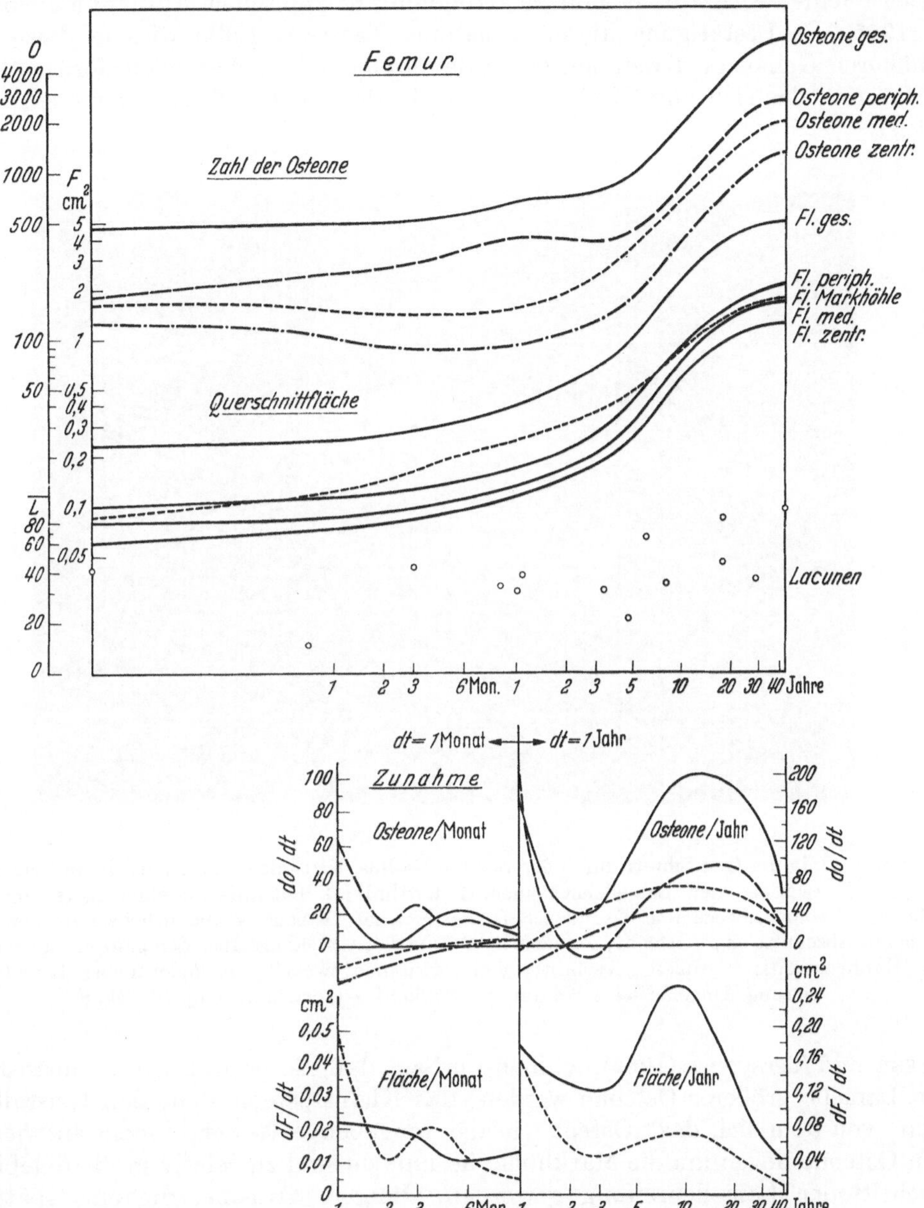

Abb. 40. Darstellung der Osteonvermehrung und des Flächenwachstums eines mittleren Femurquerschnittes von der Geburt bis zum 43. Jahr. Aufteilung beider auch für die Querschnittsbreiten. Entwicklung des entsprechenden Markhöhlenquerschnittes. Angabe der absoluten Anzahl der Lacunen. Unterer Teil: Differenzenquotient nach der Zeit für Osteon- und Flächenzunahme: Im ersten Lebensjahr $dt = 1$ Monat, dann $dt = 1$ Jahr. (Aus: KNESE und TITSCHAK, 1962; mit Erlaubnis der Akademischen Verlagsgesellschaft Leipzig)

(v. EBNER, 1875; AEBY, 1876; MEYBURG, 1904; DEMETER und MÁTYÁS, 1928; GROSS, 1934; KNESE, 1956a; LEA und PONLOT, 1958). Ihre Wand erscheint im polarisierten Licht schwach doppelbrechend und entspricht in der Struktur annähernd den sog. Faserfilzen. Eine gleichartige Struktur läßt die unmittelbar um den Haversschen Kanal gelegene innere flache Lamelle sehr vieler Osteone erkennen. Der abweichende Aufbau dieser

Lamelle wurde immer wieder betont (TOMES und DE MORGAN ,1853; KÖLLIKER, 1889; MATSCHINSKY, 1892; GEBHARDT, 1906; W. J. SCHMIDT, 1933; DALLEMAGNE und MELON, 1945; RUTH, 1947; AMPRINO und ENGSTRÖM, 1952; KNESE, VOGES und RITSCHL, 1954). KNESE (1956a, 1958b) sprach die Vermutung aus, daß dieser Lamelle die Ausreifung der Fasern fehle; er findet in den elektronenmikroskopischen Aufnahmen von FRANK et al. (1955) die Bestätigung dieser Annahme. TANAKA (1961) wies in dieser Lamelle einen höheren Gehalt an Kristallen als in den anderen Lamellen nach, ferner ein organisches Material, das sich vom Kollagen unterscheidet, dessen Natur aber noch nicht aufgeklärt ist.

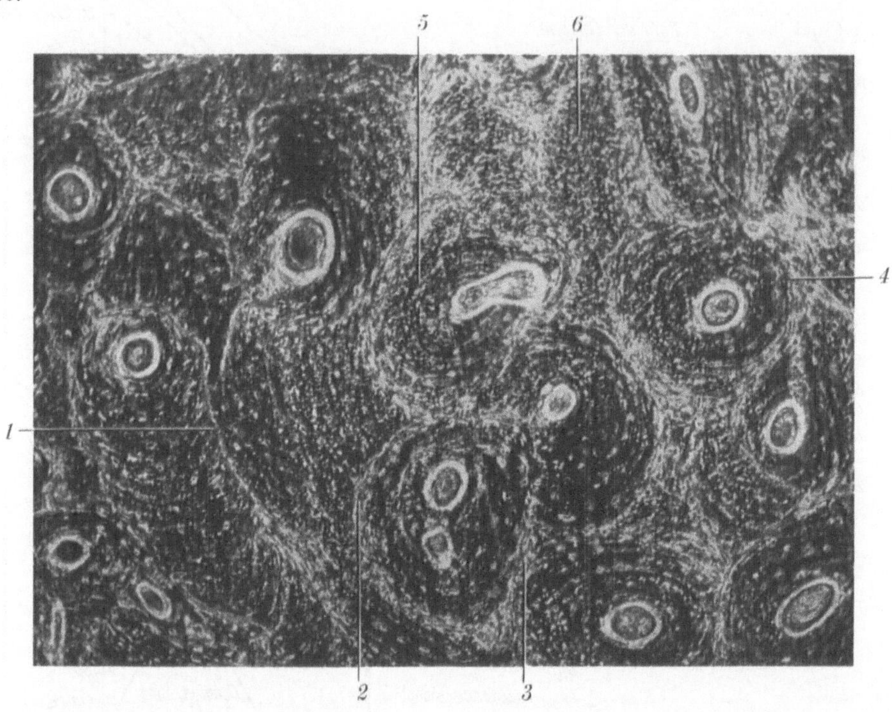

Abb. 41. Mann, 43 Jahre. Querschnitt durch den rechten Radius. Kittlinie und undeutlich lamellär gegliedertes Zwischengewebe zwischen den Lamellensystemen. *1* Kittlinie; *2* Kittlinie an einer Seite eines Osteons; *3* Zwischengewebe an der gegenüberliegenden Seite des gleichen Osteons; *4* undeutliche Lamellenbegrenzung im peripheren Abschnitt eines Osteons; *5* undeutliche Lamellenausbildung über den ganzen Querschnitt eines Osteons (Hantelosteon); *6* größere Abschnitte von „Zwischengewebe" mit undeutlicher Lamellendifferenzierung. Ungefärbtes Präparat, Phasenkontrastverfahren, Obj. 10, Ok. 8

KNESE und TITSCHAK (1962) nehmen nun an, daß die periostalen Kleinstosteone zur inneren Lamelle größerer Osteone werden; das Kleinstosteon stellt den Kristallisationskern dar, von dem sich das „Osteon" in das umgebende Gewebe hinein entwickelt. Die ältesten Osteone liegen um die Markhöhle herum, sie sind zu relativ großen Gebilden mit fortgeschrittener Lamellenreifung geworden. Jüngere Osteone, die erst später durch Apposition entstehen, liegen mehr dem Periost zu, sind kleiner, ihre Lamellen sind weniger scharf begrenzt. Die Autoren verfolgten im einzelnen quantitativ die Größe der Appositionsrate und die Anzahl der Osteone je Flächeneinheit und kommen zu dem Schluß, daß durch Apposition von periostalen Kleinstosteonen und deren Wachstum die vielfach beschriebene Verteilung der Strukturen über den Querschnitt im Hinblick auf die Osteongröße, die Lamellenreifung usw. entsteht.

Als Folge des zentrifugalen Osteonwachstums vom Haversschen Kanal aus entstehen dann bei Berührung zweier Systeme die Kittlinien, die in Marknähe gut, subperiostal weniger deutlich ausgebildet sind oder gar fehlen (Abb. 41). v. EBNER (1875) hatte bereits gefunden, daß nur beim Erwachsenen, d.h. bei voll ausgereiften Osteonen, Kittlinien vorhanden sind. W. J. SCHMIDT (1959) erklärt die Erscheinung der Kittlinien in gewöhnlichen Präparaten dadurch, daß die aneinander stoßenden doppelbrechenden Elemente, Kollagenfasern und Kristalle, zweier Lamellensysteme eine unterschiedliche räumliche Orientierung haben. Diese Ausführungen von W. J. SCHMIDT (1959) bestätigen die von KNESE und TITSCHAK (1962) vertretene Auffassung über die Entstehung der Kittlinien.

Nach sehr verschiedenen, auch autoradiographischen Beobachtungen, ist nicht zu bezweifeln, daß Osteone weiterhin durch Ausfüllung größerer Räume, der Haversschen Lacunen, entstehen. Hierbei kann die Frage der Bildung dieser Lacunen zunächst außer acht bleiben. Zur Errechnung der Anzahl der auf diesem Wege entstandenen Osteone haben KNESE und TITSCHAK (1962) festgestellt, wie groß die Zahl der Osteone ohne innere abweichend gebaute Lamelle ist. Bereits TOMES und DE MORGAN (1853) hatten bemerkt, daß diese Lamelle „fast" stets vorhanden ist. Nach Erhebungen an sehr unterschiedlichem Material (KNESE et al. 1954; AUERBACH 1957; KNESE und TITSCHAK 1962) fehlt die innere Lamelle etwa 4—5 % aller Osteone. Daraus wurde geschlossen, daß durch Ausfüllung von Lacunen nur etwa 5—10 % der Haversschen Systeme entstehen, die restlichen aber auf anderem Wege. Obwohl keine Zahlen über das Verhältnis von durch Isotopen markierten und nicht markierten Haversschen Systemen bekannt sind, ist aus Übersichtsbildern der Literatur ebenfalls ein Verhältnis von 1:10 zu erschließen.

Recht unklar ist noch, auf welchem Wege ein „Ersatz" der Tangentiallamellen durch Osteone vor sich geht, wie er verschiedentlich beschrieben wurde (s. S. 361, AMPRINO und GODINA 1954).

Vermutlich sind damit vier Wege der Osteonbildung zu unterscheiden (KNESE und TITSCHAK, 1962; KNESE, 1963b): 1. Einengung von überwiegend in der Fetalzeit gebildeten intertrabeculären Spalten; 2. zentrifugales Wachstum periostaler Kleinstosteone; 3. Ersatz von Tangentiallamellen; 4. Ausfüllung von Lacunen verschiedener Entstehungsform.

Die Frage der Baugeschichte des Knochengewebes wurde neuerlich auch mit Hilfe der Tetracyclinmarkierung untersucht. Die Tetracycline (vgl. JOHNSON, 1964) konnten von MILCH, RALL und TOBIE (1957) auch als fluorescierende Ablagerung im Knochengewebe nachgewiesen werden. Von den vielen darauffolgenden Untersuchungen können wir hier nur auf einige eingehen. Die „Tetracyclin-Physiologie" haben FROST et al. (1961) diskutiert. Auf Grund der Markierung der osteoiden Säume hat FROST (Übersichten: 1963a, 1963b, 1964, 1966) mathematische Modelle für die Dynamik des Knochenumbaues entwickelt. Hierbei wird die Knochenbildungsrate, die Resorptionsrate und das Skeletgleichgewicht (Skeletal balance $BSK = R_f - R_r$) beschrieben. Diese Umbaudynamik wird im Hinblick u.a. auf die Osteoporose, Osteomalacie und die Alterung verfolgt. Gesteuert wird der Umbau durch eine angenommene, derzeit noch hypothetische Code-Dynamik im Sinne des Gen-Codes. Der Gen-Code wird in einer ebenfalls hypothetische Mesenchymzelle realisiert. Daraus resultiert am einzelnen Skeletort die relative Anzahl von Osteoclasten und Osteoblasten sowie die jeweilige individuelle Aktivität dieser Zellen. Die Aktivierung führt erst zur Bildung einer Resorptionshöhle, dann zu einem osteoiden Saum. Von besonderem Interesse ist, daß FROST (1963c) nach 9 Jahren und SEDLIN und FROST (1963a) nach 11 Jahren noch eine Tetracyclinmarkierung nachweisen konnten. Weiterhin haben SEDLIN und FROST (1963b) eine biologische Halbwertzeit von Osteonen bis zu 17,1 Jahren errechnet.

Die Markierung von Osteonen durch Tetracycline haben AMPRINO und MAROTTI (1964) bei Hunden von 2—36 Monaten (3,8—28 kg) mit Tötung 7 Tage nach Applikation untersucht. Die Zahl der jeweils markierten Osteone nimmt mit dem Lebensalter ab und ist in den sich entsprechenden Skeletstücken beider Körperseiten sehr ähnlich. Die Autoren sehen in dieser Beobachtung eine Bestätigung der Auffassung von KNESE et al. (1954) und BAHLING (1958), daß innerhalb der Skeletstücke die Osteonverteilung topographischen und nicht statistischen Prinzipien folgt, d.h. daß eine spezifische Struktur zweiter Ordnung vorhanden ist. In diesem Zusammenhang sind die Befunde von MAROTTI und MAROTTI (1966) und MAROTTI (1968) über die Osteonmarkierung bei operativ ruhig gestellten Extremitäten zu nennen. Die Markierung ist nicht abhängig von mechanischer Beanspruchung und ist auf der ruhig gestellten Seite der bewegten praktisch gleich. Amprino und Marotti (1964) fanden neben der Osteonmarkierung eine periostale Ablagerung. Die Menge des markierten Knochens nimmt von der Schaftmitte zur Metaphyse hin zu und dann zur Epiphyse ab. Dabei verhalten sich die proximalen und distalen Teile desselben Skeletstückes etwas unterschiedlich. In der 5. Rippe ist die Markierung am Sternalende am höchsten, nimmt zur Mitte der Rippenlänge ab und zum Köpfchen hin wieder zu. Die Tetracyclinablagerungen sind jenen der Radioisotopen sehr ähnlich. Weiterhin ist die Stabilität des Knochengewebes in Femur und Humerus größer als z.B. in der Ulna.

d) Die Riesenzellen (Chondro- und Osteoclasten)

Bei einer Darstellung der Knochenstruktur sind auch die sog. Osteoclasten zu erörtern, da ihnen von verschiedenen Autoren eine bedeutsame Rolle im Rahmen der Strukturentwicklung zugesprochen wird. Kölliker (1872, 1873) hat für die Riesenzellen von sehr unterschiedlicher Gestalt mit einer wechselnd großen Kernzahl den Namen Osteoclasten geprägt. Kölliker (1889) bezeichnet seine Annahme, diese Zellen übten eine resorptive Tätigkeit aus, zwar als eine Hypothese, hat aber in der Detailbeschreibung (1873) aus dem Vorhandensein von Osteoclasten auf eine Resorption von Knochengewebe geschlossen. Die Osteoclastenlehre wurde z.T. bedingungslos angenommen, z.T. scharf abgelehnt. Arey (1920) meint, in der Beurteilung der Osteoclasten spiele „the prestige of their originator“ eine große Rolle; vielleicht war die Namensgebung für eine vorurteilsfreie Untersuchung noch verhängnisvoller (Knese, 1957). Kassowitz (1897) bezeichnet die Osteoclastenlehre als eine Behauptung; sie biete keine Erklärungen, sondern gebe nur neue Rätsel auf und rätselhafte Strukturen (Hancox, 1949) sind diese Zellen geblieben.

Erstaunlich ist die Tatsache, daß man in der Beurteilung der Aufgaben der Osteoblasten — mit Ausnahme der Hypothesen im Zusammenhang mit dem Vorhandensein von alkalischer Phosphatase — sehr vorsichtig war. Über die Bedeutung der Osteoclasten glaubte man aber, klare Aussagen machen zu können. Bei der Diskussion um die Riesenzellen werden eine Reihe verschiedener Fragestellungen nicht voneinander getrennt. Die Frage, ob im Laufe der Skeletentwicklung ein Wechselspiel von Apposition und Resorption vorliegt, hat zunächst mit den Riesenzellen wenig zu tun; die Beantwortung dieser Frage kann nicht von der cytologischen Dimension der Riesenzellen her erfolgen, sondern nur durch Untersuchung des Skeletorganes (Knese, 1957). Auch die Baugeschichte, die Histogenese des Knochengewebes, stellt ein unabhängiges Untersuchungsgebiet dar.

Die Notwendigkeit einer Resorption von Knochengewebe während des Skeletwachstums wurde häufig mit dem Vorhandensein der Skeletmineralien begründet (Kölliker, 1873; Weidenreich, 1930; Lacroix, 1951; Amprino, 1963). Durch den mit der ersten Knochenbildung beginnenden Umbau sollte sich der Knochen den wechselnden Beanspruchungen im Laufe des Lebens anpassen. Allerdings meinte Petersen (1927, 1930) hierzu, es liegt ein „hoffnungsloses Hinterherrennen der immer wieder zerstörten und veränderten Strukturen“ hinter dem ausweichenden Spannungszustand vor. Die ausführlichen Untersuchungen der Molekularbiologie der Gewebekomponenten, vor allem mit Hilfe der Radioisotopen, sprechen aber dafür, daß die Mineralien an einem lebhaften Stoffwechsel teilnehmen, das Kollagen aber stoffwechselträge ist. Der Ionenaustausch setzt nicht immer einen Knochenan- und -abbau (Armstrong, 1955) voraus, wie häufig in früheren Untersuchungen angenommen wurde.

Die Tätigkeitsform der Osteoclasten stellte man sich zunächst rein mechanisch vor, d.h. sie sollten den Knochen anfressen; die Resorptionsränder des Knochens würden dementsprechend wie angenagt aussehen. Zur Entstehung der sehr verwickelten Struktur nahm man an, daß sich Riesenzellen in mehreren Fronten hintereinander durch den Knochen hindurchfressen (Petersen, 1930). In ähnlicher Form würde der Knochen durch die äußere oder modellierende Resorption wie ein Bildwerk rein mechanisch ausgearbeitet.

Hierbei wurde nicht selten mit POMMER (1881) angenommen, daß das Knochengewebe keine aktiven Veränderungen durchmacht und sich gegenüber der lacunären Resorption rein passiv verhält.

Außer der lacunären und modellierenden Resorption wurden noch einige andere Formen des Abbaues beschrieben. ZAWISCH (1926) gibt eine vasculäre Resorption an, LIPP (1956) berichtet von einer „interlacunären" Resorption und Apposition, durch die die Form der Osteocytenhöhlen umgestaltet wird (vgl. BÉLANGER et al., 1965). KASSOWITZ (1881) hatte noch eine glatte Resorption in Erwägung gezogen, bei der die angefressenen Knochenränder fehlen.

Im Zusammenhang mit der Freßtätigkeit der Osteoclasten dachte man an echte Phagocytose, die aber lichtmikroskopisch nicht oder nicht sicher nachgewiesen werden konnte. Nach Verabreichung toxischer Dosen von Parathormon beteiligen sich viele Zellen des Knochenmarkes an der Phagocytose der zerstörten Knochensubstanz, aber nicht die Riesenzellen (MCLEAN und URIST, 1955).

Auch ein nicht „cellulärer", d.h. an eine spezifische Zellform, gebundener Knochenabbau wurde beschrieben. Einen schleichenden Abbau des Geflechtknochens nahm JAFFÉ (1929) an, von interstitiellen Veränderungen sprach BRASH (1934). An Vorgänge der Osteolyse haben BENOIT und CLAVERT (1943), STARR (1947), FELL und MELLANBY (1952) gedacht, z.T. auch im Zusammenhang mit Riesenzellen (HELLER et al., 1950).

Ein großer Teil der Hypothesen über die Osteoclastentätigkeit beruht wohl auf der Annahme, daß die Histogenese und das Wachstum in den „sichtbaren" Strukturen 4.—2. Ordnung ablaufen. Das Knochengewebe wurde als eine einheitliche steinähnliche Substanz angesehen. Da aber die Knochenbildung aus einer Reihe von Teilvorgängen besteht, sind auch für den Knochenabbau mehrere Einzelprozesse anzunehmen. Es wurde daher die Möglichkeit des Abbaues der einzelnen Gewebekomponenten, voran der Kollagenfasern und der Mineralien, erörtert (unter anderem MCLEAN, 1956; HANCOX, 1956).

Unbestritten ist, daß im Knochen wie in anderen Organen auch Abbauvorgänge auftreten, vor allem unter pathologischen oder experimentellen Bedingungen (Parathormon, Vitamin A, Altersatrophie). Schwieriger sind die Verhältnisse im Hinblick auf die regelrechte, normale Entwicklung zu beurteilen, da sich die experimentellen Ergebnisse nicht ohne weiteres auf die ungestörte Entwicklung übertragen lassen.

α) *Verbreitung der Riesenzellen*

Über die Verbreitung der Riesenzellen ist relativ wenig bekannt. Sie fehlen oder sind ungewöhnlich selten an vielen Orten erheblicher Umgestaltungen des Knochengewebes, vor allem im Verlauf der Histogenese.

KÖLLIKER (1873) hat die Verteilung von Riesenzellen an Röhrenknochen beschrieben. Riesenzellen treten in einigem Abstand von der Eröffnungszone des Epiphysenknorpels, in der sog. Metaphyse auf (KÖLLIKER, 1873; ZAWISCH, 1931; DODDS, 1932; GARDNER, 1956; KNESE, 1957; KNESE und KNOOP, 1961b). Eine ähnliche Lokalisation beschrieb BARNICOT (1947) am Schädel; die Riesenzellen erscheinen in einigem Abstand von den Nähten, d.h. hinter der Knochenbildungsfront. Weiterhin sind Riesenzellen im sog. enchondralen Zapfen zu beobachten. Bekanntlich dringt durch eine Öffnung der Diaphysenschale periostales Gewebe in die primäre Markhöhle ein; außer Gefäßen und verschiedenen skeletogenen Zellen treten hier auch Riesenzellen auf. Schließlich sind Riesenzellen in größerer Zahl am Ende der Diaphysenschale in dem Gebiet der sog. freien chondralen Flächen zu finden (KNESE, 1957; BAHLING, 1958). In diesen Gebieten fehlt der periostale Knochen und der chondrale tritt unmittelbar mit dem Periost in Verbindung; KÖLLIKER (1873) nannte diese Flächen Resorptionsflächen, STRELZOFF (1873) aplastische Flächen.

MAIR (1929) wies auf die Riesenzellen an der Schädelbasis hin, wo man sich wegen der durchtretenden Nerven und Gefäße resorptive Vorgänge schlecht vorstellen könnte. KNESE (1959a) hat an Hand des Vergleiches peruanischer Turmschädel mit nicht verformten Schädeln die Vermutung ausgesprochen, daß sich die Schädelbasis durch die

Beziehungen zu Sinnesorganen und Nerven einer künstlichen Verformung „entzieht". Barnicot (1947) hat bei Mäusen die Verteilung der Riesenzellen nach supravitaler Neutralrotfärbung besonders am Parietale verfolgt. An der Tabula interna nimmt die Anzahl der Riesenzellen bis zum 7. Tage nach der Geburt zu und sinkt dann bis zum 28. Tage fast auf Null ab. Die Riesenzellen treten an der Tabula externa des Parietale nicht vor dem 10. Tage auf und erreichen ihre größte Zahl zwischen dem 14.—18. Tage.

Dieser Befund von Barnicot (1947) spricht gegen die weit verbreitete Meinung, daß Riesenzellen mit der ersten Knochenbildung erscheinen und zeitlebens vorhanden sind (vgl. Knese, 1963c). Tonna (1960) stellt bei Untersuchung der Verteilung der Riesenzellen im Periost des distalen Femurendes von Mäusen und Ratten in verschiedenen Lebensaltern ebenfalls eine wechselnde Menge von Riesenzellen fest. Bei Ratten erscheinen Riesenzellen in der 5.—8. Woche und fehlen späterhin, bei Mäusen sind sie in der 2.—10. Woche zu beobachten und dann nur noch vereinzelt anzutreffen. Innerhalb der genannten Zeiten ist die größte Anzahl von Riesenzellen jeweils an verschiedenen Punkten des Knochenumfanges gelegen; vermutlich hängen diese Verschiebungen mit der Umgestaltung der freien chondralen Flächen zusammen, die Tonna aber nicht erwähnt. Ähnliche Altersdifferenzen werden für die Metaphyse angegeben. Für den Menschen fehlen derartige systematische Erhebungen. Knese (1957) hat darauf hingewiesen, daß Riesenzellen bei den ersten Stadien der Markraumbildung und bei der starken Erweiterung der Markhöhle in der zweiten Hälfte der Schwangerschaft praktisch fehlen. Riesenzellen im Markraum wurden in größerer Menge nur bei Feten zwischen 58—105 mm SSL aufgefunden.

Die vorliegenden Untersuchungen über die Verbreitung der Riesenzellen sind unzureichend, lassen aber doch vermuten, daß nur in bestimmten Entwicklungsphasen eine größere Anzahl von Riesenzellen vorliegt. Demgemäß können Riesenzellen kaum als Gebilde bezeichnet werden, die für die Strukturbildung in allen Lebensphasen unbedingt erforderlich sind. Auf das Auftreten von Riesenzellen unter pathologischen und experimentellen Bedingungen möge nur hingewiesen werden (Parathormon: Jaffé und Bodansky, 1930; Heller et al., 1950; Barnicot, 1948; Vitamin A: Mellanby, 1947; Barnicot, 1950; Barnicott und Datta, 1956).

β) Die Herkunft der Riesenzellen

Über die Herkunft der Riesenzellen wurden sehr verschiedene Ansichten geäußert (Arey, 1920; Haythorn, 1929; Jaffé, 1930; Weidenreich, 1930; Zawisch, 1931; Glättli, 1947; Hancox, 1949, 1956). Eine Entstehung aus indifferenten Zellen wurde von Dantschakoff (1909), Barnicot (1941), Bloom et al. (1941) und Heller et al. (1950) angenommen. Bloom et al. (1941) und Bloom et al. (1958) stützen sich auf Untersuchungen des Markknochens der Vögel und geben an, daß aus Osteoblasten Osteocyten, Spindelzellen oder Osteoclasten werden. Bei der Auflösung des Markknochens verschmelzen auch Osteocyten mit Riesenzellen. Aus diesen Riesenzellen werden unter entsprechenden hormonellen Bedingungen wiederum Osteoblasten und Reticulumzellen. Die Autoren (vgl. McLean und Urist 1955) kommen zu einem Stammbaum oder besser wohl Gestaltscyclus der Skeletzellen, der die verschiedenen funktionellen Zustände der Zellen beschreibt (ähnlich Ham 1932). Die Abkunft der Riesenzellen von Osteoblasten wurde auch von Kölliker (1873), Pommer (1883) und Arey (1920) vertreten. Eine Abstammung von Gefäßendothelien geben Pommer (1883) und Zawisch (1931) an. Schließlich nehmen Benoit und Clavert (1952) die Herkunft aus sehr verschiedenen Zellformen an, womit der Vielfalt der Riesenzellen Rechnung getragen wird.

Untersuchungen der Riesenzellen in vitro wurden von Kirby-Smith (1933), Hancox (1946 u. 1956) durchgeführt.

Bei elektronenmikroskopischen Untersuchungen der Eröffnungszone des Epiphysenknorpels beobachteten Knese und Knoop (1961b) zwei Zellformen (Abb. 42). „Helle" Zellen mit einer geringen Dichte des Grundplasmas sind wahrscheinlich aus ihren Höhlen befreite Knorpelzellen, die sich weiterhin zu Markosteoblasten entwickeln. Daneben treten „graue“ Zellen auf, deren Grundplasma sehr dicht ist und reichlich Granula und Mitochondrien enthält; ihr Kern ist im Vergleich zum Cytoplasma relativ klein. Graue und helle Zellen liegen häufig paarweise in engem Kontakt nebeneinander. In einigem Abstand von der Eröffnungszone (s. dort) werden aus den grauen Zellen vermutlich durch Zellverschmelzung Riesenzellen (Abb. 43). Die Struktur der grauen Zellen ist jener der perivasculären fibroblastenähnlichen Elemente oder aus dem Verband getretenen

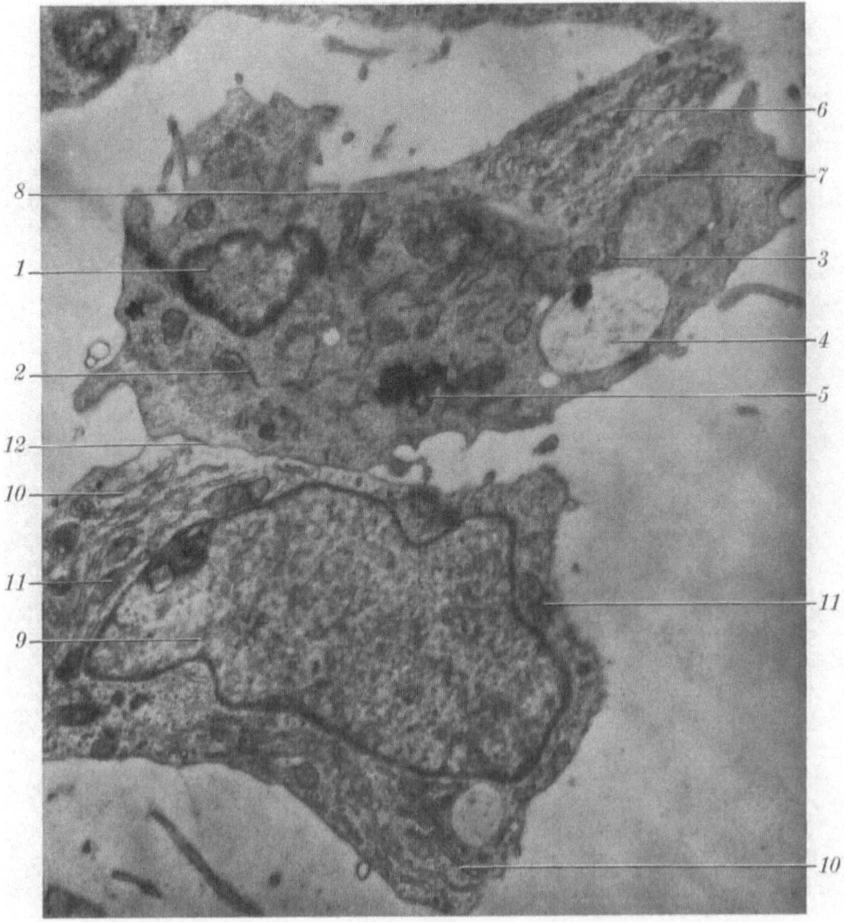

Abb. 42. Graue und helle Zelle. Graue Zelle: *1* Zellkern mit verklumptem Chromatin; *2* granuläres Grundplasma mit einzelnen Doppelmembranen; *3* Mitochondrien; *4* Vacuolen; *5* osmiophile Einlagerungen; *6* Zellabschnitt, der voraussichtlich mit der grauen Zelle verschmilzt; *7* Zellmembran; *8* Verschmelzungsbereich. Helle Zelle: *9* Zellkern; *10* endoplasmatisches Reticulum; *11* Mitochondrien; *12* Kontaktbereich. Vergr. 7500. (KNESE und KNOOP, 1961 b)

Endothelzellen sehr ähnlich. Daneben wurden auch Zellen gefunden, die ihrer Struktur nach als Übergangsformen zwischen hellen und grauen Zellen anzusehen sind. Die Entstehung der Periostriesenzellen konnte nicht aufgeklärt werden.

Als Stammform der Riesenzellen sind vermutlich alle skeletogenen Zellen in ihren verschiedenen Funktionszuständen anzusehen. Es wurde auch die Vermutung ausgesprochen, daß mehrere Formen von Riesenzellen zu unterscheiden sind (BIDDER, 1906; AREY, 1920; KNESE, 1957). So können mehrkernige Gebilde zwischen Bälkchen enchondralen Knochens, aber auch an anderen Orten als Brückenbauer auftreten (WALDEYER, 1865; BIDDER, 1906; HARTMANN, 1910; AREY, 1920; KNESE, 1957). KOJIMA et al. (1960) haben bei Kaninchen nach Behandlung mit Cortison die Bildung von reichlich Osteoid und Riesenzellen beobachtet, wobei die Riesenzellen häufig die Stelle des Osteoids einnehmen. Eine ähnliche „Stellvertretung" hat KNESE (1957) bei Untersuchungen der diaphysären chondralen Osteogenese beim Menschen in Erwägung gezogen. Für einen Teil der mehrkernigen Zellen wurde eine osteogene Potenz für möglich gehalten.

Im Hinblick auf das weitere Schicksal der Riesenzellen wurde im allgemeinen eine Rückverwandlung in die Stammzellen angenommen, aber auch ihr Zerfall bzw. die Aufnahme in Gefäße vermutet (AREY, 1919; JAFFÉ, 1930).

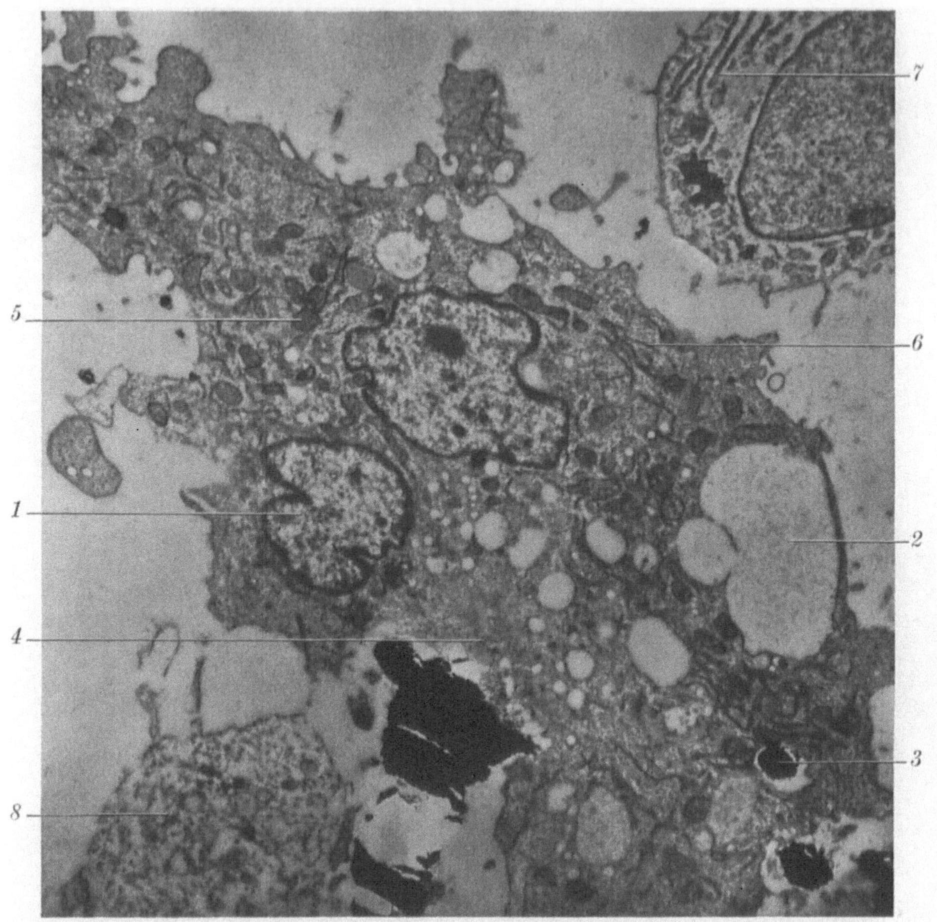

Abb. 43. Riesenzelle an Knorpelkalk angelagert. *1* Zellkern; *2* Vacuolen; *3* eingeschlossener Knorpelkalk; *4* homogene Zone in Nachbarschaft eines Resorptionsgebietes; *5* Mitochondrien; *6* Membranpaare; *7* helle Zellen mit wohlausgebildeten Membranen; *8* helle Zelle mit granulärer Struktur. Vergr. 6000. (KNESE und KNOOP, 1961b)

Riesenzellen entstehen in relativ kurzen Zeiträumen; sie treten in der Ohrkammer nach 48 Std (SANDISON, 1928), nach Verabreichung von Parathormon innerhalb 12 Std auf (HELLER et al., 1950). Im Markknochen entwickeln sie sich in weniger als 36 Std (BLOOM et al., 1941).

γ) Die Morphologie der Riesenzellen

Die Beziehung der Riesenzellen zum Knochen ist unterschiedlich, die Lagerung in Howshipschen Lacunen nicht die Regel, eher sogar die Ausnahme. Die Zellen können als flache Gebilde dem Knochen aufliegen, den Bälkchen in der Metaphyse, aber auch den Trabekeln des periostalen Knochens am Ende kappenartig aufsitzen; sie bilden weiterhin Brücken zwischen den Bälkchen enchondralen Knochens oder lassen jede Verbindung zum Knochen vermissen. Von der Lage abgesehen, ergeben sich ähnlich unterschiedliche

Beziehungen zum Knochen wie bei den Osteoblasten. Die Verbindung der Riesenzellen mit den Knochen kann so locker sein, daß sie sich bei der Fixierung wie die inaktiven Osteoblasten durch Schrumpfung vom Knochen ablösen. Bei einer innigen Verbindung mit dem Knochen erscheint häufig ein sog. Bürstensaum (s. S. 386).

Die Gestalt der Riesenzellen ist entsprechend ihrer unterschiedlichen Beziehung zum Knochen sehr wechselnd. Die Anzahl der im allgemeinen kleinen rundlichen und sich ungleichartig färbenden Kerne erreicht die Zahl 10—20 oder gar 100. Ch'Uan (1931) und Tonna (1960) beschrieben auch einkernige Osteoclasten, die in Howshipschen Lacunen liegen; die Frage liegt nahe, ob es sich hierbei nicht um Osteoblasten handelt, die als Osteocyten im Knochen eingeschlossen werden.

Die Reaktion des Cytoplasmas wurde als basophil (Askanazy, 1902) oder oxyphil (Weidenreich, 1930; Jaffé, 1930) beschrieben. Benoit und Clavert (1952) halten die basophilen Zellen für eine unreife, die oxyphilen für die reife, tätige Form (s. S. 386, endoplasmatisches Reticulum). Die Riesenzellen an verschiedenen Orten des Skeletstückes zeigen ähnlich wie die periostalen und Markosteoblasten (Pritchard, 1952; Knese, 1957) eine voneinander abweichende Farbreaktion.

Knese (1957) gibt ein annähernd gleichartiges färberisches Verhalten von periostalen Osteoblasten sowie Periost-Riesenzellen einerseits und Markosteoblasten und Markriesenzellen andererseits an. Der Unterschied der Reaktionsformen zwischen Mark- und Periostzellen ist aber nur gradueller Natur. Tonna und Cronkite (1959) und Tonna (1960) bestätigen diesen Befund für die periostalen Zellformen mit dem Zusatz, daß die Osteoclasten im Gegegensatz zu den Osteoblasten mit zunehmendem Alter keine Änderung des histochemischen Verhaltens aufweisen. Periostale Osteoblasten und Riesenzellen reagieren mit Toluidinblau metachromatisch; z.T. ist die Metachromasie an Granula gebunden. Heller-Steinberg (1951) beschrieb zuerst PAS-positive Granula. Periostale Osteoblasten und Riesenzellen speichern in gleicher Form ^{35}S. Die Metachromasie der Markosteoblasten und Riesenzellen ist schwächer als die der periostalen; mitunter reagieren sie auch orthochromatisch. Beide sind im allgemeinen stärker mit PAS-positiven Granula beladen, die allerdings in Riesenzellen auch fehlen können (Knese, 1957). Kroon (1954) beobachtet in Riesenzellen herantretende

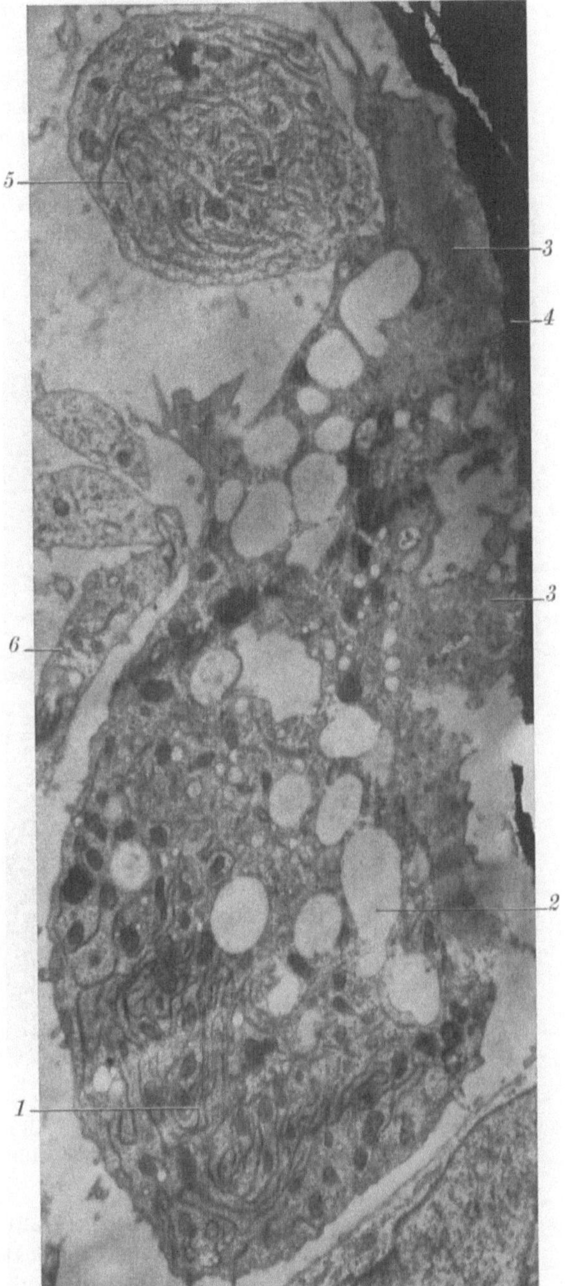

Abb. 44. Riesenzelle in flächenhaftem Kontakt mit Knorpelkalk. *1* Kalkferner Zellabschnitt mit Membranen und Mitochondrien; *2* vacuoläre Zone; *3* homogener Zellabschnitt mit Buchten; *4* Knorpelkalk; *5* helle Zelle; *6* Gefäßendothel. Vergr. 6000. (Knese und Knoop, 1961 b)

argyrophile Fasern des Knochens (s. unten), denen sich im Zelleib gleichartig reagierende Granula anschließen (vgl. Jaffé, 1930; Knese, 1957).

Die Reaktion auf alkalische Phosphatase fällt bei Osteoblasten und Osteoclasten gleich stark aus (Greep et al., 1948; Majno und Rouiller, 1951). Das Vorhandensein saurer Phosphatase muß wohl als charakteristisch angesehen werden (Changus, 1957; Fullmer, 1964, 1965). Schließlich tritt eine Aminopeptidase auf (Lipp, 1959). Über Succino-Dehydrogenase berichten u.a. Fullmer (1966) und Takada (1966). Riesenzellen lagern kein ^{3}H-Thymidin ein, so daß keine Synthese von DNS stattfindet und demgemäß auch keine Mitosen zustande kommen (Tonna, 1960).

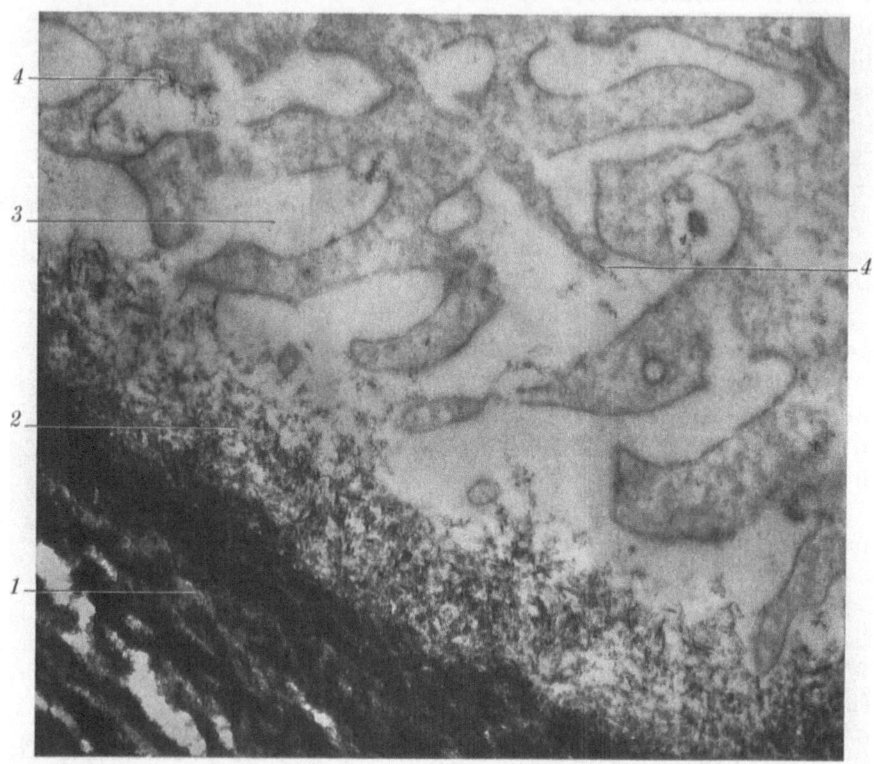

Abb. 45. Teil einer Riesenzelle mit Buchten der Zelloberfläche. *1* Dichter Knorpelkalk; *2* Knorpelkalk in Auflösung; *3* Buchten der Zelloberfläche; *4* Kalknadeln in Kontakt mit der Zellmembran. Vergr. 22000. (Knese und Knoop, 1961b)

Nach den Beobachtungen von Kölliker (1873) besitzt ein Teil der Osteoclasten einen sog. Bürstensaum. Die variable Gestalt dieser Bildung und die Abhängigkeit ihres Aussehens von der Untersuchungsmethodik hat Hancox (1956) dargestellt. Jaffé (1930) und Ham (1952) halten diesen Saum für Fibrillen des Knochens. Nach Kroon (1954) treten argyrophile Fasern des Knochens in den Bürstensaum ein, der selbst aus cytoplasmatischen Fortsätzen besteht; in der Zelle schließen sich dann argyrophile Granula an. Ähnliche Beobachtungen liegen von Knese (1957) vor.

Scott und Pease (1956) fanden elektronenmikroskopisch Zellen, die reich an Vacuolen und Mitochondrien sind, denen aber ein endoplasmatisches Reticulum fehlt. Auf der dem Knochen zugewandten Seite zeigen diese Zellen Einstülpungen der Plasmamembran, so daß eine Reihe gewundener Kanälchen mit einem Zwischenraum von 65—85 Å entsteht. Diese Bildung halten die Autoren für den Bürstensaum. Der Saum liegt Kalkmassen an, in denen Kollagenfasern fehlen; die Verfasser nehmen an, das Kollagen sei zuvor herausgelöst worden. Nach Knese und Knoop (1961b) handelt es sich auf Grund der von Scott und Pease vorgelegten Abbildungen aber nicht um Knochenkalk, sondern Knorpelkalk. Für den Knorpelkalk wurden bisher keine engeren Beziehungen zu Fibrillen nachgewiesen. Weitere Beschreibungen des Bürstensaumes liegen von DUDLEY und SPIRO (1961), KNESE (1963c), CAMERON, PARSCHALL und ROBINSON (1964) und SCOTT (1967) vor. KNESE und KNOOP (1961b) konnten Riesenzellen im Markraum nur in Nachbarschaft von Knorpelkalk beobachten (Abb. 44), ein gleiches gilt für die periostalen Riesenzellen der freien chondralen Flächen (s. dort). Zum Knorpelkalk hin besitzen die Riesenzellen eine verschieden stark gebuchtete Zelloberfläche, den „Bürstensaum" (Abb. 45).

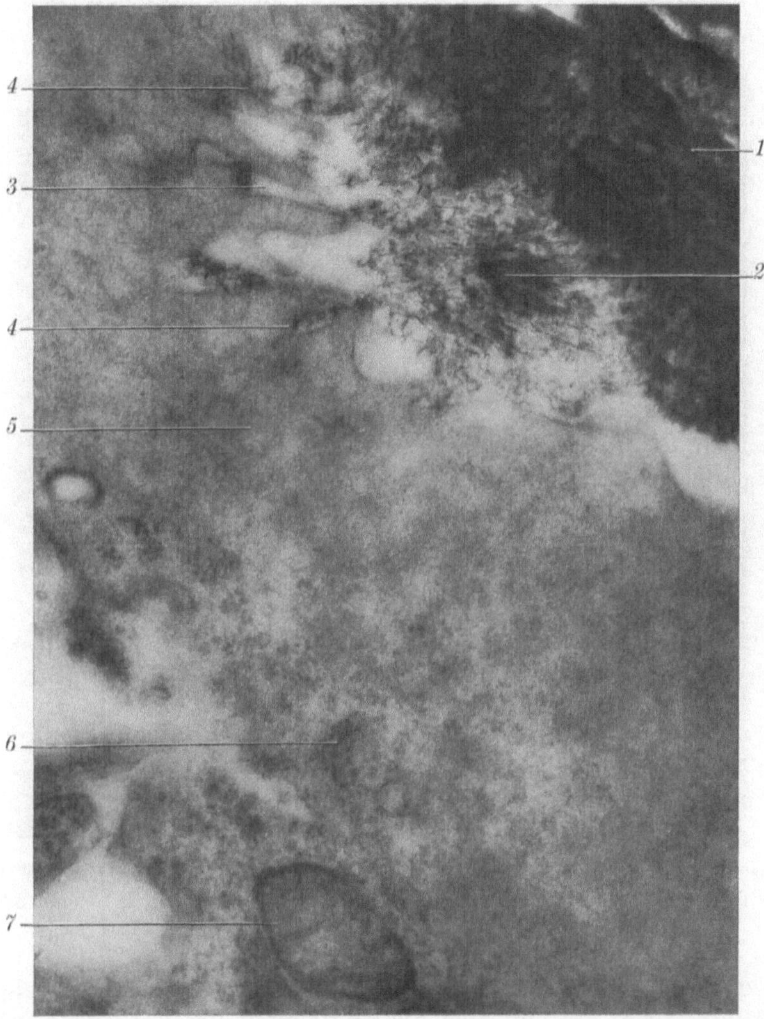

Abb. 46. Teil einer Riesenzelle mit homogenem Randsaum. *1* Dichter Knorpelkalk; *2* Kalk in Auflösung; *3* Buchten der Zelloberfläche; *4* Kalknadeln in Kontakt mit der Zellmembran, zum Teil wie in Vacuolen (Buchten ?) eingeschlossen; *5* homogener Randsaum; *6* granuläres Grundplasma; *7* Mitochondrien. Vergr. 45000. (KNESE und KNOOP, 1961b)

Dem Plasmalemm liegen Kalknadeln an und der benachbarte Knorpelkalk erscheint „aufgelockert" (Abb. 46). Auf diesen Zellabschnitt mit Ausbuchtungen folgt im allgemeinen ein zweiter mit homogenem dichtem Grundplasma, in einem weiteren treten dann verschieden große Vacuolen und vereinzelt Mitochondrien auf. In dem von Knorpelmineral abgewandten Zellteil befindet sich ein endoplasmatisches Reticulum und eine relativ große Zahl kleinerer Mitochondrien mit einer dichten Matrix. Das endoplasmatische Reticulum ist das Äquivalent der Cytoplasmabasophilie. Das Vorhandensein von RNS wurde von MORSE und GREEP (1960) nachgewiesen. Über das Schicksal der Kristallnadeln konnten KNESE und KNOOP (1961b) keine Beobachtungen machen.

GONZALES et al. (1961) haben eine fast gleichartige Beschreibung für die Riesenzellen im Frakturcallus von Ratten gegeben. Weiterhin werden Granula, aufgebaut aus feinsten Partikelchen, erwähnt; diese Granula erscheinen z.T. in Vacuolen, die auch eine geringe Zahl von Filamenten unklarer Natur enthalten. Die Filamente könnten Reste aufgelöster Kollagenfibrillen oder ein Fixierungsprodukt sein. Die Autoren weisen ausdrücklich auf das Fehlen von Kollagenfibrillen hin. Da in anderen Abschnitten des Präparates aber Fibrillen vorliegen, schließen sie ein Kunstprodukt aus und nehmen eine vorangegangene Auflösung des Kollagens an. Dem Kollagenabbau folgt eine Phagocytose, genauer gesagt eine Pinocytose der Kristalle. So zwingend zunächst die Schlußfolgerung der Verfasser

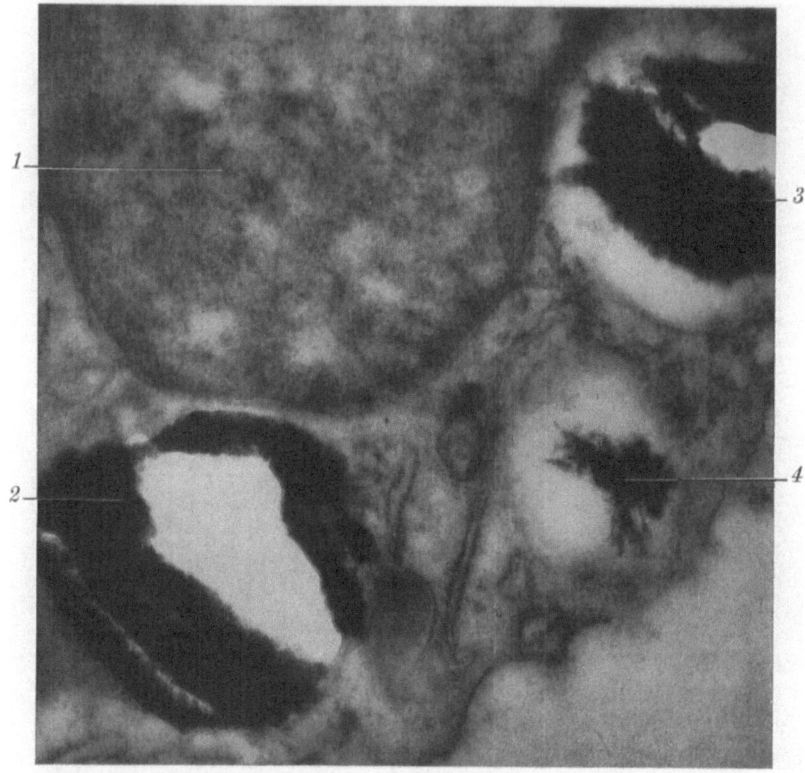

Abb. 47. Kalkeinschlüsse in einer Zelle. *1* Zellkern; *2* Kalkeinschlüsse ohne kenntliche umhüllende Membran; *3* Kalkeinschluß mit teilweiser Membranumhüllung; *4* Kalk in Auflösung (?). Vergr. 32000. (KNESE und KNOOP, 1961b)

scheint, darf doch nicht übersehen werden, daß Callus auch Knorpelgewebe enthält (HAM und HARRIS, 1956). So läßt sich die Möglichkeit des Vorliegens von Knorpelkalk nicht mit Sicherheit ausschließen. Auffällig ist, daß die Riesenzellen nach allen bisherigen elektronenmikroskopischen Beobachtungen relativ breiten Kalkzonen ohne Kollagenfibrillen anliegen.

Der von GONZALES et al. (1961) beschriebene Einschluß von Kalknadeln in Vacuolen erfolgt nach KNESE und KNOOP (1961b) nicht nur in Riesenzellen, sondern auch in anderen einkernigen Zellen (Abb. 47). Den Einschluß von Kristallnadeln in Vacuolen beobachteten weiterhin CAMERON und ROBINSON (1958), KNESE und KNOOP (1961b) sowie DUDLEY und SPIRO (1961). Immer wieder wurde auf die Mitwirkung weiterer Zellformen bei der „Resorption" hingewiesen. In der Eröffnungszone der Knorpelhöhlen nehmen nach den elektronenmikroskopischen Befunden von KNESE und KNOOP (1961b) alle dort auftretenden Zellelemente Verbindung mit Knorpelkalk auf, die „hellen" Zellen als Abkömmlinge der Knorpelzellen, die einkernigen „grauen" Zellen als Vorläufer der Riesenzellen und die Gefäßendothelien sowie perivasculäre Elemente. In den „hellen"

Zellen finden sich in sehr verschieden gestalteten Vacuolen, z.T. in Kernnähe oder im Golgifeld, Kalkeinschlüsse. Ähnliche Beobachtungen machten CAMERON und ROBISON (1958) an menschlichem Untersuchungsgut. Der Erhaltungszustand dieses Materials ließ eine genaue Bestimmung der vorliegenden Zellart nicht zu, doch dachten die Verfasser an Riesenzellen. Über das Schicksal dieser Kalkeinschlüsse liegen keine Angaben vor. Schließlich fand KNESE (1963c) an entmineralisierten Knochen, neuerlich auch an nicht entmineralisierten Knochen, eine Verdünnung der zuvor 500—600 Å dünnen Kollagenfibrillen auf 200 Å. Demzufolge müßte das morphologische Bild des Kollagenabbaues der Fibrillogenese genau spiegelbildlich ablaufen.

Im Hinblick auf die Resorption von Knochen ist nun zu diskutieren, ob die Riesenzellen die „Potenz" zum Abbau der einzelnen Gewebekomponenten, vor allem der Kollagenfibrillen und der Mineralien, besitzen. Nach älteren lichtmikroskopischen Beobachtungen treten Riesenzellen besonders in der Markhöhle nur dann auf, wenn Mineralablagerungen vorhanden sind, aber nicht bei unverkalktem Osteoid (DODDS, 1932; WOLBACH, 1947; WEINMANN und SCHOUR, 1945; BENOIT und CLAVERT, 1947). Diese Feststellung stimmt mit den elektronenmikroskopischen Befunden überein. Im Hinblick auf den Mechanismus der Kalkauflösung dachte man an Substanzen, die den chelating agents ähnlich sind (MCLEAN, 1954, 1956)..

HANCOX (1956) kommt nach Würdigung der vorliegenden Literatur zur Auffassung, Riesenzellen sind bei der Bewältigung (removal, DODDS, 1932) von Kalk beteiligt; für eine Auflösung von Kollagen sprechen aber die bisherigen Beobachtungen nicht. Keine der vorliegenden elektronenmikroskopischen Untersuchungen kann diese Feststellung entkräften. Im Hinblick auf das Kollagen liegt ein gewisser Gegensatz zwischen den Ansichten der Untersucher der Fibrillenbildung und -reifung und jenen des Knochenabbaues vor. Als Ziel der Faserbildung wird die Entwicklung unlöslicher Fibrillen angesehen, wobei sich das Knochenkollagen nicht einmal in den gewöhnlichen Lösungsmitteln für das Kollagen aus Haut und Sehnen löst (NEUMAN und NEUMAN, 1958). Dieser Auffassung wurde die Hypothese eines Abbaues auch von Kollagen und Mucopolysacchariden durch den Mechanismus der chelating agents gegenübergestellt (MCLEAN 1954), der auch bei dem pH des Organismus möglich ist. MCLEAN (1956) meint, dieser Annahme widerspreche keine bekannte Tatsache, allerdings sei bisher auch kein entsprechender Nachweis für das Vorhandensein solcher Stoffe gelungen. Im übrigen bewahrt MCLEAN bei der Übertragung der Ergebnisse von Untersuchungen mit toxischen Dosen von Parathormon auf physiologische Verhältnisse große Vorsicht. Der Verfasser sieht die Osteoclasten als eine Nebenerscheinung des Knochenabbaues an.

Die Feststellung, daß auch andere Zellen an der Resorption von Knochen (vgl. BÉLANGER et al., 1965) teilnehmen, hilft uns wenig zum Verständnis der Osteoclastentätigkeit (HANCOX, 1956). Die Riesenzellen bleiben zunächst weiterhin rätselhafte Strukturen. Allerdings wird durch diese Feststellung die Erforschung der Histogenese und des Knochenwachstums kaum beeinflußt, da für diese Phänomene die Kenntnis der Molekularbiologie der Gewebekomponenten von größerer Bedeutung ist als der z.Z. nicht zu entscheidende Streit, ob die Riesenzellen nun auch wirklich Osteoclasten sind oder nicht oder ob sie nur im Bereich von transistorischen Kalkablagerungen auftreten.

e) Das Periost

Im bisherigen Sprachgebrauch wird die „Bindegewebshülle" des knorpeligen Skeletstückes Perichondrium, die des knöchernen Periost genannt. Demzufolge wurden die ersten Vorgänge zur Bildung der Diaphysenschale als perichondrale Osteogenese bezeichnet. Elektronenmikroskopische Untersuchungen (KNESE und KNOOP, 1961c) zeigten aber, daß dieses sog. Perichondrium Knochenbildungszellen aufweist, die sich eindeutig von den Chondroblasten unterscheiden. Daher wurde vorgeschlagen, bei Vorliegen von Chondroblasten von einem Perichondrium und von Osteoblasten von einem Periost zu sprechen.

Aus einem Mesenchym, dessen Zellen einen annähernd gleichen Abstand voneinander haben, entwickelt sich in der Form einer Zellanhäufung das Vorknorpelblastem. Eine syncytiale Verbindung der Zellen besteht nicht, d.h. die Zellen sind nicht durch Cytoplasmabrücken kontinuierlich miteinander verbunden (KNESE und KNOOP, 1961a). Mit der Entwicklung des Vorknorpels entsteht in den peripheren Schichten dieser Zellansammlungen das Perichondrium. Die Zellen des Perichondriums unterscheiden sich morphologisch zunächst nicht von den umliegenden Mesenchymzellen, weisen aber durch ^{35}S-Ablagerungen eine andere Reaktionsform auf (AMPRINO, 1955). Ähnliche Mesenchymverdichtungen treten auch bei der desmalen Osteogenese auf (GRAUMANN, 1951). In einem nächsten Schritt werden Periost und Perichondrium in zwei Schichten gegliedert. Die äußere Schicht wird zur Fibroelastica und enthält den Fibroblasten ähnliche Zellen; in den schmalen Intercellularräumen liegen nur wenige Kollagenfibrillen (KNESE und KNOOP, 1961a). Nach KNESE (1966a) setzt sich bei Rinderfeten die Anlage der Gelenkkapsel über die äußere Schicht des Perichondriums in die Fibroelastica fort, wobei die zugehörigen Zellelemente PAS- und BTS-positive Substanzen enthalten. Eine besondere Cambiumschicht entsteht erst im Periost. Weiterhin ergeben sich Unterschiede in der Gliederung der Fibroelastica bei jüngeren und älteren Feten. In späteren Entwicklungsstadien scheint die Fibroelastica nur geringe oder gar keine Beziehungen zur inneren zellreichen Schicht, der Cambiumschicht, zu besitzen. An der Grenze zur Fibroelastica liegen in der Cambiumschicht die Stammzellen. Dabei ist zweifelhaft, ob diese Stammzellen als einziges Reservoir zur Bildung von Osteoblasten anzusehen sind. Über die weiteren Zellformen des Periostes haben wir bei Erörterung der Osteogenese kurz berichtet (s. S. 351; vgl. KNESE, 1966a, 1967a, b).

Der Übergang vom Perichondrium zum Periost ist lebenszeitlich sehr unterschiedlich gestaltet (KNESE, 1968). Zunächst liegt bei kleineren Feten eine schmale Schicht „cytoplasmaarmer" Osteoblasten vor. Es treten wenig später „runde Osteoblasten", z.T. eingeschlossen in ein wabiges Knochenwerk hinzu. Kurz vor Entstehung der faserigen encoche d'ossification bildet sich eine ringförmig das Skeletstück umgebende Lage von „encoche-Zellen" aus. Ein Teil der Berichte über verdämmernde Zellen und nackte Kerne (vgl. KNESE, 1956a) beruht offensichtlich auf Beobachtungen in dieser Region. Nach elektronenmikroskopischen Untersuchungen schildert KNESE (1968) dieses Verdämmern als eine Bildung von Kollagenfibrillen, verbunden mit einer Degradation des Zellmaterials, voran des ribosomalen Apparates und der Membranen. Damit liegen dann Kerne, umgeben von wenig Membranen, inmitten von Knochenfibrillen.

Die Unterscheidung zwischen Chondroblasten und Osteoblasten bereitet elektronenmikroskopisch keine Schwierigkeiten, ist aber im Lichtmikroskop besonders am Ende der Diaphysenschale nicht immer einfach. Die Gestalt der Chondroblasten ist in Höhe der einzelnen Zonen des Epiphysenknorpels recht wechselnd, wie ja auch die Gestalt der Osteoblasten entlang der Diaphyse ungleichartig ist. Im allgemeinen sind die Chondroblasten durch verschieden breite Intercellularspalten voneinander getrennt, während zwischen den Knochenbildnern lichtmikroskopisch keine Intercellularspalten zu erkennen sind. Bei Färbung mit Gallocyanin, das zum Nachweis von Desoxyribonucleinsäure und Ribonucleinsäure dient, lassen Chondroblasten eine Reaktion des Cytoplasmas vermissen, ein Befund, der dem gering entwickelten endoplasmatischen Reticulum entspricht. Dagegen ist das Cytoplasma der Osteoblasten grau bis schwarz tingiert (KNESE und KNOOP, 1961a, c).

Die rein morphologische Unterscheidung zwischen Perichondrium und Periost sagt über die Potenz der vorliegenden Zellen nichts aus. Bekanntlich sind die Periostzellen bipotent, da sie unter gewissen Bedingungen, z.B. im Frakturcallus, nicht nur Knochen, sondern auch Knorpel bilden (KASSOWITZ, 1879; SCHAFFER, 1916; FELL, 1933; STUDITSKY, 1933; ROULET, 1935; MURRAY, 1936; LACROIX, 1949).

Die Cambiumschicht besitzt im Gegensatz zur Fibroelastica keine elastischen Fasern (BIERMANN, 1957) (Abb. 48). Die Dicke der Cambiumschicht ist wechselnd; sie kann bei Kleinstkindern bis zu 600 μ erreichen, mißt beim 7jährigen noch 30—50 μ und fehlt

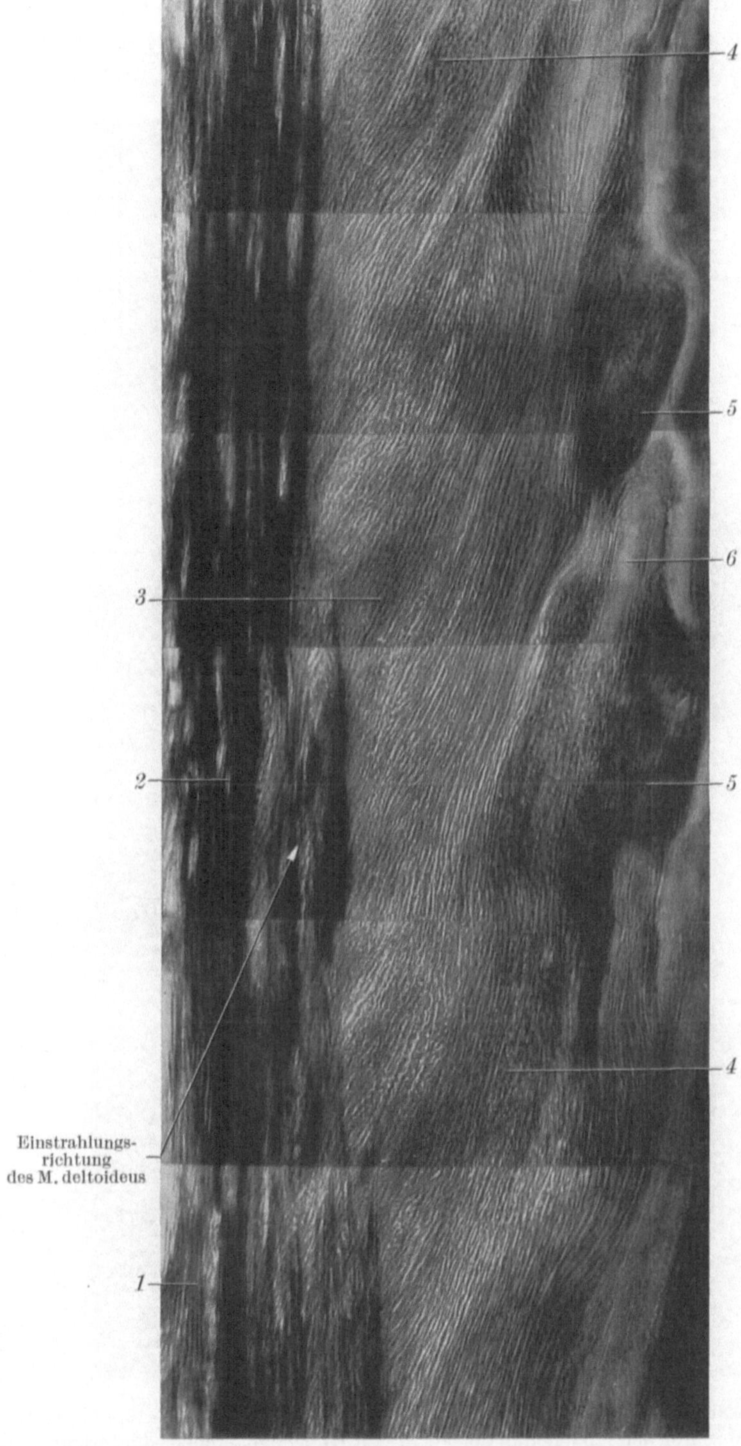

Abb. 48. Kind, 3 Monate. Tuberositas deltoidea, Längsschnitt in Einstrahlungsrichtung des M. deltoideus. *1* M. deltoideus; *2* Fibroelastica; *3* Cambiumschicht; *4* Inseln reich an Zellen, aber arm an Fasern („Blasteminseln"); *5* neugebildete Knochenbälkchen; *6* Gefäßräume. Resorcin-Fuchsin. Obj.Ph 10, Ok. 8. Photomontage. (BIERMANN, 1957)

beim 25jährigen (BIERMANN, 1957). Das Periost stellt dann in großen Bereichen des Skeletes eine Membran von unterschiedlicher Dicke dar. Die Verbindung mit dem darunter liegenden Knochen ist verschieden fest. An manchen Orten läßt sich das Periost leicht ablösen, an anderen dagegen nicht. Nach BLUNTSCHLI (1925) ist die Verbindung der Dura mater encephali mit den Schädelknochen zunächst recht innig. Sie läßt sich vom 2., spätesten 10. Jahr im Bereich des Parietale gut ablösen; nur die Verbindung an

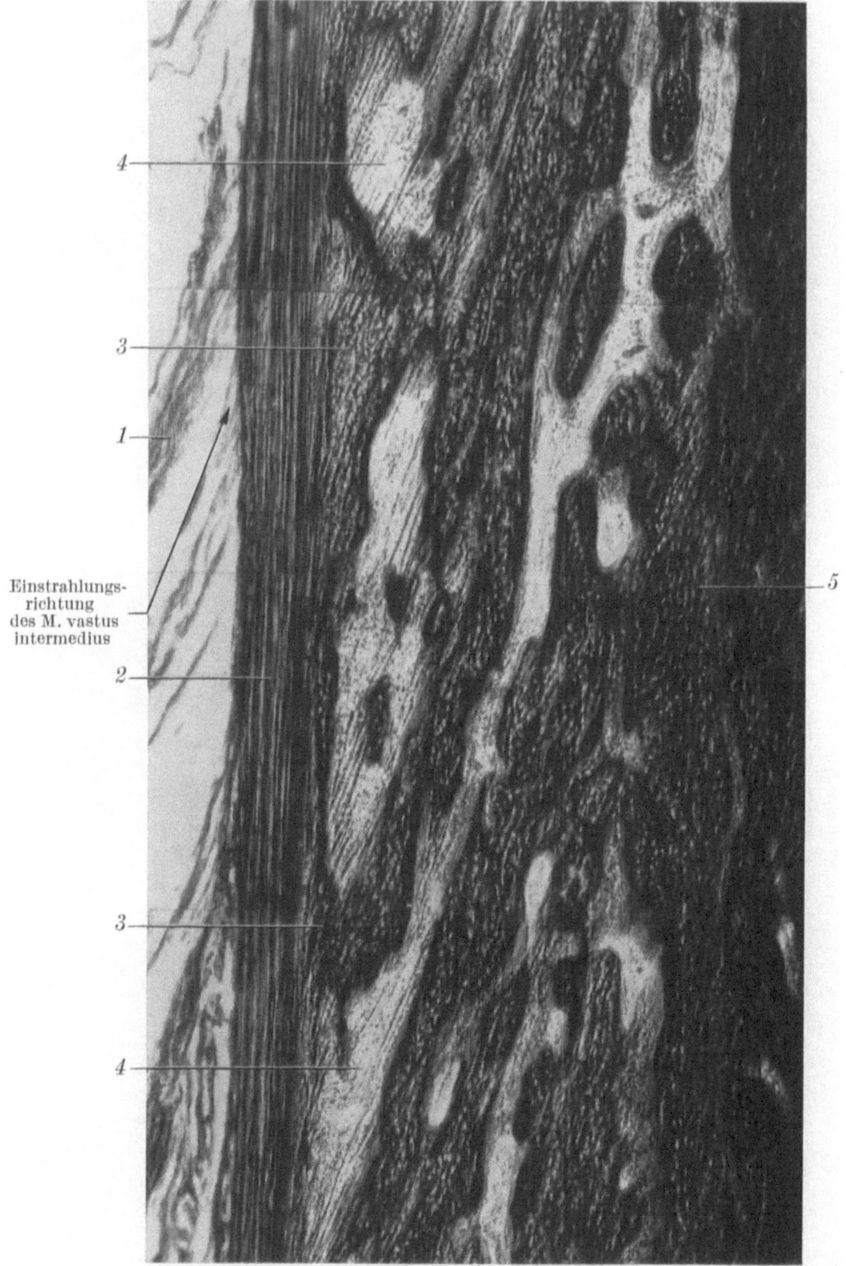

Abb. 49. Neonatus. Ansatz des M. vastus intermedius, längs. *1* Ursprungsfasern des M. vastus intermedius; *2* Periost; *3* Bildung von zellreichen Knochen in der Form von Knochenbälkchen; *4* intertrabeculäre Faserung; *5* „verdichtetes" Knochengewebe, überwiegend mit Längsgefäßen. Azan. Obj.Ph 10, Ok. 8. Photomontage. (BIERMANN, 1957)

den Nähten und an der Basis bleibt fester. Beschreibungen des Faserverlaufs im Periost liegen nicht vor. BIERMANN (1957) hat auf Grund der Untersuchung abgelöster Periost-streifen die Vermutung ausgesprochen, daß im Periost der Knochenflächen die elastischen Fasern mehr in Längsrichtung des Skeletstückes verlaufen, während an den Kanten eine Gitterordnung vorliegt.

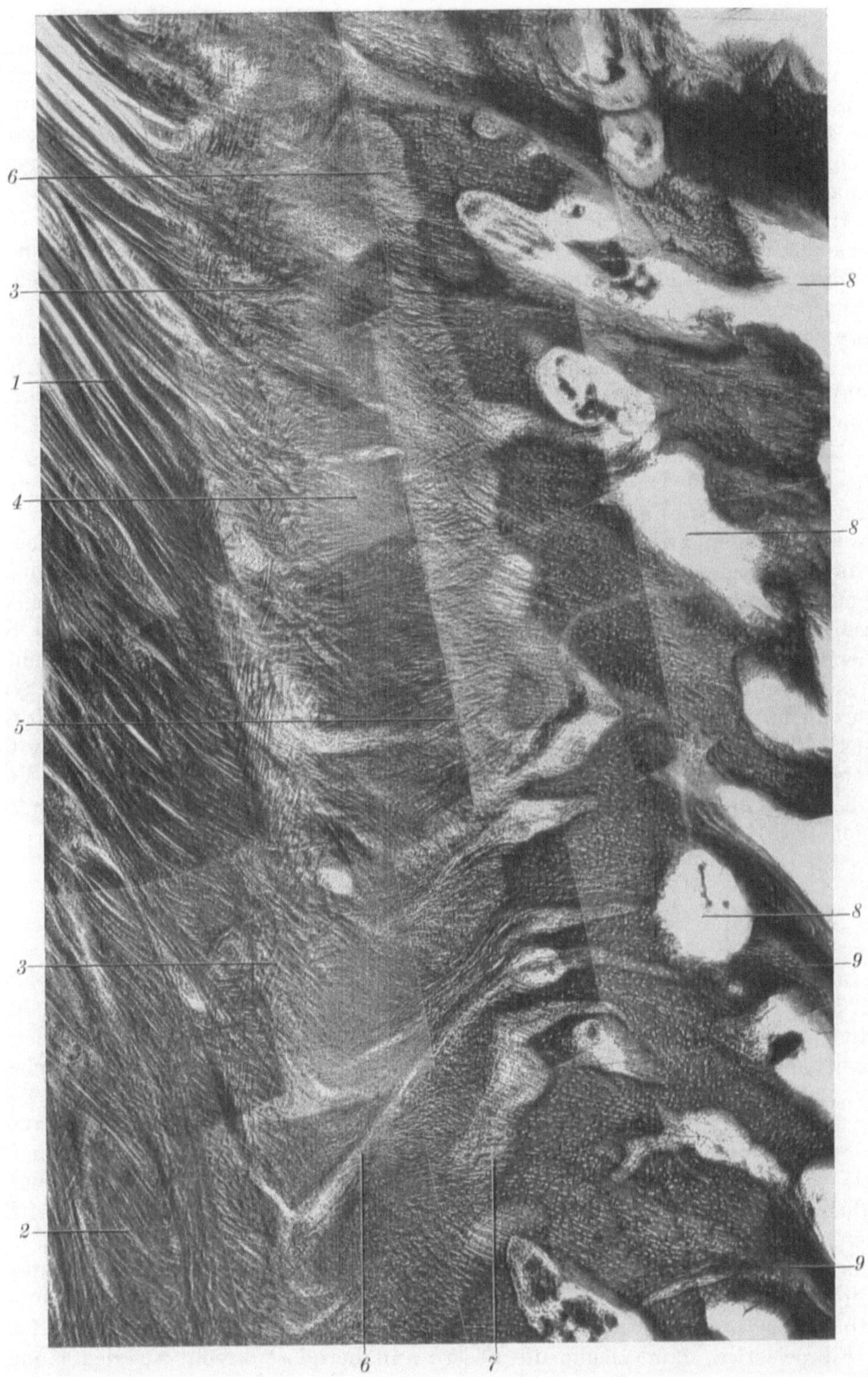

Abb. 50. Kind, 1 Jahr, 2 Monate. Tuberositas ulnae, längs. *1* Proximale Ansatzfaserung des M. brachialis; *2* distale Ansatzfaserung des M. brachialis mit beginnendem Übergang in das Periost unter Vermehrung der radiären, sowie der Knochenoberfläche parallelen elastischen Netze; *3* äußeres Netz der Ansatzstruktur; *4* Bildungsschicht mit geringfügiger Verquellung der Kollagenfasern und Vermehrung der Zellen; *5* inneres Netz der Ansatzstruktur; *6* Knochenbildung durch Einmauerung vorgebildeter Fasern; *7* aus dem Periost stammende radiäre in den Knochen ziehende Gefäße; *8* lacunäre Räume; *9* Knochengewebe mit beginnender Lamellierung um Markräume herum. Azan. Obj.Ph 10, Ok. 8. Photomontage. (Biermann, 1957)

Das Periost dient in großem Umfange Muskeln zum Ursprung. Bekanntlich wird im Diaphysenbereich zwischen einem fleischigen Ansatz am Periost und einem sehnigen an Kanten und Leisten gesprochen; DOLGO-SABUROFF (1929/30) unterscheidet periostale und tendinöse Ansätze. BIERMANN (1957) schlägt vor, flächenhafte und circumscripte Ansätze zu unterscheiden, da bei dem sog. fleischigen Ansatz in der mikroskopischen Dimension ebenfalls Sehnen vorliegen. Den Mechanismus der Kraftübertragung bei flächenhaften Ansätzen hat PETERSEN (1930) mit den Worten charakterisiert; „wenn ich die Hose habe, so habe ich auch das Bein, das darinsteckt" (s. S. 489).

Spezielle Untersuchungen über die Faserbeziehungen zwischen Periost und Knochen fehlen. Man begnügt sich mit der Feststellung, die Verbindung zwischen beiden würde durch Sharpeysche Fasern hergestellt; diese Beschreibung ist nicht gerechtfertigt (s. S. 324). BIERMANN (1957) hat in flächenhaften und circumscripten Ansätzen eine ähnliche Faserordnung aufgefunden. Die Sehnenfasern treten spitzwinklig in die Fibroelastica ein (Abb. 49), in der sie unter Änderung der Verlaufsrichtung zunächst verbleiben. Dann verlassen die Kollagenfasern das Periost und gehen in den Knochen über. Die Knochenbildung läuft ähnlich wie bei der Osteogenese unter Vorbildung von Fasern ab (v. Korffsche Fasern, s. S. 343). Die in den Knochen eingemauerten Fasern zeigen z. T. eine von der Sehne abweichende Faserordnung.

Die Beziehungen zwischen Periost und Knochen während des Wachstums waren Gegenstand experimenteller Untersuchungen. WARWICK und WILES (1934) haben nach Tuschemarkierung das Periostwachstum beim Kaninchen verfolgt. Sie kommen zu der Auffassung, daß das Periost interstitiell wächst wie alle anderen Organe des Körpers mit Ausnahme des Knochens (vgl. HEŘT, 1960). Demgemäß erfolgt eine Verschiebung des Periostes gegenüber dem Knochen. Die Befestigung an dem darunter liegenden Knochen muß durch eine „schnelle" Fixierung von neuen perforierenden Fasern hergestellt werden. LACROIX (1948, 1949, 1951) hält die Tuschemarkierung für unsicher und hat deshalb röntgenologisch verfolgbare Metallmarkierungen beim Kalbe angebracht. Der Verfasser meint, auf das Periost würde von der Epiphyse her ein Zug ausgeübt, so daß es über die Oberfläche des Knochens hinweggleitet (s. S. 398).

f) Die Struktur der Sehnen- und Bandansätze

Die Struktur der Sehnen- und Bandansätze an Kanten, Leisten und Höckern der Diaphyse wurde verschiedentlich untersucht (KASSOWITZ, 1879; WEIDENREICH, 1930; PETERSEN, 1930; DOLGO-SABUROFF, 1929/30, 1935; SCHABADASCH, 1935; AMPRINO und CATTANEO, 1937; WEINMANN und SICHER, 1955; LACROIX, 1951; BIERMANN, 1957). Knochen und Muskeln haben in ihrer ersten Anlage keine Beziehung zueinander. In der Gliedmaßenanlage differenziert sich zunächst ein Mesenchymkern als Anlage des Skeletorgans (CAREY, 1920; BIERMANN, 1957). Nach Ausdehnung des Skeletorgans wird eine Verbindung zu den Sehnen hergestellt. Im weiteren Verlauf der Entwicklung sind die Beziehungen zu den Sehnen sowie die Konstruktion der einzelnen Ansatzgebiete von einer unendlichen Vielfalt, worauf BIERMANN (1957) nach Untersuchung von 89 Ansatzpunkten bei sieben Individuen vom Neugeborenen bis zum Erwachsenen hinweist. Ähnlich wie bei Periostansätzen treten die Fasern spitzwinklig in die Fibroelastica ein, verbleiben z. T. in ihr oder verlassen sie sofort wieder. Die Kollagenfasern durchziehen die Cambiumschicht und werden in den Knochen eingemauert. In der Fibroelastica bilden die Sehnen- und Periostfasern zusammen ein spitzwinkliges Fasergitter. Mitunter liegt ein erstes Fasernetz in der Fibroelastica, dann ziehen die Fasern annähernd senkrecht auf den Knochen zu und bilden hier ein zweites Netz (Abb. 50).

Das durch die Cambiumschicht hindurchtretende Faserwerk wird zum Bestandteil des Skeletstückes. Diese Bildung wurde mitunter als geflechtartiger Knochen angesprochen (DIBBELT, 1911; PETERSEN, 1919; WEIDENREICH, 1923). Die Faserstruktur der Sehnenansätze entspricht jedoch nicht der des sog. grobfaserigen geflechtartigen Knochengewebes (Abb. 51). PETERSEN (1930) wird den Strukturunterschieden mit dem Terminus

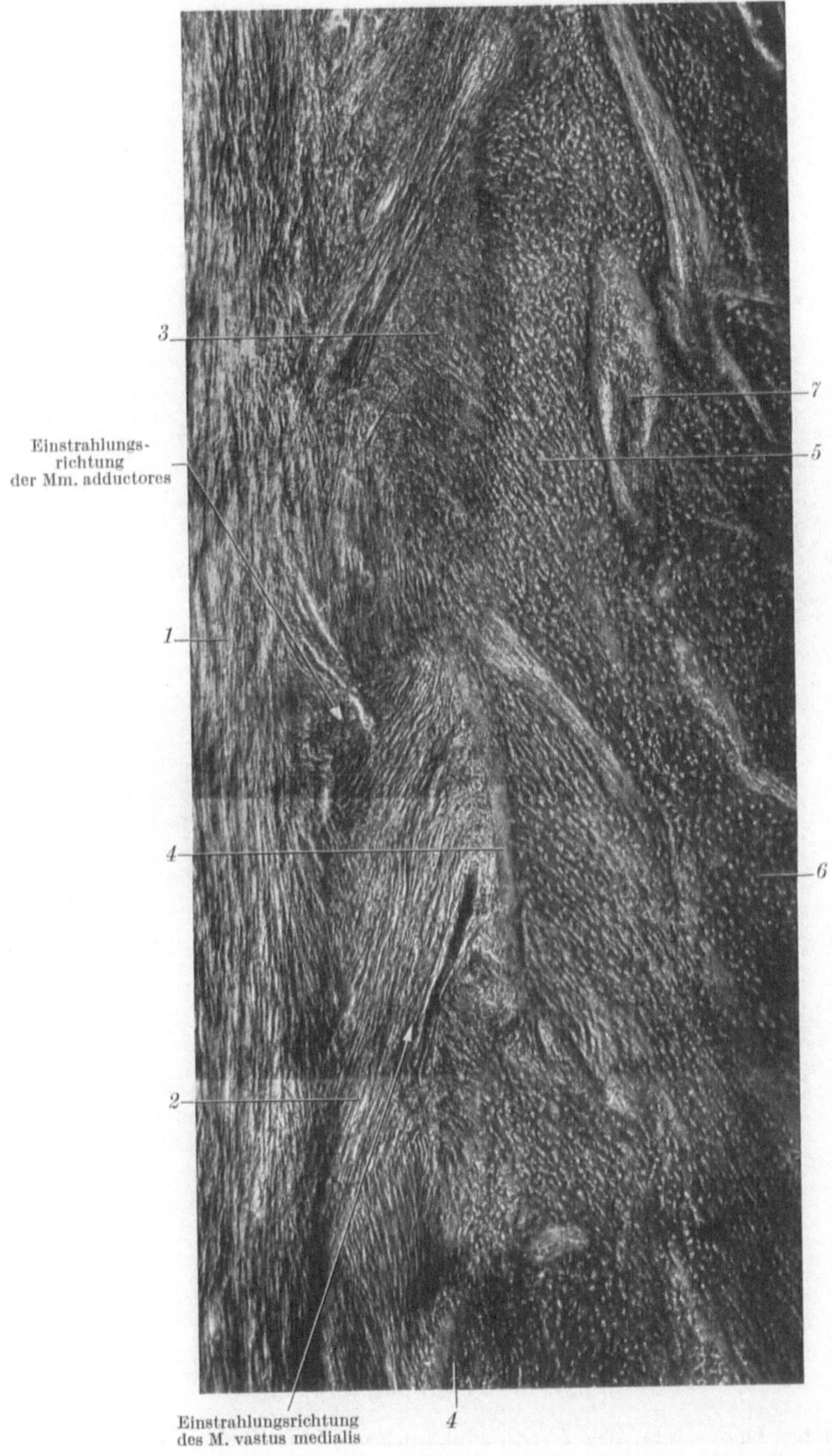

Abb. 51. Kind, 3 Monate. Linea aspera, Längsschnitt in Einstrahlungsrichtung der Mm. adductores et vastus medialis (bezeichnet). *1* Fibroelastica; *2* Ausscheren von Faserbündeln aus der Fibroelastica und deren Kreuzung in der Bildungsschicht; *3* Zwickel mit nicht deutlich erkennbarer Faserrichtung; *4* hyalin verquollene Streifen; *5* zellreicher Knochen; *6* zellarmer Knochen mit verdichteter Intercellularsubstanz; *7* Gefäße. Azan. Obj.Ph 10, Ok. 8. Photomontage. (Biermann, 1957)

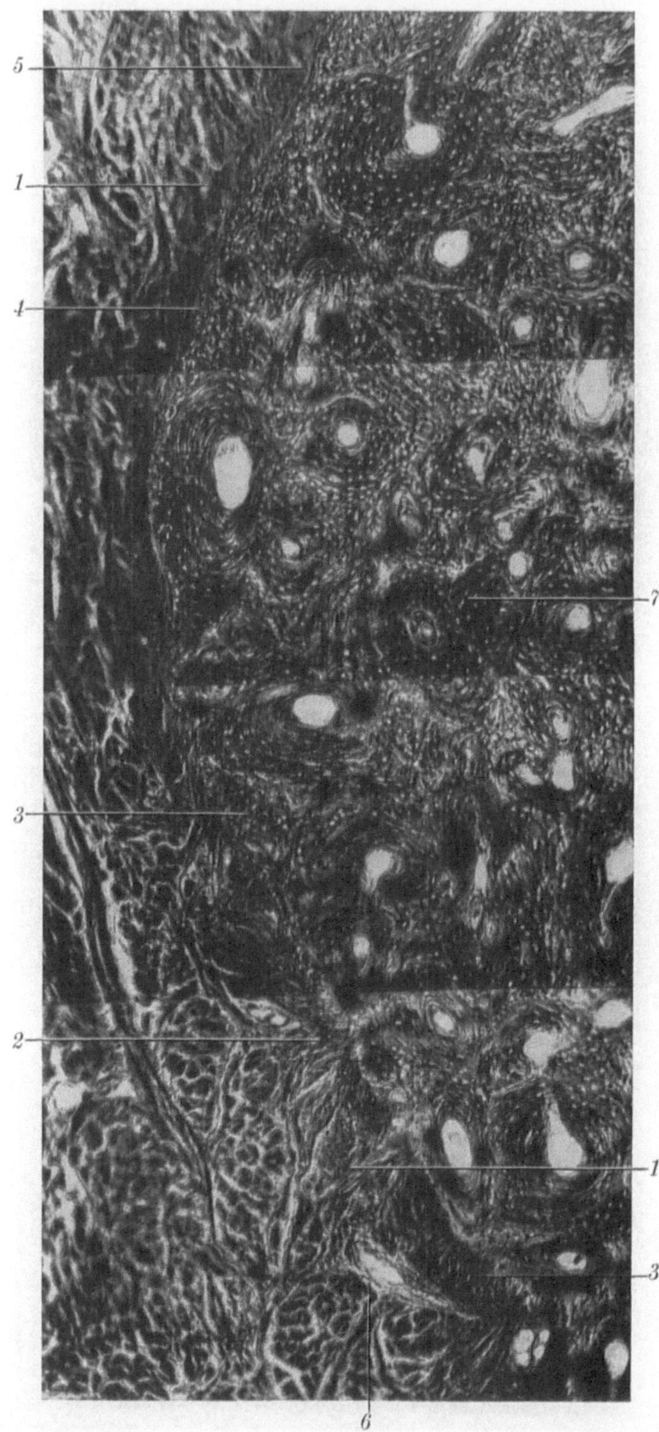

Abb. 52. Mann, 25 Jahre. Linea aspera, quer. *1* Verflechtungszone der Sehnenfasern; *2* Eindringen des Ansatzgewebes zwischen lamellären Knochenstrukturen; *3* allmählicher Übergang von Ansatzgewebe in Knochengewebe; *4* schmaler Streifen eines knöchernen Ansatzgewebes mit scharfem Übergang in „echtes" Knochengewebe; *5* Grenzstreifen; *6* größere längs verlaufende periostale Gefäße; *7* Knochengewebe mit verschieden weit differenzierten Osteonen. Azan. Obj.Ph 10, Ok. 8. Photomontage. (Biermann, 1957)

Einstrahlungsknochen gerecht. Die Faserordnung im Ansatzgebiet ist zunächst nicht „knochenspezifisch". Im weiteren Verlauf der Entwicklung nimmt diese Übergangszone an Dicke ab.

Die Struktur eines circumscripten Ansatzes weist in der endgültigen Ausprägung starke individuelle Unterschiede auf. Die Tuberositas glutea z.B. kann kompakt sein oder spongiöse Einschaltungen enthalten (Dolgo-Saburoff, 1935; vgl. Filogamo, 1945). Der Processus mastoideus ist pneumatisiert, enthält daneben Markräume, besteht nur aus Markhöhlen oder ist kompakt (Diamant, 1940). Spongiöse Einschaltungen in Ansätzen sind sehr häufig, auch an der Tuberositas deltoidea (Schabadasch, 1935; Knese, Ritschl und Voges, 1954). Derartige Hohlräume werden von den Kollagenfasern korbartig umschlossen (Biermann, 1957).

Die Annahme, daß die Osteonordnung unter Sehnenansätzen eine Störung erfährt (Gebhardt, 1901; Filogamo, 1946; Amprino und Cattaneo, 1937), läßt sich nur z.T.

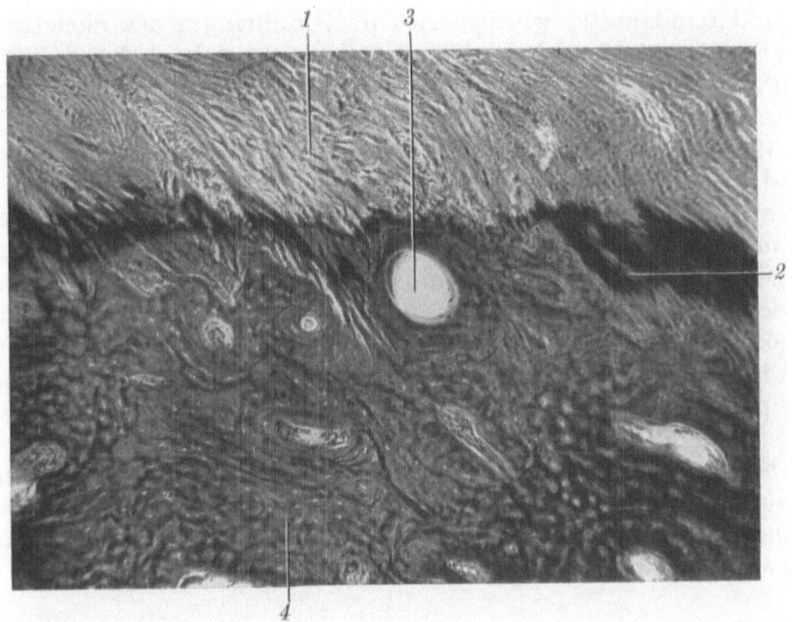

Abb. 53. Mann, 43 Jahre. Crista tuberculi majoris et minoris humeri. *1* Sehne mit teilweise blasig vergrößerten, reihenförmig gelagerten Sehnenzellen; *2* eingemauerter, knöcherner Anteil der Ansatzstruktur jenseits der Grenzlinie; *3* Randosteon; *4* überwiegend lamellärer Knochen. Azan. Obj.Ph 10, Ok. 8. (Biermann, 1957)

bestätigen. Schon Solger (1899) konnte an den Ansätzen der Ligg. flava keine Beeinflussung der Knochenstruktur beobachten. Allerdings ist es bisher nicht gelungen, die Beziehungen zwischen den Kollagenfasern der Sehnen sowie des Periostes und des Knochens beim Erwachsenen befriedigend aufzuklären. Biermann (1957) konnte an der Linea aspera zeigen, daß relativ grobe Bündel nach vielfältiger Durchflechtung wie abgeschnitten zwischen Osteonen enden, z.T. aber auch an eine scheinbar glatte Fläche herantreten (Abb. 52). An vielen Ansatzzonen wird die Sehne unter sog. „Verkalkung" Teil des Skeletstückes. Die Einpflanzung der Faserbündel zwischen Haversschen Systemen erfolgt erst in einem gewissen Abstand von der Knochenoberfläche (Abb. 53).

Die Frage, ob in diesen Ansatzgebieten ein Periost vorhanden ist oder nicht, wurde sehr unterschiedlich beantwortet (Literatur bei Schneider, 1956). Biermann (1957) und Knese und Biermann (1958) nehmen ein Periost besonderer Bauweise mit osteogenen Potenzen an, das sie die Ansatzstruktur nennen. Bidder (1906) und McLean und Bloom (1940) waren der Meinung, Sehnenzellen übernehmen die Rolle der Osteoblasten.

Jipp (1960) hat die Faserordnung in den Ansatzstrukturen präparatorisch untersucht und konnte wie z.T. auch Mollier (1937) und Biermann (1957) eine Aufteilung der an den Knochen herantretenden Sehnenbündel in Primärbündel beobachten. Die Primärbündel teilen sich in Sekundärbündel, die dann paarweise zu Tertiärbündeln verschmelzen und sich mit einer pinselförmigen Aufzweigung dem Knochen anlegen. Weiterhin hat JIPP (1960) die Verhältnisse des Periostes im Bereich der Ansätze untersucht. Das Periost spaltet sich bei Erreichen einer Ansatzsehne in zwei Anteile. Der periphere Teil geht in das Peritenonium externum der Sehne über, der andere liegt dem Knochen auf, verliert erheblich an Faserdichte und wird sehr weitmaschig. Diese Periostfasern über- und unterkreuzen sich mit Sehnenfasern, wobei auch ein Faseraustausch zwischen Sehne und Periost erfolgt. Wenn unter Periost eine ablösbare Membran verstanden wird, so fehlt in den Ansatzgebieten ein Periost; wird das Periost dagegen als umgebendes Bindegewebe des Skeletstückes definiert, das bei einer spezifischen Faserordnung osteogene Potenzen besitzt, muß auch an Sehnenansätzen von einem Periost besonderer Bauart gesprochen werden.

Sehnen- und Bandansätze wurden auch im Hinblick auf das Skeletwachstum untersucht. Muskelansätze im Bereich der Diaphyse behalten bekanntlich während des Wachstums ihre proportionale Lage zueinander und im Vergleich zum ganzen Skeletstück (WOLF, 1868; KREUZER, 1932). KASSOWITZ (1879), KAPSAMER (1897) und LACROIX (1948, 1949, 1951, 1960) nehmen an, daß während des Wachstums Höcker usw. an der einen Seite ab- und an der andern angebaut werden. Die Struktur der Ansätze soll mit dieser Annahme vereinbar und der Umbau nicht größer als im Verlauf der Dickenzunahme des Knochens sein. Bereits DOLGO-SABUROFF (1935) hat auf die Einheit des Knochen-Muskelsystems hingewiesen. Mit dem Abbau des Höckers verlieren Muskeln ihren Ansatz, am anderen Ende sind aber neue Muskelfasern erforderlich, d.h. der Umbau betrifft nicht nur den Knochen, sondern in gleichem Umfange den Muskel. Da aber durch die sog. motorische Einheit eine Beziehung zum Nervensystem besteht, ist eine ähnliche Revolution für den peripheren und zentralen Teil des Nervensystems die unvermeidbare Folge (KNESE und TITSCHAK 1962). Von derartigen Umbauten des Zentralnervensystems ist aber nichts bekannt. Eine Untersuchung des Skeletwachstums unter Berücksichtigung des Systemzusammenhanges Skelet-Muskel-Nerv-Zentralnervensystem wird vermutlich zu Vorstellungen über die Histogenese im Bereich der Sehnenansatzzonen kommen, die von den bisherigen abweichen.

g) Die Gefäßversorgung des Knochens

Die Untersuchung des Gefäßsystemes des Knochens erfolgte im Hinblick auf die Herkunft der Gefäße, die Verbindungen der Gefäße verschiedener Quelle, die Verteilung im Knochen und schließlich die Veränderungen im Laufe des Lebens. Weiterhin wurden die Beziehungen zwischen Gefäßverteilung und Knochenbildung diskutiert. RUTISHAUSER et al. (1954) kommen zum Abschluß ihres umfangreichen Überblickes allerdings zur Feststellung, daß unsere Kenntnisse über die Gefäßversorgung des Knochens fragmentarisch sind; viele Punkte seien noch unklar, wenn nicht sogar vollkommen dunkel.

In den langen Knochen sind vier Gefäßzuflüsse zu unterscheiden: A. nutricia, periostale Arteriolen, metaphysäre und epiphysäre Arterien. Die Versorgung der kurzen Knochen ist denen der Epiphysen ähnlich.

Nach LEXER (1904) liegen bei Kindern drei Stromgebiete vor, das epiphysäre, metaphysäre und diaphysäre. In der sog. primären, prähaversschen Compacta der Tibia des Menschen fand HEŘT (1960) im enchondralen Knochen ein Gefäßnetz mit langen Maschen. Im periostalen Knochen verlaufen die Gefäße fächerförmig zum Wachstumszentrum hin, im endostalen nach innen und schräg gegen die Metaphyse. Zwischen diesen Gefäßen bestehen Anastomosen. Eine Verbindung zum Periost und Mark ist vorhanden. Nach BROOKES (1958) werden Tibia und Femur menschlicher Feten vom Knochenmark her versorgt. Eine Verbindung zu den periostalen Gefäßen ist nur im Bereich der Capillaren vorhanden. TILLING (1958) gibt jedoch an, daß die peripheren Diaphysengefäße vom Periost abstammen. Damit liegen nach wie vor (vgl. RUTISHAUSER et al., 1954) einander widersprechende Angaben über die Versorgung der Compacta vor.

Seit SCHWALBES (1876) Untersuchungen wird der Lage und Richtung der Foramina nutricia ein besonderes Augenmerk gewidmet. Man nahm an, daß sich aus der Richtung des Canalis nutricius eine verschiedene Aktivität der Epiphysen und damit ein unterschiedlicher Beitrag zum Längenwachstum der Diaphyse ergibt (DIGBY, 1916; BISGARD et al., 1935; LACROIX, 1948; LÜTKEN, 1950; HUGHES, 1952). HEŘT (1957), HEŘT und NOVAK (1957) haben für die menschlichen Extremitätenknochen, SHULMAN (1959) für Radius und Ulna die Variation der Lage der Foramina nutricia untersucht. HUGHES (1952) konnte zeigen, daß anomale Kanäle am Femur beim Menschen selten, bei Tieren jedoch häufig vorkommen. Die A. nutricia teilt sich in einen auf- und einen absteigenden Ast. Als Versorgungsgebiet wird das Knochenmark und die innere Schicht der Compacta oder die ganze Compacta angesehen (BROOKES, 1958; Abb. 54, 55).

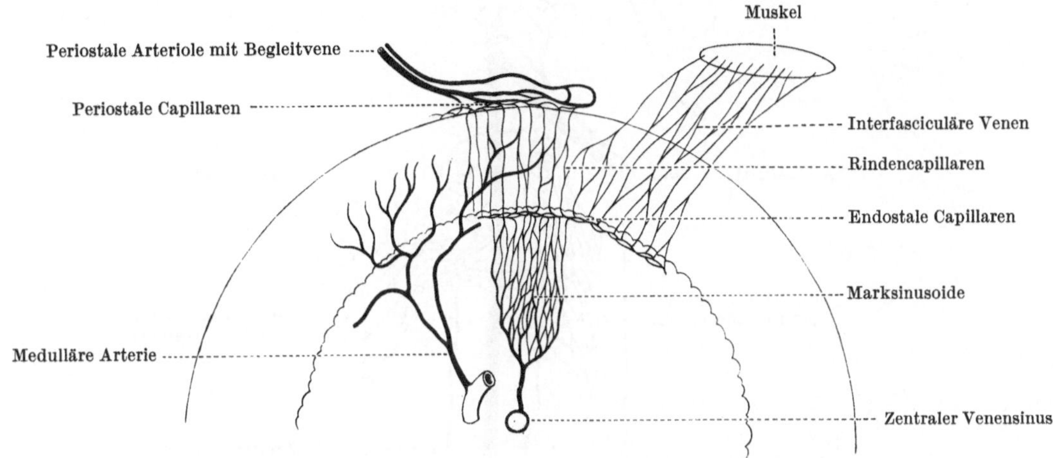

Abb. 54. Die Blutversorgung der Diaphyse, dargestellt an einem Querschnitt. (Aus: BROOKES; 1958, mit Erlaubnis des Autors und des Verlages)

HEŘT (1959) hat aus seinen Untersuchungen über die Ernährungskanäle den Anteil der proximalen und distalen Epiphyse an der Bildung der Diaphyse in Prozenten angegeben: Humerus: 80,2:19,8; Radius: 20,0:80,0; Ulna: 15,2:84,8; Femur: 25,4:74,6; Tibia: 50,7:49,3; Fibula: 58,9:41,1.

Die Knochenenden werden von einer verschieden großen Anzahl von Gefäßen versorgt, deren Querschnitt bedeutend größer als jener der A. nutricia ist (BROOKES 1958). Aus den metaphysären Gefäßen und der A. nutricia wird ein medulläres Arteriensystem gespeist. Umfangreiche Untersuchungen über die Versorgung des proximalen Femurendes liegen von TRUETA und HARRISON (1953) vor. Im Verlaufe der Entwicklung tritt eine Veränderung der Versorgung auf (TRUETA, 1957): bis zum 4.—5. Jahr fehlt ein Blutzufluß über das Lig. capitis femoris, der erst nach dem 8. oder 9. Jahr einsetzt; bis zu diesem Zeitpunkt erfolgt die Ernährung über metaphysäre Gefäße, die dann an Bedeutung verlieren. Epiphysäre Gefäße versorgen zunächst den Epiphysenknorpel und verlaufen in Knorpelkanälen (BIDDER, 1906; HINTZSCHE, 1927; HAINES, 1934). Die Beziehungen zum Knochenkern bilden sich erst später aus.

LANGER (1876), LEXER (1904) und BIDDER (1906) waren der Meinung, daß durch die Epiphysenplatte hindurch eine Verbindung zwischen epiphysären und metaphysären Gefäßen besteht. Spätere Untersucher (HARRIS, 1930; DE MARNEFFE, 1951) sahen die Epiphysenplatte als eine Gefäßbarriere an. Nach RUBASCHEWA und PRIWES (1932) treten Anastomosen erst im Laufe der Entwicklung auf; ähnliche Angaben liegen von TRUETA (1957) für das proximale Femurende vor. TILLING (1958) fand bei menschlichen Feten und beim Kalbe im Epiphysenknorpel lange vor der Entwicklung des Knochenkernes eine große Anzahl von Gefäßen. Die Beobachtungen von DE MARNEFFE (1951) und DALE

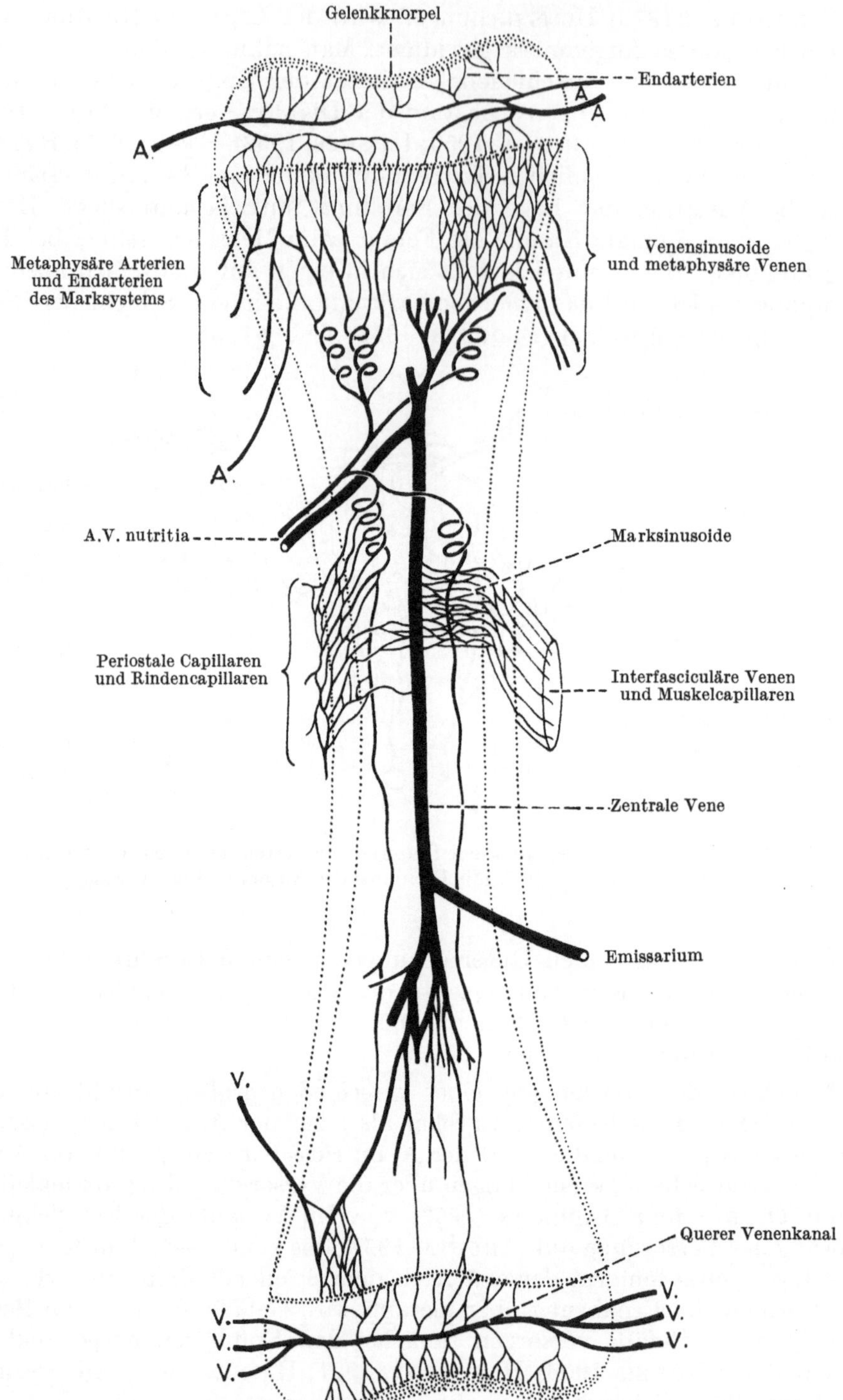

Abb. 55. Diagramm der Gefäßversorgung eines Knochens der Ratte in Längsschnitt. (Aus: Brookes, 1958; mit Erlaubnis des Autors und des Verlages)

und Harris (1958) lassen vermuten, daß in der Gefäßversorgung nicht nur Lebensaltersdifferenzen, sondern auch Unterschiede zwischen den einzelnen Skeletstücken bestehen.

Umfangreiche Untersuchungen über die Venen führte Hashimoto (1935, 1936) aus. Der Autor beschreibt einen zentralen Venenstamm von Metaphyse zu Metaphyse, dessen Ableitung über die Vena nutritia und die Metaphysenvenen erfolgt. Nach Ecoiffie et al.

(1957) haben die Venen eine doppelte Aufgabe, nämlich die Ableitung aus dem Knochen und Sammlung der Knochenmarkprodukte. Das Venenvolumen übersteigt das der Arterien um das 6—8fache (SCHOLDER, 1953).

Im Hinblick auf die Verteilung der Gefäße im Knochen selbst liegt die Frage nahe, ob Beziehungen zur Knochenbildung bestehen. Im Gegensatz zu der verbreiteten Auffassung vom provisorischen Charakter des sog. primären Knochens fällt auf, daß dieser Knochen eine bestimmte Ordnung aufweist. Die erste Knochenbildung ist nicht nur eine Gewebebildung, sie führt auch zur Anlage des Skeletstückes mit einer spezifischen Struktur (KNESE 1956b, 1959a). Es werden Bälkchen von bestimmter Dicke und vermutlich auch bestimmtem Abstand voneinander gebildet (BAHLING 1958; PINARD 1952). VONWILLER (1923) wies auf die engen Beziehungen von Gefäßen und Knochen in den knorpelig vorgebildeten Wirbeln hin. Die Gefäßarchitektur des Periosts in Beziehung auf die Knochenbildung hat HINTZSCHE (1926) diskutiert. Für die Deckknochen des Schädels beschrieb DZIALLAS (1952, 1954, 1958) das Aussprossen der Diploevenen aus Stammgefäßen. Das Verbreitungsgebiet jeder Vene entspricht einem Skeletelement. Zwischen den Venen werden die Knochenbälkchen abgelagert und schließlich in den Knochen eingeschlossen. Die Venen behalten während der Zunahme des Schädelumfanges ihre Lage in der Diploe bei.

Die Erforschung der Struktur und Ultrastruktur des Knochengewebes blickt auf eine hundertjährige Geschichte zurück. Ohne viele sog. ältere Befunde sind neuere Arbeiten undenkbar und unverständlich. Nach wie vor gilt aber PETERSENS (1927) Ausspruch: „Ein eingehendes Studium der Knochenstruktur des Menschen selbst, nicht so sehr der darüber geschriebenen Arbeiten, zeigte, welche Fülle ungelöster Fragen auch diese Organe mmer noch bieten.“

Literatur

ACHARD, J.: Physikochemische Untersuchungen am lamellären Knochen. Z. Zellforsch. **23**, 573—588 (1935).

AEBY, C.: Über Knochenwachstum. Tagebl. 49, Verslg dtsch. Naturf. Hamburg 1876, Beil., S. 126.

AMPRINO, R.: Transformations histologiques pendant l'accroissement et la remaniement du col du fémur après la naissance. C.R. Ass. Anat. **32**, 19—35 (1937).

— A contribution to the functional meaning of the substitution of primary by secondary bone tissue. Acta anat. (Basel) **5**, 291—300 (1948).

— Rapporti fra processi di ricostruzione dei minerali nelle ossa. I. Ricerche esiguite col metodo di studio dell' assorbimento dei raggi roentgen. Z. Zellforsch. **37**, 144—183 (1952a).

— Rapporti fra processi di ricostruzione e distribuzione dei minerali nella ossa. II. Ricerche con metodo autoradiografico. Z. Zellforsch. **37**, 241—273 (1952b).

— Struttura microscopica e rinovamento delle ossa. Atti Soc. ital. Pat. **4**, 9—68 (1955).

— On the growth of cortical bone and the mechanismus of the osteon formation. Acta anat. (Basel) **52**, 177—187 (1963).

—, e A. BAIRATI: Processi di riconstruzzione e di riassorbimento nella sostanza compatta delle ossa dell'uomo. Ricerche su cento soggetti della nascita sino a tarda età. Z. Zellforsch. **24**, 439—511 (1936).

AMPRINO, R., e R. CATTANEO: Il substrato istologico delle varie modalità di inserzioni tendinee alle ossa nell'uomo. Ricerche su individui di varia età. Z. Anat. Entwickl.-Gesch. **107**, 680—705 (1937).

—, and A. ENGSTRÖM: Studies on x-ray absorption and diffraction of bone tissue. Acta anat. (Basel) **15**, 1—22 (1952).

—, e G. GODINA: La struttura delle ossa nei vertebrati. Ricerche comparative negli anfibi e negli amnioti. Pontif. Acad. Sci., Acta. Commentationes **11**, 329—462 (1947).

— — Osservationi sul rinnovamento strutturale dell'osso in Pesci teleostei. Pubbl. Staz. zool. Napoli **28**, 62—71 (1956).

—, and G. MAROTTI: A topographic quantitative study of bone formation and reconstruction. In: Bone and tooth. Proc. 1st. Europ. Sympos. 1963 (ed. by H. J. J. BLACKWOOD), p. 21—48. Oxford-London-New York-Paris: Pergamon Press 1964.

AREY, L. B.: The origin, growth and fate of osteoclasts and their relation to bone resorption. Amer. J. Anat. **26**, 315—337 (1920).

ARMSTRONG, W. D.: Phosphorus metabolism in the skeleton. In: Phosphorus metabolism; A symposioum on the role of phosphorus in the metabolism of plants and animals (W. D. MCELROY and B. GLASS, eds), vol. 2, p. 698—731. Baltimore: Johns Hopkins Press 1952.

— Radiotracer studies of hard tissues. Ann. N.Y. Acad. Sci. **60**, 670—684 (1955).

ASCENZI, A.: La struttura dell'osseo umano osservata al microscopio elettronico. R. C. Ist. sup. Sanità 12, 893—902 (1949).
— Die Knochengewebestruktur, untersucht mit dem Elektronenmikroskop. Sci. medica ital. 8, 701—730 (1955).
— The relationship between mineralization and bone matrix. In: Bone and tooth (ed. by H. J. J. BLACKWOOD), p. 231—243. Oxford: Pergamon Press 1964.
—, e E. L. BENEDETTI: Osservazioni sistematiche sulla struttura del metaplama osseo esequite mediante il microscopio elettronico. Arch. Sci. biol. (Bologna) 38, 234—248 (1954).
— — An electron microscopic study of the foetal membranous ossification. Acta anat. (Basel) 37, 370—385 (1959).
— E. BONUCCI, and D. S. BOCIARELLI: An electron microscope study of osteon calcification. J. Ultrastruct. Res. 12, 287—303 (1965).
ASKANAZY, M.: Über das basophile Portoplasma des Osteoblasten, Osteoklasten und anderer Gewebszellen. Zbl. allg. Path. path. Anat. 13, 369—378 (1902).
ASTBURY, W. T.: Adventures in molekular biology. The Harvey Lectures, Ser. XI, VI, p. 3—44. Springfield (Ill.): Ch. C. Thomas 1950—1951.
AUERBACH, E.: Untersuchungen über die Variation der Knochenstruktur, dargestellt an der Tibia. Inaug.-Diss. der Med. Fakult. Kiel (1957).
AYER, J. P.: Elastic tissue. Int. Rev. connect. Tissue Res. 2, 33—100 (1964).
BAHLING, G.: Entwicklung des Querschnittes der großen Extremitätenknochen bis zum Säuglingsalter. Morph. Jb. 99, 109—188 (1958).
BAHR, G. F.: The reconstitution of collagen fibrils as revealed by electronmicroscopy. Exp. Cell Res. 1, 603—606 (1950).
— Ergebnisse elektronenmikroskopischer Untersuchungen des kollagenen und elastischen Gewebes. Arch. Derm. Syph. (Berl.) 193, 518—526 (1951).
BAIRATI, A.: Submikroskopische Struktur des Kollagens. III. Silberfärbung der Bindegewebe. Sci. med. ital., dtsch. Ausgabe 7, 273—320 (1958).
BALAZS, A., and H. HOLMGREN: Wound extracts and their effects on the growth of the fibroblasts. Nature (Lond.) 163, 488—489 (1949).
— — The basic dye uptake and the presence of a growth inhibiting substance in the healing tissue of skin wounds. Exp. Cell Res. 1, 206—216 (1950).
—, and R. W. JEANLOZ: The amino sugars, vol. IIA (1965); vol. IIB (1966). New York and London: Pergamon Press.
—, and H. J. ROGERS: The amino sugar-containing compounds in bones and teeth. In: The amino sugar (ed. by E. A. BALAZS and R. W. JEANLOZ), vol. IIA, p. 281—307. New York and London: Academic Press 1965.
BALOGH, K., H. R. DUDLEY, and R. B. COHEN: Oxidative enzyme activity in skeletal eartilage and bone. A histochemical study. Lab. Invest. 10, 839—843 (1961).
BANGA, I., and J. BALO: The structure and chemical composition of connective tissue. Connective tissue, ed. by R. E. TUNBRIDGE, M. KEECH, J. F. DELAFRESNAYE and G. C. WOOD, p. 254—263. Oxford: Blackwell Sci. Publ. 1957.
BARGMANN, W.: Histologie und mikroskopische Anatomie des Menschen, 3. Aufl. Stuttgart: Georg Thieme 1959.
BARNICOT, N. A.: Studies on the factors involved in bone absorption. I. The effects of subcutaneous transplantation of bones of the grey-lethal house mouse into normal hosts and of normal bones into grey-lethal hosts. Amer. J. Anat. 68, 497—531 (1941).
— The supravital staining of osteoblasts with neutralred: their distribution on the parietal bone of normal, growing mice, and a comparison with the mutants grey-lethal and hydrocephalus-3. Proc. roy. Soc. B 134, 467—485 (1947).
— The local action of the parathyroid and other tissues on bone in intracerebral grafts. J. Anat. (Lond.) 82, 233—248 (1948).
— The local action of vitamin A on bone. J. Anat. (Lond.) 84, 374—387 (1950).
—, and S. P. DATTA: Vitamin A and bone. In: BOURNE, The biochemistry and physiology of bone, p. 507—537. New York: Academic Press 1956.
BASSETT, D. L.: Current concepts of bone formation. J. Bone Jt Surg. A 44, 1217—1244 (1962).
BAUD, C. A.: Morphologie et structure inframicroscopique des ostéocytes. Acta anat. (Basel) 51, 209—225 (1962).
— The fine structure of normal and parathormone-treated bone cells. In: Calcified tissues. 4th Europ. Sympos. (ed. by P. J. GAILLARD, A. VAN DEN HOOFF, and R. STEENDIJK), p. 4—6. Amsterdam-London-New York: Excerpta Medica Foundation 1966.
BEAR, R. S.: X-ray diffraction studies on protein fibers. I. The large fiber axis period of collagen. J. Amer. chem. Soc. 66, 1297—1305 (1944).
— X-ray diffraction study. A review of recent researches which concern collagen. J. Amer. Leather Chemistri Ass. 46, 438—445 (1951).
— The structure of collagen fibrils. Advanc. Protein Chem. 7, 69—160 (1952).
—, and R. S. MORGAN: The composition of bands and interbands of collagen fibrils. In: Connective Tissue, ed. by R. E. TUNBRIDGE, p. 321—333. Oxford: Blackwell Sci. Publ. 1957.
BECHER, H., K. HOEGEN u. G. PFEFFERKORN: Sublichtmikroskopisch-morphologische Untersuchungen des anorganischen Knochenanteils. Acta anat. (Basel) 20, 105—115 (1954).
BEEK jr., J.: The carbohydrate content of collagen. J. Res. nat. Bur. Standards 27, 507—517 (1941a).

BEEK jr., J.: The carbohydrate content of collagen. J. Amer. Leather Chemists' Ass. 36, 696—710 (1941b).
BÉLANGER, L. F., T. SEMBA, S. TOLNAI, D. H. COPP, L. KROOK, and C. GRIES: The two faces of resorption. In: Calcified tissues. Proc. 3rd Europ. Sympos. (ed by H. FLEISCH, H. J. J. BLACKWOOD and M. OWEN), p. 1—10. Berlin-Heidelberg-New York: Springer 1965.
BENOIT, J., et J. CLAVERT: Étude histologique de l'ossification folliculinique chez les oiseaux. Bull. Histol. Techn. micr. 20, 25—42 (1943).
— — Comportement des ostéoclastes vis-à-vis de travées osseuses non calcifiées chez le canard domestiques. C.R. Soc. Biol. (Paris) 141, 911—912 (1947).
— — Différenciation et comportement des ostéoclastes chez les oiseaux. Arch. Anat. (Strasbourg) 34, 63—70 (1952).
BERTELSEN, A.: Experimental investigations into post-foetal osteogenesis. Acta orthop. scand. 15, 139—181 (1944).
BEVELANDER, G., and P. L. JOHNSON: A histochemical study of the development of membrane bone. Anat. Rec. 108, 1—21 (1950).
BIDDER, A.: Osteobiologie. Arch. mikr. Anat. 68, 137—213 (1906).
BIEDERMANN, W.: Physiologie der Stütz- und Skeletsubstanzen. XI. Knochengewebe. In: Handbuch der vergleichenden Physiologie, Bd. III/1/1, S. 1085—1188. Jena 1914.
BIERMANN, H.: Die Knochenbildung im Bereich periostaler-diaphysärer Sehnen- und Bandansätze. Z. Zellforsch. 46, 635—671 (1957).
BISGARD, J. D., and M. E. BISGARD: Longitudinal growth of long bones. Arch. Surg. 31, 568—578 (1935).
BLECHSCHMITDT, E.: Mechanische Genwirkung. Göttingen 1948.
BLOOM, M. A., L. V. DOMM, A. V. NABBANDOV, and W. BLOOM: Medullary bone of laying chickens. Amer. J. Anat. 102, 411—453 (1958).
BLOOM, W., M. A. BLOOM, and F. C. MCLEAN: Calcification and ossification. Medullary bone changes in the reproductive cycle of female pigeons. Anat. Rec. 81, 443—475 (1941).
BLUNTSCHLI, H.: Zur Frage nach der funktionellen Struktur und Bedeutung der harten Hirnhaut. Arch. Entwickl.-Med. Org. 106, 303—319 (1925).
BOGDASCHEW, N.: Funktionelle Unterscheidungsmerkmale im anatomisch-histologischen Bau der Röhrenknochen bei Haustieren. Anat. Anz. 79, 242—248 (1935).
BORASKY, R.: Guide to the literature on collagen. Philadelphia: Eastern Regional Laboratory 1950, 135p.
BOURNE, G. H.: Phosphatase and bone. The biochemistry and physiology, ed. by G. H. BOURNE, p. 251—284. 1956.
BOWES, J. H., R. G. ELLIOT, and J. A. MOSS: Some differences in the composition of collagen and extracted collagens and their relation to fiber formation and dispersion. In: Nature and structure of collagen, ed. by RANDALL, p. 199—207. London 1953.
BOWES, J. H., R. G. ELLIOT, and J. A. MOSS: The composition of some protein fractions isolated from bovine skin. In: Connective tissue, ed. by R. E. TUNBRIDGE, p. 264—280. Oxford: Blackwell Sci. Publ. 1957.
BOYDE, A., and M. H. HOBDELL: Scanning electron microscopy of lamellar bone. Z. Zellforsch. 93, 213—231 (1969).
BRACHET, J.: Chemical embryology. Translated by L. G. BARTH, p. 1—547. New York: Inkr. Publ. Inc. 1950.
BRADFIELD, J. R. G., and E. KODICEK: Abnormal mucopolysaccharide and "precollagen" in vitamin C-deficient skin wounds. Biochem. J. 49, 17—49 (1951).
BRANDENBERGER, E., u. H. R. SCHINZ: Über die Natur der Verkalkung bei Mensch und Tier und das Verhalten der anorganischen Knochensubstanz im Falle der hauptsächlichen menschlichen Knochenkrankheiten. Helv. med. Acta, Ser. A, 12, Suppl. 16, 1—63 (1945).
BRASH, J. C.: Some problems in the growth and developmental mechaniscs of bone. Edinb. med. J. 41, 305—319 (1934).
BROESICKE, G.: Über die feinere Struktur des normalen Knochengewebes. Arch. mikr. Anat. 21, 695—715 (1882).
BROOKES, M.: The vascularization of long bones in the human fetus. J. Anat. (Lond.) 92, 261—267 (1958).
— The vascular architecture of tubular bone in the rat. Anat. Rec. 132, 25—47 (1958).
BURKHARDT, L.: Über den Aufbau der menschlichen Osteone. Verh. anat. Ges. (Jena), Erg-H. zu Anat. Anz. 38, 97—102 (1929).
CABRINI, R. L.: Histochemistry of ossification. Rev. Cytol. 11, 283—306 (1961).
CAMERON, D. A., H. A. PASCHALL, and R. A. ROBINSON: The ultrastructure of bone cells. In: Bone biodynamics (ed. by H. M. FROST), p. 91—104. Boston, Mass.: Little, Brown & Co. 1964.
—, and R. A. ROBINSON: The presence of crystals in the cytoplasm of large cells adjacent to sites of bone absorption. J. Bone Jt Surg. A 40, 414—418 (1958).
CAPPELLIN, M.: Contributo alla citologia funzionale degli osteoblasti. Boll. Soc. ital. Biol. sper. 24, 1228—1229 (1948a).
— Azzione delle fosfatasi ossee sulla osteogenesi in vitro. Sperimentale 99, 133—145 (1948b).
CAREY, E. J.: Differential growth forces as stimuli to bone and muscle origin. Amer. Ass. Anat. Rec. 18, 224—225 (1920).
CARLSTRÖM, D.: X-ray crystallographic studies on apatites and calcified structures. Acta radiol. (Stockh.), Suppl. 121, 1—59 (1955).
—, and A. ENGSTRÖM: Ultrastructure and distribution of mineral salts in bone tissue. In: The biochemistry and physiology of bone (Ed. G. H. BOURNE), p. 149—176. New York: Academic Press Inc. 1956.

Carneiro, J., and C. P. Leblond: Role of osteoblasts and odontoblasts in secreting the collagen of bone and dentin, as shown by radioautography in mice given tritium-labelled glycine. Exp. Cell Res. **18**, 291—300 (1959).
Carver, J. P., and E. R. Blout: Polypeptide models for collagen. In: Treatise on collagen (ed. by G. N. Ramachandran), vol. 1, p. 441—523. London and New York: Academic Press 1967.
Caspersson, T. O.: Cell growth and cell function. A cytochemical study, p. 1—185. New York: W. W. Norton & Co. Inc. 1950.
Changus, G. W.: Osteoblastic hyperplasia of bone, a histochemical appraisal of fibrous dysplasia of bone. Cancer (Philad.) **10**, 1156—1161 (1957).
Chievitz, O., and G. Hevesy: Radioactive indicators in the study of phosphorus metabolism in rats. Nature (Lond.) **136**, 754 (1935).
Ch'uan, C. H.: Mitochondria in osteoclasts. Anat. Rec. **49**, 397—401 (1931).
Clark, S. M., and J. Iball: The x-ray crystal analysis of bone. Progr. Biophys. **7**, 225—253 (1957).
Clavert, J.: Contribution à l'étude de la formation des œufs-tilolécithiques des oiseaux. Mécanismes de l'édification de la coquille. Bull. biol. France et Belg. **82**, 289—330 (1948).
— Sur la teneur en acide ribonucléique des cellules de l'os. C.R. Acad. Sci. (Paris) **231**, 998—999 (1950).
Cohen, J., and W. H. Harris: The three-dimensional anatomy of Haversian systems. J. Bone Jt Surg. A **40**, 419—434 (1958).
—, and P. Lacroix: Comparison of microradiographic and histologic patterns in bone. Lab. Invest. **2**, 447—450 (1953).
Cohn, W. E., E. T. Cohn, and J. C. Aub: Calcium and phosphorus metabolism clinical aspects. Ann. Rev. Biochem. **11**, 415—440 (1942).
Comar, C. L., and F. Bronner: Mineral metabolism, vol. 1. New York and London: Academic Press 1960.
Dale, G. G., and W. R. Harris: Prognosis of epiphysial separation. An experimental study. J. Bone Jt Surg. B **40**, 116—122 (1958).
Dallemagne, M. J., et J. Mélon: La calcification des lamelles osseuses constitutives du système Haversiem. Arch. Biol. (Paris) **56**, 243—259 (1945).
Damas, H.: Le dévelopment de la tête de la lamproie (Lampetra fluviatilis L.). Ann. Soc. roy. zool. Belg. **73**, 201—211 (1942).
— Recherches sur le développement de lampetra fluviatilis L. Contribuion à l'étude de la céphalogénèse des vertébrés. Arch. Biol. (Liège) **55**, 1—284 (1944).
Dantschakoff, W.: Über die Entwicklung des Knochenwachstums bei den Vögeln und über dessen Veränderung bei Blutentziehung und Ernährungsstörungen. Arch. mikr. Anat. **74**, 855—894 (1909).
Davies, H. G., and A. Engström: Interferometric and x-ray absorption studies of bone tissue. Exp. Cell Res. **7**, 243—255 (1954).
Deakins, M.: Changes in the ash, water and organic content of pig enamel during calcification. J. dent. Res. **21**, 429—435 (1942).
—, and R. L. Burt: The deposition of calcium, phosphorus and carbon dioxide in calcifying dental enamel. J. biol. Chem. **56**, 77—83 (1944).
Demeter, G., u. J. Mátyás: Mikroskopisch vergleichend-anatomische Studien an Röhrenknochen mit besonderer Rücksicht auf die Unterscheidung menschlicher und tierischer Knochen. Z. Anat. Entwickl.-Gesch. **87**, 45—99 (1928).
Diamant, M.: Otitis and pneumatisation of the mastoid bone. Lund: Akademisk Avhandling 1940.
Dibbelt, W.: Beiträge zur Histogenese des Skeletgewebes und ihren Störungen. Beitr. path. Anat. **50**, 411—436 (1911).
Digby, K. H.: The measurement of diaphysial growth in proximal and distal directions. J. Anat. (Lond.) **50**, 187 (1916).
Dische, Z., A. Danilczenko, and G. Zelmanes: The neutral heteropolysaccharides in connective tissue. In: Ciba Found. Symp. Chemistry and biology of mucopolysaccharides, p. 116—135, ed. by G. E. W. Wolstenholme and M. O'Connor. London 1958.
—, and M. Osnos: Neutral mucopolysaccharides from various animal tissues. Fed. Proc. **9**, 165—166 (1950).
—, and G. Zelmanes: Polysaccharides of vitreous fibers. Arch. Ophthal. **54**, 528—538 (1955).
Dodds, G. S.: Osteoclasts and cartilage removal in endochondral ossification of certain mammals. Amer. J. Anat. **50**, 97—127 (1932).
Dolgo-Saburoff, B.: Über Ursprung und Insertion der Skeletmuskeln. Anat. Anz. **68**, 80—87 (1929/1930).
— Über einige Eigentümlichkeiten der Knochenstruktur an den Anheftungsstellen der Sehnen. Gegenbaurs morph. Jb. **75**, 393—411 (1935).
Dorfman, A.: The effects of adrenal hormones on connective tissues. Ann. N. Y. Acad. Sci. **56**, 698—703 (1953).
— Metabolism of the mucopolysaccharides of connective tissue. Connective tissue in health and disease, ed. by Asboe-Hansen. Kopenhagen 1954.
— Metabolism of the mucopolysaccharides of connective tissue. Pharmacol. Rev. **78**, 1—31 (1955/1956).
— Polysaccharides of connective tissue. J. Histochem. Cytochem. **11**, 2—13 (1963).
—, and M. B. Mathews: The physiology of connective tissue. Ann. Rev. Physiol. **18**, 69—88 (1956).
Dudley, H. R., and D. Spiro: The fine structure of bone cells. J. biophys. biochem. Cytol. **11**, 627—649 (1961).
Duran-Reynals, F.: The ground substance of the mesenchyme and hyaluronidase. Ann. N. Y. Acad. Sci. **52**, 943—1196 (1950).

DZIALLAS, P.: Die Entwicklung der Venae diploicae beim Haushunde und ihr Einfluß in das knöcherne Schädeldach. Gegenbaurs morph. Jb. **92**, 500—576 (1952).
— Zur Entwicklung des menschlichen Schädeldaches. Anat. Anz. **100**, 236—242 (1954).
— Über das Verhalten der Diploëvenen zu den Anlagen der Deckknochen des Schädels. Acta anat. (Basel) **34**, 35—52 (1958).
EASTOE, J. E.: The amino acid composition of mammalian collagen and gelatin. Biochem. J. **61**, 489—600 (1955).
— The organic matrix of bone. The biochemistry and physiology of bone, ed. by G. H. BOURNE, p. 81—103. New York: Academic Press 1956.
— Composition of collagen and allied proteins. In: Treatise on collagen (ed. by G. N. RAMACHANDRAN), vol. 1, p. 1—67. London and New York: Academic Press 1967.
— Chemical aspects of the matrix concept in calcified tissue organisation. Calc. Tiss. Res. **2**, 1—19 (1968).
—, and B. EASTOE: The organic constituents of mammalian compact bone. Biochem. J. **57**, 453—459 (1954).
EBNER, V. v.: Untersuchungen über das Verhalten des Knochengewebes im polarisierten Licht. S.-B. Akad. Wiss. Wien, math.-nat. Kl., III, **70**, 105—143 (1874).
— Über den feineren Bau der Knochensubstanz. S.-B. Akad. Wiss. Wien, math.-nat. Kl., III, **72**, 49—138 (1875).
— Sind die Fibrillen des Knochengewebes verkalkt oder nicht? Arch. mikr. Anat. **29**, 213—236 (1887).
ECOIFFIE, J., D. PROT, R. GRIFFIE et D. CATACH: Etude du réseau veineux dans les os longs du lapin. Rev. Chir. orthop. **43**, 29—37 (1957).
EGGELING, H. v.: Der Aufbau der Sekeletteile in den freien Gliedmaßen der Wirbeltiere. Jena: Gustav Fischer 1911.
ENGEL, M. B., N. R. JOSEPH, and H. R. CATCHPOLE: Homeostasis of connective tissues. I. Calcium-sodium equilibrium. Arch. Path. **58**, 26—29 (1954).
ENGSTRÖM, A., and B. ENGFELDT: Lamellar structure of osteon demonstrated by microradiography. Experientia (Basel) **9**, 19 (1953).
—, and J. B. FINEAN: Low-angle x-ray diffraction of bone. Nature (Lond.) **171**, 564 (1953).
— — Biological ultrastructure. New York: Academic Press 1958.
ERTELT, W.: Untersuchungen über Körpergröße und Knochenstruktur bei Säugetieren. Zool. Jb., Abt. Anat. u. Ontog. **74**, 588—638 (1955).
FELL, H. B.: Experiments on the differentiation in vitro of cartilage and bone. Arch. exp. Zellforsch. **7**, 390—412 (1928/29).
— Chondrogenesis in cultures of endosteum. Proc. roy. Soc. B **112**, 417—427 (1933).
— Skeletal development in tissue culture. The biochemistry and physiology of bone, ed. by G. H. BOURNE, p. 401—440. New York: Academic Press 1956.
FELL, H. B., and E. MELLANBY: Effect of hypervitaminosis. A on embryonic limb-bones cultivated in vitro. J. Physiol. (Lond.) **116**, 320—349 (1952).
FILOGAMO, G.: Contributo alla conoscenza della minuta struttura dell'osso. Osservazioni sulla zona d'attaco di tendini allo skeleto. R.C. Ist. lombardo Sci. pt. **78**, 425—448 (1945).
— La forme et la taille des ostéones chez quelques mammifères. Arch. Biol. (Paris) **57**, 137—143 (1946a).
— Forma e lunghezza degli osteoni della compatta delle ossa lunghe nell'uomo. Rec. morf. **22**, 91—98 (1946b).
— Precisazzioni sulla disposizione e sull'orientamento delle fibre collagene degli osteoni nell'uomo. Ric. morf. **22**, 99—104 (1946c).
FLEMMING, W.: Morphologie der Zelle. Ergebn. Anat. Entwickl.-Gesch. **6**, 184—283 (1896).
FOLLIS jr., R. H.: Some histochemical observations on normal and diseased cartilage and bone. Tr. Conf. Metab. Interrelat. **1**, 27—32 (1949).
— Histochemical studies on cartilage and bone. Ascorbic acid deficiency. Bull. Johns Hopk. Hosp. **89**, 9—20 (1951).
—, and M. BERTHRONG: Histochemical studies on cartilage and bone. Amer. J. Path. **24**, 685 (1948).
— — Histochemical studies on cartilage and bone. The normal pattern. Bull. Johns Hopk. Hosp. **85**, 281—297 (1949).
FOOTE, J. S. A.: The comparative histology of the femur. Smithsonian Miszellaneous collections **61**, Publ. 2232 Washington, p. 1 (1913).
FRANK, R., P. FRANK, M. KLEIN et R. FONTAINE: L'os compact humain normal au microscope électronique. Arch. Anat. micr. Morph. exp. **44**, 191—206 (1955).
FREY-WYSSLING, A.: Submicroscopic morphology of protoplasm. Amsterdam-Houston-London-New York: Elsevier Publ. Co. 1953.
FROST, H. M.: Halo Volume. Part IV. Measurement of the diffusion pathway between osteocyte lacuna and blood. Henry Ford Hosp. Bull. **9**, 137—144 (1961).
— Specific surface and specific volume of normal human lamellar bone. Henry Ford Hosp. Bull. **8**, 35 (1962).
— Mean formation time human osteons. Canad. J. Biochem. **41**, 1307—1310 (1963a).
— Bone remodeling dynamics. Springfield (Ill.): Ch. C. Thoms 1963b.
— Measurement of human bone formation by means of tetracycline labelling. Canad. J. Biochem. **41**, 31—42 (1963c).
— Dynamics of bone remodeling. In: Bone biodynamics (ed. by H. M. FROST), p. 31r—333. Boston, Mass.: Little, Brown & Co. 1964.
— A. R. VILLANUEVA, H. ROTH, and S. STANISAVLJEVIC: Tetracycline bone labeling. J. New Drugs **1**, 206—216 (1961).
— — J. R. RAMSER u. L. ILNICKI: Knochenbiodynamik bei 39 Osteoporose-Fällen, gemessen durch Tetracyclinmarkierung. Internist (Berl.) **7**, 572—578 (1966).

Fullmer, H. M.: The histochemistry of the connective tissues. Int. Rev. connective tissue Res. **3**, 1—76 (1965).
Furuta, W. J.: Demonstration of fibers in the decalcified bone matrix by enzymatic digestion. Anat. Rec. **104**, 309—317 (1949).
Gallop, P. M., O. O. Blumenfeld, and S. Seifter: Subunits and special structural features of tropocollagen. In: Treatise on collagen (ed. by G. N. Ramachandran), vol. 1, p. 339—365. London and New York: Academic Press 1967.
Gardner, E.: Osteogenesis in the human embryo and fetus. In: Bourne, The biochemistry and physiology of bone, p. 359—397. New York: Academic Press 1956.
Gebhardt, W.: Über qualitative und quantitative Verschiedenheiten der gestaltenden Reaktion des Knochengewebes. Verh. anat. Ges. Halle. 16. Vers. 1902. Erg.-H. zu Anat. Anz. **21**, 65—92 (1902).
— Über funktionell wichtige Anordnungsweisen der feineren und gröberen Bauelemente des Wirbeltierknochens. II. Spezieller Teil: 1. Der Bau der Haversschen Lamellensysteme und seine funktionelle Bedeutung. Arch. Entwickl.-Mech. Org. **20**, 187—322 (1906).
— Über funktionell wichtige Anordnungsweisen der gröberen und feineren Bauelemente des Wirbeltierknochens. Arch. Entwickl.-Mech. Org. **11**, 383—498; **12**, 1—52, 167—223 (1901).
Gegenbaur, C.: Über die Bildung des Knochengewebes. I. Jena. Z. Naturw. **1**, 343—369 (1864).
— Über die Bildung des Knochengewebes. II. Jena. Z. Naturw. **3**, 206—246 (1867).
Gersh, I., and H. R. Catchpole: The organization of ground substance and basement membrane and its significance in tissue injury, disease and growth. Amer. J. Anat. **85**, 457—521 (1949).
— — The nature of ground substance of connective tissue. Perspect. Biol. Med. **3**, 282—319 (1960).
Gibian, H.: Der Beitrag des Chemikers zur Struktur- und Funktionsaufklärung der mesenchymalen Grundsubstanz mit besonderer Bezugnahme auf die Hyaluronidase und ihre Substrate. Kapillaren und Interstitium. Stuttgart: Georg Thieme 1954.
— Mucopolysaccharide und Mucopolysaccharidasen. Einzeldarstellungen aus dem Gesamtgebiet der Biochemie (Herausg. O. Hoffmann-Ostenhof), Bd. 3, S. 1—319. Wien 1959.
Glättli, W.: Die Osteoklastenlehre. Inaug.-Diss. Univ. Bern 1947.
Glegg, R. E., and D. Eidinger: A method for fractionating the carbohydrate components of bone. Arch. Biochem. **55**, 19—24 (1955).
— — and C. P. Leblond: Some carbohydrate components of reticular fibers. Science **118**, 614—616 (1953).
— — — Presence of carbohydrates distinct from acid mucopolysaccharides in connective tissue. Science **120**, 839—840 (1954).
Glegg, R. E., and C. P. Leblond: Pressure as a possible cause of dissolution and redeposition of bone and tooth crystals. Canad. J. med. Sci. **31**, 202—206 (1953).
Glimcher, M. J.: Molecular biology of mineralized tissues with particular reference to bone. Rev. Modern Physics **31**, 359—393 (1959).
— Specificity of the molecular structure of organic matrices in mineralization. Calcific. Biol. System **64**, 421—487 (1960).
—, and S. M. Krane: The organization and structure of bone, and the mechanism of calcification. In: Treatise on collagen (ed. by G. N. Ramachandran), vol. 2 B, p. 68—241. London and New York: Academic Press 1968.
Glücksmann, A.: Studies on bone mechanics in vitro. I. Influence of pressure on orientation of structure. Anat. Rec. **72**, 97—113 (1938).
— The role of mechanical stresses in bone formation in vitro. J. Anat. (Lond.) **76**, 231—239 (1942).
Gonzales, F., and M. J. Karnovsky: Electron microscopy of osteoclasts in healing fractures of rat bone. J. biophys. biochem. Cytol. **9**, 299—316 (1961).
Gould, B. S.: Collagen biosynthesis. In: Treatise on collagen (ed. by G. N. Ramachandran), vol. 2 A, p. 139—183. London and New York: Academic Press 1968.
Grassmann, W., K. Hannig u. M. Plöcki: Eine Methode zur quantitativen Bestimmung der Aminosäurezusammensetzung von Eiweißhydrolysaten durch Kombination von Elektrophorese und Chromatographie. Hoppe-Seylers Z. physiol. Chem. **299**, 258—276 (1955).
— U. Hofmann, K. Kühn, H. Hörmann, H. Endres, and K. Wolf: Electronmicroscope and chemical studies of the carbohydrate groups of collagen. Connective tissue, ed. by R. E. Tunbridge, p. 157—171. Oxford: Blackwell Sci. Publ. 1957.
—, u. H. Schleich: Über den Kohlehydratgehalt des Kollagens. II. Mitt. zur Kenntnis des Kollagens. Biochem. Z. **277**, 230—328 (1935).
Graumann, W.: Topogenese der Bindegewebsknochen. Untersuchungen an Schädelknochen menschlicher Embryonen. Z. Anat. Entwickl.-Gesch. **116**, 14—26 (1951).
— Untersuchungen zum zytochemischen Glykogennachweis. 1. Mitteilung: Chemische Fixation auf Alkoholbasis. Acta histochem. (Jena) **4**, 29—40 (1957).
Greep, R. O., C. J. Fischer, and A. Morse: Alkaline phosphatase in odontogenesis and osteogenesis and its histochemical demonstration after demineralization. J. Amer. dent. Ass. **36**, 427—442 (1948).
Gross, J.: A study of certain connective tissue components with the electron microscope. Ann. N. Y. Acad. Sci. **52**, 964—970 (1950).
— In vitro fibrogenesis of collagen. Tr. Conf. Metab. Interrelat. **4**, 32—57 (1952).
— The behavior of collagen units as a model in morphogenesis. J. biophys. biochem. Cytol. **2**, Suppl. 261—273 (1956).

GROSS, J.: Studies on the formation of collagen. III. Time-dependent solubility changes of collagen. J. exp. Med. **108**, 215—226 (1958).
— J. H. HIGHBERGER, and F. O. SCHMITT: Extraction of collagen from connective tissue by neutral salt solutions. Proc. nat. Acad. Sci. (Wash.) **41**, 1—7 (1955).
—, and F. O. SCHMITT: The structure of human collagen as studied with the electron microscope. J. exp. Med. **88**, 555—568 (1948).
— — and J. H. HIGHBERGER: In vitro fibrogenesis of collagen. Tr. Conf. Metab. Interrelat. **4**, 32—57 (1952).
GROSS, O.: A study of the aging of collagenous connective tissue of rat skin with the electron microscope. Amer. J. Path. **26**, 708 (1950).
GROSS, W.: Die Typen des mikroskopischen Knochenbaues bei fossilen Stegocephalen und Reptilien. Z. Anat. Entwickl.-Gesch. **103**, 731—764 (1934).
GUSTAVSON, K. H.: The function of hydroxyproline in collagens. Nature (Lond.) **175**, 70—74 (1955).
— The chemistry and reactivity of collagen 1956. New York and London: Academic Press 1956.
HAGUENAU, F.: The ergastoplasm: its history, ultrastructure and biochemistry. Rev. Cytol. **7**, 425—484 (1958).
HAINES, R. W.: Cartilage canals. J. Anat. (Lond.) **68**, 45—64 (1933).
HALL, D. A.: Connective tissue fibers. Rev. Cytol. **8**, 212—252 (1959).
HAM, A. W.: The variability of the planes of cell division in the cartilage columns of the growing epiphyseal plate. Anat. Rec. **51**, 125—133 (1931).
— Some histophysiological problems peculiar to calcified tissues. J. Bone Jt Surg. A **34**, 701—728 (1952).
—, and W. B. HARRIS: Repair and transplantation of bone. The biochemistry and physiology of bone, ed. by G. H. BOURNE, p. 475—505. New York: Academic Press 1956.
HANCOX, N. M.: On the occurrence in vitro of cells resembling osteoclasts. J. Physiol. (Lond.) **105**, 66—71 (1946).
— The osteoclast. Biol. Rev. **24**, 448—471 (1949).
— The osteoclast. The biochemistry and physiology of bone, ed. by G. H. BOURNE, p. 213—247. New York: Academic Press 1956.
HANNIG, K., and A. NORDWIG: Amino acid sequences in collagen. In: Treatise on collagen (ed. by G. N. RAMACHANDRAN, vol. 1, p. 73—98. London and New York: Academic Press 1967.
HARKNESS, R. D., A. M. MARKO, H. M. MUIR, and A. NEUBERGER: Metabolism of collagen and other proteins of skin of rabbit. Biochem. J. **56**, 558—569 (1954).
HARRIS, H. A.: The vascular supply of bone with special references to the epiphysial cartilage. J. Anat. (Lond.) **64**, 3—4 (1929/1930).
HARRISON, R. G.: Heteroplastic grafting in embryology. Harvey Lect. 1933—1934, 116—157 (1935).
HARTMANN, A.: Zur Entwicklung des Bindegewebsknochens. Arch. mikr. Anat. **76**, 253—287 (1910).
HASHIMOTO, M.: Über das gröbere Blutgefäßsystem des Kaninchenknochenmarks. Trans. Soc. path. jap. **25**, 371—378 (1935).
— Über das kapilläre Blutgefäßsystem des Kaninchenknochenmarks. Trans. Soc. path. jap. **26**, 300—307 (1936).
HAWK, P. B., and W. J. GIES: Chemical studies of osseo mucoid with determinations of the heat of conbustion of some connective tissue glucoproteids. Amer. J. Physiol. **5**, 387—425 (1901).
HAYTHORN, S. R.: Multinucleated giant cells. Arch. Path. **7**, 681—713 (1929).
HELLER, M., F. C. MCLEAN, and W. BLOOM: Cellular transformation in mammalian bones induced by parathyroid extract. Amer. J. Anat. **87**, 315—347 (1950).
HELLER-STEINBERG, M.: Ground substance, bone salts and cellular activity in bone formation and destruction. Amer. J. Anat. **89**, 347—379 (1951).
HENLE, J.: Allgemeine Anatomie. Lehre von den Mischungs- und Formbestandteilen des menschlichen Körpers. Leipzig: Leop. Voss 1841 (nach WASSERMANN 1956).
HERRING, G. M., and P. W. KENT: Some studies on mucosubstances of bovine cortical bone. Biochem. J. **89**, 405—414 (1963).
HEŘT, J.: Lokalisazo foramen nutricium na dlouhých kostech dospělého člověka. Čs. Morfol. **5**, 94—110 (1957).
— Das Längenwachstum der Röhrenknochen beim Menschen. Das Aktivitätsverhältnis der Epiphysenknorpel. Anat. Anz. **106**, 399—413 (1959).
— The growth of periosteum and bone marrow in long bones. Experimental study on the tibia of the rabbit. Čs. Morfol. 8, 238—250 (1960).
—, u. V. NOVÀK: Die Lokalisation der Ernährungslöcher an den Mittelhandknochen, Mittelfußknochen und Fingerknochen. Čs. Morfol. **5**, 151—166 (1957).
HIGHBERGER, J. H., J. GROSS, and F. O. SCHMITT: The interaction of mucoprotein with soluble collagen; an electronmicroscope study. Proc. nat. Acad. Sci. (Wash.) **37**, 286—291 (1951).
HINTZSCHE, E.: Die Osteoblastenlehre und die neueren Anschauungen vom normalen Verknöcherungsvorgang. Ergeb. Anat. Entwickl.-Gesch. **27**, 413—463 (1927).
— Untersuchungen an Stützgeweben. II. Über Knochenbildungsfaktoren, insbesondere über den Anteil der Blutgefäße an der Ossifikation. Z. mikr.-anat. Forsch. **14**, 373—440 (1928).
HISAMURA, H.: Biochemical studies on carbohydrates. 37. On the carbohydrates moiety of chondromucoid. J. biochem. (Tokyo) **28**, 217—226 (1938a).
— Biochemical studies on carbohydrates. 39. Carbohydrates in the molecule of osseomucoid. J. Biochem. (Tokyo) **28**, 473—478 (1938b).

HODGE, A. J.: Principles of ordering in fibrous system. 4. Kongr. Elektronenmikroskopie, S. 119—139. Springer 1960.
— Structure at the electron microscopic level. In: Treatise on collagen (ed. by G. N. RAMACHANDRAN), vol. 1, p. 185—204. London and New York: Academic Press 1967.
HOFMANN, N., TH. NEMETSCHEK u. W. GRASSMANN: Über die Querstreifung von Kollagenfibrillen und ihre Veränderung im Elektronenmikroskop. Z. Naturforsch. 76, 509—513 (1952).
HOWATSON, A. F., and A. W. HAM: Electron microscope study of sections of two rat liver tumors. Cancer Res. 15, 62—69 (1955).
HUBER, L., et C. ROUILLER: Les fibrilles collagénes de l'os. (Etude au microscope électronique). Experientia (Basel) 7, 338—340 (1951).
HUGGINS, M. L.: Hydrogen bond in proteins. 120. Meeting Abstr. of papers, Amer. chem. Soc. New York, 3 Q, 1951.
HUGHES, H.: The factors determining the direction of the canal for the nutriant artery in the long bones of mammals and limbs. Acta anat. (Basel) 15, 261—280 (1952).
IRVING, J. T.: Calcium metabolism. London: Methuen & Co. Ltd. and New York: John Wiley & sons Inc. 1957.
JACKSON, D. S.: Chondroitin sulfuric acid as a factor in the stability of tendon. Biochem. J. 54, 638—641 (1953).
— The nature of collagen-chondroitin sulphate linkages in tendon. Biochem. J. 56, 699—703 (1954).
—, and J. P. BENTLEY: Collagen-glycosaminoglycan interactions. In: Treatise on collagen (ed. by G. N. RAMACHANDRAN), vol. 2A, p. 189—211. London and New York: Academic Press 1968.
—, and J. T. RANDALL: The reconstruction of collagen fibrils from solution. In: Nature and structure of collagen (ed. by J. T. RANDALL), p. 181—191. New York and London 1953.
JACKSON, S. F.: The formation of connective and skeletal tissues. Proc. roy. Soc. B 142, 536—548 (1954).
— Cytoplasmic granules in fibrogenic cells. Nature (Lond.) 175, 39—40 (1955).
— The morphogenesis of avian tendon. Proc. roy. Soc. B 144, 556—572 (1956).
— Structural problems associated with the formation of collagen fibrils in vivo. Connective tissue, ed. by R. E. TUNBRIDGE, p. 77—85. Oxford: Blackwell Sci. Publ. 1957.
—, and R. H. SMITH: Studies on the biosynthesis of collagen. I. The growth of fowl osteoblasts and the formation of collagen in tissue culture. J. biophys. biochem. Cytol. 3, 897—911 (1957).
JAFFÉ, H. L.: The structure of bone. With particulare reference to its fibrillar nature and the reaction of function to internal architecture. Arch. Surg. 19, 24—52 (1929).
— The resorption of bone. A consideration on the underlying processes particularly in pathologic conditions. Arch. Surg. 20, 355—385 (1930).
JAFFÉ, H. L., and A. BODANSKY: Experimental fibrous osteodystrophy (osteitis fibrosa) in hyperparathyroid dogs. J. exp. Med. 52, 669—694 (1930).
JEANLOZ, R. W.: The nomenclature of mucopolysaccharides. Arthr. and Rheum. 3, 233—237 (1960).
JEE, W. S. S., and J. S. ARNOLD: Indianik-Gelatin vascular injektion of skeletal tissues. Stain Technol. 35, 59—65 (1960).
JIPP, P.: Die Sehnenstruktur an punktförmigen Muskelansätzen. Morph. Jb. 101, 236—262 (1960).
JOHNSON, R. H.: The tetracyclines: a review of the literature — 1948 through 1963. J. oral Ther. 1, 190—217 (1964).
JOSEPH, N. R., M. B. ENGEL, and H. R. CATCHPOLE: Homeostasis of connective tissues. Arch. Path. 58, 40—58 (1954).
JOWSEY, J., B. L. RIGGS, and P. J. KELLY: Mineral metabolism in osteocytes. Proc. Mayo Clin. 39, 480—484 (1964).
KAJIKAWA, K., T. TANII, and R. HIRONO: Electron microscopic studies on skin fibroblasts of mouse, with special reference to the fibrillogenesis in connective tissue. Acta path. jap. 9, 61—80 (1959).
KAPSAMER, G.: Die periostale Ossifikation. Arch. mikr. Anat. 50, 315—350 (1897).
KASSOWITZ, M.: Die normale Ossifikation und die Erkrankung des Knochensystems bei Rachitis und hereditärer Syphilis. Med. Jb. I. Teil, 145—223, 293—457 (1879).
KIRBY-SMITH, H. T.: Bone growth studies. A miniature bone fracture observed microscopically in a transparent chamber introduced into the rabbit's ear. Amer. J. Anat. 53, 377 (1933).
KNESE, K.-H.: Die periostale Osteogenese und Bildung der Knochenstruktur bis zum Säuglingsalter. Z. Zellforsch. 44, 585—643 (1956a).
— Knochenbildung und Knochenaufbau unter Berücksichtigung der Histopathologie. Regensburg. Jb. ärztl. Fortbild. 5, 177—189 (1956b).
— Die diaphysäre chondrale Osteogenese bis zur Geburt. Z. Zellforsch. 47, 80—113 (1957).
— Über anatomische Grundlagen der Konstitution. Z. Morph. Anthrop. 49, 29—42 (1958a).
— Knochenstruktur als Verbundbau, Versuch einer technischen Deutung der Materialstruktur des Knochens. Zwangslose Abhandlungen aus dem Gebiet der normalen und pathologischen Anatomie (Herausg. W. BARGMANN u. W. DOERR), H. 4. Stuttgart: Georg Thieme 1958b.
— Neuere Untersuchungen über die Knochenbildung und ihre Beeinflussungsmöglichkeiten. Dtsch. zahnärztl. Z. 14, 925—932, 990—1000 (1959a).
— Die Ultrastruktur des Knochengewebes. Dtsch. med. Wschr. 84, 1640—1644, 1649—1650 (1959b).

KNESE, K.-H.: The ultra-structure of bone. Germ. med. mth. 4, 411—412, 427—431 (1959c).
— Über die Mineralablagerungen im Knorpel- und Knochengewebe unter Berücksichtigung elektronenmikroskopischer Befunde. Acta histochem. (Jena), Suppl. 3, 31—56 (1963a).
— Zell- und Faserstruktur des Knochengewebes. Acta anat. (Basel) 53, 369—394 (1963b).
— Knochenbildung und Entwicklung der Knochenstruktur. Verh. dtsch. Ges. Path. 47, 35—54 (1963c).
— A histochemical study of the polysaccharides in osteogenic areas. In: Bone and tooth (ed. H. J. J. BLACKWOOD), p. 283—287. Oxford: Pergamon Press 1964a.
— Zytogenese und topochemische Reaktion der frühen und späten epitheloiden Osteoblasten. Z. Zellforsch. 69, 93—128 (1966a).
— Zytologische Aspekte der Knochenbildung. Internist (Berl.) 7, 581—590 (1966b).
— Cytogenesis of osteoblasts. In: L'ostéomalcie (ed. by D. J. HIOCO), p. 65—75. Paris: Masson & Cie. 1967a.
— Topographic and temporal correlation of processes of osteogenesis discussed according to electronmicroscopic findings. In: Callus formation. Symposium on the biology of fracture healing (ed. by ST. KROMPECHER and E. KERNER), p. 165—177. Budapest: Akadémiai Kiadó 1967b.
— Über verdämmernde Zellen im Periost und die Entwicklung der encoche d'ossification. Verh. Anat. Ges., 52 Vers. 1967. Anat. Anz. 121, Erg.-H., 561—569 (1968).
—, u. H. BIERMANN: Die Knochenbildung an Sehnen- und Bandansätzen im Bereich ursprünglich chondraler Apophysen. Z. Zellforsch. 49, 142—187 (1958).
—, u. M. v. HARNACK: Über die Faserstruktur des Knochengewebes. Z. Zellforsch. 57, 520—558 (1962).
—, u. A.-M. KNOOP: Elektronenoptische Untersuchungen über die periostale Osteogenese. Z. Zellforsch. 48, 455—478 (1958).
— — Elektronenmikroskopische und histochemische Untersuchungen am Knorpelgewebe über den Ort der Bildung des Mucopolysaccharid-Protein-Komplexes. Z. Zellforsch. 53, 201—258 (1961a).
— — Elektronenmikroskopische Beobachtungen über die Zellen in der Eröffnungszone des Epiphysenknorpels. Z. Zellforsch. 54, 1—38 (1961b).
— — Chondrogenese und Osteogenese, elektronen- und lichtmikroskopische Untersuchungen. Z. Zellforsch. 55, 413—468 (1961c).
— I. RITSCHL u. D. VOGES: Quantitative Untersuchung der Osteonverteilung im Extremitätenskelet eines 43jährigen Mannes. Z. Zellforsch. 40, 519—570 (1954).
—, u. S. TITSCHAK: Untersuchungen mit Hilfe des Lochkartenverfahrens über die Osteonstruktur von Haus- und Wildschweinknochen sowie Bemerkungen zur Baugeschichte des Knochens. Morph. Jb. (1962).
KNESE, K.-H., D. VOGES u. I. RITSCHL: Untersuchungen über die Osteon- und Lamellenformen im Extremitätenskelet des Erwachsenen. Z. Zellforsch. 40, 323—360 (1954).
KÖLLIKER, A.: Über die große Verbreitung der perforating fibers von Sharpey. Würzb. Naturwiss. Z. 1, 306—316 (1860).
— Die Verbreitung und Bedeutung der vielkernigen Zellen der Knochen und Zähne. Verh. phys.-med. Ges. Würzb. 2, 243—252 (1872).
— Die normale Resorption des Knochengewebes und ihre Bedeutung für die Entstehung der typischen Knochenformen. Leipzig 1873.
— Der feinere Bau des Knochengewebes. Z. Zool. 44, 644—680 (1886).
— Handbuch der Gewebelehre des Menschen, 6. Aufl., Bd. 1. Leipzig: Wilhelm Engelmann 1889.
KOJIMA, M., and M. OGATA: On the nature of the so-called osteoclasts. Tohoku J. exp. Med. 71, 373—384 (1960).
KOLTZE, H.: Studie zur äußeren Form der Osteone. Z. Anat. Entwickl.-Gesch. 115, 584—596 (1951).
KORFF, K. v.: Die Analogie in der Entwicklung der Knochen- und Zahnbeingrundsubstanz der Säugetiere nebst kritischen Bemerkungen über die Osteoblasten- und Osteoklastenbefunde. Arch. mikr. Anat. 69, 515—543 (1906).
— Zur Histologie und Histogenese des Bindegewebes, bzw. der Knochen- und Dentingrundsubstanz. Ergebn. Anat. Entwickl.-Gesch. 17, 247—299 (1907).
KRAMER, H., and K. LITTLE: Nature of reticulin. Nature and structure of collagen, ed. by J. T. RANDALL. London 1953.
KRATKY, O., and A. SEKORA: Defection of large distances between lattice planes in kangaroo-tail tendons. Molecular structure of fiber proteins. M. makromol. Chem. 1, 113—121 (1943).
KREUZER, O.: Über Wachstum und Festigkeit langer Röhrenknochen im Laufe des postembryonalen Lebens. Arch. Entwickl.-Mech. Org. 126, 148—184 (1932).
KROON, D. B.: The bone-destroying function of the osteoclasts (Kölliker's Brush-Border). Acta anat. (Basel) 21, 1—18 (1954).
KÜHN, K., U. HOFMANN u. W. GRASSMANN: Über die Verteilung der sauren Aminosäuren in der Tropokollagenmolekel. Naturwissenschaften 47, 15—16 (1960).
KÜNTZEL, A., u. F. PRAKKE: Die Struktur der Kollagenfaser. Kolloid-Z. 90, 273—284 (1941).
KUHNKE, E.: Destruktionsformen der Kollagenfibrille. Ärztl. Forsch. 12, 471—475 (1958).
— Neuere Ergebnisse zum Feinbau der kollagenen Fibrille. Z. Rheumaforsch. 17, 259—274 (1958).
—, u. K. E. WOHLFARTH-BOTTERMANN: Neue Befunde zur Struktur der Sehnenfibrille an Hand von Dünnschnitten. Proc. Stockholm Conf. on Electr.-microsc. 1956, S. 223—225.

Lacroix, P.: Le mode de croissance du périoste. Arch. Biol. (Liège) **59**, 379—390 (1948).
— Comment le perioste et la moelle des os grandissent ils? Rev. Orthop. **3—4**, 141—145 (1949).
— The organisation of bone. Translated from the amended French edition by St. Gilder, p. 1—235. London: Churchill 1951a.
— L'os et les mécanismes de sa formation. Etude morphologique. J. Physiol. (Paris) **43**, 385—424 (1951b).
— Ca 45 autoradiography in the study of bone tissue. Bone as a tissue, ed. by K. Rodahl, p. 262—279. New York-Toronto-London: McGraw-Hill Book Co. 1960.
— Bone and cartilage. The cell, ed. by J. Brachet and A. E. Mirsky, vol. 5, p. 219—266. New York and London: Academic Press 1961.
Langer, K.: Über das Gefäßsystem der Röhrenknochen mit Beiträgen zur Kenntnis des Baues und der Entwicklung des Knochengewebes. Denkschrift Wien. Akad. **36**, 1—40 (1876).
Lea, L. M., et R. Ponlot: Sur les autoradiographies au Ca 45 des os longs en croissance. Les mécanismes de l'apposition osseuse sous periostée. Arch. Biol. (Liège) **69**, 455—465 (1958).
Leblond, C. P., and L. F. Bélanger: Mineralization of bones and teeth as shown with radiophosphorous autographs. Anat. Rec. **106**, 216—217 (1950).
— G. W. Wilkinson, L. F. Bélanger, and J. Robichon: Radio-autographic visualization of bone formation in the rat. Amer. J. Anat. **86**, 289—341 (1950).
Lerch, H.: Über den Aufbau des Sehnengewebes. Morph. Jb. **90**, 192—204 (1951).
Leriche, R., et A. Policard: Les problèmes de la physiologie normale et pathologique de l'os. Paris: Masson Cie. 1926.
Lentz, W.: Die Grundlagen der Transplantation von fremdem Knochengewebe. Stuttgart: Georg Thieme 1955.
Levander, G.: Tissue induction. Nature (Lond.) **155**, 148—149 (1945).
Lewis, M. R.: Development of connective tissue fibers in tissue culture of chick embryos. Contr. Embryol. Carneg. Inst **6**, 45 (1917).
Lexer, E., u. P. Kuliga: Untersuchungen über Knochenarterien mittels Röntgenaufnahmen injizierter Knochen und ihre Bedeutung für einzelne pathologische Vorgänge am Knochensysteme. Berlin: August Hirschwald 1904.
Lichtwitz, A., et R. Parlier: Calcium et maladies métaboliques de l'os. Tome I: Os et métabolisme du calcium á l'état normal. Paris: L'expansion scientifique française.
Lipp, W.: Neuuntersuchungen des Knochengewebes, Morphologie, Histochemie und Beeinflussung durch das periphere, vegetative Nervensystem, durch Fermente und Hormone. Acta anat. (Basel) I, **20**, 162—200 (1954); II, **22**, 151—201 (1954).
Lipp, W.: Neuuntersuchungen des Knochengewebes. III. Histologisch erfaßbare Lebensäußerungen der Osteozyten im embryonalen Knochen des Menschen. Anat. Anz. **102**, 361—372 (1956).
— Aminopeptidase in bone cells. J. Histoch. Cytochem. **7**, 205 (1959).
— Blood serum proteins and the mineralization of bone ground substance. Histochemie **9**, 339—353 (1967).
Lorentz, K.: Histochemische Aspekte bei der Azanfärbung des Knochens. Histochemie **2**, 136—142 (1960).
Lütken, P.: Investigation into the position of the nutrient foramina and the direction of the vessel canals in the shafts of the humerus and femur in man. Acta anat. (Basel) **9**, 57—68 (1950).
Mair, R.: Untersuchungen über das Wachstum der Schädelknochen. Z. Anat. Entwickl.-Gesch. **90**, 293—342 (1929).
Majno, G., u. C. Rouiller: Die alkalische Phosphatase in der Biologie des Knochengewebes. Histochemische Untersuchungen. Virchows Arch. path. Anat. **321**, 1—61 (1951).
Mall, F. P.: On the development of the connective tissues from the connective tissue syncytium. Amer. J. Anat. **1**, 329—365 (1902).
Marneffe, R. de: Recherches morphologiques et expérimentales sur la vascularisation osseuse. Acta chir. belg. **50**, 469—488, 568—599, 681—704 (1951).
Marotti, G.: The dynamics of osteon formation in inert bones. Calc. Tiss. Res. **2**, Suppl. 86 (1968).
—, and F. Marotti: Topographic-quantitative study of bone tissue formation and reconstruction in inert bones. In: Calcified tissues. Proc. 3rd Europ. Sympos. 1965 (ed. by H. Fleisch, H. J. J. Blackwood and M. Owen), p. 89—93. Berlin-Heidelberg-New York: Springer 1966.
Marshall, J. H.: Microscopic metabolism of calcium in bone. In: Bone as a tissue, ed. by K. Rodahl, p. 144—162. New York-Toronto-London: McGraw-Hill Book Co. 1960.
— J. Jowsey, and R. E. Rowland: Microscopic metabolism of calcium in bone. IV. Ca 45 deposition and growth rate in canine osteones. Radiat. Res. **10**, 243—257 (1959c).
— R. E. Rowland, and J. Jowsey: Microscopic metabolism of calcium in bone. II. Quantitative autoradiography. Radiat. Res. **10**, 213—233 (1959b).
— — — Microscopic metabolism of calcium in bone. V. The paradox of diffuse activity and long-term exchange. Radiat. Res. **10**, 258—270 (1959a).
— V. K. White, and J. Cohen: Microscopic metabolism of calcium in bone. I. Three-dimensional deposition of Ca 45 in canine osteones. Radiat. Res. **10**, 197—212 (1959a).
Martin, A. V. W.: Electron microscope studies of collagenous fibers in bone. Biochim. biophys. Acta (Amst.) **10**, 42—48 (1953).

MASUME, L. J., and M. MAKI: Paper partitions chromatograms of sugar components in glycidamins and glycoproteins. Tôhoku J. exp. Med. **53**, 237 (1951).
MATSCHINSKY, N.: Über das normale Wachstum der Röhrenknochen des Menschen. Arch. mikr. Anat. **39**, 151—215 (1892).
MCLEAN, F. C.: Biochemical and biomechanical aspects of the resorption of bone. J. Periodont. **25**, 176—182 (1954).
— The parathyroid glands and bone. The biochemistry and physiology of bone, ed. by G. H. BOURNE, p. 705—724. New York: Academic Press 1956.
—, and W. BLOOM: Calcification and ossification. Calcification in normal and growing bone. Anat. Rec. **78**, 333—359 (1940).
—, and M. R. URIST: Bone: an introduction to the physiology of skeletal tissue. Chicago: Chicago University Press 1955, sec. ld. 1961.
MCMANUS, J. F. A.: Histochemistry of connective tissue. In: ASBOE-HANSEN, Connective tissue in health and disease, p. 31—53. 1954.
MCMASTER, P. D., and R. J. PARSONS: The movement of substances and the state of the fluid in the introdermal tissue. Ann. N. Y. Acad. Sci. **52**, 992—1003 (1950).
MECKAUER, M.: The penitiori cartilaginum structure symbolae. Inaug.-Diss. Wratislaviae 1836 (nach WASSERMANN 1856).
MELCHER, A. H.: Gingival reticulin: identification and role in histogenesis of collagen fibers. J. dent. Res. **45**, 426—439 (1966).
MELLANBY, E.: The experimental production of deafness in young animals by diet. J. Physiol. (Lond.) **94**, 380—398 (1938).
— Further observations on bone overgrowth and nerve degeneration producted by defective diet. J. Physiol. (Lond.) **96**, 1—36 (1939).
— Vitamin A and bone growth: the reversibility of vitamin A-deficience changes. J. Physiol. (Lond.) **105**, 382—399 (1947).
MERCER, E. A.: The biosynthesis of fibers. Sci. Monthly **75**, 28—287 (1952).
MEYBURG, H.: Beitrag zur Kenntnis des Stadiums der „primären in toto konzentrischen" Knochenbildung. Arch. mikr. Anat. **54**, 627—652 (1904).
MEYER, K.: Summary of recent progress in the chemistry of connective tissue. Amer. J. Med. **1**, 676—679 (1946).
— The mucopolysaccharides of the interfibrillar substance of the mesenchyme. Ann. N. Y. Acad. Sci. **52**, 961—963 (1950).
— The mucopolysaccharides of mesodermal tissues. Tr. Conf. Metab. Interrelat. **4**, 63—73 (1952).
— The chemistry of the ground substance of connective tissue. In: ASBOE-HANSEN, Connective tissue in health and disease, p. 54—69. Copenhagen 1954.
— The mucopolysaccharides of bone. Ciba foundation, bone structure and metabolism. London: J. & A. Churchill, Wolstenholme and O'Connor 1956.
MEYER, K., E. A. DAVIDSON, A. LINKER, and P. HOFFMAN: The acid mucopolysaccharides of connective tissue. Biochim. biophys. Acta (Amst.) **21**, 506—518 (1956).
— A. LINKER, E. A. DAVIDSON, and B. S. WEISSMANN: The mucopolysaccharides of bovine cornea. J. biol. Chem. **205**, 611—616 (1953).
MILCH, R. A., D. P. RALL, and J. E. TOBIE: Bone localization of the tetracyclines. J. nat. Cancer Inst. **19**, 87—93 (1957).
MOLLIER, G.: Beziehungen zwischen Form und Funktion der Sehnen im Muskel-Sehnen-Knochensystem. Morph. Jb. **79**, 161—199 (1937).
MONESI, B., e G. BETTINI: L'indagine istochimica applicata alla fisiopatologia del tessuto osseo. Parte primci: Ossificazione normale. Arch. Putti Chir. Organi Mov. **10**, 326—372 (1958).
MORSE, A., and R. O. GREEP: Histochemical observations on the ribonucleic acid and glycoprotein content of the osteoclasts of the normal and ia rat. Arch. oral. Biol. **2**, 38—45 (1960).
MORSE, K. T.: Calcium and phosphorus metabolism in man and animals with special reference to pregnancy and lactation. Ann. N. Y. Acad. Sci. **64**, 279—462 (1956).
MOSS, J. A.: The carbohydrate of collagen. Biochem. J. **61**, 151—153 (1955).
MURRAY, P. D. F.: Bones: A study of the development and structure of the vertebrate skeleton. Cambridge: Cambridge University Press 1936.
NAGEOTTE, J.: Essai sur la nature et la génèse des substances conjunctives. C.R. Soc. Biol. (Paris) **79**, 1121—1126 (1916).
— Formation de pieces squelettiques surnuméraires, provoquée par la présence de griffons morts dans l'oreille du lapin adulte. C. R. Soc. Biol. (Paris) **81**, 113—118 (1918).
NEMETSCHEK, TH.: Zur Morphologie von Kollagen: Querstruktur, Elementarfibrillen und Anordnung im Zellverband. Z. Naturforsch. **13b**, 225—234 (1958).
NEUBERGER, A.: Metabolism of collagen under normal conditions. Symp. Soc. exp. Biol. **9**, 72—84 (1955).
—, and H. G. B. SLACK: The metabolism of collagen from liver, bone, skin and tendon in the normal rat. Biochem. J. **53**, 47—52 (1953).
NEUMAN, R. E.: The amino acid composition of gelatins, collagens and elastins from different sources. Arch. Biochem. **24**, 289—298 (1949).
NEUMAN, W. F., and M. W. NEUMAN: The chemical dynamics of bone mineral. Chicago: Chicago University Press 1—209 (1958).
NEUMANN, G.: Ein Beitrag zur Kenntnis des normalen Zahnbein-Knochengewebes. Leipzig 1863.
NODA, H., and R. W. G. WYCKOFF: The electron microscopy of reprecipiated collagen. Biochim. biophys. Acta (Amst.) **7**, 494—506 (1951).

NUTTING, G. C., and R. BORASKY: Electron microscopy of collagen. J. Amer. Leather Chemists' Ass. **43**, 96—110 (1948).
OREKHOVITCH, V. N.: Les procollagènes, leur structure chimique et leur rôle biologique. Intern. Congr. Biochem. Paris **2**, 106 (1952).
— The procollagens, chemical composition, properties, and biological role, 2nd Congr. intern. biochim. Chim. Biol. II., Symp. biogénèse des protéines Paris 1952.
—, and V. O. SHPIKITER: Procollagens as biological precursors of collagen and the physicochemical nature of these proteins. Connective tissue, ed. by R. E. TUNBRIGDE, p. 281—293. Oxford 1957.
— A. A. TOUSTANOVSKI, K. D. OREKHOVITCH, and N. E. PLOTNIKOVA: The procollagen of hide. Biokhimiya **13**, 55 (1948), quoted from Chem. Abstr. **42**, 7805 (1948).
OWEN, M.: Cell differentiation in bone. In: Calcified tissues. Proc. 2nd Europ. Sympos. 1964 (ed. by L. J. RICHELLE and M. J. DALLEMAGNE), p. 11—22. Collect. Colloqu. L'Université de Liége 1965.
PALADE, G. E.: The endoplasmic reticulum. J. biophys. biochem. Cytol. **2**, Suppl. 85—97 (1956).
PARK, E. A.: The influence of severe illness on rickets. Arch. Diss. Childh. **29**, 369—380 (1954).
PARTRIDGE, S. M.: The chemistry of connective tissues. I. The state of combination of chondroitin sulphate in cartilage. Biochem. J. **43**, 387—397 (1948).
PAULING, L., and R. B. COREY: The structure of fibrous proteins of the collagen-gelatin group. Proc. nat. Acad. Sci. (Wash.) **37**, 272—281 (1951).
PERRONE, J. C., and H. G. B. SLACK: The metabolism of collagen from skin, bone and liver in the normal rat. Biochem. J. **49**, 72—73 (1951).
PETERSEN, H.: Studien über Stützsubstanzen. I. Über die Herkunft der Knochenfibrillen. S.-B. Heidelberg. Akad. Wiss., math.-nat. Kl. Abt. B, 1—28 (1919).
— Über den Feinbau der menschlichen Skeletteile. Arch. Entwickl.-Mech. Org. **112**, 112—141 (1927).
— Die Organe des Skeletsystems. In: MÖLLENDORFF, Handbuch der mikroskopischen Anatomie des Menschen, Bd. II, 3, 5, S. 521—678. 1930.
— Histologie und mikroskopische Anatomie. München: J. F. Bergmann 1935.
—, u. L. BURKHARDT: Über den Umbau im wachsenden Knochen. Z. Zellforsch. **7**, 55—61 (1928).
PFEIFFER, H. H.: Polarisationsmikroskopische Messungen an Kollagenfibrillen in vitro. Arch. exp. Zellforsch. **25**, 92—100 (1943).
PIEZ, K. A.: Soluble collagen and the components resulting from its denaturation. In: Treatise on collagen (ed. by G. N. RAMACHANDRAN), vol. 1, p. 207—248. London and New York: Academic Press 1967.
PINARD, A.: Structure des vaisseaux de la diaphyse des os long chez le foetus humain. Acta anat. (Basel) **15**, 188—216 (1952).
POMMER, G.: Über die lakunäre Resorption in erkrankten Knochen. S.-B. Akad. Wiss. Wien, math.-nat. Kl., Abt. III, **83**, 17—140 (1881).
PONLOT, R.: Le radiocalcium dans l'étude des os. Bruxelles: Arscia S. A. 1960.
PORTER, K. R.: Observations on a submicroscopic basophilic component of cytoplasm. J. exp. Med. **97**, 727—750 (1953).
—, and G. D. PAPPAS: Collagen formation by fibroblasts of the chick embryo dermis. J. biophys. biochem. Cytol. **5**, 153—165 (1959).
PRATT, C. W. M.: Observations on osteogenesis in the femur of the foetal rat. J. Anat. (Lond.) **91**, 533—544 (1957).
— Postnatal changes in the shaft of the rat's femur. J. Anat. (Lond.) **93**, 310—322 (1959).
PRITCHARD, J. J.: A cytological and histochemical study of bone and cartilage formation in the rat. J. Anat. (Lond.) **86**, 259—277 (1952).
RAMACHANDRAN, G. N.: Structure of collagen at the molecular level. In: Treatise on collagen (ed. by G. N. RAMACHANDRAN), vol. 1, p. 103—179. London and New York: Academic Press 1967.
RANDALL, J. T., R. D. B. FRASER, S. F. JACKSON, A. V. W. MARTIN, and A. C. T. NORTH: Aspects of collagen structure. Nature (Lond.) **169**, 1029—1033 (1952).
— — and A. C. T. NORTH: The structure of collagen. Proc. roy. Soc. B **141**, 62—66 (1953).
RANVIER, L.: Traité technique d'histologie. 1875.
REIFENSTEIN jr., E. C.: Rationale for use of anabolic steroids in controlling adverse effects of corticoid hormones upon protein and osseus tissues. Sth. med. J. (Bgham, Ala.) **49**, 933—960 (1956).
— Anabolic steroid therapy for the protein depletion osteoperosis inducted corticoid hormones. Clin. Orthop. **9**, 75—84 (1957).
ROBB-SMITH, A. H. T.: Normal morphology and morphogenesis of connective tissue. Connective tissue in health and disease, ed. by G. ASBOE-HANSEN, p. 15—30. Copenhagen 1954.
— What is reticulin? Connective tissue, ed. by R. E. TUNBRIDGE, p. 177—185. Oxford: Blackwell Sci. Publ. 1957.
ROBERTSON, B. W. VAN: Influence of ascorbic acid on N 15 incooperation into collagen in vivo. J. biol. Chem. **197**, 495—501 (1952).
ROBINSON, R. A.: Electron micrography on bone. Tr. Conf. Metab. Interrel. **3**, 271—289 (1951).
— An electron microscopic study of the crystalline inorganic component of bone and its relationship to the organic matrix. J. Bone Jt Surg. A **34**, 389—435 (1952).
— Chemical analysis and electron microscopy of bone. Bone as a tissue, ed. by K. RODAHL, p. 186—250. New York-Toronto-London: Mc Graw-Hill Book-Co. 1960.
— Observations regarding compartments for tracer calcium in the body. In: Bone, bio-

dynamics (ed. by H. M. FROST), p. 423—439. Boston, Mass.: Little, Brown & Co. 1964.

ROBINSON, R. A., and D. A. CAMERON: Electron microscopy of cartilage and bone matrix at the distal epiphysial line of the femur in the newborn infant. J. biophys. biochem. Cytol. **2**, Suppl. 253—260 (1956).

— — Bone. In: Electron microscopic anatomy (ed. by ST. KURTZ), p. 315—340. New York and London: Academic Press 1964.

—, and ST. R. ELLIOTT: The water content of bone. I. The mass of water, inorganic crystals, organic matrix and "Co_2 space" component in a unit volume of dog bone. J. Bone Jt Surg. A **39**, 167—188 (1957).

—, and M. L. WATSON: Collagencrystal relationships in bone as seen in the electron microscope. Anat. Rec. **114**, 383—410 (1952).

— — Electron micrography of bone. Tr. Conf. Metab. Interrelat. **5**, 72—104 (1953).

— — Crystalcollagen relationships in bone as observed in the electronmicroscope. III. Crystal and collagen morphology as a function of age. Ann. N. Y. Acad. Sci. **60**, 596—629 (1955).

ROGERS, H. J.: Concentration and distribution of polysaccharides in human cortical, bone and the dentine of teeth. Nature (Lond.) **164**, 625—626 (1949).

— The polysaccharide associated with the organic matrix of bone. Biochem. J. **49**, 12—13 (1951).

— S. M. WEIDMANN, and A. PARKINSON: Studies on the skeletal tissues. II. The collagen content of bones from rabbits, oxen and human. Biochem. J. **50**, 537—542 (1952).

ROLLET, A.: Von den Bindesubstanzen. In: STRICKER, Handbuch der Lehre von den Geweben. Leipzig 1871.

ROLLHÄUSER, H.: Untersuchungen über den submikroskopischen Bau kollagener Fasern. Morph. Jb. **92**, 1—28 (1952).

ROUGET, C.: Note sur les corpuscules des os et sur le dévelopment des os secondaires. J. Physiol. (Lond.) **1**, 764—775 (1958).

ROUILLER, C., L. HUBER, E. KELLENBERGER et E. RUTISHAUSER: La structure lamellaire de l'ostéone. Acta anat. (Basel) **14**, 9—22 (1952).

ROULET, F.: Studien über Knorpel- und Knochenbildung in Gewebekulturen, zugleich ein Beitrag zur Lehre der Entstehung der sogenannten Grundsubstanzen. Arch. exp. Zellforsch. **17**, 1—42 (1935).

RUBASCHEWA, A., u. M. G. PRIWES: Blutversorgung der langen Röhrenknochen des Hundes. Z. Anat. Entwickl.-Gesch. **98**, 361—374 (1932).

RUTH, E. B.: Bone studies. I. Fibrillar structure of adult human bone. Amer. J. Anat. **80**, 35—53 (1947).

RUTISHAUSER, E., L. HUBER, E. KELLENBERGER, G. MAJNO et C. ROUILLER: Étude de la structure de l'os au microscope électronique. Arch. Sci. (Genève) **3**, 175—180 (1950).

—, u. H. KIND: Probleme der Osteolyse. Schweiz. med. Wschr. **80**, 182—183 (1950).

RUTISHAUSEN, E., et G. MAJNO: Lésions osseuses par surcharge dans le squelette normal et pathologique. Bull. schweiz. Akad. med. Wiss. **6**, 333—342 (1949) 1950.

— — Physiopathology of bone tissue. The osteocytes and fundamental substance. Bull. Hosp. Jt Dis. **12**, 469—490 (1951).

— C. ROUILLER et R. VEYRAT: La vascularisation de l'os: Etat actuel de nos conaissances. Arch. Putti Chir. Organi Mov. **5**, 9—40 (1954).

SANDISON, J. C.: A method for the microscopic study of the growth of transplanted bone in the transparent chamber of the rabbits ear. Anat. Rec. **40**, 41—49 (1928).

SCATCHARD, G., J. L. ONCLEY, J. W. WILLIAMS, and A. BROWN: Size distribution in gelatin solution. Preliminary report. Amer. J. chem. Soc. **66**, 1980—1981 (1944).

SCHABADASCH, A.: Beiträge zur synthetischen Erforschung des Mikroaufbaues des Röhrenknochens. Morph. Jb. **76**, 203—258 (1935).

SCHAFFER, J.: Ossifikationsfragen (Transplantation und Unterkieferernährung). Wien. klin. Wschr. **29**, 669—674 (1916).

— Lehrbuch der Histologie und Histogenese, III. Aufl. Leipzig: Wilhelm Engelmann 1933.

SCHMIDT, W. J.: Der Feinbau der anorganischen Grundmasse des Knochengewebes. Ber. oberhess. Ges. Natur- u. Heilk., Naturwiss. Abt. **15**, 219—247 (1933).

— Polarisationsoptische Analyse des submikroskopischen Baues von Zellen und Geweben. In: ABDERHALDENS Handbuch der biologischen Arbeitsmethoden, Abt. 5, Teil 10, S. 435—665. Berlin: Urban & Schwarzenberg 1934.

— Über homogene und sphäritische Verkalkung bei den verschiedenen Arten des Knochengewebes. Naturwissenschaften **34**, 273—277 (1947).

— Strukturelles und Polarisationsoptisches zum Verständnis der Volkmannschen Kanäle des Knochengewebes. Neue Ergebn. u. Probl. Zoologie (Klatt-Festschrift) 854—866 (1950).

— Polarisationsoptische Analyse tierischer Zellen und Gewebe. Naturwissenschaften **7**, 196—203 (1957).

— Grenzscheiden der Lakunen und Kittlinien des Knochengewebes. Polarisationsoptische Analyse kollagenfreier kongorot gefärbter Schliffe. Z. Zellforsch. **50**, 275—296 (1959).

SCHMITT, F. O.: Symposium on biomolecular organization and life-processes, chairman's prefatory remarks. Proc. nat. Acad. Sci. (Wash.) **42**, 789—791 (1956).

— J. GROSS, and J. H. HIGHBERGER: States of aggregation of collagen. Symp. Soc. exp. Biol. **9**, 148—162 (1955).

— — — States of aggregation of collagen, in fibrous proteins and their biological significance. Symp. Soc. exp. Biol. **9**, 148—162 (1958).

— C. E. HALL, and M. A. JAKUS: Electron microscope investigation of the structure of collagen. J. Cell Physiol. **20**, 11—33 (1942).

Schneider, F.: Über die Bedeutung des Kohlehydrats im Kollagen. Kolloid. Z. **111**, 136—137 (1948).
Schneider, H.: Zur Struktur der Sehnenansatzzonen. Z. Anat. Entwickl.-Gesch. **119**, 431—456 (1956).
Scholder, P.: Vascularisation osseuse et pseudokystes du poignet. Thèse de Genève 2100, 1953. Parne dans Rev. Chir. orthop. **39**, Suppl. 1, 1—56 (1953).
Schütte, E.: Stoffwechsel des Knochengewebes. 7. Colloquium der Ges. für physiol. Chemie, S. 77—102. Berlin-Göttingen-Heidelberg: Springer 1956.
Schultze, H. E.: Über Glykoproteine. Dtsche med. Wschr. **83**, 1742—1752, 1733 (1958).
Schwalbe, G.: Über die Ernährungskanäle der Knochen und das Knochenwachstum. Z. Anat. Entwickl.-Gesch. **1**, 307—352 (1876).
Schwarz, W.: Die Zwischensubstanzen des Bindegewebes. In: Kapillaren und Intersitium. Hamburger Symposion 1954 (Herausg. H. Barteilheimer u. H. Küchmeister). Stuttgart: Georg Thieme 1955.
Schwarz, W.: Morphology and differentiation of the connective fibres. Connective tissue, ed. by R. E. Tunbridge, p. 144—156. Oxford: Blackwell Sci. Publ. 1957.
—, u. H. J. Merker: Elektronenmikroskopische Untersuchungen über die Innenversilberung der Sehnenfibrillen. Histochemie **1**, 225—240 (1959).
—, u. G. Pahlke: Elektronenmikroskopische Untersuchungen an der Interzellularsubstanz des menschlichen Knochengewebes. Z. Zellforsch. **38**, 475—487 (1953).
Scott, B. L.: The occurence of specific cytoplasmic granules in the osteoclast. J. Ultrastruct. Res. **19**, 417—431 (1967).
—, and D. Pease: Electron microscopy of the epiphyseal apparatus. Anat. Rec. **126**, 465—495 (1956).
Sedlin, E. D., and H. M. Frost: Variations in rate of human osteon formation. Canad. J. Biochem. **41**, 19—22 (1963a).
— — The half-life of the osteon: a method of determination. J. Surg. Res. **3**, 82—83 (1963b).
Seifert, C., and W. J. Gies: On the distribution of osseomucoid. Amer. J. Physiol. **10**, 146—148 (1904).
Sharpey: In: Quains anatomy, 6. Aufl. 1856.
Shaw, J. H.: Effect of nutritional factors on bones and teeth. Ann. N. Y. Acad. Sci. **60**, 733—762 (1955).
Sheldon, H., and R. A. Robinson: Electron microscope studies of crystal-collagen relationships in bone. IV. The occurrence of crystales within collagen fibrils. J. biophys. biochem. Cytol. **3**, 1011—1015 (1957).
— — Studies on rickets. I. The fine structure of uncalcified bone matrix in experimental rickets. Z. Zellforsch. **53**, 671—684 (1961a).
— — Studies on rickets. II. The fine structure of the cellular components of bone in experimental rickets. Z. Zellforsch. **53**, 685—701 (1961b).
Shulman, S. S.: Observations on the nutrient foramica of the human radius and ulna. Anat. Rec. **134**, 685—697 (1959).
Sjöstrand, F. S.: The ultrastructure of cells as revealed by the electronmicroscope. Int. Rev. of Cytology, ed. by G. H. Bourne and J. F. Danielli, vol. V, p. 466—533. New York: Academic Press. 1956.
Slack, H. G. B.: Metabolism of collagen in the rat. In: Natur and structure of collagen, ed. by J. T. Randall, p. 51—60. New York and London 1953.
Smith, J. W.: Collagen fibre patterns in mammalian bone. J. Anat. (Lond.) **94**, 329—344 (1960a).
— The arrangement of collagen fibres in human secondary osteones. J. Bone Jt Surg. B **42**, 588—605 (1960b).
Smith, R. H., and S. F. Jackson: Studies on the biosynthesis of collagen. II. The conversion of 14-C,L-proline to 14-C-hydroxyproline by fowl osteoblasts in tissue cultures. J. biophys. biochem. Cytol. **3**b, 913—922 (1957).
Sobel, A. E.: The local factor in calcification. Tr. Conf. Metab. Interrelat. **2**, 113—143 (1950).
— Local factors in the mechanism of calcification. Ann. N. Y. Acad. Sci. **60**, 713—731 (1955).
—, and M. Burger: Studies of chondroitin sulfate in relation to the mechanism of calcification. Fed. Proc. **13**, 300—301 (1954a).
— — The biochemical behavior of lead. II. The influence of calcium, phosphorus and vitamin D on lead in blood and bone after withdrawal of lead from the diet. Office of Naval Res., Washington, Technical report NR. 180025 1—17 (1954b).
— A. Hirschman, H. Goldenberg, E. Scherzler, and I. Fankuchen: Composition of mineral deposited in vitro calcification in relation to fluid composition. Fed. Proc. Balt. **12**, 270 (1953).
— P. A. Laurence, and M. Burger: Nuclei formation and crystal growth in mineralizing tissue. Trans. N. Y. Acad. Sci., Ser. II, **22**, 233—243 (1960).
Sobel, E. H., L. C. Clark jr., Ph. Fox, and M. Robinow: Rickets, deficiency of "alkaline" phosphatase activity and premature loss of teeth in childhood. Pediatrics **11**, 309—322 (1953).
Sobel, H., and A. Moscane: Cultivation of embryonic organ rudiments on a nutrient derived entirely form adult tissues. Experientia (Basel) **10**, 502—504 (1954).
Sognnaes, R. F.: Microstructure and histochemical characteristics of the mineralized tissues. Ann. N. Y. Acad. Sci. **60**, 545—572 (1955).
Solger, B.: Der gegenwärtige Stand der Lehre von der Knochenarchitektur. Unterlagen zur Naturlehre des Menschen und der Tiere, Bd. 16, S. 187—218. 1899.

Spuler, A.: Beitrag zur Histogenese des Mesenchyms. Anat. Anz. **16**, Erg.-H. 13—16 (1899).

Stack, M. V.: Organic constituents of dentine. Brit. dent. J. **90**, 173—181 (1951).

Starck, D.: Vergleichende Entwicklungsgeschichte der Wirbeltiere. (1941, 1942 und teilweise 1943). Fortschr. Zool., N. F. **8**, 17—97 (1942—1944). Jena: Gustav Fischer 1947.

Starr, K. W.: Delayed unions in fractures of the long bone. St. Louis: C. V. Mosby Co. 1947.

Stefano, V. di, W. F. Neuman, and G. Rouser: The isolation of a phosphate ester from calcifiable cartilage. Arch. Biochem. **47**, 218—220 (1953).

Streeter, G. L.: Developmental horizons in human embryos (fourth issue). A review of the histogenesis of cartilage and bone. Contr. Embryol. Carneg. Inst **33**, 149—168 (1949).

Strelzoff, J.: Zur Lehre von der Knochenentwicklung. Zbl. med. Wschr. **1**, 273—278 (1873).

Studitsky, A. N.: Über das Wachstum des Knochengewebes und Periostes in vitro und auf der Allantois. Arch. exp. Zellforsch. **13**, 390—406 (1932).

— Experimentalanalyse der Differenzierungsfaktoren primärer Skelette. Z. Zellforsch. **24**, 269—302 (1936).

Studnička, F. K.: Über kollagene Bindegewebsfibrillen in der Grundsubstanz des Hyalinknorpels, im Dentin und im Knochengewebe. Anat. Anz. **29**, 334—344 (1906).

— Über einige Grundsubstanzgewebe. Anat. Anz. **31**, 497—522 (1907).

Sylvén, B.: Über das Vorkommen von hochmolekularen Esterschwefelsäuren im Granulationsgewebe und bei der Epithelregeneration. Acta chir. scand. **86**, Suppl. **66**, 1—151 (1941).

Takada, K.: Enzyme histochemistry in bone tissue. Acta histochem. (Jena) **23**, 40—70 (1966).

Tanaka, K.: Zur polarisationsoptischen Analyse der Knochenlammellensysteme des Menschen. Z. Zellforsch. **53**, 438—443 (1961).

Thiele, H., u. H. Krönke: Geordnete Kristallisation in ionotropen Gelen. Naturwissenschaften **13**, 389 (1955).

Thompson, R. C., and J. E. Ballon: Studies on metabolism turnover with tritium as a tracer. V. The predominantly non-dynamic state of body constituants in the rat. J. biol. Chem. **223**, 795—809 (1956).

Tilling, G.: The vascular anatomy of long bones. A radiological and histological study. Acta radiol. (Stockh.) **161**, Suppl. 5—105 (1958).

Tischendorf, F.: Die mechanische Reaktion der Haversschen Systeme und ihrer Lamellen auf experimentelle Belastung (nebst Bemerkungen zur Histogenese des lamellären Knochengewebes). Arch. Entwickl.-Mech. Org. **146**, 661—704 (1952—1954).

Tomes, J., and C. de Morgan: Observations on the structure and development of bone. Phil. Trans. B **143**, 109—139 (1953).

Tomlin, S. G.: Struktur von Kollagenfasern. Angew. Chem. **68**, 219—220 (1956).

Tonna, E. A.: Osteoclasts and the aging skeleton: a cytological, cytochemical and autoradiographic study. Anat. Rec. **137**, 251—270 (1960).

— The cellular complement of the skeletal system studied autoradiographically with tritiated thymidine (H3TDR) during growth and aging. J. biophys. biochem. Cytol. **9**, 813—824 (1961a).

—, and E. P. Cronkite: Histochemical and autoradiographic studies on the effects of aging on the mucopolysaccharides of the periosteum. J. biophys. biochem. Cytol. **6**, 171—178 (1959).

Trueta, J.: The normal vascular anatomy of the human femoral head during growth. J. Bone Jt Surg. B **39**, 358—394 (1957).

—, and M. H. M. Harrison: The normal vascular anatomy of the femoral head in adult man. J. Bone Jt Surg. B **35**, 442—461 (1953).

Urist, M. R.: Recent advances in physiology of calcification. J. Bone Surg. A **46**, 889—900 (1964).

— Origins of current ideas about calcification. Clin. Orthop. **44**, 13—39 (1966).

Vaes, G.: Hydrolytic enzymes and lysosomes in bone cells. In: Calcified tissues. Proc. 2nd Europ. Sympos. 1964 (ed. by L. J. Richelle and M. J. Dallemagne), p. 51—62. Collect. Colloqu. L. université de Liége 1965.

— Acid hydrolases, lysosomes and bone resorption induced by parathyroid hormone. Calcified tissues. Proc. 3rd Europ. Sympos. 1965 (ed. by H. Fleisch, H. J. J. Blackwood and M. Owen), p. 56—59. Berlin-Heidelberg-New York: Springer 1966.

Vanamee, P., and K. R. Porter: Observations with electron microscope on the subration and reconstitution of collagen. J. exp. Med. **94**, 255—268 (1951).

Veis, A.: Intact collagen. In: Treatise on collagen (ed. by G. N. Ramachandran), vol. 1, p. 367—432. London and New York: Academic Press 1967.

Veit, O.: Die Veränderung der Zahl der Knochenzellausläufer während der embryonalen Entwicklung. Med. Inaug.-Diss. Freiburg i. Br. 1934.

Verzár, F.: Aging of the collagen fiber. Int. Rev. Connect. Tissue Res. **2**, 244—296 (1964).

Vincent, J.: Recherches sur la constitution du tissue osseux compact. Arch. Biol. (Liège) **65**, 531—569 (1954).

Virchow, R.: Über Bildung und Umbildung von Knochengewebe im menschlichen Körper. Berl. klin. Wschr. **12**, 1—3, 13—16 (1875).

Vonwiller, P.: Anatomische Untersuchungen über die Wirbelsäule mit besonderer Berücksichtigung des Problems der Form der Knochen. 1. Der Einfluß der Venen auf die Form der Wirbelkörper. Z. Anat. Entwickl.-Gesch. **69**, 264—303 (1923).

Waldeyer, W.: Über den Ossifikationsprozeß. Arch. mikr. Anat. **1**, 354—375 (1865).

Wallgren, G.: Biophysical analysis of the formation and structure of human fetal bone. A microradiographic and x-ray crystallographic study. Acta paediat. (Uppsala) **46**, Suppl. 113, 7—80 (1957).

Warwick, W. T., and P. Wiles: The growth of periosteum in long bones. Brit. J. Surg. **22**, 169—174 (1934).

Wassermann, F.: Wachstum und Vermehrung der lebendigen Masse. In: Handbuch für mikroskopische Anatomie, Bd. I/2, S. 1—807. 1929.

— Electron microscopic study of the formation of fibers in the regenerating Achilles tendon of the rat. Anat. Rec. **115**, 443—444 (1953).

— The intercellular components of connective tissue: origin, structure and interrelationship of fibers and ground substance. Ergebn. Anat. Entwickl.-Gesch. **35**, 240—333 (1956).

—, and L. Kubota: Observations on fibrillogenesis in the connective tissue of the chick embryo with the acid of silver impregnation. J. biophys. biochem. Cytol. **4**, 67—70 (1956).

Wassermann, F., and J. A. Yaeger: Fine structure of the osteocyte capsule and of the wall of the lacunae in bone. Z. Zellforsch. **67**, 636—652 (1965).

Weidenreich, F.: Knochenstudien. I. Teil: Über Aufbau und Entwicklung des Knochens und den Charakter des Knochengewebes. II. Teil: Über Sehnenverknöcherungen und Faktoren der Knochenbildung. Z. Anat. Entwickl.-Gesch. **69**, 382—466, 558—597 (1923).

— Das Knochengewebe. In: Möllendorff, Handbuch der mikroskopischen Anatomie des Menschen, Bd. II/3, S. 391—520. 1930.

Weinmann, J. P., and I. Schour: Experimental studies in calcification. III. The effect of parathyroid hormone in the alveolar bone and teeth of the normal and rachitic rat. Amer. J. Path. **21**, 857—875 (1945).

—, and H. Sicher: Bone and bones, fundamental of bone biology. St. Louis: C. V. Mosby Co. 1947; sec. ed. 1955.

Wilhelm, G.: Elektronenoptische Untersuchungen zur Verknöcherung. Z. Kinderheilk. **76**, 73—78 (1955).

Wilkins, L.: Hormonal influences on skeletal growth. Ann. N. Y. Acad. Sci. **60**, 763—775 (1955).

Windrum, G. M., P. W. Kent, and J. E. Eastoe: Constitutuion of human renal reticulin. Brit. J. exp. Path. **36**, 49—59 (1955).

Wislocki, G. B., J. C. Aub, and C. M. Waldo: The effects of gonadectomy and the administration of testosterone propionate on the growth of antlers in male and female deer. Endocrinology **40**, 202—224 (1947).

— H. Bunting, and E. W. Dempsey: Metachromasie in mammalian tissues and its relationship to mucopolysaccharides. Amer. J. Anat. **81**, 1—37 (1947).

Wislocki, G. B., H. C. Weatherford, and M. Singer: Osteogenesis of antlers investigated by histological and histochemical methods. Anat. Rec. **99**, 265—295 (1947).

Wjereszinski, A. O.: Vergleichende Untersuchungen über Explantation und Transplantation von Knochen, Periost und Endosteum. Virchows Arch. path. Anat. **251**, 268—280 (1924).

Wolbach, S. B.: Vitamin-adeficiency and excess in relation to skeletal growth. J. Bone Jt Surg. A **29**, 171—192 (1947).

Wolff, J.: Über Knochenwachstum. Berl. klin. Wschr. **6**, **7**, **8**, 62—64, 76—77 (1868).

Wolpers, C.: Kollagenstreifung und Grundsubstanz. Klin. Wschr. **40/41**, 624 (1943).

— Die Querstreifung der kollagenen Bindegewebsfibrillen. Virchows Arch. path. Anat. **312**, 292—302 (1944).

— Das Sarkolemm. Klin. Wschr. **45/46**, 724—726 (1948).

— Elektronenmikroskopische Untersuchungen bei der Degeneration kollagener Fasern. Verh. der Dtsch. Ges. für Pathol. 33. Tgg Kiel. Stuttgart: Piscator-Verlag 1949a.

— Elektronenmikroskopische Kollagenbefunde. Tagg des Vereins für Gerberei-Chemie und Technik, Düsseldorf 1949b.

— Elektronenmikroskopie der Plasma-Derivate. Grenzgeb. Med. **2**, 527—535 (1949c).

Wyckoff, R. W. G.: The fine structure of connective tissue. Connective tissues 38—91, Trans, 3rd Conf. New York: Joshia Macy jr. Found. 1952.

Young, R. W.: Cell proliferation and specialization during endochondral osteogenesis in young rats. J. Cell Biol. **14**, 357—370 (1962a).

Zawisch, C.: Historisch-kritisches und Neues zur Frage der Ostoklasten, ihrer Entstehung und der Resorption im Knochen. Z. mikr.-anat. Forsch. **27**, 106—210 (1931).

— Die Verknöcherung der knorpelig vorgebildeten Platten-Knochen. Acta anat. (Basel) **19**, 384 (1953).

— Der Ossifikationsprozeß des Occipitale und die Rolle des Tectum posteriums beim Menschen. Acta anat. (Basel) **30**, 988—1007 (1957).

Zawisch-Ossenitz, C.: Histologische Untersuchungen über Gefäßeinschluß und Gefäßentwicklung im Knochen. Z. mikr.-anat. Forsch. **6**, 76—161 (1926).

— Die basophilen Inseln und andere basophile Elemente im menschlichen Knochen. I. Teil: Allgemeiner Überblick und die Entwicklung des menschlichen Femurs. Z. mikr.-anat. Forsch. **17**, 41—110 (1929).

Ziegler, D.: Studien über die feinere Struktur des Röhrenknochens und dessen Polarisation. Dtsch. Z. Chir. **85**, 248—263 (1906).

VI. Mechanik und Festigkeit des Knochengewebes

Von

K.-H. Knese

Mit 70 Abbildungen

Die Untersuchungen über die Mechanik des Skeletsystems haben eine Reihe unterschiedlicher Fragestellungen verfolgt. Sehr umfangreich ist das Schrifttum über die Gelenk- und Muskelmechanik (Fick, 1904—1911; Strasser, 1908—1917; Steindler, 1935; Dempster, 1955). Die Form des „normalen" Knochens, die Formänderungen bei bestimmten Erkrankungen, z. B. der Rachitis, und vergleichend-anatomische Beobachtungen führten zu Untersuchungen über die vermutlichen Beziehungen zwischen Form und Leistung der Skeletelemente. Die mechanischen Eigenschaften des Knochengewebes, seine Festigkeit, wurden dagegen nur von wenigen Autoren untersucht.

In diesem Artikel sollen die Festigkeit und die „Statik" der Skeletstücke auf Grund experimenteller Studien abgehandelt werden.

Die mechanischen Vorgänge im Stütz- und Bewegungsapparat werden nach den Gesetzen der allgemeinen Mechanik behandelt; häufig begnügte man sich allerdings mit einem Vergleich zwischen organischen und technisch ähnlichen Konstruktionen. Aber bereits A. Fick (1856) wies darauf hin — wenn er auch eine andere Formulierung gebrauchte —, daß für organische und anorganische Maschinen wohl die gleichen physikalischen Gesetze gelten, die jeweilige technische Lösung aber unterschiedlicher Natur ist. So ist es nicht verwunderlich, daß sich auch Techniker immer wieder für „tierische Mechanismen" interessierten (Reuleaux, 1900; Klöppel, 1958). Die speziellen mechanischen Verhältnisse der Organismen wurden in einer sog. Medizinischen Physik abgehandelt (A. Fick, 1856; Fischer, 1919). Auf den von Currey (1967) durchgeführten Vergleich zwischen den mechanischen Verhältnissen des Exoskeletes und des Endoskeletes können wir hier nur verweisen.

Die Physik benutzt die Mathematik als Handwerkszeug (Joos, 1945) zur Formulierung des Zusammenhanges von Erscheinungen. Die besonders von Fischer (1919) vorgelegten Bewegungsgleichungen sind entsprechend den zu damaliger Zeit üblichen mathematischen Hilfsmitteln für eine praktische Rechnung sehr unhandlich. Infolgedessen gelang Fischer auch keine befriedigende mathematisch-physikalische Bearbeitung des Ganges (vgl. Fick, 1929; Knese, 1955a). R. Fick (1910; vgl. Triepel, 1902) versuchte, die Ergebnisse der vorangegangenen Untersuchungen über die Gelenk- und Muskelmechanik zu popularisieren, um — wie er sagt — sie den an „literarischen" („humanistischen") Gymnasien ausgebildeten Ärzten verständlich zu machen. So glaubte man auch in der Folgezeit häufig, ohne Meßwerte und entsprechende mathematische Formulierungen bei Untersuchungen des Bewegungsapparates auskommen zu können.

Die Anzahl der Hypothesen über die mechanischen Verhältnisse des Skeletsystems ist fast unübersehbar, die der Messungen erschreckend gering. Daher ist es nicht verwunderlich, daß Spezialuntersuchungen über die mechanischen Eigenschaften des Knochengewebes kritische, allgemein gehaltene Äußerungen vorangestellt wurden: „Nicht die Vermutung großer Widerstandskräfte, die den beständigen merkwürdig gefahrlosen Gebrauch der Knochen im Leben begründet, genügt dem wissenschaftlichen Denken; sondern die Gesetze ihrer Widerstandskraft sind zu ermitteln und in Zahlen auszudrücken" (Rauber, 1876). „Mehr als uns im allgemeinen bewußt wird, treiben wir Pathologen an unserer wichtigsten Arbeitsstätte, im Seziersaal, ärztliche Kunst und nicht Wissenschaft.

Denn Wissenschaft ist die Anwendung der der persönlichen Erfahrung und Abschätzung übergeordnete, zu objektiven Feststellungen führenden Methoden; sie allein führen zu Maß und Zahl" (Rössle, 1927).

Viele mechanische Vorgänge lassen sich mit niederen mathematischen Mitteln darstellen, bei anderen sind höhere nicht zu vermeiden. In der Statik werden neben numerischen Methoden gern graphische angewandt, weil sie gut zu überschauen und Fehler leichter zu erkennen sind. Ein Minimum an mathematischem Handwerkzeug geben die klassischen Darstellungen von Föppl (1951, 1922) sowie Föppl und Föppl (1944/1947); anspruchsvoller sind die Werke unter anderem von Stüssi (1946/1962), Saliger (1949), Hirschfeld (1959); an Nachschlagewerken seien die „Hütte I" (1955) und das „Taschenbuch für Bauingenieure" (1955) genannt. Häufig wird mit sog. Näherungslösungen der Versuch unternommen, den Eigenschaften des jeweiligen Baumaterials und der Konstruktion gerecht zu werden (Föppl, 1920; Mörsch, 1923; vgl. Knese, 1956a, 1958b). Theoretisch vollständige Lösungen sind demzufolge auch im Hinblick auf die Mechanik des Skeletsystems nicht zu erwarten. Der Versuch, eine klassisch vollendete Lösung zu entwickeln, hat vermutlich die Diskussion über die Struktur der Spongiosa stark eingeengt (s. S. 473). Eine lehrbuchmäßig vollständige Darstellung der Theorie der Statik und Festigkeitslehre ist hier nicht am Platze, da für viele Erscheinungen die erforderlichen Untersuchungen am Skeletsystem noch fehlen. So soll nur kurz auf jene physikalisch-mathematischen Zusammenhänge eingegangen werden, die für das Verständnis der vorliegenden experimentellen Untersuchungen erforderlich sind.

1. Festigkeit des Knochengewebes

Im Hinblick auf die Bewegungsaufgaben können die Skeletstücke wie auch andere Körper als starr angesehen werden. Zur Beschreibung eines Bewegungszustandes kann von dem Körper auch nur dessen Massenmittelpunkt (Schwerpunkt) im Sinne der Punktemechanik (Newton) verfolgt werden. Knese (1955a, 1956b; s. S. 487) hat versucht, die Bewegungen der unteren und oberen Extremität nach den Regeln der Punktemechanik zu behandeln.

Jedoch liegen weder bei technischen noch organischen Maschinen starre, in der Form unveränderliche Körper vor. Die bei Bewegungen auftretenden Kräfte wirken auf den Körper deformierend und das Material des bewegten Körpers setzt diesen Kräften einen Verformungswiderstand entgegen. Die Gesetze der Verformung werden in einer Mechanik deformierbarer Körper oder Elastizitätslehre zusammengefaßt. Die belastenden Kräfte werden als „äußere Kräfte" bezeichnet, die der Verformung entgegenwirkenden Kräfte des belasteten Materials als „innere Kräfte" oder „Spannungen".

Eine Festigkeits- oder Belastungsaufgabe läßt sich nach diesen Angaben in mehrere Teile zerlegen. Damit ist auch der methodische Weg der Untersuchung vorgezeichnet:

1. Die mechanischen Eigenschaften, die sog. Festigkeit des Materials muß bekannt sein.
2. Die Größe und Richtung der belastenden Kräfte muß bestimmt werden.
3. Die Art der Einwirkung der äußeren Kräfte auf den Körper ist zu untersuchen.
4. Aus Form und Festigkeit des Körpers und der Art der Belastung sind die Spannungen zu errechnen.

a) Formen der Festigkeit

Als Festigkeit eines Körpers wird jene Spannungsgrenze bezeichnet, bei der seine Zerstörung beginnt. Die Festigkeit eines Bauteiles hängt vom Material, der Körperform und der Art der Einwirkung der äußeren Kräfte ab (s. unten). Mitunter wird in der Technik auch nur nach einer Grenzbeanspruchung, d.h. dem Auftreten bleibender Formänderungen, oder der Tragfähigkeit eines Konstruktionsteiles gefragt. Als einfache Festigkeitsfälle werden die Normalfestigkeit, Zug- und Druckfestigkeit, Biegefestigkeit, Scherfestigkeit, Torsionsfestigkeit, angesehen; wir schließen die Knickfestigkeit, die im engeren Sinne ein Stabilitätsproblem darstellt, und die sog. Härte an.

Die Baustoffe auch des Organismus können nur bestimmten Belastungsformen einen Widerstand entgegensetzen, z.B. sind die Kollagenfasern nur zugfest, sie knicken bei Druckbelastung aus.

Die inneren Kräfte stehen mit den äußeren im Gleichgewicht. Legt man nun einen Querschnitt durch den belasteten Körper (Abb. 1), so müssen sich auch die Kräfte auf den beiden entstehenden Schnittflächen im Gleichgewicht befinden. Bei einem einachsigen (s. S. 479) Spannungszustand ergibt sich die Spannung dann als Kraft P (kg) je Flächeneinheit F (cm²): $\sigma = \frac{P}{F} \frac{\text{kg}}{\text{cm}^2}$ (kg · cm⁻²) (Abb. 2). Bezieht man sich auf ein Flächenelement F und nähert sich damit einem Punkt an, ist $\sigma = \lim\limits_{\Delta F \to 0} \frac{\Delta P}{\Delta F}$ kg · cm⁻². Da nun

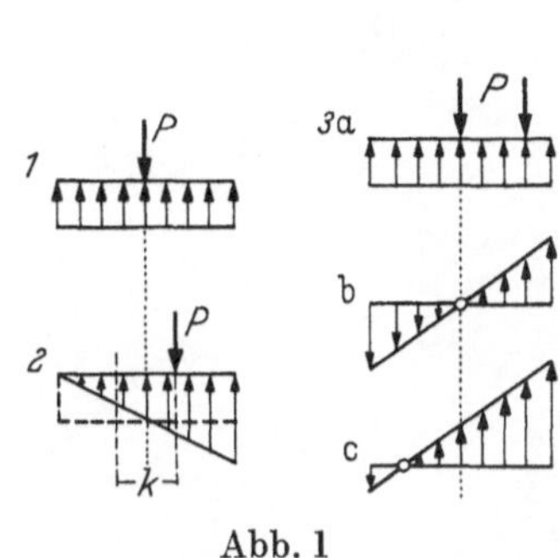

Abb. 1

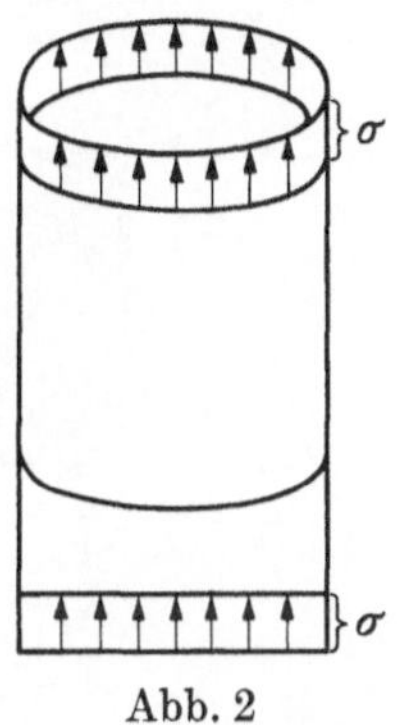

Abb. 2

Abb. 1. Spannungsverteilung für verschiedene Laststellungen. *1* Lastangriff im Schwerpunkt; *2* Lastangriff am Kernrande (*k*): Gleichsinnige Spannungen aber von verschiedener Größe; *3* Lastangriff außerhalb des Kernes: Zur Bestimmung der Spannungen wird zunächst (*a*) die Last in den Schwerpunkt zur Errechnung der Druckspannungen verschoben; danach (*b*) werden die Biegespannungen durch den ausmittigen Ansatz errechnet und schließlich (*c*) die Spannungen *a* und *b* zu den resultierenden Spannungen addiert. (Umzeichnung nach KNESE et al., 1955)

Abb. 2. Spannungsdiagramm (unten) und Spannungskörper (oben) auf einem kreisförmigen Querschnitt

Spannungen Kräfte sind, lassen sie sich als Vektoren graphisch durch einen Pfeil wiedergeben, wobei die Pfeilrichtung die Richtung der Kraft und die Länge des Pfeiles nach einem entsprechenden Kräftemaßstab die Größe der Kraft angibt. Errichtet man auf den Flächenelementen eines Querschnittes diese Spannungspfeile, so ergibt sich ein Spannungskörper $V = F \cdot \sigma = P$, dessen Inhalt den Widerstand gegen die äußeren Kräfte angibt.

Unter der Belastung erleidet der Körper auch eine Verformung, und zwar in Kraftrichtung eine Dehnung ε und senkrecht dazu eine Querkürzung ε_p. Man spricht von einer Dehnung bzw. Querkürzung, da der mathematischen Formulierung zunächst die Verhältnisse bei Zugbelastung zugrundegelegt werden. Bei einer Druckbelastung ist dann die Dehnung (Verkürzung) und Querkürzung (Verbreiterung) negativ.

Wird die ursprüngliche Länge des Körpers mit l und die Längenänderung als Δl bezeichnet, beträgt $\varepsilon = \frac{\Delta l}{l} \frac{\text{cm}}{\text{cm}}$. Nimmt die Dehnung proportional der Spannung zu (Hookesches Gesetz), kann man die Beziehung durch folgende Gleichung wiedergeben:

$$\Delta l = \frac{l}{E} \frac{P \cdot l}{F};$$

dabei ist E eine Materialkonstante, der Elastizitätsmodul, der von P, l, F unabhängig ist. Durch Umformung ergibt sich aus vorstehender Gleichung für den Elastizitätsmodul:

$$E = \frac{P}{F} \frac{l}{\Delta l} \text{kg} \cdot \text{cm}^{-2}.$$

Ist der ursprüngliche Durchmesser d und die Änderung Δd, beträgt die Querkürzung $\varepsilon_q = \frac{\Delta d}{d} \frac{\text{cm}}{\text{cm}}$. Der Zusammenhang zwischen Längsdehnung ε und Querkürzung ε_p wird durch die Poissonsche Zahl $m = \frac{\varepsilon_q}{\varepsilon}$ wiedergegeben. m ist die zweite Materialkonstante, die einen isotropen Stoff kennzeichnet. Für eine große Zahl von Materialien ist $m =$ 0,25—0,5. Sehr viele Stoffe verhalten sich in den verschiedenen Belastungsrichtungen nicht gleichartig, sie sind anisotrop. Zur Charakterisierung anisotroper Stoffe können bis zu 36 elastische Konstanten erforderlich sein.

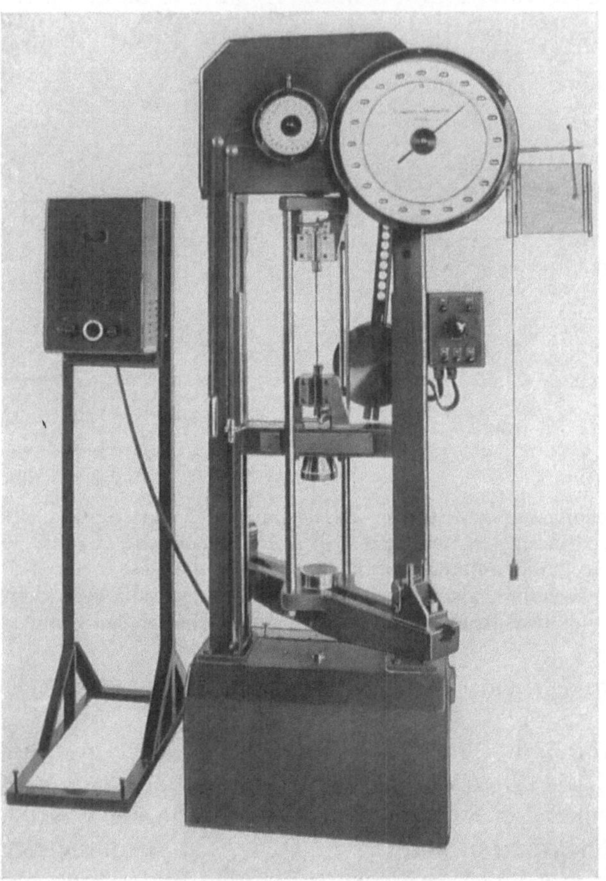

Abb. 3. Universal-Prüfmaschine (aus MELCHIOR und EMSCHERMANN, 1958)

b) Durchführung der Festigkeitsuntersuchungen

Der vorbereitete Prüfkörper wird in einer Werkstoffprüfmaschine untersucht. Über die Methoden der Werkstoffprüfung und die verschiedenartigen Maschinen unterrichten SIEBEL (1958), LUEGER (1961) und HETÉNY (1960). Neben Maschinen, die nur zur Prüfung einer Festigkeitsform dienen, gibt es sog. Universalmaschinen (Abb. 3), die sowohl Zug-, Druck- und Biegeversuche zulassen (MELCHIOR und EMSCHERMANN, 1958). Die belastende Kraft wird entweder hydraulisch oder durch ein Pendelwerk erzeugt. Für Versuche an Skeletstücken sind Maschinen zu empfehlen, die auf verschiedene Kraftbereiche einzustellen sind. Bei Biegeversuchen und Prüfung kleinerer Probekörper werden geringere Kräfte benötigt, etwa 20—500, seltener 1000 kg. Für Druckversuche an Stücken der großen kompakten Röhrenknochen muß eine Laststeigerung bis zu 6—7000 kg möglich sein.

Für die Messungen der im allgemeinen sehr geringen Längenänderungen wurde eine ganze Reihe von Geräten entwickelt (HUGGENBERGER und SCHWAIGERER, 1958). Meßuhren (Abb. 4) gestatten die Messung von Längenänderungen von 1/100 mm. Optische Spiegelgeräte sind bei Versuchen an Knochenproben nicht angebracht, da die Geräte bei dem plötzlich auftretenden Sprödbruch (s. S. 423) leicht Schaden erleiden. Bei elektrischen

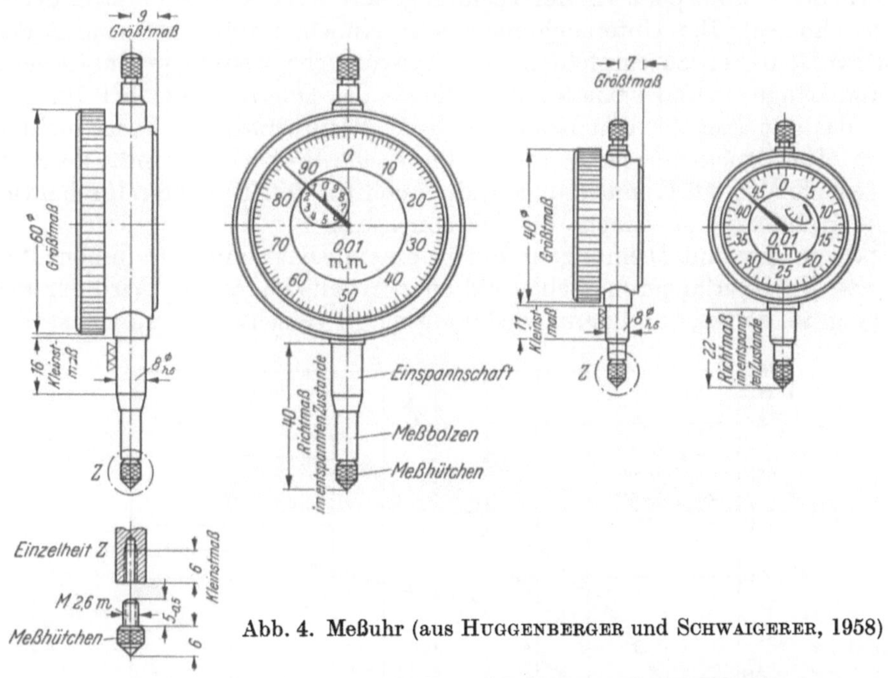

Abb. 4. Meßuhr (aus HUGGENBERGER und SCHWAIGERER, 1958)

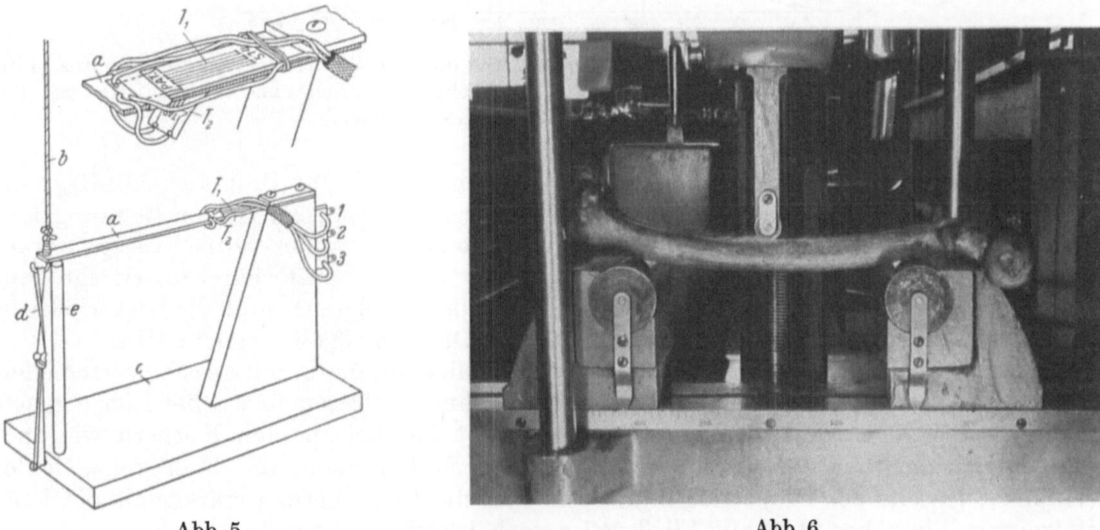

Abb. 5 Abb. 6

Abb. 5. Dehnungsmeßstreifen (aus HUGGENBERGER und SCHWAIGERER, 1958)

Abb. 6. Femur in einer Prüfmaschine mit Lagerung für Biegung von dorsal her. Die rollenförmigen Auflagerungen bewirken einen annähernd linearen Kraftangriff

Dehnungsmessern wird durch Änderung der Meßstrecke ein Widerstand, eine Induktivität oder Kapazität geändert. Die Dehnungsmeßstreifen (Abb. 5) enthalten einen dünnen Draht aus Konstantan oder Chromnickel, der mäanderartig in eine Papier- oder Kunststoffolie eingebettet ist. Mittels eines Klebelackes werden die Streifen unverrückbar auf die Meßstrecke aufgeklebt. Die Widerstandsänderung ist der Längenänderung bis zu einer Dehnung von 0,4—1 % proportional.

Besondere Sorgfalt ist bei der Zurichtung der Prüfstücke anzuwenden. Die Endflächen von Druckkörpern sind planparallel zu schleifen, um „Fehlhebel“ zu vermeiden. Recht schwierig ist die Lagerung von ganzen Skeletstücken bei Biegeversuchen (Abb. 6).

Die Form der Prüfkörper ist in der Technik genormt (DIN: Normblätter des Deutschen Normenausschusses). Bei Untersuchungen von Knochenproben ist eine Anlehnung an diese Normvorschriften zu empfehlen. Für Zugversuche werden prismatische Stäbe gewählt, deren Länge entweder das 5- oder 10fache des Querschnittes beträgt. Bei spröden Stoffen — das gilt auch für den Knochen — ist die prismatische Form nicht unbedingt erforderlich. Für Druckversuche werden zylindrische Proben verwandt, deren Höhe dem Durchmesser gleicht, bei Feinmessungen, die auch für den Knochen durchzuführen sind, beträgt die Höhe das 2,5—3fache des Durchmessers.

Die Spannungen und Dehnungen sind in einem Diagramm zusammenzufassen, dem Zerreiß- bzw. Kraftverlängerungsschaubild oder Arbeitsdiagramm. Wird der Probekörper von 0 an langsam belastet und dann wieder entlastet, verschwindet zunächst die Dehnung

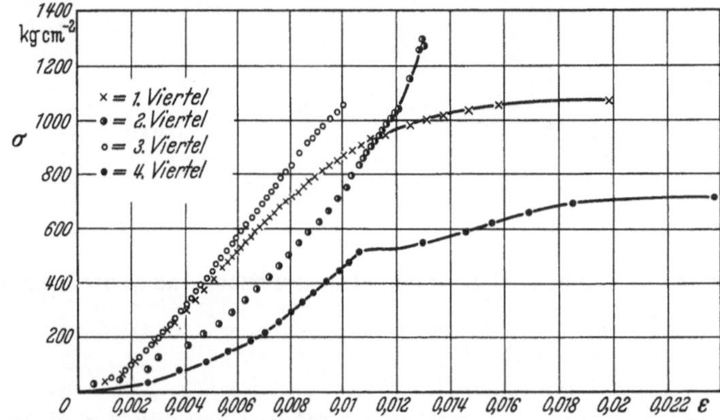

Abb. 7. Spannungs-Dehnungsschaubild im Druckversuch für die vier Viertel eines rechten Femurschaftes von einem 70jährigen Mann. Erstes und viertes Viertel mit Fließbereich, zweites und drittes Viertel verhalten sich annähernd spröde (aus KNESE, 1956a)

wieder. Spannung und Dehnung (Abb. 7) verhalten sich bis zur Proportionalitätsgrenze σP gemäß dem Hookeschen Gesetz. Bis zur Elastizitätsgrenze σE ist der Dehnungsrest, d.h. die nach Entlastung verbleibende Dehnung, so gering, daß er vernachlässigt werden kann. An der Fließgrenze σF (Zug: Streckgrenze, Druck: Quetschgrenze) erfolgt dann eine Dehnung ohne weitere Laststeigerung. Jenseits der Fließgrenze muß die Last wiederum gesteigert werden, bis die sog. Zugfestigkeit oder Druckfestigkeit erreicht wird.

Die einzelnen Stoffe verhalten sich nun im Hinblick auf die Dehnung sehr verschieden. Bei einem spröden Stoff kann die Last bis P_{max} ohne Auftreten einer Fließgrenze gleichmäßig gesteigert werden. In Druckversuchen tritt nur bei spröden Körpern wie auch dem Knochengewebe ein Bruch auf. Bei zähen Stoffen kann die Fließgrenze fehlen (Kupfer); jenseits der Proportionalitätsgrenze ist die Verlängerung stärker als die Laststeigerung. Ein zäher Stoff mit Fließgrenze verhält sich wie oben beschrieben.

Von manchen Autoren wird die technische Prüfung von organischen Materialien als unphysiologisch abgelehnt (STEVENS und RAY, 1962). Diese Verfasser übersehen, daß alle biologisch-medizinischen Prüfungen auf der Entnahme von Proben beruhen, die anschließend mit physikalischen oder chemischen Methoden untersucht werden. Versuche unter Verhältnissen, die denen in vivo in keiner Weise entsprechen (s. S. 444), können über das Material und die konstruktive Gestaltung wertvolle Aussagen zulassen; entsprechende Beispiele ließen sich auch aus der Technik aufführen (vgl. EVANS, 1964). Materialprüfverfahren haben in ihrer verwickelten Technik und der von den jeweiligen Prüfverfahren abhängigen Aussagemöglichkeit viel Ähnlichkeit mit der histologischen Technik.

Untersuchungen der Knochenfestigkeit liegen leider noch nicht in genügend großer Zahl vor (WERTHEIM, 1847; RAUBER, 1876; MESSERER, 1880; HIRSCH, 1895; HÜLSEN, 1898; KOCH, 1917; RÖSSLE, 1927, 1930; LEXER, 1928; HALLERMANN, 1934; HAASE, 1936, 1937b; HAASE und RICHTER, 1936; MAJ, 1938, 1940, 1942; EVANS et al., 1951, 1952; EVANS, 1957; CALABRISI et al., 1951; CAROTHERS et al., 1949; DEMPSTER und LIDDICOAT, 1952; KNESE et al., 1955). Unter Verwendung eigener Versuche und der von RAUBER und MESSERER haben KNESE et al. (1955) die Knochenfestigkeit variationsstatistisch untersucht; umfangreiche Zusammenstellungen der Literatur geben TRIEPEL (1902), EVANS (1957, 1967) und KUMMER (1959a).

Einige Autoren haben ihre Versuche an fixierten Knochen bzw. trockenen und macerierten Sammlungsstücken durchgeführt. Durch die Fixierung oder Maceration treten vermutlich Veränderungen, vor allem am organischen Anteil und in den Beziehungen zwischen den organischen und anorganischen Komponenten auf. Versuche an nicht nativem Material können vielleicht aufklären, wie die Komponenten des Knochengewebes zusammenarbeiten. Wir erörtern die Versuche an frischem und vorbehandeltem Material gesondert.

c) Experimentelle Untersuchungen des kompakten Knochens

α) Die Druckfestigkeit des kompakten Knochens

αα) Versuche an frischen Knochen. Beim Druckversuch werden entweder würfelförmige Körper oder Stäbe verwandt, deren Höhe das 2,5- bis 3fache des Durchmessers beträgt. Mit zunehmender Höhe des Probekörpers nimmt bei technischen Stoffen die Druckfestigkeit ab, bei zu langen Körpern können die Bedingungen des Knickens auftreten (s. S. 500). Durch die sog. Endflächenreibung sind bei Würfeln die Spannungen an der Angriffsfläche der Kraft von jenen im übrigen Körper etwas verschieden. Bei dreifacher Höhe des Probekörpers spielt diese Endflächenreibung keine Rolle mehr. Die Prismenfestigkeit wird zu etwa 70% der Würfelfestigkeit angesetzt (s. S. 426; RAUBER, 1876; KNESE et al., 1955).

Im Spannungs-Dehnungs-Schaubild eines Druckversuches (Abb. 8) von kompaktem Knochen ist zu erkennen, daß sich Spannung σ und Dehnung ε nur annähernd proportional verhalten (GOECKE, 1925; HALLERMANN, 1934; EVANS et al., 1951; DEMPSTER und LIDDICOAT, 1952; KNESE et al., 1955). Nach RAUBER (1876) reicht die Proportionalität etwa bis zur Grenze des 1. zum 2. Viertel der Festigkeit. KNESE et al. (1955) fanden, daß die Proportionalitätsgrenze — je nach Art des Prüfkörpers — höher liegt. KNESE et al. (1955) und KNESE (1956a) beobachteten ähnlich wie HALLERMANN (1934) weiterhin eine mangelnde Proportionalität im Anfangsteil des Spannung-Dehnungs-Diagramms. Da das für einen exakten Versuch erforderliche Zuschleifen der Compactaproben an den Endflächen recht schwierig ist, könnten bei Belastung zunächst Materialverschiebungen auftreten (s. S. 425). Jedoch ist auch von anderen spröden Stoffen, z.B. Gußeisen, bekannt, daß die Proportionalität von Spannung und Dehnung zu Beginn des Versuches fehlt.

Bei weiterer Laststeigerung verlaufen jedoch beim kompakten Knochen Spannung und Dehnung proportional, z.T. bis zum Bruch. Im Augenblick des Bruches verhält sich die Compacta mitunter wie ein sprödes Material und zerspringt in Bruchteilen von Sekunden in eine Fülle größerer und kleinerer Stücke, die wie bei einer Explosion herumfliegen. Andere Probekörper, wie z.B. aus dem proximalen Viertel des Femurschaftes, zeigen eine Fließgrenze, d.h. die Stauchung ist stärker als die Lastzunahme. GOECKE (1925), HAASE (1936) und LINGGI (1951) bezeichnen infolgedessen das kompakte Knochengewebe als ein Material, das zwischen jenen mit (Eisen) und ohne (Stein) Fließgrenze liegt. Während des Versuches an kompaktem Knochen können auch wie bei der Spongiosa stärkere Materialverschiebungen auftreten, nach denen eine weitere Laststeigerung möglich ist.

Die von verschiedenen Autoren ermittelten Werte der Druckfestigkeit der Compacta zeigen erhebliche Größendifferenzen. HÜLSEN (1898) bestimmte die Druckfestigkeit in

Richtung der Schaftachse am Humerus zu 2040, an der Tibia zu 2090 und am Femur zu 2110 kg · cm^{-2}. KNESE et al. (1955) und KNESE (1956a) haben Messungen an den vier Vierteln aus dem Femurschaft von vier Individuen (frisch, Raumtemperatur) vorgenommen, deren Höhe etwa das 2,5- bis 3fache des Durchmessers betrug (Tabelle 1). Die Druckfestigkeit vom proximalen zum distalen Viertel war bei einem 48jährigen Mann 971, 1057, 1058, 752, einer 53jährigen Frau 1198, 1148, 1223, 1176, einem 54jährigen Mann 1000, 1275, 1247, 877 und einem 70jährigen Mann 1072, 1292, 1048, 509 kg · cm^{-2}. Die Druckfestigkeit nimmt demzufolge vom proximalen zu den mittleren Vierteln zu und zum distalen wieder ab.

Die geringe Zahl der in der Literatur mitgeteilten Festigkeitswerte macht es schwer, zu entscheiden, ob die Festigkeit des Knochengewebes Unterschiede im Hinblick auf das Geschlecht, Lebensalter und die einzelnen Skeletstücke aufweist. Vor einer ähnlichen Aufgabe steht häufig der Techniker, der z.B. die Güte einer Produktion verfolgen soll,

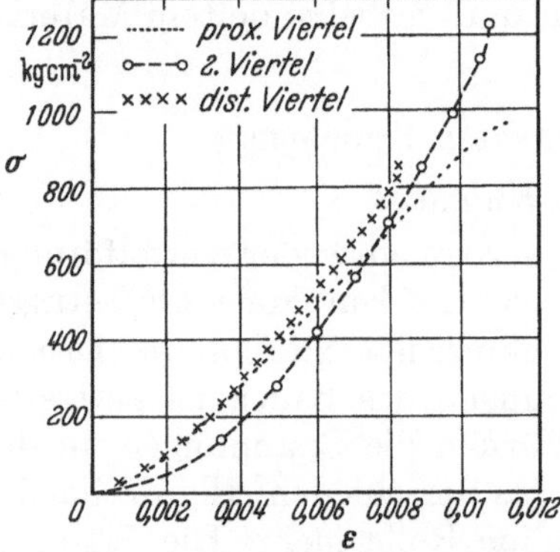

Abb. 8. Spannungs-Dehnungsschaubild für Druckversuch an drei Stücken aus dem Femur eines 54jährigen Mannes: annähernd sprödes Verhalten (aus KNESE, HAHNE und BIERMANN, 1955)

Tabelle 1. *Festigkeit der Compacta des Femurs (kg · cm^{-2})*

	Proximal	Mitte		Distal
		Frisch[1]		
Druckfestigkeit σ_d	1060	1193	1145	829
		Fixiert[2]		
Zugfestigkeit σ_z				
feucht	792	848		825
trocken. . . .	1059	1136		1057
Scherfestigkeit τ_s				
feucht	673	737		657
trocken. . . .	585	573		546

[1] KNESE (1956a).
[2] EVANS et al. (1951).

d.h. der zu prüfen hat, ob alle von verschiedenen Maschinen hergestellten Werkstücke gleichwertig sind.

Von DAEVES und BECKEL (1948) wurde infolgedessen eine graphische Methode, die sog. Großzahlforschung, entwickelt, die eine Aufgliederung eines „Urmaterials" bei Vorliegen von Mischverteilungen in mehrere Kollektive gestattet. Für jedes der Teilkollektive können der prozentuale Anteil am Urmaterial, der zugehörige Zentral-(Median-)wert und die Grenzwerte bestimmt werden. Dieses Verfahren der graphischen Kollektivanalyse wird in seinem Wert sehr unterschiedlich beurteilt, stellt aber ein Hilfsmittel zur Analyse eines Materials dar, wenn andere statistische Verfahren noch nicht anwendbar sind. EVANS (1964) und EVANS und BANG (1967) haben neuerlich eine Varianzanalyse mit Hilfe des Computers durchgeführt, worüber wir bei dem Kapitel Zugfestigkeit berichten werden.

KNESE et al. (1955) haben das von DAEVES und BECKEL (1948) entwickelte graphische Verfahren zur Untersuchung der Unterschiede der Festigkeit in bezug auf das Geschlecht, Alter usw. in ihrem eigenen Material und dem von MESSERER (1880) und RAUBER (1876) angewandt. RAUBER (1876) hat an 86 Würfeln die Druckfestigkeit ermittelt, diese Werte haben KNESE et al. (1955) in vier Teilkollektive (Tabelle 2) aufgliedern können: I 1210 $\pm$ 100 (29,1%), II 1425 $\pm$ 110 (25,6%), III 1730 $\pm$ 140 (28,4%), IV 2015 $\pm$ 85 kg · cm^{-2} (6,98%). Die größere Zahl der 81 männlichen Probanden, 40,7%, gehört zu Kollektiv III, von den 5 untersuchten weiblichen 3 zu Kollektiv I und 2 zu II. Wir kommen bei den anderen Festigkeitsprüfungen auf diese Differenzen zurück.

SCHMIDT (1915) hat die Druckfestigkeit an 20 mm hohen Knochenzylindern aus der Mitte des Femur, dem unteren Drittel der Tibia und der Mitte des Metacarpus 4 von Schweinen untersucht und fand eine Proportionalität zwischen σ und ε. Wegen des zur Messung der Dehnung verwandten Spiegelgerätes (s. S. 421) konnten die Versuche nicht bis zum Bruch fortgesetzt werden. Die Dehnungsrückstände waren zu Beginn der Belastung größer als im weiteren Verlauf des Versuches, so daß an eine teilweise Verfestigung des Materials zu denken ist. HALLERMANN (1934) gibt für Rinderknochen eine Dehnung

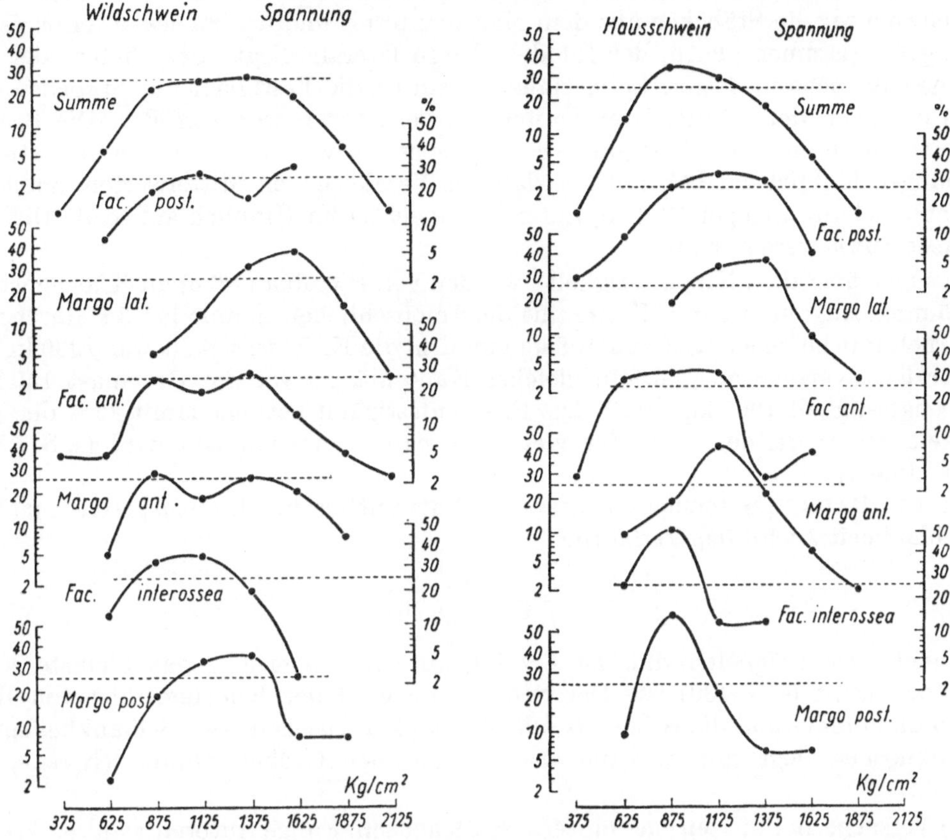

Abb. 9. Häufigkeitsverteilung der ermittelten Bruchspannungen im Druckversuch von sechs Stäben aus dem Metacarpus von Haus- und Wildschweinen: Summe = alle Proben, darunter die einzelnen Regionen (aus KNESE und TITSCHAK, 1962)

Tabelle 2. *Festigkeit* ($kg \cdot cm^{-2}$) *der Compacta in Kollektive aufgeteilt* (nach KNESE et al., 1955)

Druckfestigkeit σ_d[1]	1210 ± 100 (29,1 %)	1425 ± 110 (25,6 %)	1730 ± 140 (28,4 %)	2015 ± 86 (6,98 %)	
Zugfestigkeit σ_z[2]	660 ± 120 (20,73 %)	1025 ± 110 (64,6 %)	1320 ± 70 (14,58 %)		
Biegefestigkeit σ_b[3]	930 ± 150 (8,2 %)	1230 ± 170 (34,4 %)	1540 ± 160 (29,5 %)	1825 ± 155 (15,6 %)	2110 ± 230 (12,3 %)
Elastizitätsmodul E_b[3] für Biegung	570 ± 23000 (11,2 %)	129000 ± 33000 (82,3 %)	219000 ± 37000 (6,5 %)		

Erläuterung: Zentralwert ± Grundstreuung; in ( ) prozentualer Anteil des Kollektivs am Gesamtmaterial.

[1] Werte von RAUBER (1877): Compactawürfel.
[2] Werte von RAUBER (1877): Knochenstäbchen.
[3] Werte von MESSERER (1880) und KNESE et al. (1955): Ganze Knochen

von 1,3—1,4 % an, davon sind 0,2—0,5 % bleibende Dehnung. Bruch und Proportionalitätsgrenze fallen zusammen, die scheinbar plastische Veränderung beruhe auf einem Zusammenbruch der Struktur.

KNESE und TITSCHAK (1962) haben die Druckfestigkeit an sechs Abschnitten des Metacarpus von Haus- und Wildschweinen untersucht, die den Kanten und Flächen dieses Skeletstückes entsprechen. Die Bruchspannungen aller untersuchten Proben (Abb. 9) umfaßten beim Wildschwein die Spanne von 318—2100 und dem Hausschwein von 420—1824 kg · cm^{-2}, wobei der Medianwert etwa bei 1100 bzw. 900 kg · cm^{-2} liegt. Die Variationsbreite für die Festigkeit jedes der sechs Stäbchen ist von annähernd gleicher Größe wie alle Proben zusammengefaßt. Der Medianwert für die Festigkeit ist beim Wildschwein für die Stäbchen aus dem Margo anterior und der Facies anterior dem aller Prüfungen zusammen gleich, der für den Margo lateralis liegt etwas höher, der für die restlichen Bereiche niedriger. Beim Hausschwein ist die Festigkeit der Stäbchen aus der Facies posterior, dem Margo lateralis und Margo anterior wenig größer. Die Beachtung der Variationsbreite von Festigkeitswerten zeigt — wie ja aus anderen statistischen Erhebungen hinreichend bekannt —, daß der Vergleich von Mittelwerten, gebildet aus der Untersuchung weniger Proben, nur sehr vorsichtig im Hinblick auf reelle Differenzen hin ausgewertet werden kann.

Versuche über die „Knickfestigkeit" wurden von Rauber (1876) an Knochenstäbchen von 45 mm Länge und 3 mm Kante aus dem menschlichen Femur bei 38° durchgeführt. Der Bruch trat bei einer Last von 108 kg ein, d. h. die Knickfestigkeit war 1200 kg · cm^{-2}. Im Vergleichsversuch an Würfeln gleicher Kantenlänge war die Bruchlast 150 kg und die Druckfestigkeit 1667 kg · cm^{-2}. Die Prismenfestigkeit beträgt damit 72 % der Würfelfestigkeit, ein Wert, der heute für viele Materialien angenommen wird (s. S. 423; vgl. Knese, 1956a).

Die von Rauber untersuchten Stäbe sind als mittelschlank anzusprechen (s. S. 500). Als Schlankheit λ wird das Verhältnis

$$\lambda = \frac{l}{i} = \frac{\text{Knicklänge}}{\text{Trägheitsradius}}$$

bezeichnet. Der Trägheitsradius ist $i = \sqrt{I_{min}/F}$ cm, wobei I_{min} das kleinste Flächenträgheitsmoment (s. S. 430) ist. Der Schlankheitsgrad der Knochenstäbe von Rauber ist 51,9 und damit sind die Stäbe als mittelschlank anzusehen. Der Schlankheitsgrad der Röhrenknochen liegt mit 50—100 etwa in gleicher Größenordnung (Knese, 1956a; vgl. Abb. 52).

ββ) Versuche an fixierten oder macerierten Knochen. Einige Autoren wählten als Untersuchungsgut fixierte Knochen oder macerierte Sammlungsstücke. Carothers et al. (1949) untersuchten Präpariersaalmaterial (Femur, Tibia), das Altersmittel war 51 Jahre (30—75). Die Fixierung erfolgte mit Alkohol 95 %, reinem Glycerin und Formalin 10 % zu gleichen Teilen. Das spezifische Gewicht der Femurproben war im Mittel 1,959, das aus der Tibia 1,984 und das einer Fibulaprobe 1,825. Ganze Stücke aus dem Femurschaft zeigten eine mittlere Festigkeit von 1765, der Tibia 1850 und der Fibula 1630 kg · cm^{-2}, zylindrische Proben aus dem Femur 1617 kg · cm^{-2}. Als Elastizitätsmodul wurde für den Femur 187 700, die Tibia 199 700 und die Fibula 223 000 kg · cm^{-2} errechnet, für die Femurprismen 142 000 kg · cm^{-2}. Aus diesen Ergebnissen schließen Carothers et al. (1949) für den kompakten Knochen auf ein mittleres spezifisches Gewicht von 1,967, eine Druckfestigkeit von 1787 kg · cm^{-2} und einen Elastizitätsmodul von 192 000 kg · cm^{-2}.

Dempster und Liddicoat (1952) haben bei Untersuchung der Druckfestigkeit an Sammlungsfemora die Proportionalitätsgrenze etwa zur Hälfte der Bruchfestigkeit bestimmt. Wiederholte Versuche unterhalb dieser Grenze zeigen ein gleichbleibendes Verhältnis von Spannung und Dehnung. Die Autoren haben ihre Proben trocken und nach Befeuchtung untersucht. Die Druckfestigkeit trockener Knochen beträgt 1805 ± 333, die feuchter 1109 ± 273 kg · cm^{-2}, der Elastizitätsmodul trockener 183000 ± 11 740, feuchter Knochen 144 800 ± 8230 kg · cm^{-2}. Der Elastizitätsmodul ist bei trockenem Knochen für Druck und Zug mit 176 000—211 000 kg · cm^{-2} etwa gleich, bei feuchtem bei Druck etwa 35 000 kg · cm^{-2} kleiner als bei Zug. Die Verfasser meinen, daß der mittlere Elastizitätsmodul des lebenden Knochen etwa in Höhe des angefeuchteten oder wenig darüber liege (s. S. 445).

EVANS und LISSNER (1957) haben die Druckfestigkeit des Parietale von fixierten Leichen untersucht. Die Druckfestigkeit in der Ebene des Parietale errechnet aus 69 Versuchen beträgt 1553 kg · cm^{-2} (872—3360) und senkrecht zur Fläche (56 Versuche) 1706 kg · cm^{-2} (316—3298). Die Druckfestigkeit in der Ebene ist links und rechts gleich, senkrecht dazu auf der linken Seite 16% größer als auf der rechten. Die Druckfestigkeit des Parietale entspricht etwa dem anderer kompakter Knochen.

β) *Die Zugfestigkeit des kompakten Knochens*

αα) Versuche an frischem Knochen. Zugversuche an frischem Material wurden nur von WERTHEIM (1847), RAUBER (1876) und HÜLSEN (1898) durchgeführt. Die Mittelwerte der Zugfestigkeit betragen für den Femur nach WERTHEIM ♂ 889, ♀ 663, RAUBER ♂ 973, ♀ 634, für die Tibia nach RAUBER ♂ 1240, HÜLSEN ♂ 1057, für die Fibula nach WERTHEIM ♂ 968, ♀ 678, für den Humerus nach RAUBER ♂ 1024 und HÜLSEN ♂ 1054 kg · cm^{-2}. Das Material von RAUBER (1876) haben KNESE et al. (1955) in drei Kollektive (Tabelle 2, Abb. 10) zerlegen können: I 660 ± 120 (20,73%), II 1025 ± 110 (64,6%), III 1320 ± 70 (14,58%). Die Zugfestigkeit von Rinderknochen beträgt nach HALLERMANN (1934) 1200—1400 kg·cm^{-2}. HIRSCH und EVANS (1965) haben frische Femora von 8 Säuglingen (Neugeborenes bis 6 Monate) und den Femur eines 14jährigen auf Zugfestigkeit untersucht. Die Zugfestigkeit ist bei den Säuglingen mit durchschnittlich 1000 kg·mm^{-2} höher als die des Erwachsenen; diejenige von dem 14jährigen erreichte mit 17625 kg·mm^{-2} einen noch größeren Wert. Ebenso ist die Verlängerung stärker als bei Erwachsenen (1,850 bzw. 1,918%), der Elastizitätsmodul betrug 1012 kg·mm^{-2} bzw. 2244 kg·mm^{-2}.

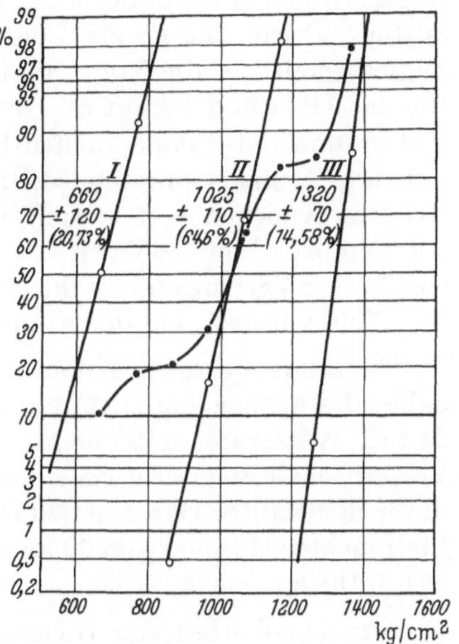

Abb. 10. Zugfestigkeit σ_z der Rauberschen Versuche mit Knochenstäbchen im Wahrscheinlichkeitsnetz: drei Kollektive (aus KNESE, HAHNE und BIERMANN, 1955)

Trotz der geringen Zahl der Versuche liegt die Vermutung nahe, daß die Zugfestigkeit geringer als die Druckfestigkeit ist. Weiterhin ergibt sich eine unterschiedliche Festigkeit der Skeletstücke, auch ist an Sexualdifferenzen zu denken.

ββ) Versuche an fixiertem Knochen. Die Zugfestigkeit von fixiertem Knochen wurde von einer ganzen Reihe von Autoren untersucht. Bei Versuchen an Stücken aus dem proximalen Drittel des Femurs haben CAROTHERS et al. (1949) nur die Festigkeit, aber nicht die Verlängerung gemessen. Die mittlere Zugfestigkeit aus elf Versuchen war 1547 kg·cm^{-2}. EVANS und LEBOW (1951) haben 242 Proben aus sechs Femora fixierter Leichen der Altersspanne 47—81 Jahre untersucht und hierbei auch den Einfluß des Wassergehaltes auf die Festigkeit verfolgt. Die Femora wurden in ein proximales, mittleres und distales Drittel und dann wieder in einen vorderen, hinteren, mittleren und lateralen Quadranten aufgeteilt. Für die feuchten Proben ergab sich in der Reihenfolge von proximal nach distal (Tabelle 1) die Zugfestigkeit von 792, 848, 825 kg · cm^{-2}, eine Verlängerung von 1,25, 1,27, 1,15% und ein Elastizitätsmodul von 137800, 148400, 145500 kg · cm^{-2}. Für die Quadranten in der obigen Reihenfolge: Zugfestigkeit 800, 817, 820, 852 kg · cm^{-2}, die Verlängerung 1,2, 1,06, 1,35, 1,34% und der Elastizitätsmodul 149000, 146300, 141300, 142700 kg · cm^{-2}. Das mittlere Drittel des Femur weist demzufolge die höchste Zugfestigkeit, den größten Elastizitätsmodul und die stärkste Verlängerung auf. Die höchste Zugfestigkeit hat der laterale, den größten Elastizitätsmodul der vordere und die stärkste Verlängerung der mediale Quadrant gezeigt.

Für alle genannten Proben haben EVANS und LEBOW (1951) einen Vergleich zwischen trockenen und feuchten Proben durchgeführt. Wir geben hier nur den Mittelwert für feucht/trocken wieder: Zugfestigkeit 832/1078 kg · cm^{-2}, Elastizitätsmodul 159500/187700 kg · cm^{-2}, Verlängerung 1,20/0,66%. Damit nehmen bei Trocknung die Zugfestigkeit und der Elastizitätsmodul zu, die Verlängerung aber ab. Das Spannungs-Dehnungsdiagramm zeigt bei getrocknetem Knochen das Verhalten eines spröden Stoffes, bei feuchtem aber eine Fließgrenze. Die Autoren haben weiterhin nachgewiesen, daß die Energieaufnahme (inch.lbs./cubic inch.) der Verlängerung proportional und bei feuchten Proben größer ist.

EVANS und LEBOW (1952) haben die gleiche Aufteilung der Proben bei Untersuchung der Tibia und Fibula von einem 36jährigen und 47jährigen Weißen und einem 72jährigen Neger vorgenommen. Bei allen drei Skeletelementen Femur, Tibia und Fibula hat das mittlere Drittel die größte Zugfestigkeit. Die drei Drittel der Tibia haben eine größere Zugfestigkeit als die von Fibula und Femur. Die Verlängerung nimmt in der Reihe Fibula, Tibia und Femur ab. Innerhalb eines Skeletstückes sinkt die Verlängerung beim Femur und der Fibula in der Reihe proximales, mittleres, distales bei der Tibia aber mittleres, distales, proximales Drittel ab. EVANS und BANG (1967) haben die Zugfestigkeit fixierter Knochen von 15 Individuen zwischen 33 und 98 Jahren untersucht, und zwar 405 Femurproben, 193 von der Tibia und 37 von der Fibula. Mit Hilfe des Computers wurde eine Varianzanalyse durchgeführt; sie ergab eine Zugfestigkeit des Femurs von 826, der Tibia von 980 und der Fibula von 945 kg·cm^{-2}.

Die Zugfestigkeit in Knochenlängsachse von macerierten Femora, Tibiae und Humeri haben DEMPSTER und LIDDICOAT (1952) geprüft. Die Proben wurden trocken und nach 24 Std Wässerung untersucht. Im Zugversuch an trockenem Knochen ergibt sich die Proportionalitätsgrenze etwa zur Hälfte der Festigkeit, bei feuchtem Knochen dagegen unter der Hälfte. Der Elastizitätsmodul für trockenen Knochen beträgt 189200 $\pm$ 29540, für feuchten 121700 $\pm$ 9000 kg · cm^{-2}, die Zugfestigkeit trocken 1200 $\pm$ 277 und feucht 804 $\pm$ 108 kg · cm^{-2}.

Aus den Werten von WERTHEIM (1847), RAUBER (1876), HÜLSEN (1898), CAROTHERS et al. (1949), EVANS und LEBOW (1951), DEMPSTER und LIDDICOAT (1952) sowie aus noch unveröffentlichten Versuchen hat EVANS (1957) ohne Rücksicht auf frisch oder fixiert die mittlere Zugfestigkeit zu 634—1057 kg · cm^{-2} errechnet. Diese beiden Zahlen entsprechen etwa den Medianwerten der zwei ersten Kollektive, die KNESE et al. (1955; Tabelle 2) aus den Messungen von RAUBER (1876) bestimmten; jedoch dürften auch höhere Werte auftreten. Die Zugfestigkeit ist geringer als die Druckfestigkeit.

Die Zugfestigkeit von Proben aus dem Parietale fixierter menschlicher Leichen bestimmten EVANS und LEBOW (1957) aus 16 Versuchen zu 719 kg · cm^{-2} (424—1110), sie ist damit etwas geringer als die von anderen kompakten Knochen. Die Zugfestigkeit des rechten Parietale war 12% größer als die des linken.

γ) *Die Biegefestigkeit des kompakten Knochens*

Eine Biegebelastung liegt vor, wenn auf einen stabförmigen Körper (Balken), der z.B. auf zwei Stützen ruht, eine Querkraft einwirkt. Diese Bedingungen dürften bei Skeletstücken nur bei Unfällen an Maschinen, in Fahrzeugen usw. streng erfüllt sein. Jedoch gewinnt die Biegung dadurch an Interesse, daß die häufig auftretende Knickbelastung in ihrer mathematischen Behandlung auf die Biegetheorie zurückgeführt wird. Daher sollen zunächst die theoretischen Grundlagen der Biegung erörtert werden.

αα) Vorbemerkungen über die Biegebelastung. Der einfachste Fall der Biegung liegt bei einem Balken vor, der auf zwei Stützen liegt, und senkrecht zur Längsachse durch die Querkraft (Q) P belastet wird (Abb. 11). Durch die Auflagerung an den Punkten A und B ergeben sich bestimmte Stützkräfte oder Lagerreaktion. Soll die Einwirkung der drei Kräfte A, B und P auf den Körper dargestellt werden, kann dies in Form eines Diagramms geschehen. Dem Balken entsprechend wird eine Horizontale angenommen. An ihrem Anfangspunkt wird die Stützkraft A in einem Kräftemaßstab aufgetragen. Die Beanspruchung des Balkens bleibt gleich bis zum Angriffspunkt der Kraft P. In dem Diagramm ist die Veränderung der Beanspruchung in der Form darzustellen, daß P in seiner Richtung und Größe an die Horizontale, bestimmt durch A, anzutragen ist. Dann bleiben die Querkräfte wiederum gleich bis zu der Kraft B. Hier tritt wiederum ein entsprechender Sprung ein. Durch die Kraftpfeile wird eine Fläche umschrieben, die als Querkraftfläche bezeichnet wird.

Diese Querkräfte spielen im allgemeinen eine geringe Rolle, so daß sie vernachlässigt werden können. Dagegen ist zu berücksichtigen, in welcher Entfernung von einem Unterstützungspunkt die Kraft ansetzt. Diese Strecke tritt als Hebelarm auf. Damit hat die Kraft ein Biegemoment, das in seiner Größe abhängig ist von der Größe der Kraft und der Länge des Hebelarmes. Das Biegemoment ist also wie alle anderen Momente ein Produkt aus einer Kraft in kg und einer Länge in cm und hat die Dimension kg·cm. Daraus ergibt sich, daß an den gestützten Enden eines Stabes das Biegemoment Null ist, da ein Hebelarm fehlt.

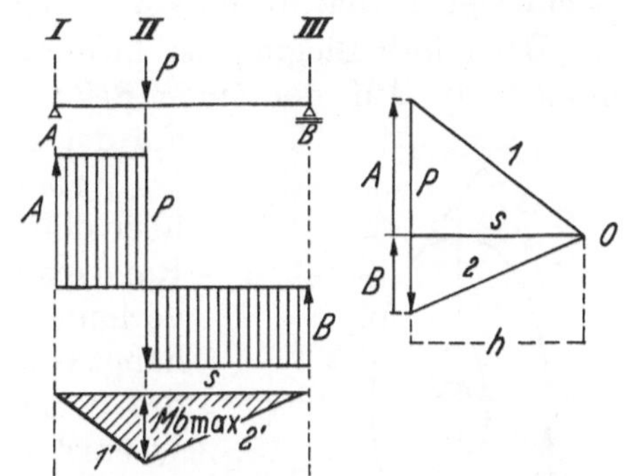

Abb. 11. Graphische Untersuchung der Belastung eines Balkens mit einer Einzellast P. A festes Lager; B bewegliches Lager. I Querschnitt von A; II von P; III von B. Rechts Seileck mit dem Polabstand h zur Bestimmung von A und B. A, P und B bestimmen die Querkraftfläche (senkrecht gestrichelt). Durch die Seilstrahlen 1, 2 und den Schlußstrahl s zwischen den untersuchten Querschnitten (hier als 1′ und 2′) wird die Momentenfläche (schräg gestrichelt) bestimmt. Mb_{max}: größtes Biegemoment (aus KNESE, 1955b)

Zur Querkraft bestehen folgende Beziehungen: 1. Das Biegemoment für einen Querschnitt ist dem Vorzeichen und der Größe nach gleich der algebraischen Summe der Inhalte aller Querkraftflächen links von einem betrachteten Querschnitt. Um die Möglichkeit zu haben, die inneren Kräfte in einem Körper näher zu untersuchen, wird der Körper „frei“ gemacht. Es wird ein gedachter Querschnitt angenommen, um dann zu berechnen, welche inneren Kräfte der abgeschnittene Anteil aufbringen muß, damit Gleichgewicht herrscht. Am linken und rechten Teil des Balkens werden dementsprechend die Kräfte mit entgegengesetztem Vorzeichen versehen. An sich bestünde die Möglichkeit, unendlich viele Querschnitte zu untersuchen. Dies ist jedoch nicht erforderlich, da eine weitere wichtige Beziehung zur Querkraft besteht: 2. Das maximale Biegemoment liegt in dem Querschnitt, in dem $Q = 0$ ist bzw. Q das Vorzeichen wechselt. Bei punktförmiger Belastung steigt das Biegemoment bis zu diesem Maximum an und fällt dann wieder geradlinig zum zweiten Unterstützungspunkt ab. In der graphischen Darstellung wird damit wiederum eine Fläche umschrieben, die als Momentenfläche bezeichnet wird. Der Querschnitt des größten Biegemomentes ist der „gefährliche“ Querschnitt.

Setzt die Belastung nicht an einem Punkt an, sondern verteilt sie sich auf eine längere Strecke, so liegt eine Streckenlast vor. Die Streckenlast ist bestimmt durch $p =$ Belastung pro Längeneinheit (Dimension kg/cm). Die gesamte Belastung ist dann Belastung pro Längeneinheit mal Länge l der belasteten Strecke: $P = p \cdot l$. Die Querkraftfläche ist von einer geneigten Geraden begrenzt, die die Horizontale durch den Endpunkt von A mit der Horizontalen durch den Anfangspunkt von B verbindet. Die Momentenfläche wird durch eine Parabel begrenzt, deren Scheitel Mb_{max} angibt. Dabei ist an sich erforderlich, die Querschnitte am Anfang und Ende einer Streckenlast und den mit Mb_{max} zu untersuchen. Es genügt jedoch für viele Fälle, die Streckenlast durch P zu ersetzen mit Angriff in demjenigen Querschnitt, der durch den Schwerpunkt der Kraftfläche bestimmt ist. Es ist dann nur eine entsprechende parabelförmige Begrenzung der Momentenfläche zu wählen.

Wirken auf einen Stab die verschiedensten Biegemomente ein, so muß für jede Kraft das Biegemoment zunächst einzeln berechnet werden. Anschließend werden die Biegemomente addiert.

Die hiermit in ihrem Wesen skizzierte Biegungsbeanspruchung ist in ihrer rechnerischen Durchführung an sechs Voraussetzungen gebunden: 1. gerade Stabachse, 2. symmetrischer Querschnitt, 3. alle äußeren Kräfte wirken in der Symmetrieebene des Stabes senkrecht zur Stabachse, 4. der Baustoff verhält sich nach dem Hookeschen Gesetz, 5. die Querschnitte behalten ihre ebene Gestalt bei, 6. Schubspannungen dürfen gegenüber den Biegungsspannungen vernachlässigt werden. Diese Voraussetzungen sind in der Praxis meist nicht erfüllt. Ihre Erfüllung wird dann häufig zunächst angenommen, man berechnet „scheinbare" Spannungen, um sich anschließend durch Korrekturen den tatsächlichen Verhältnissen anzunähern.

Bei reiner Biegung ist in einer Schicht des Balkens, der Neutralschicht, die Spannung = 0. Auf der einen Seite der Nullschicht ergeben sich Druckspannungen (σ_{bd}), auf der anderen Zugspannungen (σ_{bz}), die Maximalspannungen ($\sigma_{b\,max}$) betreffen die Randfasern. Die Verteilungen der Spannungen über den Querschnitt wird derart angenommen, daß die beiden Randspannungen durch die Nullschicht geradlinig miteinander verbunden werden (s. S. 452). Die Größe der Biegespannung hängt von dem Biegemoment Mb und der Form des Querschnittes des belasteten Stabes ab, d.h. dem Widerstandsmoment des Querschnittes W.

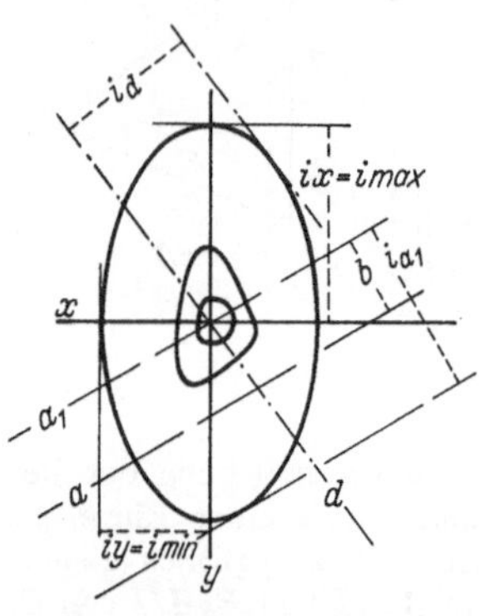

Abb. 12. Querschnitt einer rechten Tibia mit Zentralellipse, Hauptträgheitsradien $i_x = i_{max}$ und $i_y = i_{min}$; sowie Bestimmung von zwei weiteren Trägheitsradien (aus KNESE, HAHNE und BIERMANN, 1955)

Bekannt ist, daß ein T- oder Doppel-T-Träger mit einer geringen Masse eine besonders große „Tragfähigkeit" verbindet. Alle Röhrenknochen besitzen einen dreikantigen Schaft, wie auch in den Pariser Nomina anatomica (vgl. KOPSCH-KNESE, 1957) betont wird, und eine rundliche Markhöhle. Damit ist zu vermuten, daß dieser Querschnittsform im Hinblick auf die „Tragfähigkeit" eine besondere Bedeutung zukommt. Für den Querschnitt werden Flächenmomente (s. unten) bestimmt, die den Widerstand gegen die Biegung angeben. Flächenmomente von Knochenquerschnitten wurden von MESSERER (1880), GRUNEWALD (1920), KNESE et al. (1955) und EHLER (1963) berechnet, weitere Hinweise auf die Querschnittsform geben RAUBER (1875, 1876, 1877), GRAF (1894), HIRSCH (1899), GHILLINI (1899), GHILLINI und CANEVAZZI (1901), GEBHARDT (1910), KOCH (1917), KREUZER (1932), KUHN (1933), WERMEL (1935), MARIQUE (1945), PAUWELS (1950, 1953/54) und ERTELT (1955).

Das Moment der inneren Kräfte muß gleich dem der äußeren sein. Das Widerstandsmoment W hängt vom (geometrischen, im Gegensatz zum physikalischen Massen-)Trägheitsmoment I (Abb. 12) und dem Abstand e der Randfaser von der Nullinie ab: $W = \frac{I}{e}\ \mathrm{cm}^3$. Das Trägheitsmoment I ist für jede durch den Querschnitt des Körpers gelegte Achse verschieden, denn es ist die Summe aller Produkte aus unendlich kleinen Flächen dF und dem Quadrat ihrer Abstände von der Bezugsachse. Als Hauptträgheitsmomente werden das größte I_{max} und kleinste I_{min} bezeichnet. Durch die Hauptträgheitsmomente wird die Zentralellipse bestimmt, die die Bestimmung der anderen Trägheitsmomente ermöglicht (vgl. KNESE et al., 1955). Für in der Technik verwandte Profile liegen entsprechende Zusammenstellungen der Flächenmomente vor (z.B. HÜTTE I, 1955).

KNESE et al. (1955) haben zur Aufklärung der Bedeutung der dreikantigen Gestalt der Röhrenknochen regelmäßige geometrische Flächen von gleichem Flächeninhalt miteinander verglichen, und zwar den vollen Querschnitt, einen mit geometrisch gleichgestalteter (Mark-)Höhlung und den mit einer kreisförmigen Höhlung. Bei gleichem Flächeninhalt des Querschnittes weist das Dreieck mit Kreishöhlung ein relativ hohes Widerstandsmoment auf. Der Flächeninhalt beträgt 62,7%, das Widerstandsmoment 83,3% des vollen Querschnittes, d.h. daß eine vergleichsweise kleine Fläche ein sehr großes Widerstandsmoment aufweist. Ein dreikantiges Prisma hat darüber hinaus — gegenüber einem Kreiszylinder — eine große Oberfläche (128%) und damit eine größere Fläche für den Ursprung von Muskeln. Da nun Muskeln an der Oberfläche und nicht in der Stabachse ansetzen, liegen die Bedingungen des ausmittigen Ansatzes (s. S. 502) vor, der zu einer Biegebelastung führt. Die Spannungserhöhung ist durch den ausmittigen Ansatz bei dem dreikantigen Prisma an den Kanten relativ hoch, an den Flächen geringer.

Die mathematische Behandlung des Biegevorganges setzt eine ursprünglich gerade Stabachse voraus. Während der Biegung wird die Stabachse zu einer schwach gekrümmten ebenen Kurve, der elastischen Linie. Die Schubspannungen τ können im allgemeinen vernachlässigt werden, da diese Schubspannungen τ in den Randfasern verschwinden. Bei kurzen Stäben können jedoch die Schubspannungen in der Stabmitte, der Neutralschicht, von größerer Bedeutung als die Normalspannungen in den Randfasern sein. Werden bei Berechnung der Durchbiegung die Schubspannungen nicht berücksichtigt, so spricht man nicht mehr von der elastischen Linie, sondern von der Biegelinie. Durch die Formänderung (Abb. 13) bilden zwei ursprünglich parallele Querschnitte im Abstand dx voneinander einen Winkel $d\varphi$ miteinander: $d\varphi = dx \frac{M}{E \cdot I}$, wobei E der Elastizitätsmodul, I das Trägheitsmoment und M das Biegemoment ist. Das Produkt $E \cdot I$ ist das Maß für den Widerstand, den der Stab der Biegung entgegensetzt, und wird daher auch als Biegesteifigkeit bezeichnet. Nun kann man für die Biegelinie noch den Krümmungsradius bestimmen: $\varrho = \frac{E \cdot I}{M}$ cm oder den Kehrwert als Krümmung: $\frac{l}{\varrho} = \frac{M}{E \cdot I}$ cm^{-1}. Schließlich kann die allgemeine Differentialgleichung für die elastische Linie entwickelt werden, wenn für einen beliebigen Punkt der Biegelinie die Koordinaten x, y in einem rechtwinkligen System angenommen werden:

$$E \cdot I \frac{d^2y}{dx^2} = -M.$$

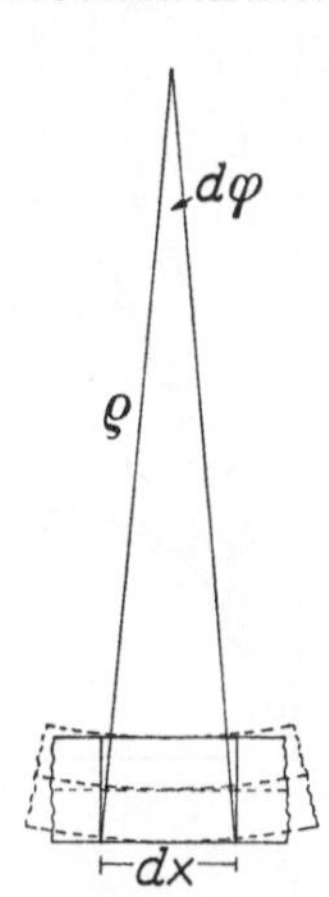

Abb. 13. Elastische Linie und Krümmung bei Biegung (vgl. Text)

Die elastische Linie wird für den Spezialfall zeichnerisch oder rechnerisch bestimmt. Für in der Technik häufig vorkommende Lagerungen und Lastformen liegen entsprechende Tabellen vor (z.B. HÜTTE I, 1955).

ββ) Biegefestigkeit des kompakten Knochens. Biegeversuche wurden an ganzen Skeletstücken und zubereiteten Proben vorgenommen. Bei Untersuchung der Biegefestigkeit wurde z.B. von MESSERER (1880), HIRSCH (1895) und RAUBER (1876) nur die Bruchlast in kg angegeben. Eine Zusammenstellung des Verhältnisses von P in kg und der Durchbiegung f in mm von 18 Biegeversuchen an ganzen Skeletstücken, Humeri (Material MESSERER, 1880 und KNESE et al., 1955) ergibt eine Variation der Bruchlast von etwa 100—300 kg (Abb. 14). Werden die Versuche nach männlich und weiblich getrennt untersucht, so liegt die Bruchlast bei Frauen niedriger als bei Männern, um 200 kg gibt es einen Überdeckungsbereich.

Zur Beurteilung der Biegefestigkeit ist die Bruchlast allein uncharakteristisch. KNESE et al. (1955) haben das Bruchmoment MbBr $= \frac{P \cdot l}{4}$ kg/cm für die Versuche von MESSERER (1880) und die eigenen errechnet, wobei l die Stützweite zwischen den Auflagerungen A und B bedeutet. Die Bruchmomente für den Humerus lassen sich in zwei Kollektive (Abb. 15) aufgliedern: I 780 $\pm$ 270 kg/cm, II 1470 $\pm$ 305 kg/cm. Das Kollektiv I wird überwiegend von Frauen und II nur von Männern gebildet, bei I sind 58,4% über 50 Jahre alt, bei II nur 28,6%.

KNESE et al. (1955) haben in gleicher Weise die Bruchmomente der großen Extremitätenknochen untersucht (Tabelle 3).

Tabelle 3. *Biegebruchmomente der Extremitätenknochen*

Femur. I: 1525 ± 725 (40%); II: 3175 ± 862,5 (55%); III: 5160 ± 410 (5%)
Tibia. I: 1310 ± 640 (76,5%); II: 2615 ± 160 (23,5%)
Fibula. I: 122 ± 51 (17,6%); II: 178 ± 58 (29,4%); III: 268 ± 85 (53%)
Humerus. I: 780 ± 270 (63,2%); II: 1470 ± 305 (36,8%)
Ulna. I: 325 ± 87,5 (75%); II: 585 ± 115 (25%)
Radius. 330 ± 250

Erläuterung: Die Biegebruchmomente wurden in Kollektive zerlegt, für die der Median-(Zentral-)wert, die Variationsbreite und der prozentuale Anteil am Urmaterial angegeben wird.

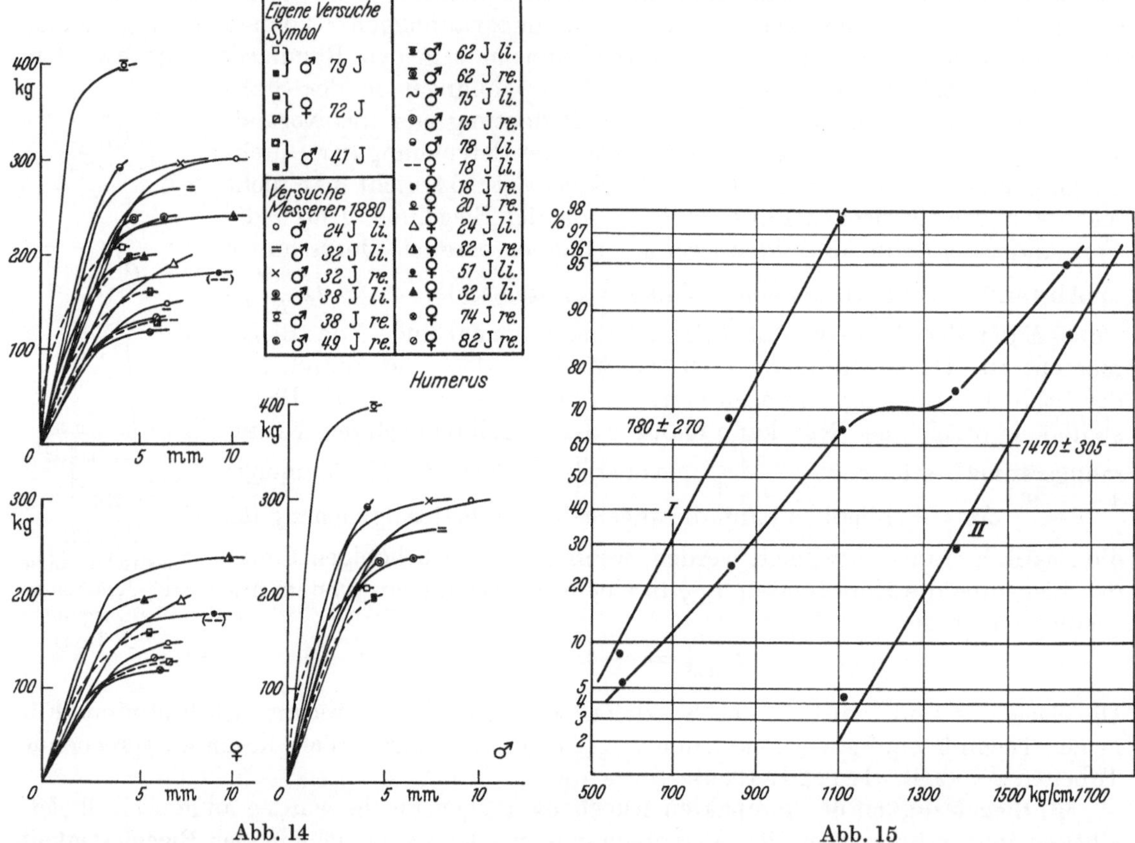

Abb. 14 Abb. 15

Abb. 14. Zusammenstellung der P—f-Diagramme der Messererschen und der eigenen Biegeversuche für den Humerus. Aufschlüsselung in ♂ und ♀ Individuen. Last P in kg, Durchbiegung f in mm. Eigene Versuche gestrichelt. Diagramme nach Messererschen Angaben gezeichnet (aus Knese, Hahne und Biermann, 1955)

Abb. 15. Bruchmomente der Messererschen und eigenen Versuche im Wahrscheinlichkeitsnetz von Daeves-Beckel, zwei Kollektive (aus Knese, Hahne und Biermann, 1955)

Die Biegebruchmomente der großen Extremitätenknochen lassen sich auf zwei Kollektive, bei Femur und Fibula auf 3, aufteilen; beim Radius liegt eine einfache Verteilung vor. Der Größe des Momentes nach folgen sich Femur, Tibia, Humerus, Ulna, Radius und Fibula. Die Frauen besetzen ausschließlich oder überwiegend die Kollektive: Femur I, Tibia I, Fibula II und I, Humerus I und Ulna I. Beim Radius liegen die Bruchmomente der Frauen im Bereich 330—250, die der Männer im Bereich 330 + 250. Die Variationsgröße des Bruchmomentes ist bei Männern größer; die größere Anzahl der Werte von Männern treten in den Kollektiven auf: Femur II, Tibia I und II, Fibula III, Humerus II. Die Bruchmomente sind bei Probanden über 50 Jahre kleiner als bei denen unter 50. Knese et al. (1955) haben ihre Biegeversuche mit Lastangriff in den verschiedenen Ebenen und in verschiedener Richtung (vorn-hinten und umgekehrt) durchgeführt; die vorliegende Zahl der Versuche ist zu gering, um eine Aussage über ein unterschiedliches Verhalten der Skeletstücke zu ermöglichen.

KNESE et al. (1955) haben für das gleiche Material — 64 Versuche ohne Fibula — den Elastizitätsmodul errechnet:

$$E = \frac{P \cdot l^3}{f \cdot I \cdot 48} \text{ kg} \cdot \text{cm}^{-2},$$

wobei P Kraft, f Durchbiegung, I Trägheitsmoment und l die Stützweite bedeutet. Für den Proportionalitätsbereich läßt sich das Material auf drei Kollektive (Tabelle 2) verteilen: I 57000 ± 23000 (11,2%), II 129000 ± 33000 (82,3%), III 219000 ± 37000 kg · cm^{-2} (6,5%). Die größere Zahl der Werte tritt damit im mittleren Kollektiv auf, das Kollektiv III wird von Skeletelementen der oberen Extremität gebildet. Über die Hälfte (52,9%) der Werte der Männer übersteigt den Zentralwert 129000 kg · cm^{-2}, bei den Frauen bleiben 53,6% unter dem Medianwert. Dem Lebensalter nach liegen bis 45 Jahre 70,8% über 129000 kg · cm^{-2}, von den Probanden über 60 Jahre 71,8% unter diesem Wert. Eine Aufschlüsselung der Werte nach rechts-links ergibt für rechts eine größere Zahl unter und links über 129000 kg · cm^{-2}.

Kurz vor dem Bruch besteht bei Biegung keine Proportionalität mehr zwischen der Spannung σ und der Dehnung ε, es tritt eine Art Fließbereich auf (KNESE et al., 1955). Da die Spannung σ annähernd gleichbleibt, die Dehnung aber zunimmt, ist der Elastizitätsmodul E^* im Augenblick des Bruches kleiner als im Proportionalitätsbereich. Die Proportionalitätsgrenze bei Biegung von Hundeknochen hat LINGGI (1951) zu $^1/_2$, $^3/_4$ und $^4/_5$ der Festigkeit angegeben, für Rattenfemora führt BELL (1956) $^3/_4$ auf. Der Elastizitätsmodul im Augenblick des Bruches E^* ist nach KNESE et al. (1955) bei menschlichen Knochen 50000 bzw. 84000 kleiner als im Proportionalitätsbereich.

Die sog. Biegefestigkeit $\sigma_{\max} = \frac{Mb}{W}$ kg · cm^{-2} zeigt eine große Variationsbreite, für die KNESE et al. (1955) fünf Kollektive wahrscheinlich machten (Tabelle 2), von denen das Kollektiv IV als Hauptkollektiv anzusehen ist: I 1020 ± 200 (6,2%), II 1200 ± 100 (10,5%), III 1500 ± 140 (25%), IV 1780 ± 180 (48,3%), V 2150 ± 250 kg · cm^{-2} (10%). Diese Kollektivanalyse zeigt nun, daß von den Männern 45,5% und von den Frauen 40,75% dem Kollektiv IV angehören, von den Frauen aber 51,81% und den Männern nur 30,33% den Kollektiven I—III und 7,41% bzw. 24,2% V. Die Biegefestigkeit der Knochen von Männern ist demzufolge höher als die von Frauen.

Im Hinblick auf die Altersklassen ergeben sich ebenfalls Veränderungen der Festigkeit. Zu den Kollektiven IV und V gehören unter 30 Jahren 72,6, zwischen 30 und 45 Jahren 91,66, zwischen 45 und 60 Jahren 33,32 und jenseits 60 Jahren 48,35% der Probanden. Zwischen 45 und 60 Jahren sind 66,6% im Kollektiv III und jenseits 60 Jahren 51,6% in den Kollektiven I—III vertreten.

KNESE et al. (1955) haben weiterhin festgestellt, daß die Maximalspannungen bei Biegungen überwiegend (58,3%) Zugspannungen sind und meinen daher, daß der Knochen im Augenblick des „Bruches" reißt (s. S. 518).

Die Untersuchung der Verteilung der Meßwerte beim Biegebruch mit Hilfe der graphischen Kollektivanalyse führten KNESE et al. (1955) zum Schluß, daß die Festigkeit der Knochen zum mittleren Alter (30—45 Jahre) hin zunimmt und dann individuell verschieden stark sinkt. Bei den Frauen ist die Festigkeit im Vergleich mit den Männern zu niedrigeren Werten hin verschoben.

Biegeversuche an ganzen Knochen von Ratten bei Lastangriff in der Mitte des Femur führten BELL et al. (1941) durch. Die Biegefestigkeit betrug 1900 kg · cm^{-2} und ist damit etwa von gleicher Größe wie bei jungen Hunden und Schafen (BELL und WEIR, 1949) und dem Menschen (KNESE et al., 1955; s. S. 432). Der Elastizitätsmodul der Rattenfemora war 110000 kg · cm^{-2}.

Bei den bisher mitgeteilten Versuchen waren die Skeletstücke in der Mitte belastet und an den Enden gestützt. Nun wurden auch Versuche an Knochen kleinerer Tiere durchgeführt, bei denen eine Einspannung an einem Ende und die Belastung am anderen erfolgte (Abb. 16); d.h. die Proben wurden im Sinne eines Balkon- oder Kragträgers belastet. Bei Einspannung an einem Ende tritt hier eine Auflagerkraft und ein Einspannmoment auf. In dem Einspannquerschnitt ist das Biegemoment am größten.

KREUZER (1932) hat Femora von Meerschweinchen einseitig eingespannt und erhielt im allgemeinen in der Einspannung den Bruch. Im Laufe des Lebens nimmt die Biegebruchfestigkeit von 413 auf 635 kg · cm^{-2} zu. Die Steigerung der Bruchfestigkeit geht sehr unregelmäßig vor sich. Bereits bei Tieren von 145—192 g treten recht hohe Werte auf und bei Exemplaren von 330—395 g ergeben sich fast die gleichen Zahlen wie bei erwachsenen Meerschweinchen von 607—750 g. Ähnlich sind die Beziehungen zwischen Femurlänge und Bruchfestigkeit.

Eine umfangreiche Untersuchung der Biegefestigkeit von Knochen des Hundes liegt von LINGGI (1951) vor. Die mittlere Festigkeit aus allen Versuchen beträgt 2003,9 kg · cm^{-2}, den höchsten Wert hatte ein Radius mit 3151 und den niedrigsten ein Femur mit 1181 kg · cm^{-2}. Den höchsten Durchschnittswert erreichten die Knochen eines 8 Jahre alten

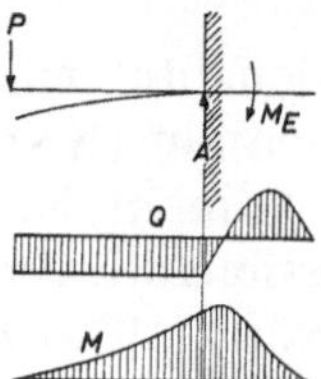

Abb. 16. Balken an einer Seite eingespannt (Kran- oder Balkonträger). P Kraft am Ende des Balkens; A Auflagereaktion an der Einspannung; M_E Einspannmoment; Q Querkraftfläche; M Momentenfläche

Tabelle 4. *Altersgang der Festigkeit beim Hunde* (nach LINGGI, 1951)

Alter	Biegung	Torsion
6 Monate bis $1^1/_2$ Jahre (11)	1881	485
2—8 Jahre (12)	2223	664
9—14 Jahre (17)	1930	600

In Klammern Anzahl der untersuchten Tiere.

Schnauzerbastards ♂ mit 2677, den niedrigsten eine $^1/_2$ Jahre alte Hündin, 1306 kg · cm^{-2}. Die mittlere Biegefestigkeit der einzelnen Knochen berechnet aus 40 Versuchen war: Radius 2193, Tibia 2108, Humerus 1919, Femur 1791 kg · cm^{-2}. Weiterhin fand LINGGI — ähnlich wie beim Menschen (s. oben) — eine Zunahme der Festigkeit zum mittleren Alter hin und dann wiederum eine Abnahme; wobei wir hier auch die Werte der Torsionsfestigkeit (s. S. 436) mitaufführen (Tabelle 4).

Es ergab sich, daß die Biegefestigkeit bei kleineren Tieren größer als bei größeren Hunden ist. LINGGI meint nun, daß der Unterschied in der Biegefestigkeit zwischen menschlichen und Hundeknochen ein Unterschied der absoluten Größen (Allometrie) sei. Dieser Schluß muß angezweifelt werden, da z.B. BELL et al. (1941) die Biegefestigkeit von Rattenfemora zu 1900 kg · cm^{-2} und HALLERMANN (1934) für Rinderknochen zu 2000 kg · cm^{-2} bestimmten (über Körpergröße und Knochenform: unter anderem ERTELT, 1955). Rassenunterschiede wurden an Lauf- und Schrittpferden von EICKHOFF (1927), von Haus- und Wildschwein von SCHMIDT (1915) sowie KNESE et al. (1962) und von Hunden von LINGGI (1951) erörtert.

LINGGI (1951) hat auch die Geschlechtsdifferenzen bei Hunden verfolgt. Die Festigkeit der Knochen von Rüden betrug für Biegung 2020 und Torsion 612, von Hündinnen 1975 bzw. 555 kg · cm^{-2}. Bei Untersuchung der Seitendifferenzen von 44 Knochenpaaren ergab sich bei Biegung und Torsion, daß viermal die Knochen beider Seiten gleich stark waren, 19mal war der rechte und 21mal der linke stärker, d.h. daß wie beim Menschen keine sicheren Seitendifferenzen bestehen (MESSERER, 1880; KNESE et al., 1955).

Die Biegefestigkeit wurde auch an zugerichteten Proben untersucht. RAUBER (1876) benutzte 80 mm lange, frische und feuchtgehaltene Stäbchen aus dem Femur und der Tibia. Die mittlere Biegefestigkeit aus drei Versuchen vom Femur und zwei von der Tibia eines 46jährigen Mannes bei 38^0 (in der Umrechnung von TRIEPEL, 1902) war 1837 kg · cm^{-2}, aus drei Versuchen bei 15—25^0 2223 kg · cm^{-2}.

An frischen und feuchtgehaltenen Stäbchen aus der Tibia und dem Femur von Haus- und Wildschweinen hat SCHMIDT (1915) die Biegungselastizität, besonders im Hinblick auf eine Restdehnung untersucht. Unmittelbar benachbarte Stücke aus dem Femur verhalten sich in ihrer Elastizität sehr verschieden. Der Autor hat infolgedessen Mittelwerte aus den Versuchen an verschiedenen Tieren gebildet. In dem Lebenszeitraum von einem $^3/_4$ bis zu 3 Jahren steigt der Elastizitätsmodul beim Wildschwein von 176000 auf 241000 und beim Hausschwein von 162000 auf 190000 kg · cm^{-2}, und zwar steigt der Elastizitätsmodul in jugendlichem Alter stärker als in fortgeschrittenem. Ein Deformationsrückstand tritt beim Wildschwein bei einer Spannung von 150—200, beim Hausschwein von 60—100 kg · cm^{-2} auf.

OLIVO, MAJ und TOAJARI (1937) stellten an Spänen aus dem Metacarpus und Metatarsus von Rindern und menschlichen Femora fest, daß keine konstante Beziehung zwischen Dehnung und Bruchlast besteht. MAJ (1942) bestimmte die Bruchlast bei Biegung von Stäben aus dem Humerus, Femur, Tibia und Ulna von 40 Individuen vom 5. bis 90. Jahr; die Spannungen werden leider nicht angegeben. Die Blöcke stammen aus den vier Quadranten des jeweiligen Skeletstückes.

δ) Die Schlagfestigkeit des Knochens

Festigkeitsversuche werden im allgemeinen unter sog. statischen Bedingungen durchgeführt, d.h. die Laststeigerung erfolgt derart, daß die Zeit keinen Einfluß hat.

Die gleichen Versuche können auch unter „dynamischen" Bedingungen als Schlagzugversuch, Stauchversuch und Schlagbiegeversuch durchgeführt werden; die Last wirkt plötzlich und von Beginn der Belastung an annähernd in voller Größe (s. S. 499). Die Untersuchung von KILLMER (1966) des Bruchvorganges beim Schlag mit dem Oszillographen ergab 2 Phasen. In der ersten, 0,5 msec währenden, biegt sich der getroffene Knochen mit einer Geschwindigkeit aus, die höher ist als jene des Schlagkörpers, die dann aber auf Grund der Elastizität wieder abnimmt. Knochen und Schlagkörper trennen sich dabei voneinander. In der zweiten Phase bleiben Knochen und Stoßkörper miteinander in Berührung und die kinetische Energie des Stoßkörpers wird in Biegeenergie übersetzt, wobei Schwingungen des Knochens hinzutreten. Während dieser Phase steigt die Dehnung des Knochens bis zur Bruchdehnung an. Die den Bruch erzeugende Kraft in der zweiten Phase kann mitunter nur 30% der maximalen Kraft der ersten Phase erreichen. In Pendelschlagwerken (Abb. 17, 18) wird der Arbeitsverbrauch zum Durchschlagen der Probe aus der Höhe des Durchschwingens nach Zertrennen der Probe errechnet und in kgm/cm^2 angegeben.

RÖSSLE (1930) hat an 60—62 mm langen Stücken aus dem zweiten distalen Viertel mit Hilfe eines Pendelschlagwerkes die Schlagfestigkeit des Knochens geprüft. Da das Material beim Zerschlagen zerspringt, wurden in einer Versuchsserie 32 Stück „kurze" Zeit in Formalin aufbewahrte Stücke verwandt, in einer zweiten Serie 109 Proben nach verschieden langer Maceration und Entfettung und bei 25 wurde nach der Maceration auf die Entfettung verzichtet. Alle präparatorischen Maßnahmen, auch die Trocknung, hatten einen geringen Einfluß auf die Schlagfestigkeit. Durch Trocknung erleiden 62 mm lange Stäbchen einen Gewichtsverlust von 2,5 g. Die Schlagfestigkeit war bei Serie 1: 0,35; 2: 0,4; 3: 0.376, d.h. im Mittel 0,375 kgm/cm^2. RÖSSLE nimmt die normale Schlagfestigkeit des Knochens infolgedessen zu 0,4—0,5 kgm/cm^2 an; die Schlagfestigkeit von Flußeisen beträgt 9,3.

Bereits 6jährige können den endgültigen Wert der Schlagfestigkeit erreichen; bei vier Kindern schwankte der Wert zwischen 0,19 und 0,4 kgm/cm^2. Die Schlagfestigkeit ist unabhängig von der Form der Probe und dem spezifischen Gewicht des Knochens. Bei älteren Leuten finden sich sehr hohe und niedrige Werte, aber die mittleren fehlen. Bei grazilen Mädchen wurden ebenfalls hohe und niedrige Zahlen gefunden. RÖSSLE konnte zwei durch Unfall verstorbene 20jährige Männer vergleichen; bei dem einen von

35,5 kg Gewicht war die Schlagfestigkeit 0,27, bei dem anderen von 57 kg Gewicht 0,68 kgm/cm².

Hallermann (1934) hat Rinderknochen im Pendelschlagversuch getestet und fand die Werte 0,086—0,092—0,125 kgm/cm² und meint, die Schlagfestigkeit sei wegen der fehlenden Plastizität des Knochens sehr gering.

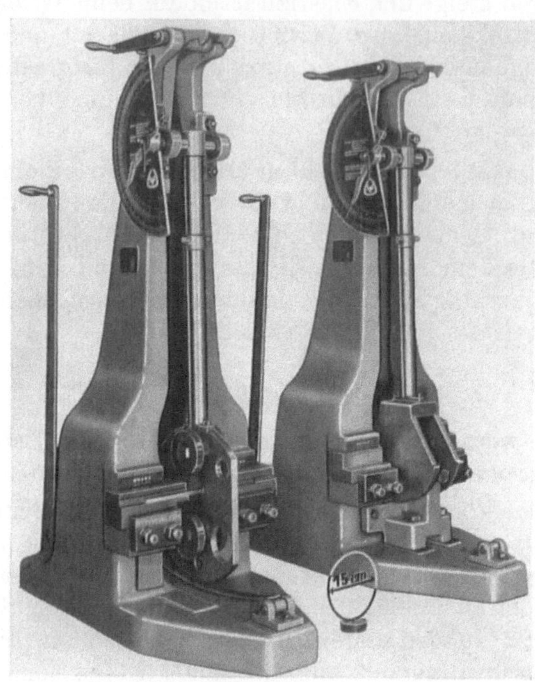

Abb. 17. Pendelschlagwerk (aus Amedick und Bussmann 1958)

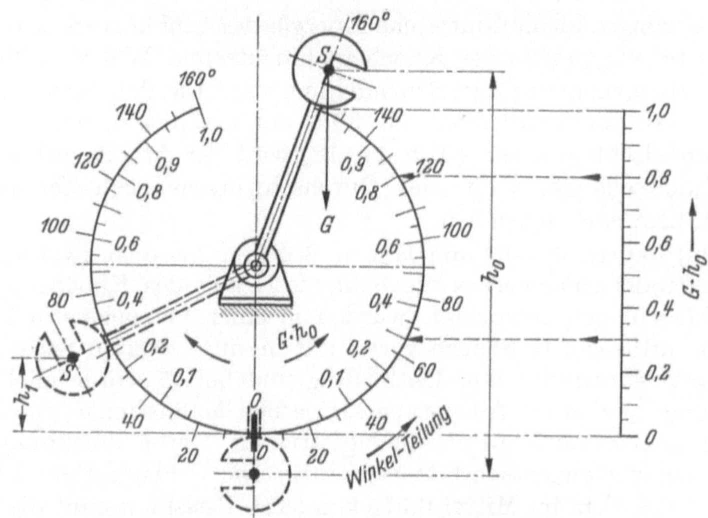

Abb. 18. Pendelschlagwerk (aus Amedick und Bussmann 1958)

ε) *Die Torsionsfestigkeit des kompakten Knochens*

Eine Drehbelastung liegt vor, wenn an einem Stabe senkrecht zur Stabachse ein Kräftepaar oder eine Kraft P mit einem entsprechenden Hebelarm r wirkt. Dann entsteht ein Torsionsmoment $M_t = P \cdot r$ kg/cm. Eine Torsion ist bei ein- oder beidseitiger Einspannung möglich. An der Einspannung liegen Einspannmomente vor. Bei beidseitiger Einspannung — wie sie für Skeletstücke zu erwägen ist (s. S. 501) — eines Stabes von der Länge l und einem Kraftangriff in dem Abstand a vom Lager A und b vom Lager B, betragen die Einspannmomente:

$$M_A = \frac{M_t \cdot b}{l}, \quad M_B = \frac{M_t \cdot a}{l} \text{ kg/cm}.$$

Der Torsion setzt die Querschnittsform des Stabes ähnlich wie bei Biegung ein Widerstandsmoment entgegen.

Die Torsionsfestigkeit hat MESSERER (1880) an großen Röhrenknochen geprüft. Die Bruchbelastung bei einem Torsionshebel von 16 cm betrug in kg: Clavicula 8 (5—11), Humerus 40 (25—51), Radius 12,5 (8,5—17,5), Ulna 8 (5—13,5), Femur 89 (50—142), Tibia 48 (30—70), Fibula 6 (4—10). Die Bruchstellen lagen beim Humerus, Femur und der Fibula im oberen bzw. unteren, beim Radius im oberen Drittel, bei Ulna und Tibia im unteren Viertel und bei der Clavicula in der Mitte. Die Bruchlinien verliefen schräg schraubenförmig in einem Winkel von 45° im Sinne der Drehrichtung um den Knochen herum, wobei dann ein Längsriß Anfangs- und Endpunkt der Schraubenlinie miteinander verbindet. Der Torsionswinkel bis zum Bruch für das beobachtete Mittelstück, das die halbe Länge des ganzen Skeletstückes maß, war: Humerus 7,6—17,2°, Radius 9,0—23,4, Ulna 6,8—7,9, Femur 5,0—16,2, Tibia 5,4—13, Fibula 7,2—23,9°. Für die Versuche an den Femora eines 29jährigen Mannes hat MESSERER die Torsionsfestigkeit zu 580 bzw. 570 und den Torsionsmodul zu 53420—46660 kg · cm^{-2} errechnet.

Einzelversuche an ganzen fixierten Knochen wurden unter Angabe des Torsionsmomentes von PEDERSEN et al. (1949), CAROTHERS et al. (1949) und EHLER (1966b) veröffentlicht.

RAUBER (1876) hat an vier frischen Stäbchen von 80 mm Länge aus dem Oberschenkel eines 30jährigen Mannes die Torsionsfestigkeit zu 790 kg · cm^{-2} bestimmt. DEMPSTER und LIDDICOAT (1952) haben aus Versuchen mit trockenen Stäbchen aus sechs Tibiae die Torsionsfestigkeit zu 748 ±80 kg · cm^{-2} errechnet.

LINGGI (1951) bestimmte als Durchschnittswert aller Torsionsversuche an Hundeknochen die Torsionsfestigkeit 595 kg · cm^{-2}, d.h. die Torsionsfestigkeit beträgt weniger als $^1/_3$ der Biegefestigkeit. Für die einzelnen Knochen ergaben sich folgende Durchschnittswerte: Radius 672, Humerus 599, Femur 583 und Tibia 527 kg · cm^{-2}. Ein 8 Jahre alter Rüde erreichte den höchsten Mittelwert mit 808, eine 6 Monate alte Hündin den niedrigsten Wert mit 257 kg · cm^{-2}. Die größte Torsionsfestigkeit zeigte der rechte Radius eines 14 Jahre alten deutschen Schäferhundes von 1049 kg · cm^{-2}, die kleinste, 222 kg · cm^{-2}, der linke Humerus einer $^1/_2$jährigen Hündin (Tabelle 4).

Die Torsionsfestigkeit von Rattenfemora bestimmten BELL et al. (1941) zu 670 kg · cm^{-2}, d.h. auch etwa zu 35% der Biegefestigkeit.

ζ) *Die Scherfestigkeit des kompakten Knochens*

Die Technik unterscheidet heute zwischen Schubspannungen und Scherspannungen. Schubspannungen entstehen z.B. in den Längsschichten eines Balkens (Abb. 19), in denen

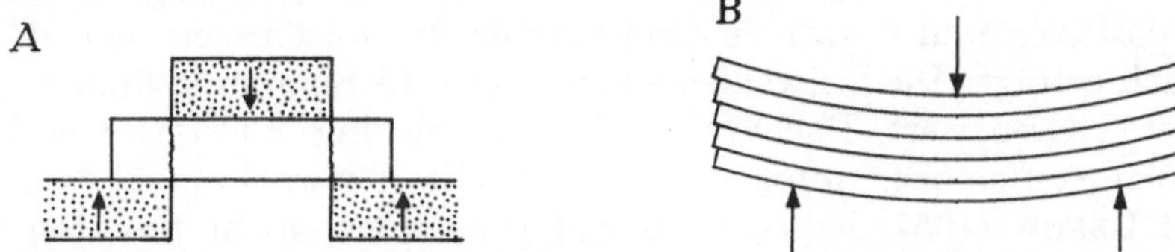

Abb. 19. A Scherbeanspruchung; B Schubbeanspruchung bei Biegung, dargestellt durch die Verschiebung getrennt gedachter Schichten des Biegebalkens

sich die Schichten bei Biegung gegeneinander verschieben (s. S. 431). Bei Scherkräften ist an das Bild der Schere zu denken, deren Branchen dicht aneinander vorbeigleiten. Derartige Belastungen liegen unter anderem bei Nieten vor. Bei dieser Scherbeanspruchung können auch kleine Biegemomente auftreten, die aber im allgemeinen wegen ihrer Kleinheit unberücksichtigt bleiben, ähnlich wie die Schubspannungen bei Biegung (s. S. 431). Die Scherspannung wird berechnet nach:

$$\tau = \frac{P}{F} \text{kg} \cdot \text{cm}^{-2}.$$

Rauber (1876) hat die Scherfestigkeit an Proben aus dem Femur eines 30jährigen Mannes untersucht. Die lange Achse von fünf Stäbchen entsprach der Längsachse des Femurs und damit erfolgte die Abscherung senkrecht zum „Faserverlauf". Die mittlere Scherfestigkeit war 1185 kg · cm^{-2}. Sechs Stäbchen desselben Femurs wurden senkrecht zur Femurachse entnommen und damit die Scherkraft parallel zur „Faser" ausgeübt, wobei sich eine Scherfestigkeit von 503 kg · cm^{-2} ergab.

Evans und Lebow (1951) haben an 242 Proben aus fixierten Knochen trocken bzw. feucht die Scherfestigkeit geprüft (Tabelle 1). Die mittlere Scherfestigkeit der trockenen Stücke war 563, der feuchten 689 kg · cm^{-2}, d.h. die feuchten Stücke hatten eine größere Scherfestigkeit als die trockenen, während die Zugfestigkeit trockener Proben (1078) größer als die feuchter (832) ist (s. S. 427). Topographisch ergaben sich folgende Differenzen: Von den trockenen Stücken erreichte das proximale Drittel (585), von den feuchten das mittlere (762) die höchste Scherfestigkeit; die Stücke aus dem distalen Drittel hatten die niedrigste Scherfestigkeit, trocken 546, feucht 658. Von den vier Quadranten aus den Femurquerschnitten besaß in trockenem Zustande der laterale (624), in feuchtem der mediale (726) die höchste Scherfestigkeit. Sowohl trocken (503) als auch feucht (662) wies der vordere Quadrant die kleinsten Werte auf. Mit Hilfe des Computers haben Evans und Bang (1967) die mittlere Scherfestigkeit für fixierte Knochen errechnet, und zwar für den Femur 700, die Tibia 805 und die Fibula 800 kg·cm^{-2}.

η) Die Wechselfestigkeit des kompakten Knochens

Bei den bisherigen Erörterungen wurde eine ruhende (statische) oder stoßartige (dynamische) Belastung angenommen. Unter diesen Belastungen tritt ein sog. Gewaltbruch auf. Nun kann auch eine Wechselbeanspruchung vorliegen, bei der die Last ständig von unterschiedlicher Größe, unter Umständen auch von verschiedener Art ist. Bei solchen Wechsellasten kommt es zu Verschiebungen oder zum Gleiten der Materialteile, die entweder zu einer Verfestigung oder zu einer Zerrüttung führen. Wenn nach unendlich vielen Lastspielen sich Verfestigung und Zerrüttung die Waage halten, d.h. kein Bruch auftritt, so spricht man von der Dauerschwingfestigkeit des Stoffes. Nach einer Anzahl von Lastspielen kann die Zerrüttung überwiegen und es kommt zum Dauerbruch. Die Bruchlinie beginnt an der Oberfläche und dringt in die Tiefe ein, bis der Querschnitt soweit geschwächt ist, daß zum Schluß ein Gewaltbruch die vollständige Durchtrennung bringt. Ausgangspunkt des Versagens sind häufig mikroskopisch kleine Unregelmäßigkeiten oder Fehler der Oberfläche. Das Lastspiel beträgt Millionen.

Dauerschwingversuche können mit Zug, Biegung und Verdrehung durchgeführt werden. Als Wechselfestigkeit σ_W wird jener Halbwert der Spannungsänderung zwischen gleich großen positiven und negativen Grenzwerten der Last bezeichnet, den der Werkstoff ohne Bruch erträgt. Die Schwellfestigkeit σ_{Sch} ist die Spannungsänderung zwischen 0 und einem oberen Grenzwert. Das Verhältnis von Schwing- zu statischer Festigkeit ist bei den einzelnen Stoffen sehr unterschiedlich, im Mittel etwa 1:3.

Evans und Lebow (1957) haben an feucht gehaltenen, nicht fixierten Stücken aus Femur und Tibia von amputierten Extremitäten die Schwingfestigkeit bei einer Belastung von 350 kg · cm^{-2} untersucht, die etwa der Hälfte der mittleren Zugfestigkeit feuchter Knochenproben entspricht. Bei 15 Femurproben ergab sich bis zum Bruch ein mittlerer Lastwechsel von 1188453 (84000—5332000), bei 47 Tibiastücken 1982650 (47000—6541000). Bei den 47 Tibiaproben wurde auch das Verhalten der Stücke aus den verschiedenen Abschnitten des Skeletstückes untersucht. Der Lastwechsel betrug:

proximales Drittel 914583 (57000—2564000), mittleres Drittel 2800117 (47000 bis 6191000), distales Drittel 1775623 (86000—6541000). Die Schwingfestigkeit des mittleren Drittel übersteigt um 57% das distale, um 206% das proximale, das distale Drittel wiederum um 94% des proximalen. Bei den Quadranten der Tibiaquerschnitte ergab sich folgendes Lastspiel: vorderer 1519799 (47000—5493000), hinterer 2283615 (154000 bis 6541000), lateraler 2120181 (128000—6191000) und mittlerer 1850608 (58000 bis 5546000). Damit ist die Schwingfestigkeit des hinteren Quadranten um 7% größer als jene des lateralen, 23% größer als des medialen und 50% größer als des vorderen, die Festigkeit des lateralen übersteigt den medialen um 14% und den vorderen um 39%, der mediale den vorderen um 21%. Fünf Fibulaproben ergaben bis zum Bruch einen Lastwechsel von 2841400. Bei einem Paraplegiker war die Schwingfestigkeit um 194% kleiner als bei den anderen; werden die Werte dieses Probanden ausgeschaltet, ergeben die restlichen 36 Versuche ein Mittel von 2378211 Lastwechsel bis zum Bruch.

Im Hinblick auf die sog. Marschfraktur haben LEASE und EVANS (1959) an 51 Metatarsen 2—5 von 8 Männern und 3 Frauen, davon jeweils ein Neger, die Schwingfestigkeit untersucht. Zehn Knochen wurden trocken, 41 feucht geprüft. Bei einer Last von 4,81 kg (15 lb) variierte der Lastwechsel bei trockenen von 1000—10297000, bei feuchten von 150000—13908000. Metatarsus 2 und 3 zeigen die größte Schwingfestigkeit feucht, 4 und 5 trocken. Die Autoren konnten keine Beziehungen zwischen der Schwingfestigkeit, Größe der Knochen oder Alter der Untersuchten finden. Die Fraktur stellt eine schiefe Bruchlinie dar.

ϑ) Die Härte des kompakten Knochens

Als Härte eines Materials wird der Widerstand bezeichnet, den die Oberfläche dem Eindringen eines Prüfkörpers entgegensetzt. Eine theoretische Formulierung der Härte hat HERTZ (vgl. FÖPPL, 1951) durchgeführt. Die erste Beschädigung des Materials tritt aber im Gegensatz zur Theorie bei verschiedenen Spannungswerten auf, die von den Radien der jeweils aufeinander gedrückten Kugeln abhängen. Die Härte hängt noch von Oberflächenspannungen ab. Eine Beziehung zwischen Härte und den übrigen Materialeigenschaften läßt sich im allgemeinen nicht nachweisen. Bei manchen Metallen bestehen Beziehungen zwischen dem Eindringwiderstand und der Zugfestigkeit. Das Knochengewebe scheint gegenüber einer reinen Oberflächenbeanspruchung sehr empfindlich zu sein (KNESE, 1959). Sehr kleine Kräfte führen zur Drucknekrose beim Decubitus, zur Usur der Wirbelsäule beim Aortenaneurysma; diese Schädigungen des Knochengerüstes sind bei Zugrundelegung der hohen Druckfestigkeit des Knochens unverständlich. Knochenstellen unter der Haut sind häufig durch Schleimbeutel (Patella, Olecranon) oder Polster (Fußsohle) abgesichert.

Die Härteprüfungen unterscheiden sich voneinander nach dem Aufbringen der Last (statisch, dynamisch), Art des Prüfkörpers und Größe der Prüfkraft; nach der Prüfkraft ergibt sich eine Makro-, Kleinlast-, und Mikrohärte. Für den Knochen liegen sowohl Prüfungen der Makro- als auch Mikrohärte vor.

RÖSSLE (1927) hat seine Versuche an planparallelen Platten aus dem Femur durchgeführt, die zur Desinfektion „kurz“ in Fixierungsflüssigkeit gebracht wurden; Vorversuche hatten ergeben, daß unfixierte Stücke die gleichen Härtewerte ergeben. Bei der Brinellschen Kugeldruckprobe mit einer Last von 10 kg mißt der Eindruck auf dem Knochenquerschnitt etwa 600 μ, das entspricht der Härtezahl 0,035. Es besteht ein Zusammenhang zwischen spezifischem Gewicht, aber nicht Ca-Gehalt, und Härte. Bis zu einem spezifischen Gewicht von 1,87 ist der Kugeleindruck nicht kleiner als 620 μ, bei einem spezifischen Gewicht unter 1,65 stets über 650 μ. Die endgültigen Härtewerte werden bereits in der Pubertätszeit erreicht, kindliche Knochen sind weicher. Die Härte weist keine Beziehungen zur Form der Skeletteile auf. Im Alter nimmt die Härte kaum ab, selbst nicht bei seniler Knochenatrophie. Geschlechtsunterschiede bestehen nicht. Die Knochenhärte hängt auch nicht von der mechanischen Leistung der Skeletstücke ab.

Lexer (1928) hat die Brinell-Härte bei 5 und 10 kg Belastung am Humerus bestimmt und mit dem Gewicht des Musculus biceps verglichen (Tabelle 5).

Tabelle 5. *Härte des kompakten Knochens* (nach Lexer, 1929)

	5 kg μ	10 kg μ	M. biceps (g)
Normal (22)	475	604	136
Tb (15)	480	613	79
Ca (38/37/33)	435	618	75
Humerus ♂ (14)	473	606	148
♀ (5)	478	622	115
Femur ♂ (23)	—	613	
♀ (11)	—	602	
♂+ ± (81, Rössle)	436		

Zahlen in Klammern geben die Anzahl der Proben an.

Alter	Humerus (5 kg)	Femur (5 kg)
15 Jahre ♂	521	525
18 Jahre ♂	489	504
90 Jahre ♂	502	497
92 Jahre ♂	489	498
93 Jahre ♀	501	481

Lexer (1928) kommt zum Schluß, daß die Härte ein für das ganze Skelet einheitliche Eigenschaft ist, die keine Beziehungen zur mechanischen Leistung der Teile und zum jeweiligen Muskelgewicht zeigt. Die Härte ändert sich bei seniler Osteoporose und einem Krebsleiden nicht, wohl aber bei Tuberkulose.

Evans und Lebow (1951, 1952) haben an ihrem fixierten Material auch die Härte mit der Methode nach Rockwell getestet. Lufttrocknung des Knochens steigert die Härte um 54%.

Die Mikrohärte haben Amprino (1958, 1961) und Rosate (1958) mit Hilfe der Vickers-Methode untersucht, bei der eine Diamantpyramide mit dem Spitzenwinkel von 136° benutzt wird. Amprino hat die Versuche an Längs- und Querschnitten von Knochen ausgeführt. Für die Prüfung wurden Osteone verschiedenen Typus, General- und Schaltlamellen ausgewählt. Bei kleineren Osteonen von Mensch, Rind und Pferd war die Prüflast 25—50 g, bei größeren von Giraffe und Elefant 50—200 g. Die Schnitte wurden nach der Härteprüfung fixiert und in gewöhnlichem Licht, Auflicht, polarisiertem Licht und mikroradiographisch untersucht. Die Verlagerung und Verdickung der Lamellen nach Härteprüfungen sind bei trockenem Knochen irreversibel. Die Härte nimmt nach Entwässerung bei 38° um 30,6%, bei 60° um 60,5% und bei 120° um 103% zu. Die Mikrohärte hängt z.T. vom Verlauf der Kollagenfibrillen ab, da sich ein Unterschied von 20—25% ergibt, je nachdem die Belastung parallel oder senkrecht zu den Fibrillen erfolgt. Weiterhin bestehen Beziehungen zum Ca-Gehalt, die allerdings nur bei Vergleich von Gebieten gleichartiger Feinstruktur nachweisbar sind. Die Härte des „primären" Knochens ist größer als die des „sekundären" mit Haversschen Systemen. Die Beziehungen zwischen Mikrohärte und Struktur sind sehr verwickelt, da sowohl die Dichte der Fibrillenlagerung als auch der Wassergehalt von Bedeutung sind.

Rosate (1958) prüfte die Mikrohärte bei schrittweiser Trocknung in oberflächlichen und tiefen Schichten des primären Knochens des Metacarpus von Rindern verschiedenen Alters. Die Mikrohärte des subperiostalen Knochens — etwa 200 μ von der Oberfläche entfernt — nimmt von Feten zu erwachsenen Tieren zu, woraus Rosate auf einen verschieden starken Mineral- und Wassergehalt des in den einzelnen Lebensperioden neu gebildeten Knochens schließt. Der primäre periostale Knochen hat einen größeren Mineralgehalt als der „sekundäre" mit Haverschen Systemen. Die Trocknung des Knochens bei 38, 60 und 120° erhöht die Härte bei Feten stärker als bei Erwachsenen. Rosate nimmt an, daß bei jüngeren Individuen das Wasser leichter als bei älteren zu entfernen und daß die Struktur des fetal und postnatal gebildeten Knochens voneinander verschieden ist. Die Mikrohärte von älterem Knochengewebe in etwa 1200 μ Abstand von der Oberfläche zeigt eine große Variation. Auch die Zunahme der Härte durch Trocknung läuft anders als bei subperiostalem Knochen ab. Vermutlich ist der Betrag des entziehbaren Wassers bei älterem Knochen geringer. Durch erneute Befeuchtung kehrt sowohl bei jungem als älterem Knochengewebe die ursprüngliche Härte zurück. Das Wasser scheint bei Wässerung in seine vorgegebene Position einzutreten.

Weiterhin hat ROSATE (1958) die Mikrohärte in den Quadranten innerhalb verschiedener Querschnittshöhen durch den Rindermetacarpus gemessen. Die Mikrohärte ist subperiostal gering, in den mittleren Zonen hoch und fällt zur Markhöhle hin ab, wenn der primäre Knochen durch Osteonknochen ersetzt ist. Dabei sind Variationen nach dem Alter und dem untersuchten Quadranten zu beachten, die vermutlich mehr von der Rate der Apposition als dem Grad der Mineralisation abhängen. Die größte Mikrohärte liegt in den mittleren Schichten und dann wieder im vorderen Quadranten der Compacta. Die Mikrohärte nimmt von der Mitte der Diaphyse zu den Epiphysen hin ab. Diese Differenzen sind bei Feten besonders deutlich. Zum Vergleich wird auf die Befunde von STROBINO und FARR (1949) hingewiesen, nach denen der Aschegehalt in der Diaphysenmitte am größten ist und zu den Knochenenden hin abnimmt, der N-Gehalt sich aber umgekehrt verhält.

ι) *Die Zerspanbarkeit des Knochengewebes*

Die bisher erörterten Untersuchungen über die Beanspruchungen des Knochengewebes suchten das Verhalten des Knochengewebes bei „natürlichen" Beanspruchungsformen zu studieren. Bei vielen chirurgischen Maßnahmen wird das Knochengewebe „ungewöhnlichen" Beanspruchungen unterworfen, einem Sägen oder Bohren, allgemeiner: einer Zerspanung. Als Zerspanbarkeit wird das Verhalten eines Werkstoffes unter dem Schnitt verschiedener spanabhebender Werkzeuge verstanden. Bei einer Materialbearbeitung durch Zerspanen wird zwischen Drehen, Fräsen, Feilen, Sägen, Bohren usw. unterschieden. Ähnlich wie bei der Prüfung auf Härte muß demzufolge das Verhalten des Materials bei den einzelnen Bearbeitungsformen für sich untersucht werden, da keine allgemeine Gesetzmäßigkeit der Zerspanbarkeit besteht. Für die Zahnhartgewebe liegen Untersuchungen über das Bohren und Schleifen vor (FRITZEL, 1950; SCHUBERT, 1957; TITKENMEYER, 1957), die Zerspanbarkeit des Knochengewebes wurde dagegen weniger untersucht (HADENFELDT, 1930; KLAPP und RÜCKERT, 1944; THOMSEN, 1951, 1955; SACHSE, 1957; Übersicht: KNAACK, 1962). Die technische Zerspanungslehre hat noch nicht alle vorliegenden Probleme gelöst (LANG, 1949), vor allem die Bedeutung intermolekularer Vorgänge (s. S. 525), die Beziehungen zwischen Werkstoff und Werkzeug mit den auftretenden Verklebungen usw. sind unklar. Eine einfache Korrelation zur Härte, Zugfestigkeit usw. besteht nicht. Die Zerspanung erfolgt in einer Reihe von Phasen, dem Einschneiden, Aufspalten, Zusammenstauchen und Abscheren. Bei den Spanformen wird zwischen Reißspan, Scher- und Fließspan unterschieden.

Das Knochengewebe ist im Hinblick auf die Zerspanbarkeit als harter Stoff anzusehen (KNAACK 1962), der eine feine Zahnteilung und einen kleinen bis negativen Zahnwinkel der Säge fordert. Die Spanform ist ein Reißspan. Bei der Kontinuitätstrennung kommt es unter Überschreitung der Zugfestigkeit der Kollagenfaser zur Zerreißung der Fasern. Die „thermoelastische Anomalie" (WÖHLISCH, 1926) der Kollagenfaser ist für die Entstehung eines Teiles der Zerspanungswärme des Knochens verantwortlich. Eine Wärmekontraktion des Kollagens erfolgt vermutlich nicht, da das Kollagen nach KNESE (1958b) durch die Hydroxylapatitkristalle vorgespannt ist. Das Kollagen wird unter Wärmeeinwirkung kautschukähnlich und erleidet eine Herabsetzung seiner Zugfestigkeit. Der Elastizitätsmodul der Rindersehne sinkt nach LERCH (1950b) bei thermischer Umwandlung von 8500 auf 25 kg $\cdot$ cm^{-2}. Der Knochen absorbiert gegenüber den Weichteilen ein Vielfaches an mechanischer Schwingungsenergie; nach THEISMANN und PFANDER (1949) ist der Schwächungskoeffizient für Schwingungsenergie beim Knochen 15mal größer als bei der Muskulatur (Absorptionsmessungen von Ultraschall HÜTER, 1948, 1952; GÜTTNER, 1954).

Eine Wärmestauung ist beim Sägen nicht zu erwarten (KNAACK, 1962; MOLLOWITZ und KNAACK, 1962). Als spezifische Wärme wird jene Anzahl von Calorien bezeichnet, die eine Temperaturerhöhung eines Stoffes mit der Masse 1 g um 1° bewirkt. Die spezifische Wärme der Knochencompacta ist 0,3 cal/g Grad (BALAKIREW, 1932), für Fettgewebe und spongiösen Knochen 0,7 cal/g Grad (vgl. GÜTTNER, 1954). Durch Austrocknung sinkt der Wert für die Compacta auf 0,25 cal/g Grad (BALAKIREW, 1932). Die Wärmeleitfähigkeit des Knochens ist gut (ROUILLER und MAJNO, 1953) und hängt nach GRAYSON (1952) vom Wassergehalt, nach HUGGINS und BLOCKSOM (1935) von den Mineralien ab. Für trockenes Elfenbein beträgt die Leitfähigkeit nach BÜRKER (1900) $10^{-4} \frac{g}{cm/sec}$, für Knochenmark nach GRAF et al. (1957) $5 \cdot 10^{-4}$.

RÖSSLE (1927, 1930) erwähnt, daß er bei Sektionen die „Sägbarkeit" des Schädeldaches beachtet hat, berichtet aber nicht über das Ergebnis. Wir (gemeinsam mit HAHNE; unveröffentlicht) haben bei Markierungen des Knochens mit Bohrlöchern eine verschiedene Geschwindigkeit beim Eindringen des Bohrers beobachtet. Die graphische Registrierung der Eindringgeschwindigkeit des Bohrers unter konstantem Bohrdruck führte jedoch zu keinen brauchbaren Werten über die topographisch unterschiedlichen mechanischen Eigenschaften des Knochengewebes, da der komplexe Zerspanungsvorgang des Bohrens vom Durchmesser des Bohrers, seiner Schneidkante usw. abhängt.

d) Die Festigkeit des kompakten Knochens

α) Die mechanischen Eigenschaften des kompakten Knochens

Die vorliegenden experimentellen Untersuchungen der Knochenfestigkeit sind nicht allzu umfangreich, im Material und in der Untersuchungstechnik nicht immer unmittelbar miteinander vergleichbar. Schwierigkeiten bereitet ohne Zweifel die Beschaffung eines genügend großen frischen Materials, so daß bei vielen Vergleichsuntersuchungen auf tierische Knochen zurückgegriffen wird. In diesem Abschnitt fassen wir die Versuche an frischem Knochen zusammen.

Das kompakte Knochengewebe verhält sich in der Beziehung zwischen Spannung σ und Dehnung ε bei Druck z.T. wie ein sprödes Material, z.T. wie ein Material mit einer Quetschgrenze, d.h. die Dehnung ist stärker als die Spannungszunahme. Im Biegeversuch kann die Durchbiegung im Proportionalitätsbereich relativ groß sein, dann folgt ein kurzer Fließbereich. Experimentell ermittelte Festigkeitswerte stellen nur dann wahre Spannungen dar, wenn im Augenblick des Bruches der ursprüngliche Querschnitt erhalten bleibt, d.h. keine wesentliche Verformung auftritt, die die Spannungsverteilung verändert; weiterhin soll das Hokesche Gesetz gelten. Beide Bedingungen sind jedoch häufig nicht erfüllt bzw. läßt sich die Querschnittsform unmittelbar vor dem Bruch nicht bestimmen. Damit werden als Festigkeit „scheinbare" Spannungen bestimmt. Jedoch kann mit diesen scheinbaren oder konventionellen Werten gerechnet werden, da sich die Konstruktionsteile im Augenblick des Bruches vermutlich wie die Prüfkörper beim Festigkeitsversuch verhalten.

Die Festigkeit des kompakten Knochengewebes liegt bei den verschiedenen Beanspruchungsformen recht hoch (Tabelle 6). In der Zugfestigkeit kommt der Knochen in den Bereich von Kupfer und Duraluminium (Tabelle 7). Für Aluminium liegen die Grenzen der Zugfestigkeit mit 700—1100 kg · cm^{-2} denen beim Knochen sehr ähnlich. Reines Eisen hat die Zugfestigkeit 2200 und Gold 1400 kg · cm^{-2}. In der Druckfestigkeit steht der Knochen etwa zwischen den Mittelwerten von Sandstein und Diabas. Die Grenzen der Festigkeit sind beim Syenit (1500—2000) und Porphyrit (1200—2400) denen beim Knochen fast gleich. Bei sehr vielen Natursteinen übersteigt die Druckfestigkeit allerdings 2000 kg · cm^{-2}.

Das spezifische Gewicht technisch verwandter Steine beträgt zwischen 2,6—3,0, das von Knochen 1,5—2,1; ROBINSON (1962) gibt für den Knochen Erwachsener 1,5—2,1 und Neugeborener 1,5—1,8 an (vgl. WETZEL, 1910, s. S. 337). Das spezifische Gewicht von Aluminium ist 2,7, von reinem Eisen 7,876 und von Gold 19,29. Etwa das gleiche spezifische Gewicht wie Knochen haben hochporöser Ziegelstein (1,71 bis 1,81) und Klinker (1,6—1,9), deren Druckfestigkeit aber nur 100—150 bzw. 350 kg · cm^{-2} beträgt.

Von den Hölzern sind dem Knochen ähnlich der Nußbaum (σ_d 720, σ_z 1000, σ_b 1470) und die Weißbuche (σ_d 550, σ_z 1040, σ_b 1600). Die Kiefer liegt in der Biegefestigkeit viel tiefer (σ_d 820, σ_z 1040, σ_b 1000). Bei den Hölzern ist die Druckfestigkeit geringer als die Zugfestigkeit, beim Knochen die Druckfestigkeit aber größer. In der Biegefestigkeit verhalten sich Knochen und Holz etwa gleich. Weiterhin ist die Variationsbreite der Festigkeit des Knochens wesentlich kleiner als die von Hölzern.

Tabelle 6. *Festigkeit frischer Compacta*

Druck[2]		
σ_d Würfel	1210—2015	[1110—2100][1]
σ_d Prismen	1200	
Zug[2]		
σ_z	660—1320	[540—1390][1]
Biegung[3]		
σ_b max	930—2110	[780—2340][1]
σ_{zb}	975—1870	[790—2110][1]
σ_{db}	1020—2150	[820—2400][1]
Torsion[4]		
τ	575	
Elastizitätsmodul		
Druck[2]	206500—238000	[188000—251500][1]
Biegung[3]	57000—219000	[24000—256000][1]
Torsion[4]	50040	

[1] Werte geben die von KNESE et al. (1955) ermittelten Zentralwerte wieder; in [ ] der untere und obere Grenzwert.
[2] RAUBER (1876).
[3] Material MESSERER (1880) und KNESE et al. (1955).
[4] MESSERER (1880).

Von Bedeutung ist, daß der Knochen die hohen mechanischen Eigenschaften mit einem recht kleinen spezifischen Gewicht erreicht. Würde der Knochen z. B. durch Basalt ersetzt (spez. Gew. 2,93—3,15), so wäre für die Druckbelastung etwa nur $^1/_3$ des Materials erforderlich, für Biegung dagegen das 7fache; dem Gewicht nach würde bei Druck die Hälfte, bei Biegung das 10fache Gewicht anzunehmen sein. Bei hochwertigem Beton (B 600) müßte für Druck das 2,4fache, für Biegung das 20fache an Material — annähernd auch an Gewicht — für Spannbeton (s. S. 450) allerdings nur die Hälfte an Material

Tabelle 7. *Festigkeit von Hölzern, Steinen und Metallen* (aus HÜTTE I, 1955)

	δ_d	δ_z	δ_b	τ
Nußbaum[1]	‖ 720 (465—890)	1000 F	1470 (990—1780)	70
(Juglans regia)[2]	⊥ 120	35		
Weißbuche	‖ 820 (550—990)	1350 (470—2000)	1600 (580—2000)	85
(Carpinus betula)	⊥			320
Kiefer	‖ 550 (350—940)	1040 (350—1960)	1000 (410—2059)	100 (61—146)
(Pinus silvestris)	⊥ 77 (37—138)			210
Tanne	‖ 470 (310—590)	840 (480—1200)	730 (470—1180)	50 (37—63)
(Abies pectinata)	⊥ 42	23		275
Aluminium		700—1100		
Eisen (rein)		2200		
Gold		1400		
Flußstahl		3700—4500		
Gußeisen		2600		
Basalt	3160 (1000—5800)	196	248	
Buntsandstein	260	14,5	25	
Solnhofer Kalkstein	2290	104	180	
Marmor	590 (400—2800)	67	80	
Granit	800—2700			
Syenit	1500—2000			
Diabas	1300—3000			
Porphyrit	1200—2400			

[1] ‖ Parallel zur Faser. [2] ⊥ Quer zur Faser.

vorliegen (KNESE, 1958b). Das Skelet ist durch den hochwertigen Stoff „Knochen" grazil gebaut und im Gewicht gering (15—20% des Körpergewichtes), so daß eine Art Leichtbau (ROUX, 1895; PAUWELS, 1948) vorliegt. Die hohe mechanische Leistungsfähigkeit bei geringem spezifischen Gewicht beruht auf der eigentümlichen Struktur des Knochengewebes und dem Zusammenwirken von Kollagenfibrillen und Apatitkristallen, der sog. Materialstruktur des Knochengewebes.

β) Die Veränderung der Festigkeit durch Vorbehandlung des Knochens

Von technischen Materialprüfungen her ist bekannt, daß die Festigkeit von Baustoffen durch Temperatur, Wassergehalt u.a. stark beeinflußt wird. Aus diesen Gründen wurde bei Versuchen an Knochen häufig auf diese beiden Faktoren geachtet.

Der Einfluß der Vorbereitung des Materials, wie Sägen und Schleifen, wurde von SCHMIDT (1915) bei Untersuchung von Schweineknochen diskutiert (s. S. 435).

Bereits RAUBER (1876) hat über den Einfluß der Feuchtigkeit auf die Festigkeit des Knochengewebes Beobachtungen angestellt. Durch Wässerung erhalten ausgetrocknete Stäbchen ihre ursprüngliche Elastizität wieder; der Elastizitätsmodul des trockenen Materials war 231000, des feuchten 203600 kg · cm^{-2}. Zum Studium der Temperaturwirkung bewahrte RAUBER (1876) die Stäbchen in Wasser von 38^0 auf und führte den Versuch unter Wasser durch. Der Biegungsmodul betrug dann 197700, dagegen bei 10^0 217800 kg · cm^{-2}. SMITH und WALMSLEY (1959) haben angegeben, daß sich der Elastizitätsmodul umgekehrt proportional zur Untersuchungstemperatur verhält. Der Elastizitätsmodul ist bei 4,5^0 C (40^0 F) 102000 und bei 37^0 C (99^0 F) 87900 kg · cm^{-2}.

DONALDSON (1919/20) hat an Ratten und KREUZER (1932) an Meerschweinchen den Einfluß der Trocknung auf Skeletstücke verfolgt; beide Autoren haben bei Luft- bzw. Ofentrocknung stärkere Veränderungen bei jüngeren als bei älteren Tieren gefunden. Im Ofen getrocknete Knochen sind hygroskopisch (DONALDSON, 1919/20). Bei Meerschweinchen von 78—167 g hat KREUZER (1932) an den Femora einen Anstieg der Festigkeit durch Trocknung beobachtet und macht hierfür die Abnahme des Wassergehaltes verantwortlich. Zum Vergleich hat KREUZER den einen Femur eines Tieres frisch, den anderen nach Trocknung im Exsiccator untersucht und gleichfalls eine Erhöhung der Festigkeit gefunden.

SCHMIDT (1915) hat an frischen Proben von Schweineknochen, die sehr sorgfältig feucht gehalten wurden, Festigkeitsprüfungen kurz hintereinander ausgeführt und eine Abnahme der Festigkeit festgestellt. Nach SMITH und WALMSLEY (1959) ist die Elastizität des Knochens bereits 10 min nach Entnahme verändert, könnte aber vielleicht durch Einlegen in physiologische Kochsalzlösung wieder hergestellt werden. Die Wasserabnahme des Knochens ist nach diesen Autoren in den ersten 200 min sehr stark, zwischen 400 und 1600 min annähernd von gleicher Größe und recht gering.

CAROTHERS et al. (1949) stellten an über Jahre getrockneten (Sammlungs-)Knochen ein spezifisches Gewicht von 1,934 und eine Druckfestigkeit von 1743 kg · cm^{-2} fest. Bei „sorgfältig" aufbewahrtem fixiertem Material, das innerhalb eines Jahres untersucht wurde, war das spezifische Gewicht 1,977 und die Druckfestigkeit 1810 kg · cm^{-2}. Der Elastizitätsmodul des trockenen Materials betrug 211000 und des fixierten 188500 kg · cm^{-2}. Weiterhin prüften CAROTHERS et al. (1949) den Einfluß der Fixierung an den Femora von sechs weißen etwa 10 Wochen alten Rattenmännchen. Der rechte Femur wurde frisch, der linke nach 6wöchentlicher Fixierung durch Injektion untersucht. Für die Biegeversuche wird leider nur die Bruchlast angegeben. Bei den fixierten Femora steigt die Bruchlast gegenüber den unfixierten um 6—116%, im Mittel um 62,8% an.

An ganzen Stücken aus dem Femur und der Tibia Amputierter haben CALABRISI und SMITH (1951) jeweils eine Probe frisch, die andere nach etwa 7wöchentlicher Fixierung (43—56 Tage) in Alkohol 95%, reinem Glycerin, Formalin 10% zu gleichen Teilen untersucht. Der Mittelwert von je sieben Proben für die Druckfestigkeit frisch war 1913 und fixiert 1638 kg · cm^{-2}, d.h. die Abnahme der Druckfestigkeit betrug 13%. An ganzen

Diaphysenstücken war die Druckfestigkeit 1828, an zugerichteten Knochenproben 1772 kg · cm^{-2}, der Unterschied zwischen beiden Prüfungen war 4,8%.

Dempster und Liddicoat (1952) meinen, daß die von ihnen untersuchten macerierten und getrockneten Knochen bei Erhaltung der Struktur der Haversschen Systeme gegenüber dem des Lebenden grundsätzlich verändert seien. Der trockene Knochen sei vermutlich starrer, elastisch über einen größeren Bereich und fester als lebender Knochen. Die künstliche Befeuchtung mache das Material dem in vivo ähnlich, jedoch die Fixierung (deterioration) und übermäßige Wasseraufnahme setze die mechanischen Konstanten herab.

Bereits die Auswertung der Ergebnisse von Untersuchungen frischen Knochenmaterials bereitet große Schwierigkeiten, da die Versuchsbedingungen bei den verschiedenen Autoren nicht genau gleich sind. Noch größere Unsicherheit besteht bei der Diskussion der durch Fixierung, Maceration usw. erzeugten Änderungen der Festigkeit. Legt man den Erörterungen die in der Literatur mitgeteilten Mittelwerte (Tabelle 8) zugrunde, so

Tabelle 8. *Veränderung der Festigkeit durch Vorbehandlung des Knochens*

			Autor
Druckfestigkeit σ_d			
frisch	1913 kg · cm^{-2}		Calabrisi et al. (1951)
fixiert	1638		Calabrisi et al. (1951)
	trocken	*feucht*	
maceriert . . .	1805	1109	Dempster et al. (1952)
Zugfestigkeit σ_z			
maceriert . . .	1200	804	Dempster et al. (1952)
fixiert	1078	832	Evans et al. (1951)
Scherfestigkeit τ			
fixiert	563	689	Evans et al. (1951)
Elastizitätsmodul			
maceriert E_d	$\approx$ 183500	$\approx$ 148500	Dempster et al. (1952)
maceriert E_z	$\approx$ 189200	$\approx$ 121700	Dempster et al. (1952)
fixiert E_z	187700	119500	Evans et al. (1951)

setzt die Fixierung die Druckfestigkeit von 1913 auf 1638 kg · cm^{-2} (Calabrisi und Smith, 1951) herunter. Fixierte Knochen haben trocken eine größere Zugfestigkeit, 1078, als feucht, 832 kg · cm^{-2}; die Scherfestigkeit ist jedoch feucht (689) größer als trocken (563 kg · cm^{-2}) (Evans und Lebow, 1951). Die Zugfestigkeit des trockenen macerierten Knochens — 1200 kg · cm^{-2} (Dempster und Liddicoat, 1952) — ist vermutlich größer als die des fixierten trockenen — 1078 kg · cm^{-2} (Evan sund Lebow, 1951) — die des feuchten macerierten — 804 — aber nur wenig geringer als die des fixierten feuchten — 832 kg · cm^{-2}. Die Druckfestigkeit des macerierten trockenen Knochens — 1805 (Dempster und Liddicoat, 1952) — ist größer als die des fixierten — 1638 (Calabrisi und Smith, 1951) —, aber kleiner als die des frischen — 1913 kg · cm^{-2}. Evans (1964) hat die Zugfestigkeit von Tibia- und Femurproben fixiert und unfixiert, nach Bearbeitung der Werte mit dem Computer miteinander verglichen. Die Zugfestigkeit von Femurproben war unfixiert und trocken höher als fixiert und feucht. Fixierte, trockene und feuchte Proben der Tibia weisen eine höhere Zugfestigkeit als die unfixierten Proben auf. Weiterhin wurden die Eigenschaften einzelner Knochenregionen untersucht.

Durch Fixierung und Maceration nimmt der Elastizitätsmodul ab. Der Elastizitätsmodul des angefeuchteten fixierten bzw. macerierten Knochens ist geringer als der des trockenen, der von fixiertem und trockenen Knochen aber gleich. Nach Anfeuchtung ist der Elastizitätsmodul des fixierten Knochens vermutlich größer als der des macerierten.

Die Ultrastruktur des Knochengewebes (s. S. 336) läßt vermuten, daß Fixierung, Maceration, Trocknung und Durchfeuchtung eine starke Veränderung der organischen Komponenten bewirken. Die Denaturierung der Kollagenfibrillen setzt den Elastizitätsmodul gegenüber dem frischen Knochen auf 80% herab. Eine erneute Befeuchtung hebt die Strukturänderung nicht auf, sondern setzt den Elastizitätsmodul weiter auf 50—70% des frischen Knochens herab.

Die Einwirkung dieser Maßnahmen auf die organische Interfibrillärsubstanz, der sog. Grundsubstanz oder Matrix, die beim ausgewachsenen Knochen nur einen geringen Prozentsatz ausmacht (s. S. 333), ist schwer zu beurteilen. Beim lebenden bzw. überlebenden Knochen sind die hier vorhandenen MPS als Träger des Wassers und aufgrund ihrer Viscosität als die Verschiebeschichten anzusehen (s. S. 337; Vorspann). Damit ist der Elastizitätsmodul des frischen „überlebenden" Knochens größer als der des fixierten oder macerierten trockenen Knochens. Eine erneute Befeuchtung des vorbehandelten Knochens scheint durch Quellung des Kollagens bzw. der MPS (?), oder beider, das ursprüngliche Zusammenspiel der Gewebekomponenten vollständig zu zerstören, der Elastizitätsmodul sinkt weiter ab.

In einer umfangreichen Studie hat Sedlin (1965) die Veränderung der mechanischen Eigenschaften des Knochengewebes durch Vorbehandlung untersucht, um ein Modell zu entwickeln, das mit mathematischen Analogien alle mechanischen Eigenschaften des Knochengewebes beschreibt. Hierbei schließt Sedlin die Bedeutung der einzelnen Komponenten für die Festigkeit zwar nicht aus, versucht aber eine Integration zu erreichen. Untersucht wurden 663 Femurproben von 43 Individuen (14—91 Jahre). Die Proben wurden 7—96 Std. post mortem entnommen. Nur einige Ergebnisse können hier aufgeführt werden (vgl. Sedlin und Hirsch, 1966). Einfrieren hat keinen Einfluß auf die Festigkeit, die Formalinfixierung erhöht den Elastizitätsmodul für Zug, die Alkoholfixierung setzt die Größe der Deformation bei Biegung herab. Eine Trocknung erhöht den Elastizitätsmodul, die Erhitzung bis 105° führt zu einer Herabsetzung der Festigkeit, die Durchbiegung ist bei 37° größer als bei 21°. Alle diese Differenzen werden im Hinblick auf die Viscosität des Knochens interpretiert. Die Elastizität des Knochens ist feucht größer als getrocknet. Eine Altersabhängigkeit der Festigkeit konnte nicht sichergestellt werden. Weiterhin besteht nach Sedlin keine Korrelation zwischen der Größe des Volumens der Haversschen Kanäle und den physikalischen Eigenschaften des Knochens. Sedlin entwickelt nun ein mathematisches Modell, das einmal das Hooksche Gesetz berücksichtigt, dann aber auch im Hinblick auf die Plastizität die Bedingungen der Strömungslehre (Prandtl) und schließlich werden im Hinblick auf die Viscosität die Eigenschaften eines Newtonschen Körpers herangezogen. Eine endgültige Stellungnahme zu diesen Vorstellungen ist derzeit wohl noch nicht möglich. Jedoch meinen wir, daß gegenüber dem Versuch, ein einheitliches mechanisches Modell für die Behandlung der mechanischen Eigenschaften des Knochengewebes zu entwickeln, eine Interpretation im Hinblick auf die verschiedenen Komponenten dem Materialcharakter des Knochengewebes mehr entsprechen würde.

Durchbiegungen bei Biegeversuchen, bei der Fibula bis zu 14, bei anderen Knochen bis zu 5—7 mm (Knese et al., 1955), setzen erhebliche Verschiebungen zwischen den Materialkomponenten voraus. Tischendorf (1951a, 1951b) hat Winkelbalken aus der Compacta der frischen Tibia unter ständiger Benetzung mit Ringerlösung auf Biegung mit $^1/_5$, $^2/_5$, $^3/_5$ der Bruchlast beansprucht. Bei Auflichtbeobachtung wurden Dicke und Abstand der Lamellen der Haversschen Systeme gemessen. Die Abstandsänderungen liegen unter 1 μ und sind bei den äußeren Lamellen eines Osteons am größten. Bei Entlastung wird die Ausgangslage wieder eingenommen. Die Lamellen verbreitern bzw. verschmälern sich unter Last zu etwa gleichen Teilen. Weiterhin verschieben sich die Lamellen in bezug auf den Querschnitt des Haversschen Systems nach innen oder außen; sowohl steil als auch flach gewickelte verschieben sich auf der Druckseite zu $^2/_3$ nach innen und $^1/_3$ nach außen, auf der Zugseite nur wenig mehr als die Hälfte nach innen (Tischendorf, 1954). Zwischen den Lamellen erfolgen tangentiale Verschiebungen und Verdrehungen. Eine Beziehung zwischen dem Verhalten einer Lamelle und der Zugehörigkeit zur Druck- oder Zugseite des Probebalkens besteht nicht (Tischendorf, 1952/54). Im mittleren und äußeren Drittel des Osteonquerschnittes sind die Breitenänderungen der Lamellen gering. Auf der Druckseite findet eine Erweiterung und eventuell Biegungseinengung des Haversschen Kanals statt.

Das Zusammenspiel der Komponenten des Knochengewebes muß demzufolge durch Veränderung des Zustands der Teile — Fixierung, Wasserentzug oder Durchtränkung — gestört werden.

Amprino (1958, 1961) hat auf Grund seiner Untersuchungen und denen von Rosate (1958) die Änderungen der Mikrohärte durch Erhitzung diskutiert. Nach Erhitzung auf 200° ist die Härte geringer als nach Erhitzung auf 120°; der Knochen wird bei der Härteprüfung in feinste Teile zerdrückt. Die Zerbrechlichkeit der Proben nimmt bei Erhitzung auf 300 bzw. 500° zu; Amprino vergleicht den Zustand des Knochens dann mit dem von trockenem Sand. Eine Erhitzung des Knochens auf mehr als 500, auf 800° oder mehr läßt die Mikrohärte wieder ansteigen, der Knochen verhält sich nunmehr wie ein gebrannter Ziegelstein. Bei derart hohen Temperaturen kommt es vermutlich zur Verschmelzung von Apatitkristallen (Dallemagne, 1943; Carlström und Finean, 1954).

Für das Gleiten der Komponenten bei der Härteprüfung macht Amprino (1958) das Wasser verantwortlich. Durch Trocknung tritt eine Schrumpfung des Volumens um weniger als 20% ein, das Material wird solider. Der Verlust des Wassers läßt die Härte ansteigen. Erneute Durchfeuchtung von 4—48 Std führt zu einer Wasseraufnahme, die etwa dem Verlust bei Trocknung entspricht. Die Mikrohärte kehrt dabei zu dem ursprünglichen Wert zurück. Bei Durchtränkung tritt keine merkliche Schwellung auf. Eine erhöhte Wassermenge kann wohl erst bei einer schweren Schädigung der Mikrostruktur angenommen werden. Auch Wässerung einer Probe aus dem Metatarsus eines 5jährigen Rindes über 2 Monate bei Raumtemperatur hat die Mikrohärte nur wenig herabgesetzt. Durch eine derart lange Wässerung verliert der Knochen etwa den gleichen Betrag löslicher organischer Stoffe wie bei der Säureentkalkung (Rogers et al. 1952); die sich ergebenden Veränderungen betreffen weniger das Netz der Kollagenfibrillen, sondern mehr die physiko-chemischen Beziehungen zwischen den anorganischen Kristalliten und der organischen Intercellularsubstanz.

Häbler und Reiss (1936) haben Knochen von Hunden auf Biege- und Torsionsfestigkeit untersucht. Die Bruchstellen wurden chemisch analysiert und deren Wassergehalt bestimmt. Die Knochen des Hundes verhalten sich individuell sehr verschieden; die Unterschiede sind bei der Tibia größer als beim Radius. Die von den Autoren gegebenen Diagramme Kraft-Durchbiegung zeigen die gleiche Variationsbreite wie entsprechende Versuche an menschlichen Knochen von Knese et al. (1955; Abb. 14). Eine gesicherte Beziehung zwischen Biegefestigkeit und Feuchtigkeitsgehalt war nicht aufzufinden; bei der Tibia nimmt die Größe der Durchbiegung mit zunehmender Feuchtigkeit aber zu. Der Einfluß des Wassergehaltes scheint bei Torsion deutlicher zu sein. Häbler und Reiss (1936) haben zum Vergleich den rechten Radius eines Tieres im Exsiccator getrocknet, den linken unter Paraffinabschluß feucht gehalten. Der Wassergehalt der feuchten Knochen zweier Tiere betrug 11,8 bzw. 10,5% der trockenen 10,2 bzw. 9,5%. Der getrocknete Knochen besaß eine höhere Festigkeit, aber eine geringere Elastizität, so daß ein Sprödbruch auftrat; der feuchte Knochen zeigte dagegen einen Fließbereich. Die Verfasser haben weiterhin den Callus nach künstlich gesetzten Frakturen untersucht. Der Ca-Gehalt des Callus bezogen auf das Trockengewicht des heilenden Knochens entspricht dem des normalen, ist bezogen auf das Gesamtgewicht aber niedriger. Während der fortschreitenden Heilung findet eine Entquellung statt. Die Festigkeit des Callus hängt von dem Wassergehalt, aber nicht dem Ca-Gehalt ab.

Die Zunahme der Mikrohärte mit dem Lebensalter (Amprino, 1961; Rosate, 1958) hängt offensichtlich nicht mit dem Grad der Mineralisation zusammen, wie Carlström (1954) nach Untersuchung einzelner Osteone vermutete. Rowland et al. (1959) konnten auch bei einzelnen Individuen für Mensch und Hund keine Veränderung des Mineralgehaltes nachweisen. Die Steigerung der Mikrohärte wurde mit der Änderung der Ordnung der Kollagenfibrillen und einer Zunahme der Polymerisation der Grundsubstanz sowie einem abnehmenden Wassergehalt in Verbindung gebracht. Damit wird dann die Gleitfähigkeit der Kristalle herabgesetzt. Nach Rosate (1958) findet in der Fetalzeit kein wesentlicher Umbau im Metacarpus des Rindes statt; beträchtliche Teile des früh gebildeten Knochens bleiben erhalten. Die Mineralisation ist mit Ausnahme der subperiostal neu gebildeten Teile recht gleichartig. Jedoch bestehen zwischen den innersten marknahen, ältesten Knochenteilen und Schichten, die sowohl etwa 1000 μ von der Markhöhle als auch dem Periost abliegen, signifikante Härteunterschiede. Es liegt keine wesentliche Differenz in der Mineralisation und der im polarisierten Licht zu erkennenden Struktur der verglichenen Gebiete vor. So mögen Unterschiede im Wassergehalt und bzw. oder der physiko-chemischen Eigenschaften der „Grundsubstanz" vorhanden sein. Diese Veränderungen setzen ein, bevor die Mineralisation merklich zunimmt.

Differenzen in der Mikrohärte des Knochengewebes und deren Veränderung durch Vorbehandlung sind ähnlich wie die der anderen Festigkeitseigenschaften auf ein sehr komplexes Zusammenwirken der Komponenten des Knochengewebes zurückzuführen. Die Beziehungen zwischen Zug-Druck- usw. -festigkeit und Härte sind ungewöhnlich schwierig zu beurteilen. Alle bisherigen Härteprüfungen wurden an nicht natürlichen Knochenoberflächen, d.h. an Quer- oder Längsschnitten durchgeführt. Die Härteprüfungen sagen offensichtlich über die Verschieblichkeit der Komponenten in einem kleinen Bereich etwas aus. Die Befunde von Amprino (1958, 1961) und Rosate (1958) legen jedoch nahe, eine Korrelation zwischen der Zugfestigkeit und der Härte zu suchen, wie sie bei einer Reihe von technischen Materialien vorliegt. Eine Verschieblichkeit der Komponenten ist aber der Struktur nach bei allen Belastungsformen anzunehmen (s. S. 446).

γ) Die Materialstruktur des kompakten Knochens

Die Festigkeit der einzelnen Stoffe beruht offensichtlich auf deren jeweils spezifischer Materialstruktur bzw. ihrer Molekularstruktur. Allerdings ist nur z.T. geklärt, warum ein Stoff spezielle mechanische Eigenschaften besitzt und unter welchen Bedingungen dann ein Versagen, der Bruch, auftritt. Für die auffällig hohe Festigkeit des Knochens bei unterschiedlicher Belastung wurde eine Erklärung in der dem Knochengewebe eigenen Struktur gesucht (s. S. 359).

Gebhardt (1906) hat angenommen, daß in einer Lamelle des Haversschen Systems die Kollagenfasern parallel zueinander verlaufen und nur eine Steigungs- oder Wickelungsform aufweisen. Es wird zwischen einer steilen Wickelung etwa in Richtung des Haversschen Kanals und einer flachen senkrecht dazu in der Querschnittsebene des Kanals unterschieden. An entsprechenden Drahtmodellen hat Gebhardt nun bei Belastungen die Veränderung der Verlaufsweise im Sinne einer Torsion studiert. Diese Modelle konnten aber keine befriedigende Auskunft über das Verhalten der Fasern geben, da die Drähte an ihren Enden in Holzplatten eingelassen sind. Von Triepel (1907, 1922a, b) wurde kritisiert, daß bei den Versuchen von Gebhardt die Materialeigenschaften des Kollagens nicht berücksichtigt wurden (vgl. Knese, 1958b).

Das Knochengewebe enthält zwei Materialien verschiedener Eigenschaften, die Kollagenfibrillen und die Kristallite, wenn zunächst von den weiteren Komponenten des Knochengewebes abgesehen wird (s. S. 337). In der Technik wird bei einem Baukörper, der aus zwei Materialien differenter Eigenschaften besteht, von einem Verbundbau gesprochen; das bekannteste Beispiel ist der Stahlbeton. So wurde auch der Knochen verschiedentlich mit dem Stahlbeton verglichen (unter anderem Gebhardt, 1911; Petersen, 1919; Sternberg, 1925; Weidenreich, 1930; Henschen, 1936; Olivo, 1937; Maj und Toaiari, 1937; Bruno, 1950; Tischendorf, 1954; W. J. Schmidt, 1952). Knese (1958b) hat darauf hingewiesen, daß diese Bauweise im Organismus weit verbreitet ist, z.B. in den Sohlen- und Ballenpolstern, aber auch in der Wand der Eingeweide und Gefäße. Für den Knorpel hat Benninghoff (1925) den Vergleich mit dem Stahlbeton näher durchgeführt; der von BENNINGHOFF angenommene Faserverlauf im Knorpel konnte jedoch von anderen Autoren nicht bestätigt werden (s. dort). HEIDSIECK (1934) hat den Knorpel mit vulkanisiertem Kautschuk verglichen und damit dessen Struktur materialgerechter gedeutet.

KNESE (1958b) hat die Materialstruktur des Knochengewebes im Sinne des Verbundbaues unter Berücksichtigung der Strukturen verschiedener Ordnung erörtert. Dabei geht KNESE davon aus, daß in der einzelnen Lamelle mattenartige Geflechte von Kollagenfibrillen und Faserverbindungen zwischen Nachbarlamellen vorliegen (s. S. 359). Diese Voraussetzungen wurden durch elektronenmikroskopische Untersuchungen bestätigt (KNESE und v. HARNACK, 1962). Lamellen verhalten sich jedoch auch als relativ selbständige Systeme höherer Ordnung im Sinne von P. WEISS (1956, 1957). Wie bereits polarisationsmikroskopische Untersuchungen zeigten (KNESE et al., 1954), können annähernd senkrecht aufeinanderstehende Lamellen ohne Fibrillenverbindung sein. Die Lamellen brechen dann zugespitzt unter Bildung treppenartiger Strukturen ab; dieser Befund wurde durch elektronenmikroskopische Beobachtungen bestätigt (KNESE und v. HARNACK, 1962).

Beim Stahlbeton wird der druckfeste Beton mit dem zugfesten Stahl verbunden (MÖRSCH, 1923; BEYER, 1956; PUCHER, 1961; BETON-KALENDER, 1962). Die Konstruktionsteile erhalten eine Stahlbewehrung in jenen Bereichen, in denen mit Zugspannungen zu rechnen ist. Die Längsstähle erhalten eine Querbewehrung oder Umschnürung mit Ring- oder Spiralbügeln, wodurch die Knicklänge der Längsstähle herabgesetzt wird. Derartige Querbewehrungen in Form von Fibrillen, die etwa senkrecht zur Masse der Fibrillen einer Lamelle verlaufen, konnten KNESE und v. HARNACK (1962) auch im Knochengewebe nachweisen.

Die Berechnung eines Konstruktionsteiles beim Verbundbau geht von der Annahme eines sog. homogenen Zustandes aus. Damit werden für die Anordnung der Bewehrung „scheinbare" Spannungen vorausgesetzt, die dem Spannungszustand des endgültigen Bauteiles nicht entsprechen. Für die Durchführung einer Stahlbetonkonstruktion lassen sich demzufolge keine Schemata aufstellen, da die genaue Kenntnis der Baustoffe und ihres Zusammenwirkens im Bauteil bis zum Bruch die im Einzelfall erforderliche Konstruktion bedingen (MÖRSCH, 1923; LEONHARDT, 1962).

Die geometrische Struktur von Knochengewebe und Stahlbeton ist in der Ordnung der Stahlbewehrung bzw. der Kollagenfibrillen sehr ähnlich. Dem Material nach sind beide voneinander verschieden und deshalb auch in dem Zusammenwirken der Komponenten unterschiedlich zu beurteilen. Der Beton ist eine feste steinähnliche Masse, der Knochen besitzt Mikrokristalle, eingebettet in eine organische Substanz, die unter anderem MPS enthält. Die Kollagenfibrillen sind nur zugfest, der Stahl hat daneben noch eine gewisse Steife und Biegefestigkeit.

Die Erörterung der Materialstruktur beginnt KNESE (1958b) mit einer Untersuchung der Verformung der Haversschen Systeme bei Belastung (Abb. 20), um danach den Verformungswiderstand aufzusuchen. In einem Konstruktionsschema werden die Veränderungen innerhalb zweier flach und einer dazwischen gelegenen steil gewickelten Lamelle bei Belastung untersucht. Bei axialem Druck müßten sich steil gewickelte Fibrillen verkürzen, und zwar etwa um die Hälfte der Verlängerung der flach gewickelten; da sich Kollagenfibrillen nicht verkürzen können, käme es zu einem Ausknicken, einer Stauchung der steilen Fibrillen. Die Kollagenfibrillen der flach gewickelten Lamellen leisten vermöge ihrer Zugfestigkeit der Umfangsdehnung und damit der Stauchung des Osteonzylinders einen Widerstand. Damit üben die Fasern der flachen Lamellen gleichzeitig einen sog. Manteldruck auf den „Kern" des Osteons aus. Ein Manteldruck erhöht aber die Druckfestigkeit des Kernes (MÖRSCH, 1923). Von Flächenpressungen der Lamellen sprachen bereits GEBHARDT (1906) und PETERSEN (1930).

Kollagenfasern haben im allgemeinen einen welligen bzw. spiraligen Verlauf, erscheinen jedoch im Knochengewebe gestreckt. Die Änderung der Verlaufsweise der Kollagenfibrillen wird besonders deutlich in den osteogenen Zonen von Sehnen- und Bandansätzen, wobei die Sehne den welligen und der Knochen den gestreckten Fibrillenverlauf zeigen (BIERMANN, 1957; KNESE und BIERMANN, 1958). Aus dem gestreckten Verlauf schließt KNESE (1958b), daß die Kollagenfibrillen im Knochen bereits in unbelastetem Zustand angespannt bzw. vorgespannt sind.

In der Technik wird heute vermehrt ein sog. vorgespannter Beton oder Spannbeton verwandt (LÜTZE, 1948; RITTER und LARDY, 1950; MEHMEL, 1957; LEONHARDT, 1962). Beim Spannbeton wird vor dem Gießen des Betons der Stahl gespannt. Nach dem Erstarren üben diese vorgespannten Stahleinlagen auf den nicht zugfesten Beton einen Druck aus, d.h. es werden im Beton vor der Belastung Druckspannungen erzeugt. Bei einer Belastung, die im Beton Zugspannungen hervorrufen würde, tritt nunmehr eine

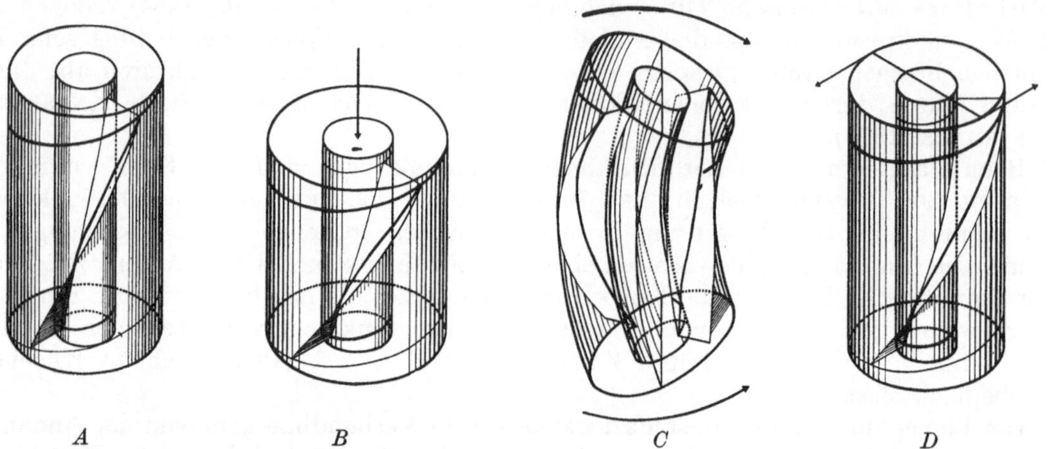

Abb. 20. Verformung eines Osteonzylinders mit einer inneren und äußeren flach gewickelten und einer dazwischen gelagerten steil gewickelten Faser. *A* Ausgangsstadium; *B* Verformung unter Druckbelastung; C Verformung unter Biegebelastung; *D* Verformung bei Torsion (aus KNESE, 1958b)

Verminderung der zuvor eingeführten Druckspannungen auf. Damit wird der Beton materialgemäß beansprucht; so kann Material gespart werden und die Konstruktionsteile sind leichter. Das Prinzip des Vorspannes ist alt; als Beispiele sollen die Holzdauben und die Stahlringe eines Fasses, die Holzfelgen und der Eisenring eines Holzrades oder die Drahtfelgen eines Rades genannt werden (MEHMEL, 1957).

Im Spannbeton wirkt der Vorspann auf den Beton, um diesem druckfesten Material die Aufnahme von Zugspannungen zu ermöglichen, die nunmehr in einer Verringerung der zuvor vorhandenen Druckspannungen besteht. Im Knochengewebe wirkt der Vorspann jedoch auf die zugfesten Kollagenfibrillen, die Kollagenfibrillen sind materialgemäß auf Zug beansprucht. Unter einer Druckbeanspruchung knicken die Fibrillen dann nicht mehr aus, sondern ihre vor der Belastung vorhandene Zugspannung wird herabgesetzt. Die Fibrillen erhalten damit eine „scheinbare" Druckfestigkeit. Die Verminderung des Vorspannes tritt auf, wenn unter der Last — wie bei den steilen Fasern des Osteonzylinders — geometrisch eine Verkürzung der Fasern erfolgen müßte. Das Ausknicken wird weiterhin durch den umgebenden Mineralmantel verhindert, der aus etwa 5—10 Schichten von Kristalliten besteht (KNESE, 1963c).

Das Knochengewebe gleicht einem straff gespannten Gewebe, das mit Kristallen prall gefüllt ist (KNESE, 1958b). Vergleichsweise könnte an steif gefrorene Wäsche gedacht werden. Durch die eingelagerten Kristalle wird das zugfeste Textilgewebe druckfest. Eine Zusammenlagerung mehrerer derartiger Wäschestücke in einer Ebene (Tangentiallamellen = Schalt- und Generallamellen) oder zu einem Rohr (Haverssches System) entspricht festigkeitstheoretisch weitgehend der Struktur des Knochens.

Der Vorspann der Kollagenfibrillen im Knochen entsteht wahrscheinlich durch Wasseraufnahme, Quellung, vermittels der MPS in den osteogenen Zonen (s. S. 348). Durch

Umlagerung der Fibrillen mit Kristallen, durch die sog. Mineralisation, wird das Wasser verdrängt (s. S. 337) und der Vorspann durch die Kristalle aufrechterhalten. Von Technikern wurde verschiedentlich erwogen, den Vorspann durch Quellung, den sog. Quellzement, zu erzeugen, da die bisher üblichen Verfahren wie Spannbrett usw. einen erheblichen Aufwand fordern. Die praktische Erzeugung eines Spannbetons durch Quellung ist aber bisher noch nicht gelungen.

Die Berechtigung zur Annahme eines Vorspanns der Kollagenfasern (KNESE, 1958b) wurde von CURREY (1964) bezweifelt. Die von KNESE (1958b) entwickelte Hypothese basiert einmal auf einer Reihe morphologischer Fakten, zum anderen auf der Überlegung, in welcher Weise die zugfesten Kollagenfibrillen an der gesamten verwickelten Beanspruchung des Knochengewebes teilnehmen könnten; dieses ist nur über einen Vorspann möglich. Nach Diskussion der Ultrastruktur des Knochengewebes kommt CURREY (1962b, 1964) zur Auffassung, daß im Knochen ein zweiphasiges Material vorliegt, das dem glasfaserverstärkten Epoxyharz entspricht, wobei die Kristalle den Glasfasern und die Kollagenfasern dem Epoxyharz gleichzusetzen wären. Damit wird zur Interpretation der mechanischen Eigenschaften des Knochengewebes eine weitere technische Anwendung des Verbundbaues herangezogen. Wir möchten bezweifeln, ob man die Kristallite den Glasfasern gleichsetzen kann. Die materiellen Unterschiede zwischen Knochengewebe und Stahlbeton wurden ausführlich diskutiert (KNESE, 1958b) und der Schwerpunkt auf die allgemeinen Regeln des Verbundbaues gelegt. Eine unmittelbare Analogie des Knochengewebes ist weder mit dem Stahlbeton noch mit dem glasfaserverstärkten Epoxyharz möglich.

Weiterhin hat KNESE (1958b) die Kollagenfibrillen mit einem Seil verglichen, das durch die Kristalle belastet wird. Durch eine Seilbelastung entsteht eine Seilspannung, so daß die Kristalle vermutlich nicht nur den Vorspann aufrechterhalten, sondern ständig neu erzeugen.

Der Vorspann und die Seilbelastung sind als „Bauprinzip" der Struktur 5. Ordnung, der Fibrillen mit ihrem Mantel, und 4. Ordnung, der Lamellen, anzusehen. Zur Erörterung der Bauprinzipien der Strukturen 3. Ordnung, den Lamellensystemen, beschäftigt sich KNESE (1958b) zunächst mit dem Faserübertritt von Lamelle zu Lamelle. Solche Faserübergänge sind als Befestigung des „Seiles" in der Nachbarlamelle anzusehen. In einem Haversschen System würden demzufolge die eine Lamelle aufbauenden Kollagenfibrillen als Seile in den beiden Nachbarlamellen befestigt sein. Durch den Seilzug üben die beiden Nachbarlamellen einen Druck auf die dazwischen gelegene Lamelle aus; es liegt eine Flächenpressung vor, die eine Festigung der gepreßten Lamelle zur Folge hat. Der Aufbau von Lamellensystemen stellt damit keine einfache Summierung von Lamellen dar, sondern bringt ein neues Bauprinzip in die Strukturhierarchie des Knochengewebes. Die in dem Knochengewebe unterschiedene Strukturordnung stellt demzufolge keine rein deskriptive Gliederung dar, sondern jede Ordnung hat ihre eigenen Bauprinzipien und entsprechende Festigkeitsaufgaben zu erfüllen.

Der Haverssche Kanal kann als ein mit Flüssigkeit gefülltes Rohr angesehen werden. KNESE (1958b) hat die Spannungsverhältnisse in einem Flüssigkeitszylinder mit geschichteter Wand diskutiert, bei der die nächst äußere Lamelle mit Zuganstrengung über die innere gezogen ist. Die äußere Lamelle ist damit vorgespannt. Die hinzutretende Wandspannung in dem belasteten Zylinder führt unter anderem zu einer Spannung in Richtung der Tangente σ_t, die vom Rohr zur Peripherie schnell an Größe abnimmt. Vorspann und Wandspannung σ_t addieren sich und erreichen vermutlich nicht jene Größe, bei der die Zugfestigkeit der Kollagenfaser überschritten wird. Aus der Spannungsverteilung in der Rohrwand errechnet KNESE den Mindestdurchmesser eines Haversschen Systems zu 70 μ und den größten zu 400 μ; beide Werte stimmen gut mit den tatsächlich zu messenden Osteongrößen überein (KNESE und TITSCHAK, 1962; s. S. 365).

Die Zugfestigkeit einzelner Osteone haben ASCENZI und BONUCCI (1965) geprüft. Die Zugfestigkeit ist trocken größer als feucht, bei steil verlaufender Wicklung, d.h. Fasern in Längsrichtung des Osteones höher als bei flacher Wicklung; die Mineralisation ist ohne Einfluß. Die Autoren kommen zu dem Schluß, daß die Zugfestigkeit überwiegend von den Kollagenfibrillen abhängt. Eine Prüfung der Druckfestigkeit einzelner Osteone ergab (ASCENZI und BONUCCI, 1968), daß diese dagegen bei flacher Wicklung größer als bei steiler ist und daß sie vom Grad der Mineralisation abhängt. Bei einer elektronenmikroskopischen Kontrolle von Bruchspalten zeigte sich eine Verformung der Kristalle und ein Reißen der Kollagenfibrillen.

Die Untersuchung des Verformungswiderstandes bei Biegung beginnt KNESE (1958b) wiederum mit Untersuchung der Verformung des Osteons (Abb. 20) und dem Verhalten der Kollagenfasern. Auf der Druckseite des Osteonzylinders würde sich rein geometrisch eine Verkürzung oder Ausknicken der steil gewickelten Kollagenfasern ergeben. Die flach verlaufenden Fibrillen werden von der Biegungsverformung nicht beeinflußt, wie das auch von der Querbewehrung beim Stahlbeton her bekannt ist. Das Haverssche System muß als stark bewehrt angesehen werden, so daß bei Biegung die Nullinie aus der geo-

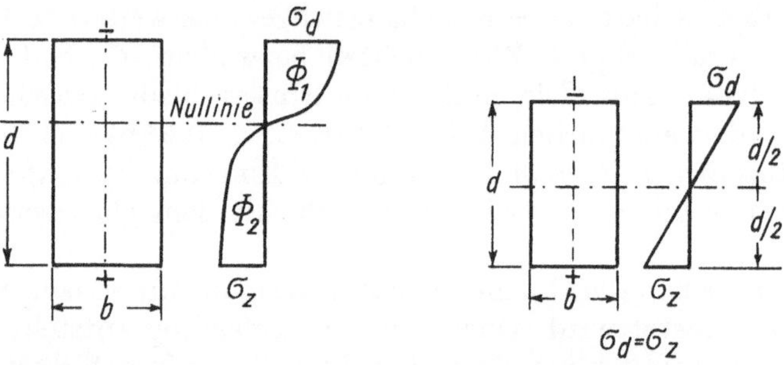

Abb. 21. Vergleich des Spannungsdiagrammes des Stahlbetons mit Verschiebung der Nullinie und parabolischer Begrenzung des Diagrammes mit dem eines homogenen Balkens (Umzeichnung nach TROCHE, 1953; aus KNESE, 1958b)

metrischen Mittellinie herausrückt und die Druckseite zusammenschrumpft. Damit würde der Kantendruck auf der Druckseite des Osteons so groß werden, daß die Kristalle herausspringen. In einem einzelnen Osteon läßt sich demgemäß kein entsprechender Verformungswiderstand bei Biegung finden, der sich aber sofort ergibt, wenn ein Osteonbündel betrachtet wird. Der gefährdeten Druckseite eines Osteons liegt dann die Zugseite des Nachbarosteons gegenüber, die die Verformung verhindert. So zwingt die Untersuchung des Biegungswiderstandes zur nächsten Ordnung, nämlich der 2., der Zusammenlagerung von Osteonen im Knochenquerschnitt, überzugehen.

Bei seinen Erörterungen der Materialstruktur des Knochens versucht KNESE (1958b), für die verschiedenen Bauprinzipien auch eine quantitative Formulierung zu finden. Hier sei nur auf den Vergleich zwischen der Druck- und Zugfestigkeit, errechnet aus den Biegeversuchen und aus der unmittelbaren Prüfung dieser Festigkeitsformen, hingewiesen. Die aus beiden Versuchsanordnungen errechnete Druckfestigkeit ist praktisch gleich groß. Die an Hand von Biegeversuchen bestimmte Zugfestigkeit ist dagegen doppelt so groß wie die aus Zugversuchen. Dieser Befund bestätigt die Annahme, daß im Knochengewebe ein Verbundbau vorliegt und die bei Biegung errechneten Spannungen „scheinbare" Spannungen sind. Im Verbundbau gebaute Teile zeigen eine Verschiebung der Nullinie zur Druckseite hin (Abb. 21). Die maximalen Randspannungen sind nicht mehr geradlinig miteinander zu verbinden, sondern parabolisch. Jeder Längenänderung entspricht eine zugehörige Spannung, wobei die Spannungsflächen für Druck- und Zugspannungen gleich sein müssen. DEMPSTER und LIDDICOAT (1952) meinen, daß bei Biegung der Knochen auf der Konvexseite plastische Eigenschaften annimmt, während auf der Konkavseite die volle Druckfestigkeit im elastischen Bereich erhalten bleibt. Die Fraktur (s. S. 518) beginnt dann im Bereich der Zugspannungen.

Beim Vergleich der mechanischen Eigenschaften des Knochengewebes mit technisch verwandten Stoffen wurde darauf hingewiesen, daß der Knochen mit hohen mechanischen Eigenschaften ein relativ geringes spezifisches Gewicht verbindet. Es ist nun zu vermuten, daß das spezifische Gewicht noch niedriger liegen würde, wenn das Prinzip des Vorspannes auch für die Struktur 2. Ordnung gilt, was voraussichtlich nicht der Fall ist.

Nach KNESE (1958b) sind in jeder Ordnung bestimmte Bauprinzipien verwirklicht. Das Bauprinzip einer Ordnung gilt aber nicht mehr für die benachbarten. Während die Struktur 5. Ordnung vom Bauprinzip des Vorspannes beherrscht wird, kommt es bei den Lamellen, den Strukturen 4. Ordnung, zur Bildung einer zweidimensionalen Netzstruktur, die sowohl Druck- als auch Zugspannungen aufnehmen kann. Von dem Lamellensystem stellen dann die Tangentiallamellen, Schalt- und Generallamellen einen gegliederten Teilkörper dar, der einen fast regelmäßigen Wechsel von steil und flach gewickelten Lamellen aufweist. Die Tangentiallamellen sind ihrem Bau nach dem Sperrholz sehr ähnlich. Allerdings wird durch die Faserverbindung von Lamelle zu Lamelle die Zusammenarbeit zwischen den einzelnen Schichten inniger als bei den verleimten Blättern des Sperrholzes. Das Bauprinzip der „primitiveren" Struktur der Tangentiallamellen ist demzufolge einfacher als das der Haversschen Systeme.

Den bisherigen funktionellen Deutungen der Knochenstruktur bereitet der Befund große Schwierigkeiten, daß die Struktur in einem Skeletstück dem Alter nach und individuell große Differenzen aufweist (s. S. 369; AUERBACH, 1957; KNESE, und TITSCHAK, 1962; KNESE, 1958b). Eine funktionelle Deutung des Feinbaues wurde daher von vielen Autoren abgelehnt. PETERSEN (1927, 1930) vertrat die Auffassung, die Unstetigkeit der Knochenstruktur strebe 0 zu, so daß ein homogenes Medium vorliege. Die experimentelle Untersuchung der Knochenfestigkeit hat jedoch gezeigt, daß sich das Knochengewebe wie ein inhomogener und anisotroper Stoff verhält. Bei einem Verbundbau kann in einer Ordnungsstufe eine große Variation der Struktur vorliegen, ohne daß dadurch die Leistung der Nachbarordnungen gestört wird, da jede Ordnung relativ selbständig ist. Die Ergebnisse experimenteller Untersuchungen des Knochengewebes stellen nach EVANS (1957) ein weiteres Argument gegen die Resultate rein mathematischer Analysen, Trajektoriendiagramme und spannungsoptischer Untersuchungen dar, die alle einen Knochen aus homogenem Material und in der Form einer „soliden Struktur" voraussetzen.

Die Deutung der nach Regionen spezifischen Verteilung der Lamellensysteme, die Struktur 2. Ordnung, ist z.Z. noch nicht gelungen; wir kommen bei Erörterung der topographischen Differenzen der Festigkeit darauf zurück.

Bei der bisherigen Diskussion der Materialstruktur wurden nur zwei Komponenten, die Fasern und Kristallite, berücksichtigt. Es liegen auch Beobachtungen über Veränderungen der Festigkeit bei verschiedenem Wassergehalt des Knochens vor. Die Untersuchungen von ROBINSON (1960) über die Wasserverteilung (s. S. 337) lassen annehmen, daß der Vorgang des Wasserentzuges oder der Wässerung nicht einfach zu deuten ist. ROLLHÄUSER (1951) hat eine Zunahme der Festigkeit der Kollagenfasern durch Trocknung beschrieben. Die Bedeutung der restlichen Komponenten, voran der MPS, für die Knochenfestigkeit ist noch unklar.

Die Feinstruktur kann heute nicht mehr unter rein mechanischen Gesichtspunkten betrachtet werden (KNESE, 1959a). Für den Knochen als Ionenpol spielt unter anderem die Größe der Kristallite eine Rolle und die davon abhängige Kristalloberfläche (vgl. ROBINSON, 1952). Eine Vergrößerung der Kristalle würde die zum Ionenaustausch zur Verfügung stehende Fläche verringern, eine Verkleinerung vielleicht die mechanische Leistungsfähigkeit des Knochens einschränken (KNESE, 1959a). Unsere Kenntnisse von der Molekularstruktur des Knochens sind jedoch noch nicht so umfangreich, daß die Aufgaben des Knochengewebes im Hinblick auf den Stoffwechsel und die mechanische Leistung befriedigend mit dem Strukturaufbau verglichen werden können. Vor allem fehlt noch eine Diskussion darüber, ob auch für den Stoffwechsel des Knochengewebes die Strukturhierarchie von Bedeutung ist; manche Befunde über die Verteilung von

Radioisotopen sprechen dafür (Knese und Titschak, 1962). Ungeklärt ist, ob diesen verschiedenartigen Aufgaben des Knochens auch zwei Knochenarten entsprechen, wie von mancher Seite angenommen wird (Vincent und Haumont, 1960; Lacroix, 1953; Marotti, 1963), ein Stoffwechselknochen (metabolic bone) und ein tragender Knochen (supporting bone). Das Vorliegen zweier Knochenarten würde zu einer eleganten Lösung für manche Schwierigkeiten führen: Der eine Knochen folgt in seiner Gestaltung den bisher vertretenen Auffassungen von der funktionellen Anpassung, der andere ist durch die Stoffwechselaufgaben des Skeletes bestimmt. Bekanntlich ergeben sich aus den derzeitigen Vorstellungen über die Mechanismen des Mineralstoffwechsels eine Reihe von Problemen (Zusammenfassung: Comar und Bronner, 1960/61; Lichtwitz und Parlier, 1964): Im Hinblick auf die Gewinnung eines entsprechenden Calciumspiegels des Blutes muß z.B. angenommen werden, daß im Knochen eine austauschbare Fraktion vorhanden ist und eine nicht austauschbare, die erst durch einen Abbau infolge der Wirkung des Parathormones frei wird. Für die Struktur des Knochengewebes wären damit die beiden konkurrierenden Prinzipien der mechanischen Leistung und des Stoffwechsels verantwortlich. Bekannt ist aber, daß bestimmte Stoffwechselstörungen die mechanische Leistungsfähigkeit des Knochens herabsetzen.

δ) Topographische Differenzen der Knochenfestigkeit

Bei Erörterung der topographischen Differenzen der Knochenfestigkeit beziehen wir uns sowohl auf die Untersuchungen an frischem als auch vorbehandeltem Material. Im Abschnitt Mechanik der Skeletelemente gehen wir auf eine Reihe weiterer Angaben über topographische Differenzen in der Festigkeit ein. Je nach Vorbehandlung scheint die Knochenfestigkeit in einem bestimmten Sinne verändert zu werden, so daß die Ergebnisse gleichartig präparierter Stücke mit einem Korrekturfaktor versehen vermutlich auch für den „überlebenden“ Knochen gelten. Bei erheblichen Unterschieden im physikalisch-chemischen Aufbau miteinander verglichener Stücke ist aber eine verschieden starke Veränderung der Festigkeit durch Vorbehandlung anzunehmen. Es sei auf den unterschiedlichen Wasserentzug bei gleicher Temperatur hingewiesen, wie ihn Amprino (1961) und Rosate (1958) an Knochen von Individuen verschiedenen Alters beobachtet haben.

Aus den bisherigen Erörterungen hat sich ergeben, daß die Zugfestigkeit (fixiertes Material: Evans et al. 1951, 1952) und die Druckfestigkeit (frisches Material: Knese et al. 1955; Knese 1956a) innerhalb eines Skeletstückes des Menschen von proximal zur Mitte hin zu- und dann nach distal wieder abnimmt (Tabelle 1). Diese Zu- bzw. Abnahme ist bei den einzelnen Skeletelementen unterschiedlich (Evans et al., 1952). Evans (1964) hat Durchschnittswerte für die Zugfestigkeit mit Hilfe des Computers errechnet. Die Zugfestigkeit der Tibia ist höher als die des Femurs und in beiden Skeletstücken im mittleren Drittel wieder größer als im proximalen oder distalen Drittel. Maj (1938) hat am Metatarsus und Metacarpus des Rindes die höchste Festigkeit ebenfalls in Diaphysenmitte gefunden.

Weiterhin wurden Unterschiede der Festigkeit in den einzelnen „Quadranten“ eines Knochenquerschnittes beobachtet, auf die wir noch im folgenden eingehen. Hierbei verhalten sich die einzelnen Stücke einer Species und dann von Species zu Species sehr verschieden, so, daß an einen strukturell verschiedenen Aufbau der Skeletelemente zu denken ist (s. S. 465).

Bei Festigkeitsuntersuchungen wurde auch die Richtung der Krafteinwirkung verschieden gewählt. Die Biegeversuche an ganzen Knochen von Knese et al. (1955) ließen wegen des geringen Materialumfanges keine Schlüsse zu (s. S. 432). Bogdaschew (1930) glaubt jedoch, am Metacarpus und Metatarsus des Pferdes Differenzen je nach Biegerichtung gefunden zu haben (s. S. 461).

Rauber (1876) fand, daß Stäbchen aus den oberflächlichen und tiefen Compactaschichten sowie bei Biegung in verschiedener Richtung den gleichen Elastizitätsmodul haben. An trockenen Knochenwürfeln fand RAUBER bei axialem Lastangriff eine größere Festigkeit als bei transversalem. KNESE et al. (1955) haben die Werte von RAUBER in ihrer Verteilung auf die Kollektive der Druckfestigkeit untersucht (s. S. 424). Die Werte der Druckfestigkeit in Knochenlängsachse zeigen folgende prozentuale Verteilung: I 1210:21,8%; II 1425:30,4%; III 1730:39,1%; IV 2015:8,7% und senkrecht zur Knochenlängsachse: I 58,8%; II 5,9%; III 35,3%. Die Verteilung der Werte auf die Kollektive läßt vermuten, daß die Druckfestigkeit in Längsachse des Skeletstückes etwas größer als quer dazu ist. Die Druckfestigkeit von Hölzern ist dagegen nach der Belastungsrichtung sehr unterschiedlich. Die Druckfestigkeit (Tabelle 7) quer zur Längsachse beträgt beim Nußbaum 16,7%, Kiefer 14%, Tanne 9%, Rotbuche 14,5% von der in Längsrichtung; noch geringer ist die Zugfestigkeit: beim Nußbaum 3,5%, Tanne 2,7%, Rotbuche 5,7%; größer dagegen ist die Scherfestigkeit, bei der Kiefer 210%, Tanne 550% und Rotbuche 425%.

DEMPSTER und LIDDICOAT (1952) haben die Festigkeit von Würfeln bei Druck in verschiedener Richtung untersucht. Die Proben stammten aus der Vorderwand der Mitte des Femurs (Sammlungsstücke!) und aus der medialen Wand des Humerus. Die Proben wurden in Längsachse, radial, d.h. vom Periost zur Markhöhle hin, und tangential belastet. Für 63 trockene Proben ergaben sich für den Elastizitätsmodul folgende Werte. Längsrichtung 123500 ± 26150; radial: 64400 ± 21170 und tangential: 64100 ± 15750 kg · cm^{-2}. Der Elastizitätsmodul für Druck in radialer und tangentialer Richtung erreicht 52% von dem in Längsrichtung. Zusätzlich wurden 21 angefeuchtete Würfel mit folgendem Ergebnis getestet: Längsrichtung: 88700 ± 16250; radial: 38400 ± 8230; tangential: 42750 ± 14280 kg · cm^{-2}. Damit beträgt der Elastizitätsmodul bei feuchten Proben nur noch 43 bzw. 48% von dem in Schaftlängsachse. Der Elastizitätsmodul des feuchten Knochens erreicht bei Last in Längsachse 72% von dem des trockenen. Die individuellen Variationen bei radialem und tangentialem Druck sind erheblich. DEMPSTER und LIDDICOAT (1952) sind der Meinung, daß der Druck in Schaftachse in Richtung der „Knochenfibrillen" und senkrecht dazu bei radialer und tangentialer Last erfolge. Der Elastizitätsmodul von Würfeln beträgt trocken 67 und feucht 60% von dem der Stäbe. Die Druckfestigkeit von trockenem Knochen in der obigen Reihenfolge war: 2080 ± 182, 1350 ± 221, 1312 ± 216 kg · cm^{-2}; von feuchtem: 1340 ± 218, 1194 ± 323, 1078 ± 197 kg · cm^{-2}. Die radiale bzw. tangentiale Druckfestigkeit erreicht bei trockenem 65 bzw. 63% und bei feuchtem 89 bzw. 82% von dem in Knochenlängsachse. Die Druckfestigkeit des feuchten mißt 64% von der des trockenen Knochens. Bei den in Schaftachse gedrückten Würfeln tritt ein Bruch auf, der in einem Winkel von 30° von einer Ecke ausgeht und die entgegengesetzt gelegene Druckfläche erreicht. Bei den anderen Prüfrichtungen tritt eine X-förmige Bruchlinie auf. Bei Prismen erfolgt bei Druck in Längsrichtung ein Quer- oder Schrägbruch; es kommen auch Längsspalten und sekundäre Quetschungen vor.

MAJ und TOAIARI (1937) haben ein Paralleliped aus der Rindertibia einer Biegelast in verschiedener Richtung ausgesetzt. Die höchste Bruchlast weisen Blöcke auf, deren Längsachse der Schaftachse entspricht. Liegt die Blockachse tangential zur Schaftachse ist die Bruchlast $^1/_3$ und bei radialer nur $^1/_6$ davon. Die Verfasser haben den Faserverlauf in ihren Proben untersucht und kommen zum Schluß, daß die größte Festigkeit dann vorliegt, wenn die größere Zahl der Fasern parallel zur Blockachse verläuft.

MAJ (1938) hat die topographischen Differenzen bei Biegung am Metatarsus und Metacarpus von Rindern und menschlichen Femora untersucht. Diaphysenabschnitte aus der Mitte dieser Skeletstücke haben eine größere Festigkeit als die proximalen und distalen Teile, und zwar ist die Abnahme nach proximal geringer als nach distal. Wird die Biegefestigkeit der einzelnen Quadranten solcher Stücke geprüft, ergibt sich eine Abnahme der Festigkeit in der Reihenfolge medialer, lateraler, vorderer und hinterer Quadrant. In den distalen Abschnitten ist die Festigkeit der vorderen und mittleren

Quadranten größer als derjenigen des hinteren und lateralen. Die Festigkeit subperiostaler Proben ist größer als die der marknahen, nur beim vorderen Quadranten verhält sie sich umgekehrt.

In weiteren Untersuchungen hat MAJ (1942) die Bruchlast bei Biegung auf kleine Stäbchen von 10—15×1,2×3 mm aus Humerus, Ulna, Femur und Tibia von 40 Individuen im Alter von 5—90 Jahren festgestellt. Die mittlere Bruchlast der Ulna war 8,36 kg, Tibia 7,7 kg, Humerus 7,17 kg und Femur 6,86 kg. Weiterhin ergeben sich Unterschiede nach dem Quadranten des Querschnittes, aus dem die Stäbchen stammten. Am Humerus weist der mittlere Quadrant die kleinste Bruchlast auf, am Femur der dorsale, an der Ulna der hintere; die höchste Bruchlast fand MAJ an der Tibia im mittleren und an der Ulna im vorderen Quadranten. Die mittlere Durchbiegung bei 5 kg Last war: Humerus 226 μ, Ulna 208 μ, Femur 232 μ und Tibia 213 μ. Die Größe der Durchbiegung nimmt mit dem Lebensalter zu. Mit dem Ansteigen der Durchbiegung ist eine Einengung der Variationsbreite der Bruchlast verbunden. Im allgemeinen nahmen Last und Durchbiegung bis zu einem Punkt proportional zu, dann folgt ein Fließbereich. Selten verhält sich der Knochen wie ein spröder Stoff und noch seltener wird mit zunehmender Last die Durchbiegung geringer. Die beiden zuletzt genannten Beziehungen zwischen Last und Deformation wurden vor allem in der ersten Hälfte des Lebens bei Vorliegen hoher Bruchlasten beobachtet.

Für die geringe Bruchlast zwischen dem 25. und 35. Jahr (s. S. 433) kann MAJ (1942) keine Erklärung geben, meint jedoch, daß weder die Dichte des Knochengewebes, noch die Struktur der Haversschen Systeme oder der Verlauf der Kollagenfibrillen für sich allein zur Erklärung hinreichen. Es muß an physikalisch-chemische Differenzen im Aufbau der Komponenten des Knochengewebes, der Kollagenfibrillen, des Osseomucoid, und der Mineralien gedacht werden.

Topographische Differenzen der Knochenfestigkeit geben Veranlassung dazu, die Beziehungen zwischen Knochenstruktur (2. Ordnung) und Festigkeit zu diskutieren. So wurde auch das Verhältnis der tragenden Intercellularsubstanz zu den Gefäß-Zellräumen untersucht, die sog. Porosität. Die ursprüngliche Formulierung der Spannung und damit Festigkeit $\sigma = \frac{P}{F}\,\mathrm{kg}\cdot\mathrm{cm}^{-2}$ ist rein geometrisch und nimmt auf die Dichte keine Rücksicht. Als Dichte ϱ eines Körpers bezeichnet man das Verhältnis der Masse m zum Volumen V: $\varrho = \frac{m}{V}$; dann ist l/ϱ das spezifische Volumen. Das spezifische Gewicht γ gibt das Verhältnis von Gewicht G zum Volumen an $\gamma = \frac{G}{V}$. Da das Gewicht $G = \mathrm{m}\cdot\mathrm{g}$ ist, kann das spezifische Gewicht auch als $\gamma = \varrho\cdot\mathrm{g}$ formuliert werden. In der obigen Erörterung (s. S. 443) wurde der Knochen als hochwertiges Gewebe angesehen, weil mit einem geringen spezifischen Gewicht eine große Festigkeit verbunden ist.

KNESE (1958b) hat versucht, die Haversschen Kanäle als mit Flüssigkeit gefüllte Rohre in das Zusammenspiel der Komponenten bei Belastung einzubeziehen. SCHMIDT (1915) vermutet, daß die Festigkeit des Knochens in vivo größer ist als die experimentell ermittelte, da der Blutdruck noch auf den Knochen wirke. ZUPPINGER (1904) meint, daß in die großen Röhrenknochen das Blut unter 160 mm Hg eintritt und unter 60 mm austritt und damit der Knochen unter einem Druck von 100 mm Hg steht; in diesem Zusammenhang erinnert ZUPPINGER an die Biegungsfraktur des erigierten Penis. Die Haversschen Kanäle sind aber auch als „Kerben" anzusehen, d.h. lochförmige Unterbrechungen des Materials, durch die örtliche Spannungserhöhungen auftreten (unter anderem WYSS 1926, 1948) und die damit zum Ausgangspunkt einer Bruchlinie werden können. So haben auch MAJ und TOAIARI (1937b) beobachtet, daß Bruchlinien häufig Haverssche Kanäle miteinander verbinden (s. S. 462). Bei der Beurteilung der Beziehungen zwischen den Haversschen Kanälen und der Knochenfestigkeit wurden sehr unterschiedliche Gesichtspunkte in Betracht gezogen; weitere experimentelle Untersuchungen sind zur Klärung abzuwarten.

Toajari (1939) hat an Knochen von holländischen und polnischen Rindern die Porosität (Anzahl der Haversschen Kanäle), die Anzahl der Kollagenfibrillen und die Biegefestigkeit untersucht. Die größere Biegefestigkeit des Metacarpus polnischer Rinder wird darauf zurückgeführt, daß der prozentuale Anteil der Fasern an der Fläche sowie der Querschnitt der Fibrillen größer als bei den holländischen ist; jedoch war bei den holländischen Rindern die Anzahl der Fasern je mm^2 größer. Maj (1938) fand keine Beziehungen zwischen der Porosität, der Anzahl der Haversschen und Volkmannschen Kanäle und der Festigkeit. Walmsley und Smith (1957) beobachteten jedoch beim Knochen, der aus Tangentiallamellen aufgebaut ist, einen höheren Elastizitätsmodul und eine höhere Bruchfestigkeit als bei Vorhandensein von Haversschen Systemen. Currey (1959) meint, daß die geringere Tragfähigkeit des Osteonknochens auf der Herabsetzung des tragenden Volumens beruhe, da etwa 3% des Volumens als Kanallumen anzusprechen sind. Nach Knese und Titschak (1962) ist der Anteil der Haversschen Kanäle 1—2% beim Femur, bei der Tibia wenig größer, 2,2%. Robinson (1960) hat die mittleren Volumenprozente des Gefäß-Mark-Osteocyten-Raumes zu 15,03% (Massen-%: 7,62%) angegeben. Currey (1959) weist aber darauf hin, daß man nicht allein die tragende Fläche für die Festigkeit heranziehen kann, denn die sekundären Haversschen Systeme haben eine geringere Mineralisation als der sog. primäre Knochen (vgl. Amprino, 1952; Vincent, 1955).

Evans (1958) hat nach histologischer Untersuchung für die ursprünglichen, d.h. geometrisch errechneten Festigkeitswerte von Evans und Lebow (1951, 1952) eine korrigierte Zugfestigkeit errechnet, die sich auf die tatsächlich tragende Fläche, d.h. abzüglich der Haversschen Kanäle, bezieht. Dieser korrigierte Wert der Zugfestigkeit ist zwischen 20% (trockene Probe aus dem Femur eines ♂ von 70 Jahren) und 28% (feuchte Probe aus der Fibula einer ♀ von 33 Jahren) größer als der ursprüngliche Wert.

Smith und Walmsley (1959) haben sich mit den Faktoren beschäftigt, die den Elastizitätsmodul des Knochens beeinflussen (s. S. 444). Bereits Kreuzer (1932) meinte, daß die reine Druck- und Zugfestigkeit im lebenden Körper keine Rolle spiele, und so ziehen auch Smith und Walmsley die Prüfung des Elastizitätsmoduls bei Biegung vor. Die Autoren haben die Biegung bei einseitiger Einspannung (Krag- oder Balkonträger) an Stücken aus der medialen Fläche der Tibia zu 80800—142000, im Mittel zu 108300 kg · cm^{-2} bestimmt. Der Elastizitätsmodul für Biegung E_b ist beim Knochen geringer als der für Zug E_z, bei einem elastisch homogenen Material sind jedoch beide gleich. Nun haben die Verfasser die Größe der tragenden Fläche vom Periost zum Mark hin verfolgt. Wenn eine gleichartige Gefäßverteilung über den Querschnitt vorliegt, ist das Verhältnis $E_z/E_b = 1$. Wenn die Fläche der Gefäßquerschnitte marknahe hoch ist und zum Periost hin abnimmt, also ein „Gefäßgradient" vorliegt, wird das Verhältnis $E_z = E_b = 1{,}46$, E_z ist größer als E_b. Bei einem hohen Gefäßgradienten ist der Knochen biegsamer als aus der Untersuchung der Zugfestigkeit anzunehmen ist.

Faßt man das Osteon als für die Festigkeit bedeutsame Struktur auf, so sind die Beziehungen zwischen Kanalweite, Osteongröße und Tragfähigkeit sicher sehr komplex. Wie die Untersuchungen von Knese et al. (1954), Auerbach (1957) und Knese und Titschak (1962) zeigten, ändert sich die Flächendichte der Osteone über den Querschnitt, d.h. die Anzahl der Osteone je Flächeneinheit und damit auch die Osteongröße. Schließlich bestehen Beziehungen zwischen Osteongröße und Kanalweite. Die Kanalweite nimmt vom Periost zur Markhöhle hin von 15,6 auf 41,2 μ zu, ist bei der Tibia subperiostal 25 und marknahe 52,3 μ. Auf die Angabe von Knese (1958b), daß mit zunehmender Festigkeit die Anzahl der Osteone je cm^2 bei Wildschweinen von 3073 auf 2214 und bei Hausschweinen von 2893 auf 2029, d.h. jeweils um etwa 1000 abnimmt, kommen wir noch zurück (s. S. 463).

Mühlemann (1962) hat an Humerus, Tibia und Mandibula von Hunden verschiedenen Alters die Größe der Hohlraumvolumina untersucht. Das Kanalvolumen mißt beim Humerus eines $^3/_4$jährigen Hundes $15{,}00 \pm 0{,}75$, beim $4^1/_2$jährigen $2{,}75 \pm 0{,}25$ Vol.-% der

Tabelle 9. *Volumen, Knochenvolumen*

	Volumen					
	♂			♀		
	Ges.[1]	Mark.[2]	%[3]	Ges.[1]	Mark.[2]	%[3]
Femur	547,4 (335,4—763,9)	79,8 (50,1—110,3)	14,6	423,4 (350,8—527,6)	74,7 (50,5—96,1)	17,6
Tibia	335,4 (205,2—419,3)	72,4 (44,3—91,4)	21,6	249,8 (206,0—297,7)	56,8 (33,6—71,7)	22,7
Fibula	50,4 (31,3—44,6)	9,7 (8,3—14,8)	19,3	38,0 (28,5—59,2)	10,4 (5,2—17,5)	27,4
Clavicula						
Humerus	184,6 (141,4—271,5)	31,8 (17,4—44,8)	17,3	125,8 (102,4—153,5)	26,6 (19,2—33,7)	21,1
Ulna	47,4 (36,4—68,8)			31,0 (25,2—49,8)		
Radius	49,0 (35,0—8,8)			35,7 (23,1—39,4)		
Rippen						
Sternum						
Oberschädel						
Unterkiefer						

[1] Gesamtvolumen errechnet nach BARTH (1940).
[2] Volumen der Markhöhle errechnet nach MECHANIK (1928, 1929, 1930, 1932): ♂ 22—58 Jahre, ♀ 21—66 Jahre.
[3] Prozentualer Anteil der Markhöhle am Gesamtvolumen.
[4] Knochenvolumen nach DAVIDA (1926).

Compacta; das Kanalvolumen wird demzufolge bei Hunden wie beim Menschen (KNESE und TITSCHAK, 1962) im Laufe des Lebens kleiner. Das größte Hohlraumvolumen hat beim Hunde der Humerus. Das Volumen der Knochenhöhlchen nimmt in der Reihe Tibia, Mandibula und Humerus an Größe ab; es beträgt im Humerus beim $^3/_4$jährigen Hunde $3{,}81 \pm 0{,}35$ und beim $4^1/_2$jährigen $3{,}40 \pm 0{,}32$ Vol.-% der Compacta. Die Größe der Kanaloberfläche im Humerus war bei den beiden gegenübergestellten Altersstufen der Hunde $7{,}17 \pm 0{,}38$ bzw. $2{,}64 \pm 0{,}20$ mm²/mm³, die Oberfläche der Knochenhöhlchen $11{,}22 \pm 0{,}75$ und $18{,}37 \pm 0{,}74$ mm²/mm³. Die Diskussion über den Einfluß der verschiedenartigen Hohlraumsysteme des Knochens auf seine Festigkeit beruht bekanntlich darauf, daß solche Kerben an der Oberfläche und im Inneren eines Baukörpers zu örtlichen Spannungserhöhungen führen. CURREY (1962a) hat sich unter diesem Gesichtspunkt nicht nur mit der Zahl, sondern auch der Verteilung der Gefäße und Knochenhöhlchen beschäftigt. Er macht darauf aufmerksam, daß Gefäße in spitzem Winkel zur Knochenlängsachse verlaufen und die kurze Achse der Knochenhöhlchen im rechten Winkel zu dieser Längsachse steht. CURREY kommt zum Schluß, daß durch diese Orientierung beider die örtlichen Spannungserhöhungen herabgesetzt, aber nicht aufgehoben werden. Experimentell erzeugte Bruchlinien bei Knochen vom Menschen und Rinde enden häufig bei Erreichen von Lacunen und Blutgefäßen.

ROBINSON (1960, Literatur) hat sich mit der Dichte des Knochengewebes sowie der Verteilung des Wassers im Knochengewebe befaßt. Für die Größe aller Intercellularräume gibt ROBINSON 15,03 Vol.-% an. An 200 Knochen der oberen Extremität bestimmten STÜWE und EHLER (1967) die mittlere Dichte für den Humerus zu 1,3, den Radius zu 1,4 und die Ulna zu 1,55.

Die bisher referierten Arbeiten gingen von Untersuchungen an Knochenschnitten oder Knochenproben aus. Die Volumina wurden auch an ganzen Skeletstücken untersucht. FRIEDRICH (1890) hat das „Porenvolumen" macerierter Knochen durch Wägung gemessen. Einmal wurden die Knochen eines 25- und eines 82jährigen Mannes vor und dann nach Füllung mit Woodschem Metall gewogen. WETZEL (1910a, b) hat aus den

und Hohlraumvolumen von Skeletstücken

Knochenvolumen[4]				Hohlraumvolumen				
Sam.[5]	♀ 16	♀ 20	♂ 21	Neon.[6]	♂ 28[6]	♂ 25[7]	♂ 82[7]	VF[8]
32—50	35	50	32	64,63		59,09	70,99	1,76
31—45	41	45	33	62,89		56,89	73,70	2,0
44—58	50	58	46			43,08	73,22	3,6
	52	60/59	52			42,30	49,25	1,41
30—50	38	50/49	42	62,41		58,61	66,82	1,46
58—61	54	61/60	52			39,01	53,91	1,8
42—59	48	59/57	48			42,25	53,84	1,6
				57,0	51,11	48,17[9]	69,7[9]	
					81,62			
				52,57	33,01			
					36,26			

[5] Sam.: unbekannte Anzahl von Sammlungsstücken.
[6] Nach TÖPPICH (1914).
[7] FRIEDRICH (1890) in der Umrechnung von WETZEL (1910).
[8] VF: Vergrößerung des Hohlraumvolumens vom 25- bis zum 82jährigen nach FRIEDRICH (1890).
[9] Mittelwert für 1., 7. und 12. Rippe.

Werten von FRIEDRICH das Hohlraumvolumen der Skeletelemente berechnet: Hohlraumvolumen $= 100 \cdot \frac{\text{Summe der Porenräume}}{\text{Knochenvolumen}}$. Hierbei legt WETZEL ein spezifisches Gewicht des Knochengewebes von 2,1445 zugrunde. Dieser Wert wurde gemeinsam mit TRIEPEL an Sägespänen der Femurcompacta bestimmt und schließt alle Hohlräume, Haverssche Kanäle, Knochenhöhlchen und -bälkchen aus, ist aber vermutlich noch etwas zu klein. Die Angaben über das spezifische Gewicht des Knochengewebes (s. S. 442) weichen stark voneinander ab, da manche Autoren die Inhomogenität und Porosität des Knochengewebes überhaupt nicht berücksichtigt haben, andere in unterschiedlicher Form errechneten.

Die von WETZEL (1910b) aus den Werten von FRIEDRICH (1890) berechneten Hohlraumvolumina (Tabelle 9) enthalten auch die Markhöhle (s. unten). Dieses Hohlraumvolumen gibt daher nicht die „Porosität" der Compacta, d.h. die Größe der tragenden Knochensubstanz an. Bei den nur aus Spongiosa aufgebauten Skeletstücken kann dagegen eine annähernd gleiche Größe von Hohlraumvolumen und „Porosität" des Materials angenommen werden (s. S. 474). Die obere Extremität verliert im Laufe des Lebens weniger an Knochensubstanz als die untere. FRIEDRICH hat auch errechnet, wievielmal größer das Hohlraumvolumen des 82jährigen gegenüber dem 25jährigen ist. Die Hohlraumvergrößerung ist am geringsten an der unteren Extremität bei der Mittelphalanx 3 (1,1), an der oberen bei der Endphalanx 2 (0,8), am größten am Arm bei der Grundphalanx 4 (3,0) und am Bein an der Fibula (3,6).

DAVIDA (1926) hat an drei Individuen (♀ 16, ♀ 20 und ♂ 21 Jahre) sowie an einer nicht angegebenen Anzahl von Sammlungsstücken das Knochenvolumen der Skeletstücke (Tabelle 9) untersucht: Knochenvolumen $= 100 \cdot \frac{\text{Volumen der Knochensubstanz}}{\text{Porenvolumen}}$. DAVIDA meint, daß die Werte des von FRIEDRICH untersuchten 25jährigen etwas zu hoch liegen; sie werden etwa von jenen der 20jährigen Frau erreicht. Die Knochenvolumina der 16jährigen Frau und des 21jährigen Mannes gleichen fast dem von FRIEDRICH untersuchten 82jährigen. Aber auch das Volumen der von DAVIDA untersuchten

Sammlungsstücke liegt recht hoch. Da die Todesursache der Probanden nicht bekannt ist, kann nicht entschieden werden, ob die vorliegenden Werte im Rahmen der Variationsbreite liegen (s. unten) oder irgendwelche Knochenveränderungen anzunehmen sind.

Die Skeletstücke der unteren Extremität sind nach Davida (1926) „poröser" als die der oberen. Femur und Humerus haben ein kleineres Knochenvolumen als die Elemente des Unterarmes und Unterschenkels. Die Fußwurzel ist poröser als die Handwurzel. Für Metacarpus, Metatarsus, Finger und Zehen konnten keine Gesetzmäßigkeiten festgestellt werden. Am Arm ist rechts das Knochenvolumen größer als links, am Bein aber links größer als rechts.

Gewicht, Volumen und Porosität des Skeletes Neugeborener hat Töppich (1914) untersucht. Der Autor gibt aber nur für einzelne Elemente die originalen Zahlen wieder, faßt sonst ganze Abschnitte (Bein, Arm usw.) zusammen. Zum Vergleich hat Töppich den Schädel, das Brustbein und die Rippen eines 28jährigen Mannes herangezogen. Die Porosität der Knochen weiblicher Neugeborener ist größer als die männlicher. Das Hohlraumvolumen von Femur, Tibia und Humerus des Neugeborenen ist größer als bei dem von Friedrich untersuchten 25jährigen, aber kleiner als jenes beim 82jährigen.

Die Untersuchungen von Friedrich (1890), Wetzel (1910), Töppich (1914) und Davida (1926) beziehen sich auf das Hohlraumvolumen der ganzen Skeletstücke ohne zwischen spongiösen und kompakten Teilen zu unterscheiden. Barth (1940) hat das gesamte Volumen von Skeletelementen gemessen. Aus den Werten von Mechanik (1928, 1929, 1930, 1932) haben wir die Größe der Markhöhle errechnet und zu den Angaben von Barth in Beziehung gesetzt. Mechanik gibt den Umfang der Markhöhle an. Unter der Annahme einer rundlichen Markhöhle läßt sich deren Volumen berechnen. Dagegen kann aus dem äußeren Umfang der Skeletstücke die Masse der Compacta nicht bestimmt werden, da die Querschnittsform stark wechselt. An Stichproben haben wir Gesamtvolumen und Volumen der Markhöhle gemessen und erhielten Werte, die denen von Barth und Mechanik entsprechen.

Der größte Wert des Gesamtvolumens und Markvolumens eines Skeletstückes ist doppelt so groß wie der kleinste (Tabelle 9). Diese große Variationsbreite beruht darauf, daß die Variation der Länge der Skeletstücke im Volumen in der dritten Potenz auftritt. Der Volumenanteil der Markhöhle am Skeletvolumen ist — mit Ausnahme der Fibula der Frauen — mit 15—20% klein. Die Markhöhle der Skeletstücke der Frauen hat einen größeren prozentualen Anteil am Volumen als bei Männern. Absolut hat der Femur die größte, die Fibula die kleinste Markhöhle. Der prozentuale Anteil des Markvolumens am Gesamtvolumen ist am Femur am kleinsten, bei der Tibia der Männer und der Fibula der Frauen am größten. Die Zunahme des Hohlraumvolumens und die Abnahme des Knochenvolumens im Senium ist an der unteren Extremität größer als an der oberen. Im Hinblick auf die Marknagelung und damit die Wahl der Nagelform zur Erzielung einer stabilen Osteosynthese haben v. Lanz, Dziallas, Lippert und Usener (1963) und Usener (1966) die Form der Markhöhle von 100 Humeri untersucht. Die Markhöhle endet proximal etwas distal der Epiphysenlinie, distal im Bereich des distalen Sechstels. Im allgemeinen (84%) nimmt die Markhöhle von proximal nach distal um 37% an Fläche ab. Die Längsachse ist für die Markhöhle und den Schaft etwa identisch und verläuft vom Tuberculum majus zur Fossa olecrani. Über die Volumenentwicklung der Skeletstücke in der Fetalzeit haben Bauer (1940) und Bahling (1958), über deren Gewicht Ingalls (1931, 1932) berichtet.

Im Hinblick auf die Statik der Skeletelemente ist die Angabe der älteren Autoren zu diskutieren, daß die Porosität der Knochen des Beines größer ist als die der Knochen des Armes. Bei Femur und Humerus ist das relative Knochen- oder Hohlraumvolumen etwa gleich groß. Der Volumenanteil der Markhöhle am Gesamtvolumen ist aber beim Femur kleiner als beim Humerus. Die scheinbar größere Porosität des Femurs gegenüber dem Humerus ist daher auf die umfangreichen spongiösen proximalen und distalen Abschnitte des Femurs zurückzuführen. Über die Größe des Volumens der spongiösen Teile der

Röhrenknochen liegen leider keine Angaben vor. Aus dem Verhältnis Markvolumen zu Gesamtvolumen ist zu schließen, daß der Femur nicht nur absolut, sondern auch bezogen auf sein Gesamtvolumen ein relativ hohes Knochenvolumen besitzt. Die absolut und bezogen auf das Gesamtvolumen große Markhöhle der Tibia könnte damit in Zusammenhang stehen, daß Tibia und Fibula statisch eine Einheit im Sinne eines Gittermastes mit dazwischen gespannter Membrana interossea bilden (s. S. 506).

Das „Hohlraumvolumen" in bezug auf das Gesamtvolumen gibt bei spongiösen Skeletstücken über die Menge der tragenden Knochensubstanz Auskunft (s. S. 474), bei Teilen mit Compacta leider nicht. Die mit unterschiedlicher Methodik gewonnenen Werte über die Hohlräume der Skeletelemente, die „Porosität", können noch nicht zu deren Festigkeit in Beziehung gesetzt werden. Jedoch geben EVANS und BANG (1967) an, daß zwischen Elastizität und Hohlräumen eine negative Korrelation bestehe, auch SEDLIN (1965) findet keinen Zusammenhang zwischen dem Volumen der Haversschen Kanäle und der Festigkeit. Jedoch ist bemerkenswert, daß das Verhältnis Markvolumen zu Gesamtvolumen, das Hohlraumvolumen im ganzen und dessen Veränderung im Laufe des Lebens von Skeletstück zu Skeletstück und bei den einzelnen Species verschieden ist. So wird die Annahme bestätigt, daß jedes Skeletstück seine mechanische Aufgabe sowohl durch eine spezifische Gestalt als auch durch ein Knochengewebe von örtlich eigener Struktur erfüllt.

Von verschiedenen Autoren wurde versucht, einen Zusammenhang zwischen der Festigkeit und dem jeweiligen Verlauf der Kollagenfibrillen aufzufinden. OLIVO (1937a) war der Meinung, daß bei Zugbelastung mehr steil verlaufende, bei Druck mehr flach verlaufende Fibrillen vorhanden sind. Nach OLIVO (1937c) ist der Bruchwiderstand proportional der Anzahl der Fibrillen. Das Auftreten von Osteonen stünde nicht mit der Blutversorgung des Knochens in unmittelbarem Zusammenhang, da die Tangentiallamellen ebenfalls gut versorgt wären; das Haverssche System stelle ein Einschachtelungssystem dar. Wenn viele Osteone mit steilen Wickelungen vorhanden sind, kann das Skeletstück einem starken und heftigen Zug unterworfen werden. Am Metacarpus und Metatarsus der Vierfüßler herrsche in den vorderen Gebieten Druck-, in den hinteren Zugbelastung (OLIVO, 1937b); so liegen in diesen Stücken vorn abwechselnd steil und flach gewickelte Osteone und in den übrigen Abschnitten mehr steil gewickelte. Nach MAJ und TOAIARI (1937a) ist die Menge der mineralisierten Intercellularsubstanz 6mal geringer als die der Kollagenfibrillen. So würde die Verteilung und Richtung der Kollagenfibrillen die mechanische Anisotropie des Knochens bedingen. Am Metatarsus des Rindes verhält sich der Elastizitätsmodul von Knochen mit Tangentiallamellen zu dem mit Osteonen wie 0,68:1, d.h. der Elastizitätsmodul des Knochens mit Grundlamellen ist kleiner als der mit Osteonen.

Die Beziehungen zwischen Struktur und Festigkeit von Metatarsus und Metacarpus des Pferdes hat BOGDASCHEW (1930) untersucht. Der Metacarpus enthält gegenüber dem Metatarsus prozentual weniger organische Stoffe und Wasser, aber mehr Asche und CaO, wie die Analyse von jeweils acht Stücken ergab. Die Druckfestigkeit des Metacarpus ist 2207, des Metatarsus 2187, die mittlere beider 2147 (1840—2805) kg · cm^{-2}. BOGDASCHEW hat auch die vier Quadranten des Querschnittes untersucht und fand für die Seitenteile 2064, dorsal und caudal 2303, caudal 2315 und dorsal 2214. Schließlich führte BOGDASCHEW Biegeversuche an den etwa 15—16 cm langen Skeletstücken bei einer Stützweite von 12 cm aus. Diese Skeletelemente haben einen elliptischen Querschnitt. Eine Biegung in Richtung von dorsal nach caudal geht in Richtung der kurzen Ellipsenachse und führt zum Bruch des Metacarpus bei 1470 und des Metatarsus bei 1740 kg · cm^{-2}. Die Biegung von medial nach lateral erfolgt in Richtung der langen Ellipsenachse; die Biegefestigkeit des Metacarpus ist dann 1260 und des Metatarsus 1730 kg · cm^{-2}. Die histologische Untersuchung ergibt, daß im Metatarsus die Haversschen Kanäle sehr dicht liegen. Anastomosen zwischen den Kanälen sind selten; im Metacarpus sind dagegen weniger Haverssche Systeme mit zahlreichen Anastomosen vorhanden. BOGDASCHEW meint nun, das dichte Netz der Haversschen Kanäle ermögliche dem Metatarsus einen besseren Ersatz der im Knochen während des Stoßens nach vorn verbrauchten Energie und stelle eine Kompensation der ständig verbrauchten Energie dar, da der Metatarsus schräg in einem Winkel von 95—100° steht. Die reichlich vorhandene organische Substanz erhöht die Elastizität des Metatarsus. Demgegenüber stellt der Metacarpus eine senkrechte Stütze dar, über die der Körper hinwegrollt; der Metacarpus ist daher mit seinem hohen Ca-Gehalt auf einen großen Druckwiderstand eingestellt. Von Interesse ist, daß Bogdaschew das Knochengewebe nicht als „totes" tragendes Material ansieht, sondern — ob mit Recht oder nicht, sei dahingestellt — als ein Material, das Energie verbraucht (vgl. S. 477).

Evans (1958) hat bei Berechnung der korrigierten Zugfestigkeit bezogen auf den Querschnitt nach Abzug der Haversschen Kanäle gefunden, daß die weniger widerstandsfähige Fibula fester als der Femur erscheint. Diese Differenz wird mit der unterschiedlichen Struktur beider Knochen in Verbindung gebracht. Die Fibula ist durch einige wenige große und unregelmäßig gebaute Osteone und Osteonfragmente gekennzeichnet, im Femur sind viele kleine typische Osteone und deren Fragmente anzutreffen. In der Fibula verlaufen die Fibrillen überwiegend steil, beim Femur mehr horizontal und schräg, d.h. flach. Damit würde die Zugfestigkeit der Fibula größer als die des Femur. Eine größere Zahl von Kittlinien je Flächeneinheit setze die Festigkeit ebenfalls herab. Evans und Bang (1967) haben den Korrelationskoeffizienten zwischen den physikalischen Eigenschaften und den histologischen Komponenten der Bruchzonen mit Hilfe des Computers bestimmt. Eine starke positive Korrelation liegt zwischen der Zugfestigkeit und dem prozentualen Anteil an Schaltlamellen vor, zwischen der Härte und der Zahl der Osteone je mm^2, zwischen der Härte und dem prozentualen Anteil der Osteone, zwischen der Scherfestigkeit und der Anzahl der Osteonfragmente, zwischen Elastizitätsmodul und prozentualem Anteil der Hohlräume. Demnach setzen Osteone die Zugfestigkeit des Knochengewebes und den Elastizitätsmodul herab, während beide durch die Anwesenheit von Schaltlamellen erhöht werden. Die Autoren führen als Grund u.a. die größere Anzahl von Kittlinien im Osteonknochen an. Bedauerlich ist, daß sich die Verfasser auf die Zug- und Scherfestigkeit beschränken, Beanspruchungsformen, die voraussichtlich für die Skeletstücke eine geringe Rolle spielen. Hert, Kucera, Vavra und Volenik (1965) geben für das Rind an, daß der Haverssche Knochen eine geringere Festigkeit als der primäre Knochen habe.

Maj und Toaiari (1937b) haben bei Biegung, Torsion und Druck die Lage der Bruchlinien an Femur, Tibia und Metatarsus von Hund, Kaninchen, Rind und Mensch untersucht. Im allgemeinen sind keine Beziehungen der Bruchlinien zu den Kittlinien und Lamellen aufzufinden. Die Frakturlinien verbinden häufig Haverssche Kanäle miteinander. Wird dagegen entmineralisiertes Gewebe einer Bruchlast unterworfen, bleiben die Haversschen Systeme unversehrt und die Bruchlinien laufen um sie herum. Die Osteone stellen damit wohl keine strukturelle Einheit dar, geben dem Knochen aber eine vermehrte Widerstandsfähigkeit. Olivo (1937c) meint demzufolge, daß in einem Knochengebiet nicht alle Teile der Feinstruktur dem gleichen Maß der Beanspruchung unterworfen sind. Currey (1959) hat sich mit dem Unterschied von primären und sekundären Osteonen befaßt, die zwar im Bau gleich sind, wobei aber die sekundären eine vollständige Kittlinie besitzen (vgl. Knese und Titschak, 1962). Die Proben aus dem Rinderfemur wurden nach der Zurichtung 24 Std in physiologischer Kochsalzlösung aufbewahrt. Es liegt eine negative Korrelation zwischen der Zugfestigkeit und dem Vorhandensein von Osteonen vor.

Knese (1958b) und Knese und Titschak (1962) haben mit Hilfe des Lochkartenverfahrens beim Wildschwein 10157 und Hausschwein 10061 Haverssche Systeme in bezug auf die Druckfestigkeit ihres Herkunftsgebietes untersucht (s. S. 425). Der Querschnitt des Metacarpus wurde in sechs Abschnitte unterteilt, für die sowohl die Druckfestigkeit als auch der Osteonaufbau ermittelt wurde. Die gemessenen Bruchspannungen wurden in Klassen aufgeteilt, wie das bei statistischen Untersuchungen üblich ist. Für jede dieser Festigkeitsklassen konnte dann die Anzahl der Osteone je cm^2 sowie deren prozentuale Aufteilung auf die verschiedenen Formen der Wicklung der Kollagenfibrillen festgestellt werden (Abb. 22); auch das Alter der untersuchten Tiere wurde berücksichtigt. Höhere Bruchspannungen treten im mittleren Alter auf (Wildschwein 20—44, Hausschwein 15—24 Monate). Die Anzahl der Osteone je cm^2 nimmt zu höheren Bruchklassen hin ab. In diesem Befund sehen die Autoren jedoch eine reine Altersdifferenz, da die Strukturentwicklung durch eine Zunahme großer und reifer Osteonquerschnitte gekennzeichnet ist. Die kleinen Osteone mit Faserfilzen, die jugendlichen (die sog. primären ohne Kittlinien) nehmen an Zahl ab. So verringert sich auch die Zahl dieser jugend-

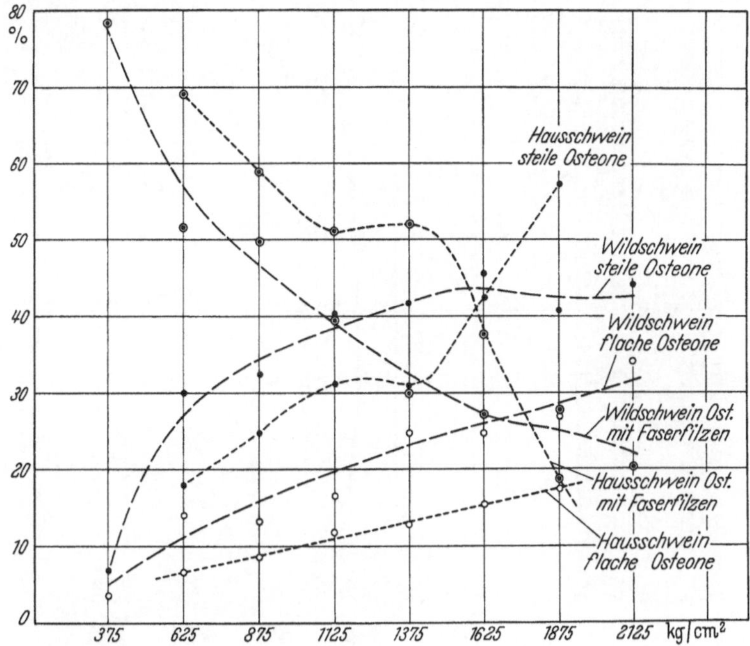

Abb. 22. Beziehung zwischen Bruchspannung (Druck) und Wickelung der Osteone: Prozentualer Anteil der Steigungsfolgen für die einzelnen Klassen der Bruchspannungen (aus Knese und Titschak, 1962)

lichen Osteone zu höheren Festigkeitsklassen hin, die reifen sind häufiger und unter ihnen wiederum die mit steiler Wickelung, die mit flacher sind seltener. Die Entwicklung der Feinstruktur mit der Bildung reifer, durch Kittlinien abgegrenzter Osteone geht bis in das höhere Alter hinauf weiter. Die Festigkeit nimmt dagegen von dem mittleren Alter an wiederum ab. Somit ist die Festigkeit nicht nur auf die Struktur, das Gefüge, sondern auch auf den physiko-chemischen Zustand der Komponenten zu beziehen, wie das immer wieder betont wurde (Maj, 1942; Amprino, 1961). Knese und Titschak (1962) meinen daher, daß erst die Analyse von etwa 100000 Osteonen, verbunden mit verschiedenartigen Festigkeitsprüfungen und physiko-chemischen Untersuchungen die Beziehungen zwischen Struktur und Festigkeit aufklären könnte.

Inwieweit der Mineralanteil bzw. andere Komponenten für die Festigkeit verantwortlich sind, läßt sich teilweise aus den Untersuchungen von Schmitt (1968) und Amtmann und Schmitt (1968) erschließen. Die Autoren haben die Materialdichte durch die Röntgenstrahlenabsorption bestimmt und diese mit der Druckfestigkeit von Femurproben fixierten Materials verglichen. Amtmann und Schmitt (1968) kommen zu der Feststellung, daß Unterschiede in der Bruchfestigkeit nur zu 40 bzw. 42% auf Unterschiede der Knochendichte zurückzuführen sind, d.h. dem Gehalt an Kalksalzen (besser Mineralien). Man muß aus den Angaben dieser Autoren schließen, daß die Struktur des Knochengewebes für die Festigkeit von wesentlich größerer Bedeutung ist als der Mineralgehalt. SCHMITT (1968) und AMTMANN und SCHMITT (1968) haben die Verteilung der Materialdichte auf Grund der Röntgenstrahlenabsorption im gesamten Femur dargestellt (Abb. 23). SCHMITT (1968) faßt die Untersuchungsergebnisse zusammen: 1. Materialdichte und Festigkeit zeigen einen Zusammenhang; 2. beide nehmen von der Schaftmitte gegen die Gelenkenden hin ab; 3. Dichte und Festigkeit sind über den Knochenquerschnitt unregelmäßig verteilt, medial und laterial größer als vorn und hinten; 4. in der Crista femoris nimmt die Dichte von innen nach außen zu. AMTMANN und SCHMITT (1968) haben mit den Mitteln der Regressions- und Covarianzanalyse nachgewiesen, daß zwei Dichte- und Festigkeitsfunktionen für Personen unter bzw. über 67,8 Jahren vorliegen. Die

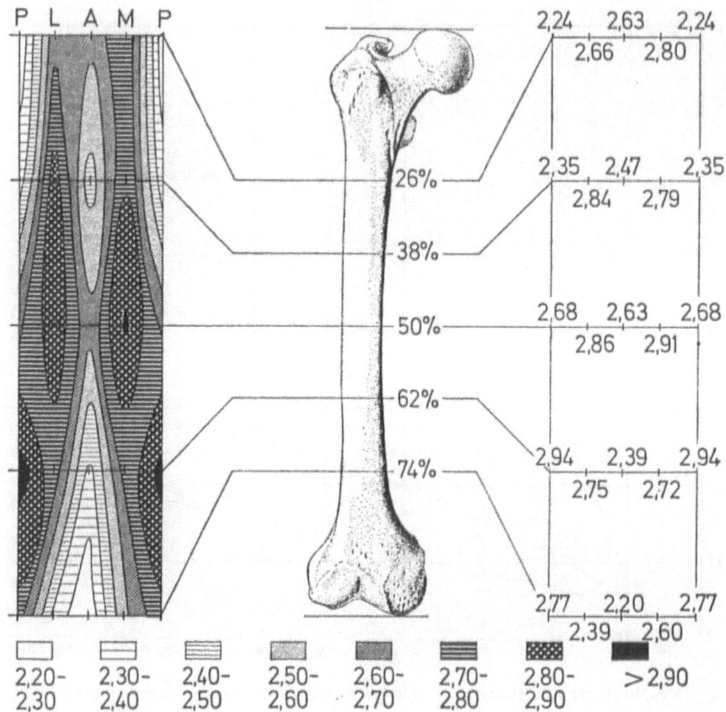

Abb. 23. Die mittleren Linien gleicher Dichte (-quadrate) der Corticalis zwischen 26 und 74% Schnitthöhe des rechten Femurschaftes bei 8 Personen zwischen 56 und 80 Jahren. Die mittlere Materialverteilung in den Probekörpern der verschiedenen Schaftpositionen ist im rechten, das daraus durch lineare Interpolation ermittelte Materialverteilungsmuster im linken Diagramm dargestellt. Die Corticalis ist dorsal aufgeschnitten und in die Zeichenebene ausgebreitet zu denken (aus AMTMANN und SCHMITT, 1968)

Dichte nimmt mit zunehmendem Alter ab, d.h. zwischen 56 und 87 Jahren. Im Abschnitt Festigkeit wurden jene Angaben der Literatur aufgeführt, die dafür sprechen, daß der höchste Festigkeitswert des Knochens etwa mit 35 Jahren erreicht wird (s. S. 433).

Weiterhin ist aber zu bedenken, daß bei einem Verbundbau sehr unterschiedliche Strukturen eine gleichartige mechanische Leistung gewähren können. Schließlich sind Eigenheiten der untersuchten Species und die jeweilige Körpergröße (Allometrie: KLATT, 1913, 1949; MÜHLMANN, 1927, 1929; HERRE, 1959) zu beachten. Für den Widerstand, den ein Skeletstück der Biegung entgegensetzt, ist nicht nur das Material, sondern auch die Querschnittsform des Skeletstückes, d.h. dessen Flächenmomente (s. S. 430) bedeutsam. Das Verhältnis der Flächenmomente, größtes I_{max} und kleinstes I_{min} Trägheitsmoment, und die Verteilung der Strukturen über den Querschnitt bei Säugetieren hat ERTELT (1955) untersucht. Dabei ist zu berücksichtigen, daß bei größeren Tieren die Faserfilzosteone (primäre) und Tangentiallamellen abnehmen; es kommt zur Ausbildung eines Osteonknochens (vgl. AMPRINO und GODINA, 1947; VIGNOLO-LUTATI, 1940). Beim Pferd z.B. sind nur Metacarpus und Metatarsus ein reiner Osteonknochen, in den anderen Skeletstücken treten auch andere Strukturelemente auf. Allein bei den Affen (vgl. SCHULTZ, 1953) findet sich ein Strukturaufbau, der dem des Menschen entspricht. So ist bei der Übertragung von an Tieren gewonnenen Ergebnissen über das Verhältnis Struktur/Festigkeit auf den Menschen Vorsicht geboten.

ERTELT (1955) hat untersucht, ob innerhalb eines Querschnittes durch ein Skeletstück bei einer Species die gleichen Strukturformen, z.B. Osteone, auftreten oder ob verschiedenartige Strukturformen in den „Quadranten" des Querschnittes vorhanden sind. ERTELT unterscheidet vier Formen der Beziehung zwischen Struktur und Flächenmomenten:

1. Den Belastungen wirkt allein die Querschnittsform entgegen, d.h. I_{max} ist bedeutend größer als I_{min}; keine auffälligen Differenzen in der Strukturverteilung über dem Querschnitt. *Femur:* Pferd, Mufflon (distal), Katze (proximal), Seehund, Hase, Emu; *Tibia:* Gibbon, Pferd, Seehund, Schwein, Katze, Emu, Hase; *Fibula:* Seehund, Gibbon; *Humerus:* Pferd, Hund, Seehund, Hase, Ziege, Orang; *Radius:* Pferd, Schwein, Ziege, Hund, Seehund, Dachs, Hase; *Ulna:* Schwein, Katze, Hase, Fuchs, Ziege, Hund, Seehund.

2. Großer Unterschied zwischen I_{max} und I_{min}; die einzelnen Abschnitte des Querschnittes sind aus verschiedenartigen Strukturformen aufgebaut. *Femur:* Gibbon, Orang, Schwein, Mufflon, Hund, Fuchs; *Tibia:* Dachs, Orang, Fuchs; *Fibula:* Schwein, Orang; *Humerus:* Schwein, Katze, Mufflon, Fuchs; *Radius:* Mufflon, Fuchs, Gibbon; *Ulna:* Dachs.

3. Kleiner Unterschied zwischen I_{max} und I_{min}; geringe Strukturdifferenzen innerhalb des Querschnittes. *Femur:* Ziege, Dachs; *Tibia:* Mufflon; *Humerus:* Dachs.

4. Kleiner Unterschied zwischen I_{max} und I_{min}; keine Strukturverschiedenheiten innerhalb des Querschnittes. *Humerus:* Gibbon; *Radius:* Orang; *Ulna:* Gibbon, Orang.

Diese Aufstellung zeigt, daß sich bei der gleichen Species die einzelnen Skeletelemente im Hinblick auf ihre Flächenmomente und ihren Strukturaufbau unterschiedlich verhalten. Ebenso different ist der Feinbau des gleichen Elementes bei verschiedenen Species. Bei Erörterung des Feinbaues eines Skeletstückes sind Beziehungen zur systematischen Stellung, Körpergröße, Art der Bewegung und Lebensform, wohl aber auch unterschiedliche Reaktionsformen auf Schäden (Rachitisverbiegung: BELL et al., 1947, s. S. 466) zu suchen. Damit werden aber die Beziehungen zwischen Struktur und Festigkeit des Knochens ungewöhnlich verwickelt.

ε) Veränderung der Knochenfestigkeit durch Ernährung, Hormone, Innervation

Der Einfluß der Ernährung auf die Knochenfestigkeit wurde verschiedentlich untersucht (MCKEOWN et al., 1932; BECKER et al., 1930; BECKER et al., 1934; CLARKE et al., 1936), doch wurde nur die Bruchlast, nicht die Festigkeit ermittelt. BELL et al. (1941) haben die Bedeutung des Ca-Gehaltes für die Knochenfestigkeit untersucht. BELL und WEIR (1949) und BELL (1956) geben die Biegefestigkeit von Rattenfemora bei Belastung der Knochen in der Mitte zu 1900 kg · cm^{-2} an. 6 Wochen alte Ratten erhielten eine vollwertige Kost, die aber wechselnde Mengen Ca 0,075—1,39 g je 100 g, enthielt. Nach 8 Wochen wurden die Femora auf Biege- und Torsionsfestigkeit untersucht. Die höchsten Festigkeitswerte ergaben sich bei einem Ca-Gehalt der Nahrung von 0,36 %, und zwar für Biegung 2460 und Torsion 667 kg · cm^{-2}. Größere Ca-Mengen in der Nahrung waren ohne Einfluß auf die Festigkeit. Bei einem Nahrungs-Ca von 0,2 % sanken Ca-Aufnahme und Festigkeit jeweils um 20 %. Bei 0,075 % Ca-Gehalt betrug die Ca-Aufnahme etwa $^1/_3$ der maximalen; die Festigkeit ging dann auf die Hälfte zurück. Die Form der Knochen blieb bei unterschiedlichem Nahrungs-Ca gleich, bei Mengen unter 0,36 % war die Knochenrinde dünner.

BELL und WEIR (1949) haben vier mit Fluor behandelte Schafe mit vier gesunden verglichen. Die Fluor-Knochen waren größer, schwerer und plumper. In dem Aschegehalt fand sich keine wesentliche Differenz gegenüber den Gesunden (69,1 bzw. 73,9 %), ebenso fehlen Differenzen in der Kristallstruktur. Der Fluor-Gehalt der befallenen Knochen betrug 1,02 %, der Kontrollen 0,028 %. Femur, Metacarpus und Metatarsus rechts wurden auf Biegung, der linke Metatarsus auf Torsion untersucht. Die mittlere Biegefestigkeit der Fluor-Knochen war 2040, der Kontrollen 1920 kg · cm^{-2}, die Torsionsfestigkeit 731 bzw. 914 kg · cm^{-2}. Der Mechanismus der Fluorwirkung ist unklar.

BELL et al. (1947) und WEIR et al. (1949) haben in vierwöchentlichen Experimenten an 50 g schweren Ratten den Einfluß einer rachitischen Diät auf die Festigkeit untersucht. Die Tiere wurden in drei Gruppen unterteilt, *R* erhielt eine rachitische Diät, *N* zu dieser Diät Vitamin D und *S* als Kontrolle eine normale Nahrung (Tabelle 10). Der Aschegehalt sinkt bei der rachitischen Kost fast auf die Hälfte, ebenso die Biegefestigkeit, der Elastizitätsmodul geht auf $^1/_3$ herunter. Die Abhängigkeit der Biegefestigkeit und des Elastizitätsmoduls von der rachitogenen Diät ist auffällig, jedoch statistisch nicht abzusichern (PERRY 1949; nach BELL 1956). Die Proportionalitätsgrenze liegt bei rachitischen Ratten niedriger als bei den anderen. Die Herabsetzung der Festigkeit kann auf Änderung des Mineralanteiles oder des organischen bzw. auf eine Veränderung der Beziehungen zwischen den Kollagenfibrillen und den Mineralien zurückgehen. Das Verhältnis Ca/P = 2/1 ist bei allen Tieren gleich; Röntgenbrechungsdiagramme zeigen bei rachitischen Ratten die gleiche Kristallordnung wie bei normalen. Auch in der Aminosäuren-Zusammensetzung verhalten sich erkrankte und gesunde Ratten gleich (PERRY, 1954; nach BELL, 1956). So kann die verminderte Festigkeit nur auf das unterschiedliche Verhältnis zwischen organischen und anorganischen Komponenten zurückgeführt werden.

Tabelle 10. *Biegefestigkeit des Femurs rachitischer Ratten* (nach BELL et al. 1947; WEIR et al. 1949)

	Rachitische Kost (R)	Rachitische Kost + Vitamin D (N)	Kontrolle (S)
Aschegehalt	36%	43%	60%
σ_b	840	1300	1900
E_b	42000	70000	112000

BELL (1956) beschäftigt sich in diesem Zusammenhang mit der rachitischen Knochenverbiegung, die bei allen rachitischen Ratten ebenso fehlte wie bei einer Ca-Mangel-Diät. BELL et al. (1947) meinen, daß die rachitische Verformung der Knochen bei Mensch und Hund nicht allein durch die mechanischen Eigenschaften der Knochen erklärt werden kann. Es liege eine abnorme Reaktion auf die Biegekräfte vor; die nach Species verschiedene Reaktion ist aber unverständlich; wir kommen bei Erörterung der Widerstandsmomente auf diese Frage zurück (s. S. 492).

BELL et al. (1943) haben Hypophysen-Vorderlappen-Hormon an Ratten verabreicht und fanden größere und stärkere Knochen; der Anstieg der Festigkeit entspricht etwa der Größenzunahme der Knochen. Östradiol, Parathyreoidea- und Schilddrüsen-Extrakt bewirken keine Änderung der Festigkeit.

Den Einfluß der Inaktivität auf die Knochenfestigkeit haben ALLISON und BROOKS (1921) bei Hunden nach einseitiger Durchschneidung des Plexus brachialis geprüft. Beim Biegebruchversuch der Metacarpen fanden die Verfasser eine Abnahme der Bruchlast. Biegebruchversuche an Prismen, die aus dem Humerus gewonnen wurden, ließen jedoch keine Differenzen der Festigkeit gegenüber den gebrauchten Gliedern erkennen. Die Biegefestigkeit des gebrauchten betrug 1200, des inaktiven Humerus 1500 kg · cm^{-2}.

Die Biegefestigkeit von Femur, Tibia und Fibula nach Nervendurchschneidung bei Katzen und weißen Ratten hat GILLESPIE (1954) geprüft. Bei der 1. Gruppe von Katzen wurde die vordere Wurzel, bei der 2. die hintere und bei der 3. wurde mit einer Durchschneidung der vorderen Wurzel eine Entfernung der sympathischen Ganglien verbunden. Die Knochen der Katzen wurden 2 Monate nach der Operation untersucht, und zwar nach Lufttrocknung über mehrere Monate, um den Einfluß des Feuchtigkeitsgehaltes auszuschalten. Femur und Tibia von 16 Rattenmännchen wurden nach vierwöchentlicher Ausschaltung von Nervus femoralis und ischiadicus in gleicher Weise untersucht. GILLESPIE fand (Tabelle 11), daß die Festigkeit der Katzenknochen auf der Seite der Durchschneidung der vorderen bzw. hinteren Wurzeln statistisch nicht signifikant größer als jene der anderen Seite ist. Dagegen ist die Festigkeit nach Durchtrennung der vorderen Wurzeln und Entfernung der Sympathicusganglien auf der aktiven, normalen Seite

Tabelle 11. *Biegefestigkeit (kg · cm⁻²) der langen Knochen der hinteren Extremität von Katzen und Ratten nach Durchschneidung der Spinalnerven* (nach GILLESPIE, 1954)

	Kontrolle	Versuche	Prozentuale Differenz %
Katzen			
Durchschneidung der vorderen Wurzeln der Spinalnerven	2670	2740	+ 2,8[1]
Durchschneidung der hinteren Wurzeln der Spinalnerven	2667	2778	+ 2,3
Durchschneidung der vorderen Wurzel und Entfernung der Grenzstrangganglien	3152	2680	—14,9
Ratten	2240	1905	—14,4

[1] + Zunahme in %; — Abnahme in %.

statistisch signifikant größer. Bei den Ratten war die Festigkeit auf der gesunden Seite ebenfalls signifikant größer. GILLESPIE nimmt an, daß die veränderte Festigkeit auf den Verlust der Muskelaktion, aber nicht auf die Blutversorgung oder einen trophischen Einfluß zurückzuführen ist.

Auf die Festigkeit heilender Frakturen im Zusammenhang mit dem Wassergehalt (HÄBLER und REISS, 1936) wurde schon hingewiesen (s. S. 447). LINDSAY et al. (1931) und McKEOWN et al. (1932a) untersuchten Frakturen der Rattenfibula. Die Fraktur wird erst nach dem 6. Tage fest, die Festigkeit nimmt bis zum 15. Tage zu, mit Bildung der Markhöhle aber ab. Jedoch steigt die Festigkeit nach dem 24. Tag durch Verdickung des Callus an, am 45. Tag war die Fraktur geheilt. McKEOWN et al. (1932b, 1932c) untersuchten den Einfluß einer an Fett bzw. Kohlenhydraten reichen Nahrung, McKEOWN, HARVEY und LUMSDEN (1932) einer Ca-armen Diät auf die Frakturheilung.

Somit liegen im Augenblick sehr wenige experimentelle Untersuchungen über die Veränderung der Festigkeit unter verschiedenartigen Einflüssen vor. Diese Ergebnisse können noch nicht im Hinblick auf die Beziehungen zwischen Struktur und Festigkeit diskutiert werden.

e) Die Festigkeit der Spongiosa

α) *Experimentelle Untersuchungen der Spongiosa*

RAUBER (1876) hat auch an einigen Proben die Festigkeit der Spongiosa geprüft und meint, daß auf Grund der sehr wechselnden Struktur der Spongiosa die Festigkeit von 0 bis zu der des kompakten Knochens reicht. RAUBER hat vier Würfel aus dem Innern eines frischen Lendenwirbels in Längsachse auf Druck untersucht und erhielt die Werte 87,5, 65, 95,5 und 87, im Mittel 83,75 kg · cm⁻². Vier Würfel aus dem Innern der Femurkondylen zeigten eine Festigkeit von 90, 120, 95 und 80, im Mittel 96,25 kg · cm⁻². Weiterhin untersuchte RAUBER die Scherfestigkeit von Spongiosa aus dem Schienbeinkopf. Einmal gewann RAUBER Stäbchen, deren längste Achse der Längsachse des Knochens entsprach und ließ die Scherkraft senkrecht zu dieser Längsachse einwirken; die Scherfestigkeit betrug 56 kg · cm⁻². Sodann entnahm RAUBER Stäbchen quer zur Knochenlängsachse, bei denen dann die Scherkraft in Knochenlängsachse wirkte; die Scherfestigkeit war 20 kg · cm⁻².

Tabelle 12. *Festigkeit der Wirbelspongiosa in kg · cm⁻²* (nach MESSERER, 1880)

Alter, Jahre, Geschlecht	Brustwirbel			Lendenwirbel		
	1	6	10	1	4	5
25, ♀	52	63	51	56	—	64
30, ♂	92	92	80	78	—	78
34, ♀	—	—	—	—	62	—
51, ♀	55	67	57	67	—	60
56, ♂	—	44	45	32	32	34
80, ♀	—	—	—	—	22	—
81, ♀	—	—	—	27	—	—

Aus Druckversuchen an Wirbeln (s. S. 509) hat MESSERER (1880) die Druckfestigkeit der Spongiosa errechnet (Tabelle 12). Die Druckfestigkeit der Spongiosa zeigt demzufolge einen Altersgang, der nach MESSERER dem der Compacta entspricht. Eine bestimmte Verteilung der Festigkeit auf die untersuchten Wirbel Th 1, 6, 10 und L 1, 4 und 5 ist nicht zu erkennen. Aus den Zahlen von MESSERER für die Individuen (25—56 Jahre) läßt sich der Mittelwert von 60 kg · cm^{-2} errechnen, für die Brustwirbel 63,5 und die Lendenwirbel 56,3 kg · cm^{-2}.

Die Festigkeit der Wirbelspongiosa wurde von LANGE (1902) für das Mannesalter zu 32—36 kg · cm^{-2}, für das Greisenalter zu 15—28 kg · cm^{-2} bestimmt. Die Elastizitätsgrenze liegt bei 5—30 kg · cm^{-2}. Die Elastizität ist bei Kindern unvollkommener als bei Erwachsenen und bei diesen wiederum geringer als bei Greisen. Die Proportionalitätsgrenze liegt bei der Hälfte der Bruchfestigkeit. Mit dem Alter nimmt die bleibende Verkürzung ab. Wenn die Belastungsdauer von 20 auf 60 sec heraufgesetzt wird, nimmt die Verkürzung um 1,3 % zu. Bei kindlichen Wirbeln beträgt die elastische Nachwirkung bei 48 kg · cm^{-2} 53 % der totalen Verkürzung und 87 % der bleibenden, bei Erwachsenen unter 26 kg · cm^{-2} 20 % der totalen und 96 % der bleibenden. LANGE kommt zum Schluß, daß der spongiöse Knochen zum Tragen eines toten (Dauer-)Gewichtes weniger geeignet sei.

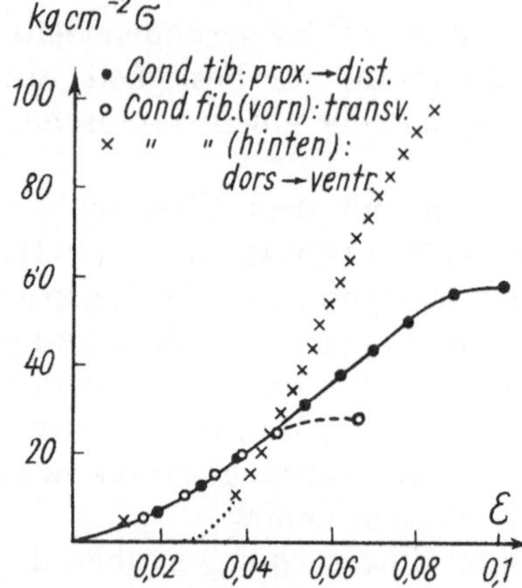

Abb. 24. Spannungs-Dehnungsschaubild für die Spongiosa der Femurkondylen eines Mannes von 70 Jahren (aus KNESE, 1958b)

GOECKE (1928) gibt die Druckfestigkeit der Wirbelspongiosa Jugendlicher zu 57—70 kg · cm^{-2}, die Dehnung zu 12,9—21,3 % an. Für die Spongiosa aus dem 2. Lendenwirbel eines 29jährigen Mannes (GOECKE, 1926, 1928) ergab sich eine Druckfestigkeit von 45 kg · cm^{-2}. Bei seniler Osteoporose liegt die Druckfestigkeit zwischen 20—30 kg · cm^{-2}, die Dehnung zwischen 9,6 und 12,3 %, d. h. die Druckfestigkeit und die Verkürzung nimmt im Alter ab. GOECKE (1926) hat weiterhin die Festigkeit in den einzelnen Bereichen des Wirbels geprüft und bei einem Probanden die Eigenschaften eines skoliotischen Wirbels (Th 7) mit einem nicht-skoliotischen (Th 12) verglichen. Bei Th 12 betrug die Festigkeit an den seitlichen Rändern 50 kg · cm^{-2}, die Verkürzung 10,7 %, für den Vorderrand lauten die Werte 45 und 10,7, den Hinterrand 47 und 8,8 und im Zentrum 40 kg · cm^{-2} und 5,7 %. Bei dem skoliotischen 7. Brustwirbel war an der Konkavseite die Druckfestigkeit 40 kg · cm^{-2}, die Verkürzung 14,6 % an der Konvexseite 30 bzw. 14,8; an der Wurzel des Bogens auf der konvexen Seite ergab sich die Druckfestigkeit zu 80 und auf der konkaven 95 kg · cm^{-2}. Die Druckfestigkeit ist demzufolge auf der konkaven Seite eines skoliotischen Wirbels größer als auf der konvexen.

Für die Festigkeit der Spongiosa ist die konstruktive Verteilung des Materials, die „Porosität", von besonderer Bedeutung. Im Druckversuch (Abb. 24) fehlt bei Beginn der Belastung die Proportionalität, offensichtlich durch ein leichtes Zusammendrücken der obersten Schichten der Probewürfel (GOECKE, 1925; KNESE, 1956a, 1958b). Bei der Spongiosa alter Leute fehlt nach GOECKE (1926) dieser Anfangsteil des Spannungs-Dehnungsdiagramms. Nachdem die Spongiosa an Endflächen des Probewürfels zusammengedrückt ist (s. S. 423), folgt ein Proportionalitätsbereich. Bei einem Höchstwert, der von KNESE (1956a, 1958b) der Berechnung der Druckfestigkeit zugrunde gelegt wurde, bricht das Gefüge der Spongiosa zusammen. Das Material verfestigt sich, so daß eine weitere Laststeigerung möglich ist, bis ein erneutes Eindrücken der Proben erfolgt; dann kann die Last wiederum gesteigert werden. Diese Beobachtung über die Tragfähigkeit der Spongiosa — offensichtlich nach Zerstörung der „Struktur" — ist für die Beurteilung eingekeilter Spongiosafrakturen von Interesse; eine solche Fraktur könnte demzufolge tragfähiger als die ursprüngliche Architektur sein. Allerdings besteht die Gefahr eines weiteren Zusammenbruches der zusammengeschobenen Spongiosa.

Für den 12. Brustwirbel eines 35jährigen Mannes fand GOECKE (1925) die Proportionalitätsgrenze bei 900 kg und den Bruch bei 1050 kg. Eine Vorbelastung von 800 kg auf

L 1 desselben Mannes ergab eine geringere Dehnung. GOECKE (1929) hat Spongiosawürfel aus dem Femur (vermutlich Kondylen) von 5 zu 5 kg $^1/_2$ min belastet und $^1/_2$ min entlastet. Bei Proben von einer 25jährigen Frau tritt bei 10 kg eine Verkürzung des 10 mm hohen Würfels um 0,12 mm ein, die bei Entlastung verschwindet. Bei 15 kg ist die bleibende Verkürzung 0,04 mm, bei 40 kg die Gesamtverkürzung 0,42 mm, die bleibende 0,25. Die Spongiosa einer 47jährigen Frau zeigt bei 60 kg eine Gesamtverkürzung von 0,20 und eine bleibende von 0,14 mm. Demgegenüber fand GOECKE bei der Spongiosa einer 59jährigen Frau mit langem Krankenlager bereits bei 20 kg · cm^{-2} eine Gesamtverkürzung von 0,70 und eine bleibende von 0,39 mm; der Bruch trat bei 25 kg · cm^{-2} ein. Bei Atrophie nimmt demzufolge die Tragfähigkeit ab und die Verkürzung zu.

Eine Untersuchung der Spongiosa des Femurkopfes führte HARDINGE (1949) durch, allerdings keine echte Festigkeitsprüfung. HARDINGE hat fünf Querschnitte von 6,35 mm Dicke von 94 Femurköpfen in verschiedenen Bereichen der Spongiosa um jeweils 3,17 mm eingedrückt; die größte Tragfähigkeit lag entlang des Trajectorium rectum. KNESE (1956a) hat die Druckfestigkeit einer Scheibe aus dem Femurkopf bei vier Individuen geprüft und erhielt die Werte: ♂ 54 Jahre: 78,9; ♂ 70 Jahre: 116,5; ♂ 48 Jahre: 97,8 und ♀ 53 Jahre: 78,9 kg · cm^{-2}, d.h. im Mittel war die Druckfestigkeit der Kopfspongiosa 93,0 kg · cm^{-2}. Von drei dieser Probanden hat KNESE die Druckfestigkeit der Kondylenspongiosa in Schaftrichtung ermittelt und als Mittel für die Probe aus dem medialen und lateralen Condylus 43,5, 48,8, 39,1 kg · cm^{-2} errechnet, für den Condylus medialis des 70jährigen Mannes 58,9 kg · cm^{-2}; damit beträgt das Mittel aller Proben aus den Femurkondylen 47,6 kg · cm^{-2}. GOECKE (1926) hatte die Festigkeit der Spongiosa aus dem distalen Femurende eines 18jährigen Mannes zu 82 kg · cm^{-2} gefunden. Die Druckfestigkeit der Spongiosa beträgt bei dem 54jährigen zwischen $^1/_{15}$ und $^1/_{30}$ und bei dem 70jährigen zwischen $^1/_{10}$ und $^1/_{40}$ von der Festigkeit der Compacta.

Bei zwei Probanden (54 und 70 Jahre) hat KNESE (1956a) die Druckfestigkeit oder Tragfähigkeit des Femurhalses zu 126 bzw. 148, im Mittel zu 137 kg · cm^{-2} bei einer Bruchlast von 1040 bzw. 1850 kg gemessen. Bei den beiden anderen Probanden (48 und 53 Jahre) wurde die Halsspongiosa in Halsrichtung nach Entfernung der Compacta gedrückt, wobei die Druckfestigkeit zu 26,9 bzw. 30,9, im Mittel 28,75 kg · cm^{-2} errechnet wurde. Die Spongiosa des Femurhalses hat demzufolge nur 21,1 % der Festigkeit des ganzen Halses. Daraus ist zu schließen, daß der Spongiosa für die Tragfähigkeit des Halses nicht jene Bedeutung zukommt, die ihr von vielen auf Grund der sog. trajektoriellen Struktur zugesprochen wird. Zum gleichen Ergebnis kommen HIRSCH und BRODETTI (1956b), die einzelne Teile der Halskonstruktion entfernt haben und dann die jeweilig verbleibende Tragfähigkeit bestimmten. Die caudale Corticalis des Halses trägt 40 % des Körpergewichtes, die craniale 20 %, craniale und caudale Spongiosa je 15 %. Caudale Compacta und anschließende Spongiosa und ebenso die cranialen Teile zusammen tragen jeweils 50 % des Körpergewichtes. Die Autoren schließen daraus, daß die Spongiosa wie die Trossen einer Brückenkonstruktion ein Verstärkungssystem darstellen, wobei das tragende Fundament die Compacta ist. Jedoch ist das Zusammenspiel zwischen Spongiosa und Compacta noch nicht endgültig geklärt (HIRSCH und FRANKEL, 1961).

Die Belastungsmöglichkeit der Spongiosa in verschiedenen Richtungen hat KNESE (1958a) auf Grund einer Nachuntersuchung der Spongiosaarchitektur (KNESE, 1956a, 1959d) geprüft. Der Verfasser beschreibt die Spongiosa als Platten (Abb. 25, 26, 27), die auf den Gelenkflächen senkrecht stehen, ähnlich wie es auch ALBERT (1900) und TRIEPEL (1908, 1922) angaben. Zwischen diesen Platten sind Bälkchen eingefügt, die im allgemeinen mit einem verbreiterten Fuß in die Platten übergehen; es handelt sich damit um die früher als Bälkchenspongiosa beschriebene Struktur. Die sog. Rundmaschenspongiosa tritt in Diaphysennähe, in Höckern, aber bei der Tibia auch in einiger Entfernung von der proximalen Gelenkfläche zwischen den Plattensystemen auf. Schnitte (KNESE, 1956a) und Röntgenaufnahmen (KNESE, 1959d) durch das proximale Femurende in verschiedener Richtung zeigen im Femurkopf ein radiäres auf der Gelenkfläche senk-

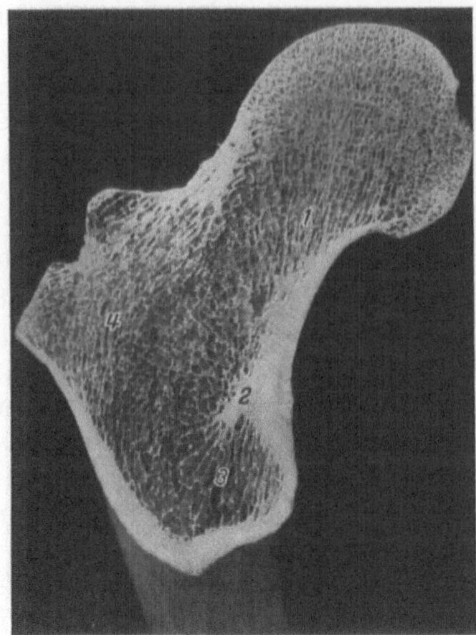

Abb. 25. Schnitt durch das proximale Ende eines linken Femurs in einer Ebene von proximal vorn nach distal hinten. *1* Trajectorium rectum; *2* Schenkelsporn; *3* hinteres frontales Plattensystem; *4* vorderes frontales Plattensystem im Übergang zur vorderen und lateralen Wand (aus KNESE, 1956a)

recht stehendes Plattensystem, das zu einem Punkt etwas unterhalb der Kopfmitte in der Gegend der Epiphysennarbe zusammenführt. Jenseits der Epiphysennarbe geht das „Trajectorium" rectum weiter, das mit seinen Platten wenig konvergierend von cranial-medial nach caudal-lateral an den unteren Umfang des Schenkelhalses und die mediale Schaftwand herantritt. An der Kopf-Halsgrenze beginnen zwei weitere Plattensysteme. Ein vorderes, annähernd frontal eingestelltes System trifft senkrecht oder spitzwinklig auf die vordere Femurwand; der größere Anteil der Platten biegt jedoch nach hinten um und erreicht die laterale Femurwand, ein kleiner Teil geht in den Trochanter major hinein. Ein hinteres Plattensystem steht im Zusammenhang mit dem Schenkelsporn und geht mit stark divergierenden Platten an die hintere Schaftwand um die Linea aspera heran. Die beiden frontalen Systeme verbinden sich im oberen Halsbereich zu dem sog. Trajectorium curvatum.

Die Spongiosa besteht demzufolge aus Platten, die in der Form von Halbröhren wie ein leicht gekrümmter Stoß Papier den Femurhals aufbauen. Von den Blättern eines Buches hatte schon ALBERT (1900) beim distalen Femurende gesprochen und GARDEN (1961) kommt auf diesen Vergleich beim Femurhals zurück. DIXON (1910) sah das tragende System des proximalen Femurendes ebenfalls als ein Röhrensystem an. GARDEN (1961) kommt nach Untersuchung von Schnitten und Röntgenaufnahmen zu einer sehr ähnlichen Schilderung der Spongiosa wie KNESE (1956a, 1958b, 1959d). Einmal

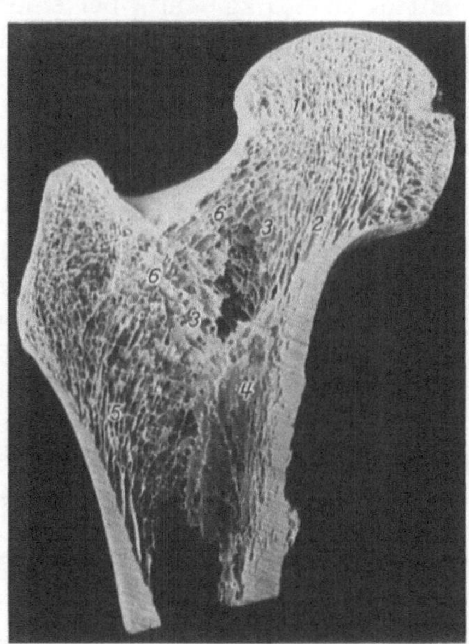

Abb. 26a

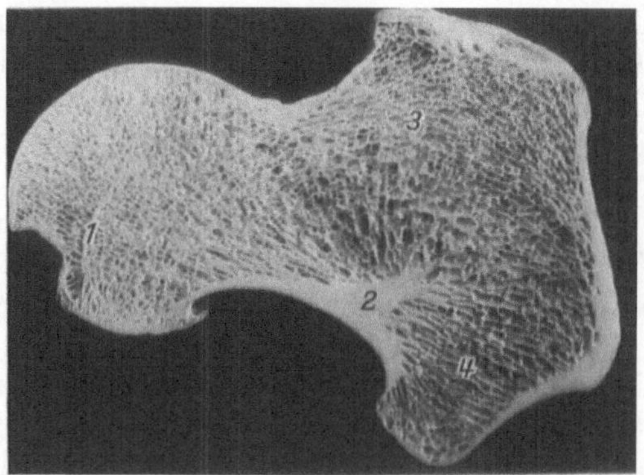

Abb. 26b

Abb. 26a. Frontalschnitt durch einen linken Femur am hinteren Umfang der Fovea capitis femoris. *1* Umbiegen der Spongiosaelemente aus der Normalen auf der Kopffläche in die Richtung des Trajectorium rectum; *2* Trajectorium rectum; *3* Anschnitte durch das hintere frontale Plattensystem; *4* Verbindung des hinteren Systems mit dem Schenkelsporn; *5* vorderes Plattensystem im Übergang in die laterale Wand; *6* Kuppelbildung zwischen vorderem und hinterem System (sog. Trajectorium curvatum) (aus KNESE, 1956a)

Abb. 26b. Längsschnitt durch Kopf und Hals eines Femurs. *1* Epiphysennarbe; *2* Schenkelsporn; *3* vorderes Plattensystem; *4* hinteres Plattensystem

gibt GARDEN wie TRIEPEL (1922b, e) für das obere Schaftende eine domartige Blattkonstruktion an. Der Schenkelsporn und die mediale Spongiosa sind als eine aufwärts gerichtete spiralige Fortsetzung der hinteren und medialen Schaftwand anzusehen; sie liegt dann am hinteren und unteren Umfang des Halses. Eine laterale Spongiosa ist eine in sich gedrehte Fortsetzung der vorderen und lateralen Schaftwand in den vorderen und oberen Teil des Halses. Ein drittes System tritt in der Trochanterregion auf, kreuzt sich mit dem lateralen und ist als Fortsetzung der Linea intertrochanterica aufzufassen. Diese Systeme sind nicht über die Epiphysennarbe hinaus in den Kopf zu verfolgen. Auch KUMMER (1962) sieht die Kopf-Hals-Spongiosa neuerlich als ein Plattensystem an.

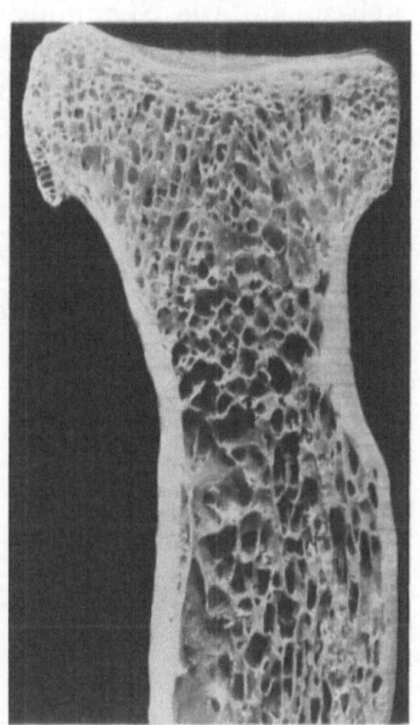

Abb. 27. Längsschnitt durch das proximale Ende des Radius. Die Spongiosaplatten stehen auf der Fläche der Fovea capituli radii senkrecht und stützen sich auf die Compacta. Zwischen den divergierenden Plattensystemen Rundmaschenspongiosa. Die Querstreben zwischen den Platten sind Bälkchen, die einen verbreiterten Fuß besitzen (aus KNESE, 1958b)

KNESE (1959b) hat darauf hingewiesen, daß die Spongiosaröhren im Röntgenbild ähnlich wie die Compacta im optischen Schnitt erscheinen, so daß nur eine Durchstrahlung in verschiedener Richtung einen Überblick über die Spongiosaarchitektur ermöglicht. Auch GARDEN (1961) beschäftigt sich mit der röntgenologischen Darstellung der Spongiosa, vor allem mit dem angeblichen Verschwinden der „Zug"lamellen bei der Coxa valga und deren Zunahme bei der Coxa vara. Diese Variation sei nicht das Ergebnis einer tatsächlichen Zu- oder Abnahme der Zahl der Lamellen, sondern beruht allein darauf, daß die Lamellen einmal en face, ein andermal im Profil erscheinen; die angenommene Veränderung der Lamellenzahl sei illusorisch und die radiologische Dichte hänge nur von der jeweiligen Rotation des Schenkelhalses ab. Nach den Ausführungen dieser beiden Autoren müßten röntgenologische Befunde über den Umbau oder die Änderung der Spongiosastruktur erneut überprüft werden. Der Verteilung des Materials auf Grund der Röntgenstrahlenabsorption und der Größe der Beanspruchung durch spannungsoptische Versuche im coxalen Femurende hat KNIEF (1967a, b) eine Studie gewidmet. Der Autor kommt zur Darstellung der Materialverteilung nach a.p. Röntgenaufnahmen in der Form eines Materialgebirges, da aus den densitometrisch ermittelten Meßstrecken nur schwer eine Vorstellung von der Verteilung der Spongiosa zu gewinnen sei. Das Wardsche Dreieck erscheint als ausgeprägte Einsenkung, die den größten Teil des Schenkelhalses einnimmt. Der Kopf stellt ein geschlossenes Materialmassiv mit Gipfel in dessen Mittelpunkt dar. In den Randpartien des Kopfes, mit Ausnahme des Adamschen Bogens, ist die Materialmenge geringer. Die laterale Corticalis wird durch einen von cranial nach caudal ansteigenden Gipfelzug dargestellt. Bei der Gegenüberstellung der Materialverteilung und der aus dem Isochromatenbild abgeleiteten Beanspruchung sowie dem Vergleich mit den Angaben von PAUWELS (1955) ergeben sich qualitative und quantitative Differenzen. Damit konnte die Annahme von PAUWELS, daß im coxalen Femurende ein Körper gleicher Festigkeit vorliegt, nicht bestätigt werden. Die Übereinstimmung zwischen der Materialverteilung und dem spannungsoptischen Bilde ist dagegen bei einer Coxa valga besser. Die Beschreibung von sog. „Trajektorien" im Schädel allein an Hand röntgenologischer Befunde durch GÖRKE (1904) und BARTH (1918) wurde bereits von KATZ (1931) und ZEIGER (1932) kritisiert. KATZ (1931) konnte an Schliffen kein Korrelat für die röntgenologisch dargestellten „Trajektorien" finden. Die von WALKHOFF (1902, 1904) röntgenologisch beschriebene Struktur des Kinnes konnte von WEIDENREICH (1904a, b) nicht bestätigt werden.

Die Untersuchung der Spongiosa-Struktur führte KNESE (1958b) dazu, die Festigkeit der Spongiosa bei Belastung in verschiedener Richtung zu prüfen. Bisher hatte nur RAUBER (1876) die Scherfestigkeit der Spongiosa in verschiedener Richtung untersucht. Die frische Spongiosa des Condylus medialis eines 70jährigen Mannes hat in Schaftrichtung eine Druckfestigkeit von 58,9 (Abb. 24), ein Würfel aus dem vorderen Anteil des Condylus lateralis in transversaler Richtung 28,3 und ein Würfel aus dem hinteren Anteil des gleichen Condylus bei Lastrichtung von hinten nach vorn 99,1 kg · cm^{-2}. KNESE (1958b) sieht infolgedessen die Spongiosa als ein Material mit drei Elastizitätsachsen an. Die Spannungs-Dehnungsschaubilder zeigen zunächst einen Verfestigungs-, dann einen Proportionalitätsbereich, der bei longitudinalem Druck 90 %, bei transversalem 45,7 % und von hinten nach vorn 85,8 % der Bruchlast umfaßt. Der Spannungsbereich st dann 49,2, 22,8 und 60,5 % der Bruchspannung und der zugehörige Elastizitätsmodul

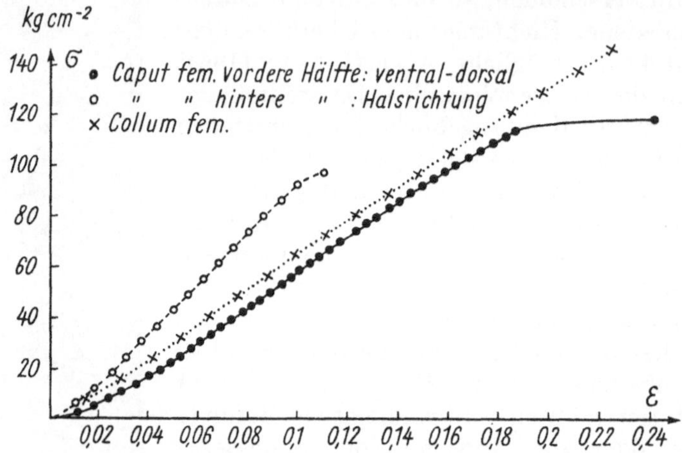

Abb. 28. Spannungs-Dehnungsschaubild für die Spongiosa des Femurkopfes und -halses eines Mannes von 70 Jahren (aus KNESE, 1958b)

623, 518 und 1565 kg · cm^{-2}. Weiterhin vermutet KNESE (1958b), daß bei angebeugtem Kniegelenk, d.h. Lastrichtung von hinten nach vorn — wie sich in einer Untersuchung der Statik des Kniegelenkes (KNESE, 1955a) ergab — die Condylen am stärksten belastet werden.

Der Femurkopf des gleichen Mannes wurde von KNESE (1958b) frontal geteilt, die vordere Hälfte von ventral nach dorsal und die hintere in Halsrichtung gepreßt (Abb. 28). Die radiäre Ordnung der Spongiosa gestattet nur bei sehr kleinen Proben eine genaue Einstellung der Last in einer bestimmten Richtung zum Plattenverlauf. Bei Druck von ventral nach dorsal war die Festigkeit des Kopfes 116,5 und der Elastizitätsmodul im Proportionalitätsbereich 580, in Halsrichtung 96,3 und 887 kg · cm^{-2}. Die Druckfestigkeit des Femurkopfes zeigt demzufolge im Vergleich mit den Femurkondylen bei Belastung in verschiedener Richtung geringere Differenzen.

Die regionalen Unterschiede der Spongiosa hat EVANS (1961) an fixiertem Material (Präpariersaal) untersucht und die Ergebnisse statistisch geprüft (Tabelle 13, 14). Die Proben entstammten den Femora von 11 Leichen (9 ♂, 2 ♀) und zwar 91 Prismen und 16 Würfel. Die Dichte der Spongiosa wurde mit einem Sr90-Dichtemesser nach EVANS, COOLBAUGH und LEBOW (1951) bestimmt. Die Proben wurden auch in unterschiedlicher Richtung belastet. Die Prismen entstammten dem Femurkopf (Längsachse anterior-posterior bzw. cranial-caudal), Hals (Halslängsachse), Trochanter major (lateral-medial), Condylus lateralis (lateral-medial) und Condylus medialis (cranial-caudal). Die Würfelfestigkeit ist bei anterior-posterior und lateral-medialer Belastung größer als die Prismenfestigkeit; damit liegt bei der Spongiosa ein ähnliches Verhältnis zwischen Würfel- und Prismenfestigkeit wie bei anderen Stoffen, auch der Compacta (s. S. 426) vor.

Die höchste Festigkeit hat nach EVANS (1961) die Halsspongiosa, 49,1 kg · cm^{-2}; es folgen Caput femoris, Condylus lateralis, Condylus medialis und mit dem geringsten Wert — 6,8 kg · cm^{-2} — der Trochanter major. Bei dem Elastizitätsmodul läßt sich die Reihe bilden: Trochanter major — 4090 kg · cm^{-2} — Collum femoris, Caput femoris, Condylus lateralis und schließlich Condylus medialis — 2110 kg · cm^{-2}. Bei der Dichte folgen sich Collum femoris, Caput femoris, Condylus medialis, Condylus lateralis und Trochanter major. Die Reihenfolge der untersuchten Spongiosaproben bei den drei physikalischen Eigenschaften ist demzufolge nicht ganz gleich. Die höchste Druckfestigkeit des Halses ist von der des Trochanter signifikant verschieden, die Energieabsorption (siehe S. 476) des Femurkopfes und medialen Condylus ist ebenfalls signifikant different.

Ein Vergleich der Mittelwerte für die einzelnen Individuen nach Alter, Geschlecht, Rasse zeigt keine deutlichen Unterschiede. Werden dagegen die Individuen von 45—70 und 71—88 Jahren zusammengefaßt, so sind Differenzen wahrscheinlich: σ_d: 38,2/18,9; E_d: 3310/1775; ϱ: 0,770/0,576).

Die Stoß- und Schwingfestigkeit der Spongiosa wurde von GOECKE (1925, vgl. Wirbelsäule S. 509) untersucht. GOECKE hat 10mal im Abstand von $^1/_4$ min auf Th 11 eines 51jährigen Mannes eine Stoßlast von 1,217 kgm einwirken lassen. Die Elastizität hat im folgenden Druckversuch abgenommen, die Bruchlast wird nicht verringert. Bei drei Schlägen von 3,04 kgm auf L 1 nimmt der Wirbel von 30 auf 27 mm an Höhe ab, die oberflächlichen Schichten werden gestaucht und gehärtet. Auf dem Längsschnitt durch den Wirbel findet man eine oberste Zone von Gewebetrümmern, dann eine Zone geknickter und ineinander geschobener Bälkchen und schließlich unveränderte Spongiosa. Ein Schlag von 6,085 kgm auf L 2 ergibt eine Verkürzung von 3,5 mm. Ein anschließender Druckversuch zeigt zunächst eine starke Dehnung, dann von 200 kg an eine Proportionalität zwischen σ und ε; die Tragfähigkeit beträgt 650 kg. GOECKE führt zum Vergleich das Verhalten von Holz an.

Tabelle 13. *Festigkeit der fixierten feuchten Spongiosaprismen* (Auszug aus Tabelle 2 von EVANS, 1961)

	σ_d (kg · cm^{-2})	E_d (kg · cm^{-2})	ϱ (g/cm^3)
Caput femoris	38,3	2930	0,748
Collum femoris	49,1	3940	0,822
Trochanter major	6,8	4090	0,590
Condylus lateralis	25,5	2880	0,658
Condylus medialis	23,4	2110	0,663

Tabelle enthält nur die Mittelwerte: σ_d Druckfestigkeit, E_d Elastizitätsmodul, ϱ Dichte.

Tabelle 14. *Festigkeit der fixierten feuchten Spongiosa bei Belastung in verschiedener Richtung* (Auszug aus Tabelle 3 von EVANS, 1961)

		σ_d (kg · cm^{-2})	E_d (kg · cm^{-2})	ϱ (g/cm^3)
Cranio-caudal	P	28,3	2500	0,682
	W	21,7	1280	0,472
Anterior-posterior	P	22,9	2140	0,672
	W	43,8	1720	0,669
Lateral-medial	P	42,2	6260	1,000
	W	118,5	4670	1,000
Halsachse	P	44,1	3940	0,822

Tabelle enthält nur die Mittelwerte: σ_d Druckfestigkeit, E_d Elastizitätsmodul, ϱ Dichte, P Prismen, W Würfel.

GOECKE (1925) hat Wirbel geteilt, die eine Hälfte zuerst auf Schwingbelastung und anschließend auf Druck, die andere zur Kontrolle nur einem Druck unterworfen. Die Schläge erfolgten zu 85—100 je Minute. 1000 Schläge verändern die Tragfähigkeit kaum, bei 2000 bildet sich eine oberflächliche Trümmerzone. Im folgenden Druckversuch tritt anfangs eine starke Dehnung auf, die Tragfähigkeit hat um 10% abgenommen. 4000 Schläge in 40 min vermindern die gesamte Elastizität des Wirbels, die Bruchlast sinkt um 100 kg, d.h. von 400 auf 300 kg.

β) *Die Materialstruktur der Spongiosa*

Experimentelle Untersuchungen haben ergeben, daß die Festigkeit der Spongiosa wesentlich geringer als die der Compacta ist. Die regionalen Differenzen der Festigkeit sind beträchtlich. Die Spongiosa ist wie die Compacta ein anisotropes und inhomogenes

Material, das bei Belastung in verschiedener Richtung auch eine unterschiedliche Festigkeit aufweist.

Seit Culmann (1866) und v. Meyer (1867, 1873) ist das obere Femurende zum „Tummelplatz mechanischer und orthopädischer Überlegungen“ (v. Bayer, 1924) geworden. Die Diskussion, ob die Spongiosa eine sog. trajektorielle Struktur besitzt (unter anderem v. Meyer, 1867; Wolff, 1869; Roux, 1895; Gebhardt, 1910a; Rhumbler, 1914; Fick, 1941; Pauwels, 1948, 1954, 1955; Kummer, 1956a, 1956b, 1959a, 1959b, 1962) oder nicht (unter anderem Mohr, 1885; Wolff, 1891; Triepel, 1903, 1904, 1908, 1922; Garden, 1961), ist bekannt. Die Kritik hat Triepel (1922) in einer Reihe (22!) von Argumenten zusammengefaßt; ihm folgen Murray (1936) und Janssen (1920). Ein Diskussionspunkt war, ob die Spongiosa auch Zugbeanspruchungen ausgesetzt ist oder nur Druck übertrage (v. Meyer, 1867; Bähr, 1898; Sudek, 1899; Hagen, 1908, 1909; Farkas et al., 1948; Garden, 1961). v. Meyer (1873) stellte schließlich fest, daß sich Spongiosa jeweils dort befindet, wo ein Skeletstück mit einer verminderten Tragfähigkeit einen größeren Umfang verbindet, wie z.B. an den Gelenkenden (Aeby, 1873; Knese, 1956a). Die Hauptschwierigkeit der rein trajektoriellen Deutung ist die Tatsache, daß ein System von Hauptspannungslinien nur für einen ganz bestimmten Belastungsfall gilt (Zeiger, 1933; Wyss, 1948), die Belastung aber sehr wechselnd ist (Knese, 1955a, 1956a, 1958b, 1959b; Garden, 1961). Zeiger (1932) führt aus: „So begnügte man sich bei der Erforschung der Spongiosastrukturen, ohne Rücksicht auf die Grundbegriffe der technischen Mechanik, mit der freien Deutung irgendwelcher anatomischer Einzelheiten. Der konstruktiven Verbundenheit aller Teile des Systems hat man kaum Beachtung geschenkt. Mitunter konnte sogar der anatomische Befund als solcher, infolge der mangelhaften Methodik, die zu seiner Ermittlung angewandt wurde, von Nachuntersuchern nicht bestätigt werden.“ Die Möglichkeit einer Belastung der Spongiosa in einer von der Hauptbelastung abweichenden Richtung wurde ebenfalls in Betracht gezogen (Culmann, 1866, v. Meyer, 1867; Wolff, 1870; Ritter, 1888; Triepel, 1908, 1922a, b).

Tabelle 15. *Volumen, Gewicht und Porenvolumen der Wirbelsäule* (nach Wetzel, 1910; sechs Individuen)

	V(cm³)	G(g)	PV
Halswirbel	10,4	8,4	59,5
	(7,6—11,8)	(5,1—11,6)	(48,7—71,3)
Brustwirbel	25,1	13,8	73,7
	(17,8—30,0)	(8,0—18,7)	(68,5—79,6)
Lendenwirbel	45,6	26,3	71,9
	(37,7—52,4)	(14,4—31,7)	(67,4—80,5)
	172,4	89,0	75,6
	(137,5—214,0)	(43,2—129,7)	(67,0—83,4)

Mittelwerte (Minimal- und Maximalwert): V Volumen, G Gewicht, PV Porenvolumen in % des Knochenvolumens.

Von Knese (1958b) und Evans (1961) wurde die Spongiosa nicht mehr für sich allein betrachtet, sondern im Zusammenhang und im Zusammenwirken mit dem Knochenmark; für die Berechtigung dieser Auffassung lassen sich weitere experimentelle Befunde anführen. Die Spongiosamaschen enthalten eine große Menge Knochenmark. Der Volumenanteil des Knochenmarkes ist nach Skeletstück und Lebensalter verschieden. Friedrich (1890) hat das „Porenvolumen“ der marcerierten Knochen eines 25jährigen und eines 82jährigen Mannes durch Wägung gemessen (s. S. 458). Wetzel (1910a, 1910b) hat das Gewicht und Volumen von Wirbeln an Europäern, Australiern, Negern und einem Orang bestimmt. Zur Volumenmessung durch Wasserverdrängung wurden die Knochen mit einer 8%igen Gelatinelösung durchtränkt. Aus Volumen und Gewicht hat Wetzel das Porenvolumen errechnet.

Von den Befunden Wetzels (1910b) geben wir nur die Werte für den Europäer wieder (Tabelle 15). Das Volumen und Gewicht nimmt von den Hals- zu den Lendenwirbeln zu. Das größte Hohlraumvolumen hat das Sacrum (75,6%), es folgen Brustwirbel (73,7%), Lendenwirbel (71,9%) und zum Schluß wegen des kleinen Wirbelkörpers und der großen Fortsätze die Halswirbel (59,5%). Da Wetzel die Bestimmung für den ganzen Wirbel vorgenommen hat, sind die Werte für die „tragenden“ Wirbelkörper nur bedingt zu verwerten. Das Hohlraumvolumen der Wirbelsäule beträgt beim Neugeborenen nach TÖPPICH (1914) 60,87%.

Aus den Werten von FRIEDRICH (1890) hat WETZEL (1910b) nach seiner Methode das Hohlraumvolumen auch für die kurzen Knochen des 25jährigen und 82jährigen Mannes errechnet (Tabelle 16). FRIEDRICH hatte bereits ermittelt, wievielmal größer das Hohlraumvolumen des Greises gegenüber dem des jungen Mannes ist. An der unteren Extremität hat das kleinste Porenvolumen die Patella (25 Jahre: 37,99; 82 Jahre: 67,42), das größte das Cuboid (25 Jahre: 68,49; 82 Jahre: 84,59), an der oberen das größte beim 25jährigen das Pisiforme (68,20), beim 82jährigen das Capitatum (74,52). POLICARD und

Tabelle 16. *Hohlraum- und Knochenvolumen spongiöser Skeletstücke*

	Neonatus[1]	Hohlraumvolumen			Knochenvolumen[4]		
		25 Jahre[2] ♂	82 Jahre ♂	VF[3]	♀ 16	♀ 20	♂ 21
Os coxae	57,84	53,31	77,64	3,04		41	32
Patella		37,99	67,42	3,4		29	29
Calcaneus		65,46	81,69	2,4	27	26	21
Talus		58,42	75,82	2,25	31	29	28
Naviculare		60,06	71,79	2,2			
Cuboideum		68,49	84,59	2,6			
Cuneiforme I		59,83	97,92	2,5			
II		53,46	75,73	2,9			
III		61,44	81,59	2,85			
Scapula	65,16	42,09	58,63	1,97	45	59/57[5]	45
Naviculare		58,07	71,02	1,8			
Lunatum		55,06	71,02	2,0			
Triquetrum		58,82	72,28	2,02			
Trapezium (Multangulum majus)		66,67	73,72	1,48			
Trapezoideum (Multangulum minus)		55,39	73,04	2,18			
Capitatum		63,42	74,52	1,7			
Hamatum		63,18	72,57	1,56			
Pisiforme		68,20	74,09	2,0			

[1] TÖPPICH (1914).
[2] FRIEDRICH (1890) in der Umrechnung von WETZEL (1910).
[3] VF: Vergrößerung des Hohlraumvolumens vom 25- zum 82jährigen nach FRIEDRICH (1890).
[4] DAVIDA (1926).
[5] Rechts-links.

ROCHE (1937) geben für den Calcaneus den Markanteil mit 80% an; diesen Wert erreic h nach FRIEDRICH der 82jährige mit 81,69%, beim 25jährigen sind es nur 65,46%. Die Vergrößerung des Porenvolumens vom jungen Manne zum Greise ist am größten an der Patella (3,4) und Trapezoideum (Multangulum minus) (2,18), am Naviculare pedis (2,2) und Trapezium (Multangulum majus) (1,48) am geringsten.

BURKHARDT (1954) und DERLATH (1958) haben eine Abnahme des spezifischen Gewichtes der Wirbelkörper (Th 12) von 1,20 in den Jahren 16—40 auf 1,14 bei über 70jährigen nachgewiesen. Das spezifische Gewicht ist bei Frauen zunächst höher als bei Männern, sinkt in der Menopause stärker und erreicht dann niedrigere Werte als bei den Männern. Die Abnahme des spezifischen Gewichtes der Schädelcalotte mit dem Lebensalter ist geringer. Wirbel mit hohem spezifischen Gewicht haben relativ dicke Spongiosabälkchen (♂ 0,222, ♀ 0,206 mm), bei mittlerem (♂ 0,184, ♀ 0,169 mm) und niedrigem spezifischen Gewicht (♂ 0,172, ♀ 0,162 mm) nimmt auch die Bälkchendicke ab. Die Stärke der Bälkchen vermindert sich mit dem Lebensalter bei Männern von 0,205 auf 0,176 mm und bei Frauen von 0,201 auf 0,167 mm, und zwar erfolgt die Abnahme bei

Frauen früher (41—60 Jahre) als bei Männern (61—80 Jahre). Mit der Veränderung der Bälkchenstärke und des spezifischen Gewichtes wechselt auch der Bälkchenabstand. Eingefügt sei der Vergleich zwischen der Zusammensetzung von spongiösen und kompakten Knochen von GONG, ARNOLD und COHN (1964). Dichte und Aschegehalt des kompakten Knochens ist höher als der des spongiösen, das Verhältnis Wasser und Asche zur organischen Substanz ist dagegen bei spongiösem Knochen höher.

Nach den mitgeteilten Befunden muß man ein spongiöses Skeletstück als einen mit Flüssigkeit gefüllten Schwamm betrachten. Die Menge der „Flüssigkeit" kann wohl nur in geringem Umfange über das Gefäßsystem geändert werden. Im Hinblick auf die Tragfähigkeit ist neben dem Knochenvolumen noch die konstruktive Verteilung der Spongiosa zu berücksichtigen, da deren Elemente in den drei Raumrichtungen von verschiedener Stärke sind.

Die Bedeutung des Knochenmarkes für die Mechanik der Spongiosa läßt sich durch den Vergleich der Festigkeit frischer und fixierter Proben darstellen. Eine Zusammenstellung der Werte von RAUBER (1876), MESSERER (1880), LANGE (1902), GOECKE (1928) und KNESE (1956a) zeigt (Tabelle 17), daß die Druckfestigkeit frischer Spongiosa etwa doppelt so groß ist wie die der fixierten (Tabelle 13, 14; nach EVANS, 1961). Nur der Wert der Halsspongiosa von KNESE (1956a) beträgt die Hälfte von dem, den EVANS (1961) angibt. Nach GOECKE (1926, 1928) ist die Dehnung der Spongiosa 10—20%; KNESE (1958b) bestimmte den Elastizitätsmodul der frischen Spongiosa zu 580—1565 kg · cm^{-2}.

Tabelle 17.
Druckfestigkeit frischer Spongiosa (kg · cm^{-2})

RAUBER (1876)	Lendenwirbel	83,75
	Femurcondylen	96,25
MESSERER (1880)	Wirbel	60,0
	Brustwirbel	63,5
	Lendenwirbel	56,3
LANGE (1902)	Wirbel	32—36
GÖCKE (1928)	Wirbel	57—70
	Femurcondylen	82
KNESE (1956a)	Femurkopf	93,0
	Femurcondylen	48,5
	Halsspongiosa	28,85
	Femurhals mit Compacta	137

Dieser Elastizitätsmodul ist nur halb so groß wie jener der fixierten Spongiosa (EVANS, 1961: 2110—4090 kg · cm^{-2}). Man kann wohl annehmen, daß die Spongiosaplatten und -bälkchen bei der Fixierung eine gleichsinnige Veränderung wie die Compacta erleiden. Bei dem kompakten Knochen nimmt durch Fixierung der Elastizitätsmodul ab (s. S. 445), die Druckfestigkeit der Compacta wird herabgesetzt. Die Druckfestigkeit der Spongiosa ist nach Fixierung ebenfalls kleiner, aber der Elastizitätsmodul erhöht. Hierfür könnte die Zustandsänderung des Knochenmarkes verantwortlich sein (s. unten).

Die Untersuchungen der Spongiosafestigkeit bei Belastung in verschiedener Richtung veranlaßten KNESE (1958b) einen Verbund zwischen der Knochensubstanz und dem Knochenmark anzunehmen. Bei einem Verbundbau wird zunächst unter Voraussetzung eines homogenen Zustandes der „scheinbare" Spannungszustand bestimmt und danach die Bewehrung angelegt; die späterhin tatsächlich auftretenden Spannungen weichen von diesen postulierten Spannungen aber ab. KNESE (1956a, 1958b) sprach in Anlehnung an die übliche Bezeichnung „scheinbare Spannungen" von einer „quasitrajektoriellen" Struktur der Spongiosa. Die Annahme eines Verbundbaues für die Spongiosa würde auch gut mit den häufig diskutierten Abweichungen der Spongiosa von einem genauen Trajektorien-Bilde vereinbar sein. Bei der Bewehrung ist aus Materialgründen ein derartiges Abweichen von dem Spannungsbild stets notwendig. So zeigen z.B. die Spongiosaplatten beim Ansatz der bälkchenförmigen Querstützen leicht Abknickungen. Die Querstützen haben einen verbreiterten Fuß. Eine Verbundkonstruktion der Spongiosa läßt die auch experimentell nachgewiesene Belastung in Richtungen zu, die dem „Trajektorien"-Verlauf nicht entsprechen.

Das Zusammenspiel der Spongiosa mit dem Knochenmark hat EVANS (1961) in der Aufgabe gesehen, Energie zu absorbieren. Der Verfasser bezieht sich auf ältere Ausführungen (EVANS, PEDERSEN und LISSNER, 1951; GURDJIAN, WEBSTER und LISSNER,

1949) über die Möglichkeit der Energieaufnahme durch Weichgewebe (s. S. 478), Schleimbeutel, Gelenkschmiere, den Trochanter major mit der Hülle aus Corticalis und einem Innern aus Spongiosa. Nunmehr sieht Evans (1961) die Spongiosa des lebenden Knochens als ein „quasihydrostatisches" System an, das Stoßenergie aufnimmt (man denke an den berühmten „Schlag ins Wasser"); ein Fall auf den Trochanter major führt wohl zu einer Collum-Fraktur, aber der Trochanter bleibt unverletzt. Die Tragfähigkeit von Talus und Calcaneus beruht nach Evans (1962) auf dem hohen Gehalt (80%) an Knochenmark.

Die Ausführungen von Knese (1958b) und Evans (1961) geben Veranlassung dazu, die Mechanik von Flüssigkeiten und deformierbaren Körpern miteinander zu vergleichen. Zur Überführung eines elastischen Körpers aus dem nicht deformierten Zustand in einen deformierten wird Arbeit benötigt. Die Arbeit ist in dem deformierten Körper als potentielle Energie enthalten. Bei Rückkehr in den ursprünglichen Zustand wird diese potentielle Energie wieder als Arbeit oder kinetische Energie einer Bewegung frei. Ein fester elastischer Körper setzt demzufolge einer Formänderung einen großen Widerstand entgegen, eine Flüssigkeit aber nicht. Dieser Unterschied läßt sich über die Laméschen Elastizitätskonstanten beschreiben, die den Elastizitätsmodul E und die Poissonsche Zahl m ersetzen:

$$\mu = \frac{E}{2(1\,m)}\,; \quad \lambda = \frac{E\,m}{(1-2\,m)\,(1+m)}\,.$$

Bei einer „idealen" Flüssigkeit wird $\mu = 0$. Im Falle des Gleichgewichtes (Hydrostatik) sind die drei Normalspannungen (s. S. 479) gleich groß und stehen auf jedem beliebigen Flächenelement senkrecht; es sind Druckspannungen (hydrostatischer Druck), Schubspannungen fehlen. Einer Volumenänderung setzt eine Flüssigkeit einen großen Widerstand entgegen. Im Zustand der Bewegung (Hydrodynamik) ist noch ein Widerstand gegen Formänderung zu beachten, der als innere Reibung, Zähigkeit oder Viscosität bezeichnet wird. Diese Viscosität wird nicht durch einen Deformationstensor (s. S. 479), sondern als ein Tensor der Deformationsgeschwindigkeit wiedergegeben.

Neben einer Stoßdämpfung durch das Knochenmark — ähnlich wie durch den Liquor cerebrospinalis oder die Amnionflüssigkeit — sind weitere Mechanismen in der Zusammenarbeit Spongiosa—Knochenmark zu erwägen: Das Knochenmark wirkt wie eine Flüssigkeitsbremse durch geringe Verschiebungen in dem engen Maschengitter der Spongiosaräume. Bei Verformung der Spongiosawaben entsteht ein Kompressionswiderstand, da das Knochenmark inkompressibel ist. Schließlich kann ein Anprall des Markes an eine Knochenlamelle mit allen Folgeerscheinungen eines „Stoßes" — Rückstoß usw. — auftreten. Das Knochenmark ist damit nicht nur ein zufälliger Bewohner eines freien Raumes, sondern hat Aufgaben im Hinblick auf die Tragfähigkeit des Skeletorganes zu erfüllen. Wenn durch Fixierung das flüssig-ölige Knochenmark in einen „festeren" Zustand überführt wird, muß der Elastizitätsmodul der Spongiosa ansteigen, während die Druckfestigkeit abnimmt.

Die experimentell ermittelten Eigenschaften frischer und fixierter Spongiosa bestätigen demzufolge die Vermutung, daß ein Verbund zwischen Spongiosaplatten und -bälkchen und dem Knochenmark vorliegt. Knese (1958b) hat darauf hingewiesen, daß ein ähnlicher Verbund in den Sohlen- und Ballenpolstern, aber auch in der Wand der Eingeweide und Gefäße vorhanden ist. In vielen Organen tritt an die Stelle der Kollagenfaser die glatte Muskelfaser. Die Organwände bilden auch eine Grenze zwischen Gebieten verschiedenen Druckes, z.B. Darm oder Uterus und Bauchhöhle oder Aorta und Thorax, wobei eine transmurale Druckdifferenz vorliegt (Attinger, 1961; Knese, 1963b).

Neuere Daten über die Bedeutung der Markfüllung für die Mechanik der Spongiosa sind den Untersuchungen von Huelke, Buege und Harger (1967) zu entnehmen. Die Autoren haben experimentell die Auswirkung eines Schusses, imitiert mit einem Bolzen, an 122 Femora geprüft. Bei einer Geschwindigkeit zwischen 427 und 509 $m \cdot sec^{-1}$ kommt es zu einer Explosion des distalen Femuranteiles und einer Kavitation mit Zerstörung der Corticalis. Fixierung des Knochenmarkes bringt keine Veränderungen, jedoch wird der Effekt der Kavitation bei Eintrocknung geringer. An getrockneten und entfetteten Femora entsteht mit der gleichen Stoßgeschwindigkeit eine Lochfraktur, wie sie sonst bei Femora mit Markfüllung nur bei einer Geschwindigkeit unter 244 $m \cdot sec^{-1}$ auftritt. Bei den getrockneten Femora fehlt das Gewebe oder die Flüssigkeit, die radial auseinander gesprengt werden kann. CALLENDER und FRENCH (1935) haben gezeigt, daß der Umfang einer Zerstörung bei identischen Geschossen von der Dichte des Gewebes und der Geschwindigkeit des Projektils abhängt. In einem Flüssigkeitssystem wie den Weichgeweben steigt der Widerstand gegen die Durchdringung mit der Stoßgeschwindigkeit. Bei genügender Höhe der Stoßgeschwindigkeit erreicht der Widerstand weniger dichter Gewebe dann jenen der dichten Gewebe bei einer geringeren Stoßgeschwindigkeit. So können bei hoher Geschwindigkeit des Projektils Eingeweide, Blutgefäße und Muskeln explodieren. Ähnlich müsse sich das Knochenmark bei hoher Projektilgeschwindigkeit verhalten. Auf die mechanischen Verhältnisse bei Verletzung innerer Organe sind EVANS und PATRICK (ohne Jahr) eingegangen. Die Untersuchungen von HUELKE et al. (1967) über die Spongiosa unter den besonderen Verhältnissen des Stoßes mit hoher Geschwindigkeit bestätigen wohl die Auffassung, daß eine materialgerechte Betrachtung der Spongiosa nur bei Berücksichtigung der Markfüllung möglich ist. Diese Interpretation wird durch das Verhalten kompakter Knochen unter entsprechenden experimentellen Bedingungen bestätigt (HUELKE, HARGER, BUEGE und DINGMAN, 1968).

2. Mechanik der Skeletelemente

In diesem Abschnitt soll die Statik oder Mechanik der Skeletelemente abgehandelt werden. Als Statik der Skeletstücke ist — wie in der Technik — die konstruktive Form der einzelnen Bauelemente anzusehen (Literatur S. 418) oder — wie in der Biologie auch gesagt wird — die funktionelle Gestalt. Der Begriff der funktionellen Struktur ist heute sicher weiter zu fassen, da unter anderem auch die Struktur im Hinblick auf die Aufgaben des Knochens als Ionenpol zu diskutieren ist; wir sprechen infolgedessen in bezug auf die mechanischen Verhältnisse von „Statik“. Die Statik des Skeletes betrifft die Compacta-Spongiosa-Verteilung, d.h. die Struktur 1. Ordnung.

In dem voraufgegangenen Abschnitt über die Materialstruktur der Compacta wurde ausgeführt, daß für jede Ordnung der Knochenstruktur ein eigenes Bauprinzip anzunehmen sein dürfte. Die in der Literatur mitgeteilten Untersuchungen lassen nicht immer erkennen, ob Ziel der Untersuchungen die Statik des Skeletes oder der Aufbau des Knochenmaterials ist (vgl. KNESE, 1958b). Die Grenze zwischen Statik und Materialstruktur ist beim Verbundbau häufig nicht scharf zu ziehen, da die Ordnung des Materials, die Bewehrung, bereits konstruktionsgerecht ausgeführt wird. Beim Knochen konnte jedoch die konstruktionsgerechte Materialordnung bisher noch nicht befriedigend nachgewiesen werden.

Dem Techniker wird im allgemeinen der Auftrag gegeben, eine Konstruktion, z.B. ein Gebäude oder eine Brücke, auszuführen, die eine bestimmte Aufgabe erfüllt. An Hand eines Konstruktionsentwurfes wird das Material ausgewählt. Die einzelnen Bauelemente erhalten dann eine Abmessung nach Form und Größe, die der gewünschten Aufgabe entspricht. Die Durchführung der Konstruktion erfolgt demgemäß in einem sog. „Bemessungsverfahren“. Umgekehrt kann die Frage aufgeworfen werden, zu welcher Leistung eine vorhandene Konstruktion fähig ist. Dann muß ein „Spannungsnachweis“ durchgeführt werden. Der Spannungsnachweis wird auch als ein Verfahren angewandt, das den fertigen Bau einmalig oder fortlaufend dahingehend überprüft, ob die Konstruktion „richtig“ durchgeführt wurde oder ob ein unbemerkter Materialfehler die Gefahr eines Versagens bringt.

In den Skeletelementen liegen fertige Bauteile vor, so daß ein Spannungsnachweis geführt werden muß (KNESE, 1955b, 1956a), um die funktionelle Struktur zu erkennen, an deren Vorhandensein wohl keiner zweifelt. Hierbei sind die auf das Skeletstück einwirkenden „äußeren Kräfte", die Last und die Beanspruchung zu ermitteln. Der Nachweis der funktionellen Struktur im Bereich der 1. Ordnung ist dann gelungen, wenn der Spannungsnachweis zur Bestimmung des Sicherheitsfaktors führt. Im Bemessungsverfahren werden nämlich die Teile nicht so berechnet, daß sie die gewünschte Leistung gerade nur erfüllen, zusätzlich wird ein Sicherheitsbeiwert berücksichtigt. Der Sicherheitsbeiwert ist nach Material und Beanspruchung verschieden groß, bei ruhender Last gegen Verformung 1,1—1,8, bei spröden Werkstoffen gegen Bruch 1,8—3,0 und Knickung 2,5—3,0, bei Wechsellasten gegen einen Dauerbruch 1,8—3,0 und Knickung 3,0—8,0. Für technische Bauten ist der Sicherheitsbeiwert durch Gesetze festgelegt. Der Sicherheitsbeiwert ist notwendig, weil eine Überschreitung der angenommenen Belastung auftreten kann, eventuell „Fehler" im Werkstoff vorliegen, die äußeren Kräfte nicht vollständig und genau zu berücksichtigen sind und mit mittleren Bruchspannungen gerechnet wird.

Für Skeletelemente kann man nach der Art des Materials wohl einen Sicherheitsbeiwert annehmen, der bei 1,8—3,0 liegt, da das Knochengewebe als annähernd sprödes Material anzusehen ist. So müßte eine Untersuchung der Beanspruchung der Skeletelemente im Vergleich zwischen ermittelter Maximalspannung und Festigkeit des Knochengewebes etwa diesen Sicherheitsbeiwert ergeben. Die damit für die Untersuchung der Statik der Skeletelemente vorliegende Aufgabe ist viel schwieriger als zunächst erscheint. Es wurden infolgedessen sehr verschiedene Wege beschritten, um Beanspruchung und Sicherheit nachzuweisen, wobei wir uns hier überwiegend auf jene Angaben beziehen, die „Maß und Zahl" anstreben.

a) Der allgemeine Spannungszustand

Bei den bisherigen Erörterungen bezogen wir uns nur auf die Normalspannungen σ senkrecht zu einer Schnittebene, die bei Zug-Druck- und Biegebeanspruchung auftreten. Bei Untersuchung des gesamten Spannungszustandes eines Körpers sind noch die Tangentialspannungen τ zu berücksichtigen. Der Spannungszustand eines Körpers (Abb. 29) läßt sich — da Spannungen gerichtete Größen sind — durch die Koeffizientenmatrix eines Tensors darstellen, der das sog. Spannungsellipsoid beschreibt. Die früher übliche Bezeichnung Tensor beruhte auf Untersuchung der mit diesen Spannungen verbundenen Dehnungen; heute wird häufig vom Affinor gesprochen:

$$T = \begin{pmatrix} \sigma_x & \tau_{xy} & \tau_{xz} \\ \tau_{yx} & \sigma_y & \tau_{yz} \\ \tau_{zx} & \tau_{zy} & \sigma_z \end{pmatrix}$$

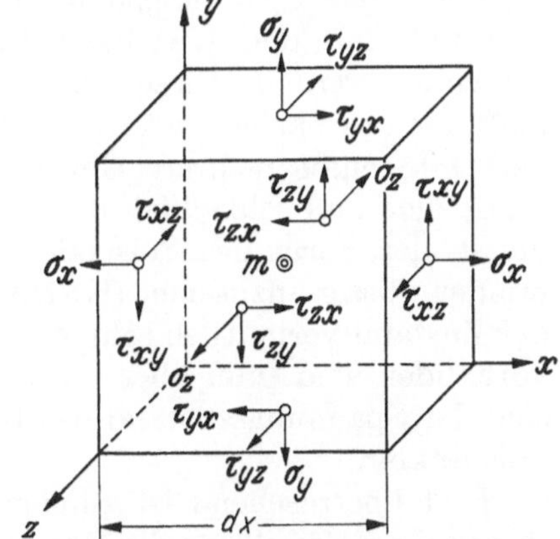

Abb. 29. Spannungskomponenten an einem würfelförmigen Körperelement (vgl. Text)

Bei Untersuchung des Spannungszustandes in einem Punkt sind durch diesen drei Ebenen zu legen, die so gewählt werden können, daß in ihnen nur Normalspannungen auftreten; dann heißen diese Ebenen Hauptebenen. Es gilt dann σ_x (maximal) $> \sigma_y$ (mittlere) $> \sigma_z$ (minimale) Spannung. Diese drei Spannungen legen das Spannungsellipsoid fest. τ_{max} halbiert den Winkel zwischen den Hauptebenen, die zu σ_x und σ_z gehören. Die maximale Tangentialspannung beträgt dann $\tau_{max} = 1/2\ (\sigma_x - \sigma_z)$. Die Ebenen der Hauptnormal- und Haupttangentialspannungen sind um 45^0 gegeneinander geneigt.

Man kann durch einen Körper die Hauptkraftlinien, die Trajektorien, verfolgen bzw. das gesamte Kraftfeld in dem Körper beschreiben. Die Kraftfelder gelten zunächst nur für ein ideal homogenes Material im vollelastischen Bereich. Kraftfelder lassen sich mit rein mathematischen Mitteln leider nur z.T. genau ermitteln (Wyss, 1926, 1948), so daß andere Methoden heranzuziehen sind (s. unten). Abweichungen ergeben sich bei Anisotropie und Inhomogenitäten des im Bau verwandten Materials. Häufig gelingt es der Technik überhaupt nicht, den gesamten Spannungszustand eines Körpers zu ermitteln; dann begnügt man sich mit der Untersuchung einzelner „gefährdeter" Querschnitte. Hierbei wird mit leicht überblickbaren graphischen Methoden gearbeitet, die einen Fehler sofort erkennen lassen.

Ziel statischer Untersuchungen der Skeletelemente war nun auch, diesen allgemeinen Spannungszustand, die trajektorielle Struktur, aufzufinden. Leider wurde für viele dieser Versuche das isolierte Skeletelement, der trockene Sammlungsrückstand (Petersen 1930) des Skeletes gewählt, z.B. der Femur unter dem Einfluß des Körpergewichtes. In Körpern bestehen nicht nur Hauptkraftfelder, sondern auch lokale Felder im Bereich des Angriffes von Kräften, z.B. der Muskeln und Bänder; Beispiele hierfür haben Knese (1958b) und J. W. Smith (1962a, b) gegeben (s. S. 490). Allerdings darf man nach dem Prinzip von St. Venant annehmen, daß sich diese lokalen Felder in der Länge des belasteten Stabes etwa nur auf die Entfernung des Querschnittsdurchmessers ausdehnen (vgl. Knese, 1955b). Weitere Veränderungen eines idealen Kraftfeldes treten durch „Kerben" auf, d.h. Materialunterbrechungen, um die Spannungslinien unter örtlicher Erhöhung der Spannung herumlaufen.

Nach den experimentellen Untersuchungen liegt im Knochengewebe nicht nur eine Anisotropie vor. Darüber hinaus ist die Festigkeit in den einzelnen Abschnitten der Diaphysenröhre, in den „Quadranten" eines Querschnittes und vom Periost zur Markhöhle hin sehr unterschiedlich. Das Knochengewebe ist inhomogen und weist eine große Zahl von Kerben auf, die Haversschen Kanäle. Als Kerben sind wohl auch die Osteocytenhöhlchen anzusehen, die in stark wechselnder Zahl auftreten (Knese und Titschak, 1962). Die Osteocytenhöhlchen besitzen z.T. auch einen Wandaufbau, der von der Struktur der Umgebung abweicht (Knese und v. Harnack, 1962). Alle aufgeführten Befunde lassen daran zweifeln, daß der Gesamtspannungszustand eines Skeletstückes zu ermitteln ist.

Wenn das Spannungsbild für die vorliegende „Form" eines Körpers bestimmt ist, muß mit einer dem jeweiligen Baumaterial gemäßen Veränderung des idealen Zustandes gerechnet werden. Diese Feststellung ist für die Beurteilung der mechanischen Verhältnisse des Skeletes während der Entwicklung von Bedeutung, da das Skelet im Laufe der Ontogenese mehrere Gewebezustände „durchläuft", dem mesenchymalen folgt der knorpelige und schließlich der ossale. Der mesenchymale Zustand ist physikalisch durch die in der Form des Sols oder Gels erscheinende Intercellularsubstanz als mehr oder minder flüssig anzusehen (Knese, 1959a). Mit dem Auftreten von Kollagenfibrillen wird der Zustand vermutlich sehr verwickelt, da z.T. noch die Eigenschaften einer Flüssigkeit vorhanden sind, nun aber mit der Flüssigkeit zugfeste Elemente kombiniert sind. Wie sich der Spannungszustand des Knorpels von dem des Knochens unterscheidet, ist ebenfalls unklar.

Fast überraschend ist zunächst die Feststellung, daß wohl eine Reihe von „idealen Spannungsplänen" für die Spongiosa entwickelt wurden, die mehr oder minder mit dem morphologischen Befund übereinstimmen, eine Aufstellung von Spannungsplänen für die Compacta (Koch, 1917; Benninghoff, 1927; Pauwels, 1950; Evans und Goff, 1957; vgl. jedoch Knief, 1967b) aber nicht gelang. Wenn eine Biegung oder Knickung für Röhrenknochen vorausgesetzt wird (s. S. 499), ist in einem homogenen Körper die bekannte Schar sich kreuzender Druck- und Zugspannungslinien anzunehmen. Für dieses Spannungsbild ist in der Ordnung der Haverschen Systeme kein Korrelat zu finden (Spaltlinien: S. 481).

Für die Spongiosa ist eine konstruktionsgerechte Ordnung des Materials sehr wahrscheinlich. Wenn es nicht gelingt, für die Compacta eine gleichartige Materialordnung nachzuweisen, so kann daraus nur geschlossen werden, daß in der Compacta andere Bauprinzipien vorliegen. Knese et al. (1954) und Pritchard (1956) lehnen das Osteon als morphologische Baueinheit ab. Die Lamellen und Lamellensysteme stellen eine „örtliche Lagerungsform von Kollagenfasern dar" (KNESE et al., 1954), die offensichtlich dem Knochen seine unterschiedlichen Festigkeitseigenschaften verleiht. Gegen die von PETERSEN (1927, 1930) und TISCHENDORF (1954) vertretene Ansicht, die Compacta verhalte sich wie ein homogenes Material, spricht die differenzierte Struktur des Knochengewebes. PETERSEN war der Meinung, die Summe der Unstetigkeiten des Knochens strebe 0 zu. Die Summe der „Unstetigkeiten" ist aber — wie die Untersuchungen der Festigkeit ergeben haben — in den einzelnen Bereichen des Knochens nicht gleich. Die Untersuchungen der Materialstruktur haben wahrscheinlich gemacht, daß die mechanischen Eigenschaften des Knochengewebes nicht nur auf eine Ordnung der Strukturhierarchie, z.B. das Osteon, bezogen werden können. Die einzelnen Ordnungen übernehmen Teilaufgaben im Hinblick auf die mechanische Leistung des Knochengewebes. So ist eine einfache Korrelation zwischen dem „Spannungsgefüge" und der Struktur einer Ordnung nicht zu erwarten, sogar unwahrscheinlich (s. unten).

Zur Bestimmung der nicht berechenbaren Spannungen kann die Dehnung (s. S. 419) gemessen werden. Mit Dehnungsmeßverfahren läßt sich die Spannung aber nur dann bestimmen, wenn die Hauptspannungsrichtungen bekannt sind. Sind die Hauptspannungsrichtungen unbekannt, müssen die Dehnungen an einem Punkte in vier Richtungen gemessen werden oder Dehnungsmeßstreifen für einen mehrachsigen Spannungszustand verwandt werden (HUGGENBERGER und SCHWAIGERER, 1958). Dehnungen haben KÜNTSCHER (1936) und MARIQUE (1945) mit mechanischen Dehnungsmessern (Hebelsysteme) gemessen. Mit Dehnungsmeßstreifen haben dann GURDIJAN und LISSNER (1944) am Schädel und EVANS (1953) und EVANS, COOLBAUGH und LEBOW nach EVANS (1957) an der Tibia des lebenden Hundes gearbeitet. Die Lage der Dehnungsmeßstreifen am Femurkopf (Abb. 30) zur Messung der Dehnungen in verschiedenen Richtungen haben HIRSCH und BRODETTI (1956a) abgebildet (s. S. 497).

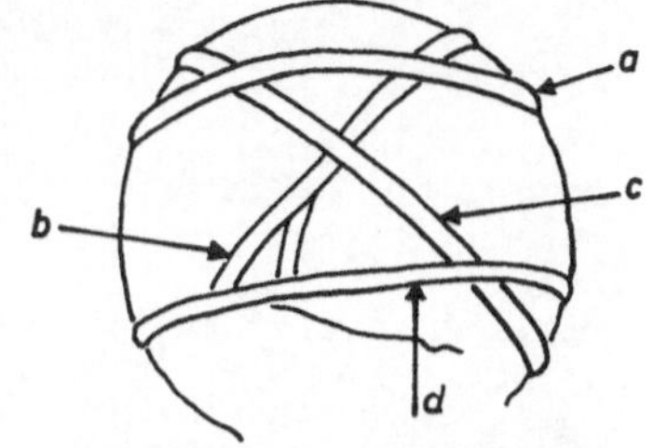

Abb. 30. Femurkopf mit Dehnungsmeßstreifen in den Richtungen *a*, *b*, *c*, *d* zur Messung der Verformung bei verschiedener Lastrichtung. (Umzeichnung nach HIRSCH und BRODETTI, 1956a)

Dehnungsmuster hat bereits ROUX (1895) an Gummimodellen mit Hilfe eines Paraffinüberzuges beobachtet. H. FICK (1941) untersuchte die Dehnungen an Gummimodellen, die dem proximalen Femurende in den einzelnen Entwicklungsstufen nachgebildet waren. Der Spannungsverlauf steht nach FICK stets senkrecht zur Epiphysenscheibe und die Spongiosa ist entsprechend eingestellt. KÜNTSCHER (1935, 1936) hat das Lackrißverfahren von DIETRICH und LEHR (1932) übernommen. Hierbei wird der zu untersuchende Teil mit einem Kollophoniumlack überzogen, der nach dem Trocknen bei Belastung an den Orten der Dehnungen Risse zeigt. Auch Stauchungen können beobachtet werden, und zwar wird der Körper erst belastet, der Lack aufgebracht und getrocknet; bei Entlastung erscheinen Risse durch Verschwinden der Stauchungen. Die „stresscoat" Technik von DE FOREST und ELLIS (1940) verwendet einen leichter zu handhabenden und genauer arbeitenden Aluminiumspray. Diese Methode übernahmen zuerst GURDIJAN und LISSNER (1945) für Untersuchungen am Schädel und EVANS, LISSNER und PEDERSEN (1948) am Femur.

Immer wieder wurde versucht, aus der Struktur auf die Beanspruchung von Skeletteilen zu schließen. Zu diesen Versuchen gehört auch die Untersuchung der Spaltlinien (BENNINGHOFF, 1925, 1927, 1931). Hierbei wird in einen entmineralierten Knochen mit einer Nadel eingestochen, der Stich verzieht sich bei Entfernung der Nadel zu einem Spalt der mit Tusche markiert wird. Diese Methode wurde am Schädel von DOWGJALLO (1932), SEIPEL (1948), TAPPEN (1953, 1957), von PAUWELS (1950/51) am normalen Femur, von MEDNICK (1955) am Ilium angewandt; BENNINGHOFF (1927) und PAUWELS (1950/51) untersuchten rachitisch verkrümmte Knochen. Dieses Verfahren kann natürlich nur über die Struktur der oberflächlichen Schichten Aussagen zulassen, die Struktur der sehr verwickelt gebauten Compacta in ihrer ganzen Breite aber nicht erfassen.

In der Compacta sollen nach Untersuchungen mittels Spaltlinien die „Osteone" überwiegend longitudinal verlaufen (BENNINGHOFF, 1927, 1931). KÜNTSCHER (1935a, b, 1936) glaubte, diesen Befund durch Lackrißuntersuchungen bestätigen zu können und meinte, daß sich die Compacta wie ein homogener Stoff verhalte. Aus den Dehnungen kann aber nur unter bestimmten Voraussetzungen auf die Spannungen geschlossen werden (s. oben; KNESE, 1958b). EVANS und GOFF (1957, vgl. EVANS, 1957) weisen darauf hin, daß das mit dem Lackrißverfahren erhaltene Dehnungsbild keinerlei Aussage über die Zusammensetzung des Materials zulasse. Dieselben Bilder sind bei gleicher Körperform sowohl von Holz, Metall als auch Knochen zu erhalten. Nur die Ausdehnung des Rißbildes (stresscoat) ist nach Material verschieden. Die Spaltlinien wiederum können nach EVANS und GOFF (1957) nicht, wie häufig angenommen wurde, dem Spannungsgefüge entsprechen, das stets sich kreuzende Scharen von Spannungslinien verlangt. Im übrigen könnten für den Knochen, der kein solider und homogener Körper ist, nicht ohne weiteres Trajektoriendiagramme gezeichnet werden; die Technik würde bei einem solchen Material auf diesen Versuch verzichten. EVANS (1965a) weist darauf hin, daß weder die quer zur Spannung liegenden stresscoat-Linien noch die Spaltlinienbilder die Spannungstrajektorien darstellen. Für den Knochen kann ein Trajektoriendiagramm nicht entworfen werden, da es sich um einen dreidimensionalen porösen Körper aus heterogenem anisotropem Material handelt. Die Spaltlinien könnten vielleicht auf die Vascularisation oder auch Wachstumsvorgänge bezogen werden; ihre mechanische Bedeutung ist unklar.

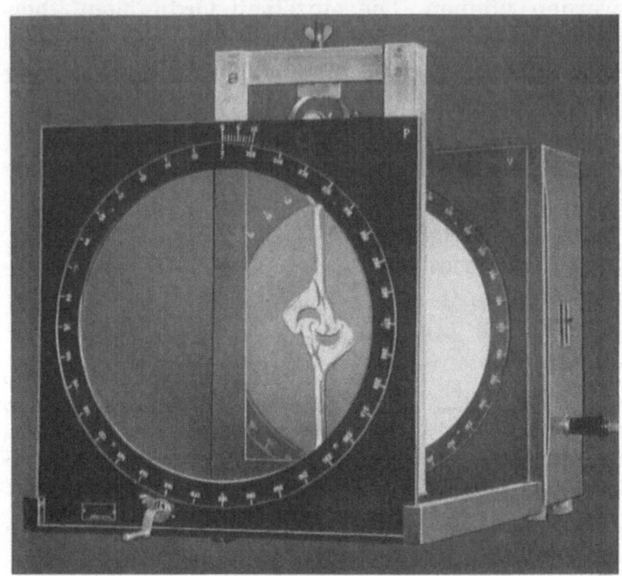

Abb. 31. Vereinfachte Apparatur zur spannungsoptischen Untersuchungen mit großen Folien (aus FÖPPL und MÖNCH, 1958)

Über den Spannungszustand einer Körperform kann auch durch spannungsoptische Modellverfahren Auskunft gewonnen werden (FÖPPL und MÖNCH, 1958; KUMMER, 1956b, 1959b; HEROLD, 1963; KNIEF, 1967a). Diese Modelluntersuchungen lassen die Untersuchung eines ebenen Spannungszustandes auch bei sehr unregelmäßigem Profil zu. Durchsichtige isotrope Materialien verhalten sich unter mechanischer Beanspruchung anisotrop, doppelbrechend. Auf eine Scheibe überall gleicher Dicke von etwa 10 mm läßt man Kräfte in der Ebene der Scheibe einwirken. Das Modell befindet sich zwischen einem Polarisator und einem Analysator (Abb. 31). Bei Verwendung von Polarisationsfolien können die Modelle in ganzer Ausdehnung untersucht werden. An Hand der auftretenden Doppelbrechungen kann der örtliche Spannungszustand bestimmt werden, d.h. aus dem Isoklinenschaubild wird der Verlauf der Spannungen ermittelt. Der Nachteil dieses Verfahrens ist, daß nur Modelle und ebene Spannungszustände erfaßbar sind. Von OPPEL (1936 nach FÖPPL und MÖNCH, 1958) wurde auch ein wenig gebrauchtes Verfahren zur Untersuchung räumlicher Spannungszustände entwickelt. Modelle vernetzter Kunststoffe behalten ihren bei höherer Temperatur eingebrachten Spannungszustand beim Einfrieren bei. Durch Zerschneiden des Modelles werden recht dünne Scheiben gewonnen, aus deren spannungsoptischer Untersuchung das gesamte räumliche Spannungsgefüge rekonstruiert wird. Die Anwendung dieser Methode für den Knochen diskutiert HEROLD (1963).

Zur Aufklärung des Spannungszustandes von Skeletstücken wurden ebenfalls spannungsoptische Modellversuche herangezogen (HALLERMANN, 1934; MILCH, 1940; PAUWELS, 1948, 1951b; KUMMER, 1956, 1959a, b, 1962; FESSLER, 1957; J. W. SMITH, 1962a, b). Die Beschränkung der Spannungsoptik hatte bereits HALLERMANN (1934) erkannt und ausgeführt, daß nur die Beziehung zwischen einem Profil, dem Umriß der untersuchten Platte und der zugehörigen Spannung beobachtet wird. Dieser Kritik haben sich KÜNTSCHER (1935), WYSS (1948), KNESE (1955b, 1956a, 1958b) und EVANS (1957) angeschlossen, vor allem deswegen, weil einige Autoren anatomische Fakten und experimentelle Befunde übergehen und die Grenzen der Aussagemöglichkeiten der Spannungsoptik überschreiten. "All of these models were quite different from a hollow bone of heterogeneous composition and complicated trabecular organization ... Thus, the various photoelastic patterns obtained by HALLERMANN, MILCH, and PAUWELS simply represent the stresses produced by loading solid models composed of homogenous material resembling a bone in outline" (EVANS, 1957). Die vorgetragenen Bedenken versuchten KUMMER (1959, 1962), HEROLD (1963) und KNIEF (1967a) zu zerstreuen. Einige Autoren haben nunmehr den spannungsoptischen Untersuchungen solche über die Knochendichte (KNIEF 1967a, b) und die Dichte und Bruchfestigkeit (SCHMITT, 1968; AMTMANN und SCHMITT, 1968) gegenübergestellt. Als Begründung hierfür wird angegeben, daß sich z.B. die Entscheidung, ob ein Körper gleicher Festigkeit vorliegt oder nicht (s. unten), nur auf quantitative Messungen stützen kann (KNIEF 1967a) bzw. daß bei den Arbeiten von PAUWELS (1948, 1950, 1954) „stillschweigend unterstellt" wurde, das Knochenmaterial besitze innerhalb des untersuchten Skeletstückes dieselben mechanischen Eigenschaften, was aber nicht zutrifft.

b) Die äußeren Kräfte: Die Belastung der Skeletstücke

Bei sehr vielen Untersuchungen der Statik der Skeletelemente wurde als Last nur das Körpergewicht angenommen; dabei ergibt sich ein ungewöhnlich hoher Sicherheitsfaktor. Aus den Werten von MESSERER (1880) hat TRIEPEL (1902) die Beanspruchung der Tibia errechnet. Bei einem Tibiaquerschnitt von 2,91 cm^2 und einer Gewichtslast von 100 kg beträgt die Spannung 34,4 kg · cm^{-2}. Bei einem Elastizitätsmodul von 200000 kg · cm^{-2} ist die Zusammendrückung 0,172%, d.h. bei einer Länge der Tibia von 40 cm etwa 0,069 mm. Wird ein zusätzliches Gewicht von 50 kg angenommen, steigt die Spannung auf 51,5 kg · cm^{-2}, damit würde $^1/_3$ der Druckfestigkeit des Knochens erreicht (vgl. TRIEPEL, 1910): Die Sicherheit des kompakten Knochens bei statischer Belastung sei sehr groß. KOCH (1917) gibt die Sicherheit des Femurs mit 5,68—30,3 an (s. S. 495). Nach DU BOIS-REYMOND (1928) trägt der Mäusefemur nach Bruchgewicht das 57fache, nach Querschnittsgröße sogar das 750fache des Körpergewichtes, der Femur der Ratte das 30- bis 35fache, der des Elefanten das 120fache des Körpergewichtes. SCHMIDT (1915) gibt den Sicherheitsfaktor für das Pferd mit 25,3, Rind 22,9, Schaf 23,6, Schwein 20—25 und den Hirsch 36,5 an, EICKHOFF (1927) für das Laufpferd 18,7 und das Schrittpferd 22,9 (vgl. WETZEL und SCHRÖDER 1925: Schädel, s. S. 517).

Der Sicherheitsbeiwert ist bei alleiniger Berücksichtigung des Körpergewichtes demzufolge sehr groß. KOCH (1917) und MICHEL (1903) meinten, eine beachtliche Auswirkung der Muskelkraft auf das Skelet sei nicht vorhanden. Andere Autoren (RAUBER, 1876; RITTER, 1888; ROUX, 1895; ZSCHOKKE, 1892; GRUNEWALD, 1912, 1916, 1920; KÜNTSCHER, 1935a, b; KREUZER, 1932; KNESE, 1955a, 1956b; KIMURA, 1966) haben dagegen die Bedeutung der Muskelkraft als Last ausführlich erörtert. GRUNEWALD (1920) kommt nach Berechnung der Kraft der Oberschenkelmuskeln an Hand deren Querschnitt (s. unten) zur Feststellung, daß als größte Belastung der Knochen die Muskeln anzusehen sind. PAUWELS (1949/50, 1950, 1951) sieht die Muskeln als Zuggurtungen an, die die Beanspruchung des Skeletes durch das Körpergewicht herabsetzen (vgl. KNESE, 1955b); trifft diese Annahme zu, würde der Sicherheitsfaktor für das Skelet noch größer als bei Berücksichtigung des Körpergewichtes allein sein. Man könnte dann aber nicht mehr von einem Leichtbau der Knochen (PAUWELS, 1948) sprechen.

Bei Berücksichtigung der Muskelkraft als Last der Knochen ist die Richtung und Größe der Kraft zu bestimmen. Die Muskelkraft wird häufig als Spannung bezeichnet. Spannung ist stets Kraft je Flächeneinheit, der Bezug auf eine bestimmte Fläche wird aber nicht angegeben. Man könnte hierbei an den physiologischen Querschnitt denken (s. unten).

Allerdings befällt den Biologen Unbehagen, wenn er bei JOOS (1945) in der „Theoretischen Physik" liest: „Wollen wir den Bewegungszustand eines Körpers, z.B. einer auf einer waagerechten ebenen Platte ruhenden Kugel ändern und bedienen wir uns dazu unserer Muskeln, so bedarf es einer gewissen Anstrengung, die um so größer ist, je größer die Geschwindigkeitsänderung sein soll. Diese Anstrengung, die wir *Kraft* nennen, ist als unmittelbare Sinnesempfindung nicht näher zu definieren. Durch die Richtung, in der wir unsere Muskeln wirken lassen, ist die *Richtung* der Beschleunigung bestimmt, die Kraft ist also eine vektorielle Größe, wie die Beschleunigung . . . zur Hervorrufung derselben Beschleunigung (ist) je nach der Natur des Körpers . . . eine sehr verschiedene Kraft erforderlich . . . Wir müssen also den einzelnen Körpern noch eine skalare Eigenschaft zuschreiben, die wir ihre *träge Masse m* nennen." Damit wird die Kraft definiert als $K = m \cdot b$, Kraft = Masse · Beschleunigung, oder „die Kraft ist gleich der auf die Sekunde bezogenen zeitlichen Änderung der Bewegungsgröße". „Nun sehen wir überall in der Natur Änderung des Bewegungszustands von Körpern, auch ohne daß wir mit unseren Muskeln eingreifen. Ihre Ursache sehen wir in „Kräften", welche in gleicher Weise auf die Körper einwirken, wie in dem erwähnten Beispiel unsere Muskeln . . . In der Mechanik nehmen wir die Kraft als gegeben hin und befassen uns mit der Berechnung der Wirkung". So kann man wohl bei Untersuchung des Urbildes der Kraft, des Muskels, deren Wirkung auf das Skelet nicht außer acht lassen.

Die Kraft eines Muskels ist von der Größe seines physiologischen Querschnittes abhängig, d.h. jenem Querschnitt, der alle Muskelfasern genau quer trifft. Die Ausmessung des physiologischen Querschnittes ist wegen der komplizierten Architektur vieler Muskeln (gefiederte, s. unten) ungewöhnlich schwierig. WEBER (1849) ging von dem Muskelgewicht und einer mittleren Faserlänge aus. An 21 Präpariersaalleichen haben SCHUMACHER und WOLF (1966a, b, c) die Trockengewichte und physiologischen Querschnitte der Muskeln untersucht. Im Hinblick auf das Gewicht kommen sie zu dem Verhältnis Körperstamm:obere Extremität:untere Extremität von 1:1,24:3,13 und im Hinblick auf den Querschnitt von 1:1,35:3,56. FICK und ROSCHDESTWENSKI (1913) preßten Muskeln in eine Meßlehre mit Lücken bekannter Flächengröße, GROHMANN (1902) wog Bleischeiben von der Form des Querschnittes, KRAHL (1947) planimetrierte Muskelabdrücke und LIPPERT (1959) errechnete den Querschnitt aus dem Umfang eines Muskels, wobei ein ellipsenförmiger Querschnitt angenommen wird. Nach SCHWARZ (1962) kann keines dieser Verfahren bei der verwickelten Muskelstruktur befriedigende Ergebnisse erzielen, weil bei Vorliegen einer Fiederung (vgl. KOLB 1937; M. tibialis anterior) nicht alle Muskelfasern erfaßt werden. Eine Reihe von Muskeln weisen sogar eine mehrfache Fiederung auf, z.B. ist der M. soleus 3fach gefiedert (DRÜNER, 1926; FALLER, 1942; UWEDA, 1926; vgl. LOETZKE, 1960). Auch scheinbar parallelfaserige Muskeln wie der M. rectus abdominis (EGGENSCHWILER, 1956; vgl. BERGENTHAL und KELLER, 1959; BERLIS und KELLER, 1959) und der M. sartorius (KANN, 1957) zeigen zugespitzte Übergänge in Endsehnen. Bei dem M. biceps brachii und M. semimembranosus liegt nach FENEIS (1935) eine Fiederung mit sehr kleinem Fiederungswinkel vor und ähnliches gilt für eine große Zahl von Muskeln.

Aus dem physiologischen Querschnitt wird mit Hilfe der „absoluten Muskelkrafteinheit" die maximale Muskelkraft errechnet. Als Muskelkrafteinheit werden sehr unterschiedliche Werte angegeben (SCHWARZ 1962). Im allgemeinen wird nach R. FICK (1910) der Wert von 10 kg/cm² angenommen, obwohl FICK feststellte, daß es sich bei der Berechnung der gesamten Kraft eines Muskels nur um eine ganz ungenaue Schätzung handelt.

Messungen mit Dynamometern (CLARKE et al., 1950; BACKMAN, 1957; PAUWELS, 1954) können nicht die Kraft der Muskeln, sondern nur die „Arbeitsfähigkeit" des aktiven und passiven Bewegungssystemes gemeinsam ermitteln. Im übrigen fallen die Werte je nach Wirkungsrichtung und Anlage der Dynamometer verschieden aus (KNESE, unveröffentlicht).

SCHWARZ hat (1962) versucht, die maximale Muskelkraft aus dem Sehnenquerschnitt zu errechnen, da ja die Sehne die Kraft auf den Knochen übertragen muß. Aus der Festigkeit der Sehne unter Berücksichtigung eines Sicherheitsbeiwertes hat SCHWARZ an 2139 Sehnen von 37 Muskelindividuen die maximale Muskelkraft und deren Variations-

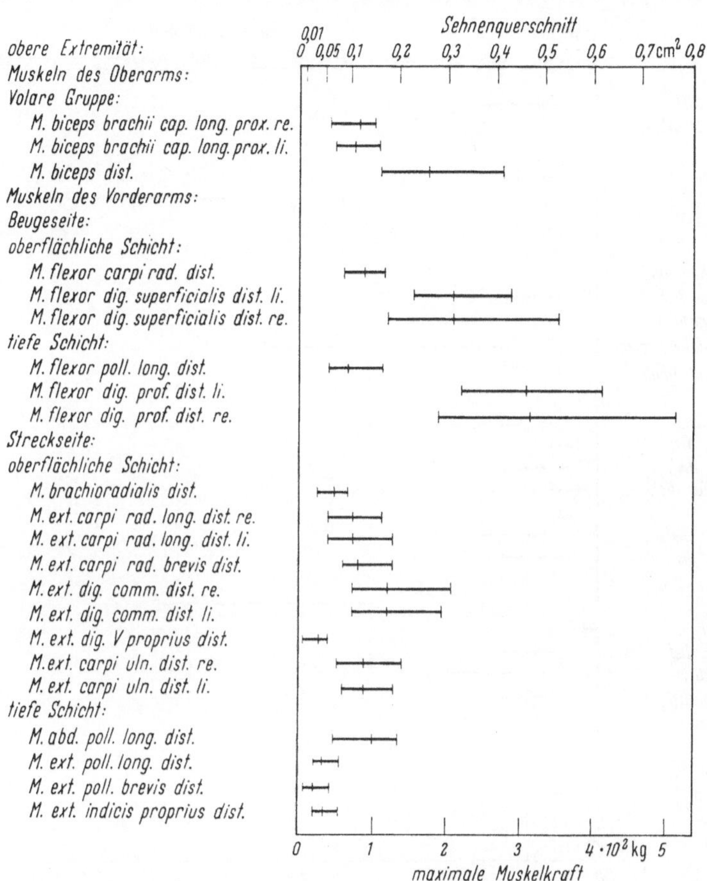

Abb. 32. Maximale Muskelkraft (untere Abszisse) und Sehnenquerschnitt (obere Abszisse) der Muskeln des Armes. Angabe des Zentralwertes (g 50), des unteren (g 5) und oberen (g 95) Grenzwertes der gemessenen Werte, bestimmt im Wahrscheinlichkeitspapier. (Umzeichnung nach SCHWARZ, 1962)

größe berechnet. Die Sehnenfestigkeit zeigt einen Altersgang (ROLLHÄUSER, 1951), für das von SCHWARZ untersuchte Material gilt etwa 1000 kg · cm^{-2}. Da die Sehne nach dem Spannungs-Dehnungs-Schaubild sich wie ein zäher Stoff verhält, kann der Sicherheitsbeiwert zu 1,1—1,8, im Mittel zu 1,5, angesetzt werden. Damit ergibt sich zur Errechnung der Muskelkraft folgender Ansatz:

$$\text{Maximale Muskelkraft} = \frac{\text{Sehnenquerschnitt} \cdot 1000}{1 \cdot 5}.$$

Bei den von SCHWARZ errechneten Werten (Abb. 32, 33) fällt auf, daß vor allem die Kraft der tiefen Unterschenkel- und Unterarmmuskeln bedeutend größer ist als bisher angenommen wurde. Es handelt sich hierbei um Muskeln, die mit einer doppelten Fiederung sehr kurze Muskelfasern unterschiedlicher Länge verbinden, d.h. eine Architektur besitzen, die sich einer direkten Bestimmung des physiologischen Querschnittes entzieht.

Bei Errechnung der Belastung der Skeletstücke kann nicht jeder Muskel mit seiner maximalen Kraft eingesetzt werden. Die Muskeln bilden nach Richtung und Kraft ein Kraftsystem, das eine Bewegung bewirkt oder eine bestimmte Stellung festhält (KNESE, 1955a, 1956e, s. unten). In der Bewegungslehre setzte man bisher voraus, daß ein Muskel nur bei Verkürzung tätig ist. Aus der Verkürzung und der Kraft hat man auch die Arbeitsfähigkeit der Muskeln errechnet (FICK, 1910, 1911). Die Muskelphysiologie (FENN, 1925a, b; REICHEL, 1960) hat aber gezeigt, daß ein Muskel ohne Längenänderung — isometrisch — Kraft entwickeln kann und daß die Kraft bei zunehmender Ausgangslänge größer ist. Diese Beziehung wird in dem Längen-Spannungsdiagramm dargestellt.

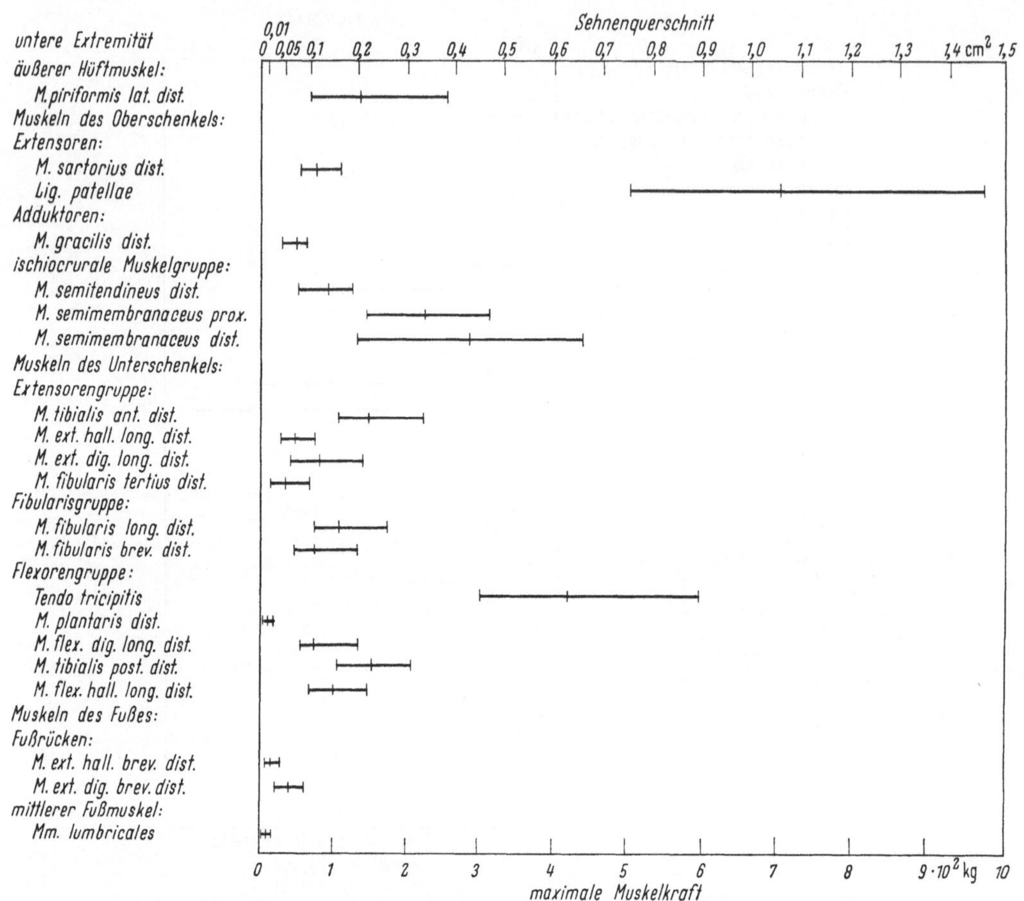

Abb. 33. Maximale Muskelkraft (untere Abszisse) und Sehnenquerschnitt (obere Abszisse) der Muskeln des Beines (vgl. Abb. 32; Umzeichnung nach SCHWARZ, 1962)

Im übrigen hat schon BRAUS (1921) erkannt, daß in der Bewegungslehre Längenänderung und Kraft des Muskels bis zu einem gewissen Grade unabhängig voneinander zu betrachten sind; die Formulierung des Zusammenhanges zwischen beiden ist Aufgabe der Physiologie (KNESE, 1963a).

Zur Untersuchung der Beanspruchung eines Skeletteiles muß jene Kraftkombination aufgesucht werden, die die maximale Belastung darstellt. Das Zusammenwirken der Muskeln und ihre jeweilig aufzubringende Kraft kann vermutlich nur experimentell ermittelt werden. Wenn für eine Stellung oder Bewegung die „jeweilige" Kraft (s. unten) bekannt wäre, könnte man rein rechnerisch nach dem Prinzip der virtuellen Arbeit vorgehen (v. LANZ und HENNIG 1957). Die Muskelkraft kann aber von 0 bis zu einer bestimmten maximalen Größe wechseln. KNESE (1955a) hat infolgedessen die Muskelkräfte, die zur Aufrechterhaltung einer Stellung des Kniegelenkes notwendig sind, durch „Muskelphantome" gemessen. An einem Gelenkpräparat der unteren Extremität wurden die Muskeln durch Drahtzüge ersetzt, in die Federwaagen eingebaut waren. Bei fixiertem

Unterschenkel hatten diese Muskelphantome ein Gewicht am Becken als sog. Körpergewicht in verschiedenen Stellungen zu halten. Richtung, Länge und Kraft der einzelnen Muskeln wurden gemessen; gleichartige Experimente wurden für die Sprunggelenke durchgeführt (KNESE unveröffentlicht, s. S. 506).

In jeder Stellung des Kniegelenkes ergibt sich durch die Lage des Massenmittelpunktes des Körpers zum Kniegelenk ein bestimmtes Kippmoment, das mit zunehmender Beugung wächst. Dem Kippmoment muß ein gleichgroßes Drehmoment der Muskeln entgegenwirken, wenn man eine Stellung halten will, wie im Eigenversuch leicht festzustellen ist. Die arithmetische Summe der am Oberschenkel aufgebrachten Kraft (Abb. 34) steigt in dem untersuchten Bereich von 300 auf 900 kg an (KNESE, 1953/54). Davon entfallen auf den M. quadriceps femoris 225 bzw. 610 kg, d.h. etwa $^2/_3$. Aus dem Querschnitt des

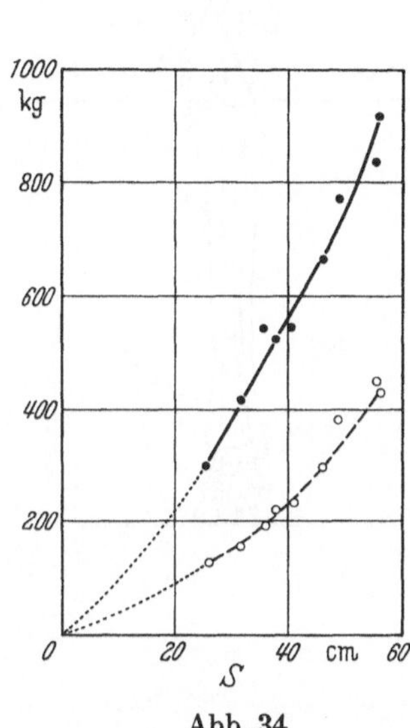

Abb. 34

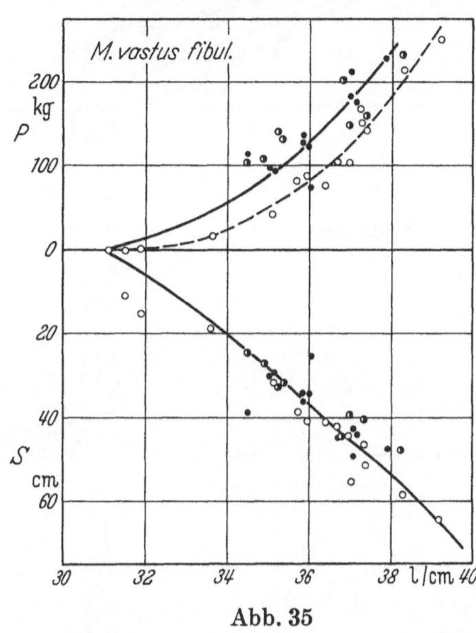

Abb. 35

Abb. 34. Kraft-Wegkurve der Muskelkraft zur Stabilisierung des Kniegelenkes in verschiedenen Beugestellungen. Kraft in Kilogramm; —●— arithmetische Summe; —○— geometrische Summe (aus KNESE, 1953/54)

Abb. 35. M. vastus fibularis: Kraft-Längendiagramme für die Kniebeuge, ermittelt mit Muskelphantomen (vgl. KNESE 1955a). Abszisse: Beugung: Weg (l) in cm; Ordinate nach unten; *s* Länge des Muskels; Ordinate nach oben = *P* Kraft des Muskels. ● Unterschenkel senkrecht; ○ vorgeneigt; ◑ rückgeneigt (KNESE, unveröffentlicht)

Ligamentum patellae hat SCHWARZ (1962) die maximale Muskelkraft des M. quadriceps zu 696,7 kg mit der Variation 497,3—975,3 errechnet; dieser Wert stimmt mit dem am Muskelphantom gemessenen gut überein. Physikalisch ist die geometrische Summe der Kräfte wirksam, sie beträgt anfangs 44, dann 36 und schließlich 53,5% der arithmetischen, d.h. mit zunehmender Beugung des Kniegelenkes wird die Wirkungsweise der Muskeln günstiger.

Rein physikalische Experimente bedürfen einer Bestätigung durch Untersuchungen am Lebenden. KNESE (1953/54) hat mit Hilfe des Elektromyogramms beobachtet, daß bei der Kniebeuge der Tätigkeitsumfang der Muskeln zunimmt und diese Zunahme annähernd der wachsenden Kraft zur Stabilisierung des Kniegelenkes parallel verläuft. Die Größe der Kraft hängt demzufolge von der jeweiligen Stellung des Gelenkes ab, so daß die Kraft als eine Ortsfunktion anzusehen ist (KNESE, 1953/54, 1955a). Während der Kniebeuge nimmt die Länge des M. quadriceps zu und zu jeder Länge gehört ein Kraftwert. Die Weg-Längen-Kraft-Kurve für die Köpfe des M. quadriceps femoris (KNESE, unveröffentlicht) entspricht dem durchhängenden Teil des Längen-Spannungsdiagramms (Abb. 35); bei Verkürzung müßte demzufolge eine entgegengesetzt aufgewölbte Kurve

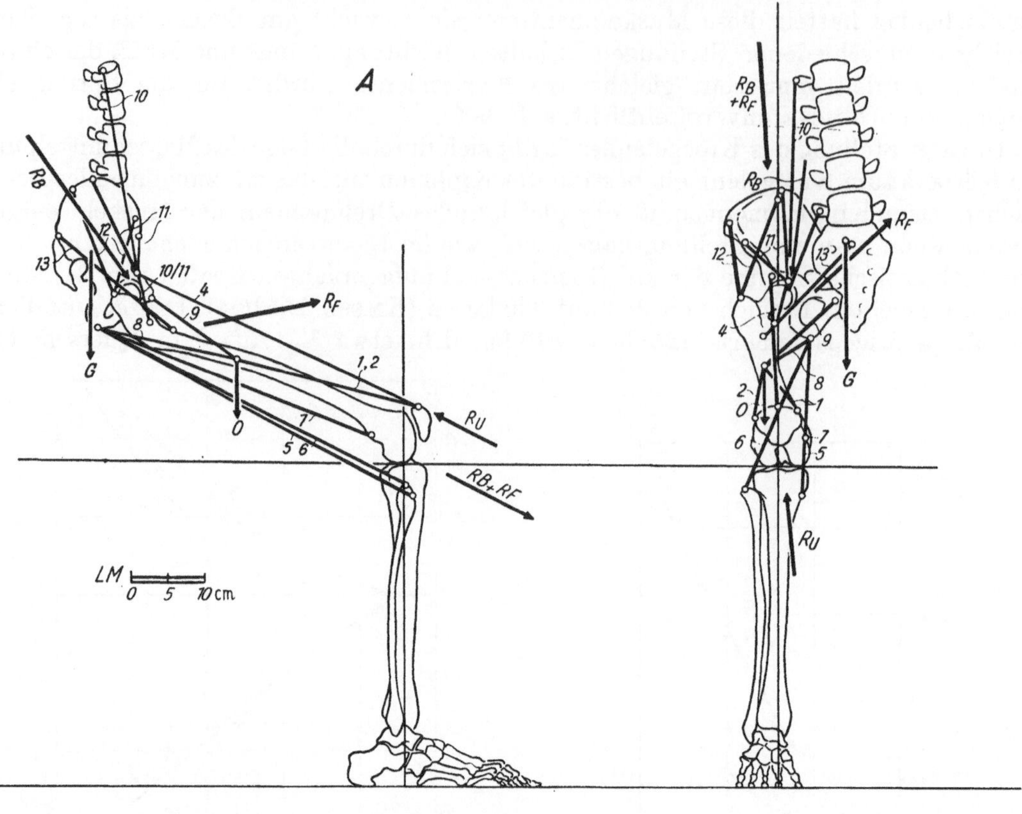

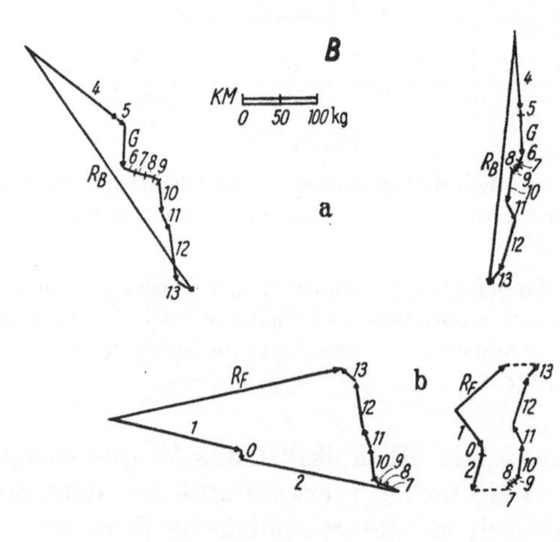

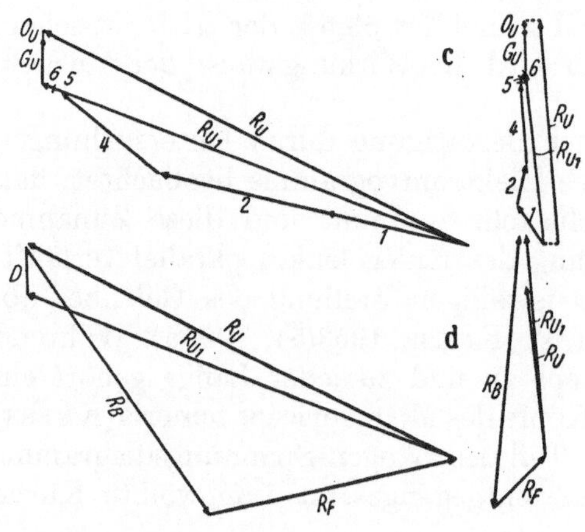

Abb. 36. A und B: Lageplan A und Kräfteplan B der Oberschenkelmuskeln bei Beugung des Kniegelenks und senkrechtem Unterschenkel. Skelet freihändig ergänzt. Lageplan in Projektion auf eine Sagittal- und Frontalebene. Meßpunkte geradlinig verbunden. Bezeichnung der Muskeln vgl. Text. G Körpergewicht = 57 kg; O Oberschenkelgewicht = 8 kg; RB Beckenresultierende; RF Femurresultierende; $RB + RF$ Becken- und Femurresultierende addiert; RU Unterschenkelresultierende. Kräfteplan B in gleicher Projektion: geometrische Addition der Muskelkräfte, die mit den im Lageplan aufgeführten Nummern bezeichnet sind. a Bildung der Beckenresultierenden; b Bildung der Femurresultierenden; c Bildung der Unterschenkelresultierenden (G_U bzw. O_U Stützreaktion durch Körper- bzw. Oberschenkelgewicht); d Addition der resultierenden Kräfte (aus KNESE, 1955)

anzunehmen sein. FLOYD und SILVER (1955) haben eine gleichartige Beziehung zwischen Länge und Kraft der Rückenmuskeln bei der Vorbeugung des Rumpfes dargestellt (vgl. KNESE, 1963a).

Bei den Experimenten mit den Muskelphantomen gelang es, den Oberschenkel bei senkrechtem Unterschenkel etwa in der Horizontalen zu halten (KNESE 1955a). Vermutlich wird in dieser Stellung (Abb. 36) jene Muskelkraft entwickelt, die als maximale Belastung anzusehen ist und KNESE (1956a) hat aus diesem Kraftsystem die Beanspruchung des Femurs errechnet (s. S. 500). Die in der deskriptiven Anatomie übliche Muskeleinteilung (Flexoren, Extensoren usw.) ist für Belastungsuntersuchungen ungeeignet. Die Einteilung erfolgte in folgende Gruppen:

I. Muskeln zwischen Oberschenkel und Unterschenkel: 1. M. vastus medialis, 2. M. vastus lateralis, 3. M. biceps Cap. breve.

II. Muskeln zwischen Becken und Unterschenkel: 4. M. rectus femoris, 5. Ischiocrurale Muskeln, 6. M. biceps Cap. longum.

III. Muskeln zwischen Becken und Oberschenkel: 7. Adduktoren mit Ansatz am Condylus medialis, 8. M. adductor magnus, 9. M. adductor longus, 10. M. psoas major, 11. M. iliacus, 12. kleine Gluteen, 13. M. gluteus maximus.

IV. Muskeln zwischen Oberschenkel und Fuß: 14. M. gastrocnemius.

Das Eigengewicht des Oberschenkels (0 = 8 kg) gehört zur Kräftegruppe I, Becken- und Körpergewicht (G = 57 kg) zur Kräftegruppe II.

Die Beziehung der Kräfte zueinander ist in einem sog. Lageplan und in einem Kräfteplan jeweils in einem bestimmten Maßstab zu untersuchen. Alle Kräfte, die auf das Becken einwirken, werden zu einer Beckenresultierenden addiert (397 kg), in gleicher Weise die Kräfte, die auf den Oberschenkel wirken (Femurresultierende: 322,5 kg) und die des Unterschenkels (592,5 kg). Diese Resultierenden sind ihrerseits zu addieren, um zu prüfen, ob Gleichgewicht besteht. Die Lage dieser Resultierenden wird dann in den Lageplan übertragen. Nunmehr kann mit diesen Kräften, die auf den Femur wirken, einschließlich jener im Hüft- und Kniegelenk die Beanspruchung des Femur ermittelt werden (s. S. 502).

Die Übertragung der Muskelkraft auf den Knochen wurde verschiedentlich untersucht. DOLGO-SABUROFF (1929/30) übernahm die in der deskriptiven Anatomie übliche Unterscheidung von zwei Ansatzformen, nämlich mittels Sehnen oder durch fleischigen Ansatz. BIERMANN (1957), KNESE und BIERMANN (1958) und JIPP (1960) fanden dagegen auch bei den fleischigen Ansätzen am Periost einen Übergang in feinste Sehnen, die im mikroskopischen Bereich senkrecht auf den Knochen zu umbiegen. KÖRNER (1939) und MACHADO DE SOUSA (1955) geben einen vorwiegend parallelen Verlauf der Sehnenfaserbündel an, WEISS und ROUVIÈRE (1914) sprechen von einem spiraligen Verlauf, MOLLIER (1937) und LUBOSCH (1937) von Vernetzungen. MOLLIER (1937) glaubte, daß das Vernetzungssystem die verschiedenartige Zugrichtung der Muskeln in unterschiedlichen Gliedstellungen ausgleicht. JIPP (1960) hält das für wenig wahrscheinlich, da das Vernetzungssystem sich nur auf den kleinen Raum von 5—20 mm erstreckt. JIPP (1960) fand bei Lupenpräparation eine Aufteilung der Sehnenbündel (Abb. 37), der sog. Primärbündel, in Sekundärbündel, von denen sich je zwei zu einem Tertiärbündel vereinen. Die Tertiärbündel gehen in Endpinsel über, die in das Periost einstrahlen oder bei apophysären Ansätzen Bestandteil des Faserknorpels an der Oberfläche der Apophyse werden.

Infolge der wechselnden Tätigkeit der motorischen Einheiten müßte das Ansatzgebiet einem Kräftehagel im Sinne der Wechsellast unterworfen sein (JIPP 1960). Durch die Vernetzung der Fasern wird die angreifende Kraft von einer Wechsellast, die zu einer Zerrüttung der Ansatzzone führen würde, zu einer Dauerlast mit halber Größe je Ansatzpunkt umgestellt. Nach BIERMANN (1957) sowie KNESE und BIERMANN (1958) ist die Zugfestigkeit des Knochens und der Sehne etwa gleich groß, der Elastizitätsmodul jedoch um fast eine Zehnerpotenz verschieden; infolgedessen ist eine Elastizitäts- oder Dehnungsdämpfung bzw. -bremsung in der Ansatzzone erforderlich. Diese Dämpfung wird in unterschiedlicher Weise erreicht, bei periostalen Ansätzen durch Netzsysteme aus Kollagen- und elastischen Fasern, bei Apophysen durch einen zugfesten Ansatzknorpel. SCHNEIDER (1955, 1956) meinte, die Sehnen wären wie ein Elektrokabel in den Knochen eingelassen, ein Bild, das nach morphologischen Untersuchungen unzutreffend ist. SCHNEIDER nimmt dann eine Biegebeanspruchung der Sehne an, Kollagenfasern sind aber nicht biegefest.

Nach KNESE et al. (1955) bringen die Abschrägungen, mit denen Muskelkanten und -leisten in den restlichen Knochen übergehen, eine Last- und Spannungsverteilung. Durch

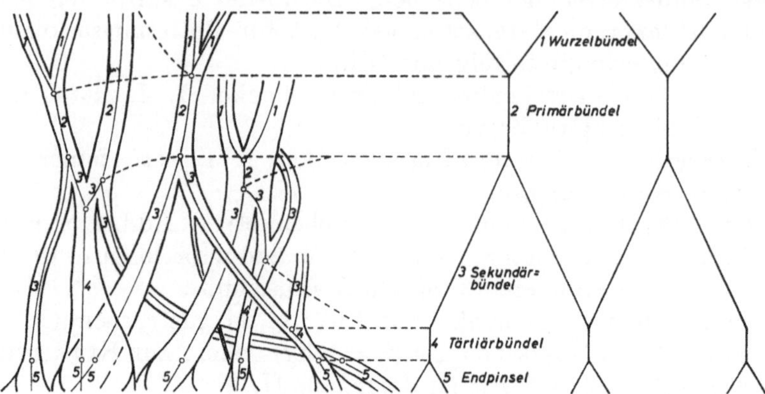

Abb. 37. Ansatz der Achillessehne am Tuber calcanei (♂ re. 60 Jahre). *A* Darstellung der präparierten Faserdurchflechtung; *B* Schema der Faserdurchflechtung. Erläuterung: Die verschiedenen Verlaufsstrecken der Fasern wurden mit den Ziffern *1—5* versehen, Wurzelbündel *1*, Primärbündel *2*, Sekundärbündel *3*, Tertiärbündel *4* und Endpinsel *5*, die Gabelungs- und Vereinigungsstellen sind mit Kreisen angezeigt. Die Höhen der einander entsprechenden Abschnitte in *A* und *B* wurden durch gestrichelte Linien verbunden (aus JIPP, 1960)

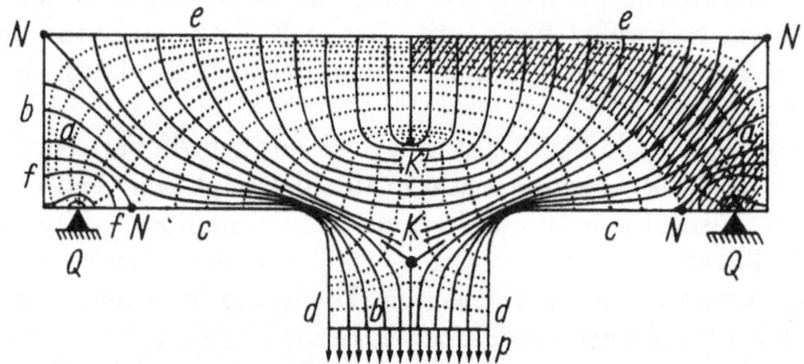

Abb. 38. Das Kraftfeld in einem Balken bei örtlichem Zug zur Darstellung der Spannungsverhältnisse an Sehnenansätzen. *a* Druckkraftlinien; *B* Zugkraftlinien von der Kraft *p* ausgehend, die an den Ecken eine Zusammendrängung zeigen. Das Verteilungssystem enthält den singulären Punkt *K*. *c* und *e* Die Spannungssysteme im Balken, am Balkenende überlagert von den Auflagerungskraftlinien, die bei *Q* entstehen und bei *N* Nullpunkte haben. Das System *c* hängt mit gleichartigen Spannungen im Zugstiel zusammen (nach BIRNBAUM aus WYSS, 1926; Umzeichnung aus KNESE, 1958b)

die Abschrägungen tritt eine Querkraftminderung ein, wobei die parabolische Schräge eine stetige Spannungsverteilung bewirkt. Eine ähnliche Auffassung vertritt CURREY (1962a). LAUX (1930) glaubte an einen Zusammenhang zwischen Richtung des Sehnenansatzes und der Spongiosaarchitektur. Der Aufbau des Knochens ist jedoch in Ansatzgebieten sehr unterschiedlich. DOLGO-SABUROFF (1935) hat gezeigt, daß z. B. die Tuberositas gluteae eine spongiöse Einschaltung ist oder als eine rein kompakte Zone auftreten kann (vgl. FILOGAMO, 1945). Der Aufbau der Sehnen- und Bandansatzzonen erfordert noch weitere Untersuchung, da nicht geklärt ist, ob Fasern in den Knochen übertreten oder nicht.

Die Dehnungsdämpfung an Sehnenansätzen ist nach KNESE (1958b) so vollständig, daß für Sehnenabrisse nur noch die Spannungsverteilung entscheidend ist. Durch den örtlichen Zug der Sehne (Abb. 38) entsteht ein sog. Zugkern, der eine Auflockerung des

Materials bewirkt; bei einem Druckkern unter örtlicher Pressung erfolgt dagegen eine Verfestigung. Die Zugspannungen werden nun durch Biegespannungen überlagert, wodurch eine Unstetigkeitszone erscheint, da die Maximalspannungen in ihrer Richtung von Punkt zu Punkt wechseln. In dieser Unstetigkeitszone reißt der Sehnen- oder auch Bandansatz keilförmig aus.

J. W. Smith (1962a und b) hat makroskopisch, mikroskopisch, röntgenologisch und an spannungsoptischen Modellen den Trochanter major, die Ilium-Ischium-Verbindung, den Calcaneus, das proximale Ende der Tibia und das distale Ende des Femurs auf Lage und Gestalt der Epiphysenscheibe hin untersucht. Smith berücksichtigt dabei, daß spannungsoptische Modelle nicht genau einen Knochenschnitt wiedergeben, die Verhältnisse in Nachbarschnitten vernachlässigt werden und die äußeren Kräfte genau in die Ebene der Scheibe verlegt werden. Smith (1962a) verfolgt die Veränderung des Spannungsbildes durch Sehnen- und Bandansätze. Wie Fick (1941) stellt der Verfasser eine Korrelation zwischen Stellung der Epiphysenplatte und dem Spannungsmuster fest. Die größeren Anteile einer knorpeligen Epiphysenplatte liegen rechtwinklig zu den Hauptdruckspannungen und parallel zu den Hauptzugspannungen. Scherspannungen, die eine Epiphysenlösung bringen könnten, sind minimal.

An der Tuberositas tibiae biegt die Epiphysenplatte in Richtung des Ligamentum patellae um. Bereits Bidder (1906) hat die Faserordnung der Tuberositas tibiae untersucht. Lacroix (1951) hat auf das Fehlen eines periostalen Ringes hingewiesen. Den Knorpel von Apophysen, den Schaffer (1930) als sekundären Knorpel ansieht, bezeichnen Knese und Biermann (1958) als zugfesten Ansatzknorpel. Von Zugepiphysen (traction epiphyses) sprechen Barnett und Lewis (1958) und Lewis (1958). Die Fasern des Ligamentum patellae treten nach Knese und Biermann (1958) an den Knorpel der Tuberositas tibiae heran und gehen nach Durchflechtung im Knorpel an den Knochen bzw. in das Periost der Diaphyse hinein; das Ansatzgebiet des M. quadriceps wird damit aus der Wachstumszone des proximalen Epiphysenendes ausgeschaltet. Nach Smith (1962b) liegen die Fasern der Tuberositas tibiae und die darunter gebildeten Knochenbälkchen in Richtung der Hauptzugspannungen.

Die Beziehungen zwischen Muskel und Knochen sind nach der geweblichen Konstruktion der Ansatzzonen (vgl. Abrißversuch von Kuhn, 1933) und in den verschiedenen Lebensaltern vermutlich unterschiedlich (Knese, 1958b). Wahrscheinlich sind Muskelansätze auch als Zwischenstützen für den Knochen anzusehen, durch die eine Unterteilung der ,,Knicklänge“ (s. S. 500) erfolgt (Knese, 1956a), so daß es damit wohl genügt, den Sicherheitsfaktor mit 1,8—3,0 anzusetzen. Schließlich erfahren Muskeln bei ihrer Tätigkeit eine Querdehnung, die an den Extremitäten durch die Fascien begrenzt wird, so daß die Muskeln mit einer Art Manteldruck auf den Knochen wirken (Knese 1958b). Das Zusammenspiel Muskel—Knochen ist damit sicher sehr komplex.

c) Die Mechanik der Röhrenknochen

Die Mechanik der Röhrenknochen wurde fast nur am Femur untersucht, vielleicht kein sehr gut gewähltes Beispiel, da der Femur in seiner Form mit einem ausgeprägten Hals von der Form aller anderen Röhrenknochen stark abweicht. Von anderen Elementen wurde nur noch die Tibia (Lorenz, 1893;, Graf, 1894; Hirsch, 1895; Hagen, 1909; Hanauseck, 1914; Grunewald 1916, 1920; Pauwels, 1950) untersucht; Hinweise auf die Konstruktion der Knochen der oberen Extremität finden sich bei Grunewald (1920) und Pauwels (1949/50, 1951).

Die übliche Deskription der Skeletelemente ist bei Untersuchung ihrer Statik durch eine festigkeitstheoretische Beschreibung zu ergänzen. Hierbei sind Verteilung und Dicke der Compacta sowie die Flächenmomente (s. S. 430) zu beschreiben. Der Konstrukteur gibt jedem Teil im Bemessungsverfahren den Umfang und die Form, die für seine Beanspruchung erforderlich ist. Ziel dieser Bemessung ist, totes, das Eigengewicht erhöhendes

Material zu vermeiden. Dabei wird ein sog. „Körper gleicher Festigkeit" angestrebt, bei dem in allen Abschnitten soviel tragendes Material vorhanden ist, daß die zulässigen Spannungen mit dem entsprechenden Sicherheitsfaktor gerade erreicht werden. Die Form ist demzufolge nach der Beanspruchung verschieden. Bei Druck oder Zug liegt an der Seite des Lastangriffes der kleinste, an der gegenüber liegenden Seite der größte Querschnitt. Ein Biegebalken auf zwei Lagern erhält eine äußere Umgrenzung in der Form einer kubischen Parabel usw. Beim Spannungsnachweis muß umgekehrt die jeweilige „Materialmenge" untersucht werden, um zu prüfen, ob vermutlich ein Körper gleicher Festigkeit vorliegt; dies gilt auch für das Skelet (RAUBER, 1877; LANGE, 1902; GEBHARDT, 1910a; KNESE, 1956a; KUMMER, 1961, 1962, 1966; KNIEF, 1967a, b; AMTMANN und SCHMITT, 1968; s. S. 506).

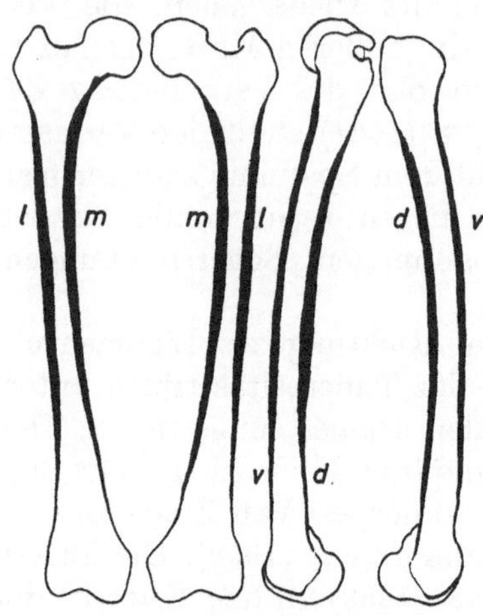

Abb. 39. Femur, Frontalschnitt und Sagittalschnitt mit Angabe der Compactadicke

Einzelne Flächenmomente haben GRUNEWALD (1920), KOCH (1917) und MARIQUE (1945) bestimmt. MESSERER (1880) hat die Trägheitsmomente nur für die durchgeführten Festigkeitsuntersuchungen und Belastungsrichtungen ermittelt. Eine systematische Untersuchung der Flächenmomente haben für menschliche Knochen KNESE et al. (1955), EHLER (1963, 1966a, 1967c) für Humerus, Radius und Ulna und ERTELT (1955) für eine Reihe von Säugetieren veröffentlicht.

Die Dicke der Compacta hat MECHANIK (1928, 1929, 1930, 1932) untersucht. Aus dem äußeren Umfang A eines Knochens und dem inneren B entsprechend der Markhöhle bildet MECHANIK einen Index:

$$C = \frac{A \cdot 100}{B}.$$

Dieser Index nimmt bei Verkleinerung der Markhöhle zu, bei Vergrößerung ab. Der Index wächst zum mittleren (32—37 Jahre) Alter hin und verkleinert sich dann wieder. Die Compacta ist bei Männern stärker als bei Frauen, der Index bei Frauen aber größer.

In den folgenden beispielhaften Angaben beziehen wir uns auf die Mitteilung von KNESE et al. (1955).

Femur. Der elliptisch gestaltete Hals hat eine Corticalis, die nach BACKMAN (1957) im oberen Bereich zwischen 0,5—1,0 und im unteren Bereich 5—6 mm mißt. Die lange Achse dieser Ellipse ist von vorn oben nach hinten-unten eingestellt (KNESE 1956a). Die Compacta (Abb. 39) nimmt in den einzelnen Wandteilen des Schaftes etwas unterschiedlich von proximal nach distal an Dicke zu und erreicht das größte Ausmaß oberhalb der Schaftmitte. Die Dickenabnahme nach distal geht langsamer vor sich. Das größte Widerstandsmoment (Abb. 40) verläuft mit geringen Abweichungen in einer Ebene von vorn-lateral nach hinten-medial. Bei einem stark verkrümmten rachitischen Femur (Abb. 41) ist die Querschnittsfläche der bei Gesunden gleich. Durch die Formänderung des Querschnittes bleibt das Flächenmoment in der Frontalen in der Größe ebenfalls dem des Gesunden ähnlich, das in der Sagittalen wird aber erheblich vergrößert. Proximal liegt das größte Widerstandsmoment in der Ebene von vorn-lateral nach dorsal-medial, in der Femurmitte fast sagittal und distal von vorn-medial nach hinten-lateral.

BELL (1956) und BELL et al. (1947) beobachteten bei Ratten keine rachitischen Verkrümmungen von Knochen, jedoch bei Hunden wie beim Menschen. Dieses differente Verhalten dürfte auf die unterschiedliche Größe der Species zurückzuführen sein. Die veränderte Querschnittsform dagegen könnte als Erhöhung des Widerstandsmomentes bei herabgesetzter Knochenfestigkeit angesehen werden. Dann läge in der Formänderung eine „funktionelle Anpassung" und keine „Belastungsdeformität" vor (s. S. 505). Ob die

Schaftkrümmung des rachitischen Femurs in gleicher Weise zu deuten ist, müßte noch näher untersucht werden (vgl. PAUWELS, 1950/51).

Anhand von Umrißzeichnungen der Querschnittsform mit einem dem Storchenschnabel ähnlichen Zeichengerät hat MICHEL (1903) den Femur des rezenten Menschen mit dem des Neandertaler und dem von Spy, sowie von Orang, Gorilla und Hylobates verglichen. Die Femora des Neandertaler und des Menschen von Spy haben mit größter Ausdehnung in der Sagittalen und einer Dreiecksform mit dorsaler Linea aspera die gleiche Form wie beim rezenten Menschen. Bei den Affen liegt dagegen eine querovale Form vor.

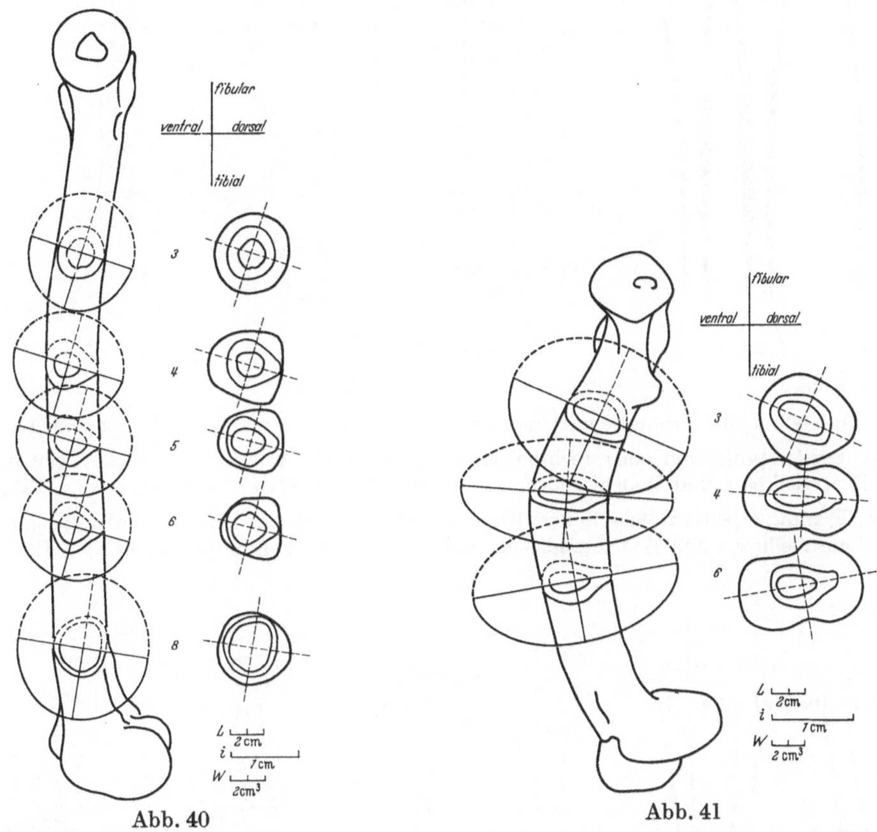

Abb. 40. Sagittalprojektion eines rechten Femurs (♂, 79 Jahre). Ansicht von tibial, eingezeichnete Zentralellipsen und Widerstandsmomente (aus KNESE, HAHNE und BIERMANN, 1955)

Abb. 41. Sagittalprojektion eines stark gekrümmten rachitischen rechten Femurs (Sammlung). Zentralellipse und Widerstandsmomente (aus KNESE, HAHNE und BIERMANN, 1955)

Tibia. Die Dickenzunahme der Compacta (Abb. 42) von proximal her und die Abnahme nach distal zu verläuft etwa gleichartig, auch im Bereich der extremen Dicke der Crista anterior. Die Widerstandsmomente (Abb. 43) sind proximal recht groß, nehmen distal erheblich an Größe ab. Die Richtung des größten Widerstandsmomentes ist etwas wechselnd wenig aus der Sagittalen herausgedreht.

Fibula. Die Widerstandsmomente der Fibula sind sehr klein.

Humerus. Innen- und Außenwand des Humerus nehmen von proximal her langsam an Dicke zu und brechen in annähernd gleicher Stärke oberhalb der Epicondylen ab. Die Dickenzunahme der Vorder- und Hinterwand beginnt etwas weiter proximal als die der beiden anderen Wände. Die von oben nach unten an Größe abnehmenden Widerstandsmomente (Abb. 44) sind in der proximalen Hälfte frontal eingestellt, distal aber entsprechend der Humerustorsion von medial-dorsal nach lateral-volar.

Radius und Ulna. Die Widerstandsmomente nehmen am Radius von oben nach unten an Größe zu und verhalten sich an der Ulna umgekehrt (Abb. 45, 46). Etwa von der

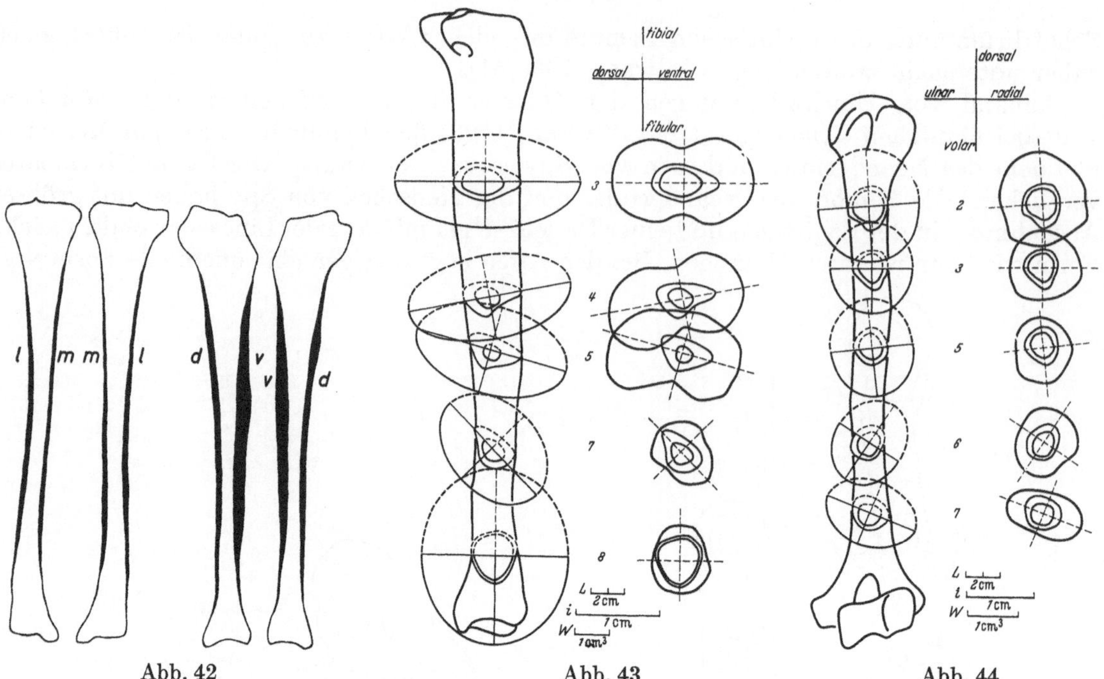

Abb. 42 Abb. 43 Abb. 44

Abb. 42. Tibia, Frontalschnitt und Sagittalschnitt mit Angabe der Compactadicke

Abb. 43. Sagittalprojektion einer rechten Tibia (♂ 79 Jahre). Ansicht von fibular, eingezeichnete Zentralellipsen und Widerstandsmomente (aus KNESE, HAHNE und BIERMANN, 1955)

Abb. 44. Frontalprojektion eines linken Humerus (♂ 79 Jahre). Ansicht von volar, eingezeichnete Zentralellipsen und Widerstandsmomente (aus KNESE, HAHNE und BIERMANN, 1955)

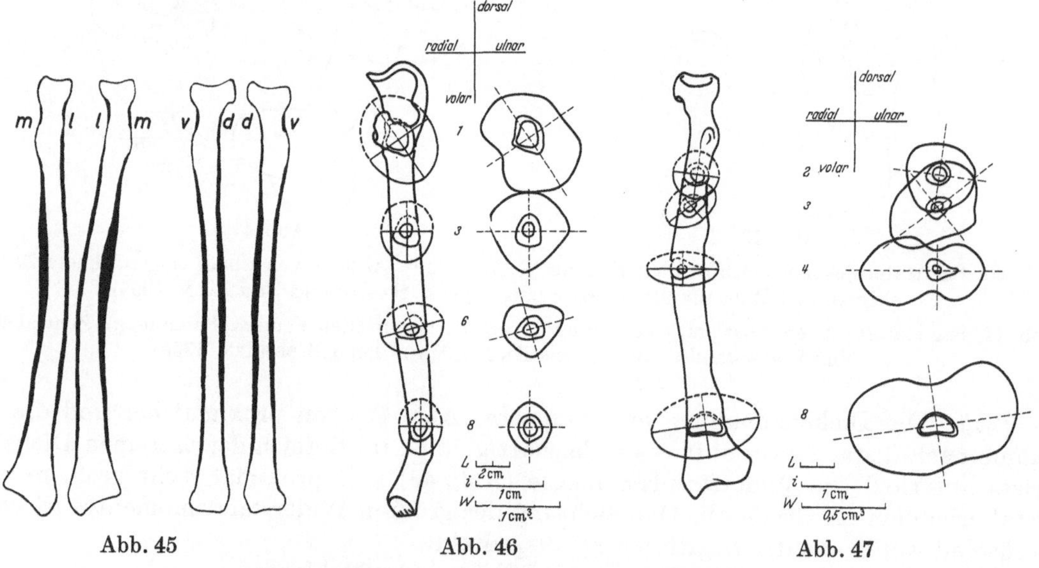

Abb. 45 Abb. 46 Abb. 47

Abb. 45. Radius, Frontalschnitt und Sagittalschnitt

Abb. 46. Frontalprojektion einer rechten Ulna (♂ 43 Jahre). Ansicht von volar, eingezeichnete Zentralellipsen und Widerstandsmomente (aus KNESE, HAHNE und BIERMANN, 1955)

Abb. 47. Frontalprojektion eines rechten Radius (♂, 43 Jahre). Ansicht von volar, eingezeichnete Zentralellipsen und Widerstandsmomente (aus KNESE, HAHNE und BIERMANN, 1955)

Hälfte der Knochenlänge ab verläuft die Richtung des größten Widerstandsmomentes fast quer, im oberen Teil sind sie symmetrisch gegeneinander eingestellt; beim Radius (Abb. 47) von medial-dorsal nach lateral-volar, bei der Ulna von lateral-dorsal nach volar-medial. Die von EHLER (1963) errechneten Zentralellipsen für Humerus, Radius und Ulna stimmen mit den angegebenen überein, im Hinblick auf die Widerstands momente ergeben sich Differenzen, weil KNESE et al. (1955) eine symmetrische und EHLER eine asymmetrische Achslage zugrunde gelegt hat.

Die einzelnen Skeletstücke haben demzufolge auch festigkeitstheoretisch betrachtet eine spezifische Gestalt, deren Bedeutung uns leider noch unbekannt ist. ERTELT (1955) zeigte, daß bei Vierfüßlern an der vorderen Extremität die Differenz zwischen I_{max} und I_{min} größer als an der hinteren ist. Weiterhin sind die Differenzen zwischen den Trägheitsmomenten am Femur bei den Säugern größer als an der Tibia. Aus dem Verhalten der Flächenmomente könnte geschlossen werden, daß die vordere Extremität als Tragextremität eine mehr gleichförmige Beanspruchung, die hintere als Abstoßextremität eine sehr wechselnde erfährt. Bei der gleichen Species besitzt die Tibia im allgemeinen auch eine höher entwickelte Struktur als der Femur.

v. MEYER (1867) und CULMANN (1866) hatten im Analogieverfahren den menschlichen Femur mit einem Kran verglichen. Bereits RITTER (1888) hat gegen diese Auffassung Bedenken vorgebracht, da die Belastung durch die Muskulatur größer als die durch das Körpergewicht sei. Da nun die Muskeln an verschiedenen Punkten und in verschiedener Richtung ansetzen, läßt sich die Beanspruchung des Femurs nicht auf eine Ebene beziehen, sondern muß als räumliche Aufgabe behandelt werden. BÄHR (1898), der den Femur als freistehenden Träger ansprach, und SUDECK (1899) kritisierten die Deutung der Spongiosastruktur (s. S. 474). GHILLINI und CANEVAZZI (1902) meinten, daß wohl in der Frontalen eine Verankerung des Femurs möglich sei — wie das für den v. MEYER und CULMANN angenommenen Kran erforderlich ist —, aber nicht in der Sagittalen. Nach HAGEN (1908, 1909) ist das obere Ende des Femurs nicht frei, sondern im Hüftgelenk geführt, so daß eine Beanspruchung auf Längsdruck mit Biegung, d.h. Knickung, erfolge. Auch GRUNEWALD (1912) sprach von einer rein äußerlichen Ähnlichkeit mit einem Kran, dem aber die Verankerung fehle, ähnlich äußert sich HANAUSECK (1914; vgl. weiter LORENZ, 1893; KORTEWEG, 1893).

Während diese Bedenken auf mehr oder minder rein mechanischen Überlegungen beruhen, gehen andere Autoren von der Struktur des Femurs aus. ROUX (1895) erkannte, daß das Kranbild des „Femurs" unvollständig ist, weil bei ihm die Vorder- und Hinterwand fehlt und die Biegung in der Sagittalen unberücksichtigt bleibt. Zur gleichen Feststellung kommt KÜNTSCHER (1935a, b, 1936). Der Nachweis, daß die Spongiosaarchitektur im oberen Femurende einen Aufbau besitzt, der von dem bisher angenommenen Bilde abweicht (KNESE, 1956a, 1958b, 1959b; GARDEN, 1961; KUMMER, 1962), fordert auf jeden Fall eine Neubearbeitung der Statik des Femurs; Trajectorium rectum, Trajectorium curvatum usw. erscheinen in der postulierten Form nur in Schnittbildern: einem Frontalschnitt oder dem optischen Schnitt im Röntgenbild.

Durch Experimente an Knochen oder mit in der Technik üblichen kombinierten Verfahren wurde versucht, die Beanspruchung des Femurs aufzuklären.

Die Belastung des Femurs haben KOCH (1917), GRUNEWALD (1920) und MARIQUE (1945) rein mathematisch untersucht, wobei sich diese Autoren der Schwierigkeit einer solchen Analyse wohl bewußt waren. KOCH (1917) fertigte von dem rechten Femur eines 35jährigen Mannes 75 Querschnitte und von dem linken Frontalschnitte an. Der Einfluß der Muskeln blieb unberücksichtigt, da ihre Einwirkung nach Meinung von KOCH gegenüber der Gewichtslast gering sei. Die höchste Zugspannung von 68,18 kg $\cdot$ cm^{-2} liegt in der Mitte des Halses, im Schaft erreicht die Zugspannung auf der Lateralseite zwischen proximalem und mittlerem Viertel nur 64,7 kg $\cdot$ cm^{-2}. Die höchste Druckbeanspruchung liegt am Hals auf der Unterseite mit 92 und an der Medialseite des Schaftes etwas unterhalb der höchsten Zugbeanspruchung mit 88,3 kg $\cdot$ cm^{-2}. Der sich bei dieser Beanspruchung durch das Körpergewicht allein ergebende Sicherheitsfaktor ist recht hoch.

GRUNEWALD (1920) hat an Hand des Körpergewichtes die maximale Zugspannung im oberen Teil des Femurs mit 63,4, die Druckspannungen zu 78,8 kg $\cdot$ cm^{-2} errechnet.

Dann bestimmte GRUNEWALD mittels der Angaben von FICK (1911) die Kraft der belastenden Muskulatur und erhielt in der Longitudinalen 2800 kg, in der Transversalen 1220 kg; die rotatorische Komponente beträgt 390 kg. Nach Diskussion der Verhältnisse an den übrigen Röhrenknochen einschließlich jener der oberen Extremität kommt GRUNEWALD zum Schluß, daß die Hauptbelastung der Knochen durch die Muskeln erfolge. Die Größe des Torsionsmomentes wird von v. LANZ und HENNIG (1962) mit 600 cm·kg angegeben. Bei einem mittleren Durchmesser des Femurs von 25 mm errechnen die Autoren eine Schubspannung τ von 200 kg · cm^{-2}. Zum Vergleich wird die Druckspannung durch mittigen Lastangriff mit 20 kg · cm^{-2} und die Biegespannung bei einem Hebelarm von 3,5 cm zu 165 kg · cm^{-2} angegeben. Die resultierende Druckspannung wird dann 235 kg · cm^{-2}. Der Sicherheitsfaktor würde demzufolge etwa 5—7,5 betragen. MARIQUE (1945) rechnet mit einer Last von 100 kg am Femurkopf und erhält dann das Verhältnis von maximalen Zug- zu Druckspannungen im Hals zu 117,14/148,81, in Höhe des Trochanter minor 105,82/148,72, in Schaftmitte 68,20/103,39 und in Höhe der Epicondylen 11,77/39,6 kg·cm^{-2}. Weiterhin sei auf die umfangreichen Arbeiten von PAUWELS (1965) und KUMMER (1959a, b) hingewiesen, die teils auf spannungsoptischen Untersuchungen, teils auf statischen Konstruktionen aufbauen.

KÜNTSCHER (1934) und EVANS (1957) haben diese rein mathematische Behandlung der Beanspruchung von Knochen kritisiert, da eine gleichartige Verteilung der Kräfte angenommen wird. Jedoch wird diese Voraussetzung in der Technik stets gemacht, wobei man dann von scheinbaren Spannungen spricht, die mit experimentell ermittelten Festigkeitswerten verglichen werden, die in der üblichen Rechenform (s. S. 442) häufig auch nur als scheinbare Spannungen anzusehen sind. Schwerer ist der Einwand von EVANS (1957) in bezug auf die Bestimmung der Flächenmomente und die Annahme eines zweiachsigen Spannungszustandes. Schließlich stimmt das Ergebnis der Rechnung nur mit der äußeren Form des Femurs, aber nicht mit der Materialverteilung überein. Die höchste errechnete Beanspruchung liegt im Femurhals und erreicht mit dem Körpergewicht allein schon dessen Festigkeit. Dagegen ist die Beanspruchung des Schaftes mit seiner dicken Compacta von hoher Festigkeit sehr gering.

Nun wurde versucht, die Tragfähigkeit der Skeletstücke durch unmittelbare Belastung zu ermitteln. Auf Versuche zur Aufklärung eines bestimmten Bruchmechanismus kommen wir in einem gesonderten Kapitel zurück (s. S. 518). Biegeversuche an ganzen Skeletstücken wurden bereits bei Erörterung der Biegefestigkeit diskutiert (s. S. 431). Die experimentellen Bedingungen bei Biegung sind vermutlich einer unmittelbaren Gewalteinwirkung in vivo recht ähnlich. Bei Druck-, Knick- oder Zugversuchen an ganzen Knochen bereitet die Experimentalanordnung zur Sicherung des Kraftangriffes an den Gelenkenden große Schwierigkeiten. MESSERER (1880) hat für zwei Humeri eine Form aus Hartblei gegossen. Im Versuch drückte sich der Schaft in den Kopf hinein, danach erfolgte ein Splitterbruch im unteren Drittel des Schaftes. Bei späteren Versuchen wurden die Gelenkenden mit Filz gepolstert, wobei im allgemeinen ebenfalls die Knochenenden zusammengedrückt wurden. Andere Untersucher verwandten auch bei Lackrißversuchen Metallpelotten (unter anderem HAASE und RICHTER, 1936; HIRSCH und BRODETTI, 1956a; EVANS, 1957; BACKMAN, 1957). Bei neun von zehn Druckversuchen, die BACKMAN (1957) durchführte, erwies sich die Fixierung als ungenügend.

MESSERER (1880) gelang im Zugversuch die Zerreißung eines Humerus unter 800 kg und des Oberschenkels bei 1550 kg Last; beide Skeletstücke stammten von einer 25jährigen Frau. Die Humerusfraktur war ein steil verlaufender Schrägbruch am oberen Ende, die Femurfraktur verlief ebenfalls schräg im unteren Viertel. Die Zugfestigkeit wurde mit 533 bzw. 674 kg · cm^{-2} errechnet; allerdings ließen sich zusätzliche Biegemomente im Versuch nicht ausschließen. Bei den Knickversuchen ganzer Knochen erhielt MESSERER selten einen Schaftbruch in der Form eines Sprödbruches. Zumeist fand ein Eindrücken an den Enden statt. Die Brüche lagen folgendermaßen: Clavicula (19 Versuche) in der Mitte oder an den Enden; Humerus (18) am Kopf oder distal, selten (1) im Schaft;

Tabelle 18. *Bruchlasten (kg) für Längsdruck ganzer Knochen* (nach MESSERER, 1880)

	Clavicula	Humerus	Femur				
			Radius	Ulna	Diaphyse	Hals	Fibula
♂	[5] 192 (125—270)	—	[6] 334 (240—430)	[3] — (180—290)	[2] — (700—875)	[5] 815 (700—1075)	[7] 61 (25—90)
♀	[7] 126 (90—210)	[1] 600	[7] 220 (105—325)	[6] 132 (90—175)	[2] (575—875)	[4] 506 (400—600)	[8] 49 (20—85)

[ ] Anzahl der Versuche. ( ) Größter und kleinster Wert.

Radius (17) Mitte des Schaftes, selten an den Gelenkenden; Ulna (17) Schaft oder unteres Ende; Femur (15) Schaftbrüche (4) oberhalb der Mitte als Splitterbrüche, im allgemeinen am Hals, selten (2) am unteren Ende; Tibia (17) keine Schaftbrüche, im allgemeinen distaler Bruch; Fibula (16) Schaftbrüche im oberen oder unteren Drittel unter starkem Ausbiegen nach innen-hinten. Nach dem Bruchgewicht (Tabelle 18) ergibt sich folgende Reihenfolge: Tibia, Femur, Humerus, Ulna, Clavicula, Fibula. BACKMAN (1957) erhielt einen Schaftbruch bei einem Femur einer 72jährigen Frau; aus seinen Versuchen errechnet er die Druckfestigkeit zu 1430 kg · cm^{-2}.

Durch unmittelbare Druckversuche an den Gelenkenden läßt sich demzufolge die Tragfähigkeit der Knochen im Hinblick auf eine Last in Längsachse des Stückes nur unter besonders günstigen Bedingungen ermitteln. Der Schluß liegt nahe, daß auch in vivo kaum mit einer reinen Längslast zu rechnen ist und im Bereich des Schaftes Querkräfte (s. S. 428) hinzutreten, die von der Muskulatur stammen. Eine Strebfestigkeit der Compacta kann weiterhin nur an herausgelösten Stücken, an Prismen gemessen werden; über diese Versuche wurde berichtet.

Mit Hilfe von Dehnungsmessern oder Dehnungsmeßstreifen wurde — im allgemeinen mit recht geringer Last — das Dehnungsbild von ganzen Skeletstücken untersucht. Ziel dieser Untersuchungen war, die sog. Spannungsspitzen bei unterschiedlichem Lastangriff aufzusuchen (vgl. GEBHARDT, 1910a; PAUWELS, 1949/50). KÜNTSCHER (1934, 1935a, 1936b), EVANS und LISSNER (1948) haben mit statischer Last am Femurkopf in Schwererichtung, EVANS, LISSNER und PEDERSEN (1948) mit dynamischer und dem Lackriß- bzw. stresscoat-Verfahren den Ort der Zug- bzw. Druckspannungen aufgesucht. Die Risse treten bei relativ geringen Lasten auf (Abb. 48), und zwar erfolgen Dehnungen durch Biegung auf der Oberseite des Halses und der Lateralseite des Schaftes, Kompressionen auf den jeweils entgegengesetzten. Bei dynamischer Belastung des Trochanter major (Abb. 49), wie bei einem Sturz (s. S. 522), erhielten PEDERSEN, EVANS und LISSNER (1949) von proximal nach distal fortschreitend an der Unterseite des Halses und den anschließenden Teilen des Schaftes Dehnungen. Diese Autoren haben den Femur auch einer Torsion unterworfen und erhielten Lackrisse, die gegen den Schaft um 45° geneigt sind (Abb. 50). EVANS, HAYES und POWERS (1953) haben eine quere Last auf die vordere, hintere und laterale Wand des Femurs einwirken lassen; es tritt eine Biegung mit Dehnung auf der dem Lastangriff entgegengesetzten Seite auf. Der Lastangriff an der Grenze oberes mittleres Viertel von lateral her ergibt die größten und in Schaftmitte von hinten die kleinsten Dehnungen. Bei diesen Versuchen wurden auch Altersdifferenzen beobachtet.

HIRSCH und BRODETTI (1956a) sowie HIRSCH und FRANKEL (1961) haben den Femurkopf in wechselnder Richtung belastet und die Dehnungen durch Dehnungsmeßstreifen registriert. Die Dehnungen sind im Lastbereich 2,5—20 kg der Last proportional (s. unten). Bei senkrechter Last kommt es zum Zusammendrücken des Halses auf der Unterseite, zur Dehnung auf der Oberseite. Dieses Dehnungsmuster wird durch andere Lastrichtungen so weit geändert, daß z. B. auf der Oberseite des Halses Stauchungen erscheinen. Versuche mit Lastangriff in verschiedener Richtung einschließlich torquierender Kräfte am Femurhals im Hinblick auf den Bruchmechanismus liegen unter anderem von BACKMAN (1957) vor (s. S. 522).

Die Versuche mit Lastangriff am Femurkopf in unterschiedlicher Richtung zeigen, daß ein Lamellensystem der Spongiosa nicht stets einer gleichen Beanspruchung unterliegt. Die Beanspruchung hängt von Lastrichtung und Lastgröße ab (unter anderem KNESE, 1956a, 1958b; SCOTT, 1957). Nach GARDEN (1961) muß der Kraft der Muskeln, die den Femurkopf am Acetabulum halten, eine gleich große entgegengesetzt gerichtete Druckkraft im Femurhals entsprechen; hinzu treten aber rotatorische Belastungen des Femur.

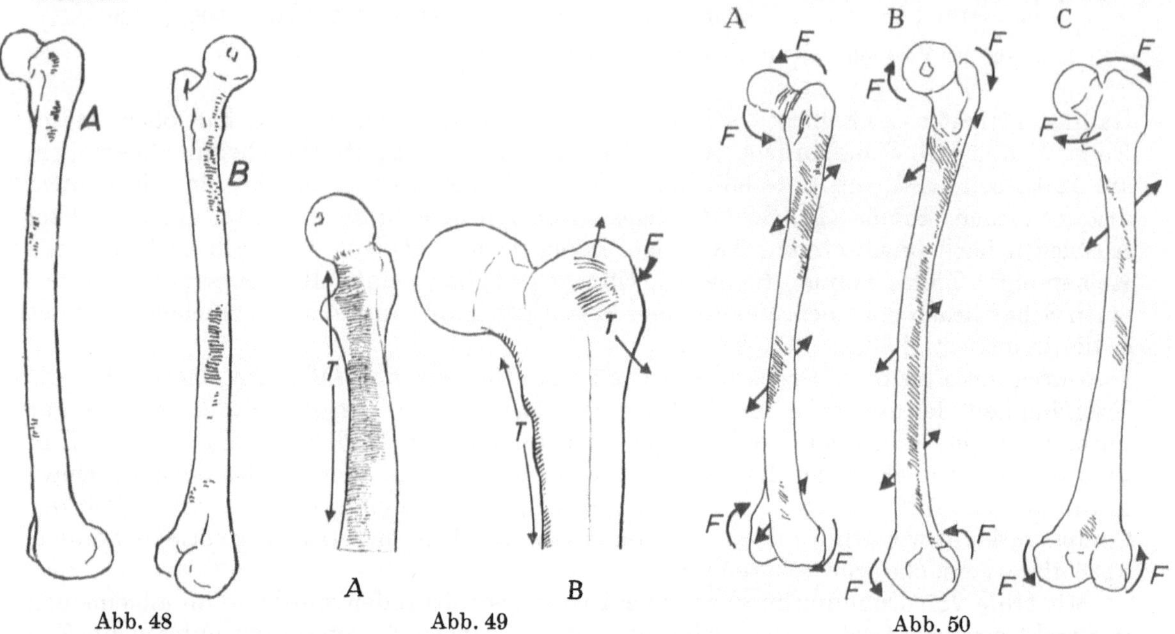

Abb. 48 A u. B. Menschlicher Femur mit stresscoat-Rissen. A durch Zugspannungen, B durch Druckspannungen bei senkrechter Last (11,35 kg) auf den Femurkopf. (Umzeichnung aus EVANS und GOFF, 1957)

Abb. 49 A u. B. Stresscoat-Risse am Femur durch Schlag auf den Trochanter major. A Stresscoat-Risse auf der Medialseite des Femurs. B *F* Lastangriff und stresscoat-Risse am Trochanter major (Umzeichnung aus EVANS, 1952)

Abb. 50 A—C. Menschlicher Femur mit stresscoat-Rissen bei Torsionsbeanspruchung. *F* Kraft; A Torsionsmoment 5,93 kgm; B 4,68 kgm; C 3,25 kgm (Umzeichnung aus LISSNER und EVANS, 1956)

Durch Messungen der Dehnungen mit mechanischen Dehnungsmessern bei verschieden hoher Last kommen KÜNTSCHER (1936) und MARIQUE (1945) zu der Feststellung, daß die Deformation der Last direkt proportional ist, d.h. der Knochen dem Hookeschen Gesetz folgt. Wird die Last zunächst gesteigert und dann wieder herabgesetzt, decken sich die beiden Last-Dehnungsschaubilder nicht (MARIQUE, 1945); es bleibt eine Restdehnung. Die Autoren haben mit recht geringen Lasten bis zu 250 kg gearbeitet, so daß die Untersuchungen wohl nur den Proportionalitätsbereich des Knochens erfaßt haben.

Mit Hilfe von Dehnungsmessungen unter relativ kleinen Lasten wurde also festgestellt, daß sich die Beanspruchung eines Knochens stark ändert. Dehnungs- und Verkürzungsseite können miteinander vertauscht werden. EVANS, COOLBOUGH und LEBOW nach EVANS (1957) konnten auch mit Dehnungsmeßstreifen an der Medialseite der Tibia des lebenden Hundes beim Laufen gegensinnige Biegungen registrieren.

Eine ganze Reihe von Untersuchungen spricht für eine stark wechselnde Beanspruchung der Skeletteile. In der Technik wird aber stets nach einer möglichen Höchstbeanspruchung gefragt. Die Technik verwendet seit ihren Anfängen auch organische Baumaterialien, z.B. Holz, und zeigte, daß im Rahmen der Statik für den Holzbau die gleichen physikalischen Gesetze unter Berücksichtigung der Materialstruktur wie für anorganische Stoffe gelten. So behandeln wir auch die mechanischen Aufgaben des

Skeletes und müssen demzufolge auch fragen: Gibt es eine „normale" Höchstbeanspruchung des Knochens? Durch eine Untersuchungsmethode allein gelingt es nicht, diese Höchstbeanspruchung aufzufinden. KNESE (1955b, 1956a) hat infolgedessen für den Femur und für den Unterschenkel (unveröffentlicht) in einem Vorgehen, das verschiedene Methoden heranzieht, die „Sicherheit" dieser beiden Elemente untersucht. An Hand des experimentell mit Muskelphantomen ermittelten Kraftsystems (KNESE 1955a, s. S. 487) wurden die Längs- und Querkräfte und das Biegemoment graphisch ermittelt. Da weiterhin die Flächenmomente der Querschnitte bekannt waren (KNESE et al., 1955), konnte in einzelnen Querschnitten die Spannung errechnet werden. Diese Spannungen wurden wiederum mit der örtlichen Festigkeit verglichen und daraus der örtliche Sicherheitsfaktor bestimmt.

Die in den statischen Experimenten zur Stabilisierung des Kniegelenkes ermittelten Kräfte (KNESE, 1955a) können unter Berücksichtigung eines Stoßkoeffizienten auch die Verhältnisse bei dynamischer Belastung wiedergeben. Häufig gelingt es nämlich auch in der Technik nicht, die Größe einer dynamischen Belastung zu messen. Dann geht man von der statischen Last aus. Durch ein plötzliches, stoßartiges Aufbringen der Last wird ein Bauteil doppelt so stark wie durch die gleiche Last unter statischen Bedingungen beansprucht (FÖPPL, 1951). Da die Kraft nicht momentan zu ihrer vollen Größe gesteigert werden kann, genügt es, den Stoßkoeffizienten im Mittel zu 1,5 (1,4—1,6) anzusetzen. Mit diesem Stoßkoeffizienten wird die statische Last multipliziert. KNESE (1955b, 1956a, 1958b) nahm den Koeffizienten zu 1,4 an.

Die gemessenen Muskelkräfte wurden mit dem Faktor multipliziert und auf einzelne Querschnitte bezogen, die der Mitte ihres Ansatzes bei linien- oder flächenförmigem Ansatz entsprechen. Das Körpergewicht, das in der Beckenresultierenden enthalten ist, und das Gewicht des Oberschenkels wurden nicht als gesonderte Kräfte behandelt. Für jeden dieser Querschnitte wurden alle dort angreifenden Kräfte in sagittale, frontale und longitudinale Komponenten aufgeteilt und während der Untersuchung wie selbständige Kräfte behandelt. Erst die sich ergebenden Spannungen wurden addiert, so daß damit ein Bild von der räumlichen Beanspruchung entsteht (Querschnitte, Muskeln und deren Komponenten s. Abbildungslegende Abb. 51).

Bei Untersuchung der Statik des Femurs ist zu berücksichtigen, daß eine Lagerung in zwei Gelenken und eine stark wechselnde Schaftkrümmung (RIED, 1928) vorhanden ist. Im Hinblick auf die Variation der Femurgestalt muß eine Beanspruchungsform vorliegen, die dieser Formenmannigfaltigkeit entspricht (KNESE, 1956a). Für die Statik der Skeletelemente ist offensichtlich von Bedeutung, daß Röhrenknochen an beiden Enden konvexe Gelenkkörper (Femur, Humerus, Phalangen) bzw. mehr oder minder flache (Tibia, Radius, Ulna) besitzen. Andere Skeletstücke, wie die Metacarpen und Metatarsen, weisen proximal ebene Flächen und distal konvexe auf; diesen Elementen fehlt dann proximal eine „größere" Beweglichkeit, da sog. Federgelenke (Articulatio plana, Amphiarthrose) vorliegen.

Bei einer Lagerung des Femurs in zwei Gelenken, einer Längsbelastung und Querkräften, kommt eine Beanspruchung auf Knickung in Frage, und zwar nach dem Euler-Fall 2 (KNESE, 1956a). An eine Knickbelastung ohne weitere quantitative Formulierung haben RAUBER (1877), MESSERER (1880), GHILLINI (1899), TRIEPEL (1908), HAGEN (1908, 1909), HANAUSECK (1914), OLIVO (1937), OLIVO, MAJ und TOAJARI (1937) gedacht. Ausführlich hat sich RAUBER (1877) mit der Knickung befaßt, dabei allerdings die ganze Beinsäule ins Auge gefaßt. Die Lagerung in organischen Gelenken ist nach RAUBER (1877) sehr verwickelt. Neben der Kapitellbildung ist eine Kuppelung durch den Bandapparat vorhanden; weiter sei der Luftdruck und die Muskulatur zu berücksichtigen. Organische Gelenke sind statisch unbestimmt, d. h. die Gleichgewichtsbedingungen reichen nicht aus, um die Lagerreaktion zu errechnen (KNESE, 1955a). Beim Knicken wird die Lagerung in Spitzengelenken vorausgesetzt, eine Bedingung, die auch bei technischen Knickstäben nicht erfüllt ist.

Bei Wiedergabe der Gleichgewichtsexperimente mit Hilfe von Muskelphantomen (KNESE, 1955a, s. S. 489) wurde eine Gruppierung der Muskulatur aufgeführt, die von der systematisch-deskriptiven abweicht. Muskeln sind bei Belastungsuntersuchungen

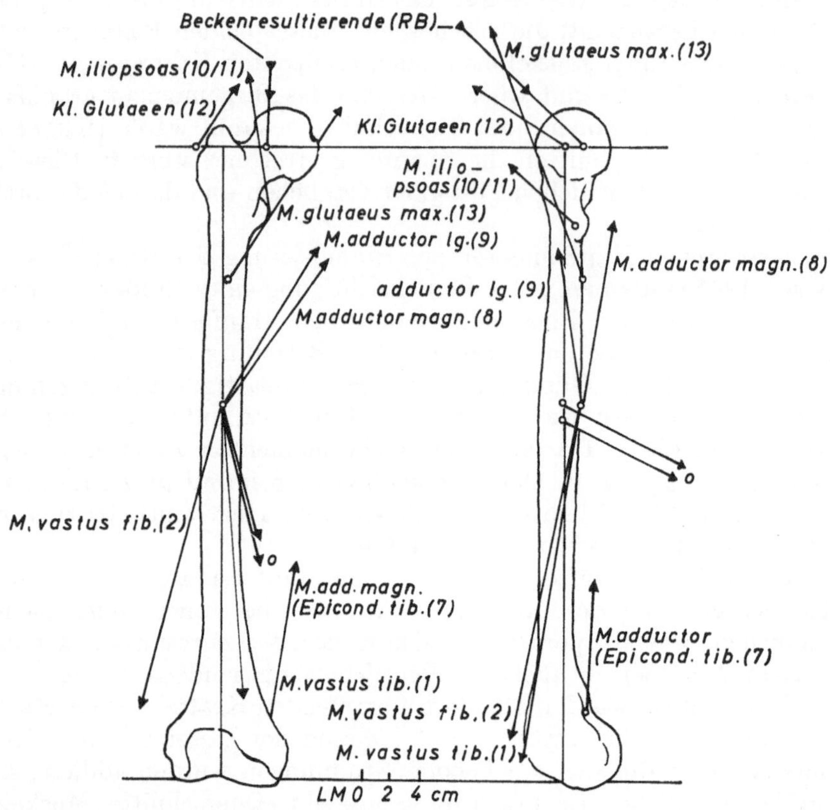

Abb. 51. Richtung der am Oberschenkel bei Kniebeuge (vgl. Abb. 36) angreifenden Kräfte bezogen auf die angenommene gerade Stabachse in der Frontal- und Sagittalprojektion. Knochenkonturen freihändig eingezeichnet (Umzeichnung nach KNESE, 1955b)

jeweils auf das Skeletstück zu beziehen, an dem sie ansetzen. Muskeln, die ein Element überspringen, wie die zweigelenkigen Beuger des Oberschenkels, wirken auf den Femur nur über die Lagerreaktion der Gelenke. Bei festigkeitstheoretischen Untersuchungen können demzufolge Gelenke nicht ausgeschaltet werden, wie es mitunter getan wurde (GRUNEWALD, 1912; PAUWELS, 1949/50, 1950, 1950/51); wir kommen darauf zurück (s. S. 507). Bei kinematischen Untersuchungen können dagegen Gliederketten zusammen betrachtet werden (v. BAYER, 1924/25; KNESE, 1955a, 1956b).

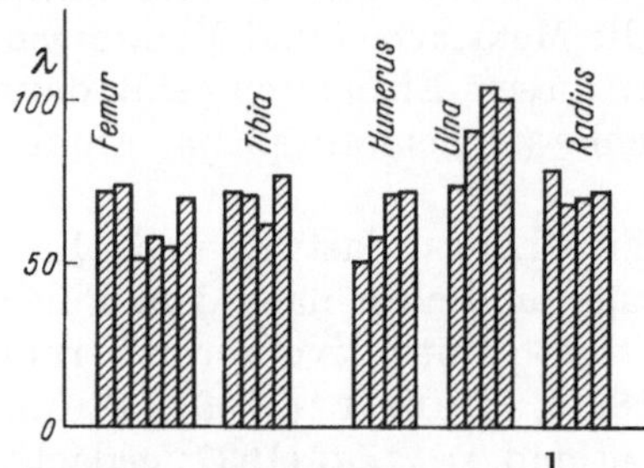

Abb. 52. Schlankheitsgrad $\lambda = \frac{1}{l}$ der Extremitätenknochen (aus KNESE 1956a)

Der Knickvorgang im engeren Sinne ist kein Problem der Festigkeitslehre, sondern eine Frage der „Stabilität". Bei Überschreiten einer Grenzspannung, der Knickspannung, kommt es zu einem plötzlichen Versagen, dem „Kollaps", des Bauteiles (KOLBRUNNER und MEISTER, 1961). Zu diesen Stabilitätsfällen gehören das Knicken, Kippen und Beulen. Ein Knicken tritt nur bei sog. schlanken Stäben auf (s. S. 426). Der Schlankheitsgrad menschlicher Röhrenknochen (Abb. 52) ist als mittelschlank zu bezeichnen (KNESE et al., 1955; KNESE, 1955a). Das starke Zurückbleiben des inneren Widerstandes gegenüber dem Kraftangriff, der Kollaps, kann durch das Verhalten des Systems oder des

Werkstoffes bedingt sein (KOLLBRUNNER und MEISTER, 1961). Zu einem Knicken kommt es unter anderem, wenn ein „Fehlhebel" wirkt. Dieser Fehlhebel kann im Kraftangriff in der Gelenklagerung oder in Seitenkräften liegen. Früher nahm man eine Summe unendlich vieler kleiner Durchbiegungsschritte an, die eine Reihe bilden. Heute wird die Verschiebung nicht mehr infinitesimal, sondern endlich groß angenommen. Eine scharfe Abgrenzung des „Kollapsproblems" von dem Spannungsproblem ist nicht leicht. Die Frage des Knickens kann demzufolge nicht allein durch Rechnung, sondern muß zu einem großen Teil durch Versuche gelöst werden, die mit Knochen kaum durchzuführen sind. Der allgemeinste Fall des Stabilitätsproblems ist das Biegedrillknicken, bei dem ein Stab eine beliebig gerichtete Querbelastung, eine Belastung durch Endmomente und eine

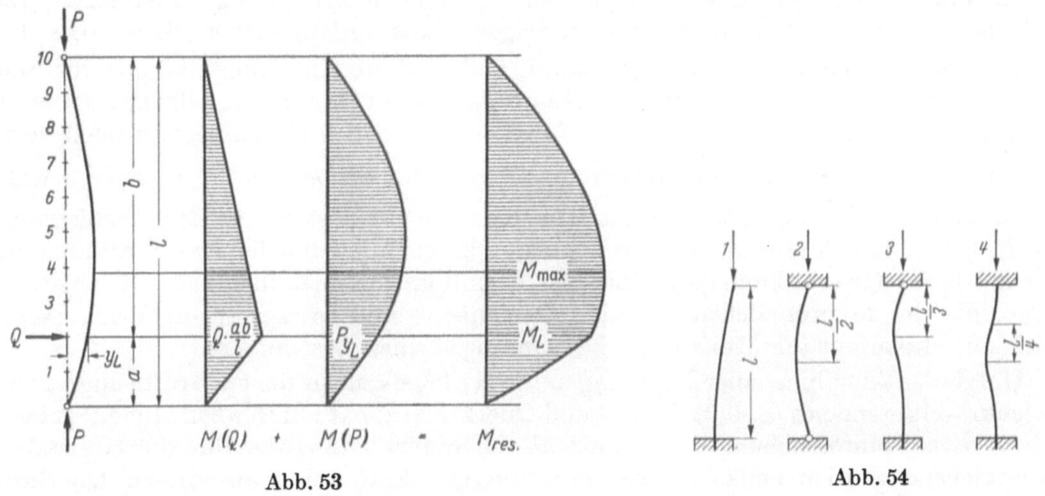

Abb. 53 Abb. 54

Abb. 53. Momentenflächen bei Knicken mit Längslast und Querkraft bei Lagerung in zwei Gelenken. Addition von M (Q): Querkraft und M (P) durch Längskraft (aus KOLLBRUNNER und MEISTER, 1961)

Abb. 54. Die vier Knickfälle nach EULER: *1* einseitige Einspannung; *2* beiderseits Gelenke; *3* einseitig eingespannt, auf der anderen Seite Gelenk; *4* beiderseits eingespannt (aus KNESE, 1956a)

exzentrische Normalkraft aufweist (Abb. 53). Diese Bedingungen gelten vermutlich für Röhrenknochen und können z.Z. nur in einer Näherungslösung untersucht werden (KNESE, 1956a). Jede theoretische Entwicklung in der Festigkeitslehre ist nach FÖPPL (1920) jedoch als Näherungslösung zu betrachten und steht nicht hinter sog. strengen Lösungen zurück.

Nach EULER werden nach der Lagerung des Knickstabes vier Fälle unterschieden (Abb. 54). In Anlehnung an die Biegetheorie hat EULER für diese vier Lagerungsformen die ideale Knicklast P_K errechnet. Hierbei tritt wieder das Produkt E · I auf, das bereits als Biegesteifigkeit (s. S. 431) erörtert wurde:

$$1 : \ 1\, P_K = \frac{\pi^2\, EJ}{4\ l^2} = \frac{2{,}5\, EJ}{l^2}\ \text{kg: Knicklast } {}^1/_4 \text{ von Fall 2}$$

$$2 : {}^1/_2\, P_K = \frac{\pi^2\, EJ}{l^2} = \frac{10\, EJ}{l^2}\ \text{kg}$$

$$3 : {}^1/_3\, P_K = \frac{2\,\pi^2\, EJ}{l^2} = \frac{2\,OEJ}{l^2}\ \text{kg: Knicklast 2mal Fall 2}$$

$$4 : {}^1/_4\, P_K = \frac{4\,\pi^2\, EJ}{l^2} = \frac{40\, EJ}{l^2}\ \text{kg: Knicklast 4mal Fall 2}$$

Die vorausgesetzte Lagerung in Spitzengelenken ist im allgemeinen auch bei Bauwerken nicht zu verwirklichen. Ein Gelenk wird als feststehend, das andere als beweglich angenommen. Für den Femur würde das Kniegelenk beim Standbein oder Stemmbein (Gehen, Laufen usw.) das feste, das Hüftgelenk das bewegliche Gelenk sein. Die

Beweglichkeit des Beckens mit der Körperlast wird durch die zweigelenkigen Muskeln, M. rectus femoris und die ischiocruralen Muskeln, gewährt (KNESE, 1956a). Elektromyographische Untersuchungen (STELGES, 1962; RAHIMI, 1962) haben gezeigt, daß stets der M. rectus femoris und der M. semimembranosus eine gleichartige Innervation aufweisen; M. semitendinosus und M. biceps Cap. longum zeigen demgegenüber ein sehr unterschiedliches Innervationsmuster. Diese Beobachtung weist darauf hin, daß physikalische Untersuchungen durch solche am Lebenden zu kontrollieren sind. BASMAJIAN (1957) hat elektromyographisch nachgewiesen, daß die zweigelenkigen Muskeln immer auf beide übersprungene Gelenke gleichzeitig einwirken. Die elektromyographische Kontrolle der Muskelaktionen ist auch bei statischen Untersuchungen unbedingt erforderlich. Leider ist die Zahl der bewegungsphysiologischen Untersuchungen gering (BASMAJIAN, 1961), diejenigen der neurophysiologischen Grundlagen etwas umfangreicher (BASMAJIAN, 1967).

Der Euler-Fall 3, eine Seite eingespannt, andere Seite ein Gelenk, könnte für Skeletelemente bei Einklemmungen in einer Maschine usw. auftreten. Im allgemeinen ist aber wohl mit dem Euler-Fall 2 zu rechnen, für den die Art der Durchbiegung noch verfolgt werden soll. Die Gleichung der Krümmungskurve des Stabes ist $f = C_1 \sin \frac{z}{l}$, wobei z die untersuchte Querschnittshöhe ist. Die Konstante C_1 ist die größte Ausbiegung bei $z = {}^1/_2\, l$. Im Bereich sehr kleiner Ausbiegungen kann C_1 jeden beliebigen Wert annehmen, solange dieser nur sehr klein gegenüber l ist. Damit gibt es unendlich viele Gleichgewichtslagen, die der ursprünglichen Geraden benachbart sind; dieser theoretischen Mannigfaltigkeit entspricht die Vielfalt der Krümmungsformen des Femurs.

Unter der Annahme einer Lagerung in zwei Gelenken, in denen Kräfte angreifen (die Gelenkresultierenden s. S. 489), Längs- und Querkräften, hat nun KNESE (1956a) graphisch die Belastungsuntersuchung des Femurs durchgeführt (Abb. 55). Für die Sagittal- und Frontalebene wurden zunächst gesondert die Querkräfte und aus diesen Querkräften die Biegemomente bestimmt. Das sagittale Biegemoment beträgt 1350, das frontale 205 kgcm. Nun setzen Muskeln nicht in der Stabachse an — wie in der Biegetheorie vorausgesetzt wird — sondern „ausmittig". Überschreitet diese Ausmittigkeit ein bestimmtes Maß, den sog. Kern des Querschnittes, treten auch durch Längskräfte Biegemomente auf. So ergibt sich ein 2. Biegemoment Mb_2, das mit Mb_1 zu einem resultierenden Biegemoment Mb zu addieren ist. Das maximale Biegemoment erreicht dann in der Sagittalen 1312, in der Frontalen 167 kgcm. Da die ermittelte Momentenfläche durch eine mehrfach geknickte Linie umgrenzt wird, wurde eine Interpolation zu einer gleichmäßig gekrümmten Kurve durchgeführt — was zulässig ist, da die Kräfte mit punktförmigen Ansätzen und nicht linien- oder flächenförmigen gemessen wurden —; dabei muß aber die ursprüngliche und die interpolierte Momentenfläche flächengleich sein. Das maximale Biegemoment würde dann 950 kgcm betragen und nach ventral weisen. Proximal und distal schließen sich je ein kleineres und entgegengesetzt gerichtetes Biegemoment von 350 kgcm an.

Schließlich wurden die in Längsachse wirkenden Kraftkomponenten addiert, wodurch etwas oberhalb der Schaftmitte eine maximale Drucklast von $P_{\max} = 926$ kg erscheint. Dieser plötzliche Anstieg der Längskräfte ist ebenfalls auf die Messung der Muskelkräfte mit punktförmigen Ansätzen zurückzuführen, die unumgänglich war, da sich Muskelphantome mit flächenförmigem Ansatz nur unter größtem Aufwand herstellen lassen. So wäre hier auch eine Interpolation wie bei den Momentenflächen angebracht, auf die aber KNESE (1956a) verzichtet hat.

Im nächsten Schritt hat nun KNESE (1956a) für einzelne Querschnitte die sich aus diesem Belastungsgefüge ergebenden Spannungen errechnet (Abb. 56). Sie wurden zunächst gesondert für das sagittale und frontale Biegemoment und die Längskräfte als Spannungsdiagramm und als Spannungskörper dargestellt. Dann wurden die drei Spannungen addiert, wobei man im mittleren Femurquerschnitt (4) die höchste Spannung als Druckspannung $\sigma_{dR} = 685\ \text{kg} \cdot \text{cm}^{-2}$ erhält. Auffällig ist die sich bei der Addition ergebende Drehung der 0-Linie, die nun von lateral-dorsal nach ventral-medial verläuft, wie das auch für die Trägheitsmomente gilt (KNESE et al., 1955). Daraus kann geschlossen werden, daß die Trägheitsmomente der Knochenquerschnitte — unter Beachtung einer Reihe von Einschränkungen — auch Aussagen über die vermutliche Hauptbelastungsrichtung zulassen.

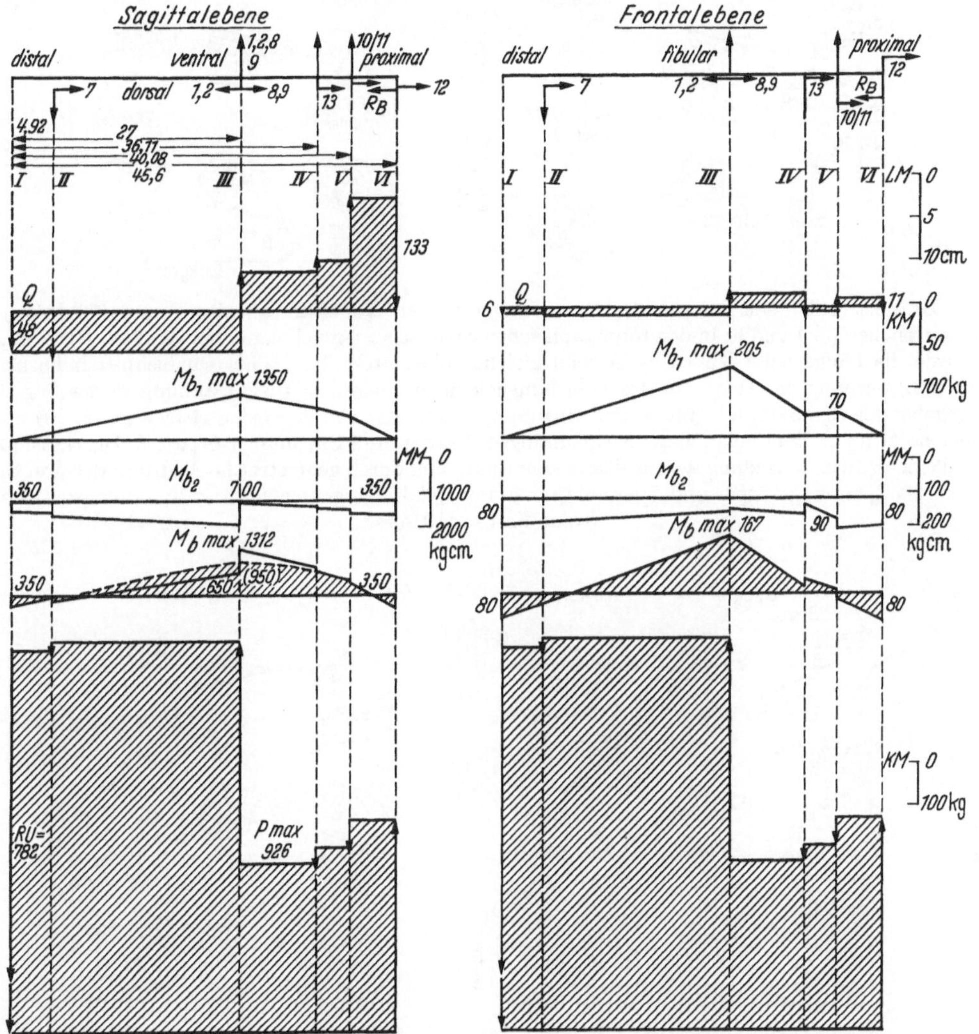

Abb. 55. Graphische Untersuchung der Oberschenkelbelastung bei Lagerung in zwei Gelenken. Darstellung in Sagittal- und Frontalebene. Zu oberst die Femurachse mit Ansatz und Richtung der Kraftkomponenten (vgl. Abb. 51, mit den Ziffern für die einzelnen Muskeln). Es folgen die Querkraftfläche Q, die Biegemomente Mb 1 durch die Querkräfte, die Biegemomente Mb 2 durch den ausmittigen Ansatz und das resultierende Biegemoment Mb mit Ausgleich der Sprünge in der Sagittalebene. Zu unterst die Druckbelastung P dargestellt als sog. lotrechte Längskräfte, d. h. die Druckkräfte werden um 90° gedreht auf der Knochenlängsachse aufgezeichnet; RU die Unterschenkelresultierende (vgl. KNESE, 1955a); LM Längenmaßstab; KM Kräftemaßstab; MM Momentenmaßstab in Sagittal- und Frontalebene verschieden (!) (Umzeichnung aus KNESE, 1956a)

Zur Aufklärung der Bedeutung der Querschnittsformen des Femurs und deren Flächenmomente wurden verschiedene Femora unter der Annahme der gleichen Belastung untersucht (Abb. 57). Ein Femur A hatte einen mehr rundlichen, B einen ausgeprägt dreieckigen (vgl. Abb. 40), C einen seitlich abgeplatteten Querschnitt und D war ein stark seitlich abgeplatteter rachitischer Femur (Abb. 41). Bei den Femora A, B, C bleiben die resultierenden Zugspannungen etwa gleich groß (205, 170, 205 kg · cm^{-2}),

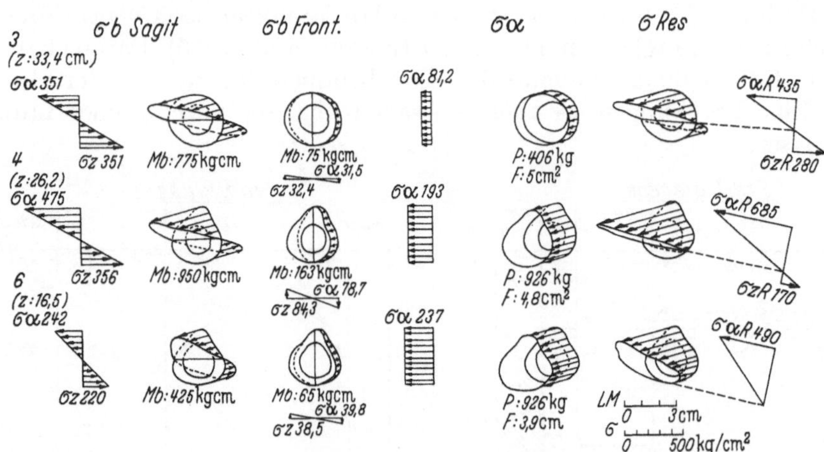

Abb. 56. Graphische Untersuchungen der Spannungen an den Querschnitten des Femur (79 Jahre) in drei Querschnittshöhen (3, 4 und 6: in den topographischen Strukturuntersuchungen von KNESE, RITSCHL, VOGES, 1954, wurde die Länge eines Knochens in zehn gleiche Teile unterteilt, die als Querschnittshöhe bezeichnet werden). z Entfernung des Querschnittes vom Kniegelenk; σ_b Sagit. = Biegespannung in der Sagittalebene wiedergegeben als Spannungsdiagramm und Spannungskörper; σ_b Front. = das gleiche in der Frontalebene; *Mb* Biegemoment; σ_d Druckspannung als Spannungsdiagramm und Spannungskörper; *P* Drucklast; *F* Querschnittsfläche; σ Res. = Bildung der resultierenden Spannung durch geometrische Addition der drei Spannungen als Spannungskörper und Spannungsdiagramm; *LM* Längenmaßstab; σ Spannungsmaßstab (aus KNESE, 1956a)

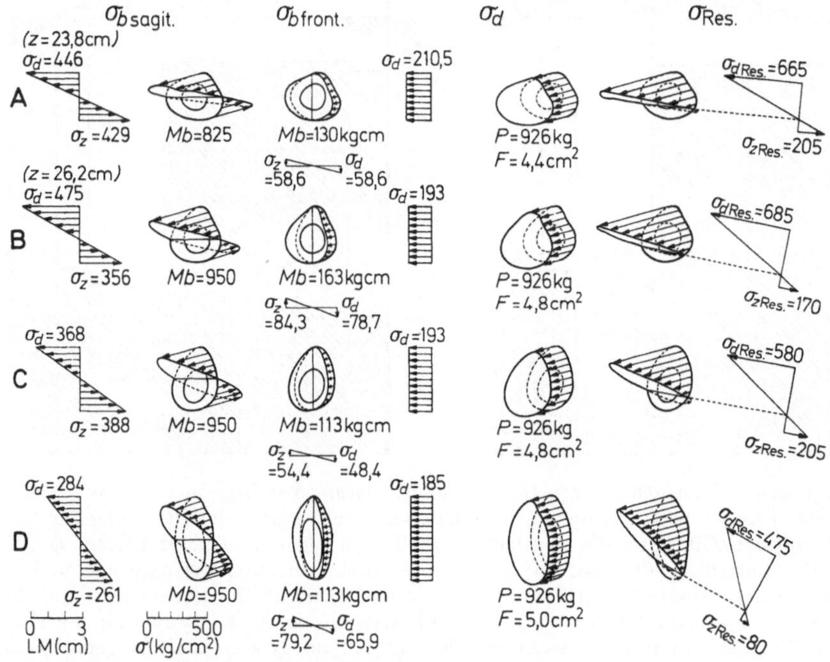

Abb. 57. Darstellung der Bedeutung der Querschnittsform und damit des Widerstandsmomentes für die Höhe der resultierenden Spannungen an den mittleren Querschnitten folgender vier Femora: *A* ♂, 43 Jahre; *B* ♂, 79 Jahre (vgl. Abb. 54); *C* (großer Sammlungsfemur, seitlich abgeplattet); *D* (rachitischer Femur) (vgl. Abb. 41). Bezeichnungen wie in Abb. 56 (aus KNESE, 1956a)

sind beim rachitischen auf 80 kg · cm^{-2} abgesunken. Die resultierenden Druckspannungen sind bei *A* und *B* wiederum von gleicher Größe (665, 685 kg · cm^{-2}), bei dem seitlich abgeplatteten und sehr großen Femur *C* auf 580 und bei dem rachitischen sogar auf 475 kg · cm^{-2} herabgesetzt. Bei dem rachitischen Femur sind bei angenommener gleicher

Belastung allein auf Grund der Querschnittsform die Spannungen relativ klein: Die Querschnittsform stellt eine „funktionelle Anpassung" bei vermutlich verminderter Festigkeit dar (s. S. 492).

Nun ist der nächste Schritt zu tun, die Bestimmung des Sicherheitsfaktors. Die maximale Spannung beträgt 685 kg · cm^{-2}. Der größere Teil der Femora (57,9%) hat eine Biegefestigkeit von 1780 ± 180 kg · cm^{-2}. Damit ergibt sich im gefährdeten Querschnitt ein Sicherheitsbeiwert von 2,6, der innerhalb des Bereiches von 1,8—3,0 liegt, der für (annähernd) spröde Stoffe auch bei Knickung gilt.

Zur Beurteilung der gesamten Form eines Röhrenknochens genügt jedoch nicht die Untersuchung des „gefährdeten" Querschnittes; es muß eine Reihe von Querschnitten und die anschließende Spongiosa auf ihre Sicherheit hin geprüft werden. Die errechnete Beanspruchung muß mit der vorhandenen Form und Festigkeit übereinstimmen (s. S. 418). KNESE (1955b) hatte zuvor zum Vergleich mit dem gleichen Kraftsystem die Belastung des Femurs im Sinne des einseitig eingespannten Kranes errechnet. Bei einer einseitigen Einspannung ist eine horizontale und vertikale Lagerreaktion sowie ein Einspannmoment zu berücksichtigen. Das größere sagittale Biegemoment nimmt vom Femurkopf zum Kniegelenk hin auf 4715 kgcm zu und entspricht in keiner Weise der Verteilung der Knochensubstanz, der Struktur.

Tabelle 19. *Biegemomente, Trägheitsmomente und Spannungen in der Sagittalebene bei der Kniebeuge* (nach KNESE, 1956a)

Querschnitt	M_b	I	$\delta_{d\ sag}$
3	775 kgcm	3,2 cm^4	351 kg·cm^{-2}
4	950	3,6	475
6	425	2,9	242

Bei Annahme der Lagerung in zwei Gelenken (KNESE, 1956a) ergibt sich dagegen bereits in der Sagittalen ein beachtliches Parallelgehen der Biegemomente, Trägheitsmomente und maximalen Spannungen (Tabelle 19).

Die Sicherheit und damit die funktionelle Gestalt kann aber nur unter Beachtung der topographisch unterschiedlichen Festigkeit des Knochengewebes ermittelt werden. KNESE (1956a) hat zunächst im Sinne einer Untersuchung der Tragfähigkeit, die ermittelten Längskräfte mit den Bruchlasten bei Druck in den vier Vierteln des Femurs verglichen (Tabelle 20). Die Bruchlast wurde dabei nur zu 70% eingesetzt, um einen Aus-

Tabelle 20. *Druckfestigkeit d, Bruchlast P der einzelnen Teile des Femurs sowie Sicherheitsfaktor ν* (nach KNESE, 1956a)

	Kopf	Hals	1. Viertel	2. Viertel	3. Viertel	4. Viertel	Kondylen
σ_d (kg · cm^{-2})	93,0	137	1060	1193	1145	829	48,5
P (kg)	1195	1445	4925	5234	4220	2553	1539
P 70% (kg)			3470	3675	2955	1787	
ν_1	*2,38*	*2,88*	8,5	3,96	3,2	*1,98*	*1,89*
ν_2			*2,44*	*1,77*	*2,34*		

σ_d, P Mittelwert aus vier Versuchen, Hals zwei Versuche. ν_1 Sicherheitsfaktor als Tragfähigkeit bei reiner Druckbelastung. ν_2 Sicherheitsfaktor an Hand der Druckspannungen.

gleich zwischen den auf Festigkeit untersuchten Prismen und der ganzen Diaphysenröhre zu erhalten (s. S. 426). Der sich ergebende Sicherheitsfaktor ν_1 ist in den proximalen $^3/_4$ des Schaftes über 3 und damit vermutlich zu groß, da die Biegespannungen unberücksichtigt blieben. Der Sicherheitsfaktor des proximalen Viertels von 8,5 ist sicher unzutreffend, da hier auf Grund der Experimentalanordnung (s. S. 486) die Längskräfte zu niedrig sind. Im distalen Viertel, in dem die Biegespannungen an Größe stark abgenommen haben, kann man den Sicherheitsfaktor von 1,98 wohl als zutreffend ansehen. Die Biegefestigkeit der einzelnen Teile der Diaphysenröhre ist nicht bekannt (vgl. MAJ, 1938). So hat sich KNESE (1956a) auf die Druckfestigkeit gestützt, da die resultierenden Spannungen Druckspannungen sind. Jedoch muß wohl angenommen werden, daß die Biegefestigkeit größer ist — etwa 25% — und demzufolge auch die Sicherheit in gleicher Größenordnung höher als die errechnete wird. Die an Hand der Druckfestigkeit errechneten Sicherheitsbeiwerte ν_2 liegen dann in den proximalen $^3/_4$ des Femurschaftes zwischen 1,77 und 2,44.

In gleicher Weise hat KNESE (1956a) den Sicherheitsfaktor der spongiösen Teile ermittelt, wobei die jeweilige Druckfestigkeit der Spongiosa mit der örtlichen Drucklast verglichen wurde. Für Kopf, Hals und Condylen ist der Sicherheitsbeiwert 1,89—2,88. Bei dieser Kalkulation wurde für die Condylen die Druckfestigkeit in Schaftlängsachse eingesetzt. Dieser Wert ist vermutlich zu klein. Bei der untersuchten Beugestellung des Femurs erfolgt der Druck von hinten auf die Condylen. Die Druckfestigkeit der Condylen von hinten nach vorn hat KNESE (1958b) später zu 99,1 gegenüber 58,9 kg · cm^{-2} in Längsachse ermittelt. Der mittlere Sicherheitsfaktor für die spongiösen und kompakten Teile des Femurs ist 2,45.

Die durchgeführte Kalkulation bezeichnet KNESE (1956a) als „Näherungslösung", da jener „Rechengang" aufgesucht wurde, der zwei gemessene Größen, die Muskelkräfte und die topographische Festigkeit, durch den Sicherheitsbeiwert miteinander verbindet. Dabei ergibt sich, daß in allen Teilen des Femurs, Spongiosa und Compacta, soviel „Material" in entsprechender Form und Festigkeit vorhanden ist, wie das für einen „Körper gleicher Festigkeit" anzunehmen ist. GEBHARDT (1910a) hatte gemeint, daß es für die Auffassung des Knochens als Körper gleicher Festigkeit nur auf eine „annähernd gesetzmäßige" Dickenzunahme der kompakten Wand ankomme, da die ideale Form nicht erreicht würde. Die Idealform eines Körpers gleicher Festigkeit für Biegung mit der äußeren Umgrenzung durch eine kubische Parabel setzt gleichartiges Material, Homogenität, voraus. „Die Knochenform ist als Idealform anzusehen, da sie dem wechselnden Spannungsgefüge nicht nur durch Form-, sondern auch Materialveränderungen gerecht wird" (KNESE, 1956a). Darüber hinaus kann man auch für den Femur einen Höchstbelastungsfall annehmen, der bei einer geringen Kniebeuge liegt, von der aus wir z.B. Lasten stemmen. Neuerlich wurde diese Auffassung von den verschiedenen Materialeigenschaften von SCHMITT (1968) an Hand von Untersuchungen der Materialdichte und der Bruchfestigkeit bestätigt. Danach wird die funktionelle Anpassung des Knochens und seine mechanische Beanspruchung nicht nur durch Änderung der Querschnittsfläche, sondern auch durch lokale Änderung der Materialdichte erreicht, die wiederum mit der Festigkeit korreliert ist. Die Frage, ob der Knochen ein Körper gleicher Festigkeit ist, wurde nunmehr von verschiedener Seite diskutiert (KUMMER, 1961, 1962, 1966; KNIEF, 1967a b; AMTMANN und SCHMITT, 1968).

Für das Sprunggelenk hat KNESE (unveröffentlicht) gleichartige Experimente mit Muskelphantomen durchgeführt. Hier sollen nur die sich bei Ermittlung der Beanspruchung der Unterschenkelknochen ergebenden Probleme, sowie die Frage erörtert werden, ob auch für diese Elemente eine gehörige Sicherheit vorliegt.

Der Unterschenkel besteht aus zwei Knochen, die durch die Membrana interossea sowie ein proximales und distales Gelenk miteinander verbunden sind. Diese Konstruktion gleicht einem stark modifizierten Gittermast, dessen einer Holm wesentlich stärker als der andere ist. Die Stäbe des Fachwerkes, der Membrana interossea, bestehen nur aus zugfesten Kollagenfasern. Die Fasern verlaufen überwiegend von der Tibia schräg distal zur Fibula (FICK, 1904). Schwächere Fasern ziehen vor und hinter dieser Schicht von der Fibula absteigend zur Tibia. Von der Fibula und der Membrana interossea entspringt eine große Zahl von Muskeln. Nach KUHN (1933) bewegt sich bei einer Dorsalflexion in den Sprunggelenken die in Ruhe nach medial gebogene Fibula nach lateral und distal. Die Membrana interossea wird gestrafft. Eine derartige Straffung der Membran muß aber auch bei jeder Muskelaktion auftreten. Jedoch muß wohl über die Bedeutung der Membrana interossea an Hand weiterer Versuche noch diskutiert werden, wie sich aus Experimenten am Unterarm ergibt. HALLS und TRAVILL (1964) haben die Druckübertragung mittels elektrischer Meßstreifen im Ellenbogengelenk gemessen. Zwischen Radius und Humerus werden 57 % und zwischen Ulna und Humerus 43 % der Last übertragen. Wird die Membrana interossea während des Versuches durchschnitten, zeigt die Kraftübertragung zwischen Ulna und Humerus zunächst eine Instabilität und geht dann zu den ursprünglichen Werten zurück. Die Autoren bezweifeln daher, daß die Membrana interossea des Unterarmes bei der Kraftübertragung eine Rolle spiele. Die Fibula als ein nachgebender Knochen (KUHN, 1933) zeigt im Biegeversuch auch eine starke Ausbiegung bis zu 14 mm (s. S. 497). So kann man wohl annehmen, daß die Muskelkraft aller Unterschenkelmuskeln überwiegend die Tibia belastet. KIMURA (1966) kommt auf Grund von elektrischen Dehnungsmessungen zum Schluß, daß der Schaft der Tibia nicht nur das Körpergewicht in Längsrichtung trägt, sondern auch den Muskelkräften beim Gehen Widerstand leistet. Die Gestalt der Tibia-Querschnitte spricht für einen Widerstand gegenüber Biegung durch Muskelkräfte, wobei der größte Durchmesser der Tibia auf die höchste Beanspruchung hinweist.

Das proximale Ende der Tibia ist Bestandteil des Kniegelenkes. Somit war zu fragen, ob die das Kniegelenk stabilisierenden Muskeln auch bei Belastungsuntersuchungen des Unterschenkels zu berücksichtigen sind. Die zum Kniegelenk gehörenden Muskeln setzen am proximalen Teil des Unterschenkels an und „drücken“ demzufolge die Tibia gegen den Femur. Sie rufen damit einen Teil der Stütz- oder Lagerreaktionen hervor, die mit entsprechenden Kräften des Oberschenkels im Gleichgewicht stehen.

Die Ursprünge der Unterschenkelmuskeln reichen bis in die Ansatzzone der Oberschenkelmuskeln hinein, so daß sich hier entgegengesetzt gerichtete Kräfte überdecken. Ähnliche Verhältnisse der Muskeltopographie mit Überdeckungszonen von in entgegengesetzter Richtung wirkenden Muskeln finden sich an allen Gelenken. Vermutlich stehen diese Kräfte derart im Gleichgewicht, daß in den übersprungenen Skeletteilen keine „Zerreißzonen“ auftreten. Dieser Überdeckungs- bzw. Verflechtungsbereich ist am Oberschenkel und Oberarm recht groß, am Unterarm und Unterschenkel dagegen kleiner.

Die „Systemgrenze“ eines Gelenkes muß bis an die proximalen und distalen Muskelursprünge und -ansätze herangelegt werden, d.h. die Grenzen des funktionellen Systems eines Gelenkes liegen mitten in den Skeletstücken. Die Systemgrenzen stellen durch die miteinander verzahnten Muskeln eine unterschiedlich breite Zone dar, die sich als Amputationshöhe der Wahl erwiesen hat. Für die Amputationshöhe ist allerdings weiterhin die Gestaltung eines prothesengerechten Stumpfes von Bedeutung.

Die Verflechtung der Muskeln benachbarter Systeme macht die Beanspruchung der Skeletteile in diesen Bereichen sehr verwickelt. Jedoch sind die Muskeln nur bei jenen Gelenken zu berücksichtigen, die sie überspringen und in denen sie entsprechende Lagerreaktionen hervorrufen. So können demzufolge die Muskeln des Kniegelenkes bei Belastungsuntersuchungen des Unterschenkels unberücksichtigt bleiben. Dagegen ist als Last das Körpergewicht einzusetzen, das dann erst mit dem Erdboden nach dem Prinzip actio-reactio im Gleichgewicht steht. Da nur senkrecht zu Flächen eine Stützungsreaktion möglich ist, haben wir das Körpergewicht mit Angriff in der Mitte des Kniegelenkes in Rechnung gesetzt. Mit der gleichen Begründung haben wir die Kraft des M. gastrocnemius als Druckkraft in Richtung des Unterschenkels angenommen.

Mit den Muskelphantomen konnten in einer Plantarflexion im Sprunggelenk bei leichter Anbeugung des Kniegelenkes die größten Kräfte gemessen werden. Der fixierte Fuß stand dabei auf einer gegen die Horizontale um 30° geneigten Ebene, d.h. in einer Stellung, die der an einem Startloch oder an einem Startklotz gleicht. Für diese Stellung wurde — wie beim Femur — die Belastungsuntersuchung graphisch durchgeführt (Abb. 58). Durch die Querkräfte in der Frontalen ergibt sich ein Biegemoment von 310 kg · cm. Wird zu diesem Moment das durch den ausmittigen Muskelansatz hinzuaddiert und die Momentenfläche mit einer durchgehenden Kurve umgrenzt, ist das maximale sagittale Biegemoment zu 400 kg · cm zu veranschlagen. Für die Frontalebene wurde in gleicher Weise ein maximales Moment von 530 kg · cm errechnet. Hinzu treten dann die Längskräfte mit 522 kg.

Die Spannungen durch die beiden Biegemomente und die Längskräfte wurden für drei verschiedene Querschnitte berechnet und zu einer resultierenden Spannung addiert. In allen Querschnitten verschiebt sich die 0-Linie weit an die Crista anterior heran und verläuft von dorsal-lateral nach ventral medial (Abb. 59). Die Maximalspannungen treten

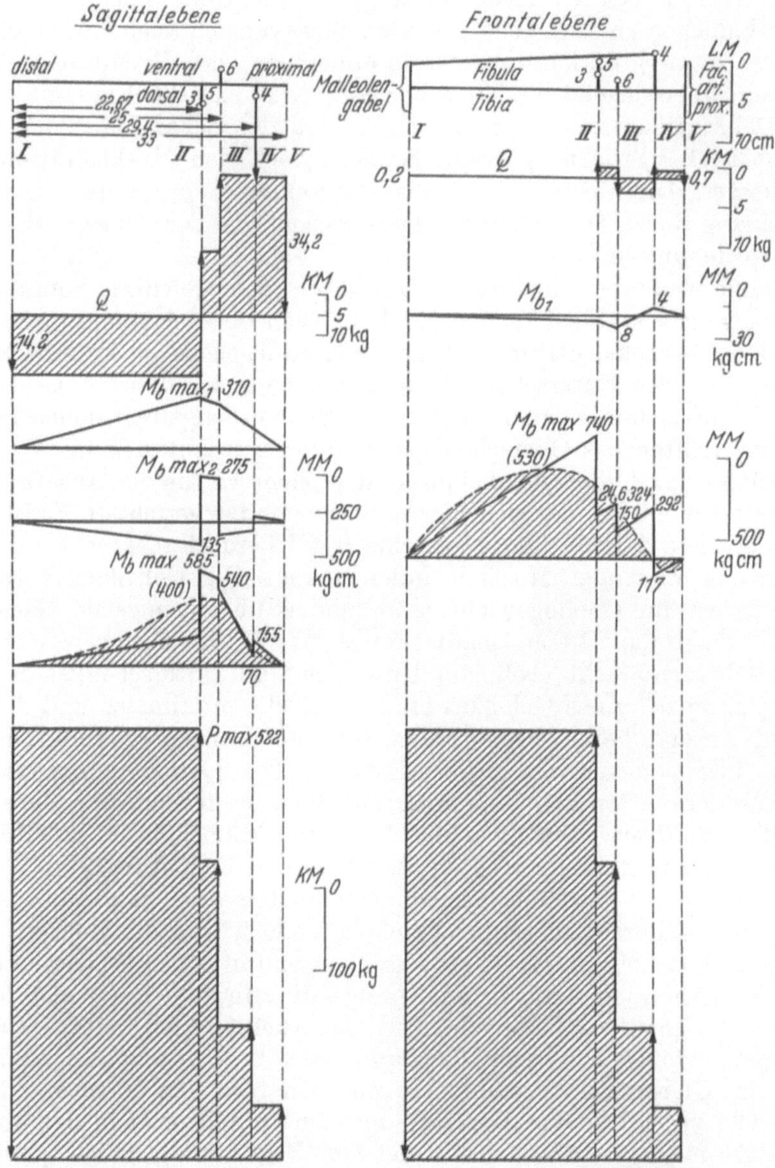

Abb. 58. Graphische Untersuchung der Belastung des Unterschenkels bei Lagerung in zwei Gelenken. Darstellung in Sagittal- und Frontalebene (vgl. Abb. 53). Querschnitt I: Sprunggelenke; Querschnitt II: Ursprung M. flexor hallucis longus (*3*), M. extensor digitorum (*5*); Querschnitt III: M. tibialis anterior (*6*); Querschnitt IV: M. fibularis longus (*4*); Querschnitt V: Kniegelenk (Knese, unveröffentlicht)

dorsal als Druckspannungen auf, denen geringere Zugspannungen auf der Ventralseite entgegenstehen. In den drei Querschnitten wurden folgende resultierenden Druck- zu Zugspannungen ermittelt: Proximal: 450/205; Mitte 640/490 und distal 728/220 kg · cm^{-2}.

Die Anlage der Versuche gestattet nur die Prüfung des Sicherheitsbeiwertes für die maximale Druckspannung von 728 kg · cm^{-2}. Die größere Anzahl der Tibien (47,1%) hat eine Biegebruchfestigkeit von 1780 $\pm$ 180 kg · cm^{-2}. So ergibt sich ein Sicherheitsbeiwert von 2,44, der dem beim Femur entspricht. Damit ist zu vermuten, daß auch die

Tibia wie der Femur ein Körper gleicher Festigkeit ist; der Nachweis dieser Vermutung erfordert allerdings einen noch größeren experimentellen Aufwand als für den Oberschenkel, ob mit Erfolg, ist schwer zu entscheiden. Für die obere Extremität (KNESE, 1956b) konnten mit Muskelphantomen keine „Maximalkräfte" gemessen werden.

Umfassende Studien zur Mechanik langer Röhrenknochen hat EHLER (1963, 1966, 1967, 1968) für Humerus, Radius und Ulna vorgelegt. Das Material entstammt mit Formalin konservierten Leichen von Individuen über 70 Jahren. Zu bedauern ist, daß von EHLER für die Experimente völlig ungeeignetes Material gewählt wurde („es war jahrelang unter ungünstigen Bedingungen trocken konserviert worden": EHLER 1967a), so daß der folgende Aufwand der Versuchsbearbeitung nicht zu eindeutig verwertbaren Ergebnissen führt. Versuchsdurchführung und Auswertung einschließlich Berücksichtigung der Flächenmomente und ausmittiger Kräfte sind nämlich von allergrößter Genauigkeit. EHLER (1963) kritisiert unter Anerkennung der hierbei zu überwindenden Schwierigkeiten in diesem Zusammenhang einige der vereinfachenden Annahmen von KNESE (1955, 1956), die zur Erzielung einer Näherungslösung den Berechnungen zugrunde gelegt wurden; sie aber ermöglichten erst den Vergleich mit experimentell ermittelten Festigkeitswerten. EHLER (1963, 1966a, 1967b) führte an den Knochen der oberen Extremität Zugversuche durch, eine Beanspruchungsform, die in vivo vermutlich eine geringe Rolle spielt. Die untersuchten Humeri verhielten sich bis zur Belastung von 100 kg sehr ähnlich, eine „Fließgrenze" wurde bei etwa 250 kg festgestellt. Als schwächste Stelle des Humerus erschien bei dieser Versuchsanordnung, das Collum chirurgicum bzw. das distale Drittel. Leider übersieht EHLER (1966a) bei seinen Versuchen, daß der kompakte Schaftteil nicht bis an die Grenze seiner Beanspruchung belastet wird und verstößt damit gegen die eigene Feststellung: „In der Form steckt die ganze Physik. Wer die Form vernachlässigt, vernachlässigt die ganze Knochenphysik!" Aus Torsions- (EHLER, 1966b) und Biegeversuchen (EHLER, 1967a) wird geschlossen, daß „Druck schlechter als Zug, aber besser als Biegung vertragen wird; am empfindlichsten ist der Knochen ... gegen Torsion." Eine äußere periodische Kraft von 100 kg hat etwa die gleiche Auswirkung wie eine statische Kraft von 400—1000 kg bei Zugwirkung (EHLER und PFAU, 1968).

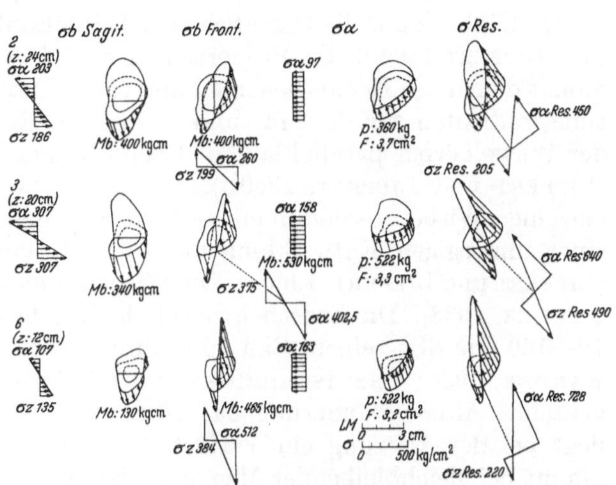

Abb. 59. Graphische Untersuchung der Spannungen in drei Tibiaquerschnitten. Bezeichnungen wie Abb. 56 (unveröffentlicht)

d) Die Mechanik der kurzen Knochen: Die Wirbelsäule

Die Mechanik der Wirbelsäule wurde vor allem im Hinblick auf die Eigenschaften der Zwischenwirbelscheiben untersucht; über die Festigkeit der Wirbelspongiosa wurde bereits berichtet. Obwohl die Mechanik der „Zwischenwirbelscheibe" nicht mehr zum Thema Knochengewebe gehört, soll das Ergebnis der vorliegenden Arbeiten referiert werden, da das im allgemeinen vernachlässigte Zusammenspiel von Knochen und Bandapparat an der Wirbelsäule experimentell untersucht wurde.

Nach v. MEYER (1873) besteht ein Widerspiel zwischen den wie Wasserkissen gebauten Bandscheiben und den zwischen den Wirbelbögen gelegenen elastischen Ligg. flava. Die

Fasern der gelben Bänder suchen eine möglichst geringe Länge einzunehmen und verformen dadurch die Bandscheiben, die ihrerseits der Verformung Widerstand leisten und damit die Bänder wieder anspannen. Durch dieses Spiel entsteht die „Eigenform“ der Wirbelsäule (VIRCHOW, 1909), dabei hat jede Wirbelsäule ihre Individualform (SULLIVAN und MILES, 1959; vgl. KNESE, 1963a). Die von den Wirbelkörpern abgetrennte Bogenreihe verkürzt sich um 3,5—4,5 cm, d.h. etwa um $^1/_7$ der Wirbelsäulenlänge und gewinnt ihre ursprüngliche Länge erst durch einen Zug von 2 kg wieder. Jedoch behält die Wirbelkörperreihe nach Abtrennung der Bogen ihre Form bei (FICK, 1904). FICK (1911) bezweifelt demzufolge die von v. MEYER und VIRCHOW angenommene Wirkung der Ligg. flava, die immerhin in der Lende eine Dicke von 0,3 cm erreichen. Neuere Untersuchungen lassen vermuten, daß das Zusammenspiel innerhalb des Bandapparates der Wirbelsäule recht verwickelt ist.

Im Hinblick auf die Eigenform der Wirbelsäule ist von Bedeutung, daß nach DZIALLAS und LIPPERT (1960) die Proportionen des einzelnen Wirbelkörpers bereits im 4. Fetalmonat denen des Erwachsenen entsprechen. LIPPERT und LIPPERT (1960a) fanden Wachstumsgradienten für die prä- und postnatale Entwicklung, die der statischen Belastung der Wirbelkörper parallel laufen. Ebenso zeigen sich fetal schon Geschlechtsunterschiede (LIPPERT und LIPPERT, 1960b). Die in der Fetalzeit vorhandenen Charakteristika der einzelnen Wirbel werden in einem kontinuierlichen Differenzierungsprozeß, z.T. im Sinne einer umwegigen Entwicklung ausgestaltet, vor allem im Cervical- und Sacralbereich (LIPPERT und LIPPERT, 1960c). Die Wirbelsäulenkrümmungen sind fetal angelegt (HASSELWANDER, 1938). Die Zwischenwirbelscheiben besitzen bei menschlichen Keimlingen von 70—140 mm SSL einen Bau, der ihrer späteren Beanspruchung entspricht (HASSELWANDER, 1938; BRETTSCHNEIDER, 1952; TÖNDURY, 1958). Die makroskopisch zu beobachtende Altersveränderung hat TÖNDURY (1955) beschrieben. Nach SYLVÉN (1951a, b) liegt bei der Alterung ein Verlust der Gelstruktur vor. Der Anteil der Kollagenfasern nimmt bei gleichbleibender Menge der Kohlenhydrate zu, so daß der Wassergehalt herabgesetzt wird (HIRSCH et al., 1953).

GOECKE (1932) fand im Spannungs-Dehnungsdiagramm, daß im kindlichen Alter eine höhere Elastizität als im Alter vorliegt. Die einzelnen Zwischenwirbelscheiben verhalten sich bei der gleichen Person sehr unterschiedlich; in der oberen Brustwirbelsäule ist die Elastizität größer als in der Lende. Die Quellbarkeit in verdünnten Säuren, Salzlösungen und Laugen ist gering. Die Wasseraufnahme erreicht bei Kindern 95% des Gewichtes, bei erwachsenen Männern 50—60%, bei Greisen nur die Hälfte dieses Wertes. VIRGIN (1951) hat an feucht gehaltenen Zwischenwirbelscheiben mit anschließenden Wirbelendplatten beobachtet, daß die Verformung nicht der Last parallel geht und bei Entlastung ein Dehnungsrest bleibt. Dabei ergeben sich starke topographische und Altersunterschiede. Bei einer Belastung mit 22,7 kg über 48 Std ist die Deformation gering und die Rückkehr zur ursprünglichen Höhe erfolgt relativ schnell. Die Zwischenwirbelscheiben haben demzufolge eine gute Erholungsfähigkeit.

INGELMARK und EKHOLM (1952) stellten an dem Discus L 3/4 fest, daß bei stehender Last die Verformung noch zunimmt und bei Entlastung ein Dehnungsrest bleibt. Bei Wiederholung des Versuches ist die Verkürzung geringer. Die Verfasser haben in die Markhöhle der benachbarten Wirbel Pferdeserum eingefüllt, fanden aber keine Veränderung der elastischen Eigenschaften der Bandscheiben. Die Zusammendrückung ist bei älteren Leuten größer als bei jungen.

LANGMAACK (1954) hat die Zwischenwirbelscheiben statisch und im Dauerschlagversuch belastet. Das Belastungsgewicht betrug bei 28 Lastwechseln in der Minute 100 kg. Die Einstellung der Wirbelsäule erfolgte derart, daß neben Druck- auch eine Biegebelastung vorlag. Der Einfluß von 135000 Lastwechseln ist gering. Eine Durchschneidung der vorderen Längsbänder stört das Gleichgewicht, die Zwischenwirbelscheiben sind elastischer und die Deformation geringer. Vermutlich haben sich die Bandscheiben in der Quere gedehnt. Bei einer Wirbelsäule wurde nach 280000 Lastwechseln das vordere

Längsband in Höhe L 3/4 und L 4/5 durchschnitten und die bleibende Zusammendrückung nahm bis zu 305000 Lastwechseln zu. Bei einer weiteren Wirbelsäule wurde vor dem Dauerschlagversuch die Durchtrennung des Längsbandes an den angegebenen Orten vorgenommen, wodurch die bleibende Verformung vom Versuchsbeginn an wuchs. Eine Zerstörung der Wirbel oder Bandscheiben wurde nicht beobachtet. LANGMAACK weist auf das „verwirrende Geflecht" der Wirbelsäulenbänder hin, die er als Kraftzerstreuer ansieht.

Die Auswirkung einer Beschleunigung von 14 g für 0,1 sec haben PATRIK, LISSNER und EVANS (1960) an 3 Leichen geprüft, die in einem Flugzeug-Schleudersitz, befestigt an Kopf, Schulter, Rumpf, Arm und Füßen, entsprechend in einem Fahrstuhlschacht bewegt wurden. Bei dieser Beschleunigung in Längsachse des Körpers treten Zugbeanspruchungen in der Halsregion und Druckbeanspruchungen in der Thorax- und Lendenregion auf. Bei beweglichem Kopf sind auch in der Halsregion Druckbeanspruchungen zu beobachten. Die Größe der Druckbeanspruchungen entspricht der Bewegungsgröße von Kopf und Thorax. Wirbelfrakturen wurden röntgenologisch bei diesen Versuchen nicht beobachtet. Die Auswirkung von Schwingungen der Wirbelsäule erzeugt von der Sitzfläche her, hat KRAUSE (1963) am lebenden Menschen durch Anbringung von Meßeinrichtungen (Dehnungsstreifen und Spiegel zur Winkelmessung) untersucht. Die Schwingungen breiten sich von der Wirbelsäule her auf die daran aufgehängten Teilsysteme aus und wirken wiederum auf die Wirbelsäule zurück, so daß ein recht komplexes Geschehen vorliegt. KRAUSE fand in der Lendenwirbelsäule hohe Biege- und Torsionswinkel, dagegen durch die Versteifung mit Hilfe des Brustkorbes nicht in der Brustregion. Hierbei erfährt die Zwischenwirbelscheibe L 3/4 die größte Deformation, und zwar durch Biegung bei 10 und 35—40 Hz, durch Torsion bei 20 und 32,5—40 Hz. Die Amplitude der longitudinalen Schwingungen liegt wiederum bei der Zwischenwirbelscheibe L 3/4 am höchsten.

WYSS und ULRICH (1954) schätzen die Druckkraft auf die Bandscheibe L 5/S 1 auf 100—250 kg. Die Zusammendrückung ist bei 300 kg Last und der Flächenlast von 15 kg $\cdot$ cm^{-2} 12—18 % der Discushöhe. Die Autoren haben die Wirbelsäule mit und ohne Gelenkreihe einer Zugbelastung unterworfen. Die Dicke des Faserringes läßt sich auf Grund seiner Struktur nicht bestimmen; die Dehnbarkeit ist aber erheblich, mit Gelenken 15 % (Last 120 kg, Flächenlast 5,4 kg $\cdot$ cm^{-2}) und ohne Gelenke 16 % der Höhe (Last 120 kg, Flächenlast 6,3 kg $\cdot$ cm^{-2}). Das hintere Längsband trägt wesentlich zur Verstärkung des dorsalen Anteils der Zwischenwirbelscheibe bei. An der von den Körpern getrennten Bogenreihe von L 1—S 1 ist die Verformung bis zu 60 kg Zug zunächst stark, bei höheren Lasten schwächer. Bei 120 kg erfolgte ein Riß der Gelenkkapsel S 1/L 5. Bis zu 60 kg war die Dehnung 11 %. Die gemessenen Werte sind vermutlich etwas zu klein, da die Fixierung in der Prüfmaschine des Präparates nicht vollständig gelang.

Mit einer Stützweite von 125 mm haben WYSS und ULRICH (1954) L 1—L 5 von ventral mit 30 kg belastet und erhielten eine Durchbiegung von 3,3 mm, bei Belastung von dorsal war sie 3,6 mm. Die Verformung erfolgt proportional zur Last. Die Neutrallinie liegt bei dieser Biegung im dorsalen Teil des Wirbelkörpers. Die Längenänderung beträgt 4—16 % bei den Zwischenwirbelscheiben und zwischen den Wirbelbögen 10—20 %. Im Torsionsversuch der Wirbelreihe L 3—L 5 ist die Verdrehung bei 1 mkg 2^0, bei 2 mkg 5^0 und dann mit einer bleibenden Verformung verbunden. Die Zerstörung am Übergang von der Bandscheibe L 3/4 in den Wirbelkörper trat bei 4,5 mkg und einer Verdrehung von 20^0 auf.

Im Scherversuch haben WYSS und ULRICH (1954) die Wirbel L 1—S 3 ohne Gelenke mit Querdruck auf L 3 untersucht, so daß die Bandscheiben L 2/3 und L 3/4 belastet wurden. Bis zur Scherkraft $P/2 = 100$ kg erfolgte die Verschiebung proportional, und zwar ohne Berücksichtigung der Drehung um 2 mm, mit Drehung von 4,5 mm. Die Bandscheiben wurden bei 370 kg zerstört. Der Nucleus pulposus reagierte bei 2 mm Verschiebung. Auf die Bedeutung der Gelenke bei Querkräften wird hingewiesen.

Die schwächste Stelle der Zwischenwirbelscheibe ist nach WYSS und ULRICH (1954) der Übergang in den Wirbelkörper und dann wiederum ist die Bandscheibe L 5/S 1 die schwächste. Auf die aus diesen Versuchen gezogenen Schlüsse zur Behandlung des Bandscheibenvorfalles kann hier nicht eingegangen werden.

HIRSCH und NACHEMSON (1954) haben in Fortsetzung älterer Untersuchungen (HIRSCH, 1951) Dicken- und Breitenveränderungen der Zwischenwirbelscheiben verfolgt. Bei einer statischen Last erfolgt die Deformation in wenigen Sekunden und nähert sich asymptotisch einem bestimmten Wert an. Eine Deformation durch 130 kg über 5 min ist reversibel. Bei längerer Krafteinwirkung ist die Erholungszeit recht erheblich und Schäden sind nicht ausgeschlossen. Jede Bandscheibe wurde drei Versuchen unterzogen, einem mit Bögen, einem nach Hemilaminektomie und einem nach vollständiger Bogendurchtrennung. Die 4. Lendenscheibe ist stärker zusammendrückbar als die 2. Bei 100 kg beträgt die Verformung der Bandscheibe 1,4 mm und die Verbreiterung nach vorn 0,75 mm. Belastungen von wenigen Sekunden ergeben volle Elastizität und können beliebig wiederholt werden. Die Durchtrennung der Bögen ändert die Tragfähigkeit nicht. Bei vertikaler Last ist demzufolge die Zwischenwirbelscheibe der allein tragende Teil. Degenerierte Bandscheiben lassen sich leichter zusammendrücken und sind empfindlicher gegen höhere Lasten. Zwischenwirbelscheiben haben die Fähigkeit, sich auf eine statische Last einzustellen, d.h. sie gewinnen eine Gleichgewichtslage. Bei einer statischen Vorlast von 10 bis 130 kg und einer zusätzlichen Schlaglast von 30 kg gerät dann die Bandscheibe in Vibration. Kurze zusätzliche Belastungen steigern damit die Deformation in hohem Grade. Diese Formänderungen haben ein Ausmaß und eine Frequenz, die durch Muskeln nicht verhindert werden kann. Die Schwingungen sind unabhängig von der statischen Gleichgewichtslage der Bandscheibe. Dorsalflexionen erhöhen nach NACHEMSON (1963) nicht nur die vertikale, sondern auch die tangentiale Beanspruchung der Zwischenwirbelscheibe.

PEREY (1957) hat in Zwischenwirbelscheiben Kontrastmittel injiziert und dessen Verhalten bei dynamischer Belastung untersucht, und zwar bei Kräften von 1050, 1200, 1250 und 1350 mkg in 6/1000 sec. Das Kontrastmittel verändert seine Lage nur bei einem gleichzeitigen Wirbelschaden. Kompressionsfrakturen traten bei 8%, Frakturen der Wirbelendplatten bei 26% der Versuche auf. Bei statischer Last auf Präparate aus zwei Wirbeln mit dazwischen gelegener Scheibe ergaben eine Bruchlast von 425 kg (290—530) bei Personen über 60 Jahren und solchen unter 40 von 780 kg (510—1100). Bei 32% der Versuche waren Endplattenbrüche zu beobachten, bei Präparaten aus drei Wirbeln bei 42%. Die Größe der Wirbelkörperendflächen wächst von 14,3 cm² bei L 1 auf 18,0 cm² bei L 5, von dieser Fläche nimmt der Nucleus pulposus etwa 26% ein.

Die ersten Untersuchungen über die Energieabsorption durch die Zwischenwirbelscheiben stammen nach EVANS und LISSNER (1959) von RUFF. Für den Abschnitt Th 10 bis L 3, einer Last von 690 kg und einer Deformation von 12 mm beträgt die Energieabsorption 4,5 kgm, für Th 7 bis L 1 und 540 kg sowie der Deformation 4,5 mm 1,4 kgm, ein Wert, der vermutlich recht klein ist. EVANS und LISSNER (1959) haben frische und fixierte Wirbelsäulen vertikaler Last und einer Biegebelastung von ventral und lateral unterworfen (Tabelle 21). Durch Fixierung steigt die Tragfähigkeit, die Deformation wird herabgesetzt. Die Verformung bei Biegung von lateral her ist größer als bei ventralem Kraftangriff. Die Deformation ist zu Beginn der Belastung gering, dann stärker anwachsend; bei lateralem Kraftangriff steigt sie dagegen schnell an. Die Energieabsorption ist am größten bei vertikaler Last (frisch 6,55, fixiert 6,95 kgm), am geringsten bei lateralem Kraftangriff (3,18 kgm). Die Energieabsorption wird durch die Fixierung nicht beeinflußt. EVANS und LISSNER (1965) fanden, daß bei feucht untersuchten fixierten Zwischenwirbelscheiben die Größe der Energieabsorption von den ersten zu den letzten Zwischenwirbelscheiben fast auf das Doppelte ansteigt. Altersbeziehungen konnten nicht beobachtet werden.

Die Untersuchungen der Mechanik der Zwischenwirbelscheiben lassen vermuten, daß die Konzeption von v. MEYER (1873) und VIRCHOW (1909) über das Zusammenspiel der

Tabelle 21. *Verformung nach Energieabsorption der Wirbelsäule* (nach EVANS, 1959)

Objekt	Last (kg)	Verformung (mm)	Absorbierte Energie (kgcm)	Biegemoment
	Senkrechte Last			
P[1]—L_1 fixiert	369	28,9	6,95	
	(276—453)	(19,1—44,8)	(2,46—13,3)	
P—Th_{12} frisch	246	39,6	6,55	
	(131—313)	(26,9—60,3)	(2,01—11,7)	
	Biegung: Kraftangriff ventral			
S[2]—L_1 fixiert	254	27,4	3,47	802
	(224—283)	(26,6—27,9)	(3,41—3,51)	(714—889)
S—Th_5 frisch	147	45,7	3,53	990
	(91—204)	(40,2—51,4)	(2,0—5,05)	(808—1170)
S—Th_7 frisch	100	49,7	2,14	890
	Biegung: Kraftangriff lateral			
S—L_1 fixiert	171	32,0	3,18	544
	(113—224)	(21,1—38,8)	(2,46—4,53)	(360—715)

[1] Pelvis: einschließlich Becken.
[2] Sacrum: einschließlich Sacrum.

Bandscheiben und elastischen Bänder zu einfach ist, obwohl sich keine der neueren Untersuchungen unmittelbar der Bedeutung der recht kräftigen Ligg. flava zugewandt hat.

e) Die Mechanik der platten Knochen

Die Plattentheorie ist ungewöhnlich schwierig. Lösungen wurden für ebene biegesteife Platten regelmäßiger Form und unterschiedlicher Einspannung, für Umdrehungsschalen als biegesteife oder biegeschlaffe Platten, für Rohre unter Innendruck usw. entwickelt. Als Ausgangspunkt dieser Lösungen wird mitunter die Membrantheorie gewählt. Man denkt sich auch einen Streifen aus einer solchen Platte herausgeschnitten. Dieser Streifen wird dann auf Biegung usw. hin untersucht. Die Plattentheorie kann hier jedoch übergangen werden, da bisher kein Versuch vorliegt, platte Knochen unter diesen Gesichtspunkten zu betrachten.

α) Das Becken

Bei der Statik des menschlichen Beckens wurde vor allem über die Beanspruchung der Symphyse diskutiert (v. MEYER, 1873; FICK, 1911; LESSHAFT, 1892; KRUKENBERG, 1928; LÜHKEN, 1935; PAUWELS, 1948). Die Spaltlinien wurden am menschlichen Becken von BENNINGHOFF (1925), an tierischen von SCHWENKENBECHER (1935; vgl. OLIVIER und LIBERSEA, 1954) untersucht. Die Konstruktion des Beckens ist sehr differenziert, da bereits das Hüftbein aus zwei aufeinander senkrecht stehenden und im Acetabulum miteinander verbundenen Rahmenkonstruktionen (vgl. WEIDENREICH, 1922) besteht, nämlich der Darmbeinschaufel und der Umrahmung des Foramen obturatum. Beide Platten dienen sowohl auf ihrer Innen- als auch Außenseite als Muskelursprungsflächen. Von der Crista iliaca geht die aponeurotische Fascie des M. gluteus medius aus, so daß dieser Muskel einerseits von der Darmbeinschaufel und andererseits von der Fascie entspringt (vgl. WEIDENREICH, 1922; KNESE, 1956a, 1958b). SMITH (1962a) hat das Spannungsbild des Hüftbeines im Vergleich zu den entgegengesetzt wirkenden Druckkräften des Femurkopfes untersucht. Die Flächenbelastung im Bereich des Ursprunges der kleinen Glutaeen schätzt JIPP (1960) auf 1 kg · cm^{-2}.

Die Hüftbeine sind einmal in der Symphyse miteinander und dann gelenkig mit dem Sacrum verbunden; hinzu treten das Lig. sacrotuberale und Lig. sacrospinosum. Das Lig. sacrotuberale dient auch dem M. gluteus maximus als Ursprung; das Lig. sacrospinale bildet gleichzeitig als M. coccygicus den hinteren Teil des Diaphragma pelvis. Die Verbindung des Hüftbeines mit dem Kreuzbein (vgl. Fick, 1911) hat eine größere Beweglichkeit als vermutet wurde (Weisl, 1954a, b; Barabás et al., 1961; vgl. Schunke, 1938). Beachtlich sind auch die Veränderungen der Festigkeit der Symphyse unter dem Einfluß von Sexualhormonen (unter anderem Crelin, 1954a, b, 1955, 1960; Crelin und Levin, 1955). Schließlich bestehen sehr enge Beziehungen zu den Eingeweiden, die sich unter anderem in der geschlechtsspezifischen Form des kleinen Beckens zeigen.

Die Statik der Knochen-Bindegewebskonstruktion „Becken“ ist z.Z. kaum befriedigend aufzuklären. Systematische Untersuchungen der Festigkeit des Beckens hat zuerst Messerer (1880) durchgeführt. Bei Druck von der Symphyse zum Kreuzbein tritt ein Bruch im horizontalen und absteigenden Ast des Schambeines auf; die Drucklast beträgt bei Männern 200—300 und Frauen 170—300 kg, für beide im Mittel 250 kg. Ein querer Druck im Mittel von 180 kg auf die Crista iliaca führt zu einer Luxation des Kreuz-Darmbein-Gelenkes. Ein querer Druck auf die Acetabula verformte den Beckeneingang zu einer Ellipse mit Hervortreten der Schambeine. In einem Falle verkürzte sich der Querdurchmesser um 27 mm und kehrte nach dem Bruch fast vollständig zur ursprünglichen Form mit einer Verkürzung von 4 mm zurück. Der Bruch des Beckens geht „in der Regel ganz ruhig und ohne Krachen“ vor sich. Nach Aufhören der Belastung und nach dem Bruch verschwindet auch die Verformung. Der Bruch bei Belastung des Acetabulums war einseitig oder doppelseitig im Schambein oder im Sacrum neben der Gelenkfläche in der Nähe der Foramina sacralia pelvina. Die Last ist im Mittel 290 kg (170—450). Nach Lesshaft (1892) tritt bei vertikalem Druck von 1254 kg (500—2338) von der Wirbelsäule zum Sitzhöcker ein Bruch im Acetabulum oder darüber auf.

Evans und Lissner (1955) und Evans (1962) untersuchten 22 Becken, davon 6 frisch, die anderen fixiert. Die Becken wurden auf eine Stahlplatte so fallengelassen, daß sie mit beiden Sitzhöckern gleichzeitig aufschlugen. An Hand des stresscoat-Musters ergibt sich: 1. Eine Lateral- oder Medialrotation des Tuber ischiadicum, 2. eine Verlagerung nach lateral oder Ausbiegung des Acetabulums, 3. Rückwärtsverlagerung der Symphyse, 4. eine Verschiebung der Darmbeinschaufel und des Beckenkammes nach medial oder lateral bzw. eine Kombination dieser Verformungen. An acht Leichen wurde nach Entfernung der unteren Extremität, der Beckenmuskeln und -eingeweide ebenfalls eine dynamische Belastung durch Sturz auf die Tubera untersucht. Das Dehnungsmuster entspricht den Beobachtungen an isolierten Becken. Bei einigen Leichen wurde eine Schicht Weichgewebe von etwa 10 mm Dicke belassen, vor allem der M. gluteus maximus; es ergab sich eine erhebliche Energieabsorption. Das Dehnungsbild wird durch die Entfernung des Lig. sacraotuberale und Lig. sacrospinale nicht geändert. Die beobachteten Dehnungsbilder lassen keinen Zusammenhang mit den von Benninghoff (1925) angegebenen Spaltlinien erkennen. Aus den Versuchen schließen die Verfasser, daß der obere Teil des Schambeinastes als eine Art Zugstange wirkt, die eine Lateralverlagerung des Acetabulums verhindert. Die beobachteten Zugspannungen im unteren Teil des Schambeinastes und den anschließenden Teilen des Sitzbeines sind auf Biegung durch eine Rotation der Tubera zurückzuführen. In der Nähe der Symphyse fehlen Dehnungen, so daß bei diesen Belastungen die Symphyse auf Druck beansprucht wird. Gleichartig verhalten sich die Dehnungen bei einem statischen Druck von der Lendenwirbelsäule zu den Sitzhöckern hin.

β) Der Schädel

Die Statik des Schädels wurde im Hinblick auf die Aufnahme des Kaudruckes, die Ausbildung von Muskelleisten und die Pneumatisation untersucht. Görke (1904), Strasser (1908/1917) und Barth (1918) haben die Fortleitung des Kaudruckes vom Kieferapparat zum Hirnschädel über drei Pfeiler beschrieben, den Eckzahn-, Jochbein- und Flügelgaumenpfeiler. Bluntschli (1926) stellte im Ober- und Unterkiefer Basalbögen dar, von denen erst diese Pfeiler ausgehen (vgl. Winkler, 1921; Bluntschli und Winkler,

1927; SCHREIBER, 1932). Weiterhin weist BLUNTSCHLI (1926) auf die Umgestaltung der Tragkonstruktion im Laufe des Individuallebens und die Entstehung der Alveolen nach Bildung der Zahnanlagen hin. Nach PAULLI (1900) steht der Umfang der Pneumatisation bei den verschiedenen Species mit der Größe des Schädels im Zusammenhang. Die konstruktive Grundform des Schädels wird nach WEIDENREICH (1924) durch Oberflächenvergrößerungen zur Bildung von Muskelursprungsflächen nicht beeinflußt. Zwischen der Grundform des Schädels und der Außenform kann damit eine Diskrepanz auftreten. Der Schädel stellt bei allen Species eine architektonische Einheit aus morphologisch und funktionell ungleichwertigen Gebilden dar, der Gehirnkapsel, dem Augentrichter, dem Nasentunnel und der Zahnplatte. Diese Elemente des Schädels können demzufolge bei verschiedenen Tiergruppen ihre gegenseitige Lage zueinander recht erheblich ändern. Bei dem Zusammenschluß dieser Teile zu einer architektonischen Einheit bleiben Räume frei, die Nebenhöhlen. Der Gesichtsschädel ist ein Fachwerkbau mit starken Platten und Balken und dickeren und dünneren Zwischenwänden. Die Verstrebungen, die Pfeiler, weichen dem Auge und der Nasenhöhle aus. Die Nebenhöhlen sind als Produkt dieser Umgehungskonstruktion funktionell „passiv". Es besteht kein grundsätzlicher Unterschied zwischen pneumatischen Räumen und Markräumen; die Cellulae mastoideae nehmen eine Mittelstellung zwischen beiden ein (vgl. DIAMANT, 1940).

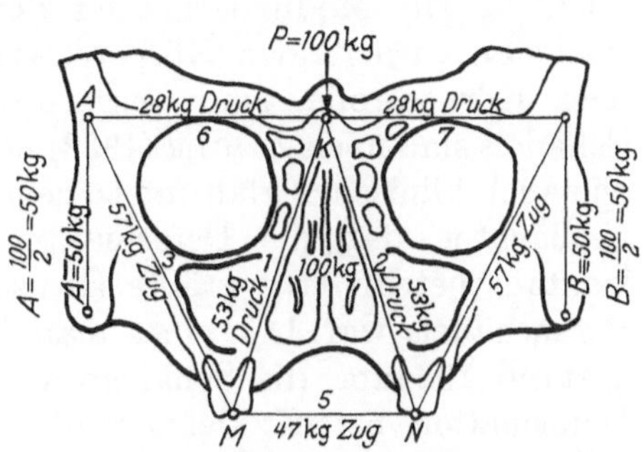

Abb. 60. Konstruktionsschema des Gesichtsschädels mit eingezeichneten Stäben nach dem Cremonaschen Kräfteplan (Umzeichnung aus STAUDENRAUS, 1939)

Nach röntgenologischer Untersuchung der Entwicklung der Kieferhöhle hat STAUDENRAUS (1939) den Aufbau des Gesichtsschädels nach dem sog. Cremona-Plan beschrieben

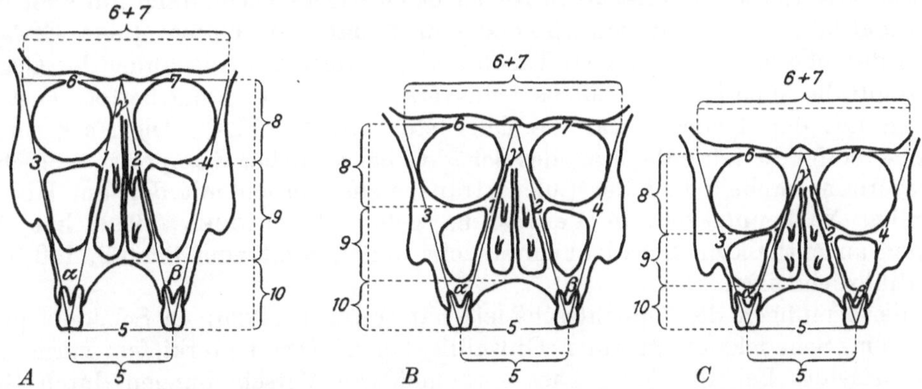

Abb. 61. Cremona-Plan für verschiedene Gesichtsformen. *A* Schmalgesicht; *B* Normalgesicht; *C* Breitgesicht. Homologe Strecken mit Ziffern bezeichnet (Umzeichnung aus STAUDENRAUS, 1939)

(Abb. 60). Bei Anwendung des Cremonaschen oder reziproken Kräfteplanes (vgl. FÖPPL, 1949) für ein Fachwerk aus Stäben wird verlangt, daß der Reihe nach für jeden Knotenpunkt von Stäben ein geschlossenes Krafteck für das Gleichgewicht der inneren und äußeren Kräfte zu entwerfen ist. Wenn gegen die Deutung von STAUDENRAUS auch morphologische und technische Einwände möglich sind, so verdient der Versuch, die verschiedenen Schädelproportionen auf einen Plan zurückzuführen, Beachtung. Nach STAUDENRAUS besteht ein Zusammenhang zwischen dem Öffnungswinkel der Zahnwurzeln und der Gesichtskonstruktion (Abb. 61). Bei kleinem Winkel der Zahnwurzeln ist der Gaumen hoch aufgewölbt, die Kieferhöhle und das Gesicht schmal und hoch, bei großem Wurzelwinkel der Gaumen flach, die Kieferhöhle und das Gesicht niedrig und breit.

Eine so einfache Korrelation zwischen Gaumenhöhe und Gesichtsform, wie sie Staudenraus (1939) annahm, besteht wohl nicht. Zeiger (1929, 1932, 1934) und Less (1934; vgl. Siemens, 1924) haben den Gaumen bei 82 gleichgeschlechtlichen Zwillingen untersucht, die etwa je zur Hälfte erbgleich und erbverschieden waren. Die Gaumenmaße gehören zu „den am stärksten umweltlabilen Meßstrecken am Kopf". Die Molarenbreite ist deutlich „umweltempfindlicher" als andere Breitenmaße des Gesichts- oder Hirnschädels. Die Modifizierbarkeit der Gaumenhöhe erreicht sogar das Doppelte des am stärksten variierenden Körpergewichtes. Die Höhenmaße, morphologische Gesichtshöhe oder Körpergröße, sind ausgesprochen „umweltstabil". Die verschiedenen Teile des Schädels sind nach Zeiger (1932) nicht in gleichem Maße durch die Umwelt modifizierbar, wie auch klinische Erfahrungen zeigen. Knese (1959a) hat an peruanischen Turmschädeln beobachtet, daß die Deformation überwiegend die Squama occipitalis und Squama frontalis betrifft. Die größte Hirnschädellänge (Glabella-Opisthocranion) des weiblichen Peruschädels war 146, eines männlichen Sammlungsschädels von gleichem Erhaltungszustand 192 mm, die Schädelbasislänge (Nasion-Basion) 97 bzw. 101 mm. Die gesetzte Deformation betrifft demgemäß nicht jenen Basisteil, der enge Beziehungen zu den Sinnesorganen, Gefäß- und Nervendurchtritten sowie zu den Kopfeingeweiden besitzt.

Untersuchungen des Spaltlinienmusters des Schädels haben Benninghoff (1925), Henckel (1931) und Tappen (1953) durchgeführt. Groth (1941) hat die Spaltlinien der Schädelbasis beschrieben und kommt zum Schluß, daß das Felsenbein statisch nicht in die Basis eingebaut ist. Endo (1965) weist darauf hin, daß die Trajektorien (Beanspruchungen) beim Kauen sehr wechselnd sind, die Spaltlinien aber ein festes System darstellen. Entsprechende Kauversuche an trockenen Schädeln ergaben, daß eine Konstruktion für das Kauen auf den hinteren und nicht auf den vorderen Zähnen vorliegt.

Wetzel (1922) faßt den Eckzahnpfeiler mit dem Gewölbe der äußeren Nase und dem vorderen Teil des Gaumens als Stirnnasenpfeiler zusammen. Er weist auch auf die Bedeutung der Dura mater, vor allem des Tentorium hin, mit der sich auch Bluntschli (1925) beschäftigt. Die Dura hat beim Neonatus eine feste Verbindung mit allen Schädelknochen und läßt sich von diesen z.T. erst vom 2. Jahr an ablösen. Beim Erwachsenen ist sie an den oberen und seitlichen Teilen des Schädels mit Ausnahme der Gegend des Sulcus sagittalis superior und Sulcus transversus nur locker angeheftet. Festere Verbindungen mit den Knochen hat die Dura stets an der Basis. Die Falx cerebri soll nach Bluntschli die Längsdehnung des Schädels bei seitlicher Kompression beschränken. Das Tentorium cerebelli und der Sulcus transversus werden mit den am Hinterhaupt ansetzenden Nackenmuskeln in Verbindung gebracht. Wetzel (1922) hat die Verformungen an entkalkten Schädeln untersucht und kommt zum Schluß, daß die Basisbrüche Rißbrüche sind.

Die Verformungen des Gesichtsschädels hat Wetzel (1925) an Schädeln gemessen, die mit dem Schädeldach in einer Gipshülle lagen. Der Unterkiefer wurde mit Gewichten belastet. Bei 10—20 kg Last sind meßbare Verschiebungen durch Straffung bzw. Dehnung der Nähte oder durch Formänderung der Knochen zu beobachten. Der Alveolarrand zwischen den oberen Schneidezähnen verschiebt sich um 0,8 mm, die knöcherne äußere Nasenöffnung erweitert sich um 0,39 mm, der Abstand der unteren Jochbogenränder nimmt um 0,1—0,2 mm ab. Die Verformung ist bei Last auf den Schneidezähnen und den Mahlzähnen etwas verschieden. Die Verformungen sind auf eine Art Torsion der Knochen zurückzuführen. Der Schädel besteht mithin aus biegsamen Formelementen, die durch zugfeste Nähte miteinander verbunden sind. Wetzel und Schröder (1925) haben auch die Sicherheit der Schädelkonstruktion geprüft. Der Querschnitt des Stirn-, Nasen-, Jochbein- und Flügelfortsatzpfeilers einer Seite mißt jeweils etwas über 50 mm^2, so daß alle Pfeiler auf beiden Seiten zusammen etwa 420 mm^2 Querschnitt haben. Die Autoren haben dann die Tragfähigkeit an macerierten Schädeln, die mit physiologischer Kochsalzlösung durchtränkt waren, zu 2214 kg gemessen. Theoretisch hatten sie etwa den 3fachen Wert bestimmt. An Hand der Muskelquerschnitte und der verschiedenen Angaben über die absolute Muskelkrafteinheit (s. S. 484) errechnen die Verfasser eine Sicherheit zwischen 22 und 144, die unwahrscheinlich ist. Nimmt man einen Stoßkoeffizienten von 1,5 (s. S. 499) und eine Sicherheit von 2,5 an (s. S. 479), kann man aus der Tragfähigkeit die maximale Last zu 590 kg annehmen. Bei Erörterung der Verformungen von peruanischen Turmschädeln betont KNESE (1959a), daß der Hirnschädel auch die Aufgabe hat, das Gehirn zu schützen. Somit ist zweifelhaft, ob eine befriedigende Kalkulation der „Sicherheit" für die natürliche Beanspruchung beim Kauakt gelingt.

Druckversuche an frischen Schädeln nach Entfernung der Weichteile hat MESSERER (1880) durchgeführt (Tabelle 22). Bei Druck auf den Schädel zwischen ebenen Platten

Tabelle 22. *Bruchlasten und Verformung des Schädels bei Flächendruck* (nach MESSERER, 1880)

Druckrichtung		Alter	Bruchlast kg	Verkleinerung in Druckrichtung mm	Vergrößerung mm	
					längs	senkrecht
Transversal	♂	42,7	489	4,26	0,43	0,75
	♀	48,1	563	5,66	0,46	0,69
					quer	senkrecht
Sagittal	♂	41,4	686	2,77	0,39	0,14[1]
	♀	41,8	610	2,76	0,19	0,19

Erläuterung: Mittelwerte.

[1] Einmal Verkleinerung um 0,36 mm; wurde bei der Mittelwertleistung nicht berücksichtigt.

fand er in Druckrichtung eine Verkleinerung, senkrecht dazu eine Vergrößerung, mitunter aber auch eine „unverständliche" Verkleinerung. Die den Platten anliegenden Teile wurden eingezogen. Bis zur Hälfte der Bruchlast fehlen bleibende Verformungen. Beim Bruch ist zunächst ein Knistergeräusch zu hören, dann erfolgt der eigentliche Bruch mit „lautem Krachen". Die Formänderung ist bei transversalem Druck größer als bei sagittalem. Die maximale Formänderung bis zum Bruch war 8,8 mm, bis zur mutmaßlichen Elastizitätsgrenze 4,5 mm, senkrecht zur Druckrichtung 1,3 bzw. 0,4 mm. Die Bruchlast betrug in sagittaler Richtung 650 kg (400—1200), in querer 520 kg (350—800). Die große Formenmannigfaltigkeit des Schädels läßt keinen Schluß auf die Bedeutung der Proportionen, Dicke der Knochen usw. zu. Der Bruch war ein Riß der Schädelbasis parallel zur Druckrichtung, bei zwei Versuchen ging der Bruch von der Druckstelle aus, bei zwei weiteren trat eine Nahtdiastase auf. Bei querem Druck verlief die Bruchlinie in der mittleren Schädelgrube von der Oberfläche einer Pyramide über den Clivus zur anderen Pyramide, bei Längsdruck von der Siebbeinplatte über das Foramen lacerum zum Foramen jugulare. Ein Druck auf die Schädelbasis vermittels der ersten vier Halswirbel führt zu einem Bruch bei der Last von 270 kg (225—300); Condylen, Sella turcica und Pyramide wurden nach innen gedrückt. Eine umschriebene Lasteinwirkung durch einen 17 mm starken Bolzen erfordert in den einzelnen Bereichen eine sehr unterschiedliche Last zum Bruch: Stirnbeinmitte 450 (280—825), Parietale 350 (180—500), Protuberantia occipitalis externa 655 (525—975), Squama temporalis 180 (170—190) und Jochbogen 30 kg (25—35). Diese letzteren Angaben hat HODGSON (1967) bestätigt.

Durch Untersuchung des Stresscoat-Musters fand EVANS (1953) bei Druck auf das Kinn am unteren Rande des Unterkiefers und am Hals der Condylen, bei querem Druck auf den Kieferwinkel parallel zur Linea mylohyoidea und am oberen Rande des Unterkieferastes Zugspannungen. Bei beiden Belastungsformen handelt es sich um Biegung. DU BRUL und SICHER (1954) haben durch Zusammendrücken der Condylen mit den Fingern mit Hilfe der stresscoat-Linien Zugspannungen entlang des Kieferkörpers beobachtet. MESSERER (1880) erhielt durch Druck auf den Kieferwinkel mit 60 kg (25—130) einen Bruch in der Unterkiefermitte, die Annäherung der Kieferwinkel betrug 6,47 mm

(4,0—10,0). Ein Druck von 190 kg (100—260) auf das Kinn erzeugte einen Bruch des Condylenhalses, ein — oder beidseitig, dabei wichen die Unterkieferwinkel 6,6 mm (3,9—13,3) auseinander. Nach BADOUX (1966) treten in der Mandibula neben vertikalen auch Torsionsbeanspruchungen auf; solche Torsionen erscheinen, wie vergleichend-anatomische Betrachtungen ergeben, bei synostosierter Symphyse, d.h. auch beim Menschen. Untersuchungen der Spaltlinien führten DOWGJALLO (1932), BENNINGHOFF (1925/26), KÜNTSCHER (1934) und SEIPEL (1948) durch.

3. Der Bruchmechanismus des Knochens

Die Untersuchungen der Mechanik und Festigkeit sollen Gestalt und Leistung der Skeletteile sowie deren Versagen, den Bruch, aufklären. Bei den Brüchen wird technisch

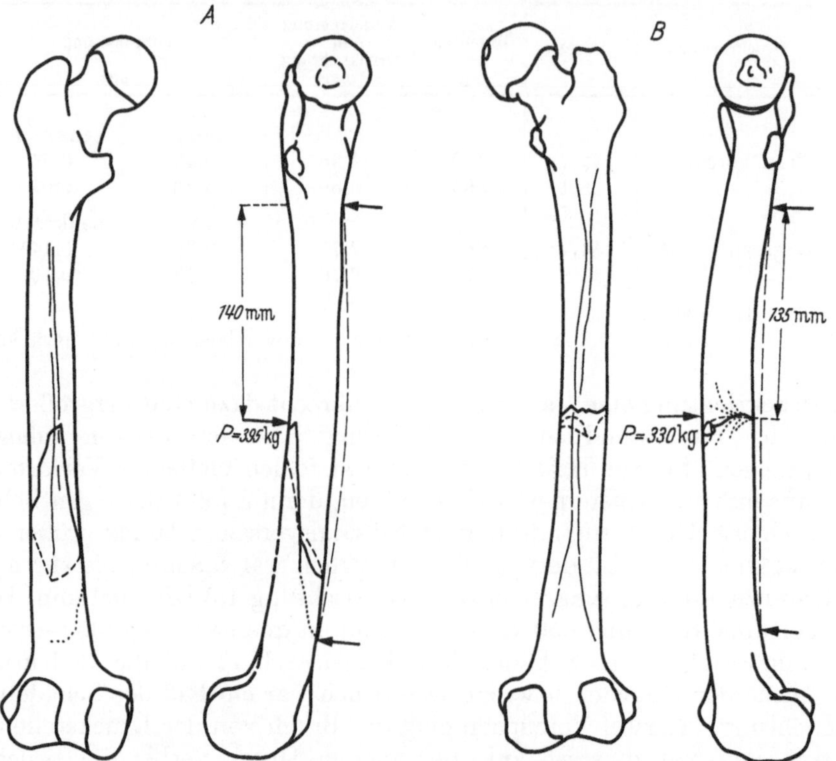

Abb. 62. Biegungsbrüche des Femurs, dargestellt in Frontal- und Sagittalprojektion: Sichtbare Bruchlinien ausgezogen, verdeckte gestrichelt; Fissuren punktiert. *A* Biegerichtung dorso-ventral (linker Femur L 14 ♂ 79 J.): MbBr = 2760 kg·cm (Stützweite 28 cm, P 395 kg); σ Druckseite: 1750 kg/cm²; σ Zugseite: 1530 kg/cm²; f (Durchbiegung) 6 mm. *B* Biegerichtung ventro-dorsal (rechter Femur L 14 ♂ 79. J): MbBr = 2225 kg·cm (Stützweite 27 cm, P 330 kg); σ Druckseite: 1120 kg/cm²; σ Zugseite 1180 kg/cm²; f: 5 mm (aus KNESE, HAHNE und BIERMANN, 1955)

zwischen einem Trenn- und einem Verschiebungsbruch unterschieden. Beim Trennungsbruch liegt die Bruchfläche etwa rechtwinklig zur Richtung der größten Zugspannung und hat eine körnige Oberfläche; zu den Trennbrüchen wird auch der Sprödbruch gerechnet. Beim Verschiebungsbruch erfolgt die Trennung entlang von Gleitflächen, die mit den Hauptspannungsebenen einen vom Spannungszustand abhängigen Winkel bilden.

In den sog. Festigkeits- oder Bruchhypothesen wird der gesamte mehrachsige Spannungszustand zu einer Anstrengung σ_v zusammengefaßt. Die Normalspannungshypothese setzt die Anstrengung den maximalen Zugspannungen gleich und bezieht sich auf Trennbrüche, die in reiner Form selten auftreten. Bei der Hauptdehnungshypothese wurde die Dehnung für den Bruch verantwortlich gemacht. Die Schubspannungshypothese setzt die Anstrengung gleich der Differenz der Hauptspannungen oder gleich der maximalen

Schubspannung ($\sigma_v = \sigma_{max} - \sigma_{min} = 2\ \tau_{max}$). Diese Hypothese wird zur Deutung des Verschiebungsbruches herangezogen, der bei plastischen Stoffen, aber auch spröden, wie Beton unter Druck auftritt. In der erweiterten Schubspannungshypothese werden Normalspannungen und Schubspannungen berücksichtigt, wobei der Bruch bei Erreichen einer „Grenzkurve" eintritt ($\tau_m = f(\sigma)$ oder $\sigma_v = \sigma_{max} - \sigma_{min}$, abhängig von $\sigma_m = (\sigma_1 + \sigma_2 + \sigma_3)/3$). Andere Hypothesen gehen von der Gestaltsänderung aus. Keine dieser Hypothesen hat allgemeine Anerkennung gefunden oder konnte experimentell voll bestätigt werden, vermutlich weil sich die Bruchbedingungen nicht rein mathematisch formulieren lassen (s. unten).

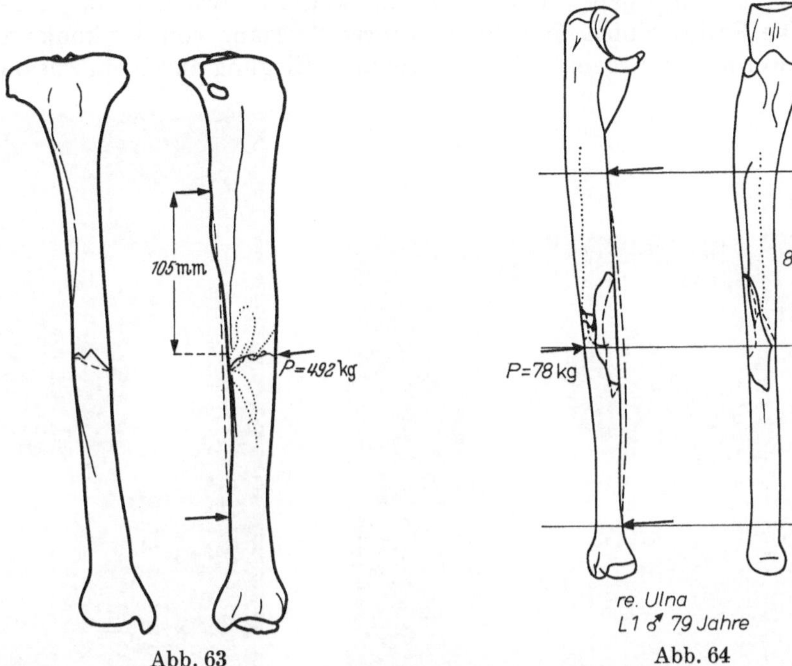

Abb. 63 Abb. 64

Abb. 63. Frontal- und Sagittalprojektion einer osteometrisch vermessenen rechten Tibia (79 Jahre). Belastungsrichtung: ventro-dorsal; P: 492 kg; Stützweite: 21 cm; Beschriftung siehe Abb. 62 (aus Knese, Hahne und Biermann, 1955)

Abb. 64. Rechte Ulna eines Mannes von 79 Jahren in der Ansicht von außen und vorn: Biegebruch. Die beiden palmaren Pfeile geben die Stützen an. $^1/_2\, l = 80$ mm, $P = 78$ kg, Bruchmoment = 312 kgcm. Auf der palmaren Seite Ausbrechen eines Keiles (sichtbare Bruchlinien ausgezogen, verdeckte gestrichelt). Punktiert: Fissuren (Versuch Knese, Hahne und Biermann, 1955) (aus Knese, 1958b)

Die Bedingungen für ein Versagen des Materials sind demzufolge heute noch nicht befriedigend anzugeben. In der Medizin interessiert noch die „Bruchursache", d.h. unter welchen äußeren und inneren Bedingung der Bruch auftritt, man könnte auch sagen der Bruchmechanismus, da wohl selten anamnestisch einwandfreie Auskünfte über den als Katastrophe eintretenden Bruch zu erhalten sind. So wird in Analogie zu technisch beobachteten Brüchen von Torsions-, Biegungs-, Stauchungsfrakturen usw. (unter anderem Zuppinger, 1904; Lauche, 1937) gesprochen. Hier kann nur von experimentellen, nicht aber von klinischen Beobachtungen berichtet werden.

Bei Biegebruchversuchen sah Messerer (1880) zuerst ein Zerreißen auf der konvexen Seite, dem mitunter ein Zusammendrücken auf der konkaven vorausgeht. Es entstehen divergierende Rißlinien, die einen Keil umgrenzen (Abb. 64), und in einem Falle sprang ein solcher Keil auch heraus. Ein Schrägbruch liegt dann vor, wenn die eine Bruchlinie fehlt. Unter 25 Biegeversuchen fanden Knese et al. (1955) bei 10 den Ausgang der Bruchlinien von der dem Kraftangriff entgegengesetzten Seite, bei 2 in der Nähe des Kraftangriffes, bei 5 keine Beziehungen zum Kraftangriff und bei 5 fehlten Fissuren überhaupt. Die Verfasser beobachteten Querbrüche (Abb. 62,63) mit einigen scharfen Graten, Schrägbrüche mit Stehenbleiben einer Knochenspitze. Die Bruchfläche war marmorartig (Abb. 65), spiegelnd kristallin oder mehr faserig (Abb. 66) und unregelmäßig zerklüftet.

Die Keilbildung bei Biegebrüchen hat auch LINGGI (1951) an Hundeknochen gefunden. Unter 140 Bruchversuchen trat bei 114 ein vollständiges dreieckiges Stück auf oder war durch Fissuren angedeutet. Bei 106 Brüchen lag die Basis an der Seite des Kraftangriffes, bei 8 an der entgegengesetzten. Bei 7 Versuchen, davon 6mal der Radius, ergaben sich Querbrüche mit Zacken und bei 5 noch anschließende Längsrisse. 12 Frakturen zeigten eine Art Querfraktur mit einer dreieckigen Knochenzacke an der konkaven Seite, von deren Spitze eine Längsspalte ausging, bei 23 weiteren Brüchen war diese Bruchform angedeutet. Die Frakturlinien nehmen stets ihren Ausgang von der konkaven Seite. Die Längsspalten werden als Ergebnis einer sekundären Biegung durch ein Zusammendrücken

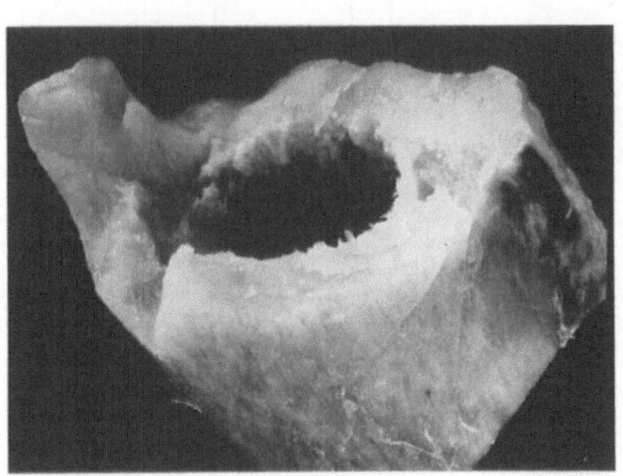

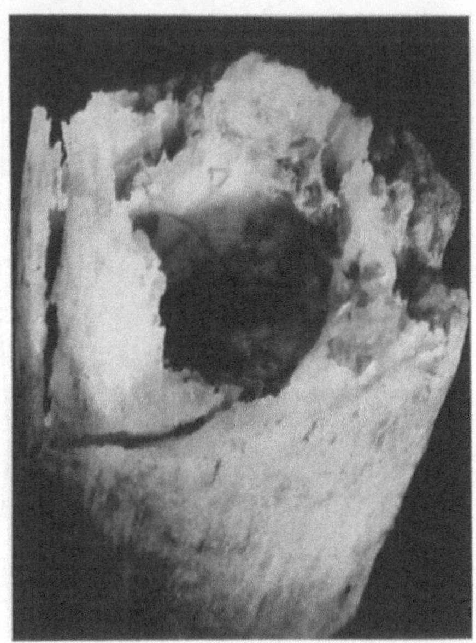

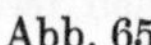

Abb. 65 Abb. 66

Abb. 65. Annähernd kristallin erscheinende Bruchfläche des proximalen Bruchendes eines rechten Femurs (♂, 79 Jahre). Bruch bei Belastung ventro-dorsal, Ansicht von tibial (aus KNESE, HAHNE und BIERMANN, 1955)

Abb. 66. Faserige Bruchfläche des proximalen Bruchendes eines rechten Femurs (♀, 72 Jahre). Ansicht von tibial, Bruch bei Belastung fibulo-tibial, *P:* 180 kg (aus KNESE, HAHNE und BIERMANN, 1955)

der Knochenröhre angesehen. Im Hinblick auf Stoßstangenverletzungen hat KILLMER (1966) mit einem Pendelschlagwerk auf menschliche Tibien, konserviert und frisch, Querkräfte einwirken lassen. Es entstand als Bruchkörper ein vollständiges oder unvollständiges Dreieck, dessen Basis an der Seite der Krafteinwirkung liegt. Der Bruchkörper ist räumlich als Pyramide anzusehen. Die entfernteren Teile der Bruchlinien erscheinen eventuell nur als Fissuren.

Die Bruchform in der Art eines Keiles wird in unterschiedlicher Weise gedeutet. HAASE (1936) vermutet Gleitebenen, die um 45° gegen die Kraftrichtung geneigt sind, und stützt sich damit auf die Schubspannungshypothese. HAASE (1937a) bildet derartige schräge Abbrüche auch bei Spongiosawürfeln aus Epiphysen des Rindes ab und zieht Vergleiche zur Bruchform des Holzes wie es auch DEMPSTER und LIDDICOAT (1952, s. S. 445) tun. ZUPPINGER (1904) nimmt den Beginn des Bruches an Stellen der höchsten Spannung an. Zug- und Schubspannungen führten direkt zum Bruch, Druckspannungen aber nur unter Vermittlung sekundärer Zug- oder Schubspannungen. Bei Biegung tritt an der Konvexseite eine Spalte auf, die sich dann divergierend teilt. EVANS (1953, 1955, vgl. 1957, 1961) sowie LISSNER und EVANS (1956) haben bei querer Belastung des Femurs die ersten Dehnungen mittels des stresscoat-Verfahrens beobachtet und stellten fest, daß die Fissuren von diesen Gebieten mit Dehnungen ausgehen; das gelte auch für Torsionsfrakturen. Demgegenüber gibt LINGGI (1951) für die Knochen des Hundes den Ausgang der Fissuren von der Seite des Kraftangriffes an. Zur Bestätigung seiner Beobachtungen hat LINGGI den Versuch bei 16 Knochen nach Erscheinen der ersten Fissuren abgebrochen. KNESE et al. (1955) sahen die Fissuren sowohl von der Seite des Kraftangriffes als auch von der Gegenseite entspringen. KNESE (1958b) weist darauf hin, daß ähnliche Bruchformen auch bei Stahlbetonbalken auftreten.

Die Art der Bruchflächen wurde bei Druck- und Torsionsbelastung nicht so eingehend wie bei Biegung beschrieben. HAASE und RICHTER (1936) erhielten im statischen Druckversuch bei Lasten bis zu 7000 kg an Femora von Rindern und Schweinen keine Schaftbrüche, obwohl die Gelenkenden in Schalen aus Zement oder Metall eingegossen waren. Schaftbrüche traten im Schlagwerk bei dynamischer Last von 60 mkg als spröde Schräg- oder Spiralbrüche auf. An Hühnerknochen erhielten die Verfasser bei Torsion Schräg- oder Spiralbrüche, bei Biegung dagegen reine Querbrüche. HIRSCH et al. (1954) haben an Hundeknochen den Bruchmechanismus untersucht. Die vertikale Längsbelastung der Tibia ruft überwiegend Brüche der Metaphyse hervor. Bei einer Last, die um 15° gegen die Längsachse der Tibia geneigt ist, treten vermehrt Schaftbrüche auf. Wird der Knochen vorher um 10° torquiert und dann in gleicher Weise belastet, ändern sich die Bruchformen nicht. Bei Torsion um mehr als 10° erscheinen in Schaftmitte Spiralbrüche. Die Bruchlast für den Femur ist geringer als jene für die Tibia; dies könnte nach der Meinung der Autoren auf der Form des Oberschenkels beruhen. Wie beim Schienbein treten Schaftbrüche des Femurs vor allem bei schräger Belastung auf. Bei dynamischer Belastung erscheint eine Fragmentierung.

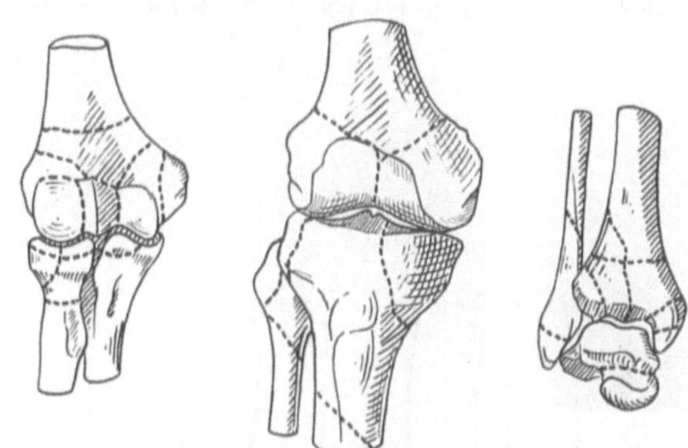

Abb. 67. Gelenknahe Frakturlinien am Ellenbogen-, Knie- und Sprunggelenk (Umzeichnung nach V. LANZ und WACHSMUTH) (aus KNESE, 1956a)

Nach HAASE und RICHTER (1936) ist für eine bestimmte Beanspruchungsform keine besondere Bruchform charakteristisch. Brüche treten auf, wenn die Beanspruchung ungewöhnlich gesteigert wird oder in einer anderen Richtung als die normale Belastung wirkt. Für die Bruchform ist auch die Struktur und Feinstruktur verantwortlich, so daß aus der Bruchform nicht auf die Art der Beanspruchung geschlossen werden kann. Auch KNESE et al. (1955) beobachteten bei gleichartiger Biegungsbeanspruchung sehr unterschiedliche Frakturen (Abb. 62, 63, 64). Für ein differentes Verhalten der Knochen auf Grund von Veränderungen in der Struktur spricht, daß bei dem männlichen Probanden von 79 Jahren die Bruchflächen kristallin schimmerten (Abb. 65). Bei den Knochen der rechten unteren Extremität einer 72jährigen Frau mit Arthrosis deformans des Hüftgelenkes erschienen aber aufgerissene, faserige Frakturenden mit mehreren einzelnen Stücken (Abb. 66). Die Knochen der linken Extremität dieser Frau und der oberen zeigten mehr glatte Bruchflächen. VOSE (1962) vertritt allerdings die Auffassung, daß für Knochenbrüche die grobe Architektur von größerer Bedeutung als die mikroskopische Mineralisation sei.

Keil- bzw. Y-förmige Bruchlinien sind auch an den Gelenkenden zu beobachten (Abb. 67). Ähnliche Y-Brüche oder Längsspalten sind von Gelenkquadern her bekannt (MÖRSCH, 1929; WYSS, 1926, 1948). Bei einer örtlichen Pressung tritt unmittelbar unter der Druckfläche ein Gebiet horizontaler Druckspannungen auf (Abb. 68). Die Druckspannungen gehen von der Druckfläche aus senkrecht ab und biegen so um, daß sie in der Entfernung h parallel zur Stabachse verlaufen. Die horizontalen Komponenten Z

der Spannungen S sind dann Zugspannungen, deren Maximum bei $h/2$ liegt. Damit entsteht eine Zone großer Unstetigkeit der Spannungen in benachbarten Elementen, die einer Abscherung sehr ähnlich ist und zum Herausspringen eines Keiles führt. Nach KNESE (1956a) lassen sich auf diesen Mechanismus viele gelenknahe Frakturen zurückführen.

Der Bruchmechanismus spongiöser Teile wurde vor allem in Hinblick auf die Schenkelhalsfrakturen untersucht, wobei wir hier nicht auf klinische Beobachtungen und Nomenklaturfragen eingehen können, sondern nur auf die Versuche zur Aufklärung des Bruchmechanismus hinweisen. Bereits MESSERER (1880) hat auch Bruchversuche am Schenkelhals ausgeführt, und zwar einmal mit Druck am Femurkopf in Schwererichtung und in Längsachse des Halses. Späterhin wurden weitere Versuche mit Druck in „Schwererichtung" (KOLODNY, 1925; GAENSLEN, 1936; COTTON und MORRISON, 1938; SPOTOFT, 1944; SPEARS und OWEN, 1949; KÜNTSCHER, 1935; EVANS, LISSNER und PEDERSEN, 1949;

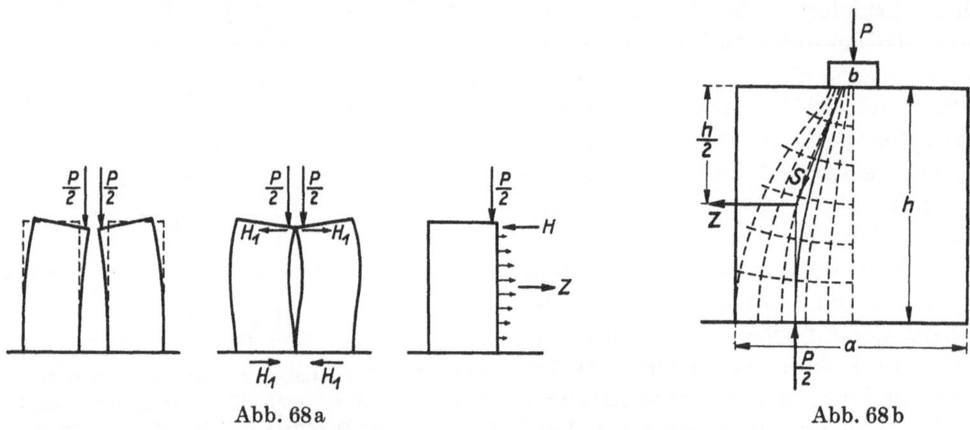

Abb. 68a

Abb. 68b

Abb. 68a. Darstellung der Druckwirkung am Stabende, Teilung des Gelenkquaders in zwei Hälften und Auseinanderrücken dieser beiden Hälften, die mit P_2 belastet sind. Zusammenrücken der beiden Hälften: Gegendruck H_1. Darstellung der Zugspannungen Z, des Gegendruckes H an der linken Hälfte des Gelenkquaders

Abb. 68b. Darstellung der Hauptspannungslinien bei Druckübertragung. S Druckspannung; Z die horizontale Komponente von S als Zugspannung. Im Abstand h laufen die Kraftlinien parallel zur Längsachse (Umzeichnung nach MÖRSCH 1923/29) (aus KNESE, 1956a)

EVANS, HAYES und POWERS, 1953; SMITH, 1953; BACKMAN, 1957) oder auf den Trochanter major durchgeführt (SPOTOFT, 1944; SPEARS und OWEN, 1949; LINTON, 1949; EVANS, 1953; SMITH, 1953; LISSNER und EVANS, 1956; BACKMAN, 1957). Das Ergebnis dieser umfangreichen Untersuchungen ist nach BACKMAN (1957), daß keine Korrelation zwischen verschiedenen Frakturtypen und bestimmten Beanspruchungsarten z.Z. festzustellen sei.

Zur Diskussion des Bruchmechanismus bei Stößen hoher Geschwindigkeit, d.h. Schußverletzungen, wurde nach HUELKE, BUEGE und HARGER (1967) bisher überwiegend klinisches und Museumsmaterial herangezogen. Die Autoren haben an 122 Femora eine Stahlnadel auf die Fossa poplitea mit der Stoßgeschwindigkeit von 213—509 $m \cdot sec^{-1}$ einwirken lassen. Bei geringerer Geschwindigkeit tritt eine Lochfraktur auf, bei höherer explodierte der Knochen mit gewaltiger radiärer Sprengung des den Geschoßweg umgebenden Materials, so daß eine Cavitation wie bei weichen Geweben erscheint. Für diese Wirkung ist das Knochenmark der Spongiosa verantwortlich (s. S. 477). Während Höhlen im umliegenden Weichgewebe zusammenfallen, bleibt die Höhle im Knochen bestehen. Die jeweilige Zerstörungsform des Knochens hängt von der Projektilgeschwindigkeit und dem Widerstand des Materials ab. Dieser Widerstand hängt wiederum nicht allein von der „Härte" (Festigkeit) und Elastizität, sondern auch von der Dichte des Gewebes ab. Im übrigen dürfte die Art der Zerstörung des Knochens nicht nur mit den jeweiligen Festigkeitseigenschaften zu korrelieren sein. Vermutlich muß ähnlich wie bei der Zerspanung usw. (s. dort) eine besondere Reaktionsform des Knochens angenommen werden, die nur bedingt auf die Festigkeit zurückgeführt werden kann.

Weder für die kompakten noch spongiösen Teile des Skeletes können demzufolge im Augenblick die „Bruchursachen" angegeben werden, obwohl alle klinisch bekannten Bruchformen auch experimentell zu erzeugen sind. Das gilt ebenfalls für den Schädel. MESSERER (1884) ließ auf einen Schädel, der auf einer Steinunterlage ruhte, einen Holzklotz fallen und fand einen Bruch bei 6 kgm oder mehr. Fällt der Schädel auf die Steinunterlage, so ist das Minimum der erforderlichen Energie zum Bruch in sagittaler Richtung 5,9 und quer 4,6 kgm. Mit einem Bolzen von 4 cm Durchmesser ist im Frontalbereich ein Lochbruch bei 3 kgm, am Parietale mit einem Bolzen von 2 cm und der Energie 3 kgm eine Impression und bei 6—14 kgm ein Lochbruch zu erzeugen. Durch das Auftreffen eines Fallklotzes auf den Schädel mit Halswirbelsäule entsteht ein Biegungsbruch der Basis. Bei nachgiebiger Unterlage ist der Energieverlust erheblich (SCHRANZ, 1881 nach MESSERER). An Schädeln mit Unterkiefer und den beiden ersten Halswirbeln auf einem Holzblock kommt es erst bei einer Energie von 7,6 kgm zur Fraktur. Ein Schädel, der mit den Condylen auf einer künstlichen Halswirbelsäule aus Holz und Kork ruht, zeigt eine Lockerung der Nähte durch 10,6 kgm, eine Fraktur erst bei 17,6 kgm. Nach MESSERER kann ein Fallgewicht von 18 kg und 24 kgm Energie von Schädeln ohne Fraktur ertragen werden. Ein 2 cm dicker Bolzen erzeugt mit 17,5 kgm eine Lochfraktur. Ein 4 cm dicker Bolzen brachte noch bei 14 kgm nur eine Knochenkontusion oder Absplitterung der Tabula interna hervor, die in einem Falle sogar erst bei 48 kgm entstand. Im Hinblick auf die Sicherheit in Fahrzeugen hat HODGSON (1967) an Leichen die Wirkung eines Stoßes auf die Gesichtsknochen, besonders den Jochbogen, untersucht. Hierbei wird die Auswirkung von Energie absorbierenden Schichten wie des Weichgewebes, die Fixierung oder Beweglichkeit der Leiche in einem schwingenden Sitz und die Kräfteverteilung diskutiert. Jedoch ist es recht schwierig, genaue Toleranzwerte zu errechnen. Es besteht weiterhin eine Abhängigkeit von der Dauer der Einwirkung. Eine Kraft von 1000 Pfund benötigt zur Fraktur 3 millisec oder weniger, eine solche von 200 Pfund etwa 4 millisec. Durch die Fraktur eines Jochbogens wird die andere Gesichtsseite nicht beeinflußt. Das Stirnbein hat eine Frakturtoleranz, die 3—4mal höher liegt als die der Mandibula und des Jochbogens.

An sechs Hunden und zwei Makaken haben GURDJIAN und LISSNER (1945) die Wirkung eines Hammerschlages auf das Schädeldach am narkotisierten und getöteten Tier sowie an skeletierten Schädeln mit Hilfe der stresscoat-Technik geprüft. Das Ergebnis ist in allen Versuchen gleich, die Rißlinien sind beim Lebenden etwas länger und am Skeletschädel an den Nähten unterbrochen. Durch den Hammerschlag wird der Knochen eingebogen, wobei radiär sich ausbreitende Spannungen und demzufolge zirkuläre Rißlinien zu beobachten sind. In etwas größerer Entfernung kommen zirkulär verteilte Spannungen mit radiären Rissen hinzu. An trockenen menschlichen Schädeln und Leichenköpfen ohne Kopfschwarte treten durch einen Hammerschlag nur zirkulär geordnete Spannungen um die Schlagstelle auf. Superpositionen von Rißlinien sprechen für eine Vibration der Schädeldecke. Frakturen durch einen Fall sind demgemäß auf Zugspannungen zurückzuführen, wobei der Ort der Krafteinwirkung von Bedeutung ist. An Schädeln, die in physiologischer Kochsalzlösung feucht gehalten wurden, wurde der Fall auf eine Stahlplatte von GURDJIAN und LISSNER (1946) untersucht. Die Energie zur Erzeugung eines Rißmusters ist nach Schädel und Schlagregion sehr unterschiedlich, für die occipitale Region kleiner als für die parietale und wesentlich kleiner als für die frontale Region. Auf der Tabula interna sind zirkuläre und an der Außenseite radiäre Dehnungen (Abb. 69) zu beobachten (GURDJIAN, LISSNER und WEBSTER, 1947). Die Einbiegung des Schädeldaches an einer Stelle ruft eine Ausbiegung in einer benachbarten im Sinne einer schwingenden Membran hervor (GURDJIAN, WEBSTER und LISSNER, 1949). Die Frakturlinien beginnen in einer gewissen Entfernung vom Ort des Kraftangriffes, da im Augenblick des Schlages hier eine Stauchung vorliegt. Die Frakturlinien dehnen sich dann zum Ort des Schlages und in entgegengesetzter Richtung aus. Beim Zurückbiegen des Knochens sind am Ort der Krafteinwirkung die höchsten Zugspannungen.

Mit Dehnungsmeßstreifen haben GURDJIAN und LISSNER (1944) die Schädeldeformation und Änderungen des intracraniellen Druckes beim narkotisierten Hunde verfolgt. Etwa $^1/_{2000}$ sec werden zur maximalen Deformation benötigt. Der Einbiegung am Ort des Schlages steht eine Ausbiegung an der entgegengesetzten Seite gegenüber. Nach zwei bis vier Schwingungen innerhalb $^1/_{2000}$ sec kehrt der Schädel in seine ursprüngliche Form zurück. Die Deformationszeit hängt nicht nur von der Schlagstärke, sondern auch von der Schädelgestalt und dem Ort des Schlages ab. Die intracraniellen Druckänderungen entsprechen dem Deformationsablauf, der höchste Druck wird nach $^1/_{1400}$ sec erreicht.

Da die gleichen Ergebnisse über den zeitlichen Ablauf der Deformation am narkotisierten Hunde und am unversehrten Kopf 24 Std nach dem Tode zu erzielen sind, führten

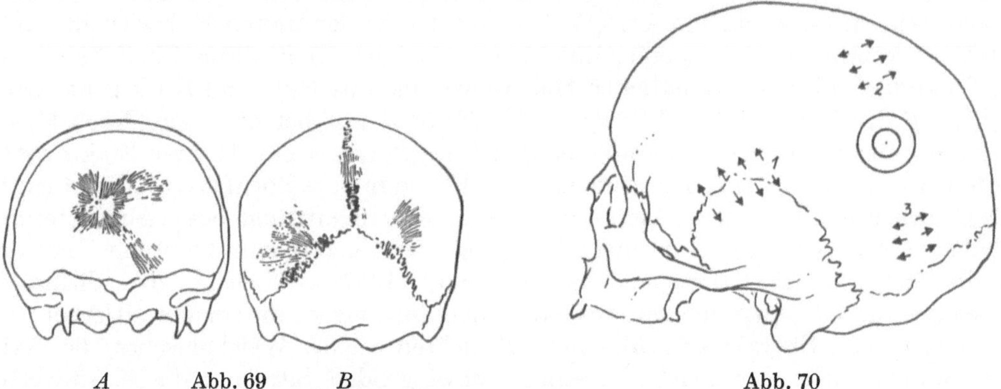

Abb. 69. Stresscoat-Muster am menschlichen Schädel. *A* Tabula interna; *B* Tabula externa (Umzeichnung aus GURDJIAN, LISSNER und WEBSTER, 1947)

Abb. 70. Spannungsgebiete am Schädel, die einem Schlag auf die hintere Parietalregion folgen (Umzeichnung aus GURDJIAN, WEBSTER und LISSNER, 1950)

GURDJIAN und WEBSTER (1947) entsprechende Versuche an menschlichen Leichenköpfen durch. Die ersten Deformationserscheinungen sind nach $^1/_{5000}$—$^1/_{2000}$, die Gesamtdeformation nach $^1/_{200}$—$^1/_{250}$ sec zu beobachten. Die Energie zur Erzeugung einer Fraktur durch Fall auf eine Stahlplatte ist sehr variabel (GURDJIAN, WEBSTER und LISSNER, 1949). Nach Auftreten einer Frakturlinie ist die Energie zur Bildung weiterer Linien oder Zertrümmerungen gering. Die Weichteile erwiesen sich als energieabsorbierendes Material. Zur gleichen Fraktur wie am Kopf mit Weichteilen wird am trockenen Schädel nur $^1/_{10}$ der Energie benötigt. GURDJIAN, WEBSTER und LISSNER (1950a) konnten zeigen, daß zwischen Auftreffen des Schädels auf der Stahlplatte und der Deformation 0,0006 und bis zur Fraktur weitere 0,0006 sec ablaufen. Nach Geschwindigkeit, kinetischer Energie und Gestalt des verletzenden Objektes werden sechs Frakturtypen unterschieden. Eine Gewehrkugel hat die höchste kinetische Energie und erzeugt eine Perforation, dann folgen Pistolenkugel, Baseball, langsame abgerundete und spitze Objekte und stumpfe Gegenstände.

Schließlich unterschieden GURDJIAN, WEBSTER und LISSNER (1950a, b) nach der zeitlichen Folge der stresscoat-Risse primäre, sekundäre und tertiäre Dehnungsgebiete (Abb. 70). Die Verfasser untersuchten zwölf Orte des Kraftangriffes. Wenn der Ort des Kraftangriffes bekannt ist, so können primäre und sekundäre Frakturen voneinander getrennt werden. Frontale Schläge führen mehr zu vertikalen Frakturlinien, vordere und hintere parietale sowie parieto-occipitale zu horizontalen (GURDJIAN, WEBSTER und LISSNER, 1953). Frakturen des Schädeldaches durch Schlag auf den Scheitel setzen sich nicht zur Basis fort.

EVANS, LISSNER und LEBOW (1958) haben die Bedingungen einer Schädelverletzung beim Auftreffen auf ein Armaturenbrett (Ford) untersucht, das im Gegensatz zu dem von GURDJIAN et al. (1949) benutzten Stahlblock eine beträchtliche Energie absorbiert. Die für Schädelverletzungen benötigte Energie und Geschwindigkeit ist demzufolge höher. Riß- oder Zertrümmerungsfrakturen entstehen bei einer Geschwindigkeit von 12,96—29,96 $msec^{-1}$ (29—45 miles/hour) und einer kinetischen Energie von 37—80 kgm (268—581 foot pounds). Die kinetische Energie zur Erzeugung der Schädelfraktur ist aber nur 4,55—10,4 kgm (33—75 foot pounds), ein Wert, der mit dem von MESSERER (1884) übereinstimmt, der Rest wird von dem Armaturenbrett absorbiert. Je länger die zur Energieabsorption zur Verfügung stehende Zeit ist, um so größer ist auch die Energie, die absorbiert wird.

An ganzen Leichen haben GURDJIAN et al. (1961) die Auswirkung eines Falles auf eine Glasscheibe von 4,7, 5,5 und 6,3 mm Dicke nach Ersatz des Gehirns durch Gelatine vom spezifischen Gewicht 1,05 untersucht. Die Geschwindigkeit beim Aufschlagen maß 1,12—15,55 m/sec, die mittlere Beschleunigung 125—90 g gemessen am Hinterhaupt während 6—12 msec beim Aufschlagen auf den Vorderkopf. Der intracranielle Druck ist temporal größer als parietal. Der mittlere temporale Druck war 1,47 kg · cm^{-2}, wenn das Glas unverletzt blieb. Zerbrach das Glas, war der Druck kleiner. Die Größe des intracraniellen Druckes wechselt von Punkt zu Punkt der Schädelhöhle. *Für eine Gehirnerschütterung ist der Druck oberhalb des Foramen magnum maßgebend, der zu einer Scherbeanspruchung des Hirnstammes führt* (CHASON et al. 1958; GURDJIAN und LISSNER 1961). Die Größe dieser Scherbeanspruchung hängt nach GURDJIAN et al. (1953) wiederum von der Größe des durch eine dynamische Belastung erzeugten Druckes und dessen zeitlicher Einwirkung ab; der Druck ist eine Funktion der Schädeldeformation (HADDAD et al. 1955); die an Hunden ermittelten Werte können infolgedessen nicht auf den Menschen übertragen werden. Durch Filmaufnahmen konnten GURDJIAN et al. (1961) bei unverletztem Glas 3—4, bei zerbrochenem $2^1/_2$ Schwingungen des Schädels beobachten. Bei dünnerem Glas treten keine Verletzungen des Schädels oder der Halswirbelsäule auf.

Am Schädel können also ebenfalls experimentell Frakturen erzeugt werden, die klinischen Beobachtungen entsprechen. Sieht man von den Frakturen am Ort des Kraftangriffes ab, so kann aber nach GURDJIAN, WEBSTER und LISSNER (1950) nicht vorausgesagt werden, wo zusätzliche Frakturen auftreten. So lassen sich eindeutige Zusammenhänge zwischen einer bestimmten Krafteinwirkung und der Fraktur von kompakten und spongiösen Teilen nicht angeben. Jedoch scheinen Frakturen überwiegend oder ausschließlich bei dynamischer Belastung, dem Stoß, aufzutreten. Vermutlich steht bei der auftretenden zusammengesetzten Belastung eine Beanspruchung auf Knicken an den langen Knochen und Beulen an den platten im Vordergrund. Die Knicktheorie bietet mit dem „Kollaps" den Ansatz für ein plötzliches Materialversagen. Das Versagen eines Bauteiles hängt damit mehr von dessen Struktur und den mechanischen Eigenschaften des Baukörpers als von der Art der äußeren Kräfte ab.

Ein Gleiten der Komponenten ist für das Knochengewebe bei Biegung und Torsion sicher nachgewiesen. Dieses Gleiten könnte sich auch in den Molekularbereich fortsetzen und damit zum Bruch führen. Schwierig ist dagegen das Zustandekommen des Sprödbruches zu deuten. Nach KOCHENDÖRFER (1953) ist für das Auftreten eines Bruches ein Mechanismus zur Entstehung eines stabilen Risses im atomaren Bereich Voraussetzung. Dieser Riß muß dann weiterhin in mikroskopische Dimensionen fortschreiten. Hierzu ist eine verhältnismäßig große Oberflächenenergie erforderlich. Beim plastischen Gleiten könnten genügend Versetzungen und Leerstellen im Kristallgitter entstehen, beim Sprödbruch ohne merkliche plastische Verformung aber nicht. Zur Aufstellung einer allgemeinen Bruchtheorie beschäftigt sich KOCHENDÖRFER daher mit den Bedingungen für das Auftreten von Versetzungen im Kristallgitter. „Damit das entscheidende Ereignis, das Zusammenwandern zweier gleichnamiger Versetzungen, stattfinden kann, müssen die Versetzungen auf etwa 90% der Schallgeschwindigkeit beschleunigt werden, damit sie das bei Annäherung auftretende starke Abstoßpotential überwinden können." Haben die Versetzungen bestimmte Abmessungen erreicht, so können sie durch langsam wandernde

Versetzungen vergrößert werden. Man muß sich wohl auch für das Knochengewebe vorstellen, daß die Bedingungen des Bruches im Bereich der Molekularstruktur liegen.

Die experimentellen Untersuchungen der Festigkeit und Mechanik der Knochen haben eine ganze Reihe spezieller technischer Lösungen physikalischer Probleme aufgezeigt, für die in der Technik keine Parallelbeispiele zu finden sind. Die Eigenheit des Skeletes liegt offensichtlich darin, daß das Knochengewebe je nach örtlicher Beanspruchung auch verschiedene mechanische Eigenschaften aufweist. Diese Differenzierung des Materials wird nicht von dem sehr spezifisch gestalteten Stahl- oder Spannbeton erreicht. Lange Zeit glaubte man bei Untersuchungen der Mechanik des Knochengewebes, dieser Schwierigkeit mit starken Vereinfachungen Herr zu werden, aber wohl auch hier gilt eine Bemerkung von P. Weiss (1955): „Simplicity, and not complexity, is the illusion".

Literatur

Aeby, C.: Zur Architektur der Spongiosa. Zbl. med. Wiss. **11**, 785—786 (1873).

Albert, E.: Einführung in das Studium der Architektur der Röhrenknochen. Wien 1900.

Allison, N., and B. Brooks: Bone atrophy. An experimental study of the changes in bone which result from nonuse. Surg. Gynec. Obstet. **33**, 250—260 (1921).

Amprino, R.: Rapporti fra processi di ricostruzione e distribuzione dei minerali nelle ossa. I. Ricerche eseguite col metodo di studio dell' assorbimento dei raggi roentgen. Z. Zellforsch. **37**, 144—183 (1952).

— Investigations on some physical properties of bone tissue. Acta anat. (Basel) **34**, 161—186 (1958).

— Microhardness testing as a means of analysis of bone tissue biophysical properties. Biomechanical studies of the musculo-skeletal system, ed. by F. G. Evans et al., p. 20—48. Springfield (Ill.): Ch. C. Thomas 1961.

—, and G. Godina: La struttura delle ossa nei vertebrati. Ricerche comparative negli anfibi e negli annioti. Commentat. Pontificia acad. sci. **11**, 329—462 (1947).

Amtmann, E., u. H. P. Schmitt: Über die Verteilung der Corticalisdichte im menschlichen Femurschaft und ihre Bedeutung für die Bestimmung der Knochenfestigkeit. Z. Anat. Entwickl.-Gesch. **127**, 25—41 (1968).

Ascenzi, A., and E. Bonucci: The measurements of the tensile strength of isolated osteons as an approach to the problem of intimate bone texture. Calcified tissues. Proc. 2nd Europ. Sympos. 1964 (ed. by L. J. Richelle and M. J. Dallemagne), p. 325—335, Collect. Colloqu. L'Université de Liège (1965).

Ascenzi, A., and E. Bonucci: The compressive properties of single osteons. Anat. Rec. **161**, 377—392 (1968).

Attinger, E. O.: Atmung und Atmungsarbeit. Dtsch. med. Wschr. **86**, 111—117, 157—160, 288—294 (1961).

Auerbach, E.: Untersuchungen über die Variation der Knochenstruktur, dargestellt an der Tibia. Inaug.-Diss. Med. Fakultät 1957.

Backman, S.: The proximal end of the femur. Acta radiol. (Stockh.), Suppl. **146**, 1—166 (1957).

Badoux, D. M.: Statics of the mandible. Acta morph. neerl. scand. **6**, 252—256 (1966).

Bähr, F.: Beobachtungen über die statischen Beziehungen des Beckens zur unteren Extremität. Z. orthop. Chir. **5**, 52—59 (1898).

Bahling, G.: Die Entwicklung des Querschnittes der großen Extremitätenknochen bis zum Säuglingsalter. Morph. Jb. **99**, 109—188 (1958).

Balakirew, P.: Die spezifische Wärme des Fettgewebes der Tiere und des Menschen. Pflügers Arch. ges. Physiol. **230**, 803—813 (1932).

Barabás, C., O. Barta, L. Z. Szabó u. T. Vizkelety: Beiträge zur funktionellen Anatomie des Sakroiliakalgelenks. Acta morph. Acad. Sci. hung. **10**, 7—20 (1961).

Barnett, C. H., and O. J. Lewis: The evolution of some traction epiphyses in birds and mammals. J. Anat. (Lond.) **92**, 593—601 (1958).

Barth, G.: Die Volumina der langen Extremitätenknochen. Anthrop. Anz. **16**, 245—259 (1940).

Basmajian, J. V.: Electromyography of two-joint muscles. Anat. Rec. **149**, 371—380 (1957).

— Electromyography of postural muscles. In: Biomechanical studies of the musculo-skeletal system (ed. by F. G. Evans), p. 136—160. Springfield, Ill.: Ch. C. Thomas 1961.

— Electromyography: Its structural and neural basis. Int. Rev. Cytol. **21**, 129—140 (1967).

Bauer, H. O. K.: Volumen und Länge der langen Gliedmaßenknochen während des fetalen Wachstums. Anthrop. Anz. **17**, 77—102 (1940).

Bayer, H. v.: Bewegungslehre und Orthopädie. Z. orthop. Chir. **46**, 24—38 (1924/25).

Becker, R. B., and W. M. Neal: Relation of feed to bone strength in cattle. Proc. Amer. Soc. Animal Production 81—88 (1930).

— — and A. L. Shealy: Effect of calcium deficient roughages upon milk yield and bone strength of cattle. J. Dairy Sci. **17**, 1—10 (1934).

Bell, G. H.: Bone as a mechanical engineering problem. The biochemistry and physiology of bone. Ed. by G. H. Bourne, p. 27—49. New York: Academic Press Inc. 1956.

BELL, G. H., J. W. CHAMBERS, and I. M. DAWSON: The mechanical and structural properties of bone in rats on a rachitogenic diet. J. Physiol. (Lond.) **106**, 286—300 (1947).

—, and D. P. CUTHBERTSON: The effect of various hormones on the chemical and physical properties of bone. J. Endocr. **3**, 302—309 (1943).

— — and J. ORR: Strength and size of bone in relation to calcium intake. J. Physiol. (Lond.) **100**, 299—317 (1941).

—, and J. B. DE V. WEIR: Physical properties of bone in fluorosis. In: Industrial fluorosis. By J. N. AGATE et al. Med. Res. Counc. Mem. London. His Majesty's Stat. Off. **22**, 85—92 (1949).

BENNINGHOFF, A.: Der funktionelle Bau des Hyalinknorpels. Ergebn. Anat. Entwickl.-Gesch. **26**, 1—54 (1925).

— Spaltlinien am Knochen, eine Methode zur Ermittlung der Architektur platter Knochen. Studien zur Architektur der Knochen, I. Teil. Verh. Anat. Ges., 34. Verslg Wien 1925. Anat. Anz., **60**, Erg.-H. 189—206 (1925/26).

— Über die Anpassung der Knochenkompakta an geänderte Beanspruchungen. (Studien zur Struktur des Knochens. 2. Teil.) Anat. Anz. **63**, 289—299 (1927).

— Über Leitsysteme der Knochenkompakta. Studien zur Anatomie des Knochens. III. Teil. Morph. Jb. **65**, 11—44 (1931).

BERGENTHAL, E., u. L. KELLER: Untersuchungen am Skelettmuskel. 1. Mitt.: Der Bau des Musculus rectus abdominis des Menschen. Morph. Jb. **100**, 265—296 (1959).

BERLIS, G., u. L. KELLER: Untersuchungen am Skelettmuskel. 2. Mitt. Der Bau des Primärbündels. Morph. Jb. **100**, 297—321 (1959).

Beton-Kalender: I und II, 21. Jg. Berlin 1962.

BEYER, K.: Die Statik im Stahlbetonbau, 2. Aufl., 2. Neudruck. Berlin-Göttingen-Heidelberg: Springer 1956.

BIDDER, A.: Osteobiologie. Arch. mikr. Anat. **68**, 137—213 (1906).

BIERMANN, H.: Die Knochenbildung im Bereich periostaler-diaphysärer Sehnen- und Bandansätze. Z. Zellforsch. **46**, 635—671 (1957).

BLUNTSCHLI, H.: Zur Frage nach der funktionellen Struktur und Bedeutung der harten Hirnhaut. Arch. Entwickl.-Mech. Org. (Berl.) **106**, 303—319 (1925).

— Die menschlichen Kieferwerkzeuge in verschiedenen Alterszuständen. Verh. Anat. Ges. Erg.-H. zu Anat. Anz. **61**, 163—176 (1926).

—, u. R. WINKLER: Kaubewegungen und Bissenbildung. In: Handbuch der normalen und pathologischen Physiologie, Bd. 3, S. 295—347. 1927.

BOGDASCHEW, N.: Der Zusammenhang der anatomischen Formen der Metacarpal- und Metatarsalknochen der Haustiere mit dem histologischen Bau und den chemisch-physikalischen Eigenschaften derselben. Anat. Anz. **70**, 143—154 (1930).

BRAUS, H.: Anatomie des Menschen. I. Bewegungsapparat. Berlin: Springer 1921.

BRETTSCHNEIDER, H.: Ein Beitrag zur normalen Anatomie der Zwischenwirbelscheibe. Z. mikr.-anat. Forsch. **58**, 381—403 (1952).

BRUNO, G.: Il tessuto osseo. Rass. clin.-sci. **26**, 8—11 (1950).

BÜRKER, H.: Experimentelle Untersuchungen über Muskelwärme. Pflügers Arch. ges. Physiol. **80**, 533—582 (1900).

BURKHARDT, L.: Über Umbau und Strukturtypen der Wirbelkörperspongiosa als Ausdruck allgemeiner Gesetzmäßigkeiten der Knochenmodellierung. Verh. dtsch. Ges. Path. **38**, 250—259 (1954).

CALABRISI, P., and F. SMITH: The effects of embalming on the compressive strength of a few specimens of compact human bone. Naval Med. Res. Inst. Project NH/R-NMO0l, 0,56.02 MR 51—2:1—3 (1951).

CALLENDER, G. R., and R. W. FRENCH: Wound ballistics: Studies in the mechanism of wound production by rifle bullets. Milit. Surg. **77**, 177—201 (1935).

CARLSTRÖM, D.: Micro-hardness measurements on single haversian systems in bone. Experientia (Basel) **10**, 171 (1954).

CARLSTROM, D., and J. B. FINEAN: X-Ray diffraction studies on the ultrastructure of bone. Biochim. biophys. Acta (Amst.) **13**, 183—191 (1954).

CAROTHERS, C. O., F. C. SMITH, and P. CALABRISI: The elasticity and strength of some long bones of the human body. Naval Med. Res. Inst. Project NM 001 056.02. 13: 1—18 (1949).

CHASON, J. C., W. G. HARDY, J. E. WEBSTER, and E. S. GURDJIAN: Alterations in cell structure of brain associated with experimental concussion. J. Neurosurg. **15**, 135—139 (1958).

CLARKE, H. H., E. C. ELKINS, G. M. MARTIN, and K. G. WAKIM: Relationship between body position and the application of muscle power to movements of the joints. Arch. phys. Med. **31**, 81—89 (1950).

CLARKE, M. F., A. L. BASSIN, and A. H. SMITH: Skeletal changes in the rat induced by a ration extremely poor in inorganic salts. Amer. J. Physiol. **115**, 556—563 (1936).

COMAR, C. L., and F. BRONNER: Mineral metabolism, vol. I (1960), vol. II (1961). London and New York: Academic Press.

COTTON, F. J., and G. M. MORRISON: Hip fractures: Valgus position — accidental or engineered. J. Bone Jt Surg. A **20**, 461—468 (1938).

CRELIN, E. S.: The effects of androgen, estrogen and relaxin on intact and transplanted pelvis in mice. Amer. J. Anat. **95**, 47—73 (1954a).

— The effects of estrogen and relaxin on the pubic symphysis and transplanted ribs in mice. Anat. Rec. **120**, 23—31 (1954b).

— A method for quantitating flexibility changes of pelvic joints in rats and mice. Proc. Soc. exp. Biol. (N.Y.) **90**, 236—238 (1955).

Crelin, E. S.: The development of bony pelvic sexual dimorphism in mice. Ann. N. Y. Acad. Sci. **84**, 479—512 (1960).
—, and J. Levin: The prepuberal pubic symphysis and uterus in the mouse. Their reponse to estrogen and relaxin. Endocrinology **57**, 730—747 (1955).
Culmann, K.: Graphische Statik. Zürich 1866.
Currey, J. D.: Differences in the tensile strength of bone different histological types. J. Anat. (Lond.) **93**, 87—95 (1959).
— Stress concentrations in bone. Quart. J. micr. Sci. **103**, 111—133 (1962a).
— Strength of bone. Nature (Lond.) **195**, 513—514 (1962b).
— Three analogies to explain the mechanical properties of bone. Biorheology **2**, 1—10 (1964).
— The failure of exoskeletons and endoskeletons. J. Morph. **123**, 1—16 (1967).
Daeves, K., and A. Beckel: Großzahlforschung und Häufigkeitsanalyse. Berlin: Chemie 1948.
Dallemagne, M. J.: La nature chimique de la substance minerale osseuse; premiers essais d'interpretation des certains phenomenes physiopathologiques de l'os à la lumiere ces notions nouvelles. Thèse agrégation Univ. Liège, Gordinne (1943).
Davida, E.: Proportionsuntersuchungen auf Grund des Knochenvolumens und der Volumindex der Extremitätenknochen. Anat. Anz. **61**, 128—136 (1926).
Dempster, W. T.: Space requirements of the seated operator. WADC Technical Report, 55—159 (1955).
—, and R. T. Liddicoat: Compact bone as a non-isotropic material. Amer. J. Anat. **91**, 331—362 (1952).
Derlath, M.: Untersuchungen über die Spongiosaarchitektur des Wirbelkörpers. Ärztl. Forsch. **6**, 309—318 (1958).
Diamant, M.: Otitis and pneumatisation of the mastoid bone. Lund: Akademisk Avhandling 1940.
Dietrich, O., u. E. Lehr: Das Dehnungslinienverfahren, ein Mittel zur Bestimmung der für die Bruchsicherheit bei Wechselbeanspruchung maßgeblichen Spannungsverteilung. VDI Zeitschrift **76**, 973 (1932).
Dixon, F.: The architecture of the cancellous tissue forming the upper end of the femur. J. Anat. (Lond.) **44**, 223—230 (1910).
Dolgo-Saburoff, B.: Über Ursprung und Insertion der Skeletmuskeln. Anat. Anz. **68**, 80—87 (1929/1930).
— Über einige Eigentümlichkeiten der Knochenstruktur an den Anheftungsstellen der Sehnen. Gegenbaurs morph. Jb. **75**, 393—411 (1935).
Donaldson, H. H.: Quantitative studies on the growth of the skeleton of the albino rat. Amer. J. Anat. **26**, 237—314 (1919/20).
Dowgjallo, N. D.: Die Struktur der Compacta des Unterkiefers bei normalem und reduziertem Alveolarfortsatz. Z. Anat. Entwickl.-Gesch. **97**, 55—67 (1932).
Drüner, L.: Über die Sehnen des Schollenmuskels und Bemerkungen über die anderen Schollenmuskeln des menschlichen Körpers. Z. Anat. Entwickl.-Gesch. **79**, 263—268 (1926).
Du Bois-Reymond, R.: Über Dicke und Festigkeit der Knochen bei großen und kleinen Tieren. Z. wiss. Zool. **132**, 1—36 (1928).
Du Brul, E. L., and H. Sicher: The adaptive chin, vol. 7, p. 3—97. Springfeld (Ill.): Ch. C. Thomas 1954.
Dziallas, P., u. H. Lippert: Über umwegige Entwicklungsvorgänge an den Wirbelkörpern des Menschen. Morph. Jb. **100**, 747—769 (1960).
Eggenschwiler, E.: Ist die Zuspitzung des Musculus rectus abdominis in seinem kaudalen Bereich durch Reduktion der Faserdicke oder der Faserzahl bedingt? Acta anat. (Basel) **26**, 175—191 (1956).
Ehler, E.: Zur Mechanik der langen Röhrenknochen der menschlichen oberen Extremität. Habilitationsarbeit, med. Fakultät der Universität Rostock (1963).
— Zur Ermittlung von Randfaserspannungen an Knochenteilen der menschlichen oberen Extremität. Gegenbaurs morph. Jb. **109**, 614—632 (1966a).
— Torsionsversuche an Knochenteilen der menschlichen oberen Extremität. Anat. Anz. **119**, 351—358 (1966b).
— Randfaserspannungen an Humeri, Radii und Ulnae. Gegenbaurs morph. Jb. **110**, 437—469 (1967b).
— Menschliche Humeri, Radii und Ulnae unter Biegebelastung. Anat. Anz. **120**, 474—491 (1967a).
— Der menschliche Humerus unter Stoßeinwirkung (Modellberechnung). Anat. Anz. **120**, 125—131 (1967c).
—, u. H. Pfau: Zur Spannungsberechnung an menschlichen Humeri bei Einwirkung axial eingeleiteter periodischer Längskräfte. Anat. Anz. **123**, 278—283 (1968).
Eickhoff, J.: Untersuchungen am Metacarpus von Lauf- und Schrittpferden besonders auf physikalisch-mechanische Eigenschaften. Diss. Göttingen 1927.
Endo, B.: Distribution of stress and strain produced in the human facial skeleton by the masticatory force. Zinruigaku Zassi **73**, 123—136 (1965).
Ertelt, W.: Untersuchungen über Körpergröße und Knochenstruktur bei Säugetieren. Zool. Jb. Abt. Anat. u. Ontog. **74**, 588—638 (1955).
Evans, F. G.: Methods of studying the biomechanical significance of bone form. Amer. J. phys. Anthropol. **11**, 413—436 (1953).
— Studies in human biomechanics. Ann. N. Y. Acad. Sci. **63**, 586—615 (1955).
— Studies on the biomechanics and structure of bone. Ass. Anatomistes **44**, 272—276 (1957).
— Relations between the microscopic structure and tensile strength of human bone. Acta anat. (Basel) **35**, 285—301 (1958).

EVANS, F. G.: Relation of the physical properties of bone to fractures. Instruction. Course lectures **18**, 110—121 (1961).
— Stress and strain of posture, expressed in the construction of man's weight-bearing skeletal structures. Clin. Orthop. **25**, 42—54 (1962).
— Significant differences in the tensile strength of adult human compact bone. Bone and tooth. 1rst Europ. Sympos. (ed. by H. J. J. BLACKWOOD), p. 319—331. Oxford-London-New York-Paris: Pergamon Press 1964.
— A commentary on the significance of stresscoat and split-line patterns on bone. Amer. J. Phys. Anthrop. **23**, 189—195 (1965).
— Bibliography on the physical properties of the skeletal system. Highway safety research institute the university of Michigan Ann Arbor (1967).
—, and S. BANG: Differences and relationships between the physical properties and the microscopic structure of human femoral tibial and fibular cortical bone. Amer. J. Anat. **120**, 79—88 (1967).
— C. C. COOLBOUGH, and LEBOW: An apparatus for determining bone sensity by means of radioactive. Science **114**, 182—185 (1951).
—, and C. W. GOFF: A comparative study of the primate femur by means of the stresscoat and the splitline techniques. Amer. J. phys. Anthropol. **15**, 59—90 (1957).
— J. F. HAYES, and J. E. POWERS: "Stresscoat" deformation studies of the human femur under transverse loading. Anat. Rec. **116**, 171—187 (1953).
—, and M. LEBOW: Regional differences in some of the physical properties of the human femur. J. appl. Physiol. **3**, 563—572 (1951).
— — The strength of human compact bone as revealed by engeneering technics. Amer. J. Surg. **83**, 326—331 (1952).
— — Strength of human compact bone under repetitive loading. J. appl. Physiol. **10**, 127—130 (1957).
—, and H. R. LISSNER: "Stresscoat" deformation studies of the femur under static vertical loading. Anat. Rec. **100**, 159—190 (1948).
— — Studies on pelvic deformations and tractures. Anat. Rec. **121**, 141—166 (1955).
— — Tensile and compressive strength of human parietal bone. J. appl. Physiol. **10**, 439—497 (1957).
— — Biomechanical studies on the lumbar spine and pelvis. J. Bone Jt Surg. A **2**, 278—290 (1959).
— — Studies on the energy absorbing capacity of human lumbar intervertebral discs. The 7th stapp car crash conference proceedings (ed. by D. M. SEVERY), p. 1—17. Springfield, Ill.: Ch. C. Thomas 1965.
— — and M. LEBOW: The relation of energy, velocity and acceleration to skull deformation and fracture. Surgery **107**, 593—601 (1958).
— — and H. E. PEDERSEN: Deformation studies of the femur under dynamic vertical loading. Anat. Rec. **101**, 225—241 (1948).
EVANS, F. G., and L. M. PATRICK: Impact damage to internal organs. Impact acceleration stress (National Acad. Sciences-National Res. Council) Public. 977 (ohne Jahr).
— H. E. PEDERSEN, and H. R. LISSNER: The role of tensile stress in the mechanism of femoral fractures. J. Bone Jt Surg. A **33**, 485—501 (1951).
FALLER, A.: Zur Deutung der akzessorischen Köpfe des Schollenmuskels. Anat. Anz. **93**, 161—179 (1942).
FARKAS, A., M. J. WILSON, and J. C. HAYNER: An anatomical study of the mechanics, pathology, and healing of fracture of the femoral neck. J. Bone Jt Surg. A **30**, 53—69 (1948).
FENN, W. O.: Die mechanischen Eigenschaften des Muskels. In: Handbuch der normalen und pathologischen Physiologie (Herausg. A. BETHE, G. v. BERGMANN, G. EMDEN, A. ELLINGER), S. 146—164. Berlin: Springer 1925a.
— Der zeitliche Verlauf der Muskelkontraktion. In: Handbuch der normalen und pathologischen Physiologie (Herausg. A. BETHE, G. v. BERGMANN, G. EMDEN, A. ELLINGER), S. 166—190. Berlin: Springer 1925b.
FENEIS, H.: Über die Anordnung und die Bedeutung des Bindegewebes für die Mechanik der Skelettmuskulatur. Morph. Jb. **76**, 161—202 (1935).
FESSLER, H.: Load distribution in a model of a hip joint. J. Bone Jt Surg. B **39**, 145—153 (1957).
FICK, A.: Medizinische Physik. Braunschweig 1856.
FICK, H.: Die Bedeutung des Epiphysenknorpels für die Entwicklung der Spongiosaarchitektur im proximalen Femurende. Morph. Jb. **85**, 115—134 (1941).
FICK, R.: Handbuch der Anatomie und Mechanik der Gelenke, Bd. I—III. Jena: Gustav Fischer 1904, 1910, 1911.
—, u. J. ROSCHDESTWENSKI: Über die Bewegungen im Hüftgelenk und die Arbeitsleistung der Hüftmuskeln. Arch. Anat. 365—456 (1913).
FILOGAMO, G.: Contributo alla conoscenza della minuta struttura dell'osso. Osservazioni sulla zona d'attaco di tendini allo scheletro. R.P. It. lombardo Sci, pt. I. **78**, 425—448 (1945).
FISCHER, O.: Medizinische Physik. Leipzig: Wilhelm Engelmann 1919.
FLOYD, W. F., and P. H. S. SILVER: The function of the erectores spinae muscles in certain movement and postures in man. J. Physiol. (Lond.) **129**, 184—203 (1955).
FÖPPL, A.: Vorlesungen über technische Mechanik, Bd. 1. München: R. Oldenbourg 1920.
— Vorlesungen über technische Mechanik, Bd.V. Die wichtigsten Lehren aus der höheren Elastizitätstheorie. München: R. Oldenbourg 1922.
— Vorlesungen über technische Mechanik, Bd.II. Graphische Statik, 10. Aufl. München: R. Oldenbourg 1949.

FÖPPL, A.: Vorlesungen über technische Mechanik, Bd. III. Festigkeitslehre, 15. Aufl. München: R. Oldenbourg 1951.
—, u. L. FÖPPL: Drang und Zwang. Eine höhere Festigkeitslehre für Ingenieure. München: R. Oldenbourg 1944/1947.
FÖPPL, L., u. E. MÖNCH: Praktische Spannungsoptik. Spannungsoptische Messungen. In: E. SIEBEL u. N. LUDWIG, Handbuch der Werkstoffprüfung, 2. Aufl., S. 520—547. Berlin-Göttingen-Heidelberg: Springer 1958.
FOREST, A. V. DE, and G. ELLIS: Brittle lacquer as an aid to stress analysis. J. Aeronaut. Sci. 7, 205—208 (1940).
FRIEDRICH, H.: Die Markräume in den Extremitätenknochen eines 25jährigen und eines 82jährigen Mannes. Inaug.-Diss. Rostock 1890.
FRITZEL, R.: Entwicklung von Reibungswärme bei der maschinellen Wurzelkanalaufbereitung mit den derzeit gebräuchlichen Aufbereitungsmitteln. Inaug.-Diss. Med. Fakultät Kiel 1950.
GAENSLEN, F. J.: Fracture of the neck of the femur. J. Amer. med. Ass. **107**, 105—114 (1936).
GARDEN, R. S.: The structure and function of the proximal end of the femur. J. Bone Jt Surg. B **43**, 576—589 (1961).
GEBHARDT, W.: Über funktionell wichtige Anordnungsweisen der feineren und gröberen Bauelemente des Wirbeltierknochens. Arch. Entwickl.-Mech. Org. **20**, 187—322 (1906).
— Die spezielle funktionelle Anpassung der Röhrenknochendiaphyse. Arch. Entwickl.-Mech. Org. **30**, 516—534 (1910a).
— Über die funktionelle Knochengestalt. Verh. Dtsch. Ges. orthop. Chir. **27**, 121—220 (1910b).
— Funktionelle Entwicklungsstufen des Knochens. Verh. dtsch. Naturforsch. Königsberg 433—461 (1910c).
— Über die funktionelle Knochengestalt. Verh. Dtsch. Ges. orthop. Chir. **9**, 121—124 (1910d).
— Über den Skelettbau mit dünnen Platten. Verh. Anat. Ges. **25**. Verslg, Anat. Anz. **38**, Erg.-H., 97—118 (1911).
GHILLINI, C.: Die Pathogenese der Knochendeformitäten. Z. orthop. Chir. **6**, 589—603 (1899).
—, u. CANEVAZZI: Über die statischen Verhältnisse des menschlichen Skelets. Z. orthop. Chir. **9**, 178—202 (1901).
— — Über die statischen Verhältnisse des Oberschenkelknochens. Z. orthop. Chir. **10**, 14—22 (1902).
GILLESPIE, J. A.: The nature of the bone changes associated with nerve injuries and disuse. J. Bone Jt Surg. Brit. **36**, 464—473 (1954).
GOECKE, C.: Das Verhalten spongiöser Knochen im Druck- und Schlagversuch. Verh. dtsch. orthop. Ges. **20**, 114—129 (1925).
— Physikalische Untersuchungen an skoliotischen Wirbeln. Verh. 21. Kongr. Dtsch. Orthop. Ges., S. 168—181. Stuttgart: Ferdinand Enke 1926.
GOECKE, C.: Die Physik des atrophischen Knochens. Verh. 23. Kongr. dtsch. Orthop. Ges., 103—112 (1928).
— Elastizitätsstudien am jungen und alten Gelenkknorpel. Verh. dtsch. orthop. Ges. **22**, 130—147 (1928).
— Beiträge zur Druckfestigkeit des spongiösen Knochens. Bruns' Beitr. klin. Chir. **143**, 539—566 (1928).
— Das Verhalten spongiösen Knochens im Druck- und Schlagversuch. Verh. 20. Kongr. Dtsch. Orthop. Ges. 1929.
— Das Verhalten der Bandscheibe bei Wirbelverletzungen. Arch. orthop. Unfall-Chir. **31**, 42—80 (1932).
GÖRKE: Beitrag zur funktionellen Gestaltung des Schädels bei den Anthropomorphen und Menschen durch Untersuchung mit Röntgenstrahlen. Arch. Anthrop. (Braunschweig), N.F. **1**, 91—108 (1904).
GONG, J. K., J. S. ARNOLD, and S. H. COHN: Composition of trabecular and cortical bone. Anat. Rec. **149**, 325—331 (1964).
GRAF, A.: Über die Architektur rachitischer Knochen. Ein Beitrag zum Wolffschen Transformationsgesetz. Z. orthop. Chir. **3**, 174—196 (1894).
GRAYSON, J.: Internal calorimetry in the determination of thermal conductivity and blood flow. J. Physiol. (Lond.) **118**, 54—72 (1952).
GROHMANN, F. W.: Über die Arbeitsleistung der am Ellenbogengelenk wirkenden Wirbel. Arch. Anat. 315—328 (1902).
GROTH, W.: Das Foramen lacerum und der Einbau des Felsenbeins beim Menschen. Anat. Anz. **91**, 97—121 (1941).
GRUNEWALD, J.: Über den Einfluß der Muskelarbeit auf die Form des menschlichen Femur. Z. orthop. Chir. **30**, 551—602 (1912).
— Die Beziehung zwischen der Form und der Funktion der Tibia und Fibula des Menschenaffen. Z. orthop. Chir. **35**, 675—780 (1916).
— Die Beanspruchung der langen Röhrenknochen des Menschen. Z. orthop. Chir. **39**, 27—49, 256—286 (1920).
GÜTTNER, W.: Die Energieverteilung im menschlichen Körper bei Ultraschall-Einstrahlung. Acustica **4**, 547—554 (1954).
GURDJIAN, E. S., and H. R. LISSNER: Mechanism of head injury as studies by the cathode ray oscilloscope. Preliminary report. J. Neurosurg. **1**, 393—399 (1944).
— — Deformation of the skull in head injuring, a study with the stress-coat technique. Surg. Gynec. Obstet. **81**, 679—687 (1945).
— — Deformations of the skull in head injury studies by the "stresscoat" technique, quantitative determinations. Surg. Gynec. Obstet. **83**, 219—233 (1946).
— — Mechanism of concussion. In: Biomechanical studies of the musculo-skeletal system, ed. by F. G. EVANS, p. 192—208. Springfield (Ill.): Ch. C. Thomas 1961.
— — F. G. EVANS, L. M. PATRICK, and W. G. HARDY: Intracranial pressure and acceleration

accompanying head impacts in human cadavers. Surgery **113**, 185—190 (1961).

GURDJIAN, E. S., H. R. LISSNER, and J. E. WEBSTER: The mechanism of production of linear skull fracture. Further studies on deformation of the skull by the "stresscoat" technique. Surg. Gynec. Obstet. **85**, 195—210 (1947).

— J. E. WEBSTER, and H. R. LISSNER: Studies on skull fracture with particular reference to engineering factors. Amer. J. Surg. **78**, 736—742 (1949).

— — — The mechanism of skull fracture. J. Neurosurg. **7**, 106—114 (1950a).

— — — The mechanism of skull fracture. Radiology **54**, 313—339 (1950b).

— — — Observations on prediction of fracture site in head injury. Radiology **60**, 226—235 (1953).

HAASE, W.: Technisch-physikalische Untersuchungen an Knochenbrüchen. Bruns Beitr. klin. Chir. **164**, 243—263 (1936).

— Schubebene und Zerrüttungszonen beim Knochenbruch. Arch. orthop. Unfall-Chir. **37**, 592—599 (1937a).

— Neue Untersuchungen menschlicher und tierischer Knochen nach den Grundsätzen technischer Werkstoffprüfung. Forsch. Fortschr. dtsch. Wiss. **13**, 130—131 (1937b).

—, u. G. RICHTER: Knochenbrüche, beurteilt nach den Grundsätzen und Erkenntnissen der technischen Mechanik. Arch. orthop. Unfall-Chir. **36**, 541—556 (1936).

HADDAD, B. F., H. R. LISSNER, J. E. WEBSTER, and E. S. GURDJIAN: Experimental concussion; relation of acceleration to physiologic effect. Neurology **5**, 798—800 (1955).

HADENFELDT, H.: Über die chirurgische Säge. Zbl. Chir. **57**, 645—646 (1930).

HÄBLER, C., u. O. REISS: Experimentelle Untersuchungen über die Festigkeit des Knochens im normalen und im Zustand der Bruchheilung. Dtsch. Z. Chir. **246**, 486—493, 760—772 (1936).

HAGEN, W.: Zur Statik des Schenkelhalses. Bruns' Beitr. klin. Chir. **56**, 627—638 (1908).

— Die Belastungsverhältnisse am normalen und pathologisch deformierten Skelett der unteren Extremität. Bruns' Beitr. klin. Chir. **63**, 761—787 (1909).

HALLERMANN, H.: Die Beziehungen der Werkstoffmechanik und Werkstofforschung zur allgemeinen Knochenmechanik. Verh. Dtsch. orthop. Ges. **62**, 347—360 (1934).

HALLS, A. A., and A. TRAVILL: Transmission of pressures across the elbow joint. Anat. Rec. **150**, 243—248 (1964).

HANAUSECK, J.: Beitrag zum statischen Problem des Skeletts der unteren Extremität. Z. orthop. Chir. **34**, 607—637 (1914).

HARDINGE, M. G.: Determination of the strength of the cancellous bone in the head and neck of the femur. Surg. Gynec. Obstet. **89**, 439—441 (1949).

HASSELWANDER, A.: Bewegungssystem. In: Handbuch der Anatomie des Kindes (Herausg. K. PETER, G. WEKEL, F. HEIDERICH), Bd. II, S. 403—589. München: J. F. Bergmann 1938.

HEIDSIECK, E.: Eine Modellvorstellung vom Knorpel. Anat. Anz. **78**, 175—182 (1934).

HENCKEL, K. O.: Vergleichend-anatomische Untersuchungen über die Struktur der Knochenkompakta nach der Spaltlinienmethode. Gegenbaurs morph. Jb. (Teil I) **66**, 22—45 (1931).

HENSCHEN, C.: Überlastungsschäden am Knochensystem. Langenbecks Arch. klin. Chir. **186**, 98—101 (1936).

HEROLD, W.: Spannungsoptische Untersuchungen an Knochenmodellen. In: Physikalische Grundlagen der Medizin. Abhandlungen aus der Biophysik, H. 4/5 (ed. von WALTER BEIER), p. 178—211. Leipzig: Georg Thieme 1963.

HERRE, W.: Über Domestikationserscheinungen bei Tier und Mensch. Dtsch. med. Wschr. **84**, 2334—2338 (1959).

HERT, J., P. KUCERA, M. VÁVRA, and V. VOLENIK: Comparison of mechanical properties of both the primary and haversian bone tissue. Acta anat. (Basel) **61**, 412—423 (1965).

HETÉNY, M.: Handbook of experimental stress analysis. New York: John Wiley & Sons, London: Chapmann & Hall Ltd. 1960.

HIRSCH, C.: Studies on the mechanism of low back pain. Acta orthop. scand. **20**, 261—274 (1951).

—, and A. BRODETTI: Methods of studying some mechanical properties of bone tissue. Acta orthop. scand. **26**, 1—14 (1956a).

— — The weight-bearing capacity of structural elements in femoral necks. Second report. Acta orthop. scand. **26**, 15—24 (1956b).

— A. CAVADIAS, and A. NACHEMSON: An attempt to explain fracture types. Acta orthop. scand. **24**, 8—29 (1954).

—, and F. G. EVANS: Studies on some physical proporties of infant compact bone. Acta orthop. scand. **35**, 300—313 (1965).

—, and V. H. FRANKEL: The reaction of the proximal end of the femur to mechanical forces. Biochem. studies of the musculoskeletal system, ed. by F. G. EVANS, p. 68—80. Springfield (Ill.): Ch. C. Thomas 1961.

—, and A. NACHEMSON: New observations on the mechanical behaviour of lumbar discs. Acta orthop. scand. **23**, 254—283 (1954).

— S. PAULSON, B. SYLVÉN, and O. SNELLMAN: Biophysical and physiological investigations on cartilage and other mesenchymal tissues. VI. Characteristics of human nuclei pulposi during aging. Acta orthop. scand. **22**, 175—183 (1953).

HIRSCH, H. H.: Die mechanische Bedeutung der Schienbeinform. Berlin 1895.

— Über eine Beziehung zwischen dem Neigungswinkel des Schenkelhalses und dem Querschnitt des Schenkelbeinschaftes. Anat. H. **11**, 671—679 (1899).

HIRSCHFELD, K.: Baustatik. Berlin-Göttingen-Heidelberg: Springer 1959.

Hodgson, V. R.: Tolerance of the facial bones to impact. Amer. J. Anat. **120**, 113—122 (1967).
Huelke, D. F., L. J. Buege, and J. H. Harger: Bone fractures produced by high velocity impacts. Amer. J. Anat. **120**, 123—131 (1967).
— J. H. Harger, L. J. Buege, and H. G. Dingman: An experimental study in bio-ballistics: femoral fractures produced by projectiles-II shaft impacts. J. Biomechanics **1**, 313—321 (1968).
Hülsen, C.: Spezifisches Gewicht, Elastizität und Festigkeit des Knochengewebes. Anz. biol. Labor St. Petersburg 1898, S. 7—37. Nach Schaffer, Jber. Anat. u. Entwickl.-Gesch., N. F. **4**, 1. Teil, S. 146 (1899).
Hüter, Th. F.: Messungen der Ultraschallabsorption in tierischen Geweben und ihre Abhängigkeit von der Frequenz. Naturwissenschaften **35**, 285—287 (1948).
— Messungen der Ultraschallabsorption im menschlichen Schädelknochen und ihre Abhängigkeit von der Frequenz. Naturwissenschaften **39**, 21—22 (1952).
Hütte: Des Ingenieurs Taschenbuch. I. Theoretische Grundlagen. 28. Aufl. Berlin: Ernst & Sohn 1955.
Huggenberger, A. U., u. S. Schwaigerer: Meßverfahren und Meßeinrichtungen für Verformungsmessungen. In: E. Siebel u. N. Ludwig, Handbuch der Werkstoffprüfung, 2. Aufl, S. 371—519. Berlin-Göttingen-Heidelberg: Springer 1958.
Huggins, C. B., and B. H. Blocksom: Temperature bone marrow in rabbits. Amer. J. Physiol. **113**, 68 (Abstract) (1935).
Ingalls, N. W.: Observations on bone weights. Amer. J. Anat. **48**, 45—98 (1931).
— Observations on bone weights. The bones of the foot. Amer. J. Anat. **50**, 435—450 (1932).
Ingelmark, E., u. R. Ekholm: Über die Kompressibilität der Intervertebralscheiben. Acta Soc. Med. upsalien. **57**, 202—217 (1952).
Janssen, M.: On bone formation: Its relation to tension and pressure, p. 1—114. London: Longmans 1920.
Jipp, P.: Die Sehnenstruktur an punktförmigen Muskelansätzen. Morph. Jb. **101**, 236—262 (1960).
Joos, G.: Lehrbuch der Theoretischen Physik, 6. Aufl. Leipzig: Akademische Verlagsgesellschaft 1945.
Kann, F.: Über Dicke und Zahl der Muskelfasern auf verschiedenen Querschnittshöhen des Musculus sartorius beim Menschen. Acta anat. (Basel) **30**, 351—357 (1957).
Katz, A.: Architektur des Unterkiefers in Zusammenhang mit der Lage der Wurzeln und Widerstandsfähigkeit des Zahnbogens beim Erwachsenen. Vjschr. Zahnheilk. **47**, 85 (1931).
Killmer, M.: Untersuchungen zur Form des Knochenbruchs in Abhängigkeit von der Energie und dem Eintreffwinkel der brucherzeugenden Gewalt. Inaug.-Diss. der med. Fakultät der Univ. Bonn (1966).
Kimura, T.: An experimental study of the form of the human tibia from the biomechanical point of view. J. Anthrop. Soc. (Tokyo) **74**, 37—45 (1966).
Klapp, R., u. W. Rückert: Die Drahtextension in der Friedens- und Kriegschirurgie, 2. Aufl. Stuttgart: Ferdinand Enke 1944.
Klatt, B.: Über den Einfluß der Gesamtgröße auf das Schädelbild nebst Bemerkungen über die Vorgeschichte der Haustiere. Wilhelm Roux' Arch. Entwickl.-Mech. Org. **36**, 387—471 (1913).
— Die theoretische Biologie und die Problematik der Schädelform. Biol. generalis (Wien) **19**, 51—89 (1949).
Klöppel, K.: Die Einheit der Wissenschaft und der Ingenieur. Dtsch. Museum, Abh. u. Ber. **26**, 1—42 (1958).
Knaack, K.: Zur Frage der Wärmeschädigung des Knochens beim Sägen. Inaug.-Diss. Med. Fakultät Kiel 1962.
Knese, K.-H.: Über physikalische und elektromyographische Untersuchungen am Bewegungsapparat. Verh. Anat. Ges., 51. Verslg 1953. Anat. Anz., Erg.-H. 301—318 (1954).
— Allgemeine Bemerkungen über Belastungsuntersuchungen des Knochens sowie spezielle Untersuchungen am Oberschenkel unter der Annahme einer Krankonstruktion. Anat. Anz. **101**, 186—203 (1955a).
— Die Statik des Kniegelenkes. Z. Anat. Entwickl.-Gesch. **118**, 471—512 (1955b).
— Elektromyographische Untersuchungen über die Muskel- und Massenwirkung bei Bewegung sowie die Frage des wechselnden Zusammenspieles der Muskeln. Pflügers Arch. ges. Physiol. **263**, 522—532 (1956a).
— Belastungsuntersuchungen des Oberschenkels unter der Annahme des Knickens. Morph. Jb. **97**, 405—452 (1956b).
— Über anatomische Grundlagen der Konstitution. Z. Morph. Anthrop. **49**, 29—42 (1958a).
— Knochenstruktur als Verbundbau, Versuch einer technischen Deutung der Materialstruktur des Knochens. Zwanglose Abh. a. d. Gebiet der norm. und path. Anatomie, von W. Bargmann u. W. Doerr, H. 4. Stuttgart: Georg Thieme 1958b.
— Neuere Untersuchungen über die Knochenbildung und ihre Beeinflussungsmöglichkeiten. Dtsch. zahnärztl. Z. **14**, 925—932, 990—1000 (1959a).
— Eine Erörterung neuerer Untersuchungen über die Bedeutung der Spongiosa-Architektur. Berichte über die 6. Tagg der Dtsch. Ges. für Anthropologie Kiel, 1958. Suppl. zu Homo. Göttingen-Berlin-Frankfurt: Musterschmidt 1959b.
— Bau und Mechanik der Wirbelsäule. In: Die Wirbelsäule in Forschung und Praxis, Bd. 26 (ed. by H. Junghanns), p. 9—19. Stuttgart: Hippokrates-Verlag 1963a.
— Topographie des Herzens. In: Das Herz des Menschen (ed. W. Bargmann und W. Doerr), p. 260—312. Stuttgart: Georg Thieme 1963b.

KNESE, K.-H.: Über die Mineralablagerungen im Knorpel- und Knochengewebe unter Berücksichtigung elektronenmikroskopischer Befunde. Acta histochem. (Jena), Suppl. **3**, 31—56 (1963c).

—, u. H. BIERMANN: Die Knochenbildung an Sehnen- und Bandansätzen im Bereich ursprünglich chondraler Apophysen. Z. Zellforsch. **49**, 142—187 (1958).

— O. H. HAHNE u. H. BIERMANN: Festigkeitsuntersuchungen an menschlichen Extremitätenknochen. Morph. Jb. **96**, 141—209 (1955).

—, u. M. v. HARNACK: Über die Faserstruktur des Knochengewebes. Z. Zellforsch. **57**, 520—558 (1962).

— I. RITSCHL u. D. VOGES: Quantitative Untersuchung der Osteonverteilung im Extremitätenskelett eines 43jährigen Mannes. Z. Zellforsch. **40**, 519—570 (1954).

—, u. S. TITSCHAK: Untersuchungen mit Hilfe des Lochkartenverfahrens über die Osteonstruktur von Haus- und Wildschweinknochen sowie Bemerkungen zur Baugeschichte des Knochens. Morph. Jb. **102**, 337—458 (1962).

— D. VOGES u. I. RITSCHL: Untersuchungen über die Osteon- und Lamellenformen im Extremitätenskelet des Erwachsenen. Z. Zellforsch. **40**, 323—360 (1954).

KNIEF, J. J.: Quantitative Untersuchung der Verteilung der Hartsubstanzen im Knochen in der Beziehung zur lokalen mechanischen Beanspruchung. Methodik und biomechanische Problematik, dargestellt am Beispiel des coxalen Femurendes. Z. Anat. Entwickl.-Gesch. **126**, 55—80 (1967a).

— Materialverteilung und Beanspruchungsverteilung im coxalen Femurende. Densitometrische und spannungsoptische Untersuchungen. Z. Anat. Entwickl.-Gesch. **126**, 81—116 (1967b).

KOCH, J. C.: The laws of bone architecture. Amer. J. Anat. **21**, 177—298 (1917).

KOCHENDÖRFER, A.: Zur Theorie der Bruchvorgänge. Naturwissenschaften **40**, 432—433 (1953).

KÖRNER, F.: Das Myon, das konstruktive Bauelement des Muskels. Z. Anat. Entwickl.-Gesch. **109**, 609—623 (1939).

KOLB, H.: Morphologie und funktionelle Analyse des M. tibialis anterior. Z. Anat. Entwickl.-Gesch. **106**, 770—781 (1937).

KOLLBRUNNER, C. F., u. M. MEISTER: Knicken, Biegedrillknicken, Kippen. Berlin-Göttingen-Heidelberg: Springer 1961.

KOLODNY, A.: The architecture and the blood supply of the head and neck of the femur and their importance in the pathology of fractures of the neck. J. Bone Jt Surg. A **7**, 575—597 (1925).

KORTEWEG, D.: Ursachen der orthopädischen Knochenmißbildung. Z. orthop. Chir. **2**, 174—179 (1893).

KRAHL, V. E.: The torsion of the humerus: Its localization, cause and duration in man. Amer. J. Anat. **80**, 275—319 (1947).

KRAUSE, H.: The mechanical oscillatory behavior of the vertebral column. Int. Z. angew. Physiol. **20**, 125—155 (1963).

KREUZER, O.: Über Wachstum und Festigkeit langer Röhrenknochen im Laufe des postembryonalen Lebens. Arch. Entwickl.-Mech. Org. **126**, 148—184 (1932).

KRUKENBERG, H.: Anatomie und Statik des Beckens. In: Biologie und Pathologie des Weibes (Herausg. HALBAN u. SEITZ), Bd. 7, Teil 2. Berlin u. Wien 1928.

KÜNTSCHER, G.: Die Darstellung des Kraftflusses im Knochen. Zbl. Chir. **61**, 2130—2136 (1934).

— Über den Nachweis von Spannungsspitzen am menschlichen Knochengerüst. Gegenbaurs morph. Jb. **75**, 427—444 (1935a).

— Die Bedeutung der Darstellung des Kraftflusses im Knochen für die Chirurgie. Langenbecks Arch. klin. Chir. **182**, 489—551 (1935b).

— Die Spannungsverteilung am Schenkelhals. Langenbecks Arch. klin. Chir. **185**, 308—321 (1936).

KUHN, B.: Untersuchungen über das menschliche Wadenbein. Anat. Anz. **76**, 289—317 (1933).

KUMMER, B.: Die Anordnung zugfesten Materials im Sphenooccipitalknorpel menschlicher Embryonen. Z. Anat. Entwickl.-Gesch. **119**, 235—250 (1956a).

— Eine vereinfachte Methode zur Darstellung von Spannungstrajektorien. Z. Anat. Entwickl.-Gesch. **119**, 223—234 (1956b).

— Die Biomechanik des Säugetierskelets. In: Handbuch der Zoologie (Herausg. J. G. HELMCKE, H. v. LEUGERKEN, D. STARK), S. 1—80. Berlin: W. de Gruyter & Co. 1959a.

— Bauprinzipien des Säugerskeletes. Stuttgart: Georg Thieme 1959b.

— Statik und Dynamik des menschlichen Körpers. In: Handbuch der Arbeitsmedizin, Bd. 1, 1. München-Berlin-Wien: Urban & Schwarzenberg 1961.

— Funktioneller Bau und funktionelle Anpassung des Knochens. Anat. Anz. **111**, 261—293 (1962).

— Photoelastic studies on the functional structure of bone. Folia biotheor. **6**, 31 (1966).

— Die Beanspruchung des menschlichen Hüftgelenks. I. Allgemeine Problematik. Z. Anat. Entwickl.-Gesch. (Jena) **127**, 277—285 (1968).

LACROIX, P.: The organisation of bone. Translated from the amended French edition by STEWART GILDER. London: Churchill 1951.

— Sur le métabolisme du calcium dans l'os compact du chien adulte. Bull. Acad. roy. Méd. Belg. **18**, 489—496 (1953).

LANG, M.: Prüfen der Zerspanbarkeit durch Messen der Schnittemperatur. München: Carl Hansen 1949.

LANGE, C.: Untersuchungen über Elastizitätsverhältnisse in den menschlichen Rückenwirbeln mit Bemerkungen über die Pathogenese der Deformitäten. Z. orthop. Chir. **10**, 47—110 (1902).

Langmaack, B.: Druck- und Schlagversuche an Leichenlendenwirbelsäulen. Z. Anat. **118**, 20—27 (1954).

Lanz, T. v., P. Dziallas, H. Lippert u. I. Usener: Zur Variabilität der Markhöhle des menschlichen Humerus. Z. Anat. Entwickl.-Gesch. **123**, 453—461 (1963).

—, u. A. Hennig: Rollwirkungen des Musculus adductor magnus am durchschnittlich geformten Schenkelbein. Acta anat. (Basel) **30**, 420—429 (1957).

— — Femurtorsion und verdrillende Muskelkräfte. Morph. Jb. **102**, 299—311 (1962).

Lauche, A.: Die Zusammenhangstrennungen der Knochen. Die Knochenbrüche, die Bruchheilung und ihre Störungen. In: Handbuch der speziellen pathologischen Anatomie und Histologie (Herausg. O. Lubarsch u. F. Henke) Bd. 9, Teil III, Knochen und Gelenke, S. 204—308. Berlin: Springer 1937.

Laux, G.: Les actions dynamiques des muscles et des ligaments sur l'architecture des os. Ann. Anat. path. **7**, 401—413 (1930).

Lease, G. O. D., and F. G. Evans: Strength of human metatarsal bones under repetitive loading. J. appl. Physiol. **14**, 49—51 (1959).

Leonhardt, F.: Spannbeton für die Praxis, 2. Aufl. Berlin 1962.

Lerch, H.: Über Wärmeschrumpfungen des Kollagengewebes. Morph. Jb. **90**, 206—220 (1950b).

Less, L.: Die erb- und umweltbedingte Variabilität der Gaumenform auf Grund von Zwillings-Untersuchungen. Morph. Jb. **74**, 105—134 (1934).

Lesshaft, D.: Grundlagen der theoretischen Anatomie. Leipzig 1892.

Lewis, O. J.: The tubercle of the tibia. J. Anat. **92**, 587—592 (1958).

Lexer, E. W.: Untersuchungen über die Knochenhärte des Humerus. Z. Konstit.lehre **14**, 227—243 (1928).

Lichtwitz, A., et R. Parlier: Calcium et maladies métaboliques de l'os. Paris: L'expansion scientifique française 1964.

Lindsay, M. K., and E. L. Howes: The breaking strength of healing fractures. J. Bone Jt Surg. A **13**, 491—501 (1931).

Linggi, A.: Die Bruchfestigkeit der Knochen des Hundes. Affoltern, Weiss, 1951 (Inaug.-Diss. Zürich).

Linton, P.: On the different types of intracapsular fractures of the femoral neck. Acta chir. scand. **90**, Suppl. 86 (1944).

Lippert, H.: Zur Methodik der Muskelquerschnittsmessung. Anat. Anz. **106**, 299—303 (1959).

—, u. E. Lippert: Über allometrisches Wachstum der Wirbelkörper des Menschen. Z. Entwickl.-Gesch. **122**, 22—41 (1960a).

— — Geschlechtsunterschiede an den Wirbelkörpern menschlicher Feten. Z. menschl. Vererb.- u. Konstit.-Lehre **35**, 445—454 (1960b).

Lippert, H., u. E. Lippert: Gestaltwandel und Wachstumsdynamik der menschlichen Wirbelsäule. Z. Anat. Entwickl.-Gesch. **12**, 63—85 (1960c).

Lissner, H. R., and F. G. Evans: Engineering aspects of fractures. Clin. Orthop. **8**, 310—322 (1956).

Loetzke, H.-H.: Über Bau und Spannungsverhältnisse am M. plantaris und Soleusbogen des menschlichen Unterschenkels. Morph. Jb. **100**, 131—162 (1960).

Lorenz, A.: Die Entstehung der Knochendeformität. Wien. med. Wschr. **6**, 198—217 (1893).

Lubosch, W.: Muskel und Sehne. Morph. Jb. **80**, 89—178 (1937).

Lueger, O.: Lexikon der Technik (Herausg. A. Ehrhardt u. H. Franke), 4. Aufl., Bd. 3, Werkstoff und Werkstoffprüfung (ed. K. Wellinger u. E. Krägeloh). Stuttgart: Deutsche Verlagsanstalt 1961.

Lühken, H.: Die Statik des menschlichen Beckens. Z. Anat. Entwickl.-Gesch. **104**, 729—738 (1935).

Lütze, M.: Spannbeton. Stuttgart 1948.

Machado de Sousa, O.: L'architecture de la substance osseuse compacte de la mandibule chez l'homme et les édentés. Rass. biol. umana **2**, 23—28 (1947).

Maj, G.: Resistenza meccanica del tessuto osseo a diversi livelli di uno stesso osso. Boll. Soc. ital. Biol. sper. **13**, 413—415 (1938a).

— Osservazioni sulle differenze topografiche della resistenza meccanica del tessuto osseo di uno stesso segmento scheletrico. Monit. zool. ital. **49**, 139—149 (1938b).

— Variazioni individuali et topografiche delle resistenza meccanica del tessuto osseo umano. Boll. Soc. ital. Biol. sper. **15**, 1151—1152 (1940).

— Studio sulle variazioni individuali e topografiche della resistenza meccanica del tessuto osseo diafisario umano in diverse eta. Arch. ital. Anat. Embriol. **47**, 612—633 (1942).

—, e E. Toaiari: La resistenza meccanica del tessuto osseo lamellare compatto misurata in varie direzioni. Boll. Soc. ital. Biol. spez. **12**, 83—86 (1937a).

— — Osservazioni sperimentali sul meccanismo di resistenza del tessuto osseo lamellare compatto alle azioni meccaniche. Chir. Organi Mov. **22**, 541—557 (1937b).

— — Osservazioni istologiche sulle fracture del tessuto osseo normale e dopo decalcificazione. Boll. Soc. ital. Biol. sper. **12**, 57—59 (1937c).

Marique, P.: Etudes sur le femur. Librairie des sciences, p. 1—180. Bruxelles 1945.

Marotti, G.: Quantitive studies on bone reconstruction. I. The reconstruction in homotypic shaft bones. Acta anat. (Basel) **52**, 291 (1963).

McKeown, R. M., S. C. Harvey, and R. W. Lumsden: Breaking strength of healing fractured fibulae of rats; observations on low calcium diet. Arch. Surg. **25**, 1011—1034 (1932).

McKeown, R. M., M. K. Lindsay, S. C. Harvey, and E. L. Howes: The breaking strength of healing fractured fibulae of rats. II. Observation on a standard diet. Arch. Surg. 24, 458—491 (1932a).

— — — and R. W. Lumsden: Breaking strength of healing fractured fibulae of rats; observations on high fat diet. Arch. Surg. 24, 467—497 (1932b).

— — — — Breaking strength of healing fractured fibulae of rats; observations on high carbohydrate diet. Arch. Surg. 25, 722—748 (1932c).

Mechanik, N.: Indices cavi medullaris et compactae femoris. Z. Anat. Entwickl.-Gesch. 86, 188—202 (1928).

— Untersuchung der Markhöhle und der kompakten Schicht des Oberarmbeines des Menschen und der Haustiere. Z. Anat. Entwickl.-Gesch. 89, 513—531 (1929).

— Die Verteilung des kompakten Knochengewebes und die Dimensionen der Markhöhle der Tibia des Menschen und der Haustiere. Z. Anat. Entwickl.-Gesch. 93, 198—222 (1930).

— Untersuchung der kompakten Schicht und der Markhöhle der Fibula des Menschen. Z. Anat. Entwickl.-Gesch. 97, 331—355 (1932).

Mednick, L. W.: The evolution of the human ilium. Amer. J. phys. Anthrop. 13, 203—216 (1955).

Mehmel, A.: Vorgespannter Beton. Berlin-Göttingen-Heidelberg: Springer 1957.

Melchior, P., u. H. H. Emschermann: Prüfmaschinen für zügige Beanspruchung. In: E. Siebel, Handbuch der Werkstoffprüfung, Bd. 1, S. 5—80. 1958.

Messerer, O.: Über Elastizität und Festigkeit des menschlichen Knochens. Leipzig: Wilhelm Engelmann 1880.

— Experimentelle Untersuchungen über Schädelbrüche. München 1884.

Meyer, H. v.: Statik und Mechanik des menschlichen Knochengerüstes. Leipzig 1873.

— Die Architektur der Spongiosa. Reicherts u. DuBoi-Reymonds Arch. 627 (1867).

Michel, R.: Eine neue Methode zur Untersuchung langer Knochen und ihre Anwendung auf das Femur. Inaug.-Diss. München 1903.

Milch, H.: Photo-elastic studies of bone forms. J. Bone Jt Surg. A 22, 621—626 (1940).

Mohr: Beitrag zur Theorie des Fachwerkes. Civilingenieur H 5 (1885).

Mörsch, E.: Der Eisenbetonbau, seine Theorie und Anwendung. Stuttgart 1923/1929.

Mollier, G.: Beziehungen zwischen Form und Funktion der Sehnen im Muskel-Sehnen-Knochen-System. Morph. Jb. 79, 161—199 (1937).

Mollowitz, G., u. D. Knaack: Zur Frage der Hitzeschädigung des Knochens durch Oszillationssägen. Zbl. Chir. 87, 1391—1396 (1962).

Mühlemann, E. M.: Experimentelle Untersuchungen über Volumina und Oberflächen des Hohlraumsystems der Knochenkompacta. Inaug.-Diss. Zahnheilk. Kiel 1962.

Mühlmann, M.: Wachstum, Altern, Tod. Ergebn. Anat. Entwickl.-Gesch. 27, 1—245 (1927).

— Neueste Forschungsergebnisse über Wachstum, Altern und Tod. Ergebn. Anat. Entwickl.-Gesch. 28, 594—653 (1929).

Murray, P. D. F.: Bones. Cambridge: University Press 1936.

Nachemson, A.: The influence of spinal movements on the lumbar intradiscal pressure and on the tensile stresses in the annulus fibrosus. Acta orthop. scand. 33, 183—207 (1963).

Olivier, G., et Cl. Libersa: L'architecture de l'os coxal des primates. C. R. Ass. Anat. 41, 12—14 (1954).

Olivo, O. M.: Rispondenza della funzione meccanica varia degli osteoni con la loro diversa minuta architettura. Boll. Soc. ital. Biol. sper. 12, 400—402 (1937a).

— Considerazioni sul significato funzionale degli osteoni. Boll. Soc. ital. Biol. sper. 12, 67—70 (1937b).

— Rapport entre la structure et la fonction dans les ostéons. C. R. Ass. Anat. 32, 334—346 (1937c).

— G. Maj e E. Toajari: Sul significato della minuta struttura del tessuto osseo compatto. Boll. Sci. med. 109, 369—394 (1937).

Patrick, L. M., H. R. Lissner, and F. G. Evans: Effects of controlled acceleration on stress-strain phenomena in the intact vertebral column. Soc. Internat. Chir. Orthop. et Traum. 781—786 (1960).

Paulli, S.: Über die Pneumaticität des Schädels bei den Säugethieren. Morph. Jb. 28, 483—565 (1900).

Pauwels, F.: Bedeutung und kausale Erklärung der Spongiosa-Architektur in neuer Auffassung. Ärztl. Wschr. 3, 379 (1948).

— Die Bedeutung der Bauprinzipien des Stütz- und Bewegungsapparates für die Beanspruchung der Röhrenknochen. Z. Anat. Entwickl.-Gesch. 114, 129—166 (1949/50).

— Die Bedeutung der Muskelkräfte für die Regelung der Beanspruchung des Röhrenknochens während der Bewegung der Glieder. Z. Anat. Entwickl.-Gesch. 115, 327—351 (1950).

— Über die mechanische Bedeutung der gröberen Kortikalisstruktur beim normalen und pathologischen verbogenen Röhrenknochen. Anat. Nachrichten 1, 53—67 (1950/51).

— Über die Bedeutung der Bauprinzipien des Stütz- und Bewegungsapparates für die Beanspruchung der Röhrenknochen. Acta anat. Basel 12, 207—227 (1951).

— Die statische Belastung der Linea aspera. Z. Anat. Entwickl.-Gesch. 117, 497—503 (1953/54).

— Kritische Überprüfung der Rouxschen Abhandlung: „Beurteilung und Erläuterung eines knöchernen Kniegelenks". Z. Anat. Entwickl.-Gesch. 117, 520—552 (1954).

— Über die Verteilung der Spongiosadichte im coxalen Femurende und ihre Bedeutung für die Lehre vom funktionellen Bau des Knochens. Gegenbaurs morph. Jb. 95, 35—54 (1955).

PAUWELS, F.: Gesammelte Abhandlungen zur funktionellen Anatomie. Berlin-Heidelberg-New York: Springer 1968.

PEDERSEN, H. E., F. G. EVANS, and H. R. LISSNER: Deformation studies of the femur under various loading and orientations. Anat. Rec. 103, 159—185 (1949).

PEREY, O.: Fracture of the vertebral endplate in the lumbar spine. Acta orthop. scand., Suppl. 25, 1—101 (1957).

PETERSEN, H.: Über den Feinbau der menschlichen Skeletteile. Wilhelm Roux' Arch. Entwickl.-Mech. Org. 112, 112—141 (1927).

— Die Organe des Skeletsystems. In: W. MÖLLENDORFF, Handbuch der mikroskopischen Anatomie des Menschen, Bd. II/3, S. 521—678. Berlin: Springer 1930.

POLICARD, A., and J. ROCHE: La formation de la substance osseuse. Essai de coordination des données histologiques et biochimiques. Ann. Physiol. Physico-chim. biol. 13, 645—703 (1937).

PRITCHARD, J. J.: General anatomy and histology of bone. The biochemistry and physiology of bone. Ed. by G. H. BOURNE, p. 1—25. New York: Academic Press Inc. 1956.

PUCHER, A.: Lehrbuch des Stahlbetonbaues, 3. Aufl. Wien: Springer 1961.

RAHIMI, M.: Elektromyographische Untersuchungen der Muskeln des Beines beim Gang. Inaug.-Diss. der med. Fakultät der Universität Kiel (1962).

RAUBER, A.: Über den mechanischen Wert einiger Querschnittsformen der Knochen. S.-B. naturforsch. Ges. Leipzig 2, 100—102 (1875).

— Elastizität und Festigkeit des Knochens. Leipzig: Wilhelm Engelmann 1876.

— Die Feststellung der Röhrenknochen in den Gelenken und die Knochenform. Morph. Jb. 3, 87—105 (1877).

REICHEL, H.: Muskelphysiologie. Berlin-Göttingen-Heidelberg: Springer 1960.

REULEAUX, F.: Lehrbuch der Kinematik, Bd. 2. Braunschweig 1900.

RHUMBLER, L.: Trajektorienmodell zur Demonstrierung einer automatischen Entstehung der Innentrajektorien eines fötalen Femurknochens durch dessen Oberflächenwachstum. Verh. Dtsch. Zool. Ges. 1914.

RIED, H. A.: Die Schaftkrümmung des menschlichen Femur. Arch. Anthrop., N.F. 21, 1—30 (1928).

RITTER, W.: Anwendungen der graphischen Statik, Teil I. Zürich 1888.

—, u. P. LARDY: Vorgespannter Beton, 2. Aufl. Zürich: Lehmann 1950.

ROBINSON, R. A.: An electron-microscopic study of the crystalline inorganic component of bone and its relationship to the organic matrix. J. Bone Jt Surg. A 34, 389—435 (1952).

— Chemical analysis and electron microscopy of bone. Bone as a tissue. Ed. by K. RODAHL, p. 186—250. New York-Toronto-London: Mc Graw-Hill Book Co. 1960.

RÖSSLE, R.: Untersuchungen über die Knochenhärte. Beitr. path. Anat. 77, 174—208 (1927).

— Versuche über die Schlagfestigkeit des menschlichen Oberschenkelknochens. Beitr. path. Anat. 83, 261—278 (1930).

ROGERS, H. J., S. M. WEIDMANN, and A. PARKINSON: Studies on the skeletal tissues. II. The collagen content of bones from rabbits, oxen and human. Biochem. J. 50, 537—542 (1952).

ROLLHÄUSER, H.: Konstitutions- und Altersunterschiede in Festigkeit kollagener Fibrillen. Morph. Jb. 90, 157—179 (1951).

ROSATE, A.: Distributzione della microdurezza del tessuto osseo nella compatta di ossa lunghe in accrescimento. Monit. zool. ital., Suppl. 67, 428 (1958).

ROUILLER, CH., u. G. MAJNO: Morphologische und chemische Untersuchungen an Knochenläsionen nach Hitzeeinwirkung. Beitr. path. Anat. 113, 100—120 (1953).

ROUX, W.: Gesammelte Abhandlungen über Entwicklungs-Mechanik, I. und II. Leipzig: Wilhelm Engelmann 1895.

ROWLAND, R. E., J. JOWSEY, and J. H. MARSHALL: Microscopic metabolism of calcium in bone. III. Microradiografic measurements of mineral density. Radiat. Res. 10, 234—242 (1959).

SACHSE, H.: Grundprobleme und Fortschritte in der Chirurgie mit Kirschnerdrähten. Bruns' Beitr. klin. Chir. 194, 158—202 (1957).

SALIGER, R.: Praktische Statik. Wien 1949.

SCHAFFER, J.: Die Stützgewebe. In: Handbuch der mikroskopischen Anatomie des Menschen, Bd. II/2, S. 1—390. 1930.

SCHMIDT, A.: Über den Einfluß der Domestikation auf die mechanischen Qualitäten der Pars compacta von Sus scrofa dom. nebst einigen Beiträgen zur Theorie der funktionellen Anpassung des Extremitätenskelets. Wilhelm Roux' Arch. Entwickl.-Mech. Org. 41, 605—671 (1915).

SCHMIDT, W. J.: Zur Polarisationsoptik des Knorpelgewebes. Z. Zellforsch. 37, 534—546 (1952).

SCHMITT, H. P.: Über die Beziehungen zwischen Dichte und Festigkeit des Knochens am Beispiel des menschlichen Femur. Z. Anat. Entwickl.-Gesch. 127, 1—24 (1968).

SCHNEIDER, H.: Die Struktur der Sehnenansatzzone und Abnutzungserkrankungen in ihrem Bereich. Münch. med. Wschr. 97, 1479—1480 (1955).

— Zur Tendovaginitis stenosans (De Quervain) und „Styloiditis radii". Wien. med. Wschr. 106, 523—526 (1956).

— Zur Struktur der Sehnenansatzzonen. Z. Anat. Entwickl.-Gesch. 119, 431—456 (1956).

SCHREIBER, H.: Anatomie. Zum funktionellen Bau des menschlichen Schädels. Fortschr. Zahnheilk. 8, 1—13 (1932).

SCHUBERT, L.: Temperaturmessungen im Zahn während des Schleif- und Bohrvorganges mittels des Lichtstrahlgalvanometers. Zahnärztl. Welt 58, 443—445 (1957).

SCHULTZ, A. H.: The relative thickness of the long bones and the vertebrae in primates. Amer. J. phys. Anthrop. **11**, 277—311 (1953).

SCHUMACHER, G. H., u. E. WOLF: Trockengewicht und physiologischer Querschnitt der menschlichen Skelettmuskulatur. I. Trockengewichte. Anat. Anz. **118**, 317—330 (1966a).

— — Trockengewicht und physiologischer Querschnitt der menschlichen Skelettmuskulatur. II. Physiologische Querschnitte. Anat. Anz. **119**, 259—269 (1966b).

— — Trockengewicht und physiologischer Querschnitt der menschlichen Skelettmuskulatur. III. Beziehungen zwischen Trockengewicht und physiologischem Querschnitt. Anat. Anz. **119**, 270—283 (1966c).

SCHUNKE, G. H.: The anatomy and development of the sacroiliac joint union. Anat. Rec. **72**, 313—331 (1938).

SCHWARZ, J.: Untersuchungen über die Größe des Sehnenquerschnittes und über die Muskelkraft. Inaug.-Diss. der med. Fakultät der Universität Kiel (1965).

SCHWENKENBECHER, W.: Untersuchungen über die Architektur des Beckens. Morph. Z. **75**, 412 (1935).

SCOTT, J. H.: Muscle growth and function in relation to skeletal morphology. Amer. J. Physic. Anthrop. **15**, 197—234 (1957).

SEDLIN, E. D.: A rheologic model for cortical bone. A study of the physical properties of human femural samples. Acta orthop. scand., Suppl. 83, **36**, 1—77 (1965).

—, and C. HIRSCH: Factors affecting the determination of the physical properties of femoral cortical bone. Acta orthop. scand. **37**, 29—48 (1966).

SEIPEL, C. M.: Trajectories of the jaws. Acta odont. scand. **8**, 81—191 (1948).

SIEBEL, E.: Handbuch der Werkstoffprüfung, Bd. I: Prüf- und Meßeinrichtungen (Ed. E. SIEBEL u. N. LUDWIG), 2. Aufl. Berlin-Göttingen-Heidelberg: Springer 1958.

SMITH, J. W.: The relationship of epiphysial plates to stress in some bones of the lower limb. J. Anat. (Lond.) **96**, 58—78 (1962a).

— The structure and stress relations of fibrous epiphysial plates. J. Anat. (Lond.) **96**, 209—225 (1962b).

—, and R. WALMSLEY: Factors affecting the elasticity of bone. J. Anat. (Lond.) **93**, 503—523 (1959).

SMITH, L. D.: Hip fractures. The role of muscle contraction on intrinsic forces in the causation of fractures of the femoral neck. J. Bone Jt Surg. **35**, 367—383 (1953).

SPEARS, G. N., and J. T. OWEN: The etiology of trochanteric fractures of the femur. J. Bone and Joint Surg. **31** A, 548—552 (1949).

SPOTOFT, J.: Osteosynthesis colli femoris. Copenhagen: E. Muksgaard 1944.

STAUDENRAUS, J.: Über die Entwicklung der Kieferhöhle nach der Geburt und ihre Bedeutung für die Entwicklung und Konstruktion des Gesichtsschädels. Med. Wiss. Würzburg 1939.

STEINDLER, A.: Mechanics of normal and pathological in man. London 1935.

STELGES, G.: Elektromyographische Untersuchungen der Muskeln des Beines bei gymnastischen Übungen. Inaug.-Diss. der med. Fakultät der Univ. Kiel (1962).

STERNBERG, C.: Über die elastischen Fasern. Virchows Arch. path. Anat. **254**, 656—661 (1925).

STRASSER, H.: Lehrbuch der Muskel- und Gelenkmechanik. Bd. I. Allgemeiner Teil 1908. Bd. III. Die untere Extremität 1917. Berlin: Springer 1908—1917.

STROBINO, L. J., and L. E. FARR: The relation to age and function of regional variations in nitrogen and ash content of bovine bones. J. biol. Chem. **178**, 599—609 (1949).

STÜSSI, F.: Vorlesungen über Baustatik, Bd. I. Basel: Birkhäuser 1946.

STÜWE, CH., u. E. EHLER: Spezifisches Gewicht und Dichte, ermittelt an menschlichen Humeri, Radii und Ulnae. Anat. Anz. **120**, 529—533 (1967).

SUDECK, P.: Zur Anatomie und Aethiologie der Coxa vara adolescentium. Langenbecks Arch. klin. Chir. **59**, 504—524 (1899).

SYLVÉN, B.: On the biology of nucleus pulposus. Acta orthop. scand. **20**, 275—279 (1951a).

— Biophysical and physiological investigations on lumbar disks. J. Bone Jt Surg. A **33**, 1034 (1951b).

TAPPEN, N. C.: A functional analysis of the facial skeleton with split-line technique. Amer. J. Physic. Anthrop. **11**, 503—532 (1953).

THEISMANN, H., u. F. PFANDER: Über die Durchlässigkeit des Knochens für Ultraschall. Strahlentherapie **80**, 607—610 (1949).

THOMSEN, W.: Über das Meißeln und Sägen in der Knochenchirurgie. Langenbecks Arch. klin. Chir. **267**, 608—610 (1951).

— Weitere Fortschritte in der Technik des Sägens und Fräsens in der Knochenchirurgie. Chirurg **26**, 189—191 (1955).

TISCHENDORF, F.: Das Verhalten der Haversschen Systeme bei Belastung. I. Mitt.: Untersuchungen über das Knochengewebe. Wilhelm Roux' Arch. Entwickl.-Mech. Org. **145**, 318—332 (1951a).

— Beobachtungen über das Verhalten der Haversschen Systeme. Verh. Anat. Ges. 49, Erg.-H. zu Anat. Anz. **98**, 204—205 (1951b).

— Quantitative Beobachtungen über das Verhalten der Haversschen Lamellen bei Belastung. II. Mitt.: Untersuchungen über das Knochengewebe. Arch. Entwickl.-Mech. Org. **146**, 1—20 (1952).

— Die mechanische Reaktion der Haversschen Systeme und ihrer Lamellen auf experimentelle Belastung (Nebst Bemerkungen zur Histogenese des lamellären Knochengewebes). Arch. Entwickl.-Mech. Org. **146**, 661—704 (1954).

TITKENMEYER, W.: Die Präparation und Versorgung lebender Zahnhartsubstanzen. Zahnärztl. Welt **58**, 187, 215, 367, 397 (1957).

Toajari, E.: Differenze nella struttura e resistenza meccanica del tessuto osseo in dul ragge di bos taurus. Arch. Sci. biol. (Bologna) **25**, 544—557 (1939).
Töndury, G.: Anatomie und Entwicklungsgeschichte der Wirbelsäule mit besonderer Berücksichtigung der Altersveränderungen der Bandscheiben. Schweiz. med. Wschr. 825—827, 835—837 (1955).
— Entwicklungsgeschichte und Fehlbildungen der Wirbelsäule. In: Wirbelsäule in Forsch. u. Praxis (Ed. H. Junghanns, Oldenburg), Bd. 7. Stuttgart: Hippokrates-Verlag 1958.
Töppich, G.: Die Porosität der Knochen des Neugeborenen mit Berücksichtigung des Verhaltens der Porosität bei Erwachsenen und Greisen. Arch. Anat. 9—24 (1914).
Triepel, H.: Einführung in die physikalische Anatomie, Bd. I, II u. III. Wiesbaden 1902 u. 1908.
— Über mechanische Strukturen. Anat. Anz. **23**, 480—486 (1903).
— Trajektorielle Strukturen. Anat. Anz. **24**, 297—300 (1904).
— Die Anordnung der Knochenfibrillen in transformierter Spongiosa. Anat. Hefte **33**, 47—78 (1907).
— Materialverbrauch bei funktioneller Anpassung. Wilhelm Roux' Arch. Entwickl.-Mech. Org. **30**, 62—73 (1910).
— Die Architektur der Knochenspongiosa in neuer Auffassung. Z. Konstit.lehre **8**, 269—309 (1922a).
— Die Architekturen der menschlichen Knochenspongiosa. München u. Wiesbaden 1922b.
Usener, I.: Ausformung der menschlichen Humerusmarkhöhle und ihre Variabilität. Morph. Jb. **108**, 607—623 (1966).
Uweda, T.: Der Bau des Schollenmuskels (M. soleus). Morph. Jb. **56**, 223—238 (1926).
Vignolo-Lutati, U.: Architettura della sostanza ossea compacta del metacarpo di grossi mammiferi e sue transformationi con l'età. Riv. Biol. **30**, 294—335 (1940).
Vincent, J.: Recherches sur la constitution de l'os adulte. Diss. med. Lowain Bruxelles 1955.
—, et S. Haumont: Identification autoradiographique des ostéones métaboliques après administration de Ca^{45}. Rev. franç. Étud. clin. biol. **5**, 348—353 (1960).
Virchow, H.: Die Eigenform der menschlichen Wirbelsäule. Verh. Anat. Ges. 23. Verslg, Anat. Anz. **34**, Erg.-H., 157—180 (1909).
Virgin, W. J.: Experimental investigations into the physical properties of the intervertebral disc. J. Bone Jt Surg. B **33**, 607—611 (1951).
Vose, G. P.: The relation of microscopic mineralization to intrinsic bone strength. Anat. Rec. **144**, 31—36 (1962).
Walkhoff, O.: Der Unterkiefer der Anthromorphen und des Menschen in seiner funktionellen Entwicklung und Gestalt. H. 9. Selenkas Menschenaffen. Wiesbaden 1902.
— Die menschliche Sprache in ihrer Bedeutung für die funktionelle Gestalt des Unterkiefers. Anat. Anz. **24**, 129—139 (1904).
Weber, W.: Mechanik der menschlichen Gehwerkzeuge. Göttingen 1836.
— Über die Längenverhältnisse der Fleischfasern der Muskeln im Allgemeinen. Ber. u. d. Verhandl. d. k. Ges. d. Wissensch. zu Leipzig (1849).
Weidenreich, F.: Die Bildung des Kinnes und seine angebliche Beziehung zur Sprache. Anat. Anz. **24**, 545—555 (1904a).
— Zur Kinnbildung beim Menschen. Anat. Anz. **25**, 314—319 (1904b).
— Über formbestimmende Ursachen am Skelett und die Erblichkeit der Knochenformen. Wilhelm Roux' Arch. Entwickl.-Mech. Org. **51**, 436—481 (1922).
— Über die pneumatischen Nebenräume des Kopfes. Z. Anat. Entwickl.-Gesch. **72**, 55—93 (1924).
— Das Knochengewebe. In: Möllendorff, Handbuch der mikroskopischen Anatomie des Menschen, Bd. II/3, S. 391—520. 1930.
Weir, J. B. de V., G. H. Bell, and J. W. Chambers: The strength and elasticity of bone in rats on a rachitogenic diet. J. Bone Jt Surg. B **31**, 444—451 (1949).
Weisl, H.: The ligaments of the sacro-iliac joint examined with particular reference to their function. Acta anat. (Basel) **20**, 201—213 (1954a).
— The articular surfaces of the sacro-iliac joint and their relation to the movements of the sacrum. Acta anat. (Basel) **22**, 1—14 (1954b).
Weiss et H. Rouviere: Sur la texture des tendons. Bibliogr. Anat. **25**, 29—33 (1914).
Weiss, P.: Nervous system (Neurogenesis). Analysis of development. Ed. by B. H. Willier, P. A. Weiss and V. Hamburger, p. 346—401. Philadelphia and London: W. B. Saunders Co. 1955.
— The compounding of complex and cellular units into tissue fabrics. Proc. nat. Acad. Sci. (Wash.) **42**, 819—830 (1956).
— Macromolecular fabrics and patterns. J. cell. comp. Physiol. **49**, Suppl. 1, 105—112 (1957).
Wermel, J.: Untersuchungen über die Kinetogenese und ihre Bedeutung in der Onto- und Phylogenetischen Entwicklung. (Experimente und Vergleichungen an Wirbeltier-Extremitäten.) III. Mitt.: Veränderungen der Widerstandsfähigkeit der Knochen. Gegenbaurs. morph. Jb. **75**, 128—149 (1935).
Wertheim, G.: Mémoire sur l'élasticité et la cohésion des principaux tissus du corps humain. Ann. Chem. Chir. Physiol. **21**, 385—414 (1847).
Wetzel, G.: Volumen und Gewicht der Knochen als Maßstab für den phylogenetischen Entwicklungsgrad. Wilhelm Roux' Arch. Entwickl.-Mech. Org. **30**, 507—537 (1910a).
— Die Wirbelsäule der Australier. I. Das Volumen der knöchernen Wirbelsäule und ihrer Abschnitte. Z. Morph. Anthrop. **12**, 313—340 (1910b).
— Studien zur Schädelstatik. Verh. Anat. Ges. Erlangen 1922, Anat. Anz. **55**, Erg.-H. 216—226 (1922).

Wetzel, G.: Versuche und Beobachtungen zur Schädelstatik. Z. Anat. Entwickl.-Gesch. **75**, 261—283 (1925).
—, u. B. Schröder: Der Sicherheitsgrad im Bau des Gesichtsgerüstes gegenüber dem Kaudruck. Arch. Entwickl.-Mech. Org. **105**, 120—148 (1925).
Winkler, R.: Über den funktionellen Bau des Unterkiefers. Z. Stomat. **19**, 401—427 (1921).
Wöhlisch, E.: Untersuchungen über elastische, thermo-dynamische, magnetische und elektrische Eigenschaften tierischer Gewebe. Verh. phys.-med. Ges. Würzb. **51**, 53—64 (1926).
Wolff, J.: Über die Bedeutung der Architektur der spongiösen Substanz. Zbl. med. Wiss. **54**, 849—851 (1869).
— Über die innere Architektur der Knochen und ihre Bedeutung für die Frage vom Knochenwachstum. Virchows Arch. path. Anat. **50**, 389—450 (1870).
— Über die Theorie des Knochenschwundes durch vermehrten Druck und der Knochenbildung durch Druckentlastung. Langenbecks Arch. klin. Chir. **42**, 302—324 (1891).
Wyss, Th.: Die Kraftfelder in festen elastischen Körpern. Berlin: Springer 1926.
Wyss, Th.: Die Kraftfelder in festen Körpern. Vjschr. naturforsch. Ges. Zürich **93**, 151—186 (1948).
—, u. S. P. Ulrich: Festigkeitsuntersuchungen und gezielte Extensionsbehandlung der Lendenwirbelsäule unter Berücksichtigung des Bandscheibenvorfalles. Vjschr. naturforsch. Ges. Zürich 1 C., Beih. 3/4 (1954).
Zeiger, K.: Zur Frage der Bedeutung der Erbmasse für das Gebiß, nach den Ergebnissen von Zwillingsuntersuchungen. Verh. Anat. Ges. 38. Verslg 1929, Erg.-H. zu Anat. Anz. **67**, 139—144 (1929).
— Entwicklungsphysiologische und konstruktionsanalytische Probleme am menschlichen Kieferapparat. Paradentium **5**, 1—20 (1932).
— Das Problem der funktionellen Struktur des Knochens. Natur u. Mus. **63**, 77—91 (1933).
Zschokke, E.: Weitere Untersuchungen über das Verhältnis der Knochenbildung zur Statik und Mechanik des Vertebratenskeletes. Zürich 1892.
Zuppinger, H.: Warum bricht der lebende Knochen leichter als der tote? Anat. Hefte **23**, 609—618 (1904).

G. Vorgänge bei der Bruchheilung und Pseudarthrosenentstehung

Von

R. Maatz und K. Haasch

Mit 101 Abbildungen

I. Die ungestörte Heilung einer Knochenwunde

1. Einleitung und geschichtlicher Überblick

Alle wie auch immer gearteten Knochenwunden heilen mit den gleichen Kräften, nur tritt nach Sitz und Art der Fraktur einmal die eine, im anderen Fall die andere Kraft mehr in den Vordergrund. Allgemeinhin kann die Heilungspotenz des Knochens — ohne Rücksicht auf Alter oder Allgemeinzustand des Patienten — als sehr gut bezeichnet werden, als so gut, daß Irrwege in der Behandlung von Frakturen bisweilen über längere Zeit beschritten und erst spät erkannt wurden. Der Knochen besitzt Reserven, mit deren Hilfe er die Vereinigung der Fragmente erreichen kann, so daß er trotz mangelnder Hilfen oder gar trotz hindernder Behandlungsfehler heilen kann.

Der verletzte Knochen bildet ein vollwertiges neues Gewebe, den lamellär aufgebauten Knochen. In Ausnahmefällen vermag er das direkt (primäre Knochenheilung, soudure autogène — Danis, 1949), meist aber geschieht das über ein Narbengewebe, den Callus (sekundäre Knochenheilung). Dieser Callus kann „primär“ entstehen (angiogener Callus — Krompecher, 1937), oder „sekundär“ auf dem Umweg über das Bindegewebe (desmaler Callus) oder über den Knorpel (chondraler Callus). Tote Knochensubstanz kann auch auf dem Wege der „schleichenden Substitution“ (Barth, 1895; Marchand, 1899) durch lebenden Knochen ersetzt werden. Da im Bereich der Fragmente stets abgestorbenes Knochengewebe vorhanden ist, ist diese Art der Knochenneubildung stets beteiligt.

Das Narbengewebe „Callus“ wird später durch lamellären Knochen ersetzt. Dabei paßt sich die Struktur des neuen Knochens der funktionellen Beanspruchung an (Roux, 1885). Je jünger ein Individuum ist, um so vollendeter vermag sich der Knochen auch in seiner äußeren Form wieder der früheren „Normalform“ anzunähern. Ausgewachsene Individuen besitzen diese Fähigkeit nur in bezug auf die innere Struktur des Knochens, wobei es offenbar mehrere Strukturarten gibt, welche der funktionellen Beanspruchung gerecht werden (Knese, 1958).

2. Feingewebliche Vorgänge bei der Knochenheilung

Jede Fraktur hat als konstantes Symptom einen Bluterguß. Der lokale Verletzungsschock führt zum Stupor der Muskulatur (Rehn, 1924). Die vorübergehende Stase im Stromgebiet macht nach Lösung einer vermehrten Blutfülle Platz. Der Bluterguß gerinnt, und sein Fibrinnetz verbindet die Fragmentenden in Form der „primären Verspannung“. Die folgende Organisation des Hämatoms entspricht ganz den Vorgängen der serofibrinösen, aseptischen Entzündung. Daran beteiligt sich der Bindegewebsapparat aller in der Umgebung vorhandenen Gewebe, Periost, Mark, Havers'sche Kanäle, Muskeln usf. Die entlang den Fibrinfasern vordringenden Gefäßsprossen sind für die spätere Anordnung der Osteoid-Bälkchen bestimmend (Bancroft, 1929). Meist wachsen sie schräg oder senkrecht zur Knochenoberfläche und bilden untereinander Querverbindungen. So entsteht ein Maschen- und Netzwerk.

Eine heilende Fraktur zeigt meist alle Formen der Callus- und Knochenbildung, wobei die eine von der anderen schwer oder gar nicht zu trennen sein kann. Besser demonstrabel sind die Vorgänge darum in Fällen mit besonders geschaffenen Bedingungen, welche nur eine Art allein oder vorwiegend zur Ausbildung kommen lassen.

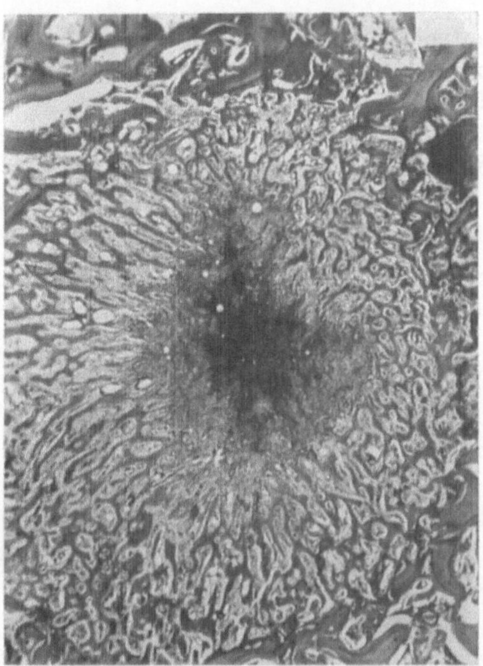

Abb. 1. Angiogene Callusbildung im zylindrischen Defekt der Spongiosa

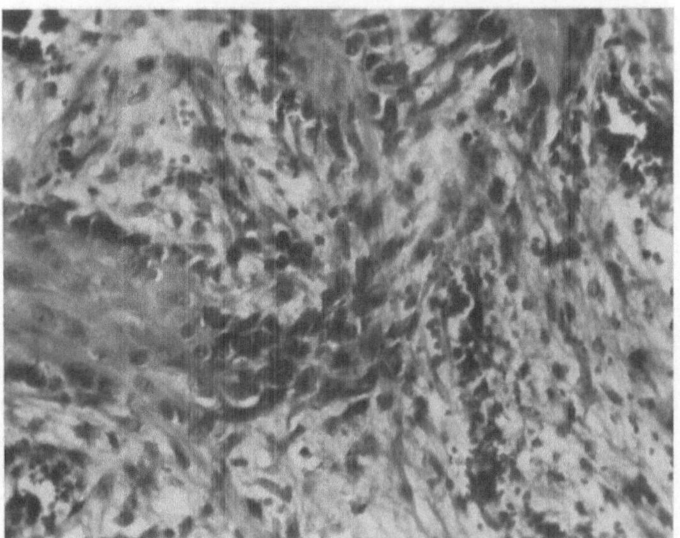

Abb. 2. Die stärkere Vergrößerung von Abb. 1 zeigt die osteoblastenreichen Spitzen der zentral verwachsenden Callusbälkchen

a) Die angiogene oder primäre Callusbildung

Die „angiogene Callusbildung“ herrscht in einem zylindrischen Defekt des Knochens vor (Abb. 1). KROMPECHER (1937) konnte nachweisen, daß die Knochenzellen aus den undifferenzierten Mesenchymzellen entstehen, welche die vordringenden Gefäßsprossen umgeben. Diese Mesenchymzellen werden zu Osteoblasten (Abb. 2), welche dank fehlender mechanischer Insulte (PAUWELS, 1941) unter diesen Bedingungen meist rundliche Gestalt haben. Diese Zellen sind morphologisch nicht sicher ansprechbar (WILTON, 1937), sie sind nur Zustandsbilder der Zellen des mesenchymalen Syncytiums (BLOCK, 1940) und determinieren je nach Beeinflussung. Darum wurde der Begriff des „pluripotenten Keimgewebes" geprägt.

Bei ungestörter Fortentwicklung geben die Osteoblasten als eine Art Sekretionsprodukt die Matrix ab. Die so auseinander gedrängten Osteoblasten wandeln sich zu Osteocyten. Das jetzt als „Osteoid" bezeichnete Gewebe wird zum jungen Knochen, zum Callus durch Einlagerung von Kalksalzen zwischen die „reticulären" (BOURNE, 1956) und in Bündeln angeordneten „kollagenen" Fasern.

b) Der schleichende Ersatz toten Knochens durch lebenden

Um eine direkte oder primäre Knochenneubildung handelt es sich auch bei dem sogenannten „schleichenden Ersatz". Es handelt sich um den zuerst von BARTH und MARCHAND

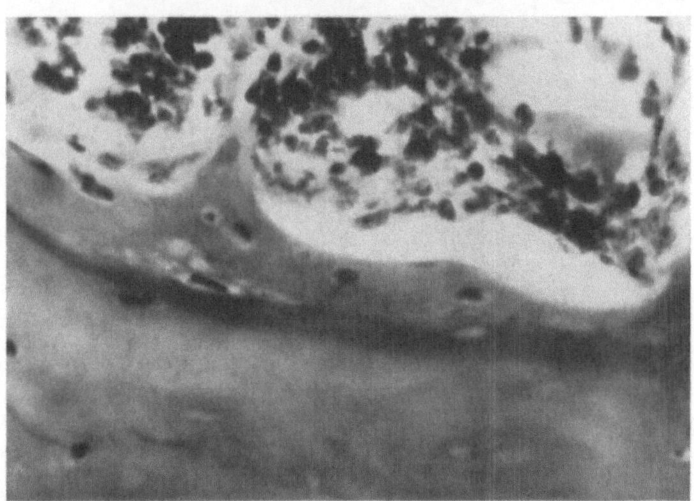

Abb. 3. Knochenneubildung auf dem Wege des „schleichenden Ersatzes"

beschriebenen Vorgang, bei dem das tote Knochengewebe durch Anlagerung von Osteoblasten, welche sich unter Abgabe der Zwischensubstanz zu Osteocyten wandeln, zu lebendem Knochengewebe umgewandelt wird (Abb. 3). Der primär schmale Osteoidsaum verbreitert sich unter gleichzeitigem Schwund des toten Knochens, diesen auf diesem Wege langsam ersetzend. Stets liegen die lebenden Zellen des neugebildeten Knochens innerhalb der Knochensubstanz und nicht etwa an der Grenze zum toten Knochen. Dieser Vorgang der Substitution „tot durch lebend" wird vor allem dort beobachtet, wo im Körper (auch nach Knochentransplantation) nekrotisches Knochengewebe entstanden ist. Teleologisch gedacht imponiert dieser Vorgang als außerordentlich zweckmäßig, da das tragende Knochengerüst auf diese Weise während der Substitution ohne Unterbrechung seine mechanische Aufgabe erfüllen kann. Während der schleichenden Substitution ist die Grenzlinie zwischen totem und lebendem Knochen meist scharf, nur manchmal verwaschen, und nur mit stärkster Vergrößerung sind kanälchenartige Strukturen erkennbar (Gitterfiguren von RECKLINGHAUSEN, 1910).

c) Die sekundäre chondrale oder desmale Callusbildung

Die chondrale und die desmale Callusbildung sind sekundär, d.h. hier entsteht das Knochengewebe über den Umweg Bindegewebe oder Knorpel. Beide Formen sind die während der Entwicklung und des Wachstums beobachteten Formen der Knochenneubildung. Die reine periostale Callusbildung zeigt die Abb. 4. Hier ist die osteogenetische

Potenz eines vom jungen Tier genommenen Cortiticalisspanes durch Konservierung abgeschwächt, so daß nach Überpflanzung ins Muskellager zunächst die periostale Neubildung dominiert. Bemerkenswert ist aber, daß die Osteoid- und Callusentstehung sich unter besonderen Bedingungen, auf die später eingegangen wird, auch aus ausgereiftem Bindegewebe entwickeln kann (Abb. 5).

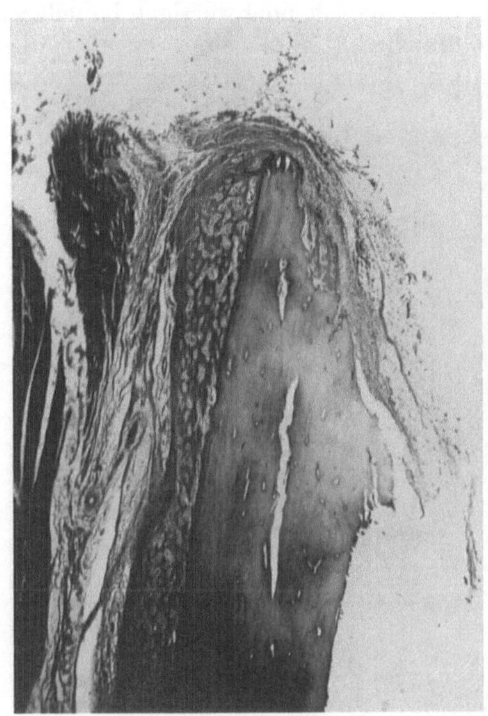

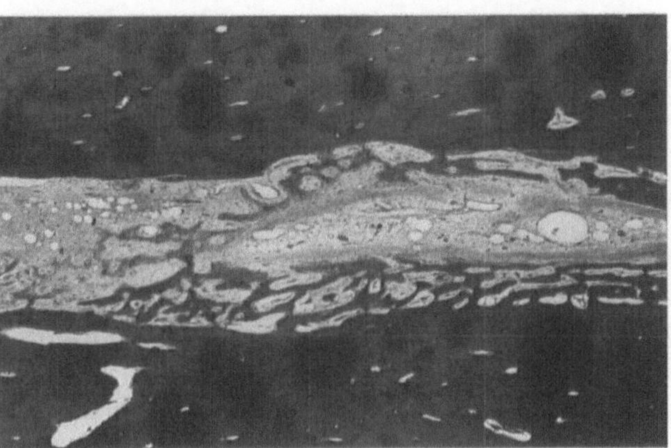

Abb. 5. Aus Bindegewebe metaplasierender Callus zwischen zwei unter Federdruck zusammengepreßten Knochen

Abb. 4. Periostale Callusbildung am autologen Span zwei Wochen nach Implantation in die Rückenmuskulatur

d) Die primäre Knochenheilung

Bei der „primären Knochenheilung“ findet eine direkte Vereinigung der lamellär aufgebauten Fragmente ohne vorübergehende Einschaltung eines Granulationsgewebes oder Narbengewebes, des Callus, statt. Abb. 6 zeigt diesen Vorgang während der Heilung der glatten Osteotomiewunde (senkrechter Spalt) der Corticalis eines Schaftknochens. Auch hier verfällt an den Enden der Fragmente die Knochensubstanz in einem schmalen Saum der Nekrose. Der Inhalt der Havers'schen Kanäle aber bleibt vital (ALLGÖWER, 1964). Von hier aus setzt der Umbau der Corticalis ein. Osteoclasten weiten den Kanal auf und treiben ihn zur Knochenwundfläche hin vor. Da dieser Vorgang von beiden Fragmenten ausgeht, vereinigen sich häufig zwei aufeinander treffende Kanälchen. Nach ausreichender Aufweitung der die Osteotomie oder Fraktur überkreuzenden Kanäle wandeln sich die Osteoclasten zu Osteoblasten und lagern neue Knochenlamellen ab. So wird die ursprüngliche Textur direkt und ohne den Umweg über Callus wieder hergestellt. Die Fragmente werden praktisch durch überbrückende Osteone miteinander verzapft. „Durch einen Regenerationsprozeß, dessen Träger die Corticalis selbst ist, erfolgt eine Vereinigung der Fragmentenden auf dem Wege der primären Wiederherstellung der ursprünglichen Corticalisstruktur“ (SCHENK, 1964). Der zeitliche Ablauf wurde durch vitale Markierung des mineralisierenden Knochens mit Tetracyclin nach der Methode von MILCH, RALL und TOBIE (1958) geprüft. Im Experiment am Hund fanden SCHENK und seine Mitarbeiter das Einsetzen der Mineralisation in der dritten Woche nach der Osteotomie. Am Ende der vierten Woche betrug die Zahl der in Erneuerung begriffenen Osteone 24%, nach sechs Wochen 54% und nach acht Wochen 64% (auf der unverletzten Kontrollseite 2,5% sämtlicher Osteone).

Die primäre Knochenheilung wird nur zwischen unverrückbar und fest und unter Druck vereinigten Fragmenten beobachtet, zwischen Fragmenten, welche ideal reponiert formschlüssig und fest aneinander liegen. Wohl drängt sich die Vermutung auf, daß der Spalt zwischen den Fragmenten so klein ist, daß ein Eindringen von Zellen oder gar Blutgefäßen ausgeschlossen ist, so daß sich ein Granulationsgewebe aus räumlichen Gründen gar nicht bilden kann (SCHENK). Überzeugender dürfte der Gedankengang sein, daß allein unter Ausschaltung jeglichen mechanischen Insults der Knochen in der Lage ist, hochwertigen lamellären Knochen zu bilden, ein Resultat, welches bei der üblichen Heilung einer Fraktur über angiogenen, chondralen oder desmalen Callus Monate bis Jahre in Anspruch nehmen kann.

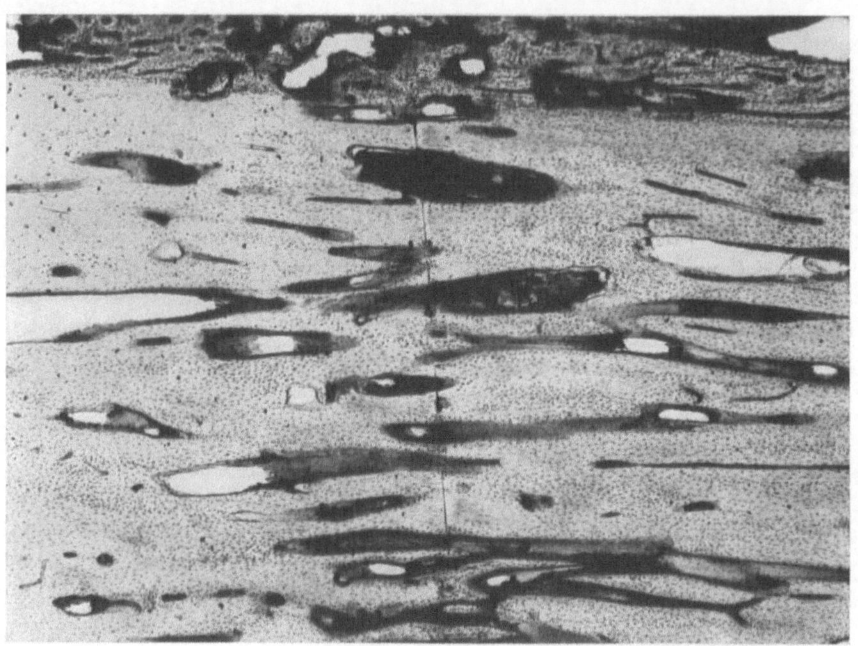

Abb. 6. Primäre Knochenheilung. Bei optimaler Reposition und optimalem Druck überbrücken regenerierende Osteone den feinen Spalt ohne Callusbildung. [Aus: SCHENK und WILLENEGGER, Langenbecks Archiv 308, 449 (1964)]

3. Theorien der Knochenneubildung

Nachdem anfänglich nur dem Periost die knochenbildende Fähigkeit zugeschrieben wurde (HEINE, 1837; OLLIER, 1867 u.a.) kam AXHAUSEN (1909) nach Transplantationsversuchen von Knochen, Periost oder Mark zu der Annahme präexistierender, spezifisch knochenbildender Zellen (Osteoblastentheorie). Die Tatsache, daß auch eine von Periost und Mark befreite Corticalis, deren Knochenzellen nach der Implantation absterben, neuen Knochen bildet (BASCHKIRZEW u. PETROW, 1912; BANCROFT, 1922; PHEMISTER, 1935 und viele andere) schwächte zwar die Bedeutung von Knochenhaut und Markgewebe ab, erschütterte aber die Gültigkeit der Osteoblastentheorie, welche von LEXER (1919) nachdrücklich gestützt wurde, keineswegs, denn an dem Vorhandensein der präexistenten Knochenbildner in sekundären Markräumen und Havers'schen Kanälchen war ja nicht zu zweifeln.

Im scharfen Gegensatz zur Osteoblastentheorie steht die Vorstellung, daß die Knochenneubildung auf dem Wege der Metaplasie vor sich geht. Unter dem Einfluß eines „Nekrohormons“ (BIER, 1923), eines „Wirkstoffes“ (LEVANDER, 1949), eines „osteogenetischen Stoffes (ANNERSTEN, 1940), eines „knochenbildenden Faktors“ (K-Faktor — OBERDALHOFF, 1947), eines von den gereizten Knochenzellen gebildeten „Aktivans“ (KÜNTSCHER, 1941) soll sich das pluripotente Keimgewebe zu Knochengewebe metaplastisch ausdifferenzieren.

Erstmalig beschrieb wohl BANCROFT (1918) die beobachtete metaplastische Ossifikation des den Span umgebenden Bindegewebes neben der Knochenbildung durch die Osteoblasten der Havers'schen Kanälchen. Erst LÉRICHE und POLICARD (1926) hielten jede Knochenneubildung für metaplastische Bindegewebsossifikation, hervorgerufen durch die im toten Knochen nach der Transplantation frei werdenden Kalksalze. BAUERMEISTER (1954) glaubt der praeformierten Form dieser Kalksalze als „fertige Bausteine" eine besondere Bedeutung beimessen zu sollen. Es besteht aber kein Zweifel daran, daß die Metaplasie in der Knochenneubildung eine beträchtliche Rolle spielt, daß bis heute aber unbekannt ist, wodurch die Metaplasie hervorgerufen wird. Nach den Untersuchungen von FUCHS, STEGEMANN und EGER (1963) sind die Kristallite allein nicht in der Lage, metaplastische Knochenbildung hervorzurufen, und nach den Untersuchungen von MAATZ, LENTZ und GRAF (1954) und BAUERMEISTER (1954) wird eine metaplastische Knochenbildung von einem präparierten Spanmaterial hervorgerufen, dessen hormonartiger Wirkstoff durch die Präparation ohne Zweifel hätte zerstört sein müssen.

W. AXHAUSEN (1952) faßte dann die „Induktionstheorie" und die „Osteoblastenlehre" zu einer einheitlichen Anschauung zusammen und URIST (1959) bekannte sich zu der „Zwei-Phasen-Theorie". Danach verläuft die Knochenregeneration in zwei osteogenetischen Phasen, von denen die erste von präexistenten, spezifischen Zellen, den Osteoblasten ausgeht, während die zweite, vom unspezifischen Bindegewebe ausgehend, metaplastisch abläuft. Erstere setzt bereits in den ersten Tagen ein, letztere nimmt bis zum Beginn mehrere Wochen in Anspruch. Beide Phasen werden durch die aktivierende Wirkung des abgestorbenen Knochensubstrats ausgelöst.

Bei der Heilung einer Fraktur lassen sich die beiden Phasen beobachtend zweifelsohne nicht trennen. Sie lassen sich immer nur im Experiment darstellen. Zusammenfassend dürfte also Gültigkeit haben, daß sich neben dem spezifisch knochenbildenden Gewebe des Periosts, des Marks und der Havers'schen Kanälchen auch der gesamte Bindegewebsapparat im Bereich der Fraktur an der Bildung des pluripotenten Keimgewebes beteiligt. Unter wessen Einfluß dieses embryonale Gewebe zu Knochen direkt oder auf dem Umweg über Knorpel oder Bindegewebe ausreift, bleibt zunächst eine offene Frage. Da der Knochen ein Stützgewebe mit einer mechanischen Funktion ist, dürfte der Gedanke sicher nicht abwegig sein, auch mechanischen Reizen bei seiner Entstehung und Regeneration eine Rolle zuzuschreiben.

4. Die Bedeutung des mechanischen Faktors in der Knochenneubildung

„Der Knochen hat eine funktionelle Gestalt und Struktur" (ROUX, 1895). „Die Callusform hat nicht das geringste mit der von den meisten Forschern so inniggeliebten Funktion zu tun, die nach ihrer Meinung alles macht" (BIER, 1923). ANNERSTEN (1940) stellt Osteogenese und Mechanik einander gegenüber. „Am Forschungsobjekt Knochen kann man weder allein mit biologisch-chemischen noch allein mit mechanisch-technischen Betrachtungsweisen zum Ziel gelangen, sondern beide gehören zu sinnvoller Synthese sich ergänzend zusammen" (GELBKE, 1953).

Es ist bezeichnend, daß der Begriff der „Biomechanik" bei Betrachtungen der Knochenbildung eingeführt wurde. Inwieweit ein mechanisch funktioneller Reiz dabei anregend oder gar differenzierend wirkt, ist noch nicht völlig geklärt, klar ist aber, daß *mechanische Insulte*, ein mechanischer *Störfaktor* schwerste Störungen in der Knochenbildung hervorrufen können. Ein mechanischer Reiz vermag ebenso wie ein thermischer oder chemischer Reiz, Knochenneubildung ohne Vorliegen einer Knochenwunde in Form periostaler Callusbildung hervorzurufen (BUSCH, 1879; KÜNTSCHER, 1941; MAATZ, 1943). Die Abb. 7 zeigt die Reaktion des Femurs beim Hund bei zusätzlicher mechanischer Belastung des Knochens in axialer Richtung mit 40 kg durch eine zentral liegende, chemisch inaktive Feder.

Eine Voraussetzung für die Bewertung des Einflusses mechanischer Kräfte auf die Knochenbildung setzt voraus, daß es möglich ist, exakt gesteuerte mechanische Kräfte wirken zu lassen. Durch die neueren Formen der Osteosynthese (Marknagel, Markraumschraube oder Feder) und die Instrumente der Schweizer Arbeitsgemeinschaft für Osteosynthese (A.O.) sind diese Voraussetzungen heute gegeben. Die von Krompecher (1937) erhobenen Befunde mußten, so richtungsweisend sie für die weitere Forschung waren, darunter leiden, daß es ihm nicht gelingen konnte, reine Druckkräfte zu erzeugen. So glaubte er, daß unter Druck allein der Callus vorwiegend auf dem Umweg über Knorpel entsteht, während wir heute wissen, daß Knorpel nur dann entsteht, wenn zusätzlich zur Druckkraft eine leichte Schleifbewegung auftritt (Benninghoff, 1938 u.a.).

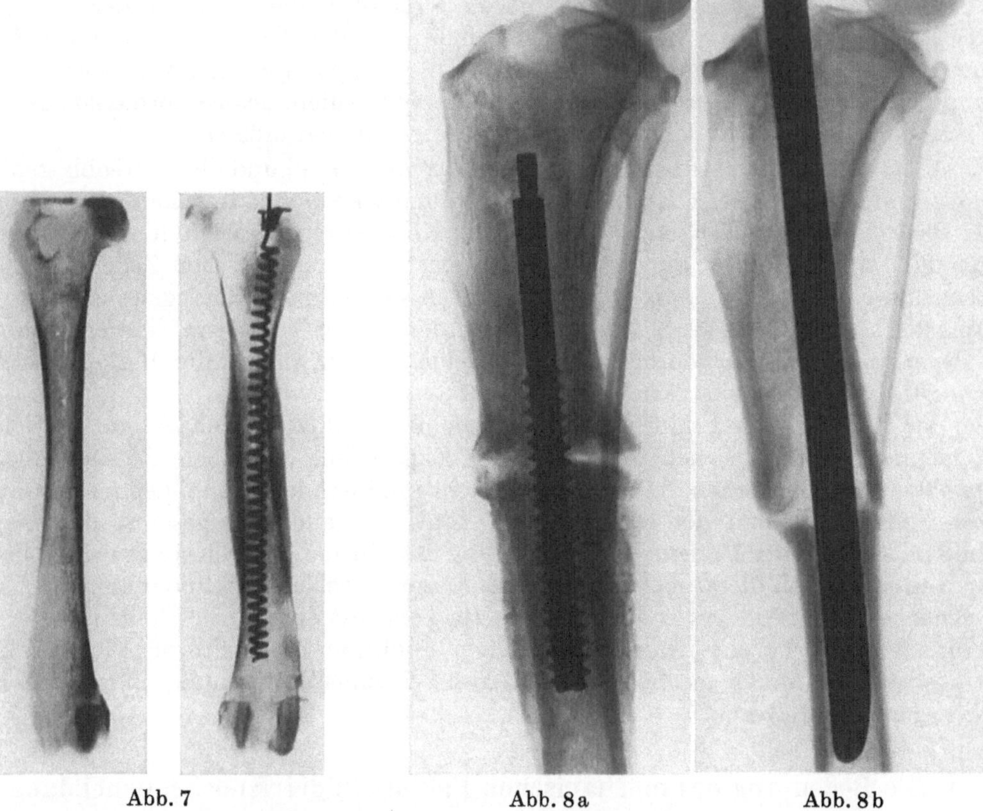

Abb. 7 Abb. 8a Abb. 8b

Abb. 7. Zusätzliche mechanische Belastung (hier durch Markraumfeder) ruft eine Verdickung des Knochens durch periostale Callusbildung hervor. (Aus: Wanke-Maatz-Junge-Lentz, Knochenbrüche und Verrenkungen. Urban & Schwarzenberg 1962, 1. Aufl. 1962, S. 9)

Abb. 8a u. b. Verzögerte Verfestigung und Heilung über den Knorpel an einer mit Sperrschraube versorgten Hunde-Tibia (a). Knöcherne Durchkonstruktion an der Kontroll-Tibia der anderen Seite. (Quelle wie Abb. 7)

Steuert man die Fragmentenden einer Osteotomie mit einer in das Knochenrohr eingeschnittenen Schraube und sorgt primär für eine vorhandene geringfügige Distraktion der Fragmentenden, so daß ein Spalt für das Aufsprossen von Granulationsgewebe frei bleibt, so differenziert sich das Keimgewebe unter dem exakten Druck mit geringfügiger Schleifbewegung zu Knorpel (Abb. 8a und Abb. 9). Fehlt diese Schleifbewegung, werden die Fragmente durch einen im Markraum liegenden Nagel stabil vereinigt (Abb. 8b), so bildet sich der Callus ohne den Umweg über den Knorpel. Werden die Fragmente unverrückbar fest und ideal aufeinander passend aneinandergefügt, so bleibt sogar jede Callusbildung aus, und es findet eine direkte Vereinigung von Knochenrohr mit Knochenrohr durch lamellären Knochen statt (siehe S. 543). So bedarf die Feststellung Krompechers, daß chondraler Callus unter Druck gebildet wird, der Ergänzung, daß diesem Druck eine Schleifbewegung zugesellt sein muß, wenn chondrale Knochenbildung stattfinden soll, und daß lückenlos und unter starkem Druck zusammengefügte Fragmente sich primär ohne den Umweg über den Callus vereinigen.

Nach KROMPECHER bildet sich dort, wo die Knochenwunde unter Dauerzug liegt, der Callus auf dem Umweg über das Bindegewebe (desmale Knochenbildung). Es sprossen dann zwischen den Reihen des kollagenen Bindegewebes undifferenzierte Mesenchymzellen auf, die sich ähnlich wie bei der chondralen Knochenbildung hier zwischen den Bindegewebszellen zu Osteoblasten wandeln, die Bindegewebsfascikel dabei auseinanderschiebend. Das Bindegewebe hat in solchen Knochenwunden von Anfang an die Richtung des Dauerzuges.

Heute besteht weitgehend Übereinstimmung in der Ansicht, daß die angiogene Callusbildung an den Orten mechanischer Ruhe auftritt (KROMPECHER, 1937; PAUWELS, 1941;

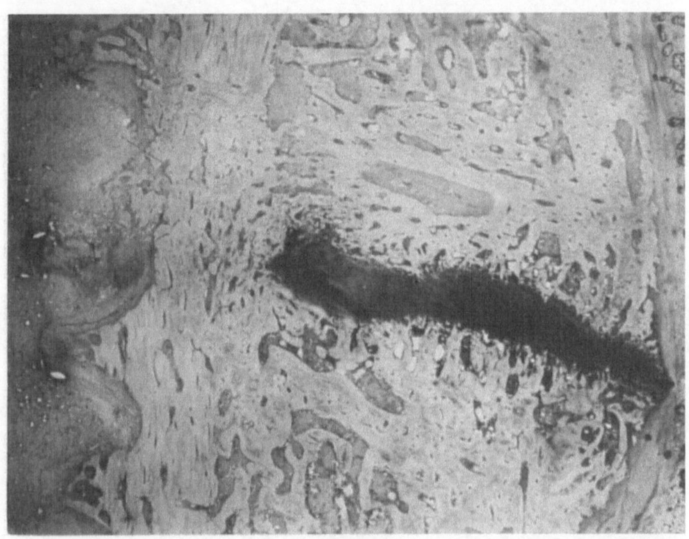

Abb. 9. Feingeweblicher Schnitt zu Abb. 8a. Links breiter Knorpelsaum, rechts Markraum mit Schraubenlager, dazwischen erste knöcherne Überbrückung des Osteotomiespalts. (Quelle wie Abb. 7, S. 546)

KÜNTSCHER, 1941 u.v.a.). Zu bedenken ist dabei aber ohne Frage, daß die Orte, für welche die Autoren mechanische Ruhe annehmen, doch nur als Orte bezeichnet werden können, in denen gröbere mechanische Einwirkungen nicht auftreten. Das Granulationsgewebe in einem seitenständigen Defekt an einem Röhrenknochen unterliegt zweifelsohne einem etwas ausgeprägteren Kräftespiel wechselnd hoher Druckspannungen bis Zugspannungen, da im Defekt als einer Kerbe im Knochen Spannungsspitzen auftreten müssen. Das von KÜNTSCHER (1935) angeführte Beispiel des Spatiums zwischen den Fragmentenden einer durch den verklemmten Nagel distrahierten Fraktur (Abb. 10) zeigt sicher noch klarer, daß dank der Elastizität des Nagels das Granulationsgewebe in dem Raum zwischen den Fragmenten etwa einem Kräftespiel ausgesetzt ist, welches als „physiologisch" für das Knochengewebe anzusehen ist. Der Gedanke, daß ein solches Kräftespiel dem werdenden Knochen adäquat sein dürfte, ist naheliegend. Damit kann nicht behauptet werden, daß dieser mechanische Reiz die Ausdifferenzierung des pluripotenten Keimgewebes in Knochengewebe bewirkt.

Der *Einfluß* der mechanischen Kräfte ist aber nicht zu leugnen. Es trifft ohne Zweifel zu, daß Richtung und Anordnung der das Hämatom organisierenden Gefäßsprossen für die spätere Anordnung der Callusbälkchen bestimmend ist (BANCROFT, 1929), die Gefäßsprossen aber wachsen an den Fibrinfasern entlang, und die Fibrinfasern bilden die primäre Verspannung zwischen den Fragmenten, und diese kann sehr wohl durch das mechanische Kräftespiel bestimmt sein.

Wie ausgeprägt die Mechanik bereits die innere Struktur des Callus bestimmt, zeigen die Untersuchungen von GRIESSMANN und REICH (1944), welche mit Nagel ausreichend stabil versorgte und allein im Gipsverband ruhiggestellte Frakturen der Tibia beim Hund feingeweblich untersuchten. Abb. 11 zeigt das wirre Flechtwerk des Callus, welcher die Fragmente im Gipsverband in allen Richtungen abzustützen hat, während Abb. 12 die

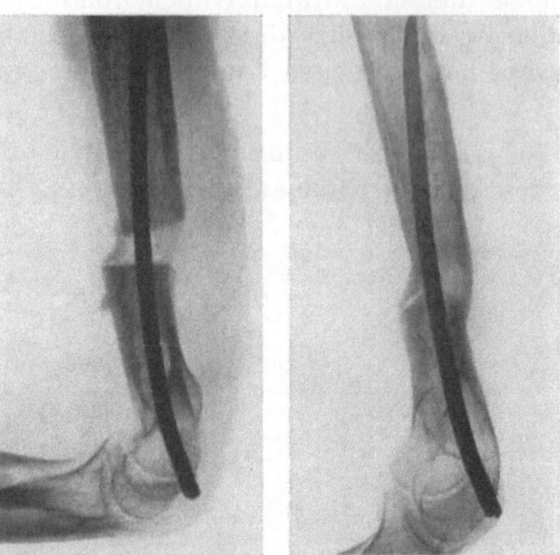

Abb. 10. Lückenfüllende Callusbildung im periostfreien Raum nach Resektion einer Humeruspseudarthrose vier Wochen und vier Monate nach der Operation. (Quelle wie Abb. 7, S. 546)

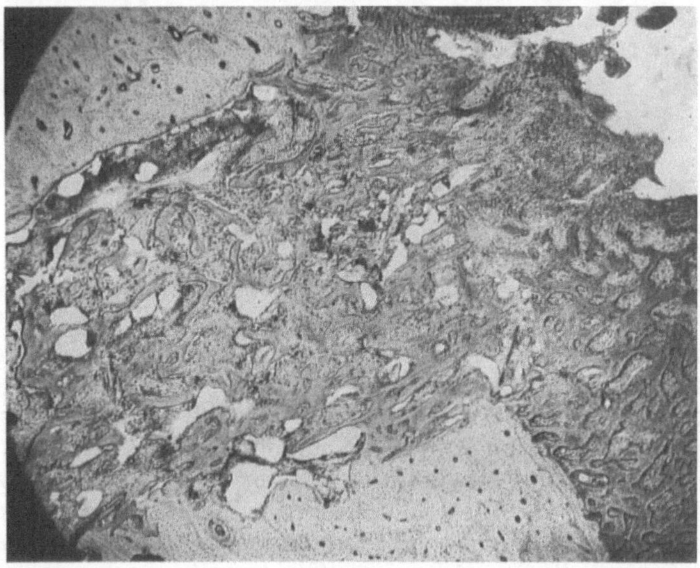

Abb. 11. Unruhiges Flechtwerk von Callus an der frakturierten und mit Gipsverband versorgten Hundetibia. [GRIESSMANN u. REICH, Arch. Klin. Chir. 205, S. 455—474 (1944)]

vorwiegend in einer Richtung angeordneten Callusbälkchen zeigt, welche unter dem vom Nagel zu einer bestimmten Richtung gesteuerten Kräftespiel entstanden sind.

Zusammenfassend ist festzustellen, daß unter hohem Druck, welcher Knochenfragmente unverrückbar zusammenhält, eine Direkt-Vereinigung der Bruchenden durch ausgereiften Lamellenknochen beobachtet wird, daß die sogenannte sekundäre Callusbildung chondral unter Druck mit Schleifbewegung und desmal unter Dauerzug beobachtet wird. Die primäre, die sogenannte angiogene Callusbildung wird dort beobachtet, wo ein für das Knochengewebe physiologisches Kräftespiel stattfindet ohne störende mechanische Faktoren. Es ist das Bestreben des Körpers, die Fragmente ruhig zu stellen. Erst dann, wenn mechanische Insulte ausgeschaltet sind, besteht für den Körper die Möglichkeit zur Bildung ausgereiften, lamellären Knochens. Um diese Ruhigstellung zu erreichen, bedient der Körper sich je nach Art der herrschenden mechanischen Insulte des Bindegewebes, des Knorpels und des (provisorischen) Callus.

Pauwels (1941) hält jede mechanische Kraft für nachteilig in der Knochenbildung. Nach seiner Meinung kann sich knöcherner Callus erst dann bilden, wenn die Bruchstelle vollkommen ruhig gestellt ist. Nach seiner Theorie geschieht die Ausdifferenzierung des „Blastoms", des Frakturhämatoms, welches primär die Ruhigstellung des Bruchortes übernimmt, unter dem allseitig wirkenden Druck, welcher nach dem anfänglichen Muskel-

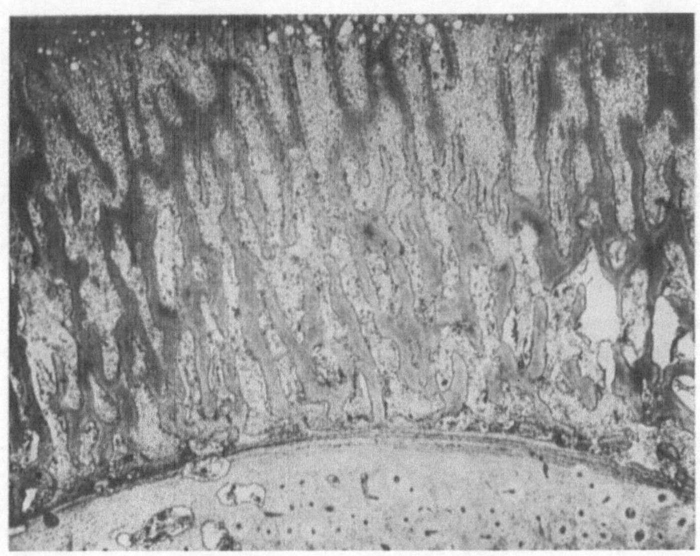

Abb. 12. Gerichteter Callus an der mit Nagel versorgten frakturierten Hundetibia. (Quelle wie Abb. 11, S. 548

stupor durch einen erhöhten Tonus der Muskulatur, den „Tetanus intermittens" nach Rehn (1924), hervorgerufen wird. Unter dem statischen Druck soll sich das Mesenchym über Knorpel zu Knochen ausdifferenzieren.

5. Röntgenologisch erfaßbare Vorgänge bei der Knochenbruchheilung

a) Die primäre Knochenheilung

Heilt eine Fraktur „primär" (siehe S. 543), so soll röntgenologisch Callus an keiner Stelle, Knochenneubildung nur im Bereich des Bruchspaltes in Form des knöchernen Durchbaus erkennbar sein (Abb. 13). Es fehlt sogar jegliche narbige Verdichtung der Corticalis, da lediglich tote Osteone durch lebende ersetzt werden. Die für diesen Umbau erforderliche Vermehrung und Erweiterung der Havers'schen Kanälchen (siehe histologischen Teil) muß zu einer leichten Auflockerung der Corticalis führen. Diese ist aber in der Mehrzahl der Fälle röntgenologisch nicht erfaßbar. Jedes Sichtbarwerden von Callus läßt auf unzureichend exakte Reposition und vor allem mangelhafte Ruhigstellung (mechanische Irritation) schließen (Abb. 14). Daraus ergibt sich, daß nur feine Sprünge im Knochen ohne Dislokation und ohne die Möglichkeit der Bewegung zwischen den Fragmenten oder Frakturen, welche durch eine besondere Form der Osteosynthese zusammengefügt werden, eine sogenannte primäre Knochenheilung zeigen können. Damit ist es auch verständlich, daß der Begriff der primären Knochenheilung (als Analogon zur primären Wundheilung) erst jüngeren Datums ist (siehe S. 541).

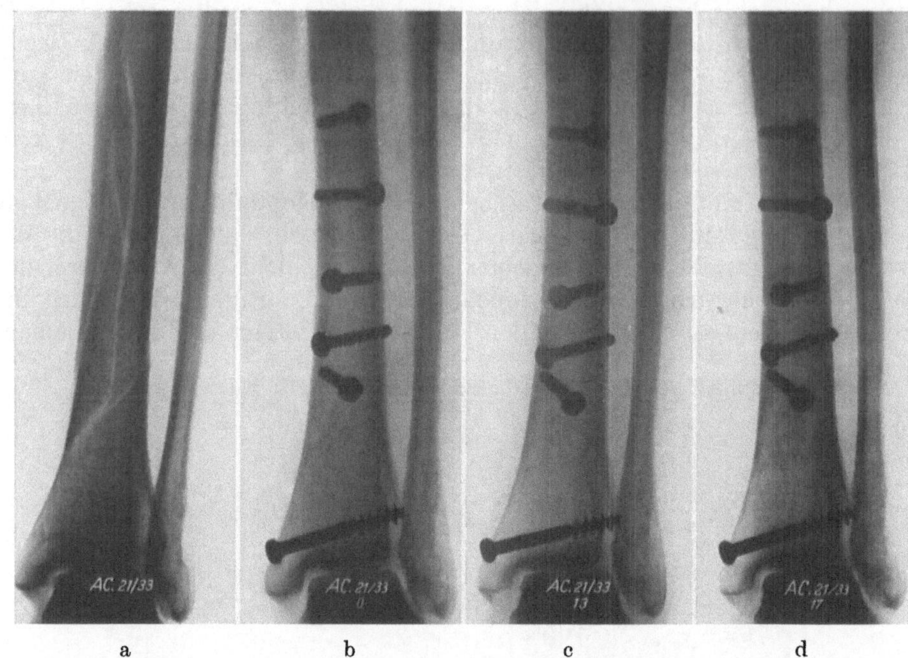

a b c d

Abb. 13a—d. Primäre Knochenheilung nach Verschraubung einer Unterschenkeltorsionsfraktur. a Frakturbild, b Kontrolle nach der Operation, c Kontrolle nach dreizehn Wochen, d Kontrolle nach siebzehn Wochen. [Aus: WIESER, Langenbecks Arch. 308, S. 435 (1964)]

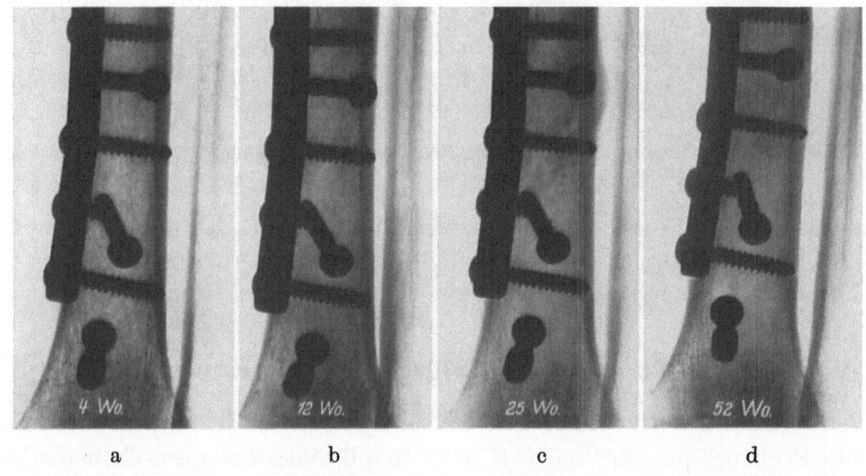

a b c d

Abb. 14a—d. Leicht gestörte primäre Knochenheilung. a Zustand vier Wochen nach der Operation. Der Bruchspalt ist fast verschwunden. b Die Patientin hat das Bein etwas zu früh belastet, Frakturspalt deutlicher. c Unter Entlastung Heilung mit Callusbildung. d Zustand 1 Jahr nach der Operation. (Quelle wie Abb. 13, S. 437)

b) Die sekundäre Knochenheilung über den Callus

Das Gros der Frakturen heilt sekundär, also auf dem Umweg über den Callus. Dieses junge Knochengewebe füllt die Lücke zwischen den Fragmenten aus oder hüllt die Fragmente in einen Callusmantel ein. Dank des größeren Radius einer solchen „Muffe“ ist die Stabilisierung der Fragmente trotz geringerer mechanischer Wertigkeit des Callus ausreichend. Im spongiösen Knochen kann der zwischen den Bälkchen sich bildende Callus als Verdichtung deutlich hervortreten (Abb. 15). Die knöcherne Heilung ist allein nach der weit später auftretenden knöchernen Durchkonstruktion zu beurteilen.

Schattengebend, also röntgenologisch sichtbar, kann das knöcherne Granulationsgewebe erst nach der Einlagerung von Kalksalzen werden, also frühestens nach zehn, meist erst nach vierzehn Tagen. Das nicht schattengebende Osteoidgewebe kann zwischen den Fragmenten als heller Saum erkennbar sein. So kann durch Umbau der Fragmentenden im Röntgenbild sogar eine Dislokation der Fragmente vorgetäuscht werden (Abb. 16).

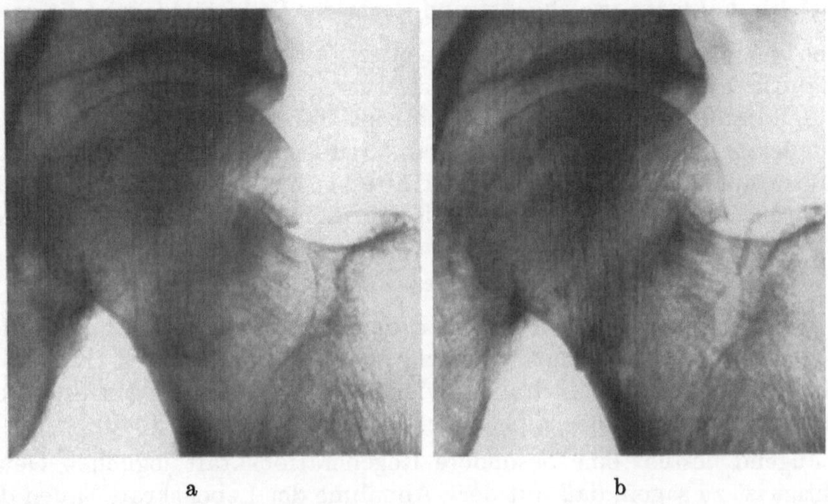

a b

Abb. 15. Zuverlässig eingekeilte Schenkelhalsfraktur bei einer 80-jährigen Patientin (a). Das Kontrollbild sechs Wochen später (b) zeigt die interspongiöse Callusbildung als Verdichtung des Knochens im Frakturbereich und seiner Nachbarschaft

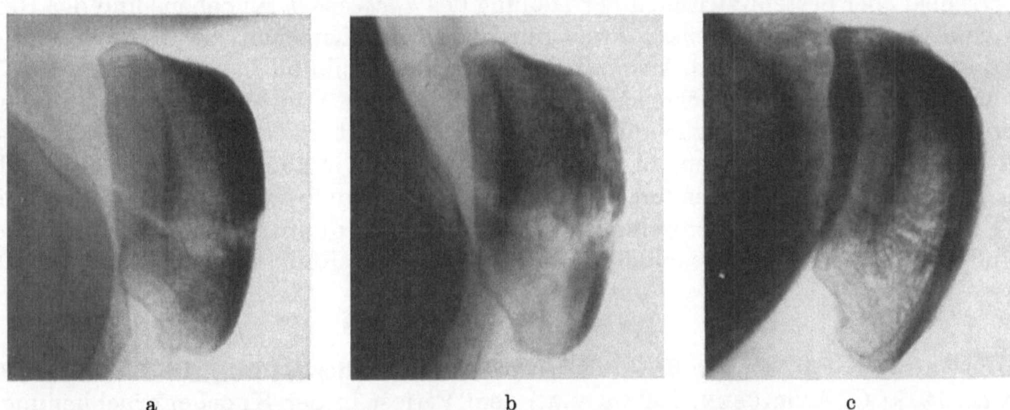

a b c

Abb. 16. Patella-Bruch bei 23jähriger Patientin (a). Bei besonders starkem Umbau im Knochen täuscht ein breiter Osteoidsaum (b) zwischen den Fragmenten eine Dislokation vor (vier Wochen). Das Kontrollbild (c) wurde fünfeinhalb Jahre nach der Verletzung gemacht. (Quelle wie Abb. 7, S. 546)

Nicht nur im Röntgenbild, sondern auch bei der feingeweblichen Untersuchung ist die Herkunft des Callusgewebes im Bereich einer heilenden Fraktur meist nicht sicher zu erkennen. Darum wählten wir im histologischen Teil vorwiegend im gezielten Experiment gewonnene Bilder, welche die Diagnose erleichtern.

Die Möglichkeit der primären Knochenheilung beleuchtet besonders eindrucksvoll die Fragwürdigkeit der in der Röntgenologie auch heute noch trotz klinischer Bedenken immer wieder verwendeten Begriffe der „guten", der „reichlichen", der „spärlichen" Callusbildung, welche allein ohne ergänzende Beiworte irreführend sein können.

Die Begriffe der „endossalen", der „intermediären" und der „parossalen" Callusbildung sollten nur mit Vorsicht verwendet werden, da der Ursprung des Callus sehr oft unsicher oder gar nicht aus dem Röntgenbild gefolgert werden kann. Die Begriffe der

„provisorischen“ und „endgültigen“ Callusbildung sollten nicht angewendet werden, weil der Callus stets ein Provisorium ist, welches in der sekundären Knochenheilung später durch den lamellären Knochen, den „endgültigen“ ersetzt wird — und bei diesem handelt es sich nicht mehr um Callus.

c) Die Faktoren, welche Art und Form der Callusbildung bestimmen

Es besteht kein Zweifel daran, daß neben der Entstehung des Callus auch seine Formgebung heute für uns noch voller Rätsel ist. Der „Nisus formativus“ (Bier), das „Wirkungsfeld“ (Debrunner, 1924), die „osteotrope Tendenz“ (Bier, 1923) sind Begriffe, welche keine letzte Klärung bringen, so daß wir resignierend feststellen müssen, daß in einem „Frakturmilieu“ die regenerativen Kräfte bis zur Heilung tätig sind. Das kann uns aber nicht daran hindern, den röntgenologisch erfaßbaren Vorgängen nachzuspüren.

α) Das Alter des Patienten

Brüche der Neugeborenen heilen wegen der enormen Knochenbildungsfähigkeit der dem Embryonalstadium eben Entronnenen außerordentlich schnell (Käfer, 1925). Eine Oberschenkelfraktur kann nach drei bis vier Tagen „plastisch“ verfestigt sein und benötigt nach acht bis zehn Tagen keinen Verband mehr (Block, 1940).

In der Jugend besteht eine besondere Regenerationskraft jeglichen Gewebes. Ob es aber berechtigt ist zu sagen, daß mit der „Abnahme der Lebenskraft“ auch die Schnelligkeit der Gewebsneubildung beim Callus nachläßt (Block, 1940), bedarf noch der experimentellen Klärung. Hat uns doch die Klinik gelehrt, daß unter zweckentsprechender Behandlung Frakturen auch im hohen Alter rasch und ungestört heilen. Ein beträchtlicher Unterschied aber besteht zwischen der Heilung des *wachsenden* Knochens und der Heilung des Knochens der *Erwachsenen*. Zwar durchläuft der Knochen der Erwachsenen eine andauernde Erneuerung, das Ausmaß der Knochenneubildung ist aber in keiner Weise mit der des wachsenden Knochens zu vergleichen. Für die Frakturheilung spielt dabei das Periost ohne Frage die überragende Rolle. Hinzu kommt die Beschaffenheit des Markes (Fettmark des alten Menschen, Burckhardt, 1925). Die mindere „Masse“ des Knochens, oder richtiger gesagt, die mindere Größe der Knochenwundfläche kann bei der Heilung der Fraktur eines altersatrophischen Knochens mit sehr dünner Corticalis oder weit auseinander liegenden Spongiosabälkchen sehr wohl eine Rolle spielen (Radasch, 1930).

β) Die Rolle des Periostes

Die Tatsache, daß eine große Zahl anerkannter Forscher (Heine, 1837; Ollier, 1867; Lexer, 1919; G. Axhausen, 1908 u.v.a.) dem Periost in der Knochenbruchheilung und damit auch in der Gestaltung des Callus die alleinige oder wenigstens überwiegende Rolle zuschrieben, während eine kaum kleinere Anzahl nicht minder anerkannter Forscher (Baschkirzew u. Petrow, 1912; Bancroft, 1929; Phemister, 1935; Leriche u. Policard, 1926 u.v.a.) dem Periost diese wichtige Rolle nicht zuerkennen wollten, zeigt, wie schwer diese Frage zu beantworten ist. Nachdem sich aber die Erkenntnis durchgesetzt hat, daß ein entscheidender Unterschied zwischen dem Periost des wachsenden und des erwachsenen Individuums besteht, lassen sich Widersprüche in den experimentellen Befunden leicht erklären, da das Alter der Versuchstiere gar nicht oder nur ungenau berücksichtigt wurde. Das Periost des Erwachsenen ist nicht dauernd „knochenbildungstätig“, es ist nur „knochenbildungsfähig“ (G. Axhausen 1909). Bei Ablösung des Periostes vom Knochen haftet an der Knochenhaut die Cambiumschicht (Duhamel, 1740). Dieses Periost in Weichgewebe verpflanzt, ergibt lebhafte Knochenneubildung (Mayer u. Wehner, 1914 u.a.), während das Periost des ausgewachsenen Individuums eine bindegewebige Grenzmembran (Bier, 1923; Martin, 1927 u.a.) bildet, welche allein verpflanzt, keinen Knochen, mit anhaftender Knochensubstanz verpflanzt, aber doch Knochenneubildung im Weichteillager ergibt (RADZIMOWSKI, 1881 u.v.a.). Das Ausmaß der periostalen Knochenneubildung nach mechanischer, chemischer oder thermischer Reizung vom Markraum aus ist altersabhängig (MAATZ, 1948). ORELL (1952) beklagte sich bei Schaffung des „os novum" durch Implantation von „os purum" in den subperiostalen Raum darüber, daß die Knochenneubildung bei dieser Technik beim Erwachsenen allzu spärlich sei.

Berücksichtigen wir die Erkenntnis, daß die Rolle des Periostes in der Frakturheilung um so mehr im Vordergrund steht, je jünger der Patient ist, daß die Knochenbildungs-

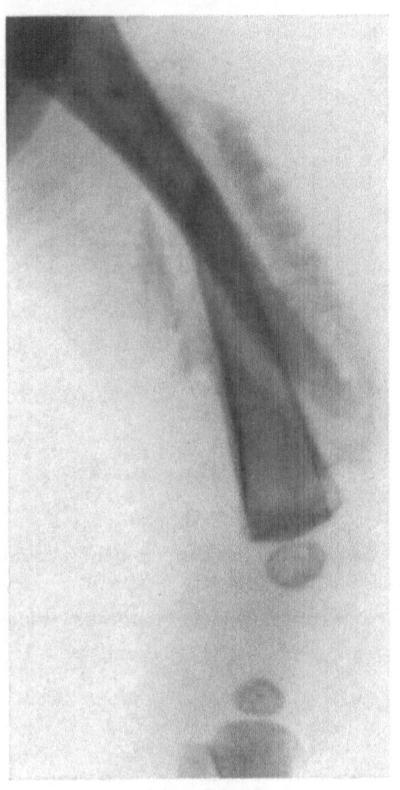

Abb. 17

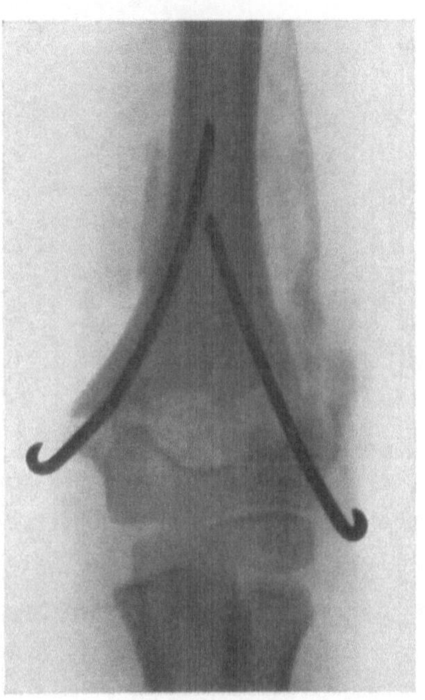

Abb. 18

Abb. 17. Enorme Mantelcallusbildung bei Oberschenkelbruch eines 3 Monate alten Säuglings. (Quelle wie Abb. 7, S. 546)

Abb. 18. Percondyläre Fraktur eines 10jährigen Knaben. Starke Callusbildung im subperiostalen Raum sechs Wochen nach der Versorgung mit Rush Pins

fähigkeit der Knochenhaut mit zunehmendem Alter entscheidend abnimmt, so werden wir an vielen Röntgenbildern leichter erkennen, welchen Ursprungs der Callus sein mag. Das Röntgenbild der Abb. 17 zeigt die geradezu gewaltige periostale Callusbildung, mit der der Oberschenkelschrägbruch eines Neugeborenen nach 2 Wochen eingehüllt ist. Auf der Abb. 18 sehen wir einen sicher vorwiegend vom Periost gebildeten Callus, da das Periost weit vom Knochen abgehoben hier im subperiostalen Raum seine eigene Leistung demonstrieren kann.

Der Satz LEXERS „der Callus wandert die Wege, die das Periost vorschreibt" trifft sicher für viele Fälle von Frakturen Jugendlicher zu, die Zahl der Ausnahmen ist aber groß, und beim Erwachsenen und besonders beim alten Menschen hat er keine Berechtigung.

Bei jungen Individuen ist das Periost eine dicke Membran, welche sich relativ leicht (mit der Cambiumschicht) vom Knochen abheben läßt. Dies geschieht entweder durch das Trauma im Augenblick der Dislokation der Fragmente oder durch eine Blutansammlung unter der Knochenhaut. Nach unserer Meinung müssen wir uns aber von der Vorstellung

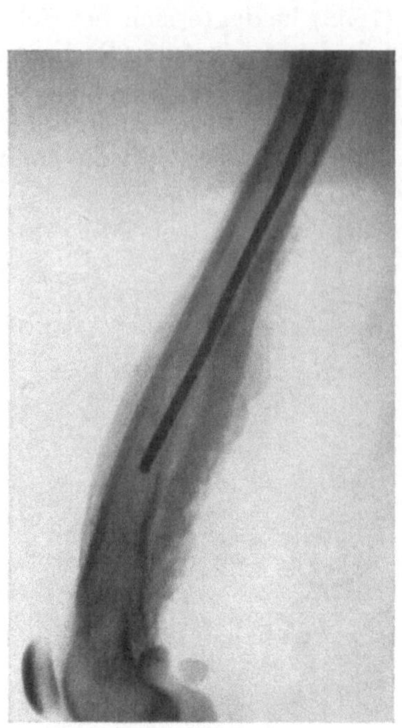

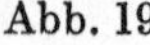

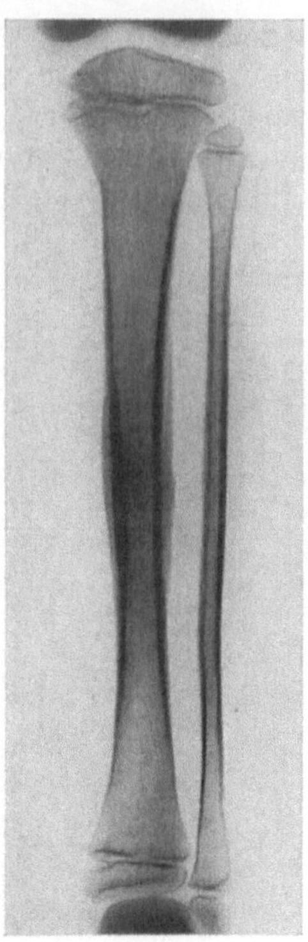

Abb. 19 Abb. 20

Abb. 19. Callus ohne Fraktur durch Markraumreiz (rostender Eisendraht). Es handelt sich um eine abacterielle Osteomyelitis

Abb. 20. Typischer periostaler Callusmantel um eine nur leicht achsenverschobene Tibiafraktur eines 12jährigen Knaben

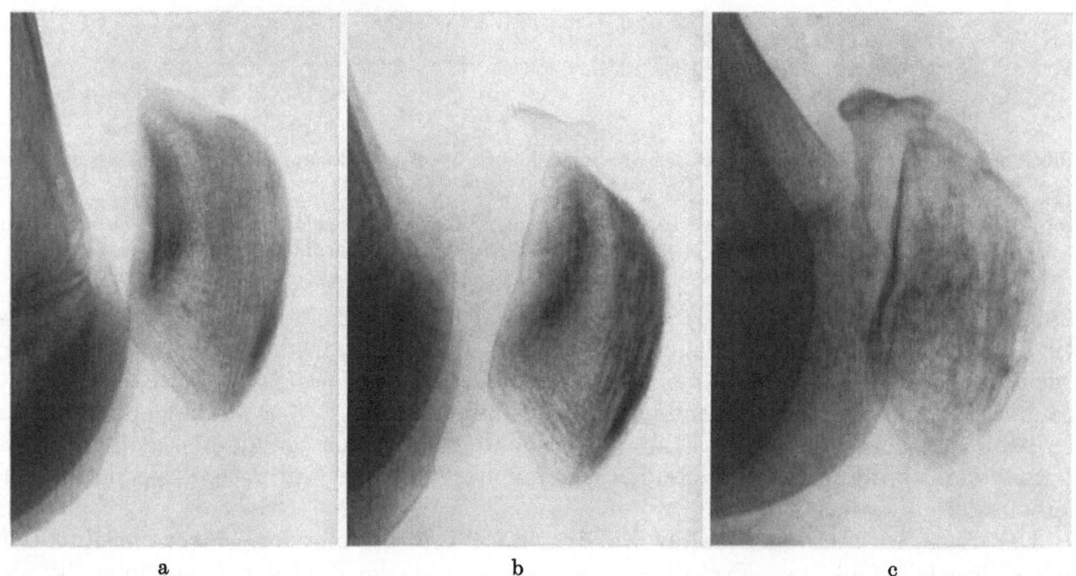

Abb. 21 a—c. Typische Callusbildung im subperiostalen Raum bei 15jährigem Knaben. a Frisch nach der Verletzung, b zwei Wochen danach, c zweieinhalb Monate später

freimachen, daß die „Ablösung des Periostes“ von entscheidender Bedeutung ist (Ollier, 1867), eine Vorstellung, die auch bei Block (1940) immer wieder hervorgehoben wird. Abb. 19 zeigt den „Callus ohne Fraktur“ (Küntscher, 1941). Hier war das Periost primär ganz sicher nicht abgehoben. Durch den Reiz, welcher vom Markraum ausgeht, antwortet der Knochen aber mit einer starken periostalen Callusbildung. Wieweit der Reiz der Fraktur ohne Abhebung des Periostes vom Knochen durch ein Hämatom zur Callusspindel führte, wie Abb. 20 sie zeigt, wird niemand entscheiden können. Mit demselben Recht werden wir aber auch annehmen dürfen, daß der Raum für den neugebildeten Knochen (Abb. 21) durch den mit Blut angefüllten subperiostalen Raum vorgeschrieben wurde. Ganz sicher aber trifft dieses nicht zu bei dem Fall der Abb. 10, da hier bei einem 32 Jahre alten Mann eine Pseudarthrose des Oberarms reseziert wurde, die Knochenenden wurden angefrischt, und der ungewollt später entstandene Raum zwischen den Fragmentenden hatte ganz sicher keine periostale Auskleidung. Hier ebenso wie bei dem Röntgenbild der Abb. 22 drängt sich wieder der Begriff des „Wirkungsfeldes" (DEBRUNNER, 1924) auf.

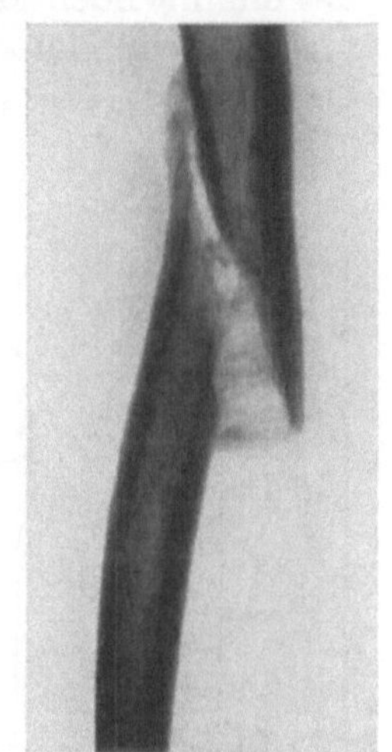

Abb. 22. Breite Callusstraße zwischen den Fragmenten eines Oberarmschrägbruches sechs Wochen nach der Verwundung. Die Schußwunde heilte primär. (Quelle wie Abb. 7, S. 546)

γ) Der Sitz der Fraktur

Der Sitz der Fraktur kann aus verschiedenen Gründen — Art — Mengen — Form — bestimmend für den Callus sein. Von großer Bedeutung ist zunächst die Blutversorgung der Fragmente, welche entscheidend werden kann, wenn eines der Fragmente durch den Sitz der Fraktur völlig aus der Ernährung ausgeschaltet ist (siehe S. 561). Liegt eine Fraktur intraarticulär, oder kommuniziert die Fraktur breit mit einer Gelenkhöhle, so kann auch die Synovialflüssigkeit entscheidende Hemmung für die Callusbildung bedeuten (siehe S. 561). Der Sitz der Fraktur kann auch dadurch die Entwicklung des Callus bestimmen, daß „typische" Fragmentdislokationen durch den Sitz der Fraktur hervorgerufen werden (z. B. subtrochantere Femurfraktur, Dislokation des proximalen Radiusfragments durch den Bicepsansatz usf.). Der Sitz kann auch eine typische und schwer auszuschaltende mechanische Irritation für die Fragmente bedeuten, sei es durch das natürliche Kräftespiel, sei es durch geradezu als typisch zu bezeichnende, häufig erforderliche Repositionsmanöver (siehe auch S. 570).

Spongiöser Knochen heilt im Vergleich zum corticalen dank seiner großen inneren Oberfläche rascher, so daß auch auf diese Weise der Sitz der Fraktur bedeutungsvoll sein kann. Im allgemeinen gilt die Heilungsneigung der Brüche in den *Metaphysen* als besonders gut. Zu der Tatsache, daß es sich um Spongiosa handelt, kommt die besonders gute Ernährung des kleinen Fragments durch Kapselgefäße unter Vermittlung des metaphysären Gefäßnetzes, während das große Fragment durch die Ausläufer der A. nutricia gut ernährt ist. Durch Muskel-, Sehnen- oder Band-Ursprünge oder Ansätze ist die Ernährung besonders gut gesichert (BLOCK, 1940). Sie wird meist auch nicht durch Lösung des Periostes unterbrochen. Das hat aber gleichzeitig zur Folge, daß Frakturen der Metaphysen im Röntgenbild meist eine periostale Callusbildung vermissen lassen.

δ) Die Form der Fraktur

Selbstredend muß die Form der Fraktur einen bestimmenden Einfluß auf die Gestalt des Callus haben, soll dieser doch die Fragmente je nach Bedarf mit oder ohne Überbrükkung zunächst provisorisch miteinander verbinden. Nur 3 Beispiele (Skizze Abb. 23) seien als Prototypen herausgegriffen. Ein langer Schrägbruch, welcher im Extensionsverband und unter dem Manteldruck der einhüllenden Weichgewebe, vor allem der Muskulatur, ausreichend ruhiggestellt ist, heilt meist unter Ausfüllung des Spatiums zwischen den großflächigen Knochenwunden durch Callusgewebe (Abb. 23a) ohne einhüllende Callusbildung, welches als eine Art Mantel sich um das gesamte Frakturgebiet legt. Diese Form des einhüllenden Mantels aus Knochen-Narbengewebe (Callus) beobachten wir aber ganz typisch beim glatten Querbruch (Abb. 23b), vorausgesetzt allerdings, daß der Patient in der Lage ist, alle ,,Reservekräfte der Frakturheilung" spielen zu lassen. Kann er das nicht, so ist die Gefahr der verzögerten Verfestigung um so größer, je weniger exakt und ruhig die Fragmente aufeinander stehen. Bei einem Trümmerbruch (Abb. 23c) kann die Intensität des ,,Frakturmilieus", das Vorhandensein vieler Knochenwundflächen, Ursache einer mächtigen, einer ausgedehnten Callusbildung sein. Die Tatsache aber, daß eine für den Skeletabschnitt vorhandene mechanische Irritation sich auf viele Bruchflächen verteilt, damit auf der einzelnen Bruchfläche weniger ausgeprägt zur Auswirkung kommt, kann wieder gegenregulierend auf eine mächtige Callusbildung wirken (siehe auch S. 545).

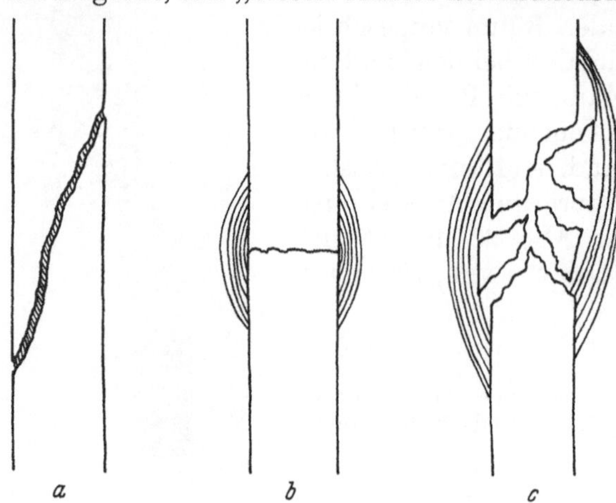

Abb. 23. Die Form der Fraktur hat mitbestimmenden Einfluß auf die Gestalt des Callus. (Siehe Text)

ε) Die Art der Kontinuitätstrennung

Bei jeder Fraktur zeigen die Enden der Fragmente einen schmalen Saum nekrotischen Knochengewebes (siehe S. 542). Mit Hitzeentstehung im Moment des Bruches muß diese Nekrose nicht erklärt werden, denn auch dann, wenn wir sehr langsam mit einer sägenden Rohrstanze Zylinder aus der Spongiosa schneiden, zeigen die Randbälkchen Knochentod (Maatz, Lentz u. Graf, 1954). Sehr wohl aber kann eine ausgedehntere Hitze-Nekrose eintreten, wenn der Knochen mit der Säge osteotomiert wird. Es ist allerdings praktisch nicht zu entscheiden, ob die häufig träge einsetzende knöcherne Vereinigung durch derartige hitze-bedingte Nekrosen oder durch die anderen Faktoren eintreten, welche ohnehin einer ,,offenen" Fraktur anhaften.

ζ) Die Stellung der Bruchenden

Vollkommene Reposition und unverrückbar feste Fixation der Fragmente können zur primären Knochenheilung ,,ohne Callus" führen. Dislozierte Fragmente, welche in nicht zu großer Entfernung voneinander stehen, werden durch ,,zielstrebigen" Callus miteinander verbunden (siehe Abb. 10 und 22). Stehen allerdings keinerlei Reserven der Heilkraft (intakter Periostschlauch, Hämatom, Muskelmantel) zur Verfügung, wie z.B. bei offenen Frakturen oder Osteotomien, so werden meist selbst kleinste Lücken nicht knöchern ausgefüllt. Stehen alle Kräfte der Knochenheilung zur Verfügung, so kann z.B. bei einem jugendlichen Menschen eine schwer dislozierte Oberschenkelfraktur im Bereich der großen Muskelmassen mit gewaltiger Callusbildung zur knöchernen Heilung kommen. Nach Osteotomien kann (auch wieder nur beim Jugendlichen) nur durch langsame Zunahme der Distraktion (Verlängerung eines Knochens) die Überbrückungsfähigkeit des Defektes erhalten bleiben (Bier, 1923).

Bemerkenswert ist die besonders rasche Vereinigung von Fragmenten, die unter Verkürzung des Gliedes auch zwischen den Knochenabschnitten eintritt, welche eigentlich keine Wundfläche zeigen (Abb. 79).

η) Der mechanische Faktor

Über die Bedeutung der mechanischen Kräfte für das Granulationsgewebe, welches sich während der Frakturheilung in Callusgewebe ausdifferenziert, wurde ausführlich auf S. 545 berichtet. Hier soll von dem *Reizcallus* gesprochen werden, welcher durch mechanische Kräfte hervorgerufen wird. „Bei einer Fraktur ist die Menge des äußeren Callus proportional zu der Dislokation und der *dynamischen* Irritation" (PAUWELS, 1941). Bei mangelhafter Ruhigstellung der Fragmente bildet sich Reizcallus. Diese Beobachtung hat einstmals zum Behämmern der Bruchstelle geführt (THOMAS, 1882) oder zum Beklopfen des Knochens in Längsrichtung (MOMMSEN, 1929). Eine alte Erfahrung ist das „Festlaufen" einer Fraktur im Gehgips.

Es gibt aber in der Klinik nur wenige Beobachtungen, nach denen man sagen kann, die Form des Callus wäre sicher durch einen mechanischen Faktor bestimmt. Am Oberarm ist der Kugelcallus als typische Folge mangelnder Ruhigstellung beschrieben (Abb. 24).

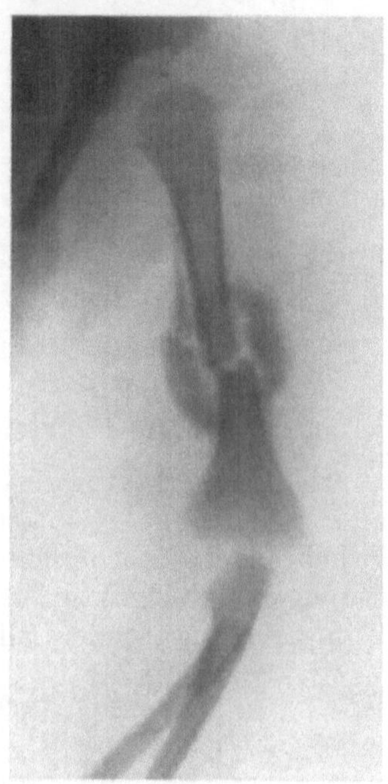

Abb. 24. Kugelcallus bei einer unvollkommen ruhiggestellten Oberarmfraktur eines ein Jahr alten Kindes fünf Wochen nach der Verletzung. (Quelle wie Abb. 7, S. 546)

Weit ausladende Calluskonsolen mit Fortsetzung der Bruchlinie im Callus sind ein sicheres Zeichen für mechanisch bedingten Reizcallus. Dann hängt es von dem Ausmaß der mechanischen Belastung und der Kraft zur Callusbildung ab, ob eine knöcherne Überbrückung oder eine Pseudarthrose resultiert.

Sehr gewagt ist es, aus Röntgenbildern der Klinik ablesen zu wollen, daß z.B. an der konkaven Seite einer Fraktur, also am Orte der Druckspannungen, sich Callus bildet, während an der konvexen Seite, dem Ort der Zugspannungen, sich Callusbildung spärlich oder gar nicht einstellt. Bereits LEXER (1919) wies darauf hin, daß die Callusvermehrung auf der konkaven Seite „periostbedingt" sei. Dann kann das Fehlen des Callus auf der konvexen Seite durch „Raumnot" (OBERDALHOFF, 1949) bedingt sein, weil hier die Weichgewebe dem Knochen fest aufliegen. Wir wollen mit diesen Erläuterungen nur zum Ausdruck bringen, daß die Bilder der Klinik zur Klärung der Frage der Bedeutung des mechanischen „Aufbaufaktors" nicht beitragen können, verweisen aber nochmals auf die experimentellen Untersuchungen (S. 545—549).

ϑ) Die Mitverletzung von Weichgeweben

Die Mitverletzung der Weichgewebe kann weniger für die Art des Callus als vielmehr für seine Form und Menge eine Rolle spielen. Bei der *offenen Fraktur* fließt die Masse des Bruchhämatoms ab. Es ist immer wieder verblüffend, wie gering die Callusbildung auch dann bei einer offenen Fraktur sein kann, wenn es durch die chirurgische Behandlung gelungen ist, aus einer „offenen" eine „geschlossene" Fraktur mit primärer Wundheilung zu machen (siehe auch S. 543 und Abb. 6).

Der Schußbruch mit seinen auf der Ausschußseite meist ausgedehnten Weichteilzerreißungen ist in der Callusbildung natürlich weitgehend davon abhängig, ob der Verletzung eine Wundeiterung folgt. Ausgedehnte Splitterung schafft mit ihren vielen Knochenwundflächen ein starkes Frakturmilieu, welches zur kräftigen Callusbildung Anlaß geben kann, wenn diese nicht durch die bekannten Nachteile der weit offenen Fraktur aufgehoben werden.

Stärkere *Muskelzerreißungen* verursachen ausgedehnte Granulationsbildungen, welche unter dem Einfluß der Frakturnähe zu vielgestaltiger und übermäßiger Callusbildung ausdifferenzieren können.

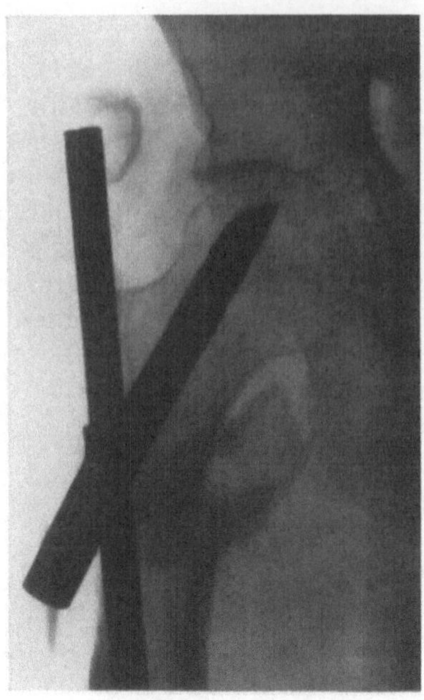

ι) Das Callushütchen

Eine besondere Form der Callusbildung stellt das sogenannte *Callushütchen* dar, welches sich am oberen Ende eines Marknagels besonders am Oberschenkel entwickelt (Abb. 25). Teleologisch gedacht ist seine Entwicklung als Bemühung des Knochens verständlich, seinen Markraum wieder abzuschließen. Bei seiner Entstehung spielen wahrscheinlich zwei Faktoren eine entscheidende Rolle, einmal die chronische Traumatisierung der Muskulatur durch das Nagelkopfende, und zum anderen der Ausfluß von Markgewebe mit kleinsten Knochenpartikeln durch die Nagelrinne nach der Operation.

Abb. 25. Callushütchen auf dem Nagelkopfende. Y-Nagelung einer pertrochanteren Fraktur eines 35jährigen Patienten ein Jahr nach der Versorgung

6. Die Beurteilung der knöchernen Verfestigung eines Bruches

Heilt eine Fraktur über den Callus — und bis heute tut dieses ohne Zweifel die Mehrzahl aller Frakturen — so ist die röntgenologische Beurteilung der „Verfestigung" eines Bruches, der „knöchernen Vereinigung", von Form und Struktur des Callus abhängig. Zielstrebiger, wohlstrukturierter Callus gestattet das Urteil der „ausreichenden Verfestigung", wabiger, luxurierender Callus legt den Verdacht auf eine Calluserkrankung nahe (siehe dort).

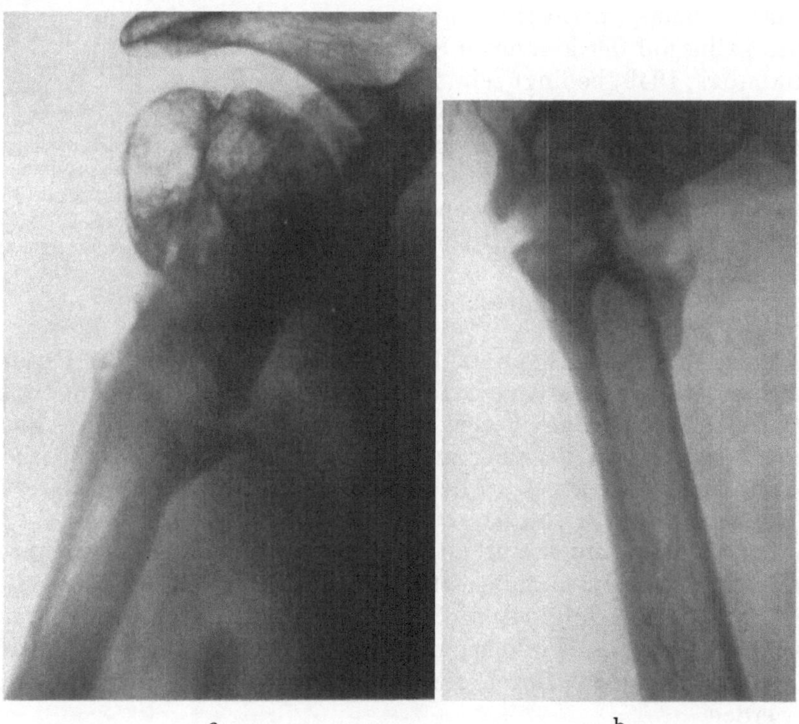

Abb. 26. Eine kopfnahe geschlossene Humerusfraktur bei einer 54jährigen Patientin wurde mit Drahtnaht versorgt, infizierte sich und führte zur schmerzhaften Pseudarthrose (a), deren Spalt allein durch gezielte Aufnahmen (b) zwei Jahre nach der Verletzung nachgewiesen wurde (siehe auch S. 671 Abb. 47)

Es besteht aber kein Zweifel, daß vom röntgenologischen Standpunkt aus eine Fraktur erst dann als zuverlässig knöchern geheilt und belastungsfähig angesprochen werden darf, wenn die Röntgenbilder eine knöcherne *Durchkonstruktion* im Bruchspalt zeigen. Durchlaufende Bälkchenstruktur bei ausreichender Kalkdichte im ganzen Frakturbereich sind bei Aufnahmen in zwei Ebenen der Beweis der knöchernen Heilung. Ist das Frakturgebiet im

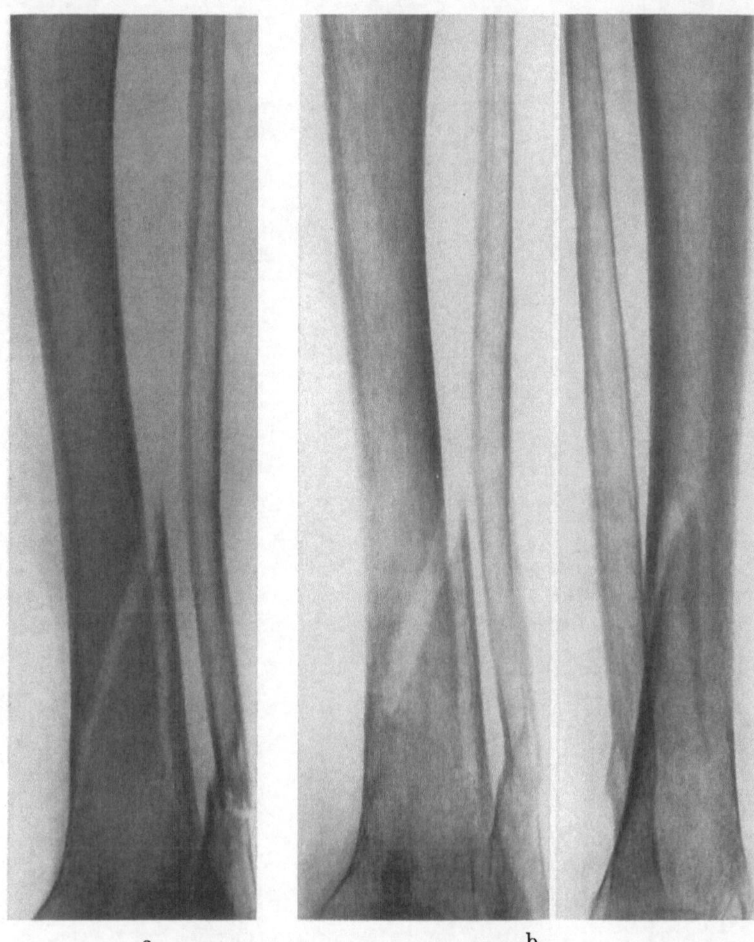

Abb. 27a u. b. Geschlossener Tibiaschrägbruch bei 65jähriger Patientin. a Die frische Fraktur, b vierzehn Wochen später ist die Fraktur klinisch belastungsfähig fest, während im sichtbaren Bruchspalt Callus nicht zu erkennen ist. Starke Kalkabwanderung

ganzen sklerotisch-kalkverdichtet, so können weitere Aufnahmen in schrägen Durchmessern, eventuell gezielte Aufnahmen und Schichtaufnahmen erforderlich sein (Abb. 26 und 59), um eine Zone mangelnder Knochenneubildung oder gar eine Pseudarthrose aufzudecken oder auszuschließen. *Klinisch* ist in solchen Fällen der vom Patienten geklagte Schmerz eine wertvolle Hilfe. Oft gesellt sich — vorwiegend am Unterschenkel — eine Anschwellung hinzu. Schmerz bei Belastung und lokale Anschwellung nach Belastung sind nahezu ein Beweis für eine noch nicht ausreichende Konsolidierung einer Fraktur.

Läßt der Callus in seiner Struktur, Form und Menge recht gute Schlüsse über die Heilung eines Knochenbruches zu, so soll dieser Callus bei der primären Knochenheilung (siehe S. 543) völlig fehlen. Damit kann röntgenologisch das Urteil der „knöchernen Heilung“ erst dann abgegeben werden, wenn der feine Bruchspalt völlig verschwunden und die Knochenstruktur wieder in ihrer alten Form aufgebaut ist.

Dieses alles weist darauf hin, daß der Termin der Belastbarkeit einer heilenden Fraktur niemals allein vom Röntgenbefund abhängig gemacht werden kann. Die seit der Verletzung verstrichene Zeit, die Art der Behandlung, der klinische Befund und die Reaktion auf erste aktive Leistungen des Gliedes sind wertvollste Hinweise. Grobe pathologische Beweglichkeit sei nicht erwähnt, aber leichtes Federn im Bruchspalt, Fehlen dieses Federns bei doch deutlicher Schmerzhaftigkeit und dieses alles eventuell in Nähe eines

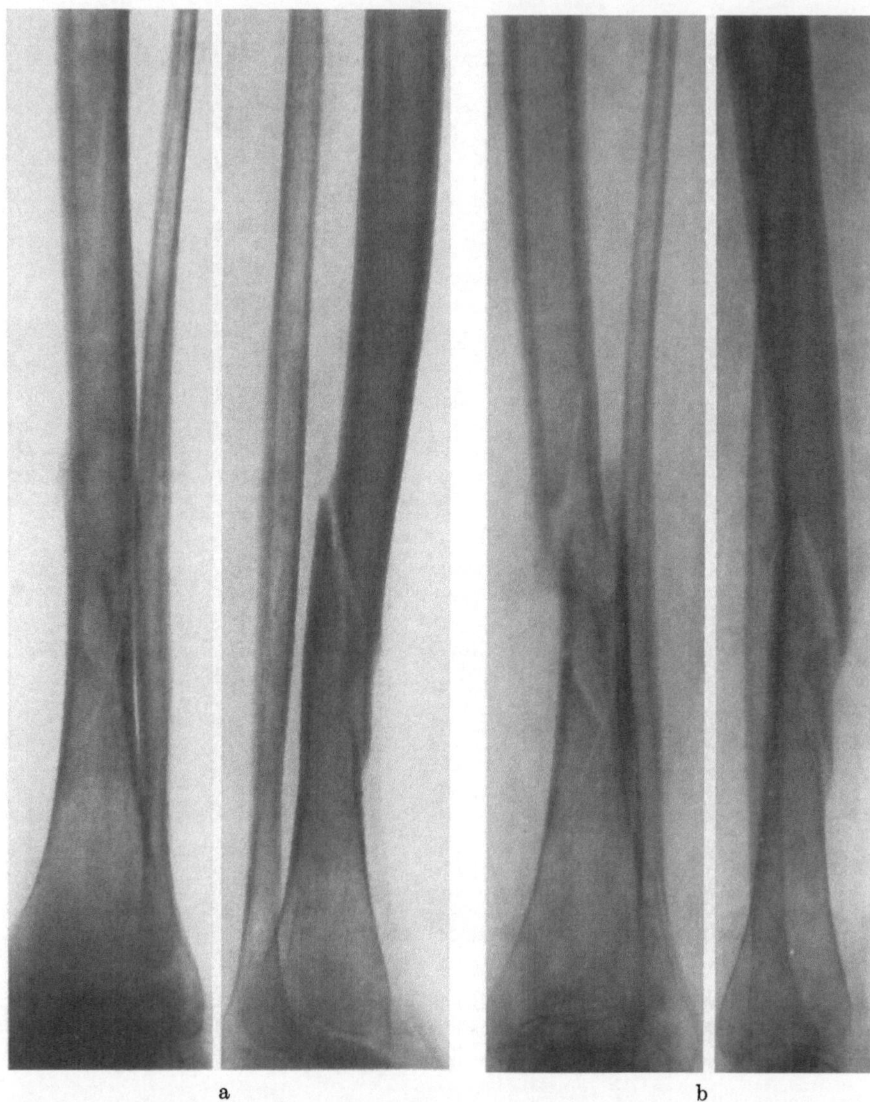

Abb. 28a u. b. Schwer zu beurteilende Tragfähigkeit im atrophischen Knochen einer 52jährigen Patientin mit Kinderlähmung. a Das Bild der Fraktur zweiundzwanzig Wochen nach der Verletzung. Klinisch und röntgenologisch durfte eine ausreichende Verfestigung angenommen werden, so daß vorsichtige Gehbelastung angezeigt erschien. b Refraktur eine Woche nach Belastung

größeren Gelenks können die Beurteilung auch im klinischen Sinne außerordentlich schwierig gestalten.

Ein völliges Versagen der röntgenologischen Untersuchung beobachten wir bei manchen langen Schrägbrüchen der Tibia, welche nach sechs oder mehr Wochen klinisch fest und belastungsfähig sind, während die Röntgenbilder im Vergleich zu den primären Bildern (ausgenommen die Kalkabwanderung) praktisch unverändert erscheinen (Abb. 27).

Besonders schwierig kann die Beurteilung im pathologisch veränderten Knochen sein (Abb. 28). Der funktionelle Reiz leichter Belastung ist für den weiteren Durchbau einer Fraktur erforderlich, der ohnehin aber mangelhaft tragfähige Knochen kann bei der versuchsweisen Belastung zur Lösung im alten Bruchspalt mit Neubruch im kranken Knochen führen.

Besondere Verhältnisse liegen dann vor, wenn die knöcherne Heilung und auch die Callusform derartig sind, daß selbst ein tragfähiger neuer Knochen im Ermüdungsbruch neu frakturiert (siehe Refraktur). Dem Patienten wird auch dieses Ereignis als das Resultat einer zu frühen Belastung erscheinen.

II. Die gestörte Knochenbruchheilung

1. Störfaktoren in der Heilung

a) Verlust des Bruchhämatoms

Mit dem Verlust des Bruchhämatoms geht ein großer Teil der Reservekräfte, welche dem Körper in der Frakturheilung zur Verfügung stehen, verloren. Es fehlt die primäre fibrinöse Verspannung, also die erste mechanische Verbindung, welche auch größere Lücken zwischen den Fragmenten primär überbrückt. Ohne Nachteil ist der Verlust des Hämatoms nur dann, wenn die Fragmente durch eine stabile Form der Osteosynthese oder bei zuverlässiger Einkeilung fest miteinander verbunden sind. Die häufig außerordentlich spärliche Callusbildung bei offenen Frakturen, welche primär gut versorgt zur geschlossenen Fraktur gemacht wurden, ist vor allem auf den Verlust des Bruchhämatoms zurückzuführen.

Kommuniziert eine Fraktur mit einer Gelenkhöhle, wie dieses bei jeder intraarticulären Fraktur, deren Fragmente nicht unverrückbar und fest miteinander verbunden sind, der Fall ist, so fehlt auch hier der geronnene Blutkuchen mit den dieser Tatsache anhaftenden Nachteilen.

b) Knochennekrosen im Frakturbereich

Während die schmalen Säume nekrotischen Knochengewebes an den Enden der Fragmente sich eher vorteilhaft für die Frakturheilung auswirken, da die lebenden Weichgewebe das tote Material zur Knochenneubildung auf dem Wege des schleichenden Ersatzes nutzen, ist die ausgedehntere Nekrose eines Fragments stets von Nachteil für die Frakturheilung. Als klassische Beispiele seien der Hüftkopf bei subcapitaler Schenkelhalsfraktur und das zentrale Fragment bei der Fraktur des Os scaphoideum genannt. Es dürfte bei letztgenanntem Knochen allerdings sehr selten eine echte Nekrose vorliegen, vielmehr nur eine vorübergehende erhebliche Mangeldurchblutung, denn die Erfahrung hat gelehrt, daß die Frakturen dieses Handwurzelknochens bei sachgemäßer Ruhigstellung praktisch alle nach acht bis zehn Wochen knöchern geheilt sind. Abb. 29 zeigt ein Beispiel der starken Kalkabwanderung im Handskelet bei relativer Dichte des einen Fragments.

Auch am Hüftkopf sind die Verhältnisse noch nicht vollständig geklärt. Sind bei einer intraarticulär gelegenen subcapitalen Fraktur in der Capsula reflexa, welche dem Knochen aufliegt, alle Arterien unterbrochen, so muß der Kopf einem autologen Transplantat vergleichbar (W. Axhausen, 1952) sein, denn die über das Ligamentum teres gehende Blutversorgung ist im höheren Alter entweder völlig unterbrochen oder vermag nur den engsten Nachbarbezirk der Fovea am Leben zu erhalten. In diesem Fall hängt das Schicksal des Kopfes vom Anschluß an das Schenkelhalsfragment ab. Finden die Capillaren ähnlich wie beim Transplantat raschen Anschluß, dann überleben die Markgewebe, während die Knochenhartsubstanz abstirbt, dann aber vom Markgewebe auf dem Wege der schleichenden Substitution durch lebenden Knochen ersetzt wird. Im Röntgenbild erkennen wir dann im Kopf kleine Aufhellungsherde als Zeichen des Umbaus, also des Lebens (Abb. 30).

Findet der capilläre Anschluß aber nicht statt, so sterben *alle* Teile des Kopfes vollständig ab, also auch das Markgewebe, und es muß dann eine Vitalisierung vom Schenkelhalsfragment aus stattfinden. In diesem Fall *heilt die Fraktur nur mit den Kräften* des einen Fragments. Bei ausreichender Ruhigstellung der Fragmente ist auch dann die knöcherne Heilung die Regel, das Schicksal des Kopfes aber hängt von den von der Fraktur

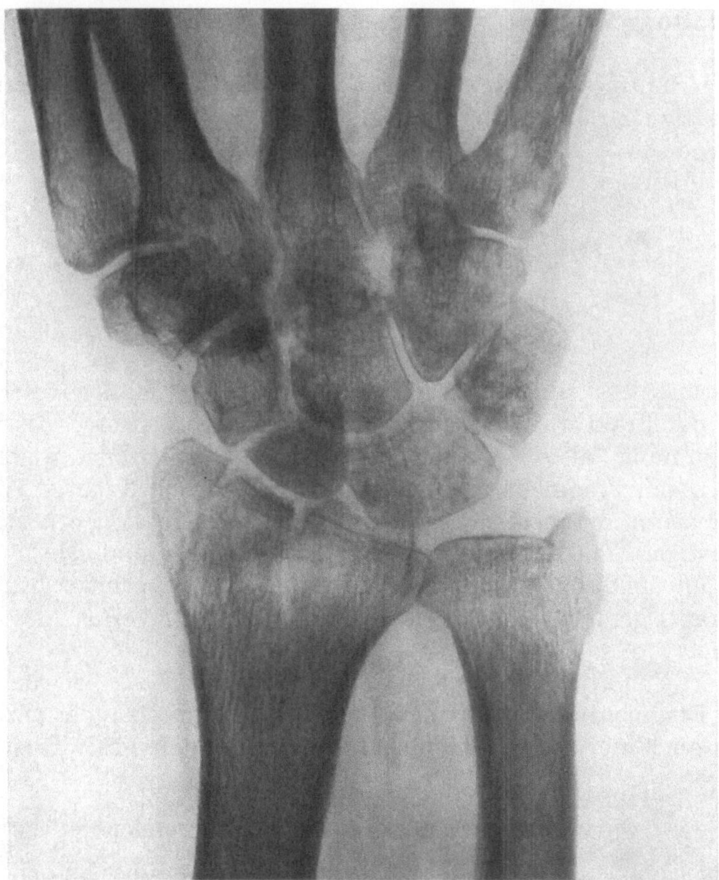

Abb. 29. Vorgetäuschte Nekrose im mangelhaft durchbluteten Fragment einer Kahnbeinfraktur bei 48jährigem Patienten zwölf Wochen nach der Verletzung

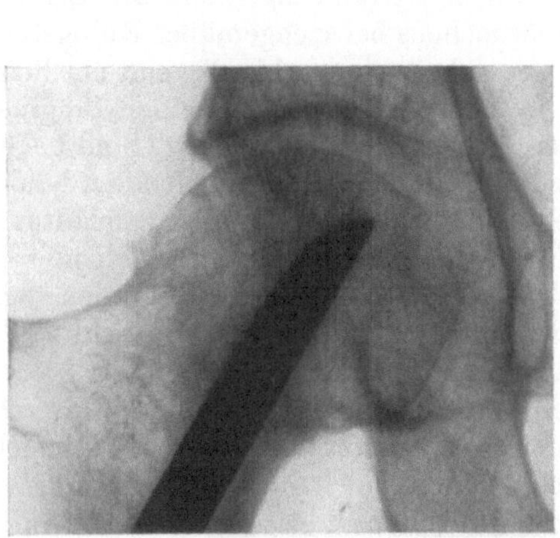

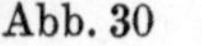

Abb. 30

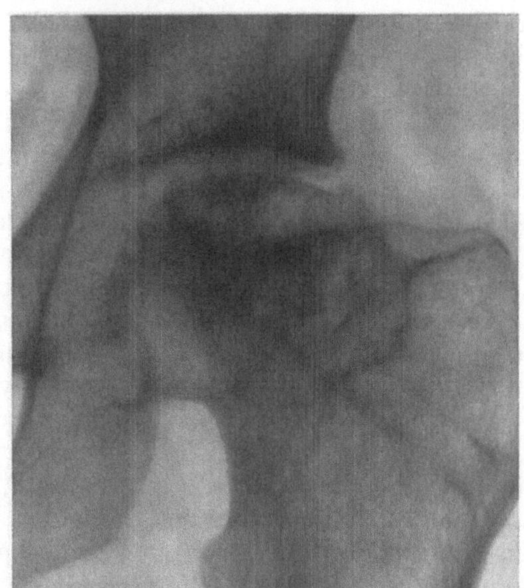

Abb. 31

Abb. 30. Kleine Aufhellungsherde im Hüftkopf einer 50jährigen Patientin drei Monate nach subcapitaler Fraktur sind ein Zeichen der Vitalität des Kopffragments

Abb. 31. Teilnekrose des Hüftkopfes an typischer Stelle nach subcapitaler Fraktur bei einer 66jährigen Patientin eineinhalb Jahre nach der Verletzung

vordringenden Weichgeweben ab. Wandelt sich das einsprossende zellreiche Gewebe in Markgewebe, so wird auch das Knochengerüst des Kopfes durch lebenden Knochen substituiert. In der Mehrzahl der Fälle aber erschöpft sich die Regenerations- und Differenzierungskraft, das vordringende fibröse Gewebe differenziert sich zu Bindegewebe aus, und es setzt in dieser Grenzzone eine bindegewebige Resorption der Bälkchen ein. Unter der mechanischen Belastung sinkt dann der noch nicht vitalisierte Teil des Kopfes unter Nachgeben der Grenzzone in den Kopf hinein. Das ist das typische Bild der Teilnekrose (Abb. 31), welche meist im Verlaufe des zweiten Jahres nach der Fraktur auftritt. Als spätester Termin wurden sieben Jahre beobachtet (SALEM, 1951).

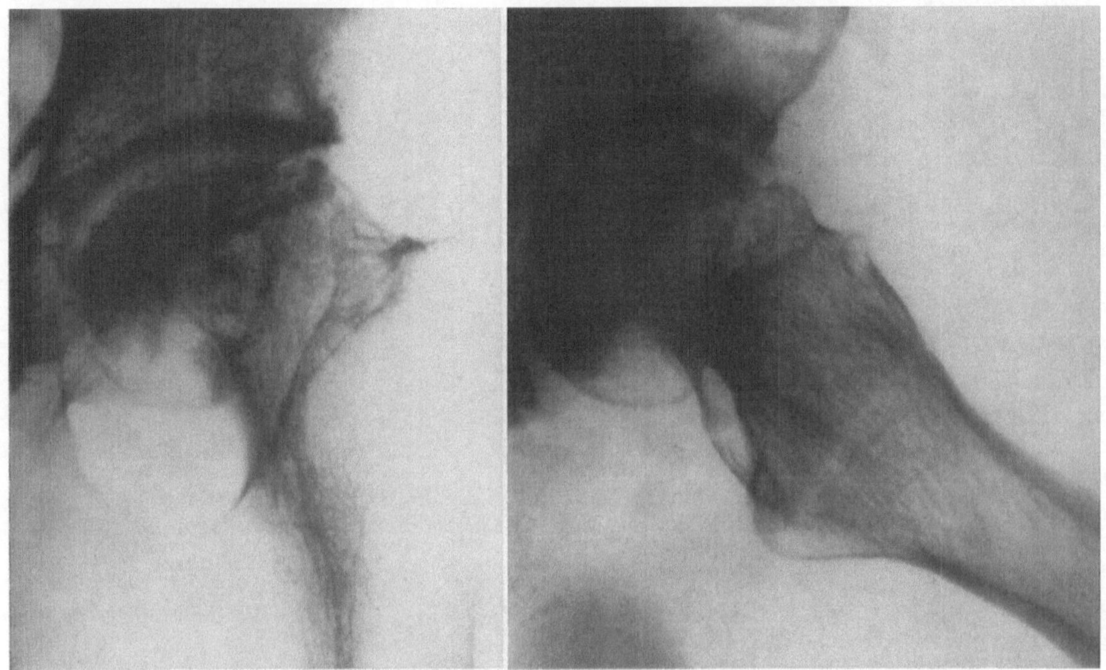

Abb. 32. Totalnekrose des Hüftkopfes bei 44jährigem Mann zwei Jahre nach subcapitaler Fraktur im Krampfanfall

Bricht nach erfolgter Frakturheilung der Kopf in seiner Gesamtheit zusammen, os handelt es sich um eine Totalnekrose des Kopfes nach subcapitaler Fraktur (Abb. 32).

Bei ungewöhnlich gelagerter Grenzzone, also dann, wenn die Vitalisierung sehr früh gestoppt wird, kann eine Pseudarthrose cranialwärts der alten Fraktur entstehen (Abb. 33). Liegen in diesen Fällen die alten Bilder nicht vor, so wird man das Ungewöhnliche der Entstehung der Pseudarthrose nicht vermuten, geschweige denn beweisen können, wird vielmehr glauben, daß die Fraktur im Bereich der Pseudarthrose vorgelegen habe.

Jeder Hüftkopf, welcher nach der Fraktur im medialen Teil des Schenkelhalses nach Monaten sehr klare und völlig ungestörte Bälkchenstruktur zeigt und dabei im Vergleich zum umgebenden Skelet kalkreicher ist, muß den dringenden Verdacht auf Nekrose des Kopfes erwecken (Abb. 34).

Sicherheit über das Schicksal des Kopfes kann das Röntgenbild während der ersten Wochen nach der Fraktur natürlich nicht geben. Aber auch nach Monaten oder sogar Jahren kann die Beurteilung durch den Röntgenologen sehr unsicher sein. Das zeigt als Beispiel das Röntgenbild der Abb. 35. Die Umbauvorgänge müssen vorgetäuscht sein, denn die feingewebliche Untersuchung des exstirpierten Kopfes ergab totale Nekrose aller Gewebe in allen Bezirken. Heilt eine subcapitale Fraktur pseudarthrotisch und zeigt der Hüftkopf nach Jahren eine zarte und sehr klare Bälkchenstruktur, so dürfen wir aus diesem Befund nicht auf eine Nekrose schließen. Der Kopf kann nekrotisch gewesen sein und wurde

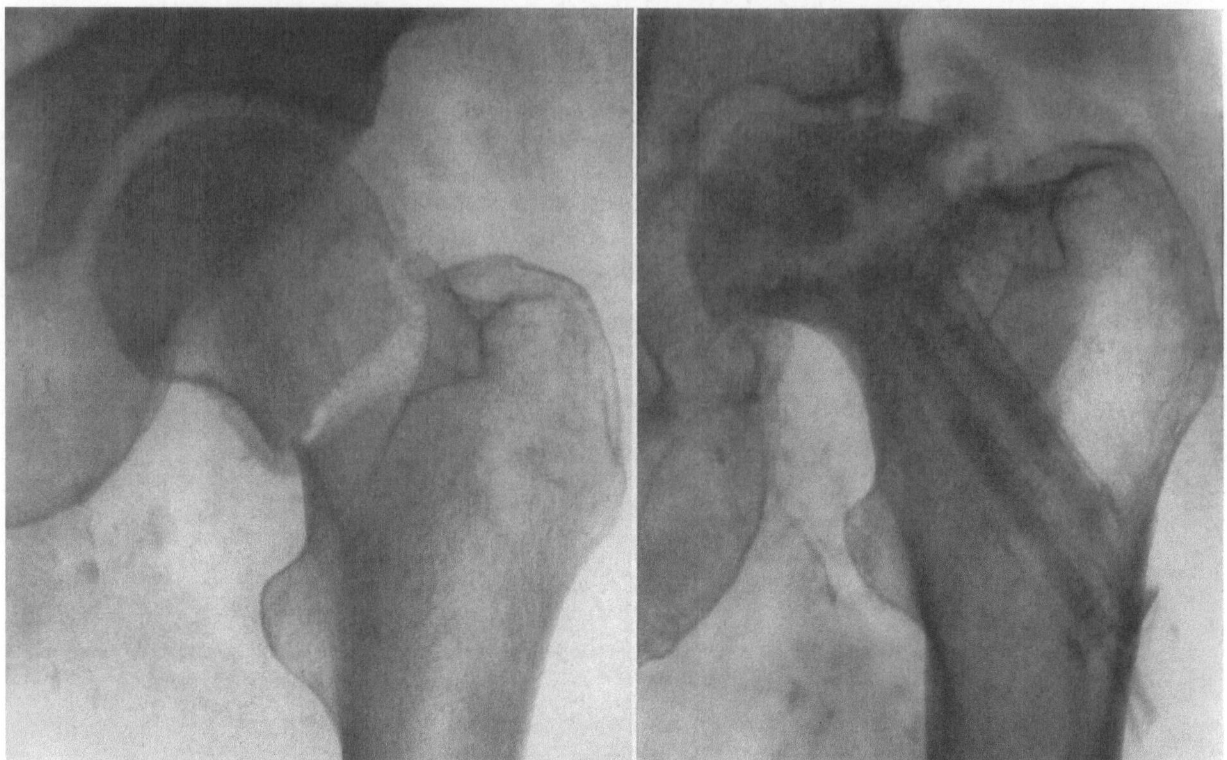

Abb. 33. Pseudarthrose cranial der basisnahen Schenkelhalsfraktur drei Jahre nach der Verletzung bei 72jähriger Frau. Die Fraktur wurde mit Nagel und Span versorgt

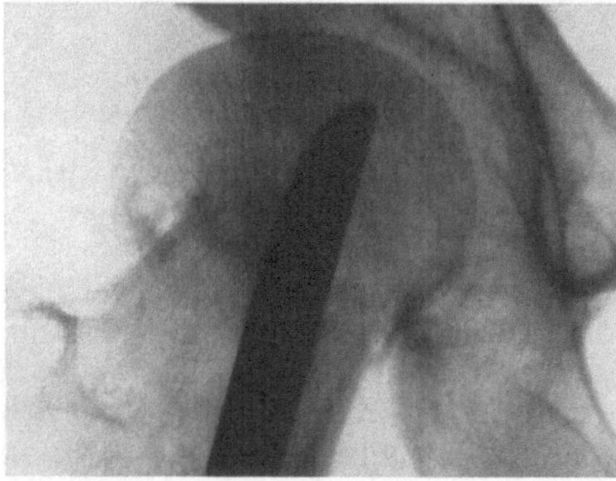

Abb. 34. Der Verdacht auf totale Kopfnekrose nach subcapitaler Fraktur bei 40jähriger Frau siebeneinhalb Monate nach Unfall und Nagelung wurde mittels Rohrstanze durch den ganzen Durchmesser des Kopfes feingeweblich bestätigt. Die Fraktur ist knöchern fest und die Patientin geht beschwerdefrei

vitalisiert. Der Körper hat bei fehlender mechanischer Belastung des Kopfes über Jahre für diesen Vorgang Zeit. Es ist jedenfalls charakteristisch, daß wir viele Jahre nach erfolgter Fraktur und pseudarthrotischer Heilung niemals totes Gewebe im Kopf, weder tote Knochensubstanz noch totes Markgewebe finden, ein Befund, der einige Monate nach der Fraktur mindestens in einigen Bezirken stets vorhanden ist.

Toter körpereigener Knochen wird unter aseptischen Bedingungen im Frakturmilieu stets in das Callusgewebe eingebaut. Er wird dabei durch lebenden Knochen ersetzt, oder er wird resorbiert, wo Callus nicht gebildet wird. Unter aseptischen Verhältnissen sind nekrotische Teile nur daran zu erkennen, daß sie länger als die Umgebung z.B. ihren corticalen, kalkreichen Charakter zeigen (Abb. 36).

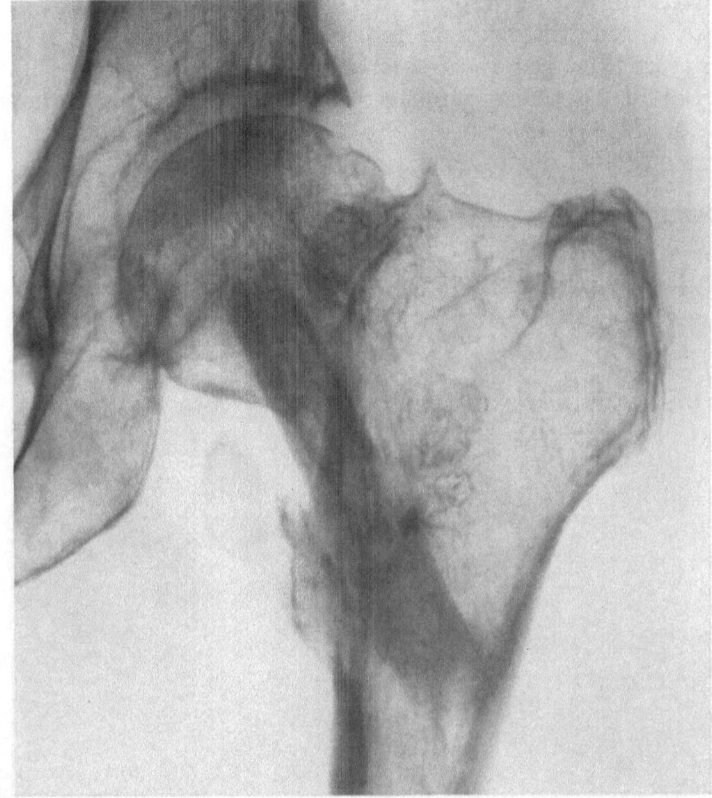

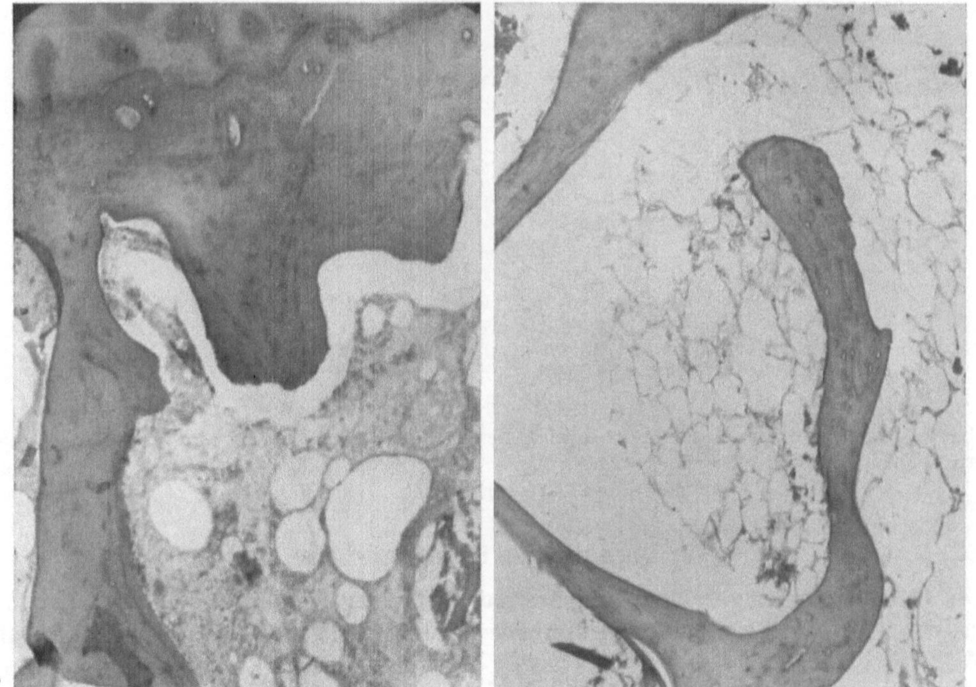

Abb. 35a—c. Die Entscheidung über Vitalität oder Nekrose kann am Hüftkopf auch nach eineinhalb Jahren sehr schwer oder unmöglich sein. 55jährige Patientin. Pseudarthrose nach Nagelung und fehlerhaft hinter dem Kopf liegendem Knochenspan (a). Die feingewebliche Untersuchung ergab unter lebendem Knorpel kräftige Spongiosabalken (b), im Zentrum des Kopfes sehr zarte Bälkchen (c). Sowohl das Knochengerüst als auch das Markgewebe sind im ganzen Kopf tot

Scharfe Grenzen eines toten Knochenteils sind typisch für septische Verhältnisse im Frakturbereich. Ein vom Eiter umspülter ,,Sequester“ zeigt bei großer Dichte typisch scharfe Grenzen (Abb. 37). Der Eiter vermag den Sequester nicht aufzulösen. Füllt sich später aber das Bett des Sequesters mit Granulationen, so vermögen diese sehr wohl den toten Knochen ,,bindegewebig resorbierend“ anzunagen oder vollständig zu resorbieren. Charakteristisch sind dabei die angenagten Ränder des Sequesters.

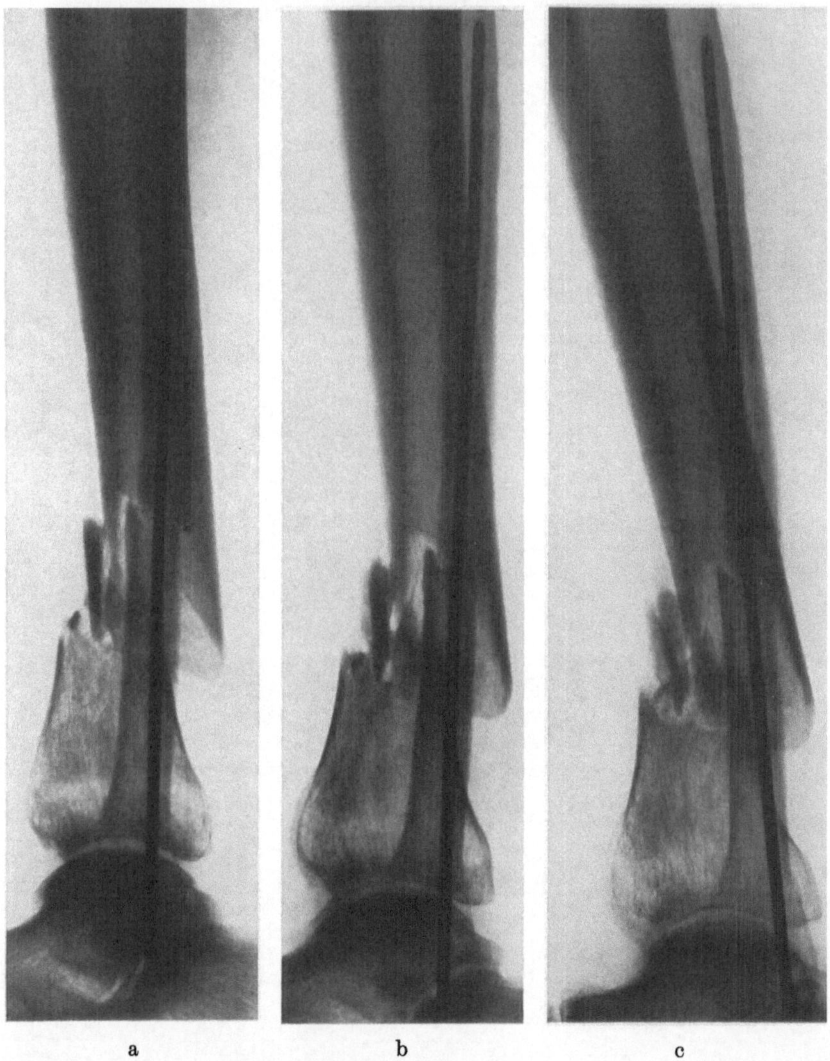

Abb. 36a—c. Einbau eines isolierten Corticalisfragments in den Callus einer geschlossenen Fraktur bei einem 66jährigen Mann. a Sechs Wochen nach der Fraktur. b Vier Wochen später. c Weitere zwei Wochen später (nur die Fibula wurde primär mit Rush Pin versorgt)

c) Die Infektion im Frakturbereich

Die Infektion einer geschlossenen Fraktur auf hämatogenem Wege ist äußerst selten (FLEMMING, 1934 u.a.). In der Regel entsteht eine solche Infektion durch Kontakt mit der Außenwelt, also bei offenen Frakturen oder durch operative, offene Versorgung einer Fraktur. Darum sprechen wir im Gegensatz zur hämatogenen Osteomyelitis von der *exogenen Osteomyelitis.* Zwar bedeutet eine Vereiterung der Wunde noch nicht in jedem Fall eine Eiterung am Knochen. Weil aber im Frakturbereich stets Knochengewebe in mehr oder minder großer Ausdehnung nekrotisch ist, greift die Infektion meist auch auf den Knochen über. Dann handelt es sich pathologisch-anatomisch praktisch stets um eine

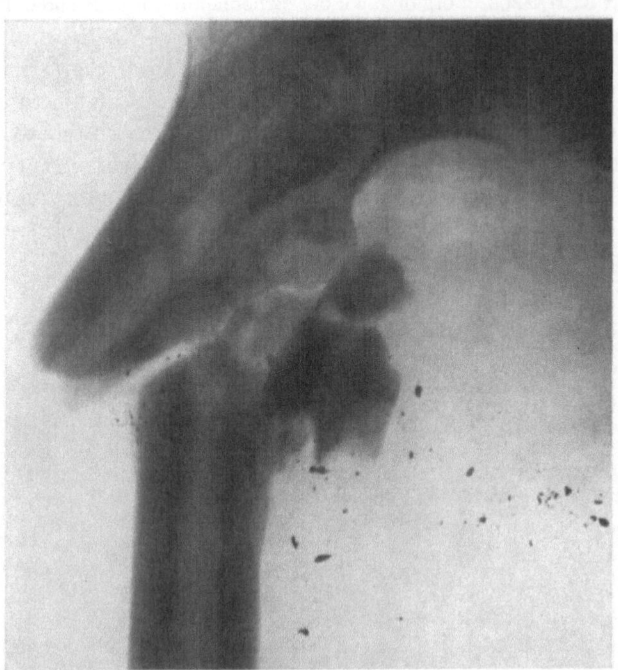

Abb. 37. Großer Sequester in eiterndem Oberschenkelschußbruch bei 22jährigem Mann

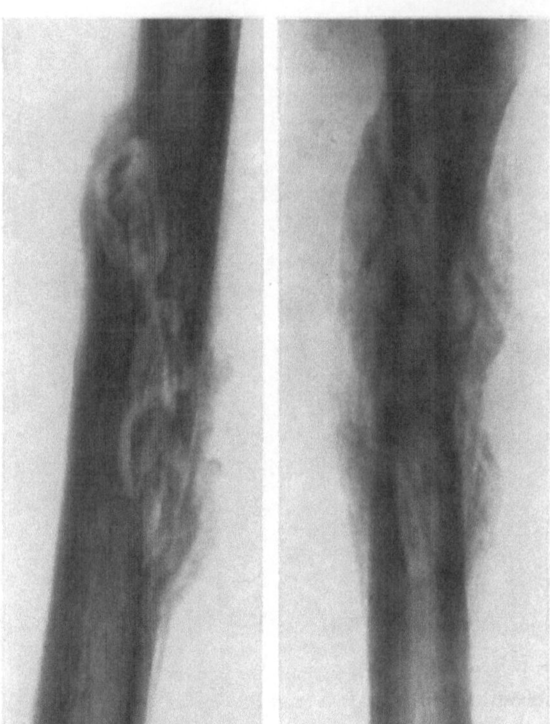

Abb. 38. Umschriebene Osteomyelitis im Bereich einer offenen Schrägfraktur des Humerus bei einem 19jährigen Mann vier Monate nach dem Unfall. Lebhafte Callusbildung, kleiner Sequester

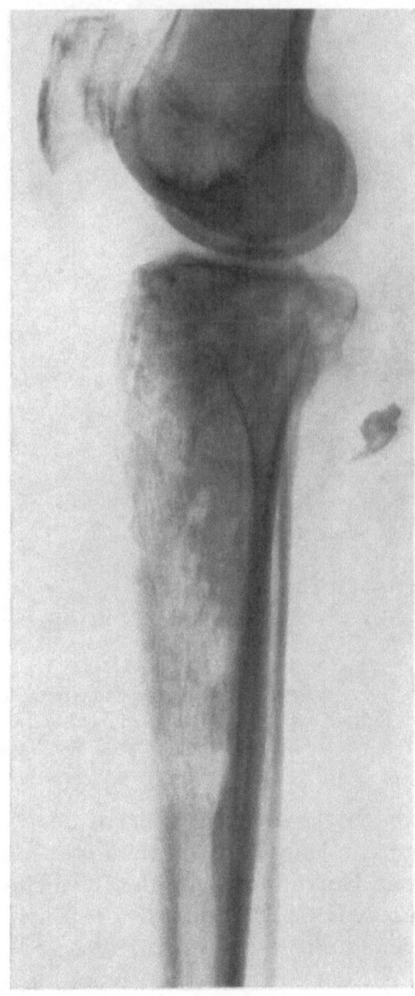

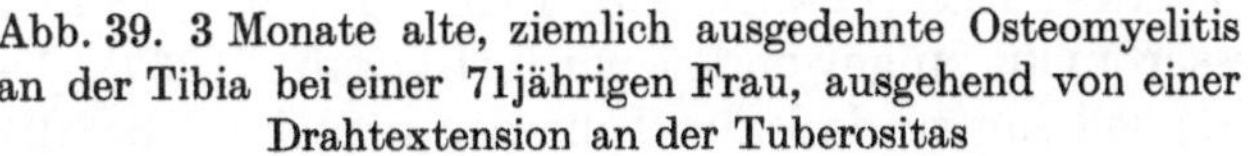

Abb. 39. 3 Monate alte, ziemlich ausgedehnte Osteomyelitis an der Tibia bei einer 71jährigen Frau, ausgehend von einer Drahtextension an der Tuberositas

Osteomyelitis, denn Markgewebe und Knochen und auch das Periost sind an der Entzündung beteiligt. Über die Nomenklatur herrscht keine vollkommene Einigkeit. Gut und klar ist sicher die Unterscheidung der hämatogenen von der exogenen Osteomyelitis. Von „traumatischer Osteomyelitis" (WITT, 1952) zu sprechen, wäre sicher irreführend, wenn nicht eine hämatogene gemeint ist, welche nach stumpfem, schweren Trauma

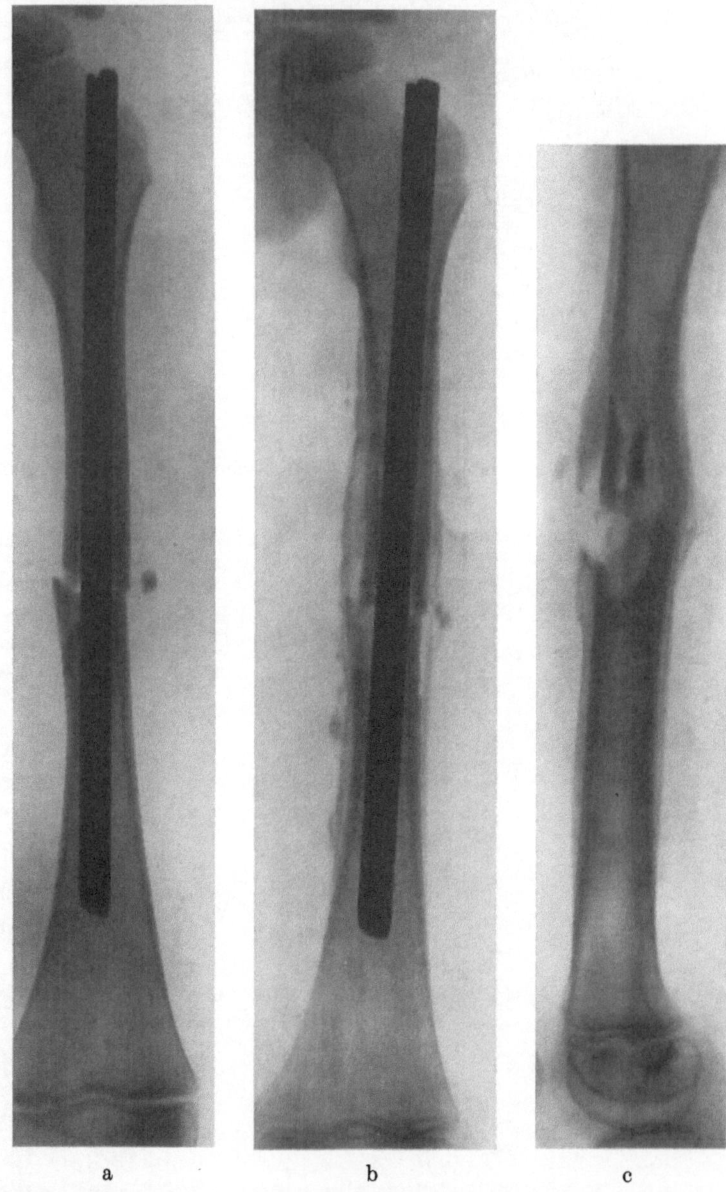

Abb. 40a—c. Das Bild der typischen juvenilen Osteomyelitis mit Totenlade und Sequester nach Marknagelung einer Femurfraktur bei 5jährigem Knaben. a Frisch nach der Nagelung (1946), b vier Wochen danach, c 6 Monate später. Die Fraktur ist geheilt und der Nagel ist entfernt. Der Ringsequester wurde später herausgenommen

beobachtet wird. Der Begriff der „Ostitis" müßte nach der sonst üblichen Nomenklatur der pathologischen Anatomie für eine Entzündung nur des Knochens reserviert sein. Eine solche Entzündung um das Weichgewebe in den Havers'schen Kanälen kommt wohl aber kaum vor (M. B. SCHMIDT, 1897; KAUFMANN, 1922; TENDELOO, 1925 u.a.), so daß diese Bezeichnung falsch sein muß und besser nicht angewendet wird (LAUCHE, 1937). Der Begriff der „Panostitis" (KOCHER, 1907) soll sagen, daß alle Teile des Knochens befallen sind. Das ist aber bei der Osteomyelitis sicher ohnehin der Fall, denn die Beteiligung des Periostes in Form einer Periostitis ist die Regel.

Der Knochen hat auf eine Infektion nur wenige Reaktionen zur Verfügung (LAUCHE, 1937). Die Ausdehnung der Entzündung aber bestimmt bei der exogenen Osteomyelitis weitgehend das klinische Bild. So ist es sicher berechtigt, von einer „lokalen Osteomyelitis" zu sprechen, wenn sich die entzündlichen Veränderungen des Knochens auf das Frakturgebiet beschränken (Abb. 38) oder, vom Infektionsherd ausgerechnet, nur eine umschriebene Ausdehnung zeigen (Abb. 39). Als „ausgedehnte Osteomyelitis" wird man stets die Entzündungen bezeichnen, welche die ganze Diaphyse des Röhrenknochens

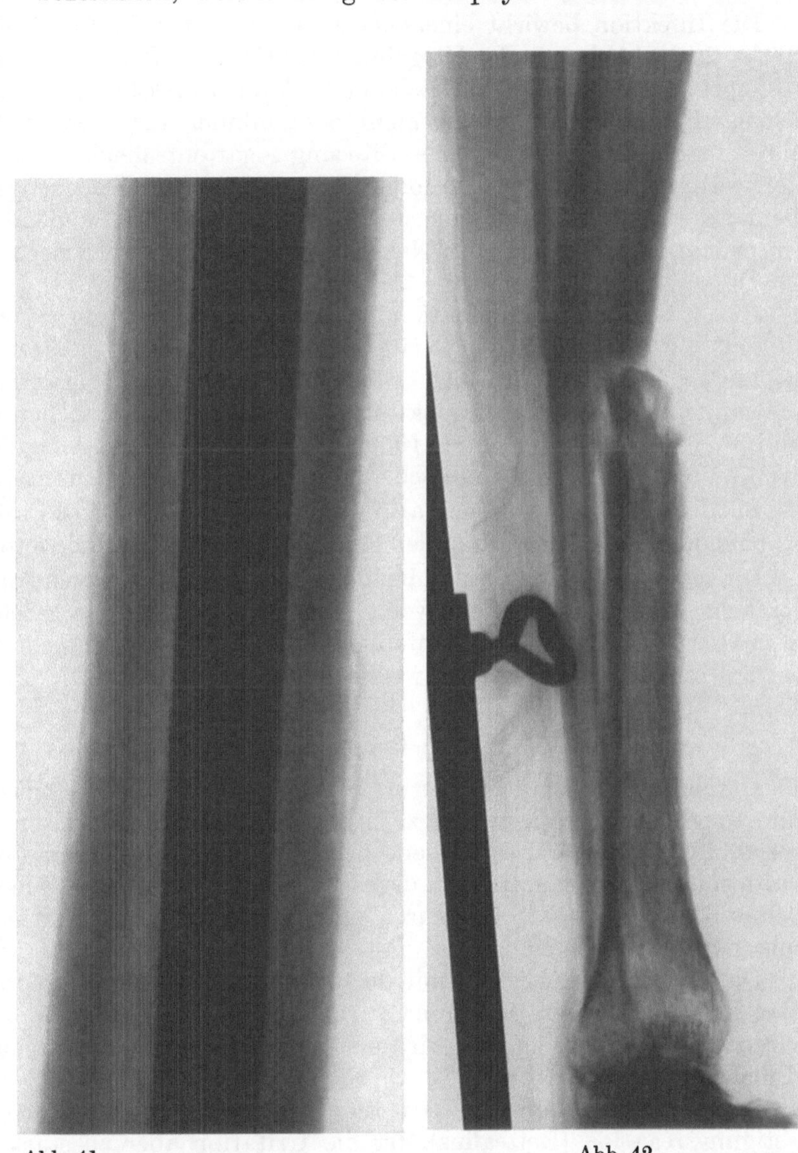

Abb. 41 Abb. 42

Abb. 41. Ausgedehnte Osteomyelitis bei 51jährigem Mann sieben Monate nach offener Nagelung einer geschlossenen Oberschenkelfraktur. Die Längsauffaserung der Corticalis und die zarte periostale Knochenneubildung sind im Kontaktausschnitt 14 cm cranial der Fraktur gut zu erkennen. Knöcherne Heilung, kein Sequester. Fistelschluß nach Nagelentfernung

Abb. 42. Kronensequester an der Tibia in offener, eiternder Fraktur eines 24 Jahre alten Mannes vier Monate nach der Verletzung

befallen. Die sich dann ergebenden Bilder entsprechen durchaus denen der „hämatogenen Ostoemyelitis", wobei das Ausmaß der Sequesterbildung und der periostalen Knochenneubildung (Totenlade) wie bei dieser weitgehend vom Alter des Patienten abhängen. Es ist sicher kein Zufall, daß diese Formen der ausgedehnten Osteomyelitis (Abb. 40 und 41) vorwiegend nach Marknagelungen beobachtet werden, weil der Nagel die Ausbreitung einer einmal eingetretenen Eiterung über den ganzen Markraum begünstigt. Es ist aber durchaus möglich, daß eine Markphlegmone nicht auf den Knochen, die sekundären Markräume und das Periost übergreift, sondern auf den Markraum beschränkt bleibt. Das ist die Form der Entzündung am Röhrenknochen, welche wohl allein durch den Marknagel oder den Rush pin hervorgerufen werden kann, und welche zweckmäßig als „Markraumeiterung" bezeichnet werden sollte.

Die Infektion bewirkt einerseits eine Anregung der Callusbildung, andererseits verstärkt sie den Abbau in der Umgebung der Fraktur. Resorption und Neubauvorgänge sind gesteigert (LAUCHE, 1937). Gravierend ist die Entstehung von Sequestern, wobei wahrscheinlich primär bereits eine mehr oder minder ausgedehnte Nekrose vorhanden war, durch welche das Angehen einer Eiterung sogar entscheidend begünstigt wird. Die Infektion verhindert dann den Ein- oder Umbau des toten Knochengewebes. Eine langwierige Demarkierung führt zum Sequester (Abb. 40 u. 42). Selbstredend kann die Eiterung auch am primär lebenden Knochen Nekrosen und damit Sequestrierung verursachen (LAUCHE, 1937).

Die Häufigkeit der Infektion nach offenen Frakturen oder operativer Frakturversorgung hängt natürlich von Keimen und Abwehrlage, primärer und operativer Gewebeschädigung und der Form der Osteosynthese ab. Nach HAEBLER und KARITZKY (1953) schwanken die Zahlen der Infektion nach aseptischen Knochenoperationen zwischen 1,5 und 37%. M. LANGE berichtete 1958 aus dem eigenen Krankengut von 2%. BLUM fand bei 720 operativ versorgten Unterschenkel- und Knöchelfrakturen 14mal eine Osteomyelitis.

Bei der Versorgung offener, also wahrscheinlich infizierter Frakturen spielt die gewebeschonende stabile Versorgung der Fragmente ohne Frage die entscheidende Rolle.

Die Heilungsaussichten sind bei der offenen Fraktur, welche operativ zur geschlossenen gemacht werden konnte, ein wenig schlechter als die der geschlossenen Fraktur (siehe S. 591). Die Zeit der Arbeitsunfähigkeit bei Frakturen mit exogener Osteomyelitis aber beträgt im Durchschnitt etwa zwei Jahre (K. H. BAUER, 1927; MITTELMEIER, 1965 u. v. a.).

d) Der mechanische Störfaktor

Durch alle Phasen der Frakturheilung ist der Körper — meist erfolgreich — bemüht, eine zunehmende Verfestigung zwischen den Fragmenten zu erreichen. Die Bildung voll ausgereiften lamellären Knochens gelingt offenbar erst dann, wenn jede „mechanische Irritation" (PAUWELS, 1941) ausgeschaltet ist, dann also, wenn die Fragmente durch Callus-Knochengewebe oder durch eine besonders stabile Form der Osteosynthese miteinander verbunden sind.

Die Verfestigung beginnt mit der primären fibrinösen Verspannung, nimmt entweder über das Osteoid zum primären Callus oder über Bindegewebe oder Knorpel zum sekundären Callus ständig zu und wird erst später in den vollwertigen Ersatz, den lamellären Knochen vollendet.

Begrenzte „mechanische Irritation" beantwortet der Körper mit vermehrter Verfestigungsreaktion (Reizcallus). Ist die Irritation aber zu stark, so vermag der Körper diese nicht zu überspielen. Ohne Zweifel ist der mechanische Störfaktor die häufigste Ursache einer verzögerten Verfestigung oder einer Pseudarthrosenbildung. Meist allerdings ist nicht er allein Ursache der Heilungsstörung, gibt aber sehr oft als entscheidender Faktor den letzten Ausschlag.

Von einer Reihe von Beispielen sei nur die „Sperr-Pseudarthrose" der Tibia im Detail besprochen, wie sie VOLKMANN bereits 1875 in ihrer Aetiologie erkannte (Abb. 43 u. 44).

Bei einem kurzen Schrägbruch an der Grenze vom mittleren zum unteren Drittel der Tibia heilt die ebenfalls gebrochene Fibula in den üblichen sechs Wochen. Das distale Fragment der Tibia ist durch Unterbrechung der A. nutricia mangelhaft mit Blut versorgt. Die Tibia ist mit nicht ganz der Hälfte ihrer Circumferenz nur von Subcutis bedeckt, es fehlt also der bedeckende Muskelmantel. Zu diesen ungünstigen Faktoren kommt ein calluszerstörender mechanischer Faktor hinzu, welcher besonders klar erkennbar wird, wenn bei knöchern geheilter Fibula das Bein im Gehgips belastet wird. Die Fibula biegt sich unter Belastung durch und federt bei Entlastung zurück. So ergibt sich ein geradezu grobes Gleiten im Frakturspalt. Der Ausdruck „Sperrpseudarthrose" ist insofern irreführend, als die geheilte Fibula nicht etwa einen ausreichenden Druckkontakt zwischen den Fragmenten verhindert. Das beweist die Tatsache, daß die Tibia ohne Resektion an der Fibula nach Ausschaltung der gleitenden Bewegungen durch einen Marknagel knöchern heilt.

Am Schenkelhals kann der mechanische Störfaktor alleinige Ursache der Pseudarthrosenbildung sein, meist handelt es sich hier aber um eine Summe störender Faktoren.

Eindrucksvoll liegen die Verhältnisse bei der Fraktur des Os scaphoideum. Trotz ungünstiger Bedingungen (intraarticulär, Mangeldurchblutung) ist die Pseudarthrosenbildung große Ausnahme, wenn die Fragmente über acht oder zehn Wochen exakt ruhiggestellt werden, also unter Einschluß des Daumengrundgliedes und eventuell auch des Ellenbogengelenks, um die Pro- und Supination auszuschalten. Nicht erkannte und damit nicht ruhiggestellte oder unzureichend ruhiggestellte Frakturen dieses Knochens führen nahezu ausnahmslos zur Pseudarthrose.

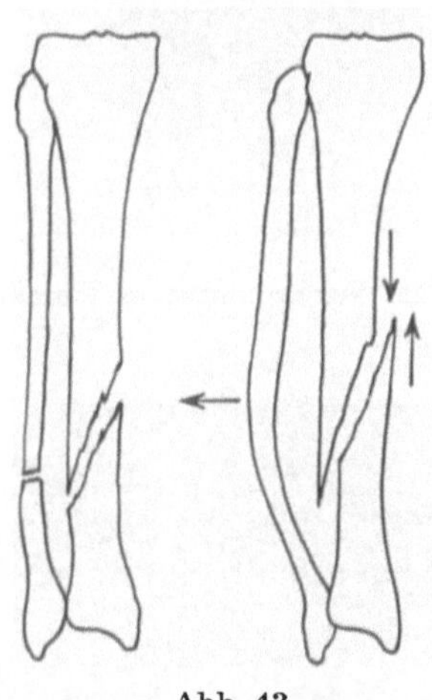

Abb. 43

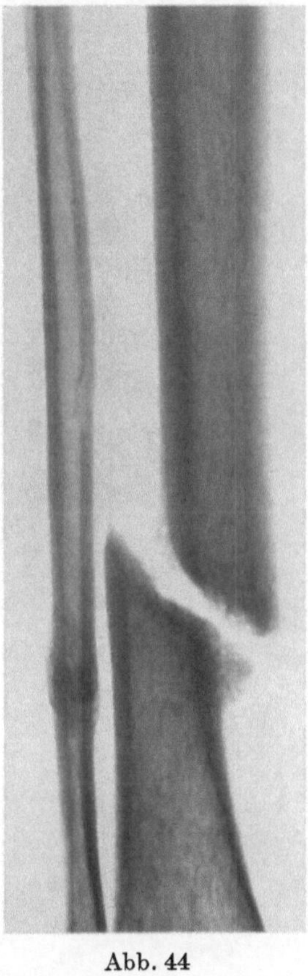

Abb. 44

Abb. 43. Sogenannte Sperrpseudarthrose der Tibia. Unter Belastung biegt sich die stets rasch heilende Fibula durch, bei Entlastung federt sie zurück, so daß am Schrägbruch ausgeprägte Schubkräfte die knöcherne Heilung verhindern. So provoziert ein Gehgips bei Schrägbruch der Tibia die Pseudarthrose

Abb. 44. Typische sogenannte Sperr-Pseudarthrose der Tibia bei 25jährigem Mann sechs Monate nach geschlossener Unterschenkelfraktur. (Siehe Legende der Abb. 43)

Eine Pseudarthrose nach Rippenfraktur gibt es praktisch nur bei neurologischen Störungen (Tabes, Syringomyelie). Beim Nervengesunden reicht die schmerzbedingt reflektorische Ruhigstellung völlig zur Heilung, meist allerdings unter Bildung eines beträchtlichen Reizcallus. Die Ruhigstellung fehlt bei Fehlen des Schmerzes und der mechanische Störfaktor überwiegt. Keineswegs ist eine trophische Störung die Ursache der fehlenden knöchernen Vereinigung, denn bei exakter Ruhigstellung heilt der Knochen des Tabikers ungestört (OELECKER, 1914; MAATZ, 1942).

e) Fremdkörper im Frakturbereich

Die Metallschädigung spielte früher als lokaler Störfaktor bei Osteosynthesen eine beträchtliche Rolle (NIKOLE, 1947; BLOCK u. BECKSTROEM, 1953; RUNNE u. MORITZ, 1961; STÖR, 1943 u.a.), ja sie hat sicher in erheblichem Maße dazu beigetragen, die operative

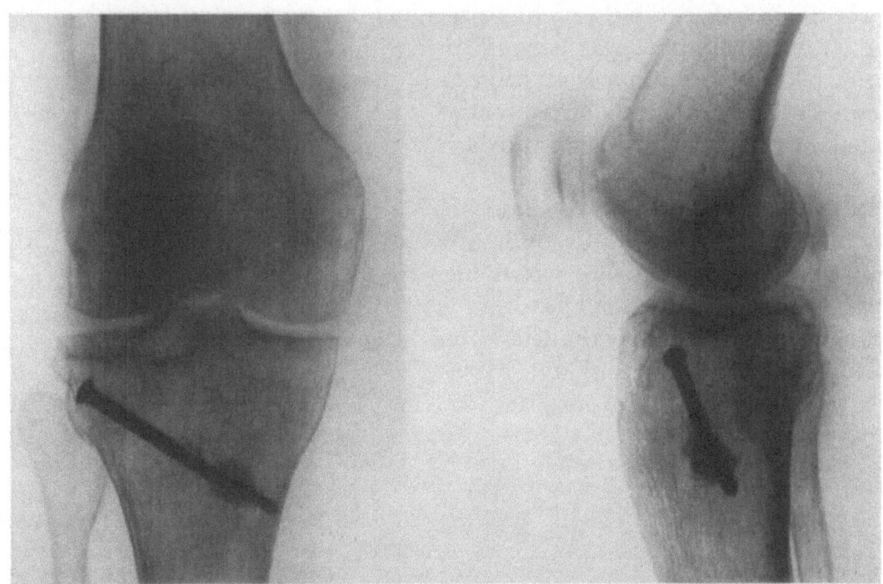

Abb. 45. Oxydation und Bruch einer Schraube fünf Jahre nach operativer Versorgung eines Tibiakopfbruches bei 45jähriger Frau

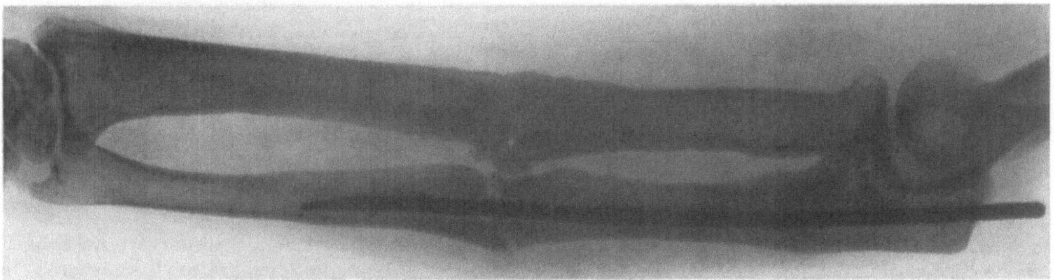

Abb. 46. Nagelbruch in der Elle ein Jahr nach Versorgung einer Ellen-Pseudarthrose mit einem allerdings etwas zu dünnen Nagel. Der Patient verspürte erst nach dem Nagelbruch erneut Schmerzen

Knochenbruchbehandlung über Jahrzehnte unter dem Motto: „Der Fremdkörper stört die Knochenneubildung“ in Mißkredit zu bringen.

Eisenfreie Legierungen (Vitallium, Triconium) oder Edelstähle wie V2a- oder V4a-Stahl, welche bei sachgemäßer Bearbeitung und Anwendung in den Gewebssäften korrosionsfest sind, stören die Heilung einer Fraktur keineswegs, während ein unzureichendes Osteosynthesematerial die Schäden hervorrufen kann, welche zusammenfassend als *Metallosen* bezeichnet werden. Dabei kann der Fremdkörper durch Abwanderung kleinster Teile *morphologisch* oder in Reaktion mit dem Gewebssaft *chemisch* wirken. Eine Kombination dieser Effekte zeigt die Abb. 45. Ein *elektrogenetischer* Effekt tritt dann ein, wenn zwei Metallkörper verschiedener Zusammensetzung einander berühren und von einer *mechanischen* Störung sprechen wir dann, wenn der Fremdkörper durch Druck oder

Bewegung auf das Lagergewebe wirkt, wie wir das in besonders eindrucksvoller Form bei den Smith-Petersen-Kappen beobachteten (GÜNTZ u. MAATZ, 1943).

Alle diese genannten Faktoren können die Bildung von Callus verhindern, bereits gebildeten Callus zerstören oder aber auch einen Reizcallus hervorrufen. Dabei spielt der

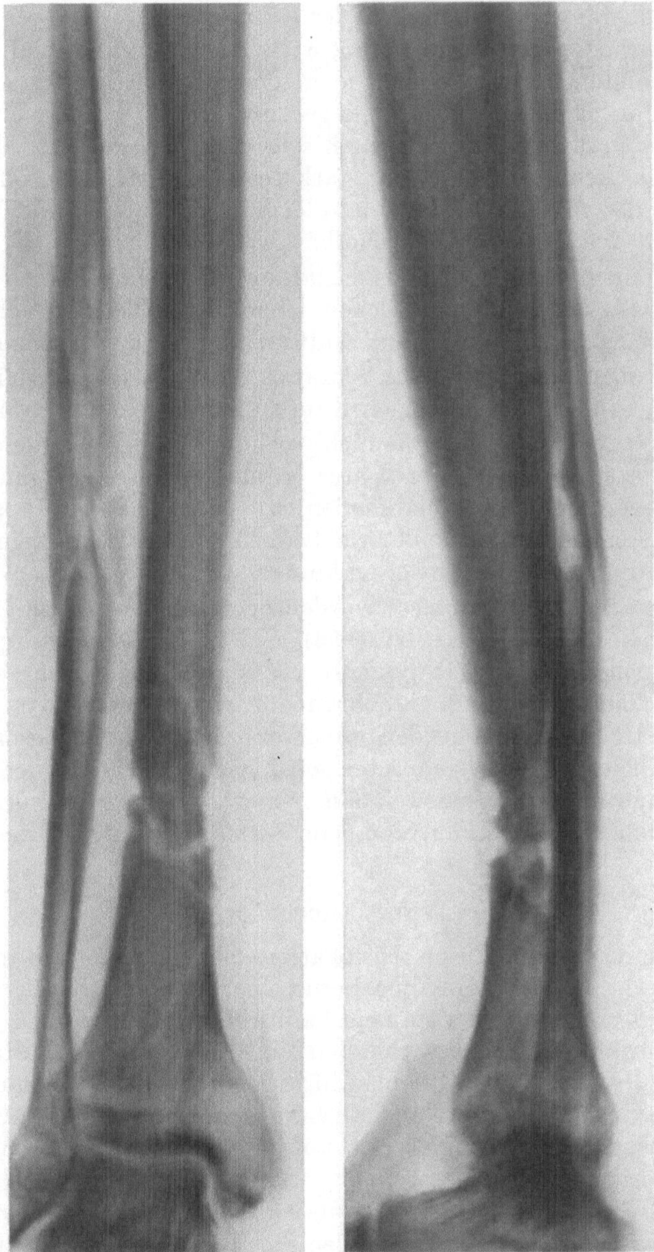

Abb. 47. Die Bilder zeigen die katastrophale Wirkung von Nylon als Knochennahtmaterial. Der geschlossene Spiralbruch des 46 Jahre alten Patienten wurde eine Woche nach dem Unfall versorgt. Zweieinhalb Monate später ausgeprägte Usuren im Knochen. Keine Eiterung, keine knöcherne Heilung. (Quelle: OSTERRIETH, Chirurg 30, S. 264, 1959)

Sitz des „Reizkörpers" allerdings eine entscheidende Rolle, wie wir aus den Versuchen von KÜNTSCHER (1941) (Callus ohne Fraktur) wissen. Im Markraum kann ein chemisch, thermisch oder mechanisch starker Reiz zur starken periostalen Callusbildung führen, im Bereich der Fraktur verhindert derselbe Reiz jegliche Knochenneubildung (MAATZ, 1943).

Welche verheerenden Wirkungen ein unsachgemäß aus eisenhaltigem V2a-Stahl offenbar unsachgemäß fabrikatorisch bearbeiteter Marknagel hervorrufen kann, zeigt der 1951 von A. W. Fischer (1951) berichtete Fall am Femur. Ein korrosionsfester metallischer Fremdkörper, am richtigen Ort im Knochen fest verankert, stört die Frakturheilung nicht.

Um eine besondere, ganz andere Art der Schädigung durch Fremdkörper handelt es sich für die Fraktur oder Osteotomie dann, wenn das Fremdmaterial der Belastung nicht gewachsen im Ermüdungsbruch bricht. Die ersten größeren Erfahrungen wurden nach der Einführung der Marknagelung an der Elle gesammelt. Wird dieser Knochen nach Osteotomie oder offener Fraktur nicht mit einem sehr dicken Nagel oder einer Feder versorgt, so zeigt er meist gar keine oder eine sehr stark verzögerte Heilung. Dann bricht der Nagel (Abb. 46) früher oder später, und das um so leichter, da Patient und Arzt sich wegen der Beschwerdefreiheit des Patienten in Sicherheit wiegten.

Ich habe bei einem 40jährigen muskelstarken Mann einen 10 mm dicken, und nach einem weiteren Jahr einen 13 mm dicken Oberschenkelnagel brechen sehen, und die Fraktur heilte erst nach Aufbohren und Einführen eines 16 mm dicken Nagels.

Schenkelhals-Nägel, die Corticalis-Schrauben an Laschennägeln oder Schrauben, Drähte, Platten, ja auch Smith-Petersen-Kappen, können in der Ermüdung brechen.

Heilt eine Fraktur oder Osteotomie nicht rechtzeitig oder gar nicht knöchern, so muß das tote Metall-Material früher oder später ermüdet nachgeben, ähnlich wie der durch Bestrahlung in seiner andauernd ablaufenden Erneuerung (Bade, 1939) gestörte Knochen schleichend zerrüttet und schleichend bricht, ohne daß wir in der feingeweblichen Untersuchung eine ,,Radionekrose" nachweisen können.

Geradezu katastrophale Ergebnisse wurden bei Knochennaht mit Kunststoffen beobachtet (Osterrieth, 1959; Schwaiger, 1953). Nylon, Perlon oder Supramid mögen beim Annähen von Knochensplittern (R. Schmid, 1958) ohne nachweisbare Nachteile sein, bei der Cerclage von Tibia-Schräg- oder Schraubenbrüchen zeigten von elf Fällen alle eine verzögerte Verfestigung, vier wurden pseudarthrotisch, und besonders eindrucksvoll waren die tiefen Usuren, welche sich unter den Ligaturen im Knochen bildeten (Abb. 47). Dabei ist die Frage ungeklärt, wieweit allein mechanische Faktoren das sehr dehnbare Supramid oder auch chemische Faktoren beim Zerfall der Kunststoffaser (Matzner, 1959) eine Rolle spielen.

f) Der Knochendefekt

Sind die Fragmentenden durch Dislokation oder Knochensubstanzverlust zu weit voneinander entfernt, so bleibt eine knöcherne Überbrückung aus. Es kommt zur Defektpseudarthrose. Eine Dislokation von 2 cm kann sehr wohl knöchern überbrückt werden, wenn sonstige Störfaktoren nicht vorhanden sind (Abb. 10 u. 22). Maßangaben über die größtmögliche Dislokation ohne Heilungsstörung gibt es nicht. Bedeutungsvoll ist sicher der Sitz des Defektes, wobei die Nachbarschaft großer Muskelansätze und ein kräftiger geschlossener Muskelmantel zweifelsohne außerordentlich callusfördernd sind. Die Erfahrungen bei Verlängerungs-Osteotomien, wie Bier (1923), Payr (1918), König (1931) und Lexer (1919) sie früher sammelten, wiesen darauf hin, daß eine langsam sich steigernde Distanz zwischen den Fragmentenden die Überbrückung bis zu 8 cm ermöglichen.

Größere Defekte müssen mit einem autoplastischen Span überbrückt werden. Am Oberschenkel empfiehlt sich eher die Verkürzungsosteotomie der gesunden Seite, welche mit einem Küntscher-Nagel leicht ausführbar ist und den Patienten nur für wenige Tage zur Bettruhe zwingt.

g) Die Interposition von Weichgeweben

Die Interposition von Weichgeweben wurde früher als Ursache verzögerter Verfestigung oder Pseudarthrosenbildung weit häufiger angesehen, als es heute — wohl mit

Recht — der Fall ist. Interponierte Muskulatur zwischen den Fragmenten einer Oberschenkelfraktur kann zwar eine ideale Reposition verhindern, die Beteiligung der Muskulatur an der parossalen Callusbildung ist aber so eindrucksvoll und stark, daß von einer Verzögerung der Verfestigung meist keine Rede sein kann.

Ganz anders liegen die Verhältnisse z.B. am Innenknöchel (Abb. 48). Schlägt sich hier das zerrissene Band in den Frakturspalt ein, so resultiert sicher eine Pseudarthrose, denn andere Faktoren (Gelenkbruch mit Hämatomverlust, Dislokation und unvollkommene Ruhigstellung) unterstützen diese Entwicklung.

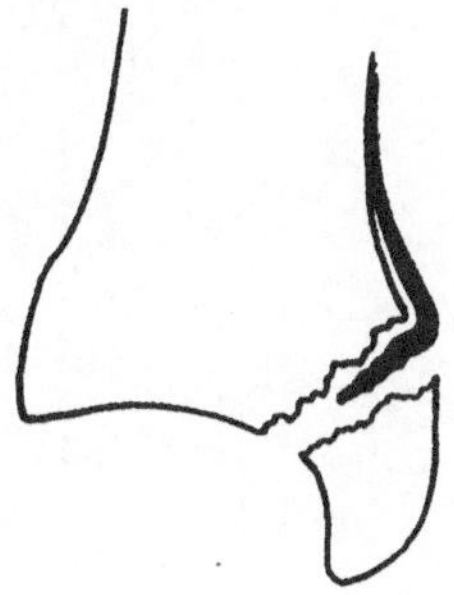

Abb. 48. Eingeschlagenes Periost und Bandgewebe sind häufig die Ursache einer Pseudarthrose am Innenknöchel

h) Trophische Störungen

Ob ein Knochen durch Inaktivität (Lähmung, Amputation u.a.) oder in irgend einer anderen Form der Osteoporose oder Atrophie weniger kalkreich und weniger tragfähig ist, der Reiz der Fraktur mobilisiert alle Kräfte und nicht selten wird beobachtet, daß ein solcher Knochen besonders rasch und störungsfrei knöchern heilt. Die Callusbildung ist allerdings meist spärlich (Abb. 49) und diese Tatsache kann die Beurteilung der Verfestigung, also der Belastungsfähigkeit der Fraktur außerordentlich erschweren. So wird man in manchem Fall ein gewisses Risiko nicht umgehen können, denn der Reiz einer vorsichtig dosierten Belastung soll zum zuverlässigen knöchernen Durchbau führen. Die Grenze der Belastbarkeit aber ist niemals bekannt. So wird man gerade in solchen Fällen dem Arzt keinen Vorwurf daraus machen, wenn es einmal zu einer Refraktur kommen sollte (siehe auch S. 558—560).

2. Die Bilder der verzögerten Verfestigung

Die verzögerte Verfestigung einer Fraktur kann sich im Röntgenbild in sehr unterschiedlichen Formen darstellen. Ein charakteristisches Bild zeigt die Abb. 50. Im Vergleich zur Aufnahme direkt nach dem Unfall hat sich kaum etwas an den Fragmenten und in ihrer Nachbarschaft verändert. Es fehlt jede den Bruchspalt überbrückende Callusbildung und eine Durchkonstruktion im Bereich der Stellen, an denen die Fragmentenden Kontakt haben, ist nicht erkennbar. Da die Patientin neben der objektiv feststellbaren leichten Schwellung Schmerzen angab, mußte unter Berücksichtigung aller Faktoren, auch der Röntgenbilder, eine verzögerte Verfestigung angenommen werden, und als Konsequenz daraus ergab sich eine weitere Ruhigstellung im Gipsverband.

Weit häufiger als dieses geschilderte Bild der „fehlenden Callusbildung“ — eine solche muß bei dislozierten Fragmenten sichtbar werden — ist die ausreichende oder bisweilen sogar reichliche Callusbildung mit Fortsetzung der Frakturlinie im Callus (Abb. 51). Derartige Bilder beweisen, daß ein mechanischer Störfaktor die knöcherne Heilung verzögert oder eventuell sogar verhindert. Die Kraft zur Callusbildung ist ausreichend vorhanden, das junge Gewebe aber wird — meist durch Schubkräfte — zerstört. Darum liegt die Zerstörungszone im Callus in Fortsetzung der Ebene der Fraktur. Das Ausmaß des Störfaktors auf der einen Seite, die weitere Möglichkeit der Callusbildung auf der anderen, entscheiden dann, ob es über das Bild der verzögerten Verfestigung zur Heilung oder zur Pseudarthrose kommt. Da die geschilderten Vorgänge auf dem Röntgenbild dem behandelnden Arzt eine sehr eindringliche Warnung geben, wird dieser meist als Folgerung eine weitere und möglichst bessere Ruhigstellung zu erreichen versuchen und damit dann erfolgreich sein.

Selbst sehr ferne und zarte Callusbrücken können für die Beurteilung des Heilungszustandes einer Fraktur von entscheidender Bedeutung sein, und zwar dann, wenn im ganzen die Callusbildung spärlich ist, und wenn die knöcherne Durchkonstruktion der Fragmente nach dem Röntgenbild gar nicht zu beurteilen ist. So beweisen sehr zarte aber völlig

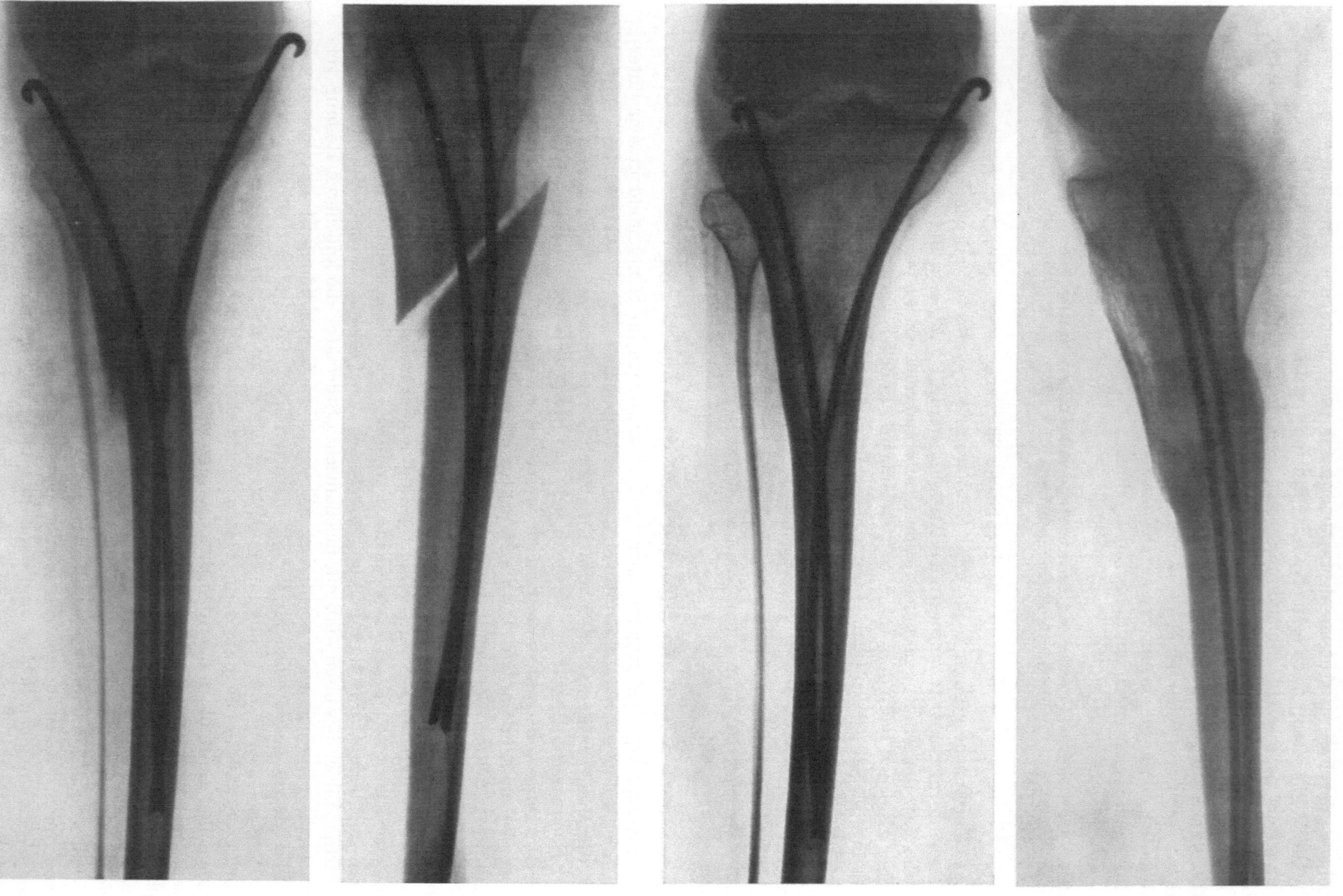

Abb. 49. Ungestörte knöcherne Heilung (b) im atrophischen Knochen bei congenitaler Lähmung des Beines. Bei dem 18jährigen jungen Mann wurde eine in X-Stellung geheilte Tibiafraktur durch Osteotomie korrigiert (a). Die Kontrollbilder wurden neun Monate später gewonnen

intakte Callusbrücken in der Abb. 52, daß die Fragmente bereits unbeweglich miteinander verbunden sind. Unter selbst vorsichtigster Gehbelastung hätten diese Brücken ohne die stärkere, aber nicht erkennbare Verbindung zerreißen müssen.

In Einzelfällen versagt das Röntgenbild vollständig. Es erscheint uns zweckmäßig, diese im Abschnitt der verzögerten Verfestigung abzuhandeln, und zwar einmal darum, weil

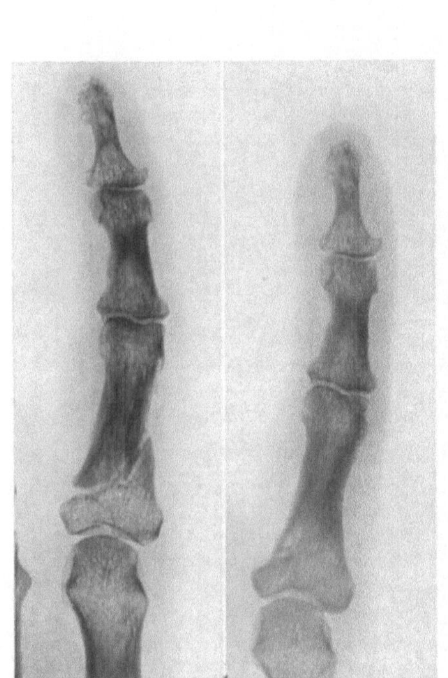

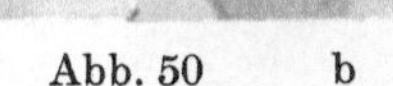

a Abb. 50 b

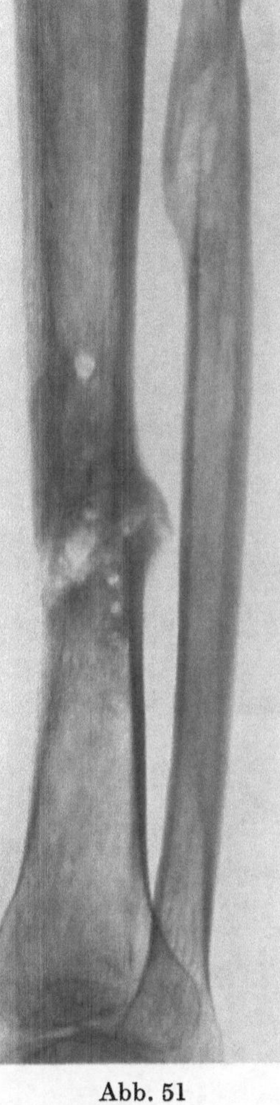

Abb. 51

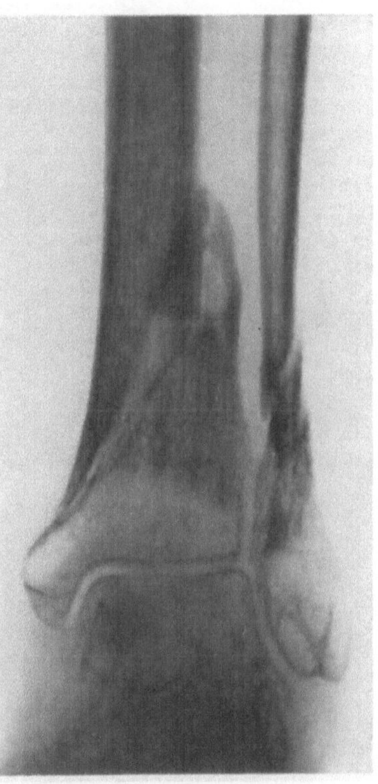

Abb. 52

Abb. 50a u. b. Stark verzögerte Heilung einer Phalangenfraktur am fünften Finger einer 53jährigen Frau. Bild a zeigt die Fraktur neun Wochen nach der Verletzung und Behandlung im Gipsverband. Bild b die abgeschlossene Heilung dreiviertel Jahr später

Abb. 51. Die Fortsetzung der Frakturlinie im Callus beweist das Vorhandensein mangelnder Ruhigstellung. Das Bild wurde von einem 18jährigen Patienten gewonnen, dessen geschlossene Fraktur mit Lane'scher Platte zehn Monate vorher versorgt worden war

Abb. 52. Die intakte zarte Callusbrücke an der Spitze des distalen Fragments beweist den Zustand mechanischer Ruhe zwischen den Fragmenten. Drei Monate alte geschlossene Unterschenkelfraktur bei 56jähriger Patientin

nicht vorauszusagen war, ob vielleicht doch noch eine knöcherne Heilung eingetreten wäre, zum zweiten, weil den Röntgenbildern jedes Kriterium der Pseudarthrose fehlte.

Die Abb. 53 zeigt die „Scheinheilung“ einer subcapitalen Schenkelhalsfraktur sieben Monate nach Versorgung mit einem Laschennagel. Vor der Nagelentfernung klagte die sicher sehr sensible Patientin über leichte Beschwerden, welche auf den großen Fremdkörper (Laschennagel) zurückgeführt wurden, da für eine beginnende Kopfnekrose kein Anhalt bestand. Nach der Nagelentfernung verstärkten sich die Beschwerden erheblich, und die Röntgenkontrolle zeigte vier Wochen später den abgerutschten Kopf. Es wurde eine Moore-Prothese eingesetzt. Die histologische Untersuchung zeigte einen total nekrotischen Kopf, d.h. sowohl die Knochenzellen als auch das Markgewebe waren abgestorben.

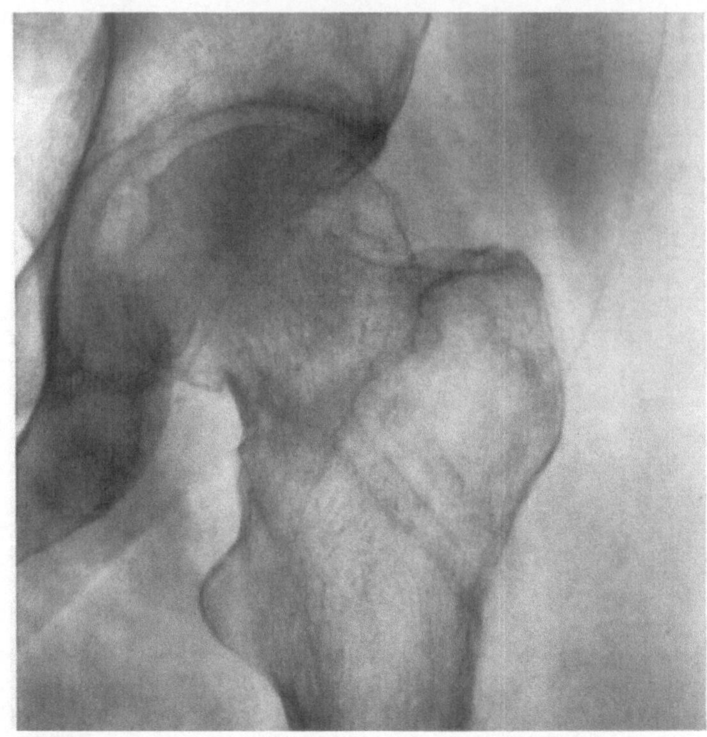

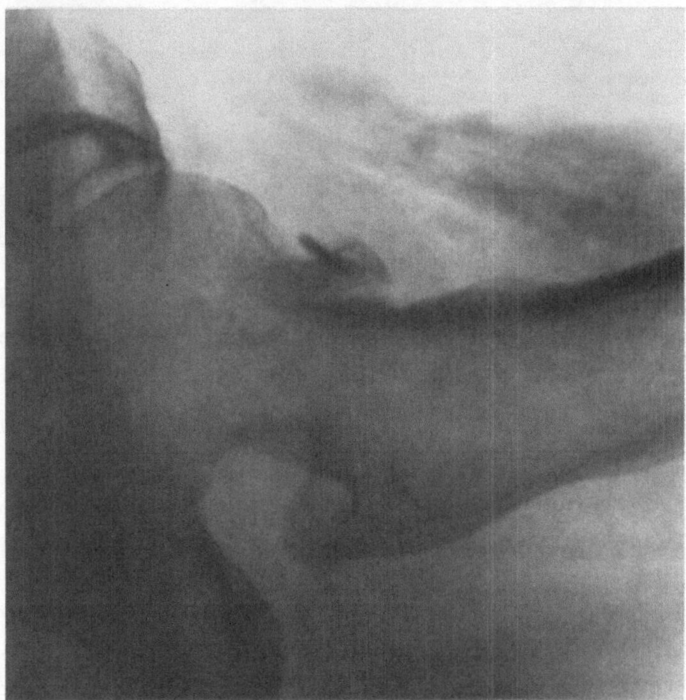

Abb. 53. Scheinheilung einer medialen Schenkelhalsfraktur bei 54jähriger Patientin neun Monate nach Versorgung mit Laschennagel. Der Kopf kippte vier Wochen nach der Nagelentfernung, welche wegen Schmerzen vorgenommen wurde, ab. Versorgung mit Moorescher Prothese. Die histologische Untersuchung ergab totale Nekrose des Kopfes in allen Gewebsteilen

Wir sehen, daß die Beurteilung der knöchernen Heilung einer Fraktur beim Fehlen jeglicher Callusbildung sehr schwer, ja unmöglich sein kann. Das zeigen auch Einzelfälle, welche nach der Methode der Schweizer Arbeitsgemeinschaft für Osteosynthese (A. O.) mit Druckplatten behandelt wurden. NEFF berichtete 1964 über mehrere Fälle bei jungen Menschen, bei denen die Platten am Oberschenkel nach mehr als einem Jahr entfernt wurden, weil der Bruchspalt durchgebaut erschien, bei denen dann aber die Fragmente „wie bei einer frischen Fraktur" auseinanderfielen.

3. Pseudarthrosen und Nearthrosen

Kommt es nicht zur knöchernen Heilung einer Fraktur, so bildet sich eine Pseudarthrose, eine Falschgelenkbildung oder eine Nearthrose, eine Neugelenkbildung. Von einer Nearthrose sprechen wir nur dann, wenn sich röntgenologisch nachweisbar eine Art Pfanne und eine Art Kopf gebildet haben. Dabei liegt erstere meist rumpfnahe. Derartige Nearthrosen entstehen nur dort, wo eine gewisse mechanische Steuerung der Fragmente vorhanden ist, sei es durch die natürlich vorhandenen Kräfte, sei es durch einen Schienenhülsenapparat, wie er bei Oberarmpseudarthrosen früher häufiger als heute getragen wurde. Nearthrosen (Abb. 54) haben an Kopf und Pfanne meist einen wenn auch dünnen Überzug von Knorpel. Sie besitzen eine regelrechte Gelenkhaut und enthalten die physiologische Gelenkschmiere.

Eine *Pseudarthrose* kann straff oder schlaff sein. Der Übergang von der verzögerten Heilung einer Fraktur zur Pseudarthrose ist nicht scharf abgrenzbar. Der Zeitfaktor allein kann zur Definition nicht ausreichen. Schon bei der verzögerten Verfestigung sahen wir, welche Schwierigkeiten die Beurteilung machen kann. Das klinische Bild des Fortbestehens der pathologischen Beweglichkeit allein sagt auch nicht genügend aus über die eventuell noch vorhandenen oder völlig erschöpften Regenerationskräfte. Mehr verrät das Röntgenbild. Zeigen die Fragmentenden bei sich verbreiterndem und geglättetem Bruchspalt beidseitige sklerotische Abdeckelung der Markräume (Abb. 55, siehe auch Abb. 44) bei einer Schaftfraktur (Sargdeckel der Regeneration. GULEKE, 1919), so haben wir das sicherste Zeichen der Pseudarthrose (BRANDT, 1937). Bei Frakturen im spongiösen Knochen finden wir analog die Sklerosierung der Fragmentenden (Abb. 56). Besteht eine solche straffe Pseudarthrose über lange Zeit, so können sich in ihren Fragmenten wie bei einer schweren Arthrosis deformans Geröllcysten bilden (Abb. 57).

Um eine Einteilung der Pseudarthrosen nach genetischen oder morphologischen Gesichtspunkten hat man sich früher sehr bemüht. BLOCK (1940) empfiehlt nur zwei Hauptgruppen:

1. Pseudarthrosen infolge Erschöpfung der Regenerationskraft durch grobe anatomische Veränderungen
   a) durch Defekte („Defektpseudarthrosen"),
   b) durch Zwischenlagerung von Weichteilen („Interpositions-Pseudarthrosen"),
2. Pseudarthrosen infolge Fehldifferenzierung des Keimgewebes, die sogenannten Spalt- oder gemeinen Pseudarthrosen, die vielfältige Ursachen haben können, die sich unterteilen lassen in solche
   a) allgemeiner Natur,
   b) örtlicher Natur.

Wir stimmen darin mit BLOCK überein, daß mit dieser Einteilung „die Gruppen sowohl nach anatomisch-biologischen wie auch gleichzeitig nach ursächlichen Gesichtspunkten" getrennt sind. Wir wollen dabei aber nicht verhehlen, daß wohl eine Defektpseudarthrose (Abb. 58) bei einem größeren Defekt als solche sicher erkannt werden kann, daß alle anderen aber in ätiologischer Hinsicht außerordentliche Schwierigkeiten bereiten können. Als Beispiel sei eine Pseudarthrose des Innenknöchels angeführt (Abb. 59). Die Dislokation, also der Defekt, kann bei der geringen Regenerationskraft „zu groß sein". Weichteile können interponiert sein. Ein mechanischer Störfaktor ist unter diesen genannten Um-

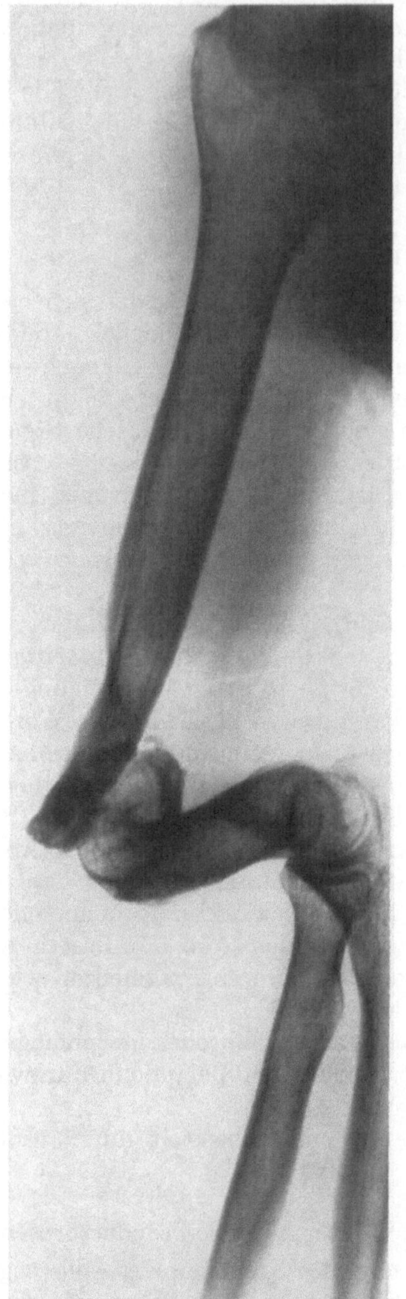

Abb. 54

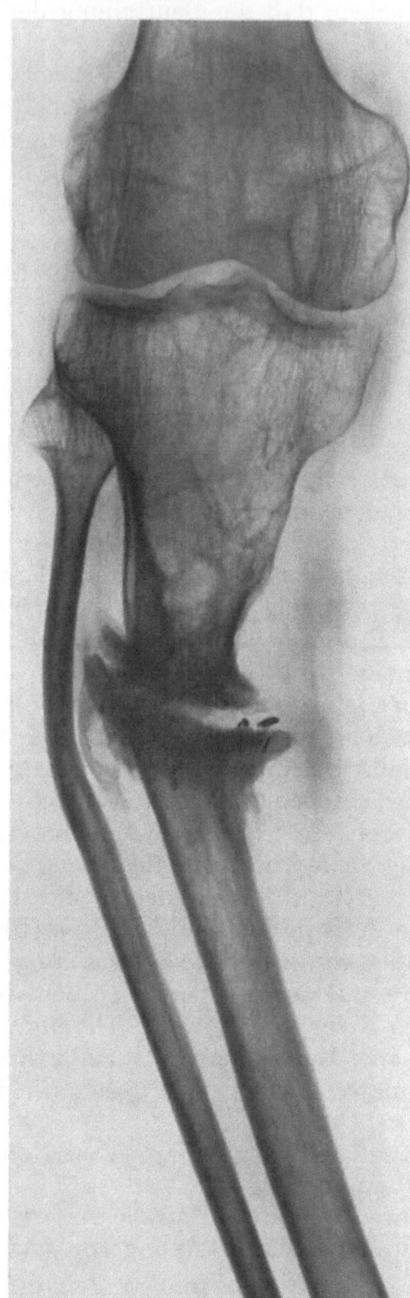

Abb. 55

Abb. 54. Nearthrose am Oberarm nach Schußbruch bei 30 Jahre altem Mann drei Jahre nach der Verwundung

Abb. 55. Dreißig Jahre alte Pseudarthrose der Tibia bei 59jährigem Mann nach Schußfraktur. Sehr ausgeprägte sklerotische Abdeckelung der Fragmente nach Jahrzehnte langem Tragen eines Schienenhülsenapparates

ständen im Gipsverband zwar nur gering, aber eventuell doch entscheidend für das Ausbleiben der knöchernen Heilung.

Frakturen im mittleren und distalen Teil der Elle neigen zur Pseudarthrosenbildung. Das hat anatomische Gründe (Maatz, 1949). Nur der Radius ist der Stützpfeiler des Unterarms. Die Elle weicht praktisch ohne Gegenhalt bei Belastung nach distal am Handgelenk aus. Bei einer Fraktur z. B. im mittleren Drittel wird das distale Fragment (Abb. 60) durch

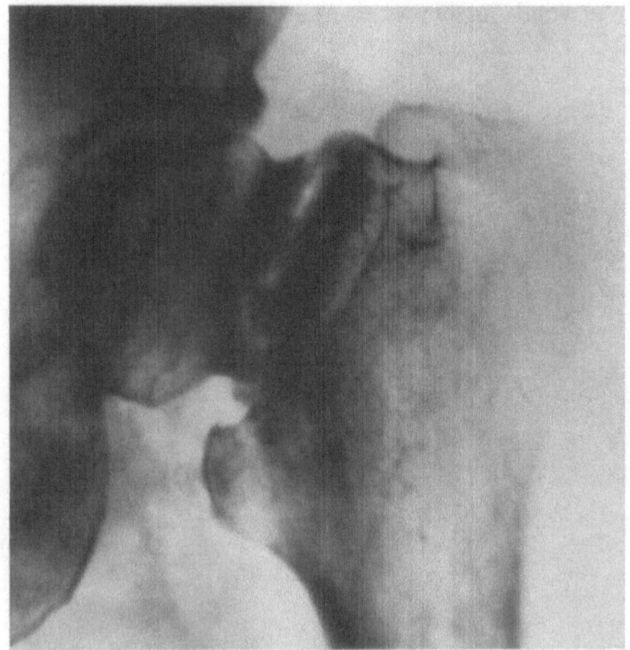

Abb. 56. Straffe Schenkelhals-Pseudarthrose bei 65jähriger Patientin mit leidlicher Gehfähigkeit drei Jahre nach der Fraktur

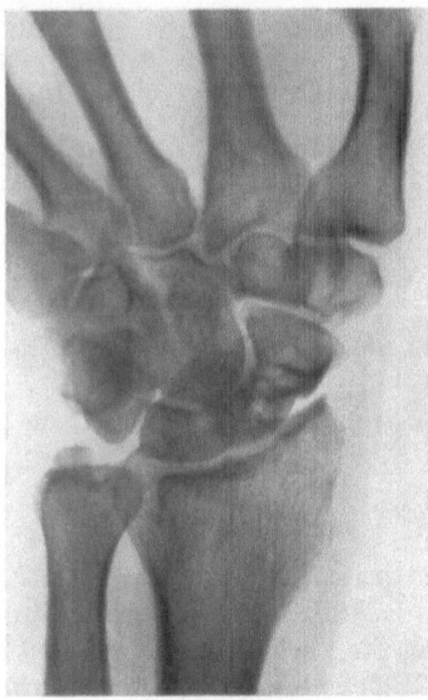

Abb. 57

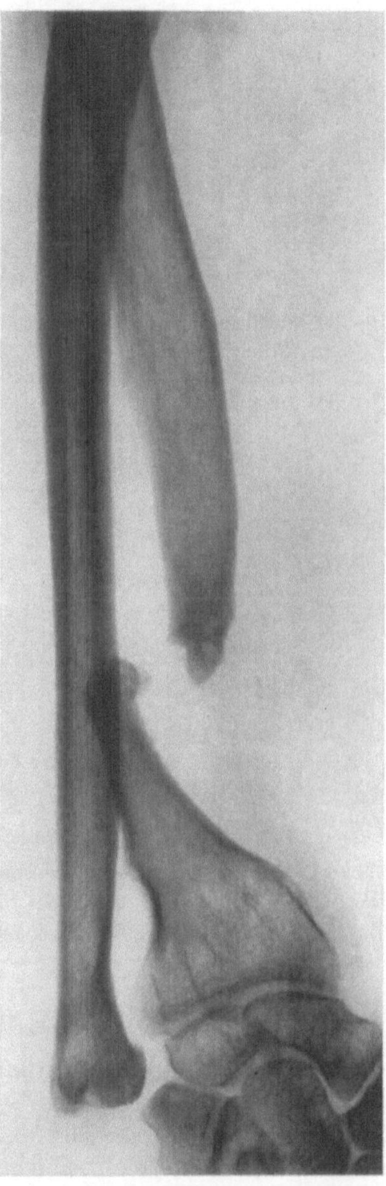

Abb. 58

Abb. 57. Os scaphoideum-Pseudarthrose wahrscheinlich zwei Jahre nach der Fraktur. Kleine Geröllcysten

Abb. 58. Defekt-Pseudarthrose am Radius nach Schußbruch vor einem Jahr. Die Größe des Defektes wird erst dann deutlich, wenn man den starken Vorschub der Elle berücksichtigt

den M. pronator teres, den M. extensor pollicis longus und M. flexor digitorum profundus nach distal gezogen. Die Zugrichtung der Bänder wirkt diesem keineswegs entgegen (Abb. 61). Es fehlt hier also jede natürliche Kraft, welche die Fragmente miteinander in Kontakt hält, ja, durch den Muskelzug kommt es zur Distraktion der Fragmente. Nach

Osteotomien ist dieser Vorgang bei Verwendung etwas dünnerer Nägel, über denen die Fragmente wie auf einer Schiene gleiten können, einwandfrei zu beurteilen.

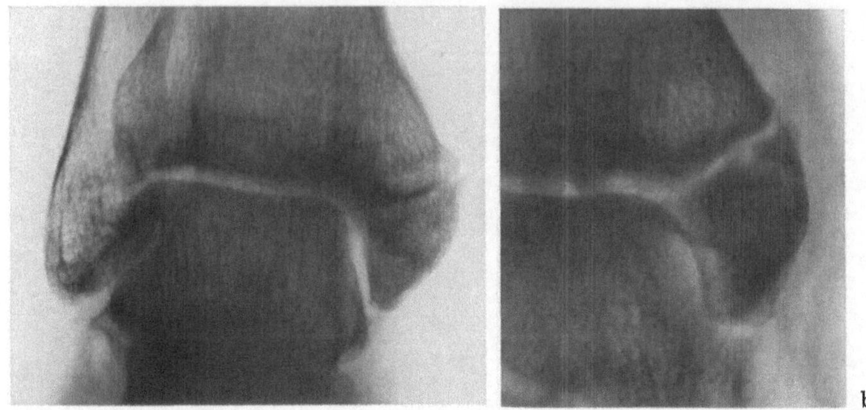

Abb. 59. 37jähriger Mann. Pseudarthrose am Innenknöchel sechs Wochen nach Luxationsfraktur (LAUGE-HANSEN: Pronations-Eversionsfraktur, Schweregrad IV). Bild a) erweckt den Verdacht, zwingt zur gezielten Aufnahme (b), welche den Verdacht bestätigt

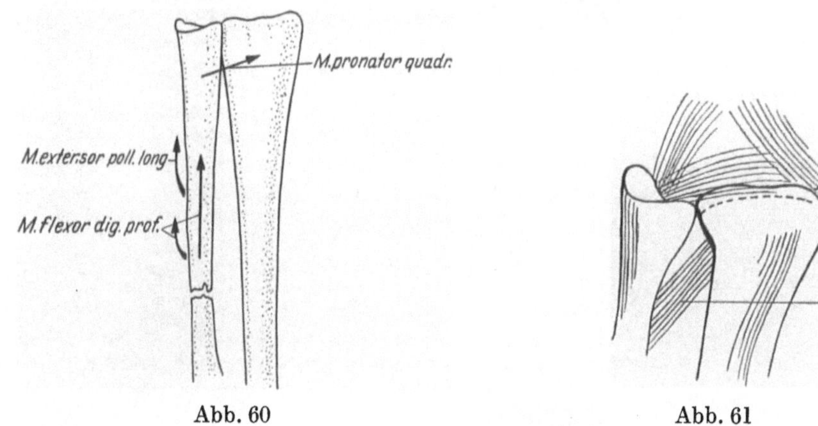

Abb. 60 Abb. 61

Abb. 60. Das distale Fragment der Elle wird durch Muskelkräfte vom proximalen Fragment entfernt [Quelle: MAATZ, Chirurg 28, 24 (1957)]

Abb. 61. Der Bandapparat am Handgelenk leistet dem Vorschub der Elle keinen Widerstand [Quelle: MAATZ, Chirurg 20, 288 (1949)]

4. Die Sudeck'sche Krankheit

Bei der Sudeck'schen Krankheit strahlt die primäre Herdstelle — z.B. die Fraktur mit ihren Heilungsvorgängen — auf vegetativen Bahnen in die benachbarten und weiteren Gefäßstromgebiete aus. SUDECK (1938) nannte es die „gesteigerte und kollaterale Heilentzündung". In den Weichteilen besteht dabei eine Schwellung, Hyperthermie und vermehrte Schmerzhaftigkeit, während erste Knochenveränderungen fünf bis acht Wochen als kleine, lückenartige Flecke an den spongiösen Gelenkenden der kleinen Röhrenknochen auftreten. Es sind die ersten Zeichen eines lebhaften Knochenumbaus, welcher das Krankheitsbild charakterisiert. Neben dem anfänglich lebhaften Abbau setzt frühzeitig Knochenneubildung ein. Das dabei gebildete osteoide Gewebe vermag zunächst bei der vorherrschenden Gewebsacidose Kalkkristalle nicht einzulagern, so daß im Röntgenbild kleine und größere Lücken vorherrschen (*fleckige Entschattung*, Abb. 62).

Die gesteigerte Heilentzündung vermag verschiedene Schweregrade zu erreichen. In leichten Fällen findet sich die fleckige Entschattung fast ausschließlich im Bereich der spongiösen Skeletabschnitte. Die typische Schmerzhaftigkeit bei passiven Bewegungen

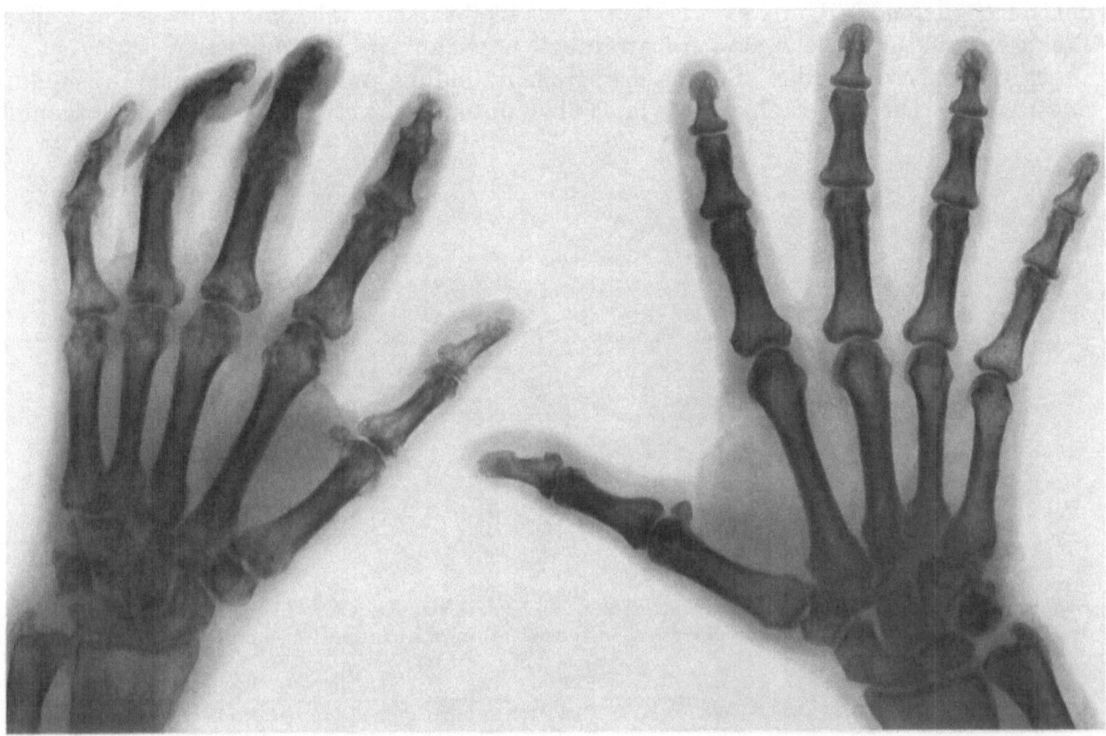

Abb. 62. 53jährige Patientin. Sudeck'sche Erkrankung nach Humeruskopffraktur vierzehn Wochen nach der Verletzung. Ausgeprägte fleckige Entschattung in den spongiösen Knochen. (Daneben die Vergleichsaufnahmen der gesunden Hand)

auch der kleinen Gelenke fern der Verletzungsstelle ist zwar vorhanden, aber weniger ausgeprägt, und kann unter zweckmäßiger Behandlung bereits nach Wochen wieder abklingen.

Nimmt diese Schmerzhaftigkeit aber zu, gesellt sich vor allem der spontane Schmerz auch in der Nacht hinzu, nimmt die Haut livide blaß-bläuliche Verfärbung mit glatter Oberfläche durch Schwellung an, so ist die Heilentzündung „entgleist". Wir sprechen von der *Dystrophie*. Die fleckige Entschattung geht stellenweise in nebelartige Aufhellung über. Jetzt zeigt auch die Corticalis längsgerichtete spaltförmige oder ovale Lücken (Abb. 63). Auch dieses Bild, welches meist nicht vor drei Monaten nach der Verletzung auftritt, ein Krankheitsbild, welches mit seinen hochgradigen Schmerzen und den charakteristischen klinischen und röntgenologischen Veränderungen außerordentlich eindrucksvoll ist, klingt meist nach weiteren drei Monaten ab, so daß auch aus der entgleisten Heilentzündung ein funktionell voll befriedigendes Heilergebnis resultiert. Als Folge

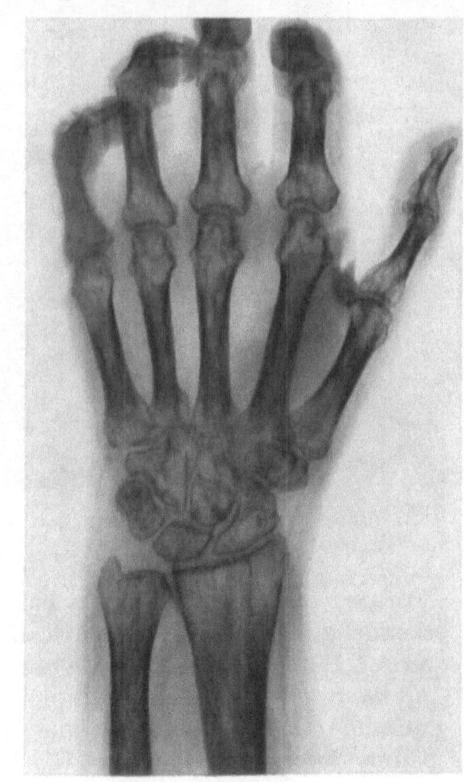

Abb. 63. Patientin wie Abb. 62 zweieinhalb Monate später. Ausgeprägte Dystrophie mit Längsauffaserung der corticalen Skeletteile und weitgehender Kalkabwanderung in der Spongiosa

des durchgreifenden Umbaus des Knochens bleibt meist allerdings eine neue, gröbere Bälkchenstruktur, welche als „grobsträhnig" bezeichnet wird (Abb. 64).

Erfreulicherweise führt die entgleiste Heilentzündung nur sehr selten zur „Ausheilung mit Defekt". Die Dystrophie geht dann über in eine schwere *Atrophie.* Im Röntgenbild

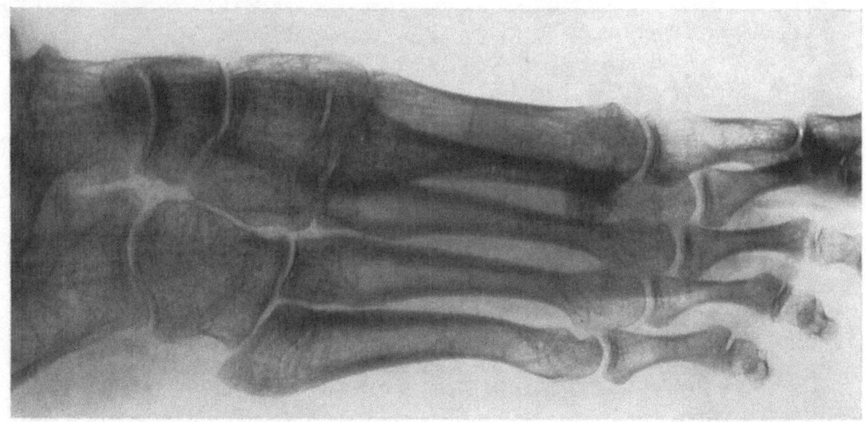

Abb. 64. Grobsträhnige Struktur der Spongiosa nach Umbau des Knochens in Sudeckscher Krankheit vor drei Jahren. Die damals 18-jährige Patientin erlitt eine schwere Luxationsfraktur im oberen Sprunggelenk

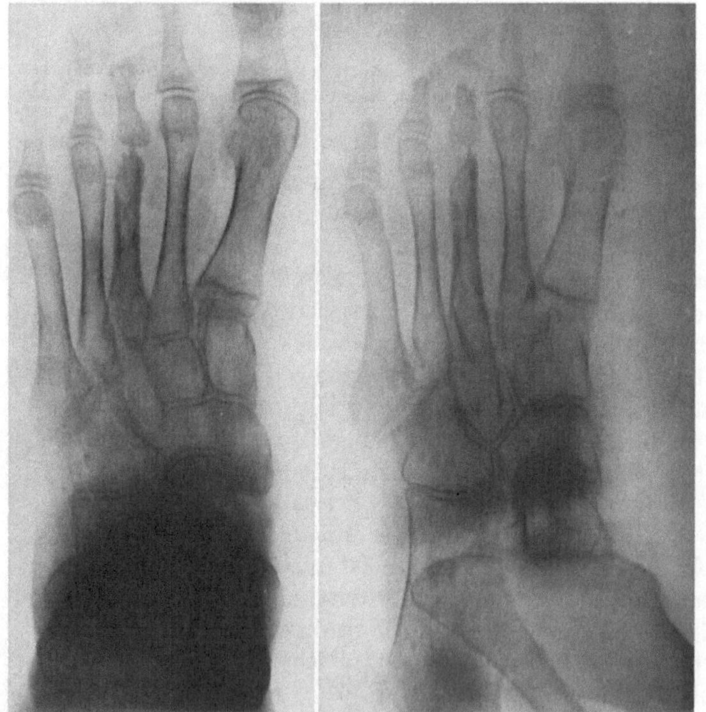

Abb. 65. Endatrophie nach Sudeckscher Dystrophie. Sogenannter Glasknochen

sehen wir den „Glasknochen", bei dem die überaus zarten Spongiosabälkchen kaum zu erkennen sind, während die Corticalis nur als feine Begrenzung „wie mit dem Bleistift nachgezogen" imponiert (Abb. 65). Klinisch sind Hand oder Fuß schwer geschädigt. Alle Gelenke sind kaum oder gar nicht beweglich, die Weichgewebe sind atrophisch, und die rosa glattglänzende Haut ist fest über die Knochen und „scheinbar" verdickten Gelenke ausgespannt. Besonders quälend ist für den Träger die hochgradige Kälteempfindlichkeit.

Eine einheitliche Nomenklatur für das Sudecksche Syndrom gibt es noch nicht. Besonders hervorzuheben aber ist an diesem Platz, daß zur Diagnose der Sudeckschen Krankheit das Röntgenbild allein nicht ausreicht. Es gibt eine ausgeprägte fleckige Entschattung in der Nachbarschaft einer heilenden Fraktur oder einer Entzündung, ohne daß das klinische Bild dieser Erkrankung besteht.

Nach den Darstellungen von SUDECK (1900) sollte man nach unserer Meinung das beschriebene Krankheitsbild nach Stadien und Schweregrad wie folgt unterteilen:

Sudecksche Krankheit

gesteigerte Heilentzündung → Heilung
↓
entgleiste Heilentzündung (Dystrophie) → Heilung (grobsträhnige Struktur)
↓
Heilung mit schwerem Defekt (Atrophie)

OEHLECKER (1948) bemühte sich sehr um die Klärung der Nomenklatur und schlug folgende Einteilung vor:

Sudecksches Syndrom (kurz: Sudeck)

Sudeck, akute Phase	Heilung
Sudeck, Dystrophie	Heilung (Endatrophie).

MAURER (1941) schlug vor, die Stadien Umbau, Dystrophie und Atrophie zu unterscheiden.

In der Praxis bürgert es sich immer mehr ein, je nach Stadium von einem Sudeck I bis III zu sprechen. BLUMENSAAT (1956) verzichtet auf eine Stadieneinteilung, und auch wir meinen, daß man dem Krankheitsbild gerecht wird und es ausreichend definiert hat, wenn wir wissen, daß diese heute so häufig vorkommende Komplikation besonders bei Frakturen im Bereich der oberen Extremität eine gesteigerte Heilentzündung ist, welche entgleist zur Dystrophie führen kann, wobei letztere erfreulich selten zur Heilung mit Defekt, zur Endatrophie führt.

5. Die Bruchheilung im kranken Knochen

Die Heilung in einem vorerkrankten Knochen kann besonders stürmisch, sie kann „normal" oder verzögert ablaufen oder praktisch aufgehoben sein. Entscheidend ist hierfür die Erkrankung des Knochens, welche, wie z.B. bei der Osteomyelitis, bereits ohne Fraktur mit einer lebhaften Knochenregeneration verläuft oder beim osteolytischen malignen Neoplasma eine Zerstörung des jungen Knochens bewirkt, so daß der starke Reiz der Fraktur zur Heilung häufig nicht ausreicht.

Der *osteomyelitisch erkrankte Knochen* bricht in der Regel spontan, nicht selten sogar im Gipsverband (Abb. 66). Hier müssen die abbauenden Vorgänge die stets nebenher laufenden reparatorischen Vorgänge beträchtlich überwiegen (LAUCHE, 1939). Die in den letzten Jahrzehnten immer seltener auftretende „Totenlade", das ist der vom Periost gebildete kräftige Callusmantel, welcher den gefährdeten Knochenabschnitt abstützend einhüllt, fehlt epiphysennahe ohnehin. So treten die Frakturen besonders gern in diesem Knochenabschnitt ein.

Bei ausreichender Ruhigstellung verläuft die Frakturheilung meist ungestört. Selten sind die Fälle, in denen große Teile des corticalen Knochenrohres völlig aufgelöst werden. Es entsteht dann ein mehr oder minder großer Defekt, und es resultiert eine Defekt-Pseudarthrose. In Unkenntnis wurde diese um die Jahrhundertwende nicht selten durch vorzeitige Entfernung des corticalen Sequesters, also vor Bildung der Totenlade, provoziert.

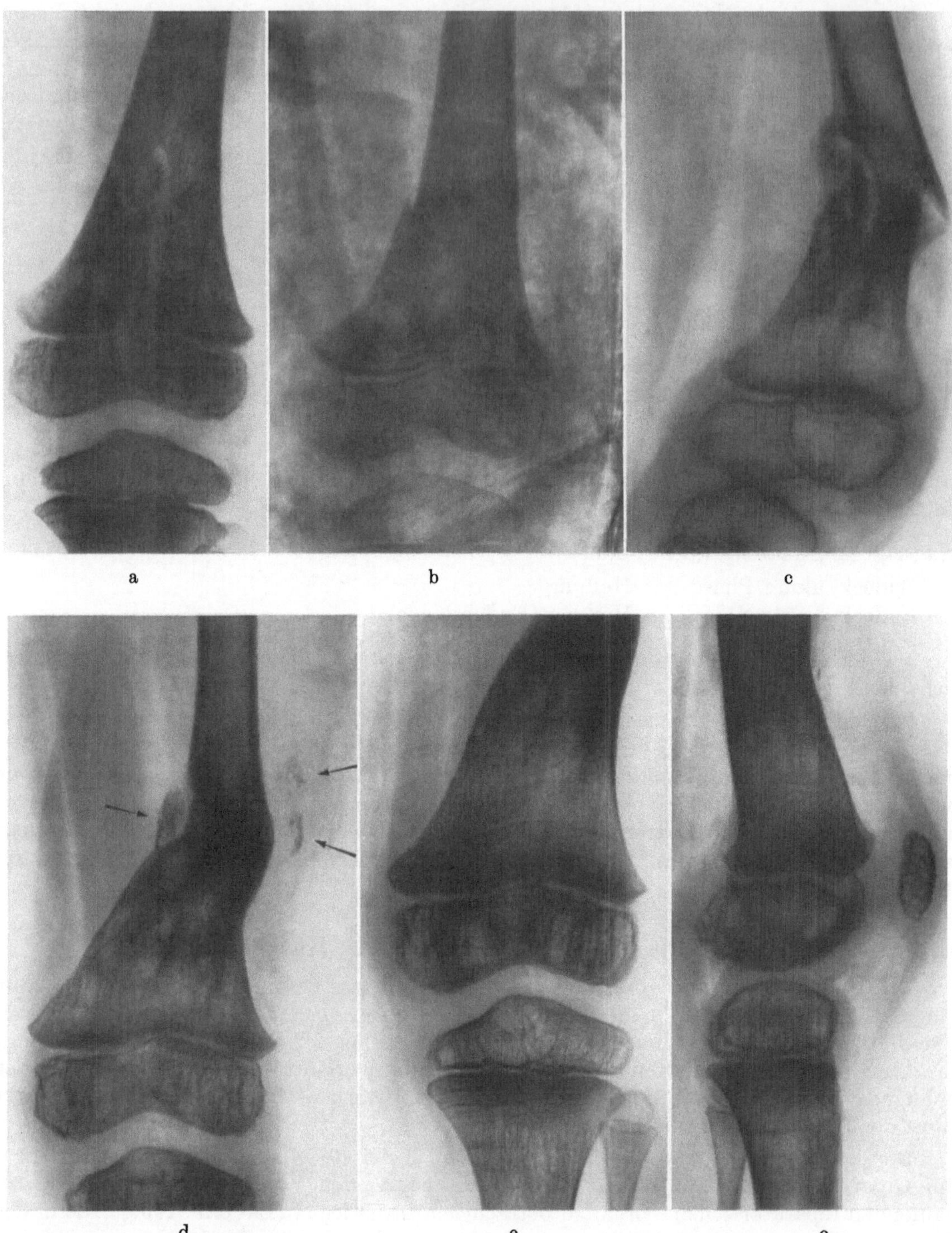

Abb. 66a—e. Verzögerte Heilung einer im Beckengips aufgetretenen Spontanfraktur im osteomyelitischen Knochen eines sechs Jahre alten Knaben. a Wurmfraß-artige Kanäle im Knochen sechs Wochen nach Beginn der Erkrankung. b Spontanfraktur des Femur drei Wochen später im Beckengips. Die Kontrollen wurden vier Monate (c), acht Monate (d) und sechzehn Monate (e) nach der Fraktur angefertigt

Die *Ostitis deformans Paget* (siehe dort) zeigt weniger Spontanfrakturen, häufiger traumatische Knochenbrüche — allerdings schon bei geringeren Traumen. Der Knochen befindet sich durch eine wahrscheinlich entzündliche Komponente in stetem stürmischen Umbau, verliert dabei an Stabilität und zeigt dann gerne zahlreiche Looser'sche Umbau-

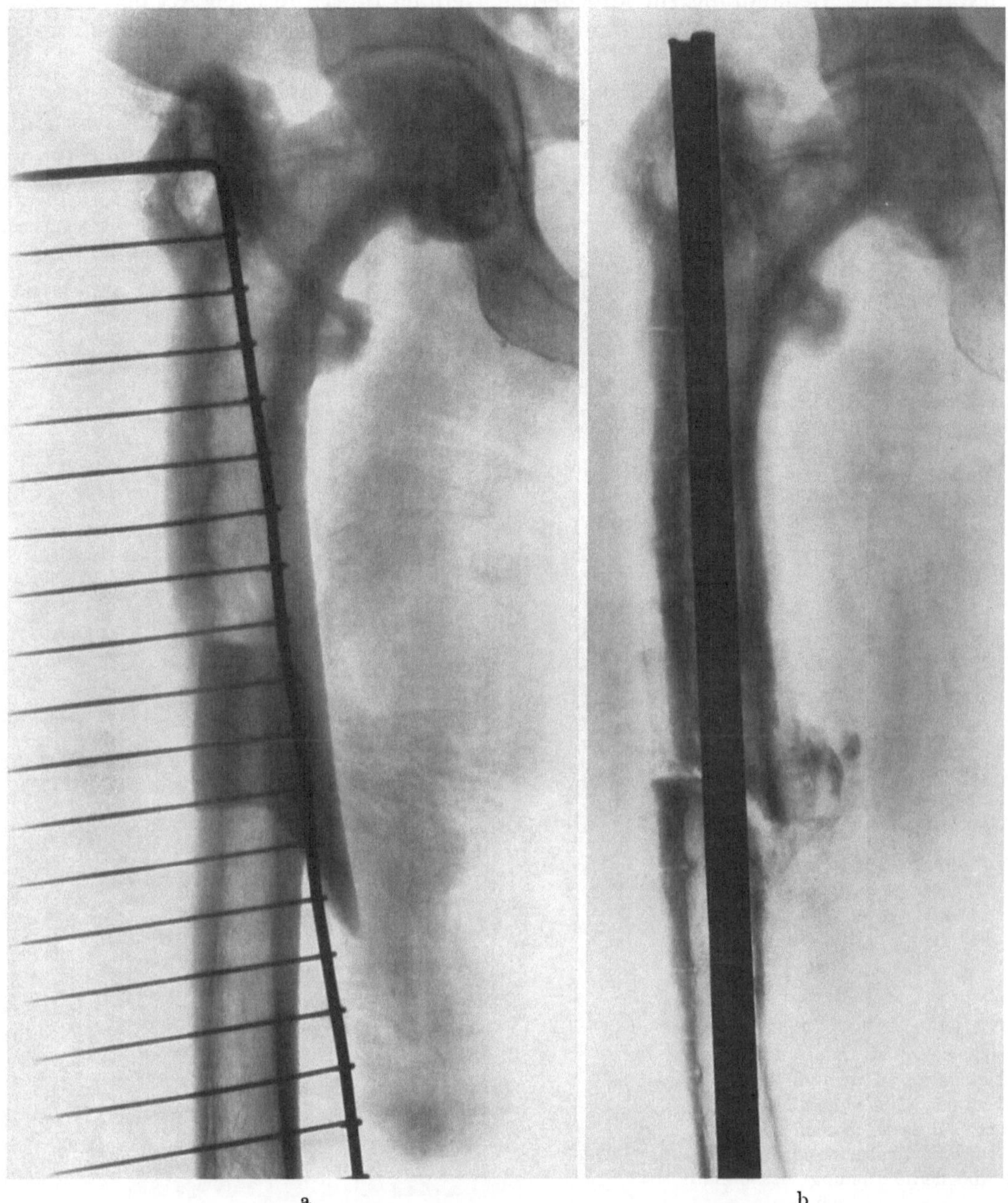

Abb. 67a u. b. 72 Jahre alte Patientin. Traumatische Fraktur im Paget-Knochen. a Typische Frakturform, welche in einer der zahlreichen Looserschen Umbauzonen quer und dann schräg verläuft. b Lebhafte ungeordnete Callusbildung bei noch deutlich sichtbarem Frakturspalt dreieinhalb Monate nach Versorgung mit Marknagel

zonen (Abb. 67). Da dem Knochen zum Umbau Zeit gelassen wird, kommt es wohl seltener zur Spontanfraktur. Die Heilung ist analog dem ohnehin stürmischen Umbau meist mit lebhafter Callusbildung verbunden. Nachdem es uns möglich ist, den Knochen mit einem Marknagel achsengerecht abzustützen, entfällt heute der Nachteil des häufig zu weichen Callus, so daß die Frakturen im Paget-Knochen befriedigend zur Ausheilung gebracht werden können.

Bei allen *gutartigen Cysten oder Tumoren* der Knochen ist die Regenerationskraft nicht nennenswert gestört, so daß der starke Reiz einer Fraktur (meist Spontanfraktur) bei entsprechender Behandlung zur knöchernen Heilung führt. Je nach Art der Erkrankung kann entweder sofort eine Ausräumung vorgenommen werden oder (meist besser) nach Abheilung der Fraktur.

Maligne, destruierende, knochenauflösende primäre Neoplasmen oder Metastasen (Abb. 68) können nach stabiler Versorgung unter Bestrahlungstherapie gut zur knöchernen Ausheilung gebracht werden. Die Verschleppung von Tumorzellen im Markraum durch einen Nagel kann eintreten (JUNGE, 1951). Die Aussicht auf knöcherne Heilung und der große

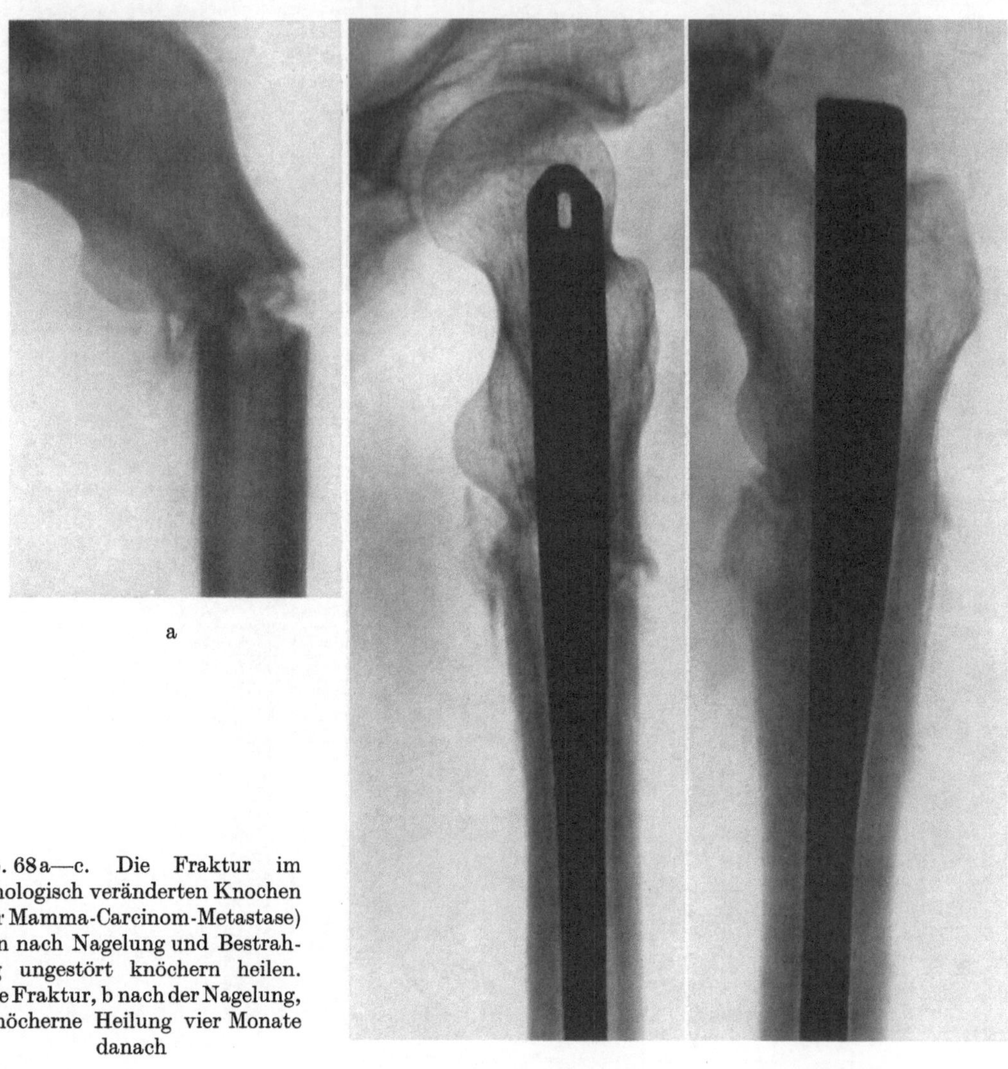

Abb. 68a—c. Die Fraktur im pathologisch veränderten Knochen (hier Mamma-Carcinom-Metastase) kann nach Nagelung und Bestrahlung ungestört knöchern heilen. a Die Fraktur, b nach der Nagelung, c knöcherne Heilung vier Monate danach

Vorteil der pflegerischen Erleichterung durch die Nagelabstützung eines Schaftknochens rechtfertigen den Eingriff aber ganz sicher.

Die erbkonstitutionellen Systemerkrankungen „*Osteogenesis imperfecta*“ und die *Marmorknochenkrankheit* zeigen beide keine Störung in der Knochenbruchheilung. Da erstere meist in frühester Jugend zu zahlreichen Frakturen führt, sind Reposition und Retention schwierig, so daß allzu leicht groteske Fehlheilungen resultieren. Das ist ein Factum, welches um so bedauerlicher ist, als das Leiden mit der Pubertät ausheilt.

Bei der Marmorknochenkrankheit brechen die Knochen ohne Trauma glatt quer und heilen — gerade unter Berücksichtigung der meist ungünstigen Bruchform — erstaunlich gut und in relativ kurzer Zeit (Abb. 69).

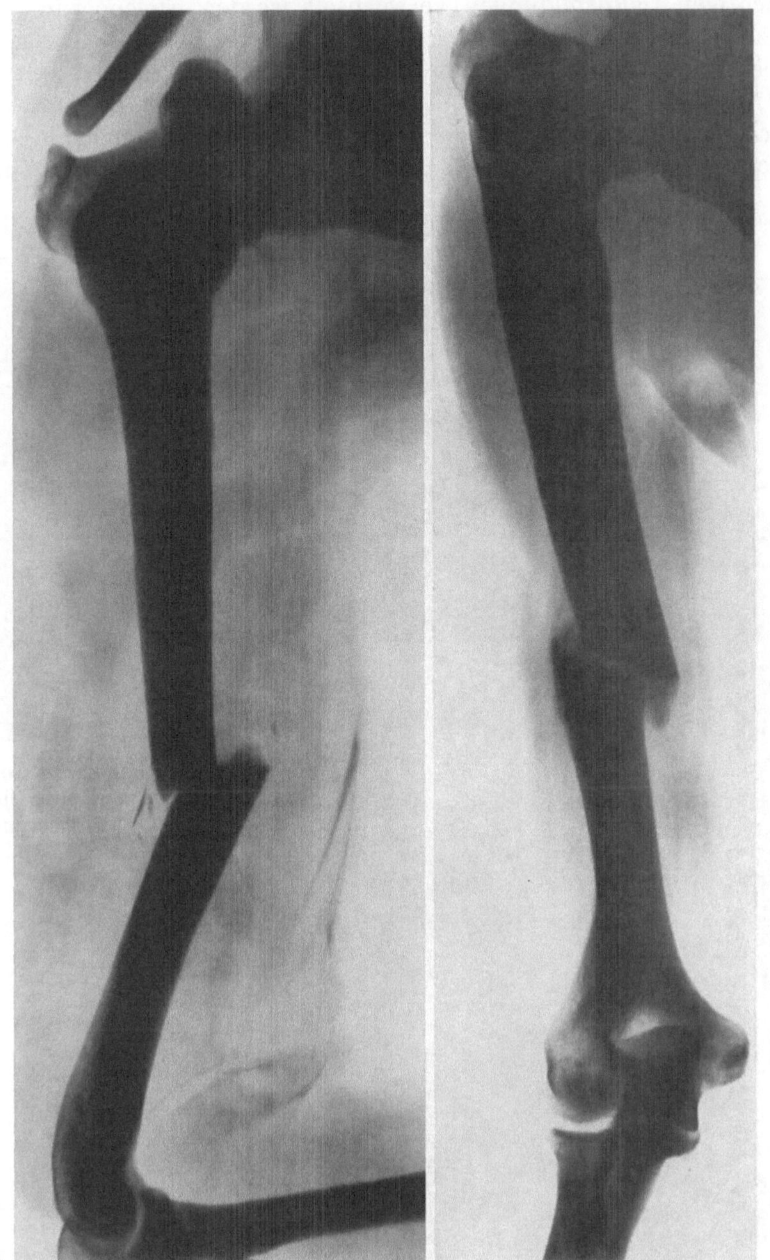

Abb. 69a u. b. 23jährige blinde Patientin mit Marmorknochen-Krankheit. a Spontanfraktur des Humerus, b zehn Wochen danach (Behandlung im Pflaster-Streckverband)

6. Besonderheiten der Callusbildung und Calluserkrankungen, auch Myositis ossificans

Von der Norm grob abweichende oder funktionelle Störungen hervorrufende Arten und Formen in der Callusbildung sind weit häufiger als das, was man eine Calluskrankheit nennen kann. Zudem sind die Übergänge fließend, so daß beides in einem Abschnitt behandelt werden soll.

Eine übermäßige und uns grundlos erscheinende mächtige Callusbildung nennen wir *Callus luxurians*. Sie ist selten, und ihre Ursache im einzelnen nicht geklärt. Sie wird mit der Narbenkeloidbildung verglichen (FRANGENHEIM, 1906 Orth.). Sie darf nicht mit den bisweilen mächtigen Callusbildungen verwechselt werden, welche wir bei ausgeprägten Trümmerbrüchen besonders am Oberschenkel im Bereich des teilweise mitzerrissenen Muskelmantels finden. Dabei kann eine bacterielle Infektion einen weiteren Anreiz zur reichlichen Knochenneubildung geben (BIER, 1923; A. W. FISCHER, 1931).

Die *überschießende Callusbildung* bei Nervenleiden (Lues, Syringomyelie) dürfte eine gesteigerte Form des „Reizcallus" sein. Er wird durch übermäßige mechanische Irritation

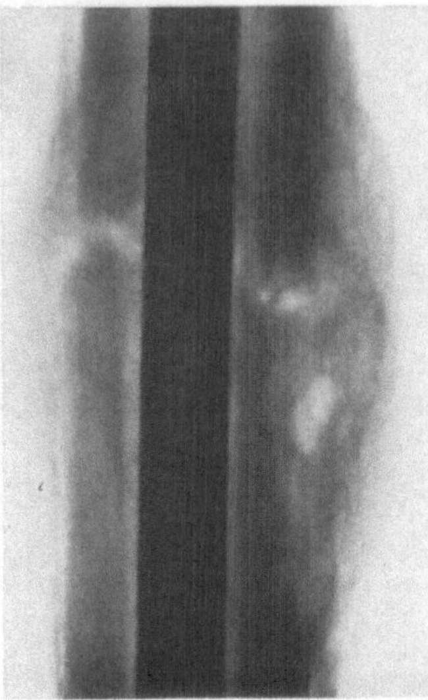

Abb. 71. Calluscysten an vier Monate alter geschlossen genagelter Oberschenkelfraktur eines 18jährigen jungen Mannes

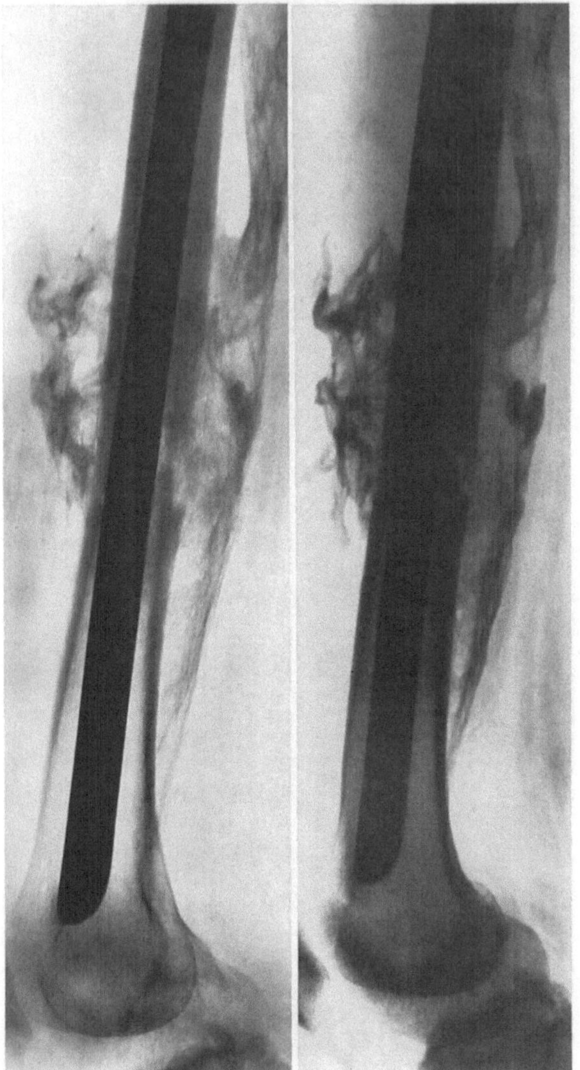

Abb. 70. Sehr ausgedehnte Callusbildung mit Myositis ossificans am Oberschenkel eines 20jährigen Mannes vier Monate nach Nagelung einer geschlossenen Fraktur

hervorgerufen. Sie fehlt jedenfalls dann, wenn es mit einer der Formen der modernen Osteosynthese gelingt, eine solche mechanische Irritation auszuschalten.

Die für die Funktion des Armes verhängnisvolle Form des *Brückencallus* zeigt besonders eindrucksvoll, wie bedenklich es ist, wenn allzuviel von Zielstrebigkeit des Callus gesprochen wird. Sind die nicht zueinander gehörenden Fragmente von Elle und Speiche einander durch ungenügende Reposition zu nahe, oder bestehen ausgedehnte Ablösungen von Periost und Muskelansätzen, so bildet sich die funktionshindernde Brücke. Auch diese ist heute bei exakter Versorgung der Frakturen ein seltenes Ereignis.

Ebenfalls erfreulich selten geworden ist das Bild der *Myositis ossificans traumatica* (Abb. 70). Sie kommt vorwiegend nach Ellenbogengelenkluxationen und supracondylären Frakturen vor. Parossale und intramusculäre Callusbildung gehen so ineinander über, daß man manchmal nicht sagen kann, ob eine Knochenneubildung innerhalb des Muskels als Callusbildung (Frakturfolge) oder unabhängig von der Fraktur entstand (v. SEEMEN,1929; v. DITTRICH, 1926; G. B. GRUBER, 1926 u.a.).

Die Tatsache, daß diese Komplikation früher häufig war, und daß posttraumatisch bewegungseingeschränkte Gelenke mit Massagen und meist gewaltsamen passiven Bewegungsübungen (Brisement) immer wieder „traumatisiert" wurden, spricht dafür, daß ausgedehntere Periostablösungen und Muskelzerreißungen nur dann zur Verkalkung und späteren Verknöcherung führen, wenn das Gewebe immer wieder neu verletzt wird. Unter völliger Ruhigstellung bildet sich diese Erkrankung meist zurück. Sollte sie es nicht tun, so darf erst nach abgeschlossener Bruchheilung, nach Abklingen jeder Neigung zur Callusbildung, eine Resektion vorgenommen werden. WATSON-JONES (1930) und L. BÖHLER (1963) zeigten als erste, daß diese Komplikation fast stets vermeidbar ist.

Neben dem Ellenbogengelenk können vor allem die Kiefergelenke durch eine ossifizierende Myositis befallen werden. Mit der operativen Lösung der Muskelansätze und der damit bedingten vorübergehenden Funktionsausschaltung erreicht man eine völlige Rückbildung (H. BECK, 1954).

Das Auftreten von *Calluscysten* (Abb. 71) sah HENSCHEN (1932) als echte „Callus-Lunker" an, erklärt also ihre Entstehung als Schwindungshohlraum bei zu rascher Auskristallisation, die metallurgisch als „Kristall-Lunker" bezeichnet werden. Nach FELSENREICH (1938), PFAB (1940), ZÖLLNER (1940) können Aufhellungszonen und Cysten durch Zerreißung von Gefäßen oder durch Eindringen von Gelenkschmiere entstehen. Am Wirbelkörper handelt es sich dann um eingedrungenes Bandscheibengewebe.

Bietet der Callus eine deutlich *wabige Struktur*, so wissen wir, daß er wenig belastungsfähig ist. Fragmente, welche durch einen solchen Callus verbunden sind, neigen zur Achsenverbiegung.

Bei zu früher Belastung kann es zur *Callusfraktur* kommen. Analog dem Überlastungsschaden am gesunden oder auch am kranken Knochen kann auch der Callus eine „schleichende Fraktur" zeigen. Da der Callus als junges Knochengewebe ohne lamellären Aufbau in seiner mechanischen Minderleistung mehr einem in seiner Festigkeit erkrankten Knochen gleicht, sollte man die Aufhellungszonen im Callus, welche durch mechanische Zerrüttung auftreten, wohl mehr den Looser'schen Umbauzonen gleichsetzen, welche bei Fortbestehen des mechanischen Störfaktors ja auch zur Pseudarthrose führen können.

7. Besonderheiten bei offenen Frakturen

Es erscheint uns berechtigt, die Besonderheiten der *offenen* Frakturen zusammenfassend herauszustellen, wenn die Einzelheiten auch an der jeweils zutreffenden Stelle besprochen wurden.

Der Begriff „komplizierte Fraktur" sollte für die Frakturen reserviert sein, welche durch Mitverletzung anderer Gewebe, Körperhöhlen oder Organe „kompliziert" sind. So ist die „offene" Fraktur dadurch kompliziert, daß sie durch eine Haut- oder Schleimhautwunde mit der Außenwelt in direkter Verbindung steht.

Ein Vorteil der offenen Fraktur ist die Tatsache, daß sie selten zur Fettembolie führt, und zwar offenbar darum, weil Bruchhämatom und Fett nach außen abfließen. Der Verlust des Bruchhämatoms hat im allgemeinen den Nachteil, daß der Blutkuchen mit der folgenden fibrinösen Verspannung der Fragmente fehlt, so daß verzögerte Verfestigungen und Pseudarthrosen häufiger auftreten als bei geschlossenen Frakturen. Dieser Nachteil bleibt auch dann bestehen, wenn es durch sachgemäße Erstbehandlung gelingt, aus der offenen eine geschlossene Fraktur mit primärer Heilung der Weichteilwunde zu machen (Abb. 72). Wirklich nachteilig aber wirkt sich dieses Moment nur dann aus, wenn es nicht gelingt, die Fragmente stabil miteinander zu verbinden. Nach stabiler Vereinigung und primärer Wundheilung wirkt sich die verzögerte Heilung klinisch nicht nennenswert aus, und Pseudarthrosen sind nicht zu befürchten.

Jede offene Fraktur ist als „infiziert“ anzusehen. Je schonender und stabiler eine solche Fraktur versorgt wird (absolute Ruhigstellung der Fragmente), um so häufiger gelingt es, das Angehen einer Infektion zu verhindern.

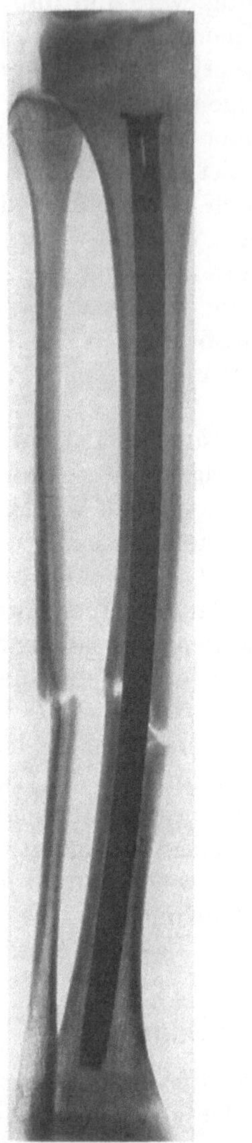

Abb. 72

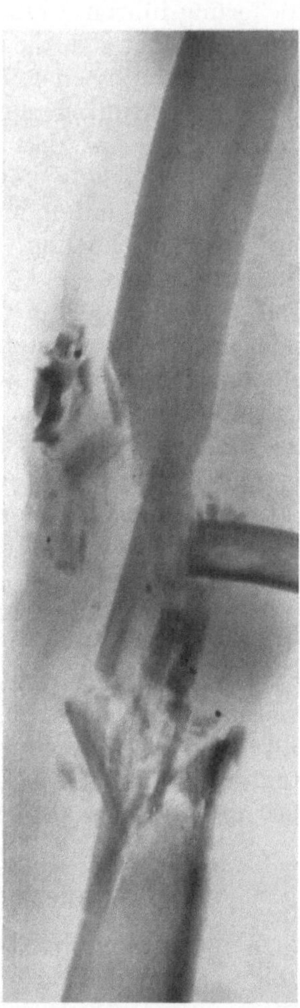

Abb. 73

Abb. 72. Bei der 15 Jahre alten Patientin wurde die offene Fraktur des Unterschenkels in der Tibia genagelt. Wundheilung komplikationslos. Das Kontrollbild wurde sieben Wochen nach dem Unfall bzw. der Nagelung angefertigt. Es zeigt in der Lücke zwischen den Fragmenten keine Spur von Callus. Der Verlauf war dank der stabilen Osteosynthese komplikationslos

Abb. 73. Wenige Tage alter Schußbruch des Femur bei 22jährigem Mann. Splitterung mit Defektbildung (Drain im Wundgebiet)

8. Besonderheiten bei Schußbrüchen

Schußbrüche sind zwangsweise offene Frakturen, und ihre Verschmutzung ist durch mitgerissene Stoff-Fetzen häufig besonders stark. Meist sind sie auch breit offen, da das den Knochen treffende Projektil diesen zersplittert (Abb. 73) und Knochensplitter als sekundäre Projektile wirken (kleiner Einschuß — großer Ausschuß). Hinzu kommt eine weitgehende Gewebszertrümmerung mit folgender Nekrose, so daß der Boden für das Angehen von Infektionen, auch der Anaerobier, günstig ist. Selbstredend sind Mitverletzung von Nerven und Gefäßen außerordentlich häufig, so daß die Mortalität besonders des Oberschenkelschußbruches (Verbluten) bereits primär außerordentlich hoch ist.

Durch Infektion und durch Substanzverlust am Knochen ist die Zahl der resultierenden Pseudarthrosen ebenfalls groß. Dabei ist allerdings besonders eindrucksvoll, daß schlecht oder gar nicht versorgte Schußbrüche des Femur, wie wir sie in den letzten Notzeiten des vergangenen Krieges sahen, unter zum Teil grotesker Verkürzung meist knöchern heilten — vergleichbar etwa der Knochenheilung in freier Wildbahn.

Schußkanäle in Spongiosa bei sonst intaktem Knochen können noch nach Monaten nachweisbar sein. Die Annahme von LAUCHE (1937), daß die Ursache für die sehr langsame Ausfüllung des Knochendefektes im Fehlen des Bewegungsreizes liege, kann nicht zutreffen, da der Loch- oder Leer-Test im Spongiosa-Test (MAATZ, 1954) sich stets rasch mit Callus füllt. Vielmehr kommt wohl ursächlich die Commotionsnekrose des umgebenden Knochens in Frage. ARNOLD (1873) beschrieb Zonen bis zu 3 cm vom Defektrand entfernt.

9. Besonderheiten bei Epiphyseolysen

Die traumatisch bedingte Lösung einer Wachstumsfuge geht regelmäßig mit einer mehr oder minder ausgedehnten Periostabtrennung einher, welche manschettenartig von der Epiphyse über die Epiphysenfuge hinweg zur Diaphyse zieht. Besonders eindrucksvoll zeigen das die Bilder der Abb. 74. Gleichzeitig demonstrieren sie die geradezu wunderbare Korrekturmöglichkeit im Wachstum im frühen Lebensalter.

Die *Chondroephiphyseolyse* ist die seltene glatte Ablösung des Epiphysenknorpels von der Knochensubstanz der Diaphyse. Hierbei haftet die Knorpelfuge ganz an der Epiphyse.

Am häufigsten ist die Epiphysenlösung mit einer Fraktur vergesellschaftet. Die Trennungslinie verläuft eine Strecke im verkalkten Fugenknorpel und biegt dann schräg in die Metaphyse um, so daß an einer Seite der gelösten Epiphyse ein keilförmiges Knochenstück der Diaphyse haftet (Osteoepiphyseolyse).

Gut reponierte Epiphysen zeigen in der Regel keinerlei Störungen im Wachstum, unzureichend reponierte sogar ein erfreulich ausgeprägtes korrigierendes Wachstum. Zu berücksichtigen ist dabei allerdings, daß die distalen Enden der Speichen eine gewisse Variationsbreite haben (EHALT 1960). Es kann vor allem der Winkel zwischen Speichenschaft und distaler Gelenkfläche, der in dorso-volarem Strahlengang gesehen, gewöhnlich 30°, radial, und seitlich gesehen 10° volar beträgt, um 5 bis 10° schwanken.

Wachstumsstörungen nach Epiphyseolyse resultieren meist nur nach vollkommen unzureichender Reposition oder nach offenen Verletzungen mit folgender Eiterung (WEBER, 1949).

10. Besonderheiten bei Frakturen am Schädel

Sowohl im Bereich der Schädelcalotte als auch an der Schädelbasis ist die Callus bildung nach Frakturen meist spärlich. Die gute Reposition einmal und die fehlende Beweglichkeit als Mangel an Reiz zum anderen wurden beschuldigt (MATTI, 1931), während das Fehlen des interfragmentären Hämatoms und mangelnde Fähigkeit der Galea zur Knochenneubildung die Hauptgründe abgeben dürften. In der Regel heilen Fissuren knöchern, beanspruchen dazu aber Monate bis über ein Jahr. Besonders Basisfrakturen neigen zum andauernden Ausbleiben der knöchernen Konsolidation. Das eingeschaltete Bindegewebe bildet allerdings einen funktionell voll ausreichenden Ersatz.

Kleine Defekte können sich knöchern schließen, und das um so leichter, je jünger das Individuum. Größere Defekte verkleinern sich zwar vom Rande her, die Regenerationskraft ist aber meist frühzeitig erschöpft. Es sollen sich handtellergroße Defekte am Schädeldach geschlossen haben (KÜSTER, 1889; SONNENBERG, 1922; STROBE, 1922). In der Knochenregeneration soll die Dura als „inneres Periost" die tragende Rolle spielen (KOCHER, 1901; BEREZOWSKI, 1899), während GÖRS (1914) der Diploe die Hauptrolle in der Regeneration zuschreiben möchte.

Wir glauben wohl, daß in dem ungünstigen Frakturmilieu am Schädeldach die Regenerationskraft der Knochenwundränder relativ früh erschöpft ist. Die Tatsache, daß bei

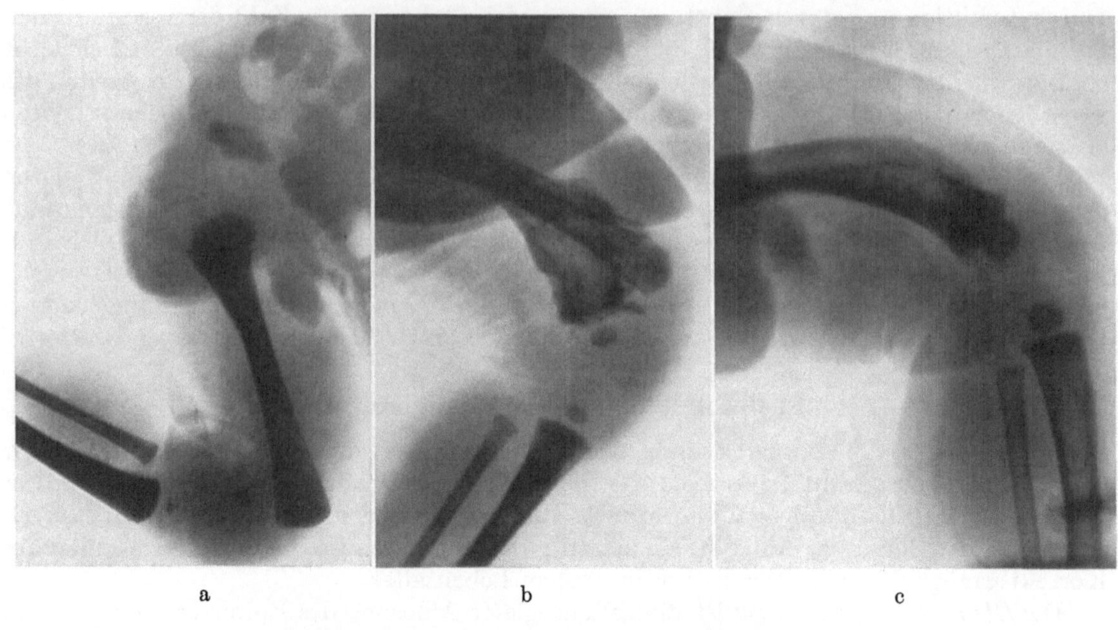

a b c

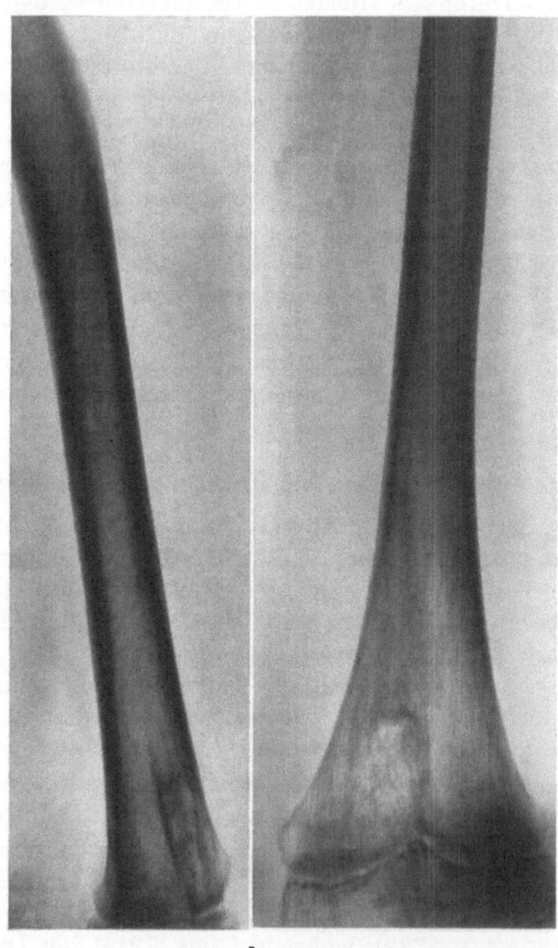

d

Abb. 74a—d. Epiphyseolyse unter der Geburt mit vollkommener Wachstums-Korrektur. a Die dislozierte Epiphyse ließ sich unblutig nicht reponieren. b ein Monat danach, c sechs Monate danach, d acht Jahre später äußerlich völlig unauffälliges Bein, keine Längendifferenz. (SCHINZ)

Defekten eine vorzeitige Vereinigung der Weichgewebe stattfindet (GREKOW, 1922), so daß eine Art Interposition von Weichgeweben vorliegt, ist zwar ein Factum, wird aber kaum als entscheidendes Moment angesehen werden dürfen.

11. Besonderheiten bei Mehrfach-Brüchen

Multiple Frakturen sind der Schwere des Unfalls und dem Trauma an mehreren Stellen entsprechend im allgemeinen von einem schweren Schock begleitet. Als zweite große Gefahr droht die Fettembolie, welche bei geschlossenen und offenen Frakturen gleichzeitig die frühzeitige endgültige Versorgung der offenen Fraktur verbietet. So werden nagelfähige Extremitätenfrakturen, welche neben Thorax- oder Beckenbrüchen bestehen, zunächst nur mit Extensions- und Gipsverbänden versorgt.

Multiple Frakturen stellen an Patienten und Pflegepersonal höchste Anforderungen. Sind die ersten Gefahren des Schocks und der Fettembolie gebannt, bieten die verschiedenen Formen der modernen Osteosynthese gerade bei diesen Verletzten außerordentliche Vorteile, da sie frühzeitig von Streck- und Gipsverbänden befreit werden können.

Doppelbrüche oder Stückbrüche bieten im allgemeinen keine besonderen Probleme, da sich die Fragmente auf Nagel oder Rush pin auffädeln lassen. Die Tibia allerdings neigt bei Doppelbrüchen in starkem Maße zur verzögerten Verfestigung einer der Frakturen, wobei einmal die proximale, häufiger aber die distale Fraktur diese Störung zeigt.

12. Die ischämische Kontraktur

Die ischämische Kontraktur, welche erstmals von v. VOLKMANN, 1881 als „Lähmung" beschrieben wurde, wird heute erfreulicherweise nur sehr selten beobachtet. Sie stellt vor allem nach supracondylärer Fraktur beim Kind die schwerste Komplikation dar. Es handelt sich um eine teilweise oder völlige Vernarbung der Muskulatur nach ischämischem scholligen Zerfall. Die starken Beuger überwiegen und ziehen die Finger zur Faust in die Hohlhand. Eine derartig verhängnisvolle Durchblutungsstörung kann bei der genannten Fraktur am ehesten dann auftreten, wenn die Fragmente unzureichend reponiert bleiben, so daß die Cubitalarterie über einem Fragment reitend gedrosselt ist, oder durch zirkuläre schnürende Verbände, oder — selbstredend — durch beide genannte Faktoren zusammen. Wie die Entwicklung bewiesen hat, läßt sich diese Komplikation bei sachgemäßer Behandlung weitgehend vermeiden. Es besteht aber doch kein Zweifel, daß sie auch unter kunstgerechter ärztlicher Betreuung auftreten kann, und zwar besonders leicht bei indolenten oder überempfindlichen Kindern, welche die Prüfung der Beweglichkeit der Finger während der ersten Stunden nach der Versorgung in Narkose erschweren oder unmöglich machen.

Frühzeitige langdauernde Quengelbehandlung ergibt in nicht schweren Fällen gute Erfolge. In Spätfällen kann bei vorhandener Restfunktion der Muskulatur durch Knochenverkürzung oder besser durch Versetzung der Muskelursprünge eine wesentliche Besserung erreicht werden.

13. Die posttraumatische Arthrosis deformans

Die posttraumatische Arthrosis deformans entsteht am häufigsten nach Gelenkfrakturen, kann aber auch „indirekt" nach Schaftfrakturen entstehen, welche in Fehlstellung geheilt zur Fehlbelastung eines Gelenkes und damit zum vorzeitigen Verschleiß des Knorpels führen (Abb. 75). Besonders gefährdet sind aus nur zu verständlichen Gründen die Gelenke der unteren Extremität wegen der stärkeren mechanischen Belastung. So wird schon bei der subcapitalen Schenkelhalsfraktur die Arthrosis deformans ohne nachweisbare Kopfnekrose mit 15% (SALEM, 1951) und 21% (MAATZ und LEMPERT, 1952) angegeben. Die Arthrosis deformans nach Tibiakopffrakturen wird als die Regel angesehen. Dabei ist an diesem Gelenk allerdings zu bedenken, daß mancher frakturbedingte „Randwulst“ nicht arthrotisch, sondern frakturbedingt ist. Entscheidend ist die Beschaffenheit des Gelenkknorpels (Maatz, 1952).

Erschreckend hoch ist die Zahl der Fälle der posttraumatischen Arthrosis deformans nach Patellafrakturen. Dabei ist eine röntgenologisch nachweisbare Arthrosis keineswegs immer mit Schmerzen verbunden. Schönbauer (1955) fand bei 274 nachuntersuchten Fällen in 21 % eine leichte und in 4 % eine schwere Arthrosis.

Überraschend waren die Angaben der österreichischen Autoren auf dem Treffen der Unfallchirurgen 1966 in Salzburg, welche darin übereinstimmten, daß Frakturen im oberen

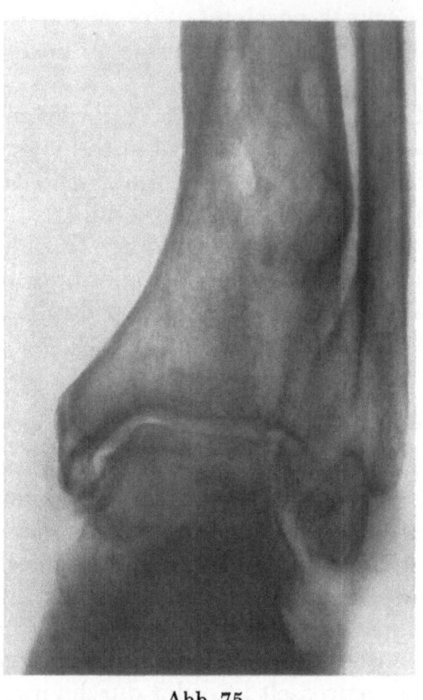

Abb. 75

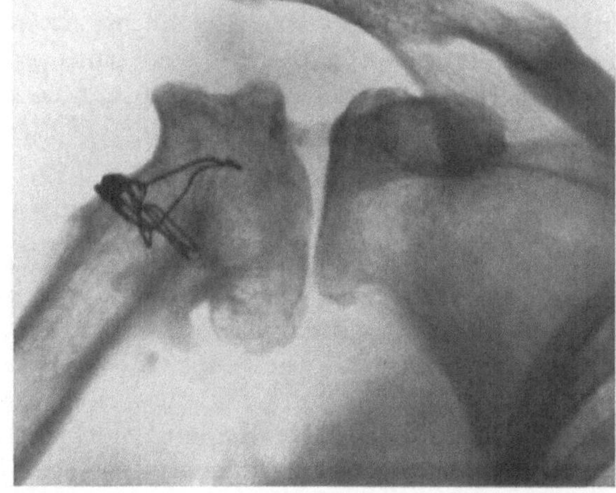

Abb. 76

Abb. 75. 75 Jahre alte Patientin. Posttraumatische Arthrosis deformans im oberen Sprunggelenk nach Heilung einer distalen Unterschenkelfraktur in Fehlstellung. Die Verletzung liegt dreieinhalb Jahre zurück

Abb. 76. Schwere posttraumatische deformierende Arthrosis nach Humeruskopffraktur, welche vor vierzig Jahren mit Drahtnaht versorgt wurde

Sprunggelenk 5 Jahre nach der Verletzung nahezu ausnahmslos eine Arthrosis deformans zeigen (Ehalt u. L. Böhler, 1966).

Allen verständlich ist die schwere posttraumatische Arthrosis deformans nach der seltenen Fraktur im anatomischen Hals des Humerus, weil hier ähnlich wie am Hüftkopf meist eine Nekrose die Folge ist (Abb. 76).

14. Die posttraumatische Osteolyse

Die Vorstellung, daß jede Fraktur mit einer geringen Verkürzung heilen muß (L. Böhler, 1963) ist durch die neuen Erkenntnisse, welche durch die moderne Osteosynthese gewonnen wurden, nicht mehr aufrechtzuerhalten (Nagelung, Küntscher, 1940; Druckplatten der Schweizer A. O.). Am Schenkelhals aber tritt nach medialer Fraktur praktisch regelmäßig ein Schenkelhalsschwund auf, ein Vorgang also, den wir mit Recht als eine posttraumatische Osteolyse bezeichnen können. An anderen frakturierten Knochen gehört dieser Vorgang zur größten Seltenheit. Uehlinger (zit. bei Alnor) führte drei Fälle von kryptogenetischer lokalisierter Osteolyse an, und zwar handelte es sich um Zustandsbilder nach Frakturen des Metacarpale 2 und der Ulna. Werder (1950) und Alnor (1951) beschrieben je einen eindrucksvollen Fall von posttraumatischer Osteolyse des lateralen Claviculaendes. Es fehlte in diesen Fällen allerdings der sichere Nachweis der Fraktur, welche nach der Art der Verletzung sehr wohl möglich und nach dem posttraumatischen Verlauf wohl doch vorgelegen haben dürfte. Die Röntgenbilder der Abb. 77 zeigen den Fall von ALNOR (1951) vierzehn Monate nach der Verletzung. Auf der erkrankten Seite besteht ein Defekt von 25 mm Länge, während direkt nach dem Trauma der Spalt im Akromio-Claviculargelenk 5 mm betrug.

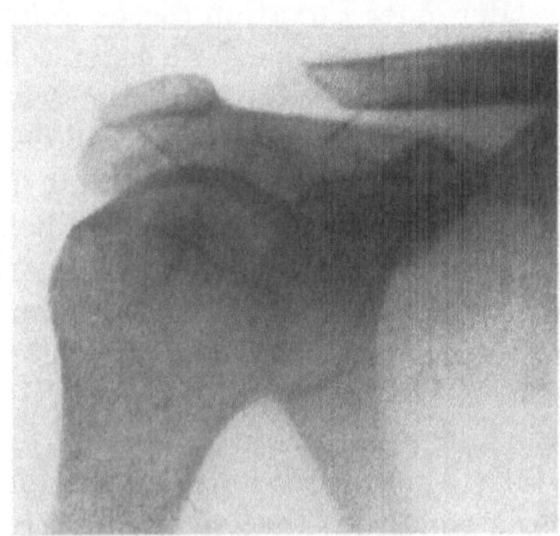

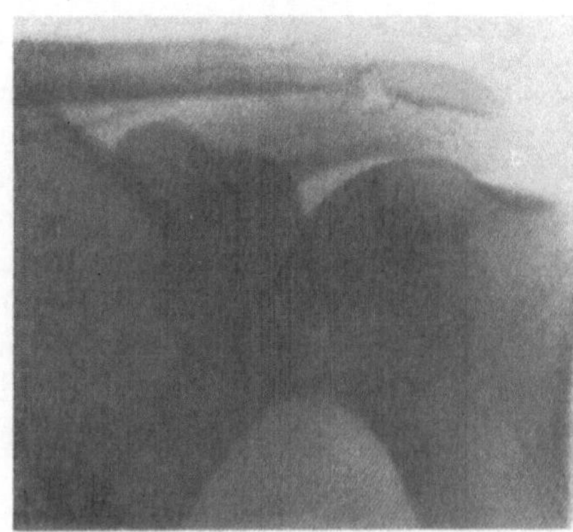

Abb. 77. Posttraumatische Osteolyse am lateralen Claviculaende. [Aus: ALNOR, Fortschritte auf dem Gebiet der Röntgenstrahlen und der Nuklearmedizin. 75, 365 (1951)]

15. Akzidentelle Schädigungen

Ungewollte Schäden, welche dem Patienten während der Behandlung einer Fraktur zusätzlich zugefügt werden, können vor allem durch *Druck*, *Schnürung* oder durch *Wärmeeinwirkung* entstehen.

Umschriebener Druck von kürzester Dauer kann eine Nervenlähmung hervorrufen, die dann meist reversibel ist. Besonders gefährdet ist der N. peronaeus bei hüftgelenknahen Frakturen alter Menschen. Vermeidbar ist diese Störung selbst bei größter Sorgfalt nicht. Es ist noch nicht geklärt, ob Repositionsmanöver, Zug am Ischiadicus oder tatsächlich nur der so leicht mögliche Druck einer Schienenkante hinterm Fibulaköpfchen die Ursache ist.

Drucknekrosen ohne oder mit Gipsverband lassen sich ebenfalls nicht immer vermeiden (BÖHLER, 1963). Besonders groß ist die Gefahr bei hinfälligen Patienten mit Durchblutungsstörungen. Beim *Heftpflaster-Streckverband*, den wir beim Kleinkind zur Behandlung der Oberschenkelfraktur am ganzen Bein anlegen und am Oberarm beim Humerussplitterbruch, besteht die Gefahr, daß der meist langsam auf der Haut rutschende Verband am Fußrücken bzw. in der Ellenbeuge sehr langsam schmerzlos einschneidend eine Drucknekrose hervorruft. Das gleitende Pflaster kann auf der Haut Blasen ziehen.

Besonders gefährlich ist die Schnürung einer Extremität, welche bei zirkulären Verbänden durch Behinderung des venösen Abflusses zu einer Art Incarceration mit Gangrän führen kann. Vorübergehende Ischämie der Muskulatur führt zu schweren Kontrakturen (siehe S. 595).

Wenig bekannt war bisher die Tatsache, daß die unter dem Gipsverband entstehende Wärme zu schweren und ausgedehnten Verbrennungen führen kann (HAASCH, 1963). Abb. 78 zeigt eine tiefgehende Verbrennung unter einem nur an den Knochenvorsprüngen gepolsterten Gipsverband. Untersuchungen ergaben, daß im Gipsverband mehr als 50° Celsius auftreten können, wenn das Eintauchwasser zu warm, die Binden nur sehr kurz eingetaucht und zu stark ausgedrückt werden und die Schicht mindestens 10- bis 12fach ist. Ein derartiger Verbrennungsschaden ist also bei entsprechender Sorgfalt wohl vermeidbar.

Zu den akzidentellen Schäden müssen wir die *„traumatisierende" Nachbehandlung* rechnen. Böhlers (1963) Grundsatz, daß jede Nachbehandlung ohne Schmerzen sein soll, trifft sicher den Kern. Matti schrieb 1918 in seinem ausgezeichneten Buch über die Frakturen und ihre Behandlung, etwa sinngemäß, „daß das weiche Herz einer Mutter für die mobilisierende Nachbehandlung einer ellenbogengelenknahen Fraktur oder einer Luxation dieses Gelenks beim Kind völlig ungeeignet sei." Zu jener Zeit war die „Myositis ossificans" eine häufig beobachtete Komplikation. Heute wissen wir, daß der Chirurg seine ganze Autorität einsetzen muß, das Kind vor jeglicher mobilisierenden Nachbehandlung durch Hausarzt, Masseuse oder „energischen" Vater zu schützen, um die Beweglichkeit möglichst ungestört sich wieder einspielen zu lassen. Als Resultat kennen wir die Myositis ossificans heute nur noch als Rarität.

Was für das Ellenbogengelenk beim Kind in so hohem Ausmaß gilt, hat an allen Extremitätengelenken seine Gültigkeit. Damit soll nicht in Abrede gestellt werden, daß in Einzelfällen zur gegebenen Zeit ein in Narkose (also schmerzfrei) durchgeführtes Brisement durchaus angebracht sein kann.

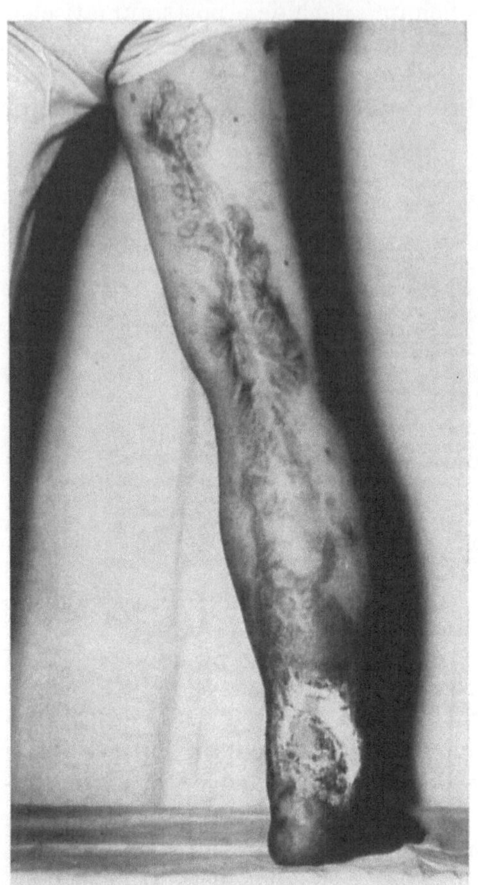

Abb. 78. Ausgedehnte Narbenbildung bei 69jährigem Mann eineinhalb Jahre nach Verbrennung unterm Gipsverband

16. Heilung in Fehlstellung, ihre Bedeutung für die Funktion, ihr spontaner Ausgleich und ihre operative Korrektur

Vor Einführung der am Knochen angreifenden Extension heilte die Mehrzahl der Schaftfrakturen in Verkürzung, aber die Frakturen heilten rasch. Durch die Extension, welche nicht selten zur Überextension gesteigert wurde und auch heute noch wird, kann die Verkürzung zwar vermieden werden, verzögerte Verfestigungen und bisweilen sogar Pseudarthrosen sind die Folge. Die Forderung von L. Böhler (1963), jede Fraktur müsse mit einer (geringen) Verkürzung heilen, besteht sicher nicht zu Recht. Das beweisen die Ergebnisse bei Nagelung und Druckosteosynthese (A. O.). Beim wachsenden Individuum aber kann eine leichte Verkürzung durchaus zweckmäßig sein, denn mit der Frakturheilung ist meist ein vermehrtes Wachstum des befallenen Knochens verbunden. Flach und Kudlich (1962) fanden es nahezu ausnahmslos und beobachteten am Femur beim Kind maximal 4 cm, allerdings bei einer mit Marknagel versorgten Patientin.

Achsenkorrekte Verkürzungen an der unteren Extremität können zu Fernschäden führen, wenn sie nicht durch Sohlenerhöhung zum mindesten teilweise ausgeglichen werden (Abb. 79).

Ein stärkerer Achsenknick führt zur *scheinbaren* Verkürzung des Beines. Stärker bemerkbar macht sich dieses vor allem am langen Oberschenkelknochen. Nachteilig ist der Achsenknick aber vor allem für die Nachbargelenke. Besonders gefährdet sind hier das Kniegelenk und das obere Sprunggelenk, wobei letzteres an erster Stelle rangiert (Abb. 75). Es ist einleuchtend, daß eine mäßige Antekurvation oder Rekurvation am

Unterschenkel vom Fußgelenk schadlos ertragen wird, während ein geringfügiger Achsenknick im O- oder X-Sinne durch die damit verbundene Fehlbelastung am oberen Sprunggelenk zur Arthrosis deformans führen kann. L. Böhler (1963) gibt als tragbare Grenze $<4°$ an.

Für das Kniegelenk können auch Antekurvation, vor allem aber Rekurvation im Femur zum arthrotischen Schaden führen, da die Patienten stets das Bemühen haben, auf einem äußerlich korrekten Bein zu gehen. Damit ergibt sich bei einem Antekurvationsfehler eine völlige Streckung beim Aufsetzen des Beines, beim Rekurvationsfehler eine zu

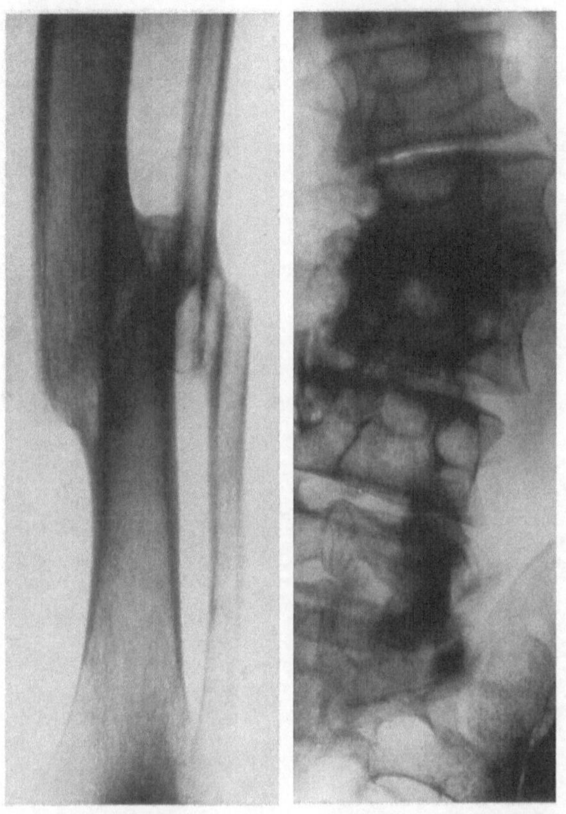

Abb. 79. Die geschlossene Unterschenkelfraktur links, welche mit 4 cm Verkürzung achsengerecht heilte, führte ohne Längenausgleich im Schuh zur Skoliose der Wirbelsäule

weitgehende Beugestellung mit entsprechender mangelhafter Standfestigkeit. Wird das Knie aber voll belastet, so bedeutet dieses eine gewaltsame Überstreckung, also eine chronische Schädigung. Am Unterarm hat selbst ein geringer Achsenknick des einen oder beider Knochen meist eine Einschränkung der Rotation zur Folge.

Der wachsende Knochen vermag Fehlstellungen in zum Teil wunderbarem Ausmaß auszugleichen, (König, 1908; Müller, 1924; Jeffery, 1929; Hohmann, 1933). Wir verweisen auch auf die Röntgenbilder der Epiphyseolyse der Abb. 74.

Abb. 80 zeigt eine supracondyläre Fraktur, welche in „typischer“ Fehlstellung konsolidierte. Der Knabe ging während der ersten sechs Monate nach Aufstehbelastung nahezu normal und unauffällig, zeigte aber eine der Fehlstellung entsprechende erschreckende Überstreckbarkeit im Kniegelenk. Diese schwand von Quartal zu Quartal durch korrigierendes Wachstum.

Gangler suchte 1934 aus 5000 Fällen der Tübinger Klinik solche aus, die in Fehlstellung geheilt waren. Alle Frakturen lagen zwanzig bis dreißig Jahre zurück. Die Gruppe der Jugendlichen bis zu achtzehn Jahren zeigte praktisch keinerlei Funktionsstörungen, obgleich ein Teil der Frakturen in extrem schlechter Stellung geheilt war. Andere

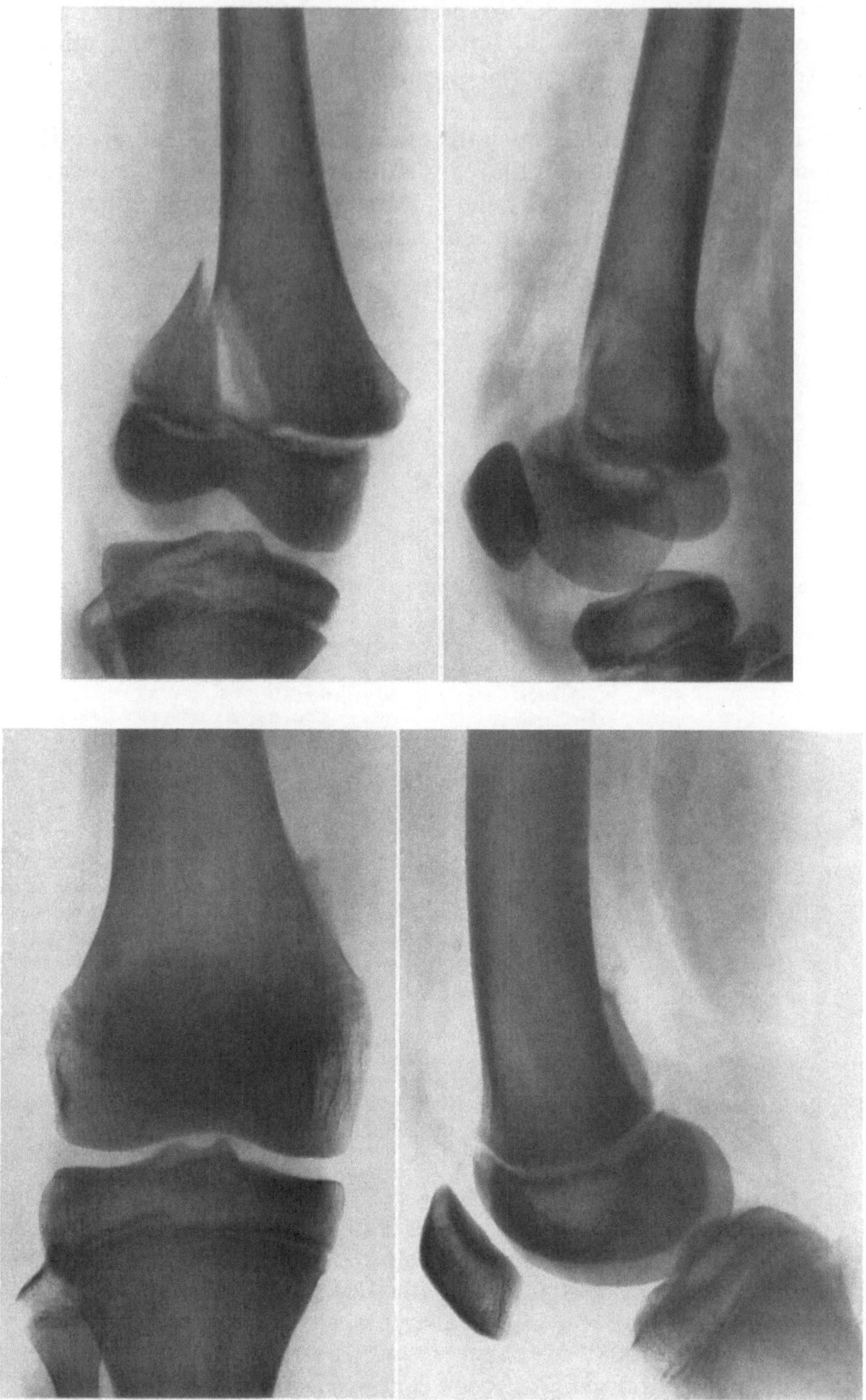

Abb. 80. Vollkommene Wachstumskorrektur im Verlauf von vier Jahren nach unvollständiger Reposition einer Osteoepiphyseolyse am Femur. Zur Zeit der Verletzung war der Knabe 9 Jahre alt

Autoren (NAUJOKS, 1934; ÖNNE u. SANDBLOM, 1949; KERN u. NENNINGER, 1954; MATZNER, 1959) bestätigen diese Beobachtung. Damit ergibt sich für uns die Verpflichtung, die Indikation zur operativen Früh- oder Spätkorrektur besonders sorgfältig zu prüfen. Eine Übersicht über alle Arten der Fehlstellungen mit kritischer Auswertung, wann wir mit Sicherheit eine spontane Korrektur erwarten können, gibt es leider noch nicht. Hinweisend ist die Tatsache, daß Fehlstellungen nach supracondylären Frakturen

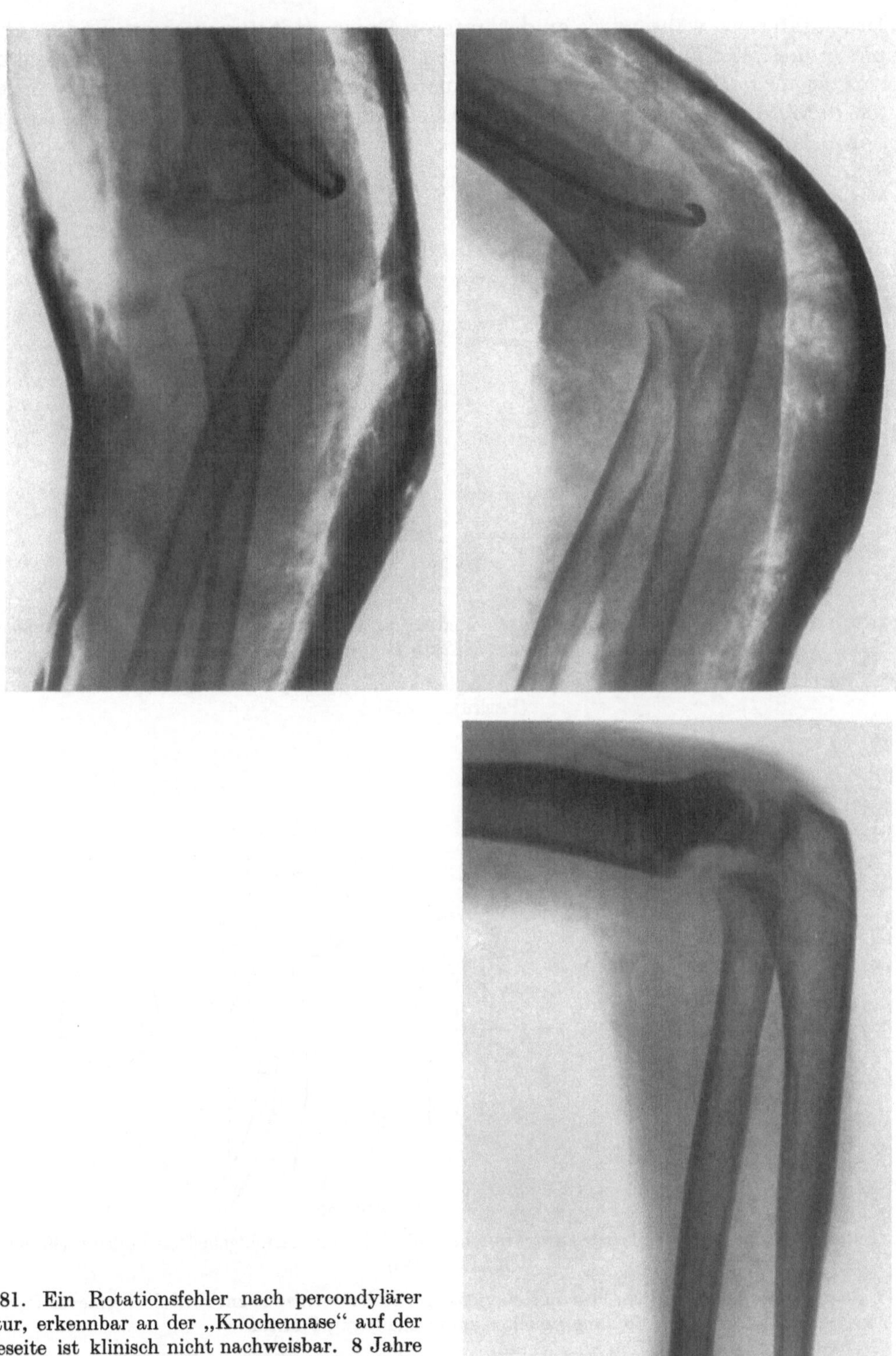

Abb. 81. Ein Rotationsfehler nach percondylärer Fraktur, erkennbar an der „Knochennase" auf der Beugeseite ist klinisch nicht nachweisbar. 8 Jahre alter Knabe. Zwischen den Aufnahmen liegen dreieinhalb Monate

des Humerus oder Condylusbrüche im kindlichen Alter mit Fehlstellung (meist O-Stellung) sich nicht spontan korrigieren. Offenbar findet die Hueter-Volkmann'sche Vorstellung (1875), daß gesteigerter Druck das Wachstum in der Fuge hemmt, verminderter Druck es steigert, hier ihre Bestätigung, denn am meist in Beugestellung gebrauchten Arm fehlt diese Druckdifferenz, während sie an der unteren Extremität und auch am Radius als dem Stützpfeiler des Unterarms sicher vorhanden ist. *Rotationsfehler* im ellenbogengelenknahen Humerus, wie er nach supracondylärer oder percondylärer Fraktur sehr häufig vorkommt und sich durch die „Knochennase" in der Ellenbeuge demonstriert (Abb. 81) ist für die Funktion belanglos.

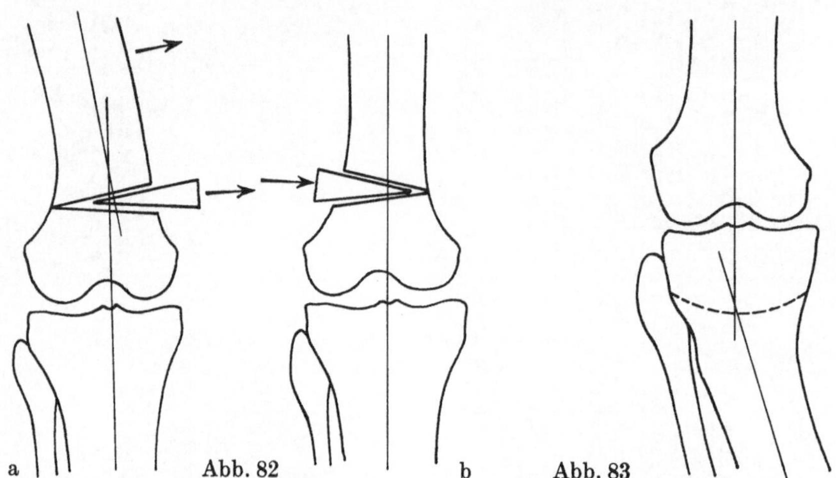

Abb. 82 a u. b. Korrektur einer in X-Stellung fehlgeheilten supracondylären Femurfraktur. a Durch Herausnahme eines Knochenkeiles (MAYER-SCHEDE 1852). b Durch Einfügen eines Knochenkeiles

Abb. 83. Korrektur einer in O-Stellung geheilten kniegelenknahen Tibiafraktur durch bogenförmige Osteotomie (PERTHES, 1923)

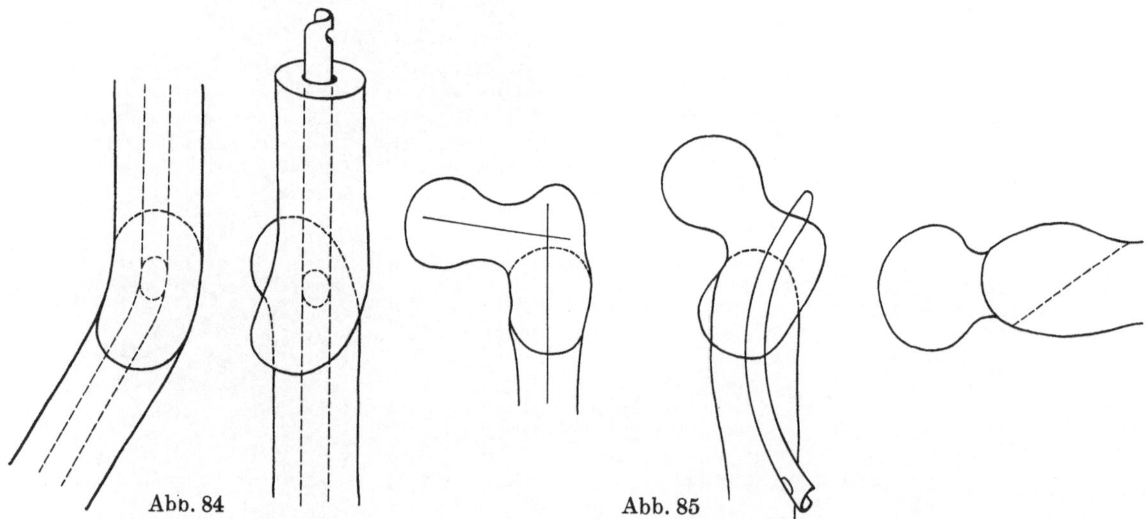

Abb. 84. Helferich'sche Osteotomie zur Korrektur einer mit Achsenknick fehlgeheilten Fraktur (KÜNTSCHER-MAATZ, 1945)

Abb. 85. Schrägosteotomie nach dem Prinzip Helferichs im Trochantermassiv zur Korrektur einer in Coxa vara-Stellung geheilten subtrochanteren Fraktur

Nur der aufmerksame Untersucher findet Rotationsfehler selbst ausgeprägteren Grades an Femur und Tibia. Während letztere sofort an der Fußstellung erkennbar ist, wenn der Patient auf planem Tisch sitzend die Unterschenkel zwanglos herabhängen läßt, verbirgt sich der Rotationsfehler am Oberschenkel, weil der Patient den Fuß beim Gehen durch Innenrotation in der Hüfte in die (wenn möglich) richtige Stellung bringt. Röntgenologisch ist diese Fehlheilung schwer oder gar nicht erfaßbar. Daß diese Rotationsfehler

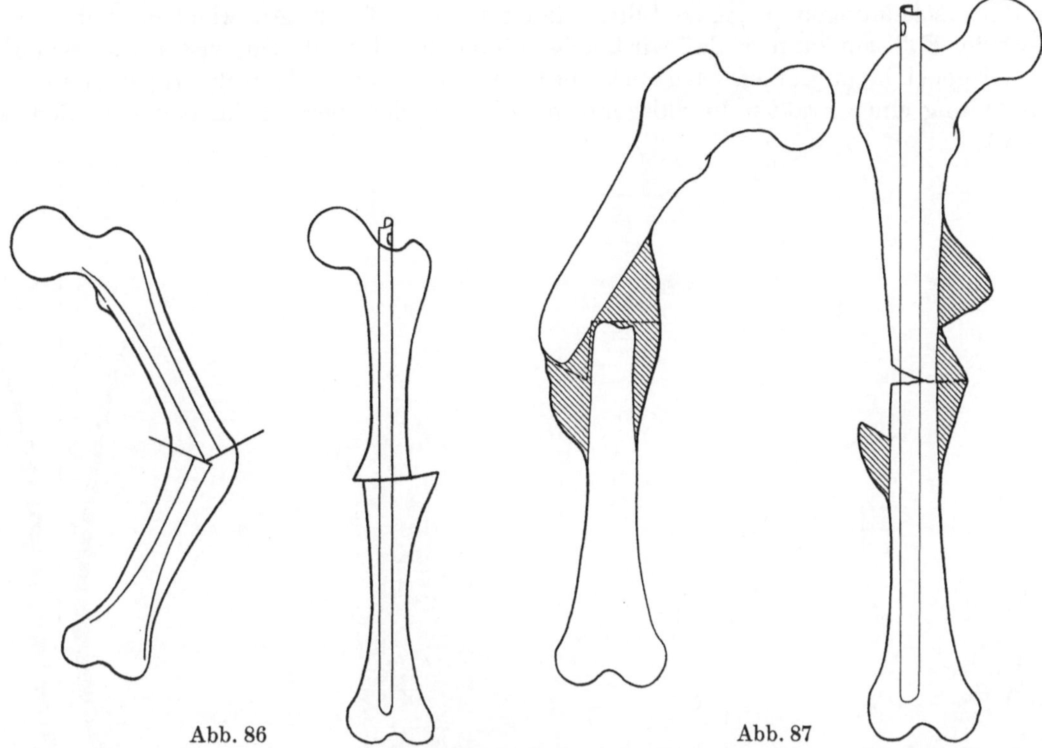

Abb. 86. Achsenkorrektur am Femur. Die Schnittflächen liegen jeweils senkrecht zu den Markraum-Achsen (KÜNTSCHER, 1945)

Abb. 87. Korrektur einer in echter Verkürzung und in Achsenknick geheilten Femurfraktur. Die von KÜNTSCHER angegebene etwas komplizierte Schnittführung gewährleistet denkbar breite Auflageflächen der Fragmente (KÜNTSCHER, 1945)

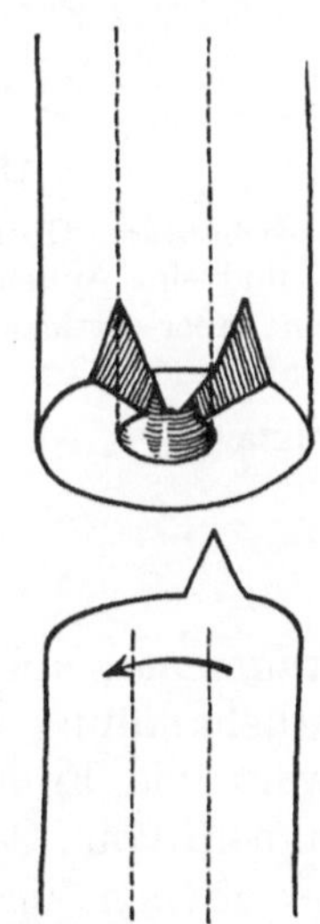

Abb. 88. Korrektur eines Drehfehlers nach Nagelung mit Zapfen und Nuten. Der Zapfen wird in die zweite Nute eingesetzt, um ein Zurückdrehen zu verhindern (KÜNTSCHER-MAATZ, 1945)

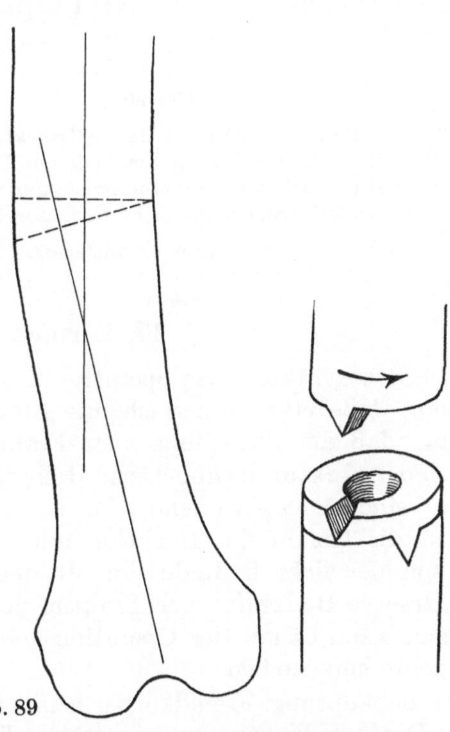

Abb. 89. Achsen- und Drehkorrektur unter Hinnahme einer geringen Verkürzung durch Herausnahme eines Keiles und Drehung und Verzapfung der Fragmente wie in Abb. 87 (MAATZ, 1965)

zu Reizerscheinungen im Knie führen können, wissen wir. Ab welchem Schweregrad dieses der Fall sein kann, so daß wir korrigierend eingreifen müssen, wissen wir noch nicht.

Wir geben einen kurzen Überblick über die heute geübten Korrekturoperationen nach Fehlheilung einer Fraktur in Skizzenform mit ausführlicherer Bildlegende in den Abb. 82—91.

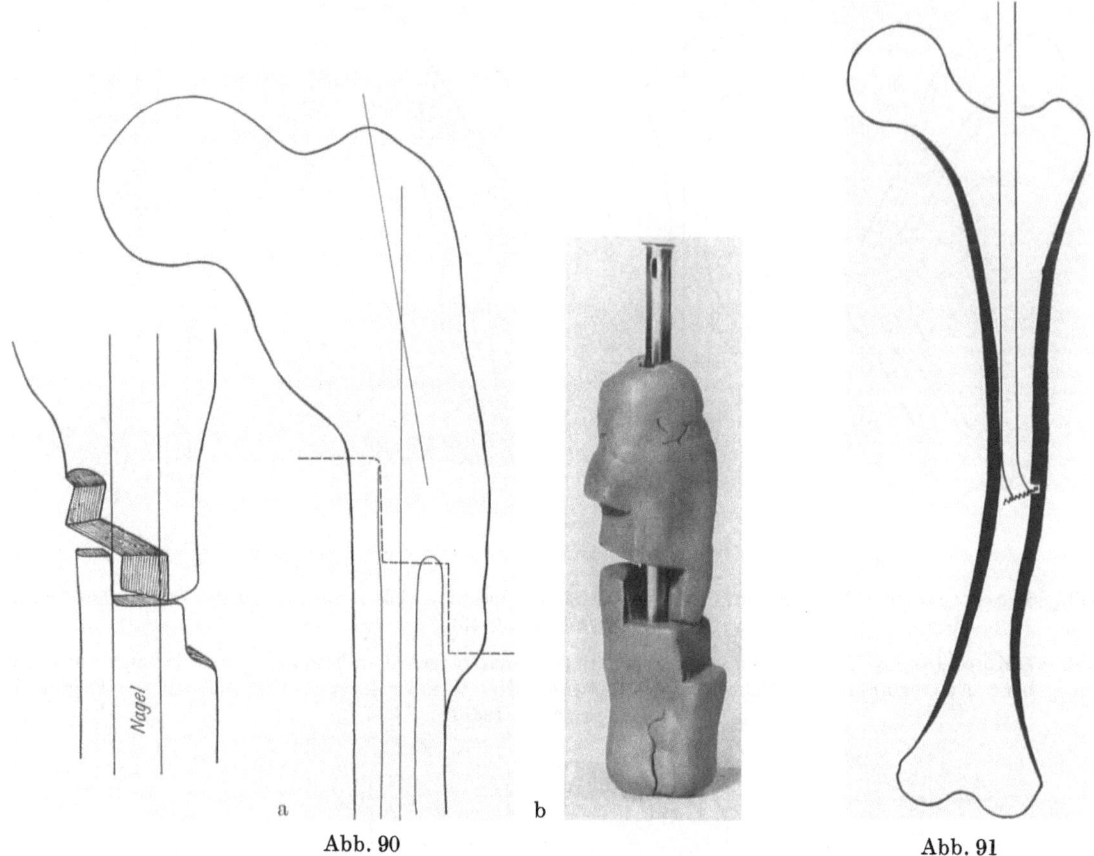

Abb. 90 Abb. 91

Abb. 90 a u. b. Drei Stufen-Osteotomie zur Korrektur einer fehlgeheilten subtrochanteren Oberschenkelfraktur. Es mußten die reelle Verkürzung von 3 cm, ein Achsenknick von etwa 15° und eine Außenrotation von 40° beseitigt werden. Nach der Korrektur stehen nur zwei verhältnismäßig kleine, aber corticalisfeste Fragmentenden aufeinander. Der dicke Nagel sorgt für eine ausreichende Stabilität (Maatz, 1964)

Abb. 91. Intraossäre Osteotomie nach Küntscher

17. Formen der Osteosynthese

Die Osteosynthese, das operative Zusammenfügen der Fragmente, nimmt in zunehmendem Maße eine vorherrschende Stellung in der Frakturbehandlung ein. Die Vorstellung, daß die Freilegung einer Fraktur und die Gegenwart von Fremdkörpern im Bereich der Fraktur die knöcherne Heilung (früher sprach man mehr von „Callusbildung") hemme, sind nicht zutreffend. Von der Tatsache, daß mit der offenen Versorgung einer Fraktur die Gefahr der Infektion mit ihren furchtbaren Nachteilen heraufbeschworen wird, soll hier nicht die Rede sein. Mit dem Ausräumen des Hämatoms aber geht ein Teil der „Reserve-Heilkraft" der Fraktur verloren. Dieser Nachteil wird vollkommen aufgehoben, wenn es mit der Operation gelingt, eine wirklich zuverlässige Verbindung der Fragmente herzustellen.

Die Behauptung, Fremdkörper hemmen die Heilung der Fraktur, hat keine Gültigkeit mehr. Das am Beginn der operativen Frakturbehandlung verwendete Material verursachte aseptisch-chemische Entzündungen. Kann man damit auch enorme Mengen von

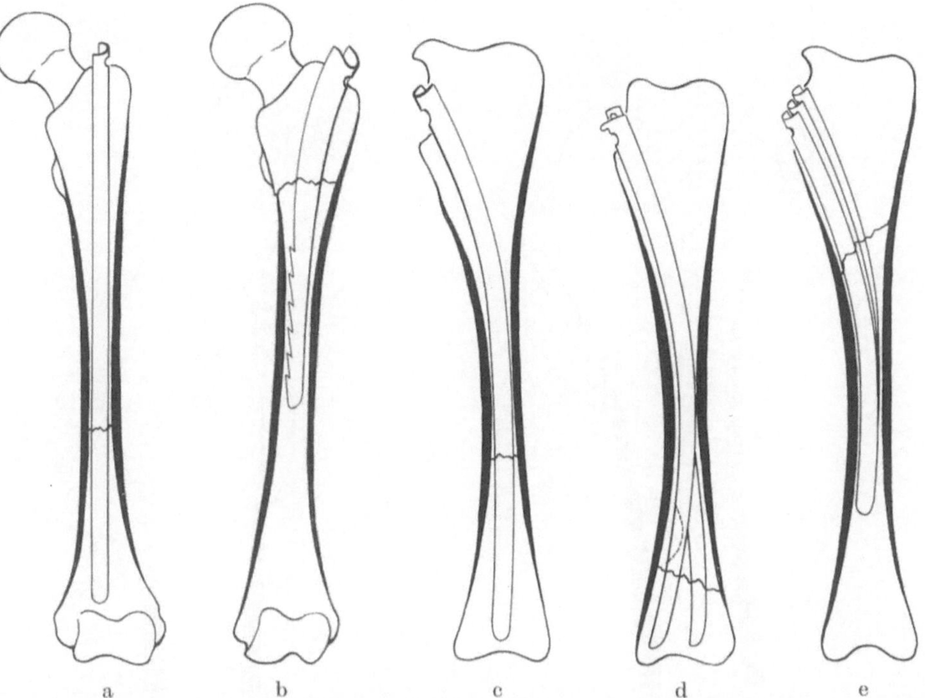

Abb. 92a—e. Osteosynthese bei Diaphysen-Schaftfrakturen: a Femurmarknagel nach KÜNTSCHER, b Trochanternagel bei subtrochanterer Fraktur (MAATZ), c Tibiamarknagel nach KÜNTSCHER, d Tibiaspreiznagel bei fußgelenknaher Fraktur (MAATZ), e Konischer Nagel bei proximalem Tibiabruch (MAATZ)

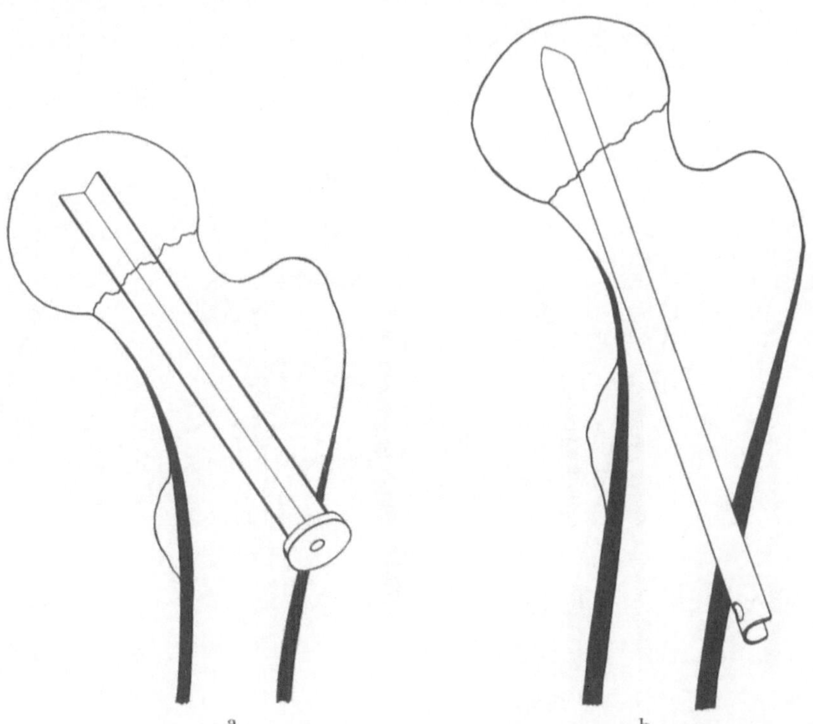

Abb. 93a—d. Osteosynthese bei medialer und subcapitaler Schenkelhalsfraktur. a SMITH-PETERSEN-Dreilamellen-Nagel, b Steiler KÜNTSCHER-Nagel

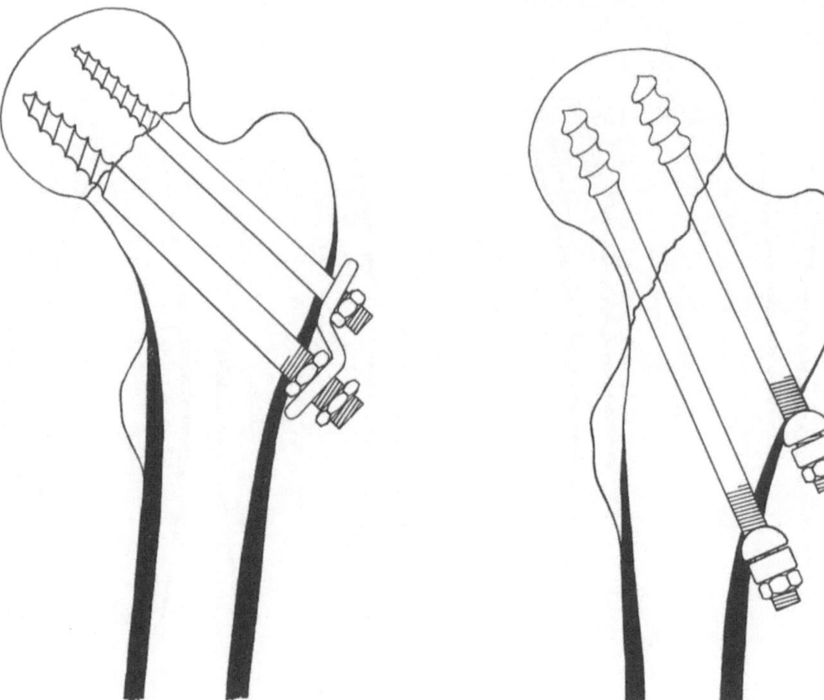

Abb. 93c. Doppel-Zug-Schraube nach POHL

Abb. 93d. Druckschraube nach REIMERS

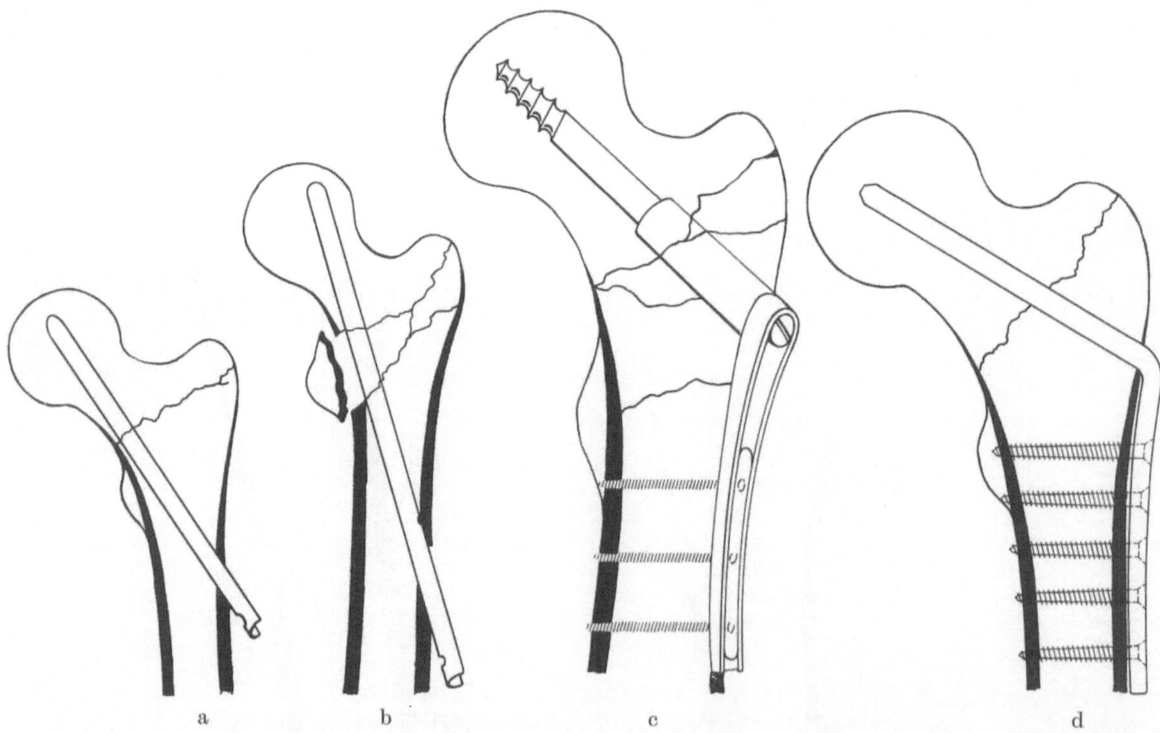

Abb. 94a—d. Osteosynthese bei pertrochanterer Fraktur: a KÜNTSCHER-Nagel bei erhaltenem Trochanter minor, b steiler KÜNTSCHER-Nagel bei abgebrochenem Trochanter minor (MAATZ), c POHL'sche Schraube bei Trümmerbruch, d Hüftbesteck der Schweizer A. O.

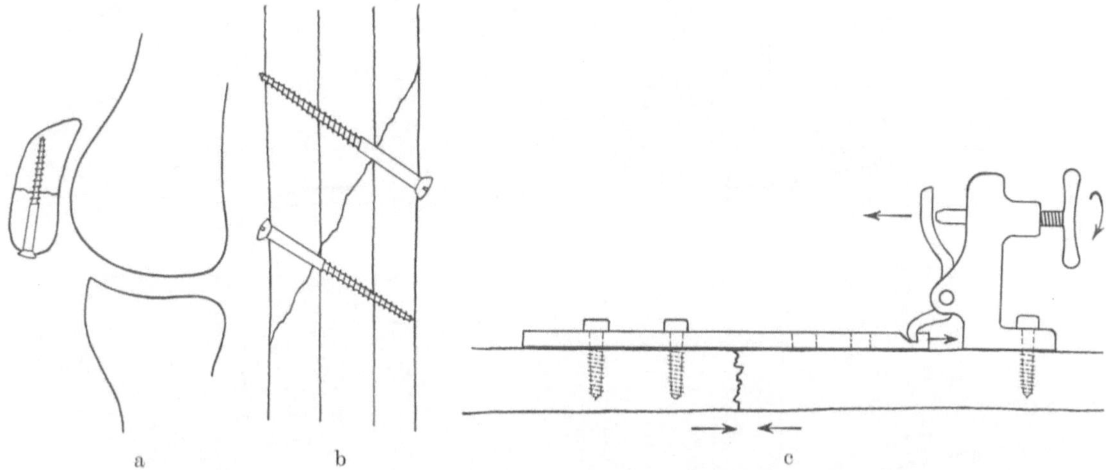

Abb. 95a—c. Druckschrauben- und Druckplatten-Osteosynthese der Schweizer A.O. a Druckschrauben bei glattem Querbruck der Patella, b Corticalis-Druckschrauben bei Schrägbruch eines Schaftknochens, c Druckplatten-Osteosynthese im Augenblick der Reposition unter hohem Druck

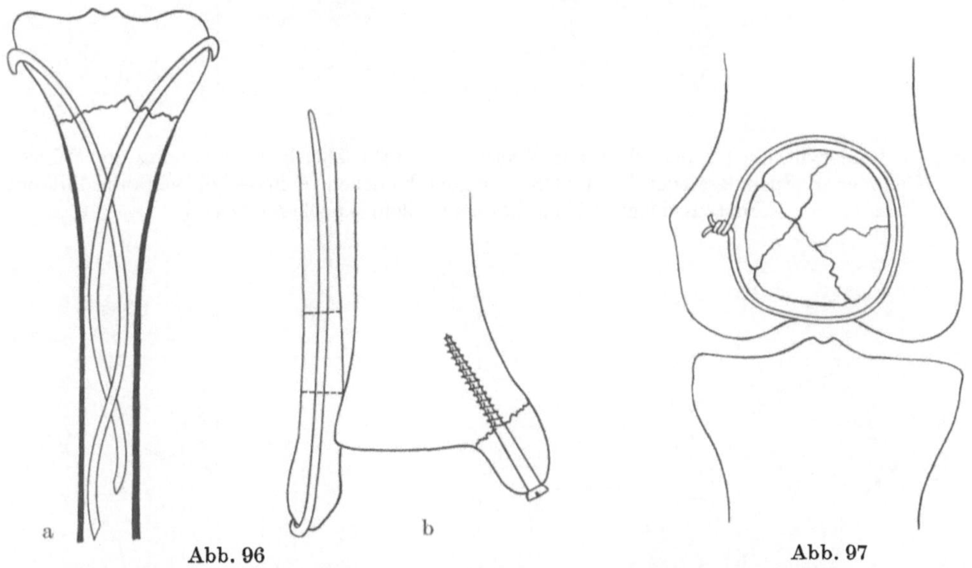

Abb. 96a u. b. Rush pin-Osteosynthese: a bei gelenknaher Tibiafraktur. b Bei einer Malleolar-Luxationsfraktur ist die Fibula mit Rush pin, der Malleolus tibialis mit Schraube versorgt

Abb. 97. Drahtcerclage bei Patella-Sternfraktur

Knochenneubildung hervorrufen, wenn dieser Entzündungsreiz *im* Markraum liegt (Küntscher, 1958), so bewirkt diese chemische Entzündung im Bereich der Fraktur selbst eine vollkommene Aufhebung der Knochenneubildung.

Heute stehen uns nicht rostende Stähle und eisenfreie Legierungen zur Verfügung, welche keinerlei Reizwirkung, so vor allem keine callushemmende Wirkungen im Frakturmilieu hervorrufen.

Eines ist dabei allerdings besonders hervorzuheben: Liegt der Fremdkörper oder liegen die Fremdkörper in dem Bereich, in dem wir Callusbildung erwarten, so kann er rein räumlich diese Bildung hemmen. Darum muß eine Osteosynthese-Druckplatte selbstverständlich die Verbindung der Fragmente so zuverlässig erreichen und die folgende Belastung der Verbindung darf nur so gering sein, daß eine Lockerung nicht möglich ist, eine zusätzliche Callusbildung also nicht erforderlich sein muß.

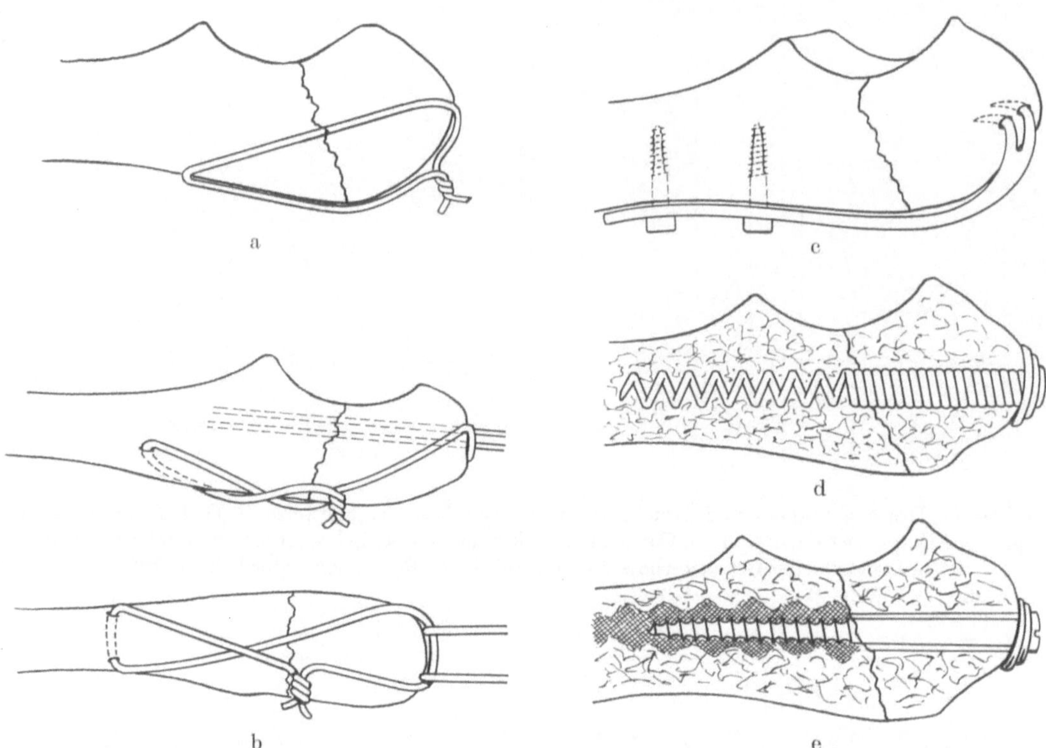

Abb. 98a—e. Osteosynthese bei der Olecranon-Fraktur: a Drahtnaht, b Zugspannung der Schweizer A.O., c Zülzer Klammer, d Spongiosafeder (MAATZ) bei jungem Knochen, e Federkopfschraube mit heterologem Schraubenlager (Schnecke) bei senilem Knochen (MAATZ)

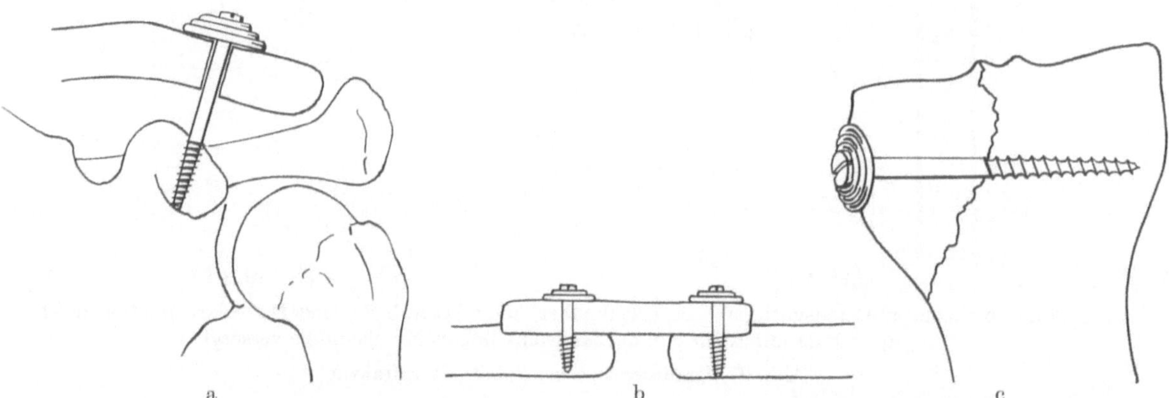

Abb. 99a—f. Osteosynthese mit der Feder (MAATZ): a Federkopfschraube bei totaler Luxation im Akromio-Claviculargelenk, b Spanfixation mit Federkopfschrauben, c Tibiakopffraktur mit Federkopfschraube, d Volkmann'sches Dreieck mit Federkopfschraube, e Fixation des herabgesetzten Trochanters mit starker Markraumfeder bei Schenkelhalseinstellplastik, f Ellenfeder mit zentralem Nagel

In den Abbildungen 92—102 geben wir in Skizzen mit entsprechender Bildlegende einen Überblick über die für den Röntgenologen sicher verwirrende Vielfalt der heute geübten Haupt- und Spielarten der Osteosynthese. Dabei macht sich nur insofern eine gewisse kritische Bewertung unsererseits bemerkbar, als wir als Beispiele selbstredend Fälle nehmen, in denen wir die Art der Osteosynthese für besonders geeignet halten, oder wenigstens als Methode bei der als Beispiel gewählten Fraktur nicht als unzweckmäßig ablehnen würden.

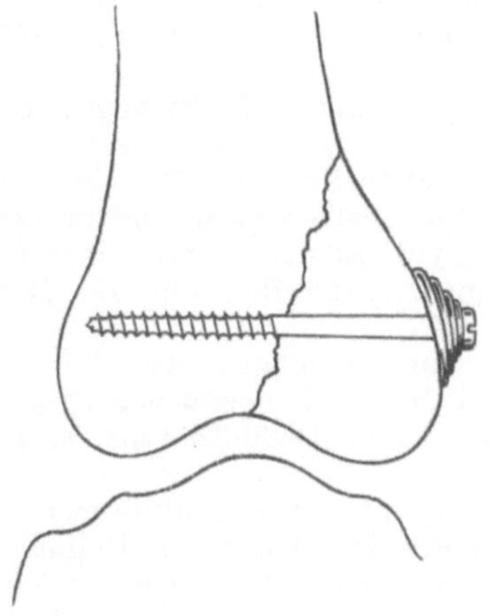

Abb. 99d

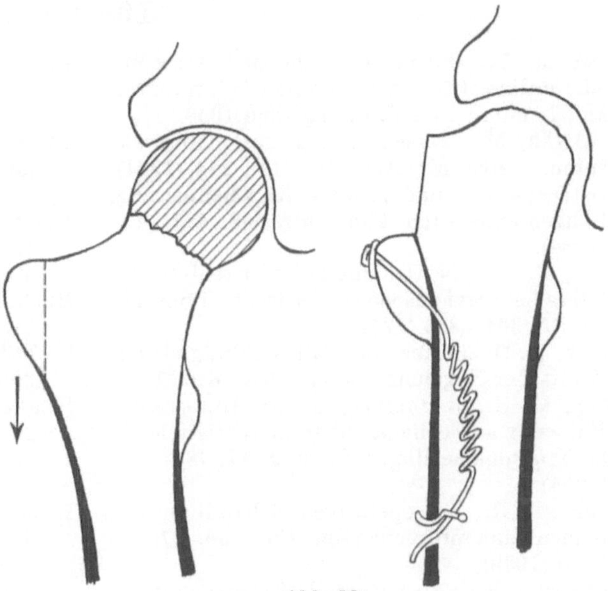

Abb. 99e

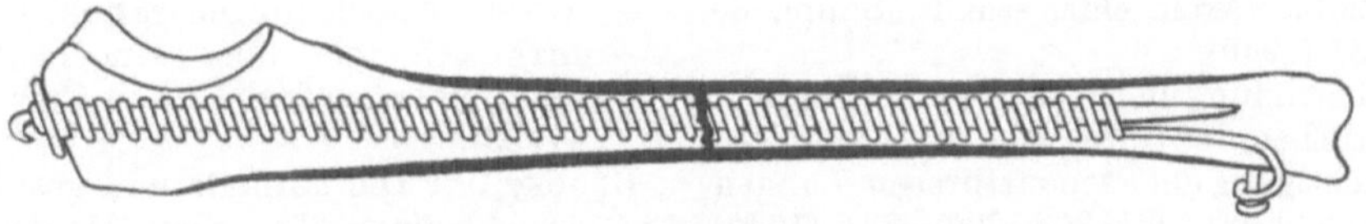

Abb. 99f

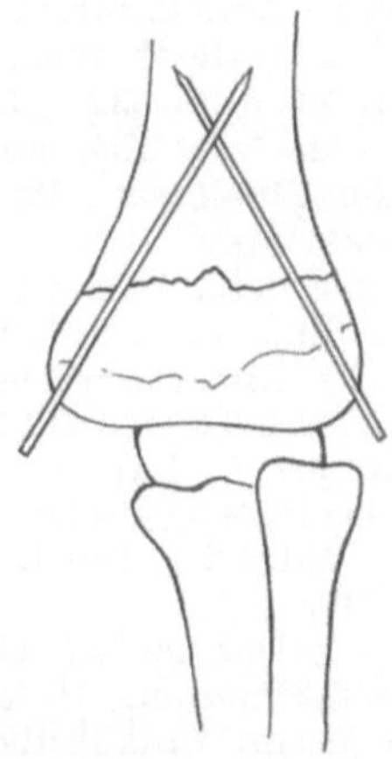

Abb. 100. Percutane Stift-Fixation einer supracondylären Fraktur beim Kind

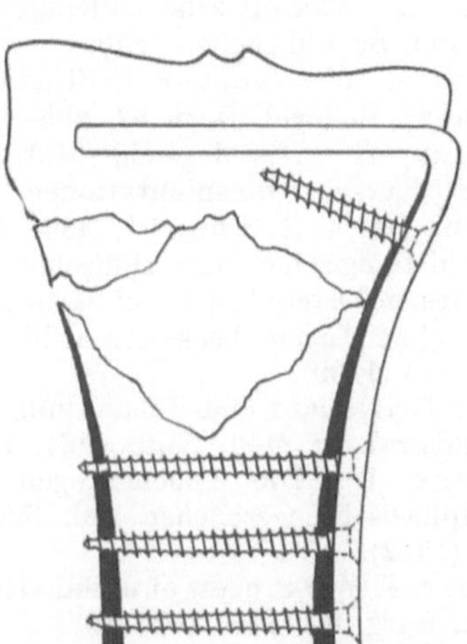

Abb. 102. Winkelplatten-Osteosynthese bei proximaler Unterschenkelfraktur (Schweizer A. O.)

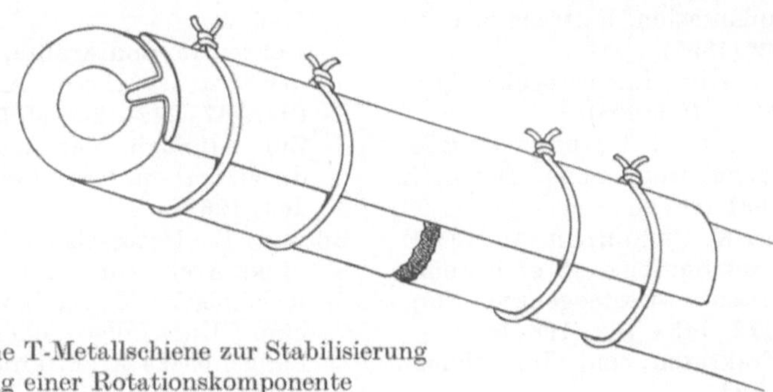

Abb. 101. Thomsen'sche T-Metallschiene zur Stabilisierung und Ausschaltung einer Rotationskomponente

Literatur

Adams, J. C.: Outline of orthopaedics second ed., outline of fractures, second ed. Edinburgh and London: E. & S. Livingstone 1958.

Allgöwer, M.: Verschraubung von Tibiafrakturen. Helv. chir. Acta **28**, 214—224 (1961).

— Osteosynthese und primäre Knochenheilung. Langenbecks Arch. klin. Chir. **308**, 423—434 (1964).

Alnor, P.: Die posttraumatische Osteolyse des lateralen Claviculaendes. Fortschr. Röntgenstr. **75**, 364—365 (1951).

Alslev, J.: Die Formen der Callusbildung bei der Küntscher-Nagelung. Inaug.-Diss. Kiel 1943.

Amler, M. H., J. Salman, and H. Bungener: Reticular and collagen fiber characteristics in human bone healing. Oral Surg. **17**, 785—796 (1964).

Andresen, R.: Zur operativen Behandlung der Schienbeinkopfbrüche. Zbl. Chir. **50**, 2759—2770 (1938).

Annersten, S.: Experimentelle Untersuchungen über die Osteogenese und die Biochemie des Frakturcallus. Arch. chir. scand., Suppl. 60, **84**, 1—181 (1940).

— Über Callusbildung und Frakturheilung bei Diaphysenbrüchen des Unterarms mit besonderer Berücksichtigung der Pseudarthrosen. Langenbecks Arch. klin. Chir. **204**, 299—331 (1943).

Arnold, L.: Anatomische Beiträge zur Lehre von den Schußbrüchen 1873.

Aubigné, M. d': Veraltete Hüftluxationen. Z. Orthop., Beilageheft zu **97**, 265—270 (1963).

Axhausen, G.: Histologische Untersuchungen über Knochentransplantationen am Menschen. Dtsch. Z. Chir. **91**, 388—428 (1908).

— Die histologischen und klinischen Geschehen der freien Osteoplastik auf Grund von Tierversuchen. Langenbecks Arch. klin. Chir. **28**, 23—145 (1909).

— Über Heilverlauf und Behandlung der Schenkelhalsfraktur. Med. Klin. **1924**, 1827—1830.

Axhausen, W.: Die Knochenregeneration, ein zweiphasisches Geschehen. Zbl. Chir. **77**, 435—442 (1952).

Bancroft, F. W.: Process of union after fracture. Ann. Surg. **90**, 546—555 (1929).

Bardenheuer, B.: Die Entstehung und Behandlung der ischämischen Muskelkontraktur. Dtsch. Z. Chir. **108**, 44—48 (1911).

Barth, A.: (1) Histologische Untersuchungen über Knochenimplantation. Beiträge z. Path. Anat. **17**, 65—142 (1895).

— (2) Über Osteoplastik. Langenbecks Arch. klin. Chir. **86**, 859—872 (1908).

Baschkirzew, N. J., u. N. N. Petrow: Beiträge zur freien Knochenüberpflanzung. Dtsch. Z. Chir. **113**, 490—531 (1912).

Basset, C. A. L., D. K. Creighton, and F. E. Stinchfield: Contributions of endosteum, cortex, and soft tissues to osteogenesis. Surg. Gynec. Obstet. **112**, 145—152 (1961).

Bauer, K. H.: Frakturen und Luxationen. Berlin: Springer 1927.

Baumann, E.: In: Nigst, Spezielle Frakturen- u. Luxationslehre, Bd. II/1, Ellenbogen. Stuttgart: Georg Thieme 1965.

Beck, A.: Die Behandlung der Pseudarthrose mit Knochenbohrung. Zbl. Chir. **56**, 2690—2692 (1929).

Beck, H.: Zur Klinik und Pathogenese der Kaumuskelverknöcherungen. Dtsch. Zahn-, Mund- u. Kieferheilk. **19**, 433—456 (1954).

Becker, E.: Ein Instrumentarium zur perkutanen Osteosynthese und extrakutanen Überbrückung mit Kunststoffen. Zbl. Vet.-Med. **4**, 205—242 (1957).

Berezowski: Untersuchungen über die Bedingungen und Methodik operativer Druckentlastung des Gehirns. Dtsch. Z. Chir. **53**, 171—194 (1899).

Bier, A.: Die Bedeutung des Blutergusses für die Heilung des Knochenbruchs, Heilung von Pseudarthrosen und von verspäteter Kallusbildung durch Bluteinspritzung. Med. Klin. **1**, 6—7 (1905).

— Über Knochenregeneration, über Pseudarthrosen und über Knochentransplantate. Langenbecks Arch. klin. Chir. **127**, 1—136 (1923).

Block, W.: Die normale und gestörte Knochenbruchheilung. In: Neue Deutsche Chirurgie, Bd. 62. Stuttgart: Ferdinand Enke 1940.

— Die perkutane Drahtfixation bei Frakturen, Luxationen und Resektionen. Arch. orthop. Unfall-Chir. **46**, 619—632 (1954).

— Reimplantation von abgesprengten Gelenkteilen. Hefte Unfallheilk. **52**, 77—81 (1955).

—, u. J. Beckstroem: Ionometrische Untersuchungen zur Metallose der Gewebe. Langenbecks Arch. klin. Chir. **277**, 89—103 (1953).

Blount, W. P.: Knochenbrüche bei Kindern. Stuttgart: Georg Thieme 1957.

Blum, E.: Zit. bei A. Lauche. In: Handbuch der speziellen pathologischen Anatomie und Histologie, Bd. IX, Teil 4, S. 1. Berlin: Springer 1939.

Blumensaat, C.: Der heutige Stand der Lehre vom Sudeck-Syndrom. Hefte Unfallheilk., Beiheft zu Mschr. Unfallheilk. **51** (1956).

Böhler, J.: Marknagel und „Kugelkallus". Zbl. Chir. **70**, 1833—1836 (1943).

— Die konservative Behandlung von Brüchen des Speichenhalses. Chirurg **21**, 687—688 (1950).

— Gekreuzte Bohrdrähte, ein einfaches Prinzip der Osteosynthese. Arch. orthop. Unfall-Chir. **47**, 242—254 (1955).

— Zur Ätiologie der Hüftkopfnekrose. Verh. dtsch. orthop. Ges., Beilagehefte zu **97**, 260—263 (1963).

Böhler, L.: Unterschenkelschaftbrüche. Langenbecks Arch. klin. Chir. **276**, 192—217 (1953).

— Ischämische Muskelkontraktur, unabwendbare Unfallfolge oder Behandlungsfolge? Langenbecks Arch. klin. Chir. **304**, 471—478 (1962).

BÖHLER, L.: Die Technik der Knochenbruchbehandlung, 13. Aufl. mit Erg.-Band. Wien: Wilhelm Maudrich 1957 u. 1963.
— Behandlung der Verrenkungsbrüche der Hüfte. Z. Orthop., Beilageheft zu **97**, 241—253 (1963).
—, u. W. EHALT: Arthrosis deformans des oberen Sprunggelenks bei konservativer Frakturbehandlung. Öst. Kongr. Unfallheilk. Salzburg 1966.
BOURNE, G. H.: The biochemestry and physiology of bone, p. 118—119. New York: Academic Press Inc. 1956.
BRANDT, G.: Verzögerte Knochenbruchheilung und Pseudarthrosenbildung. Ihre Ursachen und Behandlung. Leipzig: Georg Thieme 1937.
BRUNS, P.: Die Lehre von den Knochenbrüchen. In: Deutsche Chirurgie, Liefg 27. Stuttgart: Ferdinand Enke 1886.
BUCHBERGER, H. G.: Erfahrungen bei der Behandlung von Oberarmkopfbrüchen nach POELCHEN. Chirurg **30**, 260—263 (1959).
BÜCHNER, F.: Allgemeine und spezielle Pathologie, 4. Aufl. München u. Berlin: Urban & Schwarzenberg 1965.
BÜRKLE DE LA CAMP, H.: Fehler und Gefahren der Alloplastik in der Knochen- und Gelenkchirurgie. Langenbecks Arch. klin. Chir. **289**, 463—475 (1958).
BÜTTNER, A.: Über Refrakturen im Kindesalter. Chirurg **19**, 347—357 (1948).
BUNNEL, ST.: The surgery of the hand. Philadelphia: Lippincot & Co. 1944.
BURCKHARDT, H.: Knochenregeneration bei Tieren verschiedenen Alters, 49. Tagg Dtsch. Ges. Chir. Berlin 1925. Ref. Zentr.-Org. ges. Chir. **31**, 653 (1926).
BUSCH, F.: (1) Experimentelle Untersuchungen über Ostitis und Nekrose. Langenbecks Arch. klin. Chir. **20**, 237—260 (1876).
— (2) Die Knochenbildung und Resorption beim wachsenden und entzündeten Knochen. Langenbecks Arch. klin. Chir. **21**, 150—181 (1877).
— (3) Über den Wert der Krapp-Fütterung als Methode zur Erkennung der Anbildung neuer Knochensubstanz. Langenbecks Arch. klin. Chir. **22**, 328—342 (1878).
— (4) Beitrag zur Lehre von der experimentellen Ostitis. Langenbecks Arch. klin. Chir. **24**, 331—338 (1879).
COLLES, A.: On the fracture of the carpal extremity of the radius. Edinb. med. Surg. J. (1814).
COMPERE, E. L., S. W. BANKS u. L. C. COMPERE: Frakturenbehandlung. Stuttgart: Georg Thieme 1966.
DANCKELMANN, A. v.: Fast völlige Verknöcherung der Ellenbogengelenkkapsel nach leichtem Trauma. Langenbecks Arch. klin. Chir. **189**, 692—694 (1937).
DANIS, R.: Théorie et pratique de l'osteosynthese. Paris 1949.
DEBRUNNER, H. H., u. L. FROSCH: Experimentelle und klinische Studien zur Pseudarthrosenfrage. Arch. orthop. Chir. **23**, 10—37 (1924).
DIETHELM, L., u. W. M. HILSCHER: Der Wert des Nachweises der typischen Impressionsfraktur nach Schulterluxation. Mschr. Unfallheilk. **57**, 353—358 (1954).
DITTRICH, K. v.: Beitrag zur Lehre von der circumscripten traumatischen Muskelverknöcherung und zur Frage der Metaplasie. Virch. Arch. path. Anat. **260**, 436—456 (1926).
DOERR, W., K. KÖHN u. H. H. JANSEN: Gestaltswandel klassischer Krankheitsbilder. Berlin-Göttingen-Heidelberg: Springer 1957.
DUHAMEL (1740): Zit. bei W. BLOCK, Die normale und gestörte Knochenbruchheilung. In: Neue Chirurgie, Bd. 62, S. 19. Stuttgart: Ferdinand Enke 1940.
EHALT, W.: Die Bruchformen am unteren Ende der Speiche und Elle. Arch. Orthop. u. Unfallheilk. **35**, 397—442 (1935).
— Verletzungen bei Kindern und Jugendlichen. Stuttgart: Ferdinand Enke 1960.
FEHR, A.: Die Drahtnaht des geschlossenen Unterschenkelspiralbruches, Erfahrungen mit der grundsätzlichen und frühen Operation. Helv. chir. Acta **12**, 233—241 (1945).
FELSENREICH: Zit. bei W. BLOCK, Die normale und gestörte Knochenbruchheilung, S. 203. Stuttgart: Ferdinand Enke 1940.
FELSENREICH, F.: (1) Histologische Untersuchungen an operierten Schenkelhalsbrüchen, die Heilungsvorgänge an der Bruchfläche. Langenbecks Arch. klin. Chir. **192**, 490—544 (1938).
— (2) Histologische Untersuchungen an operierten Schenkelhalsfrakturen, das Wandern des Smith-Petersen-Nagels im Hüftkopf. Langenbecks Arch. klin. Chir. **198**, 4—29 (1940).
FISCHER, A. W.: Bakteriengifte als Knochenbildungsreiz. Langenbecks Arch. klin. Cir. **167**, 153—154 (1931).
— Ostitis durch lange liegenden Marknagel. Zbl. Chir. **76**, 815—820 (1951).
FLACH, A., u. H. KUDLICH: Das Längenwachstum des Röhrenknochens nach Schaftfrakturen an der unteren Extremität bei Kindern und Jugendlichen. Zbl. Chir. **87**, 2145—2154 (1962).
FLEMMING, C.: Suppuration in a closed fracture of clavicle. Lancet **1934I**, 346—351.
FRANGENHEIM, P.: Über die Beziehungen zwischen der Myositis ossificans und dem Callus bei Frakturheilung. Langenbecks Arch. klin. Chir. **80**, 445—459 (1906).
— Dauererfolge der Osteoplastik im Tierversuch. Langenbecks Arch. klin. Chir. **93**, 191—259 (1910).
FRANZ, H.: Kriegschirurgie, 1.—4. Aufl. Berlin: Springer 1919—1944.
FRIEHOFF, F.: Über Schlüsselbeinbrüche. Inaug.-Diss. Kiel 1949.
FUCHS, G., H. STEGEMANN u. W. EGER: Der transplantierte Knochenspan und seine Qualität nach partieller und vollständiger Enteiweißung bei erhaltener organischer Substanz. Langenbecks Arch. klin. Chir. **303**, 240—260 (1963).
GANGLER: Spätergebnisse schlecht geheilter Knochenbrüche (mit besonderer Berücksichtigung kindlicher Brüche). Chirurg **6**, 121—131 (1934).

GARRÉ, C.: Über besondere Formen und Folgezustände der akuten infektiösen Osteomyelitis. Bruns' Beitr. klin. Chir. **10**, 241—298 (1893).

GAUWERKY, F.: Traumatische Deformierungen am Humeruskopf als Folge von Schulterluxationen. Fortschr. Röntgenstr. **75**, 607—627 (1951).

GELBKE, H.: Tierversuche zum Problem der intraartikulären Knochenspanschwundes bei transartikulären Bolzungsarthrodesen (Eine Überprüfung der mechanischen Zerrüttungstheorie LEXERS und der Bierschen Hypothese von der biochemischen osteolytischen Synoviawirkung). Arch. orthop. Unfall-Chir. **46**, 159—177 (1953).

— Tierversuche zur Frage der Frakturcallus- und Pseudarthrosenentstehung. Langenbecks Arch. klin. Chir. **277**, 306—327 (1953).

GERSTEIN, D.: Über Verschluß von Defekten am Schädel mit Demonstration. Verh. dtsch. Ges. Chir. **18**, 89 (1889).

GÖRS, E.: Zur Behandlung komplizierter Splitterbrüche des Schädeldaches. Dtsch. med. Wschr. **40**, 431—434 (1914).

GRAF, R.: Der Wert der Phlebographie des Schenkelkopfes bei der Behandlung der Schenkelhalspseudarthrose. Chirurg **31**, 19—21 (1960).

GREKOW: Zit. bei H. MATTI, Die Knochenbrüche und ihre Behandlung, Bd. II, S. 41. Berlin: Springer 1922.

GRIESSMANN, H., u. H. REICH: Vergleichende Untersuchungen über den Ablauf der Knochenbruchheilung bei der Marknagelung und bei den am Gipsverband behandelten Frakturen. Langenbecks Arch. klin. Chir. **205**, 455—474 (1944).

GRUBER, G. B.: Anmerkungen zur Frage der Weichteilverknöcherungen besonders bei Myopathia osteoplastica. Virch. Arch. path. Anat. **260**, 457—465 (1926).

GULEKE, N.: Über die Pseudarthrosen der langen Extremitätenknochen nach Schußfrakturen. Arch. orthop. Unfall-Chir. **16**, 230—254 (1919).

— Die Verletzungen der Knochen und Gelenke der Gliedmaßen. In: Lehrbuch der Chirurgie, 9. umgearb. Aufl. Jena: Gustav Fischer 1931.

GURVIČ: Die histologische Grundlage der Biologie. Jena: Gustav Fischer 1930.

HAASCH, K.: Verbrennungen unter dem Gipsverband. Hefte Unfallheilk. **78**, 264—265 (1963).

HÄBLER, C.: Arthrosis deformans als Unfallfolge. Zbl. Chir. **78**, 11—13 (1953).

HALLERMANN, H.: Die Beziehungen der Werkstoffmechanik und Werkstofforschung zur allgemeinen Knochenmechanik. Beilageheft Z. orthop. Chir. **62**, 347—360 (1935).

HAMPTON, O. P., and W. T. FITTS jr.: Open reduction of common fractures. New York: Grune & Stratton 1959.

HARFF, J., u. H. W. STUTH: Zum Problem des Sudeckschen Syndroms. Z. Orthop. **84**, 359—369 (1954).

HASCHE-KLÜNDER, R.: Tierexperimenteller Beitrag zur Frage der „angiogenen" Callusbildung. Arch. orthop. Unfall-Chir. **45**, 355—362 (1952).

HEINE, B.: Recherches zur la régénération des os. Preisarbeit für Akademie der Wissenschaft, Paris 1837.

HELLNER, H.: Die Chirurgie der Knochen In: KIRSCHNER-NORDMANN, Operationslehre, Bd. 2, S. 820—840. Berlin u. Wien: Urban & Schwarzenberg 1940.

— Die Hämatogene Osteomyelitis und ihre Behandlung. Stuttgart: Ferdinand Enke 1954.

HENSCHEN, C., u. W. GERLACH: Spektrographische Untersuchungen über die von metallischen Fremdkörpern (Allenthesen) ausgehenden Metallosen der Gewebe, besonders der Knochen. Zbl. Chir. **61**, 828—837 (1934).

HENSCHEN, G., R. STRAUMANN u. R. BUCHER: Ergebnisse röntgenspektrographischer Untersuchungen am Knochen. Dtsch. Z. Chir. **236**, 485—514 (1932).

HOFFA, A.: Lehrbuch der Frakturen und Luxationen, IV. Aufl. Stuttgart: Ferdinand Enke 1904.

HOHMANN, G.: Die Behandlung der mit Verunstaltung und Funktionsstörung geheilten Knochenbrüche. Z. orthop. Chir. **58**, Beilageheft, 390—412 (1933).

— (1) Arm und Hand. München: J. F. Bergmann 1949.

— (2) Fuß und Bein. München: J. F. Bergmann 1951.

HÜBLER, A.: Ein Beitrag zur akuten Osteomyelitis des Kindesalters. Wien. med. Wschr. **1927 II**, 1456—1467.

JEFFERY, R. L.: Femoral regeneration in child. J. Bone Jt Surg. B **27**, 404—405 (1929).

JEWETT, E. L.: New approach for subtrochanteric and upper femoral shaft fractures using dual flange nail plate. Amer. J. Surg. **81**, 186—188 (1951).

JOHANNSON, S.: Die operative Behandlung der Schenkelhalsfrakturen. Leipzig: Georg Thieme 1934.

JUDET, J., and R. JUDET: Use of arteficial femoral head for arthroplasty of hop joint. J. Bone Jt Surg. B **32**, 166—173 (1950).

— — J. LAGRANGE et J. DUNOYER: Résection-réconstruction de la hanche. Arthroplastie par prothèse acrylique. Paris: L'Expansion scientifique française Ed. 1952.

JUNGE, H.: Marknagelung im abnorm brüchigen Knochen. Hefte Unfallheilk. **40**, 60—70 (1951).

JUNGHANNS, H.: Die Brüche des knienahen Unterschenkelabschnittes (Schienbeinkopfbrüche). Langenbecks Arch. klin. Chir. **276**, 242—253 (1953).

KÄFER, N.: Über Geburtshilfliche Frakturen. Verh. 3. Chir. Kongr. Odessa 1925. Ref. Zentr.-Org. ges. Chir. **37**, 230 (1926).

KAUFMANN, E.: Lehrbuch der speziellen Pathologie, 7. u. 8. Aufl. Berlin: W. de Gruyter & Co. 1922.

KIRSCHNER, M.: Verbesserungen der Drahtextension. Langenbecks Arch. klin. Chir. **148**, 651—658 (1927).

Kirschner M., u. O. Nordmann: Die Chirurgie, Bd. I—VII. Berlin u. Wien: Urban & Schwarzenberg 1940.

Klapp, R., u. W. Block: Die Knochenbruchbehandlung mit Drahtzügen. Stuttgart: Ferdinand Enke 1930.

Klose, H., u. B. Janik: Spezielle Chirurgie (H. Klose), Frakturen und Luxationen (B. Janik). Berlin: W. de Gruyter & Co. 1953.

Kocher, Th.: Hirnerschütterung, Hirndruck und chirurgische Eingriffe bei Hirnkrankheiten. In: Spezielle Pathologie und Therapie von Nothnagel, Bd. 9. Wien: Alfred Hölder 1901.

— Chirurgische Operationslehre. Jena: Gustav Fischer 1907.

König, F.: Die späteren Schicksale difform geheilter Knochenbrüche. Langenbecks Arch. klin. Chir. **85**, 187—211 (1908).

— Operative Chirurgie der Knochenbrüche. Berlin: Springer 1931.

Krompecher, S.: Die Knochenbildung. Jena: Gustav Fischer 1937.

Küntscher, G.: Nachweis der Spannungsspitzen am menschlichen Knochengerüst. Beitr. anat. funkt. Syst. **75**, 427—444 (1935).

— Experimentelle Erzeugung von Überlastungsschäden am Knochen. Zbl. Chir. **65**, 964—974 (1938).

— Die Marknagelung von Knochenbrüchen. Langenbecks Arch. klin. Chir. **200**, 443—455 (1940).

— Callus ohne Knochenbruch. Zbl. Chir. **68**, 857—868 (1941).

— Septische und aseptische Osteomyelitis. Zbl. Chir. **79**, 1430—1436 (1954).

— Aufweiten der Markhöhle bei der Behandlung der Pseudarthrose und der frischen Fraktur. Chirurg **25**, 209—213 (1954).

— „Percutane“ Knochenchirurgie. Chirurg **26**, 481—488 (1955).

— Ein Kallusmodell. Zbl. Chir. **82**, 1689—1700 (1957).

— Das Callusproblem. Arch. orthop. Unfall-Chir. **49**, 1—14 (1957).

— Der Knochen als Entzündungsmodell. Z. ges. exp. Med. **130**, 279—288 (1958).

— Praxis der Marknagelung. Wien: Wilhelm Maudrich 1958.

— Die biologischen Gesetze der Knochenbruchheilung. Chirurg **32**, 261—265 u. 312—317 (1961).

— Die geschlossene Verkürzungsosteotomie. Z. Orthop. **98**, 123—129 (1964).

— Primäre Knochenheilung. Langenbecks Arch. klin. Chir. **308**, 452—457 (1964).

—, u. R. Maatz: Technik der Marknagelung. Leipzig: Georg Thieme 1945.

Küppermann, W.: (1) Osteosynthese mit konserviertem Knochen. Mschr. Unfallheilk. **60**, 74—78 (1957).

— (2) Erfahrungen mit heteroplastischen Knochen bei der Knochenbruchbehandlung. Langenbecks Arch. klin. Chir. **298**, 246—251 (1961).

Küster, E.: Diskussionsbeitrag. Verh. dtsch. Ges. Chir. 18, 89—90 (1889).

Lacroix, P.: Sur la réparation des fractures. Les mécanismes locaux. Soc. int. Chir. 15e Congr. Lisbonne 1953, p. 553—559.

Lambotte, A.: (1) Le traitement des fractures. Paris: Masson & Cie. 1907.

— (2) Chirurgie opératoire des fractures. Paris: Masson & Cie. 1913.

Lane, W. A.: The treatment of fractures. Med. J. Rec. **121**, 261—263 (1925).

Lange, M.: Orthopädisch-chirurgische Operationslehre, 2. Aufl. München: J. F. Bergmann 1962.

Lauche, A.: Die Heilung infizierter Knochenbrüche. In: Handbuch der speziellen pathologischen Anatomie und Histologie, Bd. IX/3, S. 278—283. Berlin: Springer 1937.

— Die unspezifischen Entzündungen der Knochen. In: Handbuch der speziellen pathologischen Anatomie und Histologie, Bd. IX/IV, S. 1. Berlin: Springer 1939.

Lauge-Hansen, N.: Fractures of ankle. I. Analytic historic survey as basis of new experimental, roentgenologic and clinical investigations. Arch. Surg. **56**, 259—317 (1948).

— Fractures of ankle. II. Combined experimental-surgical and experimental-roentgenologic investigations. Arch. Surg. **60**, 957—985 (1950).

— Fractures of ankle. III. Genetic roentgenologic diagnosis of fractures of ankle. Amer. J. Roentgenol. **71**, 456—471 (1954).

— Fractures of ankle. IV. Clinical use of the genetic roentgendiagnosis and genetic reductions. Arch. Surg. **64**, 488—500 (1952).

— Fractures of ankle. V. Pronations-dorsiflexion-fracture. Arch. Surg. **67**, 813—820 (1953).

Leimbach, G.: Unfallchirurgische Operationen an Knochen und Gelenken. Stuttgart: Hippokrates 1962.

Lennert, K.: Pathologische Anatomie der Osteomyelitis. Z. Orthop. **100**, Beilageh. 27, 58—64 (1965).

Lentz, W.: Behandlungsergebnisse bei der medialen Schenkelhalsfraktur. Langenbecks Arch. klin. Chir. **282**, 260—264 (1955).

Leriche, R., et A. Policard: La physiologie de l'os. Paris: Masson & Cie. 1926.

Levander, G.: On tissue induction. Acta path. mikrobiol. scand. **26**, 113—141 (1949).

Lexer, E.: Die freien Transplantationen. I. u. II. Teil. In: Neue Deutsche Chirurgie, Bd. 26. Stuttgart 1919.

Looser, E.: Hungerosteopathie mit Umbauzonen. Zbl. Chir. **47**, 1470—1474 (1920).

— Über pathologische Formen von Infraktionen und Callusbildung bei Rachitis, Osteomalacie und anderen Knochenerkrankungen. Zbl. Chir. **47**, 1470—1474 (1920).

Maatz, R.: Wie sollen wir die Heilungsanssichten des Tabikers bei traumatischer Fraktur beurteilen? Zbl. Chir. **69**, 96—100 (1942).

— Die Bedeutung der Fettembolie bei der Marknagelung nach Küntscher. Zbl. Chir. **70**, 383—387 (1943).

— Die Küntscher-Nagelung der Unterarmfraktur. Chirurg **15**, 278—280 (1943).

MAATZ, R.: Die „chemische“ Reizwirkung des Küntschernagels. Arch. orthop. Unfall-Chir. **42**, 513—521 (1943).
— (1) Formschlüssigkeit und Kinematik bei der Küntscher-Nagelung. Zbl. Chir. **70**, 1260—1266 (1943).
— (2) Formschlüssigkeit bei der Küntscher-Nagelung (neue Nagelformen). Zbl. Chir. **70**, 1641—1649 (1943).
— Über Ursache und Verhütung der Ellenpseudarthrose. Chirurg **20**, 287—289 (1949).
— Osteosynthese mit Feder. Langenbecks Arch. klin. Chir. **263**, 201—212 (1949).
— Federosteosynthese. Kiel: K. Jansen 1951.
— Die Wundmechanik in der Federosteosynthese. Z. Orthop. **80**, 643—656 (1951).
— Die Reaktion des Knochens auf Federdruck. Arch. orthop. Unfall-Chir. **44**, 529—539 (1951).
— Die Unterschenkelfrakturbehandlung. Zbl. Chir. **79**, 165—167 (1954).
— Die Behandlung der Innenknöchel-Pseudarthrose mit einem T-Span. Bruns' Beitr. klin. Chir. **203**, 145—151 (1961).
— Drehfehler an Ober- und Unterschenkel nach Marknagelung. Zbl. Chir. **87**, 1373—1381 (1962).
— H. GRIESSMANN, H. JUNGE, H. J. HOPPE, W. SCHÜTTEMEYER u. H. LEMPERT: Ergebnisse der Marknagelung. Hefte Unfallheilk. **40** (1951).
—, u. H. LEMPERT: Zur Kopfnekrose nach medialer Schenkelhalsfraktur. Chirurg **23**, 304—306 (1952).
—, u. W. LENTZ: Gibt es eine stabile Osteosynthese am Schenkelhals? Langenbecks Arch. klin. Chir. **266**, 192—209 (1950).
— — u. R. GRAF: Der Spongiosa-Test. Frankfurt. Z. Path. **65**, 299—313 (1954).
—, u. H. REICH: Über den Verlauf der Knocheninfektion u. -regeneration nach Marknagelung geschlossener und offener Schaftbrüche sowie Osteotomien. Bruns' Beitr. klin. Chir. **174**, 358—386 (1943).
MACEWEN, W.: The growth of bone: Observations on osteogenesis, an experimental inquiry into the development and reproduction of diaphysed bone. James Maclehose & Sons 1912.
MAGNUS, G.: Frakturen und Luxationen. Berlin 1932.
MARCHAND, L.: Zur Kenntnis der Knochentransplantation. Verh. path. Ges. **2**, 368—375 (1899).
MARTIN, B.: (1) Die sympathische Knochenerkrankung. Langenbecks Arch. klin. Chir. **129**, 45—57 (1924).
— (2) Über die osteogenetische Fähigkeit des Periosts. Langenbecks Arch. klin. Chir. **144**, 489—530 (1927).
MATTI, H.: Die Knochenbrüche und ihre Behandlung, 2. Aufl. Berlin: Springer 1931.
MATZNER, R.: Lehrbuch der Chirurgie und Orthopädie des Kindesalters. Berlin-Göttingen-Heidelberg: Springer 1959.
MAURER, G.: Umbau, Dystrophie und Atrophie an den Gliedmaßen: sog. Sudecksche Knochenatrophie. Ergebn. Chir. Orthop. **33**, 476—531 (1941).
MAYER, L., u. E. WEHNER: Neue Versuche zur Frage der Bedeutung der einzelnen Komponenten des Knochengewebes bei der Regeneration und Transplantation von Knochen. Langenbecks Arch. klin. Chir. **103**, 732—762 (1914).
MEYER, H.: Die Nagelung eiternder Schußbrüche am Oberschenkel. Inaug.-Diss. Kiel 1949.
MILCH, R. A., D. P. RALL, and J. E. TOBIE: Fluorescence of tetracycline antibiotics in bone. J. Bone Jt Surg. A **40**, 897—910 (1958).
MITTELMEIER, H.: Osteomyelitis und Osteosynthese. Z. orthop. Chir., Beiheft **100**, 118—126 (1965).
MOMMSEN, F.: Mechanisch-biologische Gesichtspunkte für die unblutige Behandlung der verzögerten Frakturheilung und Pseudarthrose mit Angabe einer biologischen Behandlungsmethode. Z. orthop. Chir. **51**, 472—488 (1929).
MOORE, R. J.: Metal hip joint: new self locking vitallium prothesis. Sth. med. J. (Bgham, Ala.) **45**, 1015—1019 (1952).
—, and E. M. LUNCEFORD jr.: The self-locking hip prothesis in osteoarthritis of the hip and other conditions. J. Amer. Orthop. **2**, 155—160 (1960).
MÜLLER, M. E.: Die hüftnahen Femurosteotomien. Stuttgart: Georg Thieme 1957.
— M. ALLGÖWER u. H. WILLENEGGER: Technik der operativen Frakturbehandlung. Berlin-Göttingen-Heidelberg: Springer 1963.
MÜLLER, W.: Die normale und pathologische Physiologie des Knochens. Leipzig: Johann Ambrosius Barth 1924.
NAUJOKS, H.: Die Geburtsverletzungen des Kindes. Stuttgart: Ferdinand Enke 1934.
NEFF, G.: Aussprache zur „primären Knochenheilung“. Langenbecks Arch. klin. Chir. **308**, 459—460 (1964).
NENNINGER, H.: Über angeborene Ober- und Unterschenkelverbiegungen. Mschr. Kinderheilk. **102**, 276—278 (1954).
NIGST, H.: Spezielle Frakturen und Luxationslehre, Bd. III. Hüftgelenk und proximaler Oberschenkel. Stuttgart: Georg Thieme 1964.
NIKOLE, R.: Metallschädigung bei Osteosynthesen. Basel 1947.
OBERDALHOFF, H.: Experimente und klinische Studien zur Frage der Knochenregeneration. Langenbecks Arch. klin. Chir. **260**, 109—120 (1947).
— Der Einfluß der Funktion auf Form und Struktur des Knochenkallus. Langenbecks Arch. klin. Chir. **263**, 24—37 (1949).
OEHLECKER, F.: Ein weiterer Beitrag zur Klinik, Unfallbegutachtung und Behandlung tabischer Gelenkerkrankungen. Bruns' Beitr. klin. Chir. **92**, 599—666 (1914).
— Zur Bezeichnung „Sudecksches Syndrom“ oder kurz „Sudeck“. Chirurg **19**, 398—403 (1948).
ÖNNE, L., and P. SANDBLOM: Late results in fractures of fore-arm in children. Act. chir. scand. **98**, 549—567 (1949).

OLLIER, L.: Traité experim. et clin. de la régénération des os etc. Paris 1867.
— De l'ostéogénèse chirurgicale. Verh. X. Int. med. Kongr. Berlin 1891.
ORELL, S.: (1) Studien über Knochentransplantation und Knochenneubildung. Act. chir. scand. **74**, Suppl. 31, 1—274 (1934).
— (2) Experimentell chirurgische Studie über Knochentransplantate und ihre Anwendung in der Chirurgie. Dtsch. Z. Chir. **232**, 701—713 (1937).
— (3) Principles and experiences at the implantation of os purum, os novum and bone granulate. Act. orthop. belg. **18**, 162—173 (1952).
ORTH: Ein Beitrag zur Kenntnis des Knochenkallus. v. Leuthold-Gedenkschrift **2**, 3—22 (1906).
OSTERRIETH, D.: Zur Frage der Knochennaht mit Kunststoffen. Chirurg **30**, 263—264 (1959).
OTTE, P.: Komplikationen nach Operationen (lokale Osteomyelitis). Z. Orthop., Beiheft **100**, 111—118 (1965).
PAUVELS, F.: Grundriß einer Biomechanik der Frakturheilung. Verh. dtsch. orthop. Ges. **72**, 62—78 (1941).
— Der Schenkelhalsbruch. Stuttgart: Ferdinand Enke 1953.
— Neue Überlegungen zur kausalen Histogenese der Stützgewebe und ihre Bedeutung für die Frakturheilung und die Erzeugung echter Gelenke. Zbl. Chir. **80**, 1719—1720 (1955).
— Gesammelte Abhandlungen zur funktionellen Anatomie des Bewegungsapparates. Berlin-Heidelberg-New York: Springer 1965.
PETROKOV, W.: Die Biomechanik der Kallusbildung und experimentelle Berechnung der Druckosteosynthese. Bruns' Beitr. klin. Chir. **205**, 265—295 (1962).
PFAB, B.: Zit. bei W. BLOCK, Die normale und gestörte Knochenbruchheilung, S. 203. Stuttgart: Ferdinand Enke 1940.
PHEMISTER, D. B.: Bone groth and repair. Ann. Surg. **102**, 261—285 (1935).
POELCHEN, R.: Selbstinnervationsbehandlung geschlossener Knochenbrüche und Verrenkungen, eine biologische Behandlungsart. Stuttgart: Hippokrates 1940.
PUTTI, V.: Die operative Behandlung der Schenkelhalsbrüche. Stuttgart: Ferdinand Enke 1942.
RADASCH, H. E.: Senility of bone and its relation to bone repair. Surg. Gynec. Obstet. **51**, 42—49 (1930).
RADZIMOWSKY: Inaug.-Diss. Kiew 1881. Ref. bei MARCHAND. In: Neue Deutsche Chirurgie, Liefg 16. Stuttgart: Ferdinand Enke 1901.
RECKLINGHAUSEN, F.: (1) Die fibröse oder deformierende Arthritis, die Osteomalacie und die osteoplastischen Carcinome etc. Berlin: G. Reimer 1891.
— (2) Rachitis und Osteomalacie. Jena: Gustav Fischer 1910.
REHN, E.: Über Muskelzustände bei Knochenbrüchen und ihre Bedeutung für die Frakturbehandlung. Langenbecks Arch. klin. Chir. **133**, 410—417 (1924).
ROUX, W.: Beiträge zur Histologie der funktionellen Anpassung. Arch. Anat. Entwickl.-Gesch. 1885; — Virch. Arch. path. Anat. **209**, 168—178 (1912).
— Das Gesetz der Transformation der Knochen. Berl. klin. Wschr. **1893**, 509—533.
— Gesammelte Abhandlungen über Entwicklungsmechanik der Organismen. Leipzig 1895.
RUNNE, H. J., u. H. MORITZ: Korrosionsschäden und Metallosen nach Osteosynthesen. Zbl. Chir. **86**, 2341—2349 (1961).
RUSH, L. V., u. H. GELBKE: Atlas der intramedullären Frakturfixation nach RUSH. München: Johann Ambrosius Barth 1957.
—, and H. L. RUSH: (1) Reconstruction operation for comminuted fracture of the upper third of ulna. Amer. J. Surg. **38**, 332—333 (1937).
— (2) Medullary pinfixation of fractures near joints. Mississippi Doctor **27**, 260—267 (1949).
SALEM, G.: Erfahrungen bei 798 Schenkelhalsfrakturen. Langenbecks Archiv klin. Chir. **268**, 602—630 (1951).
SCHENK, R., u. H. WILLENEGGER: Zur Histologie der primären Knochenheilung. Langenbecks Arch. klin. Chir. **308**, 440—452 (1964).
SCHMID, R.: Beitrag zur atypischen Verwendung von Küntscher-Nägeln bei kniegelenknahen offenen Oberschenkeltrümmerbrüchen. Chirurg **29**, 470—472 (1958).
SCHMIDT, M. B.: Allgemeine Pathologie und pathologische Anatomie der Knochen. Ergebn. allg. Path. path. Anat. **4**, 531—647 (1897); **5**, 895—1004 (1898).
SCHMITT, W.: Allgemeine Chirurgie. Leipzig: Johann Ambrosius Barth 1955.
SCHNEIDER, H.-J.: Über die Möglichkeit der Bestimmung der mechanischen Wertigkeit des Skeletts beim Lebenden durch Entnahme von Knochenproben. Inaug.-Diss. Berlin 1965.
SCHÖNBAUER: Trümmerbrüche der Kniescheibe. Arch. orthop. Unfall-Chir. **47**, 266—271 (1955).
SCHÜTZ, W., R. DOHRMANN u. G. FLEMMING: Die Myositis ossificans traumatica. Chirurg **32**, 97—101 (1961).
SCHUMANN, G.: Erfolgreiche Nagelung beim Schenkelhalsbruch der Tabiker. Zbl. Chir. **69**, 1861—1868 (1942).
SCHWAIGER, M.: Frakturcerclage mit Kunststoff. Chirurg **24**, 260—261 (1953).
SCHWARZ, E.: Die Knochenbrüche und Verrenkungen und ihre Behandlung. Jena: Gustav Fischer 1958.
SCHWIER, V.: Osteosynthese von Unterschenkelschaftbrüchen mit knöchernen Schrauben. Mschr. Unfallheilk. **61**, 234—239 (1958).
SEEMEN, H. v.: Über die Entstehungsbedingungen metaplastischer Knochenbildungen. Dtsch. Z. Chir. **217**, 60—108 (1929).
SIMON, P.: Der Kahnbeinbruch der Hand und seine Komplikationen. Materia Medica Nordmark **8**, 561—572 (1965).
SMITH-PETERSEN, M. N.: Arthroplasty of the hip — A new method. J. Bone Jt Surg. A **21**, 269—288 (1939).

SMITH-PETERSEN, M. N., E. F. CAVE, and G. W. VANGORDER: Intracapsular fractures of neck of femur. Treatment by internal fixation. Arch. Surg. 23, 715—759 (1931).

— C. B. LARSON, O. E. AUFRANC, and W. A. LAW: Complications of old fractures of the neck of the femur. Results of treatment by vitallium moed arthroplasty. J. Bone Jt Surg. A 29, 41—52 (1949).

SONNENBERG: Zit. bei H. MATTI, Die Knochenbrüche und ihre Behandlung, Bd. II, S. 42. Berlin: Springer 1922.

SPEMANN, H.: Experimentelle Beiträge zu einer Theorie der Entwicklung. Berlin: Springer 1936.

STEINMANN, F.: (1) Eine neue Extensionsmethode in der Frakturbehandlung. Korresp.-Bl. schweiz. Ärzte 1, 3—13 (1907).

— (2) Die Nagelextension der Knochenbrüche. Stuttgart: Ferdinand Enke 1912.

— (3) Lehrbuch der funktionellen Behandlung der Knochenbrüche und Gelenkverletzungen. Stuttgart: Ferdinand Enke 1919.

STÖR, O.: Erfahrungen mit der Marknagelung nach KÜNTSCHER. Chirurg 15, 313—314 (1943).

STROBL: Zit. bei H. MATTI, Die Knochenbrüche und ihre Behandlung, Bd. II, S. 42. Berlin: Springer 1922.

SUDECK, P.: (1) Über die akute entzündliche Knochenatrophie. Langenbecks Arch. klin. Chir. 62, 147—271 (1900).

— (2) Die kollateralen Entzündungsreaktionen an den Gliedmaßen (sog. akute Knochenatrophie). Langenbecks Arch. klin. Chir. 191, 710—753 (1938).

TENDELOO, N. P.: Allgemeine Pathologie, 2. Aufl. Berlin: Springer 1925.

THOMAS, J.: Zit. bei W. BLOCK, Die normale und gestörte Knochenbruchheilung, S. 209. Stuttgart: Ferdinand Enke 1940.

THOMSEN, W.: Eine neue T-Schiene als wirksames Mittel für eine stabile Osteosynthese. Z. Orthop., Beilageheft zu 91, 465—468 (1959).

— Über die Technik und Indikation der Cerclage. Z. Orthop., Beilageheft zu 101, 294—298 (1966).

TROJAN, E.: Behandlungsergebnisse von 277 frischen geschlossenen Schaftbrüchen beider Vorderarmknochen. Hefte Unfallheilk. 46, 140—208 (1953).

— Hüftkopfnekrosen nach traumatischen Hüftverrenkungen und Hüftverrenkungsbrüchen. Z. Orthop., Beilageheft zu 97, 309—313 (1963).

— Knochenbruchheilung und Infektion. Z. Orthop., Beilegeheft zu 100, 155 (1965) (Diskussionsbemerkung).

—, u. A. PERSCHL: Die Behandlungsergebnisse von 79 frischen traumatischen Hüftgelenksverrenkungen und Hüftgelenksverrenkungsbrüchen. Ergebn. Chir. Orthop. 40, 90—164 (1956).

TRUETA, J.: Die 3 Typen der akuten hämatogenen Osteomyelitis. Schweiz. med. Wschr. 93, 306—312 (1963).

URIST, M. R., R. J. MAZET, and C. O. BECHTOL: Senile osteoporosis as a disorders influencing treatment and end results of fractures of the hip with a preliminary report on the use of collapatite. Amer. Surg. 25, 883—890 (1959).

VOLKMANN, R.: Handbuch der allgemeinen und speziellen Chirurgie von PITHA u. BILLROTH, Bd. 2, Abt. A, S. 694. Stuttgart: Ferdinand Enke 1869.

VOLKMANN, R. v.: Beiträge zur Chirurgie, S. 105. Leipzig: Breitkopf & Härtel 1875.

— Die ischämischen Muskellähmungen und Kontrakturen. Zbl. Chir. 8, 801—834 (1881).

VOSS, O.: Operation und Nagelung des Humeruskopfes. Bruns' Beitr. klin. Chir. 162, 190—200 (1935).

—, u. K. W. HARTMANN: Die Nagelung des Oberarmkopfbruches. Zbl. Chir. 78, 414—421 (1953).

VOSSSCHULTE, K.: Über das spätere Schicksal der im Wachstumsalter mit Verkürzung ausgeheilten Frakturen. Mschr. Unfallheilk. 41, 597—602 (1934).

WAGNER, H.: Die Einbettung von Metallschrauben im Knochen und die Heilungsvorgänge des Knochengewebes unter dem Einfluß der stabilen Osteosynthese. Langenbecks Arch. klin. Chir. 305, 28—40 (1963).

WANKE, R., R. MAATZ, H. JUNGE u. W. LENTZ: Frakturen und Luxationen, 1. Aufl. München: Urban & Schwarzenberg 1962.

WATSON-JONES, R.: Myositis ossificans of quadriceps. Brit. med. J. 1930 II, 592—598.

— In: Fractures and joint injuries, 5. ed., vol. II and I. Edinburgh: Livingstone 1956/57.

WEBER, B. G.: Epiphysen-Verletzungen. Helv. chir. Acta 31, 103—118 (1964).

WEBER, H.-W.: Wachstumsstörungen nach traumatischer Epiphysenlösung. Inaug.-Diss. Kiel 1949.

WERDER, H.: Posttraumatische Osteolyse des Schlüsselbeinendes. Schweiz. med. Wschr. 80, 912—913 (1950).

WESTHUES, H.: Eine neue Behandlungsmethode der Calcaneusfrakturen. Zbl. Chir. 62, 995—999 (1935).

WIESER, C.: Die primäre Knochenbruchheilung und ihre Störung im Röntgenbild. Langenbecks Arch. klin. Chir. 308, 434—440 (1964).

WILTON, S.: Zit. bei W. BLOCK, Die normale und gestörte Knochenbruchheilung. Stuttgart: Ferdinand Enke 1940.

WITT, A. N.: Die Behandlung der Pseudarthrosen. Berlin: W. de Gruyter & Co. 1952.

— Die transarticuläre Fixation bei Frakturen und Luxationen im Bereich des Humeroradialgelenkes. In: Chirurgie ein Fortschritt, hrsg. von MAURER. Stuttgart: Ferdinand Enke 1965.

WOLF, J.: Die innere Struktur der Knochen. Berlin 1870.

ZÖLLNER: Zit. bei W. BLOCK, Die normale und gestörte Knochenbruchheilung, S. 203. Stuttgart: Ferdinand Enke 1940.

ZUPPINGER, H., u. TH. CHRISTEN: Allgemeine Lehre von den Knochenbrüchen. Leipzig: F. C. W. Vogel 1913.

H. Radiologische Prognostik der Knochenbruchheilung

Von

A. Hulth

Mit 13 Abbildungen

1. Einleitung

a) Knochenbruchheilung und Gefäßversorgung

Für die Frakturheilung spielt die Gefäßversorgung des Frakturgebietes die größte Rolle. Frakturen in reich vascularisierten Knochen, z. B. in den Metaphysen der Röhrenknochen, in den Rippen oder in spongiösen Knochen, heilen schnell und häufig sogar ohne Ruhigstellung. Dagegen haben Tibiafrakturen, besonders die des distalen Teiles, auf Grund ihrer schlechteren Gefäßversorgung schlechtere Heilungsneigung und erfordern immer eine sorgfältige und ausreichend langdauernde Ruhigstellung. Am schlechtesten heilen gewisse, gelenknahe Frakturen, bei denen das eine Fragment durch seine intraarticuläre Lage und seine Knorpelbekleidung keine Möglichkeit hat, eine kollaterale Gefäßversorgung zu erhalten. Typische Beispiele für solche Gelenkfrakturen sind die des Naviculare carpi und die medialen Collumfrakturen, bei denen die engagierten Fragmente für ihre Ernährung auf das Vorkommen unbeschädigter synovialer Gefäße angewiesen sind.

Von den Frakturen mit ausgesprochen schlechtem Heilungsvermögen sind es nur die *medialen Schenkelhalsfrakturen*, die innerhalb des Rahmens der in diesem Kapitel vorgesehenen Darstellung liegen. Sowohl Naviculare-Frakturen als auch Unterschenkelfrakturen heilen bei adäquater Immobilisierung; außerdem hat man für ihre Behandlung keine andere Möglichkeit zur Wahl. Darum ist bei diesen Frakturen eine Frühdiagnose der gefäßgeschädigten Fragmente nicht von so großer Wichtigkeit wie bei den medialen Collumfrakturen. Auch ein Teil der dislozierten medialen Collumfrakturen kann bei adäquater Osteosynthese trotz avasculärem Caputfragment heilen, sekundär aber kommt es oft zu reparativen Prozessen im Caputfragment, die ein schlechtes funktionelles Endresultat ergeben. Diese spät hinzutretenden Komplikationen machen sekundäre Operationen notwendig, welche jedoch am besten *primär* an ausgewählten Fällen vorgenommen werden sollten. Die Voraussetzung für diese Auswahl ist das Vorhandensein einer Methode für die Frühdiagnose der Avascularität. Diese Darstellung behandelt deswegen in der Folge ausschließlich die röntgenologische Prognostik der Knochenbruchheilung bei den medialen Collumfrakturen.

b) Avasculäre Formen der Schenkelhalsfrakturen und ihre Manifestation

Früher, als die Collumfrakturen mit Gipsverband oder Extensionsbehandlung versorgt wurden, war die Zahl der Pseudarthrosen viel größer als nach der Osteosynthesebehandlung. Statt dessen ist nach der Nagelung die Zahl der sog. Caputnekrosen angestiegen. Das muß bedeuten, daß die Nagelung auch bei einem Teil der Fälle mit avasculärem Caputfragment Frakturheilungen ermöglicht hat, da es keinen Grund zu der Annahme gibt, daß sich die Frequenz der Frakturen mit avasculärem Fragment geändert hat. Im großen gesehen, dürfte die Summe aus Pseudarthrosen und Caputnekrosen in dem verschiedenen klinischen Material ziemlich konstant sein, da beide Manifestationen eines total oder partiell avasculären Caputfragments sind. Die Histopathologie der Caputnekrose wurde durch Untersuchungen von Santos (1930), Felsen-

REICH (1938—1940), PHEMISTER (1939—1940), HULTH (1961), SEVITT (1964) und HULTH und JOHANSSON (1966) klargelegt.

Diese Untersuchungen haben gezeigt, daß die klinisch-röntgenologische Diagnose Caputnekrose in Wirklichkeit verschiedenen Stadien der Regeneration des toten Knochens entspricht und daß diese Diagnose erst mehrere Monate nach der Aufhebung der Blutzirkulation gestellt werden kann. Die Regeneration des toten Knochens, der sog. schleichende Ersatz, der durch Einwachsen von Granulationsgewebe bewerkstelligt wird, kann nicht vor der Heilung der Fraktur zustande kommen (PHEMISTER). Man sieht dann röntgenologisch zuerst eine Verdichtung des Caput und danach Unregelmäßigkeiten in der Struktur, den sog. Umbaukopf. Zum Schluß kommt es zum Zusammenbruch der oberen Caputkontur. Das avasculäre Caputfragment ist somit kein absolutes Hindernis für die Frakturheilung, aber auf der anderen Seite sind bei adäquater Behandlung die meisten der entstandenen Pseudarthrosen durch einen Gefäßschaden im Caputfragment bedingt (WATSON-JONES). Bei Pseudarthrosen wird das tote Caputfragment durch das Pseudarthrosenbindegewebe für den schleichenden Ersatz unzugänglich und zeigt sich deswegen röntgenologisch intakt, abgesehen von einer Verdichtung des gesamten Fragmentes bei einzelnen Fällen. Um einen Umbau eines solchen Fragmentes zu erhalten, muß man erst eine Heilung der Fraktur erzielen (PHEMISTER).

c) Die Frühdiagnose der Avascularität

α) Die Bedeutung des Frakturtyps

Da die klinischen Manifestationen einer Caputnekrose sich erst mehrere Monate, zuweilen Jahre nach der initialen Osteosynthesebehandlung zeigen, hat man danach gestrebt, Methoden für die Frühdiagnose der Avascularität zu entwickeln. Man könnte dadurch schon primär den Patienten der definitiven Behandlung unterziehen, z. B. der Arthroplastik oder Osteotomie, und brauchte nicht erst das Resultat der gewöhnlichen Nagelosteosynthese abzuwarten. Ich will zuerst in Kürze eine Zusammenfassung geben über die Bedeutung, welche die Lage und der Verlauf der Fraktur und der Grad der Dislokation für die Prognose haben. Die schlechte Prognose gilt nur für die eigentlichen Collumfrakturen (fractura colli femoris vera), während die anatomisch naheliegenden trochanteren Frakturen beinahe ausnahmslos eine gute Prognose haben, sowohl im Hinblick auf die Heilung als auf das Fehlen der Caputnekrose.

PAUWELS zeigte, daß steiler verlaufende Frakturen (PAUWELS 3. Grad) schlechtere Heilungsbedingungen haben als mehr horizontal verlaufende (PAUWELS 1. Grad), was auf den ungünstigeren mechanischen Verhältnissen an der Bruchstelle der ersteren beruht. Diese Feststellung galt jedoch hauptsächlich bei der damals üblichen Gipsbehandlung der Collumfrakturen. Die Nagel- oder Schraubenosteosynthese dürfte in großem Ausmaße diese ungünstigen mechanischen Verhältnisse, die mit dem vertikalen Verlauf der Fraktur zusammenhängen, aufheben. Ein steiler Verlauf der Fraktur durch die Collumregion hat an sich keine Bedeutung für die Heilung, was durch die gute Heilung der sehr steil verlaufenden pertrochantären Frakturen bekräftigt wird.

Obgleich man im allgemeinen sagen kann, daß die primär stärker dislozierten Frakturen auf Grund eines größeren Gefäßschadens eine schlechtere Prognose haben als die weniger dislozierten, so ermöglicht der Grad der Dislokation allein im einzelnen Falle jedoch keine sichere Prognosestellung.

Auch bei fehlender oder geringer Dislokation gibt es verschiedene Möglichkeiten für das Entstehen von Zirkulationsschäden, z. B. individuelle Variationen der Gefäßanatomie, Kompression der Venen vom Caputfragment durch Hämatom und Schwellung. Dagegen gibt es viele stark dislozierte Frakturen, die gut heilen. Der Verlauf der Fraktur und der Grad der Dislokation sind somit Faktoren, die keine Basis für eine prognostische Beurteilung abgeben. Man muß deswegen Methoden finden, die direkt oder indirekt ein Bild der residualen Zirkulation im Caputfragment geben. Die Untersuchungen, um die es sich hier handelt, sind einerseits angiographische Methoden und andererseits Untersuchungen mit Isotopen.

β) Die Arteriographie

Die Arteriographie, die bei Zirkulationsuntersuchungen einer Extremität oder eines Organs die bedeutungsvollste angiographische Methode ist, hat bei Knochengewebe begrenzten Wert. Die Schwierigkeit, ossale Gefäße genügend kontrastgefüllt zu erhalten, ist aus verschiedenen Gründen sehr groß. Arteriographiebefunde bei Collumfrakturen wurden von Rook 1953, Müssbichler 1956 und bei Caputnekrosen von Lange und Hipp 1960 beschrieben. Hipp (1962) und Brugger (1963) haben gezeigt, daß es möglich ist, die kleinen Retinaculum-Gefäße und die Lig. teres-Gefäße darzustellen. Man scheint keine sicheren diagnostischen Werte mit Arteriographien erhalten zu haben.

γ) Die Venographie

Die Venographie, ausgeführt durch Kontrastinjektion direkt in die Caputspongiosa, ergibt eine gute Kontrastfüllung der vorhandenen Venen; gleichzeitig — bei richtiger Methode — gibt sie auch einen gewissen Überblick, ob im Fragment eine Blutzirkulation vorhanden ist oder nicht. Venographien wurden von Hulth 1953 und 1956, Rehm und Süsse 1955, de Haas und MacNab 1956, Vrbka 1957, Dahlgren 1959, Graf und Werner 1960, Palau 1961, Harrison 1962, Herzog 1962, Hulth und Johansson 1962 beschrieben.

δ) Die Untersuchungen mit Isotopen

Tucker (1950) und Boyd (1951) injizierten 1 Std vor der Probeexcision aus Caput- und Trochanter femoris ^{32}P intravenös. Um die gemessenen Durchblutungsverhältnisse im Frakturgebiet eindeutig auszudrücken, führten sie die „Trochanter-Caput-Relation" ein.

Boyd, Zilversmith und Calandruccio (1955), Boyd und Calandruccio (1963), Arden und Veall (1953) und Arden (1960) kamen zu ihren Meßergebnissen mit einem Geiger-Müller-Zähler, der durch einen nur 2 mm weiten Kanal vom Femur her in den Kopf eingeführt werden konnte. Die Radioaktivität wurde sowohl im Schenkelkopf als auch im -hals bestimmt.

Massie (1963) hat bei Frakturen mehrfache Untersuchungen des Schenkelkopfes und Schenkelhalses mit ^{32}P-markierten roten Blutkörperchen ausgeführt. Er konstruierte einen Gleitnagel mit Perforationen für das Caput und für das Trochantergebiet. Durch den hohlen Gleitnagel konnte ein Geigermesser eingeführt werden. Durch die Perforationen wurde dann die Radioaktivität gemessen. Die Messungen wurden während der Operation und nach verschieden langen Zeitintervallen vorgenommen.

Johansson (1962 und 1964) injizierte radioaktives Jod durch eine Kanüle in die Spongiosa des Schenkelkopfes und des Trochanters und bestimmte die Radioaktivität mit einem Collimator über dem Herzen. Die Steigerung der Aktivität über dem Herzen wurde nach jeder Injektion gemessen. Nach dem Verfasser gibt die Steigerung der Aktivität Aufschluß über die Zirkulationsverhältnisse im Caputfragment, respektive im Trochanter.

Diese Methode und die unten beschriebene venographische Kontrastmethode zeigen eine recht gute Übereinstimmung.

Holmquist und Alffram (1965) injizierten mit einer sehr dünnen Kanüle 0,10 ml Kochsalzlösung mit 10 Mikrocurie ^{131}I in den Femurkopf. Sie maßen dann die Radioaktivität über dem Hüftgelenk mit einem Collimator. Das Absinken der gemessenen Radioaktivität innerhalb von 5—15 min nach der Injektion wird als Indicator für die Durchblutung des Schenkelkopfes verwendet. In 25 nachuntersuchten Fällen war die Übereinstimmung zwischen gestellter Prognose und klinischem Schlußresultat sehr gut.

2. Intraossale Venographien

Es ist lange bekannt gewesen, daß eine Flüssigkeit, die ins Knochenmark oder in spongiösen Knochen injiziert wird, unmittelbar in die extraossalen Venenstämme abfließt

(HOYER 1869; LANGER 1876; JOSEFSON 1934; TOCANTINS 1941; WALLDÉN 1944; BENDA, ORINSTEIN und DEPITRE 1940; ENRIA und FERRERO 1950; DUCUING 1951; LEGER und FRILEUX 1950; DUCCI 1950; MENEGAUX 1953; SÜSSE und AURIG 1954; MÉRIEL, RUFFIÉ und FOURNIÉ 1955; GUILHEM und BEAUX 1954; BEGG 1954; SCHOBINGER 1960). Die Ursache für dieses Verhalten liegt in dem speziellen Typ der Blutversorgung des Knochens. Die arterielle Versorgung in einem Röhrenknochen besteht außer aus den Arteria nutritia-Gefäßen, die in den Diaphysen verlaufen, aus reichlicher metaphysärer Versorgung, die in der Metaphysenregion verläuft und endlich aus epiphysärer Versorgung direkt in die Epiphyse. In der Regel ist die epiphysäre Blutversorgung während der gesamten Wachstumsperiode, solange die Epiphysenscheibe erhalten ist, eine geschlossene Einheit, später aber anastomosiert sie mit der metaphysären und der Nutritiaversorgung. In allen Haversschen und Volkmannschen Kanälen sowie im Mark gibt es Gefäßzweige. Die medullären Arterienäste gehen in die großen venösen Sinus über, die den unvergleichlich größten Teil der vasculären Area der Markhöhle einnehmen. Die abführenden Venen sind an Anzahl und Kaliber den entsprechenden Arterien mehrfach überlegen. Dieser Typ der Gefäßversorgung ermöglicht, daß Kontrastmittel, die durch eine knochendicht in die Markhöhle eingesetzte Kanüle injiziert werden, leicht und unmittelbar in den großen Venenstämmen erscheinen. Die Gefäßversorgung des Knochens ähnelt in dieser Hinsicht deutlich der der Milz, bei der man auch durch direkte Punktion leicht Venographien erhalten kann. Es ist auch auffallend, daß bei normalen Knochen die intraossal injizierte Flüssigkeit den nächsten Abflußweg benutzt. Die Venen sind so weit, daß auch eine sehr schnell injizierte Flüssigkeit leicht durch die Venen abtransportiert wird, ohne falsche Wege einzuschlagen (DE MARNEFFE 1951).

Bei Kontrastmittelinjektionen in die Malleolen oder in die Tibia erhält man eine ausgezeichnete Venographie der tiefen Venen der Extremität, weil das Kontrastmittel den Knochen unmittelbar auf dem schnellsten Wege verläßt. Die Venen des Beckens füllen sich bei Injektionen ins Darmbein oder in den Trochanter major usw. Außer einem kleinen Kontrastdepot um die Kanülenspitze verschwindet das gesamte Kontrastmittel innerhalb weniger Minuten aus dem Knochen, was darauf deutet, daß die Zirkulation im Knochen normal ist. Injiziert man in die Nähe einer Fraktur, so findet man, daß das Kontrastmittel längere Zeit im Knochen verbleibt und daß es sich dabei im Frakturgebiet sammelt, was auf eine verschlechterte Zirkulation deutet (DUCCI 1950). Das gleiche Resultat erhält man, wenn man in einen osteomyelitischen Knochen spritzt (nach gleichem Verfasser). Auch bei der Arthrosis deformans coxae erhält man einen verschlechterten venösen Abfluß und erhöhte Zurückhaltung des Kontrastmittels (MÉRIEL, RUFFIÉ und FOURNIÉ 1955; HULTH 1958).

Zusammenfassend kann folgendes über den Mechanismus der intraossalen Kontrastinjektionen gesagt werden:

1. Dadurch, daß die intraossalen Gefäße zum überwiegenden Teil aus venösen Sinus mit reichen Kommunikationen zu den extraossalen Venen bestehen, wird eine intraossale Kontrastmittelinjektion einer intravenösen Injektion vergleichbar. Das Kontrastmittel fließt unmittelbar und auf dem schnellsten Wege in die großen Venenstämme ab.
2. Die Geschwindigkeit, mit welcher das Kontrastmittel verschwindet, ist unabhängig vom Injektionsdruck; innerhalb weniger Minuten ist praktisch das gesamte Kontrastmittel aus dem Knochen verschwunden.
3. Die Retention von Kontrastmittel im Knochen nach einer Injektion spricht für eine geschädigte ossale Zirkulation.

3. Intraossale Venographien bei Schenkelhalsfrakturen

a) Die Gefäßanatomie des oberen Femurteiles

Die Gefäße, die den oberen Teil des Femur versorgen, kommen hauptsächlich aus der A. circumflexa femoris medialis und lateralis und von der A. obturatoria. Die Circumflexagefäße bilden zusammen eine extracapsuläre Gefäßcorona um die Basis des Schenkelhalses herum. Die Gefäße zum Femurkopf gehen in zwei Gruppen von der A. circumflexa femoris medialis aus, in einer oberen und einer unteren Gefäßgruppe (Abb. 1 und 2). Die Gefäße durchbohren die Kapsel an ihrem Ansatz und ziehen in Synovialisfalten außerhalb des Schenkelhalses hinauf gegen die Knorpel-Knochengrenze am Caput, wo sie durch die Foramina nutritia in das Caput eintreten. Die Gefäße der oberen Gruppe (Abb. 1) werden als obere Retinaculagefäße (the lateral epiphyseal arteries nach TRUETA) bezeichnet. Sie sind für die Versorgung des Femurkopfes am wichtigsten. Die untere

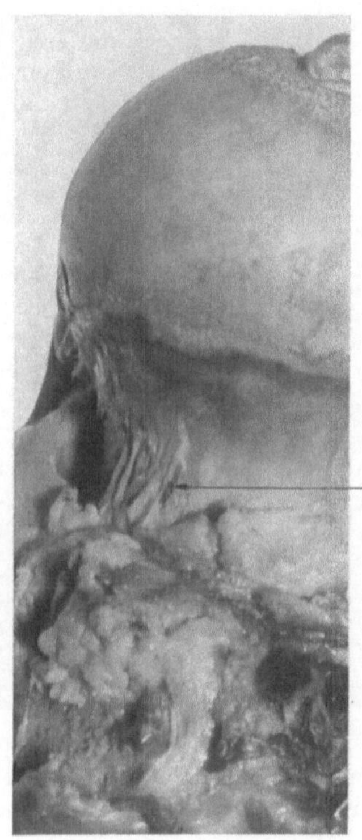

Abb. 1. Die oberen Retinaculagefäße (s. Pfeil)

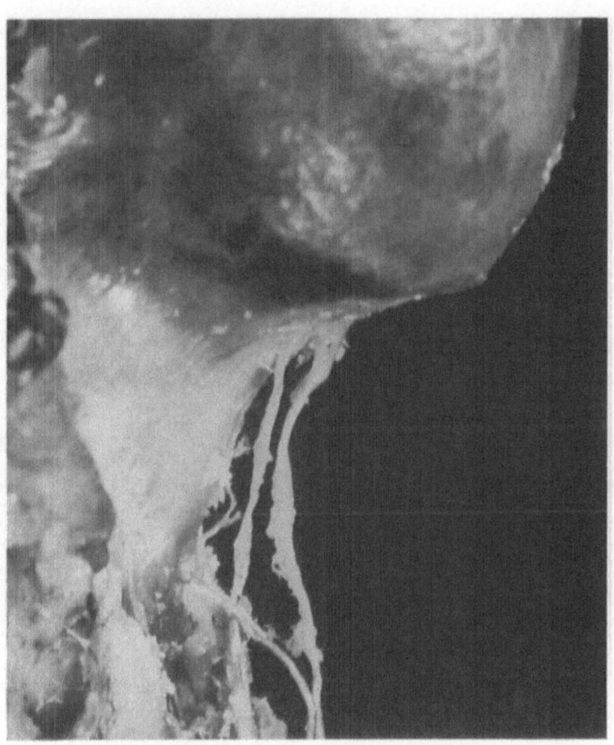

Abb. 2. Die unteren Retinaculagefäße

Gruppe, die aus zwei Gefäßen besteht, werden untere Retinaculagefäße (Abb. 2) (the metaphyseal arteries nach TRUETA) genannt. Die unteren Retinaculagefäße sind ursprünglich, wie aus dem Namen hervorgeht, metaphysäre Gefäße und ernähren hauptsächlich einen medialen unteren Keil des Caput, der metaphysären Ursprung hat. Außer von diesen beiden Gefäßgruppen wird der Femurkopf auch von Zweigen der A. obturatoria ernährt, die bei ungefähr 70—80% aller Erwachsenen durch das Ligamentum capitis femoris in das Caput zieht (the medial epiphyseal arteries nach TRUETA). Auf injizierten Gefäßpräparaten tritt deutlich hervor, daß das Caput bei Erwachsenen eine relativ selbständige Gefäßversorgung hat, die nur durch relativ kleine distale Zweige mit der rein metaphysären und reichlichen Blutversorgung des Schenkelhalses Kollateralen bildet.

Für die Gefäßversorgung des Caput ist die gruppenweise Anordnung von Gefäßen bezeichnend, die intraarticulär in den Synovialisduplikaturen (Capsula reflexa) zur Knorpel-Knochengrenze ziehen. Sie haben also einen relativ ausgedehnten intraartikulären Verlauf. Es ist außerdem bezeichnend, wie Verfasser an histologischen Studien der Retinacula bzw. des Lig. capitis femoris zeigte, daß die Arterien und Venen in den genannten Strukturen dicht nebeneinander verlaufen. Dies ist für die venographische Untersuchungsmethode und für die Schlüsse, die man aus ihr ziehen kann, von größter Bedeutung.

b) Die Gefäßversorgung des Caputfragmentes bei verschiedenen Typen von Schenkelhalsbruch

Aus der anatomischen Beschreibung und aus Abb. 3 und 4 dürfte der Unterschied der Caputversorgung bei lateralen, sog. pertrochanteren und medialen intraartikulären Frakturen klar hervorgehen. Bei den zuerst genannten verläuft die Bruchlinie lateral von den Vasa circumflexae femoris mediales, die lateral vom Kapselansatz den Schenkelhals cranialwärts kreuzen. Das Hauptgefäß und alle seine Äste befinden sich auf dem Caputfragment, und deswegen dürfte kein Risiko für seine Versorgung vorliegen. Bei

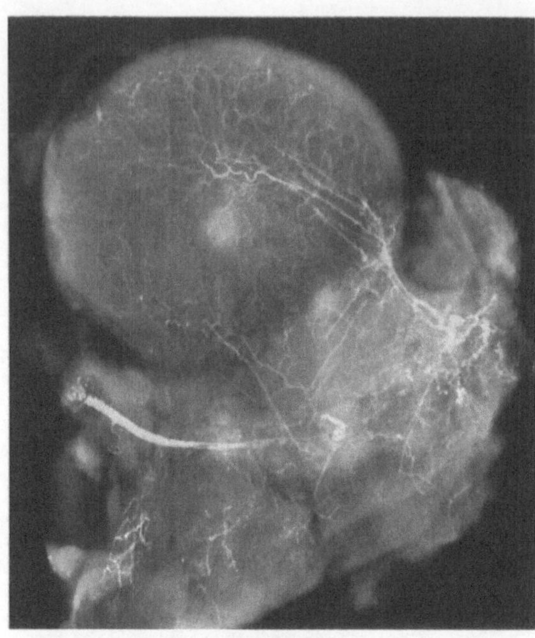

Abb. 3

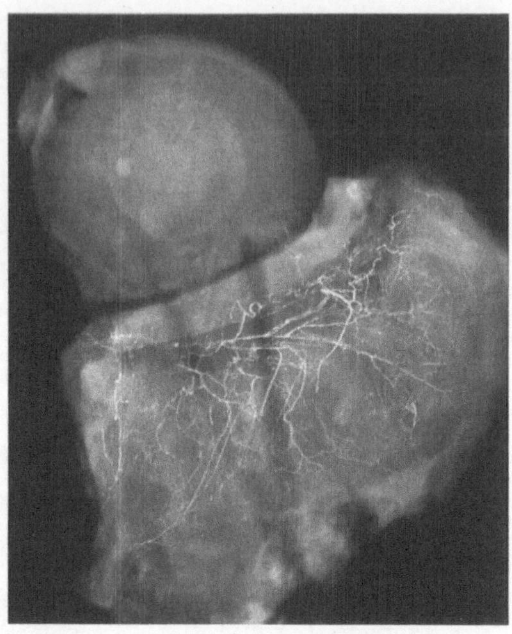

Abb. 4

Abb. 3 u. 4. Kontrastinjizierte anatomische Präparate einer pertrochanteren Fraktur (Abb. 3) und einer medialen avasculären Fraktur. Das Kontrastmittel (Zinnober) wurde in die A. circumflexa femoris medialis injiziert

den medialen Frakturen hingegen verläuft der Bruch medial von den Circumflexagefäßen. Die Folge ist, daß die Fraktur quer über die Retinaculagefäße verläuft. Bei einer vollständigen Fraktur kann nur durch Zufall der Synovialisüberzug mit Gefäßen intakt bleiben, die die Spalte überbrücken. Dies gilt besonders bei den am stärksten dislozierten Varusfrakturen, bei denen es als Folge der typischen Dislokation leicht zu einer Diastase im oberen Teil des Schenkelhalses kommt, mit der Gefahr, daß die wichtigen oberen Retinaculagefäße gedehnt oder abgerissen werden. Die Blutversorgung des Caputfragmentes bei medialen vollständigen Frakturen kann im besten Falle durch die Gefäße des Lig. capitis femoris und die oberen und unteren Retinaculagefäße erfolgen, häufig jedoch nur durch eine oder zwei dieser Gruppen, in vielen Fällen sind gar keine Gefäße erhalten. Diese Gefäße, speziell die Venen, die in den synovialen Brücken verlaufen, können, auch wenn ihre Kontinuität erhalten ist, leicht geknickt oder abgeklemmt werden. Das Lig. capitis femoris wird zwar nie bei Schenkelhalsbrüchen geschädigt, aber seine Gefäße können klein sein oder völlig fehlen. Dazu kommt, daß es keine Möglichkeit einer kollateralen Versorgung gibt, da das Fragment intraarticulär liegt und keine Muskelansätze besitzt.

c) Die Technik der venographischen Untersuchung des Femurkopfes

Zur Untersuchung wurde eine verhältnismäßig grobe Kanüle mit einem Mandrin verwendet. Diese wurde direkt von vorne oder von der Seite wie ein Collumnagel in den

Knochen getrieben. Die wichtigste Forderung ist, daß die Injektionsflüssigkeit ohne Leckage an der Nadelspitze in die Knochensubstanz eindringt. Ich habe 10 cm lange Kanülen von leicht konischer Form verwendet. Das breite Ende (5 mm äußerer Diameter) ist mit einem Gewinde versehen. Auf dieses paßt ein aufschraubbarer Handgriff. Die Kanüle hat außerdem einen Konus auf den eine Injektionsspritze paßt (Abb. 5). Man kann auch eine kürzere Kanüle verwenden, die mit einem Handbohrer direkt von vorne in das Caput getrieben wird. Dies kann mit Röntgentelevision überwacht werden. Die venographische Untersuchung wird vorgenommen, nachdem die Fraktur in gewohnter Weise auf dem Repositionstisch eingerichtet worden ist. Die Untersuchung soll nicht in den ersten 4—5 Tagen nach dem Trauma vorgenommen werden, da während dieser Zeit das Caputfragment undicht ist. Wichtig ist, daß die Kanüle nicht aufs Geradewohl eingeführt wird, weil dabei das Caput beschädigt werden kann und bei der Injektion das Kontrastmittel ins Gelenk rinnt. Die Spitze der Kanüle soll so weit medial und zentral

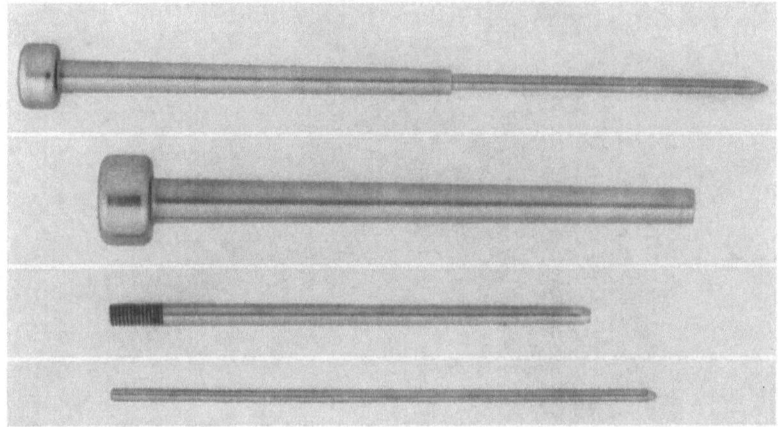

Abb. 5. Die Kanüle aufgeschraubt (oben). Handgriff, Kanüle und Mandrin (unten)

wie möglich im Fragment sitzen. Der kontralaterale Knorpel darf nicht durchbohrt werden. Nachdem die Kanüle in die gewünschte Position gebracht worden ist, injiziert man ganz langsam 2 ml Kontrastmittel, z.B. 50%iges Urografin. Wie Graf und Werner 1960 richtig angaben, darf das Kontrastmittel nicht zu schnell injiziert werden, da es dann zu unnötigen Extravasaten oder Schäden an vorhandenen Venen kommen kann. Unmittelbar nach Abschluß der Injektion wird eine Röntgenaufnahme (frontal), danach ein Seitenbild und ungefähr 2—3 min nach dem ersten Bild eine erneute Röntgenaufnahme (frontal) gemacht. Die Kassette muß richtig unter dem Patienten liegen, so daß das Foramen obturatum mit auf das Bild kommt, um die V. obturatoria sehen zu können (Dahlgren 1959). Die gesamte Untersuchung einschließlich des Entwickelns der Bilder braucht die Operation nicht um mehr als 15 min zu verlängern. Nachdem die Bilder gemacht worden sind, spült man die Kanüle mit 2 ml physiologischer Kochsalzlösung durch, um die Reste des Kontrastmittels zu beseitigen.

α) Verschiedene Venographietypen

Wenn eine Kontrastmittelinjektion eine Auffüllung und Darstellung der vom Fragment abführenden Venen zur Folge hat, nennt man dies eine *positive Venographie*.

Kontrastmittelinjektionen, bei denen die Substanz retiniert wird oder ins Gelenk ausläuft, werden *negative Venographien* genannt.

Bei der Prüfung der Methode wurden zwölf pertrochantere Frakturen untersucht. Man nahm an, daß die Gefäßversorgung bei diesen Frakturen gut erhalten war; dies wurde mittels Venographie verifiziert, die in allen Fällen positiv war (s. Abb. 6). Für die Gefäßanatomie des Caputfragmentes bei allen diesen Frakturen ist bezeichnend, daß das Circumflexagefäß medial von der Bruchlinie verläuft.

Die eigentlichen Schenkelhalsbrüche (mediale oder intraarticuläre Frakturen) wurden nach dem Grade der Dislokation aufgeteilt, indem man der gebräuchlichen Methode folgte. Valgus- oder Abduktionsfrakturen sind solche ohne oder mit geringer Dislokation. Varus- oder Adduktionsfrakturen sind die mit stärkerer Dislokation und mit größerem oder kleinerem Grad von Diastase zwischen den Fragmenten.

Beim Ausarbeiten der Venographiemethode wurden 18 Fälle von Valgusfrakturen untersucht. Von diesen ergaben 14 positive Venographien. Die negativen Venographien bei Valgusfrakturen zeichnen sich aus durch Retention des Kontrastmittels im Caputfragment eventuell bis an die Frakturlinie, jedoch ohne sie zu überschreiten. Das Kontrastmittel kann auf Grund des intimen Kontaktes zwischen den Fragmenten nicht in

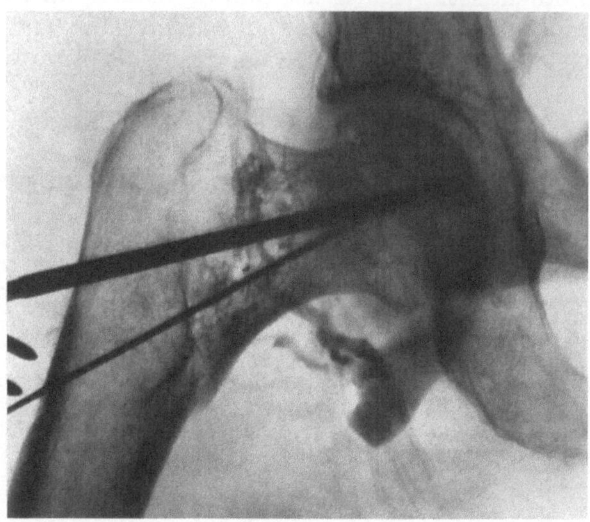

Abb. 6. Venographie bei einer pertrochantären Fraktur. Die Circumflexagefäße verlaufen medial von der Bruchlinie

die Frakturspalte oder ins Gelenk auslaufen. Die Ursache für die negative Venographie bei Valgusfrakturen ist sicher in der Abklemmung der Venen durch Schwellung zu suchen, da die Dislokation nicht so groß ist, daß sie ein Abreißen der Gefäße erklären könnte. Bei Valgusfrakturen sind Caputnekrosen nicht ganz ungewöhnlich, aber auf Grund der stabilen Frakturlage kommen Pseudarthrosen selten vor. Bei Brücken ohne oder mit nur geringer Dislokation soll man meiner Meinung nach keine intraossären Venographien machen, einerseits wegen der relativ guten Prognose dieser Frakturen und andererseits wegen der Gefahr, in dem schon vorher abgeschnürten Fragment durch die Injektion von hypertoner Kontrastlösung, die leicht retiniert wird, die Zirkulation weiterhin zu schädigen. Bei derartigen Fällen ist es sicherer, daß man sich der intraossären Injektion von ^{131}I in einer isotonen Lösung nach JOHANSSON oder HOLMQUIST et al. bedient.

Das Anwendungsgebiet der Venographie liegt bei den dislozierten medialen Collumfrakturen (d. h. Varusfrakturen). Diese haben die schlechteste Prognose; bei ihrer Behandlung hat man Anlaß, beim Verdacht auf Avascularität eine therapeutische Alternative zu erwägen. Die verschiedenen Typen von *positiven Venographien*, die bei den vollständigen Frakturen vorkommen, beruhen völlig auf den erhalten gebliebenen Gefäßverbindungen, die ein Caputfragment besitzen kann. Man kann eine Auffüllung der Teresvenen und ihrer Fortsetzung in die V. obturatoria und V. iliaca interna im Becken erhalten (s. Abb. 7 und 8). Es kann zur Darstellung der Retinaculavenen, gewöhnlich der unteren, und ihrer Fortsetzung in die V. circumflexa femoris medialis bzw. V. femoralis und V. iliaca externa kommen (s. Abb. 9). Auch eine Kombination dieser beiden Bilder kommt vor (s. Abb. 10). Nur in einigen wenigen Fällen kam es zur Darstellung der oberen Retinaculavenen; das muß seinen Grund darin haben, daß diese Venen am

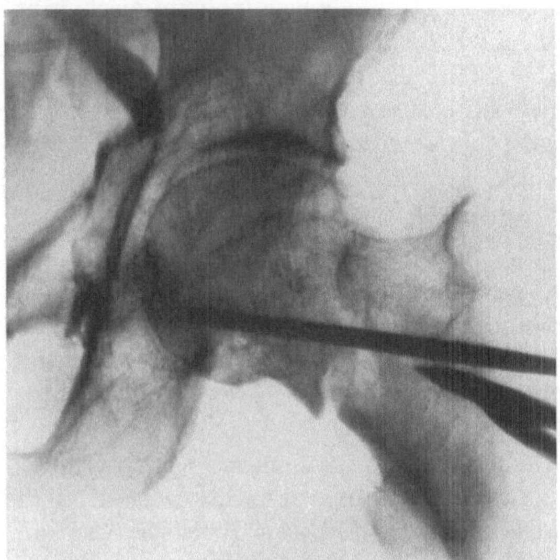

Abb. 7

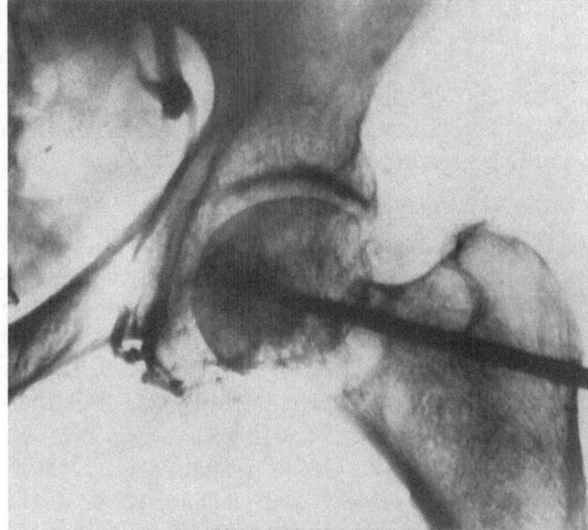

Abb. 8

Abb. 7 u. 8. Positive Venographien von zwei Varusfrakturen. Man sieht die Venen des Lig. capitis femoris und die Obturatoriavene

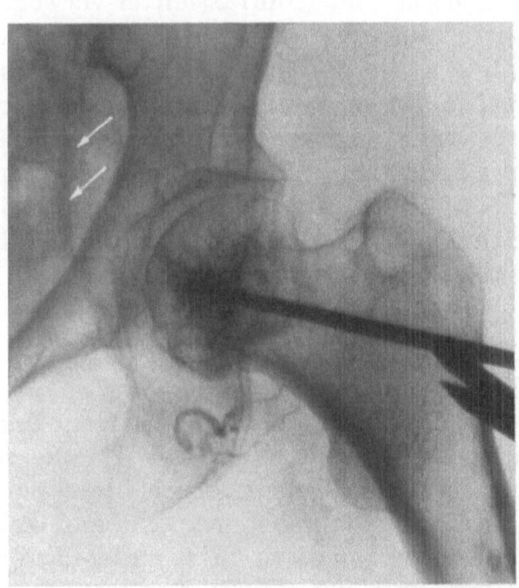

Abb. 9

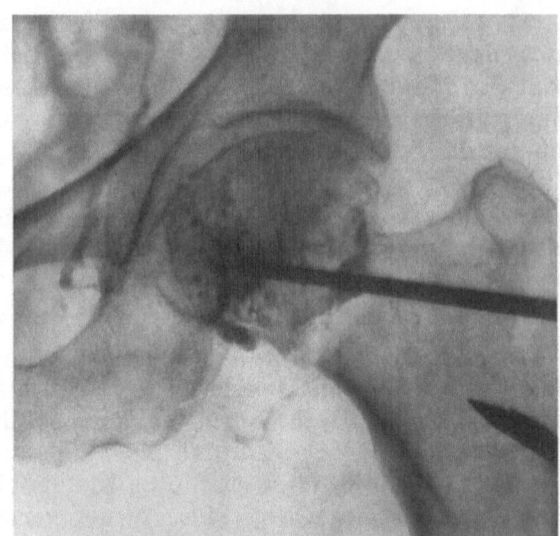

Abb. 10

Abb. 9. Positive Venographie einer Varusfraktur mit den unteren Retinaculagefäßen, Vv. circumflexae femoris mediales und V. iliaca ext. (s. Pfeile)

Abb. 10. Positive Venographie einer Varusfraktur mit Circumflexavene und Obturatoriavene

leichtesten durch Dehnung oder Abreißen geschädigt werden. In einzelnen Fällen kann eine kontrastgefüllte Retinaculavene sich durch eine Anastomose in der Fossa acetabuli in die V. obturatoria fortsetzen. Auf dem Röntgenbild ist es leicht, den Unterschied zwischen einer Obturatoria-iliaca interna-Venendarstellung und einer Femoralis-iliaca externa-Venendarstellung zu sehen. Die erstgenannte Vene zieht vom Foramen obturatum in einem konzentrischen Bogen medial um die Caputkontur herum und verläuft dann in beinahe rechtem Winkel medial-cranial mit der inneren Kontur des Beckens. Die Vv. femoralis und iliaca externa dagegen ziehen mehr gerade nach oben und medialwärts.

Wenn man zu große Kontrastmittelmengen verwendet und zu schnell injiziert, gibt es außer der Gefahr, das Fragment zu schädigen, auch noch die Möglichkeit, daß es zu *atypischen positiven Venogrammen* kommt, die darauf beruhen, daß das Kontrastmittel sich von der Frakturlinie aus in die Spongiosa des Collums verteilt und von da durch die Circumflexavenen abfließt. Einer solchen Venographie kann keine diagnostische Bedeutung zugesprochen werden.

β) Diskussion der positiven Venographien

Da die Gefäßversorgung des Caput durch parallellaufende Arterien und Venen charakterisiert ist, kann man nach positiven Venographien annehmen, daß auch die entsprechenden Arterien erhalten geblieben sind. Diese Annahme wird von der bekannten Tatsache unterstützt, daß Venen empfindlicher sind als Arterien und deswegen leichter als Arterien durch Schwellung oder Dehnung geschädigt werden.

Eine positive Venographie zeigt nur, daß Gefäßverbindungen zum Caputfragment bestehen, sie ist keine quantitative Methode zur Bestimmung der Zirkulation. Auf partielle Gewebsschäden ischämischer Natur läßt sie keine direkten Rückschlüsse zu. Das injizierte Kontrastmittel verteilt sich im Fragment, wird von der vorhandenen Zirkulation aufgefangen und fließt in die Venen ab. Man kann jedoch indirekt aus Größe und Art der Kontrastaufladung im Fragment gewisse Rückschlüsse ziehen, ob das Fragment sehr geschädigt ist oder nicht. Dies jedoch nur unter der Voraussetzung, daß die Injektion vorsichtig ausgeführt wurde und daß nicht zu viel Kontrastmittel verwendet wurde. Eine geringe Auffüllung um die Spitze der Kanüle herum, eventuell kombiniert mit feingranulierten Kontraststreifen in Richtung auf die abführenden Venen, die auf dem Frontalbild Nr. 2 verschwunden sind, sprechen für eine relativ gute Zirkulation. Eine diffuse und dichte Kontrastfüllung (Verschattung) großer Teile des Fragmentes, die auf dem anderen Bild unverändert bleibt, spricht für eine Stase und verschlechterte Zirkulation. Wenn die Kanülenlage ideal ist, d. h. die Spitze tief zentral liegt, kann das Vorkommen eines größeren Kontrastmittelaustrittes in die Frakturlinie und demzufolge schwächer dargestellte Venen auch für einen Zirkulationsschaden sprechen.

γ) Diskussion der negativen Venographien

Die negativen Venographien (s. Abb. 11 und 12) sind von Interesse, da sich unter ihnen alle Fälle von kompletter Avascularität finden. Man muß die negativen Venogramme, die auf technischen Fehlern beruhen, ausschließen. Wenn die Kanüle exzentrisch, nahe der Frakturlinie liegt, oder wenn man den Gelenkknorpel durchbohrt oder auch nur die falschgerichtete Kanüle ein Loch ins Fragment gemacht hat, kann man dem Fehlen kontrastgefüllter Venen keine Bedeutung zumessen. Eine andere Fehlerquelle entsteht, wenn man die Untersuchung zu früh nach dem Unfall ausführt, da abgerissene Gefäße dann offenstehen und bei der Injektion Kontrastmittelaustritte verursachen. Man muß mindestens 4—5 Tage warten, um mit einer einigermaßen sicheren Thrombosierung dieser abgerissenen Venen und damit mit einem dichten Fragment rechnen zu können. DAHLGREN hat 1959 die Zahl der Venographien mit Kontrastmittelaustritt in die Fraktur, die am 3. Tage nach dem Unfall gemacht wurden, mit denen verglichen, die nach dem 3. Tage gemacht wurden. Von 26 der ersteren Gruppe erhielt er 8 negative Venographien und von 24 der letzteren Gruppe nur 3 negative, was obige Annahme bestätigt. Negative Venographien können dann als gleichbedeutend mit Avascularität des Fragmentes angesehen werden, wenn folgende Forderungen erfüllt sind:

1. Untersuchung frühestens am 4.—5. Tag nach dem Unfall.

2. Die Kanüle soll tief (mindestens 2 cm) und am besten zentral im Fragment liegen. Falls das nicht der Fall ist, muß es zu einer Kontrastmittelauffüllung des Caputfragmentes kommen, die dafür spricht, daß das schattengebende Mittel mit dem Areal für mögliche Venen — wenn solche erhalten geblieben sind — in Kontakt gewesen ist.

3. Das Fragment darf nicht der Schädigung einer falsch eingeschlagenen und wieder herausgezogenen Kanüle ausgesetzt gewesen sein. Die Kanüle darf den Gelenkknorpel nicht perforiert haben.

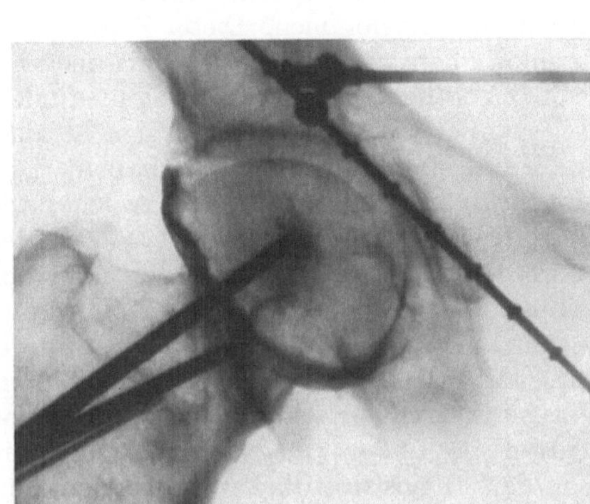

Abb. 11

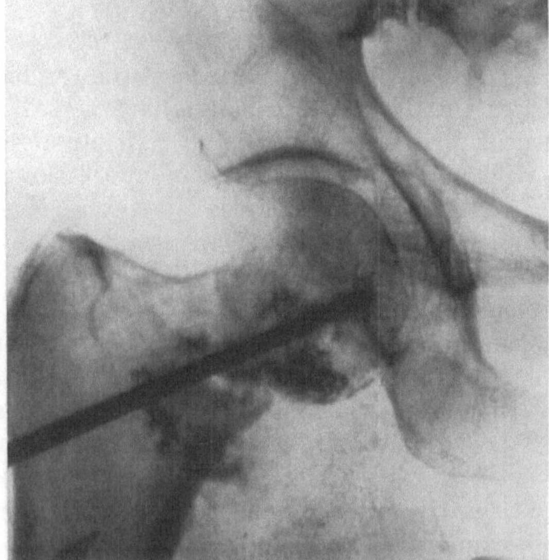

Abb. 12

Abb. 11 u. 12. Negative Venographien zweier Varusfrakturen. Venen sind nicht sichtbar. Das Kontrastmittel tritt in den Frakturspalt aus

δ) Resultat der Venographie im Verhältnis zum Grade der primären Dislokation

In meinem Material ergab sich folgende Aufteilung der Venographietypen: von 100 untersuchten Collumfrakturen waren 66 positive Venographien und 15 negative. Aus den restierenden 19 Untersuchungen konnte man keine Schlüsse ziehen. Dieses Material umfaßt sowohl Valgusfrakturen, von denen mehrere nicht disloziert waren, als auch Varusfrakturen. Bei 82 untersuchten Varusfrakturen waren 52 Venographien positiv, 13 negativ und 17 unsicher.

Meine Untersuchungen zeigten, daß sich die Valgusfrakturen vor allem durch besser erhaltene Zirkulation via Retinacula- bzw. Circumflexagefäße von den Varusfrakturen unterscheiden. Die Varusfrakturen haben verhältnismäßig weniger positive Venographien der Circumflexagefäße, haben aber statt dessen in mehreren Fällen Zirkulation via Lig. capitis femoris. Hingegen gab es keinen statistisch gesicherten Unterschied zwischen der relativen Zahl negativer Venographien in den entsprechenden Gruppen (Valgusfrakturen: von 18 untersuchten 14 positive Venographien = 78%, Varusfrakturen: von 82 untersuchten 52 positive Venographien = 63%).

Bei den Varusfrakturen gab es keinen Dislokationstyp oder -grad, der in sich selbst unbedingt Avascularität zur Folge hatte. Es fanden sich im Material Fälle mit sehr starker Dislokation, die trotzdem eine erhaltene Retinaculazirkulation hatten. Bei ausgeprägter Varusdislokation können die oberen Retinaculagefäße nicht unbeschädigt bleiben, da sie am Ort der größten Diastase verlaufen, dagegen haben aber die unteren Retinaculagefäße eine günstigere Lage. Der Verlauf der Fraktur im Schenkelhals hat keine so große Einwirkung auf die Retinaculagefäße. Nur die Frakturen, die extrem subcapital verliefen, hatten relativ weniger Fälle mit erhaltenen Retinaculagefäßen. Der Verlauf der Fraktur im Schenkelhals hat natürlich keinerlei Einwirkung auf die Teresvascularisierung, der wohl bei den subcapitalen Frakturen die größte Rolle zugeschrieben werden muß und die ein relativ kleines Caputsegment zu versorgen hat. Der Winkel zwischen der Bruchebene und dem Femurschaft wird nach Eyre-Brook u. a. (1941) gemessen, d. h., es ist im großen gesehen der Supplementwinkel zu dem von Pauwels angegebenen Winkel zwischen der Frakturebene und der Horizontalebene. Es zeigt sich, daß die Größe dieses Winkels keine Einwirkung auf die residuale Blutversorgung des Caputfragmentes hat, was interessant ist, weil PAUWELS u. a. angegeben haben, daß bei den steiler verlaufenden Frakturen schlechtere Heilungsbedingungen beständen.

ε) Nachuntersuchung

Die Nachuntersuchungen wurden in einem Zeitraum von mindestens einem Jahr nach dem Unfall, in vielen Fällen nach noch längerer Zeit, vorgenommen. Dieser Zeitraum ist nicht lang genug, um später auftretende Komplikationen aufzudecken, scheint aber voll ausreichend, um avasculäre Manifestationen in der eigentlichen Frakturregion aufzufinden. Es zeigt sich nämlich, daß während einer Zeitspanne von 1—$1^1/_2$ Jahren sich in allen Fällen mit negativem Venogramm avasculäre Manifestationen eingestellt haben. Dies gilt sowohl für mein Material als auch für das von S. DAHLGREN (1959), welches wie meines untersucht und behandelt wurde. Bei längerer Nachuntersuchungszeit werden sicherlich weitere Komplikationen festgestellt werden, besonders in Form von Einbruch der oberen Caputkontur nach der Frakturheilung. Diese spät auftretenden Manifestationen kann man jedoch nicht primär mit der Venographiemethode diagnostizieren, d. h. voraussagen, und sie beruhen sicher auf einer partiellen vasculären Schädigung.

Es wurden 43 Patienten — nur dislozierte Varusfrakturen — nachuntersucht, von denen 31 positive und 12 negative Venogramme hatten; alle 12 mit negativem Venogramm bekamen früh avasculäre Manifestationen. Von den 31 positiven bekamen 10 deutliche Zeichen einer avasculären Nekrose. Der Typ der Nekrose bei positiven Venogrammen unterscheidet sich jedoch in der Mehrzahl der Fälle von dem, den wir bei negativen Venogrammen finden. Bei den negativen Venographien kann man annehmen, daß es sich um vollständige Avascularität handelt; die Nekrose manifestiert sich in diesen Fällen im Frakturgebiet, entweder in dem es zur Pseudarthrose kommt oder auch dadurch, daß es zu einer kontinuierlichen Resorption des distalen Teiles des Caput kommt, oft bei Heilung der Fraktur. Das Caputfragment bekommt bei diesen letzteren Fällen eine charakteristische Pilzform, die besonders auf dem Seitenbild sichtbar ist. Gleichzeitig mit der Resorption kommt es zu einer erhöhten Penetration der Nägel, die zuweilen den Gelenkknorpel durchbohren. In einigen Fällen wandert der Nagel oder durchbohrt das Fragment lateral nach vorne. Bei zwölf Patienten mit negativen Venogrammen trat in fünf Fällen eine Pseudarthrose auf, in vier Fällen eine distale Resorption des Caput und in zwei Fällen eine Coxa vara mit Nageldurchbruch. Die restlichen Fälle bekamen einen Einbruch der oberen Caputkontur.

Die avasculären Manifestationen, die bei den 10 Fällen der 31 positiven Venographien auftraten, hatten ein anderes Aussehen. Da es sich hier wahrscheinlich um eine relative vasculäre Insuffizienz hauptsächlich durch Schädigung der wichtigen oberen Retinaculagefäße handelt, kommt es zu einem Einbruch des oberen Caputteiles. Der erhalten gebliebene Blutzufluß durch die unteren Retinaculum- oder Lig. teres-Gefäße war in diesen Fällen für die Ernährung des gesamten Fragmentes unzureichend, und der am entferntesten gelegene Teil des Caput, d. h. der obere Teil, leidet zuerst unter der unzureichenden Blutversorgung. Von den zehn Fällen mit avasculären Manifestationen hatten sechs einen solchen oberen Einbruch; nur ein Fall von Pseudarthrose trat auf, ein Fall von verzögerter Heilung und ein Fall von Nagelgleiten. Bei einem Patienten fand sich relative Dichte und homogene Knochenstruktur als einzige sichtbare Manifestationen der Nekrose. Alle übrigen 21 Fälle heilten ohne Schwierigkeiten.

Nach der von mir festgelegten Methode (mit 2—3 ml Kontrastmittel und Nachspülung mit physiologischer Kochsalzlösung) wurde ein weiteres schwedisches Krankengut von DAHLGREN (1959) nachuntersucht. Er hatte 25 Fälle, die er nach 1—2 Jahren nachuntersuchte. Das Resultat war folgendes:

von 8 positiven Venogrammen.	1 Nekrose
von 9 negativen Venogrammen	9 Nekrosen
von 3 atypisch positiven Venogrammen.	0 Nekrosen
von 5 unsicher negativen Venogrammen	4 Nekrosen

Eine dritte Untersuchungsreihe (Hulth und Johansson 1962) ergab etwa gleichartige Verhältnisse. Von 44 Patienten mit positiven Venographien zeigten 8 avasculäre Manifestationen. Bei 15 von 16 Fällen mit negativer Venographie wurden avasculäre Manifestationen festgestellt. Außerdem gab es 27 Venographien mit unsicheren Ergebnissen, die aus verschiedenen Gründen nicht gedeutet werden konnten, von diesen kam es bei 14 zur Nekrose.

ζ) Venographische Untersuchung der Pseudarthrosen

Bei der Behandlung einer Pseudarthrose nach einer medialen Collumfraktur ist es sehr wertvoll zu erfahren, ob das Caputfragment Gefäßversorgung hat oder nicht (s. Abb. 13). Es kann den Versuch wert sein, ein revascularisiertes Caputfragment zu

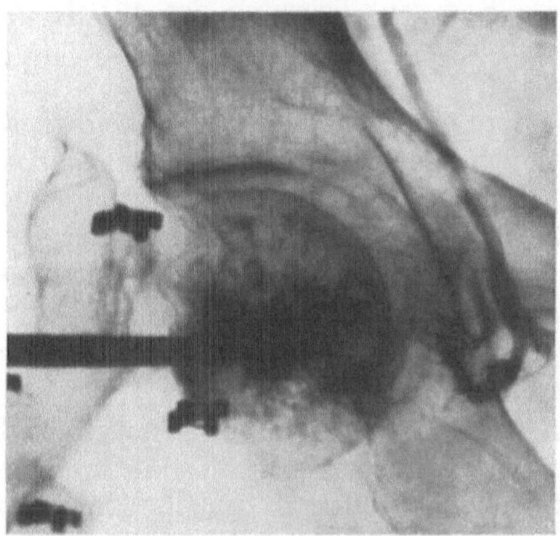

Abb. 13. Venographie einer Pseudarthrose, die eine Revascularisierung des Caput zeigt

bewahren. Bei einem Fragment ohne Gefäße ist dieser Versuch wertlos. Die Venographie scheint somit bei der Beurteilung von Pseudarthrosen wertvoll zu sein, wie auch Graf angeführt hat. Die Untersuchung soll gemacht werden, ehe eventuell Osteosynthesematerial herausgezogen wird. Alternativ kann die Kanüle via Nagelkanal eingesetzt werden.

d) Diskussion der Untersuchungsmethode

Die intraossale Kontrastmittelinjektion in das Caputfragment bei medialen Collumfrakturen ist eine Methode, die ziemlich sichere Aussagen über die restierenden Gefäßverbindungen des Caputfragmentes ergibt. Verglichen mit anderen veröffentlichten prognostischen Methoden gibt diese Untersuchung erstaunlich gleichmäßige Resultate (Arden 1960; Boyd et al. 1963; Johansson 1964). Jede der beschriebenen Methoden zeigt in etwa einem Viertel bis einem Drittel nicht verwertbare Ergebnisse infolge von Undichtigkeiten und Aussickern bei der Injektion in den spongiösen Knochen, oder weil die Trochanter-Kopf-Relation einen Grenzwert zwischen einwandfreier Durchblutung oder einwandfreier Nichtdurchblutung ergibt. Eine korrekte Voraussage war in 80—90 % möglich bei den verschiedenen Methoden, die verwertbare Ergebnisse zeigten. Bei nachgewiesener Avascularität war das Risiko einer Nekrose oder Pseudarthrose etwa 90 %. Eine gute Bruchheilung medialer Schenkelhalsbrüche nach Osteosynthese ist hauptsächlich vom Vascularisierungsfaktor abhängig. Dies ist eine wertvolle Schlußfolgerung der prognostischen Methoden, die besonders betont werden muß, weil auch heute noch das Entstehen von Pseudarthrosen anderen Ursachen, nämlich mechanischen Verhältnissen oder der Einwirkung der Synovialflüssigkeit zugeschrieben wird. Unsichere Untersuchungsergebnisse und falsche Voraussagen lassen sich meist auf die schlechten Durchblutungsverhältnisse vieler Schenkelköpfe zurückführen und sind seltener verursacht durch die angewendete Methode. Bei dislozierten Bruchstücken sind die Gefäßverbindungen — venös und/oder arteriell — meist sehr geschädigt. In vielen Fällen ist die Blutversorgung des Schenkelkopfes gerade noch an der Grenze der Lebensfähigkeit.

Histologische Untersuchungen von FELSENREICH (1938—1940) und von SEVITT (1964) zeigen partielle oder totale Nekrosen des Kopfes häufiger als man an Hand der klinisch manifesten Nekrosen annehmen konnte. Die Ergebnisse der verschiedenen Meßmethoden hängen sicher sehr davon ab, wo im Kopf die Untersuchung durchgeführt wurde. Die Durchblutungsverhältnisse der untersuchten Stelle brauchen nicht übereinzustimmen mit denen im ganzen Oberschenkelkopf. In vielen Fällen verbessert sich die Durchblutung erst allmählich. Die Untersuchungen von MASSIE sprechen für diese Annahme. Außerdem kann die sorgfältige und exakte Reposition der Fraktur und die Fixation mit einem Nagel eine bessere und schnellere Revascularisierung des Bruchgebietes bedeuten. Schlechte Reposition und Nagelung führen bei Grenzfällen zu einer größeren Zahl manifester Nekrosen und Pseudarthrosen.

Eine sichere und exakte prognostische Methode haben wir also noch nicht. Die dargelegten Untersuchungsmethoden geben jedoch recht gute Hinweise. Nicht alle Caputnekrosen zeigen schwere klinische Symptome. Die Endoprothesen ergeben nicht immer ein zufriedenstellendes Endergebnis. Sie sind deshalb nur gerechtfertigt als Ersatz bei wirklich schmerzhaften Hüften, besonders bei älteren Verletzten.

In ausgewählten Fällen ergibt die Untersuchung mit einer prognostischen Methode, die technisch leicht ausgeführt werden kann, wie die der intraossären Injektion, recht gute Hilfe. Sie wird daher empfohlen:

1. Bei Pseudarthrosen oder veralteten nicht genagelten Schenkelhalsfrakturen, die röntgenologisch ein Caput mit normaler Knochenstruktur zeigen. Hier kann entschieden werden ob das Knochengewebe lebt oder tot ist (HULTH und JOHANSSON 1966). Pseudarthrosen mit veränderter Knochenstruktur, also einem „Umbaukopf", der revascularisiert ist, haben einen zerstörten Knorpel und sind daher funktionell schlecht.

2. Bei Schenkelhalsfrakturen bei sehr alten Verletzten. Hier ist die Endoprothese eine gute Alternative gegenüber einem nekrotischen Kopf.

Die beste Lösung ist doch immer das eigene Caput zu behalten, sofern es noch lebensfähig ist. Nach richtiger Reposition und Nagelung bei Fällen mit noch erhaltener Durchblutung (50% der untersuchten Fälle) ist die Prognose gut in 90%. Die Endoprothesen können bei dem restlichen Teil verwendet werden, immer dann, wenn die Untersuchung Avascularität oder nicht verwertbare Ergebnisse gezeigt hat.

Literatur

ARDEN, G. P.: Radioactive isotopes in fractures of the neck of the femur. J. Bone Jt Surg. B **42**, 21—27 (1960).

—, and N. VEALL: The use of radioactive phosphorus in early detection of avascular necrosis in the femoral head in fractured neck of femur. Proc. roy. Soc. Med. **46**, 344—346 (1953).

BEGG, A. C.: Intraosseous venography of the lower limb and pelvis. Brit. J. Radiol. **27**, 318—324 (1954).

BENDA, R., E. ORINSTEIN et E. DEPITRE: Injection intra-médullaires osseuses de substances opaques chez l'homme. Sang **14**, 172—176 (1940/41).

BOYD, H. B.: Use of the Geiger counter in estimating the blood supply in the femoral head. J. Bone Jt Surg. B **33**, 475 (1951)

— D. B. ZILVERSMIT and R. A. CALANDRUCCIO: The use of radioactive phosphorus to determine the viability of the head of the femur. J. Bone Jt Surg. A **37**, 260—269 (1955).

BOYD, H. B., and R. A. CALANDRUCCIO: Further observations on the radioactive phosphorus (P^{32}) to determine the viability of the head of the femur. Correlation of clinical data in 130 patients with fractures of the femoral neck. J. Bone Jt Surg. A **45**, 445—460 (1963).

BRUGGER, G.: Zur Frage des prognostischen Wertes angiographischer Untersuchungen bei medialen Schenkelhalsfrakturen. Mschr. Unfallheilk. **66**, 337—344 (1963).

DAHLGREN, S.: Venography of the femoral neck. Acta chir. scand. **117**, 494—500 (1959).

DUCCI, L.: L'injection intramédullo-osseuse d'un produit de contrast pour le diagnostic des affections osseuses. Presse méd. **58**, 623—628 (1950).

DUCUING. J., P. GUILHEM, D. ENJALBERT, J. POULHES et R. BAUX: La phlébographie du pelvis par voie transosseuse pubienne. Lyon chir. **46**, 93—404 (1951).

ENRIA, G., e R. FERRERO: La flebografia degli arti par via ossa. Chirurgia (Milano) **5**, 289—296 (1900).

EYRE-BROOK, A. L., and K. H. BRIDIE: Intracapsular fractures of the neck of the femur. Brit J. Sug. **29**, 115—138 (1941).

FELSENREICH, F.: Histologische Untersuchungen an operierten Schenkelhalsbrüchen. I.—VIII. Mitteilung. Langenbecks Arch. klin. Chir. **192** (I), 490—544 (1938); (II) 96—134 (1938); (III) 584—620 (1938); (IV) 18—29 (1939); (V) 413—454 (1939); (VI) 589—610 (1939); (VII) 14—29 (1940); (VIII) 532—578 (1940).

GRAF, R.: Der Wert der Phlebographie des Schenkelhalskopfes bei der Behandlung von Schenkelhalspseudarthrosen. Chirurg **31**, 19—21 (196).

—, u. H. WERNER: Die Phlebographie des Schenkelkopfes bei der frischen medialen Schenkelhalsfraktur. Fortschr. Röntgenstr. **92**, 331—337 (1960).

GUILHEM, P., et R. BAUX: La phlébographie pelvienne par voies veineuse, osseuse et utérine. Paris: Masson & Cie. 1954.

HAAS, W. DE, and J. MACNAB: Fractures of the neck of the femur. A method of assessing the viability of the femoral head. Sth Afr. med. J. **30**, 1005—1010 (1956).

HARRISON, M. H. M.: A preliminary report of vascular assay in prognosis of the fractured femoral neck. J. Bone Jt B **44**, 858—868 (1962).

HERZOG, W.: Zur Problematik der medialen Schenkelhalsfraktur. Angiographische, histologische und tierexperimentelle Untersuchungen. Langenbecks Arch. klin. Chir. **299**, 200—227 (1962).

HIPP, E.: Die Gefäße des Hüftkopfes. Anatomie, Angiographie und Klinik. Z. Orthop. **96**, Beilageheft (1962).

HOLMQUIST, B., and P.-A. ALFFRAM: Prediction of avascular necrosis following cervical fracture of the femur based on clearance of radioactive iodine from the head of the femur. Acta orthop. scand. **36**, 62—69 (1965).

HOYER, H.: Zur Histologie des Knochenmarkes.

HULTH, A.: Injection of contrast medium in the head of intra-capsular fractures of the neck of the femur. Acta Soc. Med. upsalien. **59**, 41—51 (1953).

— Intra-osseous venographies of medial fractures of the femoral neck. Acta chir. scand. Suppl. **214** (1956).

— Femoral-head phlebography. A method of predicting viability. J. Bone Jt Surg. A **40**, 844—852 (1958a).

— Circulatory disturbances in osteoarthritis of the hip. Acta orthop. scand. **28**, 81—89 (1958b).

HULTH, A.: Necrosis of the head of the femur. A roentgenological, microradiographic and histological study. Acta chir. scand. **122**, 75—84 (1961).

— Prediction of the viability of the femoral head in femoral neck fractures. Acta chir. scand. **129**, 72—80 (1965).

—, and S. H. JOHANSSON: Venography in fractures of the femoral neck. Acta chir. scand. **123**, 287—297 (1962).

— — Structural changes of the femoral head in cases of non-union of the femoral neck. Virchows Arch. path. Anat. **340**, 320—329 (1966).

JOHANSSON, S. H.: Prognostic assessment in fractures of the neck of the femur using ^{131}I and venography. Acta chir. scand. **123**, 298—306 (1962).

— The prognostic value of the radio-iodine test in femoral neck fractures. Acta Soc. Med. upsalien. **69**, 64—82 (1964).

JOSEFSON, A.: A new method of treatment—intraossal injections. Acta med. scand. **81**, 550—555 (1934).

LANGER, E.: Über das Gefäßsystem der Röhrenknochen. Denkschr. kaiserl. Akad. Wiss. **36** (1876).

LEGER, L., et C. FRILEUX: La phlébographie par injection intra-médullo-osseuse du produit de contrast. Presse méd. **58**, 29—32 (1950).

MARNEFFE, E. DE: Recherches morphologiques et expérimentales sur la vascularisation osseuse. Bruxelles: Les Editions "Acta Medica Belgica" 1951.

MASSIE, W. K.: Fractures of the hip. J. Bone Jt Surg. A **46**, 658—690 (1964).

MENEGAUX, G., L. LEGER et P. DETRIE: La médullographie osseuse. Presse méd. **61**, 1728—1731 (1953).

MERIEL, P., R. RUFFIE et A. FOURNIE: La phlébographie de la hanche dans les coxarthroses. Rev. Rhum. **22**, 238—239 (1955).

NUSSBAUM, A.: Die arteriellen Gefäße der Epiphyse des Oberschenkels und ihre Beziehungen zu normalen und pathologischen Vorgängen. Bruns' Beitr. klin. Chir. **130**, 494—535 (1924).

PALAU, M. S.: La flebografia intraosea en las fractura del cuello de femur. Cirug. Ginec. Urol. **15**, 621—647 (1961).

PAUWELS, F.: Der Schenkelhalsbruch, ein mechanisches Problem. Stuttgart: Ferdinand Enke 1935.

PHEMISTER, D. B.: Pathology of ununited fractures of the femur with special references to the head. J. Bone Jt Surg. **21**, 681—639 (1939).

— Changes in bones and joints resulting from interruption of circulation. Arch. Surg. (Chicago) **41**, 436—446 (1940).

REHM, J., u. H. J. SÜSSE: Transossale Venographie des Kopffragmentes bei Schenkelhalspseudarthrosen. Mschr. Unfallheilk. **58**, 137—143 (1955).

SANTOS, J. V.: Changes in head of femur after complete intracapsular fracture of the neck. Arch. Surg. (Chicago) **21**, 470—511 (1930).

SCHOBINGER, R. A.: Intra-osseous venography. New York and London: Grune & Stratton 1960.

SEVITT, S.: Avascular necrosis and revascularization of the femoral head after intracapsular fractures. A combined arteriographic and histological necropsy study. J. Bone Jt Surg. B **46**, 270—296 (1964).

SÜSSE, H. J., u. G. AURIG: Über die transossale Venographie. Zbl. Chir. **79**, 596—600 (1954).

TOCANTINS, L. M., and J. F. O'NEILL: Infusions of blood and other fluid into general circulation via bone marrow. Surg. Gynec. Obstet. **73**, 281—287 (1941).

TRUETA, J., and M. H. M. HARRISON: The normal vascular anatomy of the femoral head in adult man. J. Bone Jt Surg. B **35**, 442—461 (1953).

TUCKER, F. R.: Arterial supply to the femoral head and its clinical importance. J. Bone Jt Surg. B **31**, 82—93 (1949).

— The use of radioactive phosphorus in the diagnosis of avascular necrosis of the femoral head. J. Bone Jt Surg. B **32**, 100—107 (1950).

VRBKA, M.: The early diagnosis of aseptic necrosis of the head in fractures of the neck of the femur. Univ. Carolina Med. **3**, 615—620 (1957).

WALLDEN, L.: On injuries of bone and bone-marrow after intra-osseous injection. Acta chir. scand. **96**, 152—160 (1948).

WATSON-JONES, R.: Fractures and joint injuries, 4th ed. Edinburgh: Livingstone, Vol. I (1952), Vol. II (1955).

J. Vorgänge bei der Knochentransplantation

Von

R. Maatz und K. Haasch

Mit 50 Abbildungen

I. Geschichtlicher Überblick

Wie in der Knochenbildung und Knochenwundheilung sind auch in der Transplantation des Knochens wesentliche Probleme noch nicht gelöst. So hat ein kurzer geschichtlicher Überblick über ihre Entwicklung die Fehlerquelle, daß sogenannte „Marksteine" — und nur solche können in einem kurzen Überblick gegeben werden — sich später nach Gewinnung weiterer Erkenntnisse als „weniger markant" oder sogar als Irrtümer herausstellen können. Unter Hervorhebung dieser Gefahrenquelle halten wir eine kurze Übersicht über die Entwicklung der Knochentransplantation aber doch für gerechtfertigt. Dabei bemühen wir uns in besonderem Maße darum, den Autoren Gerechtigkeit widerfahren zu lassen, welche durch die überragende Autorität von Zeitgenossen oder Nachfahren allzu sehr in den Schatten gestellt wurden. Der Heteroplastik muß zu diesem Zeitpunkt, da dieser Beitrag verfaßt wird, ein etwas ausführlicherer Raum gegeben werden, weil nach Gewinnung der Erkenntnis, daß das heterologe Spanmaterial durch weitestgehende Abschwächung seiner Antigenität in einem breiten Indikationsgebiet das autologe Spanmaterial entbehrlich macht. Da diese Fragen im Fluß sind, haben wir auch die Wege, welche wahrscheinlich nicht zweckmäßig sind, welche aber erprobt werden mußten, ebenfalls — wenn auch in äußerster Kürze — skizziert.

Die erste sicher nachgewiesene Verpflanzung eines Knochens wurde vom Hund auf den Menschen vorgenommen (van Meekren, 1682), war also *heteroplastisch.* Der russische Edelmann mußte sich den Knochen, mit dem ein durch Säbelhieb entstandener Schädeldefekt „erfolgreich" gedeckt wurde, allerdings auf Anordnung der Kirche wieder entfernen lassen. Da diese Entfernung 2 Jahre nach der Implantation mühelos gelang, gehen wir sicher nicht fehl, eine bindegewebige Einscheidung anzunehmen. Nach unseren heutigen Kenntnissen war diese Heteroplastik also nur im „Frühergebnis klinisch erfolgreich".

Die ersten *Autoplastiken* führte v. Walther (1821) durch. Es waren sicher freie Verpflanzungen, wenn auch die Implantate am Schädeldach zum Teil wieder in ihr altes Bett gelegt wurden.

Ollier (1860) prägte die Begriffe der *Auto-Homoio- und Heteroplastik.* Er sprach von einer „Spezifität der Gewebsflüssigkeit und der Gefäße", machte also als erster auf die immunologischen Fragen der Transplantation aufmerksam. Trotz dieser Erkenntnis und der Leistungen von Duhamel (1740), Knochenhaut und Markhaut als Knochenbildner zu erkennen, und der weiteren Erkenntnis von Dupuytren (1839), daß auch die umgebenden Zellgewebe sich an einer Knochenneubildung beteiligen, wurde zunächst eine Verpflanzung von Mensch auf Mensch nicht gewagt. Die Arbeiten von Barth (1895) waren für diese Entwicklung ohne Zweifel von entscheidender Bedeutung. Er behauptete, daß alle Teile eines verpflanzten Knochens stets abstürben, und daß der Ersatz des toten durch lebenden Knochen stets nur vom Lagergewebe geleistet würde. Damit sei es ganz gleich, ob auto-homoio- oder heteroplastisches Spanmaterial zur Verwendung käme. Marchand (1899) stellte diesen Irrtum dann richtig, Barth ließ sich überzeugen, und Marchand berichtete gleichzeitig über die in russischer Sprache erschienene und darum bis dahin nicht bekannte

Arbeit von RADZIMOWSKY (1881), welcher beobachtet hatte, daß nur die Knochenzellen bei einer autoplastischen Verpflanzung abstürben. Unter dem Einfluß von G. AXHAUSEN (1908), LEXER (1912) und MACEWEN (1919) ging die Entwicklung unaufhaltsam zur Vormachtstellung des autoplastisch frischen Spanes hin, wenn Tierspäne auch noch in Einzelfällen angewendet wurden, so von TUFFIER und MAGITOT (1870) nach Konservierung in der Eistruhe und von LANDERER (1894) im macerierten Zustand, wie BARTH es nach seinen ersten Arbeiten empfohlen hatte.

Erst 1912 wurde — angeregt durch die Gedankengänge von OLLIER und MACEWEN die erste *homoioplastische* Spanverpflanzung vorgenommen. Der Autor verwendete Knochenkeile, welche er bei der Korrektur rachitisch verkrümmter Beine bei Kindern gewonnen hatte, zur Ausfüllung des Defektes im osteomyelitischen Knochen nach Sequestrotomie. Trotz der früh (1820 und 1858) geäußerten Meinungen von DUPUYTREN („nicht nur Periost und Markhaut, sondern auch Zellgewebe der umgebenden Weichgewebe beteiligen sich") und VIRCHOW (1871) („und daß eigentlich alle recht haben, indem sich der neue Knochen aus dem verschiedensten Material aufbaut") konnte G. AXHAUSEN (1908) seiner *Osteoblastentheorie* weitgehend Anerkennung verschaffen, nach der die Knochenneubildung ausschließlich an spezifische Knochenbildner gebunden ist. Damit begann der „Siegeszug" des autoplastischen Spanes, dessen Leistungsfähigkeit durch die hervorragenden Erfolge LEXERS und anderer Kliniker bewiesen wurde, und dessen praktisch vorhandene Alleinherrschaft erst ein Halbjahrhundert später gebrochen werden sollte.

Nicht unerwähnt darf in dieser Schilderung der Name WOLFF (1884) bleiben, welcher in seiner Lehre von der Transformation der inneren Architektur der Knochen auf die „umgestaltende Wirkung der Funktion" hinwies, eine Tatsache, welche ja auch nach der freien Verpflanzung von Knochen von Bedeutung ist.

Im Gegensatz zur Osteoblastentheorie kamen BASCHKIRZEW und PETROW (1912) auf Grund von Tierversuchen zu der Erkenntnis, daß die Hauptquelle der Regeneration bei der Übertragung eines Knochentransplantates in ein Weichteillager bindegewebige Elemente seien, die in den Knochen einwüchsen und dort zu Osteoblasten und Osteocyten *metaplasieren.* In Übereinstimmung damit nimmt BIER (1923) an, daß der neue Knochen unter Mitwirkung aller seiner Teile „und von beliebigem Bindegewebe" gebildet wird, welches durch allerlei Reize, vor allem aber vom verletzten Knochen durch *Nekrohormone* zur Metaplasie „erregt" wird.

Für die Erfolgsaussichten einer Knochentransplantation erkennt LEXER (1924) die *Bedeutung des Lagers,* welches er als *ersatzfähig, ersatzschwach* oder *ersatzunfähig* bezeichnet. Er stützt damit gleichzeitig die Osteoblastentheorie, während LÉRICHE und POLICARD (1926) jede Knochenneubildung als metaplastisch ansehen, wobei die Anwesenheit der Kalksalze toten Knochens die Anregung geben. Unterstützung fanden die Anhänger der Metaplasielehre in der Induktionslehre von SPEMANN (1936). LEVANDER (1949) bezeichnete einen aus dem Knochen mit Alkohol extrahierten, nicht art- und individualgebundenen Wirkstoff, mit dem er (in der Kaninchenmuskulatur) metaplastische Knochengewebsbildung hervorrief, als *Osteogenin;* KÜNTSCHER glaubt dabei an eine Sekretionsleistung der gereizten Knochenzellen. Wenn auch die Wirkung von Nekrohormonen bei der Pflanze nachgewiesen sind, ist ihre Bedeutung als hormonartiger Stoff in der Knochenbildung heute doch sehr in Frage gestellt, da tote unvollkommen geglühte heteroplastische Späne in unerhört starkem Maße ein ersatzstarkes Lager zur Knochenneubildung anregen (MAATZ, LENTZ u. GRAF, 1954), und heteroplastische Späne, welche im 20—40%igen Wasserstoffsuperoxyd „ausgebrannt" werden, und welche anschließend im Ätherdampfapparat sterilisiert werden, ebenfalls diese Eigenschaft zeigen. Darüber hinaus konnten FUCHS, STEGEMANN und EGER (1963) zeigen, daß weder die organische Substanz allein noch die anorganische das Lager zur lebhaften Callusbildung anregt, sondern nur die Matrix, welcher die antigenisierende Eigenschaft genommen ist, welche aber aus Fibrillen und Kristalliten besteht. Es muß die Frage heute als offen angesehen werden, welcher Reiz die Mesenchymzellen zur Ausdifferenzierung zu Osteoblasten veranlaßt. Daß diese

Metaplasie, welche eigentlich nur eine Differenzierung ist, stattfindet, unterliegt heute allerdings keinem Zweifel mehr.

Was DUPUYTREN, BIER und auch VIRCHOW annahmen, und was durch die *Osteoblastentheorie* und die Lehre der Metaplasie auseinandergefallen war, vereinigte W. AXHAUSEN (1952) wieder in seiner *Zweiphasentheorie*. Danach wird die sofort einsetzende Knochenneubildung von praeexistenten Osteoblasten geleistet, während spätere Knochenbildung ebenfalls durch Osteoblasten entsteht, welche aber aus jungen Bindegewebszellen, undifferenzierten Mesenchymzellen, *metaplasieren*. So haben, um wieder mit VIRCHOW zu sprechen, eigentlich alle recht, nur diejenigen allerdings nicht, welche allein das eine oder das andere Gewebe als Knochenbildner verantwortlich ansehen wollten.

Wie wir gesehen haben, wurden Fremdspäne (homogen oder heterogen) in Einzelfällen immer wieder auch in den Zeiten genommen, als der lebend frische autologe Span das Feld vollkommen beherrschte. Mit der *Konservierung* der Späne begann ein neues Kapitel. TUFFIER und MAGITOT (1870) verwendeten gefrorene Späne, BARTH (1895) im Experiment macerierte, LANDERER (1894) einen mazerierten Span am Menschen und GALLIE (1918) *gekochte* Späne.

1934 berichtete ORELL über sein „Os purum", einen von den Weichgeweben befreiten, also mazerierten Tierspan. Der auf BARTH zurückgehende Gedankengang, daß die Knochensubstanz ohnehin abstirbt, veranlaßte ihn, ein „sauberes Knochengerüst" als Transplantat zu verwenden. Durch Vorverpflanzung in einen subperiostalen Raum wollte der Autor dem Span Leben und autologe Eigenschaften geben (Os novum). In der Klinik konnte sich das Spanmaterial nicht durchsetzen.

1939 berichteten O'CONNER, BROWN und DE MERE über die Konservierung homologer Späne in Merthiolat, ein Verfahren, welches MORGAN, JANNISON und POWEL 1933 für die Gewebekonservierung angegeben hatten. Dieses Verfahren konnte sich nur an wenigen Stellen bis heute halten, nachdem INCLAN (1942) über eine erste Serie klinischer Erfolge mit homologen Spänen berichtete, welche im Tiefkühlverfahren konserviert waren. BUSH prägte dann 1947 den Begriff der "Bone bank" und JUDET und ARVISET (1949) übertrugen das Verfahren auch auf die heterologen Späne. Sie verwendeten dann das von KREUZ, HYATT, TURNER und BASSET (1951) verbesserte Verfahren des Schnellgefrierens und Trocknens (freeze-dried), durch das dann auch die Aufbewahrung unabhängig von der Tiefkühltruhe in Vacuumampullen möglich wurde.

1952 prüften MAATZ, LENTZ und GRAF die Überlebensfähigkeit konservierter Späne mit autologen Spänen, welche in die Muskulatur implantiert wurden, da im Gewebzuchtverfahren stets nur Überleben der bindegewebigen Elemente nachweisbar war. Sie fanden unter günstigen Bedingungen in der Eigenblutkonserve Überleben der knochenbildenden Potenz bis zu 16 Tagen. Jeder gefroren konservierte Span hatte die osteogenetische Potenz verloren.

Mit dem von MAATZ 1951 inaugurierten Spongiosa-Test, einem Schnelltest zur Prüfung der Spanqualität, fanden MAATZ, LENTZ und GRAF 1952 die Möglichkeit, heterologe Späne von ihrer Antigenität zu befreien, so daß dieses Spanmaterial als „Calluslocker" rascher als autologe Späne substituiert wurden. Mit dem Wasserstoffsuperoxydverfahren fand BAUERMEISTER in seiner Dissertationsarbeit 1954 ein sicheres und fabrikatorisch verwertbares Oxydationsverfahren, welches die heterologen Späne für die Implantation in den Menschen geeignet machen.

1956 berichteten LOSEE und Mitarb. über einen eiweißfreien heterologen Span (Ossar). Dieses Spanmaterial bestand nach Extraktion der Eiweißkörper mit Diäthylamin praktisch nur aus Kristalliten, war entsprechend bröckelig und ließ jede Art der Anregung der Osteogenese eines ersatzfähigen Lagers vermissen.

TUCKER berichtete 1956 über "cultured calf bone", ein Spanmaterial, welches vom Kalb gewonnen, in autologem Serum lange konserviert, als Transplantat in der Humanmedizin geeignet sein sollte. DINGWALL und Mitarb. (1961) prüften dieses Material immunologisch und fanden hohe Antigenität.

RAY und HOLLOWAY gingen 1957 einen anderen Weg, indem sie den heterologen Knochen von der anorganischen Substanz befreiten. Ihr "biologic rubber" (EDTA) wurde auf Autogenität nicht geprüft, wurde im Tierexperiment substituiert, aber zeigte keinerlei Vorteile.

1959 bewies GRAF im Tierexperiment, daß ein autologer Span unter günstigsten Bedingungen (z.B. Spongiosatest) bereits 4 Tage nach der Implantation mit seinen Capillaren Anschluß an die Capillaren des Lagers gewonnen hat, so daß der Span durchblutet ist.

URIST glaubte 1959 bewiesen zu haben, daß Patienten mit Knochenatrophie einen zur Behandlung einer Schenkelhalsfraktur verwendeten Metallnagel nicht vertrugen, verwendete darum tragfähige Corticalis alter Rinder, präparierte das Material mit Chymotrypsin und nannte den Span "collapatite".

DINGWALL, ANDERSON und zahlreiche Mitarb. berichteten 1961 erstmalig über ein vom Kalb gewonnenes Spanmaterial, welches in einem besonderen Verfahren (Firma Squibb) von den Weichgeweben befreit die Antigenität verloren hat, rasch capillaren Anschluß im Lager gewinnt und rascher als autologe Corticalis vom Wirtsgewebe durch körpereigenen lebenden Span ersetzt wird. Damit zeigt dieses seit 1964 als „Boplant" bezeichnete Spanmaterial dieselben guten Eigenschaften wie das von MAATZ und BAUERMEISTER (1954) bekanntgegebene Material, welches unter dem Namen „Kieler Span" von der Firma Braun-Melsungen hergestellt wird. Beiden Spanmaterialien ist eigen, daß sie Antikörperbildung nicht verursachen und vom jungen Tier gewonnen werden. Die raschere Aufbereitung des Spanmaterials durch das Wirtsgewebe wird mit dem lockeren Gefüge des jungen Knochens erklärt, denn im Knochen des jungen Tieres sind die Haversschen Kanäle ungleich weiter als beim ausgewachsenen Tier. Als totes Implantat ist dieses Transplantationsgut selbstredend nur in einem „ersatzfähigen Lager" verwendbar.

II. Immunologie der Knochentransplantation

OLLIER (1860) vermutete für den Knochen dieselbe Individual- und Artspezifität wie bei anderen Geweben, und damit gab er MACEWEN (1912) die Anregung, homoiologe Transplantate statt wie bisher heterologe zu verwenden, da die Antigenität bei der Verpflanzung vom Tier auf Mensch ungleich größer sein mußte als bei der Verpflanzung von Mensch auf Mensch.

Diese Fragen wurden erst wieder aktuell mit der Einführung der sogenannten *Knochenbank*. Die Erfahrung lehrte, daß das Spanmaterial in der Tiefkühltruhe homoiologer Genese sein mußte und dabei erst dann mit besserer Aussicht auf Erfolg verwendet werden konnte, wenn es über die Dauer einiger Wochen konserviert war. So war der Schluß erlaubt, daß das Spanmaterial durch die Konservierung an Antigenität einbüßte. Diese Beobachtung wurde auch bei heterologem Material gemacht, da dieses z.B. als frischer Kalbsknochen in der Mehrzahl der Fälle in aseptischer Eiterung abgestoßen wurde, während es nach Konservierung immerhin in der Mehrzahl der Fälle behalten wurde, wenn auch der knöcherne Einbau nur sehr langsam ablief, wenn es nicht doch zu einer bindegewebigen Einscheidung oder Resorption kam.

Im Vergleich zur Haut-, Gefäß- und der Organtransplantation nimmt der Knochen — immunologisch gesehen — eine ungleich günstigere Stellung ein, da es möglich ist, seine Antigenität bis zur „Nichtnachweisbarkeit" abzuschwächen, während seine Morphologie und ein wichtiger Teil seiner physiologischen Funktion für die Transplantation erhalten bleibt. Der von MAATZ und BAUERMEISTER zunächst noch als „maceriert" bezeichnete, mit H_2O_2 und Ätherdämpfen präparierte Tierspan verursacht keinerlei Antikörperbildung im Empfänger (KIENHOLZ u. KEMKES, 1956).

MILLOWICH, AMREIN und BORMAN wiesen 1962 in einem besonderen Verfahren die Antigenität des Rinderknochens nach, und ANDERSON, LECOCQ und DINGWALL (1961) zeigten, daß der Kalbsknochen, den sie zunächst „processed bone" und später „Boplant" (Firma Squibb) nannten, bei den Versuchstieren (Meerschweinchen) stets einen Antititer von 0 beließ, während der Antititer bei Verwendung frischen Kalbsknochens in 10tägigen Intervallen von 1:32 über 1:128 auf 1:250 stieg. Der unbehandelte Kalbsknochen konnte bereits nach 10 Tagen die "fatal anaphylaxis" verursachen, der "processed bone" tat es zu keiner Zeit.

Von besonderem immunologischen Interesse sind die Untersuchungen von DUYFJES (1965), welcher nachweisen konnte, daß der präparierte Tierspan (hier „Kieler Span") schwach antigen-positiv ist, wenn die Zellkerne in den Knochenhöhlen nicht alle entfernt sind, daß er aber antigen-negativ ist, wenn die Knochenhöhlen leer sind, das Spanmaterial also nur aus Fibrillen und Kristalliten besteht.

Nicht unerwähnt darf bleiben, daß durch homoiologes Spanmaterial aus der Knochenbank rhesus-negative Empfänger sensibilisiert, also rhesus-positiv wurden (EHALT, 1956).

III. Feingewebliche Vorgänge bei der freien Knochenverpflanzung

Zum Studium des Einbaus und zur Prüfung der Wertigkeit von Knochentransplantaten wurden bisher 3 Wege beschritten:

1. Die Verpflanzung in Weichteile (Muskulatur, Subcutis, Bauchhöhle, vordere Augenkammer, Hahnenkamm usf.),
2. Schädeldachtrepanation und Ausfüllung des Defektes mit passender Knochenscheibe,
3. künstliche wandständige oder circuläre Defekte am Röhrenknochen mit Einfügung des mehr oder minder genau passenden Implantats.

Hinzugekommen sind der *Spongiosa-Test* am Hund (MAATZ), ein Schnelltest, und der Schädeldach-Test am unverletzten Schädel der Ratte (MAATZ), ein Testverfahren am

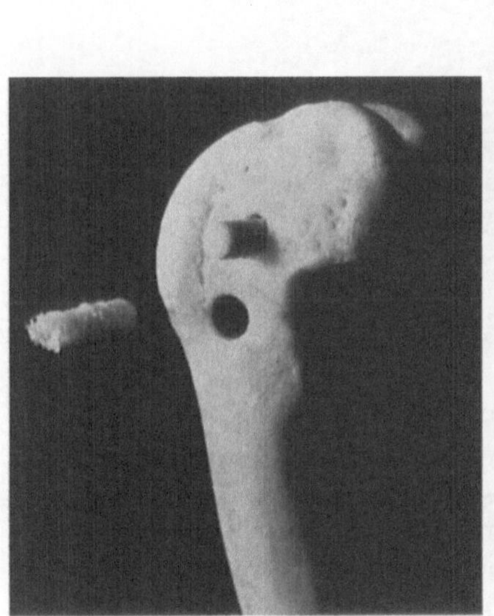

Abb. 1

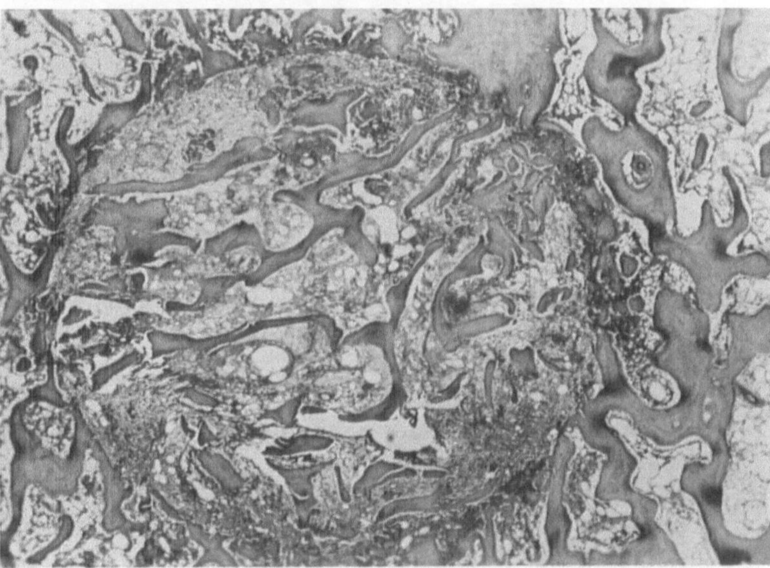

Abb. 2

Abb. 1. Im Spongiosa-Test lassen sich alle Arten von Knochenspänen im Lager gleichbleibender Ersatzfähigkeit in kurzer Zeit prüfen

Abb. 2. Lupenübersicht eines Querschnitts durch den Spongiosa-Test. Der homologe Tiefkühl-Span hemmt die Lagerleistung nur in der ersten Woche (acht Tage nach Implantation)

kleinen Versuchstier. Durch den Spongiosatest (MAATZ, 1951) wurde das Prüfungsverfahren zeitlich gerafft, weil alle Knochenvorgänge in der Spongiosa ungleich rascher ablaufen als an der Corticalis, und seine Genauigkeit wurde beträchtlich verbessert durch Ausschaltung der verdeckenden Leistung des Periostes, durch Exaktheit in der Formschlüssigkeit zwischen Lager und Span und endlich durch die Tatsache, daß an einem Hund mindestens 8 vergleichende Testungen gleichzeitig vorgenommen werden können.

Zur Erleichterung des Verständnisses zeigt Abb. 1 den Spongiosatest an einem weichteil-befreiten Hundefemur. Das 15—20 mm lange Implantat aus spongiösem Knochen ist formschlüssig in die als ersatzstarkes Lager bekannte Spongiosa eingefügt. Abb. 2 zeigt einen Querschnitt durch Lager und Span etwa in der Mitte der Länge des Spanes, dort also, wo ein periostaler Einfluß nicht anzunehmen ist. Die Lagerleistung allein kommt im Leertest (Abb. 1, S. 541) klar zum Ausdruck. Der Test gestattet eine gute Abgrenzung von Lager- und Spanleistung. Bei hoher Eigenleistung des Spanes fehlt ein merkbares Gefälle von der Peripherie zum Zentrum, bei fehlender Eigenleistung ist das Gefälle groß, und bei hemmender Wirkung des Spanes wird die Lagerleistung meßbar abgebremst.

1. Der autologe Span

Der autologe Span sitzt 2 Tage nach der Verpflanzung fest im Lager. Schon zu dieser Zeit ist etwa die Hälfte der Knochenhöhlen kernlos leer, also humoral aufgelöst. Nach 4 Tagen sind nur in wenigen Knochenzellhöhlen pyknotische Kernreste erkennbar. *Es*

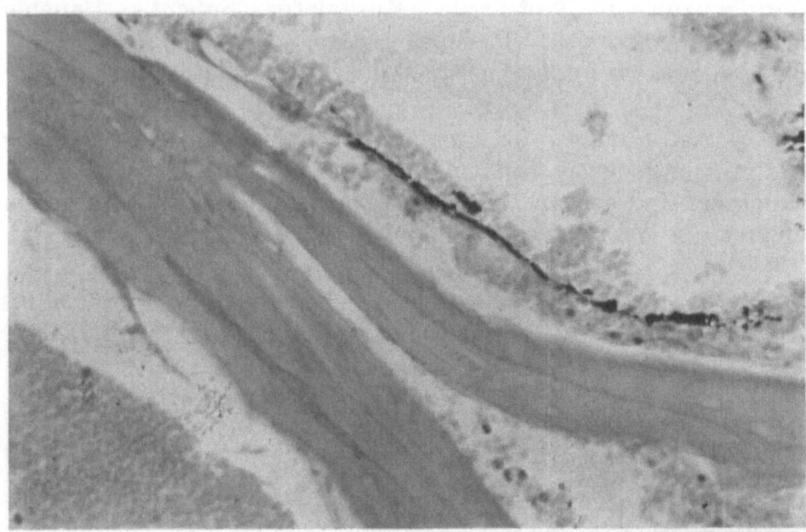

Abb. 3. Autologer Spongiosa-Span zeigt im Spongiosa-Test vier Tage nach der Transplantation im Tuschversuch (GRAF) Anschluß der Capillaren ans Lager

sterben also alle Knochenzellen bei der autologen Spanverpflanzung auch unter günstigsten Bedingungen ab. Daß diese Bedingungen im Spongiosatest die denkbar günstigsten sind, ist einleuchtend, und wurde auch von GRAF (1959) bewiesen, denn am 4. Tag nach der Transplantation hatten die Capillaren des Implantats Anschluß an die Capillaren des Lagers (Abb. 3), der Span war also durchblutet, seine Weichgewebe haben die Verpflanzung unter diesen günstigen Bedingungen überstanden, während die gegen Ernährungsstörung offenbar sehr empfindlichen Knochenzellen der Nekrose verfallen (Abb. 4).

Schon zu diesem frühen Zeitpunkt haben sich große Zellen der überlebenden Weichgewebe den toten Knochenzellen angelagert. Es ist der Beginn der „schleichenden Substitution", welche das tote Knochengewebe durch lebendes ersetzt. Die Abb. 3, S. 542, zeigt diesen Vorgang in etwas fortgeschrittenerem Stadium, und in Abb. 5 sind die überpflanzten Trabekeln bis auf kleine Reste durch den neuen Knochen ersetzt. Da dieser Vorgang im Zentrum ebenso wie am Rande des Implantats abläuft, dürfen wir — in Übereinstimmung mit allen klinischen Erfahrungen — sagen, daß der autologe, lebend überpflanzte Span seine abgestorbene Knochensubstanz zu einem großen Teil aus eigener Kraft, und zwar mit den überlebenden Weichgeweben des Spanes, durch lebendes Knochengewebe ersetzt.

Ein in die Muskulatur implantierter periostgedeckter, autologer lebender Span zeigt darüber hinaus die Leistungsfähigkeit der Cambiumschicht unter der Grundmembran

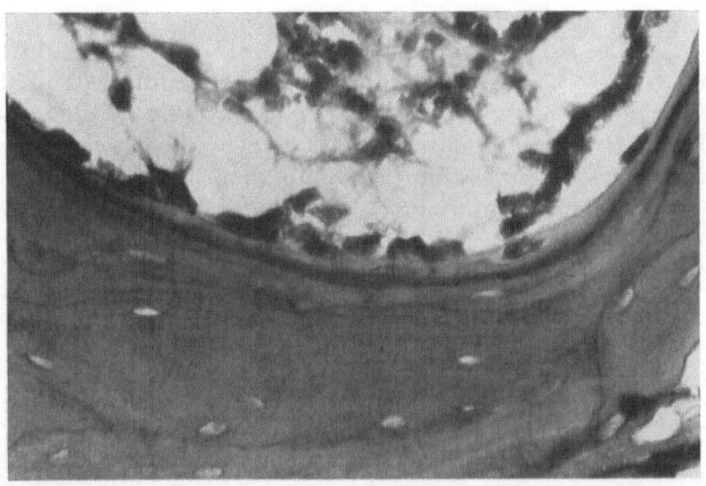

Abb. 4. Autologer Spongiosa-Span vier Tage nach der Verpflanzung. Totes Knochengerüst mit leeren Zellhöhlen, überlebende Weichgewebe, von denen erste Knochenzellbildung ausgeht

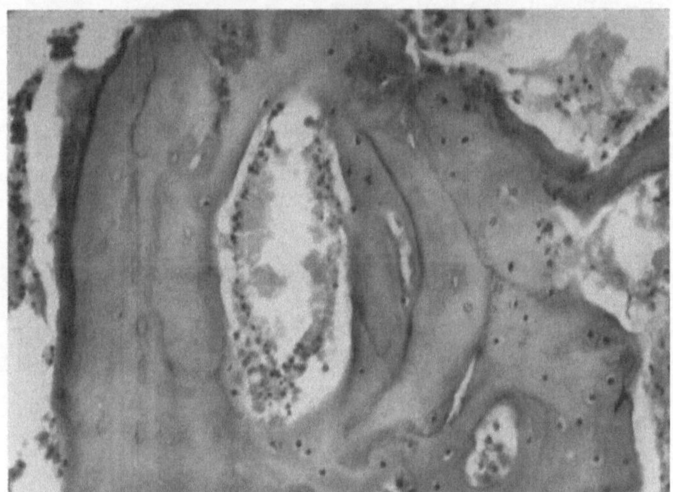

Abb. 5. Weit fortgeschrittene schleichende Substitution zwei Wochen nach der Implantation. Rechts der Mitte liegt noch eine schmale Sichel toten Knochengewebes

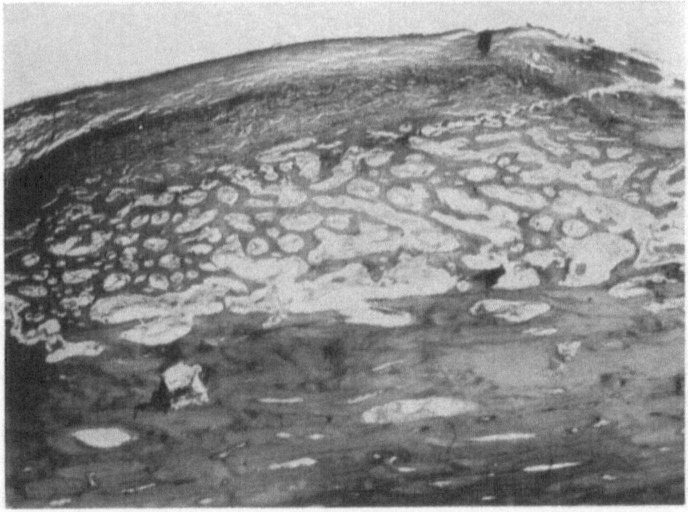

Abb. 6. Lebhafte periostale Callusbildung am autologen Span, welcher, sechs Tage in Eigenserum konserviert, in die Skeletmuskulatur implantiert wurde

Periost (MACEWEN, 1912), zeigt lebhafte periostale Callusbildung (Abb. 6), die in Abhängigkeit vom Alter des Spenders mehr oder weniger mächtig ist (MAATZ, 1948).

Neben der Knochenneubildung auf dem Wege des schleichenden Ersatzes tritt selbstredend auch angiogene Callusbildung auf, und zwar ausgehend vom Lagergewebe als auch zwischen den implantierten Bälkchen vom überlebenden Markgewebe.

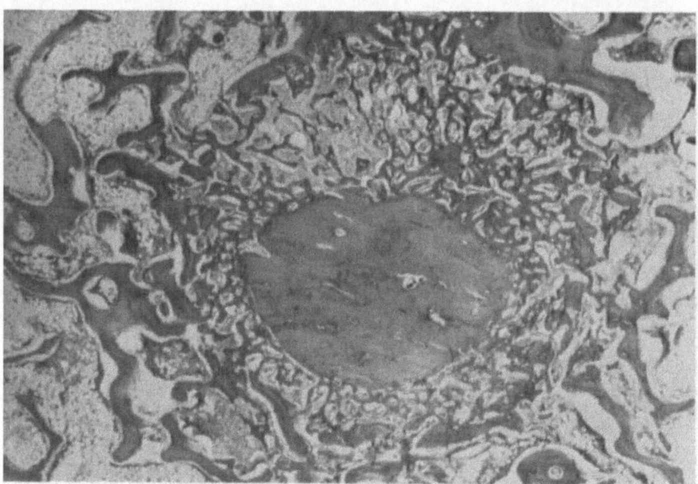

Abb. 7. Lebhafte, völlig ungestörte Callusbildung im Spongiosa-Test zwei Wochen nach Implantation eines autologen Corticalis-Spanes. In der Corticalis sind zu dieser Zeit nur erste Anfänge des Umbaus erkennbar

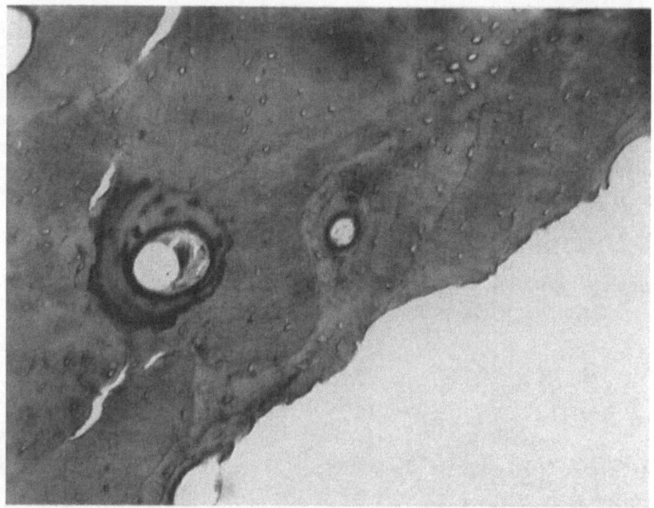

Abb. 8. Spärliche schleichende Substitution im autologen Span ein Jahr nach der Transplantation zur extraarticulären Arthrodese des Handgelenks

Vergegenwärtigen wir uns noch einmal die Tatsache, daß auch bei der autologen Transplantation die Knochenzellen absterben, so daß das Knochengerüst durch lebendes Knochengewebe ersetzt wird, so verstehen wir die Bedeutung des eklatanten Unterschiedes im Tempo der Substitution zwischen Spongiosa und Corticalis. Die Vorgänge am Knochen sind Oberflächenvorgänge. Die große innere Oberfläche der Spongiosa ermöglicht einen raschen Ablauf der Substitution, im Spongiosabolzen von 4 mm Durchmesser ist der Vorgang nach etwa 4—6 Wochen abgeschlossen. Die Corticalis muß durch Erweiterung der Haversschen Kanäle aufgelockert werden. Sie wird spongiosiert, ähnlich wie die Fragmentenden bei einer Schaftfraktur. Zwei Wochen nach der Implantation hat dieser Vorgang praktisch noch nicht eingesetzt (Abb. 7). Das Mikrofoto der Abb. 8 zeigt einen

Corticalisspan ein Jahr nach der Implantation mit nur geringer Substitution durch lebenden Knochen. Wir müssen uns merken, daß dieser Vorgang noch Jahre in Anspruch nehmen kann (MAATZ, 1956; v. SCHLEYER, 1964; ANDERSON, LE COCQ, AKESON u. HARRINGTON, 1964).

2. Der homologe Span

Der homologe Span unterscheidet sich, wie auch die Abb. 2 zeigt, ganz klar vom autologen, da die Spaneigenleistung fehlt, hier also ein starkes Gefälle vom Rande, der Zone der Lagerleistung, zum Zentrum des Spanes besteht. Im weiteren Verlauf aber zeigt sich, daß sich dieses Spanmaterial der Substitution durch das Wirtsgewebe widerstandslos hingibt. Hier herrscht dann vorwiegend die Umwandlung auf dem Wege des schleichenden Ersatzes.

3. Der heterologe Span

Ganz anders ist das Verhalten eines unbehandelten heterologen Spanes. Im Grenzgebiet zwischen Span und Lager spielt sich zunächst eine lebhafte entzündliche Reaktion mit leukocytärer Infiltration zwischen Zelldetritusmassen ab. Die Knochenbildung vom

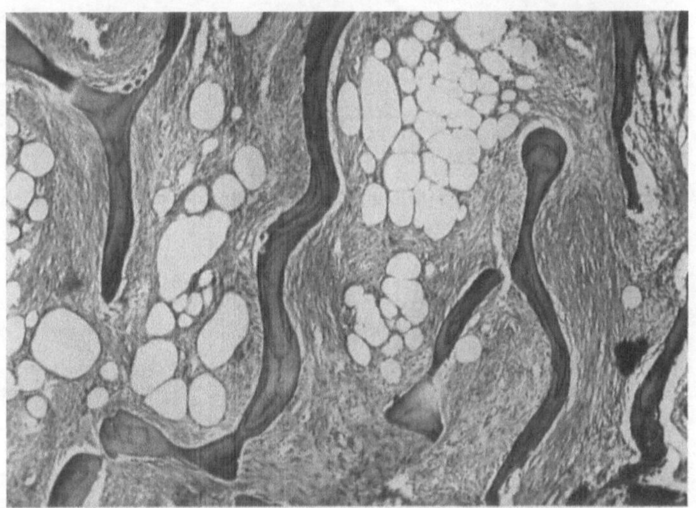

Abb. 9. Der heterologe frische Span zeigt im Spongiosa-Test zwei Wochen nach der Implantation bindegewebige Einscheidung und beginnende lacunäre Resorption, außerdem große Fettlacunen

Lager her setzt erst spät ein, nachdem die Räume zwischen den Knochenbälkchen durch Granulationsgewebe vom Lager her ausgefüllt sind (Abb. 9). Die Bälkchen, welche zu so später Zeit (2 Wochen) trotz sicheren Zelltodes noch gute Kernfärbung zeigen, sind bindegewebig eingescheidet, und im Bindegewebe liegen Fettlacunen als Reste des Fettmarkes des Implantats. Vom Bindegewebe werden die Bälkchen durch Osteoclasten lacunär resorbiert. Vom Lager her dringt dann die Knochenneubildung vor (Abb. 10) und ersetzt das Implantat vorwiegend auf dem Umweg über die bindegewebige Resorption. *Es ist nur allzu klar, daß ein solches Implantat in der Klinik entweder frühzeitig in aseptischer Eiterung abgestoßen wird, oder es wird bindegewebig eingescheidet ohne Resorption oder mit langsam folgender Resorption, und im günstigsten Fall kann in einem Lager mit starker osteogenetischer Potenz eine Substitution durch körpereigenen lebenden Knochen stattfinden.*

Es besteht Einigkeit darüber, daß das Spanmaterial im Konservierungsverfahren (Tiefkühltruhe ohne oder mit Trocknung, Merthiolat u.a.) an Antigenität verliert. Einigkeit besteht auch darüber, daß ein derartig konserviertes Spanmaterial in allen Teilen tot ist. Die Vitalität läßt sich nur in Nährlösungen über etwas länger als zwei Wochen mit osteogenetischer Potenz erhalten (MAATZ, LENTZ u. GRAF, 1953), während ein bindegewebiges Wachstum in Gewebekulturen sich auch über noch längere Zeit erhalten läßt. An Kernfärbbarkeit allein, wie TUCKER (1956) es annimmt, kann die Vitalität eines Spanes nicht erkannt werden. Darüber hinaus verlieren die in Eigenserum über Monate konservierten Späne *nicht* ihre Antigenität.

Es besteht also kein Zweifel daran, daß wir mit den Spänen der Knochenbank avitale Späne verwenden. Die Abschwächung der Antigenität heterologer Späne durch Lyophili-

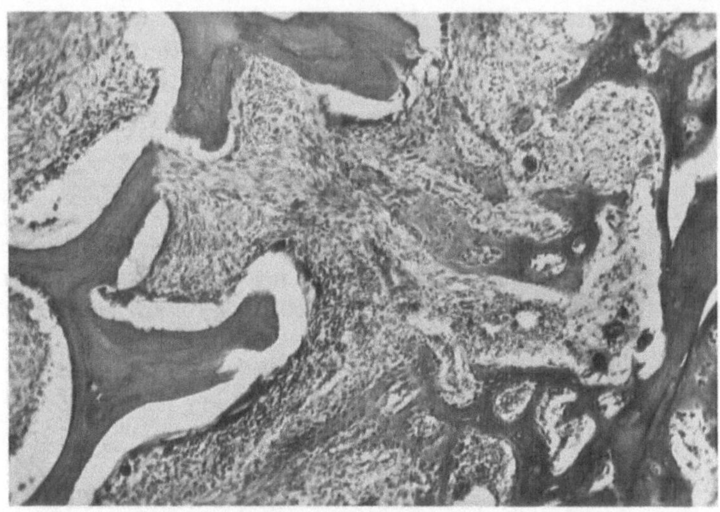

Abb. 10. Randzone von Abb. 9. Lebhafte lacunäre Resorption. Gehemmte Knochenneubildung des Lagergewebes (links)

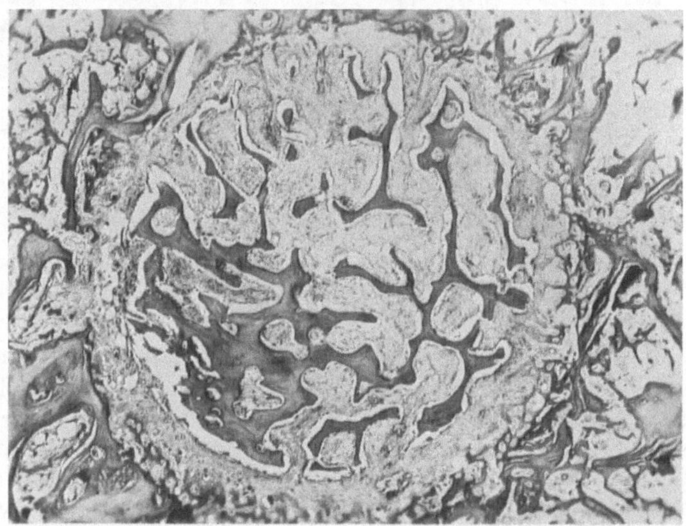

Abb. 11. Ein in Seifenlauge macerierter heterologer Span zeigt zwei Wochen nach der Implantation bindegewebige Einscheidung und vollkommene Hemmung der Knochenbildung vom Lager aus

sation, wie sie die *Lyoner Arbeitsgruppe* (GUILLEMINET, HERBERT, DUBOST, STAGNARA u. Mitarb., 1950) beim vom Kalb gewonnenen Span glaubten erreichen zu können, erwies sich aber doch als unzureichend (KINGMA, KAWAMURA u.a., 1960).

Der von MAATZ, LENTZ und GRAF und von MAATZ und BAUERMEISTER (1954) erarbeitete Tierspan, welcher als „Kieler Span“ bekannt wurde, und der "processed bone" von ANDERSON, DINGWALL und Mitarb. (1962), welcher heute als „Boplant“ bekannt ist, ähneln sich bei tierexperimenteller Prüfung in ihren Eigenschaften sehr, so daß ihre Charakteristica zusammen abgehandelt werden können.

Als geeigneter Spender dient das Kalb. Der Kalbsknochen ist poröser, hat weitere Haverssche Kanäle als das ausgewachsene Rind, wird darum rascher vascularisiert und damit auch durch wirtseigenen Knochen, vorwiegend auf dem Wege des *schleichenden Ersatzes* substituiert. Dieses Spanmaterial besitzt keinerlei Antigenität, sensibilisiert den Empfänger nicht, wird also ohne „Fremdkörperreaktion" angenommen.

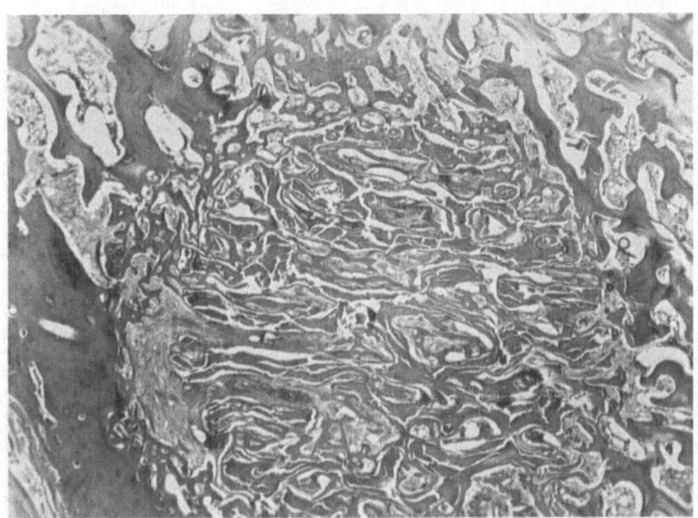

Abb. 12. Ein in 20%igem H_2O_2 gereinigter und in Ätherdämpfen entfetteter und sterilisierter heterologer Span zeigt zwei Wochen nach der Implantation planimetrisch gemessen reichlicheren Ersatz des toten Knochens durch lebenden

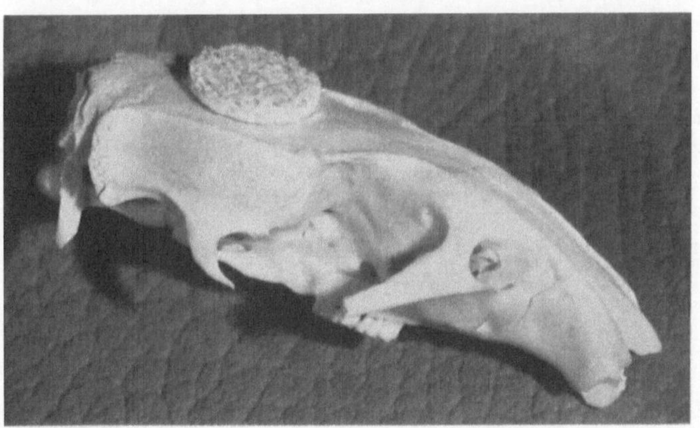

Abb. 13. Das Modell des Schädeldach-Testes an der Ratte (Kronentest)

Die Abb. 11 und 12 demonstrieren eindrucksvoll den Unterschied zwischen einem mit Seifenlauge macerierten Kalbsspan und einem in 20% H_2O_2 und Ätherdampf von allen Weichgeweben bis in die Knochenzellhöhlen hinein befreiten Span gleichen Ursprungs. Ersterer ist nach zwei Wochen in Bindegewebe eingescheidet, letzterer weitgehend durch körpereigenes, lebendes Knochengewebe ersetzt. *Dieses aus Fibrillen, Kristalliten und Matrix bestehende Material wird im ersatzfähigen Lager* ebenso rasch oder rascher als autologer lebender Knochen ersetzt. Es ruft in der Skeletmuskulatur metaplastische Knochenbildung hervor (Bauermeister, 1954; Haasch, 1961). Maatz und Mitarb. (1955) prägten darum den Begriff „Calluslocker", eine Eigenschaft, welche besonders eindrucksvoll im

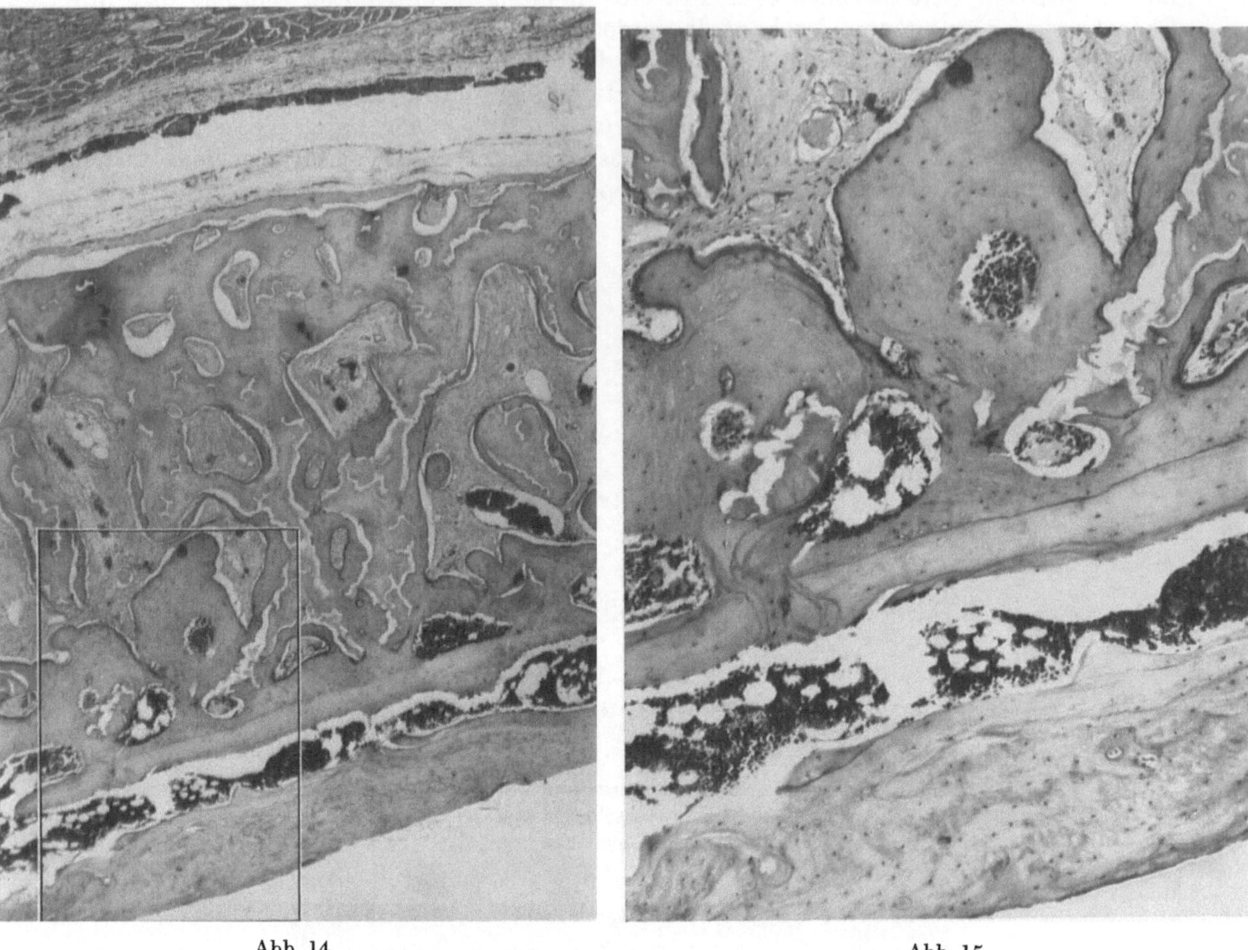

Abb. 14 Abb. 15

Abb. 14. Querschnitt durch Kronen-Test (Abb. 13) fünf Monate nach der Implantation. Der heterologe Span (wie Abb. 12) wird vom unverletzten Schädelknochen auf dem Wege des schleichenden Ersatzes durch lebenden Knochen ersetzt

Abb. 15. Der Ausschnitt aus Abb. 14. Nur rechts und links oben noch tote Span-Reste. (Das Schädeldach ist mit Bogenklammer abgegrenzt.)

Schädeldach-Test an der Ratte zum Ausdruck kommt. Hier wird der zu testende Span, eine kreisrunde Scheibe von 10 mm Durchmesser und 1,2 mm (!) Dicke aus Spongiosa unter der Galea dem nahezu planen, sehr dünnen Knochen der Ratte aufgelegt (Abb. 13). Besonders hervorzuheben ist dabei, daß der Knochen des Schädeldachs *unverletzt* bleibt. Die Galea ist sehr leicht vom Knochen zu lösen. Die Abb. 14 und 15 zeigen 5 Monate später eine teilweise Substitution des toten heterologen Implantats durch lebenden Knochen, und zwar nur vom Knochen, nicht von der Galea ausgehend. Hier *lockt* also das Implantat den Callus aus dem unverletzten Knochen an einem Skeletabschnitt, welcher keineswegs durch einen zusätzlichen funktionellen Reiz zur Knochenneubildung angeregt wird. Eine weitere Eigenheit des „Kieler Spans“ ist die sinnvolle Kombination von Spongiosa mit Corticalis (MAATZ, 1955), wobei die große innere Oberfläche der Spongiosa mit all ihren Vorteilen ausgenutzt wird, während die Corticalis als Stütze dem Span ausreichende Festigkeit gibt.

IV. Eigenheiten von Corticalis und Spongiosa

Die Abb. 7 und 8 und im Vergleich hierzu die zahlreichen Abbildungen, in denen die feingeweblichen Vorgänge an der Spongiosa gezeigt werden, demonstrieren sehr deutlich den eklatanten Unterschied im Ablauf aller Geschehnisse zwischen diesen beiden Knochenarten. Die sogenannte größere osteogenetische Potenz der Spongiosa (Matti, 1932; Fehr, 1949; Leriche, 1951) ist wohl auf die große Zahl der präexistenten Osteoblasten in den sekundären Markräumen und auch auf ihre (im Vergleich zur Knochenmasse) größere innere Oberfläche zurückzuführen. Beckenkamm-Spongiosa war schon lange als besonders gutes Transplantat in der Autoplastik beliebt. Abbot, Schottstaedt u. Saunders (1947) hoben nach tierexperimentellen Studien die besondere Qualität der Spongiosa hervor. Anderson und Mitarb. (1962) fanden nur bei autologer Spongiosa, nicht bei Corticalis, Knochenneubildung in der vorderen Augenkammer. Das Schicksal eines biologisch minder guten Spanes (heterolog lyophilisiert) ist bei Corticalis die reine bindegewebige Einscheidung (Kingma, 1949), während spongiöses Material gleicher Herkunft und Behandlung die Aussicht auf knöchernen Ersatz besitzt. Den autologen Spänen haftet der Nachteil an, daß eine besondere und sinnvolle Kombination von Corticalis und Spongiosa kaum oder nur in Grenzen gewährleistet sein kann, während das Tierskelet eine Fülle der Kombinationen gestattet, so daß dieser Vorteil beim heterologen Material vollkommen ausgenutzt werden kann.

V. Die Bedeutung der Intaktheit des Knochengerüstes

Der Empfehlung von Matti (1932), autologe Spongiosa zertrümmernd in Knochenhöhlen oder Pseudarthrosenspalten einzustampfen, ist in der Klinik über viele Jahre gefolgt worden. Maatz (1955) zeigte im Spongiosa-Test, daß die Zertrümmerung den Ersatz implantierter Knochensubstanz durch lebenden Knochen wesentlich verzögert, und Anderson, Le Cocq und Dingwall (1962) fanden bei ihren Testungen in der vorderen Augenkammer, daß ein Spanmaterial durch Zertrümmerung oder vielfache Fragmentation an osteogenetischer Potenz einbüßt, während die entzündliche Reaktion im Lager verstärkt wird.

Ohne in allen Einzelheiten diese Befunde erklären zu können, müssen wir uns heute mit der Feststellung begnügen, daß ein von einem jugendlichen Spender gewonnenes, praktisch antigenfreies Knochengerüst nur dann rasch und ungestört durch körpereigenen, lebenden Knochen ersetzt wird, wenn das Lagergewebe ein intaktes Klettergerüst vorfindet.

VI. Kombination von Spänen verschiedener Herkunft

Der Gedanke, autologe mit homoiologen, oder heterologen Spänen zu kombinieren, ist naheliegend und ist auch ohne Frage in der Praxis oft geübt worden, ohne daß darum eine Publikation erfolgte. Der Kombinationsmöglichkeiten gibt es viele. Am überzeugendsten waren bisher ohne Zweifel die Mitteilungen von Weaver (1949), welcher große Tibiadefekt-Pseudarthrosen nach Schußverletzungen mit homoiologen Spänen der Tiefkühltruhe überbrückte und den Raum zwischen den überbrückenden Spänen mit autologer Spongiosa ausfüllte (Skizze Abb. 16).

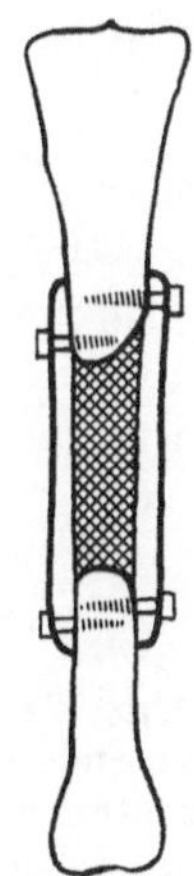

Abb. 16. Kombination von homologem Span aus der Tiefkühltruhe und autologer Spongiosa vom Beckenkamm bei großem Tibiadefekt (Weaver, 1949)

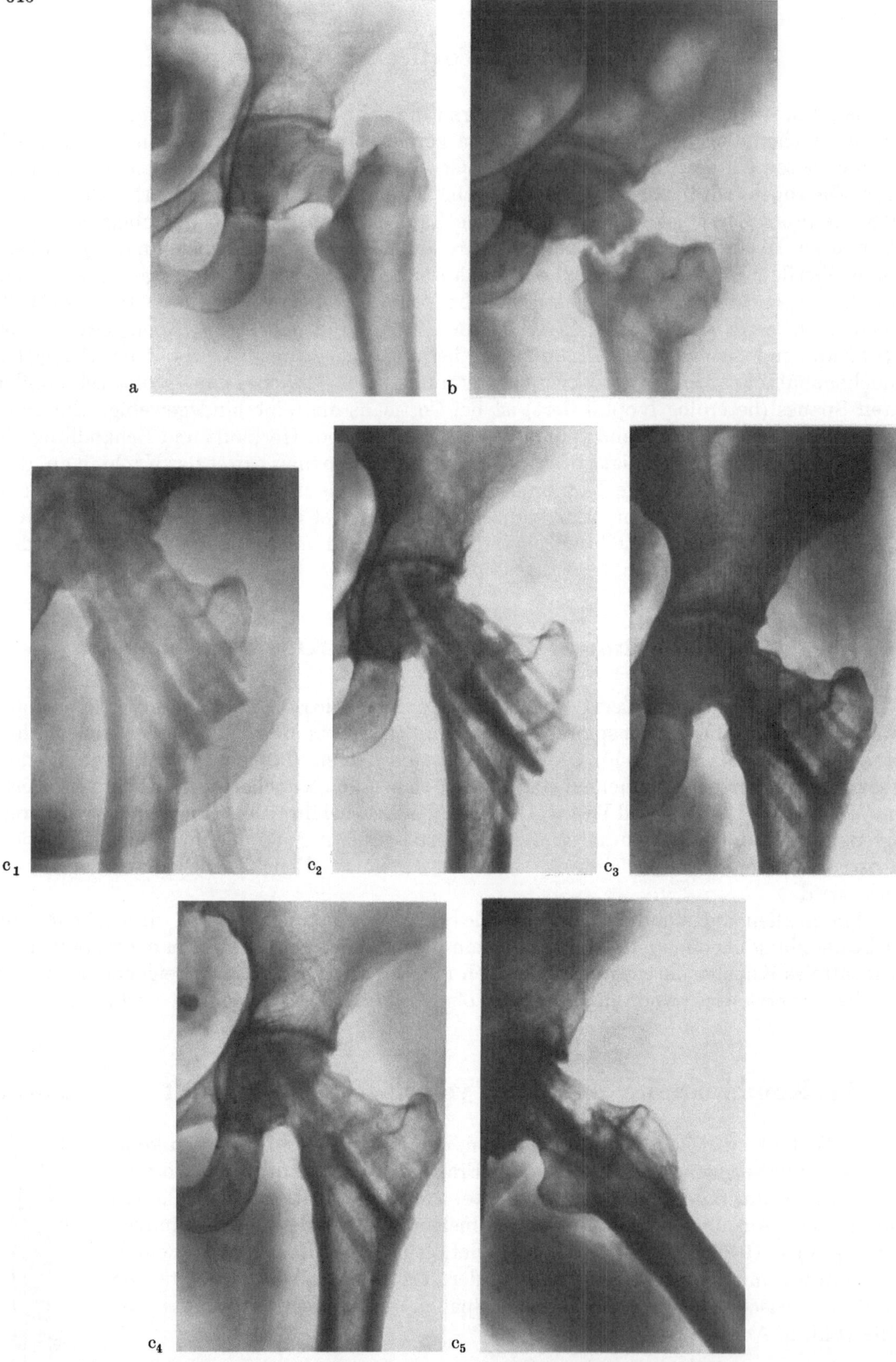

Abb. 17a—c. 43 Jahre alte Patientin. a Ermüdungsbruch des Schenkelhalses bei Coxa vara. b Verheilte valgisierende subtrochantere Osteotomie, persistierende Pseudarthrose. c Implantation von vier Knochenspänen, zentral zwei homologen Tiefkühl-Spänen, cranial und ventral je einem autologen Tibiaspan zur Verbreiterung des Schenkelhalses. Die vier folgenden Bilder zeigen den Einbau der Späne. Die Hüfte ist voll leistungsfähig

Das „Os novum" von ORELL, welches er durch Implantation von „Os purum" in den Subperiostalraum gewann, stellt ebenfalls eine Kombination von heterologem und jungen autologen Knochen dar. Der ohne Frage geniale Gedanke, ein heterologes Spanmaterial auf diese Art zum autologen umzuwandeln, litt nur unter der Tatsache, daß der subcutane Raum des Erwachsenen nach Implantation von „Os purum" häufig nur sehr spärlich Callus bildet. Ob mit den neuen heterologen Materialien („Kieler Span" oder „Boplant") bessere Ergebnisse erzielt werden können, wird die Zukunft lehren.

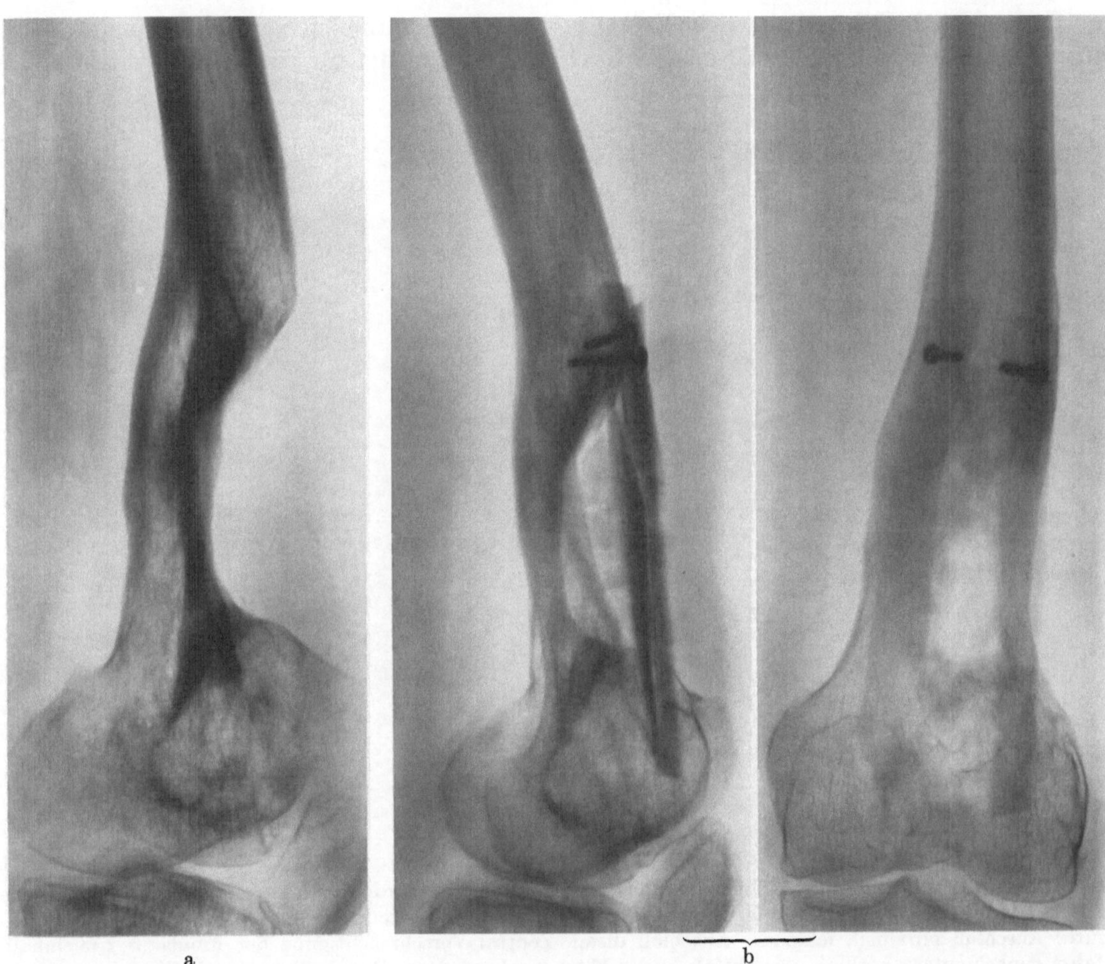

Abb. 18a u. b. 22jähriger Mann. a Ausgedehnter muldenförmiger Defekt am Femur nach offener, lange eiternder Fraktur. b Stabilisierung der gefährlichen „Kerbe" im Knochen mit zwei autologen Tibiaspänen und heterologen Spongiosablöcken drei Monate nach der Transplantation

Die Kombination von autologen Cortexspänen mit homologen Spänen zeigen die Röntgenbilder der Abb. 17. Zur Verbreiterung des Schenkelhalses wurden zwei autologe Späne, deren osteogenetische Potenz für diese Aufgabe unerläßlich schien, mit zwei intraossär gelagerten Spänen homoiologen Ursprungs aus der Tiefkühltruhe kombiniert.

In der Kombination von Spänen differenter Genese wird man stets besonders sorgfältig abwägen müssen, ob man einem autologen Material, dessen Einbau ja ohnehin niemals mit Sicherheit vorausgesagt werden kann, die Belastung durch die Nachbarschaft von Spanmaterial anderer Genese zumuten darf. Ohne Zweifel gibt es Situationen, in denen Kombinationen angezeigt sind. Stets aber wird dabei bedacht werden müssen, ob das autologe Material nicht allein rein räumlich durch die anderen Späne am raschen

Gefäßanschluß des Spanbettes gehindert wird. Zum anderen wird es stets erforderlich sein, ein nicht autologes Material zu verwenden, welches frei von Antigenität ist. Die Röntgenbilder der Abb. 18 zeigen die Kombination autologer Corticalisspäne mit ausfüllender lockerer heterologer Spongiosa unter Vermeidung eines ausgedehnten Kontaktes der Implantate verschiedener Herkunft.

VII. Besondere Spanformen

Lange Zeit beliebt, aber wenig Erfolg versprechend war bzw. ist die Verwendung der autologen Fibula als Röhrenknochen. Nach Einführung der Marknagelung erschien ihre

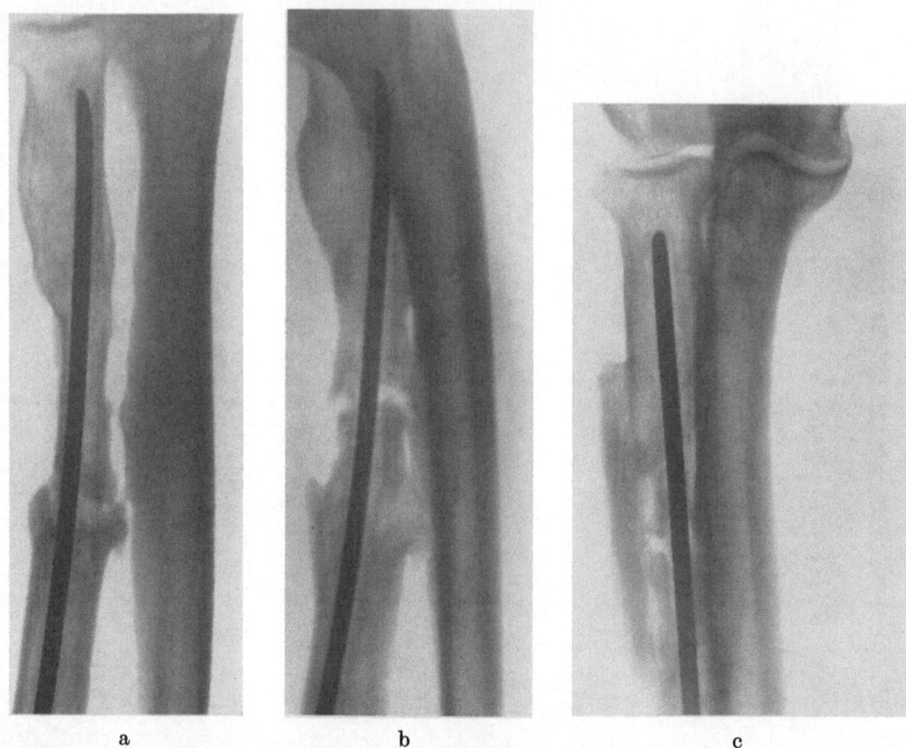

Abb. 19a—c. Ein 6 cm langer Defekt am Radius nach Schußbruch wurde durch eine „aufgefädelte" autologe Fibula ausgefüllt. (Das erste Bild ist leider verloren gegangen.) a vierzehn Monate nach der Transplantation guter Anschluß proximal, fehlender Anschluß distal. Zentral Verschmächtigung der Fibula. b zweieinhalb Jahre danach guter Anschluß nach distal. In der Mitte des Implantats Pseudarthrose nach Ermüdungsbruch. c Heilung zwölf Monate nach Verwendung eines autologen Überbrückungs-Spanes

Anwendung zunächst sehr verlockend, da sich mit dem Nagel eine gute Fixation (Auffädeln) ermöglichen ließ (Wanke, 1947). Die Röntgenbilder der Abb. 19a—c zeigen besonders instruktiv das Schicksal eines solchen Spanes. Dieser hat proximal nach sechs Monaten guten Anschluß an den Mutterknochen gefunden, distal aber bei einer geradezu einhüllenden Knochenneubildung des Mutterknochens fehlt der Anschluß zunächst. Der Span ist proximal besonders deutlich verschmächtigt, wurde also von außen her resorbiert. Acht Monate später ist der knöcherne Durchbau an der distalen Kontaktstelle zwischen Radius und Implantat vollkommen, es hat sich aber in der Mitte des Transplantats ein Ermüdungsbruch eingestellt, welcher zur breit klaffenden Pseudarthrose führte. Es ist offenbar, daß der Span von seinen Enden her vitalisiert und substituiert wurde. Im mittleren Abschnitt konnte er darum der Ermüdung erliegen. Die Zerrüttungszone hier wurde dann bei liegendem Nagel mit einem autologen Beckenkammspan erfolgreich überbrückt und zur Ausheilung gebracht. Das „aufgefädelte" Transplantat hatte nur an den Enden und damit einen zu kleinflächigen Kontakt mit dem Mutterknochen.

Der große autologe Tibiaspan aus Cortex ist der „Span der Wahl" immer dann, wenn größere Defekte zu überbrücken sind, und wenn vom Span eine beträchtliche Festigkeit verlangt wird. Die Röntgenbilder der Abb. 20 zeigen ein solches „klassisches" Transplantat, dessen Schicksal uns später noch interessieren soll (siehe Seite 672).

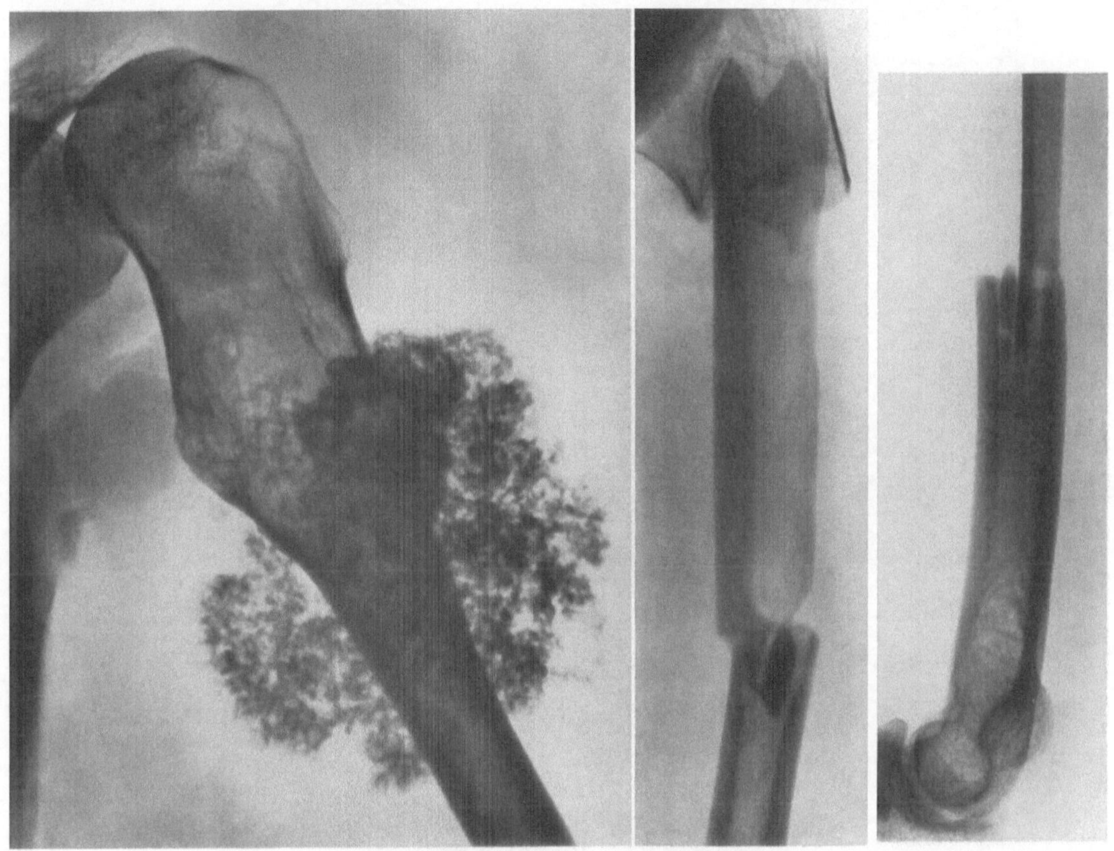

Abb. 20. 34 Jahre alter Mann. Resektion eines ausgedehnten Osteochondroms am linken Oberarm mit Implantation eines 12 cm langen autologen Tibia-Spanes, welcher proximal in die Spongiosa des Kopfes, distal in den Markraum eingebolzt wurde. (Weiteres Schicksal des Spanes siehe Abb. 49)

Autologe Transplantate vom Beckenkamm müssen zwangsläufig in der Größe und auch in der mechanischen Wertigkeit beschränkt sein. Abb. 21 zeigt ein solches Transplantat, welches extraarticulär mit Federkopfschrauben zur Ankylosierung eines tuberlulös erkrankten Schultergelenks verwendet wurde.

Der Beckenkamm ist auch Spender für Spongiosastücke, welche als Plomben verwendet werden. Ein Zerdrücken, ein Einstampfen ist nicht zweckmäßig, wie auf S. 645 ausgeführt wurde.

Es bleiben noch die kleinen Spänchen, welche — vorwiegend aus Spongiosa bestehend — einen schwachen Corticalisdeckel besitzen. Sie werden ebenfalls aus dem Beckenkamm gewonnen und eignen sich für die Blockierung der kleinen Wirbelgelenke bei Skolioseoperationen oder zur Ausfüllung des operativ geschaffenen Defektes im Os scaphoideum bei Pseudarthrose dieses Knochens.

Die autologen Rippen sind ein gutes Transplantationsmaterial. Ihre Gewinnung aber birgt den nicht geringen Nachteil, daß bei ihrer Entnahme Pleuraverletzungen nicht mit Sicherheit vermieden werden können. Abb. 22 zeigt einen großen, wegen Osteom gesetzten Schädeldefekt, welcher sofort mit autologen Rippen gedeckt wurde. Um den Transplantaten primär eine mechanisch-funktionelle Aufgabe zu geben, wurden die angeschliffenen Rippenenden in Falze zwischen Lamina externa und interna unter leichter Spannung eingefügt.

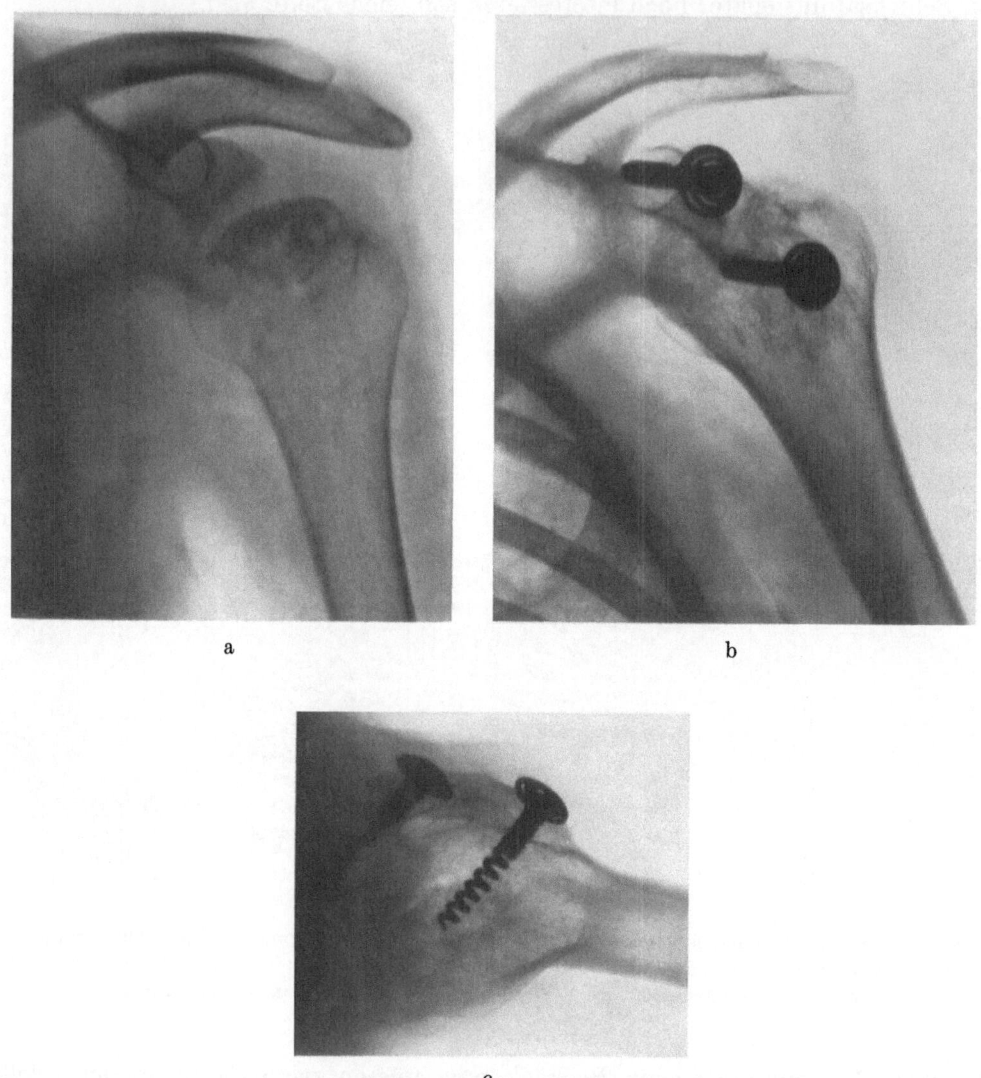

Abb. 21a—c. 16jähriger Patient. a Tuberkulose des linken Schultergelenks. Extraarticuläre Arthrodese mit autologem Beckenkamm-Span, welcher mit Spongiosafedern fixiert wurde. b u. c Die Kontrollbilder vier Jahre später zeigen die ausgeheilte Tuberkulose und den gut eingebauten Span

Bei der Verwendung homoiologer Späne sind uns in Form und Größe keine Grenzen gesetzt, wenn man die juristische Schwierigkeit der Entnahme von der Leiche außer acht läßt. Praktisch aber verbietet sich die Verwendung zu großer Spanmassen, da es sich um totes Material handelt, dessen Einbau allein durch die Größe in Frage gestellt wird.

Das Tierskelett gestattet uns die Verwendung von Spänen in gewünschter Form und Größe, es gestattet vor allem aber die Kombinationen von Corticalis und Spongiosa in einem Stück. So nutzt der *Anlegespan* (Abb. 23) die Vorteile der Spongiosa mit ihrer großen inneren Oberfläche (siehe S. 645), während die ausreichende Festigkeit durch den vom Knochen abgewandten corticalen Teil gewährleistet ist.

Der Tatsache, daß totes Spanmaterial in entscheidendem Maße von der guten Formschlüssigkeit zwischen Mutterknochen und Span abhängig ist, tragen der Stufenspan, der Füllspan und der Konkavspan dabei Rechnung (Abb. 24).

Der Schiffchenspan (Abb. 25) gleicht im Querschnitt einem T. Er eignet sich vor allem für die Pseudarthrose des Innenknöchels. Hier ist die Auflagefläche für einen Anlegespan allein zu klein. Der „Kiel" des Schiffchens wird in eine Nut der beiden Fragmente ver-

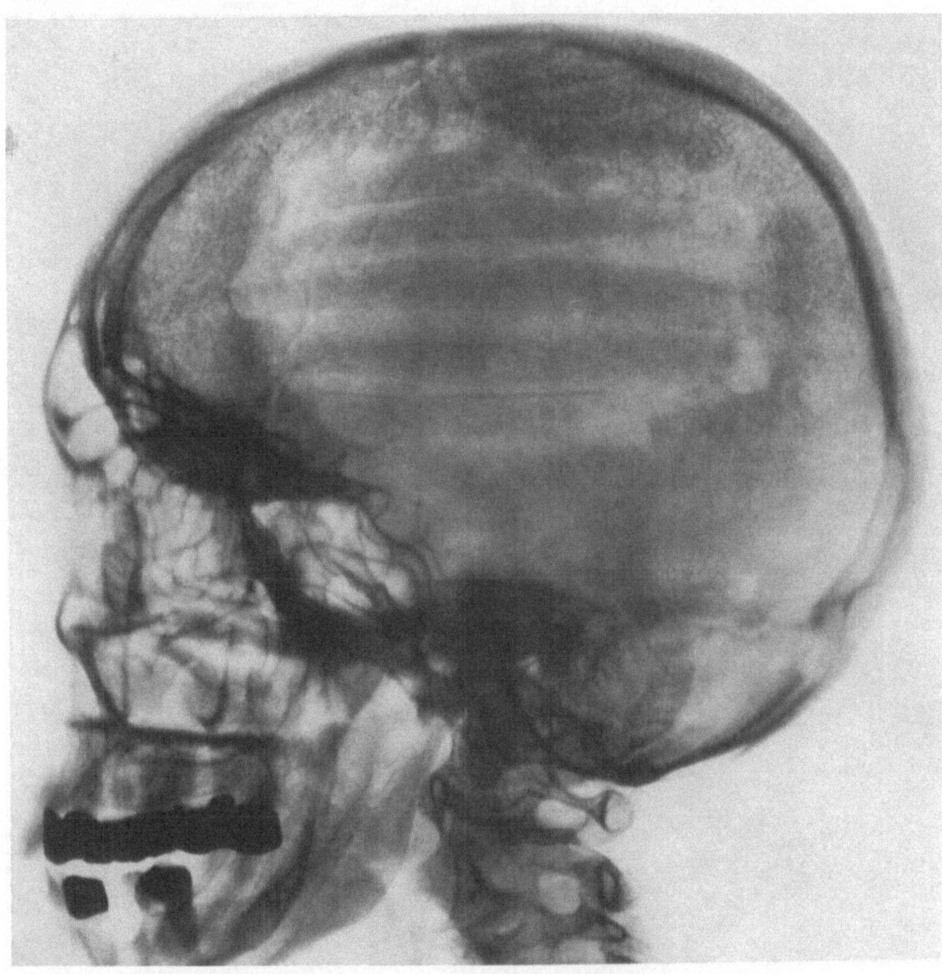

a

Abb. 22a—c. 46 Jahre alte Patientin. a Ein frischer großer Schädeldachdefekt, welcher durch Resektion eines großen Osteoms entstand, wurde mit „eingespannten" autologen Rippen gedeckt. b Kontrolle nach 3 Jahren. c Kontrolle nach 12 Jahren. (Wanke-Maatz-Junge-Lentz: Frakturen und Luxationen, 2. Aufl. Urban & Schwarzenberg 1967)

senkt. Damit besteht der gewünschte breitflächige Kontakt zwischen Span und Fragmenten. Gleichzeitig besteht eine bessere Stabilisierung der Fragmente zueinander. Ein rasches Durchwachsen mit neugebildetem Knochen ist dadurch frühzeitig möglich, daß der Span aus dichter Spongiosa besteht (siehe auch Abb. 48).

Der Osteotomiekeil (Abb. 26) besteht in seinem tragenden Teil aus sehr dichter Spongiosa mit einem dünnen Corticalisdeckel, während sein sich verjüngender Teil in lockere Spongiosa ausläuft. Eine kleine Nase verhindert das Auswandern des Keiles, bevor er die erforderliche Verflechtung mit körpereigenem neuen Knochengewebe zeigt.

Zur Verblockungsoperation an der Wirbelsäule (Cloward, 1963) eignen sich Dübel aus dichter Spongiosa (Abb. 27), deren Material ausreichende Tragfähigkeit gibt, und deren Form ein Wandern vor dem Durchwachsen mit Lagerknochen verhindert.

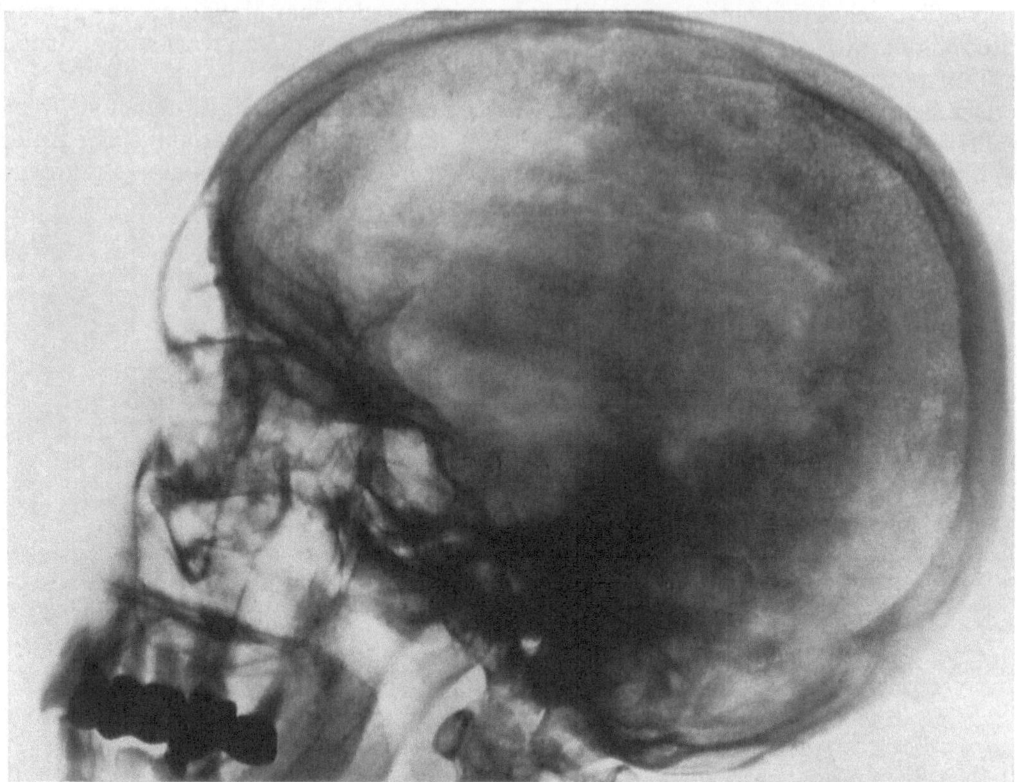

Abb. 22 b

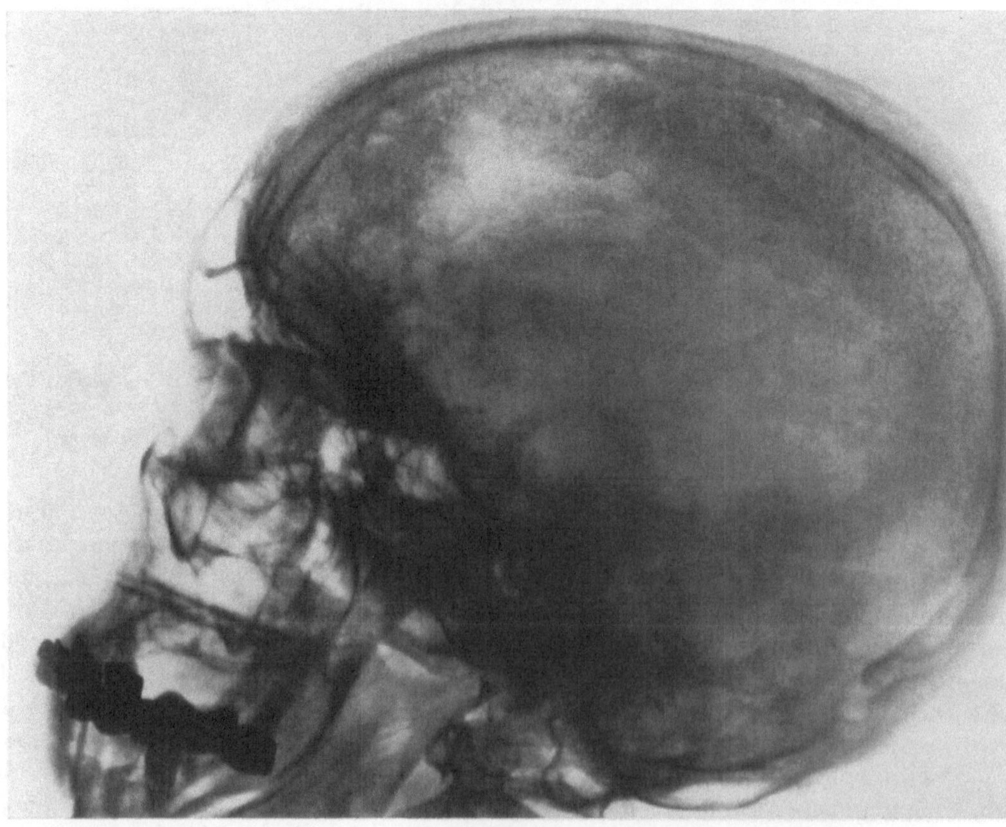

Abb. 22 c

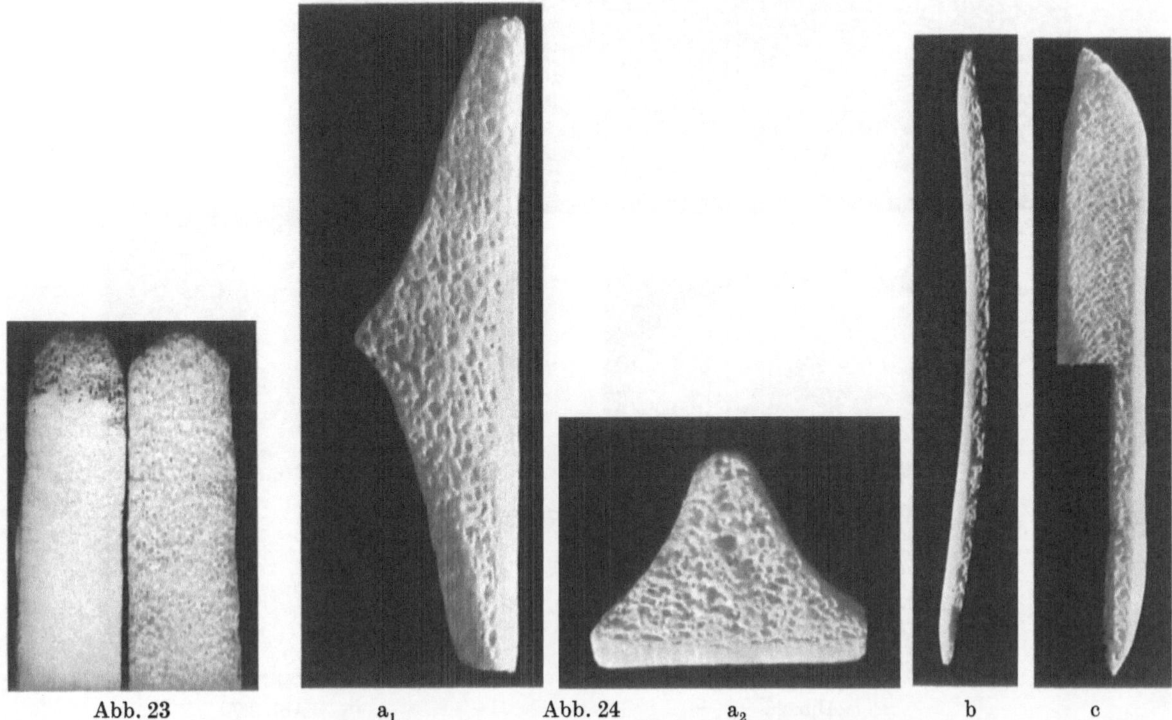

Abb. 23. Der heterologe Span besteht aus Corticalis und Spongiosa (Kieler Span)

Abb. 24a—c. Variationen des Anlegespans Abb. 23. a Füllspan, b Konkavspan, c Stufenspan

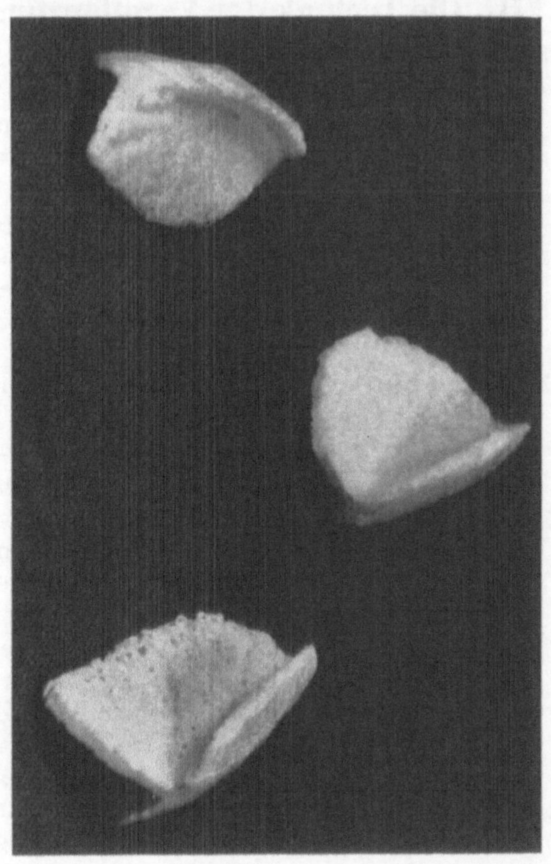

Abb. 25. Schiffchen-Span

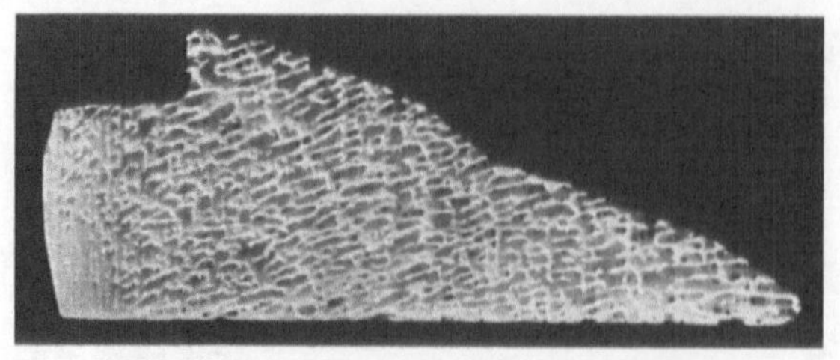

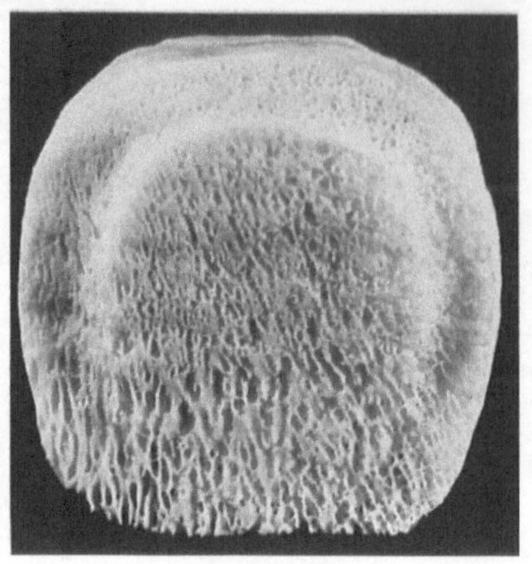

Abb. 26

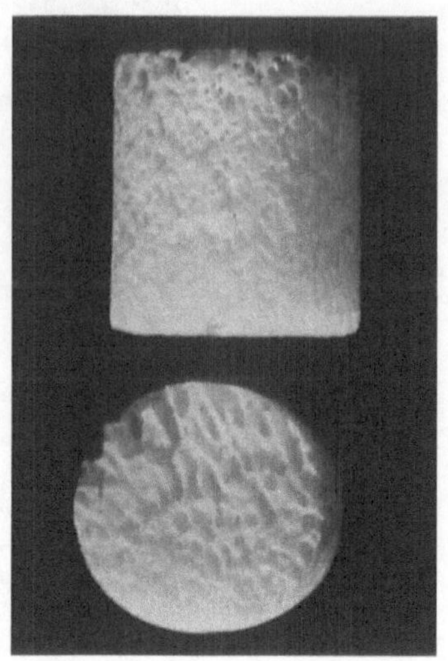

Abb. 27

Abb. 26. Osteotomie-Keil

Abb. 27. Dübel nach CLOWARD (1963) zur Verblockung zweier Halswirbel

VIII. Die Technik der Verpflanzung

Die gestielte Verpflanzung von Knochen läßt sich nur an wenigen Stellen des Körpers durchführen. Zuverlässig und einfach ist die Deckung kleinerer Defekte im Schädeldach durch flache Knochenlamellen, welche am Periost gestielt vom Rande des Defektes her auf die Lücke übertragen werden.

Abb. 28. Spanverpflanzung (aus KLEINSCHMIDT, Operative Chirurgie, 2. Aufl. Springer 1943, S. 332)

Sehr selten ist die Indikation zur Umkipp-Plastik (SAUERBRUCH, 1922) gegeben. Hier wird die Tibia mit Weichgeweben gestielt durch Kippen um 180° zum Ersatz des distalen Femur gemacht.

Die gestielte Verpflanzung der Fibula in einen sehr großen Defekt der Tibia (Hahnsche Operation, 1884) wird meist in zwei, seltener in einer Sitzung (Abb. 42) durchgeführt.

Bei der heute geübten gestielten Verpflanzung von Knochen handelt es sich meist um Gliedabschnitte, und zwar um Finger. Dabei soll vor allem das Ziel erreicht werden, einen leistungsfähigen Daumen zu gewinnen. Dazu werden entweder andere Finger (NICOLADONI, 1900 u.a.) oder die 2. Zehe (NICOLADONI), seltener die Großzehe (PAYR, 1918) verwendet.

Die *Vorpflanzung* eines Knochens (PAYR, 1908; HELLER, 1918; LIMBERG, 1928) kann auch heute noch zweckmäßig sein, wenn der Span in ein stark vernarbtes Gebiet eingepflanzt werden muß, in dem seine Aussichten auf einen guten Ernährungsanschluß in Frage gestellt sind. Der Knochen wird z. B. unter die Bauchhaut gepflanzt und von hier aus gestielt in den Defekt — z. B. am Unterarm — eingesetzt (Abb. 28). Die Röntgenbilder der Abb. 29 zeigen einen solchen Fall, bei dem trotz mehrfacher technisch einwandfreier Transplantation die Einheilung der Späne nicht erreicht werden konnte. Bei der Operation zeigte sich dann auch eine starke Vernarbung im Transplantationsbett.

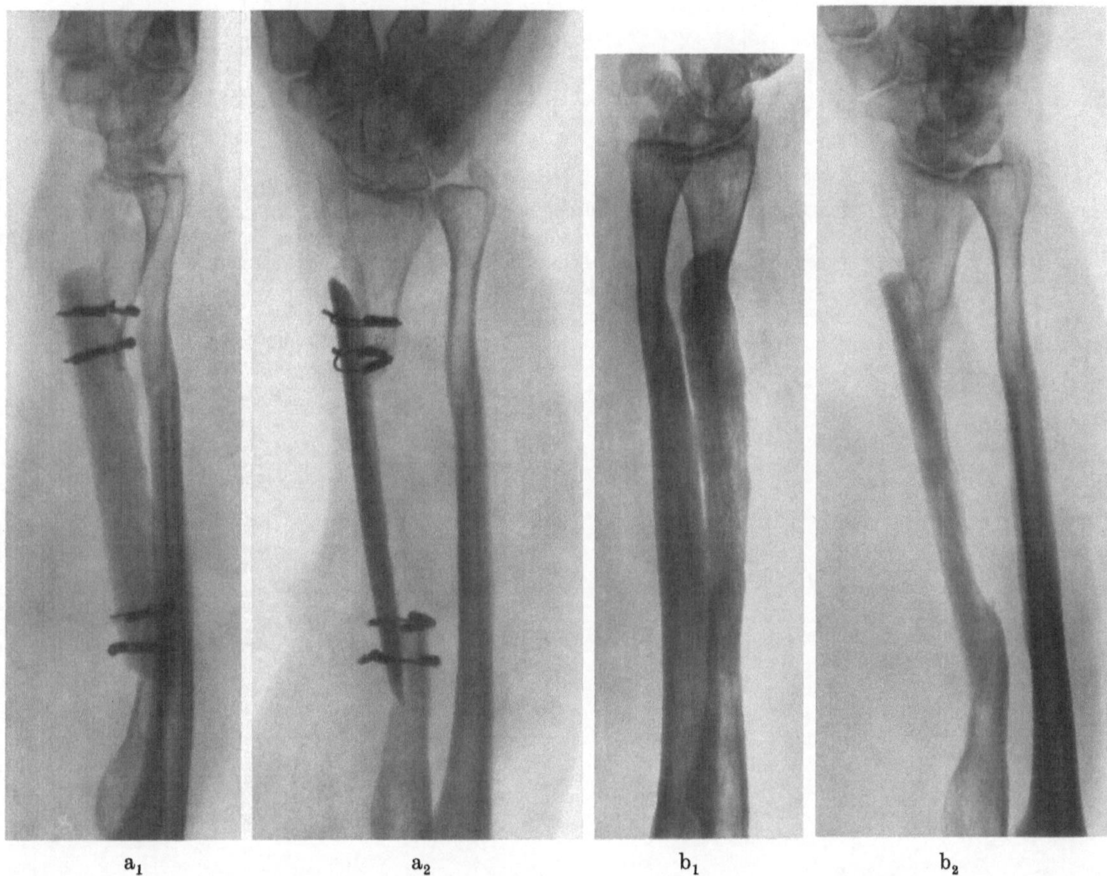

Abb. 29a u. b. 39 Jahre alte Patientin. Großer Defekt am Radius nach mehrfach operierter, nicht heilender Fraktur. a Gestielte Transplantation eines vor zwei Wochen unter die Bauchhaut vorgepflanzten autologen Tibiaspans. Befestigung mit Ligaturfedern. b Zustand ein Jahr nach der Verpflanzung

Sowohl Einbettung als Fixation spielen für die Erfolgsaussichten einer Knochentransplantation eine sehr große Rolle. Zur Ausfüllung von Knochenhöhlen bedarf es natürlich nicht einer Fixation. Durch PHEMISTER (1935) wurde das Prinzip der „tischlermäßigen" Zurichtung eines Spanes und die genaue Einpassung in das Spanbett mit exakter Fixation („Lexer-Prügel") durchbrochen. Dabei wurde die Fixation früher vorwiegend mit Drahtligaturen durchgeführt. Nachdem uns handwerklich richtige Schrauben zur Verfügung stehen, empfiehlt sich deren Anwendung, weil der Knochen subperiostal weniger weit skeletiert wird, oder bei extraperiostaler Lagerung der Drahtligaturen ebenfalls die Gefahr einer Nekrose oder Einschnürung besteht.

Die Skizzen der Abb. 30 mit ausführlicher Legende geben einen Überblick über die verschiedenen Wege, welche heute gegangen werden, oder auch als nicht mehr zweckmäßig angesehen werden müssen. Hervorzuheben ist besonders das große Verdienst PHEMISTERs, die Resektion der Pseudarthrose, die Anfrischung der Knochenenden in der überwiegenden Mehrzahl der Fälle als nicht notwendig erkannt zu haben. Die (zarten) Anlegespäne werden

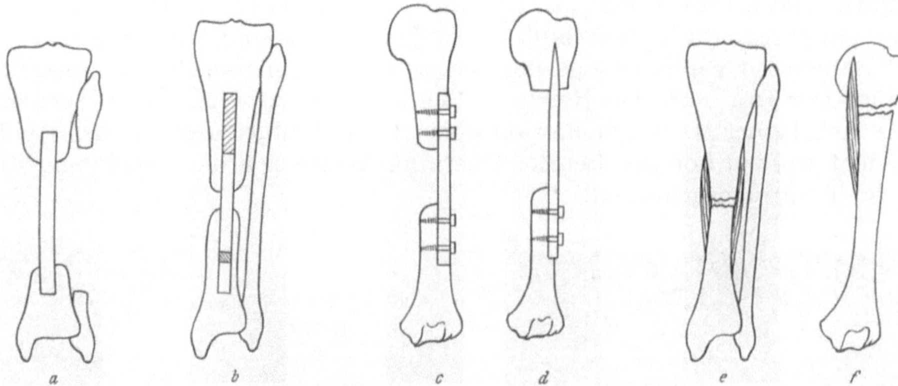

Abb. 30 I a—f. Beispiele der Knochenverpflanzung. a Gestielte Verpflanzung der Fibula (Hahn'sche Operation), b Verschiebe-Span, c Defektüberbrückung mit autologem Tibiaspan, Fixation mit Schrauben nach tischlermäßiger Spanbett-Bereitung, d wie c, aber Einbolzung des Spanes in die Spongiosa des kurzen Kopffragmentes, e Subperiostale Anlegespäne (PHEMISTER, 1947), f Einlege-Anlegespäne bei kurzem Kopffragment. (Quelle wie Abb. 22)

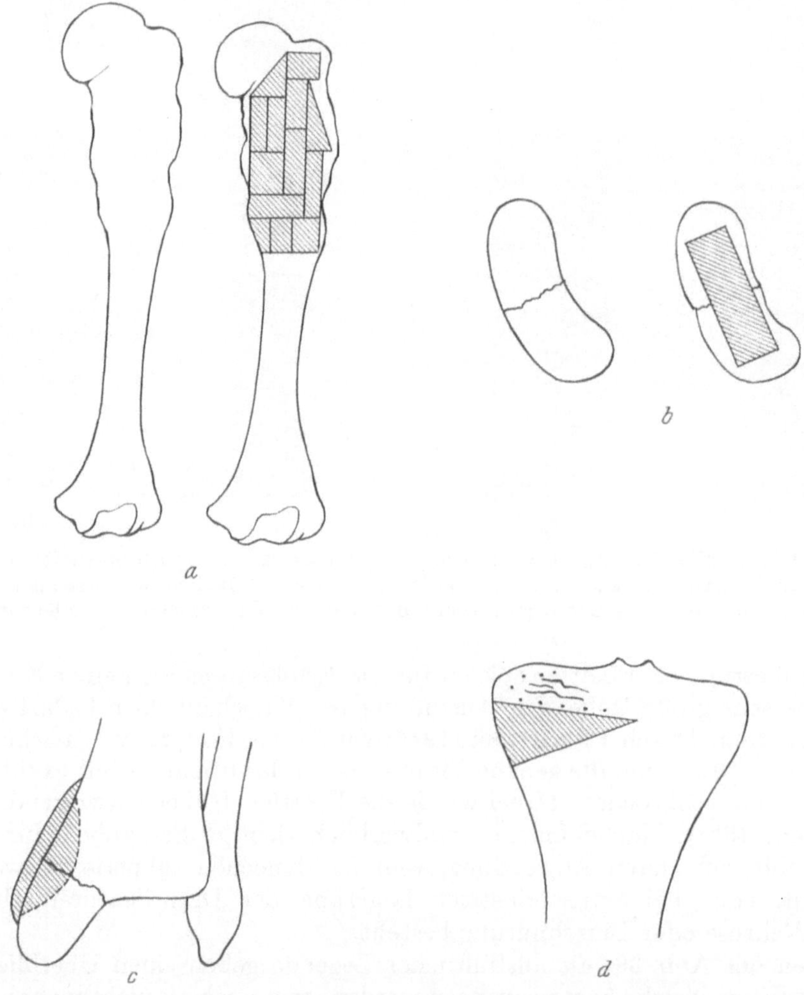

Abb. 30 II. a Ausfüllung einer ausgeräumten juvenilen Knochencyste mit Spongiosa. b Teilausräumung eines Kahnbeins bei Pseudarthrose und Füllung mit dichtem formschlüssigem Spongiosaspan. c Schiffchenspan bei Knöchelpseudarthrose. d Keil-Span zur Unterfütterung einer operativ gehobenen frakturierten Gelenkfläche am Tibiakopf

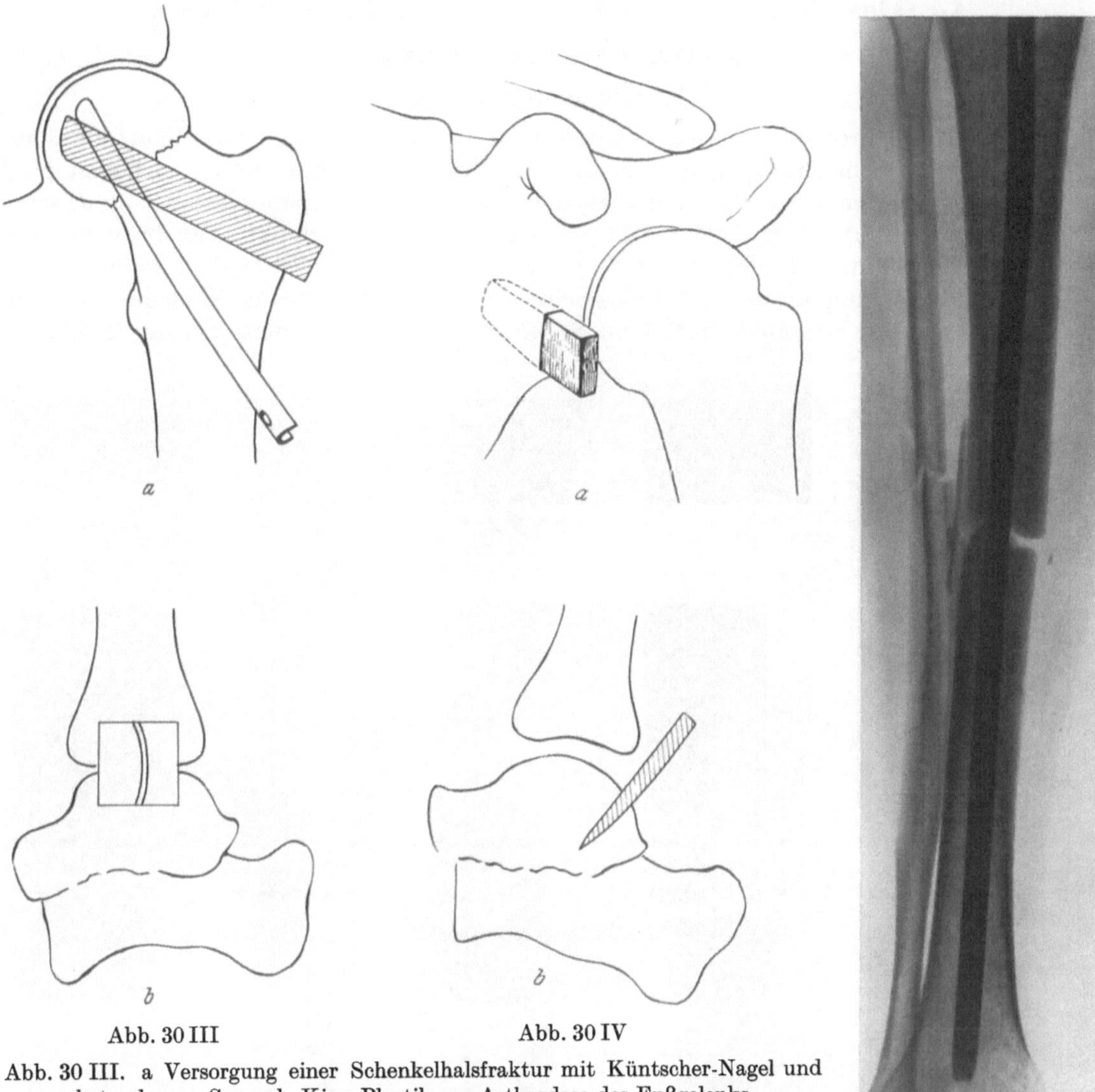

Abb. 30 III   Abb. 30 IV

Abb. 30 III. a Versorgung einer Schenkelhalsfraktur mit Küntscher-Nagel und heterologem Span. b Kipp-Plastik zur Arthrodese des Fußgelenks

Abb. 30 IV. a Eden-Plastik bei habitueller Schulterluxation. b Arthrorise am Fußgelenk bei Lähmungs-Spitzfuß

Abb. 31

Abb. 31. 47jähriger Mann. Primäre Nagelung einer offenen Unterschenkelfraktur. Anlegespan drei Monate später wegen verzögerter Verfestigung (siehe auch Abb. 48)

in eine subperiostale Tasche eingeschoben bzw. gelegt. Bei mechanischer Ruhe heilen die Späne ein, während die Pseudarthrose sich knöchern durchbaut (Abb. 31 u. 45). In Ausnahmefällen geschieht wohl letzteres, während die Späne vom röntgenologischen Standpunkt aus gesehen „unbeteiligt" dem Knochen anliegen.

Stets unzweckmäßig ist die Einbolzung eines Spanes in die Markräume bei Überbrückung einer Schaftpseudarthrose. Dieses Vorgehen ist um so verwerflicher, je kürzer der zu überbrückende Defekt ist, denn Span und Knochenrohre zusammen sind außerordentlich biegefest, der Span allein im Bereich des Knochenrohrdefektes aber wird in unerhörtem Maße mechanisch beansprucht. Hier haben wir gewissermaßen eine tiefe Kerbe in dem Skelettabschnit, und in dieser Kerbe liegen die Spannungsspitzen, welche früher oder später zum Bruch des Spanes führen müssen. Anders liegen die Verhältnisse beim Einbolzen eines Spanes in den spongiösen Knochen eines kurzen Fragments (Abb. 30 I f Skizze und Abb. 47).

IX. Das röntgenologisch-klinisch erfaßbare Schicksal des Knochentransplantats

1. Allgemeingültiges

Die Reihenfolge röntgenologisch — klinisch wählen wir bewußt, da die Beurteilung des Einbaus eines Knochentransplantats im weitesten Maße röntgenologisch geschehen muß.

Sehen wir von den beiden Extremen ab, dem Überleben des Spanes und der aseptischen Abstoßung aufgrund hoher Antigenität, so kann jede Art von „klinisch brauchbaren" Spänen Schicksale durchlaufen, die einander so ähnlich oder gleich sind, daß uns eine gemeinsame Besprechung je nach Art dieses Schicksals sinnvoll erscheint. Nach dem Studium der feingeweblichen Vorgänge (S. 637 bis S. 645) wird dem Leser diese unsere Einstellung begreiflich sein.

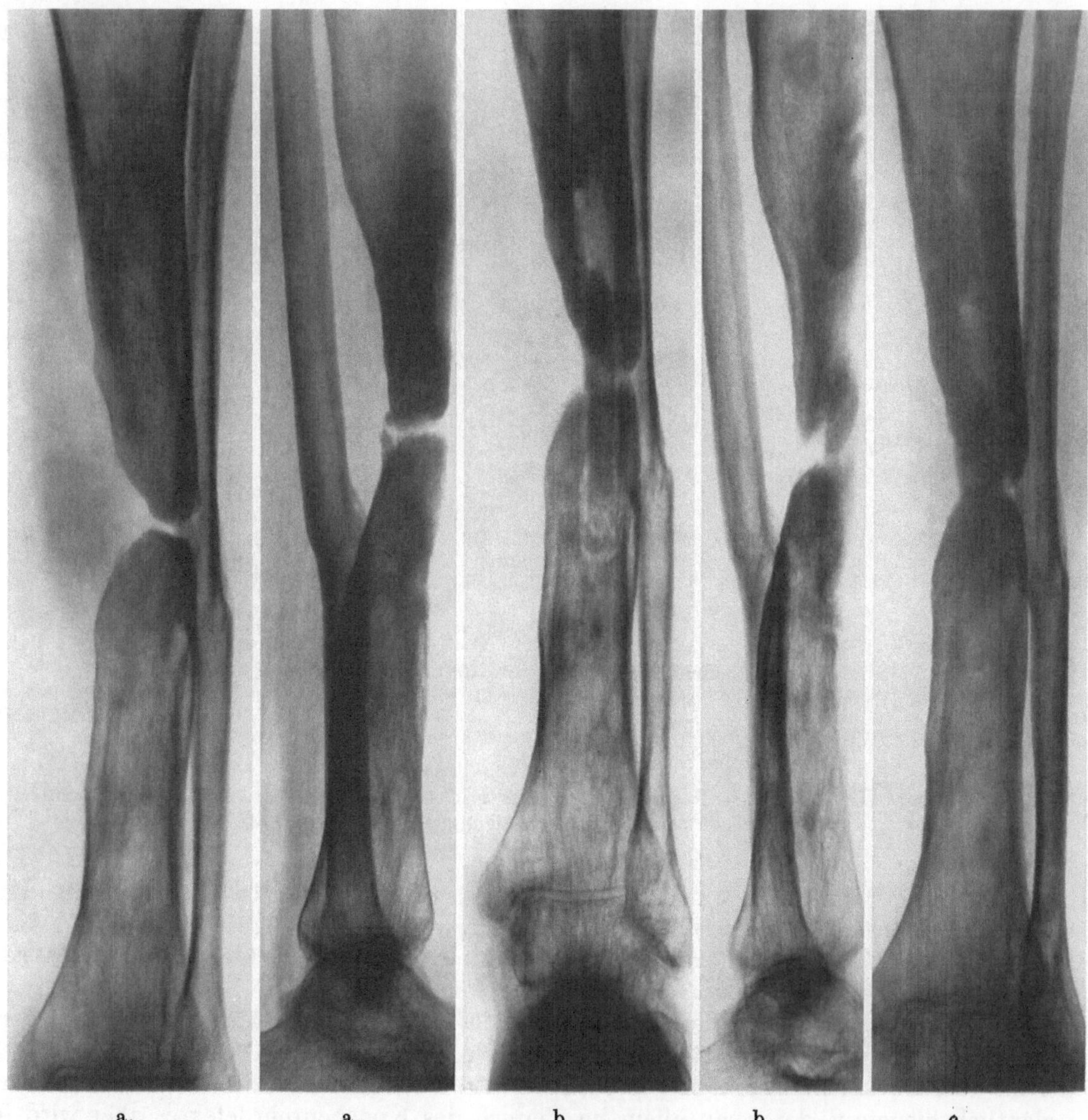

Abb. 32a—e. Am 19. März 1953 erlitt der 23jährige Mann eine offene Unterschenkelfraktur. Ende März Küntscher-Nagelung. Ende Juni Eiterung, Nagelentfernung, Sequestrotomien, Heilung. Arbeitsfähig ab März 1954. 1954, 1958 und 1959 zeitweise wegen Infektion arbeitsunfähig. Juli 1961 Ausmuldung. März 1962 Ermüdungsbruch. Ab Januar 1963 mit Schienenhülsenapparat arbeitsfähig. Im Februar 1964 Spanverschiebung. Knöcherne Heilung unter milder eitriger Sekretion. Im Mai 1965 Ermüdungsbruch, welcher wieder zur Pseudarthrose der Tibia ohne Fistelung führte

2. Das Frühschicksal eines Spanes

a) Die aseptische Abstoßung

Von einer aseptischen Abstoßung sprechen wir dann, wenn diese ohne bakterielle Beteiligung unter Eiterbildung abläuft. Diesen Vorgang beobachten wir praktisch nur bei Spänen mit hoher Antigenität. L. BÖHLER u. Mitarb. berichteten Ende der 40iger Jahre in Wien über solche Beobachtungen bei Verwendung frischen Kalbsknochens in der Klinik. Werden solche frischen heterologen Implantate in ein tiefliegendes Lager (z.B. Spongiosa — MAATZ, LENTZ und GRAF, 1954 oder Muskulatur — W. AXHAUSEN, 1952) eingebettet, so fehlt meist die Abstoßung, aber unter allen Zeichen der aseptischen Entzündung wird das Implantat zunächst abgegrenzt und später aufgesogen.

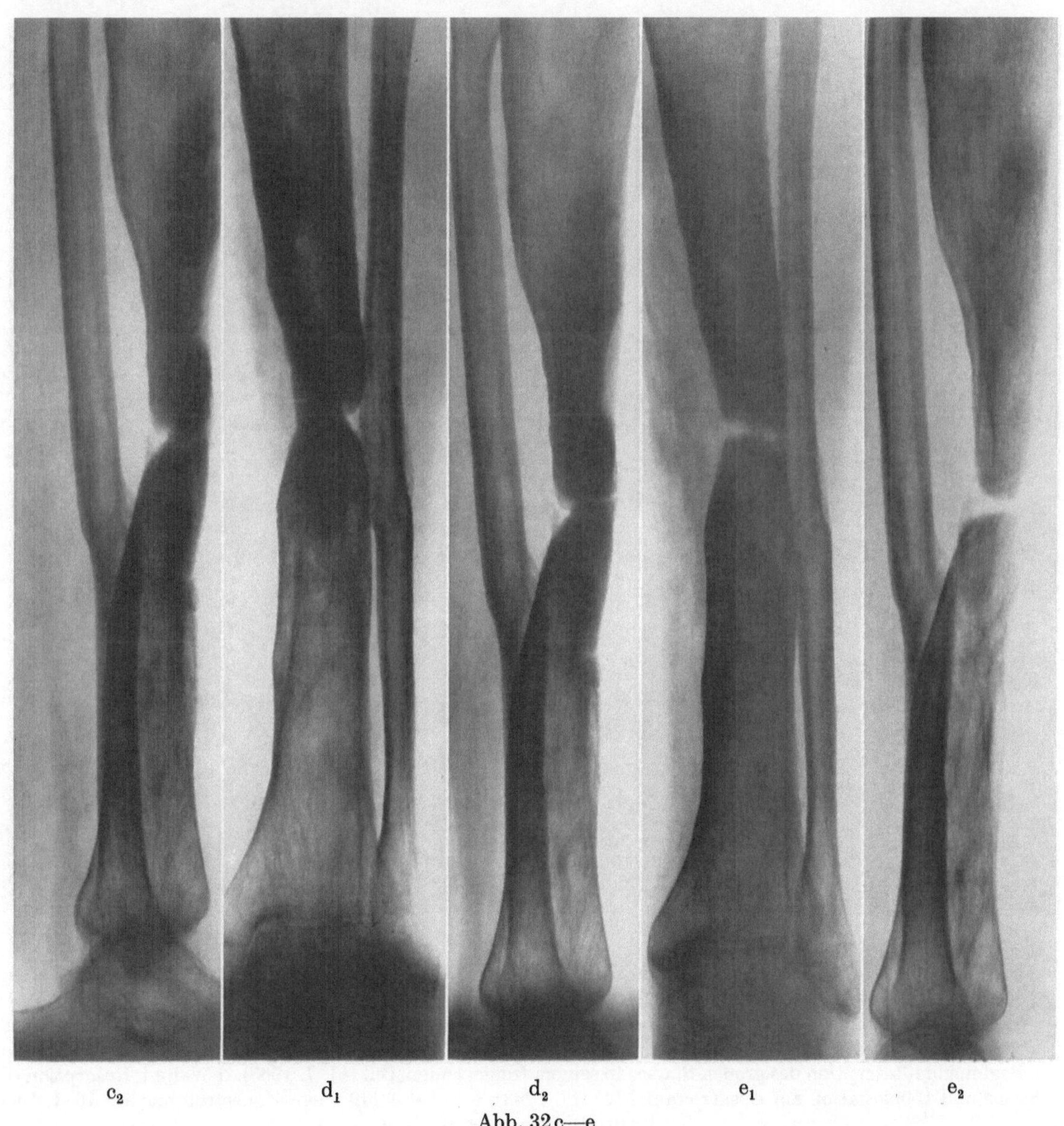

c_2 d_1 d_2 e_1 e_2

Abb. 32c—e

b) Die Infektion mit Eiterung

Auf diesem Gebiet liegt der Klinik aus nur zu begreiflichen Gründen ein reiches Krankengut vor. Dabei muß allerdings hervorgehoben werden, daß die Zahl der Infektionen durch schonenderes Operieren, Verhütung von Nekrosen, in geeigneten Fällen bessere

Osteosynthese und unter dem Schutze eines Antibioticums auf ein Minimum gesunken ist. Kriegszeiten und Nachkriegszeiten (vernarbtes Implantationsbett, ruhende Keime) haben ohnehin höhere Infektionsquoten.

Ist der Span bei einer Wundeiterung von Eiter umspült, so kann er den Ernährungsanschluß an das Muttergewebe nicht finden, er wird zum Sequester und wird sich abstoßen oder muß eines Tages entfernt werden.

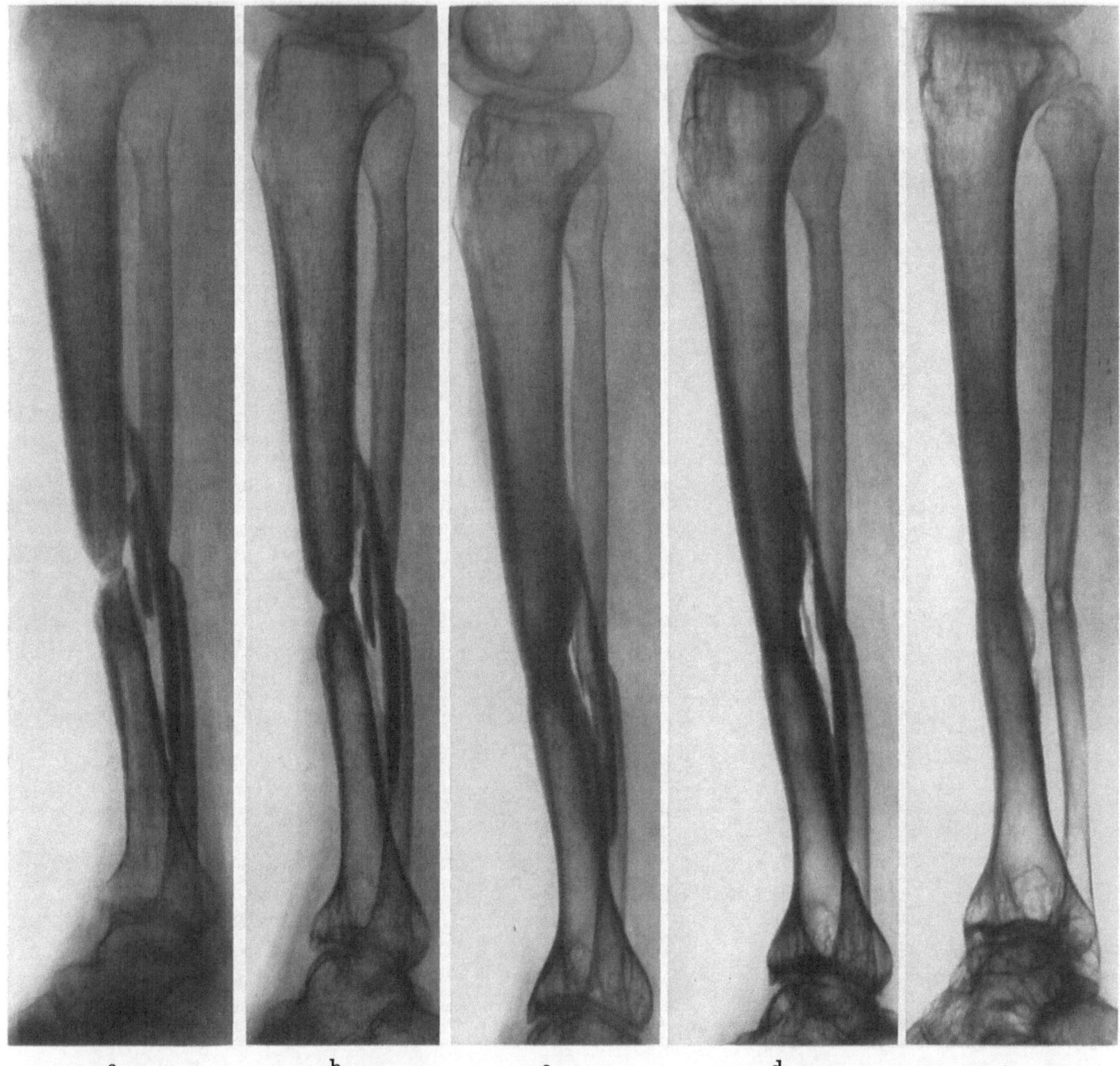

Abb. 33a—e. Am 14. 3. 1960 erlitt die 54jährige Patientin einen offenen Unterschenkelbruch, welcher am 2. 6. 1960 offen genagelt wurde. Nagelentfernung am 25. 8. 1960. Nach Abklingen der Entzündung am 3. 11. 1960 zwei Anlegespäne wegen Pseudarthrosenbildung. a Erster Anschluß der Späne am 27. 1. 1961. b Der große Span hat sehr guten Anschluß. Pseudarthrose geheilt (6. 10. 1961). Der kleine Span ist sequestriert. Fistelung. c Beginnende Resorption des großen Spanes in seinem freiliegenden Teil (11. 7. 1963). d Weitere Resorption des Spans und Demarkation am Ansatz cranial (21. 11. 1963). e Fistelschluß nach Sequestrotomie am 10. 1. 1964. Kontrollbild am 29. 10. 1964

Weder beim autologen und noch weniger beim heterologen Span (ohne Antigenität) muß eine Eiterung von einer Abstoßung gefolgt sein. Teilweiser Einbau wird am häufigsten, völliger Einbau allerdings selten beobachtet. Auch diese Verhältnisse lassen sich an einem eindrucksvollen Beispiel am besten veranschaulichen. Einzelheiten gehen aus der ausführlichen Bildlegende der Abb. 32 hervor. Epikritisch lautet hier das Schicksal in äußerster Kürze wie folgt: ein 23jähriger gesunder Mann erleidet im März 1953 einen offenen Unterschenkelbruch, welcher nach vierzehn Tagen Streckverband mit Küntscher-Nagel versorgt wurde. Es kam zur langanhaltenden Eiterung. Leider wurde der Nagel sofort entfernt. Während der folgenden neun Monate Gipsverband, Sequestrotomie, knöcherne Heilung und ab März 1954, also zwölf Monate nach dem Unfall, arbeitsfähig (Bürotätigkeit). 1955/1956 entzündliche Reizungen. Im Juli 1961 Ausmuldung wegen Fistelbildung. Im März 1962 Ermüdungsbruch des Knochens in Höhe der Ausmuldung. Pseudarthrosenbildung, Schienenhülsenapparat. Im Februar 1964 Spanverschiebung. Milde Eiterung, langanhaltende flache Fistelung, knöcherne Heilung ohne Sequester. Ab Mai 1965 arbeitsfähig. Drei Wochen später (am 20. Mai 1965) Ermüdungsbruch. Flache Ulcerationen im Narbenbereich. Ab September 1965 bei geheilten Wunden mit Schienenhülsenapparat dienstfähig.

Inwieweit der verschobene Span zur Zeit des Bruches in seiner knöchernen Substanz vital war, vermögen wir nach den Röntgenbildern nicht zu sagen (siehe auch Abb. 8). Die Tatsache des Ermüdungsbruches spricht jedenfalls dagegen, daß er bereits ausreichend substituiert war.

Besonders interessant und auf die Grenzen der röntgenologischen Beurteilungsmöglichkeit hinweisend, sind die Röntgenbilder der Abb. 33. Hier handelt es sich um zwei heterologe Anlegespäne bei Tibiapseudarthrose nach offener Fraktur. Der kleinere Span wurde in milder Eiterung abgestoßen, während der größere ganz sicher an beiden Enden vollkommenen Kontakt mit dem Mutterknochen fand und auch in seiner Struktur den Eindruck des guten Einbaus erweckte. Die Pseudarthrose war knöchern durchgebaut; nach drei Jahren aber sequestrierte der mittlere Teil des größeren Spanes in milder Eiterung und mußte später operativ entfernt werden.

c) Der mehr oder minder gute Anschluß an den Mutterknochen

Eine formschlüssige und großflächige Anlage des Spanes an den Mutterknochen ist der beste Garant für einen guten knöchernen Anschluß. Das gilt beim subperiostal angelagerten Span, mehr aber noch beim fixierten Span, welcher von Anbeginn an eine mechanische Aufgabe zu erfüllen hat. Das Röntgenbild der Abb. 34 zeigt weder guten

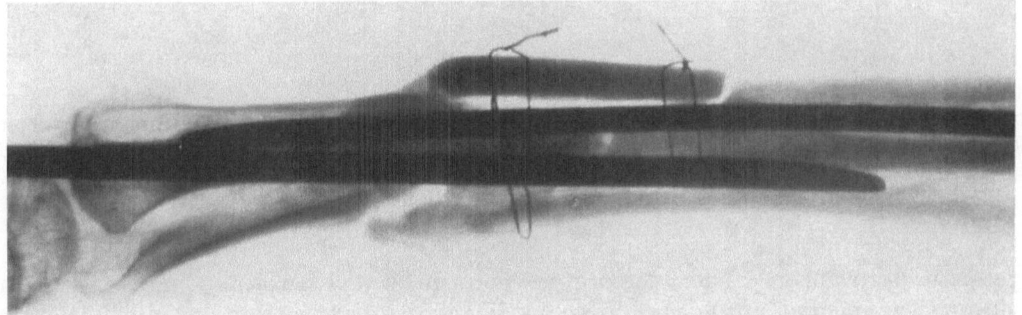

Abb. 34. 26jähriger Mann. Der autologe Span liegt weder formschlüssig im Lager, noch ist er gut fixiert. Knöcherner Anschluß zwölf Wochen nach der Transplantation nur am distalen Ende

Paß noch gute Fixation. Der (autologe) Span hat nur peripher den Anschluß an das Spanbett gefunden, und hier auch nur in dem kurzen Bereich, in dem der Span dem Knochen aufliegt.

Die homologen Späne aus der Tiefkühltruhe zeigen bei sonst guter klinischer Verwendungsfähigkeit häufig einen verzögerten Anschluß und langdauernde Substitution, wie das Röntgenbild der Abb. 35 ein Beispiel an der Elle demonstriert.

Auch die beste Formschlüssigkeit ist nutzlos, wenn ein mechanischer Störfaktor die bereits anlaufende knöcherne Verbindung zwischen Schaftknochen und Span zerstört. Dieser Vorgang stellt sich in den Röntgenbildern der Abb. 36 eindrucksvoll dar. Eine mit

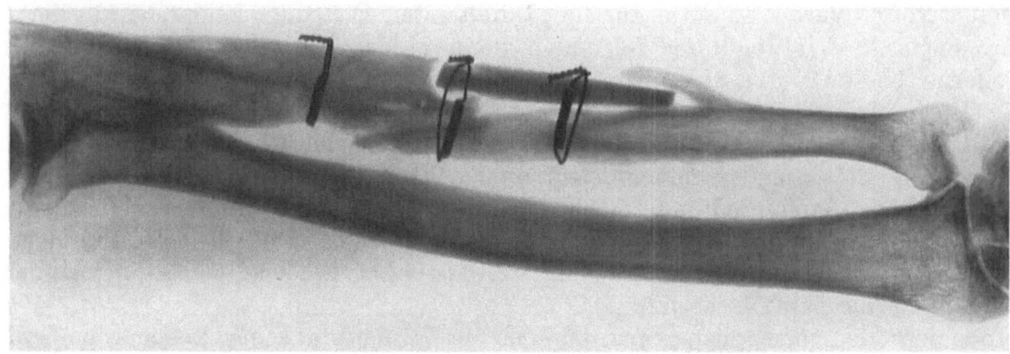

Abb. 35. 28jähriger Mann. Der homologe Span hat nach neun Monaten nur sehr unvollkommen Anschluß an den Lagerknochen gefunden

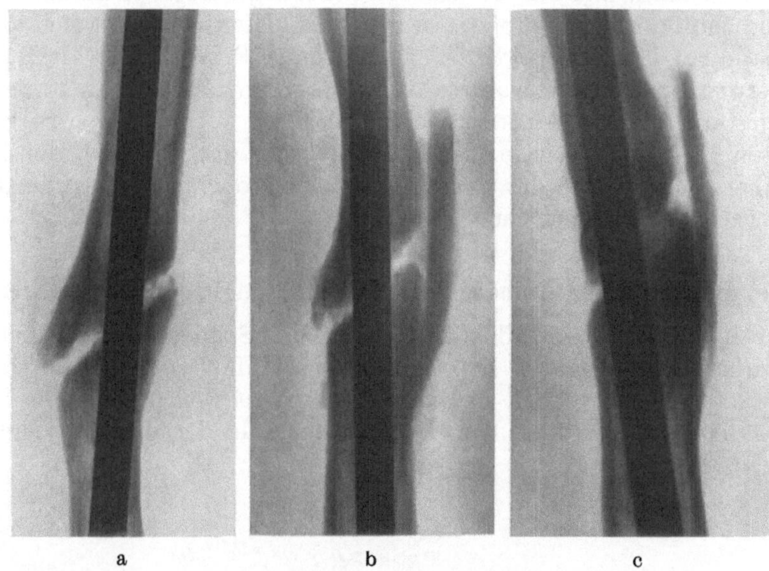

Abb. 36a—e. 34jährige Patientin. a Persistierende Pseudarthrose nach Nagel mit Feder. b Der heterologe Anlegespan hat vier Monate nach der Implantation auf beiden Fragmenten guten Anschluß. c Nach weiteren sechs Monaten hat er sich am proximalen Fragment wieder gelöst. d u. e Knöcherne Heilung durch Ausschaltung der Rotation mittels Riegelspan

Nagel und (schwacher) Feder versorgte Oberarm-Pseudarthrose — persistierend nach Markraumbolzung mit autologem Span — blieb pseudarthrotisch, da die Patientin die erforderliche Ruhigstellung im Gipsverband auf keinen Fall durchhalten wollte. Ein heterologer Anlegespan fand an beiden Fragmenten rasch guten Anschluß, wurde aber nach Gipsabnahme am proximalen Fragment durch einen Rotations-Störfaktor wieder losgerüttelt. Nach Ausschaltung der Rotationskomponente durch heterologen Riegelspan kam die Pseudarthrose zur Ausheilung.

Intraspongiös liegende Späne, wie sie z.B. beim operativen Aufbau frakturierter Gelenkflächen zur Unterpolsterung benutzt werden, finden auch bei heterologen Spänen meist früh, bisweilen etwas später den knöchernen Anschluß an das Bett. Entweder verschwimmen die anfangs scharfen Konturen des Spanes frühzeitig (Abb. 37), oder es

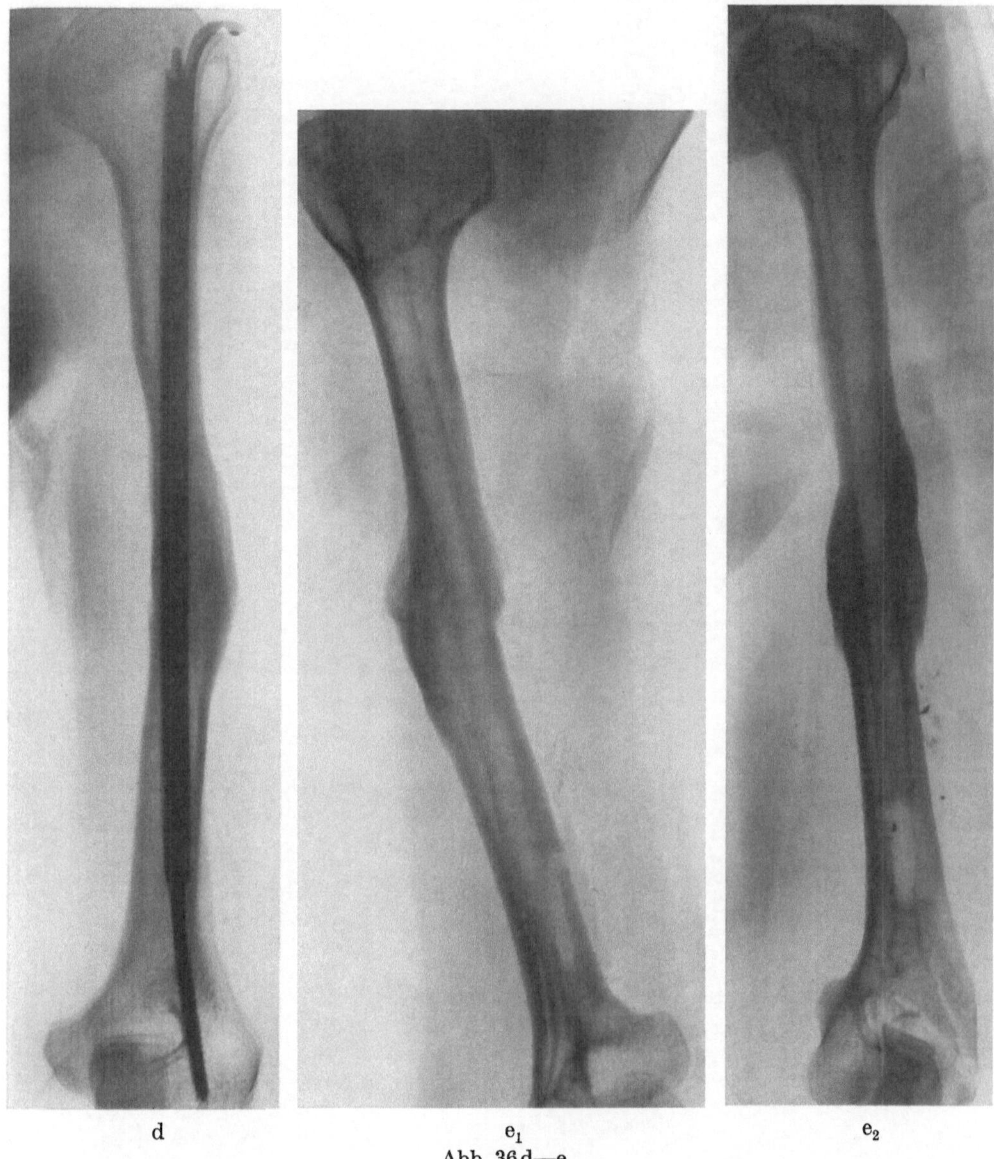

Abb. 36d—e

bildet sich um den Span eine helle Zone (Abb. 38) (im angelsächsischen Sprachgebiet „halo"). Diese Aufhellungszone darf auf keinen Fall dazu führen, eine bindegewebige Einscheidung, eine Sequestrierung des Spanes anzunehmen. Vielmehr handelt es sich fast immer um einen Osteoidsaum, welcher nach Einlagerung der Kalksalze schwindet.

3. Das spätere Schicksal des Spanes

Die Übergänge zwischen Früh- und Spätschicksal sind fließend. Hat ein Span die ersten Wochen nach der Verpflanzung gut überstanden und zeigt er Anschluß an den Mutterknochen, so treten die im Frühschicksal geschilderten Fälle der aseptischen Abstoßung praktisch nie, die Störung durch Eiterung äußerst selten auf.

a) Die bindegewebige Einscheidung

Das klassische Beispiel der bindegewebigen Einscheidung erlebte KÜTTNER (1917) mit der Affenfibula, welche er einem Kinde mit fehlender Fibula einsetzte. Sie wuchs „reaktionslos"ein, der Autor frohlockte, mußte aber nach Jahren feststellen, daß die Fibula

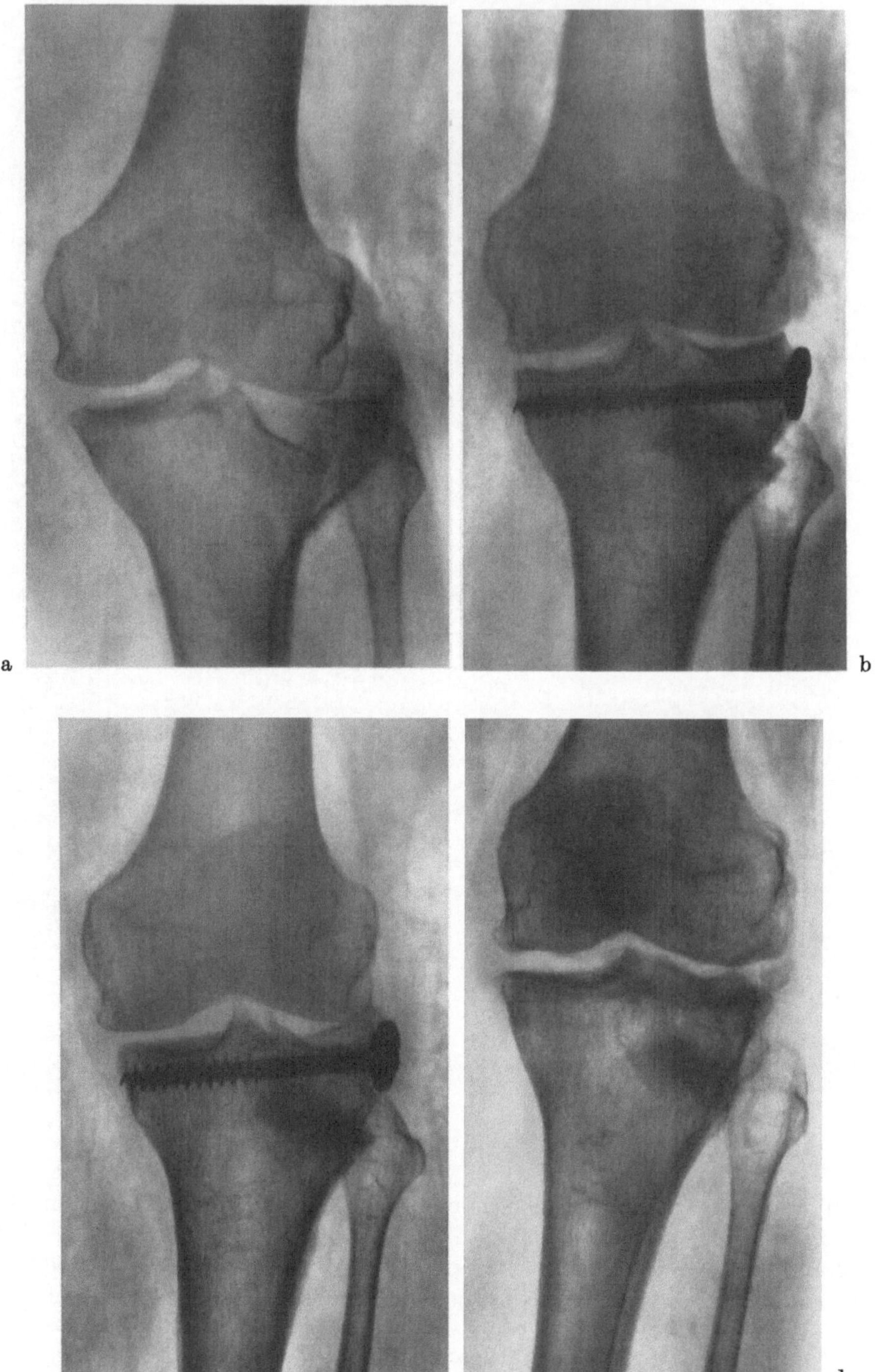

Abb. 37a—d. 52jährige Frau. a Tibiakopf-Impressionsfraktur. b Versorgung mit heterologem Span und Federkopfschraube (Überkorrektur). c Nach zwei Monaten zeigt der Span verwaschene Grenzen. d Nach zweiundzwanzig Monaten ist der Span etwa zu $^2/_3$ substituiert

völlig unverändert blieb, auch kein Wachstum zeigte. Der Autor entfernte dann nach Jahren den Fremdkörper und fand die bindegewebige Einscheidung.

Wir erleben diesen Vorgang selten, am ehesten noch am Schädeldach. Damit kann durchaus ein klinischer Erfolg verbunden sein. Meist aber verfällt ein solcher Knochen der

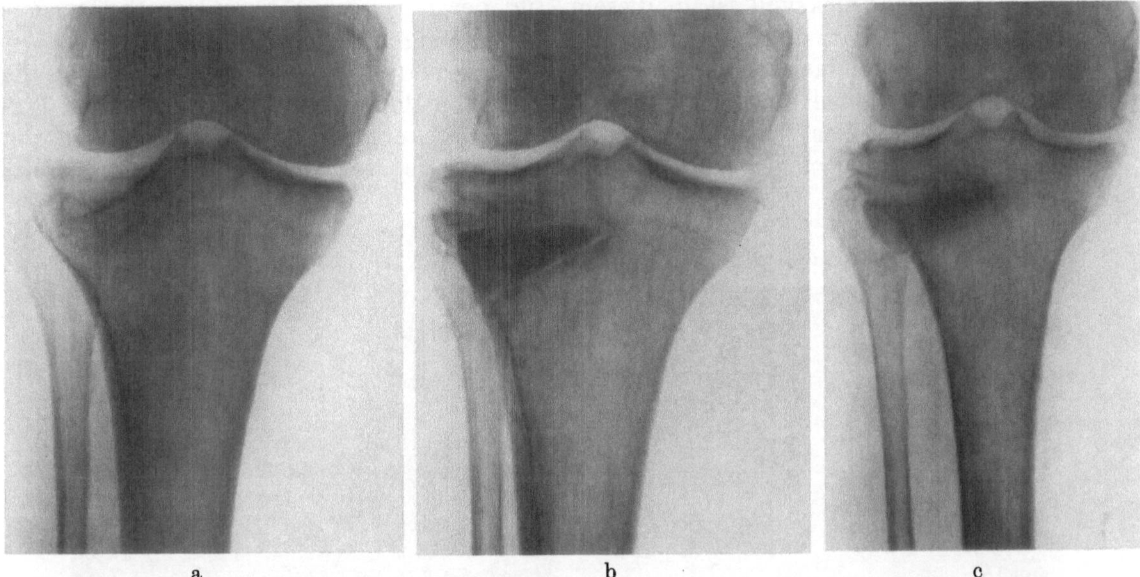

Abb. 38. a Tibiakopf-Impressionsfraktur bei 76jähriger Frau. b Der heterologe Span, welcher die gehobene Gelenkfläche trägt, ist sieben Wochen nach der Implantation von einem Osteoid-Saum umgeben. c Acht Wochen später ist der Saum weitgehend durch Kalksalzeinlagerung geschwunden. (Nach MAATZ-HAASCH in SCHINZ 1969)

bindegewebigen Resorption, wird also abgebaut und aufgesogen (siehe auch Histologie Abb. 9 und 10 und Röntgenbild Abb. 40).

b) Die Resorption des Spanes

Im ersatzstarken Lager, z.B. im Knochengewebe, kann ein Span mit Antigenität sehr wohl zunächst bindegewebig resorbiert werden. Hier setzt dann aber daneben frühzeitig Knochenneubildung ein. Diese Vorgänge lassen sich röntgenologisch nicht erfassen. Im ersatzschwachen oder ersatzunfähigen Lager aber erleidet der Span röntgenologisch eindrucksvolle Veränderungen, wie die Abb. 39 zeigt. Die technisch einwandfrei durchgeführte Operation der Spanversteifung am Hüftgelenk mußte zu einem Mißerfolg führen, weil die Indikation falsch war. Man hatte eine Tuberkulose angenommen, es handelte sich aber um eine congenitale Subluxation. So mußten die homologen Späne aus der Tiefkühltruhe früher oder später brechen; zuerst der größtenteils extraossär liegende, welcher das klassische Bild der bindegewebigen Resorption zeigt, die lacunären Arrosionen. Im Bereich der Doppelkontur liegt die Fraktur. Der intraossäre Span brach nach 14 Monaten intra-

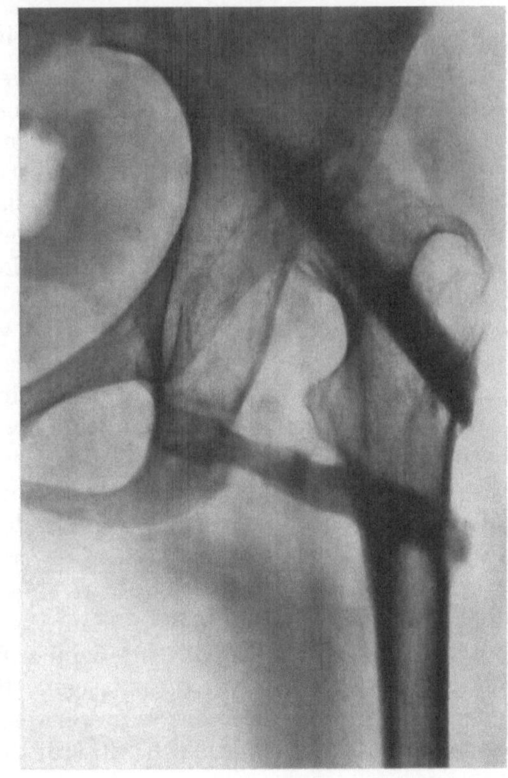

Abb. 39. 11jährige Patientin. Intra- und extraarticulare Spanarthrodese am Hüftgelenk mit homologen Spänen aus der Tiefkühltruhe. Nach acht Monaten sind die Grenzen des intraossär liegenden Spanes verwaschen. Der extraossär liegende Span zeigt bindegewebige Resorption, Lockerung im medialen Bett und Spanfraktur

articulär. Sehr eindrucksvoll ist in diesem Bild der langsame Einbau des Bankspanes intraossär im Gegensatz zur Resorption im ersatzunfähigen Weichteillager.

Auch am Schädeldach beobachten wir bei Verwendung toten Knochens meist die Resorption. Als Beispiel führen wir die Röntgenbilder der Abb. 40 an. Ein bei der Trepanation verschmutzter Schädeldachteil wurde ausgekocht. Es handelt sich also um denaturierten toten autologen Knochen. Sieben Monate später war die Resorption bereits weit fortgeschritten.

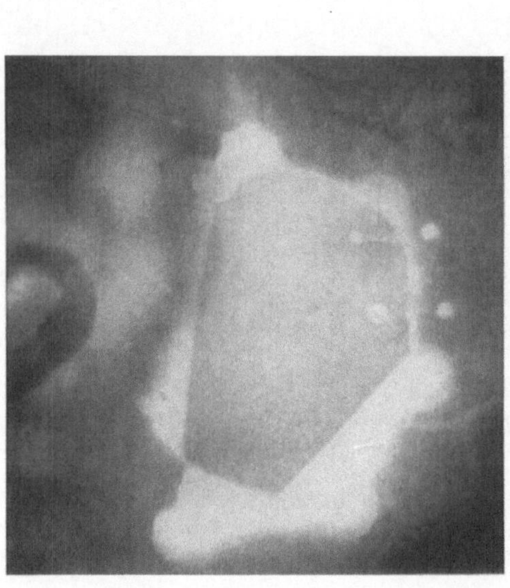
a

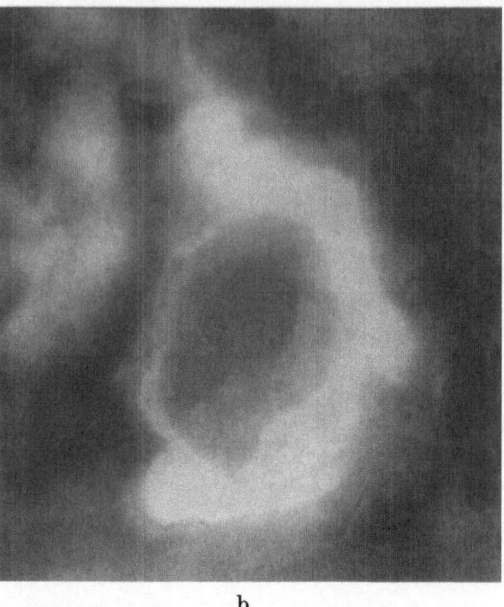
b

Abb. 40a u. b. 13jähriger Knabe. a Autologes, ortsständiges Schädeldach, welches während der Operation allerdings die Verbindung mit der Galea verlor. b Weitgehende Resorption des autologen Materials sieben Monate später

c) Substitution und Umbau

Erinnern wir uns der feingeweblichen Beobachtungen, so wissen wir, daß der überlebende autologe Span in seiner Knochensubstanz stets abstirbt und durch die überlebenden Weichgewebe durch lebendigen Knochen ersetzt werden muß. Dieser vorwiegend auf dem Wege der schleichenden Substitution (siehe Abb. 4 und 5) ablaufende Vorgang geht um so rascher vonstatten, je größer die innere Oberfläche des Spanes ist, also je spongiöser seine Struktur, während die dichte Corticalis außerordentlich lange Zeiten erfordern kann. Dieser innere Umbau des Spanes erfordert eine Auflockerung. Mehr oder minder große Umbauplätze geben dem Span eine Spongiosierung. Zeigt sich diese Auflockerung im Röntgenbild, so wissen wir, daß der Span „lebt" (Abb. 41). Mit dieser inneren Erneuerung ist dann meist eine Veränderung der inneren Struktur und je nach Alter des Patienten auch eine mehr oder minder ausgeprägte Veränderung der äußeren Form als Anpassung an die Funktion des Spanes verbunden. So sehen wir aus dem Gitterwerk der autologen Rippen am Schädeldach (Abb. 22) im Verlauf von zwölf Jahren eine Knochenplatte — mit allerdings einigen kleinen Randdefekten — sich bilden. Vollendet anzupassen allerdings vermag sich nur der kindliche Knochen (Abb. 42), wie wir es ja auch bei den Wachstumskorrekturen nach Frakturheilung in Fehlstellung sehen.

Über das endgültige Schicksal eines Knochentransplantates ist unser Wissen noch lückenhaft. Zweifelsohne wird das abgestorbene Knochengewebe in der Mehrzahl der Fälle im Laufe der Zeit durch lebenden Knochen ersetzt. In welcher Zeit aber dieser Vorgang abläuft, wissen wir nicht. Eigene Beobachtungen lassen vermuten, daß Jahrzehnte darüber vergehen können. Wir verweisen auf das histologische Bild der Abb. 8. Das zugehörige Röntgenbild (Abb. 43) läßt bei der Dichte des Spanes allerdings vermuten, daß

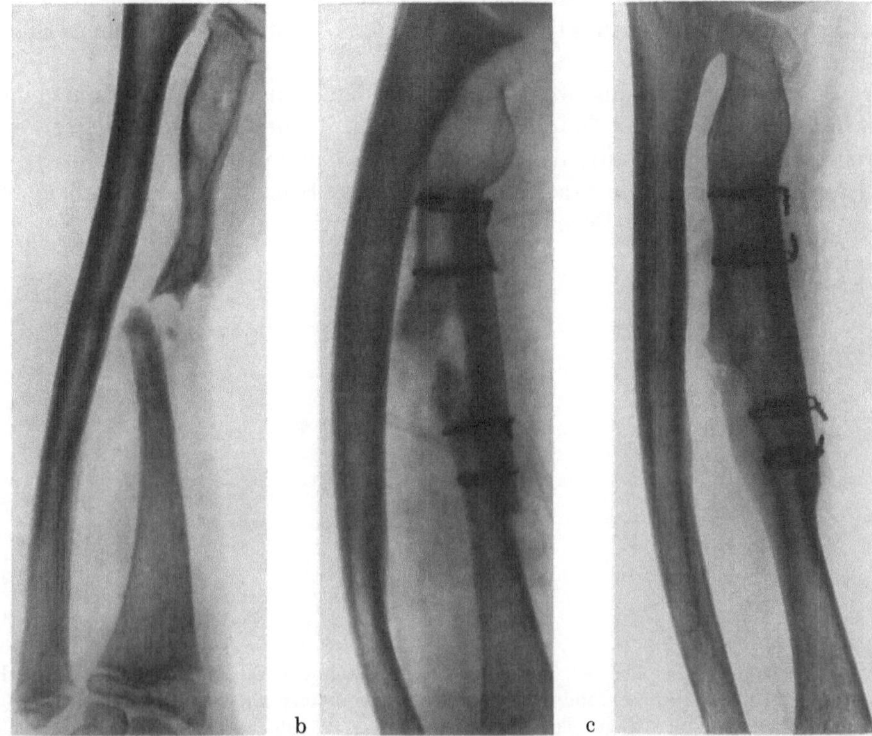

Abb. 41 a—c. 14 Jahre alter Knabe. a Defektpseudarthrose des Radius nach Schußbruch (beachte den Ellenvorschub!). b Nach Drahtextension durch Mittelhandknochen und Olecranon steht das Ellenköpfchen wieder am Platz. Der autologe Tibiaspan wurde mit vier Ligaturfedern fixiert. c Kontrollbilder nach zwei Jahren. Völliger Einbau des Spanes bei Aufbau des Radius. (Nach MAATZ-HAASCH in SCHINZ 1969)

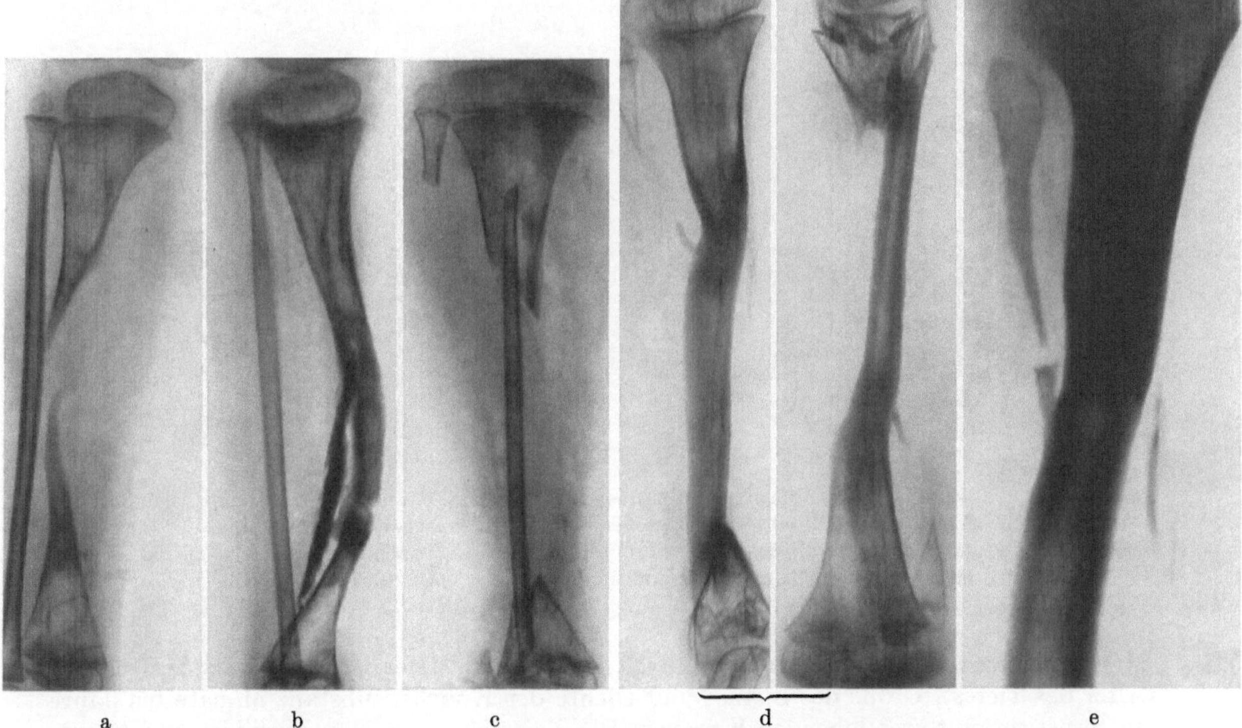

Abb. 42 a—e. Funktionelle Anpassung der gestielt überpflanzten Fibula bei 5 Jahre altem Mädchen. a Seit zwei Jahren bestehende Pseudarthrose der Tibia. b 4 Monate nach Einfügen eines Bankspanes. c Zustand nach der Verpflanzung der Fibula. d Vierzehn Monate danach (Quelle wie Abb. 22). e Neun Jahre später

ein nennenswerter Umbau ein Jahr nach der Transplantation noch nicht eingetreten sein kann. In Prozenten ausgedrückt kann man nach dem histologischen Bild unter 5% annehmen.

Überraschender ist der feingewebliche Befund bei dem Tibiaspan der Abb. 44, dreizehn Jahre nach der Verpflanzung. Nach dem Röntgenbild besteht ganz sicher kein Verdacht auf Nekrose, vielmehr muß aus der Struktur des Spanes auf guten Einbau geschlossen werden. Eine Probeentnahme am cranial gelegenen Spanteil aber ergab leere Knochenhöhlen und im übersehbaren Bereich keine Substitution.

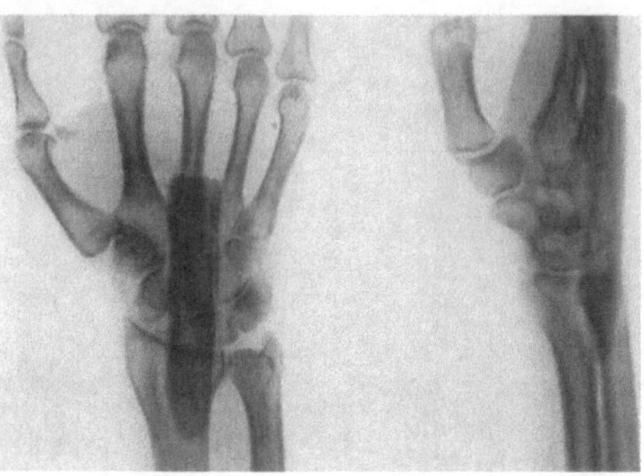

Abb. 43. Temporäre Handgelenksversteifung wegen Naviculare-Pseudarthrose ein Jahr nach dorsaler Auflage eines autologen Tibia-Spans (A. W. FISCHER). (Siehe Text S. 640 u. Abb. 8. Quelle: MAATZ, Verhdlg. Dtsch. Orthop. Ges. 43. Kongr. 1955, Verhandlgs-Band S. 44.)

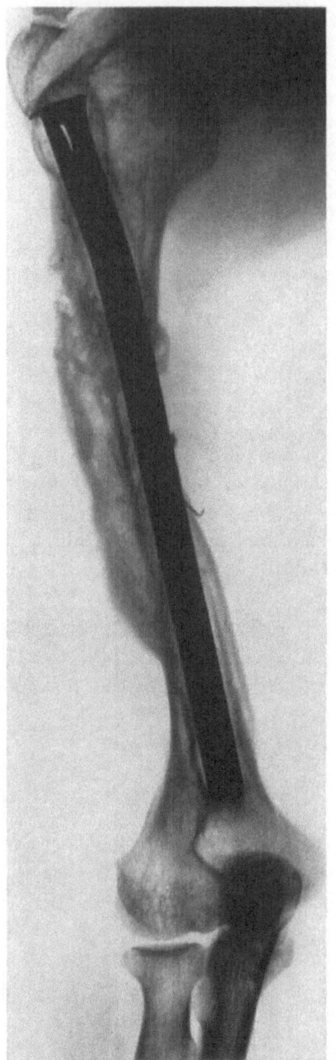

a

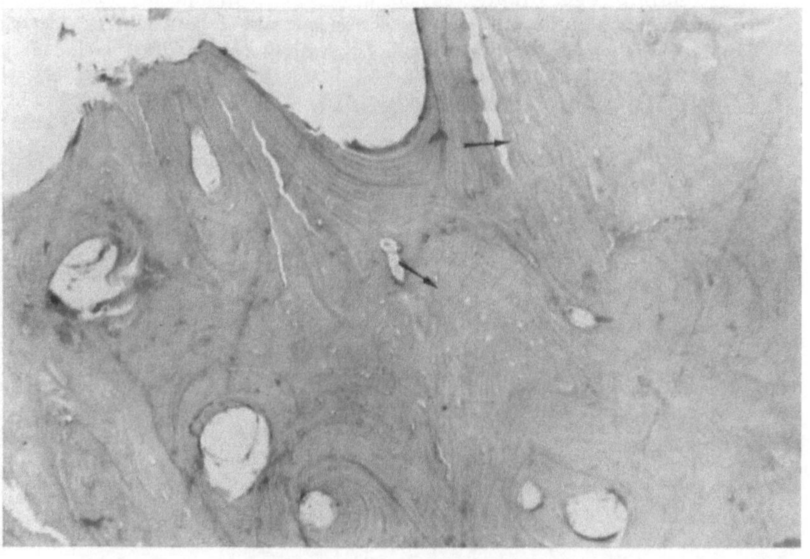

b

Abb. 44a. u b. Ein Schußbruch des Humerus 1941 führte zur Pseudarthrose, welche 1952 bei dem damals 36 Jahre alten Patienten erfolglos genagelt und 1953 mit großem autologen Tibiaspan versorgt wurde. Der Span frakturierte. Heilung durch sehr dicken Nagel (a). Eine Probeentnahme vom Spanende (b) ergab, daß die Substitution dreizehn Jahre nach der Transplantation noch nich t abgeschlossen ist (Pfeile)

Der heterologe Span (in unseren Fällen „Kieler Span") beansprucht je nach Herkunft (Alter des Tieres), Größe des Spanes und Dichte der Knochensubstanz Monate bis Jahre zur Substitution durch lebenden Knochen. Ein Beispiel zeigen Röntgenbilder und Mikrofoto der Abb. 31 u. 45. Die Entnahme wurde auf der medialen Seite vorgenommen, an der vom Span röntgenologisch nichts mehr zu erkennen war. Im feingeweblichen Schnitt finden wir geringfügige Reste des Implantats.

Die Abb. 46—49 zeigen den Einbau von heterologen Spänen unter verschiedener Indikation. Die Bildlegenden weisen auf Besonderheiten hin. Hervorgehoben sei hier nur, daß bei Knochenhöhlen im Bereich des Markraumes eines Röhrenknochens von uns immer wieder beobachtet wird, daß der Einbau recht lange Zeit in Anspruch nehmen kann. Wir führen das darauf zurück, daß hier im Markraum der Knochen später ohnehin wieder abgebaut wird, daß damit wohl der funktionelle Anreiz als Bildungskomponente fehlt.

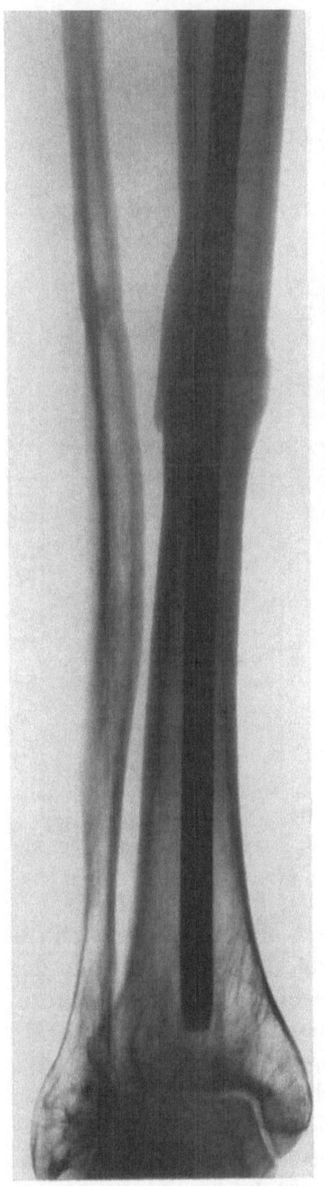

a

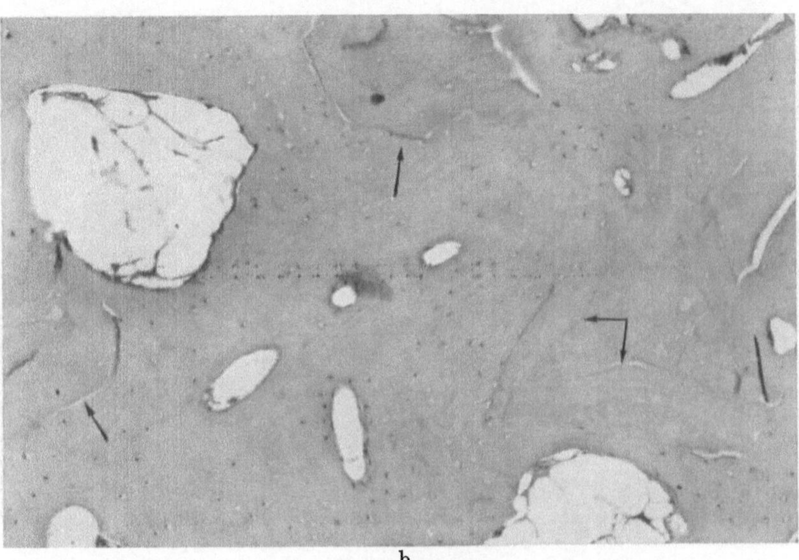

b

Abb. 45a u. b. Früheres Bild siehe Abb. 31. a Röntgenologisch vollkommener Einbau der heterologen Anlegespäne nicht ganz zwei Jahre nach der Verpflanzung wegen verzögerter Verfestigung einer genagelten offenen Fraktur. b Eine Rohrstanzenprobe, welche während der Nagelentfernung vorgenommen wurde, zeigt nur noch feine Spanreste im Callus (Pfeile)

Bei der Patientin B. der Abb. 47 (siehe primäre Bilder Abb. 26, S. 558) zeigt sich sehr schön der fortschreitende Einbau des Spanes, welcher proximal in die Spongiosa eingetrieben und distal dem Schaft formschlüssig aufliegt.

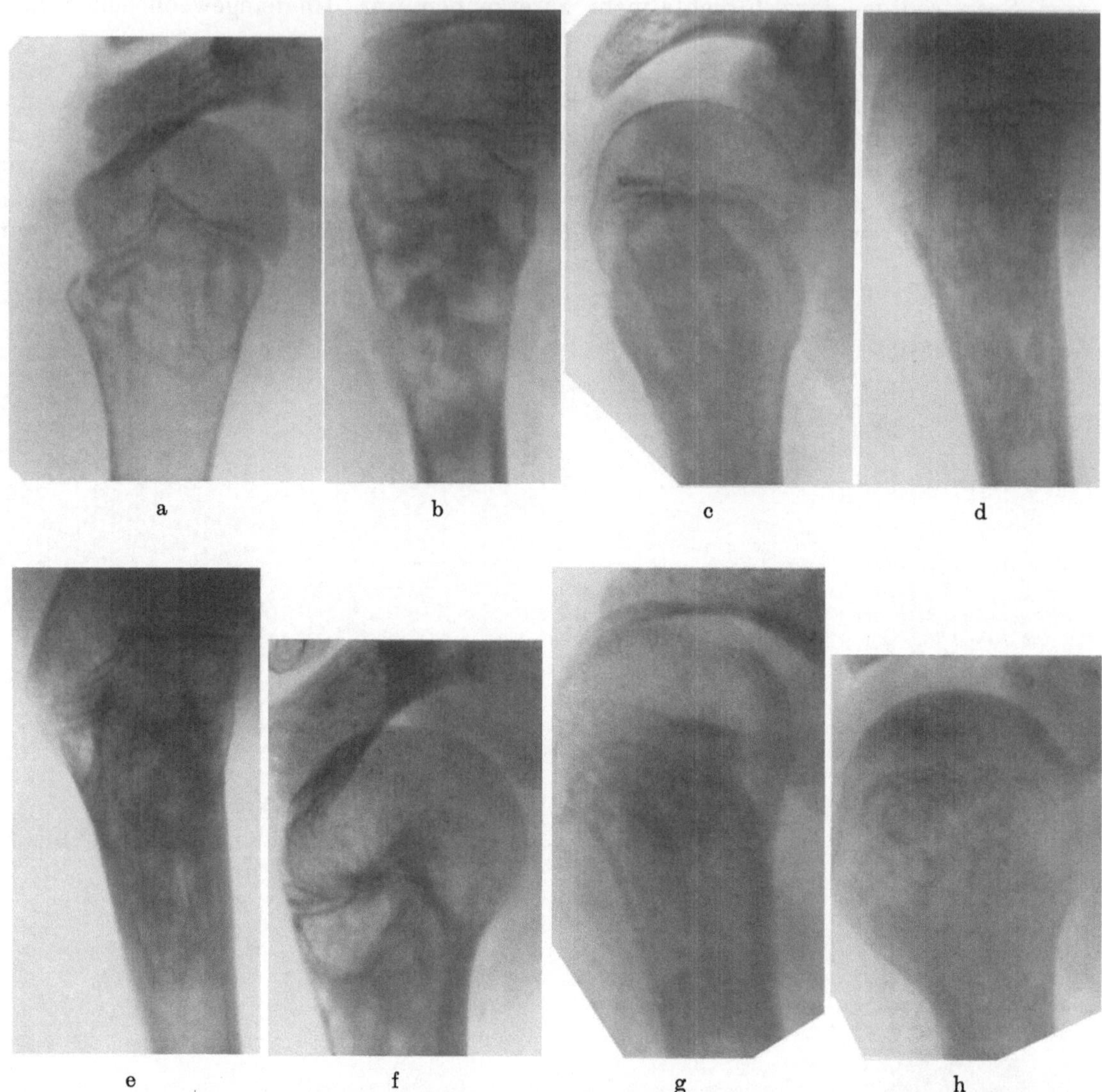

Abb. 46a—h. 11 Jahre alter Knabe. Knochencyste am Humerus. Nach Ausräumung und Ausfüllung mit heterologer Spongiosa rascher Einbau, aber nach einem Jahr erstes Zeichen eines Rezidivs (e), welches sieben Monate später evident ist (f) und nochmals ausgeräumt und wieder mit heterologer Spongiosa versorgt wurde. g und h: Kontrollen nach der zweiten Operation

Der Schiffchenspan (Abb. 48, siehe auch Abb. 25) demonstriert besonders deutlich die Schwierigkeiten, welche dem Röntgenologen in der Beurteilung der Bilder durch das heterologe Spanmaterial erwachsen können. Schon ein gut anliegender Anlegespan kann mit seinem spongiösen Teil einen knöchernen Anschluß an den Schaftknochen vortäuschen. Der Schiffchenspan kann frisch nach der Operation eine Heilung der Pseudarthrose vortäuschen, da er mit seinem „Kiel" den Pseudarthrosenspalt überbrückt. Mit zunehmender

Abb. 47a u. b. Heterologer Einlege-Anlegespan bei 54jähriger Patientin bei kopfnaher Pseudarthrose am Humerus (siehe auch Frakturen, Abb. 26, S. 558). a Spananlage eineinhalb Jahre nach der Fraktur, welche nach Drahtnaht geeitert hatte. b Nachuntersuchungsbild fünf Jahre später. Röntgenologisch vollkommener Einbau des Spanes

Abb. 48a—d. Innenknöchel-Pseudarthrose bei 46jährigem Mann $3^1/_2$ Monate nach Supinations-Eversions-Luxationsfraktur IV. a Das Kontrollbild erweckt den Verdacht, b die gezielte Aufnahme bestätigt ihn, c Kontrollbild nach Operation mit Schiffchen-Span. 5 Wochen Gips, nach 6 Wochen Gehbelastung. d Kontrollbild 10 Monate später

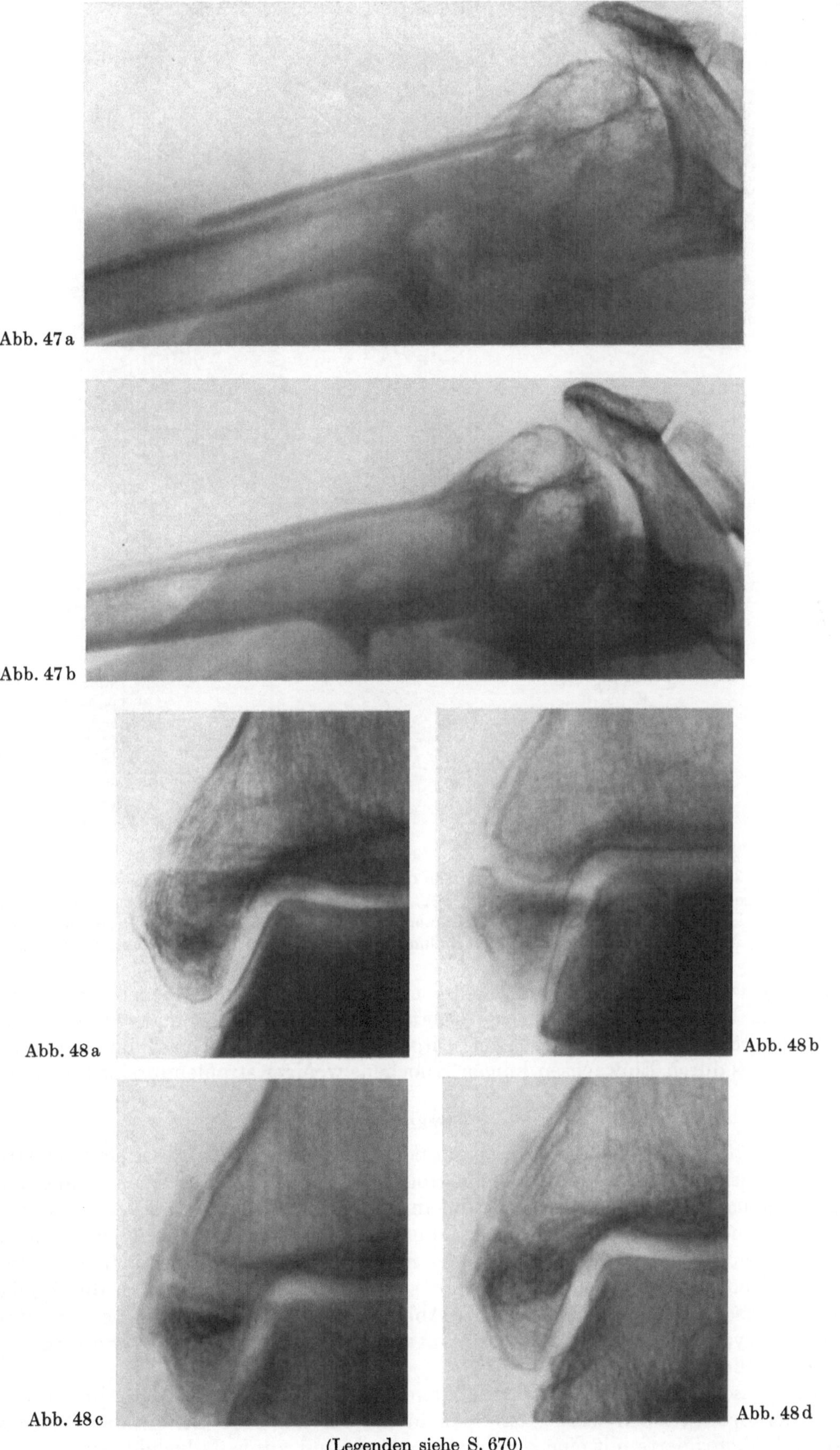

Abb. 47a

Abb. 47b

Abb. 48a

Abb. 48b

Abb. 48c

Abb. 48d

(Legenden siehe S. 670)

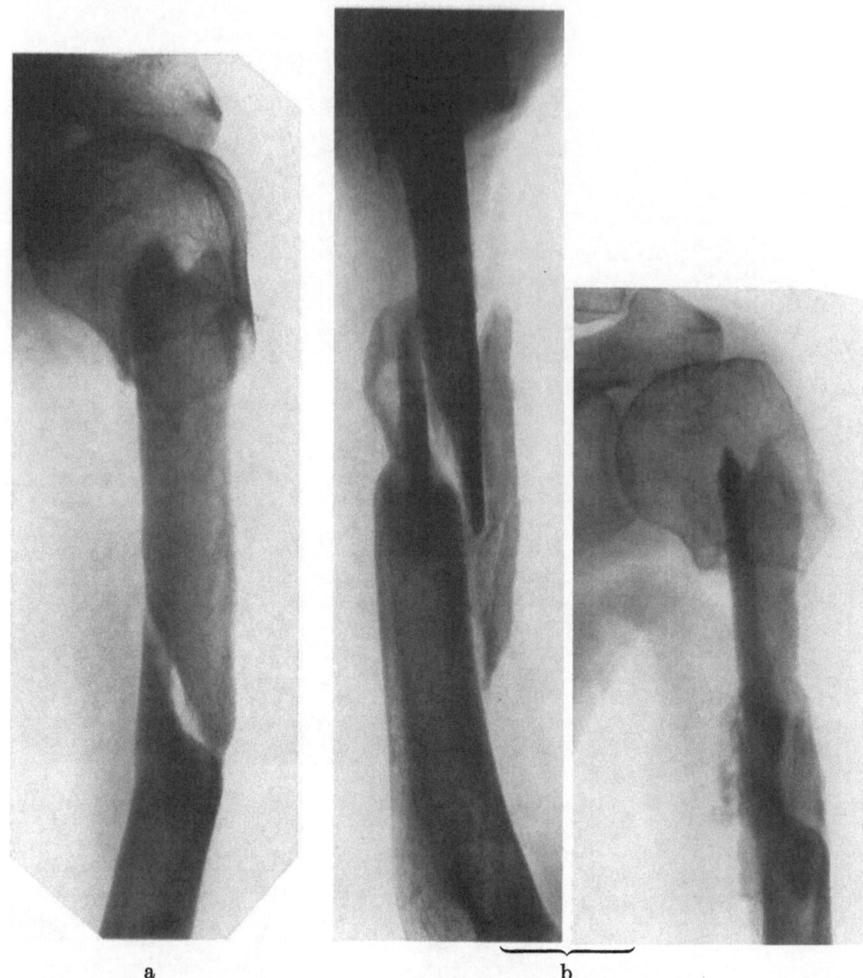

Abb. 49a—e. 35jähriger Patient. Ermüdungsbruch des großen autologen Tibiaspans, welcher nach Osteochondrom-Resektion implantiert wurde (s. Abb. 20). a Fraktur im November 1958. b Heterologer Stufen-Anlegespan bei gleichzeitiger Verkürzung des Armes am 14. 11. 58. Weitere heterologe Anlegespäne am 30. 11. 59. c und d Kontrollbilder mit knöcherner Heilung 1960 und 1961. e Kontrollbilder am 13. 4. 65

Erfahrung werden die Feinheiten leichter erkannt werden. Sehr lockeres Spanmaterial, welches zur Unterfütterung einer frakturierten Gelenkfläche eingefügt wurde, kann allerdings dem röntgenologischen Nachweis entgehen und erst dann im Bilde erkennbar werden, wenn es durch Einwachsen jungen Knochens weniger strahlendurchlässig ist.

d) Spanfraktur

Wir schätzen das Ereignis der Spanfraktur auf etwa 10%. Dabei sind selbstredend nur überbrückende, tragende Späne einbezogen. Dieser relativ hohe Prozentsatz erscheint uns durchaus verständlich. Einmal ist allein die Form des Spanes im Vergleich zu einem gesunden Knochen unzureichend (siehe Abb. 20 und 49), und zum anderen ist die Gefahr des Ermüdungsbruches — denn um solche handelt es sich fast ausschließlich — so groß, weil das Knochengerüst, nach der Verpflanzung tot, meist nur langsam durch lebenden Knochen ersetzt wird. Das Beispiel der Abb. 49 zeigt uns eine „typische" Spanfraktur, nicht die „typische" Heilung, denn es mußten heterologe Anlegespäne verpflanzt werden, um eine Heilung zu erreichen.

Die typische „normale" Frakturheilung zeigt das Röntgenbild der Abb. 50b. Durch die Federkopfschrauben wurde der Span in das mechanische Gefüge der Elle fest eingespannt. Er reagierte mit einem Ermüdungsbruch mit guter Callusbildung.

Unter ungünstigen Bedingungen bleibt die knöcherne Heilung eines Spanbruches aus. Wir verweisen auf den Verschiebespan, welcher auf S. 658 und 659 eingehend geschildert und in den Röntgenbildern der Abb. 32 wiedergegeben wurde.

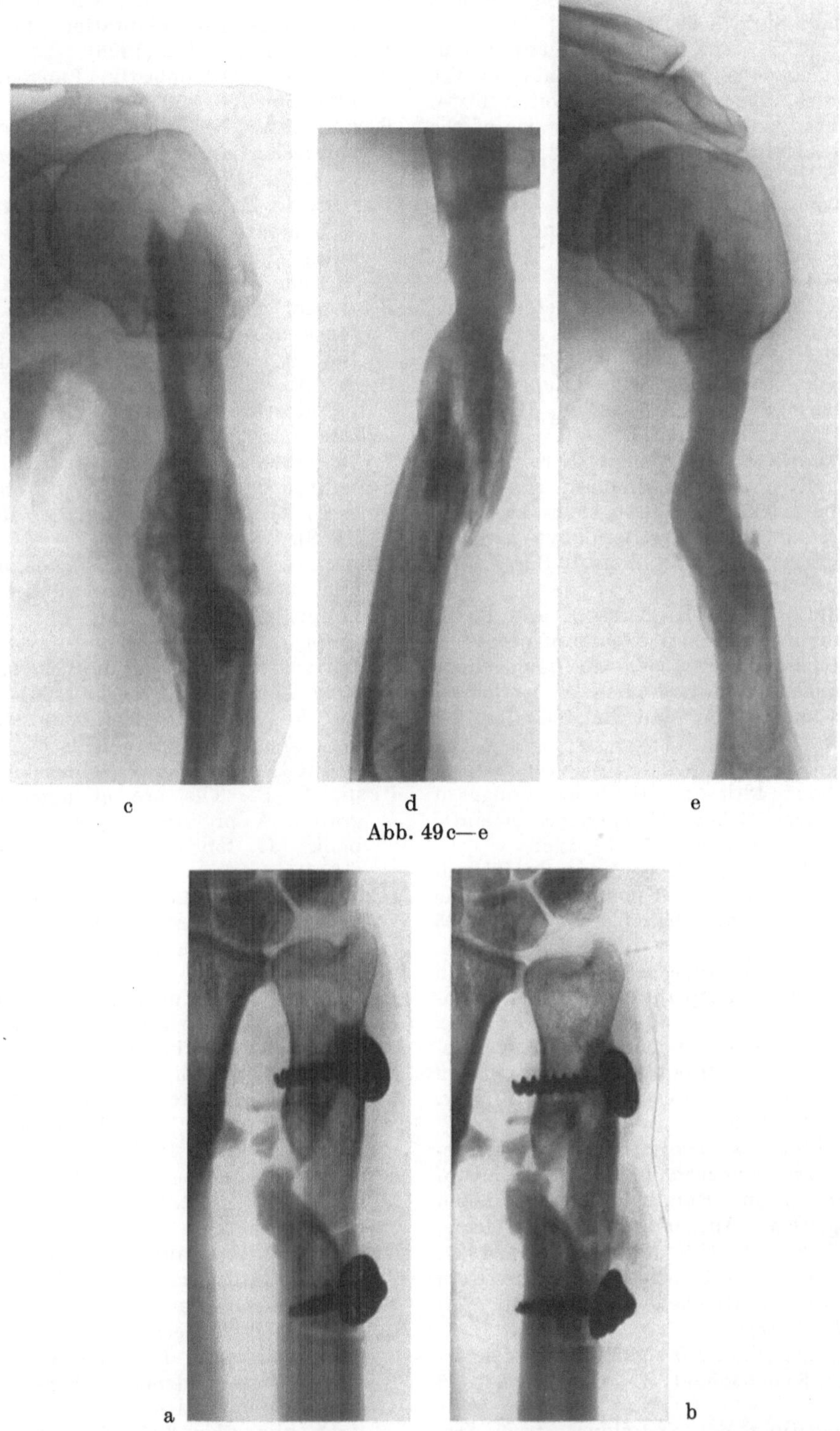

Abb. 49c—e

Abb. 50a u. b. Heilung einer Spanfraktur. a Span vom Beckenkamm mit Federkopfschrauben fixiert. b 4 Monate später hat der Span gut Anschluß an den Mutterknochen gefunden, zeigt aber eine Fraktur mit bereits lebhafter periostaler Callusbildung

Literatur

ABBOT, L. C., E. R. SCHOTTSTAEDT, J. B. SAUNDERS, and F. C. BOST: The evaluation of cortical and cancellus bone as grafting material. A clinical and experimental study. J. Bone Jt Surg. A **29**, 381—414 (1947).

ANDERSON, K. J.: The behavior of autogenous and homogenous bone transplants on the anterior chamber of the rat's eye. A histological study of the effect of the size of the implant. J. Bone Jt Surg. A **43**, 980—995 (1961).

— Experimental investigations of large and small fragment bone implants and extracts of heterogenous bone. J. Bone Jt Surg. A **43**, 996—1004 (1961).

— The development of processed heterogenous bone. II. Experimental and clinical assessment of its effectiveness as a biological transplant. Presented at the Eighth Annual Congr. of the Pan Pacific Surgical Association, Honolulu, Hawaii, November 6, 1963.

— J. A. DINGWALL, JOAN SMITH, J. F. LECOCQ, and D. K. CLAWSON: Induced connective tissue metaplasia I. Heterogenous bone extract implants in the rat anterior eye chamber. A preliminary report. J. Bone Jt Surg. A **43**, 996—1004 (1961).

— J. F. LECOCQ, W. H. AKESON, and P. R. HARRINGTON: End-point results of processed heterogenous, autogenous, and homogenous bone transplants in the human. A histological study. Clin. Orthop. and Related Res. **33**, 220—236 (1964).

— —, and J. A. DINGWALL: Processed heterogenous bone. 48th Annual Clinical Congr. of the American College of Surgeons. Atlantic City, New Jersey. Oct. 15—19, 1962.

— J. G. LE COCQ, and J. G. MOONEY: Clinical evaluation of processed heterogenous bone transplants. Clin. Orthop. **29**, 248—263 (1963).

AXHAUSEN, G.: (1) Histologische Untersuchungen über Knochentransplantationen am Menschen. Dtsch. Z. Chir. **91**, 388—428 (1908).

— (2) Die histologischen und klinischen Geschehen der freien Osteoplastik auf Grund von Tierversuchen. Langenbecks Arch. klin. Chir. **28**, 23—145 (1909).

—, u. E. BERGMANN: Die Ernährungsunterbrechungen am Knochen (traumatische Knochennekrose). In: Handbuch der speziellen pathologischen Anatomie und Histologie, Bd. IX/3, S. 146—155. Berlin: Springer 1937.

AXHAUSEN, W.: Die Knochenregeneration, ein zweiphasisches Geschehen. Zbl. Chir. **77**, 435—442 (1952).

— Die Knochenbildungsfähigkeit der frei überpflanzten Knochenhaut. Zbl. Chir. **77**, 27—36 (1952).

— Die Bedeutung der Individual- und Artspezifität der Gewebe für die freie Knochenüberpflanzung. Beiheft Mschr. Unfallheilk. **72** (1962).

BADE, H., u. G. KÜNTSCHER: Wirkungen von Röntgenstrahlen auf den Knochen. Fortschr. Röntgenstr. **60**, 235—242 (1939).

BARTH, A.: (1) Histologische Untersuchungen über Knochenimplantation. Beiträge Path. Anat. **17**, 65—142 (1895).

— (2) Über Osteoplastik. Langenbecks Arch. klin. Chir. **86**, 859—872 (1908).

BASCHKIRZEW, N. J., u. N. N. PETROW: Beiträge zur freien Knochenüberpflanzung. Dtsch. Z. Chir. **113**, 490—531 (1912).

BASSET, C. A. L., and D. K. CREIGHTON jr.: A comparison of host response to cortical autografts and processed calf heterografts. J. Bone Jt Surg. A **44**, 842—854 (1962).

BAUERMEISTER, A.: Experimentelle Grundlagen für den Aufbau einer neuen Knochenbank. Beiheft Mschr. Unfallheilk. **58** (1958).

BIER, A.: Über Knochenregeneration, über Pseudarthrosen und über Knochentransplantate. Langenbecks Arch. klin. Chir. **127**, 1—136 (1923).

BONFIGLIO, M.: Repair of bone-transplant fractures. J. Bone Jt Surg. A **40**, 446—456 (1958).

BÜRKLE DE LA CAMP, H.: Knochenkonservierung und Verwendung konservierten Knochens. Langenbecks Arch. klin. Chir. **279**, 26—37 (1954).

— Betrachtungen über die Knochenverpflanzung. Med. Welt **3**, 1—12 (1961).

BUSCH, F.: Zit. nach E. KAUFMANN, Lehrbuch der speziellen pathologischen Anatomie, 4. Aufl. Berlin: Georg Reimer 1907.

BUSH, L. F.: The use of homogenous bone grafts. A preliminary report of the bone bank. J. Bone Jt Surg. A **29**, 620—628 (1947).

CLOWARD, R. B.: Lesions of the intervertebral disks and their treatment by interbody fusion methods. (The painful disk.) Clin. Orthop. **27**, 51—77 (1963).

DEBRUNNER, H.: Zur praktischen Verwendung heteroplastischer Knochentransplantate. Arch. orthop. Unfall-Chir. **47**, 694—702 (1955).

DUHAMEL (1740): Zit. bei W. BLOCK, Die normale und gestörte Knochenbruchheilung. In: Neue Chirurgie, Bd. 62, S. 19. Stuttgart: Ferdinand Enke 1940.

DUPUYTREN: Leçons orales de clinique chirurgical, 2. ed., vol. 1, p. 378. Paris: Germez-Ballière 1839.

DUYFJES, F.: Over antigene herking van heterologe botimplaten. (Een experimtal onderzoek.) Inaug.-Diss. Leiden 1965.

ECKE, H.: Tierexperimentelle Untersuchungen zur Bestimmung der Qualität von Knochenspänen verschiedener biologischer Herkunft für Transplantationszwecke. Langenbecks Arch. klin. Chir. **307**, 169—194 (1964).

EHALT, W.: Unsere Erfahrungen mit der Knochenbank. Verh. Dtsch. Orthop. Ges. Z. Orthop., H. 91, 75—77 (1956).

FEHR, A. M.: Erste Erfahrungen mit der sog. Chips-Plastik, d.h. Spongiosaplastik nach MATTI. Helvet. chir. Acta **16**, 296—301 (1949).

FUCHS, G., H. STEGEMANN u. W. EGER: Der transplantierte Knochenspan und seine Qualität nach partieller und vollständiger Enteiweißung bei erhaltener organischer Substanz. Langenbecks Arch. klin. Chir. **303**, 240—260 (1963).

GALLIE, W. E.: The use of boiled bone in operative surgery. Amer. J. orthop. Surg. **16**, 373—383 (1918).

GRAF, R.: Gefäßversorgung autoplastischer Spongiosatransplantate und ihre Bedeutung. Bruns' Beitr. klin. Chir. **198**, 390—400 (1959).

GÜNTZ, E.: Über eine einfache Methode der Knochenkonservierung. Langenbecks Arch. klin. Chir. **279**, 56—60 (1954).

HAASCH, K.: Metaplastische Knochenbildung beim Menschen durch heterogene eiweißarme Spongiosa. Chirurg **32**, 183—186 (1961).

HAHN, E.: Eine Methode Pseudarthrosen der Tibia mit großem Knochendefekt zur Heilung zu bringen. Zbl. Chir. **1884**, 337—341.

HALLÉN, L. G.: Heterologous transplantation with kiel bone. Acta orthop. scand. **37**, 1—19 (1966).

HARMON, P. H., J. A. DINGWALL, and M. S. ABEL: Lumbar arthrosis and discopathy treated with anterior discectomy and fusion: Comparative and roentgen studies of spines fused with protein and fat extracted heterologous bone. J. Bone Jt Surg. A **46**, 1143—1144 (1964).

HEINE, B.: Über die Wiedererzeugung neuer Knochenmasse und Bildung neuer Knochen. Graefes u. Walthers J. Chir. **24**, 513 (1836).

HELLER, E.: Transplantation der Knorpelfuge. Langenbecks Arch. klin. Chir. **109**, 104—109 (1918).

HEPP, O.: KOCH und DAHMEN schildern die von HEPP angegebene Technik der Fusionsoperation an der Wirbelsäule. Arch. orthop. Unfall-Chir. **54**, 139—152 (1962).

HERGET, R.: Primäre Infarkte der langen Röhrenknochen durch lokale Zirkulationsstörungen. Zbl. Chir. **77**, 1372—1375 (1952).

INCLAN, A.: Use of preserved bone grafts in orthopedic surgery. J. Bone Jt Surg. A **24**, 81—96 (1942).

JOB-A-MEEKREN: Heilung eines Schädeldefektes nach Säbelhieb durch Einlagerung eines Schädelstückes vom Hunde (1682). Zit. bei J. WOLFF, Zur Osteoplastik. Berl. klin. Wschr. **1862**, 492—499.

JUDET, J., R. JUDET et A. ARVISET: Banque d'os et heterogreffe. Presse med. **68**, 1007—1009 (1949).

KAWAMURA, H., HOSONO, TAKAHASI TOMITA, NAKAZOE, HIRAYAMA, and KIDO: Experimental studies on heterogenous bone transplantation. J. Bone Jt Surg. A **42**, 543—571 (1960).

KIENHOLZ, M., and B. KEMKES: Untersuchungen über den immunbiologischen Wert heteroplastischer konservierter Knochenspäne. Arch. orthop. Unfall-Chir. **48**, 623—632 (1956).

KLEINSCHMIDT, O.: Operative Chirurgie, S. 332. Berlin: Springer 1943.

KLEN, R.: Methode und organisatorische Probleme der Versorgung der CSSR mit Gewebskonserven. Berlin: Volk u. Gesundheit 1965.

KOCH, W., u. G. DAHMEN: Histologische Untersuchungen über den Ein- und Umbau heterologer mazerierter Knochentransplantate. Arch. orthop. Unfall-Chir. **54**, 139—152 (1962).

KREUZ, F. P., G. W. HYATT, T. C. TURNER, and A. L. BASSET: Preservation and clinical use of freeze-dried bone. J. Bone Jt Surg. A **33**, 863—872 (1951).

KROMPECHER, S.: Die Knochenbildung. Jena: Gustav Fischer 1937.

KÜNTSCHER, G.: Eine neue Methode der Knochentransplantation. Zbl. Chir. **74**, 319—320 (1948).

— Die biologischen Gesetze der Knochenbruchheilung. Chirurg **32**, 261—265 u. 312—317 (1961).

KÜPPERMANN, W.: (1) Osteosynthese mit konserviertem Knochen. Mschr. Unfallheilk. **60**, 74—78 (1957).

— (2) Erfahrungen mit heteroplastischen Knochen bei der Knochenbruchbehandlung. Langenbecks Arch. klin. Chir. **298**, 246—251 (1961).

KÜTTNER, H.: Die Transplantation aus dem Affen und ihre Dauererfolge. Münch. med. Wschr. **45**, 1449—1452 (1917).

LAHNINGER, J., u. G. SALEM: Erfahrungen mit dem Kieler Knochenspan (32 Fälle). Chirurg **35**, 495—499 (1964).

LANDERER, A.: Über neuere Methoden der Frakturbehandlung. Münch. med. Wschr. **1894**, 1005—1120.

LENTZ, W.: Die Grundlagen der Transplantation von Knochengewebe. Stuttgart: Georg Thieme 1955.

LERICHE, R., et A. POLICARD: La physiologie de l'os. Paris: Masson & Cie. 1926.

LEXER, E.: Die freien Transplantationen. I. Teil. In: Neue Deutsche Chirurgie, Bd. 26. Stuttgart: Ferdinand Enke 1919.

— Die freien Transplantationen. I. u. II. Teil. In: Neue Deutsche Chirurgie, Bd. 26. Stuttgart 1919.

— Die freien Transplantationen. II. Teil. Stuttgart: Ferdinand Enke 1924.

LIMBERG: Zit. bei KLEINSCHMIDT, S. 332.

LOSEE, F. L., and L. A. HURLEY: Bone treated with ethylenediamine as a successful foundation material in cross-species bone grafts. Nature (Lond.) **1956**, No 4518, 1032—1033.

MAATZ, R.: Die Knochentransplantationen. Z. Orthop., Beilageheft zu **87**, 44—51 (1956).

— Die Behandlung der Innenknöchel-Pseudarthrose mit einem T-Span. Bruns' Beitr. klin. Chir. **203**, 145—151 (1961).

— Das Wesen des Kieler Spans. Langenbecks Arch. klin. Chir. **308**, 1028—1031 (1964).

MAATZ, R., u. A. BAUERMEISTER: A method of bone maceration. Results in animal experiments. J. Bone Jt Surg. A **39**, 153—166 (1957).
— — Klinische Erfahrungen mit dem Kieler Span. Langenbecks Arch. klin. Chir. **298**, 239—244 (1961).
— W. LENTZ u. R. GRAF: Die Knochenbildungsfähigkeit konservierter Späne. Zbl. Chir. **77**, 1376—1382 (1952).
— — — Experimentelle Grundlagen der Transplantation konservierter Knochen. Langenbecks Arch. klin. Chir. **273**, 850—855 (1953).
— — — Spongiosa test of bone grafts for transplantation. J. Bone Jt Surg. A **36**, 721—731 (1954).
— — — Der Spongiosa-Test. Frankfurt. Z. Path. **65**, 299—313 (1954).
MARCHAND, L.: Zur Kenntnis der Knochentransplantation. Verh. path. Ges., 2. Tagg, 368—375 (1899).
MARTIN, B.: (1) Die sympathische Knochenerkrankung. Langenbecks Arch. klin. Chir. **129**, 45—57 (1924).
— (2) Über die osteogenetische Fähigkeit des Periosts. Langenbecks Arch. klin. Chir. **144**, 489—530 (1927).
MATTI, H.: Über freie Transplantation von Knochenspongiosa. Langenbecks Arch. klin. Chir. **68**, 236—258 (1932).
MILLOWICH, A. H., B. J. AMREIN, and A. BORMAN: Antigenity of bovine cortical bone. Proc. Soc. expl. Biol. (N.Y.) **109**, 562—564 (1962).
MORGAN, L. C., W. A. JAMISON, and H. M. POWEL: Merthiolate as preservative for biological products. Production and preservation of diphtheria toxoid. J. Immunol. **25**, 121—126 (1933).
NICOLADONI, C.: Daumenplastik und organischer Ersatz der Fingerspitze (Anticheiroplastik und Daktyloplastik). Langenbecks Arch. klin. Chir. **61**, 606—614 (1900).
O'CONNER, G. B.: Merthiolate: tissue preservative and antiseptic. Amer. J. Surg. **45**, 563—565 (1939).
OLLIER, L.: Recherches expérim. sur les greffes osseuses. J. Physiol. (Paris) **3**, 88 (1860).
— Traité experim. et clin. de la régénération des os etc. Paris 1867.
— De la greffe osseuse chez l'homme. Arch. physiol. et path. **1889**, 168.
— De l'ostéogénèse chirurgicale. Verh. X. Int. med. Kongr. Berlin 1891.
ORELL, S.: (1) Studien über Knochentransplantation und Knochenneubildung. Act. chir. scand. **74**, Suppl. 31, 1—274 (1934).
— (2) Experimentell chirurgische Studie über Knochentransplantate und ihre Anwendung in der Chirurgie. Dtsch. Z. Chir. **232**, 701—713 (1937).
— (3) Principles and experiences at the implantation of os purum, os novum and bone granulate. Act. orthop. belg. **18**, 162—173 (1952).
PAYR, E.: Über osteoplastischen Ersatz nach Kiefer-Resektion (Kieferdefekten) durch Rippenstücke mittels gestielter Brustrandlappen oder freier Transplantation. Zbl. Clin. **35**, 1065—1070 (1908).
— Ersatzglieder und Arbeitsprothesen. Berlin: Springer 1918.
PHEMISTER, D. B.: Bone groth and repair. Ann. Surg. **102**, 261—285 (1935).
— Treatment of ununited fractures by onlay bone grafts without screw or tie fixation and without breaking down of the fibrous union. J. Bone Jt Surg. A **29**, 946—960 (1947).
RADZIMOWSKY: Inaug.-Diss. Kiew 1881. Ref. bei MARCHAND. In: Neue Deutsche Chirurgie, Liefg 16, Bd. 16. Stuttgart: Ferdinand Enke 1901.
RAY, A. D., and J. A. HOLLOWAY: Bone implants: Preliminary report of an experimental study. J. Bone Jt Surg. A **39**, 1119—1128 (1957).
ROTH, H.: Die Konservierung von Knochengewebe für Transplantationen. Wien: Springer 1952.
ROUX, W.: Das Gesetz der Transformation der Knochen. Berl. klin. Wschr. **1893**, 509—533.
— Gesammelte Abhandlungen über Entwicklungsmechanik der Organismen. Leipzig 1895.
SAUERBRUCH, F.: Die Exstirpation des Femur mit Umkipp-Plastik des Unterschenkels. Dtsch. Z. Chir. **169**, 1—12 (1922).
SCHLEYER, H. v.: Diskuss.-Beitr.: Zur Behandlung des juvenilen Knochensystems mit dem Kieler Span. Berl. Chir. Ges. März 1964.
SCHMID-SCHMIDFELDEN, O.: Ein weiterer Beitrag zur Transplantation von kältekonservierten Knochen (Knochenbank) mit Kritik der Spätergebnisse. Arch. orthop. Unfall-Chir. **46**, 315—329 (1954).
SCHNEIDER, H.-J.: Über die Möglichkeit der Bestimmung der mechanischen Wertigkeit des Skeletts beim Lebenden durch Entnahme von Knochenproben. Inaug.-Diss. Berlin 1965.
SCHWIER, V.: Zu den Problemen der Osteosynthese, der Knochenneubildung und der Knochenverpflanzung. Chirurg **31**, 220—236 (1960).
SPEMANN, H.: Mechanics of development of mammalian egg. Psychiatr.-neurol. Wschr. **38**, 205—207 (1936).
TUCKER, E. J.: Studies of the use of cultured calf bone in human bone grafts. Clin. Orthop. **7**, 171—188 (1956).
TUFFIER u. MAGITOT: Zit. bei A. CARREL, The preservation of tissues and its application in surgery. J. Amer. med. Ass. **59**, 523 (1912).
URIST, M. R., R. J. MAZET, and C. O. BECHTOL: Senile osteoporosis as a disorders influencing treatment and end results of fractures of the hip with a preliminary report on the use of collapatite. Amer.S urg. **25**, 883—890 (1959).

VALENTIN, F., CAPRAS, BARONE u. BOUTET: Tierexperimente mit lyophilisierten Kalbsknochen. Symposium sur l'os heteroplastique Lyon 3.—4. Mai 1958. Rev. Chir. orthop. **45**, 1—103 (1959).

VIRCHOW, R.: Die Cellularpathologie in ihrer Begründung auf physiologische und pathologische Gewebslehre, 4. Aufl. Berlin: August Hirschwald 1871.

WALTHER, PH. v.: Wiedereinheilung der bei der Trepanation ausgebohrten Knochenscheibe. (GRAEFE u. WALTHER). J. Chir. **2**, 571 (1821).

WANKE, R.: Defektpseudarthrose des Armes und ihre Behandlung. Zbl. Chir. **72**, 1157—1159 (1947).

WEAVER, S. B.: Experiences in the use of homogeneous (bone bank) bone. J. Bone Jt Surg. A **31**, 778—792 (1949).

WITT, A. N.: Wandlungen in der Behandlung der Kallusverzögerung und Pseudarthrose. Z. Orthop., Beilageheft zu **97**, 313—329 (1962).

WOLFF, J.: Zur neuesten die Knochenwachstumsfrage betreffenden Polemik. Berl. klin. Wschr. **1884**, 635—637.

K. Struktur und Ultrastruktur des Knorpels

Von

K.-H. Knese

Mit 51 Abbildungen

1. Einleitung: Allgemeine Kennzeichen des Knorpelgewebes

Das Knorpelgewebe tritt beim Menschen in sehr unterschiedlicher Gestalt auf; eine Reihe weiterer Formen ist bei niederen Chordaten zu beobachten. Ein Teil der knorpeligen Bildungen bleibt zeitlebens erhalten wie Gelenkknorpel, Rippenknorpel, Disci articulares und der Knorpel des Atmungstraktes. An anderen Orten ist das Knorpelgewebe ein sog. transitorisches Gewebe, Vorgänger und Platzhalter für das Knochengewebe. Weitere knorpelige Bildungen erscheinen im Individualleben relativ spät, mitunter nur unter gewissen Bedingungen, z. B. der Knorpel des Callusgewebes.

In diesem Artikel sind damit sehr unterschiedliche Fragestellungen zu erörtern, die der älteren Histologie weitgehend unbekannt waren. In dem vorgesteckten Rahmen können die verschiedenen Probleme nur angeschnitten werden, die vollständige Wiedergabe der umfangreichen Literatur ist unmöglich.

In unseren Lehrbüchern der Histologie des Menschen werden drei Formen des Knorpelgewebes aufgeführt, der hyaline, elastische und Faserknorpel; mitunter wird auch der Zellknorpel genannt. Im allgemeinen bleibt unberücksichtigt, daß der sog. Faserknorpel in sehr unterschiedlicher Ausprägung auftritt. Der Faserknorpel ist bisher ein Stiefkind der Histologie geblieben (Prader 1947, Knese und Biermann 1958).

Schaffer (1930) stellt seinen umfangreichen Erörterungen über das Knorpelgewebe die Betrachtung einer Reihe von Geweben voraus und kommt zu folgender Einteilung:

1. Chordagewebe
2. Das blasige Stützgewebe von chordoidem Typus
3. Das chondroide (oder vesiculöse) Stützgewebe
4. Das Knorpelgewebe
   a) Der grundsubstanzarme Zellknorpel
   b) Der Knorpel mit verzweigten Zellen
   c) Der Euhyalinknorpel
   d) Die sekundären Knorpelbildungen
   e) Der elastische Knorpel
   f) Der Faserknorpel

Schaffer (1930) hatte sich zur Aufgabe gesetzt, das Verhältnis der Gewebeelemente zueinander in den verschiedenen Stützgeweben oder mechanischen Geweben zu untersuchen. Er gelangt damit zu einer „logischen“ Systematik der Gewebe, indem er von „einfachen“ zu „verwickelten“ fortschreitet. Auf diesem Wege ist selbstverständlich kein „natürliches“ System der Stützgewebe zu gewinnen. Die Beziehungen zwischen den verschiedenen Geweben können nur durch histogenetische Untersuchungen erkannt werden, wobei an einem bestimmten Orte die Abfolge der Gewebe im Laufe des Individuallebens zu verfolgen ist (Knese und Biermann 1958). Hierbei zeigt sich, daß die Folge der Gewebe während der Histogenese nicht den „logischen“ Kategorien von einem „einfachen“ zu einem „verwickelten“ entspricht.

Die Zusammenfassung von Schaffer (1930) zeigt, daß der transitorische Knorpel und damit die frühe Histogenese des Skeletsystemes in der Vergangenheit recht wenig

Interesse gefunden hat. Der transitorische Knorpel wurde lange Zeit nur von Embryologen und Vergleichenden Anatomen im Hinblick auf die Form der knorpeligen Skeletteile und deren Beziehung zu jener der knöchernen untersucht. Die begleitenden histogenetischen Vorgänge, die vom mesenchymalen Skelet zum chondralen und schließlich ossalen führen, wurden dagegen wenig beachtet. Das erste Knorpelgewebe erscheint in der 4. Fetalwoche (Schaffer 1930) und in der 7.—8. Woche (etwa 20 mm SSL) sind alle knorpeligen Skeletteile angelegt (O'Rahilly, Gardner und Gray 1957). Die Entstehung des knorpeligen Skeletes fällt damit in die Phase der größten Empfindlichkeit des Keimes während der 4.—8. Woche (Töndury 1962).

Unter dem Gesichtspunkt der Skeletentwicklung kann man weder das Knorpel- noch das Knochengewebe isoliert im Sinne der Schafferschen logischen Kategorien betrachten. Der Anteil der jeweiligen Zellformen an der Bildung des Skeletsystemes sowie die genetischen Beziehungen der Zellen der Skeletgewebe zueinander müssen Gegenstand weiterer umfangreicher Arbeiten mit den verschiedensten Methoden sein.

Die Beurteilung der Beziehung zwischen verschiedenen, einander folgenden Formen der Stützgewebe wird dadurch erschwert, daß erst in letzter Zeit durch autoradiographische, histochemische und elektronenmikroskopische Untersuchungen die Wechselwirkungen zwischen den Zellen und den Intercellularsubstanzen einer Klärung zugängig sind. Der häufig unklare Mechanismus hormoneller Wirkungen ist ein besonders einprägsames Beispiel für die noch unbekannten Relationen Zelle-Intercellularsubstanz. Im Hinblick auf die histogenetischen Beziehungen ist damit die jeweilige „Potenz" der Zellen einer Gewebeform zu diskutieren, d. h. es ist zu klären, ob eine vorliegende Gewebeform ausdifferenziert ist oder nicht. Die Untersuchung der Potenz der Zellen wird durch das Vorhandensein der Intercellularsubstanzen erschwert. Der Begriff Potenz in seiner derzeitigen Definition ist an die Zelle als elementare Lebenseinheit gebunden und nicht auf die Intercellularsubstanz übertragbar. Das Verhalten der Zellen der Stütz- und Bindegewebsreihe (der Mechanocyten von Willmer 1960) bereitete nun bei der Diskussion über die Potenz von Zellen und deren Einschränkung im Sinne der Differenzierung erhebliche Schwierigkeiten (Needham 1950, Grobstein 1959, Willmer 1960, 1965, Brachet 1960). Im Bereich von Sehnenansätzen ist die Umwandlung von Sehnenzellen in „chondroide" und schließlich in Knorpelzellen zu beobachten. Diesen Zellen muß demgemäß eine Pluripotenz zuerkannt werden. Unklar ist, welche Vorgänge sich während dieser Umwandlung der Zellen in der Intercellularsubstanz abspielen. Mitunter wurde ein Abbau der Intercellularsubstanz als Voraussetzung zur Bildung neuer Intercellularsubstanzen angenommen. Die Bindegewebszellen und das gilt bereits für die Mesenchymzellen, können offensichtlich nicht isoliert von den zugehörigen Intercellularsubstanzen betrachtet werden. Knese (1967a) hat die Eigenheiten der Differenzierung im Stütz- und Bindegewebe im Hinblick auf die durch die Zellen produzierten Intercellularsubstanzen dargestellt. Vor allem müssen die Beziehungen der Zellen der verschiedenen Skeletgewebe zueinander noch geklärt werden. Nach den bisherigen Vorstellungen sollen nämlich diese Zellen ausdifferenziert sein und damit keine weitere Potenz mehr besitzen. Soweit Untersuchungen zu dieser Frage vorliegen, kommen wir darauf zurück.

Die Struktur bestimmter knorpeliger Bildungen wie der Sehnenansätze ist sehr verwickelt und weicht von dem „logischen" System so stark ab, daß kaum zu entscheiden ist, ob eine besondere Gewebeform vorliegt, die am Ende einer Differenzierungsreihe steht oder nicht. Das System der Stützgewebe wird auf der Beschreibung der Form und Verteilung der Zellen, Art und Ordnung der Fasern sowie des Charakters der Intercellularsubstanzen aufgebaut; hyaliner Knorpel ist dann durch die glasige Intercellularsubstanz, die Sehne als straffes Gewebe durch die dicken, parallel verlaufenden Fasern usw. gekennzeichnet. Beim Ansatz von Sehnen an knorpeligen Apophysen gewinnt man häufig den Eindruck, daß die Fasern noch wie in der Sehne angeordnet sind, die Zellen gleichen aber Knorpelzellen, Zellen und Intercellularsubstanz werden schließlich als „Einstrahlungsknochen" Bestandteil des Skeletstückes (Knese und Biermann 1958).

Bezirke derartiger Struktur wurden daher auch als Mischgewebe bezeichnet (Drahn 1922, Weidenreich 1923a, Schneider 1956). Dieser Formulierung ist entgegenzuhalten, daß die Gewebekomponenten in bezug auf den Stoffwechsel und in ihrer mechanischen Leistung eine Einheit bilden dürften.

Knese und Biermann (1958) haben sich bei Untersuchung der apophysären Sehnen- und Bandansätze mit der Frage befaßt, ob überhaupt von einem ausdifferenzierten Knorpelgewebe gesprochen werden kann, und kommen zum Schluß: „Das Knorpelgewebe besitzt zwar eine spezifische Leistungsfähigkeit, ist aber histogenetisch nicht ausdifferenziert, d. h. unipotent, sondern besitzt die Möglichkeit weiterer geweblicher Entwicklung. Dafür spricht bereits, daß das Knorpelgewebe in weiter Verbreitung im Skelet als Vorläufer des Knochengewebes auftritt ... Vielleicht ist es sogar das Schicksal des Knorpels, sich zu irgendeiner Zeit endgültig in Knochengewebe „umzudifferenzieren". Wenn im Rahmen der Arthritis deformans und der Spondylitis deformans Knochenbildung mit dazugehöriger Markraum- und Gefäßbildung auftritt (vgl. Lang 1934), muß wohl latent eine Potenz hierzu im Knorpel angenommen werden. Inwieweit die Ausbildung von „Knochen" dann schicksalsmäßig abläuft, durch Noxen ausgelöst oder begünstigt wird, ist histogenetisch gesehen sekundärer Natur."

Das Knorpelgewebe hat im Hinblick auf die sog. amorphen Intercellularsubstanzen, voran die Mucopolysaccharide (MPS), in den letzten Jahrzehnten eine ausführliche Bearbeitung erfahren. Somit sind im Rahmen dieses Kapitels die Vorstellungen über die Organisation der Intercellularsubstanzen zu erörtern. Allerdings war das Knorpelgewebe bei diesen Untersuchungen häufig nur ein Modell, d. h. ein Gewebe, das die nichtfibrillären Substanzen in größerer Menge enthält. Der Anteil des Chondroitinsulfates im Knorpel beträgt 20—30% der Trockensubstanz und etwa 5% der Frischsubstanz bei einem Wassergehalt von 75% (Einbinder et al. 1951, vgl. Knese und Knoop 1961a). Morphologische und örtliche Differenzen der Knorpelgewebe wurden bei diesen Untersuchungen leider wenig berücksichtigt. Gegenstand der Untersuchungen waren die MPS, aber nicht der Knorpel.

Die auffällige Ordnung der Zellen im Epiphysenknorpel und ihre morphologischen Differenzen führten dazu, die Einflüsse von Hormonen und Vitaminen sowie die Ablagerung von Radioisotopen an Hand der Umgestaltungen in der Epiphyse zu beschreiben. Leider beschränkte sich der größere Teil der Untersucher darauf, die gröberen Veränderungen auf Grund von Beobachtungen an Routinepräparaten zu beschreiben, so daß bei der vorliegenden Darstellung der morphologischen Fakten nur am Rande auf diese Untersuchungen verwiesen werden kann.

2. Die Komponenten des Knorpelgewebes

Bei den verschiedenen Formen des Knorpelgewebes sind dem chemischen Aufbau und der Verteilung nach die gleichen Komponenten wie bei den übrigen Stützgeweben zu unterscheiden (s. S. 318).

a) Die Zellen

α) Die chondroiden Zellen

Im Bereich von Sehnenansätzen treten zwischen den Sehnenfasern in Reihen geordnete rundliche Zellen auf, die von älteren Autoren z. T. als Knorpelzellen, von Schaffer (1930) zunächst als vesiculöse, dann als chondroide Zellen bezeichnet wurden (Abb. 1). Schaffer beschrieb diese Zellen als „hyalin" mit einer Kapsel. Wenn diese Kapsel eine basophile Beschaffenheit annimmt, ist eine Verwechselung mit Knorpelzellen möglich. Diese Zellen sind nicht durch eine Umwandlung aus „fertigen" Sehnenzellen, sondern aus indifferenten Bildungszellen entstanden. In anderem Zusammenhang meint Schaffer allerdings auch, daß Übergänge zwischen chondroidem und echtem Knorpelgewebe möglich sind.

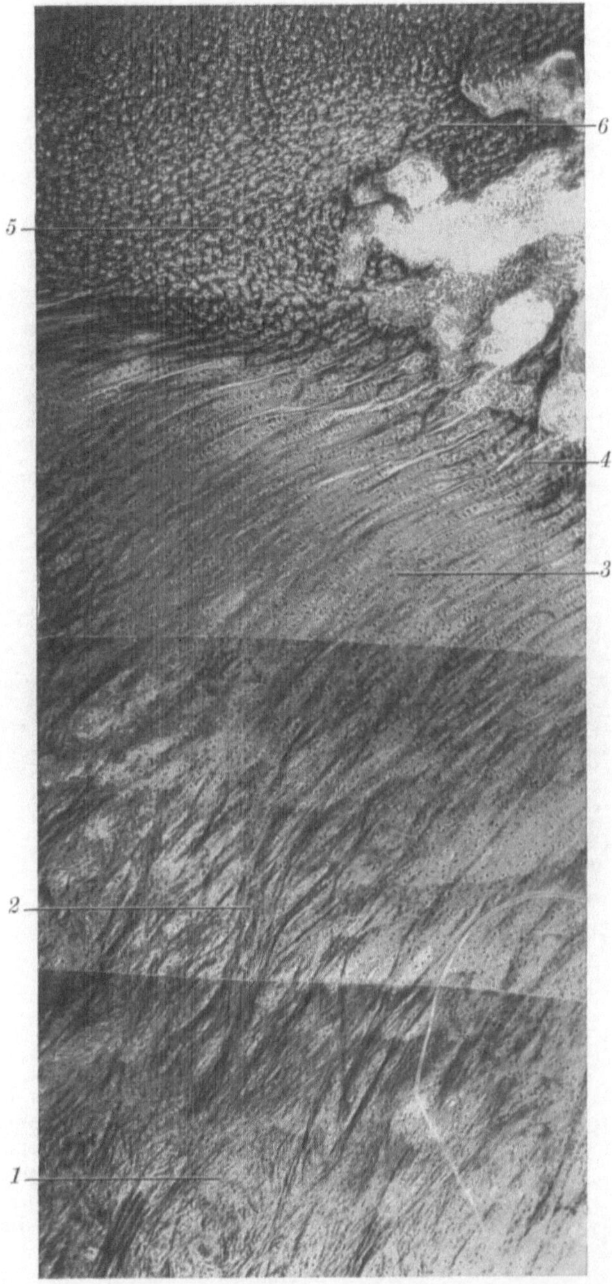

Abb. 1. Fet 282 mm SSL. Femur, Querschnittshöhe 2. Balken enchondralen Knochens mit Demaskierung der Fasern in den Knorpelresten. *1* Markraum; *2* Osteocyten; *3* demaskierte, im Azanpräparat dunkelblau gefärbte Kollagenfasern an der Grenze der Knorpelreste; *4* fädige Umwandlung der Knorpelreste. Azan. Ob. 40, Ok. 10. (KNESE u. BIERMANN, Z. Zellforsch. **49**, Abb. 21, 1958)

Derartige Zellelemente wurden in Sehnen sehr verschiedener Species beschrieben (DRAHN, 1922; WEIDENREICH, 1923a; VIS, 1957; LEUTERT, 1955, 1958, 1959, 1960; KNESE und BIERMANN, 1958), weiterhin in Sehnenfurchen (BALOGH und FÖLDES 1955; LEUTERT 1955, 1959), aber auch in den als Gleitsehnen bezeichneten Abschnitten der Sehne des M. fibularis longus und M. tibialis posterior. Die Knorpelzelle unterscheidet sich von den chondroiden Zellen nach LEUTERT (1955) durch das Vorhandensein des Hofes, der Kapsel sowie der metachromatischen Reaktion ihres Cytoplasmas. Weiterhin treten in Gleitsehnen besonders große Zellen von 20—25 μ Durchmesser ohne Kapsel, aber mit einem metachromatisch reagierendem Cytoplasma als Gleitsehnen-Riesenzellen auf; diese Zellen besitzen nur einen Kern.

Von verschiedenen Autoren wurde eine Umwandlung von Sehnenzellen in chondroide und schließlich in Knorpelzellen beschrieben (Schaffer, 1930; Weidenreich, 1923; Petersen, 1930; Dolgo-Saburoff, 1929/30; Amprino und Cattaneo, 1937; Leutert, 1955, 1959, 1960; Vis, 1957). Knese und Biermann (1958) führen aus, daß die unmittel-

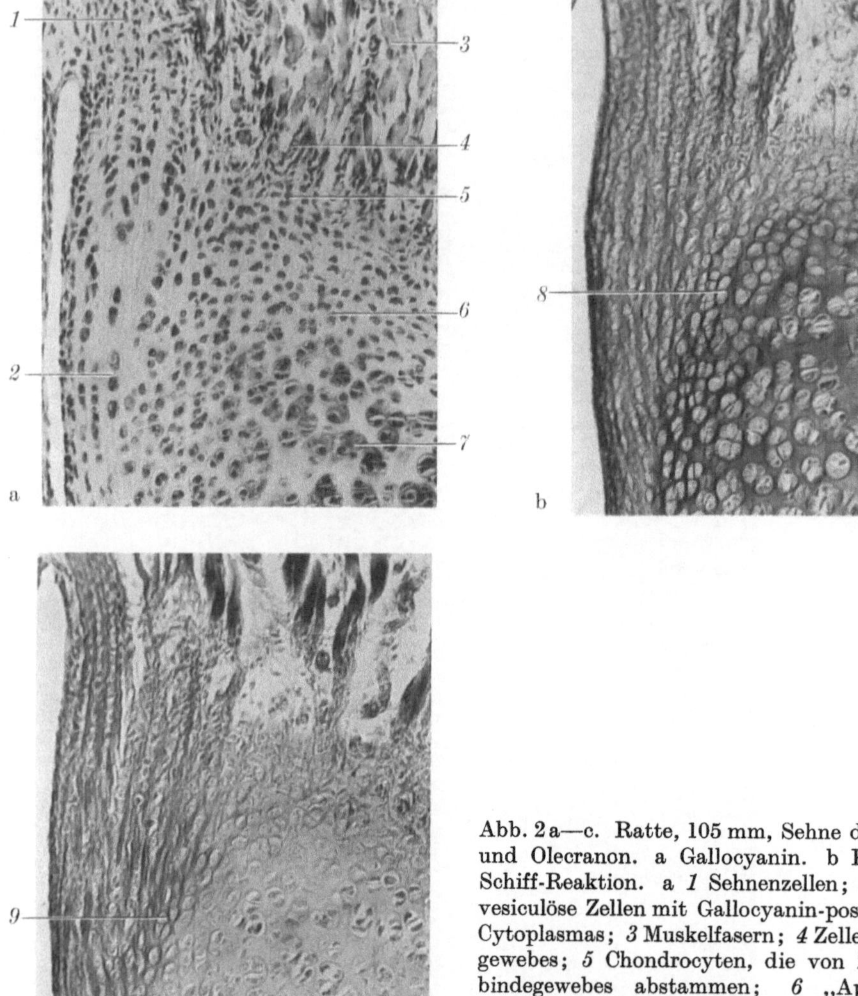

Abb. 2a—c. Ratte, 105 mm, Sehne des Musculus triceps und Olecranon. a Gallocyanin. b PAS. c Ninhydrin-Schiff-Reaktion. a *1* Sehnenzellen; *2* chondroide bzw. vesiculöse Zellen mit Gallocyanin-positiver Reaktion des Cytoplasmas; *3* Muskelfasern; *4* Zellen des Muskelbindegewebes; *5* Chondrocyten, die von Zellen des Muskelbindegewebes abstammen; *6* „Appositionsknorpel"; *7* Knorpelterritorien, Kapsel und Hof mit Chromalaun gefärbt; b *8* PAS-positive Kapseln des Appositionsknorpels; c *9* Ninhydrin-positive Kapseln am Übergang der Sehne in den Knorpel. Ob. 16, Ok. 12,5

bare räumliche Kontinuität mit direkten Übergängen bzw. mehr oder minder deutlichen Grenzschichten zwischen verschiedenartigen Geweben, nämlich Sehne, Knorpel und Knochen, auch als Zeichen genetischer Zusammenhänge zu deuten ist. Die zu den genannten Geweben gehörigen Zellen sind als Skeletzellen mit unterschiedlichem Habitus anzusehen. Zu diesem Gefälle, Sehne — Knochen, treten noch gewebliche Unterschiede im Hinblick auf die Ontogenese hinzu.

Die vorstehenden Ausführungen beruhen auf lichtmikroskopischen Beobachtungen und lassen demgemäß über die Vorgänge dieser Modifikation der Zellgestalt keine Aussagen machen. Topochemische Befunde (unveröffentlicht) legen bei Beachtung der Befunde an anderen Orten (vgl. Knese und Knoop 1961a und c) die Vermutung nahe, daß die Umwandlung der Zellgestalt mit einer Stoffproduktion verbunden ist. Die gebildeten Stoffe beeinflussen vermutlich den Zustand der Intercellularsubstanz. In der Sehne des M. triceps brachii der Ratte vergrößern sich die in Reihen zwischen den Kollagenfasern gelegenen Sehnenzellen unmittelbar vor dem Ansatz an dem knorpeligen Olecranon zu „chondroiden" Zellen (Abb. 2). Aus dem schlanken, stäbchenförmigen, bei Färbung mit Gallocyanin sehr dicht erscheinendem Kern der Sehnenzelle wird ein rundliches bzw. ovoides Gebilde. Der Kern der chondroiden Zellen ist weniger dicht als derjenige der Sehnenzellen und besitzt einen großen Nucleolus. An den Kern der Sehnen-

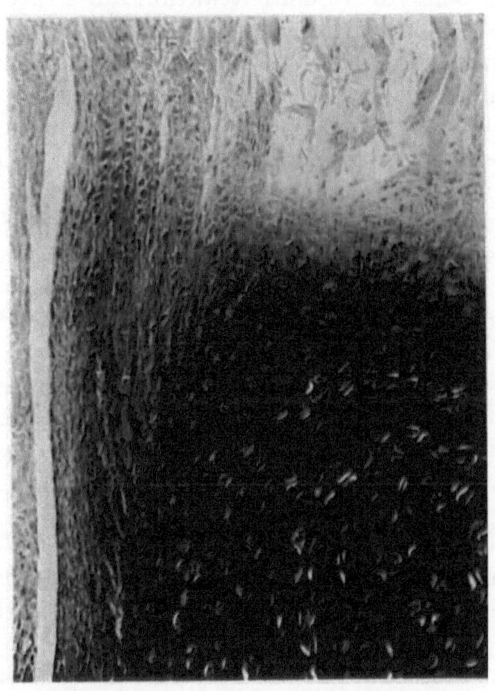

Abb. 3. Ratte, 105 mm, alkoholische Toluidinblau-Lösung. Sehnenfasern orthochromatisch blau. Sehnenfasern in Höhe der chondroiden Zellen metachromatisch violett, Metachromasie im Bereich der Apposition durch das Muskelbindegewebe. Ob. 16, Ok. 12,5

zelle schließt sich beiderseits eine mit Gallocyanin kaum angefärbte Cytoplasmahaube an; die Cytoplasmasäume beiderseits der Längsseiten des Kernes sind im Lichtmikroskop nicht zu erkennen. Der Kern der chondroiden Zellen ist allseits von einem mit Gallocyanin angefärbtem Cytoplasma umgeben. Diese Cytoplasmafärbung spricht für das Vorhandensein von Ribonucleinsäuren (RNS), die bekanntlich mit der Synthese von Proteinen in Verbindung stehen. Die Modifikation der Zellgestalt von der Sehnenzelle zur chondroiden (hyalinen nach Schaffer 1930) steht damit vermutlich mit einer Stoffproduktion in Zusammenhang.

Unter schrittweiser Vergrößerung der Zellen mit gleichzeitiger Abnahme der Intensität der Gallocyaninreaktion werden aus den chondroiden die Knorpelzellen. Diese Knorpelzellen liegen häufig zu zweit in einer Höhle und dann auch in Gruppen (Territorien) zu 3—4, eingebettet in hyaline Intercellularsubstanz, beieinander. Die chondroiden Zellen schmiegen sich den Kapseln an, die Knorpelzellen neigen dagegen zu den bekannten Schrumpfungserscheinungen (s. S. 694). Die Kapseln färben sich mit dem Chromalaun der Gallocyaninfarbflotte metachromatisch rot an. Ähnlich gestaltete Zellen treten im Bereich des musculären Tricepsansatzes am Olecranon auf. Die Reihenordnung der Zellen in bezug auf die Muskelfasern spricht für eine Abkunft dieser chondroiden Zellen aus denen des Muskelbindegewebes.

Die Art der von den chondroiden Zellen gebildeten Stoffe läßt sich, jedenfalls vermutungsweise, aus der Farbreaktion der Intercellularsubstanz erschließen. Bei Färbung mit alkoholischer Toluidinblaulösung reagieren die Zelleiber der chondroiden Zellen orthochromatisch, die dünnen Kapseln schwarz-violett und die Kollagenfasern hellviolett metachromatisch (Abb. 3). Bei der PAS-Reaktion nimmt die Anfärbung der Kollagenfasern im Bereich der chondroiden Zellen an Stärke zu und ist besonders kräftig in jener Schicht, die dem Appositionsknorpel unter dem Perichondrium (Knese und Knoop 1961a) entspricht; in der Tiefe des Olecranonknorpels ist die Reaktion geringer. Unter den musculären Ansatzpartien ist die PAS-Färbung schwächer, nur im Appositionsknorpel ausgeprägt. Die Ninhydrin-Schiff-Reaktion auf Proteine der Kollagenfasern ist schwächer als die der Muskelfasern und verliert sich im Appositionsknorpel fast vollständig. Die Sehnen- und chondroiden Zellen zeigen nur eine Kernfärbung, einzelne Chondrocyten lassen eine schwache Cytoplasmareaktion erkennen.

Topochemische Erhebungen legen somit die Annahme nahe, daß die sog. chondroiden Zellen im Bereich der Sehnenansätze während der Ontogenese Bildungszellen sind. Über Bildungszellen von abweichender Form wurde besonders im Hinblick auf die Osteogenese verschiedentlich diskutiert (Kassowitz 1897, Bidder 1906, Weidenreich 1923a, b, c, McLean und Bloom 1940, Knese 1956b, Biermann 1957, Knese und Biermann 1958). Die chondroiden Zellen entstehen aus Sehnenzellen oder Zellen des Muskelbindegewebes und bilden offensichtlich Mucopolysaccharide (MPS), wie die Reaktion der Intercellularsubstanz zeigt. Die Gallocyanin-Reaktion des Cytoplasmas läßt auch eine Proteinsynthese vermuten, da diese Reaktion dem Cytoplasma der Sehnen- und Knorpelzellen fehlt. Welcher Art diese Proteine sind, ist z. Z. nicht zu erkennen. Die Struktur der Sehnenansätze im Hinblick auf die in den Knorpel einstrahlenden Kollagenfasern läßt an Proteine denken, die mit den MPS vergesellschaftet sind.

β) Die Zellen des Zellknorpels und des Vorknorpels

Im Zellknorpel liegen große blasenartige Zellen vor, die unmittelbar aneinanderstoßen oder nur durch eine geringe Menge von Intercellularsubstanz voneinander getrennt sind. Schaper (1902) spricht daher von einem Turgorgewebe. Der Zellknorpel tritt als permanente Gewebeform bei vielen niederen Chordaten auf. Die Zellen des Ohrknorpels, unter anderem, der Maus sind weiterhin durch Fetteinlagerungen ausgezeichnet. Der transitorische Zellknorpel, der sog. Vorknorpel, ist bei vielen Species Vorläufer des grundsubstanzreichen Knorpels, in den er durch Vermehrung der Intercellularsubstanz unmittelbar übergeht. Vermutlich sind der Zellknorpel niederer Chordaten und der Vorknorpel keine gleichartigen Gewebe.

Bei Untersuchung des Vorknorpels im Lichtmikroskop entsteht nach Schaffer (1930) der Eindruck, daß eine „symplasmatische“ Masse mit dichter Lagerung der Kerne vorliegt. Es wird zunächst eine oxyphile „protochondrale Zwischensubstanz“ gebildet, die bald basophil reagiert und damit zur „prochondralen“ Zwischensubstanz wird. Fell (1925) konnte bei Färbung mit Eisenhämatoxylin im Knorpel des Hühnchens Zellgrenzen sehen; auch bei Gallocyanin-Färbung sind die Zellen gegeneinander abzugrenzen (unveröffentlicht). Amprino (1956) beschreibt die Intercellularsubstanz als acidophil mit nichtmetachromatischen Kollagenfasern; später tritt die Basophilie und die metachromatische Reaktion auf. Mit der Bildung des Vorknorpels werden die äußeren Schichten zum Perichondrium (Amprino 1956). Die Zellen zeigen innerhalb der Skeletanlage eine bestimmte Ordnung (Romeis 1911, Fell 1925, Streeter 1949; s. unten).

Die Skeletanlage stellt eine Mesenchymverdichtung dar. Nach Streeter (1949) entsteht die Armknospe bei menschlichen Embryonen von 21—29 Ursegmenten (etwa 3—4 mm, 26 Tage), und zwar in Höhe der Cervicalsomiten 5—7. Die Knospe der hinteren Extremität tritt wenig später bei Vorliegen von 30—35 Ursegmenten auf (Keibel und Elze, 1908). Über der Ansammlung der Mesoblasten verdickt sich das Ektoderm. Zwilling (1955) war der Meinung, für das Auswachsen der Extremitätenknospe sei das Ektoderm von Bedeutung. Umstritten sind die Beziehungen zwischen dieser sog. apikalen Ektodermleiste und dem Mesenchym der Extremitätenknospe. Während eine Gruppe von Autoren (Zwilling 1961) einen induktiven Einfluß auf das Mesenchym annimmt, wird von anderen (Amprino 1965) die Mesenchymdifferenzierung als eine schrittweise Selbstdifferenzierung angesehen. McKay et al. (1956) wiesen dann im Ektoderm Glykogen, RNS und alkalische Phosphatase nach. Weitere umfangreiche topochemische Unter-

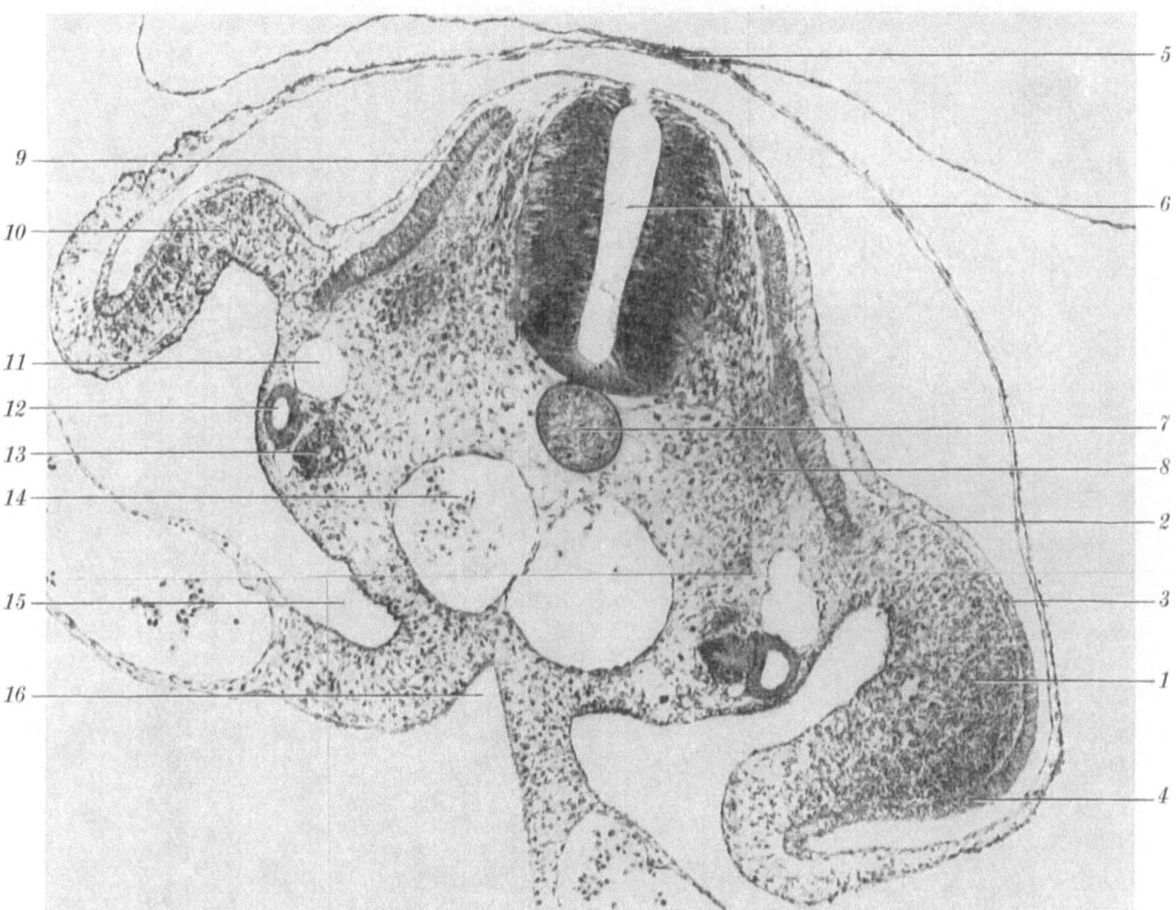

Abb. 4. Hühnerkeimscheibe, 48 Std bebrütet. *1* Mesenchym der Extremitätenknospe, Mesenchymzellen mit Gallocyanin-positivem Cytoplasma; *2* Epidermis mit Basalmembran; *3* Mitose im Epidermis; *4* vergrößerte Epidermiszellen mit Gallocyanin-positivem Cytoplasma, vermutlich ohne Basalmembran; *5* Amnionnaht; *6* Rückenmark mit periventricularen Ventosen; *7* Chorda; *8* Sklerotom; *9* Dermatom und Myotom; *10* Schnitt durch das Ende der Extremitätenknospe; *11* Vena cardinalis caudalis; *12* Wolffscher Gang; *13* Vor- bzw. Urnierenkanälchen; *14* Aorta (paarig); *15* Cölom; *16* Darmrinne. Ob. 10, Ok. 12,5 (Photomontage)

suchungen über die apikale Ektodermleiste liegen von Milaire (1962, 1963) vor. Das Ektoderm färbt sich demgemäß sowohl mit Gallocyanin (Abb. 4) als auch mit Methylenblau (pH 4,1) an und zeigt reichlich Mitosen, die im benachbarten Mesenchym gleichfalls gehäuft auftreten. Balinsky (1957) konnte am Ektoderm der Extremitätenknospe von Amphibien das Fehlen einer Basalmembran elektronenmikroskopisch nachweisen, wie das auf Grund lichtmikroskopischer Beobachtungen zuvor vermutet wurde. Viswanath und Knese (im Druck) fanden dagegen elektronenmikroskopisch bei der Extremitätenknospe des Hühnchens nach 3—7 Tagen Bebrütung eine morphologisch gleichartige Basalmembran unter der apikalen Ektodermleiste und der übrigen Epidermis. Die Ultrastruktur der Zellen in der Ektodermleiste spricht für einen hohen Protein- und oxydativen (große Zahl von Mitochondrien) Stoffwechsel.

Die Mesenchymzellen in der Umgebung der Skeletanlage bilden einen relativ lockeren Verband (Abb. 5). Die Kerne dieser Zellen sind verschieden groß, rundlich bis ovoid, haben ein oder mehrere Nucleolen. Ihr Chromatin liegt der Kernmembran in dichter Schicht an und ist im übrigen locker über das Kernareal verteilt. In der Anlage des

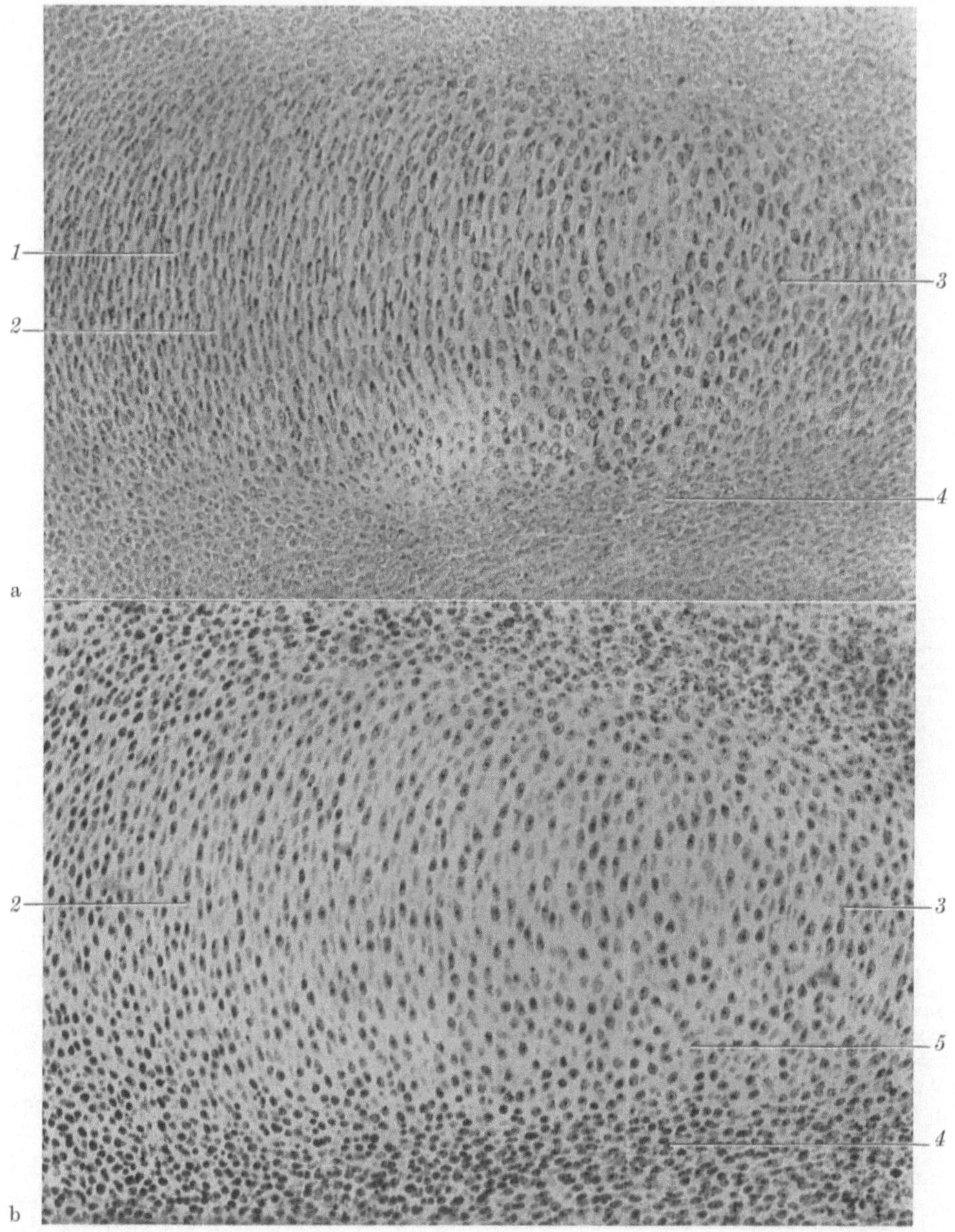

Abb. 5a u. b. Rinderfetus, 21,6 mm SSL, Anlage der Tibia. a PAS. b Gallocyanin. a *1* Vorknorpelzellen mit PAS-positiven Granula; *2* Zellreihen nach proximal konvex; *3* Zellreihen nach distal konvex; *4* Anlage des Perichondriums; b *5* Zellen in bogenförmiger Anordnung vom Periochondrium ausgehend. Ob. 16, Ok. 12,5

Perichondriums sind die Intercellularspalten relativ eng. Die Zellen sind mit ihrer Längsachse in Längenachse des Gliedes ausgerichtet. Die Kerne der Perichondriumzellen zeigen die gleichen Größen- und Formverschiedenheiten wie die der umgebenden Mesenchymzellen. Beim Übergang zum Knorpel werden die Zellen und deren Kerne rundlich, der Nucleolus nimmt an Größe zu, die Zellen rücken durch die Intercellularsubstanz auseinander. Zur Mitte der Skeletanlage hin werden die Zellen flacher und stellen sich mit ihrer Längsachse etwa quer zum Skeletstück. Dabei bilden die Zellen bogenförmige Reihen, deren Konvexität im distalen Stück nach distal, im proximalen entsprechend nach proximal weist. Weiterhin sind bogenförmige Zellreihen vom Perichondrium her in das Zentrum der Skeletanlage zu verfolgen.

Das Cytoplasma dieser jungen Knorpelzellen färbt sich nicht mit Gallocyanin an; nur bei einigen zentral gelegenen Chondrocyten ist eine schwache Graufärbung zu beobachten. Bei Färbung mit alkoholischer Toluidinblaulösung reagiert die neugebildete Intercellularsubstanz schwach metachromatisch. Die Stärke der Reaktion nimmt zur Mitte der Skeletanlage zu. Die Kerne der umgebenden Mesenchymzellen sind schwach orthochromatisch, die des Perichondriums stärker und die der Knorpelzellen wieder weniger angefärbt. PAS-positive Granula treten vereinzelt in den tiefen Schichten des

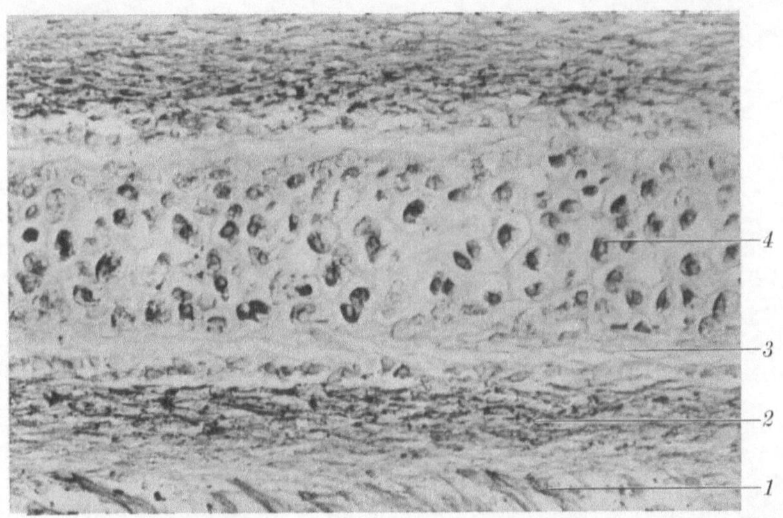

Abb. 6. Rinderfetus, 36 mm SSL, erste Rippe, PAS. *1* Muskelfasern; *2* Perichondrium, Zellen mit kleinen PAS-positiven Granula; *3* Appositionsknorpel; *4* Chondrocyten mit großen PAS-positiven Granula. Ob. 16, Ok. 12,5

Perichondriums auf. Die Chondrocyten weisen Granula in größerer Zahl auf. Die Zellen des Perichondriums und des umgebenden Mesenchyms sind bei Rinderfeten unter 30 mm SSL frei von PAS-positiven Granula (Abb. 6); einige Körnchen erscheinen in den Zellen der Coriumanlage. Die Mesenchymzellen bei Rinderfeten über 30 mm SSL enthalten stets einige PAS-positive Granula (Knese und Knoop, 1961a).

Die chemische Differenzierung der Zellen eilt der Histodifferenzierung (Huxley, 1924) bei der Vorknorpelbildung voraus. Vor der Knorpelbildung ist eine Phosphataseaktivität vorhanden, die mit der Bildung der Intercellularsubstanz verlorengeht und erst später vor Einsetzen der Osteogenese erneut auftritt (Moog, 1944). Mit dem Verschwinden der alkalischen Phosphatase treten PAS-positive Substanzen auf (Kroon, 1952). Die Zellen speichern ^{35}S, bevor sie morphologisch von den umgebenden Mesenchymzellen zu unterscheiden sind (Amprino, 1956; Verne et al., 1956, 1957; Johnston und Comar, 1957; Okada, 1959). Die Wirbelkörper von Rattenfeten zeigen nach Verabreichung von ^{35}S an die Muttertiere ^{35}S-Ablagerungen, die Zwischenwirbelscheiben aber nicht (Boström und Odeblad, 1953); die Aktivität ist im knorpeligen Humerus des Fetus 30mal größer als im Sternum der Muttertiere (Dziewiatkowski, 1951). Die Abgabe des ^{35}S von den Zellen an die Intercellularsubstanzen ist mit dem Auftreten der basophilen und metachromatischen Reaktion verbunden.

Elektronenmikroskopisch konnten Knese und Knoop (1961a) und Godman und Porter (1960) im Vorknorpelblastem nur feine Intercellularspalten zwischen den Mesenchymzellen beobachten; ein syncytialer Verband liegt nicht vor (Abb. 7). Der Kern der Blastemzellen ist relativ groß und besitzt einen Nucleolus; Mitosen sind häufig (Abb. 8). Das Cytoplasma ist dicht und granulär strukturiert, enthält ein Golgi-Feld und ein gering entwickeltes endoplasmatisches Reticulum. Die Anzahl der Mitochondrien ist beachtlich groß. Mit dem Auftreten der Intercellularsubstanz, die elektronenmikroskopisch Fibrillen erkennen läßt, erweitern sich die Zisternen des endoplasmatischen Reticulums zu sackartigen Auftreibungen (Abb. 9). GODMAN und PORTER (1960) halten diese Auftreibungen für Bestandteile des Golgi-Apparates. Erst beim Heranreifen zum hyalinen Knorpel ist auch eine Vermehrung des endoplasmatischen Reticulums festzustellen.

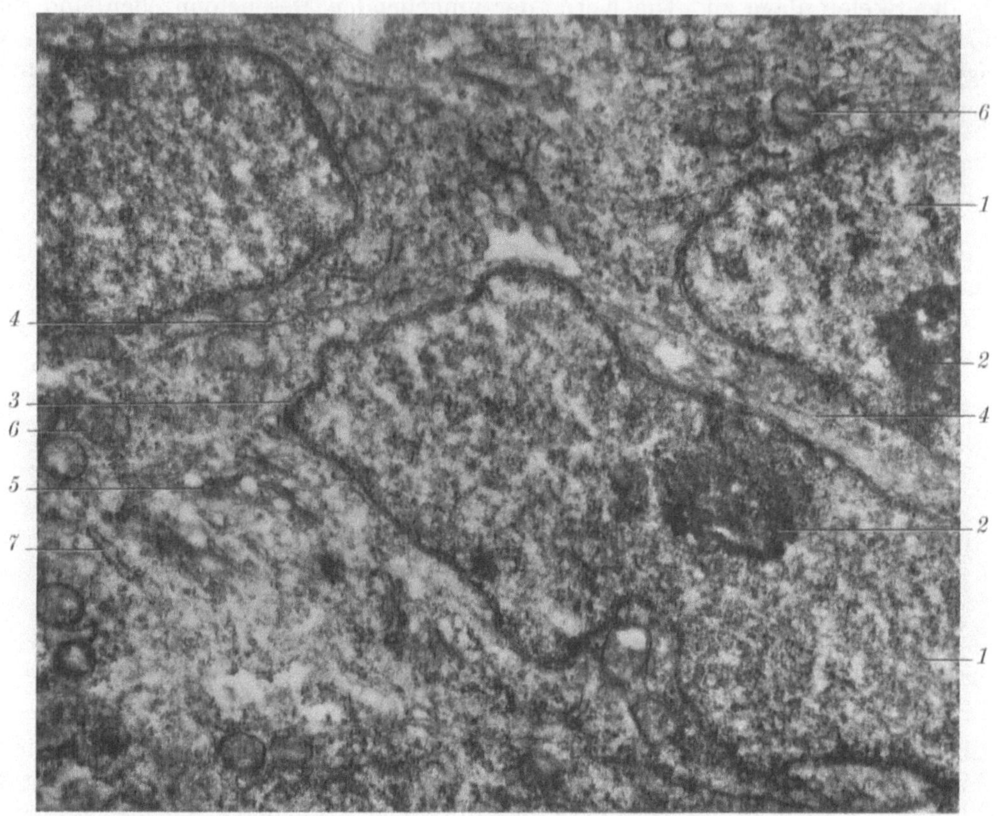

Abb. 7. Zellen des Vorknorpelblastems. *1* Kern; *2* Nucleolus; *3* Kernmembran; *4* Plasmalemm benachbarter Zellen mit schmalem Intercellularspalt; *5* Golgi-Feld mit Bläschen, dunklen Körpern und Golgi-Lamellen; *6* Mitochondrien; *7* endoplasmatisches Reticulum. Vergr. 20000. (KNESE u. KNOOP, 1961a)

Nicht immer geht die Bildung des Vorknorpels über ein Stadium des Zellknorpels vor sich, z. T. treten sternförmige Zellen auf, zwischen denen dann die knorpelige Intercellularsubstanz entsteht (SCHAFFER, 1930). Nach SENSENIG (1948) sollen bei 12 mm langen menschlichen Keimlingen diese verstreut liegenden Zellen im Wirbelkörper, nicht aber im Wirbelbogen erscheinen (vgl. TÖNDURY, 1958). Eine den Fibrocyten ähnliche spindelförmige Gestalt der Chondrocyten im Wirbelkörper sahen wir auch bei älteren menschlichen Feten. Unterhalb des Perichondriums im Appositionsknorpel sind die Zellen wie an anderen Skeletorten parallel zur Oberfläche des Wirbelkörpers ausgerichtet. In der Tiefe des Wirbelkörpers ist eine bestimmte Orientierung der Zellen nicht festzustellen. In der Nähe der Knochenkerne stellen sich die Zellen mit der Längsachse parallel zur Eröffnungszone ein. Es folgt dann eine schmale Schicht Säulenknorpel und hypertropher Zellen. Eröffnungszone und der Ablauf der enchondralen Osteogenese erscheinen wie an den langen Extremitätenknochen. Im übrigen wird auch periostaler

Knochen gebildet. Der Bildungsmodus des Wirbelbogens mit „Epiphysen“ und einer Diaphysenröhre läuft ebenfalls wie an langen Knochen ab (SCHIEDT, 1955). In den Wirbelbögen reichen die flachen Zellen mit dem Bau der Zellen des Appositionsknorpels weit in die knorpelige Anlage hinein. Dann erscheinen aber die rundlichen Zellen wie in anderen Knorpelanlagen. Bei Rinderfeten bis 37 mm SSL und Goldhamsterfeten bis

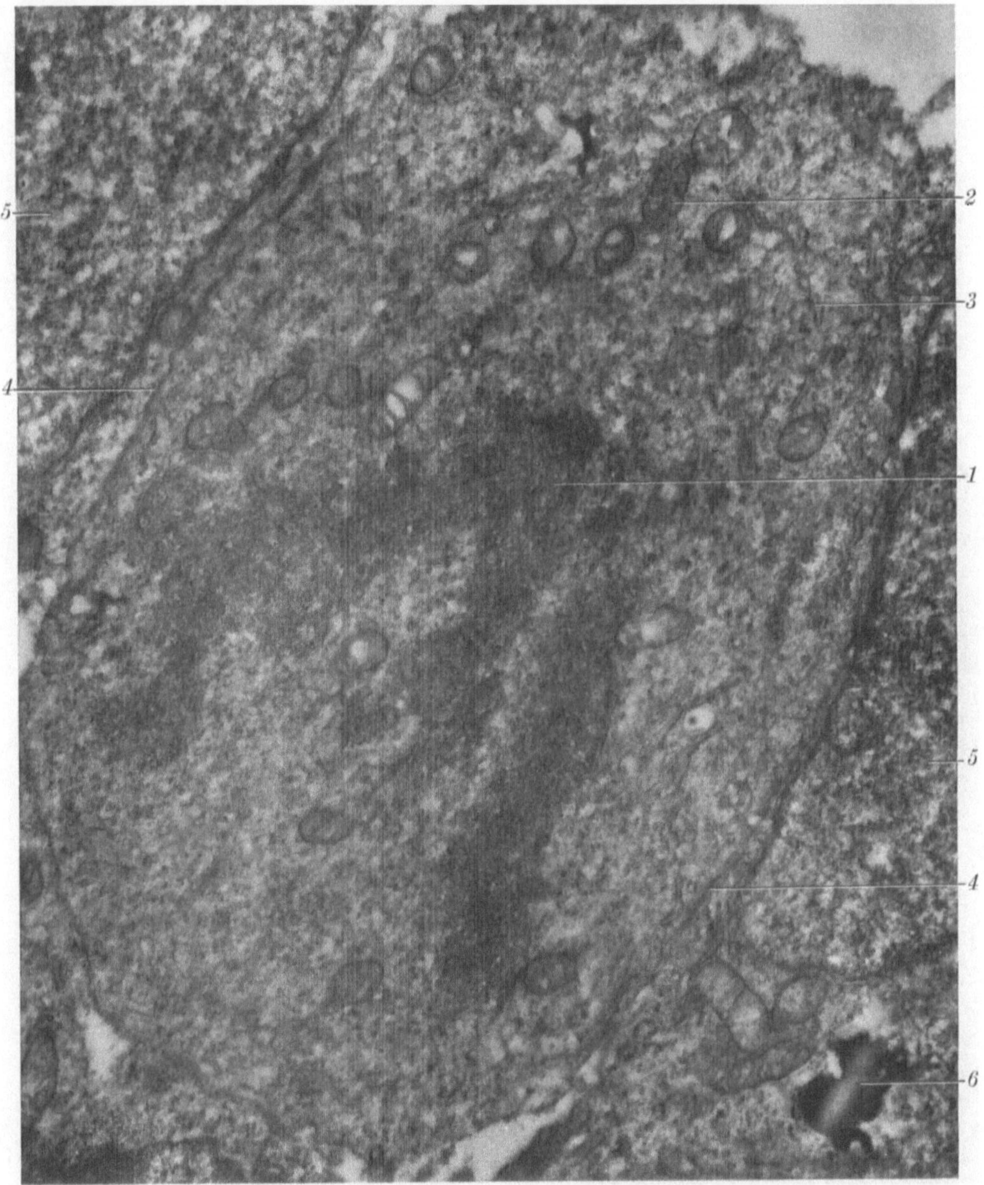

Abb. 8. Mitose einer Zelle des Vorknorpelblastems (Monaster). *1* Chromosomen; *2* Mitochondrien; *3* endoplasmatisches Reticulum; *4* Plasmalemm benachbarter Blastemzellen; *5* Zellkern der anstoßenden Blastemzelle; *6* osmiophile Einlagerung. Vergr. 18000. (KNESE u. KNOOP 1961a)

zur Geburt fanden wir in den Wirbelkörpern nur rundliche Chondrocyten, so daß in frühen Stadien das Bild eines Zellknorpels mit wenig Intercellularsubstanz vorliegt.

Wir (unveröffentlicht) beobachteten diese Form der Chondrogenese (Abb. 10) auch im Bereich der Ohrkapsel eines Rinderfetes von 37 mm SSL (vgl. ANSON und BAST, 1955). Unmittelbar benachbart fand die Chondrogenese in der weitverbreiteten Form der Mesenchymverdichtung statt. Die Knorpelanlage für die Kapsel von Utriculus, Sacculus und Bogengängen ist von Mesenchymzellen umgeben, deren Form, Größe und Ordnung der an anderen Skeletanlagen gleicht. Mit geringfügiger Verengerung der Intercellularspalten, aber nicht in einer unmittelbaren Aneinanderlagerung der Zellen, ordnen sich die Zellen mit ihrer Längsachse parallel zur Oberfläche der Ohrkapsel an. Bei Rinderfeten größer als 30 mm SSL zeigt der größere Teil aller Mesenchymzellen bereits eine

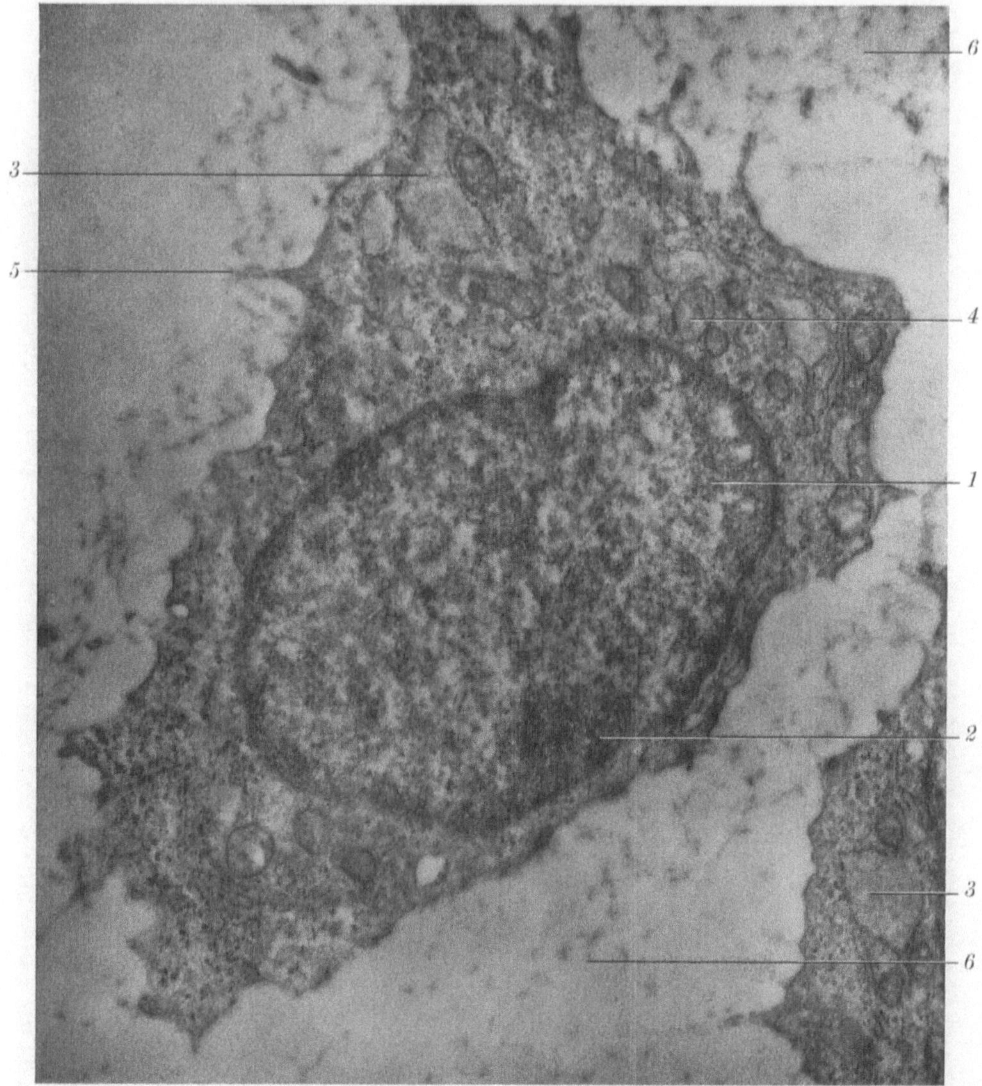

Abb. 9. Heranreifende Knorpelzelle. *1* Zellkern; *2* Nucleolus; *3* Zisterne; *4* Mitochondrien; *5* Zellfüße; *6* Intercellularsubstanz mit einer geringen Anzahl von Fasern. Vergr. 21000. (KNESE u. KNOOP, 1961a)

positive PAS-Reaktion. Die Mesenchymzellen des Perichondriums sind aber mit einer erheblichen Anzahl PAS-positiver Granula beladen, die z. T. perinucleär gehäuft auftreten. Im Appositionsknorpel weisen die Zellen neben kleineren recht große Granula auf, die den Zelleib mitunter prall anfüllen. An einigen Orten konnten wir auch eine PAS-positive Reaktion der Intercellularsubstanz beobachten. Die Bildung des Appositionsknorpels ist mit einer Abrundung der Zellen verbunden, deren Abstand voneinander etwa dem der benachbarten Mesenchymzellen gleicht. Sowohl bei Färbung mit Methylenblau (p_H 4,1) als auch mit alkoholischer Toluidinblaulösung tritt eine metachromatische Reaktion der Intercellularsubstanz auf.

An anderen Orten der Ohrkapsel und den Anlagen des Temporale tritt ein Perichondrium bzw. Periost mit sehr dichter Lagerung der Zellen auf. Die Zellgrenzen sind nicht zu erkennen. Bei PAS-Reaktion erscheint das Perichondrium als eine einheitlich stark angefärbte Schicht. Die Kerne dieser Chondroblasten sind wesentlich kleiner als die der umgebenden Mesenchymzellen. Bei Bildung des Appositionsknorpels entstehen aus

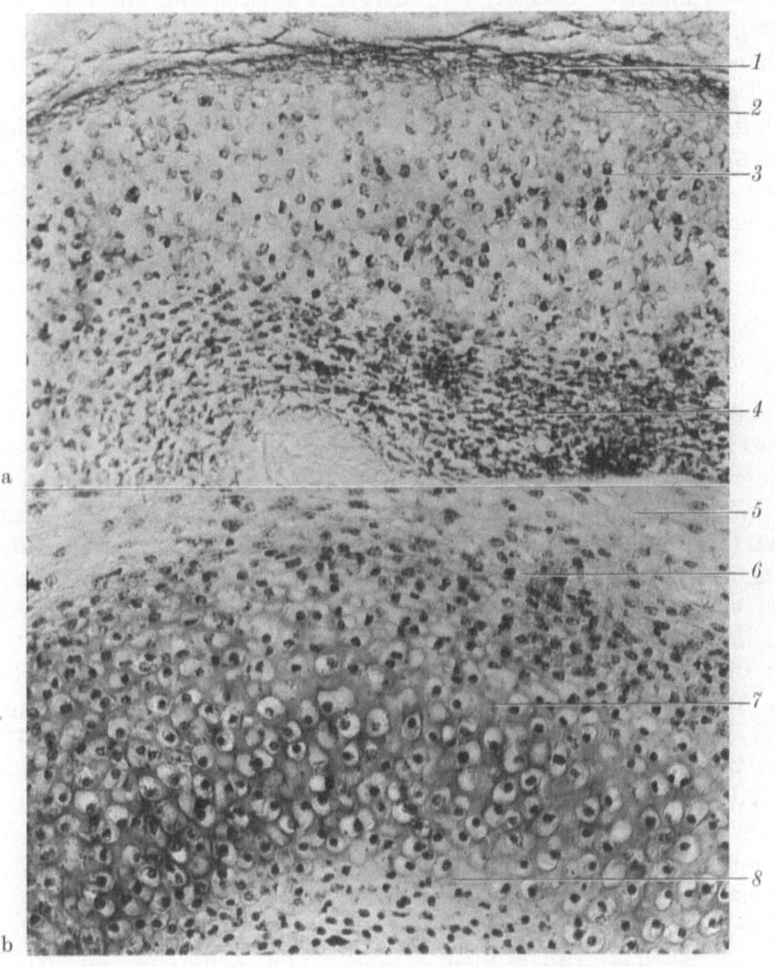

Abb. 10a u. b. Rinderfetus, 37 mm SSL, Bildung der Ohrkapsel. a PAS. b Alkoholisches Toluidinblau. a *1* Perichondrium; *2* Appositionsknorpel; *3* Knorpelzellen mit großen PAS-positiven Granula; *4* Zellen der Vorknorpelblastems in Nachbarschaft des Bogenganges, beladen mit PAS-positiven Granula, Abstand der Zellen voneinander in gleicher Größe wie im Mesenchym; b *5* Mesenchym; *6* dichte Lagerung der Zellen in der Anlage des Perichondrium; *7* zunehmende metachromatische Reaktion der Intercellularsubstanz; *8* Auftreten der metachromatischen Intercellularsubstanz an der Grenze zum Vorknorpelblastem. Vergr. Ob. 16, Ok. 12,5

den flachen Chondroblasten nicht wie sonst flache, sondern rundliche Chondrocyten mit relativ großen Kernen. Die Zellen sind von einer schmalen Schicht Intercellularsubstanz umgeben, so daß das Bild eines echten Zellknorpels vorliegt.

Die Bildung der knorpeligen Skeletanlage geht demgemäß an dicht benachbarten Orten, bei verschiedenen Skeletstücken und dem gleichen Skeletstück bei verschiedenen Species in unterschiedlicher Form vor sich. Man kann folgende morphologische Reihe bilden: Chondrogenese ohne Größenänderung des Intercellularraumes des Mesenchyms, mit Verschwinden des Intercellularraumes, aber ohne wesentliche Änderung der Zellgestalt und schließlich mit Änderung der Zellgestalt. Diesen morphologischen Differenzen entspricht eine abweichende Reaktionsform der Prächondroblasten und Chondroblasten, gleich bleibt nur das Erscheinen der metachromatischen Intercellularsubstanz in der Knorpelbildungsfront.

KNESE und KNOOP (1961c) haben beim Vergleich der Chondrogenese und Osteogenese auseinandergesetzt, daß, abgesehen von qualitativen Unterschieden der gebildeten Intercellularsubstanzen, auch der Ort der Bildung der Gewebekomponenten verschieden ist. Die metachromatisch reagierende Intercellularsubstanz entsteht beim Knorpel erst in der Bildungsfront, die Fasern aber bereits im Perichondrium. Diese Auffassung wird durch Untersuchungen von LASH et al. (1960) über die Induktion der Knorpelbildung des Wirbelkörpers in vitro bei Vorhandensein von radioaktivem Schwefel bestätigt. Die Autoren konnten Chondroitinsulfat nur bei Vorhandensein der knorpeligen Intercellularsubstanz nachweisen. Bei der Osteogenese sind färberisch MPS bereits in den Osteoblasten nachweisbar, die Fasern dagegen entstehen in der Knochenbildungsfront. Diese Angaben beruhen auf Untersuchungen des Epiphysenknorpels. Es ist z. Z. nicht zu sagen, welche Bedeutung den geschilderten verschiedenen Abläufen der Chondrogenese zukommt. Jedenfalls entsteht nicht nur das Knochengewebe, sondern auch das Knorpelgewebe auf sehr unterschiedlichem Wege.

γ) Bemerkungen über Zellgestalt und Zelleistung

Die Bildung des frühen Knorpelgewebes auf morphologisch so unterschiedlichen Wegen bereitet dem Verständnis der hier ablaufenden Vorgänge große Schwierigkeiten. Im allgemeinen setzen wir voraus, daß eine spezifische Zelleistung auch an eine bestimmte Zellform gebunden ist. Im Hinblick auf die bei der Chondrogenese auftretenden Zellen kam HANSEN (1899) zur Auffassung, daß die morphologisch unterschiedlich erscheinenden Bildungsvorgänge physiologisch gleichartig ablaufen. Für die Knochenbildung wurde ebenfalls eine osteogene Potenz für Zellen unterschiedlicher Gestalt angegeben (WEIDENREICH, 1923; MCLEAN und BLOOM, 1940; KNESE, 1956c).

MCLEAN und URIST (1955, 1961) haben zur Bestimmung von Bindegewebszellen verschiedene Kriterien angegeben, und zwar morphologische, solche der Lage, des Ursprunges, der Funktion und der Potenz. Die Potenz ist latent (s. S. 679) und kann zu einer entsprechenden Aktivität führen. Eine reversible Änderung der Zellgestalt ist eine Modulation (WEISS nach BLOOM, 1937), eine nicht reversible Differenzierung. KNESE (1956c) sprach von einer Zellmetamorphose, um die Gestaltänderung ohne Urteil über eine Veränderung der Potenz zu beschreiben. Morphologische Zeichen für die Potenz einer Zelle sind bisher nicht bekannt. Auch in Gewebekulturen läßt sich die Potenz von Zellen nicht eindeutig feststellen (BLOOM, 1937). Für das Verhalten von Zellen in Gewebekulturen ist das Anpassungsvermögen von Zellen an ein fremdes Milieu von besonderer Bedeutung. Das Kulturmilieu kann den Verhältnissen in vivo nicht vollständig entsprechen. Wir können häufig nur Zellen bestimmter Gestalt und Lagerung beschreiben, die im allgemeinen als persistierende Zellelemente erscheinen. Wir können nicht entscheiden, ob diese Zellen unter gewissen Voraussetzungen nicht doch ihre Gestalt ändern (vgl. Entstehung von Osteoclasten aus Osteocyten s. S. 382). Im Hinblick auf das Erscheinen bestimmter Zellformen mit entsprechender Potenz, die sonst auf bestimmte Lebensabschnitte beschränkt sind, z. B. Osteoblasten bei der Callusbildung, wurde angenommen, daß den pluripotenten Mesenchymzellen gleichzusetzende Schlummerzellen als Stammzellen vorhanden sind. Bei Bildung einer neuen Zellform aus einer bereits „differenzierten" glaubte man daher, daß zunächst eine Entdifferenzierung, eine Rückentwicklung zur pluripotenten Mesenchymzelle, erfolgen muß (WEIDENREICH, 1923b; FELL, 1933; vgl. KNESE und BIERMANN, 1958). WEIDENREICH (1923b) hat weiterhin regulative und korrelative Formänderungen von Zellen unterschieden. Solche Veränderungen schildern PLÖTZ (1937/38) sowie BALOGH und FÖLDES (1955) an „Gleit"-Sehnen nach deren Verlagerung und Umwandlung zu Zugsehnen. Derartige Umwandlungen „einer" Gewebeform in eine „andere" bei veränderter Umgebung wurden als Gewebeentstehung durch mechanische Ursachen angesehen (CAREY und ZEIT, 1927; KROMPECHER, 1937/38;

Plötz 1937/38). Nach intrauteriner Extremitätenamputation bei Goldhamsterfeten beobachtete Knese (1960) die Ausbildung einer Art Perichondrium am Amputationsschnitt (Abb. 11); die Knochenbildung läuft dann in der Form ab, wie sie von den distalen Enden der Nagelphalanx ohne Epiphyse her bekannt ist.

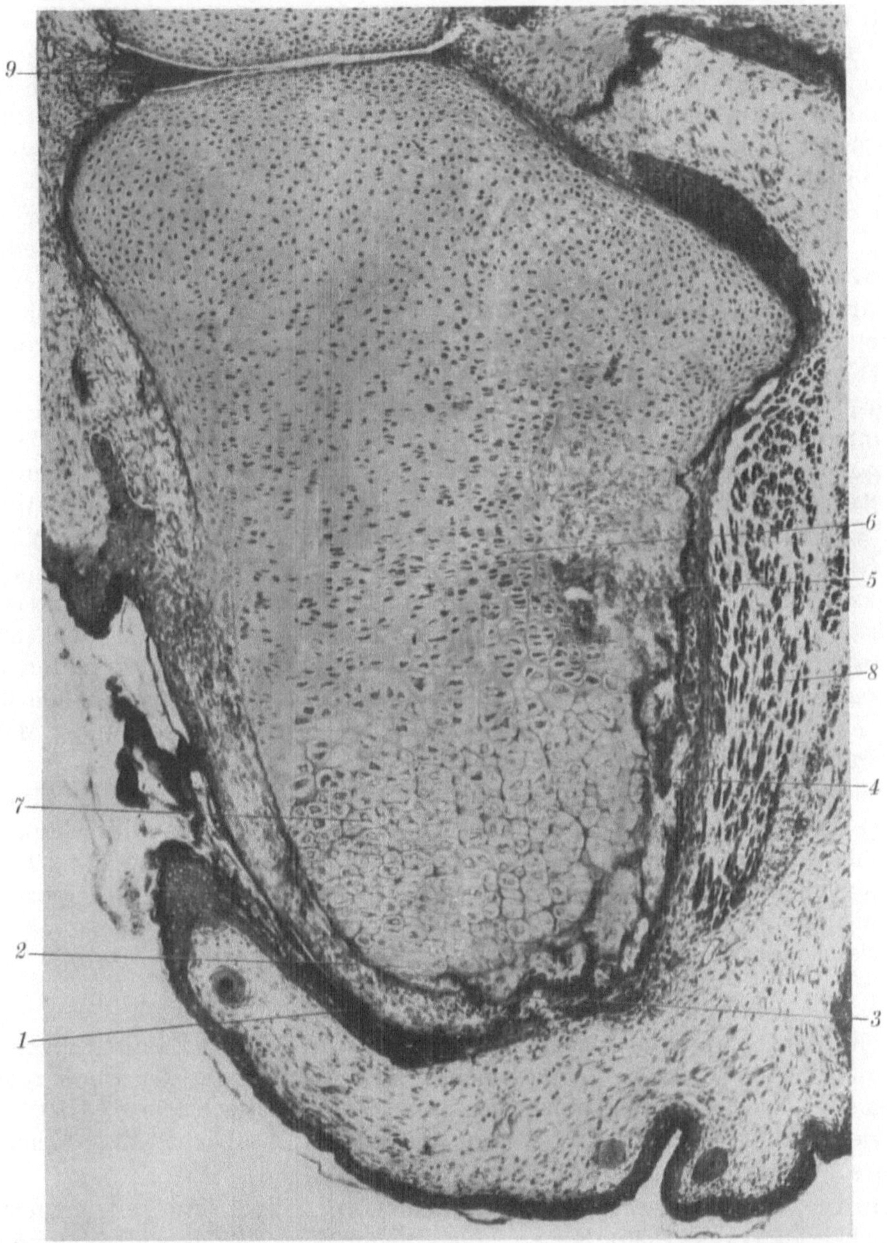

Abb. 11. Goldhamster, intrauterine Amputation der rechten Tibia eines Feten am 13. Tag der Gravidität: Tibia längsgeschnitten. *1* Mit dem Amputationsstumpf in die Tiefe gezogene Hautfalte mit zerfallender Hornschicht; *2* Übergang des Perichondriums des Schaftes auf die Amputationsfläche; *3* periostale Bälkchen am Amputationsschnitt; *4* periostaler Knochen an der Schaftseite; *5* in das Knorpelmodell einwanderndes periostales Gewebe; *6* Reihenknorpel; *7* hydropisierter Knorpel; *8* degenerierende Muskelfasern; *9* Kniegelenkspalt mit Meniscus. Azan. Ob. 10, Ok. 12,5 (Photomontage). (Knese, 1960)

Die wiedergegebenen Vorstellungen über Zellgestalt, Potenz, Differenzierung usw. beruhen auf lichtmikroskopischen Studien. Durch topochemische Untersuchungen wurde nachgewiesen, daß mit der Zellmetamorphose eine veränderte Reaktionsform der Zellen verbunden ist. Die Farbreaktionen lassen unter Beachtung von Untersuchungen mittels Radioisotopen eine Stoffproduktion vermuten, die den „Zustand" der Intercellularsubstanz verändert (Knese und Knoop 1961a). Viele Radioisotope treten zuerst in Skeletzellen auf und werden an die Intercellularsubstanz abgegeben (vgl. Leblond et al., 1955; Leblond und Greulich, 1956; Schiller et al., 1956; Dziewiatkowski, 1958; Carneiro und Leblond, 1958).

Auf Grund elektronenmikroskopischer Untersuchungen wurde bisher noch kein morphologisches System der Bindegewebszellen aufgestellt. Die vorliegenden elektronenmikroskopischen Untersuchungen (Literatur bei Gusek, 1962; Branwood, 1963; Giesekking, 1966; Ross, 1968) der Bindegewebszellen gestattet noch nicht die Aufstellung eines natürlichen Systems, das über die verwandtschaftlichen Beziehungen der Zellen Auskunft gibt. Die Beschreibung „spezifischer" Zellen nach Gestalt und Struktur wird dadurch erschwert, daß nur eine kleine Anzahl von Cytoplasmastrukturen vorhanden ist (Wolfarth-Bottermann, 1959). Chondroblasten und Osteoblasten unterscheiden sich voneinander durch ein verschieden stark entwickeltes endoplasmatisches Reticulum. Das endoplasmatische Reticulum erreicht in Osteoblasten und Pankreaszellen den gleichen Umfang (Knese und Knoop, 1961c).

Ein großer Teil der bisherigen elektronenmikroskopischen Untersuchungen wurde an mit Osmiumsäure fixiertem Material durchgeführt, so daß man von einer Osmiumhistochemie sprach (Bernhard, 1958). Die vielfach vertretene Auffassung von der ausgezeichneten Erhaltung der Strukturen durch Osmiumsäure-Fixierung ist unberechtigt (Zeiger, 1938, 1960). Bahr (1954, 1955) hat in vitro eine ganze Reihe von Substanzen auf ihre Reaktionsfähigkeit mit Osmiumtetroxyd hin untersucht. Versuche mit anderen Fixantien sind noch nicht zum Abschluß gekommen (Dalton, 1955; Lehmann et al., 1958).

Zellen mit elektronenmikroskopisch gleichartiger Struktur wie die flachen Knochenbildungszellen am Ende der Diaphyse und die polaren Osteoblasten verhalten sich gegenüber histochemischen Methoden sehr unterschiedlich; in den flachen Zellen überwiegen MPS gegenüber RNS, in den polaren Osteoblasten dagegen RNS gegenüber MPS (Knese und Knoop, 1961c; Knese, 1959a).

Unsere Kenntnisse über den Ablauf der Bildungsvorgänge wurden durch Untersuchungen mit Hilfe topochemischer Methoden, dem Elektronenmikroskop, der Autoradiographie und der Gewebezüchtung vertieft. Aussagen über die Potenz von Zellen und deren Schicksal, d. h. Modulation der Zellgestalt oder weitere Differenzierung bzw. Entdifferenzierung, stellen vielleicht gut begründete Vermutungen dar, können aber nicht bewiesen werden.

δ) Die Zellen des Hyalin-Knorpels

Die Zellen des Hyalinknorpels zeigen in der Form und ihrem Bau in Rippen-, Gelenk-, Epiphysenknorpel usw. große Unterschiede. Die Morphologie der Chondrocyten wird demzufolge bei Erörterung der einzelnen Gewebeformen beschrieben. Hier werden nur die bei vielen Chondrocyten im fixierten Zustand zu beobachtenden Schrumpfungen sowie die sog. Knorpelkapsel diskutiert.

Einschlüsse von Fett und Glykogen in Knorpelzellen sind seit langem bekannt (Literatur bei Schaffer, 1930). Neuere Untersuchungen über das Auftreten von Lipoiden liegen von Borghese (1936) vor. Schaffer (1926) wies mit Thionin metachromatisch reagierende Granula nach, die er für Kalk hielt. Weiterhin wurden ein Chondriom, d. h. die Gesamtheit der Mitochondrien einer Zelle, eine Centrosphäre (Centriolen) und ein Golgi-Apparat beschrieben. Der Schluß lag nahe, daß die Knorpelzellen im Gegensatz zu den „hyalinen" Zellen des chondroiden Gewebes eine sehr verwickelte Cytoplasmastruktur besitzen, die für ihre Empfindlichkeit gegenüber äußeren Einflüssen, z. B. der Fixierung, verantwortlich ist. Obwohl damit stets mit Fixierungsartefakten zu rechnen ist, wurde z. B. aus der Schrumpfung der hypertrophen Knorpelzellen im Epiphysenknorpel auf ein Absterben dieser Zellen geschlossen (s. S. 734).

Der hyaline Zustand der chondroiden Zellen während der Entwicklung ist auf den Reichtum an Gallocyanin-positiven Substanzen, vermutlich RNS, zurückzuführen. Die chondroiden Zellen sind als modifizierte Bildungszellen, anzusehen. Die Fixierungsschrumpfung bzw. Zerstörung durch Herauslösung von Zellbestandteilen dieser Bildungszellen ist, nach lichtmikroskopischen Untersuchungen zu urteilen, von geringem Grade.

Die Größe der Knorpelkapsel läßt das Ausmaß der Schrumpfung der Knorpelzelle im Vergleich mit derjenigen der Intercellularsubstanz angeben. Eine Fixierung ohne Zellschrumpfung ist kaum zu erreichen. KNESE (1968) gibt an, daß die hypertrophen Knorpelzellen nur etwa 7—35% ihrer Knorpelhöhle einnehmen; der verbleibende Raum enthält die Pericellularsubstanz, wodurch der tatsächliche Grad der Zellschrumpfung schwer zu beurteilen ist. Allerdings ist mitunter ein relativ guter Erhaltungszustand der Zellen, z. B. der hypertrophen Knorpelzellen im Epiphysenknorpel zu beobachten, ohne daß die Gründe hierfür erkennbar wären. Der Schrumpfungsgrad der verschiedenen Knorpelzellen ist sehr unterschiedlich, aber bei der gleichen Zellart stets von annähernd gleichem Umfang, bei den Zellen des hyalinen Epiphysenknorpels geringer als bei den hypertrophen, gering auch im Gelenk- und Ohrknorpel. Die topochemischen Reaktionen dieser Zellen und ihre Ultrastruktur sind recht unterschiedlich (s. S. 756; KNESE und KNOOP, 1961a, c). Wahrscheinlich sind Zellen, die bei der Präparation stärker schrumpfen, besonders reich an niedermolekularen, wasserlöslichen Stoffen. COELHO und CHRISMAN (1960) konnten bei Untersuchung über ^{35}S-Ablagerungen auch einen Substanzverlust bei der Präparation nachweisen (vgl. KNESE und KNOOP, 1961b). Nach Lösung der niedermolekularen Stoffe retrahiert sich der verbleibende Zellrest und ruft auf diese Weise den Eindruck des Absterbens der Zelle hervor. Im allgemeinen betrifft die Fixierungsschrumpfung überwiegend oder ausschließlich das Cytoplasma, weniger oder gar nicht den Kern. Die Desoxyribonucleinsäuren des Kernes sind relativ stabile Makromoleküle (CHARGAFF et al., 1953; SIEBERT und SMELLIE, 1957).

Zwischen dem an Ribonucleinsäuren reichen Nucleolus und dem Cytoplasma bestehen enge Beziehungen (CASPERSON und SCHULTZ, 1940; BRACHET, 1940; VINCENT, 1955; STICH, 1956). Die aus zwei Blättern aufgebaute Kernmembran weist Kernporen auf (WATSON 1955), die auch an Zellen des Vorknorpelblastems und Chondroblasten auftreten (KNESE und KNOOP, 1961a, c). Die Kernmembranen und der zwischen ihnen befindliche perinucleäre Spalt sollen zu den Membranen des endoplasmatischen Reticulums genetische Beziehungen haben (WATSON, 1955; BENETT, 1956). Erweiterungen des perinucleären Raumes und blasenartige bzw. verzweigte Ausstülpungen der äußeren Kernmembran wurden auch an Chondroblasten (Abb. 12) beobachtet (KNESE und KNOOP, 1961a, c). Die Kernstruktur ist vermutlich für die relativ geringe Schrumpfung des Kernes gegenüber der des Cytoplasmas verantwortlich zu machen. Die durch die präparatorische Vorbehandlung relativ geringe Beeinflussung der Kernstruktur in hypertrophen Knorpelzellen spricht dafür, daß die Cytoplasmaveränderungen weniger als ein morphologisches Zeichen für ein Absterben, sondern mehr als ein Fixierungsartefakt anzusehen sind. Im gleichen Sinne ist die starke Speicherung von Radioisotopen dieser Zellen zu deuten. Besonders groß ist offensichtlich der Substanzverlust bei den sog. hypertrophen Zellen. Von KNESE (1968) wurden infolgedessen sog. Doppelfixierungen entwickelt, bei denen in einem Gange die Proteine und in einem zweiten die Kohlenhydrate fixiert werden, die zu einer besseren Erhaltung der hypertrophen Knorpelzellen führen. Degenerative Veränderungen von Skeletzellen wurden vielfach beschrieben (SCHAFFER, 1930; KNESE, 1956c). Die Struktur dieser Zellen unterscheidet sich eindeutig von jener geschrumpfter Zellen (KNESE und KNOOP 1961c).

Als *Knorpelkapsel* wurden die Bezirke der Intercellularsubstanz um die Knorpelzellen bezeichnet. SCHAFFER (1930) unterscheidet verschiedene Abschnitte der Zellumhüllung: Die Kapsel ist eine die Zellhöhle unmittelbar begrenzende, gleichmäßig dünne Schicht der Intercellularsubstanz. Der Zellhof umschließt dann eine Kapsel oder einen Zellbezirk

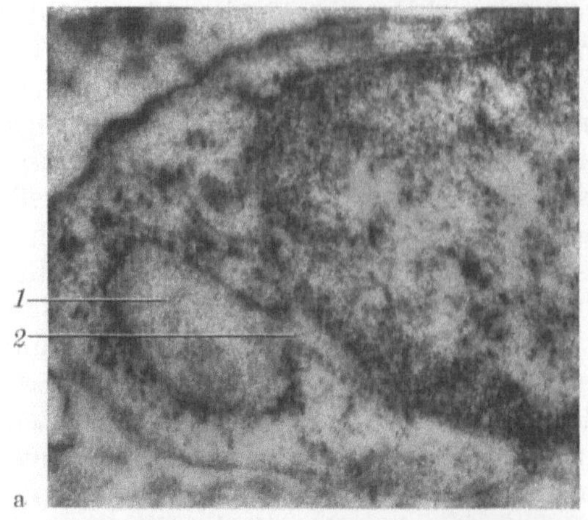

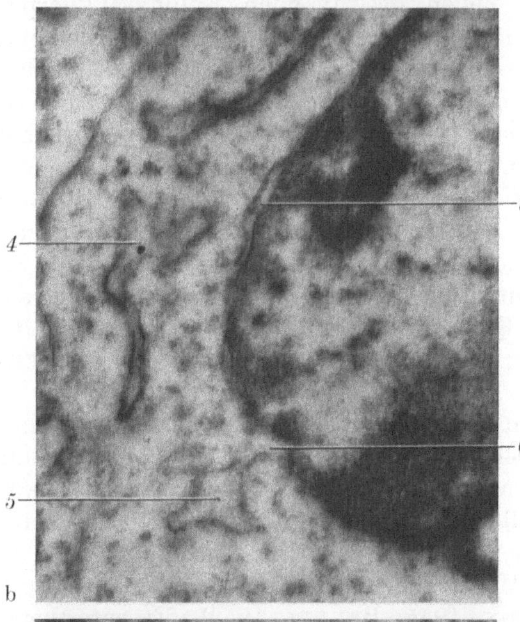

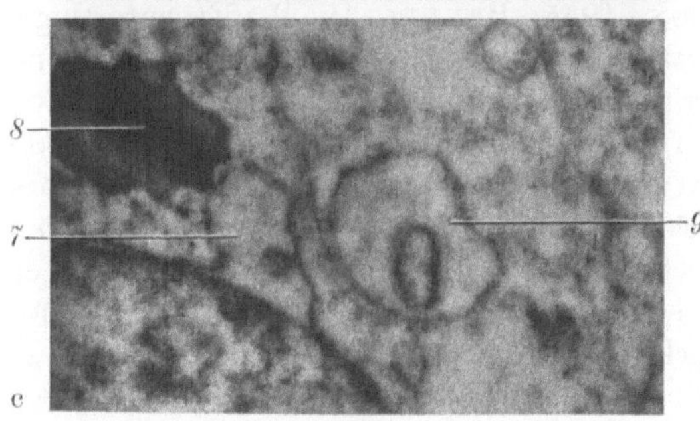

Abb. 12a—c. Erweiterungen des perinucleären Raumes in Chondroblasten und Chondrocyten. a Chondrocyt des Appositionsknorpels. *1* Perinucleäre Blase; *2* Stiel der Blase. Vergr. 56000. b Chondroblast: *3* Mäßige Erweiterung des perinucleären Raumes; *4* endoplasmatisches Reticulum; *5* verzweigte perinucleäre Ausstülpung; *6* deren Stiel. Vergr. 25000. c Chondroblast: *7* Perinucleäre Blase mit einem bläschenartigen Einschluß; *8* osmiophile Einlagerung; *9* angeschnittener Zellfuß. Vergr. 21500. (KNESE u. KNOOP, 1961c)

mit den zugehörigen Kapseln (Territorium, Chondron von BENNINGHOFF 1922). Die interterritoriale Substanz stellt ein die Zellhöfe oder Territorien verbindendes alveoläres Netzwerk dar. Weiterhin beschreibt SCHAFFER (1930) als Kapsel drei verschiedene Bildungen: Die definitive Kapsel entspricht etwa der Grenzscheide einer Knochenlacune (s. S. 322); die transitorische Kapsel ist eine neugebildete Intercellularsubstanz, die späterhin zum Zellhof wird; regressive Kapseln entstehen als stark basophile Gebilde um kataplastische (zugrunde gehende) Zellen. Die genannten Bildungen der Intercellularsubstanz unterscheiden sich voneinander durch ihre Lichtbrechung im Nativpräparat und ihr Verhalten gegenüber Farbstoffen. SCHAFFER (1930) kritisiert den Terminus „Chondron“ von BENNINGHOFF (1922), der dem „Osteon“ als Baustein gleichgesetzt werden sollte (s. S. 367); Zellhöfe und Interterritorialsubstanz sind ein Ganzes, in dem die einzelnen Teile genetisch miteinander in Beziehung stehen.

Die Umwandlung einer transitorischen Kapsel in einen Zellhof weist darauf hin, daß beide nicht Gebilde sui generis darstellen. KNESE und KNOOP (1961a) haben bei ihren topochemischen Untersuchungen der Intercellularsubstanz des Epiphysenknorpels das Augenmerk auf den färberischen Nachweis von MPS gerichtet. Reihenuntersuchungen am Metacarpus von Rinderfeten ergaben nach Anwendung der bekannten Färbungen zum Nachweis von KH und MPS (s. S. 711) voneinander abweichende Reaktionen der Intercellularsubstanz der verschiedenen Anteile des Epiphysenknorpels. Die Färbungsdifferenzen betreffen morphologisch differente Zonen des Epiphysenknorpels. Die Vermutung liegt nahe, daß mit den einzelnen Färbemethoden Gebiete verschiedener stofflicher Zusammensetzung und Struktur dargestellt werden. Den Untersuchungen dieser Autoren ist nun zu entnehmen, daß Kapseln, Zellhöfe und Interterritorialsubstanz bei manchen Farbreaktionen, eventuell nach vorheriger Enzymdigestion, deutlich voneinander zu unterscheiden sind, bei anderen dagegen nicht. Zellhöfe und Kapseln erscheinen bei den verschiedenartigen Methoden auch von ungleicher Breite. Somit kann angenommen werden, daß die Kapseln

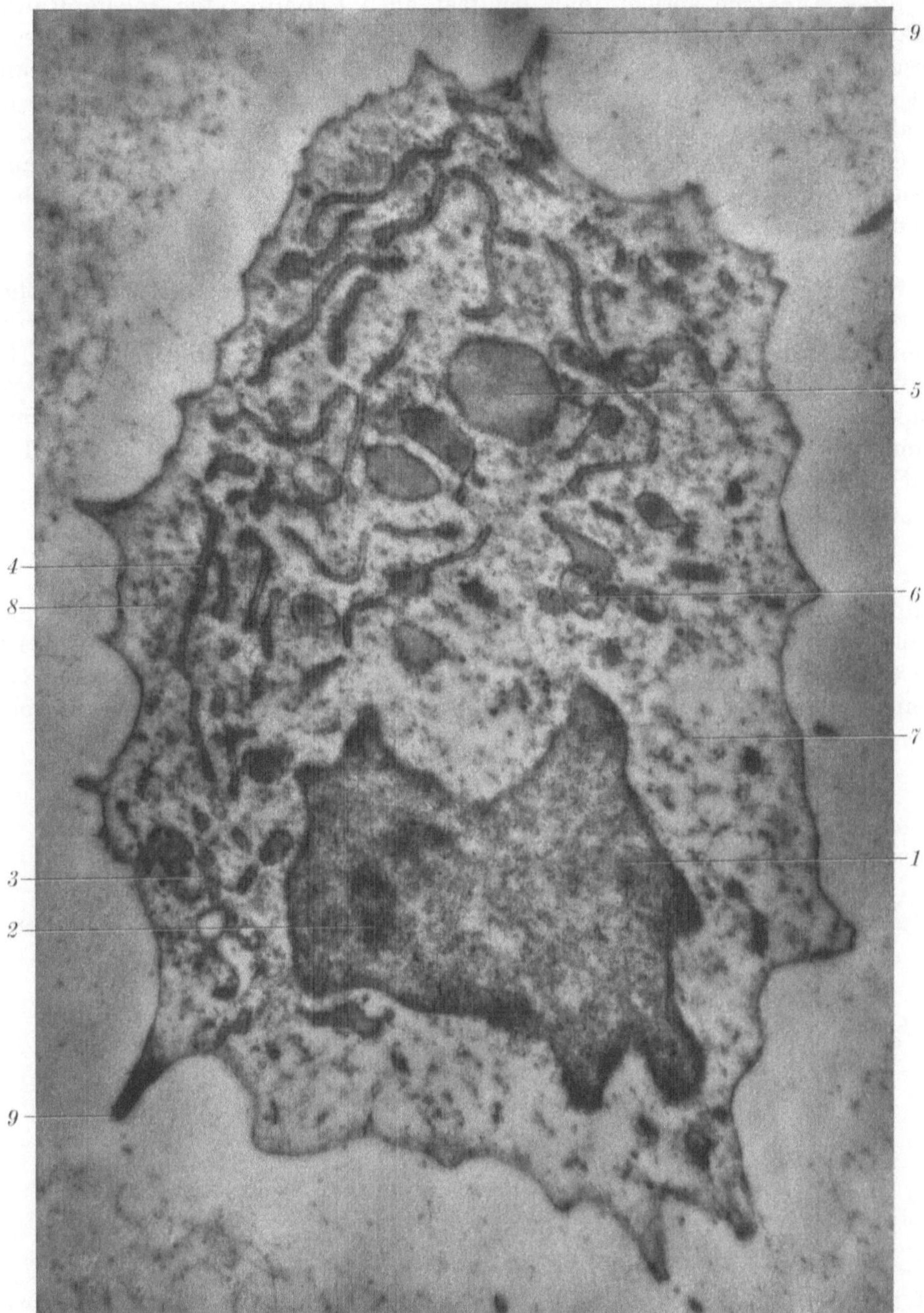

Abb. 13. Chondrocyt des hyalinen Epiphysenknorpels. *1* Zellkern; *2* Nucleolus; *3* Golgi-Lamellen; *4* endoplasmatisches Reticulum mit annähernd gleichbreiten Zisternen; *5* sackartig erweiterte Zisternen; *6* Mitochondrien; *7* Hyaloplasmabezirke mit geringer Substanzdichte; *8* Hyaloplasma mit Palade-Granula; *9* Zellfüße in Kontakt mit der Intercellularsubstanz. Vergr. 16500. (KNESE u. KNOOP, 1961a)

und Höfe nur Zonen unterschiedlicher Bauweise der Intercellularsubstanz, aber nicht morphologisch selbständige Gebilde darstellen.

Auf Grund von elektronenmikroskopischen Untersuchungen des Epiphysenknorpels wurden von einigen Autoren (SCOTT und PEASE, 1956; CAMERON und ROBINSON, 1958; ZELANDER, 1959; TAKUMA, 1960) helle Höfe um Zellen des Proliferations- und hypertrophen Knorpels beschrieben, die ein Äquivalent einer Kapsel sein sollen (Abb. 13).

Gegen diese Annahme spricht, daß bei fast allen Chondrocyten solche Räume lichtmikroskopisch nachweisbar sind. KNESE und KNOOP (1961a) meinen, daß es sich bei den beschriebenen hellen Zonen um Schrumpfräume handelt. Dieser sog. Schrumpfraum enthält die Pericellularsubstanz, die nichts mit der Knorpelkapsel zu tun hat und wohl kaum als eigentlicher Teil der Intercellularsubstanz aufgefaßt werden kann (KNESE, 1968). Offensichtlich wegen ihrer großen Empfindlichkeit gegenüber Fixierung wurde die Pericellularsubstanz relativ selten beschrieben (SCHAFFER, 1930). Diese Autoren beobachteten bei den geschrumpften Zellen ähnlich wie ZBINDEN (1952/53) und DURNING (1958) Zellfüße mit einer engen Verbindung zur Intercellularsubstanz und zwischen diesen Füßen eine ,,Retraktion" (SCHAFFER, 1930) der Zellmembran. Schließlich sahen die Verfasser nach Fixierung mit Formalin, DURNING (1958) nach Gefriertrocknung einen unmittelbaren Kontakt zwischen Plasmalemm und Intercellularsubstanz. CAMERON und ROBINSON (1958) geben eine etwas dichtere Lagerung der Fibrillen in der Wand der Zellhöhlen an. An relativ dicken Schnitten beobachteten wir (unveröffentlicht) elektronenmikroskopisch ebenfalls einen dichteren Faserring, der offensichtlich der Kapsel entspricht.

b) Die Fasern

α) Die Kollagenfibrillen

Sämtliche Formen des Knorpelgewebes enthalten Kollagenfibrillen; im elastischen Knorpel treten noch elastische Fasern hinzu. Im Epiphysenknorpel der Ratte entfallen 17—18% des Trockengewichtes auf das Kollagen (FOLLIS und TONSIMIS, 1958). Bei Hunden nimmt bis zur 21.—25. Lebenswoche der Kollagengehalt des Knorpels zu, der an Chondroitinsulfat ab (EICHELBERGER et al., 1958).

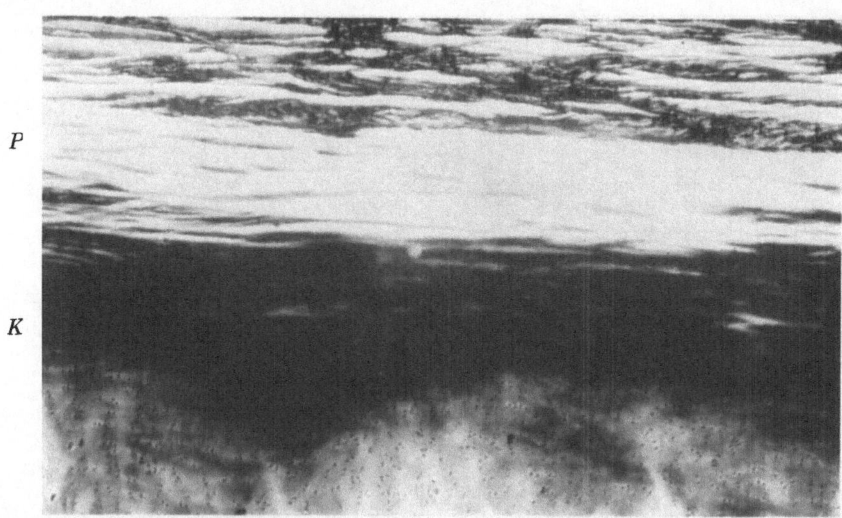

Abb. 14. Bos taurus, Nasenknorpel, Querschnitt 150:1, Pol ×, unter Wirkung des Brace-Kompensators. *P* Perichondrium; *K* subperichondrale Knorpellage, diese kompensiert (dunkel). (W. J. SCHMIDT 1952)

Die Fasern des hyalinen Knorpels sind nur im polarisierten Licht, nach Färbung, Silberimprägnation oder Maceration im Lichtmikroskop zu beobachten (AMPRINO, 1938; OBERHOLZER, 1943). Nach Färbung mit den sog. Routinemethoden bleiben die Fasern unsichtbar, sie sind maskiert (HANSEN, 1905; v. KORFF, 1914). Die Maskierung könnte auf einer physikalischen oder chemischen Veränderung der Fibrillen beruhen. Nach W. J. SCHMIDT (1952b) ist die gleiche Lichtbrechung von Fasern und der übrigen Intercellularsubstanz für die ,,optische" Maskierung verantwortlich. Neben der Eigendoppelbrechung der Kollagenfibrillen liegt eine Formdoppelbrechung vor, da die Stärke der Doppelbrechung von der Brechzahl des Einbettungsmittels abhängt (BORMUTH, 1933;

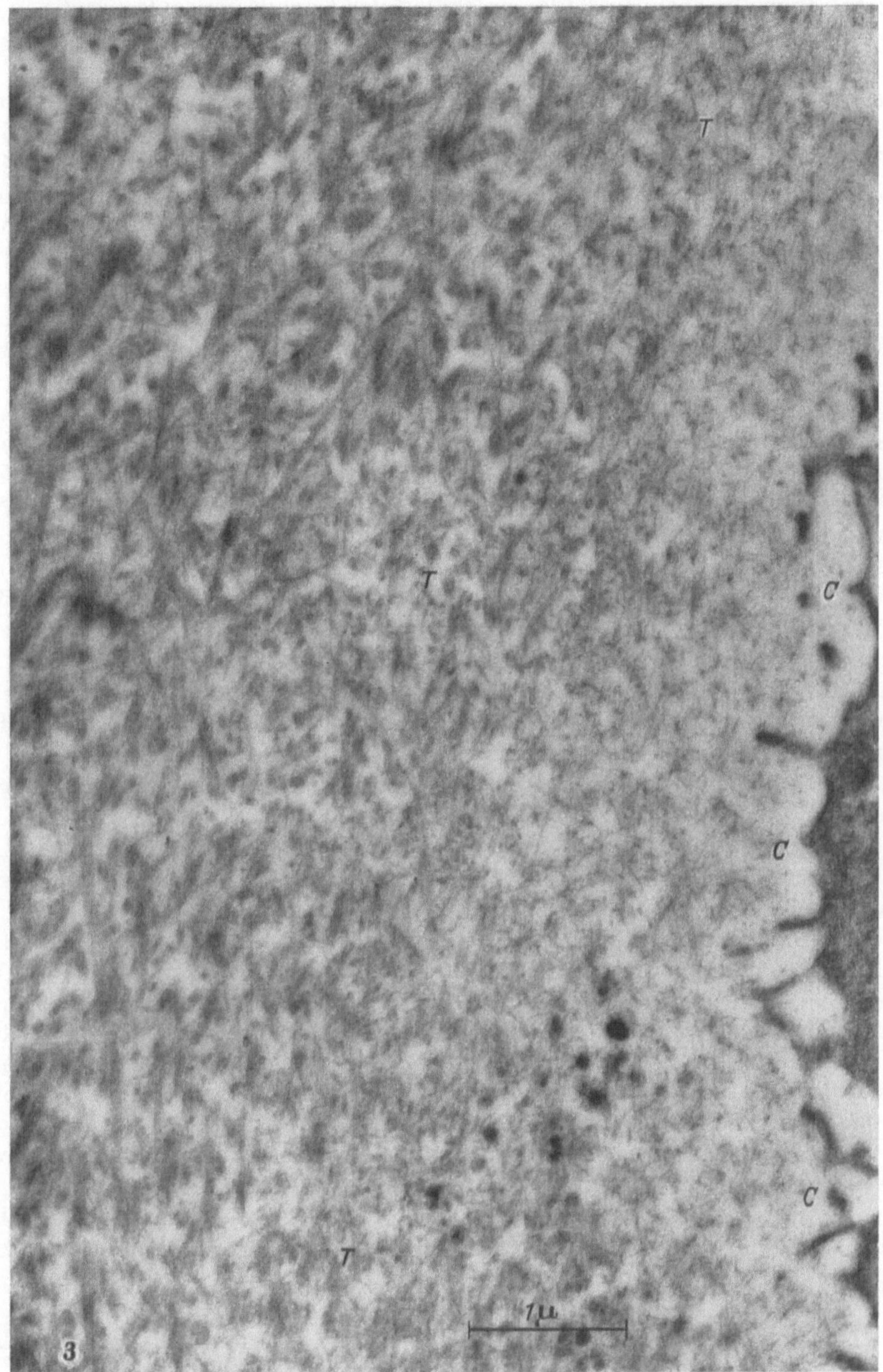

Abb. 15. Die Ordnung der Intercellularsubstanz mit der fibrillenarmen Kapsel C, die Cytoplasmafortsätze enthält, dient Territorium T mit zunehmender Anzahl von Fibrillen. Auf der linken Seite die interterritoriale Region mit Fibrillen von konstantem Durchmesser und gleichmäßiger Querstreifung. Vergr. 21000. (T. ZELANDER, 1959)

DAWSON, 1928; W. J. SCHMIDT, 1952b, 1957). Die Doppelbrechung des Appositionsknorpels ist geringer als die des Perichondriums, d. h. mit dem Auftreten der MPS wird die Doppelbrechung herabgesetzt (Abb. 14). W. J. SCHMIDT (1952b) erwägt, ob dieses Phänomen auf negativ doppelbrechenden Fadenmolekülen der Chondromucoide beruht. Diese Annahme konnte aber nicht bestätigt werden. In einiger Entfernung von den Zellen tritt das „normale" optische Verhalten auf.

BENNINGHOFF (1925) hatte eine zirkuläre knäuelartige Wickelung der Fibrillen in der Knorpelkapsel angenommen. Durch Untersuchungen im polarisierten Licht (BORMUTH, 1933; BUCHER, 1942; STAUB, 1950) und mit Hilfe des Elektronenmikroskopes (CAMERON und ROBINSON, 1958) wurde nachgewiesen, daß die Kollagenfibrillen den Zellen und Zellgruppen ausweichen. Nach den elektronenmikroskopischen Beobachtungen von MARTIN (1954) sollen aber die Fibrillen zirkulär um die Zellen herumlaufen. ZELANDER (1959) gibt für die Fibrillen in Höhe der Chondrocyten einen mehr „radiären", für die entfernter gelegenen dagegen einen mehr „tangentialen" Verlauf an (Abb. 15). Durch elektronenmikroskopische Untersuchungen konnte ebensowenig wie durch lichtmikroskopische (SCHAFFER, 1930) die Ordnung der Fibrillen im Knorpel aufgeklärt werden.

Die Angaben über die Dicke der Fibrillen sowie das Vorhandensein oder Fehlen einer Periode an Hand elektronenmikroskopischer Untersuchungen weichen ebenfalls stark voneinander ab (WOLPERS, 1944; ROUILLER et al., 1952; MARTIN, 1953, 1954; ZBINDEN, 1952/53, 1953; SCOTT und PEASE, 1956; ROBINSON und CAMERON, 1956; CAMERON und ROBINSON, 1958; ZELANDER, 1959; TAKUMA, 1960; GODMAN und PORTER, 1960; KNESE und KNOOP, 1961a und c). ZBINDEN (1953) und KNESE und KNOOP (1961a) führten die unterschiedlichen Befunde über die Struktur der Fibrillen unter anderem auf die jeweilige Fixierung zurück; NEMETSCHEK (1958) hat auf den Einfluß der Fixierung zur Darstellung der Fibrillen-Periode hingewiesen. KNESE und KNOOP (1961a) erwägen weiterhin, ob diese Fixierungsunterschiede auch auf der Vergesellschaftung der Fibrillen im Knorpel mit der relativ großen Menge MPS beruhen. Die Verfasser sahen bei Fixierung mit Formalin eine Querstreifung der Fibrillen, aber nicht bei Anwendung von Osmiumsäure; ZBINDEN (1953) konnte jedoch auch bei Osmiumfixierung eine Querstreifung erkennen.

Die Dicke der Fibrillen soll zwischen 200—1200 (—2000) Å betragen, nach ZELANDER (1959) sogar nur 85 Å und nach ROBINSON und CAMERON (1956) für den Knorpel beim menschlichen Neugeborenen 100—200 Å. Bei der Ratte nimmt die Dicke der Fibrillen von 120 Å in der zuerst gebildeten Intercellularsubstanz auf 180—300 Å am 18. Tag des Fetallebens und bis zur Geburt auf 180—500 Å zu (GODMAN und PORTER, 1960). WOLPERS (1944) hatte an isolierten Knorpelfibrillen eine Periode beobachtet. Einige Autoren konnten keine periodische Streifung feststellen (SCOTT und PEASE, 1956; TAKUMA, 1960), andere nur an bestimmten Orten (MARTIN, 1954; CAMERON und ROBINSON, 1958; ZELANDER, 1959). Die Periode der Kollagenfibrillen beträgt zunächst etwa 200 Å und wächst beim Erwachsenen auf 580—630 Å an.

Die Kollagenfibrillen sind im Knorpel im allgemeinen dünner als an anderen Orten des gleichen Untersuchungsobjektes (KNESE und KNOOP, 1961c). Für die mitunter vertretene Ansicht, die Fibrillen seien durch die Gegenwart des Chondroitinsulfates gequollen und damit maskiert, ist elektronenmikroskopisch keine Bestätigung zu finden.

β) Die elastischen Fasern

Im allgemeinen wird heute zwischen Elastin als chemischer Substanz und elastischen Fasern bzw. einem elastischen Gewebe oder einer Elastica als morphologischer Struktur unterschieden (vgl. HALL, 1955). Die lichtmikroskopische Darstellung von elastischen Fasern erfolgt durch sog. Elastica-Färbungen wie Resorcin-Fuchsin nach WEIGERT, Orcein usw. (vgl. LANSING, 1952). Diese Färbungen sind allerdings für das elastische Material nicht streng spezifisch. In formalinfixiertem Gewebe färben sich die Kollagenfasern nach Acetylierung oder Benzolierung ebenfalls mit Elastica-Farben an (FULLMER und LILLIE, 1957).

Kollagenfasern erscheinen z. B. im Unterhautbindegewebe als haarlockenartig gewellte Bündel, die elastischen Fasern als drahtartige Gebilde, die sich verzweigen und Netze bilden. Die elastischen Fasern zeigen im polarisierten Licht keine Doppelbrechung. Röntgenbrechungsdiagramme sprechen dafür, daß in unbelasteten elastischen Fasern keine Orientierung der Moleküle vorliegt (ASTBURY, 1938, 1940), dagegen tritt bei Dehnung eine Orientierung der Moleküle auf. Auf Grund dieser Befunde wurde angenommen, daß in der nicht gestreckten elastischen Fibrille gekrümmte oder gefaltete Moleküle mit einem Maximum an Entropie vorliegen.

Nach elektronenmikroskopischen Untersuchungen sind die elastischen Fasern aus Protofibrillen von 80 Å Dicke aufgebaut (WOLPERS, 1944; GROSS, 1949; BAHR, 1951; LANSING et al., 1952; HALL et al., 1955). LANSING (1952) und LANSING et al. (1952) kommen zu der Auffassung, daß die elastischen Fasern nach dem Ort des Auftretens verschieden gebaut sind.

SHELDON und ROBINSON (1958) haben im Ohrknorpel des Kaninchens außer einem Netzwerk aus feinen, nicht strukturierten Fibrillen einen gröberen Faserfilz aus elastischen Fasern beobachtet. Diese groben Fasern sind interterritorial gelegen. Nach intravenöser Verabreichung von Papain stellten SHELDON und ROBINSON (1960) das Verschwinden der elastischen Komponente und des amorphen Materials der Intercellularsubstanz fest. Die Kollagenfibrillen bleiben erhalten.

Die biochemischen Untersuchungen des Elastins wurden vor allem am Nackenband des Rindes und der Aortenwand durchgeführt. Elastin enthält weniger Hydroxylprolin und basische Aminosäuren, aber mehr Valin als Kollagen (BOWES und KENTEN, 1949; LANSING, 1952). PARTRIDGE et al. (1955, 1957) isolierten ein β-Protein aus zwei Ketten mit 21 Aminosäurenresten und ein α-Protein mit sieben Ketten und 35 Resten. Elastin enthält 0,3 % KH. HALL (1955, 1957b) nimmt an, daß die elastischen Fasern aus einem Kern und einem Mantel bestehen. Das höher polymerisierte α-Protein soll den Kern, die β-Proteine den Mantel bilden.

Die Altersveränderungen des Elastin sind dadurch ausgezeichnet, daß die Affinität für Calcium von 0,6 auf 6,8 % im 7.—8. Jahrzehnt ansteigt, mitunter sogar auf 13 %. Der Gehalt an Hydroxylprolin nimmt zu.

An anderer Stelle (s. S. 333) sind wir auf jene Befunde eingegangen, die für eine Abkunft der elastischen Fasern von Kollagenfibrillen spricht.

Auf Grund der färberischen Eigenschaften und des abweichenden Verhaltens gegenüber Enzymen haben FULLMER und LILLIE (1958) eine sog. Oxytalan-Faser beschrieben. Diese Fasern wurden im Periodontium, in Sehnen und Bändern, in der Adventitia von Gefäßen in Hautanhängen, im Epi- und Perineurium nachgewiesen; an anderen Orten fehlen sie.

c) Die organischen Inter- bzw. Perifibrillärsubstanzen

Der nicht fibrilläre (amorphe) Anteil der organischen Intercellularsubstanz wird mitunter noch als „Grundsubstanz" oder „Matrix" bezeichnet (s. S. 319). Nach der Ansicht von K. MEYER (1953) gebührt bei Erörterungen über die Interzellularsubstanzen die Führung dem Histologen und nicht dem Chemiker, da es sich zunächst um Aufklärung morphologischer und nicht chemischer Fakten handele. So meint auch LILLIE (1952) im Hinblick auf das Kollagen, daß durch anatomische Kriterien das Material ausgewählt wird, welches nunmehr mit anderen Methoden zu untersuchen ist. WYCKHOFF (bei LILLIE, 1952) fügt hinzu, daß in der morphologischen Definition eine Ursprungs-(parent)definition vorliegt. Morphologie, Chemie und Physik verwenden jeweils eigene Kriterien zur Beschreibung und Definition der Gewebselemente, so daß sich Definitionen verschiedener Disziplinen nicht völlig miteinander decken können.

Die Diskussionen um die Bedeutung (Semantik) des Terminus Grundsubstanz sind als Zeichen der Begriffsklärung mit fortschreitenden Kenntnissen über Bau und Aufgaben der Intercellularsubstanz anzusehen. Die flüssige Matrix als innere Umwelt (MCLEAN, 1960) umfaßt das Blut und die extracellulären Flüssigkeiten, damit auch den flüssigen oder halbflüssigen Teil der Intercellularsubstanz der Bindegewebe.

Die extracellulären Flüssigkeiten gewannen ein besonderes Interesse im Hinblick auf die Prozesse, die als homeostatische Regulation bezeichnet werden. Die Vorstellungen von der Selbstregulation biologischer Prozesse geht auf CLAUDE BERNARD (1878) mit der Unterscheidung zwischen einem milieu extérieur, in dem der ganze Organismus lebt, und dem milieu intérieur zurück, in dem die Zellen leben. In der Selbstregulation biologischer Prozesse sah CANNON (1929) einen für den Organismus so spezifischen Vorgang, daß er den Terminus Homeostase prägte. Unter Homeostase wird damit die Aufrechterhaltung der inneren Umwelt des Organismus im Hinblick auf eine breite Schwankung seiner eigenen Aktivität und die Veränderungen der äußeren Umwelt angesehen. Zu diesen Vorgängen gehört auch die Regulation der Körpertemperatur und des Blutzuckerspiegels. Der Steuerungsmechanismus kann im Sinne der Regeltechnik oder Kybernetik betrachtet werden (GOLDMAN, 1960).

In starker Verallgemeinerung kann die Elektrolytkonzentration der Gewebsflüssigkeit des lockeren Bindegewebes einem Ultrafiltrat des Blutes gleichgesetzt werden (McLEAN 1960). Zwischen einer kolloidreichen und wasserarmen Phase auf der einen Seite, einer kolloidarmen, aber wasserreichen auf der anderen Seite findet ein homeostatischer Ausgleich statt. Der Vorgang hängt von dem Aggregatzustand des Kolloids ab (ENGEL et al., 1954).

Der Stoffaustausch zwischen Blutbahn und Zellen wird durch die Intercellularsubstanzen vermittelt. Von DURAN-REYNALS (1942) und MEYER (1947) wurde angenommen, daß Art und Menge der MPS diesen Stoffaustausch beeinflussen. Die Stoffe sollen entlang der Oberfläche der Kollagenfasern diffundieren (McMASTER et al., 1950). DURAN-REYNALS (1942) meint, daß die örtliche Struktur der Intercellularsubstanzen für die spezifische biochemische Verfassung (make up) der entsprechenden Organe und Gewebe verantwortlich ist. ENGEL et al. (1960) sprechen von einem physiko-chemischen Profil der Intercellularsubstanzen. Somit kann unter Beachtung homeostatischer Prozesse weder die Zelle noch die Intercellularsubstanz für sich allein betrachtet werden. Homeostatische Vorgänge in der Zellumgebung, hervorgerufen z. B. durch Veränderungen der Blutzusammensetzung, bedingen ein anderes Milieu für die Zelle. Wenn „fremde" Moleküle, unter anderem Pharmaca, in die Intercellularsubstanz eintreten, wird ihr gesamtes Ladungsgefüge verändert. In gleicher Weise kann die Zelle durch Bildung entsprechender Substanzen Menge und Art der Intercellularsubstanzen beeinflussen.

DORFMAN und SCHILLER (1958) meinen, die Termini „Grundsubstanz" und „extracelluläre Flüssigkeit" seien synonym. Unter Berücksichtigung des spezifischen „make up" der Intercellularsubstanz ist wohl empfehlenswert, zwischen einem gewebeeigenen Anteil der Intercellularsubstanz und der durchwandernden extracellulären „Flüssigkeit" zu unterscheiden. Die extracelluläre Flüssigkeit ist mit gewissen Einschränkungen als ein Ultrafiltrat des Blutes anzusehen. Ob eine derartige begrifflich scharfe Scheidung den Gegebenheiten voll entspricht, ist z. Zt. noch nicht zu sagen.

Die biochemische Untersuchung der Intercellularsubstanzen stößt auf große Schwierigkeiten, da erst eine Zerstörung der Struktur ihre Herauslösung gestattet (PARTRIDGE und DAVIS, 1958). So ist häufig nicht zu unterscheiden, ob eine isolierte Substanz mit bestimmten morphologischen Strukturen, z. B. Fibrillen, in Verbindung steht bzw. selbständig auftritt oder beide Möglichkeiten verwirklicht sind.

α) *Die sauren Mucopolysaccharide (MPS)*

Die organischen Interfibrillärsubstanzen bestehen im allgemeinen aus Stoffen, die sowohl Kohlenhydrate als auch Proteine enthalten; hierbei wird von den löslichen Kollagenen abgesehen (s. S. 329). Das Vorhandensein von Kohlenhydraten und Proteinen erschwert die Klassifizierung dieser Substanzen. Mitunter wurde versucht, durch das Präfix „Glyko" anzudeuten, daß der Polysaccharidanteil für den Stoff charakteristisch ist; mit dem Präfix „Muco" wurde dann auf einen größeren Anteil (über 4%) an Hexosamin hingewiesen (vgl. GIBIAN, 1959). So wurden stark voneinander abweichende Nomenklaturen entwickelt (MEYER, 1938, 1945, 1953; STACEY, 1946; BLIX, 1951, MONTREUIL, 1957). Auf die von JEANLOZ (1960, vgl. JEANLOZ und BALAZS 1965, 1966) vorgeschlagene Nomenklatur sind wir bereits eingegangen (s. S. 334). Die bisherige Trivialnamen werden durch unmißverständliche Bezeichnungen ersetzt (s. Tabelle 1). Die Polysaccharide mit Aminozuckern werden Glykosaminoglycane genannt. Allgemein üblich sind bereits die Termini Polysaccharid- (bzw. Chondroitinsulfat-)Protein-Komplex oder indifferenter Kohlenhydrat-Protein-Komplex, wenn mit dem Vorhandensein von Oligosacchariden zu rechnen ist.

Bisher konnte nur die Struktur und das Vorkommen der sauren MPS näher aufgeklärt werden, so daß wir uns auf deren Darstellung beschränken; auf die sog. neutralen Polysaccharide sind wir beim Knochengewebe kurz eingegangen (s. S. 335). Zusammenfassende Erörterungen über Aufbau und Synthese der MPS liegen von GIBIAN (1954, 1959), DORFMAN (1955/56), RODÉN (1956), ZAMBOTTI (1957), DELAUNAY und BAZIN (1958), BAZIN und DELAUNAY (1959), STARY (1959), JEANLOZ (1963), BRIMACOMBE und WEBBER (1964), MUIR (1964), S. F. JACKSON (1964), SALTON (1965), BUDDECKE (1966), JEANLOZ und BALAZS (1965, 1966) vor, weiterhin Konferenzberichte, herausgegeben von RAGAN (1951—1954), WOLSTENHOLME und O'CONNOR (1958) und CLARK und GRANT (1961).

Die MPS sind aus Disaccharideinheiten aufgebaut, die aus einem Aminozucker und einer Hexuronsäure bestehen (LEVENE 1941, DAVIDSON und MEYER 1954, 1955). Nach Zusammensetzung und optischer Aktivität wurden von MEYER und RAPPORT (1951), MEYER et al. (1956) drei verschiedene Chondroitinsulfate unterschieden. Hinzu treten die Hyaluronsäure, das Chondroitin, Keratansulfat sowie das Heparin.

Tabelle 1. *Mucopolysaccharide der Stützgewebe*

	Aminozucker	Uronsäure	Sulfat
Hyaluronsäure	N-Acetylglucosamin	Glucuronsäure	—
Chondroitin-4-sulfat (A)	N-Acetylgalaktosamin	Glucuronsäure	+
Chondroitin-6-sulfat (C)	N-Acetylgalaktosamin	Glucuronsäure	+
Chondroitin	N-Acetylgalaktosamin	Glucuronsäure	—
Keratansulfat	N-Acetylglucosamin	(Galaktose)	+

In Tabelle 1 wurden nur jene Aminozucker aufgenommen, die in den Stützgeweben im engeren Sinne auftreten. Unberücksichtigt blieben das Dermatansulfat (Chondroitinsulfat B) der Haut, Heparin und Heparansulfat aus Lunge und Aorta. Die Unterscheidung zwischen Chondroitinsulfat A und C bereitete zunächst Schwierigkeiten. Es zeigte sich jedoch (HOFFMAN, LINKER und MEYER, 1958), daß bei A die Sulfatgruppe in der Position 4 und bei C in 6 steht (vgl. ORR 1954); dieser Unterschied wurde in der Nomenklatur berücksichtigt. Beide Stoffe werden durch Testis-, aber nicht durch Bakterienhyaluronidase hydrolisiert (MEYER und RAPPORT, 1951; MEYER, 1953, 1954; MEYER et al., 1956). Hyaliner Knorpel enthällt 20—40% des Trockengewichtes, kompakter Knochen (Rind, GLEGG und EIDINGER, 1955) 0,25% des Trockengewichtes Chondroitinsulfate.

Chondroitinsulfat C tritt in Sehnen (Schwein und Kalb), hyalinem Knorpel, im Nucleus pulposus (Mensch, 20% des Trockengewichtes; MALMGREN et al., 1952; HALL et al., 1957) und Knochengewebe auf. Die Untersuchungen über den Chondroitinsulfat-Gehalt des Knorpels (vgl. SCHUBERT und HAMERMAN, 1965) haben nun fast eine hundertjährige Geschichte, die hier nicht dargestellt werden kann. Unter der Voraussetzung, daß alle hyaline Knorpel gleich sind (MEYER 1959), wurden zur Gewinnung einer genügend großen Ausgangsmenge für die Analysen zunächst überwiegend Nasen- und Rippenknorpel, aber kaum Epiphysen untersucht (LINDENBAUM und KUETTNER, 1967). Der Vergleich zwischen verschiedenartigen Knorpeln (MEYER, 1959) ergab jedoch bei verschiedenen Knorpeln auch einen sehr unterschiedlichen Bestand an MPS. Der Nasenknorpel enthält fast nur Chondroitin-4-sulfat, Rippenknorpel dagegen auch Chondroitin-6-sulfat. Auch lebenszeitliche Veränderungen sind zu beachten, der Gehalt an Keratansulfat nimmt im Laufe des Lebens zu, gleichzeitig der von Chondroitin-4-sulfat aber ab. Leider wird immer noch nicht genügend berücksichtigt, daß die Verhältnisse der „permanenten" Nasen- und Rippenknorpel in keiner Weise representativ für alle Knorpel sind, vor allem gelten sie nicht für die Epiphyse. Im übrigen zeigen die genannten Knorpelarten strukturell erhebliche Unterschiede.

Das Vorhandensein von Chondroitin wurde im Knorpel auf Grund eines relativ niedrigen Gehaltes an S angenommen (Davidson et al., 1954), jedoch kann dieser Befund auch auf eine unvollständige Sulfurierung eines Chondroitinsulfates zurückzuführen sein (Meyer et al., 1956). Im Frakturcallus der Ratte wurde ebenfalls Chondroitin gefunden (Maurer et al., 1952).

Hyaluronsäure konnte in der Synovia von Mensch und Rind, in Kalbsknochen und Fibroblastenkulturen nachgewiesen werden.

Keratansulfat ist das einzige MPS ohne Uronsäure. Das Keratansulfat enthält N-Acetylglucosamin, Galaktose und Sulfat in aequimolaren Mengen und ähnelt damit den Glykoproteinen. Einen besonders hohen Gehalt an Keratansulfat weist der Nucleus pulposus (Glegg, Eidinger und Leblond, 1954), vor allem mit zunehmendem Alter auf. Es wurde zuerst aus der Cornea isoliert und erhielt daher seinen Namen „Keratan"sulfat. Diese Substanz wurde im Kälberknochen und Knorpel gefunden.

Die sog. Chondroitinschwefelsäure der Cornea und Herzklappen ist ein Gemisch aus Chondroitin und Keratansulfat (Davidson et al., 1954; Woodin, 1952; Meyer et al., 1953).

Das Chondroitinsulfat B wird durch Testis-Hyaluronidase nicht hydrolisiert. Es fehlt ebenso wie Heparin in den Skeletgeweben.

Die MPS zeigen beachtliche Differenzen im Hinblick auf ihre biologische Halbwertzeit. Sie beträgt 3—5 Tage für das Chondroitin-6-sulfat, ist beim Chondroitin-4-sulfat wahrscheinlich etwas kürzer und erreicht beim Keratansulfat mehr als 60 Tage (Davidson und Small, 1963a, b). Auf diese verschiedene Halbwertzeit dürfte teilweise die Zunahme des Keratansulfates bei der Alterung beruhen. Die genannten Autoren konnten auch zeigen, daß unter dem Einfluß von Wachstumshormon und Oestrogen die Halbwertzeit von Chondroitin-6-sulfat heraufgesetzt, die des Keratansulfates aber herabgesetzt wird. Cortison ändert die Halbwertzeit von Chondroitin-6-sulfat nicht, verringert die von Keratansulfat auf 5 Tage.

Einige Hinweise über das Vorkommen der Glykoproteine (bzw. proteide), der sog. neutralen MPS, mögen angefügt werden. Diesen Kohlenhydrat-Protein-Komplexen fehlen Uronsäure und Sulfat, dagegen ist die Neuraminsäure (Klenk, 1941) vorhanden, so daß chemisch Polyanionen vorliegen. Die acetylierten Derivate der Neuraminsäure werden als Sialinsäure bezeichnet und damit die Stoffgruppe mitunter auch die der Sialoproteine. Weiter treten Galaktose, Mannose, Hexosamin und Fucose auf. Glykoproteine wurden im Knorpel bereits von Glegg, Eidinger und Leblond (1954) nachgewiesen.

β) Bindung der Mucopolysaccharide an Proteine

Die Bindung der MPS an Proteine ist nach Art der MPS und deren Herkunftsort unterschiedlich. Früzeitig wurde vermutet, daß Hyaluronsäure aber auch andere MPS salzartige, leicht dissoziierbare Verbindungen mit basischen Proteinen eingehen (Meyer und Chaffee, 1939; Curtain, 1955 und Day, 1947). Die Ordnung und Verteilung der Hyaluronsäure im lockeren Bindegewebe wird durch das Filzwerk der Kollagenfasern bestimmt. Allerdings wurde die Frage der Bindung an Proteine zunächst wenig verfolgt, da Hauptziel der biochemischen Arbeiten die Aufklärung der Struktur der isolierten Aminozucker war. Durch diese Beschränkung der Fragestellung entstand offensichtlich außerhalb des biochemischen Arbeitskreises mitunter der Eindruck von einer recht einfachen Struktur der Kohlenhydrate (s. Färbung).

Die sauren MPS, die Sulfat und Uronsäure enthalten, treten im allgemeinen mit Proteinen vergesellschaftet auf (DORFMAN und MATHEWS, 1956; BETTELHEIM-JEVONS, 1958). Zunächst wurde angenommen, daß außer den MPS an Proteinen nur Kollagen vorhanden sei (u. a. PARTRIDGE 1948). Verschiedene Autoren isolierten jedoch später Proteine, die vom Kollagen verschieden sind (SHATTON und SCHUBERT, 1954; CONSDEN und BIRD, 1954; WOODIN, 1952; MATHEWS, 1956). PARTRIDGE und DAVIS (1958) gelang die Isolation eines unzerstörten MPS-Proteinkomplexes aus hyalinem Knorpel und dessen Trennung von Kollagen. Die Aminosäuren-Analyse dieser Fraktion ergab das Fehlen von Hydroxyprolin und einen hohen Gehalt an Tyrosin. Das Protein unterscheidet sich durch seinen abweichenden Gehalt an Prolin, Serin, Glycin, Lysin und Arginin auch von den Plasmaproteinen (PARTRIDGE und DAVIS, 1958).

Für die Bindung der Proteine an MPS wurden sehr verschiedene Modi angenommen (EINBINDER und SCHUBERT, 1950, 1951; BLIX, 1951; SHATTON und SCHUBERT, 1954; DORFMAN und MATHEWS, 1956; MEYER, 1956; BERNARDI, 1957; MUIR, 1958). Zunächst wurde an salzartige Bindungen gedacht (MEYER und SMYTH, 1937; PARTRIDGE, 1948; BLIX, 1951; MEYER 1952, 1953; JORPES und YAMASHINA, 1956). Der Ausdruck „salzartige Bindung“ ist nach LOEVEN (1955) nicht zu empfehlen, da er eine rein chemische Interpretation im Sinne der stöchiometrischen Bindung ausdrücken würde. Im Anschluß an Modellversuche hat LOEVEN die Schwellung des Knorpels in nativem Zustand und nach milder Extraktion der MPS untersucht. Er schließt aus seinen Versuchen, daß in dem Protein-MPS-Komplex ein kolloidales System im Sinne von BUNGENBERG DE JONG (1949) vorliegt. Der Auffassung von LOEVEN schlossen sich PARTRIDGE und DAVIS (1958) an. Weiterhin glauben die Autoren, daß die Viscosität nicht auf der Bindung von Chondroitinsulfat-Molekülen an Proteine beruhe, sondern auf der Bildung von Makromolekülen, die aus kleineren Mucoprotein-Molekülen entstehen. Inzwischen ist die Bedeutung des Serins für die Bindung der Kohlenhydrate an Proteine endgültig nachgewiesen worden (JACOBS und MUIR, 1963; BUDDECKE, KRÖZ und LANKA, 1963), wobei LINDAHL und RODÉN (1966) eine glykosydische Bindung zwischen der Xylose und der Hydroxyl-Gruppe des Serins annehmen. Die vielfältigen neueren Isolierungsmethoden (GREILING 1966) haben die Trennung einer ganzen Reihe von Fraktionen aus einem Extrakt gestattet. Durch Zentrifugieren wurde u.a. eine schwere (PPH) und eine leichte (PPL) Fraktion isoliert (GERBER, FRANKLIN und SCHUBERT, 1960; CAMPO und DZIEWIATKOWSKI, 1962). Diese Arbeiten führten schließlich dazu, sich mit der Gestalt des Makromoleküls der Kohlenhydrat-Protein-Komplexe zu beschäftigen (S. F. JACKSON, 1964; MUIR, 1964; BRIMACOMBE und WEBBER, 1964); dabei nimmt man an, daß einem Proteinkern die unterschiedlichen langen Ketten der Kohlenhydrate angefügt sind.

Nach PARTRIDGE (bei MUIR 1961) enthält ein Chondroitin-Sulfat-Protein-Komplex, aus frischem Knorpel isoliert, 20—25% Protein. Das durch Osmose bestimmte Molekulargewicht betrug $1—5 \times 10^{-6}$. Die Polysaccharidketten werden durch Proteine aneinander gebunden, und zwar erfolgt die Bindung nur an einem Punkt der Protein-Rückgrat-(backbone)ebene. Dieser Komplex stellt vermutlich in der Lösung eine Aggregation von molekularen Einheiten dar. Die Einheiten enthalten wenigstens 20 Polysaccharidketten. Entlang einer Proteineinheit von 3700 Å sind etwa 62 Chondroitinsulfatketten von je 50000 Molekulargewicht verteilt. Weitere Angaben bei S. F. JACKSON (1964).

Im Hinblick auf die Insertion von Sehnen an knorpeligen Apophysen ist bemerkenswert, daß in Sehnen andere Kohlenhydrate vorliegen als im Knorpel (GLEGG et al., 1954). Die Menge der sauren MPS ist mit 0,5% gering. MEYER et al. (1956, 1957) haben in Sehnen einen etwa gleichen Anteil Chondroitinsulfat B und C sowie eine geringe Menge Hyaluronsäure gefunden. Das Verhältnis der MPS zu den Kollagenfibrillen der Sehne ist noch umstritten (EINBINDER und SCHUBERT, 1951; JACKSON, 1953, 1954).

γ) Charakter der Mucopolysaccharide und ihre Aufgaben in der Intercellularsubstanz

Die sauren MPS sind lineare Polyelektrolyte mit einem hohen Molekulargewicht. Die MPS sind weiterhin polydispers, d. h. von wechselnder Molekülgröße. Die Kettenlänge der Fasermoleküle beträgt zwischen 3800 (MATHEWS, 1956) und 4700 Å (MEYER et al., 1948). Auf Grund elektronenmikroskopischer Untersuchungen gereinigter Hyaluronsäurepräparate wurde eine mikrofibrilläre Struktur angenommen (GROSS, 1948, 1950). Das Molekulargewicht wurde mit 260000 (BLIX und SNELLMAN, 1945) bzw. 45000 (MATHEWS und DORFMAN, 1953) und für einen Chondroitin-Sulfat-Protein-Komplex mit $5—25 \times 10^{-6}$ (MATHEWS, 1956) angegeben. Nach SCHUBERT (1964) liegt das Molekulargewicht zwischen 15000—10000000 bei 50—50000 Disaccharid-Einheiten.

DORFMAN und SCHILLER (1958) fassen die möglichen Aufgaben der Mucopolysaccharide zusammen: 1. Kontrolle der Elektrolyte und des Wassers in der extracellulären Flüssigkeit, 2. Mitwirkung bei der Mineralisation, 3. Wundheilung, 4. Widerstand gegen Infektion, 5. Schmiermittel, 6. Blutcoagulation, 7. Clearing-Aktivität, 8. Aufrechterhaltung eines stabilen transparenten Mediums (Auge). SALTON (1965) meint jedoch, daß über die sog. Funktionen der Aminozucker viele Spekulationen angestellt wurden, aber noch wenig experimentelle Erhebungen vorliegen.

Nach MATHEWS (1956) und MATHEWS et al. (1958) sind die Chondroitinsulfatketten im Knorpel durch Kovalenzbindung an Proteine gebunden und bilden einen makromolekularen Komplex von 4000000 Molekulargewicht. Da in den sich wiederholenden Einheiten sowohl Carboxyl- als auch Sulfatgruppen vorhanden sind, liegt ein Polyelektrolyt mit hoher negativer Ladung vor. Infolge der Abstoßung zwischen den negativen Ladungen kommt ein gestreckter Zustand der Ketten zustande. Die lineare Ordnung wird durch Bindung von Kationen verändert. In Gegenwart von Kationen wird die effektive Ladung herabgesetzt und die Moleküle gehen in den Zustand statistischer Knäuel (random coil) über. Durch diese Gestaltänderung der Ketten wird der Transport von Ionen und Wasser durch die Intercellularsubstanz beeinflußt. Die MPS werden damit zu einer kontrollierenden Barriere, der Bindegewebsschranke (spreading, Permeabilität; DURAN-REYNALS, 1942; MEYER, 1947). Da auf diesem Wege eine Ionenauswahl erfolgt, kann die extracelluläre Flüssigkeit innerhalb der Intercellularsubstanz nur bedingt als ein Ultrafiltrat des Plasmas angesehen werden. Weiterhin werden Viscosität und Strömungsdoppelbrechung von der Hydratation und dem Knäuelungsgrad beeinflußt (MATHEWS und DORFMAN, 1953; MATHEWS, 1953).

Das Chondroitinsulfat ist ein Ionenaustauscher und zwar sowohl für Metallionen als auch basische Ladungen von Proteinen (BOYD und NEUMAN, 1951; MATHEWS, 1953, BERSIN, 1950; BETTELHEIM-JEVONS, 1958). Das Bindungsvermögen des Rippenknorpels für Na^+, Ca^{++}, Ba^{++} entspricht dem Sulfatgehalt unter der Annahme, daß sowohl Sulfat- als auch Carboxylgruppen an der Bindung beteiligt sind. JOSEPH et al. (1959) und ENGEL et al. (1960) führen im Hinblick auf den Ionenaustausch aus, daß in der Interfibrillärsubstanz ein komplexes Ladungsmosaik mit negativ und positiv geladenen Gruppen vorliegt. Hinzu treten ungeladene polare Gruppen. Ein wesentlicher Unterschied des Mechanismus zwischen der Bindung kleiner Moleküle und Ionen und verschieden großer Makromoleküle besteht nicht. Elektrostatische Bindungen innerhalb der Interfibrillärsubstanz können zwischen den Carboxyl- und Aminogruppen und zwischen den Sulfat- und Aminogruppen erfolgen. Die erforderliche Energie zur Bildung von Sulfat-Amino-Gruppen ist größer als die für Carboxyl-Amino-Gruppen. Nach JOSEPH et al. (1959) überwiegen im Knorpel die Sulfat-Amino-Bindungen.

Vor der Mineralisation ist im präossalen Gewebe ein hoher Gehalt an MPS zu beobachten. So wurde auch angenommen, daß das Chondroitinsulfat als Ca-Fänger eine Rolle spiele (SYLVÉN, 1947; BÉLANGER, 1955; AMPRINO, 1952; s. S. 352).

ENGEL et al. (1954) und JOSEPH et al. (1952) haben auf Grund elektrometrischer Untersuchungen das Ionen-Bindungsvermögen in Abhängigkeit von der elektrischen

Ladungsdichte bestimmt. Die Autoren haben die Beziehungen zwischen Ladung und Ionenbindung für Ca^{++}, Na^{+} und K^{+} in Nomogrammen dargestellt. Die Ca-Ionen-Konzentration ist dem Quadrat, das gebundene Ca dem Kubus der kolloidalen Ladungsdichte proportional. Die Natrium-Bindung erfolgt dagegen linear, wenn ionisierte und gebundene Form zusammengefaßt werden. Im Knorpelgewebe erreicht die totale Kationenkonzentration für Na das Doppelte, K das 14fache, Ca das 7fache und Mg das 11fache der Blutkonzentration. Diese Werte stimmen mit den Ergebnissen analytischer Untersuchungen am Knorpel des Hundes von EICHELBERGER et al. (1951, 1958) gut überein. Die Elektrolytkonzentration des lockeren Bindegewebes entspricht dagegen annähernd einem Ultrafiltrat des Blutes.

In vorliegendem Zusammenhange dürfte es zweckmäßig sein, eine Reihe kritischer Stimmen über unsere Vorstellungen von der Reaktionsweise der Intercellularsubstanzen aufzuführen. Wie stehen nämlich vor der Tatsache, daß nunmehr eine Fülle von Fakten über den Aufbau und die Reaktion der Intercellularsubstanzen beschrieben wurden, die schwerlich mit den alten Vorstellungen von den „Grundsubstanzen" vereinbar sind, die sich aber andererseits noch nicht zu einem vollständigen und widerspruchslosen Bilde zusammenfassen lassen. Unsere Kenntnisse wurden durch Untersuchungen mit einer Reihe von Methoden vermehrt. So entwickelte sich zwischen den Vertretern verschiedener Disziplinen eine z.T. scharfe Diskussion über den Aussagewert ihrer Befunde.

Seit langem ist bekannt, daß ein Teil der Stützgewebe relativ dicht und wasserarm, ein anderer Teil locker und wasserreich ist. Beide stehen jedoch mit dem Blut im Gleichgewicht. Weiterhin kann eine Reihe von Gewebeformen unter verschiedenen Einflüssen, wie Hormonen, ihren Wassergehalt ändern. Wenn ein solches Gewebe als „homogene Lösung" angesehen wird, müßte eine Änderung des Wassergehaltes zu einem osmotischen Ungleichgewicht führen. So kamen JOSEPH et al. (1952) und ENGEL et al. (1954) zu dem Schluß, daß die Interfibrillärsubstanz als ein zweiphasiges System anzusehen sei. Einer kolloidreichen, wasserarmen Phase steht eine kolloidarme, aber wasserreiche gegenüber. Damit ist die Änderung der Zusammensetzung einer Phase ohne Störung des Gleichgewichtes mit dem Blutplasma möglich. Bei der Annahme zweier Phasen ist das Vorhandensein einer zusätzlichen sog. Gewebsflüssigkeit nicht mehr erforderlich. Die Auffassung über die Gewebsflüssigkeit hat sich damit bei dieser Gruppe von Autoren erheblich gewandelt. GERSH und CATCHPOLE (1949) haben zunächst Gewebsflüssigkeit und „Grundsubstanz" gesondert betrachtet. GERSH (1949/50) kam dann dazu, beide im gleichen anatomischen „Raum" zu lokalisieren. Nunmehr sprechen GERSH und CATCHPOLE (1960) nicht nur von einem zweiphasigen kolloidalen System, sondern sehen auch die Kollagenfibrillen als eine teilweise Aggregation, Aufreihung und Orientierung von monomeren Kollagenmolekülen in der dichteren Phase an.

GERSH und CATCHPOLE (1949) haben auf Grund des wechselnden Ausfalles der PAS-Reaktion an verschiedenen Geweben oder dem gleichen Gewebe unter verschiedenen Einflüssen von einer Polymerisation bzw. Depolymerisation der Grundsubstanz gesprochen. Dieser Auffassung widersprachen MCMANUS (1954) und DORFMAN (1955/56) wegen mangelnder Beweiskraft der histochemischen Methoden energisch. GERSH und CATCHPOLE (1960) nehmen heute den Terminus „Polymerisation" als inkorrekt und mißverständlich zurück und ersetzen ihn durch „Aggregation". Die Autoren führen eine ganze Reihe von Befunden an der Intercellularsubstanz unter Einwirkung von Hormonen und Vitaminen (C) usw. auf, die ihrer Ansicht nach für eine Änderung des Aggregatzustandes sprechen.

DORFMAN (bei DORFMAN und SCHILLER, 1958) meint, in der biologischen Literatur würde eine allzu große Hoffnung auf die histochemischen Methoden zum Nachweis der MPS gesetzt. „The whole story of depolymerisation, I think, is based on unsound methods." Die Anwendung einer Farbreaktion allein, wie z. B. der PAS-Reaktion, ist selbst bei Vorliegen anderer biochemischer Befunde unzureichend (s. unten). Im allgemeinen wird sowohl von den Verteidigern als auch den Kritikern topochemischer Methoden zu wenig berücksichtigt, daß diese Methoden nur in Verbindung mit rein morphologischen

Befunden Aussagen von einer gewissen Sicherheit zulassen. Die Diskussionen über Wert und Unwert einer Farbreaktion sind häufig fruchtlos, weil die verschiedenen Methoden an unterschiedlichem und morphologisch nicht vergleichbarem Material gewonnen wurden.

Die biochemischen Untersuchungen der Intercellularsubstanzen können aber ebenfalls nicht zum Maßstab der Beurteilung des Zustandes dieser Stoffe erhoben werden, wenn sie auch das Odium der exakten Methode umgibt. Jede biochemische Untersuchung fordert eine Zerstörung der Struktur des Materials (PARTRIDGE und DAVIS, 1958). Somit können biochemische Erhebungen nicht zu zuverlässigen Aussagen über den nativen Zustand der MPS, ihr Molekulargewicht, ihren Aggregatzustand, ihre Teilchenform und ihre Bindung an begleitende Substanzen führen (MATHEWS, 1956; BLUMBERG und OGSTON, 1957, 1958; WEBBER und BAYLEY 1956; BERNARDI, 1957). Jedoch müssen die Ergebnisse biochemischer Untersuchungen über den Aufbau der Interfibrillärsubstanzen daraufhin geprüft werden, wie sie die an Hand morphologischer Untersuchungen gewonnenen Vorstellungen vom Bau der Stützgewebe modifizieren. Da die Gewebselemente zu physikalisch-chemischen Untersuchungen nach morphologischen Gesichtspunkten isoliert werden, muß andererseits gefragt werden, wie durch das Ergebnis dieser Untersuchungen die morphologische Klassifikation der Gewebskomponenten beeinflußt wird.

SOLOMON (1960) hat auseinandergesetzt, daß zur Wiedergabe einer beobachteten Verteilung von Radioisotopen in biologischen Systemen abstrakte Modelle entwickelt werden. Diese Modelle setzen ein biologisches System einem Mehrkammer(compartment)-System gleich. Ein Dreikammersystem wurde unter anderem bereits von SCHADE (1927, nach NETTER, 1959) für die Wasserverteilung im Körper mit einem Zellraum, Intercellularraum und einem Blutraum angenommen (s. S. 337). Ein solches abstraktes Modell kann aber keine vollgültige Repräsentation des biologischen Systems darstellen. Das verabreichte Isotop ruft eine Störung (perturbation) im biologischen System hervor. An Hand der beobachteten Verteilung des Isotopes wird das einfachste Modell entwickelt, das zur Beschreibung des kinetischen Verhaltens des Isotopes geeignet erscheint. Das Modell wirft Fragestellungen auf, die nach entsprechenden Experimenten eine Korrektur des Modells veranlassen.

Die „Kammer" kann als Äquivalent einer anatomisch-physiologischen Region, z. B. der Zelle, zugeordnet werden. Im Hinblick auf den Reaktionsmechanismus kann die Kammer einer Phase analog gesetzt werden, wobei im Hinblick auf die Thermodynamik für diese Phase eine homogene Zusammensetzung vorausgesetzt wird. In der molekularen Dimension ist streng zwischen dem gelösten Molekül und dem des Lösungsmittels zu unterscheiden. Diese Unterschiede werden aber häufig vernachlässigt, indem das Verhalten aller Moleküle zusammengefaßt wird. Ähnliche Vereinfachungen werden auch im Hinblick auf anatomisch-physiologische Elemente gemacht. Die Zelle wird durch eine Reihe von Untereinheiten — Kern, Hyaloplasma, Ergastoplasma, Mitochondrien usw. — repräsentiert, die in ihrer Gesamtheit als eine homogene Reaktionseinheit zusammengefaßt werden. So stellt die im Modell vorausgesetzte Einheit in der anatomischen Dimension eine größere Vereinfachung als im Bereich der thermodynamisch bestimmten Phasen dar. Die Bezeichnung „Kammer" kann aber auch auf eine chemische Substanz als Reacktionseinheit bezogen werden.

Von sehr verschiedenen Seiten wird darauf hingewiesen, daß viele der Vorstellungen über ein reagierendes Substrat als Modelle anzusehen sind. DORFMAN (Diskussion DORFMAN und SCHILLER, 1958) hält z. B. die Beschreibung von MATHEWS (1956) des gestreckten oder geknäuelten Zustandes der MPS-Ketten nicht für ein getreues Abbild der physiologischen Verhältnisse, sondern nur für eine Illustration der physiko-chemischen Reaktionsform dieser Substanzen. GERSH und CATCHPOLE (1960) sehen das Zweiphasensystem als die geringste, aber ausreichende Anzahl von Phasen an, die zur Beschreibung der Eigenheiten der Intercellularsubstanzen ausreichen; das Vorhandensein polyphasischer Systeme kann physiko-chemisch nicht ausgeschlossen werden.

Den Ausführungen von SOLOMON (1960) und anderer Autoren ist demgemäß zu entnehmen, daß die auf Grund physikalisch-chemischer Untersuchungen entwickelten Vorstellungen über den Aufbau der Interfibrillärsubstanz Modelle zur Erfassung der beobachteten Reaktionsform darstellen; es sind „Rechenregeln", mit denen der funktionale Zusammenhang zwischen verschiedenen Phänomen analytisch oder graphisch wiedergegeben wird. So ist es nicht verwunderlich, daß zur Beschreibung des Verhaltens von radioaktivem Ca im Organismus eine verwirrende Vielfalt von Vorgängen (NEUMAN, BRONNER, COMAR bei MARSHALL, 1960) wie Neubildung von Substanzen, Zuwachs, kurz- oder langfristiger Austausch, Rekristallisation oder Neuverteilung (redistribution) angenommen wurde. Die intensive Untersuchung der Ablagerung von Radioisotopen hat zu der Einsicht geführt, daß dem Einbau dieser Substanzen vielfältige, zum großen Teil noch unbekannte Vorgänge vorausgehen (u. a. DORFMAN und SCHILLER, 1958). Unter diesem Gesichtspunkt müssen zahlreiche Hypothesen, z. B. über den Umbau des Knochens, überprüft werden, die an Hand von Ablagerungen markierter Stoffe Aussagen über die begleitenden oder parallelgehenden histologischen Vorgänge gemacht haben (KNESE und TITSCHAK, 1962).

Sowohl die morphologische Klassifizierung der Gewebeelemente als auch die Beschreibung des physikalisch-chemischen Verhaltens dieser Substanzen und damit ihrer molekularen Organisation sind nur unter Berücksichtigung der jeweiligen Untersuchungsmethoden gerecht zu würdigen. Dabei ist zu diskutieren, ob konkurrierende Aussagen im Hinblick auf die gleiche Dimension vorliegen oder ob verschiedene Bereiche eines Gewebes beschrieben werden. Bei dieser Diskussion kann auf die Vorstellung einer Strukturhierarchie (s. S. 317) zurückgegriffen werden, wie sie für das Knochengewebe entwickelt wurde, die aber in wenig modifizierter Form für alle Stützgewebe gilt. Die Struktur 6. Ordnung, die Ultrastruktur der Gewebskomponenten, ist vermutlich für alle Stützgewebe von gleicher oder sehr ähnlicher Organisation. So wurde auch die Ultrastruktur der Gewebekomponenten jeweils an dem Gewebe untersucht, das die entsprechende Substanz in größerer Menge oder in leicht zugänglicher Form enthält. Die Übertragung der gewonnenen Ergebnisse im Hinblick auf Struktur und Reaktionsform auf andere Gewebsformen ist wohl mit geringen Einschränkungen möglich.

Bei der weiteren Darstellung beziehen wir uns nur auf das Knorpelgewebe. Die Struktur 5. Ordnung umfaßt beim Knorpel die Beziehungen zwischen den Fibrillen und den restlichen Elementen. Als Struktur 4. Ordnung ist die Verteilung und Ordnung der Fibrillen einschließlich der weiteren Substanzen im Aufbau der Kapseln, Höfe und Interterritorien zu beschreiben. Die Struktur 3. Ordnung gibt die Beziehungen zwischen den Chondrocyten und der sie umgebenden Intercellularsubstanz wieder. Als letzte, 2. Ordnung im Bereich der mikroskopischen Anatomie ist die spezifische Gestaltung des Gelenk-, Epiphysen-, Rippen- usw. Knorpels anzusehen.

Die Beachtung einer derartigen Strukturhierarchie „fördert die gedankliche Synthese der Strukturen — und damit der Funktionen — auf den verschiedenen Größenstufen, die für biologische Einsicht unentbehrlich ist. Verfolgen der Struktur nur in Richtung auf das Kleinste — so nötig es ist! — führt letzten Endes zu Molekeln und Atomen, die als solche keinen Einblick in die Lebenserscheinungen zu geben vermögen. Vielmehr beruhen diese auf der spezifischen abgestuften Ordnung (und den damit gegebenen Wirkungsmöglichkeiten), die von den chemischen Bausteinen bis zum ganzen Organismus reicht" (W. J. SCHMIDT, 1957). Durch eine solche Ordnungseinteilung wird die Dimension angegeben, in die bestimmte Beobachtungen einzuordnen sind. Vorgänge in einer Ordnungsstufe basieren auf einem komplexen Reaktionssystem mit einer Reihe von Zwischenprozessen. Bei Untersuchung der nächsten Ordnung kann die niedere Stufe dagegen häufig als ein einheitliches System angesehen werden. Prozesse in benachbarten Ordnungen können sich nicht gegenseitig vertreten, sie sind nach verschiedenen und nicht homologen Gesichtspunkten zu diskutieren. Ein Beispiel für die Untersuchung der Aufgaben der einzelnen Strukturordnungen im Hinblick auf die mechanische Leistung des Knochengewebes hat KNESE (1958) gegeben. Entsprechende Untersuchungen, z. B. im Hinblick auf den Stoffwechsel des Knorpel- oder Knochengewebes, stehen noch aus, könnten aber vermutlich sich scheinbar widersprechende Beobachtungen über die Ablagerung von Radioisotopen aufklären.

Mit anatomischen Methoden wird die Gewebsstruktur bis zur 5. Ordnung untersucht, physiko-chemische Methoden erfassen, wenn auch nicht ausschließlich, die Molekularbiologie der Gewebselemente und damit die Struktur 6. Ordnung. Die Morphologie untersucht die Lokalisation der Gewebeelemente, die Gewebetopographie, physikalisch-chemische Methoden die Reaktionsform dieser Elemente und zwar weitgehend unabhängig von der Topographie. So werden z. B. bei Untersuchung der Wasserverteilung alle Zellen des Körpers unter Vernachlässigung ihrer morphologischen Differenzen zusammengefaßt und in gleicher Weise alle intercellulären Räume.

Morphologische und physiko-chemische Klassifikationen stehen wegen der unterschiedlichen Einteilungsprinzipien gleichberechtigt nebeneinander, können sich ergänzen, aber sich nicht gegenseitig ersetzen und sich nur in wenigen Bereichen (Dimensionen) decken. Topographisch ist demzufolge zwischen einer Perifibrillärsubstanz, die die Fibrillen umgibt, und einer Interfibrillärsubstanz zu unterscheiden. Dabei ist unter morphologischen Gesichtspunkten gleichgültig, ob beide eine verschiedene chemische Zusammensetzung aufweisen oder nicht. Eine Reihe von Erhebungen sprechen für einen differenten Aufbau von Peri- und Interfibrillärsubstanz (s. S. 336).

Allerdings sind die biochemischen Befunde über eine Reaktionsform der Intercellularsubstanzen eines Geweboortes dazu geeignet, manche anatomischen Vorstellungen zu korrigieren. Bestimmte Formen des Faserknorpels im Bereich von Sehnen- und Bandansätzen wurden mitunter als Mischgewebe bezeichnet (DRAHN, 1922; WEIDENREICH, 1923a; SCHNEIDER, 1955, 1956), da sie Charaktere verschiedener sog. „reiner" Gewebeformen aufweisen. Diese Auffassung wurde bereits unter rein histologischen Aspekten von KNESE und BIERMANN (1958) kritisiert. Auf Grund der biochemisch nachgewiesenen Reaktionseinheit innerhalb eines Gewebes ist die Vorstellung von Mischgeweben abzulehnen. Zur Zeit gelingt es allerdings noch nicht, an Hand der morphologischen Kennzeichen verwickelte Gewebeformen wie die verschiedenen Arten von Faserknorpel in das Gewebesystem von SCHAFFER (1930) einzuordnen. Die geringe Anzahl von Gewebekomponenten ermöglicht offensichtlich durch ihren komplexen Aufbau eine vielfältige und ortspezifische Gestaltung der Stützgewebe, die sich einer Klassifizierung entzieht. Hinzu kommen Änderungen des physiko-chemischen Profils (ENGEL et al., 1960) im Laufe des Individuallebens und unter veränderten hormonellen Situationen.

Besondere Schwierigkeiten bereiten „Übergangszonen", in denen eine Gewebeform in eine andere übergeht, z. B. eine Sehne in Knochengewebe. Ein „Umbau" zu einer anderen Stützgewebeform setzt eine ganze Reihe von Vorgängen voraus, die sowohl von den Zellen als auch von der Intercellularsubstanz ausgehen. Die Auswirkung derartiger lokalisiert beginnender Prozesse „stört" das gesamte Gleichgewicht und kommt damit zur Auswirkung an allen Gewebekomponenten. In diesem Zusammenhang sei an die mit gallocyaninpositiven Substanzen beladenen chondroiden Zellen und die abweichenden Reaktionsformen der dazwischen gelegenen Sehnenfasern erinnert (s. S. 683).

GERSH und CATCHPOLE (1960) meinen, die Herkunft der einzelnen Gewebekomponenten — aus dem Blut oder den Zellen bzw. aus beiden Quellen — sei von geringer Bedeutung. Unter morphologisch-topographischen Gesichtspunkten ist jedoch die Quelle der verschiedenen Substanzen von großem Interesse. Die Intercellularsubstanzen stellen nämlich nicht nur eine Anhäufung von Substanzen mit bestimmten Eigenschaften dar, sondern sind ein Glied in der Strukturhierarchie der Gewebe, d. h. eines biologischen Systems.

Für den Stoffwechsel der Intercellularsubstanzen, voran der MPS, sind demzufolge folgende Einzelprozesse anzunehmen (nach GIBIAN, 1959):

1. Änderungen in der Synthese der Ausgangsprodukte für eine MPS-Bildung; der Ort dieser Vorgänge ist vermutlich intracellulär.

2. Änderungen in der Synthese — ebenfalls intracellulär — der MPS selbst.
3. Abbau der MPS, der wahrscheinlich extracellulär abläuft.
4. Änderungen in der Zu- bzw. Abfuhr von Ausgangs- und Endprodukten des MPS-Stoffwechsels.
5. Änderungen der Ionen-Konzentration und des p_H der Intercellularsubstanzen.

Diese Vorgänge dürften überwiegend fermentativ gesteuert werden; allerdings sind die in vivo wirkenden Fermente z. T. noch unbekannt, da Beobachtungen in vitro nicht ohne weiteres auf die Verhältnisse in vivo übertragen werden können. So ist auch der Wirkungsmechanismus bzw. der Angriffspunkt von Hormonen und Pharmaca im Stoffwechsel der MPS noch unklar (DORFMAN und SCHILLER, 1958; ASBOE-HANSEN, 1966).

δ) Die Darstellung von Kohlenhydraten und Mucopolysacchariden durch Färbung im Schnitt

LILLIE (1952) hat den Wirkungsmechanismus älterer Bindegewebsfärbungen (VAN GIESON, AZAN, MASSON) erörtert. Neuere sog. topochemische Färbemethoden haben zum Ziel, bestimmte Substanzen oder reaktionsfähige Gruppen in Gewebeelementen nachzuweisen. Der Färbetechnik gewidmete Werke (PEARSE, 1960; LILLIE, 1965; LIPP, 1954; CASSELMANN, 1959; ROMEIS, 1948; MCMANUS und MOWRY, 1964) enthalten auch theoretische Angaben über den Wirkungsmechanismus der einzelnen Methoden. Eingehende Darstellungen über die Spezifität der Färbungen geben unter anderem MCMANUS (1954), HALE (1957) und CURRAN (1961, 1964). Der Einfluß der Fixierung (vgl. ZEIGER, 1960), des p_H der Farbflotte sowie die unterschiedliche Natur der Farbstoffe verschiedener Firmen (vgl. auch HARMS, 1957) werden z.Zt. diskutiert.

Die bisher bekannten Bindegewebsfärbungen erwiesen sich als nicht spezifisch für bestimmte, chemisch zu definierende Substanzen, nicht einmal immer für bestimmte Gruppen. Jedes Färbungsergebnis ist daher an Kontrollpräparaten derselben Schnittserie nach einer Vorbehandlung mit Enzymen wie Hyaluronidase, Diastase, aber auch Pepsin, Ribonuclease, Desoxyribonuclease zu vergleichen. Allerdings enthalten auch die angebotenen hochgereinigten Enzympräparate noch Beimengungen, vor allem wohl Proteasen. Auf derartige Stoffe sind vermutlich unerwartete Enzymwirkungen zurückzuführen, z. B. die Veränderung der Metachromasie der Intercellularsubstanz des Knorpels durch Ribonuclease (KNESE und KNOOP, 1961a).

Perjodsäure-Schiff-Reaktion (PJS, PAS). Die von MCMANUS (1946), LILLIE (1947) und HOTCHKISS (1948) angegebene Reaktion wird in der Literatur im allgemeinen in der englischen Abkürzungsform PAS aufgeführt. Die durch Perjodsäure gebildeten Aldehydgruppen werden mit Schiffschem Reagens (Leukofuchsin) nachgewiesen. Die Reaktion ist demgemäß weder für Kohlenhydrate noch MPS spezifisch. Niedermolekulare Substanzen sollen sich wegen der hohen Anzahl von Endgruppen stärker anfärben als hochmolekulare. Auf Grund der unterschiedlichen Anfärbungen wurden demzufolge Rückschlüsse auf den Polymerisationsgrad gezogen (GERSH und CATCHPOLE, 1949, 1960; s. S. 707). JOEL et al. (1956) haben im Vergleich mit der Hale-Reaktion für den Knorpel an Hand der zunehmenden PAS-positiven Reaktion auf eine Abnahme an Glykogen und sauren MPS gegenüber den neutralen Polysacchariden im Verlaufe der Alterung geschlossen. Die Oxydation mit Perjodsäure kann auch durch eine solche mit Bleitetraacetat ersetzt werden (GRAUMANN, 1953); das Färbungsergebnis weicht dann aber von dem der Originalmethode ab.

Basophilie. Saure MPS können auch durch Prüfung der Basophilie nachgewiesen werden. Hierzu verwendet man Methylenblau in einer Lösung von verschiedenem p_H. Eine Kontrolle mit Orange G, das sich in der Anfärbbarkeit bei verschiedenem p_H zu Methylenblau spiegelbildlich verhält, gestattet die Bestimmung des isoelektrischen Punktes. Zur Abgrenzung gegen Nucleinsäuren ist ein doppelter Test mit Ribonuclease und Hyaluronidase erforderlich. Nicht selten zeigt die Intercellularsubstanz, aber auch das Cytoplasma, mit Methylenblau eine metachromatische Farbreaktion.

Durch STEEDMAN (1950) wurde Alcianblau zur Schleimfärbung eingeführt und in der Zukunft von einer Reihe von Autoren auch bei Knorpel angewandt (QUINTARELLI, SCOTT und DELLOVO, 1964a, b; QUINTARELLI und DELLOVO, 1965). QUINTARELLI, SAJDERA und DZIEWIATKOWSKI (1968) haben versucht, den Färbungsmechanismus und die Spezifität der Alcianblau für bestimmte MPS-Protein-Fraktionen aufzuklären.

Metachromasie. Als Metachromasie bezeichnen wir die Anfärbung von Gewebeelementen in einem Farbton, der von dem der Farbflotte abweicht. Von den vielen bekannten Farbstoffen werden vor allem Toluidinblau und Azur A verwandt (vgl. HARMS, 1957; KNESE, 1966a). Die metachromatische Farbe ist rot bis violett und hat damit eine größere Wellenlänge als das orthochromatische Blau. Je nachdem, welche Adsorptionsbande erscheint, wird auch zwischen γ-(rot)- und β-(violett)-Metachromasie (MICHAELIS, 1947) unterschieden.

Über die Bedeutung der Metachromasie liegt eine umfangreiche Literatur vor (u. a. LISON, 1935; MICHAELIS 1947; WISLOCKI et al., 1947; SYLVÉN, 1947, 1948; LILLIE, 1950; VITRY, 1958; SZIRMAI und BALAZS, 1958; SZIRMAI, 1963). SYLVÉN (1954) hat eine große Reihe von Substanzen auf ihre Reaktion hin geprüft und kommt zu der Auffassung, daß zum Auftreten einer Metachromasie eine entsprechende Anzahl von elektronegativen Ladungen mit einem Abstand geringer als 5 Å erforderlich ist. Bei diesen Ladungen kann es sich um Sulfate, Phosphate, aber auch um Carboxylgruppen handeln. Zum Nachweis von sauren MPS vermittels der Metachromasie ist eine enzymatische Kontrolle mit einer Hydrolyse durch Hyaluronidase notwendig, die auch auf Chondroitinsulfat einwirkt. Durch Testishyaluronidase tritt eine stufenweise Desaggregation und Depolymerisation zu Tetrasacchariden, durch Bakterienhyaluronidase zu Oligo- und Monosacchariden ein (MEYER, 1947; GIBIAN, 1954, 1959; DORFMANN, 1955/56).

Durch eine Variation des p_H der Farbflotte wird die metachromatische Reaktion der verschiedenen Strukturen spezifischer (SMITH und ATKINSON, 1956; KNESE und KNOOP, 1961a; KNESE, 1966a). Diese Methode hat sich bei Untersuchung der einzelnen Abschnitte der Intercellularsubstanz des Knorpels sowie der Chondrocyten als vorteilhaft erwiesen (KNESE und KNOOP, 1961a, c).

Die metachromatische Reaktion ist durch eine ganze Reihe von Maßnahmen, unter anderem Zugabe von Salzlösungen, zu beeinflussen. Da in situ die MPS selten isoliert auftreten, können durch die Gegenwart von Proteinen anionische Gruppen blockiert werden, wodurch auch die Metachromasie herabgesetzt wird (KELLY, 1958; HAMERMAN und SCHUBERT, 1953; FRENCH und BENDITT, 1953).

Eisenhydroxyd-Berliner Blau-Reaktion. Diese Reaktion beruht auf der Bindung von kolloidalem Eisen-III-hydroxyd an saure Gruppen, wobei diese Bindungen durch Berliner Blau sichtbar gemacht werden (HALE, 1946). Auch diese Methode ist für MPS nicht spezifisch, da neben sauren Gruppen der Polysaccharide auch Polynucleotide und Phospholipide eine gleiche Reaktion zeigen (IMMERS, 1954). Von MÜLLER (1955/56, 1959) und GRAUMANN (1958) wurden Modifikationen der Hale-Technik empfohlen. Nach KNESE und KNOOP (1961c) sind vermutlich durch die Methode von GRAUMANN mehr intercellulare, durch die von MÜLLER (1955/56) dagegen extracelluläre saure MPS darzustellen. GRAUMANN hatte aus der negativen Farbreaktion der Intercellularsubstanz des Appositionsknorpels geschlossen, daß an die Polysaccharide noch keine Sulfatgruppen gebunden sind; das Vorhandensein von Sulfatgruppen in diesen Gebieten ist aber durch autoradiographische Untersuchungen gesichert.

Die Spezifität topochemischer Reaktionen. Der Streit um die Spezifität topochemischer Methoden ist ungewöhnlich heftig, die Kritik an diesen Methoden zur Untersuchung von Intercellularsubstanzen z. T. vernichtend (DORFMAN bei DORFMAN und SCHILLER, 1958). Im Rahmen einer solchen kurzen Übersicht kann in keiner Weise erschöpfend zu diesem Streit Stellung genommen werden. Ohne Zweifel haben einige Autoren die Spezifität der von ihnen angegebenen Methoden überschätzt. Im allgemeinen wird übersehen, daß topochemische Farbreaktionen von Gewebestrukturen nicht auf derselben Ebene stehen wie chemische Reaktionen in vitro. SPICER, LEPPI und STOWARD (1965) haben auf Grund histochemischer Reaktionen eine Klassifikation der „Mucosubstanzen" aufgestellt. Die Kritik von K. MEYER (1966) an dieser Klassifikation verdient besondere Beachtung, da dieser Autor in vielen Äußerungen den Wert histologischer Untersuchungen am Schnitt voll anerkannt hat. MEYER weist auf die bereits vorliegenden Schwierigkeiten auf Grund der komplexen, polydispersen und heterogenen Struktur der „Mucosubstanzen" hin. Es sei auch nicht berechtigt, eine histologische Reaktion auf eine spezifische chemische Gruppe zu beziehen, die mit chemischen Methoden an isolierten und abgebauten Substanzen nachgewiesen wurde. Auf der anderen Seite würde aber der Biochemiker durch topochemische Untersuchungen auf Beobachtungen hingewiesen, die eine weitere Untersuchung erforderlich machten.

Weiterhin darf nicht vergessen werden, daß zu jeder chemischen Analyse ein recht umfangreiches Ausgangsmaterial erforderlich ist. So liegen recht umfangreiche Untersuchungen über den Nasenknorpel und das Hautbindegewebe vor. Histologen beschäftigen sich demgegenüber mit sehr kleinen und recht different aufgebauten Regionen, wie z.B. dem Epiphysenknorpel, die derzeit einer biochemischen Untersuchung noch nicht zugänglich sind. Der Wunsch, die aufgefundenen Differenzen qualitativ zu interpretieren, ist verständlich, die Berechtigung hierzu aber an Hand der angewandten Methoden zu bezweifeln. Auf der anderen Seite wollen wir auf den interessanten Versuch von LINDENBAUM und KUETTNER (1967) hinweisen, die mit analytischen Methoden die Differenzen der einzelnen Zonen des Epiphysenknorpels untersuchten. Sie wählten hierzu das Schulterblatt des Kalbes, um genügend Material zur Verfügung zu haben. Morphologisch muß aber festgestellt werden, daß die Knorpelknochenverbindung der Scapula nicht den Aufbau der Epiphyse eines langen Röhrenknochens aufweist, wie wir an Mensch und Ratte beobachteten und wie es die Bilder der Autoren zeigen. Die Verhältnisse der Scapula sind morphologisch jenen im Bereich eines Knochenkernes recht ähnlich.

In der angewandten Topochemie muß gefordert werden, daß im allgemeinen für jede Färbungsdifferenz auch ein morphologisches Äquivalent vorhanden ist. KNESE und KNOOP (1961a) haben z. B. am Metacarpus von Rinderfeten mit den Methoden zum Nachweis von Kohlenhydraten und MPS an Schnittserien die Anfärbbarkeit der Intercellularsubstanz des Knorpels geprüft. Die Autoren kommen zu dem Schluß, daß mit den verschiedenen Methoden mitunter ein Färbungsergebnis von gleicher Deutungsmöglichkeit zu erhalten ist. In anderen Fällen treten aber starke Differenzen auf, die jedoch auch morphologisch voneinander abweichende Zonen des Epiphysenknorpels betreffen. Fast verwirrend wird das Färbungsergebnis, wenn ein Vergleich mit den enzymatischen Kontrollen herangezogen wird, da Ribo- und Desoxyribonuclease die Färbung der Intercellularsubstanzen beeinflussen. Unter Beachtung der verwickelten, nur z. T. aufgeklärten Ultrastruktur der Intercellularsubstanzen kann aus einer Färbungsdifferenz nur dann auf einen unterschiedlichen stofflichen und strukturellen Aufbau geschlossen werden, wenn hierfür weitere morphologische Fakten sprechen. Worauf diese Differenzen aber beruhen, kann selbst vermutungsweise nicht gesagt werden. Auf Grund der verschiedenen Form und Lagerung der Zellen wurde im Epiphysenknorpel eine Reihe von Zonen unterschieden. Wenn nun zusätzlich durch Färbung ein differenter Aufbau der Intercellularsubstanz wahrscheinlich gemacht werden kann, liegt darin eine wesentliche Erweiterung unserer Kenntnisse. Mit anderen Methoden kann man dann versuchen, die Grundlage der unterschiedlichen Färbung aufzuklären.

Topochemische und analytisch chemische Untersuchungen stehen im Hinblick auf ihre „Naturtreue" eigentlich auf einer Ebene. Die Topochemie erhält den Organverband, kann aber keine klaren stofflichen Aussagen machen, die analytische Chemie zerschlägt den Gewebeverband und ist dann fähig, sog. saubere Analysen durchzuführen.

ε) *Bildung des Mucopolysaccharid-Protein-Komplexes*

Die Biosynthese der MPS kann unter biochemischen und morphologischen Gesichtspunkten untersucht werden. Der Aufbau aus einer Hexuronsäure und einem Hexosamin fordert zunächst die Bildung dieser monomeren Bestandteile, die dann zu der Disaccharideinheit zusammentreten. Ausgangspunkt für beide ist vermutlich die Glucose der jeweiligen Zelle (DORFMAN, 1955/56; ZAMBOTTI, 1957; BAZIN und DELAUNAY, 1959; GIBIAN, 1959; BRIMACOMBE und WEBBER, 1964; BUDDECKE, 1966; BOSTRÖM und RODÉN, 1966), wobei allerdings noch nicht alle Schritte dieser Synthese gesichert sind.

Die Biosynthese der Hyaluronsäure und des Chondroitinsulfates (Tabelle 2) verlangt die Bildung einer β-Bindung, einer Polymerisation und den Wechsel von Uronsäure und

Tabelle 2. *Voraussichtlicher Stoffwechsel bei der Glykosaminoglycan-Biosynthese* (nach BOSTRÖM und RODÉN 1966)

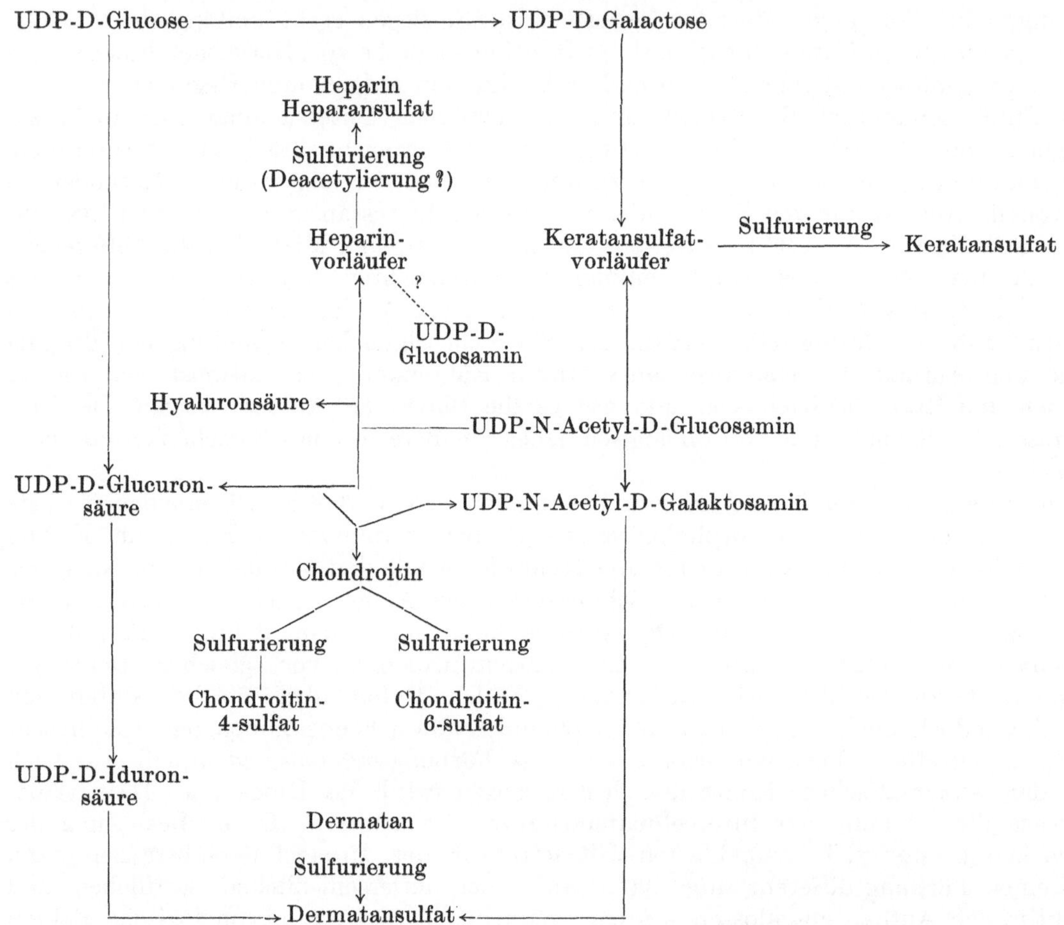

Aminozuckern in der Molekülkette (MARKOVITZ et al., 1959). Bei der Hexosamin-Bildung sind vier Schritte anzunehmen (vgl. BAZIN und DELAUNAY, 1959): 1. Phosphorylation (C_6), 2. Amination, 3. Acetylation, 4. Bindung an UTP; bei der Hexuronsäurebildung drei Schritte: 1. Phosphorylation (C_1), 2. Bindung an UTP und 3. Oxydation. Über das Verhalten der Uridindiphosphatzucker bei der MPS-Synthese und den entsprechenden Stoffwechsel der Uridinnucleotide unterrichten DORFMAN (1963) und STROMINGER (1964). Die Polymerisation wird als eine nucleophile Substitutionsreaktion aufgefaßt (BUDDECKE, 1966). Bei dem viel diskutierten Sulfateinbau wird heute angenommen, daß er offensichtlich sowohl in der Stufe des Oligosaccharides als auch Polysaccharides durchgeführt werden kann (KENT, 1961). Der Sulfateinbau erfolgt über ein aktives Sulfat (PAPS:

3-Phosphoradenosin-5-Phosphosulfat; ROBBINS und LIPMANN, 1956). Für cytologische Untersuchungen ist von besonderem Interesse, daß D'ABRAMO und LIPMANN (1957) ein partikelfreies Multienzymsystem aus Hühnchenknorpel isolierten, so daß die Chondroitinsulfatsynthese in einem löslichen System, d.h. im Zellsaft oder Hyaloplasma anzunehmen ist (s.u.). Mit weiteren zellfreien Systemen gelangt die Synthese der Bindungsregionen für die Protein-Polysaccharidbindung (TELSER, ROBINSON und DORFMAN, 1965; TELSER, ROBINSON und DORFMAN, 1966), ebenso die Steuerung der Alternativeinwanderung von N-Acetylgalaktosamin und Uronsäure (PERLMAN, TELSER und DORFMAN, 1964; TELSER und ROBINSON und DORFMAN, 1966).

Bei einer Untersuchung der Morphologie der MPS-Bildung erhebt sich die Frage, sind diese Substanzen 1. ein Sekretionsprodukt von Zellen, 2. ein „transformiertes" Cytoplasma oder 3. sind sie unabhängig von Zellen entstanden. Alle drei Hypothesen der Entstehung extracellulärer Substanzen wurden diskutiert (s. S. 332). Die Rolle der Zellen bei Bildung der Intercellularsubstanzen kann in situ aus topochemischen Reaktionen durch Beobachtung der Ablagerung von Radioisotopen und aus elektronenmikroskopischen Untersuchungen erschlossen werden. Bei Untersuchungen von Gewebekulturen ergibt sich auch die Möglichkeit, die gebildeten Stoffe biochemisch zu analysieren.

Eine einfache Umwandlung von Teilen des Cytoplasmas in Intercellularsubstanz kann heute auf Grund elektronenmikroskopischer Untersuchungen ausgeschlossen werden. Die Tätigkeitsform der Bildungszellen des Stützgewebes wurde seit langem mit der von Drüsenzellen verglichen (Lit. bei KNESE, 1956a, 1967a; KNESE und KNOOP, 1961c). Als Begründung für diese Auffassung wurde angeführt, daß in diesen Zellen mit Radioisotopen markierte Substanzen gebildet werden, die in den Extracellularraum abgegeben werden (GREULICH und LEBLOND, 1953; BÉLANGER, 1956a, b; AMPRINO, 1955, 1956). Weiterhin wurde auf die sehr ähnliche Morphologie von Drüsenzellen und Bildungszellen, besonders im Hinblick auf die Ausbildung des endoplasmatischen Reticulums, hingewiesen (SHELDON und ROBINSON, 1957; KNESE und KNOOP, 1958). KNESE und KNOOP (1961c) haben gezeigt, daß ein Vergleich zwischen Drüsenzellen und skeletogenen Zellen nur im Hinblick auf die Struktur der Zellen, aber nicht mit Rücksicht auf die gebildeten Stoffe berechtigt ist. Die sekretorische Tätigkeit der Drüsenzellen spielt sich in einem ausdifferenzierten Organverband ab, das Sekret wird aus dem Organ abgeführt. Die von den skeletogenen Zellen gebildeten Stoffe werden dagegen zu extracellulären Komponenten des Gewebes; die Stoffproduktion ist ein entscheidender Anteil der Strukturbildung und Gewebedifferenzierung.

Die Untersuchung der Zelleistung bei Bildung des MPS-Protein-Komplexes bereitet große Schwierigkeiten, da diese Stoffe zu den „amorphen" Teilen der Intercellularsubstanz gehören. Von ASBOE-HANSEN (1957) wurde die Bildung von Hyaluronsäure durch Mastzellen angegeben; heute bringt man die Mastzellen nur noch mit der Bildung von Heparin in Zusammenhang. Die Synthese von Hyaluronsäure durch Fibroblasten konnte von CURRAN (1953), GROSSFELD et al. (1955), KLING et al. (1955) und anderen nachgewiesen werden. GROSSFELD et al. (1957), MANCINI et al. (1956), BERENSON et al. (1958) beobachteten die Bildung von Sulfo-MPS durch Fibroblasten. MOORE et al. (1957) und SCHOENBERG et al. (1957, 1958) stellten die Bildung von Oligosacchariden als Vorläufer der MPS durch Fibroblasten sicher. Der Nachweis der Bildung von MPS durch Chondroblasten gelang dann BÉLANGER (1954) und AMPRINO (1955) mit Hilfe von ^{35}S. Die Ablagerung von ^{35}S ist nach Behandlung mit Hyaluronidase nicht mehr nachzuweisen, so daß der Einbau des Radiosulfates in Chondroitinsulfat als gesichert anzunehmen ist (DZIEWIATKOWSKI, 1951, 1958; BOSTRÖM et al., 1952; BÉLANGER, 1954; GREULICH, 1956).

Die topochemischen Untersuchungen über die MPS-Bildung gehen auf Beobachtungen von PAS-positiven Granula in einer Reihe von Zellen der Stützgewebe zurück (GERSH et al., 1949; MANCINI et al., 1951; FOLLIS und BERTHRONG, 1949; HELLER-STEINBERG, 1951; PRITCHARD, 1952). McMANUS (1954), KNESE (1959a) und KNESE und KNOOP (1961a, c) zeigten, daß diese Granula nicht in allen Zellen nachweisbar sind, die vermutlich mit einer MPS-Synthese in Verbindung stehen. Die PAS-Reaktion fällt auch an Zellen aus vergleichbarem Untersuchungsgut unterschiedlich aus. Vor allem fehlen PAS-positive Granula in Chondroblasten, für die eine MPS-Synthese in großem Umfange anzunehmen ist. Chondroblasten verhalten sich im übrigen gegen eine größere Zahl von Farbstoffen

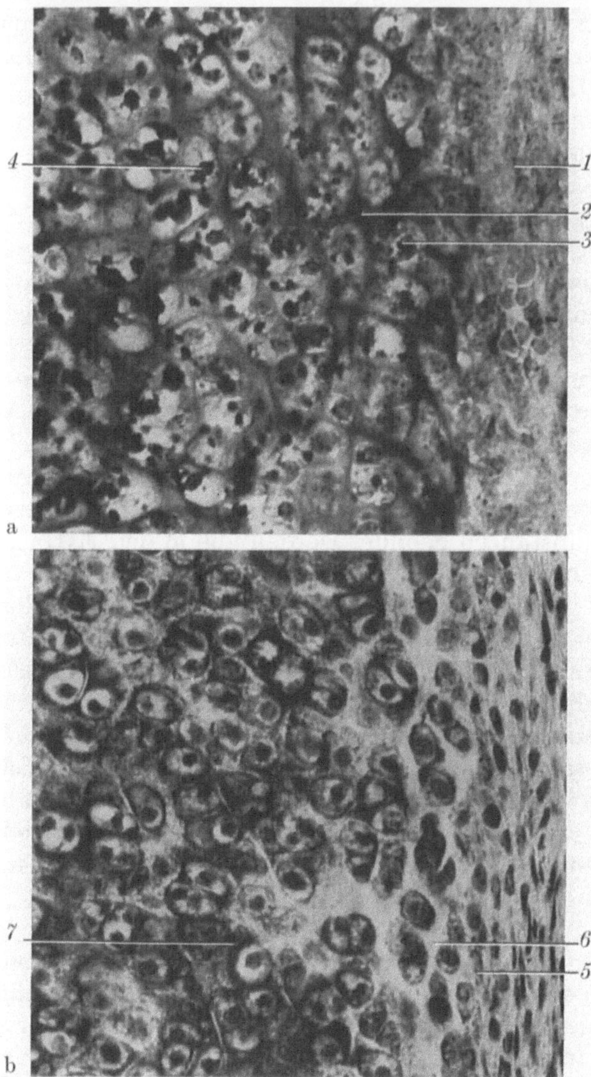

Abb. 16a u. b. Perichondrium und Knorpel. a Färbung mit HALEs kolloidaler Eisenlösung. b Polysaccharid-Eisenreaktion nach GRAUMANN. a *1* Perichondrium; *2* Intercellularsubstanz des Appositionsknorpels, tief dunkelblau; *3* Chondrocyten des Appositionsknorpels mit kleinen blauen Granula; *4* Zellen des hyalinen Epiphysenknorpels mit verschieden großen Granula. b *5* Perichondrium, zentrale Chondroblasten mit geringer Cytoplasmafärbung; *6* Appositionsknorpel, Intercellularsubstanz fast farblos, schmale Knorpelkapseln; *7* hyaliner Epiphysenknorpel. Färbung der Intercellularsubstanz nimmt mit dem Abstand von den Knorpelkapseln ab. Metacarpus eines Rinderfeten von 126 mm SSL. Vergr. 480. (KNESE u. KNOOP, 1961a)

refraktär. Die Verteilung und Größe der Granula in Periostzellen ist mit der BTS-Reaktion (GRAUMANN, 1953) von der mit PAS verschieden (KNESE und KNOOP, 1961c). Die mit Färbemethoden in Zellen nachweisbaren Kohlenhydrate unterliegen am gleichen Ort bei verschiedenen Individuen der gleichen Spezies großen Schwankungen (FOLLIS und BERTHRONG, 1949; PRITCHARD, 1956; TONNA und CRONKITE, 1959; KNESE und KNOOP, 1961a, c).

Die Basophilie der Chondroblasten, d. h. ihre Anfärbbarkeit mit Methylenblau in einem p_H unter 4,0, ist gering, so daß sie sich eindeutig von den stark basophilen Osteoblasten unterscheiden. Auch die metachromatische Reaktion der Chondroblasten mit Toluidinblau ist geringer als die der Osteoblasten. Bei Färbung mit Toluidinblau ist in den Osteoblasten ein dunkelblau-violett tingiertes Netzwerk zu beobachten; die Netzmaschen enthalten mehr hellrot-violettes Material (KNESE und KNOOP, 1961c; TONNA und CRONKITE, 1959). Mit der Polysaccharid-Eisen-Reaktion von GRAUMANN (1958)

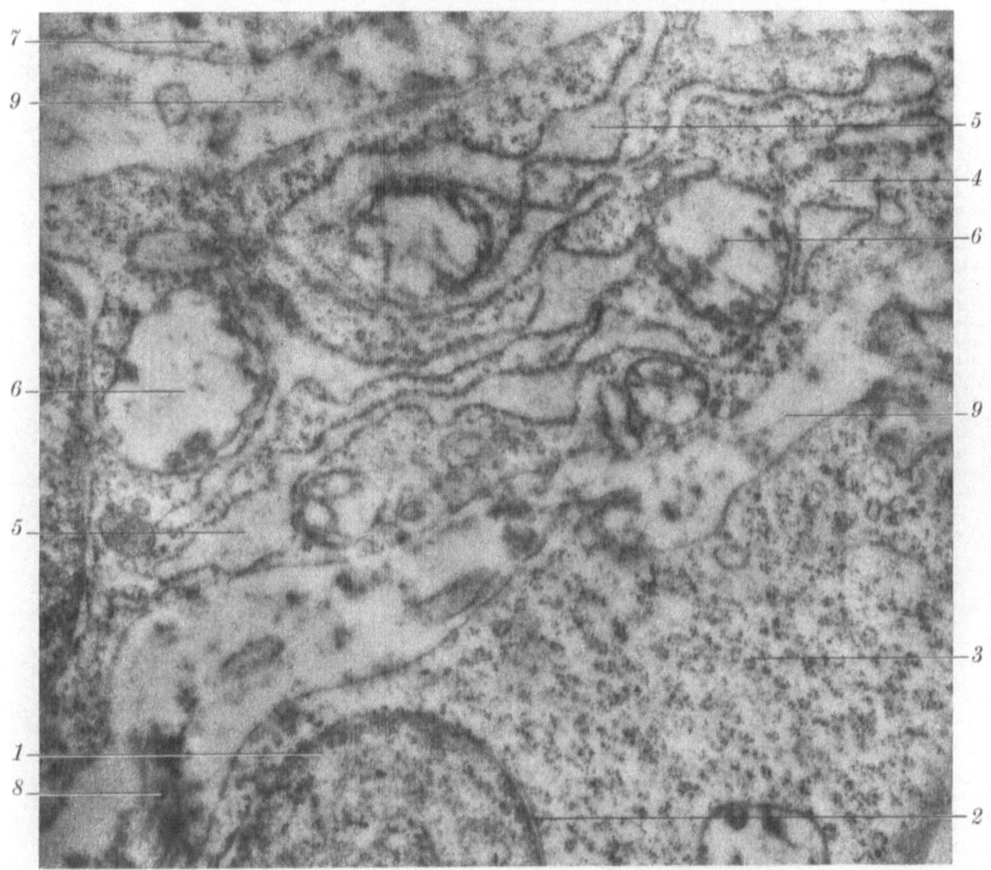

Abb. 17. Chondroblast aus dem Perichondrium der Ratte. *1* Zellkern; *2* Kernmembran; *3* Hyaloplasma des einen Chondroblasten angefüllt mit Palade-Granula ohne Membranen des endoplasmatischen Reticulum; *4* intermembranöses Hyaloplasma mit Palade-Granula; *5* perlschnurartig erweiterte Zisternen; *6* Mitochondrien in engem Kontakt mit Membranen des endoplasmatischen Reticulum; *7* angeschnittene Zellfortsätze; *8* intercelluläre Fibrillen; *9* Intercellularraum. Vergr. 30000. (KNESE u. KNOOP, 1961a)

färbt sich das Cytoplasma der knorpelnahen Chondroblasten zart an, mit der Modifikation der Hale-Reaktion von MÜLLER (1955/56) dagegen die Intercellularsubstanz (Abb. 16).

Die bisher beschriebenen Farbreaktionen der skeletogenen Zellen lassen eine intracelluläre Bildung des MPS-Protein-Komplexes vermuten. Bemerkenswert ist allerdings die geringe Anfärbbarkeit der Chondroblasten bei allen entsprechenden Reaktionen. Elektronenmikroskopische Untersuchungen der Bildungszellen können diese Färbungsdifferenzen aufklären. KNESE und KNOOP (1958) haben in jenem Abschnitt der Osteoblasten, der dem präossalen Gewebe zugewandt ist, Auftreibungen der Zisternen des endoplasmatischen Reticulums beobachtet und angenommen, daß diese Erweiterungen des intermembranösen Spaltraumes mit der Produktion der sog. amorphen Substanzen in Verbindung stehen. Ähnliche Erweiterungen der Zisternen konnten in Chondroblasten und einem Teil der Chondrocyten des Epiphysenknorpels nachgewiesen werden (KNESE und KNOOP, 1959, 1961a). In den Prächondroblasten sind die Zisternen perlschnurartig erweitert, in den Chondroblasten erreichen die Zisternensäcke einen Durchmesser von 3—4000 Å (Abb. 17). Eine eventuelle Anfärbung des in den Zisternen enthaltenen Materials kann sich damit der lichtmikroskopischen Beobachtung entziehen. Vergleich-

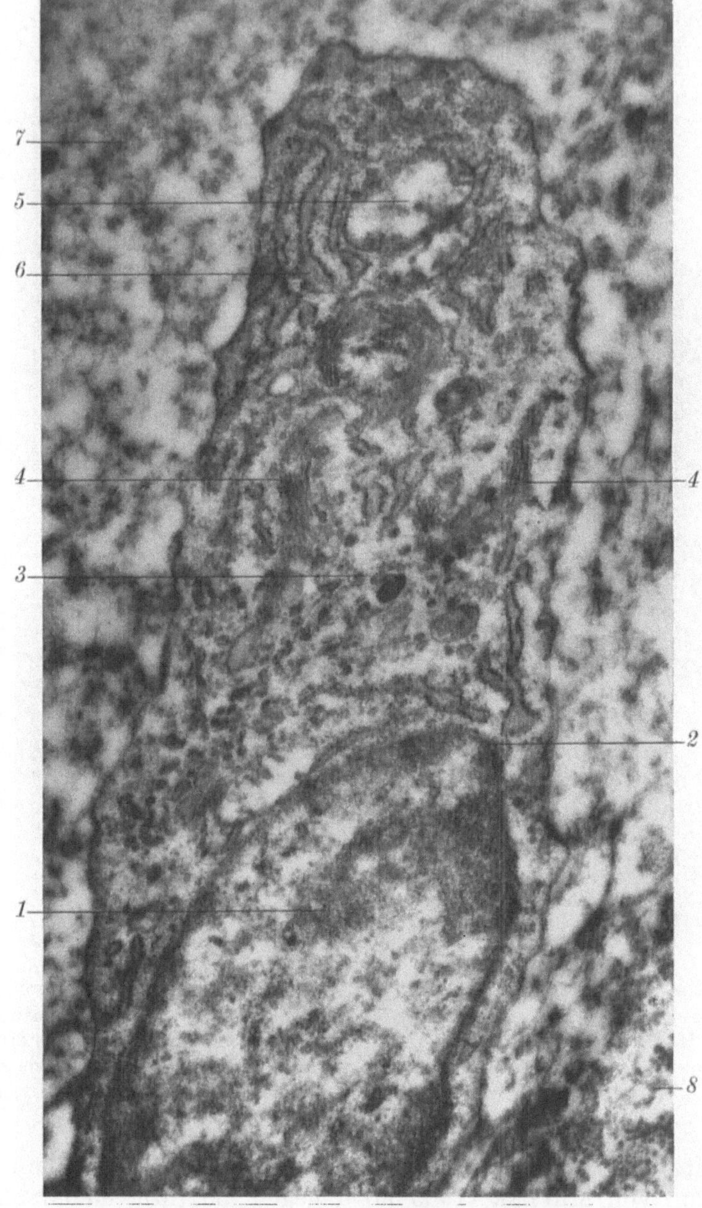

Abb. 18. Junger Chondrocyt aus der Appositionszone. *1* Zellkern; *2* Kernmembran; *3* Golgi-Feld mit dunklen Körpern; *4* Golgi-Lamellen; *5* Mitochondrien; *6* gering erweiterte Zisternen; *7* Intercellularsubstanz mit überwiegend längsgeschnittenen Fibrillen; *8* Intercellularsubstanz mit Faserquerschnitten. Vergr. 52000. (KNESE u. KNOOP, 1961a)

bare Zisternenerweiterungen fehlen den Zellen des Appositionsknorpels, d. h. bei der Umwandlung von Chondroblasten in Chondrocyten gehen die Zisternenerweiterungen verloren (Abb. 18). Da nun in dieser Knorpelbildungsfront die extracellulären MPS auftreten, wie durch autoradiographische und topochemische Untersuchungen nachgewiesen wurde, haben KNESE und KNOOP (1959, 1961a) einen Zusammenhang zwischen Zisternerweiterung und Bildung des MPS-Protein-Komplexes angenommen.

In den Chondrocyten des Epiphysenknorpels entstehen in Richtung auf den Säulenknorpel hin erneut Erweiterungen des intermembranösen Spaltraumes in der Form einzelner größerer Zisternensäcke mit einem Durchmesser von 1—3, ja sogar 5 μ. Granula entsprechender Größe lassen sich färberisch mit der PAS-Reaktion und der Hale-Reaktion nachweisen, ferner mit wäßriger Touluidinblaulösung in niederem p_H (Abb. 19). Bereits SCHAFFER (1930) hat bei Färbung mit Thionin metachromatische Granula in Chondrocyten des Frosches beobachtet, die er für Kalk hielt. KNESE und KNOOP (1959, 1961a) nehmen an Hand dieser elektronenmikroskopischen und topochemischen Befunde an,

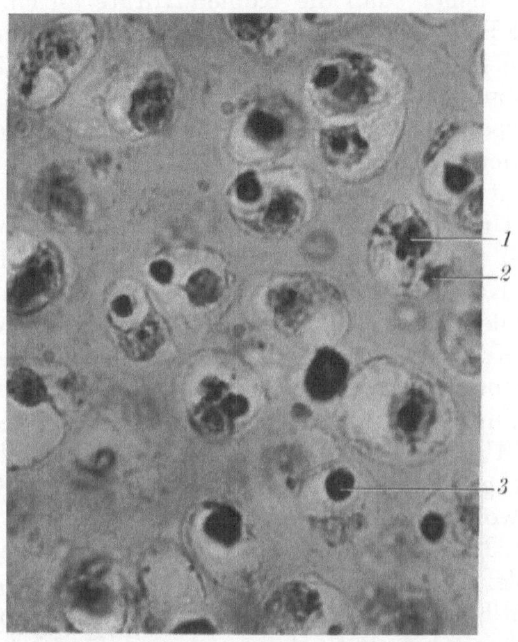

Abb. 19. Hyaliner Epiphysenknorpel. *1* Zellkern mit Nucleolus; *2* Cytoplasma (geschrumpft); *3* metachromatische Granula verschiedener Größe. Metacarpus eines Rinderfeten von 126 mm SSL. Toluidinblau, wäßrige Lösung p_H 3,6. Vergr. 1240. (KNESE u. KNOOP, 1961a)

daß von den Chondrocyten Substanzen gebildet und an die Intercellularsubstanz abgegeben werden; hierauf beruhe die unterschiedliche Färbbarkeit der Intercellularsubstanz in den einzelnen Regionen des Epiphysenknorpels. SHELDON (1960) beschrieb ähnliche Zisternenerweiterungen an Osteoblasten bei Rachitis. GODMAN und PORTER (1960) halten diese „Vesicel" für Abkömmlinge des Golgi-Apparates. MERKER (1961) hat in Fibroblasten der Haut im Zusammenhang mit dem endoplasmatischen Reticulum ähnliche Bildungen beobachtet und sie ebenfalls mit der MPS-Bildung in Zusammenhang gebracht.

Die Lokalisation der MPS-Synthese wurde weiterhin z.T. an Zellfraktionen, z.T. am Schnitt auch mit Hilfe von Radioisotopen nicht nur an der Knorpel-, sondern auch an der Leberzelle untersucht. Dem Golgi-Apparat wird hierbei von einigen Autoren (REVEL und HAY, 1963; PETERSON und LEBLOND, 1964a, b; NEUTRA und LEBLOND, 1966a, b) eine besondere Bedeutung zugesprochen. NEUTRA und LEBLOND (1966), die Ratten untersucht haben, meinen, daß Glykoproteine und MPS in der Golgi-Region, alle anderen Polysaccharide außerhalb dieses Gebietes gebildet würden. Dieser Ansicht widersprechen bereits die oben wiedergegebenen Untersuchungen mit zellfreien Multienzymsystemen. Weiterhin ist eine grundsätzlich unterschiedliche Lokalisation der verschiedenen Kohlenhydratsynthesen in der Zelle schwer vorstellbar, da bei allen diesen Vorgängen das Glucose-6-phosphat am Anfang steht. Ein elektronenmikroskopischer Vergleich verschiedener MPS-bildender Zellen bei Rind und Ratte hat gezeigt, daß nur die Knorpelzellen der Ratte über einen ausgedehnten Golgi-Apparat verfügen, ein solcher aber bei den Knorpel- und Periostzellen der Rinderfeten fehlt, die ohne Zweifel ebenfalls ein MPS-Synthese durchführen (KNESE).

Die Beschäftigung mit den Kohlenhydrat-Protein-Komplexen hat dazu geführt, zu untersuchen, ob und welche Zusammenhänge während der Synthese beider Komponenten bestehen. Durch gleichzeitige Verabreichung von ^{35}S und ^{14}C markierten Aminosäuren konnten GROSS, MATHEWS und DORFMAN (1960) und CAMPO und DZIEWIATKOWSKI (1962) nachweisen, daß die Chondrocyten den gesamten Komplex bilden. TELSER, ROBINSON und DORFMAN (1965) meinen, daß die Kohlenhydrate an ein Protein als Acceptor gebunden werden, da die Polysaccharidsynthese durch Puromycin gehemmt wird. LAWFORD und SCHACHTER (1966) sind der Auffassung, daß das Hexosamin in der Leber im Bereich der Polyribosomen gebunden wird, obwohl kein Code-Wort in den messenger-RNA vorhanden ist. Die Incorporation von ^{14}C-Glucosamin soll in den Kanälen des granulären und agranulären Reticulums erfolgen. Nach HORWITZ und DORFMAN (1968) ist die Sulfotransferase-Aktivität im agranulären Reticulum viermal größer als im granulären, ebenso der Gehalt an Uronsäure. Die Autoren lehnen infolgedessen ebenso wie LAWFORD und SCHACHTER (1966) die Annahme einer Beteiligung des Golgi-Apparates bei der Synthese von komplexen Kohlenhydraten ab. Es dürfte weiterhin nicht berechtigt sein, die Beobachtungen an Schleim produzierenden Epithelzellen, die von vielen Autoren herangezogen wurden, auf Knorpelzellen zu übertragen (vgl. KNESE).

Der elektronenmikroskopische Vergleich zwischen Knorpelzellen von Rinderfeten und Ratten, sowie Cambiumzellen des Periostes von Rinderfeten führte KNESE zu der Auffassung, daß die MPS-Synthese ähnlich wie die des Glykogenstoffwechsels an das Kohlenhydratpolymer gebunden ist, d.h. in wesentlichen Schritten im Hyloplasma lokalisiert ist. Den Kohlenhydrat-Granula stehen häufig Ribosomen des granulären Reticulums gebenüber. In den entstehenden Kontaktbereichen müßten dann die Kohlenhydrat-Protein-Komplexe gebildet werden. In diesen Zonen treten stark kontrastierbare Granula auf, die sich in Form und Größe von den übrigen Glykogengranula unterscheiden. Die elektronenmikroskopischen Befunde sprechen dafür, daß in den miteinander verglichenen Zellen recht unterschiedliche Kohlenhydrat-Protein-Komplexe gebildet werden. Die Beteiligung des endoplasmatischen Reticulums, an dessen Membranen die Glucose-6-Phosphatase gebunden ist, an der Synthese der verschiedenartigen Kohlenhydraten ist heute gesichert, wenn auch im einzelnen noch ungeklärt. Besonders muß über die Bedeutung des Zisternensystems und die Zisternenerweiterungen in manchen MPS-bildenden Zellen (KNESE und KNOOP, 1959, 1961a; FÖLDES et al., 1963) noch weiter diskutiert werden.

Untersuchungen mit sehr unterschiedlichen Methoden und an verschiedenartigem Material haben damit klargestellt, daß Zellen unmittelbar an der Bildung des MPS-Protein-Komplexes beteiligt sind. Jedoch ist z. Zt. noch umstritten, in welchem „Zustand" die MPS von der Zelle abgegeben werden. MEYER (1956) und RODEN (1956) haben eine Sulfat-Veresterung in hohem Polymerisationsgrad angegeben; ^{35}S-Einlagerungen sind bereits in den Zellen zu beobachten (BÉLANGER, 1954; AMPRINO, 1955; VERNE, et al. 1956). Die Diskussion über den Zustand des MPS bei Abgabe durch Zellen beruht darauf, daß die verschiedenen Arbeitsgruppen Untersuchungen mit unterschiedlichen Methoden durchgeführt haben. Zur Beschreibung des Zustandes der Intercellularsubstanz wurden die Termini Polymerisation und Aggregation verwandt. Dem Gebrauch dieser wohl definierten Begriffe zur Deutung beobachteter färberischer Unterschiede (u. a. GERSH und CATCHPOLE 1949, 1960) wurde von MCMANUS (1954) und DORFMAN (1955/56) wegen mangelnder Beweiskraft der topochemischen Methoden energisch widersprochen.

Die erzielten Ergebnisse lassen den Schluß zu, daß von der Zelle Stoffe abgegeben werden, die mit voller Berechtigung als MPS anzusehen sind. Die Ausschüttung morphologisch unveränderter Kohlenhydratgranula im großen Umfange wurde im Periost beobachtet, der Durchtritt von stark kontrastierten Kohlenhydratgranula durch das Plasmalemm bei Chondrocyten (KNESE). Im übrigen sind die Extrusionsmechanismen für die Kohlenhydrate wohl ebenso vielfältig wie ihre vermutlich recht unterschiedliche Struktur. Die extracellulären MPS lassen sich nach verschiedenartiger Kontrastierung im Elektronenmikroskop nachweisen (Knese, 1966b; Matukas, Panner und Orbison, 1967). Allerdings dürften die aufgefundenen Granula nicht die „natürliche" Form der Kohlenhydrat-Protein-Komplexe in vivo wiedergeben, sondern das Produkt der jeweiligen Fixierung und Entwässerung sein. Dabei können in der Nähe von Zellen mitunter recht große Granula erscheinen (Knese). Der Übertritt dieser Substanzen in die Intercellularsubstanz bringt vielleicht eine erste Änderung des „Zustandes" mit sich, da intracelluläre MPS sich topochemisch mit der Eisen-Reaktion von Graumann, extracelluläre aber mit der von Müller darstellen lassen (Knese und Knoop, 1961c). Mit chemisch-analytischen Methoden ist der Zustand der MPS in derartig kleinen Volumina wie der Zelle, ihrer unmittelbaren Umgebung und den einzelnen Zonen des Epiphysenknorpels z. Zt. noch nicht zu untersuchen. So scheint die Beurteilung des Zustandes der MPS auf Grund des färberischen Verhaltens der Intercellularsubstanz als eine Art Zwischenlösung unvermeidbar. Die Untersuchungen mit einer Reihe entsprechender Färbemethoden zeigen, daß abweichende Färbungen auch mit morphologisch wohl definierten Zonen zusammenfallen (Knese und Knoop, 1961a). Damit dürften grundsätzliche Bedenken wegen der mangelnden Spezifität topochemischer Methoden bzw. ihres komplexen Reaktionsmechanismus kaum angebracht sein. Dagegen ist jede Kritik berechtigt, die sich dagegen wendet, daß aus der Farbreaktion auf einen bestimmten physikochemischen Zustand geschlossen wird, weil damit die Aussagegrenze der Methode überschritten wird.

Der inzwischen vielfältig gesicherte Nachweis einer lebhaften Stoffproduktion durch die Knorpelzellen hat dazu geführt, die bisherigen „Chondrocyten" nunmehr auch als „Chondroblasten" zu bezeichnen (unter anderem Godman und Lane, 1964; Fullmer 1965). Die Zellen der knorpeligen Epiphyse entsprechen durch die lebhafte Stoffproduktion in keiner Weise mehr der alten Vorstellung von jenen Zellen (Chondro„cyten"), die nur noch den Stoffwechsel des Gewebes aufrechterhalten. Auf der anderen Seite bilden die im Perichondrium gelegenen Zellen (Chondro„blasten") nicht die gesamte Menge der Intercellularsubstanzen. Diese wesentliche Erkenntnis wird vielleicht in der Zukunft dazu beitragen, die Bedeutung der Epiphyse für das Skeletorgan weiter aufzuklären. Man sollte aber berücksichtigen, daß durch die Tätigkeit der Chondroblasten der hyaline Knorpel entsteht, der dann allerdings noch durch die Aktivität der Knorpelzellen vielfach umgestaltet wird. Schließlich geben die alten Bezeichnungen auch topographische Bestimmungen wieder. Um Verwechselungen zu vermeiden, ist zu empfehlen, weiterhin alle Zellen im Knorpel selbst Chondrocyten und alle an dessen Oberfläche Chondroblasten zu nennen, wenn auch das Wesen und die Bedeutung dieser Zellen neu bestimmt werden muß.

ζ) Die Mucopolysaccharide während der Ontogenese

In allen Geweben nimmt während der Ontogenese die Menge der MPS, bezogen auf die Fasern, ab (Campani et al., 1950; Angevine, 1950; Mauer et al., 1952; Seelich, 1952; Banfield, 1954). Auch für den Rippenknorpel wurde eine Verminderung an Chondroitinsulfat nachgewiesen (Loewi, 1953; Kuhn et al., 1958; Shetlar et al., 1955). Kuhn et al. (1958) und Stidworthy et al. (1958) wiesen für den Knorpel vom Menschen bis zum 6. Jahr eine bedeutende, zwischen dem 10. und 90. Jahr eine geringfügige Abnahme des Galaktosamin nach. Das Glucosamin nimmt von der Geburt bis zum 40. Jahr gering zu und bleibt dann konstant. Die Menge des Keratansulphates steigt im Knorpel während des Lebens an (Meyer et al., 1958). Im Nucleus pulposus bleibt der Volumenanteil der MPS konstant, der des Kollagens wird aber erhöht (Hirsch et al., 1953); ein gleiches gilt für den Knochen (Sobel et al., 1954). Allerdings liegen nicht nur quantitative, sondern auch qualitative Veränderungen der Intercellularsubstanzen vor (Angevine, 1950; Meyer et al., 1956). Loewi (1953) gibt auch eine Depolymerisation der MPS mit zunehmendem Alter an. Die Viscosität von Chondroitinsulfatextrakten aus Knorpel wird zwischen dem 3. und 20. Jahr geringer. Durch die Depolymerisation soll die Anzahl der freien sauren Gruppen erhöht werden und damit die Fixierung von Ionen ermöglicht sowie die Mineralisation gefördert werden.

d) Die Mineralablagerungen im Knorpel

Die Mineralablagerung im Epiphysenknorpel ist eine Erscheinung deren Bedeutung für die Skeletentwicklung noch völlig ungeklärt ist. Die Mineralablagerung ist keine Knochenbildung und keine ,,Verknöcherung" des Knorpels, wie immer wieder auch in den neuesten Arbeiten zu lesen ist. Eine (enchondrale bzw. metaphysäre) Knochenbildung tritt erst unterhalb der Epiphyse auf und führt zur Bildung der primären Spongiosa. Vor allem bei analytischen Untersuchungen wird aus dem Nachweis von Calcium oder Mineralien auf das Vorhandensein von Knochengewebe geschlossen. Knochengewebe und mineralisierter Knorpel haben aber eine grundsätzlich verschiedene Struktur (Knese 1963b; s.u.). Die mangelnde Beachtung dieser Tatsachen hatte allerdings die Folge, daß die an der Epiphyse beobachteten Erscheinungen (Glykolyse, Enzyme) als essentieller Anteil des Vorganges der Mineralisation angesehen wurden. Die verschiedenartigen Theorien der Mineralisation müßten infolgedessen dahingehend überprüft werden, ob sie für die Mineralisation des Knorpels oder des Knochengewebes Gültigkeit haben.

Die Mineralablagerungen im Knorpel haben bei den Röntgenographen wenig Interesse gefunden. Mineralablagerungen treten während der regelrechten Entwicklung in den Epiphysen auf und werden an anderen Orten, so im Rippenknorpel, als regressive Erscheinung angesehen. Nach Brandenberger und Schinz (1946) handelt es sich um einen Hydroxylapatit in kryptokristalliner Form. In einem Rippenknorpel fanden die Autoren nach dem Glühen noch eine nicht näher bestimmbare Kristallart, vermutlich ein $CaCO_3$.

Zu den älteren histologisch-färberischen Untersuchungen über Mineralablagerungen im Knorpel (Weidenreich, 1930) sind neuerlich vermehrt solche mit Versilberung (Kossa, 1901) hinzugetreten (Bloom und Bloom, 1940; McLean und Bloom, 1940; McLean und Urist, 1955). Eine wesentliche Bereicherung der Kenntnisse wurde durch Untersuchung der Ablagerung von Radioisotopen gewonnen, und zwar zunächst mit ^{32}P (Leblond et al., 1950), später mit ^{45}Ca (Comar, 1952; Ponlot, 1960). Weitere Untersuchungen erfolgten mit Hilfe der Mikroradiographie (Wallgren, 1957) und des Elektronenmikroskopes (Robinson und Cameron, 1956; Scott und Pease, 1956; Durning, 1958; Knese, 1959; Zelander, 1959; Knese und Knoop, 1961b u. c.).

Die Mineralablagerungen des Epiphysenknorpels erscheinen in den Längsbalken, so daß von einer besonderen Mineralisationszone gesprochen wird. Zunächst sind nur einzelne Kristallnadeln in regelloser Lagerung (Abb. 20) zu beobachten (vgl. Knese, 1959b, c, 1963a), die dann zu größeren Komplexen und schließlich zu colonähnlich gestalteten Gebilden heranwachsen (Abb. 21). Die Nadeln haben ein mittleres Ausmaß von 90 zu 20 Å und sind demzufolge länger und dünner als die Kristallnadeln des präossalen Gewebes (184,5 zu 54 Å, Knese und Knoop, 1958). Eine Beziehung zu den Kollagenfibrillen wie im Knochengewebe besteht nicht. Reste von Knorpelsubstanz, umgeben von enchondralem Knochen, weisen nach Entkalkung mit Versen (Titriplex: Äthylen-diamintetraessig-Säure) eine Hülle von Kollagenfibrillen auf (Knese und Knoop, 1961b u. c), die auch im polarisierten Licht zu erkennen ist (Knese, 1957). Im Bereich der Knorpelsubstanz sind nur noch einige fädige Gebilde zu beobachten, deren Natur unklar ist (Abb. 22), jedoch könnte angenommen werden daß es sich bei den Fäden um präcipitierte MPS handele. Die Mineralablagerungen sind vermutlich wegen der unterschiedlichen Beziehungen zu den Kollagenfibrillen von verschiedener Gestalt (Knese, 1959b, c, 1963a). In jungem Knochengewebe liegt eine netzartige Orientierung der Kollagenfibrillen und der entsprechend ausgerichteten Kristalle vor. Dabei ist der Kristallmantel etwa aus 5—10 Schichten aufgebaut. Die Nadeln sind kettenförmig gelagert, zwischen je zwei Kettenlinien bleibt

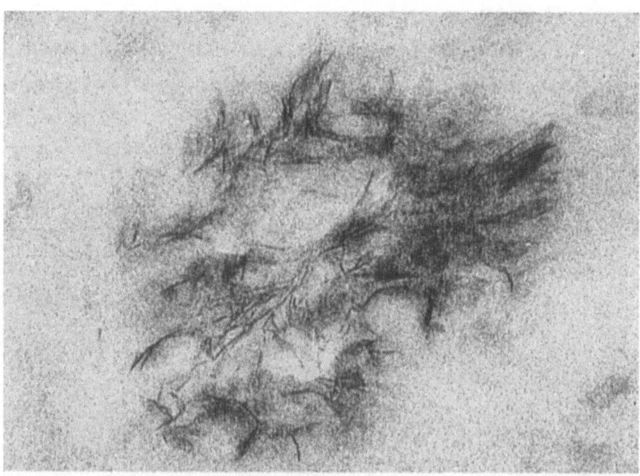

Abb. 20. Kleine Kalkablagerungen in der Form von Kristallnadeln ohne Beziehung zu Fasern im Epiphysenknorpel eines Rattenfetus. In der Umgebung einige Fasern, die in die amorphe Interfibrillärsubstanz eingelagert sind. (Elektronenmikroskopische Aufnahme, Vergr. 110000.) (KNESE, 1959)

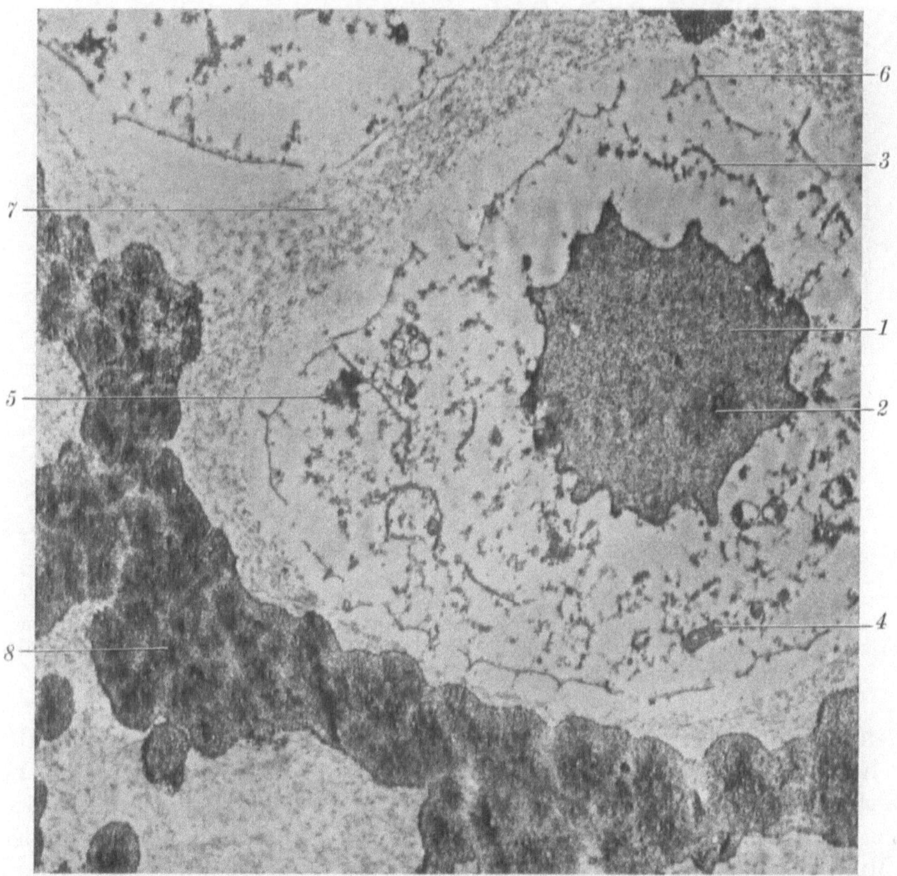

Abb. 21. Zelle aus der Mineralisationszone. *1* Zellkern; *2* Nucleolus; *3* Membranen des endoplasmatischen Reticulum; *4* Mitochondrien; *5* osmiophile Einlagerungen; *6* Zellmembranen mit Füßen; *7* faserige Intercellularsubstanz; *8* Kalkeinlagerung mit scharfer Umgrenzung. Vergr. 5000. (KNESE u. KNOOP, 1961 b)

ein freier Raum, dessen Breite etwas geringer als die Nadeldicke ist. Die Mineraldepots des Knorpels stellen dichte Ballen dar, an deren Umfang die regellose Lagerung der Kristallnadeln weiterhin zu erkennen ist.

Über die Biochemie der Mineralablagerungen im Knorpelgewebe liegt eine umfangreiche Literatur vor (vgl. ZAMBOTTI, 1957). Von vielen Autoren wurde angenommen, daß für die Kristallbildung im Knorpel- und Knochengewebe gleiche Bedingungen herrschen. Der Knorpel als mineralisationsfähiges Gewebe wurde für Versuche in vitro gewählt, da das geringe Volumen der mineralisierenden präossalen Zone sich derartigen

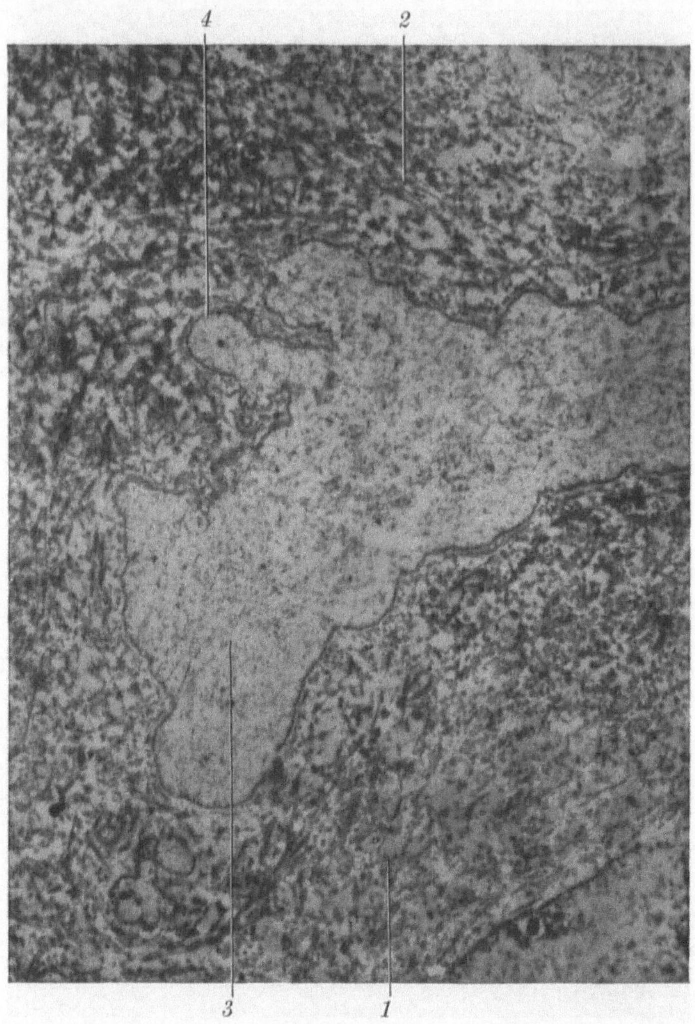

Abb. 22. Entkalkter enchondraler Knochen. *1* Quergeschnittene Fibrillen; *2* längsgeschnittene Fibrillen des Knochens; *3* Gebiet des Knorpelkalkes mit granulärer bzw. fibrillärer Struktur; *4* Grenze der Kalkeinlagerungen. Entkalkung Titriplex (= Versen). Vergr. 7500. (KNESE u. KNOOP, 1961b)

Untersuchungen entzieht. Viele Angaben über die Biochemie mineralisationsfähiger Zonen gelten demzufolge nur für den Knorpel. Ob eine Übertragung auf die Verhältnisse im präossalen Gewebe möglich ist, wurde bisher nicht geklärt. GLIMCHER (1960) glaubt allerdings, daß auch im Knorpelgewebe die Kollagenfibrille als induzierendes Element bei der Mineralisation auftritt. ROBINSON und CAMERON (1956), NEUMAN und NEUMAN (1958), KNESE (1959b, c, 1963a) sowie KNESE und KNOOP (1958, 1961b) neigen dazu, beide Kristallisationsvorgänge in der Beziehung zu den Kollagenfibrillen als voneinander verschieden anzusehen. Beide Prozesse könnten allerdings dann auf eine Stufe gestellt werden, wenn für die Kristallkernbildung die MPS verantwortlich sind. THIELE und KRÖNKE (1955, 1959) untersuchten ionotrope Gele, die auch als Symplexe aus zwei Makromolekülen bestehen können (THIELE und LANGMAACK, 1957) und wie die MPS als Polyelektrolyte anzusehen sind. In ionotrope Gele als Leitstruktur können Kristalle schwerer löslicher Verbindungen wie Bleijodid, Blei- bzw. Calciumhydroxylapatit eingelagert werden. Es liegt eine geordnete, anisotrope, intermicellare Kristallisation vor, die auf einem Ionenaustausch mit den am Gelgerüst gebundenen Gegenionen beruht. Der Vorgang ist rerversibel, ein Befund, der im Hinblick auf den Abbau von Knorpelmineralien von Bedeutung ist. Als eine entsprechende Leitstruktur im Knochen und Knorpelgewebe könnten die Fadenmoleküle der MPS mit ihren ionischen Gruppen auftreten. Es muß dann angenommen werden (Knese, 1963a), daß die MPS-Fadenmoleküle im Knochengewebe durch die Kollagenfibrillen ausgerichtet sind, im Knorpelgewebe jedoch nicht; damit ist die Entstehung der unterschiedlichen Kristallstruktur bei gleichem Ablagerungsmechanismus möglich.

Die Bedeutung und das Schicksal der Mineralablagerungen im Epiphysenknorpel ist noch nicht endgültig aufgeklärt.

Jedoch kann wohl angenommen werden, wie viele elektronenmikroskopische Untersuchung gezeigt haben (s. S. 386), daß die Knorpelmineralien unter Mitwirkung der Riesenzellen in der Metaphyse abgebaut werden. Diese Zellen sind damit eigentlich Mineraloklasten, keine Chondroklasten (s.u.) aber auch keine Osteoklasten. Der Mechanismus des Mineralabbaues ist im einzelnen allerdings noch unklar.

3. Die Beziehungen zwischen Knorpel- und Knochengewebe im Skeletsystem

Ein größerer Teil der Skeletstücke besteht zunächst aus Knorpelgewebe. Die Bildung knöcherner Skeletstücke erfolgt histogenetisch auf vier Wegen: 1. Periostale Osteogenese, 2. enchondrale Osteogenese, 3. diaphysär-chondrale Osteogenese (Knese, 1957) und 4. sog. „Metaplasie“. Durch die periostale Knochenbildung wird das Knorpelmodell von einer Knochenmanschette umgeben. Histogenetische Beziehungen zwischen Knorpel- und Knochengewebe bestehen hierbei wahrscheinlich nicht. Die desmale Osteogenese im Bereich der Deckknochen des Schädels läuft wohl wie die periostale ab. Im folgenden sind die chondralen Bildungsformen zu erörtern, in deren Verlauf Knorpelgewebe durch Knochengewebe „ersetzt“ wird.

Über die Vorgänge im Epiphysenknorpel liegt eine große Zahl von Veröffentlichungen vor, auch über die durch Hormone, Vitamine und Ernährung erzeugten Störungen. Die Morphologie, Histochemie, Biochemie und — nach Untersuchungen mit Isotopen — der Stoffwechsel sind gut bekannt. Die histogenetische Bedeutung dieser Vorgänge im Hinblick auf die enchondrale Osteogenese ist aber völlig unklar. In der Beurteilung der Vorgänge in der Epiphyse, besonders derjenigen in der Eröffnungszone, und der enchondralen Osteogenese besteht eine bisher nicht erörterte Diskrepanz (Knese, 1936b). Die Umwandlung der Zellgestalt der Chondrocyten innerhalb der verschiedenen Zonen des Epiphysenknorpels und dessen Stoffwechsel werden einerseits als Vorbereitung für eine Mineralisation bzw. einer „Verknöcherung“ betrachtet. Auf der anderen Seite wird fast allgemein angenommen, daß die Zellen der hypertrophen bzw. Mineralisationszone sterbende Knorpelzellen sind. Die Fülle der Prozesse im Epiphysenknorpel müßte demzufolge eine Vorbereitung auf diesen Zelltod sein. Die Knochenbildung soll dann durch Osteoblasten erfolgen, die von Periostzellen und anderen „indifferenten“ Zellen abstammen. Von einigen Autoren wurde allerdings erwogen, ob ein Teil der im Knorpel gebildeten Substanzen, voran das Chondroitinsulfat, bei der Osteogenese eine Rolle spielen (Siffert, 1951; Godard, 1951; Neuman et al., 1952; Dziewiatkowski, 1958; Davies und Young, 1954; Bélanger, 1954; Amprino, 1955). Weiterhin wurde als selbstverständlich vorausgesetzt, daß die enchondral gebildete primäre Spongiosa sofort einer Resorption anheimfalle, d. h. daß etwas nur zu einer folgenden Zerstörung gebildet wird, ein für den Organismus einmaliger Vorgang. Weiterhin wird der Epiphyse eine Organisatorwirkung zur Bildung des periostalen Ringes zugesprochen (Lacroix, 1951a, b).

Die bisherigen Arbeiten gingen infolgedessen von zwei einander widersprechenden Hypothesen aus: entweder die epiphysären Prozesse sind eine Vorbereitung für eine

Knochenbildung, oder Knorpelzellen und Intercellularsubstanz des Knorpels verschwinden, um einem transitorischem enchondralen Knochen Platz zu machen.

Sehr viele Befunde lassen vermuten, daß die epiphysären Prozesse für die Organogenese des Skeletes (KNESE, 1957) eine größere Bedeutung als für die Histogenese des Knochengewebes haben. Jedoch müssen periostale und chondrale Osteogenese miteinander verglichen werden, um festzustellen, welche gleichartigen Vorgänge bei beiden zu beobachten sind. Vor allem ist die Entwicklung der knochenbildenden Zellen zu verfolgen (KNESE, 1963b, 1967b, 1968). Bei der chondralen Osteogenese ist weiterhin das Schicksal des Knorpels und seiner Mineralien zu diskutieren.

a) Die diaphysäre-chondrale Osteogenese

Die Entwicklung eines knorpeligen Skeletelementes hat STREETER (1949) am Beispiel des Humerus von einem Keimling mit 21—29 Ursegmenten an geschildert. STREETER gibt die Ausbildung verschiedener Zellformen und deren Verteilung über das Skeletstück an. Hierbei unterscheidet er folgende Stadien in der Knorpelentwicklung: I. Stadium des Vorknorpels, II. Stadium der vermehrten Intercellularsubstanz und Anordnung der Zellen in queren Reihen, III. Stadium der vergrößerten und kugeligen Zellen mit Vacuolen im Cytoplasma, IV. Stadium der maximalen Größe der Knorpelzellen, V. Stadium der Desintegration der Knorpelzellen. Die Bildung der einzelnen Zonen ist mit einer unterschiedlichen Kohlenhydratspeicherung in den Zellen verbunden (unveröffentlicht): Zur Mitte des hyalinen Epiphysenknorpels hin enthalten die Zellen zunehmend kleine Kohlenhydratgranula, sie nehmen an Menge in den Zellen des Säulenknorpels ab und die Zellen des hypertrophen Knorpels weisen wenige recht große Granula auf. KASSOWITZ (1879) hat sieben Zonen angegeben und zwar Zone A des allseitig wachsenden Knorpels, B der einseitigen Zellproliferation, C der Zellvergrößerung, D der Knorpelverkalkung, E der Gefäßraum -und Markraumbildung, F der metaplastischen Knochenbildung und G der neoplastischen Knochenbildung. KNESE und KNOOP (1961a) haben bei ihren elektronenmikroskopischen und histochemischen Untersuchungen mit einigen Ergänzungen auf diesen Einteilungen aufgebaut und kommen zu folgender Gliederung: 1. Perichondrale Appositionszone, 2. Gelenkknorpel. 3. hyaliner Epiphysenknorpel (etwa das Gebiet des späteren Epiphysenkernes), 4. Zone der einseitigen Zellproliferation, 5. Säulenknorpel, 6. Zone der hypertrophen Knorpelzellen, 7. Zone des mineralisierten Knorpels und 8. Eröffnungszone der Knorpelhöhlen mit folgender Zone der enchondralen Knochenbildung. Das zuletzt genannte Gebiet wird heute häufig als Metaphyse bezeichnet. Diese Bezeichnungen wurden in das Schema der Skeletzellen übernommen (KNESE, 1964c, 1966a; s. S. 342, Abb. 9). Da allerdings der Terminus „Proliferation" auch für den Säulenknorpel gebraucht wird, schlagen wir jetzt die Bezeichnung „Transformationszone" vor.

Die ersten Vorgänge der chondralen Osteogenese treten in Entwicklungsstadien auf, in denen das knorpelige Skeletstück bereits eine einfache periostale Knochenschale besitzt (KNESE, 1957). Mitunter sind dieser periostalen Schale bereits radiäre und Teile von zirkulären Bälkchen angefügt (Abb. 23). In der periostalen Schale befindet sich eine Lücke, durch die periostale Elemente in den Knorpel als sog. enchondraler Zapfen eindringen. Zunächst werden einzelne Knorpelhöhlen unter Erhaltung der Intercellularsubstanz eröffnet; damit wird eine Art Kanalsystem gebildet (Abb. 24). Schließlich werden die Höhlen größer und gewinnen Verbindung miteinander. Eine Knorpelschicht legt sich der periostalen Grundschicht von innen her an (Abb. 25). Mitunter ziehen noch Knorpelbalken durch die Markhöhle. Mit der Bildung der Markhöhle sind gleichzeitig zwei voneinander getrennte Epiphysen entstanden. Diese Vorgänge im Knorpelschaft leiten die Ausbildung der Form des knöchernen Skeletstückes ein. So liegt ein organogenetischer Prozeß vor, neben dem die Histogenese eine untergeordnete Rolle spielt.

Die dem periostalen Knochen angeschmiegte Knorpelsubstanz erhält auf der Markhöhlenseite einen Überzug von Osteoblasten (Abb. 26). KNESE (1957) hat diese Vorgänge,

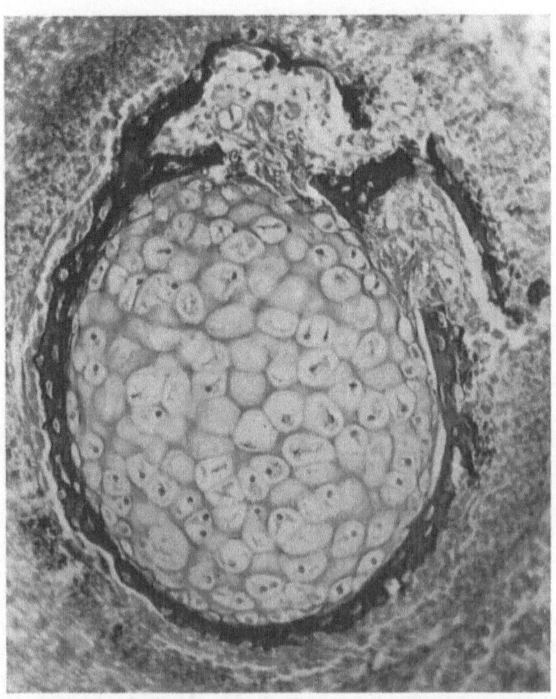

Abb. 23. Fet, 34 mm SSL. Humerus, Querschnittshöhe 4. Knorpelmodell umgeben von einer Schicht periostalen Knochens mit Zellen, sowie Bildung radiärer Bälkchen auf der Dorsalseite und einer zweiten Schale. Dorsal zwei Öffnungen in der periostalen Knochenschicht. Azan, Ob. 20, Ok. 8. (KNESE, 1957)

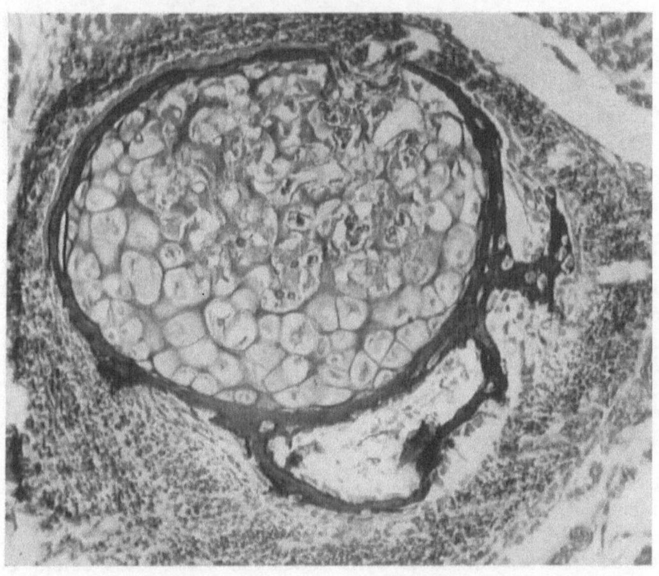

Abb. 24. Fet, 34 mm SSL. Ulna, Querschnittshöhe 6. Auf der ersten periostalen Schale sind palmar und radial radiäre und tangentiale Bälkchen aufgebaut. Die Höhlen des Knorpelmodells sind zu zwei Drittel mit osteogenem Gewebe erfüllt. In der Nähe der Lücke im periostalen Knochen hat sich ein System von Spalten entwickelt. Hier erscheinen die Knorpelbalken verdickt und stärker angefärbt. Azan, Ob. 20, Ok. 8. (KNESE, 1957)

die bisher nur geringe Beachtung fanden (STEUDENER, 1875; STRELZOFF, 1875; KAPSAMMER, 1897) als diaphysär-chondrale Osteogenese bezeichnet. LEBLOND et al. (1950, 1955, 1956) haben im Femur junger Tiere auf Grund der Ablagerung von Radioisotopen eine endostale Knochenbildung festgestellt. In späteren Entwicklungsstadien fehlt diese Form der

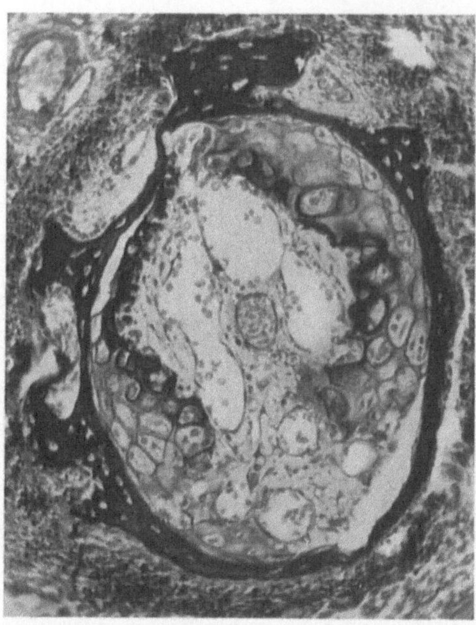

Abb. 25. Fet, 58 mm SSL. Fibula, Querschnittshöhe 4. Beginn der diaphysären chondralen Osteogenese. Der periostale Knochen wird auf der dorsal-tibialen Hälfte durch Bälkchen weitergebaut. Primitive Markhöhle. Bildung des diaphysär chondralen Knochens durch Markosteoblasten (tibial) bzw. Umwandlung der Intercellularsubstanz um Knorpelhöhlen. Azan. Ob. 20, Ok. 8. (KNESE, 1957)

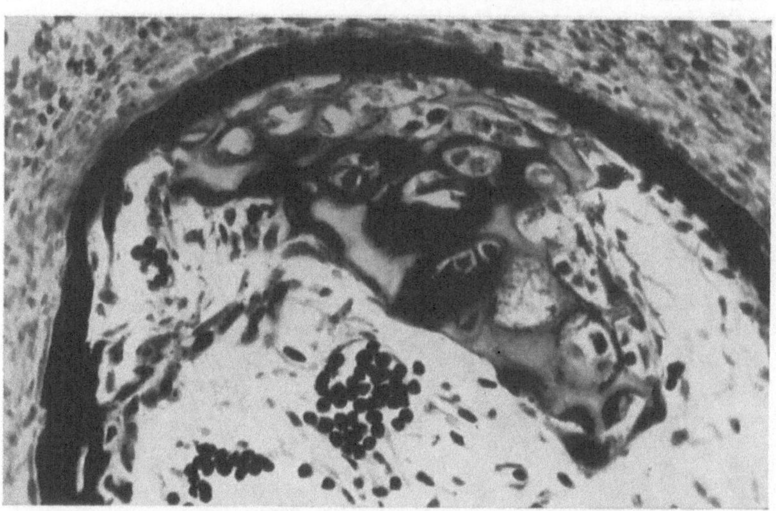

Abb. 26. Fet, 74 mm SSL. Fibula, Querschnittshöhe 4. Der einfachen periostalen Schale ist ein Knorpelteil mit diaphysärer chondraler Osteogenese angelagert. Im Anlagerungsbereich enthalten die Knorpelhöhlen mehrere kleine Zellelemente, die den Markosteoblasten gleichen. Der Markhöhle zugewandt findet eine Umwandlung der knorpeligen Intercellularsubstanz in knöcherne statt. Aus einem Zellstrom der Markhöhle scheren Markosteoblasten aus. Azan. Ob. 40, Ok. 8. (KNESE, 1957)

Knochenbildung. Die diaphysäre chondrale Osteogenese ist nicht nur dem Ort nach, sondern auch in der Beziehung zwischen Knorpel- und Knochengewebe von der enchondralen verschieden. Bei der enchondralen Osteogenese liegen, wie besonders deutlich Querschnitte durch Knochenstücke zeigen, enge Knorpelröhren vor, die von innen her mit einem Knochensaum überzogen werden. Knorpelzellen bleiben hierbei nicht erhalten. Dagegen entstehen durch die diaphysäre chondrale Osteogenese Knochentapeten auf unverändertem (?) Knorpel, der auch Zellen enthält.

In diesem Zusammenhang soll kurz der Begriff „Endost" diskutiert werden. Nach Kölliker (1889) ist das Endost die bindegewebige Auskleidung von Markräumen und Haversschen Kanälen. In ähnlicher Form wird das Endost noch heute beschrieben (Ham und Harris, 1956; McLean und Urist, 1961). Das Endost besteht aus Zellen des Markreticulums, die sich in einfacher Lage, mitunter als flache osteogenetische Zellen, dem Knochen anlegen. McLean und Urist (1961) erkennen diesen Zellen sowohl osteogenetische als auch hämatopoetische Potenzen zu. Ham (1953) weist darauf hin, daß

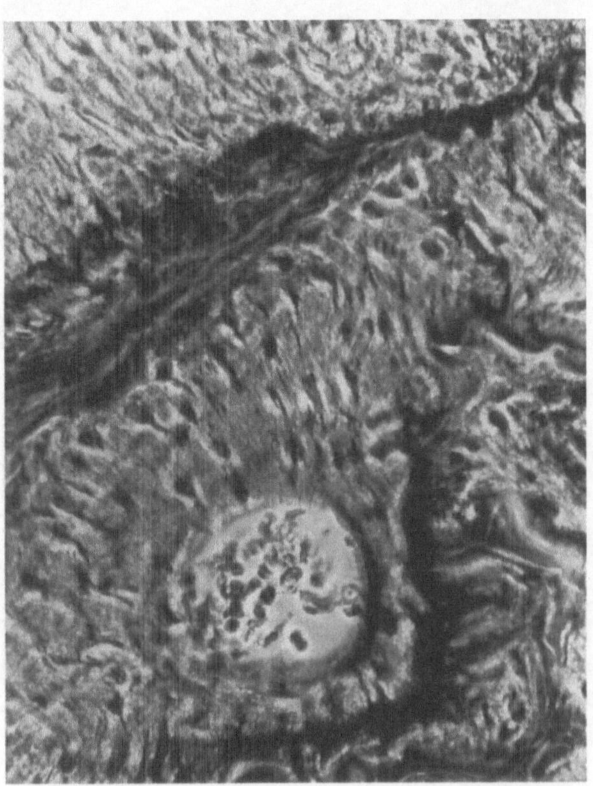

Abb. 27. Fet, 282 mm SSL. Humerus, Querschnittshöhe 7. Bildung der perienchondralen Grenzlinie durch Erschöpfung der zwischen periostalem und chondralem Knochen gelegenen Zellschicht. Im chondralen Knochen Reste von Knorpelgrundsubstanz. Hämatoxylin Eosin. Phasenkontrastverfahren. Ob. 40, Ok. 8. (Knese 1957)

die Endostzellen der Haversschen Kanäle Abkömmlinge des Periostes sind, da die Bildung der Haversschen Kanäle vom Periost her erfolgt. Petersen (1935) und Weidenreich (1930) lehnen die Bezeichnung Endost ab, da keine geschlossene membranartige Bekleidung des Knochens vorliegt. Auf jeden Fall werden als Endost Zellen sehr verschiedener Gestalt und Bedeutung sowie unterschiedlicher Herkunft zusammengefaßt.

Die Bildung des diaphysär-chondralen Knochens schreitet zentrifugal von der Markhöhle her auf den periostalen Knochen zu fort. Der Knochen umschließt Inseln von knorpeliger Intercellularsubstanz, die auch Zellen enthält. Chondraler und periostaler Knochen sind durch eine peri-enchondrale Grenzlinie voneinander getrennt (Strelzoff, 1873). Knese (1957) führt diese Grenzlinie auf Reste der Intercellularsubstanz des Knorpels zurück (Abb. 27). Die Markhöhle weitet sich unter Erhaltung der peri-enchondralen Grenzlinie bis zur Geburt erheblich. Die Querschnittfläche der Markhöhle mißt dann in der Mitte des Femur 14, der Tibia 15 und des Humerus 19 mm^2, im distalen Teil des Femur erreicht sie sogar 67 mm^2 (Bahling 1958). Die Beobachtungen von Bahling über die Dickenentwicklung der Diaphyse und den Zeitpunkt der Vergrößerung der Markhöhle stimmen mit den Angaben von Kölliker (1873) überein, der im 3. Monat noch keine Markhöhle sah. Die Vergrößerung der Markhöhle erfolgt im 5.—6. Monat. Nach BAHLING (1958) setzt das Wachstum der Markhöhle beim Humerus, der Fibula und den mittleren Abschnitten von Femur und Tibia erst bei Feten von 240 mm SSL, in den distalen Teilen von Femur und Tibia etwas früher ein.

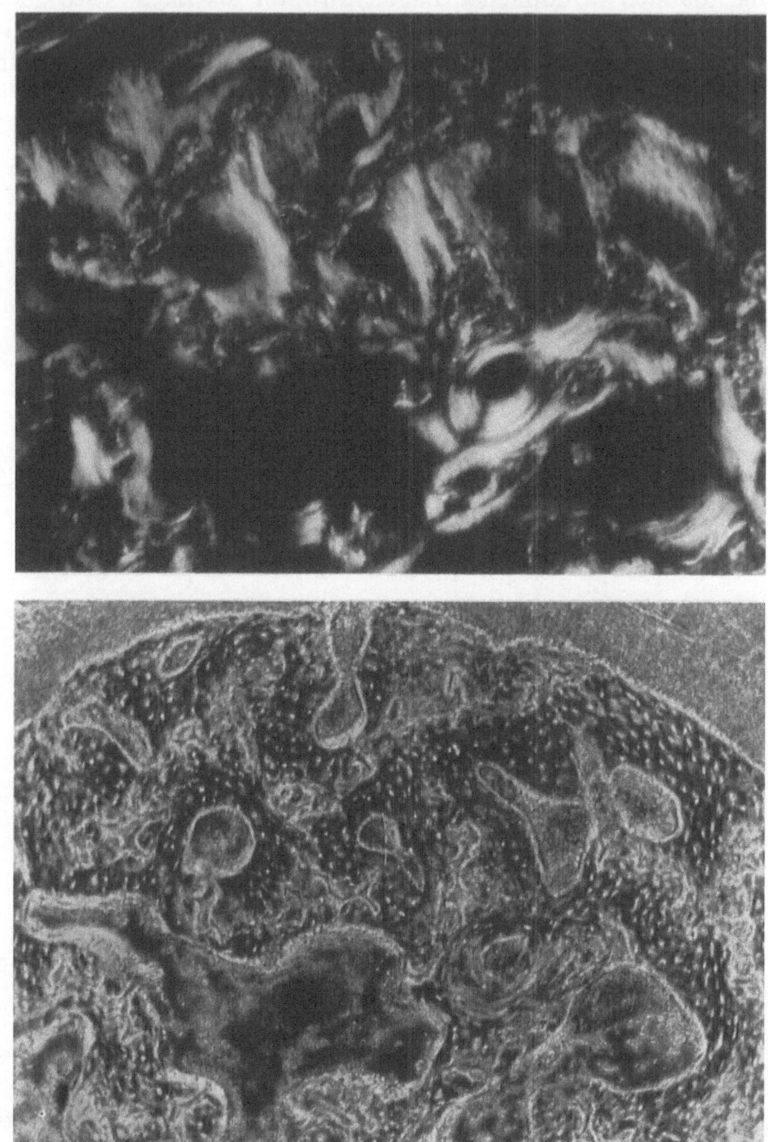

Abb. 28. Fet, 282 mm SSL. Humerus, Querschnittshöhe 8. Ausbildung von Kollagenfaserstrukturen in Form von Faserfilzbezirken und Osteonen mit noch undeutlich abgegrenzten Lamellen. Dazwischen Reste von Knorpel mit Demaskierung der Fasern. Darstellung in polarisiertem Licht und mit Phasenkontrastverfahren. O. 10, Ok. 8. (KNESE, 1957)

Der chondrale Knochen ist längere Zeit an Resten von knorpeliger Intercellularsubstanz zu erkennen (Abb. 28). Diese von Knochen umschlossenen Knorpelreste und die peri-enchondrale Grenzlinie verschwinden im Laufe des ersten Lebensjahres, so daß sich die Herkunft dieser Knochengebiete späterhin morphologisch nicht mehr bestimmen läßt. Auf welchem Wege diese Knorpelreste verschwinden, ist noch nicht endgültig geklärt. KNESE (1957) beschreibt, wie diese Knorpelteile am Ende der Schwangerschaft an Breite verlieren, wobei im polarisierten Lichte eine Umrandung durch dichte Packungen

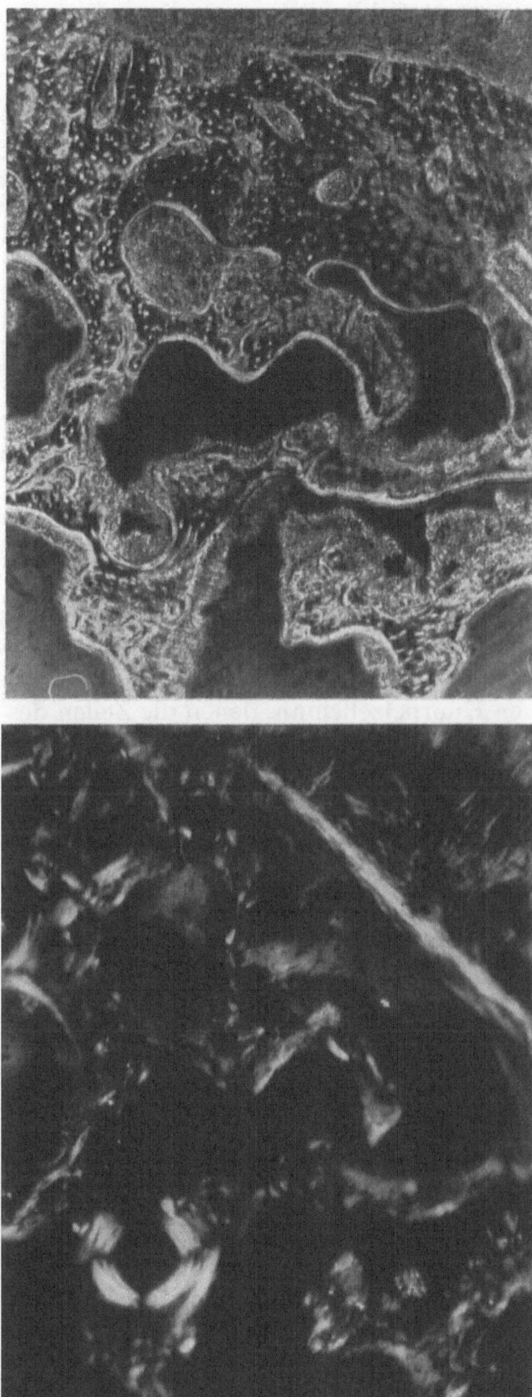

Abb. 29. Fet, 282 mm SSL. Tibia, Querschnittshöhe 7. Ausbildung von Kollagenfaserstrukturen in Form von Faserfilzbezirken und Osteonen. Knorpelreste im chondralen Knochen. Perienchondrale Grenze. Periostaler Knochen, aufgebaut aus einem präkollagenen Faserwerk mit überwiegend radiärer Ausrichtung der Fasern. Bezirk einer freien chondralen Fläche. Darstellung in polarisiertem Licht und Phasenkontrastverfahren. Ob. 10, Ok. 8. (KNESE, 1957)

von Kollagenfibrillen sichtbar wird. Elektronenmikroskopische Untersuchungen lassen vermuten, daß diese Knorpelreste im Knochen Mineraleinlagerungen besitzen, die an eine geringe Menge fädiger Gebilde, aber wohl nicht an Kollagenfibrillen gebunden sind.

(Knese und Knoop, 1961c). Schließlich sind diese Knorpelreste lichtmikroskopisch nicht mehr aufzufinden.

Knese (1957) konnte bei Untersuchungen desselben Schnittes mit dem Phasenkontrastverfahren und im polarisiertem Licht nachweisen, daß noch bei Vorhandensein der Knorpelreste im Knochen bereits eine lamelläre Struktur vorliegt. Die mehr oder minder gut gegeneinander abgegrenzten Lamellen umgeben Gefäßkanäle oder sog. Markräume (Abb. 29). Diese Lamellierung ist im chondralen Knochen weiter vorangeschritten als in dem benachbarten periostalen. Die Breite der Lamellenanlagen beträgt im periostalen Knochen 2—4 μ, im chondralen 5—8 μ (Knese und Knoop, 1961c).

b) Die Epiphysen und die enchondrale Osteogenese

In der Einleitung zu diesem Kapitel wurde darauf hingewiesen, daß die Vorgänge in der Epiphyse relativ gut bekannt sind, während die Beziehungen dieser Prozesse zur enchondralen Osteogenese noch einer eingehenden Diskussion bedürfen. Der Lebenscyclus einer Zelle des Epiphysenknorpels beginnt mit der Umwandlung von den fibroblastenähnlichen Elementen zu Prächondroblasten und zu Chondroblasten, die dann als flache Zellen in den Appositionsknorpel eingeschlossen werden. Die Zellen runden sich in der Tiefe des Epiphysenknorpels ab. Am Übergang vom Proliferations- zum Säulenknorpel nehmen die Zellen eine flache Gestalt an und ordnen sich in Reihen an (Abb. 30). In einem relativ schmalen Abschnitt der Epiphyse schwellen die Zellen nun zu den sog. hypertrophen Knorpelzellen an, denen die Zellen des mineralisierten Knorpels morphologisch nur z.T. gleichen (Knese, 1968).

Eeg-Larsen (1956) hat für die Dauer des Entwicklungscyclus der Epiphysenzellen 30—45 Std errechnet. Dabei verbleibt die einzelne Zelle 20—30 Std in der Proliferations-, 7—15 Std in der hypertrophen und 3—5 Std in der Mineralisationszone. Dodds (1930) hat die Teilung der Zellen senkrecht zur Wachstumsrichtung ausführlich untersucht. Er weist darauf hin, daß nicht immer eine Säulenordnung, sondern häufig auch eine Ballenordnung auftritt. Kember (1960) hat bei Ratten den Teilungsvorgang und die Wanderung der Zellen mit Hilfe von ^{3}H-markiertem Thymidin verfolgt, das als Vorläufer von Desoxyribonucleinsäure (DNA) nur in sich teilenden Zellen aufgenommen wird (Abb. 31). Die Tiere wurden in einem Abstand von 1 Std bis zu 7 Tagen nach intraperitonealer bzw. intravenöser Injektion untersucht. Zur Bestimmung der Zellage zählt Kember rückwärts von der letzten hypertrophen Zelle aus, die die Nummer 1 erhält. Nach 1 Std sind die markierten Zellen in der Position 12—25, nach einem Tage in 6 und nach 2 Tagen in der Stellung 2 aufzufinden. Damit beträgt der Nachschub zur Eröffnungszone 5 Zellen je Tag. Sissons (1955) hatte $7^1/_2$ Zellen angegeben. Kember (1960) errechnet aus dem Durchmesser der hypertrophen Zellen von 25 μ multipliziert mit 5 einen Wachstumsbetrag der Epiphyse von 125 μ je Tag.

Die Form und Struktur der Chondrocyten ändert sich während ihres Lebenscyclus beträchtlich. Diese Veränderungen wurden auch elektronenmikroskopisch untersucht (Knese und Knoop, 1961a; Godman und Porter, 1960; Knese). Die Zellen des Appositionsknorpels besitzen eine lange, schmale Gestalt, ein relativ dichtes Grundplasma, ein mäßig entwickeltes endoplasmatisches Reticulum, Mitochondrien und einen gut ausgebildeten Golgi-Apparat mit glatten Lamellen und Bläschen. Bei der Umwandlung zu Zellen des hyalinen Epiphysenknorpels erscheinen die Zellen im Schnitt dreieckig, späterhin in der Tiefe des Knorpels ovoid oder rundlich. Diese Formänderung ist auf eine Vergrößerung des hyaloplasmatischen Raumes zurückzuführen; daneben erscheinen einzelne blasenartige Auftreibungen des endoplasmatischen Reticulums. Elektronenmikroskopische Untersuchungen (Knese, 1969) haben gezeigt, daß zur Transformationszone hin (s. S. 726), d.h. am Übergang von hyalinen Epiphysenknorpel zum Säulenknorpel, die Menge der Glykogeneinlagerungen vermehrt wird (Knese).

Gleichzeitig setzt eine erhöhte MPS-Synthese ein, die elektronenmikroskopisch durch das Auftreten intracellulärer größerer, stark kontrastierter Granula, die auch durch das Plasmalemm hindurchtreten, gekennzeichnet ist. Die Metamorphose der Zellen des Proliferationsknorpels zu denen des Säulenknorpels vollzieht sich unter Verkleinerung

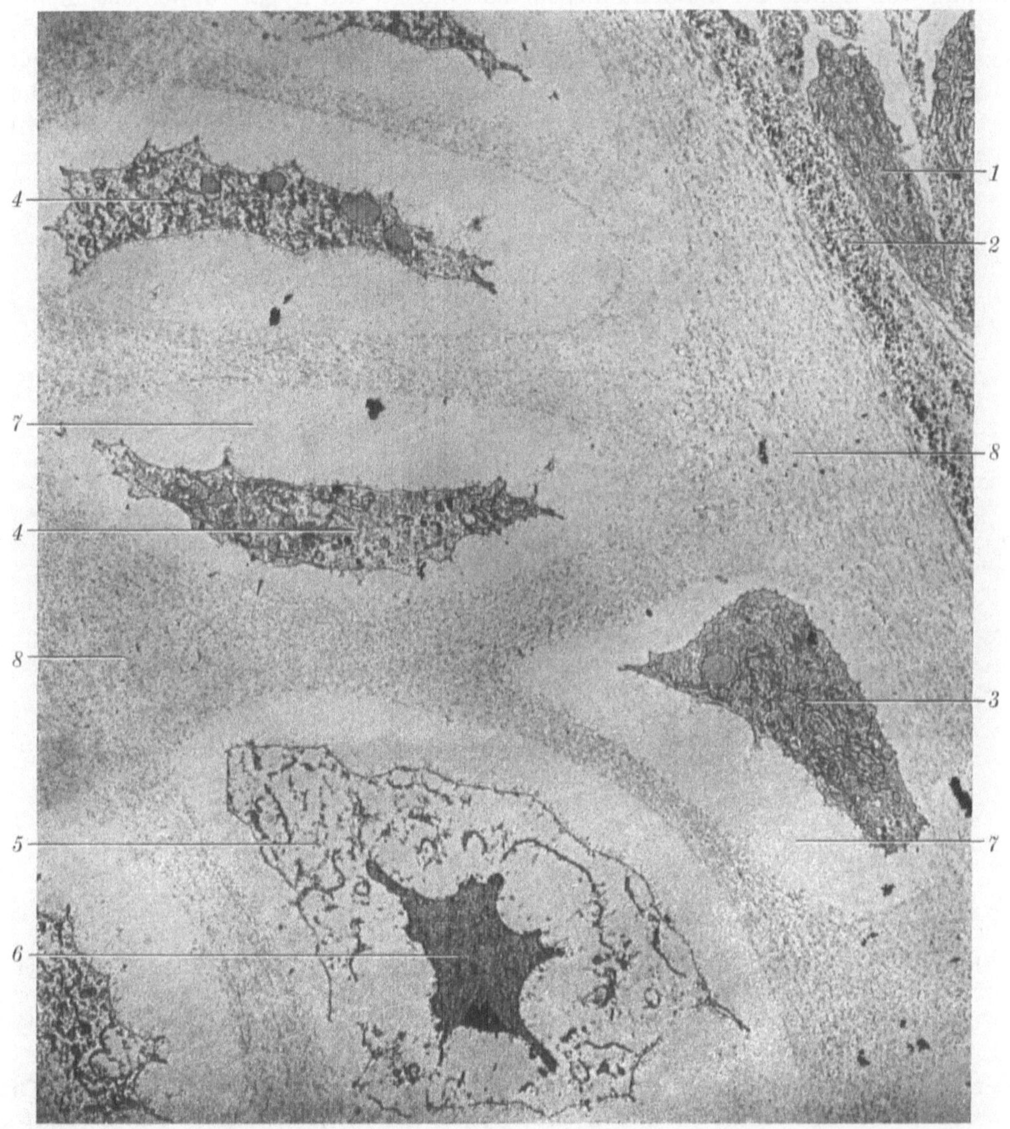

Abb. 30. Chondrocyten am Übergang vom Säulenknorpel zum hypertrophen Knorpel. *1* Osteoblast; *2* präossales Gewebe; *3* im Schnitt dreieckige Knorpelzelle mit dichtem Cytoplasma und blasenartiger Erweiterung einer Zisterne; *4* Zellen des Säulenknorpels mit einer Reihe von Zisternenerweiterungen sowie von der Kapsel abgerissenen Zellfüßen; *5* hypertrophe Knorpelzelle mit einzelnen Ergastoplasmamembranen; *6* Kern mit Nucleolus dieser Zelle; *7* Schrumpfraum; *8* Intercellularsubstanz. Vergr. 4700. (Knese u. Knoop 1961a)

und Abplattung der Chondrocyten, jedoch kann z. Zt. nicht festgestellt werden, worauf diese Volumenabnahme beruht. Die Chondrocyten des Säulenknorpels enthalten in ihrem Zelleib eine Fülle unterschiedlich gestalteter „Vacuolen"; sie sind entweder mit elektronenmikroskopisch dichtem Inhalt versehen oder optisch fast leer (Abb. 32). Der größere Anteil dieser Gebilde ist als stark erweiterte Zisternen des endoplasmatischen Reticulums mit einem wolkig erscheinenden Inhalt anzusehen. Die Elemente mit dichterem Inhalt stellen das stark zusammengedrückte Hyaloplasma dar, in dem auch Mitochondrien liegen. Kleinere Vacuolen, die optisch leer erscheinen, gehören wohl dem Golgi-Apparat an. Ein umfangreicher Golgi-Apparat erscheint nur bei Ratten, aber nicht Rinderfeten (KNESE, 1969). Die Menge der Kohlenhydrate nimmt in den Säulenknorpelzellen ab, das endoplasmatische Reticulum ist gut entwickelt. Der Mechanismus der Umwandlung von Zellen des Säulenknorpels zu solchen des hypertrophen ist nicht leicht zu klären (KNESE und KNOOP, 1961a). Die Umwandlung zu hypertrophen Zellen (KNESE, 1968, 1969) beginnt mit einer vermehrten Einlagerung von Kohlenhydraten. Das endoplasmatische Reticulum bildet ein kanalartiges mit einander kommunizierendes Röhrensystem. Die Röhren stehen mit den großen sackartigen Erweiterungen der Zisternen

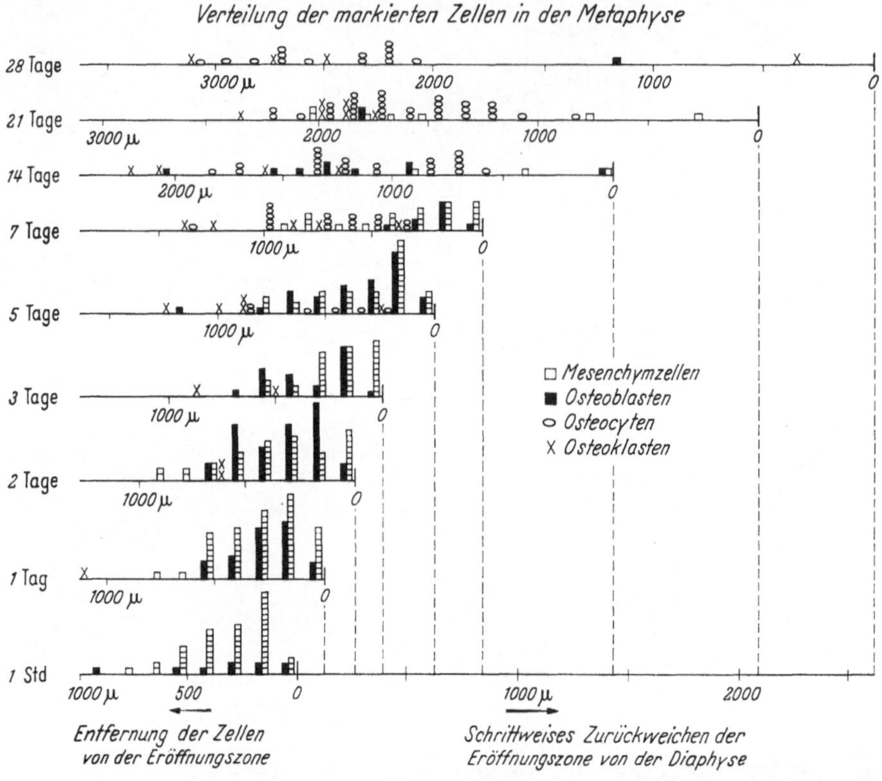

Abb. 31. Verteilung der mit Thymidin ^{3}H markierten Mesenchymzellen, Osteoblasten, Osteocyten und Osteoclasten in der Tibia-Metaphyse von Ratten zu verschiedenen Zeiten. Mit 0 wird die Eröffnungszone angegeben. Abstand der markierten Zellen von dieser Eröffnungszone in μ. (Nach KEMBER 1960)

in Verbindung. In der weiteren Entwicklung lassen sich elektronenmikroskopisch Granula nur noch in geringer Zahl in den hypertrophen Zellen nachweisen. Die Chondrocyten sind jetzt größere rundliche Gebilde mit einem ähnlich gestalteten, mitunter gelappten Kern. Im Zelleib sind elektronenmikroskopisch einzelne Membranen des endoplasmatischen Reticulums und Mitochondrien zu beobachten (Abb. 33). Im übrigen erscheint die Zelle leer. Dieser Befund wurde auch von elektronenmikroskopischen Untersuchern als ein Zeichen des Absterbens angesprochen (SCOTT und PEASE, 1956; ZELANDER, 1959; TAKUMA, 1960). KNESE und KNOOP (1961a—c) vermuten, daß die Zellen niedermolekulare, bei der Präparation leicht lösliche Stoffe enthalten. Das Material der Zellen läßt sich aber durch Doppelfixierung, d.h. getrennte Fixierung der Proteine und Kohlenhydrate (KNESE, 1968), für lichtmikroskopische Untersuchungen erhalten. Die Zellen nehmen nur etwa 7—35% der zugehörigen Höhlen ein, was z.T. auf Fixierungsschrumpfung beruht. Im übrigen sind die Zellen von einer Pericellularsubstanz umgeben (s. S. 698). Eine starke Ninhydrin-Schiff-Reaktion der Zellen weist auf das Vorhandensein von basischen Proteinen hin (s.u.).

Die Befunde über die Biochemie und Topochemie des Epiphysenknorpels stimmen in vielen Punkten überein (Lacroix, 1951a u. b; Follis und Berthrong, 1949; Monesi und Bettini, 1958; Zambotti, 1957; Knese und Knoop, 1961a). Eine Reihe voneinander abweichender Angaben beruht wohl z. T. auf artlichen Differenzen, aber auch auf unterschiedlicher Technik (z. B. Phosphatase: Borghese, 1957). Weiter spielt das Lebensalter der entsprechenden Individuen eine Rolle (Knese, 1959; Knese und Knoop, 1961a).

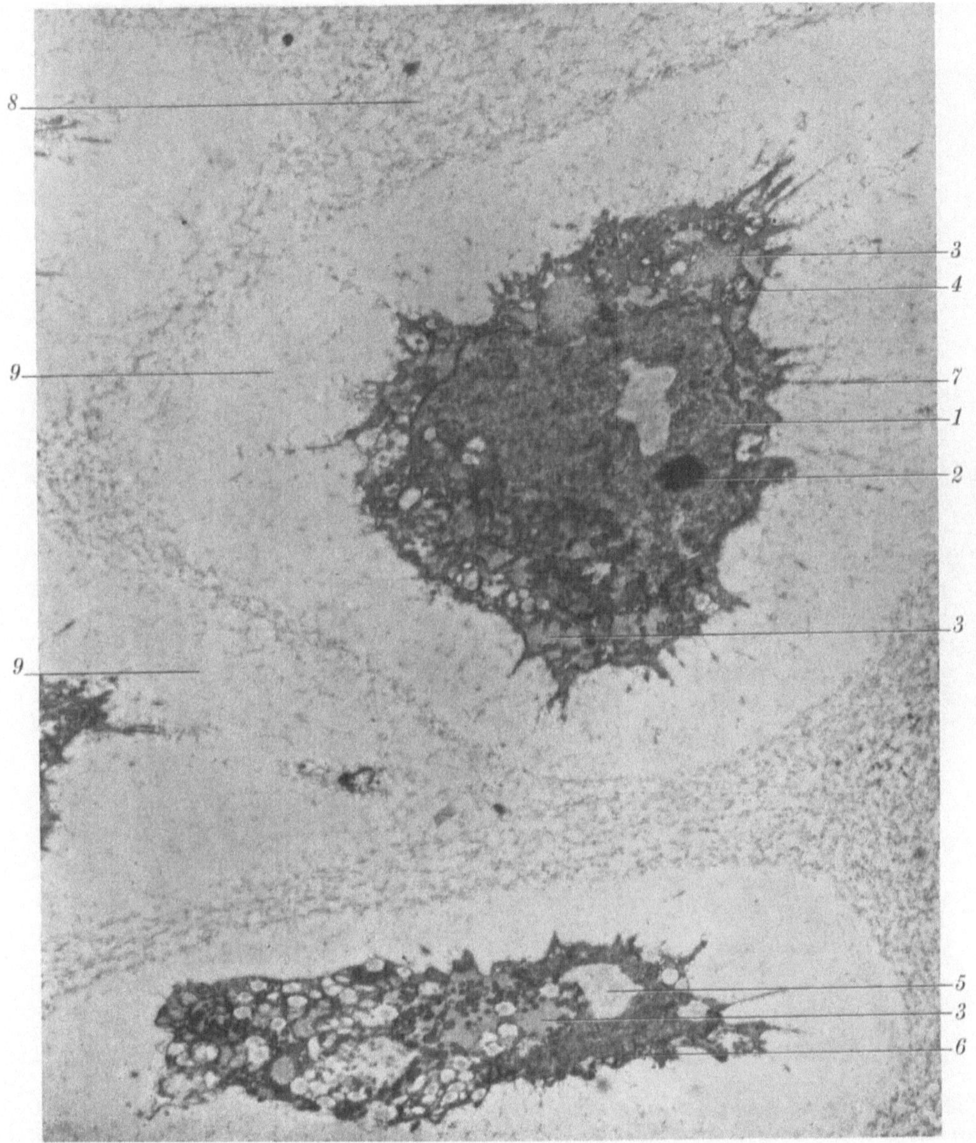

Abb. 32. Chondrocyten am Übergang vom Proliferations- zum Säulenknorpel. *1* Zellkern; *2* Nucleolus; *3* Zisternen mit homogenem Inhalt; *4* Mitochondrien; *5* Vacuolen; *6* Hyaloplasma; *7* Zellfüße mit Sekundärfüßen; *8* Intercellularsubstanz; *9* Schrumpfraum. Vergr. 10000. (Knese, u. Knoop, 1961a)

An Serienschnitten haben Knese und Knoop (1961a) mit verschiedenen Methoden zur Darstellung von Polysacchariden, verbunden mit einer enzymatischen Kontrolle, die Anfärbung der Intercellularsubstanzen und Chondrocyten im Epiphysenknorpel geprüft. Mit den zur Verfügung stehenden Methoden ergibt sich ein wechselndes Färbungsmuster, das an die morphologisch differenten Zonen gebunden ist. Die Grenzzonen zwischen zwei Gebieten verhalten sich färberisch derart, daß sie einmal der einen, zum anderen der Nachbarzone ähneln. Mit Methylenblau färbt sich die Intercellularsubstanz leicht metachromatisch an. Die Zone des Epiphysenknorpels tingiert sich in einem größeren p_H-Bereich der Farbflotte annähernd gleichartig. Im Säulenknorpel liegt das Maximum der Färbbarkeit zwischen dem p_H 4,7 und 5,3, im hypertrophen Knorpel bei 5,3. Bei Färbung mit alkoholischer Toluidinblaulösung wird die metachromatische Reaktion zum hypertrophen Knorpel hin stärker. Durch Behandlung mit wäßriger Toluidinblaulösung

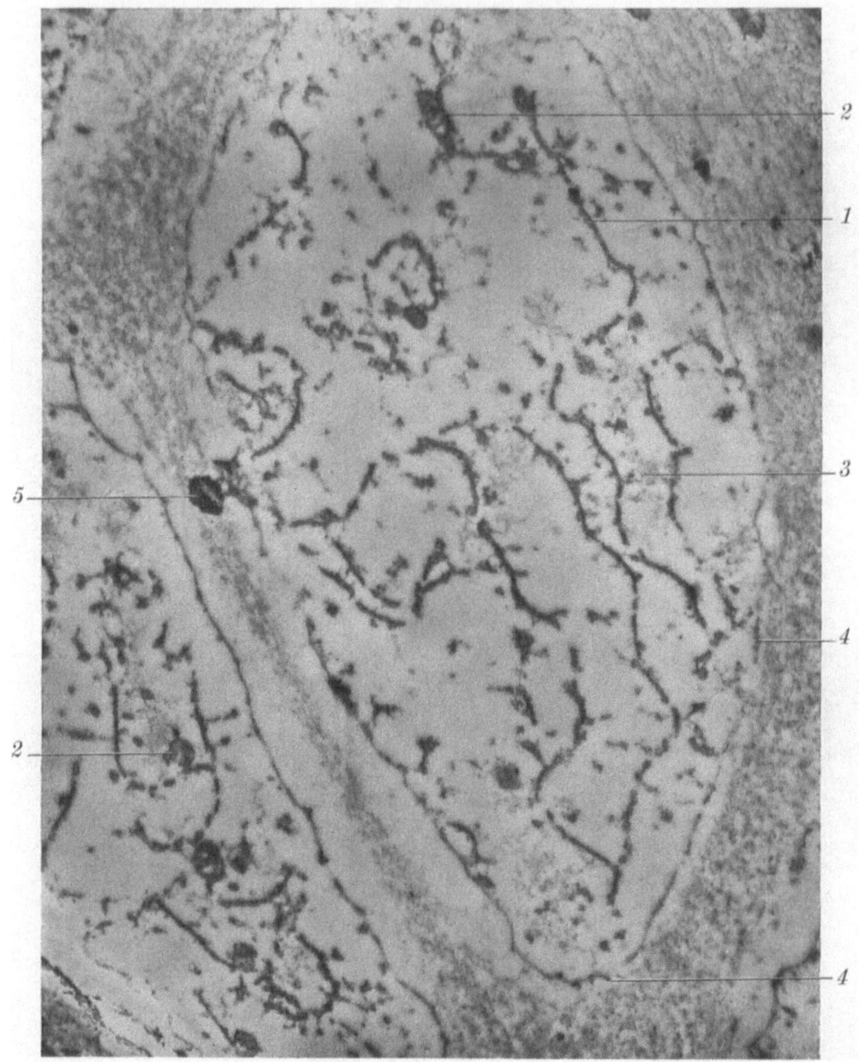

Abb. 33. Hypertrophe Knorpelzelle. *1* Membranen des endoplasmatischen Reticulum; *2* Mitochondrien; *3* Reste des Grundplasmas; *4* Zellmembranen mit Füßen in Verbindung mit der Intercellularsubstanz; *5* Kalkeinlagerung in enger Verbindung mit der Zellmembran. Vergr. 7200. (KNESE u. KNOOP, 1961 b)

in verschiedenem p_H wird der Säulenknorpel durch eine stärkere Reaktion gegenüber allen anderen Zonen hervorgehoben. Eine starke PAS-positive Reaktion zeigt die Intercellularsubstanz des hypertrophen Knorpels. Die Anwendung der Hale-Methode führt zu einer Blau-schwarz-Färbung des hyalinen Epiphysen- und Proliferationsknorpels, bei Rinderfeten über 100 mm SSL auch der Intercellularsubstanz des Säulen- und hypertrophen Knorpels. Bei Rinderfeten unter 100 mm SSL werden in diesen beiden Zonen nur die Kapseln und Zellhöfe dunkel gefärbt; die interterritoriale Substanz reagiert dagegen nicht mit dem kolloidalen Eisen.

Die Einlagerung von Glykogen in Knorpelzellen wurde verschiedentlich beschrieben (Glock, 1940; Follis und Berthrong, 1949 u. a.). Nun konnten Knese und Knoop (1961a) zeigen, daß zunächst kleinere, dann an Größe zunehmende, mit der Hale-Methode nachweisbare Granula bereits im Appositionsknorpel erscheinen. Diese Hale-färbbaren Granula sind in allen Chondrocyten zu beobachten und fehlen nur in den Anfangsabschnitten des Säulenknorpels. PSA-positive Granula treten erst in den peripheren Schichten des hyalinen Epiphysenknorpels auf; sie fehlen in allen Zellen des Säulenknorpels. Das Areal von Zellen mit BTS-positiven Granula ist größer und reicht weiter in die Peripherie des Epiphysenknorpels hinein. Nur wenige Zellen in der Mitte der Reihen des Säulenknorpels lassen BTS-positive Körnchen vermissen. Mit wäßriger Toluidinblaulösung von einem pH von 2,6 sind in den Chondrocyten mit Ausnahme jener der Appositionszone Granula mit einem roten Farbton (γ-Metachromasie) nachzuweisen. In den Zellen des Säulen- und hypertrophen Knorpels reagiert fast das gesamte Cytoplasma stark metachromatisch. Im Säulenknorpel sind weiterhin orthochromatisch blaugefärbte Elemente eingelagert.

Die mit verschiedenen Methoden zum Nachweis von Polysacchariden anfärbbaren Granula in Chondrocyten halten Knese und Knoop (1961a) für ein lichtmikroskopisches Äquivalent der elektronenmikroskopisch zu beobachtenden Zisternensäcke. Die Autoren machen wahrscheinlich, daß diese Granula mit einer Produktion von Substanzen in Zusammenhang stehen, die den Zustand der Intercellularsubstanz verändert; hierauf beruht deren unterschiedliche Anfärbbarkeit. Um welche Stoffe es sich handelt, kann z. Zt. nicht gesagt werden. Auch eine enzymatische Kontrolle der Granula-Färbung führt zu keinem klaren Ergebnis. Die Anfärbung der Granula mit Toluidinblau bleibt nach Vorbehandlung mit Hyaluronidase und Diastase aus. Die PAS-positive Reaktion ist nur durch Diastase aufzuheben. Im übrigen ist zu berücksichtigen, daß mit den Färbemethoden vermutlich nicht nur physikalisch-chemisch voneinander verschiedene Stoffe erfaßt werden, sondern auch deren morphologische Struktur.

Der Stoffwechsel des Epiphysenknorpels ist sehr lebhaft, und zwar sowohl im Hinblick auf Kohlenhydrate als auch Proteine. Die Glykolyse sollte den von Robison und Rosenheim (1934) angenommenen „zweiten" Mechanismus der Mineralisation neben der alkalischen Phosphatase darstellen (Gutman, 1946; Gutman und Yu, 1950). Die Glykogenverteilung wurde von Harris (1932), Gendre (1938), Glock (1940) und Eeg-Larsen (1956) untersucht; letzterer hat sich auch mit dem Auftreten von Milchsäure befaßt. Die Enzyme der Glykolyse wiesen Gutman et al. (1941) und Albaum et al. (1952) nach. Die NADP (TPN) abhängigen Enzyme treten vorwiegend im hypertrophen Knorpel auf (vgl. Balogh, Dudley und Cohen, 1961). Da die zur MPS-Synthese erforderliche Glucose vom Glykogen der einzelnen Zelle abstammt, wurde neuerlich (Knese, im Druck) die Beziehung zwischen der Glykogenverteilung und der MPS-Bildung untersucht. Bereits Gendre (1938) hatte eine Beziehung zwischen dem Glykogen und dem Aufbau der Intercellularsubstanz diskutiert. Dabei ist zu berücksichtigen, daß die Bildung des Glucose-6-Phosphates der initiale Schritt für die Bildung des Hexosamins und der Hexuronsäure aber auch der Glykogensynthese und der Glykolyse ist. Auf einige Ergebnisse dieser Untersuchungen wurde bei der MPS-Synthese eingegangen. Nach Bona und Stănescu (1966) ist die Glucose-6-Phosphatase im Säulenknorpel stärker vertreten als im hypertrophen. Takada (1966) weist darauf hin, daß die NAD (DPN) abhängigen Dehydrogenasen vor allem im Säulenknorpel erscheinen.

Die Bildung von Sulfo-MPS im Epiphysenknorpel ist wohl durch die Untersuchungen mit ^{35}S gesichert (Dziewiatkowski 1951, 1958, Bélanger 1954, Amprino 1956). Die ^{35}S-Einlagerung wird in Richtung auf den hypertrophen Knorpel hin stärker, ist aber bei der Katze im Säulenknorpel am größten (Verne et al. 1956).

Der Proteinstoffwechsel der Zellen des Säulenknorpels beträgt 33%, des Gelenkknorpels 2% derjenigen der Pankreaszellen mit der höchsten Stoffwechselrate aller Körperzellen (Niklas et al., 1956; Koburg, 1961), ^{35}S-Methionin und ^{35}S-Cystin sind in den hypertrophen Knorpelzellen nachzuweisen und auf eine Glyko-Protein-Fraktion zu beziehen (Bélanger 1956a, b). Ablagerungen von ^{14}C treten im Proliferationsknorpel auf und werden zum hypertrophen hin stärker, fehlen aber in der Eröffnungszone (Greulich und Leblond, 1953). Durch die Untersuchungen von Gross, Mathews und Dorfman (1960) sowie Campo und Dziewiatkowski (1962) ist die Synthese eines Kohlenhydrat-Protein-Komplexes durch Knorpelzellen gesichert. Weiterhin konnten durch elektronenmikroskopische Autoradiographie von Cooper und Prockop (1968) und Salpeter (1968) die Bildung von Kollagen und dessen direkte Ausschleusung aus den Chondrocyten nachgewiesen werden.

Die Zunahme der Phosphataseaktivität zu den hypertrophen Knorpelzellen hin wurde von einer großen Zahl von Autoren beschrieben (Robison, 1932; Übersichten von Moog, 1946; Majno und Rouiller, 1951; Bourne, 1956; Burstone, 1960). Aminopeptidase, Cytochromoxydase, Succinodehydrogenase sind sowohl in „ruhenden" Knorpelzellen als auch in den hypertrophen vorhanden; ihre Aktivität ist im Perichondrium allerdings noch stärker (Burstone, 1960). Eine Amylo-1,4→1,6-Transglucosidase im Säulenknorpel ermöglicht die Bildung gekoppelter Polysaccharide (Takeuchi, 1958). Drei Glucosidasen wurden von Takada, Yoshiki und Okamoto (1962) nachgewiesen. Balogh und Cohen (1961) fanden die Uridin-Diphosphat-Glucose-Dehydrogenase, durch die aus der UDP-Glucose die Glucuronsäure gebildet wird. Eine hohe Aktivität an Hexosamin-Synthetase im Epiphysen-, aber nicht im Gelenkknorpel wird von Cipera und Willmer (1962) angegeben. Ein gegensinniges Verteilungsmuster der ATPase und der '5-Nucleotidase wurde von Gibson und Fullmer (1967) aufgedeckt; bereits die Zellen des hyalinen Knorpels reagieren stark, die des Säulenknorpels und die hypertrophen etwas schwächer. Eine Glutamin-Asparagin-Transaminase gestattet die Synthese von Peptidbindungen (de Bernard und Schubert, 1955 nach Zambotti, 1957, dort auch weitere Literatur).

Die Intensität aller Stoffwechselvorgänge im Epiphysenknorpel widerspricht der Vorstellung vom Untergang der hypertrophen Knorpelzellen. Die höchsten Enzymaktivitäten liegen im unteren Anteil des Säulenknorpels und im oberen Anteil des hypertrophen (Takada, 1966). An Hand der Enzymverteilung kommen Bona und Stănescu (1966) zum Schluß, daß im hyalinen Epiphysenknorpel Glykoproteine, wenig Sulfopolysaccharide und kein Kollagen gebildet wird, in dem Säulenknorpel dagegen Tropokollagen, die Masse der Sulfo-MPS. In den hypertrophen Zellen würde die Synthese von Glykoproteinen neu einsetzen (s.u.). An Hand der Verteilung weiterer Enzyme meinen die Autoren, daß zwei Verteilungsmuster vorliegen, eines für jene Enzyme, die den Stoffwechsel aufrechterhalten und dann ein weiteres mit hohen Aktivitäten nur in einzelnen Regionen. Die Annahme vom Absterben der Knorpelzellen beruht auf der im fixierten Zustand zu beobachtenden Schrumpfung der hypertrophen Knorpelzellen (s. S. 734), dem refraktären Verhalten der Zellen der Eröffnungszone gegenüber vielen Färbemethoden und dem Verschwinden markierter Substanzen in dieser Zone. Knese und Knoop (1961b) vermuten, daß alle drei Phänomene als Artefacte anzusehen sind, die durch die Lösung niedermolekularer Stoffe erst bei der Präparation auftreten. Mit Fluorescein markierten Antikörpern der Protein-Polysaccharide untersuchten Hirschman und Dziewiatkowski (1966) Ratten- und Kälberepiphysen. In der Zone der Mineralisation ist ein starkes Abfallen der leichten MPS-Fraktion (PPL) zu beobachten. Es könnte einmal möglich sein, daß die Polysaccharide nicht mehr kovalent gebunden sind oder daß zum anderen die Proteine drastisch verändert erscheinen. Lindenbaum und Kuettner (1967) fanden an der Kälber-Scapula die höchste Konzentration der MPS und Mucoproteine in der 2 mm breiten hypertrophen Zone. Weiterhin zeigte sich in Richtung zur Knorpel-Knochengrenze hin eine Zunahme des Äquivalentgewichtes und eine Abnahme der austauschbaren Sulfatgruppen. Unter Berücksichtigung der topochemischen und elektronenmikroskopischen (s.u.) Befunde müssen wir wohl entscheidende Veränderungen der Zellen in ihrer Struktur und in ihren Bestandteilen annehmen, wobei das Auftreten basischer Proteine von besonderer Bedeutung ist, die vermutlich den Globulinen zuzurechnen sind.

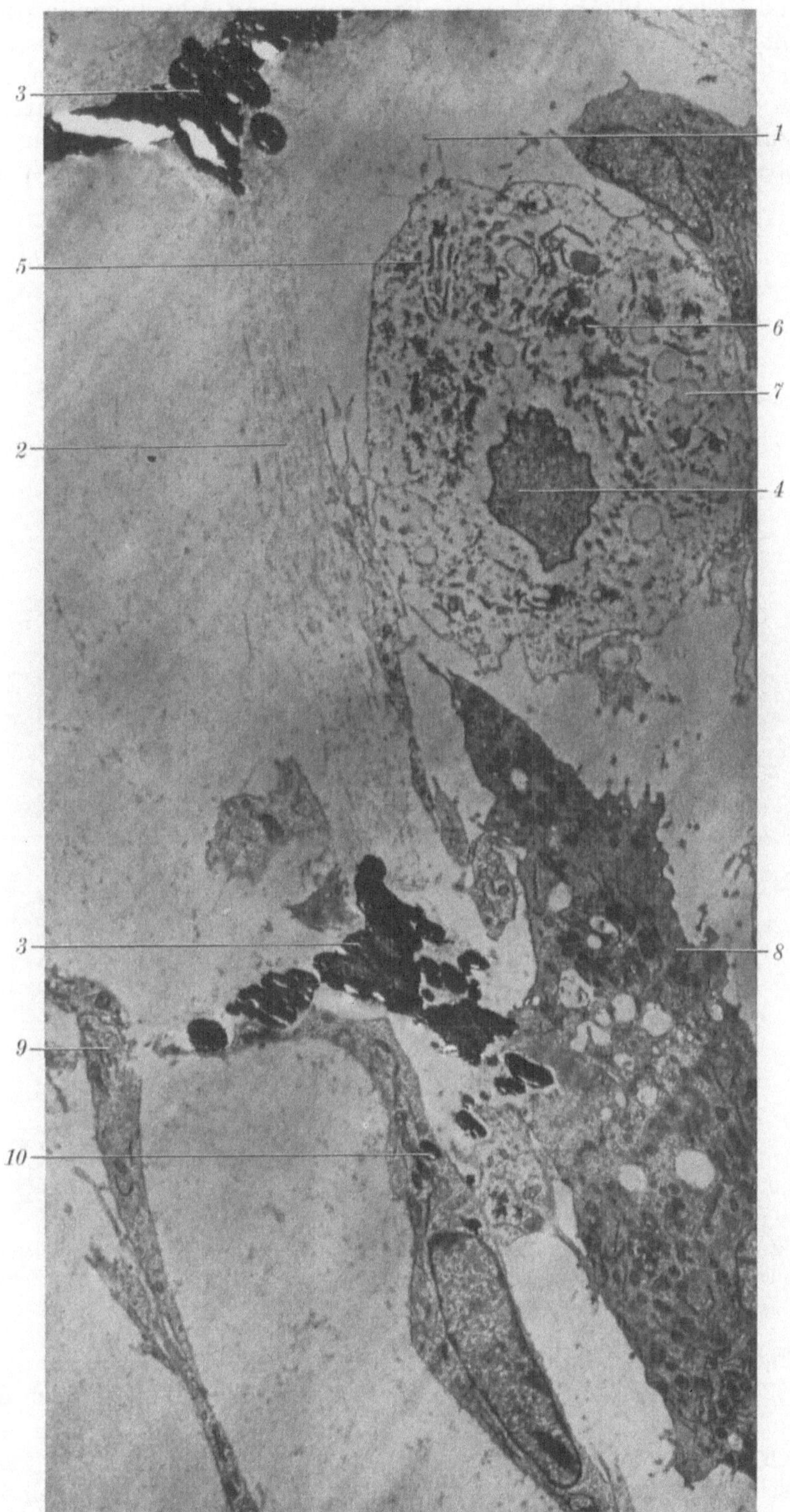

Abb. 34. Eröffnungszone. *1* Knorpelhöhle; *2* Längsbalken aus organischer Interfibrillärsubstanz; *3* Knorpelkalk; *4* Chondrocytenkern; *5* endoplasmatisches Reticulum; *6* osmiophile Einlagerungen; *7* Vesicel (erweiterte Zisternen?); *8* graue Zellen; *9* Endothelzelle, eine Querwand durchbrechend; *10* Endothelzelle mit Kalkeinschlüssen. Vergr. 3500. (KNESE u. KNOOP, 1961b)

KNESE und KNOOP (1961 b) haben die Eröffnungszone elektronenmikroskopisch untersucht, da mit lichtmikroskopischen Methoden keine zuverlässigen Aussagen über das Schicksal der Knorpelzellen zu gewinnen sind. Bei der Eröffnung der Knorpelhöhlen verschwinden zunächst die Querbalken der Intercellularsubstanz, während die Längsbalken stehenbleiben und einen Überzug von enchondralem Knochen erhalten. Die Autoren beobachten das Herantreten von Gefäßsprossen bzw. aus dem Verband heraus-

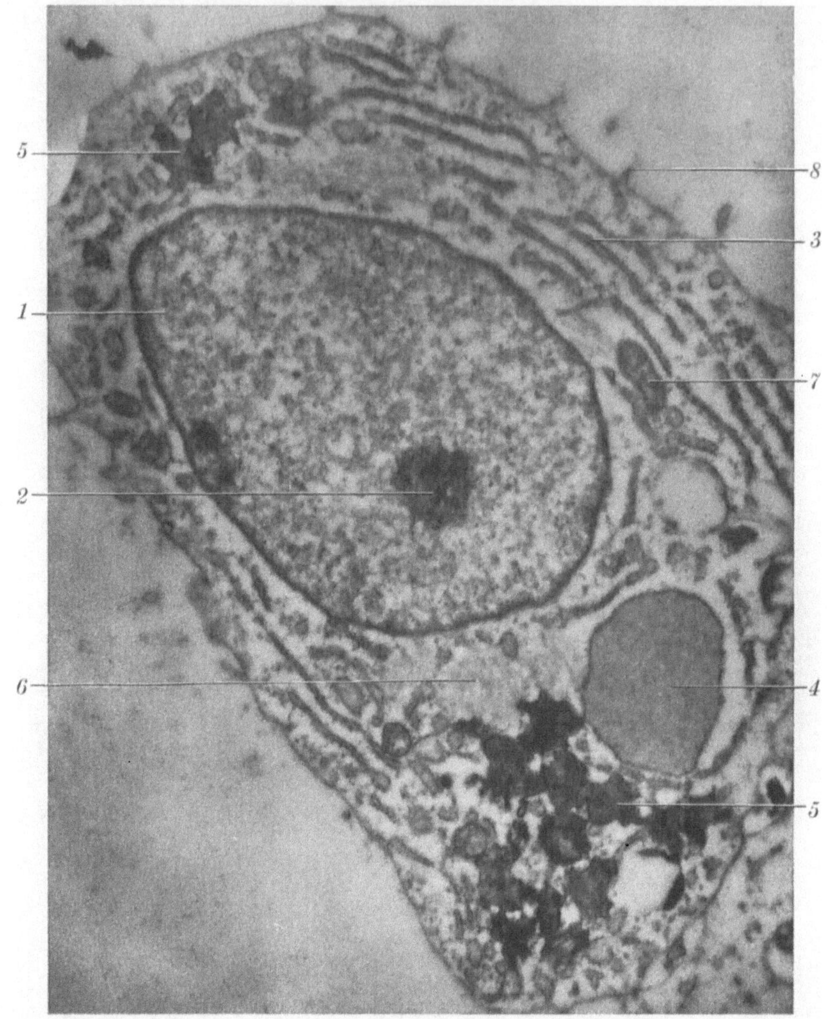

Abb. 35. Helle Zelle. *1* Zellkern; *2* Nucleolus; *3* Membranen des endoplasmatischen Reticulum; *4* Zisternensack; *5* osmiophile Einlagerung; *6* Bezirke homogenen Grundplasmas; *7* Mitochondrien; *8* Zellwand mit Füßen. Vergr. 3500. (KNESE u. KNOOP, 1961 b)

getretener Endothelzellen oder von Elementen, die die Gefäße begleiten, wie es ähnlich TAKUMA (1960) beschrieb (Abb. 34). Gleichzeitig verschwindet aber auch die organische Intercellularsubstanz der Längsbalken, so daß nur die Mineralmassen stehenbleiben. Damit werden die lichtmikroskopischen Untersuchungen von DODDS (1932) bestätigt, nach denen sehr verschiedene Zellformen an der Eröffnung der Knorpelhöhlen beteiligt sind. Riesenzellen, d. h. mehrkernige Zellen („Chondroclasten") treten erst in einem gewissen Abstand von der Eröffnungszone auf (u. a. KÖLLIKER, 1873; ZAWISCH, 1931; KNESE, 1957).

Außer Gefäßendothelien und perivasculären, den Fibroblasten ähnlichen Zellen fanden KNESE und KNOOP (1961b) jenseits der Eröffnungszone zwei Zellformen, die sie als helle und graue Zellen bezeichnen. Die hellen Zellen (Abb. 35) entsprechen in ihrer Cytoplasmastruktur den Knorpelzellen der Mineralisationszone und werden demzufolge als Abkömmlinge von Chondrocyten angesehen. Diese Zellen unterliegen anschließend einer Metamorphose und werden zu Markosteoblasten, indem das endoplasmatische Reticulum stärker ausgebildet wird und das Hyaloplasma sich verdichtet.

Die sog. grauen Zellen dringen in eröffnete Knorpelhöhlen ein; häufig liegen jeweils eine helle und graue Zelle paarweise nebeneinander. Die grauen Zellen haben im Vergleich zur Größe des Zelleibes einen relativ kleinen Kern (Abb. 36), ein dichtes Grundplasma mit isoliert liegenden Ribosomen (Palade-Granula), reichlich Mitochondrien, aber nur

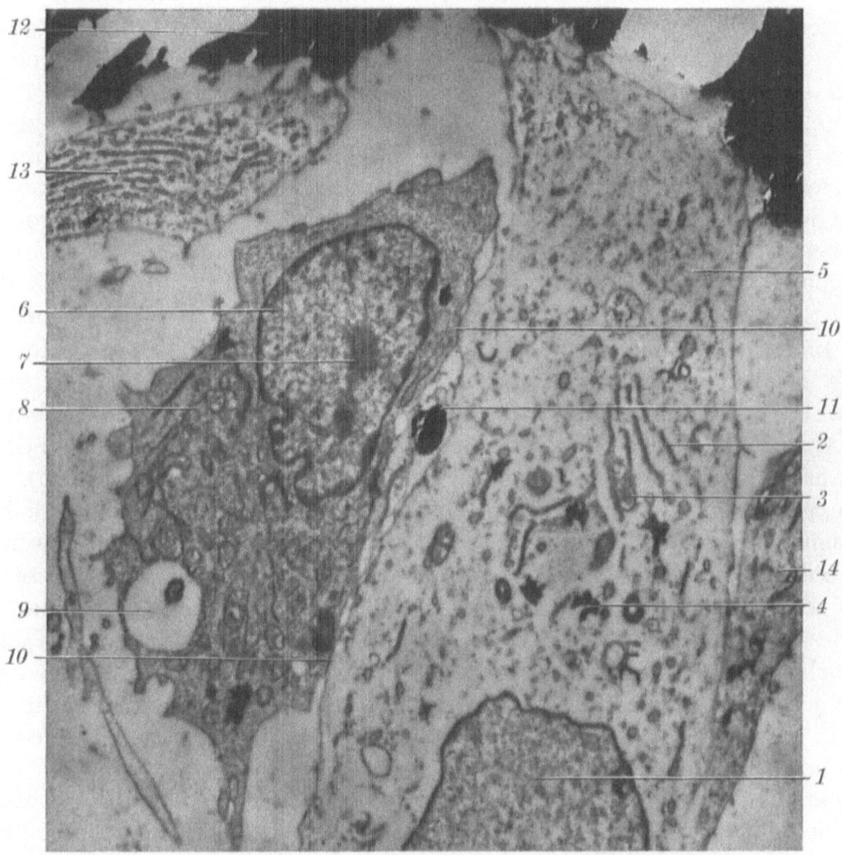

Abb. 36. Helle und graue Zellen in Kontakt miteinander. Helle Zelle: *1* Kern mit locker angeordnetem Chromatin; *2* endoplasmatisches Reticulum; *3* Mitochondrien; *4* osmiophile Einlagerungen; *5* Grundplasma mit wenig Granula. Graue Zelle: *6* Zellkern mit randständigem Chromatin; *7* Nucleolus; *8* feinkörniges, dichtes Grundplasma mit Mitochondrien, einigen Membranen und osmiophilen Einlagerungen; *9* Vacuole; *10* Kontakt zwischen grauer und heller Zelle; *11* Kalkbrocken zwischen beiden Zellen; *12* Knorpelkalk; *13* helle Zelle mit größerer Anzahl von Doppelmembranen; *14* Fibroblast. Vergr. 5800. (Knese u. Knoop, 1961b)

ein spärlich ausgebildetes endoplasmatisches Reticulum. Die Abkunft dieser Zellen konnte morphologisch nicht aufgeklärt werden. Sie ähneln in der Cytoplasmastruktur den Fibroblasten oder Endothelzellen. Jedoch sind auch Zellen aufzufinden, die als Übergangsformen zwischen hellen und grauen Zellen angesehen werden können. Aus den grauen Zellen werden, vermutlich durch Zellverschmelzung, Riesenzellen. Bei einer neuerlichen elektronenmikroskopischen Untersuchung der Eröffnungszone (unveröffentlicht) konnte einmal die Eröffnung der Knorpelhöhlen, zum anderen das Ausschlüpfen von Zellen beobachtet werden. Diese geschlüpften Zellen zeigen lichtmikroskopisch nach Doppelfixierung eine starke Ninhydrin-Schiff- und PAS-Reaktion. Elektronenmikroskopisch treten dagegen z.T. Bilder einer Desintegration auf, wie sie bereits früher beschrieben wurden (Knese und Knoop, 1961b), wobei in einer granulären Masse wohlerhaltene

Zellorganellen liegen. Die Entwicklung der grauen Zellen geht offensichtlich im Bereich der Trichterregion (funnel: LEBLOND et al., 1950) von Fibroblasten aus, die eine Fülle fingerförmiger Fortsätze entwickeln. Sobald diese Zellen frei zwischen der primären Spongiosa liegen, treten eine große Zahl von Mitochondrien auf und damit entsprechen die Zellen dem beschriebenen Bild der grauen Zellen.

TONNA (1961) konnte durch Markierung der DNA mit ^{3}H-Thymidin den Nachweis erbringen, daß als Zellreservoir für das Wachstum der Epiphyse das Perichondrium auftritt. Allerdings reicht dieser Zellnachschub nicht aus; so erscheinen weiterhin mitotische Teilungen in der Proliferations- und hypertrophen Zone. Während die Proliferationsrate im Periost zwischen der 1. und 5. Lebenswoche der Mäuse abnimmt, bleibt sie in der Epiphysenscheibe zunächst unverändert und sinkt erst nach der 5. Woche ab.

KEMBER (1960) hat das Schicksal mit ^{3}H-Thymidin markierter Zellen jenseits der Eröffnungszone, in der Metaphyse der Tibia von Ratten im Zeitraum von 1 Std bis zum 28. Tag nach Markierung verfolgt (Abb. 31). Der Autor unterscheidet vier Zellformen, Mesenchymzellen, Osteoblasten bzw. Präosteoblasten, Osteocyten und Riesenzellen. Der größere Teil der markierten Zellen wird als primitive Mesenchymzelle angesprochen; sie sind die Stammzellen für alle anderen Formen. Wie KNESE und KNOOP (1961b) elektronenmikroskopisch nachgewiesen haben, können in der Metaphyse mehrere Zellformen als „primitive" Stammzellen angesehen werden. Die von KEMBER (1960) beobachtete Verteilung der markierten Zellen in der Epiphyse und Metaphyse spricht dafür, daß es sich bei den sog. Mesenchymzellen um ehemalige Chondrocyten handelt. Die von KEMBER angewandte Hämatoxylinfärbung reicht im übrigen für eine cytologische Diagnostik nicht aus. Angesichts des Entwicklungszustandes des Gewebes ist außerdem der Gebrauch des Terminus „Mesenchymzelle" kaum noch angebracht (KNESE, 1963b). Die in der Epiphyse markierten Zellen verschieben sich bis zum 3. Tag von der Proliferations- zur Mineralisationszone. In der Metaphyse sind nach 1 Std fast nur Mesenchymzellen und einige Osteoblasten in einem Abstand bis zu 1000 μ von der Eröffnungszone markiert. Die Anzahl der markierten Osteoblasten nimmt nun so stark zu, daß eine gleich große Zahl von Mesenchymzellen und Osteoblasten eine Markierung besitzen. Nach 28 Tagen sind nur noch Osteoblasten und Riesenzellen markiert, die beide in einem Abstand von 2000—3000 μ von der Eröffnungszone liegen. TONNA (1961) hat dagegen nur sehr wenig ^{3}H-Thymidin-markierte Riesenzellen beobachtet und schließt daraus, daß diese Zellen sich nicht mehr mitotisch teilen.

Im allgemeinen werden in der Eröffnungszone alle Knorpelhöhlen eröffnet; ferner sind die verbleibenden Längsbalken ohne Zellen. Am Metacarpus des Rindes konnten KNESE und KNOOP (1961b) eine Modifikation der enchondralen Osteogenese beobachten (Abb. 37). In der Eröffnungszone werden nämlich nicht alle Höhlen eröffnet. so daß in den Längsbalken noch Chondrocyten vorhanden sind. Damit liegt eine Bildungsform vor, die eine Zwischenstellung zwischen der enchondralen und diaphysär-chondralen einnimmt. Die Chondrocyten in den Längsbalken zeigen bei der Ninhydrin-Schiff-Reaktion auf Proteine eine schwache Anfärbung des Cytoplasmas. Die Knorpelhöhlen werden nun von der Längsseite her eröffnet; erst anschließend verschwinden auch die Querwände. Die nun frei in der Markhöhle liegenden Zellen behalten zunächst ihre seriale Lage wie im Knorpel bei, aber ihre Struktur ändert sich. Der Kern wird relativ klein und erscheint dunkel. Der ebenfalls verkleinerte Zelleib färbt sich stark mit Gallocyanin an, d. h. es sind Ribonucleinsäuren aufgetreten. Mit dieser Modifikation der Zellstruktur ist offensichtlich die Metamorphose von Knorpelzellen zu Markosteoblasten vollzogen. KNESE (1963b) konnte bei Rinderfeten in der subepiphysären Zone einzelne den Knorpelzellen ähnliche Elemente beobachten, die eine starke Kohlenhydratreaktion, aber auch einzelne Granula bei der Eisenreaktion zeigen. Auf Grund der Kohlenhydratreaktion und der topographischen Verteilung der Zellen schließt KNESE (1963b), daß die subepiphysären Osteoblasten von Chondrocyten abstammen. Die zur Markhöhle hin unmittelbar benachbarten Osteoblasten sind dagegen von perivasculären Fibroblasten abzuleiten.

Das Schicksal der aus ihren Höhlen befreiten Knorpelzellen wurde sehr verschieden beurteilt. Die Annahme, daß die Chondrocyten absterben, ist weit verbreitet und wurde neuerlich auch auf Grund elektronenmikroskopischer Untersuchungen vertreten (KÖLLIKER, 1873; LACROIX, 1951a; SCOTT und PEASE, 1956; ZELANDER, 1959; TAKUMA, 1960). Die

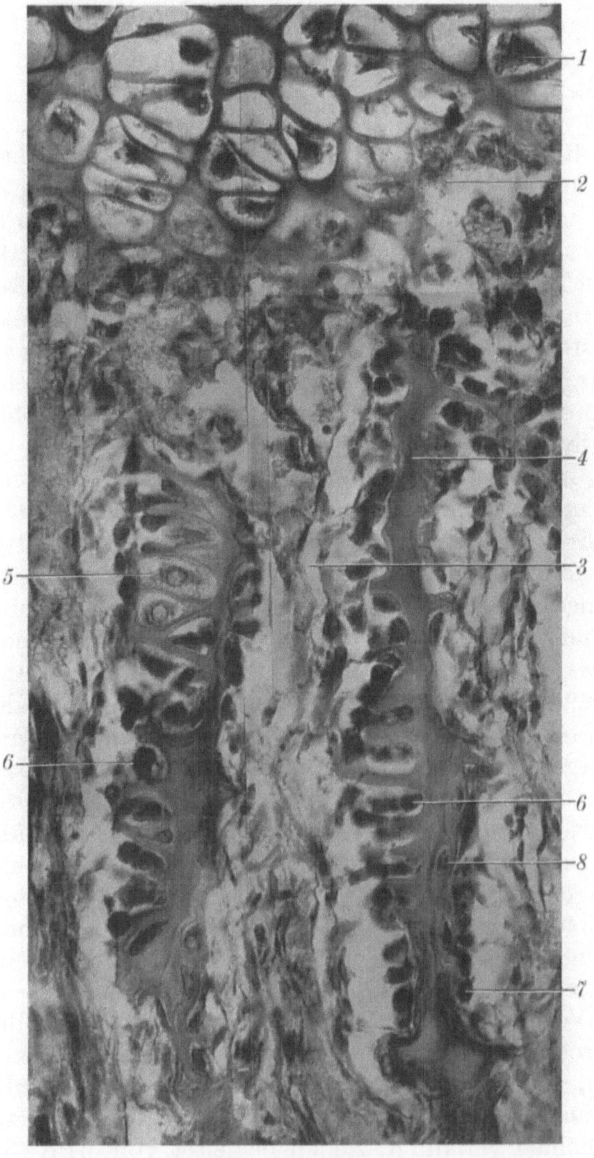

Abb. 37. Eröffnungszone aus dem Metacarpus eines Rinderfetus von 151 mm SSL. *1* Knorpelzellen der Mineralisationszone; *2* Eröffnungszone; *3* Gefäße; *4* Längsbalken von knorpeliger Intercellularsubstanz; *5* noch nicht eröffnete Höhlen; *6* soeben eröffnete Knorpelhöhlen mit noch erhaltenen Querwänden; *7* Osteoblasten; *8* Osteocyten in enchondralem Knochen. Ninhydrin-Schiff-Reaktion. Ob. 40, Ok. 12,5 (Photomontage). (KNESE u. KNOOP, 1961b)

Markosteoblasten wurden als Abkömmlinge indifferenter Zellen angesehen (GEGENBAUR, 1864; FELL, 1925; GARDNER, 1956). Von anderen Autoren wurde die Abkunft der Osteoblasten von Knorpelzellen angenommen (MÜLLER, 1858; HANSEN, 1899; SPULER, 1899; DEINEKA, 1916). HOLTROP (1966) hat die Herkunft von Osteoblasten aus Chondrocyten experimentell untersucht. Dazu hat HOLTROP zunächst Knorpelrippen bei Mäusen intramusculär transplantiert und fand nach 2 Wochen enchondrale Knochenbildung, Osteoblasten, Osteocyten und Osteoclasten. Weiterhin hat HOLTROP Spendermäuse mit

^{3}H-Thymidin markiert und konnte nach der Transplantation in einem nicht markierten Gast markierte Osteoblasten und Osteocyten nachweisen. Zur Entscheidung, ob die Knochenzellen von Knorpelzellen oder vom Perichondrium abstammen, hat HOLTROP bei Ratten die vom Perichondrium befreiten Rippen, z.T. markiert, transplantiert und fand ebenfalls eine enchondrale Knochenbildung. Die Abkunft von Knochenzellen von Knorpelzellen ist damit nach HOLTROP gesichert.

Untersuchungen mit sehr unterschiedlichen Methoden lassen demgemäß annehmen, daß die Knorpelzellen in der Eröffnungszone nicht absterben. STREETER (1949) sowie FELL und ROBINSON (1933) sehen den Gestaltwandel der Chondrocyten innerhalb der Epiphyse als einen Reifungsprozeß an, der nach KNESE und BIERMANN (1958) zunächst mit der Metamorphose zu Markosteoblasten endet. Die knorpelige Epiphyse ist nicht nur ein Platzhalter, sondern auch ein Zellreservoir (KNESE und KNOOP, 1961b) für die Osteogenese. Hierfür sprechen auch die Beobachtungen an mit ^{3}H-Thymidin markierten Zellen (KEMBER, 1960; TONNA, 1961). So wurde dann (KNESE, 1967b, 1968) die Umgestaltung der Zellformen in der Epiphyse als ein Vorgang angesehen, der teilweise der Entwicklung der Osteoblasten im Periost (KNESE, 1966a) analog verläuft. Hierbei dürfte vor allem ein Wechsel der Zelleistungen bei der Abfolge der verschiedenen Zelltypen eine Rolle spielen, z.B. die Ablösung der Synthese komplexer Kohlenhydrate durch eine Protein-(Kollagen-)Synthese. Mit dieser Auffassung gewinnen aber auch die Untersuchungen der epiphysären Wachstumsstörungen unter hormonellen Einflüssen einen neuen Ansatz. Bei ungewöhnlichen hormonellen Situationen muß mit einer erheblichen Änderung der Zellstruktur gerechnet werden (Parathormon und Chondrocyten: KNESE 1969). Demzufolge können die Chondrocyten der Epiphysen nicht mehr als ausdifferenzierte Zellen mit eingeschränkter Potenz angesehen werden; ob ein gleiches für Knorpelzellen anderer Elemente gilt, bedarf der Untersuchung (vgl. Knochenbildung im Kehlkopf des Rehwildes, BEJSOVEC, 1954). KNESE und BIERMANN (1958) bezeichnen Chondroblasten, Chondrocyten, Osteoblasten und Osteocyten als Modifikationen von Skeletzellen. WILLMER (1960), der von Untersuchungen des Verhaltens von Zellen in Gewebekulturen ausgeht, spricht von der Familie der „Mechanocyten“ und stellt ihnen die Epitheliocyten und Amoebocyten gegenüber. Beide Auffassungen müssen erneut überprüft werden, wie wohl überhaupt ganz neue Vorstellungen über die Differenzierung der Stützgewebe zu entwickeln sind, worauf wir in der Einleitung hingewiesen haben. Hierbei sind die Ergebnisse entwicklungsgeschichtlicher und der verschiedenartigsten cytologischen Untersuchungen zu berücksichtigen. Auf der anderen Seite steht eine weitere Untersuchung der Bedeutung der Epiphyse für die Skeletentwicklung noch bevor, einschließlich der vielfältigen Störungen in dieser Region (vgl. ASBOE-HANSEN, 1966). Bisher wurden nur Vermutungen über das Schicksal der Intercellularsubstanz geäußert. Im Elektronenmikroskop (unveröffentlicht) konnte die Desintegration der hyalinen Intercellularsubstanz und die Resorption durch in ihrer Struktur stark veränderte Knorpelzellen beobachtet werden. Die Kollagenfibrillen, die ursprünglich parallel zur Wand der Knorpelhöhlen verlaufen, ziehen begleitet von MPS-Granula jetzt senkrecht auf die Zellen zu und gehen hier in eine feingranuläre Substanz über. Zur Ausbildung eines echten Bürstensaumes kommt es bei diesen Zellen nicht.

Periostale und Markosteoblasten verhalten sich gegenüber topochemischen Reaktionen nicht gleichartig, obwohl die Unterschiede mehr gradueller Natur sind (PRITCHARD, 1952; KNESE, 1957). Auch elektronenmikroskopische Untersuchungen lassen vermuten, daß enchondrale (Abb. 38) und periostale Osteogenese zwar sehr ähnlich, aber nicht vollständig gleichartig ablaufen (SCOTT und PEASE, 1956; KNESE und KNOOP, 1961b), doch sind die Differenzen bisher nicht weiter untersucht worden. Das von den metaphysären Osteoblasten gebildete Flechtwerk der Kollagenfibrillen hat nicht die gleiche Dichte wie jenes bei der periostalen Ostogenese.

Durch die enchondrale Osteogenese wird eine sog. primäre Spongiosa gebildet. Nach älteren Vorstellungen soll diese primäre Spongiosa sofort wieder resorbiert werden.

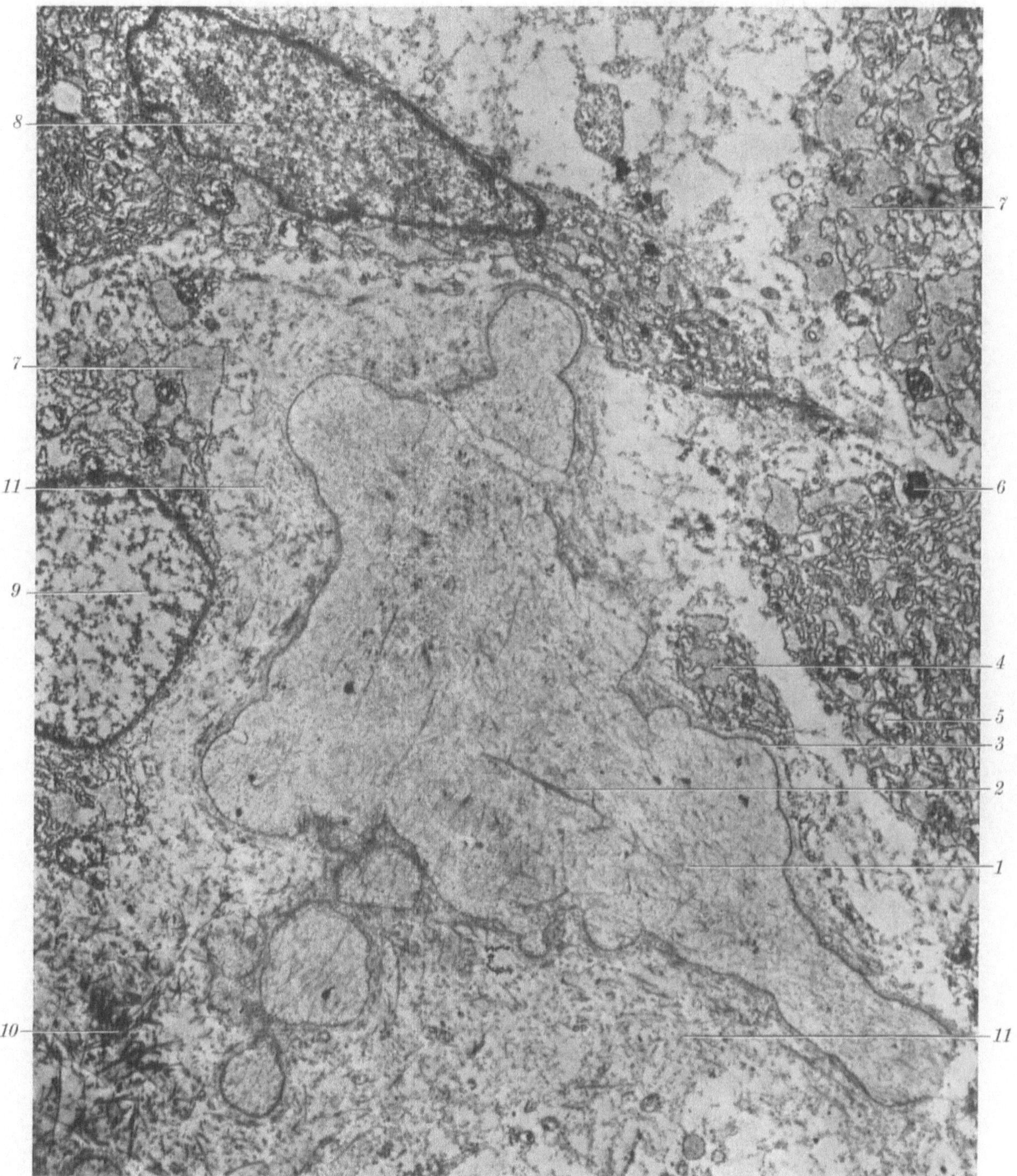

Abb. 38. Markosteoblasten um ein Bälkchen von Knorpelsubstanz, entmineralisiert (Titriplex = Versen). *1* Gebiet der Knorpelmineralien, die durch Titriplex entfernt sind, mit fädigen Gebilden (MPS?); *2* quergestreifte Kollagenfibrille; *3* Umhüllung des Mineralgebietes; *4* Teil eines Markosteoblasten in unmittelbarer Anlagerung an das Knorpelmineral, vom restlichen Teil des Osteoblasten durch Schnitt abgerissen; *5* Mitochondrium; *6* osmiophile Einlagerung; *7* stark erweiterte Zisternen des endoplasmatischen Reticulums; *8* Kern eines Markosteoblasten mit randständigem Chromatin und Nucleolus sowie dichte Chromatinbrocken, verteilt über das ganze Kernareal; *9* Kern eines zweiten Markosteoblasten, relativ chromatinarm; *10* präossales Gewebe mit größerer Anzahl von Kollagenfibrillen; *11* Reste der hyalinen Intercelluarsubstanz. Vergr. 15500

LEBLOND et al. (1950) zeigten mit Hilfe von ^{32}P, daß die Bälkchen als Trichter (funnel) ein Teil des Schaftes werden (Abb. 39). Auf diese Einverleibung chondralen Knochens sind wohl die seit langem bekannten freien chondralen Flächen zurückzuführen (KÖLLIKER, 1873; STRELZOFF, 1873; KNESE, 1957; BAHLING, 1958).

Im Zentrum des Epiphysenknorpels werden bei den einzelnen Skeletelementen in bestimmten Zeiträumen Mineralien abgelagert; es entsteht der sog. Knochenkern. Die folgenden Vorgänge mit Bildung eines Hohlraumsystems (Abb. 40) und chondralen

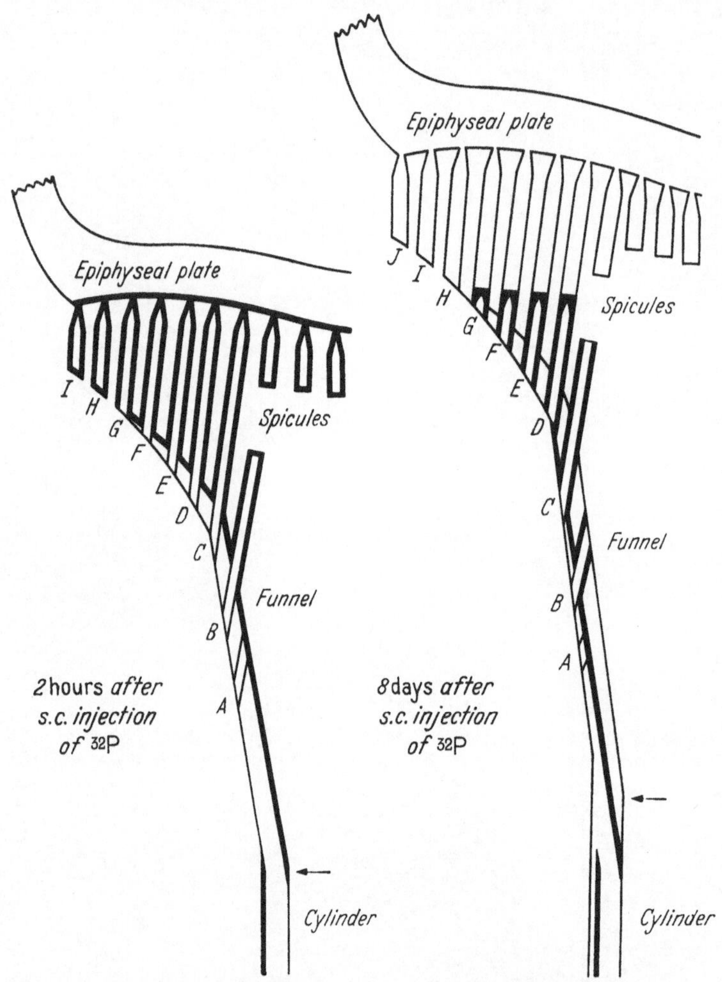

Abb. 39. Diagramm der Ablagerung von ^{32}P-Phosphat im proximalen Ende der Tibia von 50 g schweren Ratten; links 2 Std, rechts 8 Tage nach subcutaner Injektion. Die dunklen Linien geben die Ablagerungen von ^{32}P an. Die Ablagerung erfolgt an der unteren Fläche der Epiphysenplatte (links) und bleibt als gebrochene Linie an den subepiphysären Bälkchen erhalten (rechts). Die Ablagerungen an der Bälkchenoberfläche (links) werden in den Trichter einbezogen (rechts). Die endostale Ablagerung im Trichter wandert nach peripher, die subperiostale Ablagerung in der Diaphyse (Cylinder) wandert markwärts. (Nach LEBLOND, WILKINSON, BÉLANGER und ROBICHON, 1950)

Knochens entsprechen etwa jenen bei der enchondralen Osteogenese (Gefäße s. S. 764). Bei den präparatorischen Veränderungen im Knorpel fehlt allerdings die Ausbildung einer Schicht von Säulenknorpelzellen (KNESE, unveröffentlicht). Aus den rundlichen Chondrocyten werden sofort hypertrophe Knorpelzellen, deren Kapseln aber auch eine stärkere Anfärbung mit dem Chromalaun bei Gallocyanin-Färbung und ebenso eine PAS-positive Reaktion zeigen. Die Osteoblasten des Epiphysenkernes weisen bei Gallocyanin-Behandlung eine kräftige Cytoplasmafärbung auf und enthalten demnach wohl auch reichlich Ribonucleinsäuren.

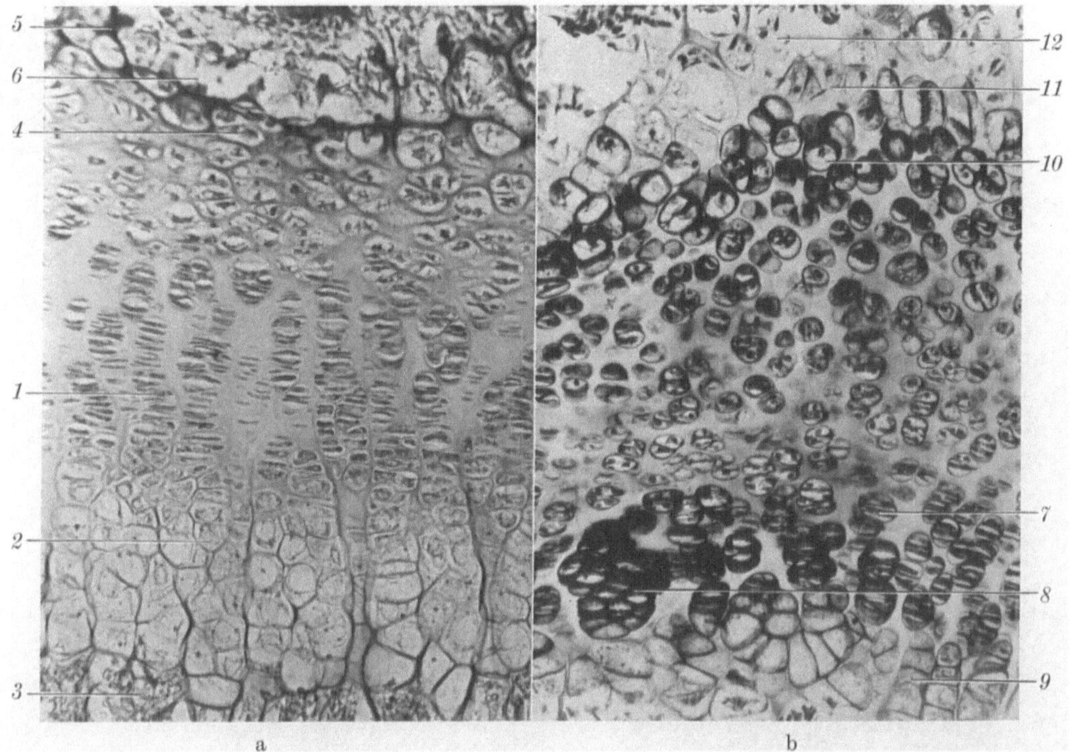

Abb. 40a u. b. Ratte, 105 mm, Epiphysenknorpel mit Übergang zur enchondralen Verknöcherung und zum Knochenkern. a Proximale Humerusepiphyse, PAS. b Distale Humerusepiphyse, Gallocyanin. a *1* Zellen des Säulenknorpels; *2* hypertrophe Knorpelzellen; *3* Eröffnungszone; *4* unregelmäßige Anordnung hypertropher Knorpelzellen, in der Peripherie des Knorpelkernes; *5* PAS-positive Reaktion der Intercellularsubstanz; *6* eröffnete Knorpelhöhlen zum Knochenkern hin. b *7* Zellen in Reihenanordnung; *8* Zellen in Ballenanordnung; *9* hypertrophe Knorpelzellen vor der Eröffnungszone der enchondralen Verknöcherung; *10* hypertrophe Knorpelzellen um den Epiphysenkern mit zum Teil Gallocyanin-positiver Reaktion des Cytoplasma und Anfärbung der Kapsel; *11* hypertrophe Knorpelzellen mit geringer oder fehlender Anfärbung des Cytoplasmas und der Kapsel; *12* Eröffnungszone im Bereich des Knochenkernes mit einzelnen spindelförmigen Osteoblasten. Ob. 16, Ok. 12,5

c) Die Knochenbildung in Apophysen und die Bildung des Faserknorpels

Als Apophysen werden sich zunächst wie Epiphysen selbständig entwickelnde, knorpelige Anteile des Skeletes bezeichnet, die im knöchernen Zustand mit den übrigen Abschnitten des Skeletstückes verbunden sind. Sie dienen Muskeln zum Ansatz. Über den Aufbau der knorpeligen Apophysen und die hier ablaufende Knochenbildung ist wenig bekannt, da sich mit diesen Zonen seit Kassowitz (1879) kaum mehr als ein Dutzend Arbeiten an wahllos herausgegriffenen Beispielen beschäftigt hat. Die einzige systematische Untersuchung von 89 periostalen und apophysären Ansatzgebieten an sieben Individuen vom Neugeborenen bis zu einem 43jährigen Manne liegt von Biermann (1957) sowie Knese und Biermann (1958) vor. Eine historische Darstellung der Entwicklung der Vorstellungen über die Knochenbildung kann im Rahmen dieses Artikels nicht gegeben werden. So muß nur auf die Tatsache hingewiesen werden, daß unsere Kenntnisse über die Osteogenese auf Untersuchungen weniger Skeletelemente beruhen. Auf der Suche nach dem „Typus" der Knochenbildung hat man einfach verabsäumt, die verschiedenen Orte der Knochenbildung miteinander zu vergleichen. Hierbei handelt es sich durchaus nicht um irgendwelche weniger bedeutsame und damit zu vernachlässigende Vorgänge, wie der Hinweis auf Exostosen im Bereich von Sehnenansätzen zeigt. Die Frage, ob es verschiedene Möglichkeiten der Knochenbildung gibt,

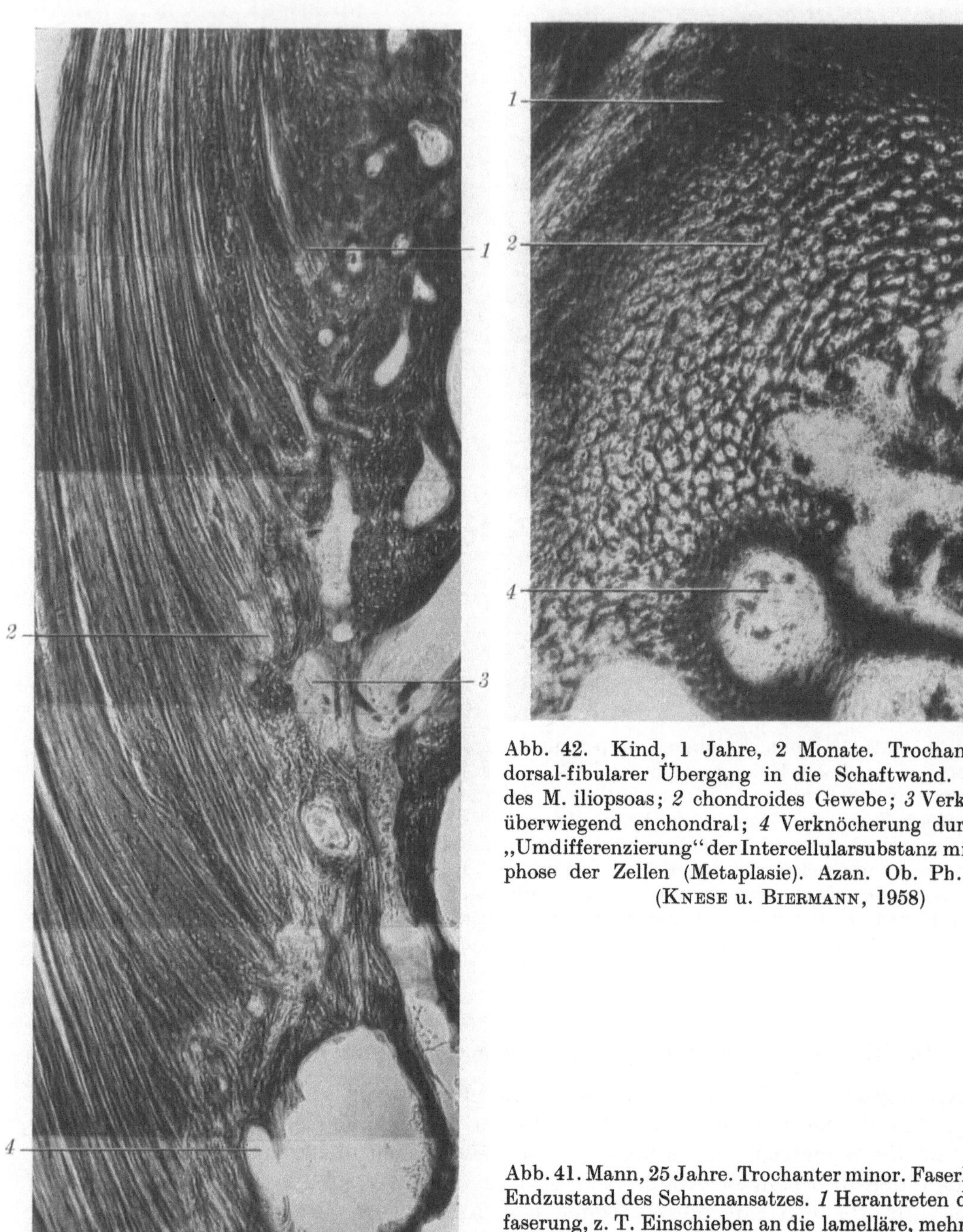

Abb. 42. Kind, 1 Jahre, 2 Monate. Trochanter minor, dorsal-fibularer Übergang in die Schaftwand. *1* Faserung des M. iliopsoas; *2* chondroides Gewebe; *3* Verknöcherung, überwiegend enchondral; *4* Verknöcherung durch direkte „Umdifferenzierung" der Intercellularsubstanz mit Metamorphose der Zellen (Metaplasie). Azan. Ob. Ph. 10, Ok. 8. (KNESE u. BIERMANN, 1958)

Abb. 41. Mann, 25 Jahre. Trochanter minor. Faserknorpeliger Endzustand des Sehnenansatzes. *1* Herantreten der Sehnenfaserung, z. T. Einschieben an die lamelläre, mehr kompakte Knochenmasse; *2* Einlagerung von knöcherner Interfibrillärsubstanz zwischen Sehnenfasern; *3* Insel echten Knochengewebes; *4* an die knöchern veränderte Sehne Anlagerung eines Streifens lamellären Knochengewebes. Azan. Ob. Ph. 10, Ok. 8 (Photomontage). (KNESE u. BIERMANN, 1958)

ist nach CAREY und ZEIT (1927) nur durch Untersuchung der verschiedensten Skeletorte sowie zeitlich in verschiedenen Entwicklungsstadien (KNESE, 1956b, 1966a) zu entscheiden.

Die Knochenbildung an Apophysen wurde bisher nur lichtmikroskopisch untersucht. Topochemische und elektronenmikroskopische Untersuchungen stehen noch aus. Ein besonderes Interesse haben die sog. verknöcherten Sehnen bei Säugetieren, Vögeln und fossilen Reptilien erregt (LIEBERKÜHN, 1863; BROILI, 1922; WEIDENREICH, 1923a, 1930; FILOGAMO, 1945; AMPRINO, 1948). Die Sehnenknochen bestehen aus lamellärem Knochengewebe in der Form von Osteonen, die AMPRINO (1948) auch in Rekonstruktionen dargestellt hat.

Die Sehnen zeigen kurz vor ihrem Ansatz am Apophysenknorpel eine Änderung der Struktur durch erhebliche Vergrößerung der Zellen und einen nicht mehr gewellten, sondern gestreckten Verlauf der Kollagenfasern (BIERMANN, 1957; KNESE und BIERMANN, 1958). Die damit vorliegende Gewebeform wurde z. T. als Chondroidgewebe, z. T. als eine Art Faserknorpel angesprochen (Abb. 41). SCHAFFER (1930) meint, bei beiden Gewebeformen besäßen die Zellen eine Kapsel. Jedoch liege ein Faserknorpel nur dann vor, wenn die Zellen eine Retractilität, d. h. eine Fixierungsschrumpfung (s. S. 694) aufweisen. Ob eine derartige Unterscheidung heute aufrechterhalten werden kann, ist zweifelhaft.

Das Knorpelgewebe der Apophysen ist nach der Einteilung von SCHAFFER (1930) den sog. sekundären Knorpelbildungen zuzurechnen. Der primäre Knorpel bildet die Skeletanlage im engeren Sinne und gehört histologisch zum hyalinen Knorpel. Die sekundären Knorpelbildungen treten nach SCHAFFER später als die primären auf, mitunter erst postnatal oder sogar nur unter besonderen Bedingungen, wie z. B. im Knorpelcallus. Das hyaline Knorpelgewebe des Skeletes stellt nicht nur eine Gewebeanlage,

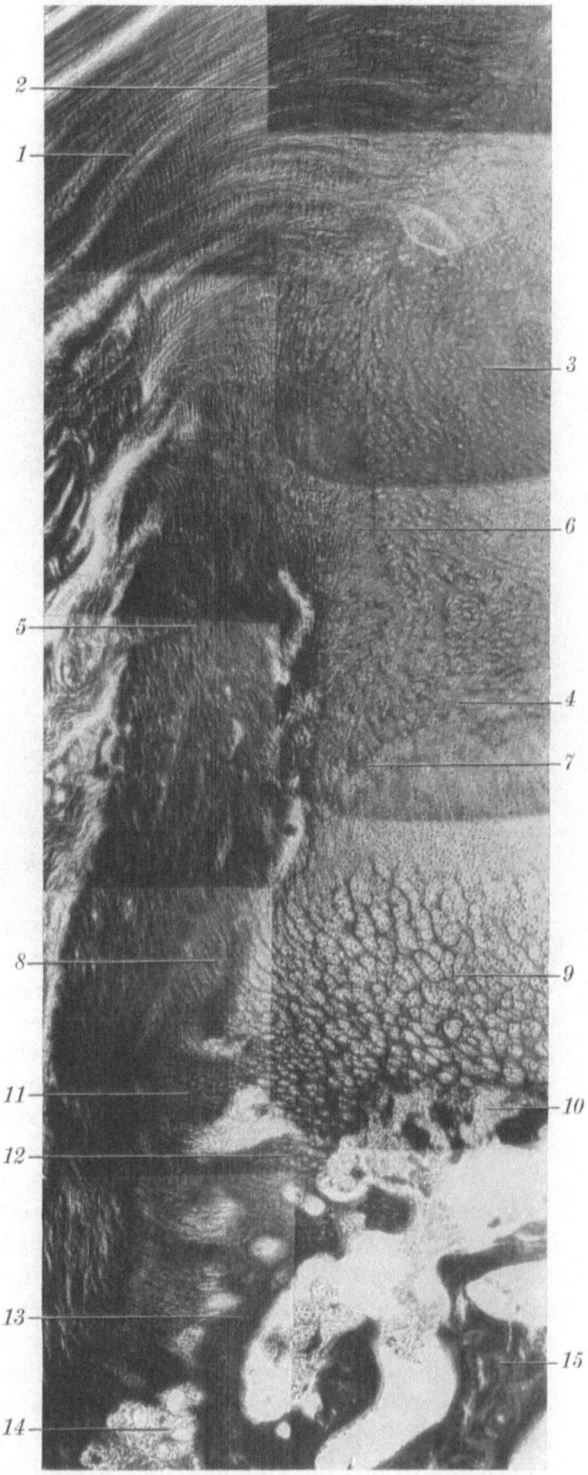

Abb. 43. Neonatus, ventraler Teil des Trochanter minor mit angrenzender Schaftwand. *1* Sehne des M. iliopsoas, Fasern gewellt; *2* Zone der gestreckten Sehnenfasern; *3* knorpelige Apophyse; *4* Zwischenschicht zur knorpeligen Schaftwand; *5* Periost; *6* ventrale Apposition an die knorpelige Apophyse, vom Perichondrium ausgehend; *7* knorpelige Apposition der Schaftwand aus einem abgegrenzten Wachstumsgebiet heraus; *8* knorpelige Apposition des Schaftes aus einer subperiostalen Faserlage; *9* Säulenknorpel; *10* Eröffnungszone und enchondrale Verknöcherung; *11* periostale Knochenbildung unter Vorbildung von Fasern; *12* unmittelbare Verbindung zwischen periostalem Knochen und Knorpelknochen, d. h. einem Gewebe, das in seinem Zellbestand weitgehend Knorpelzellen gleicht, in der Intercellularsubstanz dagegen weitgehend knöcherne Eigenheiten aufweist; *13* periostale Knochenbalken; *14* eingeschlossene Gefäßgruppe, das obere Gefäß wird durch zwei sich gegenüberstehende Zapfen von den übrigen abgetrennt; *15* chondraler Knochenbalken mit z. T. lamellärer Struktur und Resten von Knorpelgrundsubstanz. Azan. Ob. Ph 10, Ok. 8 (Photomontage). (KNESE u. BIERMANN, 1958)

sondern auch eine Organanlage dar (KNESE und BIERMANN, 1958). Die sog. sekundären Knorpelbildungen erscheinen in der Form mehr oder minder isolierter Gebilde. Allerdings ist der sekundäre Knorpel mitunter zeitlich auch vor dem hyalinen zu beobachten, z. B. an der Clavicula (ZAWISCH, 1953).

In ihrer Struktur, vor allem in der Faserordnung, unterscheiden sich der sog. ,,typische“ Hyalinknorpel z. B. in Epiphysen und im Rippenknorpel und der Ansatzknorpel in Apophysen voneinander. Beide sind aber wegen der Maskierung der Fasern als hyaliner

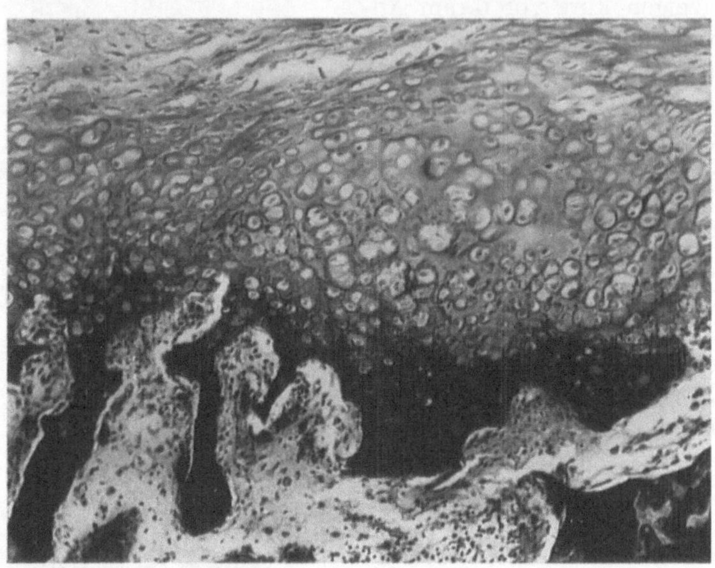

Abb. 44. Kind, 3 Monate (421 mm SSL). Femur, Schaftwand unterhalb des Trochanter minor. Unmittelbare Umbildung von Knorpel in Knochen (Metaplasie) und Bildung von Knochenbälkchen durch enchondrale Verknöcherung. Versilberung nach BODIAN. Ob. 10, Ok. 12,5. (KNESE 1957)

Knorpel anzusehen (KNESE und BIERMANN, 1958). Die Kollagenfasern — zum größeren Teil als unmittelbare Fortsetzung der Sehnenfasern — bilden im Ansatzknorpel Netze mit rhombischen Maschen (Abb. 42). In den Netzlücken liegt jeweils nur eine spindelförmige Knorpelzelle; Ballen aus mehreren rundlichen Zellen wie in anderen hyalinen Knorpeln fehlen. Damit liegen zwar bemerkenswerte morphologische Differenzen zwischen beiden Geweben vor, die im Zusammenhang mit der unterschiedlichen mechanischen Leistung stehen (s. S. 766), die aber kaum dazu hinreichen, die Existenz zweier verschiedener Gewebeformen zu behaupten.

Mehrfach wurde darauf hingewiesen, daß eine Klassifizierung der Stützgewebe in Formen, die eindeutig voneinander zu unterscheiden sind, nicht möglich ist. Die fließenden Übergänge zwischen den Formen der Stützgewebe konnten KNESE und BIERMANN (1958) bei histogenetischen Untersuchungen an Apophysen nachweisen. Ein Schnitt durch den Trochanter minor des Neugeborenen weist die ganze Spielbreite der Stützgewebe mit entsprechenden Übergängen auf. An den Trochanter minor treten die Sehnenfasern des M. iliopsoas in der bekannten Wellung heran (Abb. 43, 1), strecken sich (2) und gehen in den Epiphysenknorpel hinein (3), der durch eine Zwischenschicht (4) vom Schaft abgesetzt ist. Die faserige Hülle dieses Femurabschnittes ist z. T. Periost, z. T. Perichondrium, da von hier aus sowohl Ansatzknorpel (6), Säulenknorpel zum Schaft hin (7, 8) als auch periostaler Knochen (11) gebildet wird. In den Femurschaft aus periostalem Knochen (13) ist ein knorpeliger Anteil (9) eingelassen. Von diesem knorpeligen Schaftabschnitt wird durch eine Art enchondraler Osteogenese bzw. durch Metaplasie (vgl. KNESE 1957) Knochen gebildet (Abb. 44). Damit liegen in enger Nachbarschaft im Trochanter minor eine Reihe von unterschiedlichen Stützgeweben nebeneinander und gehen auch ineinander über. So muß ein enger genetischer Zusammenhang zwischen

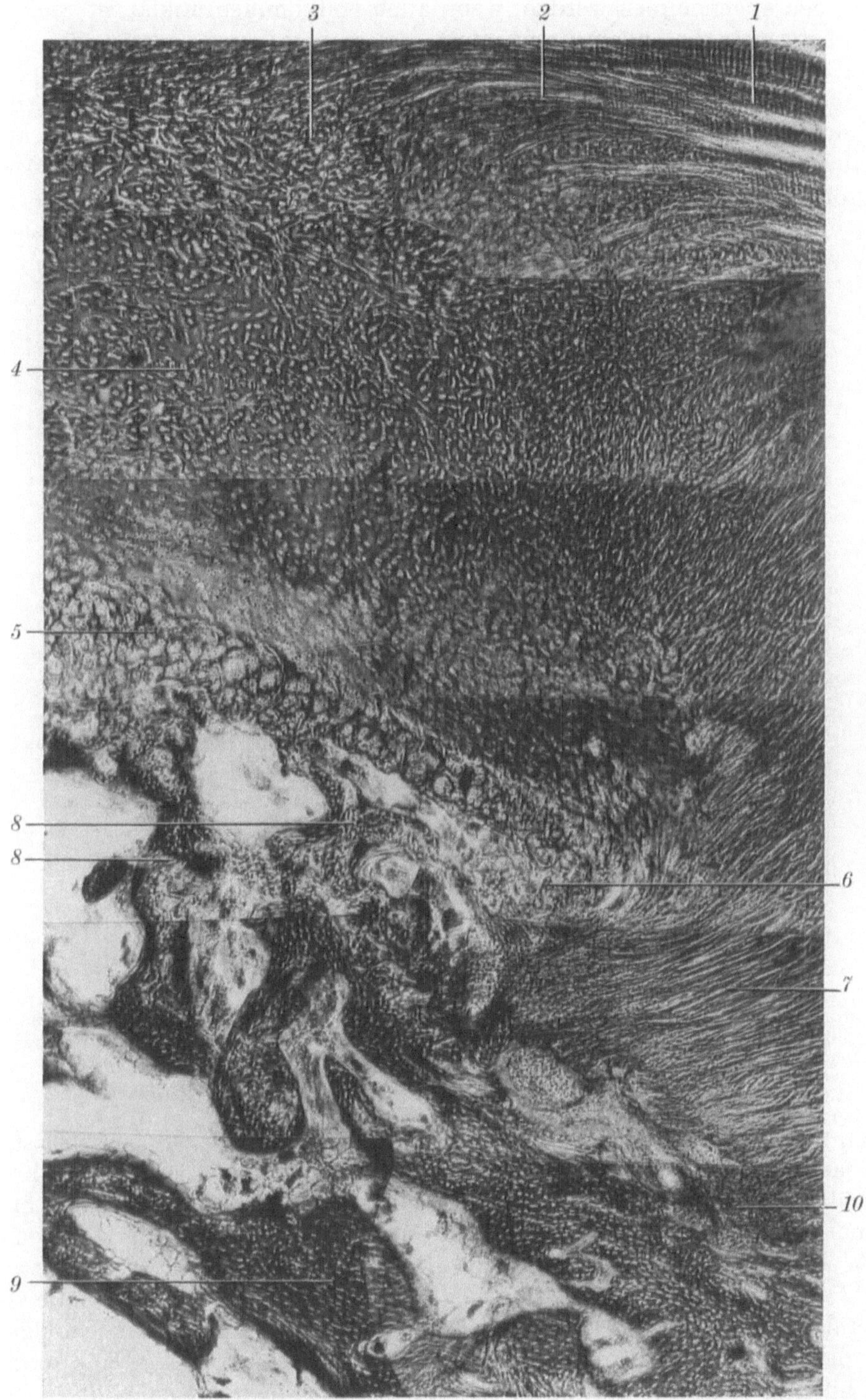

Abb. 45. Kind, 7 Jahre. Ventraler Teil des Trochanter minor. *1* Sehne des M. iliopsoas; *2* Zone der gestreckten Sehnenfasern; *3* faserknorpelige Ansatzzone; *4* knorpelige Apophyse; *5* präparatorische Veränderung des Knorpels zur Verknöcherung; *6* Differenzierungsgebiet, aus dem nach oben ein abgewandelter Säulenknorpel, nach unten periostaler Knochen gebildet werden; *7* periostale Faserung; *8* Knochenbalken in Verbindung mit Knorpel, in Knorpelnähe Reste von Knorpelgrundsubstanz, die etwas weiter entfernt davon fehlt; *9* periostale Knochenbalken mit teilweiser Lamellierung; *10* periostale Knochenbalken mit hyalinen Streifen. Azan. Ob. Ph. 10, Ok. 8 (Photomontage). (KNESE u. BIERMANN, 1958)

diesen Formen angenommen werden, wenn auch vollkommen unklar ist, welche Prozesse eine Gewebeform in die andere umwandeln.

In der Peripherie vieler Ansatzgebiete ist während der Ontogenese eine Appositions- oder Nachschubzone zu beobachten, die wohl der encoche d'ossification homolog ist (KNESE und BIERMANN, 1958). Diese Appositionszonen (Abb. 45) bestehen aus morphologisch nicht differenzierten Zellen, die vermutlich „pluripotent" sind, da von hier aus Ansatzknorpel, eine Art Epiphysenknorpel und periostaler Knochen gebildet wird. Von einer solchen Nachschubzone zwischen der Apophyse der Tuberositas tibiae und dem Schaft werden wohl zu beiden Seiten hin neue Gewebeteile gebildet.

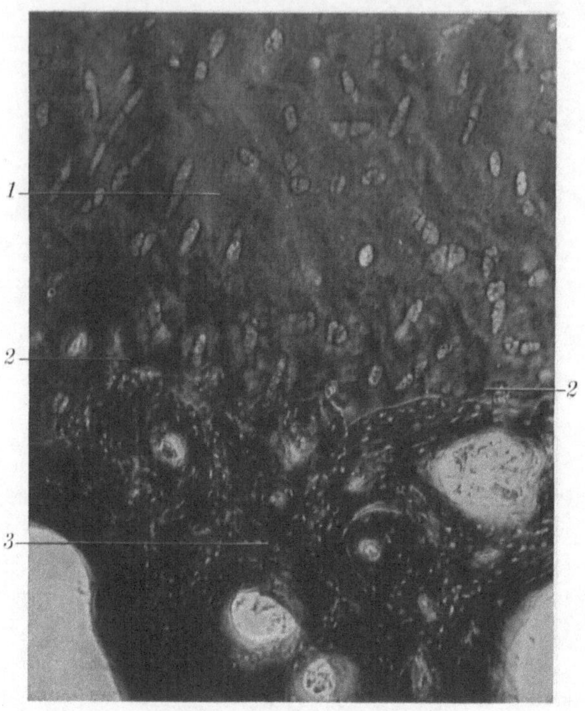

Abb. 46. Mann, 25 Jahre. Condylus lateralis femoris. *1* Knorpel überwiegend mit Kettenanordnung der Zellen, teilweise Ballenanordnung; *2* Eintauchen von Knorpelzellen in Knochen; *3* lamellärer Knochen. Azan. Ob. Ph. 10, Ok. 8. (KNESE u. BIERMANN, 1958)

In den zentralen Abschnitten der Apophysen bilden die den Sehnen entstammenden Kollagenfasern ein Netzwerk mit rhombischen Maschen. Zum Knochen hin folgt ein mehr paralleler Faserverlauf, so daß eine Art chondroides Gewebe bzw. ein modifizierter Säulenknorpel anschließt, der zum Markraum hin in eine Zone mit Knochenbildung übergeht. Bei dieser Form der Osteogenese fehlt die Ausbildung der hypertrophen Zellzone (vgl. MCLEAN und BLOOM, 1940). Eine solche abgewandelte enchondrale Osteogenese tritt überall dort auf, wo im Endzustand Spongiosa vorliegt. In den Randgebieten der Ansatzzonen ist ein chondroides Gewebe zu beobachten, von dem eine metaplastische Knochenbildung ausgeht. Häufig erscheinen Metaplasie und enchondrale Osteogenese unmittelbar nebeneinander.

Eine Reihe von Beobachtungen, derzeit nur mit den üblichen lichtmikroskopischen Routinemethoden, spricht für eine Art Umwandlung eines Stützgewebes in ein anderes. Spezifische Bildungszellen im Sinne der Chondroblasten oder Osteoblasten liegen ebensowenig vor, wie eine Knorpel- bzw. Knochenbildungsfront. Da Untersuchungen mit spezielleren Methoden, z.B. histochemische bzw. elektronenmikroskopische fehlen, ist unbekannt, welche Vorgänge sich bei dieser sog. Umwandlung von Geweben abspielen. Es handelt sich überwiegend um Gebiete der Knochenbildung, die kaum näher untersucht wurden, z.B. Sehnen- und Bandansätze, aber auch Teile der Schädelbasis. Wir weisen auf solche Befunde hin und benutzen zu ihrer Kennzeichnung den bisher verwandten Terminus „Metaplasie", da ein besserer derzeit nicht vorgeschlagen werden kann. „Metaplasie" ist ein unglückseliges Wort, wie ZAWISCH (1953) meint, allerdings mehr deswegen, weil dieser Terminus postuliert, daß jeder Gewebezustand der Stützgewebe auch ein endgültiger ist, woran heute zu zweifeln ist. Von einer Metaplasie ist dann zu sprechen, wenn das Knorpelgewebe in breiter Front in Knochengewebe übergeht, ohne daß eine Eröffnung von Knorpelhöhlen mit Verschwinden von knorpeliger Intercellularsubstanz zu beobachten ist. In der Literatur liegen viele zuverlässige Zeugnisse für eine metaplastische Knochenbildung vor (vgl. KNESE und BIERMANN, 1958). An Täuschungen, wie POMMER (1881) meint, ist dabei kaum zu denken. In umfangreichen Gebieten nimmt die Intercellularsubstanz die färberischen Eigenheiten des Knochengewebes unter Verlust derjenigen des

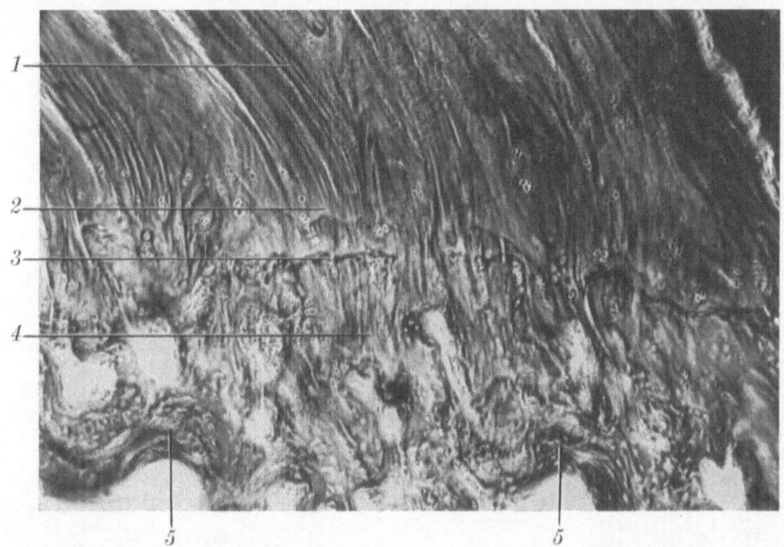

Abb. 47. Mann, 25 Jahre. Tuberositas radii. *1* Sehne des M. biceps; *2* Zone mit vereinzelten, aufgereihten Knorpelzellen; *3* Grenzlinie; *4* Einstrahlungsknochen mit knorpelähnlichen Zellen zwischen lamellären (5) Knochenstrukturen. Azan. Ob. Ph. 10, Ok. 8. (KNESE u. BIERMANN, 1958)

Knorpels an (Abb. 46). Die Knorpelzellen verändern ihre Gestalt derart, daß sie jungen, rundlichen Osteocyten gleichen.

An der Tuberositas radii und Tuberositas ulnae wird ein parallelfaseriger Faserknorpel unmittelbar zu einem Einstrahlungsknochen (Abb. 47). Dabei wechseln die färberischen Eigenschaften der Intercellularsubstanz in einer Schicht, die von vielen Autoren als Verkalkungsgrenze bezeichnet wurde (MATSCHINSKY, 1892; WEIDENREICH, 1923b; SCHNEIDER, 1955, 1956). Vermutlich ist aber die Änderung der Färbbarkeit auf eine Reihe von Zustandsänderungen der Intercellularsubstanzen zurückzuführen. Eine weitere Form der Knochenbildung liegt an der Tuberositas tibiae (Abb. 48) vor, da aus dem Apophysenknorpel Fasern austreten, die dann durch eine rein periostale Osteogenese Bestandteil des Knochens werden.

Bei der Bildung des Hirschgeweihs haben WISLOCKI et al. (1947) auch mit topochemischen Methoden die Umwandlung eines chondroiden Fasergewebes in Knochen beobachtet (chondroidal bone formation).

Einige Bemerkungen über die Bildung der Clavicula sind hier anzuschließen, da unter anderem die Ansicht vertreten wurde, daß sie im ganzen oder an ihren Enden eine Osteogenese auf Grund von Chondroidgewebe oder Pseudoknorpel aufweist (SCHAFFER, 1930; ZAWISCH, 1953). Andere Autoren sprachen von einer desmalen Osteogenese (u. a. HANSON, 1920). KOCH (1960) hat gezeigt, daß die Clavicula bei Embryonen von 12 mm SSL in der Form eines verdichteten Mesenchyms angelegt wird. Bei Embryonen von

12—22 mm SSL liegt dann ein Knorpelgewebe mit einer geringen Menge basophiler Intercellularsubstanz vor, das Koch als Wabenknorpel, d. h. als eine Art Zellknorpel beschreibt. Ab 22 mm SSL beginnt die Bildung der Diaphyse durch periostale Osteogenese. Infolge der frühen Entwicklung einer Knochenschale bleibt nach Koch die Ausbildung eines echten Hyalinknorpels aus. Der Knorpel zeigt im übrigen die von Streeter (1949) beschriebenen Entwicklungsstadien und eine periostale Knochenbildung in der von Knese (1956b) für lange Knochen angegebenen Form.

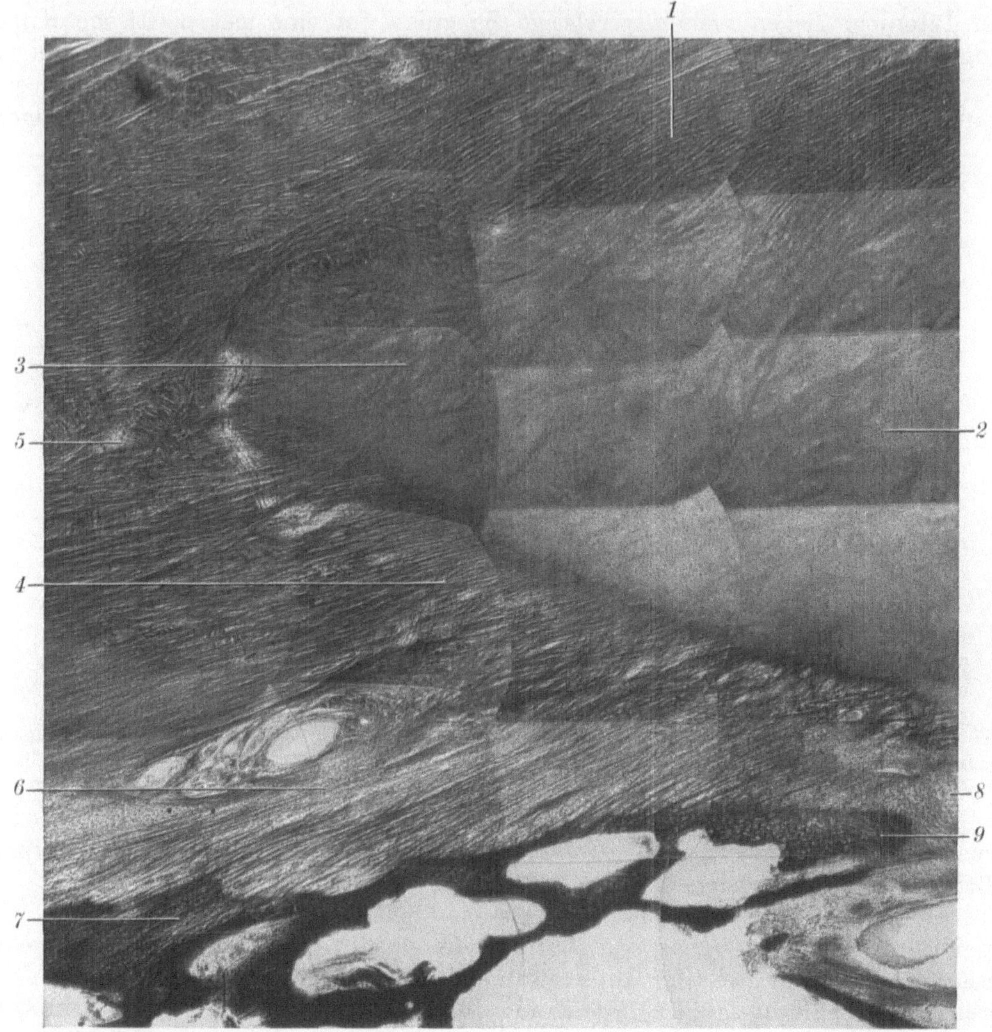

Abb. 48. Kind, 1 Jahr 2 Monate. Tuberositas tibiae. *1* Lig. patellae; *2* knorpelige Apophyse; *3* unvollständige Maskierung der Kollagenfasern am Ende der Apophyse mit deutlich erkennbarer Richtungsänderung des Faserverlaufes; *4* aus der Apophyse entlassene Faserung des Lig. patellae; *5* Faserstrom in Richtung der Fibroelastica; *6* Bildungsschicht mit dichten Zellansammlungen und Gefäßen; *7* periostale Knochenbildung unter Einschluß vorgebildeter Fasern; *8* distales Ende der Blasteminsel zwischen Apophyse und Säulenknorpel; *9* zellreicher Knochen, gebildet von der Blasteminsel her mit wenig vorgebildeten Fasern. Azan. Ob. Ph. 10, Ok. 8 (Photomontage). (Knese u. Biermann, 1958)

4. Die Formen des Knorpelgewebes und die Struktur knorpeliger Skeletstücke

a) Der Hyalinknorpel

Der frische Hyalinknorpel ist durch sein bläulich-weißes, milchglasähnliches Aussehen gekennzeichnet. Die Chondrocyten sind von unterschiedlicher Gestalt, rundlich bis ovoid und liegen allein oder zu mehreren in einer Knorpelhöhle, die eine Kapsel besitzt. Mehrere

Höhlen werden durch sog. Höfe zu Territorien zusammengefaßt. Zwischen den Territorien liegt die interterritoriale Substanz, die den hyalinen Charakter dieser Knorpelform bestimmt. Form und Ordnung der Zellen, Verteilung und Mächtigkeit der Intercellularsubstanz sind bei den verschiedenen knorpeligen Elementen sehr unterschiedlich.

α) Der Epiphysenknorpel

Die Morphologie der Chondrocyten wurde bei Erörterung der MPS-Bildung und der enchondralen Osteogenese bereits dargestellt (s. S. 715). Die Intercellularsubstanz ist in den einzelnen Zonen unterschiedlich aufgebaut. Diese Differenzen beruhen wahrscheinlich auf einer verschiedenen stofflichen Zusammensetzung im Hinblick auf den Kohlenhydrat-Proteinanteil (KNESE und KNOOP 1961a). Die Faserstruktur der einzelnen Zonen dürfte ebenfalls für die unterschiedliche topochemische Reaktion verantwortlich sein. In der älteren Literatur liegen einige Mitteilungen über die Faserordnung in den Epiphysen vor, die sich aber in entscheidenden Punkten widersprechen (ROMEIS, 1911; MOLLIER, 1910; GEBHARDT, 1911; SCHAFFER, 1911; PAUWELS, 1960).

β) Der Rippenknorpel

Der Rippenknorpel ist ein stabförmiges Gebilde, dessen Konstruktion dem des mehrfach untersuchten Trachealknorpels sehr ähnlich ist. Unter dem Perichondrium sind schmale, spindelförmige Chondrocyten mit ihrer Längsachse parallel zur Skeletoberfläche zu beobachten. Da weiterhin die Intercellularsubstanz noch nicht alle färberischen Eigenschaften eines voll ausgebildeten Hyalinknorpels zeigt, entspricht diese Schicht dem Appositionsknorpel der Epiphyse. Im Innern des Rippenknorpels liegen die Chondrocyten in Ballen, Territorien, die reihenförmig und senkrecht zur Skeletoberfläche angeordnet sind. Zwischen diesen Zellreihen befinden sich etwas breitere Balken von interterritorialer Substanz. AMPRINO und BAIRATI (1934) zeigten, daß diese Ordnung im Rippenknorpel erst im 5. Jahre, im Trachealknorpel im 10. Jahre erscheint. Gleichzeitig treten aber auch die ersten kataplastischen, d. h. degenerativen Veränderungen auf. Eine Studie über die Altersveränderung des Knorpels von Rippen, Trachea und Bronchien an Hand ihres färberischen Verhaltens haben QUINTARELLI und DELLOVO (1966) vorgelegt.

Im Knorpel sind sog. regressive oder kataplastische Erscheinungen häufig zu beobachten (Literatur bei SCHAFFER 1930), deren Wesen nur z. T. bekannt ist. Es handelt sich um eine einfache Atrophie oder Hypoplasie, das Auftreten von Asbestfasern, eine körnige „albumoide" Entartung, eine Erweichung und Verflüssigung, Mineralablagerungen und auch um Knochenbildung. Nach AMPRINO und BAIRATI (1934) beginnt die albumoide Metamorphose bereits zwischen dem 10. und 24. Jahr und nimmt weiterhin an Stärke zu. Asbestfasern sind nur im Rippenknorpel zu beobachten. Die Mineralablagerung setzt jenseits des 40. Jahr ein. Beim Menschen ist eine Knochenbildung und dann auch nur im Trachealknorpel selten zu beobachten (vgl. Knochenbildung im Kehlkopf des Rehwildes, BEJSOVEC 1954). Neben regressiven Vorgängen kommt es aber auch zur Neubildung. Unter dem Perichondrium des Trachealknorpels wird jenseits des 40. Jahres wiederum Knorpel gebildet. Auch in Erweichungsherden findet eine Chondrogenese statt.

Die Faserstruktur stabförmiger Knorpelgebilde, voran des Trachealknorpels, hat BENNINGHOFF (1925) ausführlich untersucht. Den von BENNINGHOFF geprägten Begriff „Chondron", der häufig, aber nicht immer einem Territorium entspricht, haben SCHAFFER (1930) und W. J. SCHMIDT (1957) als unberechtigt abgelehnt. Innerhalb eines solchen Chondrons soll nach BENNINGHOFF eine zirkuläre Wicklung der Fasern vorliegen. BORMUTH (1933), BUCHER (1942) und STAUB (1950) konnte solche zirkulären Wicklungen nicht auffinden; die Kollagenfasern weichen den Zellhöhlen aus. Nun sollen nach BENNINGHOFF (1925) ähnliche Wicklungen höherer Ordnungsstufen als Zweier-, Vierer- usw. Packung folgen; die letzte Packung ist dann das Perichondrium. Unter dem Perichondrium enthält ein Knorpelstab periphere tangentiale, der Oberfläche parallele Fasern. Diese Fasern biegen um und verbinden dann senkrecht die Oberflächen des Knorpelstückes. Nach den weiterhin vorliegenden polarisationsmikroskopischen und elektronenmikroskopischen Beobachtungen ist anzunehmen, daß BENNINGHOFFs (1925) Beschreibung des Faserverlaufes im Knorpel eine sehr starke Vereinfachung zum Zwecke einer funktionellen Deutung (s. S. 765) darstellt. BORMUTH (1933), BARGMANN (1939) und BUCHER (1942) haben weder bei Selachierknorpeln noch Rippenknorpeln einen gestreckten Faserverlauf beobachten können. In diesen Knorpeln liegen zwei steile, sich in einem Winkel von 30° kreuzende, S-förmig gekrümmte Fasersysteme vor, die durch zwei flache, sich in ähnlicher Form kreuzende Systeme ergänzt werden. Die Fasersysteme laufen in das Perichondrium ein oder sind bei Selachiern mit den Kalkplatten verbunden, die unter dem Perichondrium liegen.

γ) *Der Gelenkknorpel und die Gelenke*

Im Rahmen dieser summarischen Darstellung sollen den Erörterungen über den Gelenkknorpel einige Bemerkungen über die Biologie der Gelenke angeschlossen werden. Von GARDNER und GRAY (1950, 1953), GRAY und GARDNER (1950, 1951) sowie GRAY, GARDNER und O'RAHILLY (1957) liegen umfangreiche Untersuchungen über die Entwicklung des Knie- (vgl. SONNENSCHEIN, 1952), oberen Sprung- und Ellenbogengelenkes vor. Menisken und Kreuzbänder werden in der 8. Woche gebildet, bevor eine Gelenkhöhle vorhanden ist, die erst in der 9. Woche entsteht. Zwischen den aus Vorknorpel aufgebauten Epiphysen des Ellenbogengelenkes befindet sich bei Feten von 17 mm eine Zwischenzone, die sich bei solchen von 20 mm in drei Schichten gliedert. Keimlinge ab 22 mm weisen einige voneinander getrennte Höhlen auf, die bei 39 mm Länge zu einer einheitlichen Gelenkhöhle zusammenfließen. Die Form der Gelenkteiie ähnelt bereits bei Feten von 30 mm der bei Erwachsenen. Nach KNESE (1966b) beginnt histogenetisch die Entwicklung der Gelenke mit Ausbildung der Tangentialschicht. Die Säulenknorpelzellen innerhalb des Skeletstückes bilden Bogenreihen, deren Konvexität auf das Gelenk hin gerichtet ist. Zwischen den entgegengesetzt gekrümmten Bogenreihen zweier benachbarter Skeletstücke liegt eine Zellschicht mit dem Charakter des „Mesenchyms", aus der im Kniegelenk z.B. auch die Menisken und Kreuzbänder entstehen. Bei weiterer Entwicklung des Skeletstückes mit Ausbildung des hyalinen Epiphysenknorpels bilden sich an der Stelle des zukünftigen Gelenkspaltes tangential eingestellte Reihen von Zellen, die kaum noch Glykogen-Einlagerungen aufweisen. Geringe Mengen von Intercellularsubstanz sind vorhanden. Dann entsteht in einzelnen Teilen, im allgemeinen zentral beginnend, der Gelenkspalt. MUNARON (1954) nimmt an, daß sich der Gelenkspalt durch Auflösung der Intercellularsubstanz vermittels Hayluronidase bildet. ANDERSEN und BRO-RASMUSSEN (1961) wiesen im Gelenkbereich die Bildung von Chondroitinsulfat A und C, aber nicht von Hyaluronsäure nach. Die Verfasser meinen, daß die Bildung des Gelenkspaltes von zentral her einsetzt, wenn der zukünftige Gelenkknorpel seine Tätigkeit als knorpelbildende Zone einstellt. Späterhin wird Knorpel nur noch von den peripheren Abschnitten her zur appositionellen Vergrößerung der Gelenkfläche gebildet.

FELL und CANTI (1934) konnten in der Kultur von Hühnchengliedmaßen die Entwicklung von Gelenken beobachten und nachweisen, daß in dem Extremitätenmosaik der Ort der Gelenkbildung nicht strikt lokalisiert ist. Eine Gelenkbildung ist nämlich auch dann möglich, wenn die präsumptive Gelenkregion fehlt, aber genügend undifferenziertes Material vorhanden ist. Die charakteristische Gestalt der Gelenkflächen ist jedoch ein Teil des Extremitätenmosaiks. LELKES (1958) meint, daß sich in der Kultur nur dann Gelenkflächen ausbilden und erhalten, wenn die Kulturstücke entsprechend bewegt werden.

Der Gelenkknorpel ist während der Entwicklung ein Abschnitt der knorpeligen Epiphyse und stellt erst nach Ausbildung der knöchernen Epiphyse eine gesonderte Knorpelschicht unterschiedlicher Dicke dar. In der oberflächlichen Tangentialfaserschicht

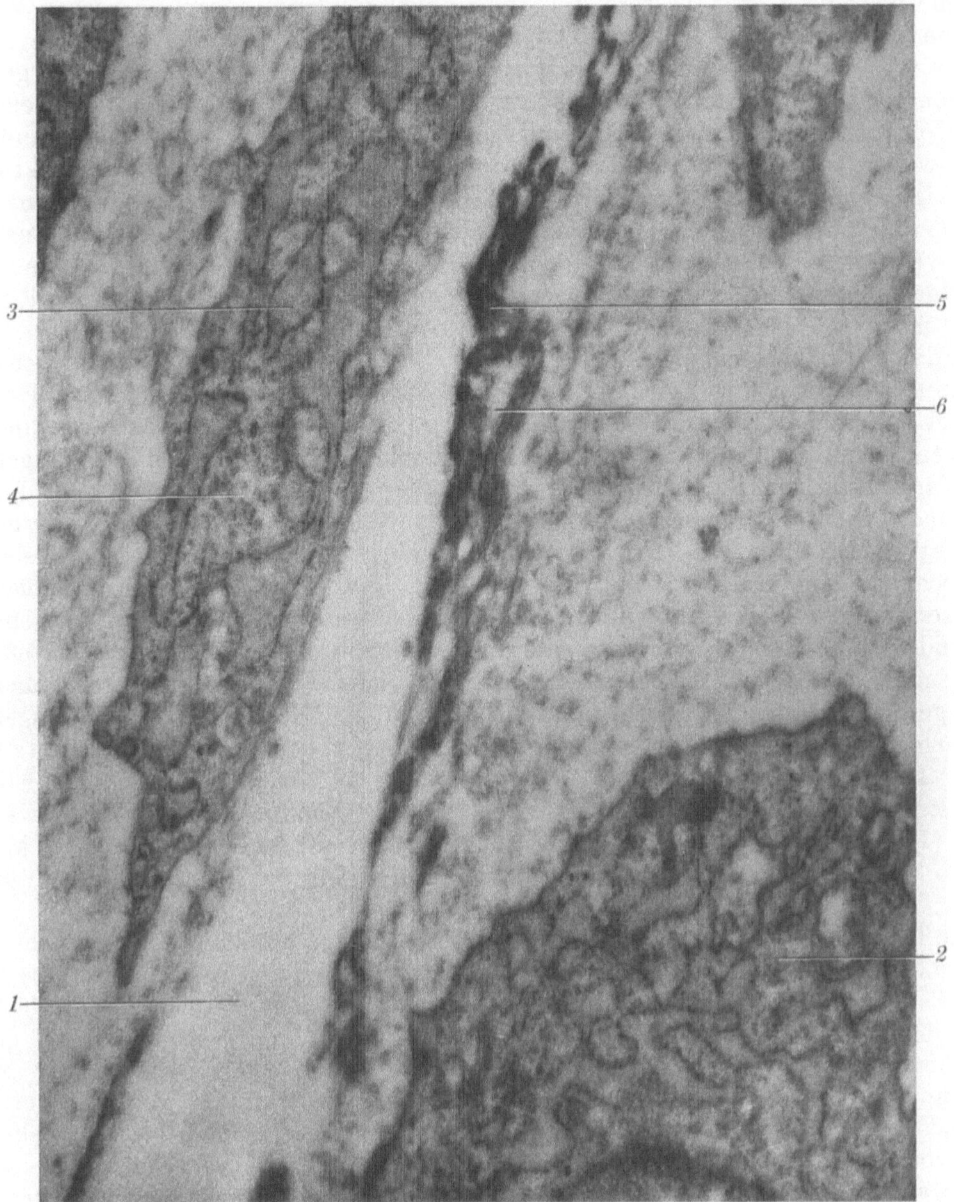

Abb. 49. Gelenkknorpel. *1* Gelenkspalt; *2* rundlicher Chondrocyt mit erweiterten Zisternen, dichtem Grundplasma und osmiophilen Einlagerungen; *3* Zisternen eines länglichen Chondrocyten, der nur von einer dünnen Schicht Intercellularsubstanz zum Gelenkspalt hin überkleidet ist; *4* Grundplasma dieses Chondrocyten mit relativ großen (300 Å und mehr) Granula. Degenerierende Zellen; *5* Reste des Grundplasmas; *6* leere Zisternenräume (?). Vergr. 26500. (KNESE u. KNOOP, 1961c)

liegen flache Zellen, in den tieferen Chondrocyten, die denen des Epiphysenknorpels auch bei Vorhandensein einer knöchernen Epiphyse gleichen. Diese tiefer gelegenen Zellen nehmen ^{35}S auf, die oberflächlichen nicht (AMPRINO, 1955; VERNE et al., 1956). Die metachromatische Farbreaktion der Tangentialschicht ist gering (VERNE et al., 1956).

Elektronenmikroskopische Untersuchungen der Gelenke von Rattenfeten führten KNESE und KNOOP (1961b) zur Unterscheidung von drei Zelltypen. Flache Chondrocyten können mit ihrem dichten Grundplasma, dem mäßig entwickelten endoplasmatischen Reticulum, aber stark erweiterten Zisternen (vgl. TAKUMA, 1960) den Chondrocyten des eigentlichen Epiphysenknorpels gleichen (Abb. 49). Von diesem Zellhabitus lassen sich rein morphologisch zwei weitere Zelltypen ableiten, deren morphologisches Verhalten an einen Zelluntergang denken läßt. Bei der einen Art von Zellen bleiben zunächst weitere von Membranen umgrenzte Zisternen erhalten; ihr Inhalt ist aber von geringerer elektronenmikroskopischer Dichte als der in den Zisternen anderer Knorpelzellen. Bei unmittelbar in der Gelenkoberfläche gelegenen Zellen nimmt die intermembranöse Substanz weiter an Dichte ab und das Grundplasma fließt zu dichten, unstrukturierten, verzweigten Bändern zusammen (Abb. 50). Diese Reste des Grundplasma werden dann zu undefinierbaren Massen. Bei anderen Zellen bleiben noch einzelne Zellorganellen mit kaum veränderter Struktur erhalten, z. B. Mitochondrien und Granula (Palade-Granula, Ribosomen ?). Diese Zellen haben eine Breite von 3000 Å oder weniger und gelangen damit an die Grenze der „Sichtbarkeit", sie „verdämmern" (SCHAFFER, 1930).

In den ersten Fetalmonaten durchziehen die Fasern den Gelenkknorpel in wechselnder Richtung (AMPRINO, 1938), nehmen später an Zahl zu und verlaufen mehr oder minder parallel zueinander. LIT TLEund PIMM (1956) haben elektronenmikroskopisch und durch Röntgenbrechung in der Oberfläche des Oberschenkelkopfes von Feten und Neugeborenen eine Tangentialfaserschicht gefunden, die annähernd radiär vom Ansatz des Lig. teres ausgeht. Darunter liegt ein dreidimensionales Netzwerk von Fasern. Im mittleren Lebensalter sind im inneren Drittel des Gelenkknorpels in Knochennähe parallele Fasern senkrecht zur Knochenoberfläche zu beobachten. Bei artritischen Gelenken reicht diese Faserzone bis unter die Tangentialfaserschicht; die interfibrilläre Substanz ist gleichzeitig vermindert. Die Faserorientierung entspricht annähernd dem von BENNINGHOFF (1925) gegebenen Schema, d. h. es liegen senkrecht aufsteigende Faserzüge vor, die bügelförmig umbiegen und damit die Tangentialfaserschicht bilden. Die Einstellung der Bügelebenen ist nach Gelenk verschieden und im einzelnen nicht genügend aufgeklärt (PAUWELS 1959). In den Gewicht tragenden Knorpelteilen ist die Menge des Chondroitinsulfats im Verhältnis zum Kollagen größer als in den nicht Gewicht tragenden (MATHEWS, 1953). Nach MAKOWSKY (1949) zeigen Druckgebiete einen geringeren Wassergehalt als Gleitgebiete, aber eine größere Fähigkeit zur funktionellen Schwellung durch Wasseraufnahme.

Die Dicke des Gelenkknorpels schwankt zwischen 2—5 mm. Für das Kaninchen haben HOLMDAHL und INGELMARK (1948) eine Reihe von Prinzipien für den Bau des Gelenkknorpels aufgestellt: 1. Der Gelenkknorpel ist dicker im zentralen als im peripheren Teil der Gelenkfläche, dicker an den konvexen als an den konkaven Teilen, an größeren Gelenken dicker als an kleineren, in den Berührungsgebieten während der Normalstellung wiederum dicker als im restlichen Teil der Gelenkfläche. 2. Eine Korrelation zwischen der Dicke des mineralisierten und des nicht mineralisierten Knorpelteiles ist nicht vorhanden. 3. Der prozentuale Gehalt des Knorpels an Zellen ist in Gelenkköpfen größer als in Gelenkpfannen, in größeren Gelenken aber niedriger als in den kleinen. 4. Die Anzahl der Zellen je Chondron ist in sich gegenüberliegenden Gelenkköpfen und Gelenkpfannen etwa gleich, in den großen Gelenken ist die Zahl der Zellen je Chondron größer als in den kleinen, vor allen bei den Gelenkpfannen. Nach ANDERSON et al. (1964) besteht eine relativ eindeutige Beziehung zwischen chemischem Aufbau des Knorpels und Lebensalter. Der Anteil des Kollagens beträgt im Mittel vom 10. bis 90. Lebensjahr 56,4 %, der an Mucopolysacchariden 90,3 %, der an Nicht-Kollagen-Proteinen 22,8 % der Trockensubstanz. Unabhängig vom Alter, der klinischen Diagnose und der Herkunft des Knorpels finden sich große Schwankungen der Werte. Diese Variation macht es schwierig, Veränderungen statistisch gesichert festzustellen. Die Autoren meinen, daß keine signifikanten Unterschiede zwischen normalem, verletztem oder degenerativem Knorpel bestehen. Dagegen nehmen im Laufe des Lebens die Mucopolysaccharide an Menge ab, das Kollagen dagegen zu. Eine elektronenmikroskopische Studie über die Altersveränderund des Gelenkknorpels am Femurkopf der Maus vom ersten Lebenstage bis zu mehr als 2 Jahren haben SILBERBERG, SILBERBERG, VOGEL und WETTSTEIN (1961) veröffentlicht. In einer weiteren Arbeit (SILBERBERG, SILBERBERG und FEIR, 1964) werden die Lebens-

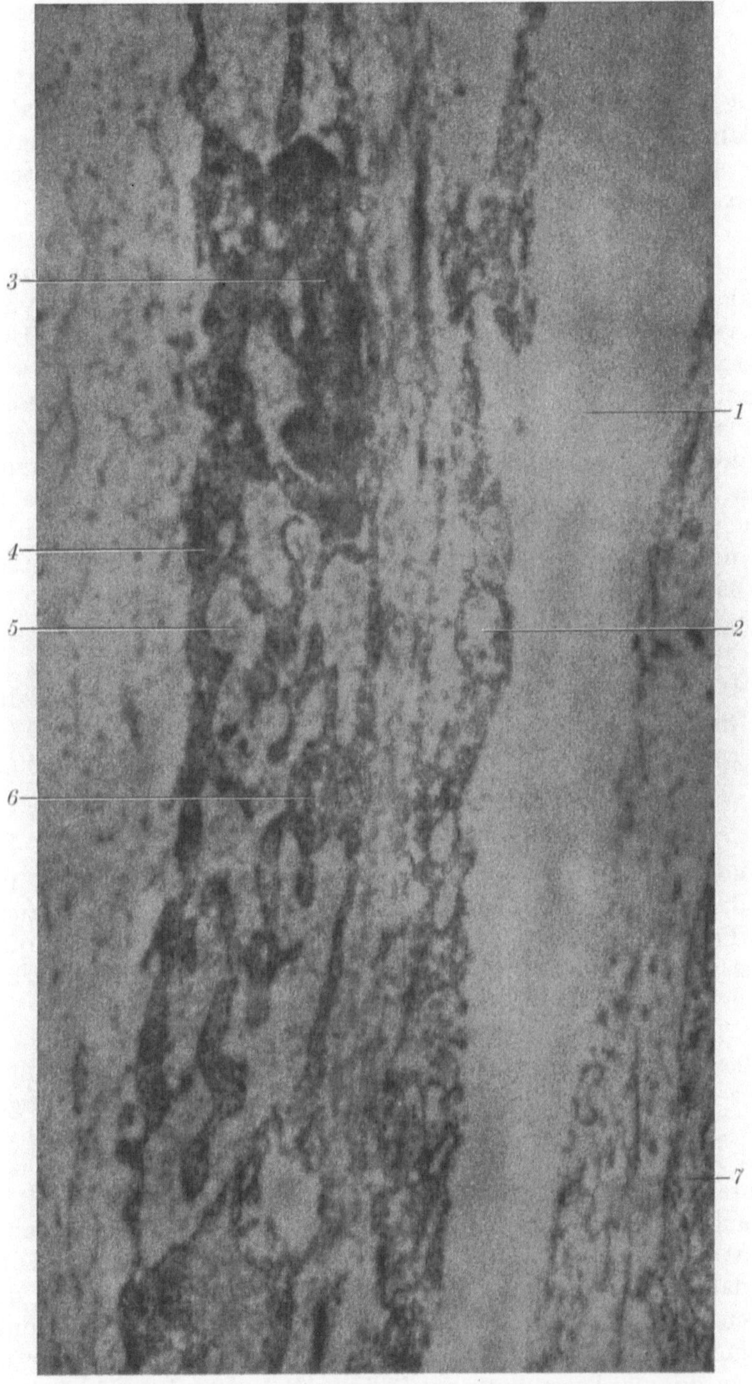

Abb. 50. Gelenkknorpel. *1* Gelenkspalt; *2* Mitochondrien in einer verdämmernden Zelle, degenerierende Zelle; *3* Zellkern; *4* Grundplasma; *5* erweiterte Zisternen; *6* Mitochondrium; *7* Chondrocyt. Vergr. 24000. (KNESE u. KNOOP 1961c)

cyclen der Knorpelzellen beschrieben. Der aufsteigende Teil der Kurve ist durch eine zunehmende Organisation der Zellen gekennzeichnet, der absteigende Teil durch zeitweise Zunahme von Mitochondrien und einer folgenden Degeneration der Organellen mit Erscheinen von Glykogen und Lipiden sowie Schwellung und Zerfall der Zellen. Dem Zelltod folgt eine Knochenbildung oder der Ersatz durch eine Fasernarbe.

HOLMDAHL und INGELMARK (1948) haben den Gelenkknorpel wachsender Kaninchen auch nach einem verschieden langen Lauftraining untersucht. Der nicht verkalkte Gelenkknorpel ist bei trainierten Tieren dicker. Durch Training tritt wohl auch eine Zellvermehrung und eine Vermehrung der Zellen je Chondron auf, aber die Zunahme an Intercellularsubstanz ist viermal größer. Über die absolute Zellgröße können die Autoren keine sicheren Aussagen machen, meinen aber, daß mit gesteigerter Tätigkeit auch die Zellen an Größe zunehmen.

Umfangreiche Literaturübersichten zur Biologie der Gelenke geben BAUER (1940), GARDNER (1950) und RUCKES (1961). Die Pariser Nomina Anatomica unterscheiden bei der Gelenkkapsel zwischen einem Stratum fibrosum und Stratum synoviale. HIDVÉGI (1954) und LANG (1957) halten diese Gliederung auf Grund der Untersuchung der Gefäßarchitektur für nicht ausreichend. Synovialzotten enthalten korkzieherartig aufgeknäulte Capillaren, die von gestreckt herantretenden Arteriolen versorgt werden. Von diesen Zotten aus wird der sog. unspezifische Anteil der Synovia gebildet, der aus Wasser und niedermolekularen Stoffen besteht. Weiterhin sind Fettzotten mit einem weitmaschigem Capillarnetz vorhanden (LANG 1956). Histochemische und elektronenmikroskopische Untersuchungen haben die Bildung von Hyaluronaten durch die oberflächlichen Synovialzellen sichergestellt (LEVER et al., 1958; RINONAPOLI et al., 1958; HAMERMAN, 1959); hierbei gehen auch Zellen zugrunde.

Die Synovia (vgl. ROPES et al., 1947, 1953) enthält etwa 96% Wasser und 4% feste Bestandteile. Die Viscosität der Synovia ist 10—200mal größer als die von Wasser (SUNDBLAD, 1953; FESSLER et al., 1954). Der Einfluß des Proteins auf die Viscosität ist noch unklar. Die Synovia enthält 25% Protein (OGSTON et al., 1952). Weiterhin wurden Albumin und wenig Globulin, aber kein Fibrinogen in der Synovia aufgefunden.

b) Der Faserknorpel

Als Faserknorpel bezeichnen wir ein Gewebe, dessen Kollagenfasern nicht oder wenig maskiert und damit auch im Lichtmikroskop ohne besondere Präparation sichtbar sind. Zwischen den Fasern liegen in Reihen angeordnet die Knorpelzellen, die basophile und metachromatische Kapseln haben. Die Begriffsbestimmung des Faserknorpels ist umstritten (SCHAFFER, 1930; KROMPECHER, 1938; KNESE und BIERMANN, 1958). SCHAFFER, (1930) widmet in seinem Artikel von 374 Seiten dem Faserknorpel 6 Seiten und das Interesse für dieses Gewebe ist auch heute noch nicht viel größer (PRADER, 1947a, b). Die Beurteilung des Faserknorpels bereitet bereits im Hinblick auf die Histogenese besondere Schwierigkeiten. Die Frage, ob Faserknorpel primär oder sekundär aus hyalinem Knorpel entsteht, kann in dem Sinne beantwortet werden, daß beide Bildungsformen je nach Ort zu beobachten sind (PRADER, 1947a, b; KNESE und BIERMANN, 1958). Weiterhin zeigt die Faserordnung in den einzelnen Elementen so erhebliche Unterschiede, daß morphologisch kaum vergleichbare Gewebe vorliegen. Der hyaline Anteil kann so stark ausgeprägt sein, daß manche Autoren von einem hyalinen Knorpel mit durchdringenden Fasern sprechen (SCHNEIDER, 1955). Der „knorpelige Teil" tritt mitunter derart weit zurück, daß eine Art „Knorpelsehne" vorliegt (PETERSEN, 1930). Der unterschiedliche Faserverlauf wurde als besonders sinnfälliges Beispiel einer funktionellen Struktur angesehen.

BAER (1949) hat die Symphyse menschlicher Feten von der 6. Woche an bis zu Kindern von 7 Jahren untersucht und die Angabe von ZULAUF (1901) bestätigt, daß aus dem hyalinen Knorpel erst im Kindesalter Faserknorpel wird. An die Facies symphysialis des Schambeines schließt sich hyaliner Knorpel mit einem dreidimensionalen Gitterwerk aus sich spitzwinklig kreuzenden Fibrillenzügen mit häufig S-förmigem Verlauf an. Dieser Faserverlauf entspricht der von BUCHER (1942) unter anderem in Nasen- und Trachealknorpel aufgezeigten Ordnung. Genauere Angaben über die gesamte Faserordnung der Symphyse kann der Autor an Hand der untersuchten Schnitte allerdings nicht machen.

Die Faserstruktur ist aber bereits in der 7. Fetalwoche in der Form festgelegt, die dem späteren Bauprinzip entspricht. Der faserknorpelige Anteil der Symphyse besteht in der 8. Woche aus transversalen Fasern, die beide hyalinen Knorpel miteinander verbinden. Durch das starke Wachstum der Schambeine stellen sich in der 10. Woche die Fasern in der Sagittalen ein. Der eigentliche Faserknorpel wird erst von der Geburt an gebildet und zwar so, daß an der Symphyse von außen nach innen das fibrilläre Gewebe allmählich in Faserknorpel übergeht. Die Fasern sind nach außen bogenförmig ausgebuchtet. Der Symphysenspalt erscheint in der 10. Woche, ist bei Frauen meist größer und wird von den Fibrillen des Faserknorpels konzentrisch umfaßt. Oestrogene veranlassen den Ersatz des Symphysenknorpels durch Bindegewebe (SILBERBERG und SILBERBERG 1956).

Blutgefäße dringen vom 5. Fetalmonat an vom Lig. arcuatum pubis her aus der A. penis in die Symphyse ein und stehen durch den hyalinen Knorpel mit Gefäßen des Knochenmarkes in Verbindung (HINTZSCHE, 1928a, b; PUTSCHAR, 1931). Die Vascularisation ist beim Neugeborenen am stärksten und bildet sich zwischen dem 5. und 17. Jahr zurück (PUTSCHAR, 1931). Die Gefäße überschreiten nicht die dicht gewebte Grenze zwischen hyalinem und Faserknorpel.

Angaben zur Frühentwicklung des Achsenskeletes hat KNESE (1964b, 1965) gemacht. Die späteren Sklerotomzellen sind bereits bei ihrer Auswanderung aus dem Primitivstreifen durch einen besonderen Reichtum an Kohlenhydraten gekennzeichnet (KNESE 1965). Die Chorda ist späterhin von radiären Filamenten umgeben, die nach ihrem färberischen Verhalten vermutlich aus MPS-artigen Substanzen bestehen (KNESE, 1964b). Diese Filamente bilden die Leitstruktur bei der Auswanderung der Sklerotomzellen aus den Ursegmenten, die zuvor ihre Kohlenhydrate verlieren. Anschließend wird die radiäre Ordnung durch eine zirkuläre um die Chorda ersetzt. Die Teilung des skleletogenen Mesenchymes in Wirbel und Zwischenwirbelscheiben ist histogenetisch mit der Entwicklung von hyalinem Knorpel und Faserknorpel verbunden. Zunächst ist in beiden Teilen die Ordnung der Zellen gleich, die langen Zellen in der Anlage der Wirbelkörper runden sich ab und bilden metachromatisch reagierende Intercellularsubstanzen. In den Zwischenwirbelscheiben werden die Zellen spindelförmig und zeigen nun in ihrer Lagerung bereits die zukünftige Faserstruktur der Zwischenwirbelscheibe an.

Die Entwicklung der Zwischenwirbelscheibe wurde von TÖNDURY (1958) und seinen Schülern (u. a. PRADER, 1947; THEILER, 1950, 1951) sowie BRETTSCHNEIDER (1952) untersucht. Bei menschlichen Feten von 12 mm SSL ist die Gliederung Wirbelkörper — Zwischenwirbelscheibe ausgeprägt und die Chorda durchsetzt in gleichbleibender Stärke die ganze Anlage. Bei 20—50 mm langen Keimlingen sind die Zwischenwirbelscheiben bikonkave Gebilde mit einer Außen- und Innenzone. Die Chorda bildet nun in der Zwischenwirbelscheibe ein Chorda„segment“ und im Wirbelkörper einen dünneren Chordastrang. Die Außenzone besitzt bei Feten unter 20 mm Fibrillen und sie begleitende längliche Zellen, die in gegeneinander versetzten, Zwiebelschalen vergleichbaren Lamellen liegen. Die Inenzone besteht aus Knorpel. Späterhin (70—130 mm) sind die Fasern kräftiger und verlaufen in einer Lamelle mehr steil, in der folgenden mehr flach. Bei Feten von 70 mm dringen von dorsolateral in die Zwischenwirbelscheibe Gefäße ein. Die Gefäße stammen von Intersegmentalarterien ab; nur an der Grenze zwischen Bandscheibe und Wirbelkörper kommen auch Gefäße aus dem Wirbelkörper vor (BRETTSCHNEIDER, 1952). Die Rückbildung der Gefäße beginnt im 2. Jahr; sie ist im 4. vollendet (TÖNDURY, 1955).

SYLVÉN (1951) hat die Biologie des Nucleus pulposus als dem Knorpel ähnliches avasculäres Gewebe untersucht. Die vier Komponenten der Intercellularsubstanz — Kollagenfasern, Polysaccharide und an sie gebundene Proteine sowie Wasser — bilden ein dreidimensionales Gel-Gitter. Der Wassergehalt beträgt 83%. Das dichte Netzwerk der Kollagenfibrillen wird von dem Polysaccharid-Protein-Komplex überzogen und bildet damit die Perifibrillärsubstanz (s. S. 336). Dazwischen liegen Maschen oder Poren,

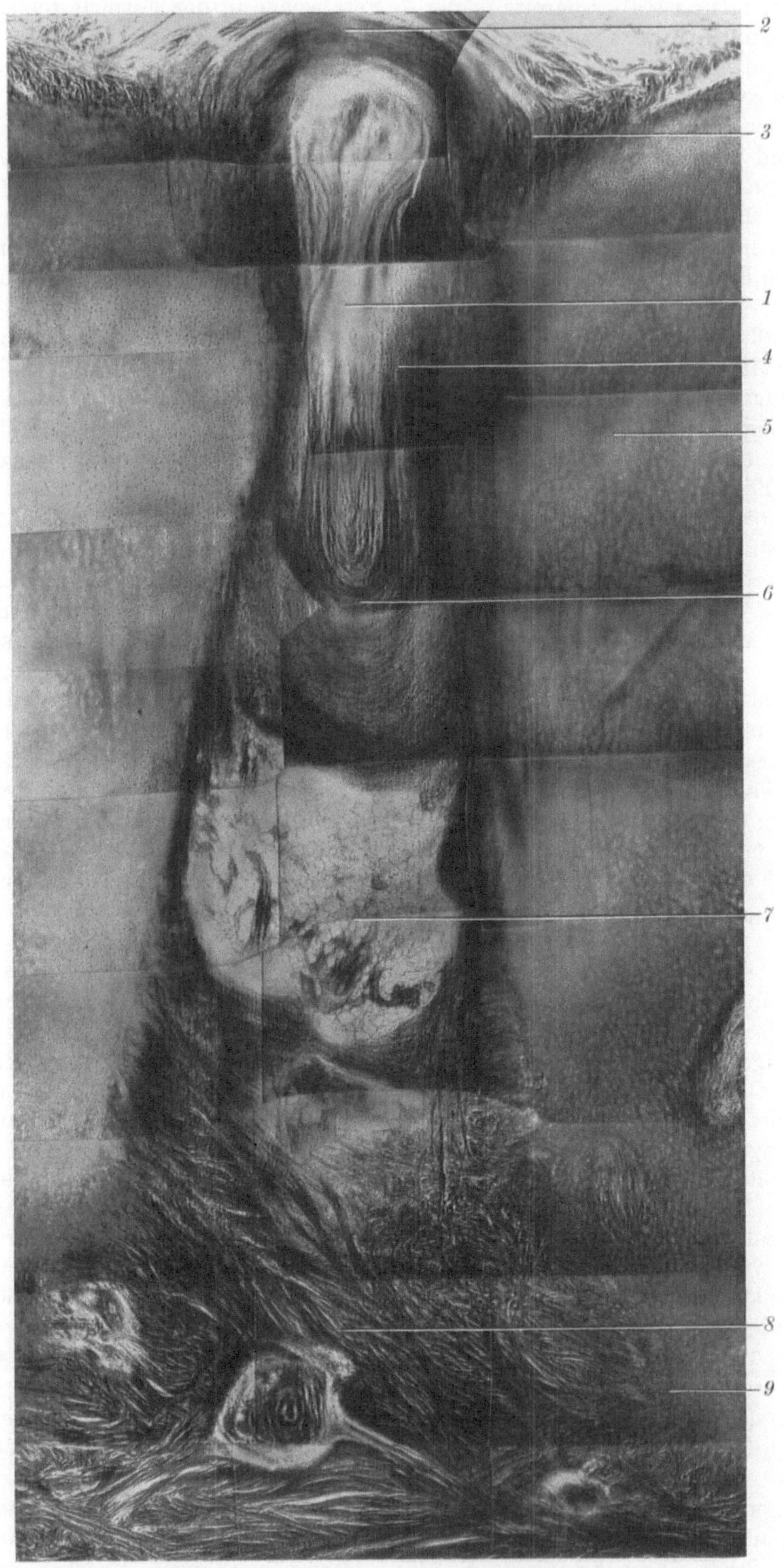

Abb. 51 (Legende s. S. 763)

deren Größe elektronenmikroskopisch nicht zu messen ist. Der Polysaccharid-Protein-Komplex enthält 5,5—6% N des Trockengewichtes und große Mengen Ester-Sulfat. Der Polysaccharidanteil ist in diesem Komplex dreimal größer als der des Proteins. Das Polysaccharid ist ein Chondroitinsulfat C (MALMGREN und SYLVÉN, 1952; HALL et al., 1957). Das hohe Wasserbindungsvermögen führt SYLVÉN (1951) auf die polaren OH-Gruppen des Polysaccharids zurück. Die molekulare Bindung der Komponenten scheint derart zu sein, daß die Polysaccharide durch chemische Bindung an die Oberfläche der Kollagenfibrillen gekettet sind. Das freie Protein ist an das Ende der Polysaccharide gebunden. Polysaccharide und Protein lassen sich leicht extrahieren, die Kohlenhydratreste sind dagegen schwer von den Kollagenfibrillen zu isolieren. Zwischenwirbelscheiben werden durch Hyaluronidase-Einwirkung härter und unelastischer und zwar, wie HARTMANN et al. (1954) vermuten, durch Ödembildung und eine vermehrte Faserspannung.

Der Anlageplan der Zwischenwirbelscheiben entspricht in frühfetaler Zeit dem späteren Aufbau. Die sog. Alterserscheinungen verändern nicht den Plan, aber das Gefüge, und bestehen in einer Faserverstärkung an den ventralen und lateralen, aber nicht den dorsalen Abschnitten (BRETTSCHNEIDER, 1952). Es treten weiterhin Spalten auf, die früher für Gelenke gehalten wurden, vor allem zwischen C 5/6 und C 6/7 (TÖNDURY, 1955). Im Nucleus pulposus erscheinen sog. degenerative Veränderungen im 3. Jahrzehnt (SYLVÉN, 1951). Sie bestehen in einer Abnahme der Zellzahl und einem Verlust an mucoidem Material. Den großen Kollagenfaserbündeln fehlt späterhin z. T. ein Überzug von mucoiden Stoffen. HIRSCH et al. (1953) konnten zeigen, daß die MPS je Volumeneinheit konstant bleiben, aber der Kollagengehalt steigt. Im Gefolge dieser Veränderungen geht die Gel-Struktur des Gallertkernes verloren (SYLVÉN, 1951).

Von den faserknorpeligen Gebilden haben weiterhin die Menisken des Kniegelenkes eine ausführliche Bearbeitung erfahren. Die Menisken erscheinen vor Ausbildung des Gelenkspaltes bei Keimlingen von 26—32 mm SSL (HESSER, 1926; LANGER, 1929; GRAY und GARDNER, 1950). Bei Feten von 37 mm gleicht der Meniscus in der Form bereits dem des Erwachsenen (LANGER, 1929). EBERL-ROTHE und SONNENSCHEIN (1951) bezeichnen das Gewebe der Menisken bereits bei Feten von 54 mm als Faserknorpel. McDERMOTT (1943) meint, der Faserknorpel würde erst jenseits des 3. Lebensjahres gebildet. BENETT et al. (1942) fanden bei Kindern von 8—10 Jahren stets Faserknorpel.

Die Menisken besitzen in der 12. Fetalwoche in ihrem äußeren Teil eine gute Gefäßversorgung (GRAY und GARDNER, 1950; TOBLER, 1936; REINBACH, 1954).

REINBACH (1954) hat den Faserverlauf im Meniscus untersucht und dessen Bedeutung im Zusammenhang mit der Gelenkbewegung diskutiert. Die Fasern sind überwiegend zirkulär angeordnet und liegen in der Peripherie des Meniscus besonders dicht. Ein zweites Fasersystem geht von den Ansatzpunkten aus und überkreuzt sich mit dem anderen System spitzwinklig.

Relativ wenige Untersuchungen liegen über Knochenverbindungen vor, in denen als Gelenkknorpel nicht hyaliner, sondern Faserknorpel wie in den Clavicula-, Sternochondralgelenken usw. auftritt. LUSCHKA (1858) hat bei diesem Gelenktyp von Halbgelenken gesprochen. Sternochondralgelenke können vollkommen geschlossen sein bzw. teilweise oder vollständig eine Gelenkhöhle besitzen (GRAY und GARDNER, 1950; WILLIAMS, 1957). Im Sternoclaviculargelenk besaßen 44% der von BEAM et al. (1956) untersuchten Gelenke einen vollständigen, 52% einen unvollständigen und 4% keinen Discus articularis. Die PNA (Pariser Nomina Anatomica; vgl. KNESE, 1956) unterscheiden

Abb. 51. Kind, 1 Jahr 2 Monate. Horizontalschnitt durch die Symphyse (vgl. KNESE u. BIERMANN, 1958, Abb. 1). *1* Cavum symphyseos; *2* dorsaler Faserbogen; *3* Übergang der dorsalen Fasern in Faserknorpel und anschließenden hyalinen Knorpel; *4* Faserknorpel um den Symphysenspalt; *5* hyaliner Knorpel; *6* ventraler Faserbogen; *7* Fettgewebe mit Gefäßen; *8* ventrales Bindegewebe mit Gefäßen; *9* Verbindung des Bindegewebes mit dem Knorpel mit Hilfe einer Faserknorpelzone. Azan. Phasenkontrast, Ob. 10, Ok. 8 (Photomontage)

zwischen Junctura synovialis, cartilaginea und fibrosa und berücksichtigen damit die sog. Halbgelenke nicht. KÜNZEL (1956) schlägt daher folgende Einteilung vor: Diarthrosis, Hemidiarthrosis und Synarthrosis.

5. Die Ernährung und das Gefäßsystem des Knorpels

Gefäßkanäle im Epiphysenknorpel und kurzen Knochen treten in relativ früher Fetalzeit auf (HINTZSCHE, 1928a, b; HINTZSCHE und SCHMID, 1935; BÖHMIG, 1930; PUTSCHAR, 1931; GRAY und GARDNER, 1950), im Rippenknorpel aber erst während der Kindheit (LINBERG, 1925). Nach HAINES (1933) dringen die Gefäße nicht aktiv in den Knorpel ein, sondern werden beim Knorpelwachstum mit dem sie umgebenden Gewebe eingeschlossen. Jedoch muß unter anderem nach GRAY und GARDNER (1950) der Knorpel in irgendeiner Weise angegriffen werden, da die Anzahl der Gefäße zunimmt und sich Verzweigungen und Anastomosen ausbilden. Aufteilungen und Verzweigungen der einzelnen Kanäle sind in der distalen Femurepiphyse häufig, Verbindungen zwischen den verschiedenen Kanalsystemen dagegen selten (HINTZSCHE 1928a). Der Gelenkknorpel bleibt in einer Schichtdicke von $^3/_4$—$1^1/_4$ mm gefäßlos. Die epiphysären Gefäßkanäle biegen senkrecht in Richtung auf die Knorpelknochengrenze um und verbinden sich mit diaphysären Gefäßen. Diese Verbindungen zwischen Gefäßbereichen können aber kaum durch Einschluß entstehen (GRAY und GARDNER, 1950). Beim Erwachsenen werden die Epiphysen von der Markhöhle her versorgt (vgl. RUTISHAUSER et al., 1954).

In einer umfangreichen Studie hat TRUETA (1957) die Blutversorgung des Femurkopfes im Laufe des postnatalen Lebens untersucht. Von den 3 verschiedenen Gefäßquellen des Erwachsenen fehlt von der Geburt bis zum 3.—4. Jahr die Versorgung durch das Ligamentum teres. Nach dem 4. Jahr verlieren die metaphysären Gefäße an Bedeutung und verschwinden. Mit dem 8.—9. Jahr setzt der Blutstrom durch das Ligamentum teres ein. Nach dem Schluß der Epiphysennarbe nehmen die epiphysären Gefäße und jene des Ligamentum teres wiederum Verbindung mit den metaphysären Gefäßen auf.

Die Knorpelkanäle bilden sich schrittweise zurück und werden durch chondroides oder Knorpelgewebe verschlossen (UEBERMUTH, 1929; BÖHMIG, 1930; PUTSCHAR, 1931). Im Bereich derartiger Kanäle zwischen Markhöhle und Epiphysenknorpel kommt es wahrscheinlich auch zur Knochenbildung; der Knochen färbt sich dann mit Thionin im p_H 3,2 orthochromatisch blau, die knorpelige Intercellularsubstanz metachromatisch (unveröffentlicht, vgl. KNESE, 1957). Hierbei sind auch lange spindelförmige Bildungszellen zu beobachten.

Die Knorpelgefäße stehen in der Epiphyse nicht unmittelbar mit der Knochenbildung in Zusammenhang. Die Osteogenese setzt zu sehr unterschiedlichen Zeiten postnatal ein. Aber erst nach Bildung eines umfangreichen Markraumes durch die Gefäße kommt es zu einer Knochenbildung (HINTZSCHE, 1928).

Eine umfassende Literaturdarstellung der verschiedenen Ansichten über die Ernährung des Gelenkknorpels gibt EKHOLM (1951). Er unterscheidet drei Wege: Ernährung durch Gefäße der Kapsel, durch Gefäße des unter dem Knorpel liegenden Knochens und von der Synovia her. EKHOLM (1951, 1955) hat die Ernährung des Gelenkknorpels unter Verwendung von ^{198}Au und ^{32}P beim Kaninchen untersucht und kommt zum Schluß, daß die Ernährung überwiegend von der Epiphysenseite her erfolgt, aber auch von der Synovia. HOLMDAHL und INGELMARK (1950) konnten bei Gelenken des Kaninchens kanalförmige und ampulläre Verbindungen zwischen Markhöhle und Knorpel beobachten; die kanalförmigen Verbindungen treten bei Gelenken mit starker Druckbelastung auf. BRODIN (1955) wies einen fluorescierenden Farbstoff 30 sec nach Injektion im Gelenkknorpel nach. Die Menge des Farbstoffes ist bei Tötung der Tiere $3^1/_2$ min nach der Verabreichung wesentlich geringer.

BRODIN (1955) hat auch die Verteilung des fluoreszierenden Farbstoffes in der Zwischenwirbelscheibe verfolgt. Die hyaline Knorpelplatte nimmt den Farbstoff schnell auf, die

Faserringe weniger und dann vor allem in den peripheren Abschnitten. PAULSON et al. (1951) und SYLVÉN (1951) haben interferometrisch die Diffusionsgeschwindigkeit verschiedener Stoffe durch frische Schnitte des Nucleus pulposus von Kälbern gemessen. NaCl, $CaCl_2$, Na_2SO_4, eine Reihe organischer Substanzen wie Harnstoff, Aminosäuren und einfache Zucker (Trauben-, Rohrzucker) haben eine Diffusionsgeschwindigkeit, die halb so groß wie im Wasser ist. Die Diffusionskonstanten sind von gleicher Größenordnung wie in einer Gelatine mit dem Wassergehalt des Nucleus pulposus. Die Verfasser nehmen eine effektive Porengröße von etwa 15 Å an; d. h. daß nur Moleküle kleiner als 15 Å durch die Intercellularsubstanz hindurchdiffundieren können. Ein derartiges „passives" Ernährungssystem durch Diffusion reicht aber für die Ernährung des Gallertkernes nicht aus, so daß noch andere Mechanismen eine Rolle spielen müssen. In diesem Zusammenhang ist der Hinweis von AMPRINO (1955) von Bedeutung, daß die ^{35}S-Aufnahme durch Zellen des Epiphysenknorpels von inneren Bedingungen und nicht von äußeren, wie z. B. der Blutversorgung, abhängt. Die ^{35}S-Aufnahme kann sogar dem Umfang der Gefäßversorgung widersprechen. Die gefäßlose Metaphyse nimmt mehr ^{35}S als die Epiphyse auf, die beim Hühnchen wenige Tage vor dem Schlüpfen vascularisiert wird.

6. Materialstruktur und Mechanik des Knorpelgewebes

Das Knorpelgewebe besitzt eine auffällige Faserstruktur, die mit der Leistung, der Belastung oder der sog. Funktion in Zusammenhang gebracht wurde. Zur Aufklärung der Bedeutung einer solchen Struktur ist die genaue Kenntnis des Faserverlaufes erforderlich. Eine Reihe von Diskussionen beruht wohl darauf, daß die erforderlichen morphologischen Befunde mit unterschiedlichen, z. T. unzureichenden Methoden erhoben wurden. Die für die mechanischen Eigenschaften eines Gewebes verantwortliche Ordnung der Komponenten ist in der mikroskopischen Dimension oder gar der der Ultrastruktur zu suchen, d. h. es handelt sich um Strukturen 3.—6. Ordnung. Die Rekonstruktion des räumlichen Gefüges der Teile aus dem Schnittbild ist ungewöhnlich schwierig, z. T. fast unmöglich.

BENNINGHOFF (1925) hat sich mit dem Aufbau stabförmiger Knorpelstücke am Beispiel des Trachealknorpels beschäftigt. Bei einer Biegebelastung soll auf der konvexen Seite das Perichondrium die Zugspannungen, auf der konkaven Seite der druckfeste Knorpel die Druckspannungen aufnehmen. LANGE (1934) faßt das Perichondrium als zugfesten Schlauch auf, in den die druckfeste, besser druckelastische (BUCHER, 1942) Masse des Knorpels eingefügt ist. Nach BENNINGHOFF sollte das Chondron in seiner Peripherie zirkulär verlaufende Fasern enthalten, während in der Interterritorialsubstanz beide perichondrale Seiten durch senkrechte Fasern miteinander verbunden sind. LUBOSCH (1927, 1938), DAWSON und SPARK (1928), BORMUTH (1933), LEPPERT (1933, 1934), BUCHER (1942) und STAUB (1950) konnten an sehr verschiedenem Untersuchungsgut eine derartige spezielle Wicklung in den Knorpelkapseln nicht beobachten (s. S. 756). Diese Autoren fanden übereinstimmend Fibrillen von S-förmigem Verlauf, die sich kreuzen, wobei zwei Systeme vorhanden und um 45° gegeneinander versetzt sind. Das Bild des Faserverlaufes ist von der Schnittrichtung unabhängig, d. h. es liegt ein dreidimensionales Fasergitter vor (BUCHER, 1942). Die auslaufenden Schenkel des S gehen in das Perichondrium über. In Richtung der Winkelhalbierenden und damit senkrecht zum Perichondrium sind die Zellreihen angeordnet (BUCHER, 1942).

BUCHER (1942) hat den Spannungsverlauf für Biegung bei S-förmiger Ordnung der Knorpelfibrillen kurz skizziert. Das Perichondrium auf der Konvexseite kann durch die zugfesten Kollagenfasern nicht nachgeben und drückt auf die Knorpelmasse. Weiterhin werden aber die mit dem Perichondrium verbundenen Knorpelfibrillen angespannt. Die S-förmigen Fasern suchen sich zu strecken und üben damit auf ihrer Konkavseite einen Druck auf die Intercellularsubstanz und die Zellen als druckelastische Elemente aus (BORMUTH, 1933). Die mechanischen Eigenschaften beruhen demzufolge auf der Zusammenarbeit zweier Materialien unterschiedlicher Festigkeitseigenschaften, d. h. es liegt ein sog. Verbundbau vor (GEBHARDT, 1911; BENNINGHOFF, 1925; KNESE, 1958).

Für den Gelenkknorpel hat BENNINGHOFF (1925) Faserbügel angegeben, die mit ihrem einen Schenkel aus dem verkalkten Knorpel aufsteigen, unter Bildung einer sog. Tangentialfaserschicht an der Oberfläche in den anderen senkrechten Schenkel umbiegen BENNINGHOFF (1925) hat am Gelenkknorpel 4 Schichten unterschieden: 1. die oberflächliche Tangentialschicht mit Ausrichtung der länglichen Zellen parallel zur Oberfläche des Knorpels, 2. die Übergangszone mit unregelmäßig rundlichen Zellen, 3. die Radiärzone mit wiederum etwas länglichen Zellen, deren Längsachse senkrecht zur Oberfläche des Knorpels steht, und schließlich 4. den mineralisierten Streifen, der mit dem Knochengewebe verbunden ist. Diesem Zellbild sollte die Ordnung der Fasern in Form von Faserbügeln entsprechen. Rein senkrecht verlaufende Fasern, wie sie BENNINGHOFF (1925) angenommen hatte, sind poralisationsoptisch in der Radiärschicht nicht zu beobachten (KNESE 1966b). Es liegen sich überkreuzende Fasersysteme vor, deren Kreuzungswinkel von Gelenk zu Gelenk etwas wechselnd zwischen 20 und 30° beträgt. Nach Untersuchung der Schultergelenkpfanne mit Hilfe der Spaltlinienmethode glaubte BENNINGHOFF für die Ordnung der Bügel eine trajektorielle Deutung geben zu können. Eine Nachuntersuchung von PAUWELS (1959) konnte eine Reihe individueller Varianten der Spaltlinien nachweisen, die aber nach spannungsoptischen Untersuchungen dem Dehnungsbild der individuell gestalteten Schulterpfanne entsprechen. Jedoch hat bereits BUCHER (1942) gezeigt, daß mit Hilfe der Spaltlinien der Faserverlauf im Knorpel nicht befriedigend geklärt werden kann.

Die Frage, worauf die Elastizität des Gelenkknorpels beruht, hat SOKOLOFF (1963) experimentell an der Tibia von Hunden geprüft. Der Gelenkknorpel befand sich hierbei in einem Bad, das verschiedenartige Ionen enthält, und wurde statisch belastet. SOKOLOFF kommt zum Schluß, daß offensichtlich die anionischen Gruppen für die physikalischen Eigenschaften des Knorpels entscheidend sind. Wenn die elektrostatische Ladung durch Kationen herabgesetzt wird, nimmt nämlich die Elastizität ab und die Deformation ist durch Abgabe von Wasser während der Belastung größer. Der Autor nimmt an, daß durch Kationen die Größe der kolloidalen Aggregate herabgesetzt wird; damit werden dann auch die osmotischen Eigenschaften der polianionischen Intercellularsubstanz verändert. Es sind 2 bzw. 3 Komponenten der Elastizität zu unterscheiden (SOKOLOFF, 1966): Die unmittelbare Elastizität und der Deformationseffekt durch Abgabe von Flüssigkeit oder durch einen inneren viscösen Fluß der „Grundsubstanz". Im Speziellen gibt SOKOLOFF (1966) an, daß Rippenknorpel starrer als Gelenkknorpel ist. Der Elastizitätsmodul vom menschlichen Gelenkknorpel beträgt 70 g/mm^2, für Rippenknorpel vom 9. bis 22. Jahre 402 und für das 42.—66. Jahr 724 g/mm^2.

Das Knorpelgewebe wird fast ausschließlich als druckelastisches Material angesehen, d. h. als ein Stoff, der sich unter Druckbelastung verformt und anschließend zu seiner ursprünglichen Gestalt zurückkehrt. KNESE und BIERMANN (1958) haben nun den Ansatzknorpel in Apophysen als zugelastisches Material näher untersucht. Sehnen- und Knochengewebe haben etwa die gleiche Zugfestigkeit von 1000 kg · cm^{-2}, der Elastizitätsmodul des Knochengewebes ist aber zehnmal größer als der der Sehne und damit die Verformung des Knochengewebes geringer. Zwischen Sehne und Knochengewebe ist als sog. „Ansatzstruktur" eine Dehnungs- oder Elastizitätsbremse eingeschaltet. In dieser Ansatzstruktur wird die Dehnung durch Verhinderung der Querkürzung herabgesetzt.

Jede Dehnung in der Längsrichtung eines Körpers ist mit einer Veränderung des Querschnittes, einer Querkürzung verbunden. Wird die Querkürzung verhindert, setzt sich auch die Längsdehnung herab. Bei einer Querkürzung der Sehne nähern sich die Sehnenfasern unter Zusammendrücken des Peritenonium internum einander an. In einem faserknorpeligen Ansatz setzen die in Reihen zwischen den Sehnenfasern eingelagerten druckelastischen chondroiden Zellen die Querkürzung herab. Im Ansatzknorpel bilden die Fasern ein Netzwerk mit rhombischen Maschen, in denen längliche

Knorpelzellen liegen. Diese Zellen und der Einbau der Fasern in die hyaline Intercellularsubstanz wirken der Formänderung des Maschennetzes entgegen. Der sog. „sekundäre“ Knorpel der Ansatzgebiete unterscheidet sich in seiner Struktur demzufolge als zugelastisches Gewebe von dem druckelastischen „primären“ Knorpel in Gelenken usw. Der Dehnungsausgleich im Bereich von Muskelansätzen ist derart, daß für Sehnenabrisse nur noch die Spannungsverteilung, aber nicht mehr der unterschiedliche Elastizitätsmodul eine Rolle spielt. Es treten Unstetigkeitsflächen in der Spannungsverteilung auf, so daß die Sehne mit einem sog. Zugkeil aus dem Knochen ausreißt (KNESE 1958). Ähnliche Gewebeformen wie in den Apophysen an anderen Orten des Körpers erfordern noch eine eingehende Untersuchung der Bedeutung ihrer Struktur.

SCHNEIDER (1955, 1956) hat den Sehnenansatz mit der Einpflanzung eines Elektrokabels in ein Gerät verglichen und an diesen Stellen Biegungsspannungen angenommen. Ein Faserverlauf im Sinne der Einpflanzung der Sehne in den Knochen konnte jedoch von KNESE und BIERMANN (1958) und JIPP (1960) nicht beobachtet werden, so daß schon an Hand der morphologischen Befunde die Deutung von SCHNEIDER abzulehnen ist. Im übrigen stellen Sehnen ein zugfestes und nie ein biegungsfestes Material dar. Beim Umbiegen von Sehnen um Hypomochlien usw. sind nur Reibungskräfte anzunehmen. Demzufolge ist hier das Bild der sog. Gleitsehnen (PLÖTZ, 1937/38; STILWELL und GRAY, 1954) sowie häufig die Einlagerung in Sehnenscheiden zu beobachten (über die Fabella vgl. BIERMANN, 1957, das Os peroneum WEIDENREICH, 1923d).

Mit technischen Prüfverfahren wurden die mechanischen Eigenschaften der Wirbel und Zwischenwirbelscheiben untersucht (LANGMAACK, 1954; EVANS und LISSNER, 1959). INGELMARK und EKHOLM (1952) haben hierbei auch den wechselnden Flüssigkeitsgehalt der Bandscheiben berücksichtigt. Alle genannten Autoren kommen zu dem Schluß, daß die Festigkeit der Wirbelkörper und die Elastizität der Zwischenwirbelscheiben mit zunehmendem Lebensalter abnimmt. WYSS und URLICH (1954) haben ihre Untersuchungen über die Belastung der Wirbelsäule auch im Hinblick auf die Behandlung von Bandscheibenschäden ausgewertet und empfehlen neben Extension eine gezielte Kyphosierung durch Pelottendruck. PEREY (1957) hat das Verhalten von injizierten Kontrastmitteln in der Zwischenwirbelscheibe während der Belastung röntgenologisch kontrolliert und eine Verschiebung des Kontrastmittels nur bei gleichzeitigem Wirbelschaden beobachtet.

HIRSCH (1955) und HIRSCH und NACHEMSON (1957) stellten einmal die statische, über längere Zeit hingehende Verformung der Zwischenwirbelscheibe fest. Unter dynamischer, d. h. plötzlich auftretender Belastung kommt es zu Schwingungen bzw. zu einem Vibrieren. Die in Bruchteilen von Sekunden einwirkende Kraft kann relativ klein sein, aber eine große Belastung darstellen. Die Autoren glauben jedoch, daß die in der Ontogenese auftretenden Änderungen in der chemischen Zusammensetzung der Zwischenwirbelscheiben für die Möglichkeit von Verletzungen bedeutsamer als mechanische Einwirkungen sind.

Die vorliegende Darstellung zeigt, daß uns das Knorpelgewebe beim Menschen, besonders bei Berücksichtigung der Ontogenese, in sehr vielfältiger Gestalt entgegentritt. Neben permanenten Knorpelbildungen wie Gelenk- und Rippenknorpeln, verdienen die transitorischen Bildungen, Epiphysen, Apophysen usw. eine eingehende Diskussion. In diesen Teilen ist der Knorpel ein Übergangsglied in der Reihe der Stützgewebe zum Knochengewebe. Viele der mit dieser Entwicklung verbundenen histogenetischen Fragen sind noch ungeklärt. Die transitorischen Knorpel spielen beim Wachstum und der Formbildung des Skeletes, aber vermutlich auch im Stoffwechsel, eine große Rolle.

Literatur

ALBAUM, H. G., A. HIRSCHFELD and A. E. SOBEL: Calcification. VIII. Glycolytic enzymes and phosphorylated intermediates in pre-osseous cartilage. Proc. Soc. exp. Biol. (N. Y.) **79**, 682—686 (1962).

AMPRINO, R.: La struttura delle ossa de'lluomo sottrate alle sollecitazioni meccaniche. Considerazioni sul significato funzionale delle strutture della sostanza compatta. Wilhelm Roux' Arch. Entwickl.Med. Org. **138**, 365—422 (1938).

AMPRINO, R.: A contribution to the functional meaning of the substitution of primary by secondary bone tissue. Acta anat. (Basel) 5, 291—300 (1948).
— Radiographic research on the S-35-sulfate metabolism in cartilage and bone differention and growth. Acta anat. (Basel) 24, 121—163 (1955).
— Uptake of S^{35} in the differentiation and growth of cartilage and bone. In Ciba Found. Symposion on bone structure and metabolism, S. 89—102. London: J. u. A. Churchill 1956.
— Aspects of limb morphogenesis in the chicken. In: Organogenesis (ed. by R. L. DEHAAN and H. URSPRUNG), p. 255—281. New York: Holt, Rinehart & Winston 1965.
—, and A. BAIRATI: Studi sulle transformazioni delle cartilagini dell'uomo nell'accrescimento e nella senescenza. III. Cartilagini fibrose. Z. Zellforsch. 21, 448—482 (1934).
—, and R. CATTANEO: Il substrato istologico delle varie modalità di inserzioni tendinee alle ossa nell'uomo. Ricerche su individui di varia età. Z. Anat. Entwickl.-Gesch. 107, 680—705 (1937).
ANDERSEN, H., and F. BRO-RASMUSSEN: Histochemical studies on the histogenesis of the joints in human fetus with special reference to the development of the joint cavities in the hand and foot. Amer. J. Anat. 108, 111—122 (1961).
ANDERSON, C. E., J. LUDOWIEG, H. A. HARPER, and E. P. ENGLEMAN: The composition of the organic component of human articular cartilage. Relationship to age and degenerative joint disease. J. Bone Jt Surg. A 46, 1176—1183 (1964).
ANGEVINE, D. M.: Structure and function of normal connective tissue. Connective Tissues, 1. Conf. Ed. by CH. RAGAN, S. 13—41. New York: Josiah Macy Foundation 1950.
ANSON, B. J., and TH. H. BAST: The ear and the temporal bone development and adult structure. Otolaryngology 1, 1—111 (1955).
ASBOE-HANSEN, G.: On the structure and function of the mast cells. Connective tissue, ed. by R. E. TUNBRIDGE, p. 12—26. Blackwell: Publ. Oxford 1957.
— Hormones and connective tissue. Munksgaard: Scandinavian-University-Books 1966.
ASTBURY, W. T.: Protein structure from the viewpoint of x-ray analysis. Lab. Carlsberg 22, 45—53 (1938).
— The molecular structure of the fibres of the collagen group. J. int. Soc. Leath. Chem. 24, 69—92 (1940).
BAER, J. P.: Der funktionelle Bau der Symphyse im Embryonal- und Kindesalter auf Grund von Untersuchungen im polarisierten Licht. Acta anat. (Basel) 7, 273—301 (1949).
BAHLING, G.: Die Entwicklung des Querschnittes der großen Extremitätenknochen bis zum Säuglingsalter. Morph. Jb. 99, 109—188 (1958).
BAHR, G. F.: Ergebnisse elektronenmikroskopischer Untersuchungen des kollagenen und elastischen Gewebes. Arch. Derm. Syph. (Berl.) 193, 518—526 (1951).
BAHR, G. F.: Osmium tetroxide and ruthenium tetroxide and their reaction with biologically important substances. Electron staines. III. Exp. Cell Res. 7, 457—479 (1954).
— Continued studies about the fixation with osmium tetroxide. Electron staines. IV. Exp. Cell Res. 9, 277—285 (1955).
BALINSKY, B. J.: New experiments on the mode of action of the limb inductor. J. exp. Zool. 134, 239—273 (1957).
BALOGH, G., u. I. FÖLDES: Die funktionelle Gewebestruktur der Sehnenfurchen. Acta morph. Acad. Sci. hung. 5, 355—368 (1955).
BALOGH, K., JR., and R. B. COHEN: Histochemical localization of uridine diphosphoglucose dehydrogenase in cartilage. Nature (Lond.) 192, 1199—1200 (1961).
— H. R. DUDLEY, and R. B. COHEN: Oxidative enzyme activity in skeletal cartilage and bone. A histochemical study. Lab. Invest. 10, 839—845 (1961).
BANFIELD, W.: Aging in connective tissues. In: ASBOE-HANSEN, Connective tissue in health and disease, p. 151—158. 1954.
BARGMANN, W.: Zur Kenntnis der Knorpelarchitekturen. (Untersuchungen am Skeletsystem von Selachiern.) Z. Zellforsch. 29, 405—424 (1939).
BAUER, H. O. K.: Volumen und Länge der langen Gliedmaßenknochen während des fetalen Wachstums. Anthrop. Anz. 17, 77—102 (1940).
BAZIN, S., et A. DELAUNAY: Le métabolisme des mucopolysaccharides. Biol. et Méd. 48, 351—441 (1959).
BEAMS, A. W., T. N. TAHMUSIAN, R. DEVINE and E. ANDERSON: Ultra structure of the nuclear membrane of a gregarine parasitic in grass-hoppers. Exp. Cell Res. 13, 200—204 (1957).
BEJŠOVEC, J.: Die Ossifikation des Schildknorpels beim Rehbock (Capreolus capreolus capreolus). Čs. Morfol. 2, 169—178 (1954).
BÉLANGER, L. F.: Autoradiographic visualization of the entry and transit of S^{35} in cartilage, bone, and dentine of young rats and the effect of hyaluronidase in vitro. Canad. J. Biochem. 32, 161—169 (1954).
— Autoradiographic visualization of Ca^{45} intake by normal and pathological cartilage in vitro. Proc. Soc. Exp. Biol. (N. Y.) 88, 150—152 (1955).
— Autoradiographic visualization of the entry and transit of S^{35} methionine and cystine in the soft and hard tissues of the growing rat. Anat. Rec. 124, 555—580 (1956a).
— Autoradiographic studies of the formation of the organic matrix of cartilage, bone and the tissues of teeth. Ciba Found. Symposion on bone structure and Metabolism (CF). London: J. u. A. Churchill, Wolstenhalme and O'Connor 1956b.
BENNETT, G. H., H. WAINE and W. BAUER: Changes in the knee joint at various ages. Commonwealth Fed. N. Y. 1942.

BENNETT, ST.: The concepts of membrane flow and membrane vesiculation as mechanisme for active transport and ion pumping. J. biophys. biochem. Cytol. **2**, 99—104 (1956).

BENNINGHOFF, A.: Über den funktionellen Bau des Knorpels. Verh. anat. Ges. 31. Vers. Erlangen 1922, S 250—267.

— Der funktionelle Bau des Hyalinknorpels. Ergebn. Anat. Entwickl.-Gesch. **26**, 1—54 (1925).

BERENSON, G. S., W. M. LUMPKIN and W. G. SHIPP: Study of the time-course production of acid mucopolysaccharides by fibroblasts in a synthetic medium. Anat. Rec. **132**, 585—596 (1958).

BERNARD, C.: Leçons sur les phénomènes de la vie communs aux animaux et aux végétaux, p. 121. Paris: Baillière 1878.

BERNARDI, G.: The molecular size, shape and weight of mucoprotein from cartilage. Biochim. biophys. Acta (Amst.) **26**, 47—52 (1957).

BERNHARD, W.: Ultrastructural aspects of nucleo-cytoplasmic relationship. Exp. Cell Res. **6**, 17—50 (1958).

BERSIN, TH.: Die biochemische Bedeutung der Austauscher. Forsch. Fortschr. dtsch. Wiss. **26**, 251—253 (1950).

BETTELHEIM-JEVONS, F. R.: Protein-carbohydrate complexes. Advanc. Protein Chem. **13**, 1—105 (1958).

BIDDER, A.: Osteobiologie. Arch. mikr. Anat. **68**, 137—213 (1906).

BIERMANN, H.: Die Knochenbildung im Bereich periostaler-diaphysärer Sehnen- und Bandansätze. Z. Zellforsch. **46**, 635—671 (1957).

BLIX, G.: Glykoproteide. In: Physiologische Chemie I von B. FLASCHENTRÄGER u. E. LENNARTZ, S. 751—767. Berlin-Göttingen-Heidelberg: Springer 1951.

—, and O. SNELLMAN: On chondroitin sulfuric acid and hyaluronic acid. Ark. Kemi. Mineral. Geol. A **19**, 1—19 (1945).

BLOOM, W.: Cellular differentiation and tissue culture. Physiol. Rev. **17**, 589—617 (1937).

—, and M. A. BLOOM: Calcification and ossification. Calcification of developing bones in embryonic and newborn rats. Anat. Rec. **78**, 497—523 (1940).

BLUMBERG, B. S., and A. G. OGSTON: The effects of proteolytic enzymes on the hyaluronic acid complex of synovial fluid. Biochem. J. **66**, 342—346 (1957).

— — Further evidence on the protein complexes of some hyaluronic acids. Biochem. J. **68**, 183—188 (1958).

BÖHMIG, R.: Die Blutgefäße der Wirbelbandscheiben, das Verhalten des intervertebralen Chordasegments und die Bedeutung beider für die Bandscheibendegeneration. Langenbecks Arch. klin. Chir. **158**, 374—424 (1930).

BONA, C., et STÁNESCU: Cytoenzymologie du chondrocyte dans le cartilage de conjugaison humain en conditions normales et pathologiques. Rev. roum. Embroyol. Cytol. Sér. Embryol. **3**, 59—74 (1966).

BORGHESE, E.: I lipidi nel processo di ossificazione. Z. Zellforsch. **25**, 622—654 (1936).

— Recent histochemical results of studies on embryos of some birds and mammals. Int. Rev. Cytol. **6**, 289—341 (1957).

BORMUTH, H.: Die trajektoriellen Strukturen im Knorpel der Haifische auf Grund von Untersuchungen im polarisierten Licht. Z. Zellforsch. **17**, 767 (1933).

BOSTRÖM, H., and E. ODEBLAD: Autoradiographic observations on the incorporation of S^{35}-labelled sodium sulfate in the rabbit fetus. Anat. Rec. **115**, 505—510 (1953).

— — et U. FRIBERG: A quantitative autoradiographic study of the incorporation of S^{35} in tracheal cartilage. Arch. Biochem. **38**, 283—286 (1952).

—, and L. RODÉN: Metabolism of glycosaminoglycans. In: The amino sugars, vol. IIB (ed. by R. W. JEANLOZ and E. B. BALAZS), p. 46—79. New York and London: Academic Press 1966.

BOURNE, G. H.: Phosphatase and bone. In: The Biochemistry and Physiology, ed. by G. H. BOURNE, p. 251—284. 1956.

BOWES, J. H., and R. H. KENTEN: The amino acid composition and titration curve of collagen. Biochem. J. **43**, 358—365 (1948).

BOYD, E. S., and W. F. NEUMAN: The surface chemistry of bone. V. Ion-binding properties of cartilage. J. biol. Chem. **193**, 243—251 (1951).

BRACHET, J.: La détection histochimique des acides pentose nucléiques. C.R. Soc. Biol. (Paris) **133**, 88—90 (1940).

— The biochemistry of development. VII. The biochemistry of differentiation. London-New York-Paris-Los Angeles: Pergamon Press 1960.

BRANDENBERGER, E., u. H. R. SCHINZ: Über die Natur der Verkalkung bei Mensch und Tier und das Verhalten der anorganischen Knochensubstanz im Falle der hauptsächlichen menschlichen Knochenkrankheiten. Helv. med. Acta, Ser. A, **12**, Suppl. 16, 63 (1945).

BRANWOOD, A. W.: The fibroblast. Int. Rev. Connect. Tissue Res. **1**, 1—28 (1963).

BRETTSCHNEIDER, H.: Ein Beitrag zur normalen Anatomie der Zwischenwirbelscheibe. Z. mikr.-anat. Forsch. **58**, 381—403 (1952).

BRIMACOMBE, J. S., and J. M. WEBBER: Mucopolysaccharides. Amsterdam - London - New York: Elsevier Publ. Comp. 1964.

BROILI, F.: Über den feineren Bau der verknöcherten Sehnen (= verknöcherten Muskeln) von Trachodon. Anat. Anz. **55**, 465—475 (1922).

BUCHER, O.: Zur Architektur des hyalinen Knorpels. Anat. Anz. **93**, 306—313 (1942).

— Beitrag zum funktionellen Bau des hyalinen Knorpels auf Grund von Untersuchungen im polarisierten Licht. Z. Zellforsch. **32**, 281—300 (1943).

BUDDECKE, E.: Polysaccharide und Polysaccharidsulfate des Bindegewebes. In: D-Glucose und verwandte Verbindungen in Medizin und Biologie (Hrsgb. H. BARTELHEIMER, W. HEYDE und W. THORN), S. 573—603. Stuttgart: Ferdinand Enke 1966.

BUDDECKE, E., W. KRÖZ u. E. LANKA: Chemische Zusammensetzung und makromolekulare Struktur von Chondroitinsulfat-Proteinen. Hoppe-Seylers Z. physiol. Chem. **331**, 196—218 (1963).

BUNGENBERG DE JONG, H. G.: Complex colloid systems. Kruyt, H. R. Colloid Science II. Amsterdam: Elsevier Publ. Co. 1949.

BURSTONE, M. S.: Histochemical observations on enzymatic processes in bones and teeth. Ann. N. Y. Acad. Sci. **85**, 431—444 (1960).

CAMERON, D. A., and R. A. ROBINSON: Electron microscopy of epiphyseal and articular cartilage matrix in the femur of the newborn infant. J. Bone Jt Surg. A **40**, 163—170 (1958).

CAMPANI, M., and O. REGGIANINI: Observations in the experimental animal on the nature of the metachromatic ground substance in granulation tissue. J. Path. Bact. **62**, 563—568 (1950).

CAMPO, R. D., and D. D. DZIEWIATKOWSKI: Intracellular synthesis of protein-polysaccharides by slices of bovine costal cartilage. J. biol. Chem. **237**, 2729 (1962).

CANNON, W. B.: Organization for physiological homeostasis. Physiol. Rev. **9**, 399—431 (1929).

CAREY, E. Z., and W. ZEIT: The early postnatal development of the patella of the dog (Canis familiaris). Anat. Rec. **36**, 51—67 (1927).

CARNEIRO, J., and C. P. LEBLOND: Role of osteoblasts and odontoblasts in secreting the collagen of bone and dentin, as shown by radioautography in mice given tritium-labelled glycine. Exp. Cell Res. **18**, 291—300 (1959).

CASPERSON, T., and J. SCHULTZ: Ribonucleic acids in both nucleus and cytoplasm; and the function of nucleolus. Proc. nat. Acad. Sci. (Wash.) **26**, 507—515 (1940).

CASSELMAN, B.: Histochemical technique. London: Methuen u. Co. Ltd. 1959.

CHARGAFF, E., C. F. CRAMPTON and R. LIPSHITZ: Separation of calf thymus desoxyribonucleic acid into fractions of different composition. Nature (Lond.) **172**, 289—292 (1953).

CIPERA, J. D., and Y. S. WILLMER: Composition of epiphyseal cartilage. III. Differences in enzymatic activities of epiphyseal and articular cartilage of rachitic chicks. Canad. J. Biochem. Physiol. **40**, 419—423 (1962).

COELHO, R. R., and O. D. CHRISMAN: Sulphate metabolism in cartilage. II. S^{35}-sulphate uptake and total sulphate in cartilage slices. J. Bone Jt Surg. A **42**, 165—172 (1960).

COLLINS, D. A., H. BECKS, C. W. ASLING, M. E. SIMPSON and H. M. EVANS: Changes in the ossification of the third metacarpal occurring at progressively longer intervals following hypophysectomy in the female rat. Anat. Rec. **101**, 13—16 (1948).

COLLINS, D. A., H. BECKS, C. W. ASLING M. E. SIMPSON and H. M. EVANS: The growth of hypophysectomized female rats following chronic treatment with pure pituitary growth hormone. V. Skeletal changes: Skull and dentition, vol. 13, p. 207—220. Philadelphia: Growth 1949.

COMAR, C. L.: Skeletal metabolism studies with radiocalcium. In: The role of atomic energy in agricultural research. Proceedings of the fourth annual Oak Ridge summer symposium August 25—30, 1952. (Comar, C. L., and Hood, S. L. comps.) Oak Ridge, Tenn. Technical Information Service 1953, p. 225—329.

CONSDEN, R., and R. BIRD: Carbohydrate of connective tissue. Nature (Lond.) **173**, 996—997 (1954).

COOPER, G. W., and D. J. PROCKOP: Intracellular accumulation of protocollagen and extrusion of collagen by embryonic cartilage cells. J. Cell Biol. **38**, 523—537 (1968).

CURRAN, R. C.: Observations on the formation of collagen in quartz lesions. J. Path. Bact. **66**, 271—282 (1953).

— The histological demonstration of connective-tissue mucopolysaccharides. In: The biochemistry of mucopolysaccharides of connective tissue (ed. by F. CLARK and J. K. GRANT), p. 24—38. Cambridge: University Press 1961.

— The histochemistry of mucopolysaccharides. Int. Rev. Cytol. **17**, 149—202 (1964).

CURTAIN, C. C.: Nature of the protein in the hyaluronic-complex of bovine synovial fluid. Biochem. J. **61**, 688—696 (1955).

D'ABRAMO, F., and F. LIPMANN: The formation of adenosine-3'-phosphate 5'-phosphosulfate in extracts of chick embryo cartilage and its conversion into chondroitin sulfate. Biochim. biophysica Acta (Amst.) **25**, 211—213 (1957).

DALTON, A. J.: A chrome-osmium fixation for electron microscopy. Anat. Rec. **121**. 281 (1955).

DAVIDSON, E. A., and K. MEYER: Chondroitin, a new mucopolysaccharide. J. biol. Chem. **211**, 605—611 (1954).

— — Structural studies on chondroitin sulfuric acid. II. The glucuronidic linkage. J. Amer. chem. Soc. **77**, 4796—4798 (1955).

—, and W. SMALL: Metabolism in vivo of connective tissue mucopolysaccharides. I. Chondroitinsulfate C and keratansulfate of nucleus pulposus. Biochim. biophys. Acta (Amst.) **69**, 445—452 (1963a).

— — Metabolism in vivo of connective-tissue mucopolysaccharides. II. Chondroitinsulfate B and hyaluronic acid of skin. Biochim. biophys. Acta (Amst.) **69**, 453—561 (1963b).

DAVIES, D. V., and I. YOUNG: The distribution of radioactive sulphur (^{35}S) in the fibrous tissues, cartilages and bones of the rat following its administration in the form of inorganic sulphate. J. Anat. (Lond.) **88**, 174—183 (1954).

DAWSON, A. B., and CH. SPARK: The fibrous transformation and architecture of the costal cartilage of the albino rat. Amer. J. Anat. **42**, 110—137 (1928).

DAY, T. D.: The nature and significance of the cementing substance in interstitial connective tissue. J. Path. Bact. **59**, 567—573 (1947).
DEINEKA, D.: Die Entwicklung der Knochenzellen im perichondralen Prozeß. Anat. Anz. **46**, 97—126 (1914).
DELAUNAY, A., et S. BAZIN: Metabolisme des mucopolysaccharides. Ann. Histochim. **4**, 259—278 (1958).
DODDS, G. S.: Row formation and other types of arrangement of cartilage cells in endochondral ossification. Anat. Rec. **46**, 385—399 (1930).
DOLGO-SABUROFF, B.: Über Ursprung und Innervation der Skeletmuskeln. Anat. Anz. **68**, 80—87 (1929/30).
DORFMAN, A.: Metabolism of the mucopolysaccharides of connective tissue. Pharmacol. Rev. **78**, 1—31 (1955/56).
— Polysaccharides of connective tissue. J. Histochem. Cytochem. **11**, 2—13 (1963).
—, and M. B. MATHEWS: The physiology of connective tissue. Ann. Rev. Physiol. **18**, 69—88 (1956).
—, and S. SCHILLER: Effects of hormones on the metabolism of acid mucopolysaccharides of connective tissue. Recent Prog. Hormone Res. **14**, 427—481 (1958).
— — Effects of hormones on the metabolism of acid mucopolysaccharides of connective tissue. In: Hormone research (ed. by G. PINCUS), vol. 14, p. 427—481. London and New York: Academic Press 1958.
DRAHN, F.: Über den histologischen Bau der Gleitsehne des Musc. biceps brachii beim Pferd. Arch. mikr. Anat. **96**, 39—52 (1922).
DURAN-REYNALS, F.: Tissue permeability and spreading factors in infection; contribution to host: parasite problem. Bact. Rev. **6**, 197—252 (1942).
DURNING, W. C.: Submicroscopic structure of frozen-dried epiphyseal plate and adjacent spongiosa of the rat. J. Ultrastruct. Res. **2**, 245—260 (1958).
DZIEWIATKOWSKI, D. D.: Radioautographic visualization of Sulfur-35 disposition in the articular cartilage and bone of suckling rats following injection of labeled Sodium sulfate. J. exp. Med. **93**, 451—458 (1951).
— Autoradiographic studies with S^{35}-sulfate. Rev. Cytol. **7**, 159—194 (1958).
EBERL-ROTHE, G., u. A. SONNENSCHEIN: Die autogenetische Ausbildung des Kniegelenkes beim Menschen. Z. Anat. Entwickl.-Gesch. **115**, 251—272 (1951).
EEG-LARSEN, N.: An experimental study on growth and glycolysis in the epiphyseal cartilage of rats. Acta physiol. scand. **38**, Suppl. **128**, 1—77 (1956).
EICHELBERGER, L., W. H. AKESON and M. ROMA: Biochem. Studies of articular cartilage. I. Normal Values. J. Bone Jt Surg. B **40** (17), 142—152 (1958).
— F. D. BOROWER and M ROMA: Histochemical characterization of inorganic constituents, connective tissue and chondroitinsulfate of extracellular and intracellular compartments of hyaline cartilage. Amer. J. Physiol. **166**, 328—330 (1951).
EINBINDER, J., and M. SCHUBERT: Separation of chondroitin sulfate from cartilage. J. biol. Chem. **185**, 725—730 (1950).
—, and U. SCHUBERT: Binding of mucopolysaccharides and dye by collagen. J. biol. Chem. **188**, 335—341 (1951).
EKHOLM, R.: Articular cartilage nutrition. How radioactive gold reaches the cartilage in rabbit knee joints. Acta anat. (Basel) **11**, Suppl., No 15 (1951).
— Nutrition of articular cartilage. A radioautographic study. Acta anat. (Basel) **24**, 329—338 (1955).
ENGEL, M. B., N. R. JOSEPH, D. M. LASKIN and H. R. CATCHPOLE: A theory of connective tissue behaviour: its implication in periodontal disease. Ann. N. Y. Acad. Sci. **85**, 399—420 (1960).
ENGEL, U., N. R. JOSEPH and H. R. CATCHPOLE: Homeostasis of connective tissues. I. Calcium-sodium equilibrium. Arch. Path. **58**, 26—29 (1954).
EVANS, G., and H. R. LISSNER: Biomechanical studies on the lumbar spine and pelvis. J. Bone Jt Surg. A **2**, 278—290 (1959).
FELL, H. B.: Chondrogenesis in cultures of endosteum. Proc. roy. Soc. B. **112**, 417—427 (1933).
— The histogenesis of cartilage and bone in the long bones of the embryonic fowl. J. Morph. **40**, 417—459 (1925).
—, and R. ROBISON: Glycogen in cartilage. Nature (Lond.) **131**, 62 (1933).
FESSLER, J. H., A. G. OGSTON and J. E. STANIER: Some properties of human and other synovial fluids. Biochem. J. **58**, 656—660 (1954).
FILOGAMO, G.: Contributo alla conoscenza della minuta struttura dell'osso. Osservazioni sulla zona d'attaco di tendini allo scheletro. Rend. ist. lombardo Sc. e Pt I, **78**, 425—448 (1945).
FÖLDES, I., I. ZS. NAGY, K. BENKÖ, G. LEVAI u. P. ARY-BALOGH: Elektronenmikroskopische Untersuchungen am postembryonalen Epiphysenknorpel der Albinoratte. Acta morph. Acad. Sci. hung. **13**, 283—299 (1963).
FOLLIS jr., R. H., and M. BERTHRONG: Histochemical studies on cartilage and bone. The normal pattern. Bull. Johns Hopk. Hosp. **85**, 281—297 (1949).
—, and A. J. TONSIMIS: Experimental lathyrism in the rat; nature of the defect in epiphysial cartilage. Proc. Soc. exp. Biol. (N. Y.) **98**, 843—848 (1958).
FRENCH, J. E., and E. P. BENDITT: The histochemistry of connective tissue: II. The effect of proteins on the selective staining of mucopolysaccharides by basic dyes. J. Histochem. Cytochem. **1**, 321—325 (1953).
FULLMER, H. M.: The histochemistry of the connective tissues. Int. Rev. Connect. Tissue Res. **3**, 1—76 (1965).

Fullmer, H. M., and R. D. Lillie: The staining of collagen with elastic tissue stains. J. Histochem. Cytochem. 5, 11—14 (1957).
— — The oxytalan fiber: a previously undescribed connective tissue fiber. J. Histochem. Cytochem. 6, 425—430 (1958).
Gardner, E.: Physiology of movable joints. Physiol. Rev. 30, 127—176 (1950).
— Osteogenesis in the human embryo and fetus. In: Bourne, The biochemistry and physiology of bone, p. 359—397. New York: Academic Press 1956.
—, and D. J. Gray: Prenatal development of the human hip joint. Amer. J. Anat. 87, 163—211 (1950).
— — Prenatal development of the human shoulder and acromioclavicular joints. Amer. J. Anat. 92, 219—276 (1953).
Gebhardt, W.: Diskussion zum Vortrag Schaffer: Trajektorielle Strukturen im Knorpel, S. 162—168. Verh. Anat. Ges. 25. Verslg Leipzig. Anat. Anz. 38 Erg.-H., 169—172 (1911).
Gegenbaur, C.: Über die Bildung des Knochengewebes. I. Jena. Z. Med. Naturw. 1, 343—369 (1864).
Gendre, H.: Le glycogène dans les cartilages en voie d'ossification. Bull. Histol. Techn. micr. 15, 165—178 (1938).
Gerber, B. R., E. C. Franklin, and M. Schubert: Ultracentrifugal fractionation of bovine nasal chondromucoprotein. J. biol. Chem. 235, 2870—2875 (1960).
Gersh, I.: Ground substance and the plasticity of connective tissues. Harvey Lect. 45, 211—241 (1949—1950).
—, and H. R. Catchpole: The organization of ground substance and basement membrane and its significance in tissue injury, disease and growth. Amer. J. Anat. 85, 457—521 (1949).
— — The nature of ground substance of connective tissue. Perspect. Biol. Med. 3, 282—319 (1960).
Gibian, H.: Das Hyaluronsäure-Hyaluronidase-System. Ergebn. Enzymforsch. 13, 1—84 (1954).
— Mucopolysaccharide und Mucopolysaccharidasen. Einzeldarst. aus dem Ges. Gebiet der Biochemie, herausg. O. Hoffmann-Ostenhof, Bd. 3, S. 1—139. Wien 1959.
Gibson, W., and H. M. Fullmer: Demonstration of 5'-nucleotidase activity in decalcified bones and teeth. J. Histochem. Cytochem. 14, 934—935 (1967).
Gieseking, R.: Mesenchymale Gewebe und ihre Reaktionsformen im elektronenoptischen Bild. Veröff. Morphol. Path., H. 72. Stuttgart: Gustav Fischer 1966.
Glegg, R. E., and D. Eidinger: A method for fractionating the carbohydrate components of bone. Arch. Biochem. Biophys. 55, 19—24 (1955).
— — and C. P. Leblond: Presence of carbohydrates distinct from acid mucopolysaccharides in connective tissue. Science 120, 839—840 (1954).
Glimcher, M. J.: Specificity of the molecular structure of organic matrices in mineralization. Calcif. Biol. Syst. 421—487 (1960).
Glock, G. E.: Glycogen and calcification. J. Physiol. (Lond.) 98, 1—11 (1940).
Godard, H.: L'os de croissance épiphysaire et les mucopolysaccharides. Arch. Anat. micr. Morph. exp. 40, 223—245 (1951).
Godman, G. C., and N. Lane: On the site of sulfation in the chondrocyte. J. Cell Biol. 21, 353—366 (1964).
—, and K. R. Porter: Chondrogenesis, studies with the electron microscope. J. biophys. biochem. Cytol. 8, 719—760 (1960).
Goldman, S.: Cybernetic aspects of homeostasis. In: Mineral Metabolism, ed. by C. L. Comar and F. Bronner, p. 61—100. 1960.
Grant, J. K., F. Clark and J. K. Grant: The biochemistry of mucopolysaccharides of connective tissue. Biochem. Soc. Symp. Bd. 20, S. 1—124. Cambridge: University Press 1961.
Graumann, W.: Die histochemische Reaktion der Knorpelgrundsubstanz mit Perjodsäure und Bleitetraacetat. Mikroskopie 8, 218—225 (1953).
— Weitere Untersuchungen zur Spezifität der histochemischen Polysaccharid-Eisenreaktion. Acta histochem. (Jena) 6, 1—7 (1958).
Gray, D. J., and E. Gardner: Prenatal development of the human knee and superior tibiofibular joints. Amer. J. Anat. 86, 235—288 (1950).
— — Prenatal development of the human elbow joint. Amer. J. Anat. 88, 429—470 (1951).
— — and R. O'Rahilly: The prenatal development of the skeleton and joints of the human hand. Amer. J. Anat. 101, 169—224 (1957).
Greiling, H.: Bestimmungsmethoden von Mucopolysacchariden und Glycoproteiden. In: D-Glucose und verwandte Verbindungen in Medizin und Biologie (Hrsg. H. Bartelheimer, W. Heyde u. W. Thorn), S. 158—182. Stuttgart: Ferdinand Enke 1966.
Greulich, R. C.: Microradiographic studies of the organic matrices of dentine and enamel. J. dent. Res. 35, 963 (1956).
—, and C. P. Leblond: Radioautographic visualization of radiocarbon in the organs and tissues of newborn rats following administration of C^{14}-labelled bicarbonate. Anat. Rec. 115, 559—585 (1953).
Grobstein, C.: Differentiation of vertebrate cells. In: The cell, vol. I (ed. by J. Brachet and A. E. Mirsky), p. 437—496. New York and London: Academic Press 1959.
Gross, J.: Electron microscope studies of sodium hyaluronate. J. biol. Chem. 172, 511—51 (19448).
— The structure of elastic tissue as studied with the electron microscope. J. exp. Med. 89, 699—708 (1949).
— Aging changes in the collagenous connective tissue of rat skin. A study with the electron microscope. J. nat. Cancer Inst. 10, 1353 (1950).

GROSS, J. I., M. B. MATHEWS, and A. DORFMAN: Sodium chondroitin sulfate protein complexes of cartilage. II. Metabolism. J. biol. Chem. **235**, 2889—2892 (1960).

GROSSFELD, H., K. MEYER and G. GODMAN: Differentiation of fibroblasts in tissue culture as determined by mucopolysaccharide production. Proc. Soc. exp. Biol. (N. Y.) **88**, 31—35 (1955).

— — — et A. LINKER: Mucopolysaccharides in tissue culture. J. biophys. biochem. Cytol. **3**, 391—396 (1957).

GUSEK, W.: Submikroskopische Untersuchungen zur Feinstruktur aktiver Bindegewebszellen. Stuttgart: Fischer 1962.

GUTMAN, A. B.: Relation of phosphorylase and phosphatase to calcification in cartilage. Trans. Conf. Metab. Aspects Convalesc. 1946, 14. meet. p. 20—24.

—, and E. B. GUTMAN: A phosphorylase in calcifying cartilage. Proc. Soc. exp. Biol. (N.Y.) **48**, 687—691 (1941).

—, and T. F. YU: A concept of the role of enzymes in endochondral calcification. Trans. Conf. Metab. Interrelat. 1950, 2. meet., p. 167—190.

HAINES, R. W.: Cartilage canals. J. Anat. (Lond.) **68**, 45—64 (1933).

HALE, A. J.: The histochemistry of polysacharides. Int. Rev. of Cytology, ed. by G. H. BOURNE and J. F. DANIELLI, vol. VI, p. 194—263. New York: Academic Press 1957.

HALE, C. W.: Histochemical demonstration of acid polysaccharides in animal tissues. Nature (Lond.) **157**, 802 (1946).

HALL, D. A.: The reaction between elastase and elastic tissue. I. The substrate. Biochem. J. **59**, 459—465 (1955).

— Collagen and elastine: the effect of age on their relationship. J. Geront. **1**, 347—363 (1957).

— Connective tissue fibers. Rev. Cytol. **8**, 212—252 (1959).

— R. REED and R. E. TUNBRIDGE: Electron microscope studies of elastic tissue. Exp. Cell Res. **8**, 35—48 (1955).

HALL, D. H., C. F. LLOYD, E. HAPPY and W. HORTON: Mucopolysaccharides of human nuclei pulposi. Nature (Lond.) **179**, 1078—1079 (1957).

HAM, A.W.: Histology, 2nd Ed. Philadelphia: Lippincott 1953.

—, and W. R. HARRIS: Repair and transplantation of bone. The Biochemistry and Physiology of Bone, ed. by G. H. BOURNE, p. 475—505. New York: Academic Press 1956.

HAMERMAN, D., and M. BLUM: Histologic studies on human membrane. II. Localization of some oxidative enzymes in synovial membrane cells. Arthr. and Rheum. **2**, 553—558 (1959).

—, and J. RUSKIN: Histologic studies on human synovial membrane. I. Metachromatic staining and the effects of streptococcal hyaluronidase. Arthr. and Rheum. **2**, 546—552 (1959).

HAMERMAN, D., et M. SCHUBERT: A quantitative study of metachromasy in synovial fluid and mucin. J. gen. Physiol. **37**, 291—300 (1953).

HANSEN, F. C. C.: Über die Genese einiger Bindegewebsgrundsubstanzen. Anat. Anz. **16**, 417—438 (1899).

HANSEN, F. C. C.: Untersuchungen über die Gruppe der Bindesubstanzen. I. Der Hyalinknorpel. Anat. H. **23**, 535—820 (1905).

HANSON, F. B.: The history of the earliest stages in the human clavicle. Anat. Rec. **19**, 309—325 (1920).

HARMS, H.: Handbuch der Farbstoffe für die Mikroskopie. Kamp-Lintfort: Staufen-Verlag 1957.

HARRIS, H. A.: Glycogen in cartilage. Nature (Lond.) **130**, 996—997 (1932).

HELLER-STEINBERG, M.: Ground substance, bone salts, and cellular activity in bone formation and destruction. Amer. J. Anat. **89**, 347—379 (1951).

HESSER, C.: Beitrag zur Kenntnis der Gelenkentwicklung beim Menschen. Morph. Jb. **55**, 489—567 (1926).

HIDVÉGI, E.: On the finer structure and blood supply of the synovial membrane, with special regard to its physiological circulation. Acta morph. Acad. Sci. hung. **4**, 319—331 (1954).

HINTZSCHE, E.: Die Osteoblastenlehre und die neueren Anschauungen vom normalen Verknöcherungsvorgang. Ergebn. Anat. Entwickl.-Gesch. **27**, 413—463 (1927).

— Untersuchungen an Stützgeweben. I. Über die Bedeutung der Gefäßkanäle im Knorpel nach Befunden am distalen Ende des menschlichen Schenkelbeines. Z. mikr.-anat. Forsch. **12**, 61—126 (1928a).

— Untersuchungen an Stützgeweben. II. Über Knochenbildungsfaktoren, insbesondere über den Anteil der Blutgefäße an der Ossifikation. Z. mikr.-anat. Forsch. **14**, 373—440 (1928b).

—, and M. SCHMID: Untersuchungen an Stützgeweben. IV. Weitere Befunde über die Gefäßkanäle im Knorpel. Nach Untersuchungen am Armskelet menschlicher Embryonen. Z. mikr.-anat. Forsch. **32**, 1—41 (1933).

HIRSCH, C.: The reaction of intervertebral discs to compression forces. J. Bone Surg. A **37**, 1188—1196 (1955).

—, and A. NACHEMSON: New observations on the mechanical behaviour of lumbar discs. Acta orthop. scand. **23**, 254—283 (1954).

— S. PAULSON, B. SYLVÉN and O. SNELLMAN: Biophysical and physiological investigations on cartilage and other mesenchymal tissues. VI. Characteristics of human nuclei pulposi during aging. Acta orthop. scand. **22**, 175—183 (1953).

HIRSCHMAN, A., and D. D. DZIEWIATKOWSKI: Protein-polysaccharide loss during endochondral ossification: Immunochemical evidence. Science **154**, 393—395 (1966).

HOFFMAN, PH., A. LINKER, and K. MEYER: The acid mucopolysaccharides of connective tissue. III. The sulfate linkage. Biochem. biophys. Acta (Amst.) **30**, 184 (1958).

Holmdahl, D. E., and B. E. Ingelmark: Der Bau des Gelenkknorpels unter verschiedenen funktionellen Verhältnissen. Acta anat. (Basel) 6, 309—375 (1948).

— — Der Kontakt zwischen Gelenkknorpel und Knochenmarkhöhle. Acta Soc. Med. upsalien. 55, 147—171 (1950).

Holtrop, M. E.: The origin of bone cells in endochondral ossification. Calcified Tissues, 3rd Europ. Sympos. (ed. by H. Fleisch, H. J. J. Blackwood, and M. Owen), p. 32—35. Berlin-Heidelberg-New York: Springer 1966.

Horwitz, A. L., and A. Dorfman: Subcellular sites for synthesis of chondromucoprotein of cartilage. J. Cell Biol. 38, 358—368 (1968).

Hotchkiss, R. D.: A microchemical reaction resulting in the staining of polysaccharide structures in fixed tissue preparations. Arch. Biochem. 16, 131—141 (1948).

Huxley, J. S.: Early embryonic differentiation. Nature (Lond.) 113, 276—278 (1924).

Immers, J.: Chemical and histochemical demonstration of acid esters by acetic iron reagent. Exp. Cell Res. 6, 127—133 (1954).

Ingelmark, B. E., u. R. Ekholm: Über die Kompressibilität der Intervertebralscheiben. Acta Soc. Med. upsalien. 57, 3—4, 202—217 (1952).

Jackson, D. S.: Chondroitinsulfate as a factor in the stability of tendon. Nature and Structure of Collagen, ed. by T. J. Randall, S. F. Jackson, p. 177—180. London 1953.

— The nature of collagen-chondroitin sulphate linkages in tendon. Biochem. J. 56, 699—703 (1954).

Jackson, S. F.: The development of connective and skeletal tissue in the embryonic fowl. Proceedings of the 3. internat. conf. on electron microscopy, London 1954a, vol. 137, p. 585—587.

— The formation of connective and skeletal tissues. Proc. roy. Soc. B 142, 536—548 (1954b).

— Connective tissue cells. In: The cell (ed. by J. Brachet and A. E. Mirsky), vol. VI, p. 387—520. New York and London: Academic Press 1964.

Jacobs, S., and H. Muir: A heparan sulphate-peptide from human aorta. Biochem. J. 87, 38 p (1963).

Jeanloz, R. W.: The nomenclature of mucopolysaccharides. Arthr. and Rheum. 3, 233—237 (1960).

— Mucopolysaccharides (acidic glycosaminoglycans). Compr. Biochem. Physiol. 5, 262—296 (1963).

—, and E. A. Balazs: The amino sugars. New York and London: Academic Press, vol. II A (1965), vol. II B (1966).

— P. J. Stoffym and M. Frémège: Sulphated galactosamine — containing mucopolysaccharides. Ciba Foundation Symp. Chem. and Biol. mucopolysaccharides. London 1956.

Jipp, P.: Die Sehnenstruktur an punktförmigen Muskelansätzen. Morph. Jb. 101, 236—262 (1960).

Joel, W., Y. F. Masters and M. R. Shetlar: Comparison of histochemical and biochemical methods for the polysaccharides of cartilage. J. Histochem. Cytochem. 4, 476—478 (1956).

Johnston, P. M., and C. L. Comar: Autoradiographic studies of the utilization of S^{35} sulfate by the chick embryo. J. Biophys. Biochem. 3, 231—238 (1957).

Jorpes, E., u. I. Yamashina: Die Mucopolysaccharide und Glykoproteide des Bindegewebes, S. 25—42. 7. Coll. der Ges. für physiol. Chemie. Berlin-Göttingen-Heidelberg: Springer 1956.

Joseph, N. R., H. R. Catchpole, D. M. Laskin and M. B. Engel: Titration curves of coloidal surfaces. II. Connective tissues. Arch. Biochem. Biophys. 84, 224—242 (1959).

— M. B. Engel and H. R. Catchpole: Interaction of ions and connective tissue. Biochim. biophys. Act. (Amst.) 8, 575—587 (1952).

— — — Homeostasis of connective tissues. Arch. Path. 58, 40—58 (1959).

Kapsammer, G.: Die periostale Ossifikation. Arch. mikr. Anat. 50, 315—350 (1897).

Kassowitz, M.: Die normale Ossifikation und die Erkrankung des Knochensystems bei Rachitis und hereditärer Syphilis. Med. Jb. I. Teil, 145—223, 293—457 (1879); II. Teil, Rachitis 315—466 (1881).

Keibel, F., u. C. Elze: Normentafeln zur Entwicklungsgeschichte der Wirbeltiere. Jena: Gustav Fischer 1908.

Kelly, J. W.: The use of metachromasy in histology, cytology and histochemistry. Acta histochem. (Jena) 1, 85—102 (1958).

Kember, N. F.: Cell division in endochondral ossification. A study of cell proliferation in rat bones by the method of tritiated thymidine autoradiography. J. Bone Jt Surg. B 42, 824—839 (1960).

Kent, P. W.: Some biochemical aspects of sulphates mucosubstances. In: The biochemistry of mucopolysaccharides of connective tissue (ed. by F. Clark and J. K. Grant), p. 90—108. Cambridge: University Press 1961.

Klenk, E.: Neuraminsäure, das Spaltprodukt eines neuen Gehirnlipoids. Hoppe-Seylers Z. physiol. Chem. 268, 50 (1941).

Kling, D. H., and G. Cameron: Morphological and physiological study of tissue cultures of human and mammalian synovial membranes. Anat. Rec. 121, 472 (1955).

Knese, K.-H.: Knochenbildung und Knochenaufbau unter Berücksichtigung der Histopathologie. Regensburg. Jb. ärztl. Fortbild. 5, 177—189 (1956a).

— Die periostale Osteogenese und Bildung der Knochenstruktur bis zum Säuglingsalter. Z. Zellforsch. 44, 585—643 (1956b).

— Die diaphysäre chondrale Osteogenese bis zur Geburt. Z. Zellforsch. 47, 80—113 (1957).

— Knochenstruktur als Verbundbau, Versuch einer technischen Deutung der Materialstruktur des Knochens. Zwanglose Abhandlungen auf dem Gebiet der normalen und pathologischen Anatomie von W. BARGMANN u. W. DOERR, H. 4. Stuttgart: Georg Thieme 1958.

KNESE, K.-H.: Neuere Untersuchungen über die Knochenbildung und ihre Beeinflussungsmöglichkeiten. Dtsch. zahnärztl. Z. 14, 925—932, 990—1000 (1959a).

— Die Ultrastruktur des Knochengewebes. Dtsch. med. Wschr. 84, 1640—1644, 1649—1650 (1959b).

— The ultra-structure of bone. Germ. med. Mth. 4, 411—412, 427—431 (1959c).

— Untersuchungen über die Reaktion der Gewebe von Säugetierfeten (Mesocricetus aureatus) auf intrauterine operative Eingriffe. Wilhelm Roux' Arch. Entwickl.-Mech. Org. 152, 455—490 (1960).

— Über die Mineralablagerungen in Knorpel- und Knochengewebe unter Berücksichtigung elektronenmikroskopischer Befunde. Acta histochem. (Jena), Suppl. III, 31—56 (1963a).

— Knochenbildung und Entwicklung der Knochenstruktur. Verh. dtsch. Ges. Path. 47, 35—54 (1963b).

— Zur Topochemie des Ektomesenchyms. Anat. Anz. 115, 123—127 (1964a).

— The early development of the skeletal blastema. Calcified tissues, ed. L. J. RICHELLE and M. J. DALLEMAGNE, p. 285—290. Liège 1964b.

— A histochemical study of the polysaccharides in osteogenic areas in bone and tooth, ed. by H. J. J. BLACKWOOD, p. 283—287. Oxford: Pergamon Press 1964c.

— Zur Topochemie der Ursegmente. Verh. Anat. Ges. 60, Vers. 1964. Anat. Anz. 115, Erg.-H., 205—210 (1965a).

— Zytogenese und topochemische Reaktion der frühen und späten epitheloiden Osteoblasten. Z. Zellforsch. 69, 93—128 (1966a).

— Feinbau und Belastungsmöglichkeiten des Knorpels. Sportarzt u. Sportmed. 17, 444—458 (1966b).

— Cytogenesis of osteoblasts. In: L'Ostéomalacie (ed. by D. J. HIOCO). Paris: Masson & Cie. 1967a.

— Topographic and temporal correlation of processes of osteogenesis discussed according to electronmicroscopic findings. In: Callus formation symposium the biology of fracture healing (ed. by ST. KROMPECHER and E. KERNER), p. 165—177. Budapest: Akadémiai kiadó 1967b.

— The ultrastructure of the hypertrophic cartilage cells. Calcified Tissues, 5th Europ. Sympos. (ed. by G. MILHAUD), p. 409—415. Paris: Société d'édition d'enseignement supérieur 1968.

— Zur Ultrastruktur der Skeletzellen. Hippokrates (Stuttg.) 7, 241—247 (1969).

— Cytologische Beobachtungen an Skeletzellen über die Bildung der Kohlenhydrat-Protein-Komplexe. Z. mikr.-anat. Forsch. (im Druck).

—, u. H. BIERMANN: Die Knochenbildung an Sehnen- und Bandansätzen im Bereich ursprünglich chondraler Apophysen. Z. Zellforsch. 49, 142—187 (1958).

KNESE, K.-H., u. A. M. KNOOP: Elektronenoptische Untersuchungen über die periostale Osteogenese. Z. Zellforsch. 48, 455—478 (1958).

— — Elektronenmikroskopische Befunde über die Mucopolysaccharidbildung. Dtsch. Ges. für Elektronenmikr. Freiburg i. Br. 9. Tagg 18. bis 21. Oktober. Programm und Autorenreferat 1959.

— — Elektronenmikroskopische und histochemische Untersuchungen am Knorpelgewebe über den Ort der Bildung des Mucopolysaccharid-Protein-Komplexes. Z. Zellforsch. 53, 201—258 (1961a).

— — Elektronenmikroskopische Beobachtungen über die Zellen in der Eröffnungszone des Epiphysenknorpels. Z. Zellforsch. 54, 1—38 (1961b).

— — Chondrogenese und Osteogenese, elektronen- und lichtmikroskopische Untersuchungen. Z. Zellforsch. 55, 413—468 (1961c).

—, u. S. TITSCHAK: Untersuchungen mit Hilfe des Lochkartenverfahrens über die Osteonstruktur von Haus- und Wildschweinknochen sowie Bemerkungen zur Baugeschichte des Knochens. Morph. Jb. 102, 337—458 (1962).

KOBURG, E.: Autoradiographische Untersuchungen zum Eiweißstoffwechsel der Zellen des Knorpels und Knochens. Beitr. path. Anat. 124, 108—135 (1961).

KOCH, A R.: Die Frühentwicklung der Clavicula beim Menschen. Acta anat. (Basel) 42, 177—212 (1960).

KÖLLIKER, H.: Die normale Resorption des Knochengewebes und ihre Bedeutung für die Entstehung der typischen Knochenformen. Leipzig 1873.

— Handbuch der Gewebelehre des Menschen, 6. Aufl. Leipzig: W. Engelmann 1889.

KORFF, K. v.: Über den Geweihwechsel der Hirsche, besonders über den Knorpel- und Knochenbildungsprozeß der Substantia spongiosa der Baststangen. Anat. H. 51, 691—731 (1914).

KOSSA, J. v.: Über die im Organismus künstlich erzeugbaren Verkalkungen. Beitr. path. Anat. 29, 163—202 (1901).

KROMPECHER, S.: Die Entstehungsbedingungen des Faserknorpels. Anat. Anz. 85, 229—236 (1938).

KROON, D. B.: Phosphatase and the formation of protein-carbohydrate complexes. Acta anat. (Basel) 15, 317—328 (1952).

KÜHN, K., U. HOFFMANN u. W. GRASSMANN: Veränderung der Intensität der Querstreifen des Kollagens durch Einlagerung von Phosphorwolframsäure. Naturwissenschaften 21, 521 (1958).

— — — Über die Verteilung der basophilen Aminosäuren in der Tropokollagenmolekel. Naturwissenschaften 46, 512 (1959).

KÜNZEL, E.: Ein Beitrag zur Frage der Halbgelenke. Verh. Anat. Ges. 53. Vers. Anat. Anz. 103, Erg.-H., 207—218 (1956).

KUHN, R., u. H. J. LEPPELMANN: Galaktosamin und Glucosamin im Knorpel in Abhängigkeit vom Lebensalter. Justus Liebigs Ann. Chem. 611, 254 (1958).

LACROIX, P.: The organisation of bone. Translated from the amended French edition by STEWART GILDER. London: Churchill 1951a.
— L'os et les mécanismes de sa formation. Étude morphologique. J. Physiol. (Paris) **43**, 385—424 (1951b).
LANG, F. J.: Arthritis deformans und Spondylitis deformans. In: Handbuch der speziellen pathologischen Anatomie und Histologie, Bd. IX/2, S. 252—376. 1934.
LANG, J.: Bau und Funktion der Gefäße des Stratum synoviale. Anat. Anz. **103**, 13—19 (1956).
— Die Gelenkinnenhaut, ihre Aufbau- und Abbauvorgänge. Morph. Jb. **98**, 387—482 (1957).
LANGE, K. H.: Rippen und Brustbein in ihren funktionellen Verknüpfungen. Morph. Jb. **73**, 355—384 (1934).
LANGER, M.: Über die Entwicklung des Kniegelenkes. Z. Anat. Entwickl.-Gesch. **89**, 83—101 (1929).
LANGMAACK, B.: Druck und Schlag an Leichenlendenwirbelsäulen. Z. Anat. **118**, 20—27 (1954).
LANSING, A. I.: Chemical morphology of elastic fibers. Connective Tissues, 2. Conf. 1951, ed. by CH. RAGAN, p. 45—84. New York: Josiah Macy Jr. Found. 1952.
LANSING, A. I., T. B. ROSENTHAL, M. ALEX and E. W. DEMPSEY: The structure and chemical characterizing of elastic fibers as revealed by elastase and by electron microscopy. Anat. Rec. **114**, 555—576 (1952).
LASH, J. W., and M. W. WHITEHOUSE: An unusual polysaccharide in the chondroid tissue of the snail Busycon: polyglucose sulfate. Biochem. J. **74**, 351—355 (1960).
LAWFORD, G. R., and H. SCHACHTER: Biosynthesis of glycoprotein by liver. J. biol. Chem. **241**, 5408—5418 (1966).
LEBLOND, C. P.: Distribution of periodic acid-reactive carbohydrates in the adult rat. Amer. J. Anat. **86**, 1—49 (1950).
— L. F. BÉLANGER and R. C. GREULICH: Formation of bones and teeth as visualized by radioautography. Ann. N. Y. Acad. Sci. **60**, 629—659 (1955).
—, and R. C. GREULICH: Autoradiographic studies of bone formation and growth. The biochemistry and physiology of bone, ed. by G. H. Bourne, p. 325—342. 1956.
— G. W. WILKINSON, L. F. BÉLANGER and J. ROBICHON: Radio-autographic visualization of bone formation in the rat. Amer. J. Anat. **86**, 289—341 (1950).
LEHMANN, F. E. und V. MANCUSO: Der fibrilläre Feinbau des Mitoseapparates von Tubifex nach Behandlung mit verschiedenen Fixiermitteln. Rev. suisse Zool., 360—371 (1958).
LELKES, G.: Experiments in vitro on role of movement in the development of joints. J. Embryol. exp. Morph. **6**, 183—186 (1958).
LEPPERT, F.: Untersuchungen über die funktionelle Struktur des Schulterblattknorpels des Pferdes. Morph. Jb. **72**, 309—340 (1933).
LEPPERT, F.: Beitrag zur funktionellen Struktur der Trachea und des Kehlkopfes des Pferdes. Morph. Jb. **74**, 581—624 (1934).
LEUTERT, G.: Über den Bau der Sehne des Musculus fibularis longus im Bereich des äußeren Fußrandes. Z. mikr.-anat. Forsch. **61**, 512—532 (1955).
— Über den histologischen Aufbau des Os peronaeum. Z. mikr.-anat. Forsch. **64**, 639—651 (1958).
— Über den Bau der Sehne des Musculus tibialis posterior im Bereich des Malleolus medialis und des Caput tali. Anat. Anz. **106**, 50—61 (1959).
— Über den Bau der Sehne des Caput longum musculi bicipitis brachii beim Menschen, Hund und Rind. Z. mikr.-anat. Forsch. **66**, 4, 445—455 (1960a).
— Über die Entwicklung der Struktur der Sehne des Musculus peronaeus longus. Anat. Anz. **106**, 90—95 (1960b).
— Die Biomorphose der Gewebe aus der Sicht der normalen Anatomie. Z. Alternsforsch. **14**, 1—17 (1960c).
LEVENE, P. A.: On chondrosin. J. biol. Chem. **140**, 267—277 (1941).
LEVER, J. D., and E. H. R. FORD: Histological, histochemical and electron microscopic observations on synovial membrane. Anat. Rec. **132**, 525—539 (1958).
LIEBERKÜHN, N.: Weitere Beiträge zur Lehre von der Ossifikation. Arch. Anat. 614—634 (1863).
LILLIE, R. D.: Reticulum staining with Schiff reagent after oxidation by acidified sodium periodate. J. Lab. clin. Med. **32**, 910—912 (1947).
— Further exploration of the HIO-Schiff reaction with remarks on its significance. Anat. Rec. **108**, 239—253 (1950).
— Connective tissue staining. Trans. 3rd. Conf. Connective Tissues, p. 11—35. New York (N. Y.): Josiah Macy Jr. Found. 1952.
— Histopathologic technic and practical histochemistry, 3rd ed. New York-Toronto-Sydney-London: McGraw-Hill Book Co. 1965.
LINBERG, B. E.: Zur Pathologie der posttyphösen Rippenchondritis. Virchows Arch. path. Anat. **258**, 367—404 (1925).
LINDAHL, U., and L. RODÉN: The chondroitin-4-sulfate-protein linkage. J. biol. Chem. **241**, 2113—2119 (1966).
LINDENBAUM, A., and K. E. KUETTNER: Mucopolysaccharides and mucoproteins of calf scapula. Calc. Tiss. Res. **1**, 153—165 (1967).
LIPP, W.: Neuuntersuchungen des Knochengewebes. Morphologie, Histochemie und Beeinflussung durch das periphere, vegetative Nervensystem, durch Fermente und Hormone. Acta. anat. (Basel) **20**, 162—200 (1954).
LISON, L.: Études sur la métacromasie; colorants métacromatique et substances chromotropes. Arch. Biol. (Liège) **46**, 599—668 (1935).
— Alcian blue 8 G with chlorantine fast red 5 B. Stain Technol. **29**, 131—138 (1954).

LITTLE, K., and L. H. PIMM: Osteoarthritis of the hip joint. Electron Microscopy. Proc. of the Stockholm Conf. (F. S. Sjöstrand and I. Rhodin), p. 233—234. 1956.
LOEVEN, W. A.: The binding collagen — mucopolysaccharide in connective tissue. Acta anat. (Basel) **24**, 217—244 (1955).
LOEWI, G.: Changes in the ground substance of aging cartilage. J. Path. Bact. **65**, 381—388 (1953).
LUBOSCH, W.: Das perennierende Kalkskelet der Wirbeltiere und der fibrilläre Bau der knorpeligen Skeletteile. Z. mikr.-anat. Forsch. **11**, 67—171 (1927).
— Die permanenten knorpeligen Skeletteile. In: Handbuch der vergleichenden Anatomie der Wirbeltiere (BOLK, G PPERT, KALLIUS-LUBOSCH), Bd. 5, S. 249—274. 1938.
LUSCHKA, H.: Die Halbgelenke des menschlichen Körpers. Berlin 1858.
MAJNO, G., and C. ROUILLER: Die alkalische Phosphatase in der Biologie des Knochengewebes. Histochemische Untersuchungen. Virchows Arch. path. Anat. **321**, 1—16 (1951).
MAKOWSKY, L.: Experimentelle Studien zur Pathogenese der degenerativen Gelenkknorpelveränderungen. Langenbecks Arch. klin. Chir. **263**, 118—163 (1949).
MALMGREN, H., and B. SYLVÉN: Biophysical and physiological investigations on cartilage and other mesenchymal tissues. V. Identification of the polysaccharide of bovine nuclei pulposi. Biochim. biophys. Acta (Amst.) **9**, 706—707 (1952).
MANCINI, R. E., E. S. LUSTIG and C. NUNEZ: Radiosulfur intake by mucopolysaccharides of embryonic and cultured connective tissues. Anat. Rec. **124**, 493—494 (1956).
—, and E. SACERDOTE DE LUSTIG: Accion de la desoxicorticosterona y cortisona sobre las mucoproteinas de los fibroblastos in vitro. Rev. Soc. argent. Biol. **27**, 86—94 (1951).
MARKOVITZ, A., J. A. CIFONELLI and A. DORFMAN: Biosynthesis of hyaluronic acid by group A streptococcus. VI. Biosynthesis from uridine nucleotides in cell-free extracts. J. biol. Chem. **234**, 2343—2350 (1959).
MARSHALL, J. H.: Microscopic metabolism of calcium in bone. Bone as a Tissue, ed. by K. Rodahl, p. 144—162. New York-Toronto-London: McGraw-Hill Book Comp. Inc. 1960.
MARTIN, A. V. W.: Fine structure of cartilage matrix. Nature and Structure of Collagen, ed. J. T. Randall, S. 129—139. London: Butterworth & Co. 1953.
— An electron microscope study of the cartilaginous matrix in the developing tibia of the fowl. J. Embryol. exp. Morph. **2**, 38—48 (1954).
MATHEWS, M. B.: Chondroitinsulfuric Acid. — A linear polyelectrolyte. Arch. Biochem. **43**, 181—193 (1953).
— Interactions of mucopolysaccharides and some protein components of connective tissue. Circulation **14**, 972—973 (1956).
MATHEWS, M. B., and A. DORFMAN: The molecular weight and viscosimetry of chondroitin-sulfuric acid. Arch. Biochem. **42**, 41—53 (1953).
—, and J. LOZAITYTE: Sodium chondroitin sulfateprotein complexes of cartilage. I. Molecular weight and shape. Arch. Biochem. **74**, 158—174 (1958).
MATSCHINSKY, N.: Über das normale Wachstum der Röhrenknochen des Menschen. Arch. mikr. Anat. **39**, 151—215 (1892).
MATUKAS, V. J., J. B. PANNER, and J. L. ORBISON: Studies on ultrastructural identification and distribution of proteinpolysaccharide in cartilage matrix. J. Cell Biol. **32**, 365—377 (1967).
MAURER, P. H., and S. S. HUDACK: The isolation of hyaluronic acid from callus tissue of early healing. Arch. Biochem. **38**, 49—53 (1952).
MCDERMOTT, L. J.: Development of the human knee joint. Arch. Surg. **46**, 705—719 (1943).
MCKAY, D., E. C. ADAMS, A. T. HERTIG and S. DANZINGER: Histochemical horizons in human embryos. II. 6 and 7 millimeter embryos Streeter horizon XIV. Anat. Rec. **126**, 433—463 (1956).
MCLEAN, F. C., and W. BLOOM: Calcification and ossification. Calcification in normal growing bone. Anat. Rec. **78**, 333—359 (1940).
— Introduction: Homeostasis in mineral metabolism. In: Mineral metabolism (ed. by C. L. COMAR and F. BRONNER, vol. IA, p. 1—10. New York and London: Academic Press 1960.
—, and A. M. BUDY: Connective and supporting tissues: bone. Ann. Rev. Physiol. **21**, 69—90 (1959).
—, and M. R. URIST: Bone; an introduction to the physiology of skeletal tissue, 182 p. Chicago: University of Chicago Press 1955. 2. Ed. 1961.
MCMANUS, J. F. A.: Histological demonstration of mucin after periodic acid. Nature (Lond.) **158**, 202 (1946).
— Histochemistry of connective tissue. In: Asboe-Hansen, Connective Tissue in Health and Disease, p. 31—53. 1954.
—, and R. W. MOWRY: Staining methods. Histologic and histochemical. New York-Evanston-London: Harper & Row; Tokyo: J. Weatherhill 1964.
MCMASTER, PH. D., and R. J. PARSONS: The movement of substances and the state of the fluid in the intradermal tissue. Ann. N. Y. Acad. Sci. **52**, 992—1003 (1950).
MERKER, J. H.: Elektronenmikroskopische Untersuchungen über die Fibrillogenese in der Haut menschlicher Embryonen. Z. Zellforsch. **53**, 411—430 (1961).
MEYER, K.: The chemistry and biology of mucopolysaccharides and glycoproteins. Symp. Quant. Biol. **6**, 91—102 (1938).
— Mucoids and glycoproteins. Advanc. Protein Chem. **2**, 249—273 (1945).
— The biological significance of hyaluronic acid and hyaluronidase. Physiol. Rev. **27**, 335—359 (1947).

Meyer, K.: Chemistry of connective tissue, polysaccharides. Trans. Conf. Connective Tissues 1, 88—100 (1951).
— The mucopolysaccharides of mesodermal tissues. Trans. Conf. Metab. Interrelations 4, 63—73 (1952).
— Hyaluronic acid, chondroitin sulphates and their protein complexes. Discuss. Faraday Soc. No 13, 271—275 (1953).
— The chemistry of the ground substance of connective tissue. In: Asboe-Hansen, Connective Tissue in Health and Disease, p. 54—69. 1954.
— The mucopolysaccharides of bone. Bone structure and metabolism (Ciba Foundation). London: J. A. Churchill, Wolstenholme and O'Connor 1956.
— Chondroitin sulfates. In: Polysaccharides in biology (ed. by G. F. Springer), 4. Conf., p. 9—56. New York: Josiah Macy, jr. Foundation 1959.
— Problems of histochemical identification of carbohydrate rich tissue components. J. Histochem. Cytochem. 14, 605—606 (1966).
—, and E. Chaffee: Hyaluronic acid in pleure fluid associated with malignant tumor involving pleure and peritoneum. J. biol. Chem. 133, 83—91 (1939).
— E. Davidson, K. A. Linker and Ph. Hoffmann: The acid mucopolysaccharides of connective tissue. Biochim. biophys. Acta (Amst.) 21, 506—518 (1956).
— R. Dubos and E. M. Smyth: Hydrolysis of polysaccharide acids of vitreous humor, of umbilical cord, and of streptococcus by autolytic enzyme of pneumococcus. J. biol. Chem. 118, 71—78 (1937).
— Ph. Hoffmann and A. Linker: Mucopolysaccharides of costal cartilage. Science 128, No 3329, 896 (1958).
— A. Linker, E. A. Davison and B. S. Weissmann: The mucopolysaccharides of bovine cornea. J. biol. Chem. 205, 611—616 (1953).
—, and M. M. Rapport: The mucopolysaccharides of the ground substance of connective tissue. Science 113, 596—599 (1951).
—, and E. M. Smyth: On glycoproteins. VI. The preparation of chondroitinsulfuric acid. J. biol. Chem. 119, 507—510 (1937).
Meyer, K. H., M. E. Odier and A. E. Siegrist: Constitution de l'acide chondroitine sulfurique. Helv. chim. Acta 31, 1400—1419 (1948).
Michaelis, J.: The nature of the interaction of nucleic acids and nuclei with basis dyestuffs. Cold Spr. Harb. Symp. quant. Biol. 12, 131—142 (1947).
Milaire, J.: Détection histochemique de modifications des ebauches dans les membres en formation chez la souris oligosyndactyle. Bull. Cl. Sci. 48, 505—528 (1962).
— Étude morphologique et cytochimique du développement des membres chez la souris et chez la taupe. Arch. Biol. (Liège) 74, 131—317 (1963).
Mollier, S.: Über Knochenentwicklung. S.-B. Ges. Morph. u. Physiol. Münch. 22, 1—18 (1910a).
— Referat über Romeis. S.-B. Ges. Morph. u. Physiol. München 22, 12—18 (1910b).
Monesi, B., e G. Bettini: L'indagine istochimica applicata alla fisiopatologia del tessuto osseo. Parte prima ossificazione normale. Arch. Putti Chir. Organi Mov. 10, 326—372 (1958).
Montreuil, J.: Glycoprotéides. Chimie et Biochimie. Bull. Soc. Chim. biol. (Paris) 3, 1—83 (1957).
Moog, F.: Localizations of alkaline and acid phosphatases in the early embryogenesis of the chick. Biol. Bull. 86, 51—80 (1944).
— The physiological significance of the phosphomonoesterases. Biol. Rev. 21, 41—59 (1946).
Moore, R. D., and M. D. Schoenberg: Studies on connective tissue. I. The polysaccharides of umbilical cord. Arch. Path. 64, 39—45 (1957).
Müller, G.: Über die Vereinfachung der Reaktion nach Hale (1946). Acta histochem. (Jana) 2, 68—70 (1955/56).
Müller, H.: Über die Entwicklung der Knochensubstanz nebst Bemerkungen über den Bau rachitischer Knochen. Z. Zool. 9, 147—233 (1858).
Muir, H.: The nature of the link between protein and carbohydrate of a chondroitin sulphate complex from hyaline cartilage. Biochem. J. 69, 195—204 (1958).
— Chondroitin sulphates and sulphated polysaccharides of connective tissue. In: The biochemistry of mucopolysaccharides of connective tissue, ed. by F. Clark and J. K. Grant, p. 4—23. Cambridge: Univ. Press 1961.
— Chemistry and metabolism of connectiv tissue glycosaminoglycans (Mucopolysaccharides). Int. Rev. Connect. Tissue Res. 2, 101—154 (1964).
Munaron, G.: Rilievi istochimici es istofisici sul mesenchima intermedio delle articolazioni embrionali e sui suoi derivati. Atti Soc. ital. Anat., Suppl. zu Monit. zool. ital. 63, 347—349 (1954).
Needham, J.: Biochemistry and morphogenesis. Cambridge: Univ. Press 1950.
Nemetschek, Th.: Zur Morphologie von Kollagen: Querstruktur, Elementarfibrillen und Anordnung im Zellverband. Z. Naturforsch. 13b, 225—234 (1958).
Netter, H.: Theoretische Biochemie, S. 1—816. Berlin-Göttingen-Heidelberg: Springer 1959.
Neuman, W. F., and B. J. Mulryan: The surface chemistry of bone. VI. Recrystallization in vivo. J. biol. Chem. 195, 843—848 (1952).
Neutra, M., and C. P. Leblond: Synthesis of the carbohydrate of mucus in the Golgi complex as shown by electronmicroscope radioautography of goblet cells from rats injected with glucose-H^3. J. Cell Biol. 30, 119—136 (1966a).
— — Radioautographic comparison of the uptake of galactose-H^3 and glucose-H^3 in the

Golgi region of various cells secreting glycoproteins or mucopolysaccharides. J. Cell Biol. **30**, 137—150 (1966b).

Niklas, A. W., Oehlert u. R. Roesch: Autoradiographische Untersuchung der Größe des Eiweißstoffwechsels verschiedener Organe, Gewebe und Zellarten. Beitr. path. Anat. **116**, 92—123 (1956).

Oberholzer, R. J. H.: Beitrag zur Kenntnis der fibrillären Struktur des Hyalinknorpels, gewonnen am Bronchialknorpel des Kaninchens. Z. Zellforsch. **32**, 517—534 (1943).

Ogston, A. G., and J. E. Stanier: Further observations on the preparation and composition of the hyaluronic acid complex of synovial fluid. Biochem. J. **52**, 149—156 (1952).

Okada, T. S.: Tracer study on the reconstitution of cartilage from dissociated cells. Exp. Cell Res. **16**, 437—440 (1959a).

— Regeneration of cartilaginous matrix from the dissociated chondrocytes in vitro. Experientia (Basel) **15**, 147—149 (1959b).

O'Rahilly, R., D. J. Gray, and E. Gardner: Chondrification in the hands and feet of staged human embryos. Contr. Embryol. **36**, 183—192 (1957).

Orr, S. F. D.: Infra-red spectroscopic studies of some polysaccharides. Biochem. biophys. Acta (Amst.) **14**, 173—181 (1954).

Partridge, S. M.: The chemistry of connective tissues. I. The state of combination of chondroitin sulphate in cartilage. Biochem. J. **43**, 387—397 (1948).

—, and H. F. Davis: The chemistry of connective tissues. IV. The presence of a non-collagenous protein in cartilage. Biochem. J. **68**, 298—305 (1958).

— — and G. S. Adair: The chemistry of connective tissues. II. Soluble proteins derived from partial hydrolysis of elastin. Biochem. J. **61**, 11—21 (1955).

— — — The composition of mammalian elastin. Connective Tissues, ed. by R. E. Tunbridge, p. 222—237. 1957.

Paulson, S., B. Sylvén, C. Hirsch and O. Snellman: Biophysical and physiological investigations on cartilage and other mesenchymal tissues. III. The diffusion rate of various substances in normal bovine nucleus pulposus. Biochim. biophys. Acta (Amst.) **7**, 207—213 (1951).

Pauwels, F.: Die Struktur der Tangentialfaserschicht des Gelenkknorpels der Schulterpfanne als Beispiel für ein verkörpertes Spannungsfeld. Z. Anat. Entwickl.-Gesch. **121**, 188—204 (1959).

— Eine neue Theorie über den Einfluß mechanischer Reize auf die Differenzierung der Stützgewebe. Z. Anat. Entwickl.-Gesch. **121**, 478—515 (1960).

Pearse, A. G. E.: Histochemistry; theoretical and applied, 2nd Ed., p. 1—998. London: J. & A. Churchill 1960.

Perey, O.: Fracture of the vertebral endplate in the lumbar spine. Acta orthop. scand., Suppl. 25 (1957).

Perlman, R. L., A. Telser, and A. Dorfman: The biosynthesis of chondroitin sulfate by a cell-free preparation. J. biol. Chem. **239**, 3623—3629 (1964).

Petersen, H.: Die Organe des Skeletsystems. In: Möllendorff, Handbuch der mikroskopischen Anatomie des Menschen, Bd. II/3, S. 521—678. 1930.

Petersen, Hans: Histologie und mikroskopische Anatomie. München: J. F. Bergmann 1935.

Peterson, R., and C. P. Leblond: Synthesis of complex carbohydrates in the Golgi region, as shown by radioautography after injection of labeled glucose. J. Cell Biol. **21**, 143—149 (1964a).

— — Uptake by the Golgi region of glucose labeled with tritium in the 1 or 6 position, as an indicator of synthesis of complex carbohydrates. Exp. Cell Res. **34**, 420—423 (1964b).

Plötz, E.: Präparate bei Bearbeitung der Frage nach der Umwandelbarkeit von „Gleitsehnen" in Zugsehnen. Verh. Anat. Ges. 45. Vers. Anat. Anz. **85**, Erg. H., 266—273 (1937/38).

Pommer, G.: Über die lakunäre Resorption in erkrankten Knochen. S.-B. Akad. Wiss. Wien, math.-nat. Kl. **83**, 17—140 (1881).

Ponlot, R.: Le radiocalcium dans l'étude des os. Ed. Arscia, S. A. Bruxelles. 1960.

Prader, A.: Die frühembryonale Entwicklung der menschlichen Zwischenwirbelscheibe. Acta anat. (Basel) **3**, 68—83 (1947a).

— Die Entwicklung der Zwischenwirbelscheibe beim menschlichen Keimling. Acta anat. (Basel) **3**, 115—152 (1947b).

Pritchard, J. J.: A cytological and histochemical study of bone and cartilage formation in the rat. J. Anat. (Lond.) **86**, 259—277 (1952).

— The osteoblast. The Biochemistry and Physiology of Bone, ed. by G. H. Bourne, p. 179—211. New York: Academic Press 1956.

— J. H. Scott and F. G. Girgis: The structure and development of cranial and facial sutures. J. Anat. (Lond.) **90**, 73—86 (1956).

Putschar, W.: Über Fett im Knorpel unter normalen und pathologischen Verhältnissen. Beitr. path. Anat. **87**, 526—539 (1931).

Quintarelli, G., and M. C. Dellovo: The chemical and histochemical properties of alcian blue. IV. Further studies on the methods for the identification of acid glycosaminoglycans. Histochemie **5**, 196—209 (1965).

— — Age changes in the localization and distribution of glycosaminoglycans in human hyaline cartilage. Histochemie **7**, 141—167 (1966).

— J. E. Scott, and M. C. Dellovo: The chemical and histochemical properties of alcian blue. II. Dye binding of tissue polyanions. Histochemie **4**, 86—98 (1964a).

— — — The chemical and histochemical properties of alcian blue. III. Chemical blocking and unblocking. Histochemie **4**, 99—112 (1964b).

Quintarelli, G., S. Sajdera, and D. Dziewiatkowski: Modifications of connective tissue matrices by an enzyme extracted from cartilage. Histochemie **15**, 1—20 (1968).

Ragan, Ch.: The physiology of the connective tissue (loose areolar). Ann. Rev. Physiol. **14**, 51—72 (1952).
— Connective tissues. Trans. 1—5 Conf. **1** (1951); **2** (1952); **3** (1952); **4** (1953); **5** (1954).
Reinbach, W.: Die kollagenen Fibrillen in den Kniegelenkmeniscen; die Ursachen ihrer Entstehung und Anordnung. Arch. orthop. Unfall-Chir. **46**, 485—498 (1954).
Revel, J. P., and E. D. Hay: An autoradiographic and electronmicroscopic study of collagen synthesis in differentiating cartilage. Z. Zellforsch. **61**, 110—144 (1963).
Rinonapoli, E., e C. Sanguinetti: Contributo istochimico allo studio della sinoviale normale e patologica. Arch. Putti Chir. Organi Mov. **10**, 118—132 (1958).
Robbins, P. W., and F. Lipmann: Identification of enzymatically active sulfate as adenosine-3′-phosphate-S′-phosphosulfate. J. Amer. chem. Soc. **78**, 2652—2653 (1956).
Robinson, R. A., and D. A. Cameron: Electron microscopy of cartilage and bone matrix at the distal epiphyseal line of the femur in the newborn infant. J. biophys. biochem. Cytol. **2**, Suppl., 253—260 (1956).
Robison, R.: The significance of phosphoric esters in metabolism. New York: New York University Press 1932.
—, and A. H. Rosenheim: Calcification of hypertrophic cartilage in vitro. Biochem. J. **28**, 684—698 (1934).
Rodén, L.: Effect of glutamine on the synthesis of chondroitin sulphuric acid in vitro. Ark. Kemi **10**, 333—344 (1956).
Romeis, B.: Die Architektur des Knorpels vor der Osteogenese und in der ersten Zeit derselben. Wilhelm Roux' Arch. Entwickl.-Mech. Org. **31**, 387—422 (1911).
— Histologische Technik. München: Leibniz 1948.
Ropes, M. W., and W. Bauer: Synovial fluid changes in joint disease. Commonwealth Fed. Cambridge (Mass.): Harvard University Press 1953.
—, W. Robertson, B. Rosmeisl, E. Peabody and W. Bauer: Synovial fluid mucin. Acta med. scand. **128**, Suppl. 196, 700—744 (1947).
Ross, R.: The connective tissue fiber forming cell. In: Treatise on collagen (ed. by G. N. Ramachandran), vol. A 2, p. 1—75. London and New York: Academic Press 1968.
Rouiller, C., L. Huber et E. Rutishauser: Les fibrilles de la substance fondamentale du cartilage hyalin. Étude au microscope électronique. (Note préliminaire.) Arch. ac. (Genève) **5**, 215—218 (1952).
Ruckes, J.: Experimentelle Untersuchungen über die Resorptionsfähigkeit des Stratum synoviale. Z. Zellforsch. **55**, 313—369 (1961).
Rutishauser, E., Ch. Rouiller et R. Veyrat: La vascularisation de l'os: État actuel de nos connaissances. Arch. Putti Chir. Organi Mov. **5**, 9—40 (1954).
Salpeter, M. M.: H^3-proline incorporation into cartilage: electron microscope autoradiographic observations. J. Morph. **124**, 387—422 (1968).
Salton, M. R. J.: Chemistry and function of amino sugars and derivatives. Ann. Rev. Biochem. **34**, 143—175 (1965).
Schaffer, J.: Trajektorielle Strukturen im Knorpel. Anat. Anz. **38**, Erg.-H., 162—168 (1911).
— Knorpelgewebe. In: Enzyklopädie mikroskopischer Technik v. R. Krause, 3. Aufl., Bd. 2, S. 1205. 1926.
— Die Stützgewebe. In: Handbuch der mikroskopischen Anatomie des Menschen, Bd. II/2, S. 1—390. Berlin: Springer 1930.
Schaper, A.: Beiträge zur Analyse des tierischen Wachstums. Eine kritische und experimentelle Studie. I. Quellen, Modus und Lokalisation des Wachstums. Arch. Entwickl.-Mech. Org. **14**, 307—400 (1902).
Schiedt, E.: Beitrag zur Ossifikation der Wirbelsäule. Langenbecks Arch. klin. Chir. **280**, 241—260 (1955).
Schiller, S., M. B. Mathews, J. A. Cifonelli and A. Dorfman: Metabolism of mucopolysaccharides in animals; further studies on skin utilizing C^{14}-glucose, C^{14}-acetate and S^{35}-sodium sulfate. J. biol. Chem. **218**, 139—145 (1956).
Schmidt, W. J.: Über die Verkalkung des Knorpelgewebes der Haie. Z. Zellforsch. **37**, 377—388 (1952a).
— Zur Polarisationsoptik des Knorpelgewebes. Z. Zellforsch. **37**, 534 (1952b).
— Polarisationsoptische Analyse tierischer Zellen und Gewebe. Naturwissenschaften **7**, 196—203 (1957).
Schneider, H.: Die Struktur der Sehnenansatzzone und Abnutzungserkrankungen in ihrem Bereich. Münch. med. Wschr. **97**, 1479—1480 (1955).
— Zur Struktur der Sehnenansatzzonen. Z. Anat. Entwickl.-Gesch. **119**, 431—456 (1956).
Schneider, M.: Homogenous epiphyseal-cartilage graft. An experimental study. J. Bone Jt. Surg. A **38**, 601—610 (1956).
Schoenberg, M. D., and R. D. Moore: Studies on connective tissue. II. Histochemical differences in the connective tissue polysaccharides of the mature and immature human umbilical cord. Arch. Path. **64**, 167—170 (1957).
— — Studies on connective tissue. III. Enzymatic studies on the formation and nature of the carbohydrate intermediate of the connective tissue polysaccharides in the human umbilical cord. Arch. Path. **65**, 115—124 (1958).
Schubert, M.: Intercellular macromolecules containing polysaccharides. Biophys. J. **4**, 119—138 (1964).
—, and D. Hamerman: Amino sugar containing compounds in cartilage, tendon, and intervertebral disc. In: The amino sugars, vol. IIA (ed. by R. W. Jeanloz and E. A. Balazs), p. 257—279. New York and London: Academic Press 1965.

SCOTT, B. L., and D. PEASE: Electron microscopy of the epiphyseal apparatus. Anat. Rec. **126**, 465—495 (1956).

SEELICH, F.: Zur Biochemie der Gewebsalterung. Wien. klin. Wschr. **64**, 593—595 (1952).

SENSENIG, E. C.: Note on the formation of cartilage. Anat. Rec. **100**, 615—620 (1948).

SHATTON, J., and M. SCHUBERT: Isolation of mucoprotein from cartilage. J. biol. Chem. **211**, 565—573 (1954).

SHELDON, H.: Observations on the production of matrix by bone and cartilage cells. Proc. Eur. Reg. Conf. on Electron Microsc. Delft **2**, 786—790 (1960).

—, and R. A. ROBINSON: Electron microscope studies of crystal-collagen relationships in bone. IV. The occurrence of crystals within collagen fibrils. J. biophys. biochem. Cytol. **3**, 1011—1015 (1957).

— — Studies on cartilage: Electron microscope observations on normal rabbit ear cartilage. J. biophys. biochem. Cytol. **4**, 401—406 (1958).

— — Studies on cartilage. II. Electron microscope observations on rabbit ear cartilage following the administration of papain. J. biophys. biochem. Cytol. 8, 151—163 (1960).

SHETLAR, M. R., and Y. F. MASTERS: Effect of age on polysaccharide composition of cartilage. Proc. Soc. exp. Biol. (N. Y.) **90**, 31—33 (1955).

SIEBERT, G., and R. M. S. SMELLIE: Enzymatic and metabolic studies on isolated nuclei. Int. Rev. of Cytology, ed. by G. H. BOURNE and J. F. DANIELLI, vol. IV, p. 383—424. New York: Academic Press 1957.

SIFFERT, R. S.: The role of alkaline phosphatase in osteogenesis. J. exp. Med. **93**, 415—426 (1951).

SILBERBERG, M., and R. SILBERBERG: Steroid hormones and bone. In: The biochemistry and physiology of bone, ed. by G. H. BOURNE, p. 622—668 (1956).

SILBERBERG, R., M. SILBERBERG, A. VOGEL, and W. WETTSTEIN: Ultrastructure of articular cartilage of mice of various ages. Amer. J. Anat. **109**, 251—275 (1961).

— — and D. FEIR: Life cycle of articular cartilage cells: An electron microscope study of the hip joint of the mouse. Amer. J. Anat. **114**, 17—47 (1964).

SISSONS, H. A.: Experimental study on the effect of local irradiation on bone growth. In: Progress in Radiobiology. Proc. of the fourth intern. conf. on radiobiology, ed. by J. S. MITCHELL, B. E. HOLMES and C. L. SMITH. Edinburg and London: Oliver & Boyd 1955.

SMITH, E. W., and W. B. ATKINSON: Simple procedure for identification and rapid counting of mast cells in tissue sections. Science **123**, 941—942 (1956).

SOBEL, A. E., and U. BURGER: Studies of chondroitin sulfate in relation to the mechanism of calcification. Fed. Proc. **13**, 300—301 (1954).

SOBEL, H., and A. MOSCANA: Cultivation of embryonic organ rudiments on a medium derived entirely from adult tissues. Experientia (Basel) **10**, 502—504 (1954).

SOKOLOFF, L.: Elasticity of articular cartilage: Effect of ions and viscous solutions. Science **141**, 1055—1057 (1963).

— Elasticity of aging cartilage. Fed. Proc. **25**, 1089—1095 (1966).

SOLOMON, A. K.: Compartmental methods of kinetic analysis. Mineral Metabolism, ed. by F. C. COMAR and F. BRONNER, vol. Ia, p. 119—168 (1960).

SONNENSCHEIN, A.: Biologie, Pathologie und Therapie der Gelenke, dargestellt am Kniegelenk. Die Entwicklung des Kniegelenkes beim Menschen. Basel: Benno Schwabe & Co. 1952.

SPICER, S. S., T. J. LEPPI, and P. J. STOWARD: Suggestions for a histochemical terminology of carbohydrate-rich tissue components. J. Histochem. Cytochem. **13**, 599—603 (1965).

SPULER, A.: Beitrag zur Histogenese des Mesenchyms. Verh. Anat. Ges. 13. Verslg. Anat. Anz. **16**, Erg.-H., 13—16 (1899).

STACEY, M.: The chemistry of mucopolysaccharides and mucoproteins. Advanc. Carbohyd. Chem. **2**, 161—201 (1946).

STARY, Z.: Mucosaccharides and glycoproteins, chemistry and physiopathology. Ergebn. Physiol. **50**, 174—408 (1959).

STAUB, W.: Über den funktionellen Bau des elastischen Knorpels. Acta anat. (Basel) **9**, 309—329 (1950).

STEEDMAN, H. F.: Alcian blue 8 GS: A new stain for mucin. Quart. J. micr. Sci. **91**, 477—479 (1950).

STEUDENER, F.: Beiträge zur Lehre von der Knochenentwicklung und dem Knochenwachstum. Abh. naturforsch. Ges. zu Halle **13**, 207—236 (1875).

STICH, H.: Bau und Funktion der Nukleolen. Experentia (Basel) **12**, 7—14 (1956).

STIDWORTHY, G., Y. MASTERS and M. SHETLAR: The effect of aging on mucopolysaccharide composition of human costocartilage as measured by hexosamine and uronic acid content. J. Geront. **13**, 10—13 (1958).

STILWELL, D. L., and D. J. GRAY: The microscopic structure of periosteum in areas of tendinous content. Anat. Rec. **120**, 663—677 (1954).

STREETER, G. L.: Developmental horizons in human embryos (Fourth Issue). A review of the histogenesis of cartilage and bone. Contr. Embryol. Carneg. Inst **33**, 149—168 (1949).

STRELZOFF, J.: Über die Histogenese der Knochen. Untersuchungen an dem Pathol. Institut Zürich, Herausg. EBERTH, S. 1—94, 1873.

— Über Knochenwachstum. Arch. mikr. Anat. **11**, 33—74 (1875).

STROMINGER, J. L.: Nucleotide intermediates in the biosynthesis of heteropolymeric polysaccharides. Biophys. J. **4**, 139—153 (1964).

SUNDBLAD, L.: Studies on hyaluronic acid in synovial fluids. Acta Soc. Med. upsalien. **58**, 113—238 (1953).

Sylvén, B.: Cartilage and Chondroitin sulphate. I. The physiological role of chondroitin sulphate in cartilage. J. Bone Jt. Surg. **29**, 745—752 (1947).
— Biological aspects of the physiology of hyaline cartilage. Acta orthop. scand. **18**, 21—27 (1948).
— On the biology of nucleus pulposus. Acta orthop. scand. **20**, 275—279 (1951).
— Metachromatic dye-substrate interactions. Quart. J. micr. Sci. **95**, 327—358 (1954).
— Cartilage and chondroitin sulphate. I. The physiological role of chondroitin sulphate in cartilage. J. Bone Jt Surg. B **29**, 745—752 (1947).
Szirmai, J. A.: Quantitative approaches in the histochemistry of mucopolysaccharides. J. Histochem. Cytochem. **11**, 24—34 (1963).
—, and E. A. Balazs: Metachromasia and the quantitative determination of dye binding. Acta histochem. (Jena), Suppl. I, 56—79 (1958).
Takada, K.: Enzyme histochemistry in bone tissue. I. Histochemical detection of oxidative enzymes in developing knee joints of rats. Acta histochem. (Jena) **23**, 40—52 (1966).
— S. Yoshiki, and J. Okamoto: Histochemistry of various enzymes in developing knee joint of rodent animals. Arch. histol. jap. **22**, 317—327 (1962).
Takeuchi, T.: Histochemical demonstration of branching enzyme in animal tissues. J. Histochem. Cytochem. **6**, 208—216 (1958).
Takuma, S.: Electron microscopy of the developing cartilaginous epiphyses. Arch. oral. Biol. **2**, 111—119 (1960).
Telser, A., H. C. Robinson, and A. Dorfman: The biosynthesis of chondroitin-sulfate protein complex. Proc. nat. Acad. Sci. (Wash.) **54**, 912—919 (1965).
— — — The biosynthesis of chondroitin sulfate. Arch. Biochem. **116**, 458—465 (1966).
Theiler, K.: Die Auswirkung von partiellen Chordadefekten bei Triton alpestris. Beitrag zur Entwicklungsmechanik der Wirbelsäule. Wilhelm Roux' Arch. Entwickl.-Mech. Org. **144**, 476—490 (1950).
— Die Entwicklung der Zwischenwirbelscheiben bei der Short-Danforth-Maus. Rev. suisse Zool. **58**, 484—488 (1951).
Thiele, H., u. H. Krönke: Geordnete Kristallisation in ionotropen Gelen. Naturwissenschaften **13**, 389 (1955).
— — Zweistoffsysteme durch geordnete Kristallisation. Z. Naturforsch. **14**b, 92—98 (1959).
—, u. L. Langmaack: Strukturbildung durch Ionendiffusion, Symplexionotropie. Z. Naturforsch. **12**b, 1, 14—23 (1957).
Tobler, T.: Zur normalen und pathologischen Histologie des Kniegelenkmeniscus. Langenbecks Arch. klin. Chir. **177**, 483—495 (1933).
Töndury, G.: Anatomie und Entwicklungsgeschichte der Wirbelsäule mit besonderer Berücksichtigung der Altersveränderungen der Bandscheiben. Schweiz. med. Wschr. **1955**, 825—827, 835—837.
Töndury, G.: Entwicklungsgeschichte und Fehlbildungen der Wirbelsäule. Wirbelsäule in Forschung und Praxis, Ed. H. Junghanns, Oldenburg, Bd. 7. Stuttgart: Hippokrates-Verlag 1958.
— Embryopathien. Berlin-Göttingen-Heidelberg: Springer 1962.
Tonna, E. A.: The cellular complement of the skeletal system studied autoradiographically with tritiated Thymidine (H3TDR) during growth and aging. J. biophys. biochem. Cytol. **9**, 813—824 (1961).
—, and E. P. Cronkite: Histochemical and autoradiographic studies on the effects of aging on the mucopolysaccharides of the periosteum. J. biophys. biochem. Cytol. **6**, No 2, 171—178 (1959).
Trueta, J.: The normal vascular anatomy of the human femoral head during growth. J. Bone Jt Surg. B **39**, 358—394 (1957).
Uebermuth, H.: Über die Altersveränderungen der menschlichen Zwischenwirbelscheibe und ihre Beziehung zu den chronischen Gelenkleiden der Wirbelsäule. Ber. sächs. Akad. Wiss. Leipzig, math.-nat. Kl. Bd. 81, Sitzg v. 22. 7. 1929.
Verne, J., J. Bescol-Liversac, B. Droz et L. Olivier: Aspects de la fixation du 35-S dans les cartilages. Corrélations histophysiologiques. Ann. Histochim. **1**, 191—198 (1956).
—, et M. Marois: Un territoire de choix pour l'étude histochemique du tissu conjonctif. La symphyse pubienne. Annales histochim. **4**, 284—299 (1957).
Vincent, W. S.: Structure and chemistry of nucleoli. Int. Rev. of Cytology, ed. by G. H. Bourne and J. F. Danielli, vol. IV, p. 269—298. New York: Academic Press 1955.
Vis, J. H.: Histological investigations into the attachment of tendons and ligaments to the mammalian skeleton. Koninkl. Ned. Akad. Wetenschap. Proc., Ser. C, **60**, 148—157 (1957).
Viswanath, J. R., and K.-H. Knese: The ultrastructure of the apical ectodermal ridge of the limb buds of chick embryo. (Im Druck.)
Vitry, G.: La réaction metachromatique et son utilisation pour l'étude des polysaccharides. Ann. Histochim. **4**, 277—307 (1958).
Wallgren, G.: Biophysical analyses of the formation and structure of human fetal bone. A mikroradiographic and x-ray crystallographic study. Acta paediat. (Uppsala) **46**, Suppl. 113, 7—80 (1957).
Watson, M. L.: The nuclear envelope. Its structure and relation to cytoplasmic membranes. J. biophys. biochem. Cytol. **1**, 257—270 (1955).
Webber, R. V., and S. T. Baley: Some observations on the molecular form of chondroitin sulfate. Canad. J. Biochem. **34**, 933—1005 (1956).
Weidenreich, F.: Knochenstudien. II. Über Sehnenverknöcherungen und Faktoren der Knochenbildung. Z. Anat. Entwickl.-Gesch. **69**, 558—597 (1923a).
— Über die Differenzierung und Entdifferenzierung. Arch. mikr. Anat. **97**, 227—250 (1923b).

WEIDENREICH, F.: Über den Begriff der „Knochen" und die Beziehungen des Knochengewebes zu Bindegewebe und Knorpel. Erg.-H. Anat. Anz. **57**, 138—153 (1923c).

— Das Knochengewebe. In: Handbuch der mikroskopischen Anatomie des Menschen, Bd. II/3, S. 391—520. Berlin: Springer 1930.

WILLIAMS, M.: Morphology of the sternochondral joints of mammals. J. Morph. **101**, 275—305 (1957).

WILLMER, E. N.: Cytology and evolution, p. 1—430. New York u. London: Academic Press 1960.

— Morphological problems of cell type, shape and indification. In: Cells and tissues in culture, vol. 1 (ed. by E. N. WILLMER), p. 143—176. London and New York: Academic Press 1965.

WISLOCKI, G. B., H. L. WEATHERFORD and M. SINGER: Osteogenesis of antlers investigated by histological and histochemical methods. Anat. Rec. **99**, 265—295 (1947).

WOHLFAHRT-BOTTERMANN, K. E.: Gestattet das elektronenmikroskopische Bild Aussagen über Dynamik in der Zelle? Z. Zellforsch. **50**, 1—27 (1959).

WOLPERS, C.: Die Querstreifung der kollagenen Bindegewebsfibrillen. Virchows Arch. path. Anat. **312**, 292—302 (1944).

WOLSTENHOLME, G. E. W., and M. O'CONNOR: Chemistry and biology of mucopolysaccharides. Ciba Found. London: J. and A. Churchill Ltd. 1958.

WOODIN, A. M.: The corneal mucopolysaccharide. Biochem. J. **51**, 319—330 (1952).

WYSS, TH., u. S. P. ULRICH: Festigkeitsuntersuchungen und gezielte Extensionsbehandlung der Lendenwirbelsäule unter Berücksichtigung des Bandscheibenvorfalles. Vjschr. naturf. Ges. Zürich C **1**, Beih. 3/4 (1954).

ZAMBOTTI, V.: Die Biochemie des Knorpels, der zum Knochen umgebaut wird und die Verknöcherung. Sci. med. ital. **5**, 630—660 (1957) (Dtsch. Ausg.)

ZAWISCH, C.: Historisch-kritisches und Neues zur Frage der Ostoklasten, ihrer Entstehung und der Resorption im Knochen. Z. mikr.-anat. Forsch. **27**, 106—210 (1931).

— Die Verknöcherung der knorpelig vorgebildeten platten Knochen. Acta anat. (Basel) **19**, 384 (1953).

ZBINDEN, G.: Über Feinstruktur und Altersveränderungen des hyalinen Knorpels im elektronenmikroskopischen Schnittpräparat und Beitrag zur Kenntnis der Verfettung der Knorpelgrundsubstanz. Schweiz. Z. allg. Path. **16**, 165—189 (1953a).

— Der hyaline Knorpel im elektronenmikroskopischen Bild. Z. wiss. Mikr. **61**, 231—238 (1953b).

ZEIGER, K.: Elektronenmikroskopische Präparationstechnik in der Biologie. I. Fixieren und Einbetten. 4. intern. Kongr. für Elektronenmikroskopie 1958, S. 17—26. Berlin-Göttingen Heidelberg: Springer 1960.

ZELANDER, T.: Ultrastructure of articular cartilage. Z. Zellforsch. **49**, 720—738 (1959).

ZULAUF, C.: Die Höhlenbildung im Symphysenknorpel. Arch. f. Anat. 95—116 (1901).

ZWILLING, E.: Ectoderm-mesoderm relationship in the development of the chick embryo limb bud. J. exp. Zool. **128**, 423—441 (1955).

— Limb morphogenesis. In: Advances in morphogenesis, vol. 1 (ed. by M. ABERCROMBIE and J. BRACHET), p. 301—330. New York and London: Academic Press 1961.

XI. Biological bases of the radioisotope investigation of the skeleton

By

Rodolfo Amprino

With 26 Figures

Bone serves two distinct functions, viz., (1) it aids to protect part of the body, to support it in rest and in locomotion, and (2) it plays the role of a store of inorganic matter helpful in the mineral homeostasis in the blood and in the extracellular fluids. Bone owes most of its functional characteristics to its mineralization, i.e., to the presence within an organic matrix — gel-like polysaccharides which form a continuous phase and embed collagen fibres — of a system of discrete submicroscopic particles built of a complex mineral substance chiefly composed of calcium, phosphate and carbonate. The mineral phase gives a Roentgen-ray diffraction pattern characteristic of a structure called by the minerologists hydroxyapatite crystal lattice.

Both functions of bone are favored by the heterogeneity of the material at various levels of organization. The inner cancellous architecture of bones does not only add greatly to their physical strength at the minimum cost of material but represents a fabric which provides an extremely large area of contact — favorable for the diffusion of substances of molecular and atomic size — between bone tissue proper and the adjacent soft tissues which fill in bone spaces and cavities. Likewise, a dual value seems to possess the microscopic network of the vascular channels of bone compacta. At the submicroscopic level the discontinuity of the mineral phase built of discrete mineral crystals embedded in the organic matrix contributes to the elasticity of the tissue and also favors the diffusion of fluids indispensable for the mineral ion exchange involved in the buffering function of bone. Irregular and randomly distributed discontinuities seem to be present even within the structure of the single apatite crystals, i.e., Ca-deficient apatite in which Ca is replaced by H bonding. The crystals, described as tiny hexagonal tablets or rods or needle-like formations, are only a few until cells thick; their surface is therefore large in proportion to the mass.

Each crystal is regarded as including interior unit cells, surface unit cells, ions bound by surface forces and a surface hydration shell containing ions in equilibrium both with the surrounding milieu and with the surfaces (Neuman and Neuman, 1958). From $^1/_{10}$ to $^1/_4$ of all the ions present could reside in the crystal surface or in the layers immediately beneath. 1 gm of bone mineral is said to have a surface area of 100 sq.m; the total surface area of the bone crystals in the skeleton of an average man of 70 kg (about 1.200 gm of calcium) would amount to more than 100 acres. Through this enormous surface bone mineral is in equilibrium with the surrounding fluids.

The amount of mineral for unit volume of bone (degree of calcification) tends to increase with the age of the tissue; as a consequence, the latter becomes more and more hard and rigid. Part of the highly calcified material is gradually substituted by new-forming bone which is more flexible and permeable. This patchy microscopic reconstruction due to destruction of old material and neoformation is a unique feature of bone among supporting tissues and is continuous from fetal to senile age. The reconstruction rate, however, varies in the various regions of the skeleton and according to the age of the individual and the animal species (cf. i. a., Amprino and Godina, 1947). In general, when the bones do no longer change size or shape as after the end of body growth under normal conditions, the rates of formation and resorption of bone tissue balance each other. During body growth the over-all formation of bone tissue dominates on the resorption. This positive balance may have a very high value: e.g., the infant rat increases its skeletal weight of 15% in a single day. However, the rate of formation of new bone tissue is not a precise indicator of the amount of mineral deposited in the skeleton because of the different concentration of the mineral in structures laid-down at different times and coexisting in each skeletal piece.

Recently formed less calcified bone has a higher water content; it permits fast diffusion and rapid fixation of additional minerals. Besides, in young bone tissue the crystals are smaller and probably less "perfect", thus permitting rapid surface ion-exchange, dissolution and redeposition of crystals (recrystallization) and intracrystalline exchange. The increment in the calcification seems to impart a progressive irreversibility to the exchanges. The ions migrated into the interior of the crystal lattice of the forming crystals become buried under layers of subsequently added mineral; their back-migration to the surface and escape from the crystal to reenter the circulation is hindered (NEUMAN and NEUMAN, 1958).

1. Use of bone-seeking radioactive elements in the study of the skeleton

In general terms it can be said that the skeleton is available to ions from the circulation and that ionic interchanges within the bone occur at fast rates; minerals can also be drawn from the skeleton and return into circulation.

Minerals, e.g. calcium normally absorbed through the intestine may be found in various positions in the body: in solution in the extra- and intracellular fluids, bound to organic components, and fixed in the crystal lattice of bone mineral. The calcium deposited in the skeleton may be made available for physiological activities; a part of this calcium while circulating is excreted through the kidney and the intestine, a part may be reincorporated into the bone mineral. The same route of the calcium is followed by phosphorus, magnesium, sodium, carbonate, etc., and may also be taken by ions which are not normal constituents of the skeleton, e.g., radioactive transuranic elements and fission products entering the body. Apparently, bone is unable to distinguish between the atoms which normally form the crystal lattice of the apatite and extraneous radioactive ions. As the uptake of the latter is rapid and their release comparatively slow, their permanence in the skeleton may be life-long and represent a potential health hazard for the individual on account of the radiation emitted by decay.

Radioisotopes of the physiological mineral elements with a relatively short half-life are on the contrary useful tools when applied to the study of bone metabolism. In early researches of this kind, radioisotopes were administered orally or parenterally and the entry of the ions into the blood, their fixation to the bone, the general pattern of their distribution in the skeleton, and the time required for their release from bone and excretion from the body analyzed. To get a deeper insight into bone physiology the distribution of radioisotopes in the skeleton was later studied at the microscopical level by means of histological procedures. This was possible after the discovery and refinement of autoradiographic techniques by means of *in vivo* experiments or treatment of bone sections *in vitro*.

The biochemical and the histological approaches to the study of the skeletal metabolism by means of radioisotopes though aiming at the analysis of two different aspects of bone physiology are complementary to each other and are often sought concurrently. Only a few elementar concepts and data on the autoradiographic methods are summarized in the following pages; for details and special techniques, cf. i. a., YAGODA (1949), BOYD (1955), SACKS (1956), HARBERS (1958), BUDY (1963). Informations on the biochemical approach to the radioisotope study of bone mineral turnover will be reported in section 4 (p. 826); for special methods and techniques, see HEVESY (1948), SIRI (1949), COMAR (1955), NORDIN (1962), HEANEY (1963), RAY *et al.* (1965).

a) Autoradiography

Pioneers of the studies on radioactivity discovered that radiations from uranyl-sulfate and thorium compounds could activate a photographic emulsion and give rise to discernible localized images after development. The tree major types of radiations emitted in the decay of radioactive elements — the *alpha* and *beta* particles and the *gamma* rays — may be detected by means of particular emulsions. The *alpha* particle is much more effective in producing localized ionization and chemical action in the photographic emulsion than the *beta* particle. The *gamma* rays are most penetrating of all but they are useless for autoradiography because their long path and the randomness of their interactions with matter result in diffuse images detectable only in fast, coarse-grained emulsions. However, many *gamma*-emitters produce also low-energy *beta* particles. Of the synthetic radioactive isotopes only those of the transuranium elements emit *alpha* particles; the latter can be detected by the use of special nuclear type emulsions containing a large percentage of silver bromide in extremely small grains.

The tracers of greatest interest in the study of bone, such as ^{14}C, ^{35}S, ^{32}P and ^{45}Ca decay with the emission of *beta* particles or *gamma* radiations. Their autoradiographic localization can be effected by the use of photographic emulsions sensitive to the energies of the *beta* particles. High-energy *beta* particles give longer tracks than *alpha* particles and a diffuse grain distribution; low-energy *beta* particles such as those from ^{14}C permit a much better autoradiographic resolution.

Macroscopic autoradiography. May be used when studying only the gross distribution of radioactive material at the surface of fairly large specimens. When the surface of the specimen is not flat the *contour autoradiography* technic may be applied. In this case a permeable-base stripping film may be floated on the object or liquid emulsion painted on its surface. This method has found limited application in the study of radioactivity distribution at the surface of the calvarium bones of small animals or of whole teeth (Jodrey and Wilbur, 1951; Martin and Slater, 1951). Wider application has the *apposition autoradiography* in the study of specimens which can be cut in parts according to flat planes. Entire laboratory animals are cut while frozen or bones are divided longitudinally or cut in thick sections after embedding in plaster-of-Paris or in plastics; the flat surface of cutting is laid on the photographic film or plate directly or through a thin sheet of material permeable to radiations.

Macroscopic autoradiographs have a poor definition. When autoradiographs are needed sufficiently sharp to permit exact correlation with corresponding regions in the tissues and to differentiate activity variations corresponding to variations in photographic density, free-hand slices or sections from embedded specimens are used and exposed in contact with the emulsion *(contact autoradiography)*. The embedding material is usually removed but the sections are stained only after exposure. The sections are separated from the autoradiographic plate or film before photographic processing. The advantage of this procedure is that the same section may be exposed repeatedly until autoradiographs of the desired density or contrast are obtained.

Automicroradiography. In contact autoradiography the image is not frequently sharp. Attempts at improved resolution have centered chiefly in the use of thin tissue sections and in the perfection of contact by permanent adhesion of the tissue to the emulsion. An emulsion layer temporarely bonded to a film or plate support by means of a water permeable base of gelatin or an impermeable film base may be stripped off, floated onto the tissue sections over which it dries and remains during exposure and photographic processing. The advantage of the *stripping-film* technique (Pelc, 1947, 1956), viz. of a uniformly thin emulsion layer adherent to the section is also obtained with *liquid emulsions* which must be melted and painted over the sections (Bélanger and Leblond, 1946); this *coating technique* has been further improved (Kopriwa and Leblond, 1962).

In general, the sections are stained before exposure. By the introduction of this "integrated" method of autoradiography images are obtained so sharp as to serve for analysis at the cellular level. Bélanger (1950) has proposed a technique of coating and inverting by which the developer does not penetrate into the tissue. When used for undecalcified microtome or ground sections of mineralized tissues, the removal of a part of the mineral during staining before coating of the emulsion may thus be prevented. Methods for dry-mounting tissue sections can be used to the same purpose (cf. Hammarström *et al.*, 1965).

The total resolving power of the autoradiographs is depending on emulsion characteristics, radiation energy, tissue thickness and perfection in cutting and mounting. High sensitivity and high resolution of the emulsion cannot be satisfied by one film only and when possible several types of emulsions should be exposed. Macroscopic autoradiographs may be usefully examined only at low magnification as may be overexposed automicroradiographs from rather thick sections *(contrast autoradiographs)*. With thin sections and a thin emulsion layer the images may be examined under high power with the bright-field microscope in case of stained sections or with phase-contrast microscope if the section is unstained for the analysis of tracks or random grain distribution and of their relative concentration. The microscopic examination reveals whether the track departs from, or the grains overlay cells or any special structure of the preparation.

Quantitative autoradiography. A precise study of the metabolism of bone at a microscopical level requires techniques by which the amount of radioactive element present in an extremely small volume of tissue may be measured. Several procedures are available:

Direct measurement of the radioactivity of the sample with a Geiger counter designed to scan areas of nearly microscopic magnitude. A metal plate bearing a hole of 0.5 to 1.00 mm in diameter is placed over the section; the radiation passing through the hole which is centered over the regions of the section whose radioactivity must be evaluated is recorded by the counter.

Photometric determination of emulsion blackening of the autoradiograph carried out at low magnification. DUDLEY and DOBYNS (1949) described the use of a thick plaster-of-Paris block containing known amounts of ^{45}Ca to produce on the autoradiographic film calibration exposures to be developed simultaneously with the tissue section. The autoradiographic blackenings are compared microphotometrically. A useful improvement of the technique of quantitation has been suggested (JOWSEY *et al.*, 1965). Sections of dimensions greater than the maximum range of the radiation particles are required. TOMLIN *et al.* (1953, 1955) determined by microdensitometry of autoradiographs by means of a photomultiplier the ^{45}Ca specific activities in the cortex of rat long bones. Autoradiographs corresponding to a range of exposure times were measured to establish a density-exposure time relationship for the reaction of the film to the ^{45}Ca *beta* particles. ARNOLD *et al.* (1956) evaluated the ratio of ^{45}Ca concentration in newly formed bone of haversian systems to that of old primary bone in the tibial shaft of rabbit. ODEBLAD (1956) presented a theory of quantitative autoradiography (matrix theory) focused on the calculations and handling of geometric exposure integrals, each of which forms an element in a matrix. A simple method for quantitative assessment of the density of *beta* particles autoradiographs by comparative histophotometry was more recently applied by BÉLANGER (1958) to the study of regional differences in the synthesis of proteins and sulfated mucopolysaccharides in supporting tissues labelled *in vivo* with ^{35}S.

MARSHALL *et al.* (1959c) have recently extended the radiation calibration technique of DUDLEY and DOBYNS to densitometric measurements of the activities of *beta*-emitters in radioactive sources in which the distribution of activity is invariant in at least one dimension for a distance more than 5 to 10% of the maximum particle range. By this procedure, MARSHALL *et al.* (1959a) attempted autoradiographic measurements of the total ^{45}Ca content of individual osteons in the bone cortex of dogs after administration of a single dose of the radioisotope. Autoradiography has been used, e.g., by VAUGHAN and OWEN (1959) to measure the dose-rate of radiation in rabbit bone which had received ^{90}Sr. A quantitative estimate of the dose-rate at any point of bone was made by comparing the measurements of the autoradiographs with those of the density from a known ^{90}Sr standard.

With the use of thin sections, thin emulsions and shorter exposure times than those used for contrast autoradiography, relative counts may be made in a microscopic field at high magnification of the silver grains or the *alpha* tracks overlying given regions of the radiation sample. This method has been applied also in experiments of concurrent administration of an *alpha* and a *beta*-emitter (ARNOLD and JEE, 1954). The ratio of the *alpha*-track to the silver grain number may offer in such case an approximate evaluation of similarities or differences in the distribution of the two isotopes in bone. Methods have been proposed for the correction of grain count (cf. STILLSTRÖM, 1963, 1965).

2. Autoradiographic pattern of bone formation, growth and reconstruction

a) Bone matrix formation, calcification, resorption

Most of the autoradiographic evidence of the formation of organic bone matrix was obtained with the use of ^{14}C given as bicarbonate and of ^{35}S administered as inorganic sulfate or ^{35}S-labeled methionine or cystine.

The tagged carbonate appears widely distributed in bone of fast growing newborn rats (GREULICH and LEBLOND, 1953) and is most probably incorporated into the collagen and/or the carbohydrates of the matrix (GREULICH, 1953). Earlier investigations on adult rats had shown incorporation of radiocarbon into the mineral phase of bone tissue (ARMSTRONG *et al.*, 1948; BLOOM *et al.*, 1947; SKIPPER *et al.*, 1951), though a slight labeling of bone proteins had been also detected (SCHUBERT and ARMSTRONG, 1949). A tentative explanation of the difference in uptake of radiocarbonate by the mineral in the adult and the newborn animal respectively could be that the mineral of young bone is naturally low in carbonate content (GREULICH, 1956) and thus little radiocarbonate would enter young bone either by new crystal formation or by isoionic exchange.

In the diaphysis of growing long bones the higher ^{14}C activity is apparent directly under the periosteum as a narrow band in autoradiographs made shortly after radiocarbonate injection. With time this tagged layer appears displaced from the periosteum more and more inward toward the marrow cavity by newly formed unlabeled layers of bone tissue. The uptake of radiocarbonate decreases with age; in older animals the subperiosteal radioactive band is less intense and is more slowly displaced from the surface in parallel with the slower appositional growth.

Autoradiographs from the bone shaft of young growing mammals treated with ^{35}S-sulfate show a pattern of distribution of the isotope which is very similar to that recorded with radiocarbonate. A thin radioactive band in the region of periosteal apposition correlates with a metachromatic layer of newly formed matrix (DZIEWIATKOWSKI, 1952). BÉLANGER (1954), DUTHIE and BARKER (1955), and others showed the displacements

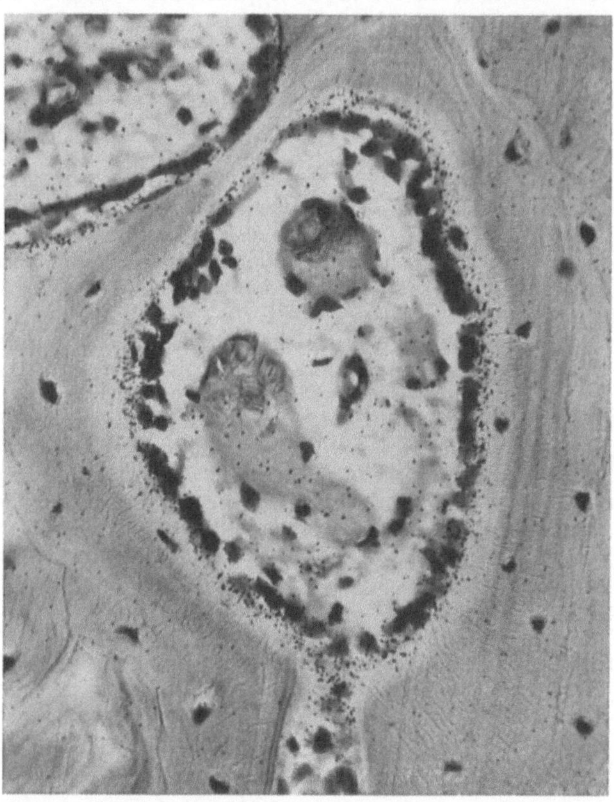

Fig. 1. Autoradiograph left on the section of bone compacta from a 109-day old dog one hour after injection of ^{3}H-glycine. Silver grains nearly equally distributed over the osteoblasts and the more recently laid-down and lightly stained layer of preosseous matrix in a forming osteon. [Courtesy of C. P. LEBLOND *et al.*, Bull. Acad. roy. Méd. Belg. 25, 421 (1929)]

undergone by this reactive layer in consequence of the continued appositional growth. The labeled sulfate is incorporated in bone tissue into a chondroitinsulfate; the label disappears after hyaluronidase digestion *in vitro* (BÉLANGER, 1954). Ribonuclease removes the ^{35}S from the matrix of bone and other mineralized tissues; this may suggest the existance of a close relationship between chondroitinsulfuric acid and ribonucleic acid in the organic matrix of calcified tissues and this association has been supposed to be of importance in the process of mineralization (GREULICH and FRIBERG, 1957). Also the osteoblastic layer of periosteum binds large quantities of radiosulfate (DZIEWIATKOWSKI, 1951*a*; AMPRINO, 1955); according to the latter author, the periosteal uptake preceeds the labeling of the adjacent bone matrix proper. BÉLANGER (1956) has shown uptake of ^{35}S-methionine in very young osteoblasts (preosteoblasts). The amount of radiosulfate accumulated by the periosteum seems to decrease progressively throughout life (TONNA and CRONKITE, 1959). The early concentration of ^{35}S-methionine tagged material is apparently proportional to the growth rate in bone, but the ^{35}S-methionine seems to label a different fraction than the ^{35}S-sulfate; the former predominates in mineralized tissues by accumulation in the calcified portion (BÉLANGER, 1956). The main data on the fate of ^{35}S in mineralized tissues have been reviewed by DZIEWIATKOWSKI (1958, 1962), and JOHNSTON (1961).

The first autoradiographic demonstration of the participation of osteoblasts in the matrix formation has been offered by CARNEIRO and LEBLOND (1959) and LEBLOND *et al.* (1959) in adult mice and dogs after injection of glycine-2-^{3}H. Very soon after injection the osteoblasts are overlaid by an intense autoradiographic reaction (Fig. 1); at 4 to 6

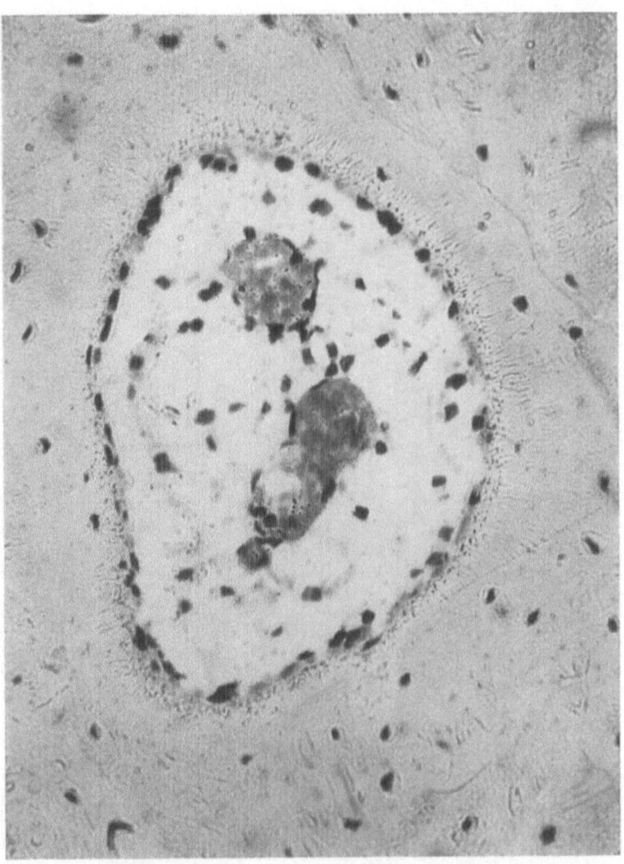

Fig. 2. Autoradiograph left on the section of bone compacta from a 109-day old dog six hours after injection of ^{3}H-glycine. The grains lay over the recently formed preosseous matrix. [Courtesy of C. P. LEBLOND *et al.*, Bull. Acad. roy. Méd. Belg. **25**, 421 (1959)]

hours, the radioactivity has largely disappeared from the osteoblasts and the adjacent preosseous matrix has become intensely radioactive (Fig. 2). The reactive layer is later found farther and farther from the osteoblast layer without apparent decrease in intensity (Fig. 3). The labeled glycine taken up by the osteoblasts is apparently built into a precursor of the collagen later found in the matrix.

More recently, by combining histological and autoradiographical analysis, and using various ^{3}H-labeled amino acids or ^{3}H-thymidine, the origin, proliferation rate, differentiation, selective synthesizing activity, and fate of bone cells in relation with their microenvironment have been accurately studied in small laboratory mammals under normal or experimentally modified conditions (OWEN, 1963, 1965; OWEN and MACPHERSON, 1963; TONNA, 1961*b*, 1964; TONNA and CRONKITE, 1961*b*, 1962*a*, 1962*b*, 1964; YOUNG, 1962*a*, 1962*b*, 1962*c*, 1963, 1964). In the periosteum of 2-week-old rabbits the pre-osteoblasts show the highest proliferative rate (about 33 %/day), while the fibroblasts seem to be relatively unimportant for the increase of the bone cell population (OWEN, 1963, 1965). Also incorporation of ^{3}H-glycine is much greater in osteoblasts than in fibroblasts or in osteocytes; osteoclasts fail to utilize this aminoacid. Osteoblasts begin to secrete the labeled glycine one hour after injection (YOUNG, 1962c), and they would produce up to 2 to 3 times their own volume of matrix in their most active period (OWEN, 1963). The incorporation of these cells into bone proper is not a random process; in fact, the periosteal osteoblast remains a certain time at the bone surface before becoming an osteocyte, or a relatively inactive osteoblast lining an haversian canal (OWEN, 1963).

Soon after the organic matrix of bone tissue has been laid down, mineral ions become fixed to it. Electron microscope evidence suggests that there are specific regions in the collagen microfibrils which probably act as nucleation centers: small (20 to 150 A) dense particles giving the electron-diffraction pattern of apatite are deposited regularly spaced along the microfibrils (GLIMCHER, 1959). No preferential orientation of these crystallites

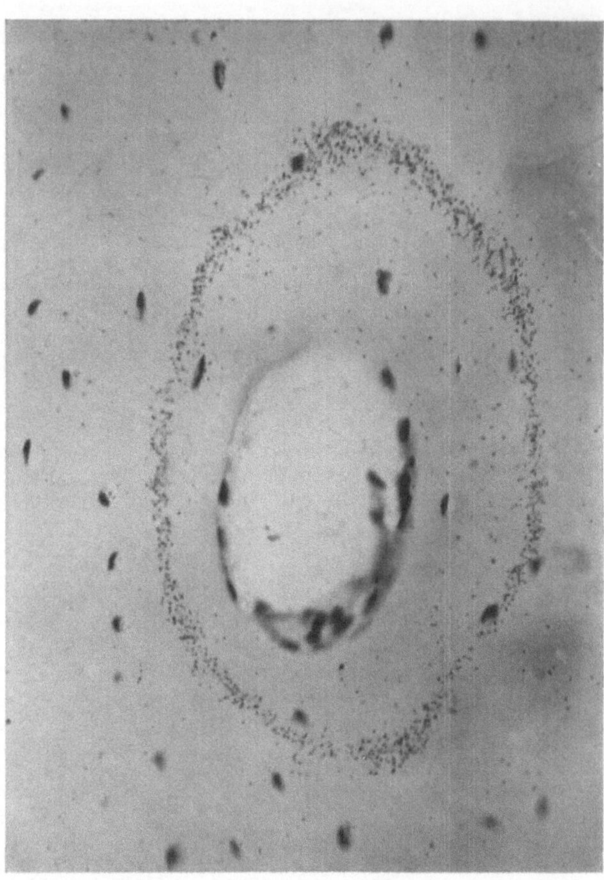

Fig. 3. Dog treated with H^3-glycine at the age of 109 days and sacrificed fifteen days later. The line of reduced silver grains over the forming osteon is separated from the lumen of the latter by an unlabeled thick layer of bone tissue laid-down after isotope injection. [Courtesy of C. P. LEBLOND *et al.*, Bull. Acad. roy. Méd. Belg. **25**, 421 (1959)]

relative to the fibril axis has been observed (FITTON-JACKSON and RANDALL, 1956). Further crystal growth results in asymmetric crystals with one axis elongated; this process seems to occur primarily within the fibrils and to be associated with orientation of the crystals (GLIMCHER, 1959). The problem of mineral accretion, namely of the increase in size of the crystals and of new crystal formation, has been approached by Roentgen-ray absorption technique (microradiography) and by autoradiography using ^{32}P, ^{45}Ca, and radiostrontium; the latter isotope seems to behave like ^{45}Ca in bone. It has been shown by means of microradiography that bone matrix does not calcify immediately after it has been laid-down (VINCENT, 1954). However, in adult bone the layer of uncalcified preosseous matrix revealed by microradiography and histochemical staining seems to be much thicker than that detected with the electron microscope in rapidly growing regions of bone (KNESE and KNOOP, 1958).

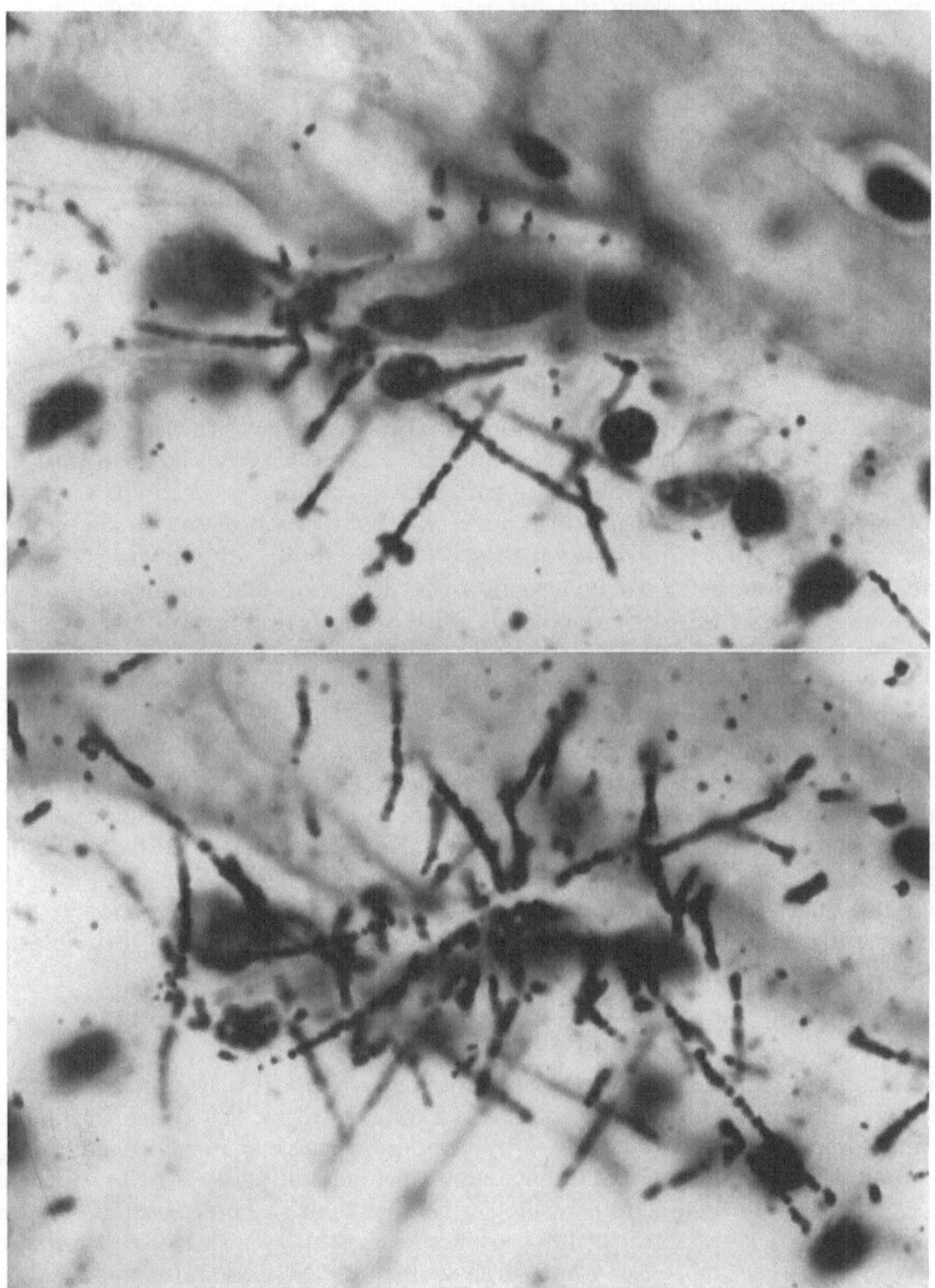

Fig. 4. The tissue and the α-track level of the autoradiograph of an osteoclast laying at the surface of a trabecula in a vertebra of a rat sacrificed 24 hours after ^{239}Pu injection. [Courtesy of J. S. ARNOLD and W. S. S. JEE, Amer. J. Anat. **101**, 367—417 (1957)]

Within the first few hours after ^{32}P, ^{45}Ca or radiostrontium injection at least 60% of the dose administered to growing and mature laboratory mammals is fixed in the skeleton. As it has been shown by the pioneer work of LEBLOND *et al.* (1951) by the use of ^{32}P, the activity is deposited in a diffuse uniform manner in mature bone and in concentrated layers on bone surfaces where growth is occurring. During the first few days after isotope administration there seems to occur a rapid, and thereafter slower, decrease in the ^{32}P concentration in the material diffusely deposited in mature bone.

A strongly reactive band along the periosteal surface has been described in autoradiographs of the cortex of long bones in young growing mammals sacrificed at early intervals after ^{45}Ca administration. This band is thin or thick depending on whether is related to slow or rapid apposition (LEA and PONLOT, 1958), it is not sharply limited but it fades into a weaker diffusely reacting portion of the cortex extending through all its thickness. The current interpretation of such image is that the more radioactive subperiosteal band is correlated with a region of rapidly increasing calcification, viz., of addition of new mineral ions to the preexisting crystals or to formation and growth of new crystals, while the diffuse less reactive portion is due to the activity of ^{45}Ca atoms which entered by exchange (see further on, p. 821) the crystals of the matrix which was already highly calcified at the time of radiocalcium administration. The higher fixation of radiostrontium as that of radiocalcium takes place in sites of bone mineralization.

No new knowledge on bone resorption was derived from the use of radioisotopes. Apparently, the bone matrix and the mineral are destroyed simultaneously but the resolution of the autoradiographs is insufficient to permit a thorough analysis of the rim of bone resorption surfaces. An interesting observation was made, however, by ARNOLD and JEE (1957) in young rats given plutonium. Plutonium localizes at the periosteal surface and in higher concentration at the endosteal surface of growing bones but without apparent selective deposition with respect to the presence of osteoblastic activity. In the mentioned experiments all the bone tissue formed post-injection showed a diffuse labeling; when resorption occurred, plutonium derived from the resorbing bone progressively concentrated in the osteoclasts (Fig. 4). The plutonium was later transferred from the osteoclasts to macrophages. ARNOLD and JEE assume that the osteoclast fragments and then digests the ingested bone particles in its cytoplasm where it concentrates the liberated Pu. Evidence has been offered in favour of the view that osteoblasts may serve as precursors for osteoclasts (TONNA and CRONKITE, 1961*a*), though several specific proteins appear to differ in these two types of cells (YOUNG, 1964). In PTE-injected rats, both osteoclasts and osteoblasts seem capable of reversion to the osteoprogenitor state during recovery from the PTE treatment, and the osteoblasts regain the ability for DNA synthesis (YOUNG, 1964).

b) Intramembranous ossification

The formation of membrane bone is preceded by the transformation of connective spindle cells into osteoblasts. The uptake of radiosulfate by the dense fibrillar tissue in which membrane bone differentiates is well apparent in early developmental stages and higher than that of mesenchymal blastemata which will give rise to fibrous tissues (capsules, tendons and ligaments), but lower than that of the precartilaginous primordia. A remarkable increase of radioactivity occurs when the spindle cells differentiate into osteoblasts and even more so when preosseous intercellular substance is laid down (AMPRINO, 1955) (Fig. 5). This sulfate uptake should depend on the synthesis of sulfated polysaccharides (FRIBERG and RINGERTZ, 1955). The formation of intercellular matrix during intramembranous ossification was detected also in autoradiographs from newborn rats injected with ^{14}C-carbonate. A positive reaction is apparent on the edges of the bone spicules surrounded by osteoblasts and in contact with the latter. Later the reaction is seen also within the spicules which have progressively formed (LEBLOND and GREULICH, 1956). Later mechanisms of flat bones growth have been analyzed by YOUNG (1962*c*) in the parietal bones of rats injected ^{3}H-glycine.

The calcification of forming membrane bone seems to be a rapid process occurring in a rather uniform manner as shown by ^{32}P autoradiographs. In older animals the ^{32}P uptake is apparently limited to the layers subjacent to the osteoblasts (LEBLOND and GREULICH, 1956).

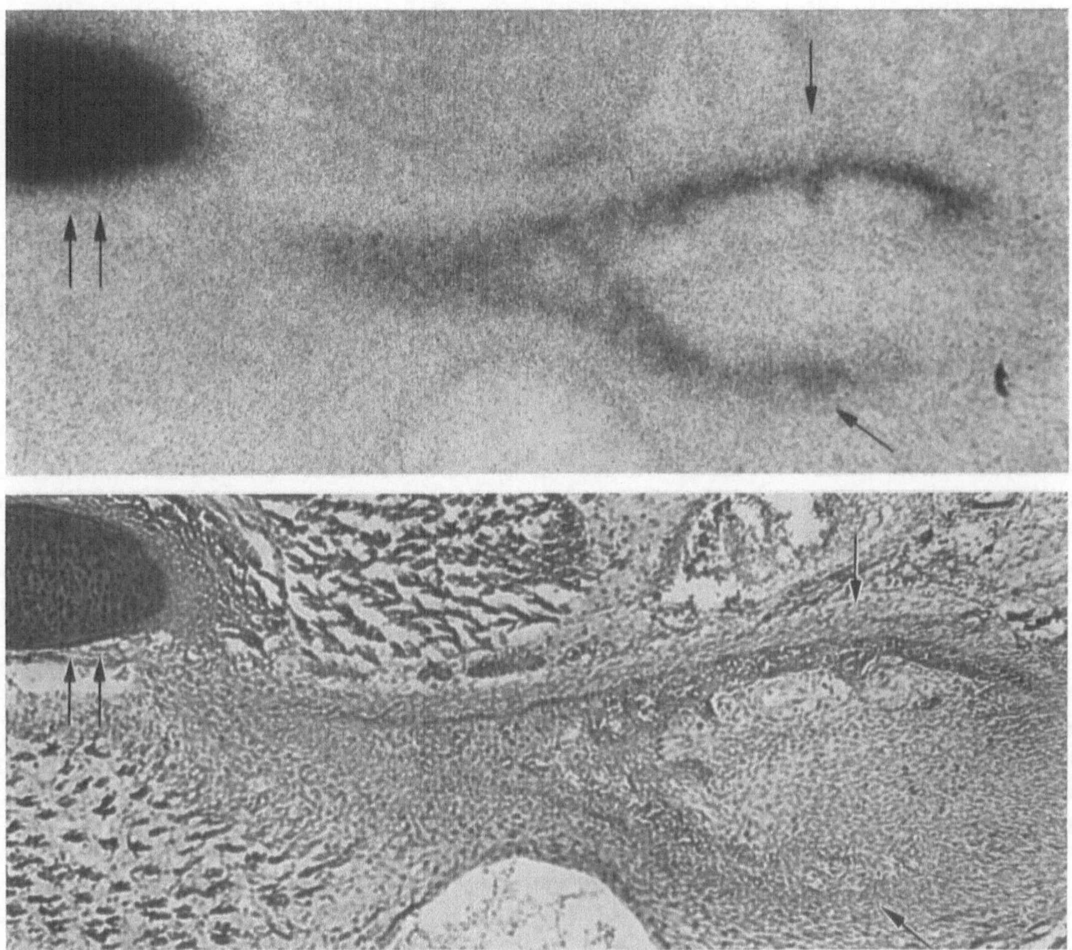

Fig. 5. Autoradiograph and microphoto of the stained section of a region of intramembranous bone formation in an embryo 24 hours after ^{35}S-sulfate treatment. The activity of the forming thin bone trabeculae *(arrow)* and of the clusters of osteoblasts is considerably lower than that of the adjacent cartilaginous bar *(double arrow)*. [From R. AMPRINO, by permission of Acta anat. (Basel) **24**, 121 (1955)]

c) Endochondral ossification

α) Cartilage differentiation and growth

The cartilaginous model of the bones differentiates and grows through processes very similar to those which take place in all the hyaline cartilage of the embryo and fetus. With the use of ^{14}C and ^{35}S new informations have been gained on the role played by the cells in matrix formation. The mesenchymal forerunners of the cartilaginous primordia take up larger amounts of radiosulfate than the mesenchyme which will form loose or dense connective tissues. A considerable activity is autoradiographically appreciable before a basophilous and metachromatic intercellular substance is histologically detectable. Conclusive evidence was offered by BÉLANGER (1954) and in mature cartilage by PELC and GLÜCKSMANN (1955) showing that accumulation of radiosulfate takes place in the cells within one or two hours after isotope administration and later passes to the surrounding matrix. Utilization of inorganic sulfate by the cells in the synthesis of chondroitin-sulfate seems to occur almost as rapidly as the sulfate enters the cartilage (CAMPO and DZIEWIATKOWSKI, 1961). This rapid shift of radioactivity from the cells to the matrix has been shown also in the initial differentiation *in vitro* of precartilage into cartilage with metachromatic matrix (OKADA, 1960). Double label experiments on pure cultures of chondrocytes (PROCKOP *et al.*, 1964) indicate that collagen synthesis occurs concurrently with sulfate incorporation. Chondrocytes grown for several generations on fibrin clots, dedifferentiate and do no longer incorporate sulfate or synthesize hydroxyproline, although they take up as much labeled proline as the freshly liberated chondrocytes. It appears also that interactions between associated chondrocytes are important in inducing and maintaining chondroitinsulfate synthesis; when chondrocytes are cultivated as monodisperse cells, they cease synthesizing chondroitin-sulfate and collagen, they synthesize DNA and divide (ABBOTT and HOLTZER, 1966).

With time, in parallel to the increase of the amount, basophilia and metachromasia of the matrix, an increment of the radiosulfate uptake seems to occur in cartilage. Also the perichondrium, which in embryos is particularly rich in cells differentiating into chondroblasts, takes up considerable amounts of ^{35}S.

^{14}C in differentiating cartilage is incorporated mainly if not exclusively in the formation of the matrix collagen; it concentrates first in the chondrocytes then moves out in the intercellular substance (LEBLOND and GREULICH, 1956). Some time after administration of ^{14}C-carbonate or of ^{35}S-sulfate the matrix appears uniformly labeled and the cells are no longer reactive. Most of the ^{35}S-sulfate fixed by cartilage is incorporated into chondroitinsulfate in *in vivo* experiments (DZIEWIATKOWSKI, 1951*b*) as well as in slices of cartilage preserved *in vitro* (BOSTRÖM and MÅNSSON, 1953). The radioactivity of cartilage which has incorporated ^{35}S-sulfate disappears after treatment of the sections with hyaluronidase (BÉLANGER, 1954; GREULICH, 1956); the enzyme seems not to extract the sulfate taken up by the cells (CURRAN and KENNEDY, 1955). Treatment of the sections with hyaluronidase does not diminish the ^{14}C radioactivity over cartilage. The rate of incorporation of ^{35}S decreases with rising age probably as a consequence of the progressive diminution of chondroitinsulfate synthesis and turnover (LAYTON, 1950; BOSTRÖM and MANSSON, 1953; DZIEWIATKOWSKI, 1953, 1954*a*, 1962, and others). Other tissues which incorporate radiosulfate show the same behavior (GLÜCKSMANN *et al.*, 1956).

β) Cartilage replacement by trabecular bone

According to the extensive researches of DZIEWIATKOWSKI, in very young epiphyses of the rat the ^{35}S uptake is high especially in the region which foreruns the epiphyseal plate. Later, the ^{35}S reaction disappears relatively more rapidly from the region of the plate than from the rest of the epiphysis; the distribution of the isotope in the whole epiphysis is then nearly uniform. The radioactivity decreases when an ossification center develops. If the tracer is administered when the epiphyseal center has partially formed, ^{35}S gets fixed in relatively greater amount in the layer of cartilage adjacent to the bone nucleus and in the epiphyseal plate (Fig. 6); the rate of chondroitinsulfate synthesis seems therefore to be higher in the cartilage which will soon calcify and be later resorbed. Apparently, the radiosulfate uptake is quantitatively correlated to the rate of substitution of the cartilage with trabecular bone.

In the epiphyseal plate the greatest uptake of ^{35}S-sulfate and ^{14}C-carbonate occur in the zone of proliferation and of cell hypertrophy. The cartilaginous trabeculae undergoing mineralization do not fix these isotopes if the latter are injected when the calcification process has commenced, they appear radioactive if the treatment is made before mineralization starts. When the chondrocytes become inactive and presumably die the incorporation of radiocarbonate and radiosulfate is interrupted.

Evidence has been produced with the use of ^{35}S in rabbits that the epiphyseal plate undergoes expansion transversely to the bone long axis in the layer of the reserve cells, especially in its peripheral region (LANGENSKIJÖLD *et al.*, 1967). According to TONNA (1961), this expansion is ensured by the continuous apposition of new cartilage differentiating from a pool of chondroosteogenic cells of the adjacent periosteum.

CAMPO and DZIEWIATKOWSKI (1963) deduced from their autoradiographic observations that a portion of the chondroitin-sulfate of the epiphyseal plate is retained in the cores of the metaphyseal spicules of bone, while the protein-polysaccharide is somehow removed before calcification of cartilage.

The pattern of labeling in the cells located at the various levels of the epiphyseal plate of young growing rats was analyzed by KEMBER (1960) for intervals of one hour to 28 days after injection of

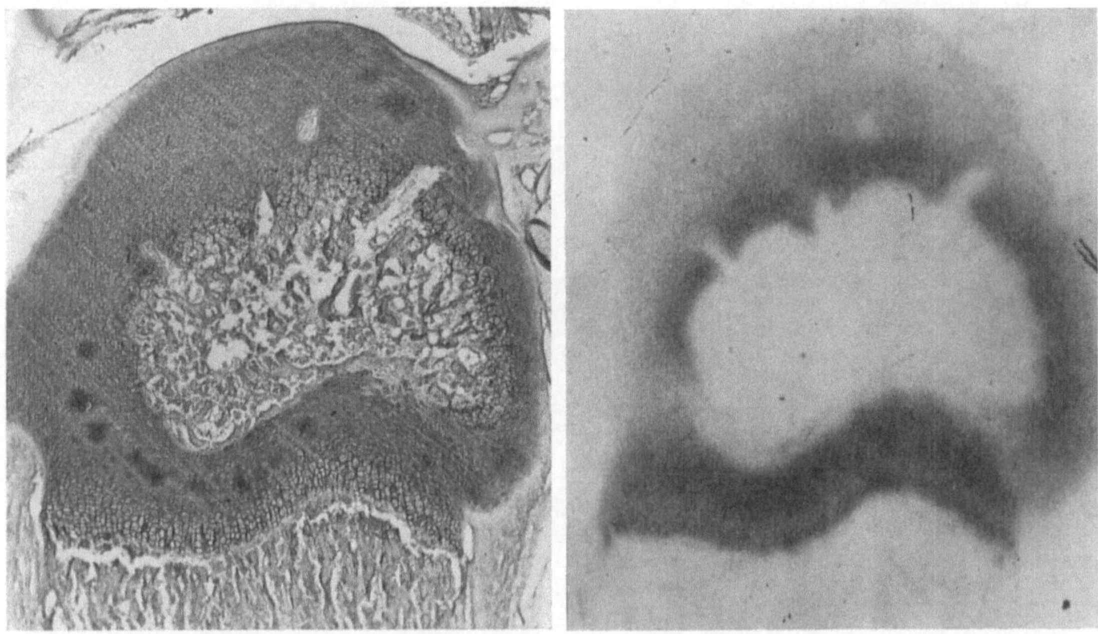

Fig. 6. Uneven distribution of ^{35}S-sulfate in an epiphysis undergoing endochondral ossification. Stained section and autoradiograph. Guinea-pig full term fetus 48 hours after ^{35}S treatment. [From R. AMPRINO, by permission of Acta anat. (Basel) **24**, 121 (1955)]

^{3}H-thymidine. The region of more active cell division was thus better defined, and the existence of a zone of *reserve cells* on top of the cell columns objectively proved. The sites of cell division have been shown in the epiphyseal anlage and in the growth cartilage through ^{3}H-thymidine labeling also in *in vitro* explanted bone rudiments of rat and rabbit (RIGAL, 1962). BONI and RAMPOLDI (1958) with the use of ^{35}S-sulfate observed that the entire life cycle of the cells in the growth cartilage of young rabbits may unfold within a period of 36 to 40 hours.

Following administration of ^{32}P or ^{45}Ca a highly reactive band appears at the lower surface of the epiphyseal plate (Fig. 7) where the cartilaginous trabeculae of the hypertrophic cell region calcify; this was shown by various authors and definitely demonstrated by PONLOT (1960) in puppies. Also the thin layers of bone tissue which soon coat the remnant spicules of calcified cartilage are first reactive in ^{14}C and ^{35}S autoradiographs; when they calcify they become autoradiographically detectable after ^{32}P or ^{45}Ca administration. By comparing autoradiographs made at progressively longer intervals of time from the injection of the radiotracer, the resorption of the preexisting bone trabeculae and the continuous formation of new ones has been evidenced (LEBLOND *et al.*, 1950). In this region a redistribution of mineral of previously formed to newly laid-down bone structures seems to occur. The metaphyseal trabeculae formed some time after administration of the radiotracer are faintly tagged, the less labeled the more recently formed (Fig. 8). A progressive decrease in the destruction of the initially labeled trabeculae and an increase in the formation of new

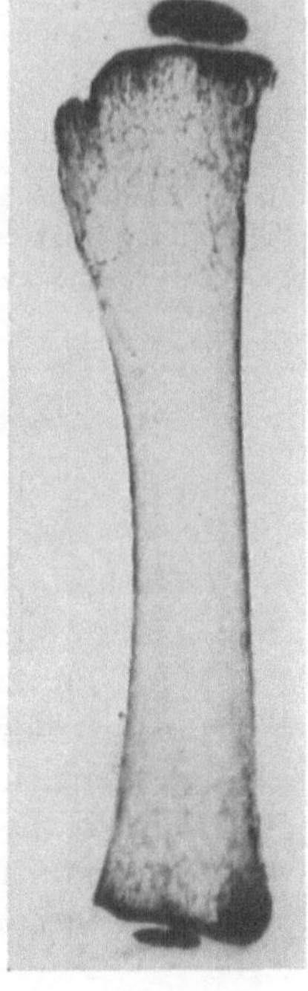

Fig. 7. Distribution of ^{45}Ca in an autoradiograph of the tibia of a three-week old puppy five hours after isotope injection. The greatest activity is located in the subperiosteal layer of the shaft, in the metaphyseal zone of trabecular growth and in the calcified region of the cartilaginous epiphyseal plate. [Courtesy of R. PONLOT, Le radiocalcium dans l'étude des os. Masson, 1960)

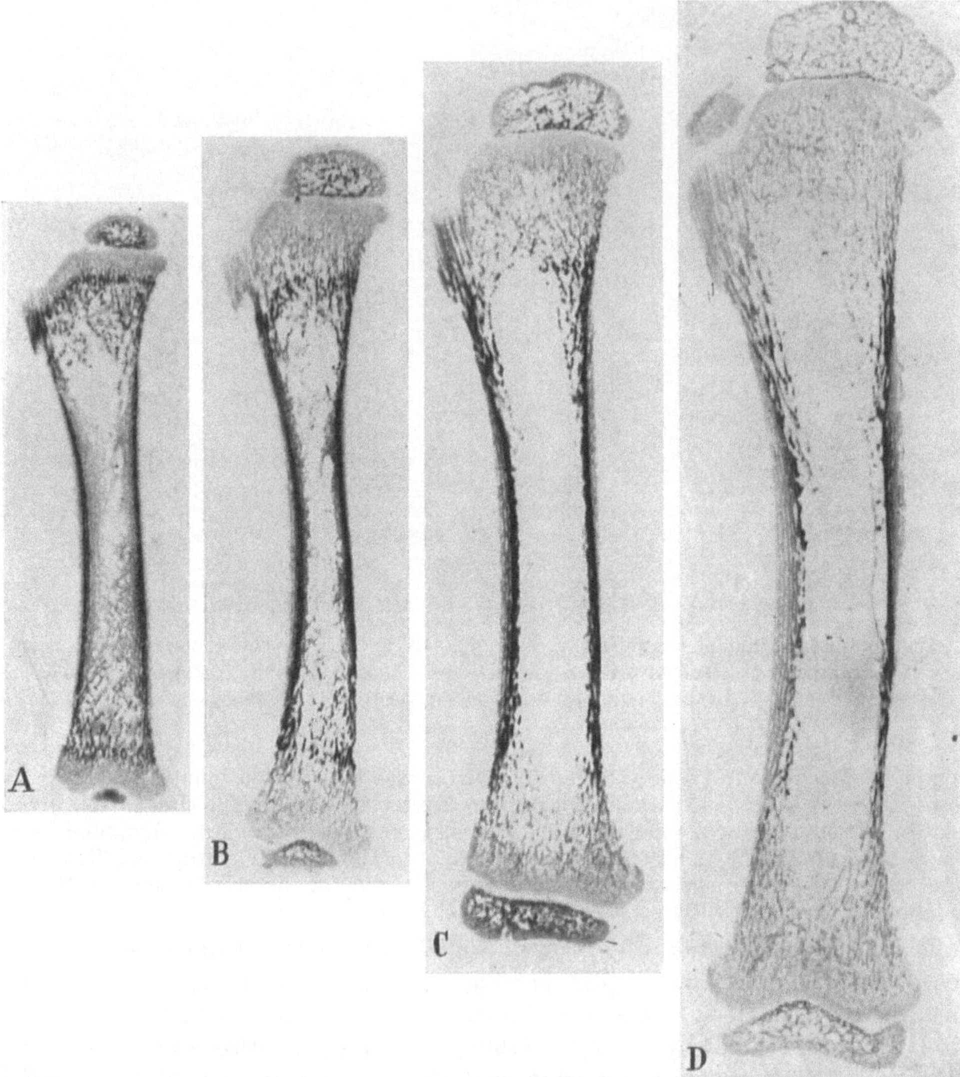

Fig. 8. Autoradiograph of the tibia of puppies injected with ^{45}Ca when three-week old and sacrificed one (A), two (B), three (C), and four weeks (D) after isotope treatment. The changes in the distribution of the activity in the shaft compacta are due to appositional growth and remodeling. Gradual decrease with time of the activity in the newforming metaphyseal trabeculae (Courtesy of P. LACROIX, by permission from Bone as a Tissue, edit. by Rodahl, Nicholson and Brown. Copyright 1960. Blakiston Div., McGraw-Hill Book Co.)

ones occur; a gradient of decreasing radioactivity from the older to the newer post-injection bone becomes therefore detectable in the metaphyseal region (LACROIX 1960).

γ) Periosteal bone formation and growth

A few data from the researches of LEBLOND *et al.* (1950) on rat bones (^{32}P), COMAR *et al.* (1952) on pig bones (^{32}P, ^{45}Ca, and ^{89}Sr), TOMLIN *et al.* (1953) and the LACROIX group (cf. PONLOT 1960) in rats and respectively in puppies treated with ^{45}Ca will be reported in addition to those mentioned at page 792.

The formation of the first perichondral bone collar and its subsequent appositional growth have been analyzed in ^{35}S and ^{14}C autoradiographs. The first osseous lamina which appears highly radioactive when the isotope is injected a short time before its formation, becomes separated from the osteoblastic layer of periosteum by the laying-

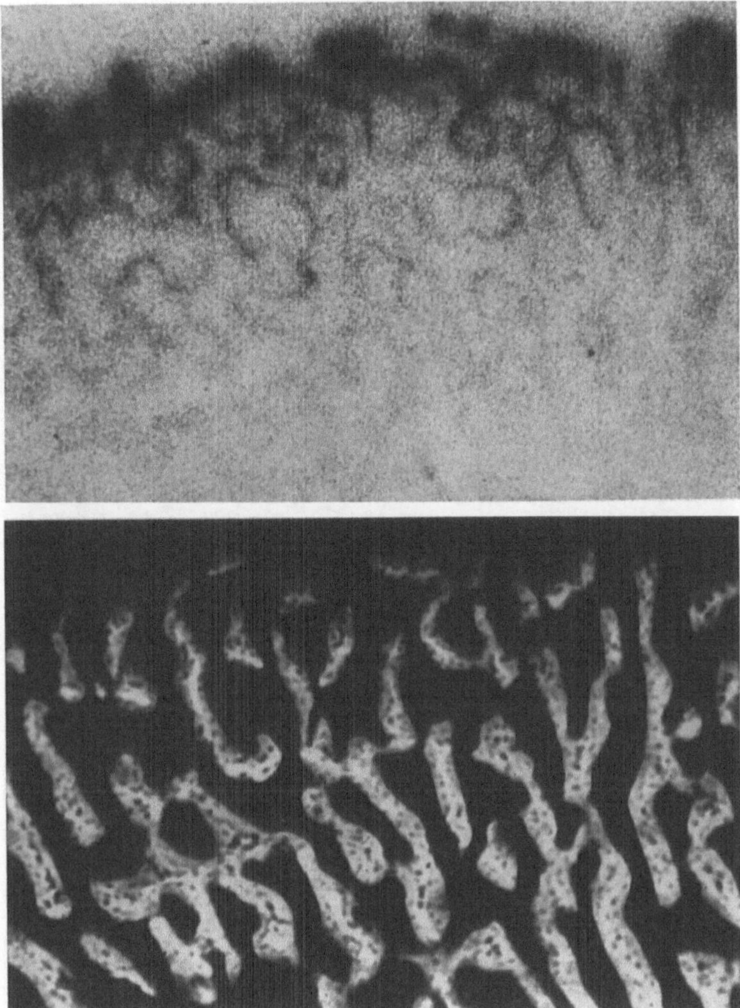

Fig. 9. Autoradiograph and microradiograph of the compacta of the tibia of a three-week old dog five hours after ^{45}Ca injection. Cross section of the diaphysis. Higher activity in the more recently formed and rapidly calcifying bone tissue: outer spicules of the trabecular network and thin layers deposited on the wall of the haversian spaces (Courtesy of R. PONLOT, Le radiocalcium dans l'étude des os. Masson, 1960)

down of progressively thicker strata of less and less reactive bone deposited when the activity of the isotope in the blood has already decreased considerably from the time of injection. This pattern repeats throughout fetal and postnatal life till the appositional growth ceases.

In newborn and young growing mammals the radioactivity appears more diffuse through the whole cortex in ^{32}P and ^{45}Ca autoradiographs than in the adult in which only the subperiosteal layer appears highly reactive. The autoradiographic researches of the LACROIX group (LEA and PONLOT, 1958; LACROIX, 1960, and PONLOT, 1960) on puppies sacrificed at various times from birth a few hours after one injection of radiocalcium show that in cross section of the diaphysis the subperiosteal zone appears highly reactive in the first days of life while the rest of the bone network formed during the later part of fetal life does not take up a sufficient amount of tracer to be detectable. A few weeks after birth the outer zone of the cortex still reacts intensely (Fig. 9) but its thickness is already quite different in the various sectors in connection with a various rate of appositional growth. According to LEA and PONLOT (1958), the autoradiographic expression of a fast appositional growth is a chain-like sequence of complete or

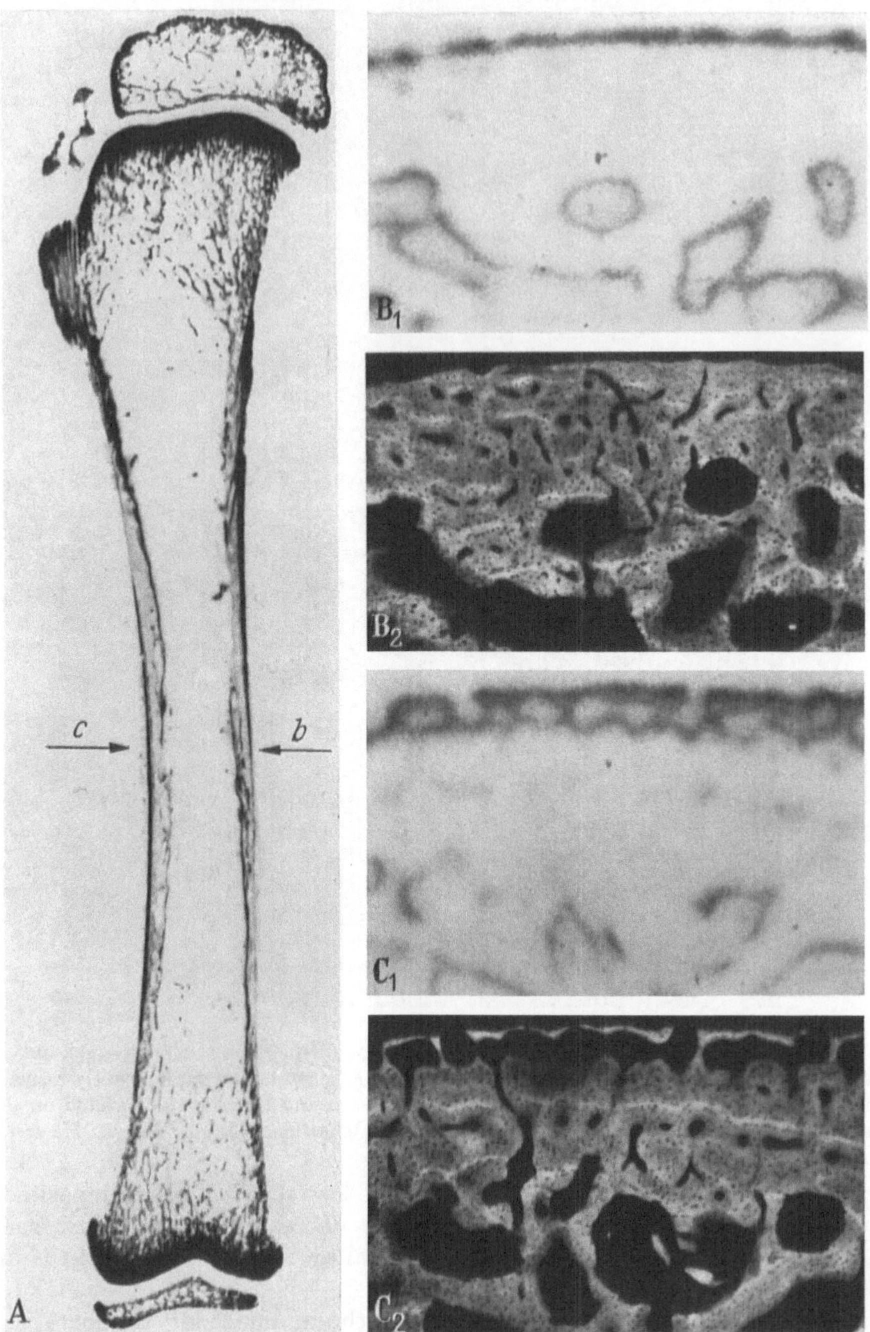

Fig. 10. Autoradiograph (A) of the tibia of a 75-day old dog ten hours after ^{45}Ca injection. The thickness of the highly reactive subperiosteal layer is different in various regions of the shaft. Autoradiograph (B_1) and microradiograph (B_2) of a cross section of the tibia compacta of a 63-day old dog 48 hours after injection of ^{45}Ca. The highly radioactive thin upper line corresponds to periosteal bone formation in a sector undergoing slow appositional growth. The radioactive circular profiles in the lower half of fig. B_1 are due to the ^{45}C incorporated in thin layers of bone tissue which are being deposited on the wall of large resorption cavities. Autoradiograph (C_1) and microradiograph (C_2) of the same cross section as in fig. B in a sector of rapid appositional growth. [Courtesy of L. M. LEA and R. PONLOT, Arch. Biol. **69**, 455 (1958)]

incomplete radioactive rings in the subperiosteal layer. This is due to the laying-down of a more or less thin trabecular network which encloses large haversian spaces; the first laid down axial core of these trabeculae calcifies rapidly and takes up a relatively large amount of radiotracer. The grooves in between the trabeculae are subsequently filled in by concentric deposition, viz., the so called primary osteons (or addition osteons, according to LACROIX, 1960) are built; the latter by their progressive mineralization determine the presence of the radioactive rings in the autoradiographs (Fig. 10, C_1). In this way, rows of radioactive osteons laying side by side form in the subperiosteal layer. The differences in the intensity of the autoradiographic reaction seems to suggest that the calcification rate is higher in the fast growing outer spicules of the periosteal bone than in the layers deposited on the wall of the haversian spaces to form the primary osteons. A smooth radioactive band is apparent under the periosteum in the cross section of the cortex in the sectors and at the age in which the appositional growth rate is low (Fig. 10, B_1).

δ) *Secondary bone changes*

They include altogether the results of the processes of reconstruction, namely of osteoblastic deposition and osteoclastic resorption which determine (1) the remodeling of the bone shape, and (2) the microscopical renewal of its compact and spongy constituents. The outer remodeling is nearly completed at the end of the body growth period, the process of inner reconstruction unfolds throughout life with a continuous formation and substitution of secondary haversian systems, osteons, which are bounded from the

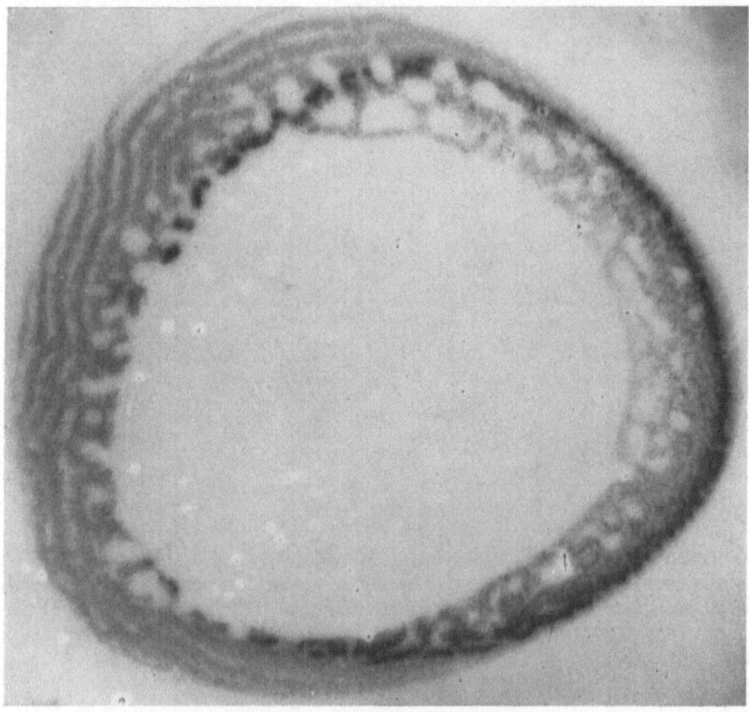

Fig. 11. Autoradiograph of the cross section of the middle diaphysis of a dog injected ^{45}Ca when three-week old and sacrificed one month later. The arrangement of the highly radioactive zone depends on the excentric growth and remodeling undergone by the shaft in the period following the isotope injection. The rate of periosteal apposition and respectively of endosteal resorption was much higher in the quadrants laying at the left than on those at the right in the autoradiograph. (Courtesy of R. PONLOT, Le radiocalcium dans l'étude des os. Masson, 1960)

surrounding preexisting material by the so-called cementing line. The rate of reconstruction varies considerably in connection with various factors, but steadily the newly laid-down matrix acquires slowly and progressively the chemical and physical characteristics of mature bone tissue through an increment of mineralization which probably runs parallel to a progressive reduction of the water content of the matrix.

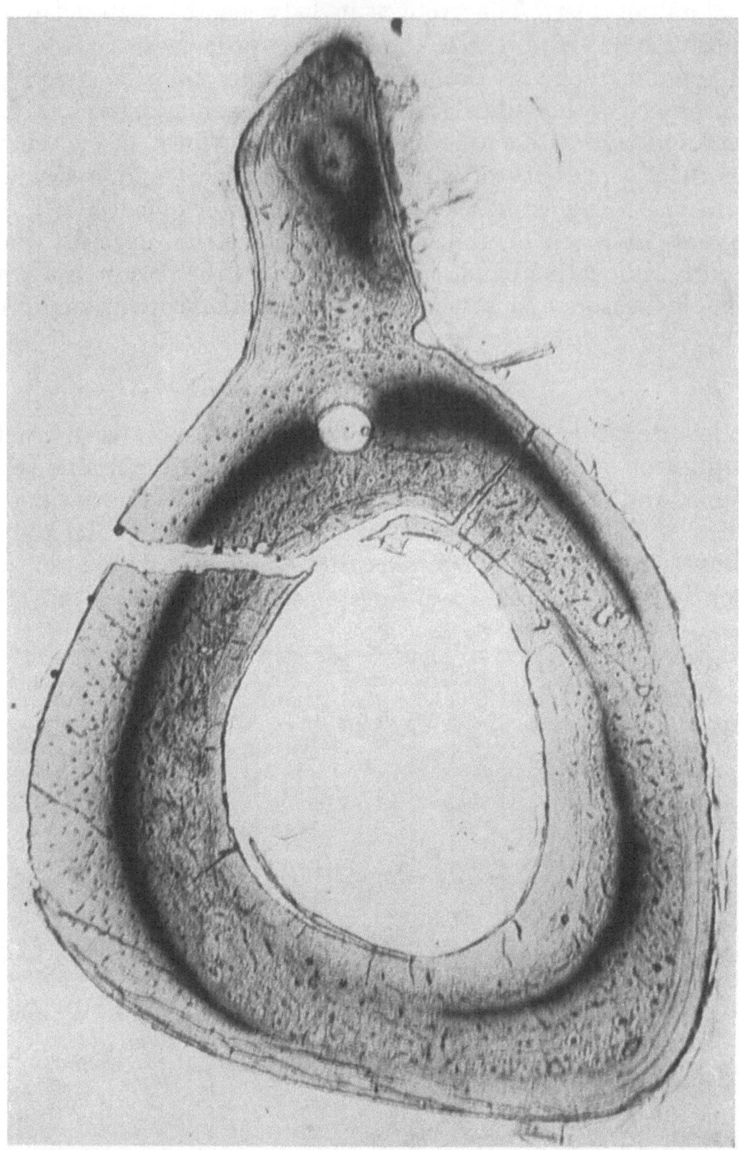

Fig. 12. Autoradiograph left on the cross section of the diaphysis of a tibia of a rabbit injected ^{90}Sr at five to seven weeks and sacrificed 24 weeks later. The remnants of the periosteal bone in the anterior wall and of the endosteal bone in the posterior wall formed directly after the isotope treatment are highly radioactive. The bone tissue more recently deposited at the periosteal and endosteal surface of the shaft does not show an appreciable radioactivity. [Courtesy of M. OWEN *et al.*, J. Bone Jt Surg. B **37**, 324—342 (1955)]

Remodeling of the form (1). The processes of resorption on the inner and outer aspect of the compacta in the diaphyseal and metaphyseal regions have been evidenced autoradiographically. The appearance in cross and longitudinal sections of the shaft may vary from bone to bone and in various mammals in connection with a different mechanism of growth of the shaft, viz., a more or less excentric transverse growth and more or less profound changes of its primitive shape (TOMLIN *et al.*, 1953). The distribution of the sites of concentration of the radiotracer in cross sections of the shaft may vary especially when the animal is sacrificed some time after administration of one single dose of the radioactive marker. In some sectors the more intense reaction may appear in the subperiosteal region if no apposition occurred in the interval of time passed from the injection; in other sectors the reactive layers may be buried in the intermediate or in the inner zone of the compacta and covered toward the periosteum by variously thick strata of bone tissue formed after radioisotope treatment. Where the transverse growth of the shaft is very excentric the reactive layers formed under the periosteum at the time of the injection may have been displaced inward toward the marrow cavity and disappeared in consequence of endosteal resorption in that sector (PONLOT, 1960) (Fig. 11). Similar evidences have been obtained with the use of radiostrontium in rabbit (OWEN *et al.*, 1955) (Fig. 12). Altogether, the autoradiographic pattern of diaphyseal growth coincides with the pattern that was already known from older experiments in which madder was used as a marker. Autoradiographic and alizarin techniques are fully complementary as shown in the study of skull bones growth in rodents (DIXON and HOYTE, 1959; DIXON, 1961). The metaphyses undergo the greatest remodeling during growth. The neck of the epiphysis widens faster than the diaphysis proper and the metaphyseal region acquires a funnel-like shape (LEBLOND *et al.*, 1950). This part of the bone is progressively reshaped through outer resorption and inner deposition of endosteal bone; thus the metaphyseal spicules which may enclose remnants of the calcified cartilage plate are embedded into the new-forming endosteal bone and may persist within the compacta during the further growth in length of the shaft. The increase in length of the diaphysis is due to a gradual remodeling and assimilation of the funnel regions. It has been suggested that a various extension of the funnel toward the diaphysis proper might depend on the mineral content of the diet: in rats fed on a low-Ca diet the funnel extended further into the diaphysis than it did in control rats fed on a high-Ca diet (TOMLIN *et al.*, 1953).

Processes of inner reconstruction (2). *Compact bone.* The reconstruction processes determine the formation in compacta of tunnel-like cavities mainly arranged according to the longitudinal axis of the shaft. The resorption cavities are progressively filled through concentric laying-down of bone matrix which undergoes calcification. Thus the secondary haversian systems or osteons (replacement osteons, according to LACROIX, 1960) are formed. The deposition occurs in two steps, viz., (1) formation of a PAS-positive layer, and (2) its transformation into a PAS-negative layer. The PAS-positive material, so-called preosseous layer or prebone, is orthochromatic, contains akaline phosphatese and takes up radiosulfate (VINCENT, 1954; ENGFELDT *et al.*, 1954; LACROIX, 1954, 1956; LEA and VAUGHAN, 1957). In the opinion of LEA and VAUGHAN, the ^{35}S present in the preosseous matrix is in a different chemical form to the ^{35}S present later in calcified bone tissue. Subsequently, when another layer of preosseous matrix is laid concentrically to the preexisting one, the latter takes up radiocalcium, its Roentgen-ray absorption increases rapidly, viz., it undergoes a rapid and high mineralization. Radiosulfate is incorporated in the bone matrix which is forming not in the material which is already calcified at the time of the ^{35}S-sulfate treatment. Radiosulfate seems thus to be a valuable marker for the evaluation of the rate of bone matrix formation in the process of bone reconstruction. According to VINCENT (1955) it takes about six weeks for an osteon of average size to be laid-down in the compacta of the adult dog.

^{32}P-phosphate is apparently incorporated in the bone tissue which is being deposited and also in the bone undergoing mineralization (ENGFELDT *et al.*, 1952). ^{45}Ca gets fixed exclusively to the bone matrix which undergoes calcification (ARNOLD, 1951; COMAR *et al.*, 1952; TOMLIN *et al.*, 1953). Also this process occurs in two steps: at first a rapid and heavy mineralization of the recently formed organic material then a much slower fixation of mineral takes place, as it has been shown by means of the method of study of the Roentgen-ray absorption (AMPRINO and ENGSTRÖM, 1952). According to VINCENT (1955) it may take more than three months for an osteon of the adult dog to reach its full mineralization. Till the optimal degree of calcification has been attained, the osteon takes up radiocalcium. A correlation seems to exist between the actual overall degree of calcification of each osteon and its radiocalcium uptake: the younger less calcified osteons fix a very large amount of radiocalcium per unit volume of tissue, they fix progressively less ^{45}Ca with the increase of the degree of mineralization (Fig. 13). In animals sacrificed a few days after ^{45}Ca injection the densest imprints *(hot spots)* of the autoradiographs correspond to the osteons which are not yet fully laid-down but have already started to calcify. From these to the less radioactive spots, imprints of different density correspond to osteons nearly completely laid-down or to completely laid-down but not yet fully mineralized systems (LACROIX, 1960). Also radiostrontium and radium concentrate in newforming and rapidly calcifying osteons (Fig. 14). JOWSEY *et al.* (1953)

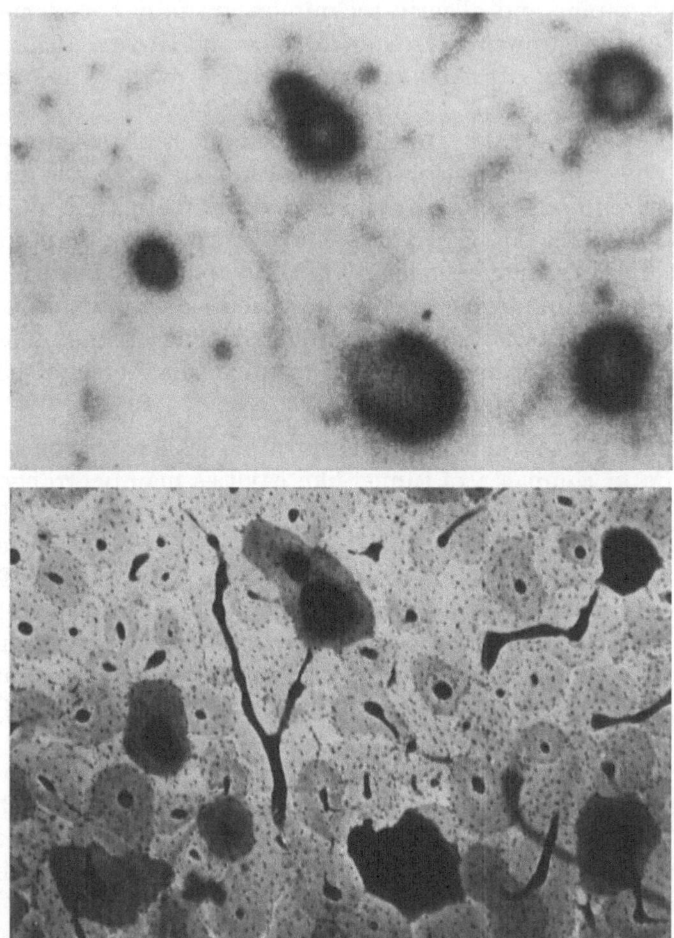

Fig. 13. Autoradiograph and microradiograph of a cross section of the compacta of a tibia of adult dog seven hours after ^{45}Ca injection. The highly radioactive areas are related to rapidly calcifying layers of bone tissue in forming osteons. The weaker spots correspond to the inner lamellae of older and nearly fully calcified osteons. (Courtesy of R. PONLOT, Le radiocalcium dans l'étude des os. Masson, 1960)

by the use of ^{90}Sr in monkeys sacrificed 24 hours after isotope administration showed that the densely radioactive zone of some osteons was separated from the lumen of the concentric systems by a narrow rim of much less reactive bone tissue, and they attribute the latter to bone matrix deposited when the blood level of the ^{90}Sr was already too low for a significant uptake. As it appears from the few examples reported, autoradiography after ^{45}Ca or radiostrontium treatment offers — much as historadiography (AMPRINO, 1952*c*; JOWSEY, 1960) — an easy means to investigate the time sequence in the formation of the osteons in compact bone.

Attempts have been made by various authors to assess quantitatively the differences of radioisotope fixation in newly formed and old bone tissue respectively. DUDLEY and DOBYNS (1949) measuring the radiation dosage distribution of ^{45}Ca in the bones of dogs found an average ratio of 10 to 1 between the activity of the most reactive areas (in the epiphyses) and the less reactive areas in the cortex of long bones. According to COHEN *et al.* (1957) the ratio between the specific activity in sites of high concentration of ^{45}Ca to the diffuse component specific activity in the compacta of dogs given one dose of radiocalcium averaged 20 to 1 but ranged from 12 to 1 to 35 to 1. The ^{32}P specific activity of recently laid-down endosteal bone may be occasionally 200 times that of the bone average in small mammals, as shown by WEIDMANN (1956). By means of quantitative autoradiography of the tibia cortex of growing rabbits sacrificed from one hour to three weeks after one dose

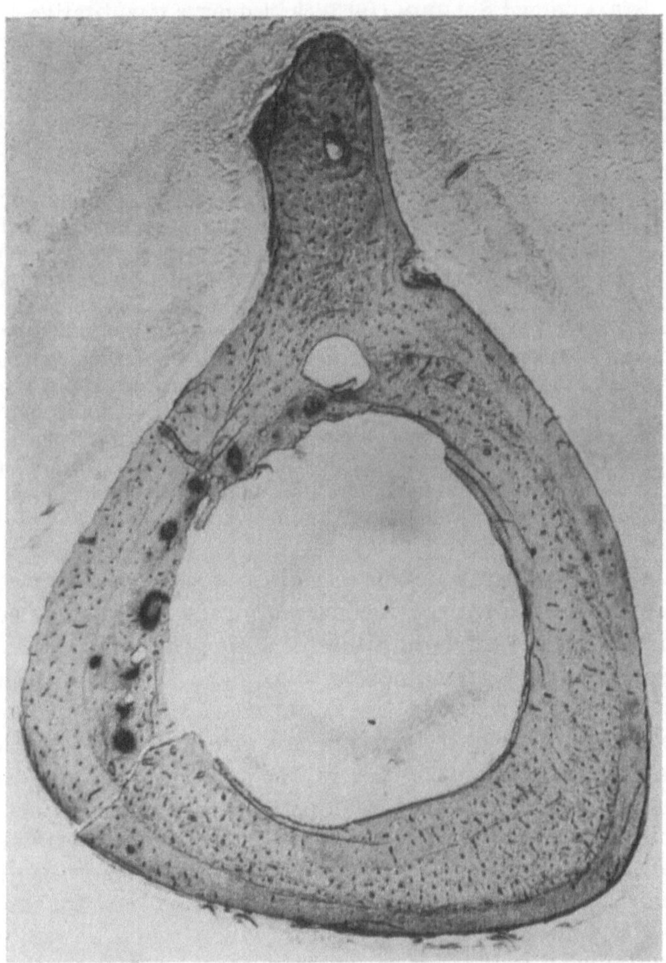

Fig. 14. Autoradiograph left on the cross section of the diaphysis of a tibia of rabbit injected ^{90}Sr when six-month old and sacrificed seventeen days later. Highly reactive osteons in the inner zone of compacta of the anterior wall of the shaft. [Courtesy of M. OWEN *et al.*, J. Bone Jt. Surg. B **37**, 324—347 (1955)]

of radiocalcium, ARNOLD *et al.* (1956) estimated the ratio of the radioactivity in newly formed osteons to that of fully calcified old primary bone. In the latter the distribution of the isotope appears rather uniform while forming osteons present a continuous distribution of avidity for ^{45}Ca up to 10 times that of old bone. The concentration of ^{45}Ca was five times greater on an average in new than in old bone and a slight increase in the ratio of the isotope concentration in new to old bone took place between one and 24 hours following ^{45}Ca treatment; from 24 hours to three weeks no further change was observed. Concentration changes were not recorded in the old bone during 21 days; the fixation of the isotope to old bone is virtually complete after one half to one hour from the isotope administration and apparently irreversible. In general, the intense ^{45}Ca concentration in forming osteons is limited to a few rapidly calcifying lamellae and not evenly distributed; the rate of deposition of the osteons appears to be higher during the formation of the outer half of each haversian system. In 21 days from 20 to 30% of the osteons which had started to form when the ^{45}Ca was injected completed their deposition (JEE and ARNOLD, 1954).

After *in vivo* administration of ^{45}Ca and ^{32}P to dogs, the rate of uptake in haversian systems isolated by means of a dissection technique in cross sections of compact bone was calculated. The rates of uptake showed a close correlation with the degree of mineralization studied by applying microchemical procedures. Only portions of periosteal and endosteal lamellar bone located close to the surfaces of the bone shafts showed higher rates of uptake, and the periosteal lamellar bone a higher rate than the endosteal lamellar bone although they had the same degree of mineralization. The uptake of ^{45}Ca and ^{32}P occurred in a proportion equal to the Ca/P ratio in bone tissue (STRANDH, 1961). The rate of ^{32}P uptake varied between 1.3 and 12×10^{-3}% P/hour (STRANDH and BENGTSSON, 1961*a*), and that of ^{45}Ca between 5.6 and 159×10^{-3}% Ca/hour in haversian systems (STRANDH and BENGTSSON, 1961*b*). STRANDH and SOLHEIM (1963) carried out a quantitative analysis of ^{32}P distribution in the various microscopical structures of the right and left 4th metacarpal bone taken from one dog at 8 and respectively 13 months of age, two days after ^{32}P injection. At the age of 8 months, the radiophosphorus uptake was found to be twice as high in highly mineralized periosteal and osteonic bone and 8 times as high in highly mineralized endosteal bone as at the age of 13 months. These age-dependent differences have been tentatively related to differences of vascularity and of bone tissue density.

MARSHALL *et al.* (1959a) measured in the autoradiographs the ^{45}Ca content of individual osteons in dogs given one dose of the isotope and correlated it with the diameter of their lumen. The formation of a resorption cavity would take approximately three weeks in the adult dog and an osteon may contain up to 10^{-6} of the injected activity, its total activity being nearly proportional to the square of its lumen diameter at the time of the injection. The calcium accretion rate per unit length in an osteon with a 100 μ diameter of the lumen has been evaluated in about 0.2 μg of calcium per millimeter/day. The same authors estimate that the mean time of bone turnover through resorption and osteon formation typical of the midshaft of long bones in a normal adult dog would be about 70 years (0.004% per day), but has been found to be 2.3 years (0.32% per day) in another adult dog. MARSHALL *et al.* (1959b) have also attempted to study the rate of osteon formation by means of autoradiography in serial sections after one injection of ^{45}Ca. In one middle-aged dog from 10 to 20 forming osteons were counted in one cross section of the shaft of a long bone and several hundred in a corresponding long bone cross section in a young adult dog. The most active regions of radiocalcium uptake had lengths of the order of one millimeter.

Altogether, the autoradiographic investigation has demonstrated the existance of conspicuous differences in the rate of reconstruction in the various sectors and levels of bone compacta, in the various skeletal pieces of a given individual, in subjects of various age. However, reconstruction seems not to take place at random; this well known fact has been pointed out again recently by LACROIX (1960): the various regions of each bone have a different stability and some are not attained by resorption for a long time. If radioactive material gets incorporated in the regions of bone whose reconstruction rate is comparatively low it may exert for a long time its harmful effect on the surrounding living matter. The mentioned variations of bone microscopical turnover can be at present analyzed very carefully by the use of a non-radioactive fluorescent marker, viz., the tetracycline antibiotics, which get fixed in the mineralizing parts of the skeleton (cf. MILCH *et al.*, 1958; FROST *et al.*, 1960; HARRIS, 1960). This method of study gives results very similar to those obtained by the use of autoradiography after radiocalcium treatment.

Spongy bone. As it has been known from older researches, the reconstruction processes in cancellous bone are qualitatively identical to those occurring in compact bone. The distribution of ^{45}Ca and ^{35}S seem to obey the same laws in both whole extremities of long bones compared with the diaphysis as an average. The over all rate of reconstruction is much higher in cancellous than in compact bone; ENGFELDT *et al.* (1954) from activity measurements of bone powder from long bones of young growing dogs treated with ^{35}S-sulfate estimate that the activity of the spongiosa is nearly twice that of the compacta. In cancellous as in compact bone the higher uptake of radiocalcium and radiostrontium occurs in the younger, less mineralized structures. The rate of reconstruction seems to be higher in the metaphyses proper than in the epiphyses (Fig. 15).

The ^{45}Ca specific activity of the extremities of an adult dog bone are, according to LACROIX (1960), from 2 to 3 times higher than that of the diaphysis. Such differences are already detectable during the period of growth of the long bone and they seem not to undergo changes in a period of over 6 months in the adult rabbit (LONTIE, 1953). BAUER (1954*a*, 1954*b*) maintains that the ratio of the ^{45}Ca specific activities of diaphyseal to epiphyseal bone in young rats undergoes a progressive increase from below to above unity in a period of two months; with time, the specific activity of the extremity of long bones which undergoes a more rapid elongation becomes lower than that of the opposite end of the same bone. The redistribution of the isotope in different parts of the skeleton seems thus to vary with the rate of growth of these parts.

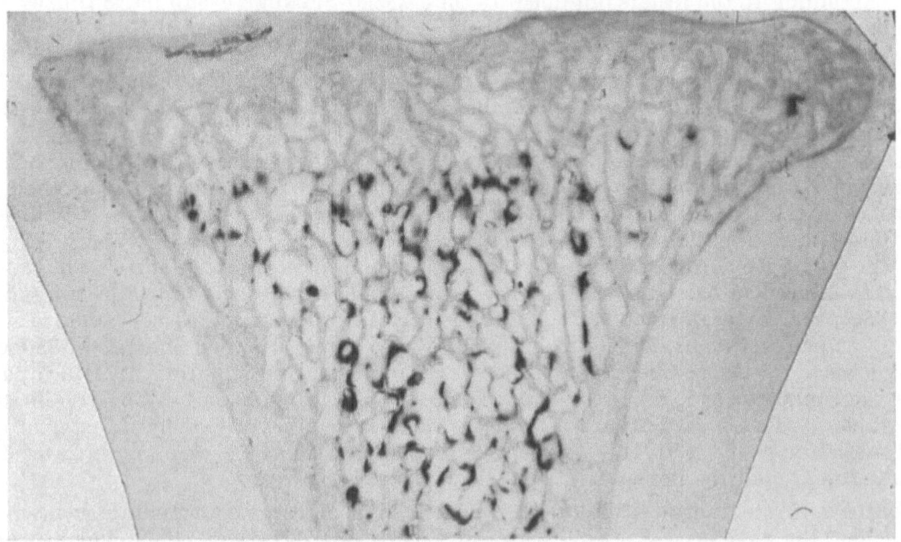

Fig. 15. Autoradiograph of a longitudinal section of the upper end of the tibia of an adult dog seven days after injection of ^{45}Ca. Radioactive bone in the trabecular network of the metaphysis not of the epiphysis proper. (Courtesy of P. LACROIX, by permission of Bone structure and metabolism, Ciba Foundation Symposium, ed. by G. E. W. WOLSTENHOLME and C. M. O'CONNOR. Churchill Ltd., 1956)

d) Distribution and redistribution of radioactive elements in the skeleton

The site of fixation of radioisotopes in the skeleton greatly depends on the distribution pattern and the rate of bone growth and remodelling; it varies according to the species, the body size and age of the individual, the type of bone and the time interval from the administration of the isotope, not in connection with the route of introduction of the radioactive element in the body. The distribution in general is much more uniform in the fetal period (cf. PLUMLEE *et al.*, 1952) than in young or mature postnatal life; this should depend on the more uniform structure of the fetal than of the adult bone.

Altogether, all radioactive substances fall into two patterns of distribution in the skeleton: (1) calcium, phosphorus, strontium, radium, etc. are primarily deposited in areas of active bone growth, below the epiphyseal plate in the primary spongiosa, under the periosteum and endosteum, in forming and calcifying haversian systems, in the spongiosa of the vertebrae, of the metaphyses of long bones. A lower concentration of these elements is distributed in a diffuse manner throughout the whole skeleton. (2) Plutonium, thorium, mesothorium, yttrium, etc. localize preferentially on endosteal surfaces and on the wall of the vascular channels in compacta. ^{91}Y for instance concentrates in rabbit bone in the sites of trabecular bone growth beneath the epiphyses but not beneath the endosteum and periosteum and in a patchy way in the shaft in association with the connective tissue around blood vessels (RAYNER *et al.*, 1953; RAMSDEN, 1961).

The distribution of radionuclides in the skeleton undergoes changes with time, viz., a *redistribution* takes place of the fraction of the isotope retained by the skeleton which is set free through resorption from the regions of bone which previously held it, it reenters circulation but is not excreted from the body and is incorporated again in bone. Through reconstruction, therefore, a various concentration of radioactive material is fixed to bone tissue in relation to the specific activity of the isotope in the blood. The final distribution of the radioactive element in the skeleton long time after its introduction into the body may be rather different from that which is observed a few hours or a few days after treatment.

A few more detailed informations on the fate of ^{45}Ca, ^{85}Sr, ^{226}Ra in the human skeleton will be reported. According to the results obtained by the LASZLO-SPENCER group (cf. SHULERT *et al.*, 1959) on terminal cancer patients, ^{85}Sr and ^{45}Ca given simultaneously in tracer amount in a single dose show an almost identical distribution. The isotopes are nearly equally distributed between bone and soft tissues during the first few days; 4 months after administration more than 99% of the isotopes retained in the body is in the skeleton. The greater retention was found in vertebrae and ribs, the lowest in the diaphysis of long bones and in cranial bones. The concentration of the isotopes varies in each bone; even in a flat bone like a rib the concentration of ^{85}Sr was found to decrease more than twice from the sternal end to the axillary region. The concentration varied also in the various zones of the femoral cortex at different time intervals from the isotope administration. In a man exposed to radium intake for 34 years with a terminal mean skeletal burden less than 0.3 μg radium, the distribution resulted to be very uneven in the skeleton (HINDMARSH and VAUGHAN, 1956): Ra was concentrated almost entirely in osteons, in periosteal and endosteal bone and in calcified joint cartilage, the trabecular bone of the head of a metacarpal examined contained less Ra than in other sites. In one section of the femur only 25% of 335 highly calcified and 7% of 880 less calcified osteons contained Ra; a similar distribution was found in a section from a metacarpal. LOONEY (1955) in the compact bone of humans from 25 to 40 years after use of radioactive material found that the values of Ra concentration in a number of bone samples varied by a factor of two and respectively of six and of ten in three patients; in some instances Ra was concentrated in only one or two lamellae around the lumen or at the periphery of the osteons.

The pattern of retention of Radium, and the doses in microscopic volumes of bone in the human and canine skeleton have been studied, i.a., by ROWLAND and MARSHALL (1959) and ROWLAND (1961). Dosimetry results in different parts of the skeleton of young and adult rabbits given an injection of $^{90}Sr + ^{90}Y$ and sacrificed at different times, have been reported by OWEN (1962). An experimental and theoretical study made by ROWLAND (1962) aims to offer a method for calculating the concentration of an alkaline earth radioisotope existing in a given site of the skeleton at any previous time from a terminal autoradiograph from which the quantity of the isotope per unit mass of bone in the same site has been determined. Moreover, a method of specific gravity fractionation has been proposed for the quantitative evaluation of the distribution of bone-seeking radioisotopes in the skeleton (HERMAN and RICHELLE, 1961). Samples of ground bone are separated by centrifugation into fractions of different specific weight: bone particles should not exceed 5 micra. As the isotope uptake in calcified tissues appears to be approximately an inverse exponential function of the degree of calcification of the tissue, the method may enable a closer direct analysis of the distribution pattern of, e.g., radiocalcium in the various bone structures after *in vivo* administration of the tracer and under normal as well as experimental conditions (cf. LEMAIRE, 1966).

e) Bone repair and transplantation

The use of radioisotope tracers in fractured bones has served so far to confirm the uneven distribution of the bone-seeking radionuclides, viz., their preferential concentration in areas of active bone formation but might represent in the future an easy and valuable tool in the investigation of the capacity for regeneration in the fracture sites by external counting methods (cf. pag. 828). Most of the work has been done experimentally on small mammals with the use of ^{35}S, ^{32}P and ^{45}Ca.

In fractured bones of albino rats given ^{35}S-sulfate 24 hours before sacrifice, the metachromatic matrix laid down under the periosteum adjacent to the fracture area contains radiosulfate within 48 hours from the fracturing; the radiosulfate uptake increases till the seventh day in parallel with the formation of the periosteal and medullary cartilaginous callus. The distribution of ^{35}S may be correlated to the localization of alkaline phosphatase in the newforming chondrogenic and osteogenic tissues, but the presence of alkaline phosphatase seems not to be necessary for the earlier phases of chondroitinsulfuric acid metabolism (DUTHIE and BARKER, 1955*b*). In rats about six weeks of age treated with ^{32}P and ^{35}S when the bones are fractured, the same authors (1955*a*) did not observe any preferential uptake of ^{35}S in the healing fracture site over 28 days while the sulfate metabolism of the epiphyseal plate of the fractured bone appeared normal. This failure to show a greater sulfate incorporation in the fracture area has been related to the early lack of blood supply in the fracture region because of hematoma formation; when the blood vessels invade this area the ^{35}S blood level is probably already too low for an autoradiographically detectable uptake of the isotope.

In the fractured humerus of adult rats the radiosulfate incorporation of bone proper would be 2.2 times higher as in intact bone; according to OSBORNE and KOWALEWSKI (1956) the uptake is limited to an area immediately adjacent to the fracture site. ^{32}P is deposited in the fracture site in two phases (DUTHIE and BARKER, 1955*a*); during the first 48 hours the uptake is diffuse, at 17 days there follows another increased deposition of radiophosphate which accompanies the first radiographic appearance in bony union. BOHR (1955) studied the uptake of ^{32}P at various intervals from one week to one year after fracturing in the mid-diaphysis the rat femur. A marked increase of the uptake was observed not only at the fracture site but also in the extremities of the femur and to a lesser degree in the adjacent epiphysis of the tibia; the increase in the epiphyses was limited to the first eight weeks while it was detectable six months after fracturing in the fracture site. In the latter region the vascularity seemed to be an important factor of the high ^{32}P uptake. However, the ^{32}P fixation seems to be indipendent of the degree of fracture healing: fractures with good and poor healing showed the same rate of bone formation though resorption was increased in fractures which failed to heal.

Also CARTIER *et al.* (1956) maintain that the bone salt formation in the repair of femoral fractures in adult rats studied with the use of ^{32}P is accomplished in two steps, viz., during the first 20 days the uptake is small and it increases rapidly from the 20th to the 25th day on; 75% of the full mineralization is attained in the successive ten day. In the ends of the fractured bone a 20% of the ^{32}P content was recorded in the first ten days after fracturing; then demineralization starts in the extremities and in the diaphysis at some distance from the fracture site to reach a value of — 30% toward the 25th day in parallel with the rapid calcification of the callus. Later the mineralization increases and a normal phosphorus content is attained at the stage of bony union. According to CARTIER *et al.*, the existance of an increase of excretion in stools and urine of radiophosphorus previously fixed to the skeleton, would indicate that the evolution of a fracture does not unfold as a merely local process but with a more general participation of the whole skeleton.

RUF (1955) showed that the specific activity of the ^{45}Ca in the blood of rabbit decreases from the time of fracturing during five days and increases again to a steady but lower value till healing is complete. Reciprocally, an increased uptake of ^{45}Ca occurs in the fracture site from the fourth day and reaches its maximum between 12 to 15 days in the rabbit (RUF, l.c.), during the second or third week from fracture in the rat (LEMAIRE, 1966); when the callus is resorbed the ^{45}Ca uptake returns to normal values though the ^{45}Ca activity of the fractured bone remains high for a long time. In mature rats injected ^{45}Ca one week after fracturing one femur, BAUER (1954*c*) could determine from the Ca content and radioactivity of the blood serum and of various portions of long bones the rate of bone salt formation during the healing process. Bone is more quickly resorbed in the metaphyses of the fractured than of the intact femur and changes of bone turnover take place also in the tibia of the fractured side (cf. BAUER and CARLSSON, 1955). The rate of bone mineral formation in the seven-day callus was evaluated by BAUER (1954*c*) to 0.04 mg Ca per hour; the newly laid-down bone tissue of the callus would persist four to five days before undergoing resorption. If a mixture of ^{45}Ca, ^{35}S and ^{91}Y is injected into rats bearing tibial fractures at various stage of repair from 3 to 18 days and the distribution of the isotopes is studied 24 hours after injection (MACDONALD et al., 1957) it appears that the injured bone takes up more of the three isotopes than the contralateral bone up to the tenth day; but the maximum 24 hours retention declines rapidly for ^{35}S, does not undergo detectable changes for ^{91}Y and continues to rise though at a reduced rate for ^{45}Ca after the tenth day. These facts show that ^{35}S and ^{91}Y are fixed in the formation of the fibrocartilaginous callus and of the bone matrix, ^{45}Ca is taken up during the mineralization process.

The reaction of the periosteal cell population to bone fracture has been studied in some detail by TONNA and CRONKITE (1961*b*, 1962*b*, 1964) with the use of ^{3}H-thymidine. In the femur of mice, the cell proliferation commences 16 hours after fracture in the periosteum and adjacent soft tissues, and it extends along the entire shaft. The maximum increase in the labeled cell population in the periosteum (25% ca) was recorded at 32 hours; 14 days after fracture, the labeled population is still above the control values. An increased cell proliferation with DNA synthesis as the one depending on bone fracture or disruption of the periosteum, is elicited by extraperiosteal injection of saline, serum or whole blood. The differences in the proliferative response of the periosteum of the fractured femur recorded in 18-month-old and young growing mice is merely quantitative.

Radioisotopes have been applied also in the study of the mineral turnover of pieces of bone auto- and homoplastically transplanted. RUF (1955) carried out an extensive analysis in rabbits by means of ^{45}Ca and ^{32}P: fresh bone grafts show an increase of the ^{32}P uptake already from the second week to three months after transplantation. The uptake is higher in heteroplastic than in homoplastic grafts; a much lesser increment in the ^{32}P incorporation was recorded from grafts preserved in autologous blood or kept at low temperature. Fresh autogenous grafts implanted intramuscularly in dogs take up five times as much ^{32}P as do boiled grafts and twice as much as frozen bone (ODELL *et al.*, 1951). Fresh grafts of iliac bone inserted subcutaneously in dogs incorporate in the first 24 hours 60 % of the ^{32}P which gets fixed in the same time to the intact control ilium; after ten days the percentage tends to increase. Boiled grafts show an uptake of only 7 % and frozen grafts would take up nearly as much ^{32}P as fresh grafts (KIEHN *et al.*, 1948). From experiments of grafting on rat bones with the use of ^{90}Sr RAY *et al.* (1955) come to the conclusion that the viability of bone cells seems not essential in the process of inorganic salt incorporation in bone when is well preserved the normal organic matrix; therefore, the uptake of radioisotopes cannot be considered a reliable index of bone cell viability. The mobilization of the inorganic salt from bone is, on the contrary, favored by the presence of living cells.

COHEN *et al.* (1957, 1962) studied the fate of homogenous bone grafts in dogs by implanting (1) perfrigerated (—20° C) radioactive bone from donors previously injected one dose of ^{45}Ca, and (2) perfrigerated non-radioactive bone into hosts injected with one dose ^{45}Ca before, during or after the operation. The Ca of the radioactive grafts entered the blood and was apparently redistributed in a manner similar to that of the Ca entering the blood from other sources; no evidence was found for a local preferential transfer of Ca to the surrounding callus from the graft or from the bone regions adjacent to the graft site. In dogs receiving nonradioactive grafts and treated with ^{45}Ca, the specific activity of the bone callus was over 100 times that of the diffuse component of the host cortical bone, and depended on the relation between time of injection and time of grafting. The callus formed apparently with the same ^{45}Ca specific activity as that of the blood serum during the period of deposition, i. e., when the serum specific activity is higher than the average specific activity of cortical bone. Similar conclusions were drawn by URIST *et al.* (1958) from a study of bone grafts taken from animals previously given ^{45}Ca, ^{90}Sr and ^{91}Y: during resorption of the graft no concentration of the isotope was observed locally in the callus forming about the graft.

f) Vitamins and bone

Vitamin A. The uptake of radiosulfate and radiophosphate by femurs and tibiae of vitamin A-deficient rats is less than in normal controls and it increases following vitamin A administration. The incorporation of radiosulfate is particularly enhanced in the epiphyseal cartilage, that of radiophosphorus in the metaphyseal trabeculae subjacent to the cartilage plate. The specific activity of the ^{35}S in the chondroitinsulfate extracted from the skeleton of vitamin A-deficient rats decreases progressively as the deficiency continues to increase up over the normal value following administration of vitamin A (DZIEWIATKOWSKI, 1954*b*); this observations suggests an influence of vitamin A on the synthesis of chondroitinsulfate (DZIEWIATKOWSKI, 1958).

Vitamin D. The rate of synthesis of chondroitinsulfate in bone of rachitic rats is similar to the rate in normal control animals. In vitamin D-deficient rats there seems to be an impairment of the utilization of chondroitinsulfate; administration of vitamin D accelerates the latter process. In rickets the rate of break-down of the mature cartilage cells is poor, therefore the epiphyseal plate increases in thickness (DZIEWIATKOWSKI, 1954*c*). The skeleton in rachitic animals contains less mineral. This may depend on a defective intestinal absorption of Ca; in fact, parenteral administration of Ca in sufficient amount may maintain bone formation in proportion to the rate of body growth. When vitamin D is given to rachitic animals injected with radiocalcium, radiophosphorus or radiosulfate there is a rapid rise in the uptake of the isotope in bone; however, according to HARRISON and HARRISON (1950) the increment of the mineral metabolism of the skeleton under these conditions seems to be independent from the Ca intestinal absorption which is enhanced by vitamin D treatment. The distribution of radiocalcium is altogether very similar in the normal and rachitic animal, though in the latter the fixation rate is considerably lower (five times lower in rats, according to MILHAUD *et al.*, 1960). The decrease in the ossification process seems to be the same in the whole skeleton, but the calcium content of the various bones is unevenly reduced: in the skull it is nearly normal while in the ends of long bones it is less then one half of the normal amount. A rapid uptake of radiostrontium in the skeleton occurs in the rachitic as in normal young rats, but in the former a rapid elimination through urine of the isotope accumulated in bone takes place within the first 24 hours (JONES and COPP, 1951). BAUER *et al.* (1957) maintain that bone salt accretion rate in children affected by resistant rickets studied by means of ^{140}Ba before treatment with vitamin D is nearly the same as in normal children (i.e., 1.20 gm Ca/day); after treatment with high doses it rises to about five times this value. In deficient rickets studied with P^{32} the accretion rate of bone salt is lower than in normal children of the same age; vitamin D restores the accretion rate of bone salt to normal (BAUER *et al.*, 1956). According to BAUER *et al.* (1955) even in physiological doses vitamin D has a pronounced stimulating influence on bone resorption; CARLSSON and LINDQUIST (1955) have shown that in young rats the intestinal absorption of Ca is increased in the same degree by the administration of 10 as of 1.000 I.U. of vitamin D, but the effect on bone resorption is much more marked after the higher dose. BOHR (1961) observed that the uptake of ^{47}Ca and ^{85}Sr in bone during the first hour after injection is the same in normal and in vitamin D deficient rats, although the activity in the latter decreases within 8 hours to about half the maximal value. The primary uptake would thus depend on a reversible exchange between blood and bone tissue; accretion would take place through a secondary, slower uptake.

The calcifying influence of vitamin D as detectable through increase of radiocalcium uptake in the skeleton has been shown also in the healing of fractures in rachitic and osteoporotic bone (RUF, 1955). An interesting finding was observed by KODICEK (1956): tracer experiments made with ^{14}C-tagged vitamin D injected to rats showed that bones contained 4% of the administered ^{14}C; about half of this activity was present as vitamin D.

Long bone autoradiographs of rachitic rats given [1α-^{3}H] vitamin D by mouth, show the label in the cytoplasm of metabolizing flattened chondrocytes of the metaphyseal plate. Little or no radioactivity was found in the older, hypertrophic chondrocytes in the zone where mineralization occurs. No radioactivity was detected in osteoblasts and osteoclasts (KODICEK and THOMPSON, 1965).

g) Hormones and bone

Thyroxine. It is known that a deficient secretion of the thyroid gland results in retardation of growth and development in young animals. DZIEWIATKOWSKI (1957) has shown that the synthesis of sulfomucopolysaccharides is probably depressed in thyroidectomized rats and in rats in which the thyroid is made non-functional by a single dose of ^{131}I. Daily administration of 5 to 10 γ of I-thyroxine in these animals favors an increase of the ^{35}S sulfate incorporated into the chondroitinsulfate of the skeleton. The decremental rate of ^{35}S concentration in cartilage is slower in thiouracil-treated and faster in thyroxine-treated animals. A nearly 100% increase of pre-osteoblasts was observed in young rats receiving thyroxine and given a dose of ^{3}H-thymidine 40 minutes before sacrifice (UEHLINGER, 1965).

Parathyroid hormone. Its precise action on bone tissue has not been elucidated through radiotracer studies, but several interesting new data have been acquired on changes of bone mineral metabolism affected by this hormone. TALMAGE *et al.* (1953) showed autoradiographically that more ^{32}P than ^{45}Ca is removed from the metaphyseal trabeculae of long bones in rats under the influence of parathyroid extract. ^{32}P but not ^{45}Ca is removed from young sheep long bones after five to seven days of parathyroid extract administration: the serum level of phosphate undergoes an increment not that of Ca. ^{32}P is taken from the primary spongiosa subjacent to the epiphyseal plate and from the endochondral bone of the metaphyseal funnel (LOTZ *et al.*, 1954). According to WHITEHEAD and WEIDMANN (1959) parathormone reduces the uptake of ^{32}P in all the districts of the skeleton in young kittens but its effect is greater in the areas with a high specific activity. Also the incorporation of ^{32}P into cartilage adenosine-triphosphate is reduced by the hormonal treatment. Parathyroid hormone modifies the renewal of bone phosphate (^{32}P) in rats and dogs through an acceleration of the normal process of bone destruction: in young animals the rate of renewal of phosphate in the skeleton is decreased, while is increased in old animals. The ratio between resorption of newly formed and old bone tissue seems to be the same as in normal animals; the overall decrease in the amount of bone tissue would lead to an increased rate of bone formation, which is less apparent in young animals because the increased destruction covers a proportionally larger amount of newly formed bone in comparison to the older animals (ENGFELDT and ZETTERSTRÖM, 1954). Also according to WEIKEL and NEUMAN (1961) a prolonged administration of parathyroid hormone to adult rats fed a diet of constant ^{45}Ca specific activity for protracted periods, despite an increased bone resorption, does not affect materially the level of skeletal radioactivity. The bone mineral would be formed at a growth rate near to or greater than the normal but resorbed under the stimulus of PTH.

JOWSEY *et al.* (1958) have beautifully shown by the use of radiocalcium that in the compacta of parathyroidectomized adult dogs the rate of reconstruction is reduced, though resorption is not completely prevented. The increased bone resorption determined in female dogs by pregnancy and lactation is reduced by parathyroidectomy; however, under the latter conditions the incidence of resorption is still from three to four times that found in the parathyroidectomized male. According to BRONNER (1957), though the level of ^{35}S in the blood, urine and stools increases after parathormone treatment, no difference of the ^{35}S content is detectable in the skeleton in comparison with the normal conditions. Chemical analysis shows that administration of parathyroid extract to immature rats induces a higher than normal metabolic activity through bone resorption and formation in the end of long bones expressed by a 14% increase in the ratio between the ^{35}S content of the humerus ends and shaft; in these animals the ^{35}S plasma level increases about 30%, the increase in the excretion of ^{35}S in urine and pelts is respectively 25% and 17% higher than in control litter mates (BRONNER, 1960, 1961, 1962).

Parathyroid extract administered before, with or after ^{35}S-sulfate would enhance the incorporation of sulfate into the mucopolysaccharides of rachitic cartilage and its subsequent release; this evidence seems in favour of the view that the action of the hormone on bone is mediated by its direct or indirect influence on the metabolism of bone mucopolysaccharides (BERNSTEIN and HANDLER, 1958). SHETLAR *et al.* (1961) hold the view that parathormone increases the release of sulfated mucopolysaccharides, mainly chondroitinsulfate, probably through cellular activity. In *in vitro* conditions, PTE would depress the uptake of ^{14}C-glycine in fragments of rat metaphyseal bone and its incorporation into hexosamine of the matrix (HENNEMAN, 1966).

Some evidence has been offered of the fact that parathyroid extract may induce demineralization of stable bone. This was shown through a rise in the excretion of ^{45}Ca determined by hormone injection long time after ^{45}Ca treatment, viz., when all the skeletal ^{45}Ca had already been buried in fully mineralized, unavailable bone (WOODS and ARMSTRONG, 1956). A similar view has been advanced by ELLIOTT and TALMAGE (1958; cf. also TALMAGE and ELLIOTT, 1958) who maintain that endogenous parathyroid hormone — as well as near-physiological levels of citric acid — apparently mobilize calcium from the deep areas of bone mineral and not from those which come into contact with radiocalcium during the first 24 hours after its administration. This action should be mediated through metabolic processes in bone cells which enable calcium to be dissolved in concentration greater than the solubility of apatite crystals. In this connection, BRONNER (1957) and other authors (v.s.) maintain that parathormone favours rather resorption of recently deposited bone mineral at the metaphyseal level of long bones in growing animals. RICHELLE and BRONNER (1963) have more recently shown that the percentage of *in vitro* exchangeable calcium in bone samples from rats treated with PTE increases in comparison to normal controls; they hypothesize that this may depend on an alteration of the normal relationships between bone organic matrix and mineral which would take place prior to osteoclastic resorption of high density bone. On the other hand, GORDON (1963) has advanced the suggestion that PTE-induced release of radiocalcium from boiled, dried ^{45}Ca-labeled adult mouse bone in the presence of human serum albumin, as well as the osteolytic activity apparently exerted by sera from patients with hyperparathyroidism could be the result of a binding of divalent cations by an albumin-parathyroid peptide complex.

As to the activity of parathormone on bone cells, YOUNG (1963) has shown by his beautiful autoradiographic work that when treatment with PTE immediately follows ^{3}H-thymidine administration to young rats, specialization of osteoprogenitor cells appears to be chiefly oriented to formation of osteoclasts. If administration of labeled-thymidine is withheld until the maximum histological effect of PTE has been obtained, specialization of osteoprogenitor cells during the recovery phase seems almost entirely directed toward osteoblast formation. In this phase, osteoclasts also would be capable of reversion to the osteoprogenitor state. TALMAGE (1966) from an autoradiographic study with the use of ^{3}H-cytidine concludes that one of the actions of parathormone is to increase the rate of bone resorption through the stimulation of the rate of formation of osteoclasts not deriving from osteoblasts. However, this effect on bone cells would not be necessarily correlated with the calcium homeostatic function of the hormone.

Calcitonin. Evidence for the existance of a new plasma calcium lowering hormone, called calcitonin, was first offered by COPP *et al.* (1962). Originally thought of parathyroid origin, its production from the thyroid (parafollicular, C-cells) was later demonstrated (cf. FOSTER *et al.*, 1964). It has been extracted so far from the thyroid of rat, rabbit, pig, goat, cow, dog, monkey and man. Injection of this hormone, now called thyrocalcitonin, produces a marked and rapid drop in plasma calcium and phosphate. Bone seems to be the site of action as it has been shown that thyrocalcitonin causes radiocalcium uptake by perfused isolated bone (MACINTYRE *et al.*, 1967), and a shift toward bone production and/or inhibition of resorption of long bone rudiments of mouse embryos cultivated *in vitro* (GAILLARD, 1966).

Estradiol. High doses of estrogens affect the bone turnover to a various extent and through different mechanisms from species to species. An autoradiographic analysis of the proximal ends of tibiae from immature rats given estradiol benzoate and injected with ^{35}S-sulfate at weekly intervals or ^{45}Ca-chloride shows that both ^{35}S and ^{45}Ca are deposited in strata in higher amount than normal. The autoradiographic stratification of ^{35}S in the metaphysis is evidence of its periodic administration. The last dose of ^{35}S given 24 hours before sacrifice is not autoradiographically detectable in the metaphysis: the trabecular network adjacent to the epiphyseal plate has taken up very little ^{35}S while it is heavily tagged in the case of ^{45}Ca administration. The different arrangement of ^{35}S and respectively of ^{45}Ca labeled strata suggests that most of the ^{35}S in the metaphysis is derived from the chondroitinsulfate of the epiphyseal plate replaced by the metaphyseal bone (DZIEWIATKOWSKI et al., 1957). If estradiol benzoate is administered weekly and ^{35}S given 24 hours before sacrifice, no ^{35}S is detectable in the metaphyseal spongiosa and the activity of the epiphyseal plate is slightly weaker than that of litter mate controls. A high single dose of estradiol benzoate (e.g., 10 mg) and repeated weekly doses of ^{35}S-sulfate give the same autoradiographic pattern as when 2 mg of estradiol benzoate and

^{35}S-sulfate are administered weekly. A single 10 mg dose of 17-β-estradiol valerate does not inhibit the resorption of the metaphyseal spongiosa (DZIEWIATKOWSKI, 1958).

^{45}Ca kinetic and autoradiographic studies in estrogen-treated immature rats (0.5 mg estradiol n-valerate weekly) indicate according to LINDQUIST *et al.* (1960) a 50% reduction in the rate of resorption of the upper end of the tibia; however, the resorption seems not to be greatly affected by estradiol treatment in the regions of bone which undergo extensive growth and remodeling. According to SIMMONS (1963), the primary effect of estradiol in the metaphysis of young growing mice is the stimulation of undifferentiated bone marrow cells to form osteoblasts: an increased population of ^{3}H-thymidine-labeled mitotic osteoblasts has been detected autoradiographically in sites of endochondral ossification during two weeks after estrogen treatment. An increase over 100% of the preosteoblasts was recorded after one week treatment in two-month-old male rats (UEHLINGER, 1965).

A 7 to 8 times higher uptake of ^{32}P takes place in the medullary than in the cortical bone of estrogenized male pigeons (GOVAERTS and DALLEMAGNE, 1948, and others). Similarly, the ^{45}Ca uptake in medullary bone of egg-laying fowls is nearly 10 times greater than in cortical segments of the femur and tibia (HURWITZ, 1965): the femur first takes up then it releases more radiocalcium than tibia.

The ^{45}Ca uptake in pigeons bones, especially in the femur, after daily injection of estrogen occurs not only in the newly laid-down medullary bone but also in the old cortical bone; the rate of replacement of the Ca in the diaphysis is increased. The same behaviour is apparent in the tibia, not in the other bones. The equilibrium between the ^{45}Ca specific activity of blood and of bone is attained much more rapidly in the femur and tibia of pigeons treated with estrogen than in control pigeons. Estradiol enhances the mineral metabolism also when given in supplementary doses to pigeons in spontaneous sexual activity (DALLEMAGNE *et al.*, 1950). The excretion of ^{45}Ca is decreased in estradiol-treated pigeons and the overall retention of ^{45}Ca increased (GOVAERTS *et al.*, 1951). In hens treated with Nicarbazin, which prevents ovulation and egg-shell formation, the percentage of exchangeable calcium in femur ends, cortical and medullary segments was evaluated at 3.3, 0.5, and 5.2% respectively. Results of a long-term radiocalcium feeding indicate that in a 12-day period at least 70% of calcium was replaced in the medullary bone (HURWITZ, 1965). Nearly 4.5 g of the skeletal calcium participate in the egg-shell formation in laying hens, and about 1 g is turned over daily (MUELLER *et al.*, 1964). The size of the exchangeable calcium pool seems related to the quantity of egg-shell produced, and it is larger in pullets with a negative than with a positive calcium balance.

Testosterone appears to increase the uptake of ^{35}S by costal cartilage grafted to hypophysectomized rats; thus it would act sinergistically with growth hormone (cf. further on). Castration seems to decrease the uptake of ^{35}S, but treatment with testosterone does not exert a significant effect on bone ^{35}S uptake of normal and castrated animals. ^{35}S uptake would be increased instead in the healing fractured bones of normal and castrated rats treated with synthetic 17-ethyl, 19-nortestosterone (cf. GESCHWIND, 1961).

Growth hormone. Hypophysectomy in young rats decreases the uptake of ^{32}P by the skeleton: the concentration of P in bone ash is not different from normal, but the ash content of whole bone is decreased. The concentration of plasma ^{32}P is higher in the operated than in the normal animal. This effect on P appears to be accompanied by effects on renal tubular transport and on transport of phosphate from the extracellular to the intracellular fluid compartments. Also the high ^{45}Ca serum level of the hypophysectomized rat seems related to a decreased radiotracer uptake by bone. ^{32}P bone uptake increases to normal levels after administration of growth hormone to the hypophysectomized rat, especially in the growing metaphyseal region of the bone shaft (GESCHWIND *et al.*, 1951; GESCHWIND, 1961).

Following growth hormone administration, the relative ^{35}S specific activity of the costal cartilage of the hypophysectomized animals increases three- to five-fold (ELLIS *et al.*, 1953). The same behaviour has been shown in the costal cartilage transplanted subcutaneously in the hypophysectomized rat (BERGENSTAL *et al.*, quoted by GESCHWIND, 1961). Incorporation of radiosulfate into cartilage of growing rats is greatly reduced by hypophysectomy, and restored by growth hormone administration. Whether the reduced sulfate uptake after hypophysectomy can be restored by growth hormone not only *in vivo* but in *in vitro* conditions as well, is still a matter of discussion although evidence has been produced in favour of the view that growth hormone controls a serum factor which stimulates the *in vitro* sulfate incorporation by cartilage. In fact, increased uptake of ^{35}S-sulfate by rudiments of 9-day chick embryo femur maintained several days *in vitro* on a medium containing physiological concentrations of growth hormone has been observed; overdoses would, however, inhibit growth and radiosulfate incorporation of the explant (ITO *et al.*, 1960).

An autoradiographic study with the use of ^{3}H-thymidine has defined the distribution and the percentage of dividing chondrocytes in the epiphyseal plate and joint cartilage of the proximal tibial end in growth-hormone-treated hypophysectomized compared with normal control rats (ASLING and NELSON, 1962). This analysis provides rigorous conditions for the demonstration of the proliferation-inducing ability of the hormone in endochondral osteogenesis.

Cortisone. The uptake of ^{35}S in the chondroitinsulfate of the costal cartilage of guinea-pigs is inhibited by cortisone; noninhibition is exerted by the natural adrenal hormone hydrocortisone

(LOTMAR, 1960). BOSTRÖM (1953) showed a slight reduction of the ^{35}S content of chondroitinsulfate in cortisone-treated as compared with control rats. BOSTRÖM and ODEBLAD (1953) maintain that the decrease of the incorporation of ^{35}S in the chondroitinsulfuric acid of cortisone-treated animals depends probably on a decrease of the rate of renewal of the ester sulfate group of this compound. DUTHIE and BARKER (1955*b*) autoradiographically showed that ^{35}S is used earlier and less ^{35}S is metabolized in the cartilaginous callus of fractured rat bone treated with 1 mg daily of cortisone acetate; radiographically detectable calcification occurred but true consolidation of the fracture by bone formation did not take place. In young adult male rats, diminution of the rate of ^{45}Ca fixation in the skeleton and a less marked decrease of Ca release from bone was found after cortisone treatment: the result is a negative calcium balance (MILHAUD *et al.*, 1960*b*). An overall body Ca depletion by diminution of the intestinal absorption and increase in the renal and intestinal excretion was recorded only in animals receiving cortisone acetate for a long period (i.e., 21 days).

According to BOHR and DAWIDS (1964), adult rats given dexamethasone (cortisone) show decreased retention of both radiocalcium and radiostrontium. These effects would not be counteracted by additional injections of nortestosterone, although rats treated with the latter compound only show

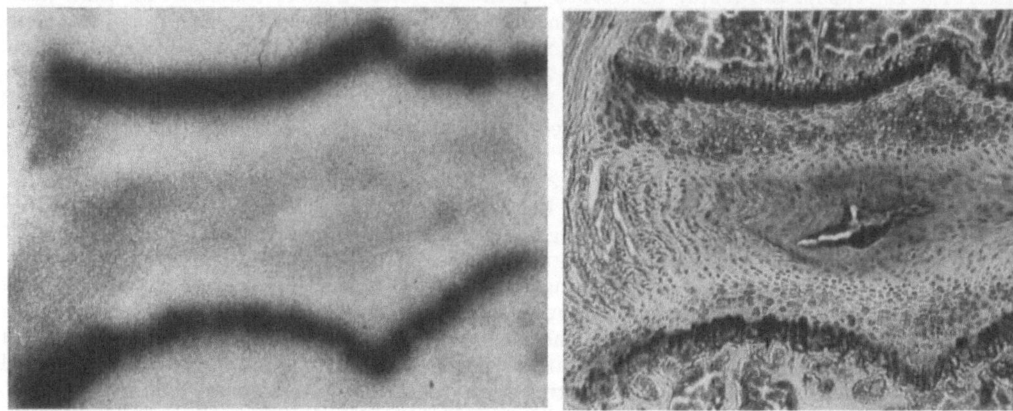

Fig. 16. Autoradiograph and stained section of an intervertebral disc of a 50-day old rat, 48 hours after injection of ^{35}S-sulfate. [From R. AMPRINO by permission of Acta anat. (Basel) **24**, 121 (1955)]

increased retention of radiocalcium as compared with controls. GARRETT *et al.* (1964) on the basis of the calcium data and of ^{47}Ca kinetic analysis following administration of cortisone to young dogs, suggest that adrenal steroid regimen inhibits the capacity of the compartment which may be associated partly with bone matrix, and the rates of transfer to a "deep compartment" to be probably identified as bone. Recently, autoradiographic evidence has been produced of a significant reduction of the pre-osteoblasts in the endochondral ossification of growing rats after a 10-day cortisone treatment (UEHLINGER, 1965).

Other corticoids (e.g., 9 *alpha*-fluoro, 16 *alpha*-methylprednisolone, 6 *alpha*-methylprednisolone, and 6 *alpha*-prednisolone) tested for their influence on the utilization of radiocalcium (^{47}C) in young dogs, showed a decreased uptake by bone and an increased fecal and urinary radiocalcium excretion, although no direct effect on bone formation and resorption was detected (COLLINS *et al.*, 1963).

h) Cartilage and fibrous tissues of joints

In the intervertebral disc of young growing mammals treated with ^{35}S-sulfate the radioactivity of fibrocartilage proper appears not uniform throughout: it is higher in the ventral than in the dorsal half of the disc. Altogether, the uptake of radiosulfate by the fibrocartilage of the disc seems to be higher than that of the faintly basophilous cartilage which covers the upper and lower surfaces of the adjacent vertebral bodies but lower than that of hypertrophic cartilage undergoing resorption and substitution with bone tissue (Fig. 16). In fibrocartilage as in hyaline cartilage, the ^{35}S uptake seems to be quantitatively related to the denseness of the tissue, and especially to the amount of basophilous and metachromatic staining component of the ground substance.

The distribution of ^{35}S in the articular cartilage in synovial joints undergoes remarkable changes with age. As long as an active resorption of the deeper zone of the cartilage and its substitution with endochondral bone takes place, this region maintains its ability to incorporate a large amount of radiosulfate. This layer is continuous with a middle zone in which the radioactivity decreases abruptly and considerably; the thickness of the latter zone varies greatly in various joint cartilages, being in general thicker the greater is the overall thickness of the cartilage. A relatively high fixation of radiosulfate is detectable for a long period of the body growth in the more superficial zone of the joint cartilage, where growth processes probably continue even in young adult individuals (Fig. 17).

The fibrous capsules, the ligaments and the menisci take up for unit volume of tissue less radiosulfate than the joint cartilage and undergo a progressive decrement of their

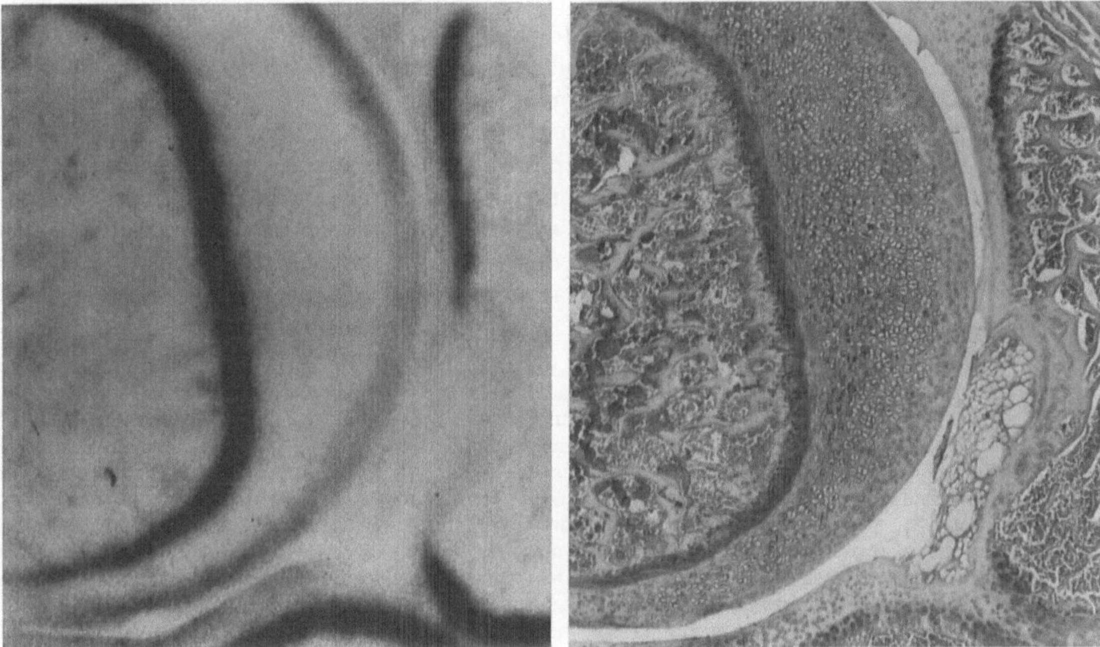

Fig. 17. Autoradiograph and stained section of the decalcified head of a femur of a 50-day old rat, 48 hours after injection of ^{35}S-sulfate. [From R. AMPRINO, by permission of Acta anat. (Basel) **24**, 121 (1955)]

ability for ^{35}S uptake with age. A relatively high incorporation in young adults occurs only in the regions of the menisci in which fibrocartilage and not merely fibrous tissue differentiates. The ^{35}S-sulfate uptake is lesser in white fibrocartilage such as the menisci than in elastic fibro-cartilage (DAVIES and YOUNG, 1954). The tendons show a higher radioactivity after ^{35}S-sulfate treatment in the region near their insertion to the bone than in other portions (DAVIES and YOUNG, 1954; BÉLANGER, 1956); the treatment of the radioactive sections with hyaluronidase does not produce a detectable loss of activity. These areas, which do not stain previously with toluidine bleu stain metachromatically after hyaluronidase digestion; according to BÉLANGER (1956) these localizations should be interpreted as concentration sites of hyaluronidase-resistant chondroitinsulfate, type B. Tendons and ligaments incorporate to some extent ^{35}S-methionine (BÉLANGER, 1956).

3. Bone mineral metabolism

a) Bone inner milieu and bone-seeking radioactive elements

The physical continuity of the extracellular fluid phase of the organism serves in bone as in other tissues and organs for the diffusion processes and the exchanges at the molecular or atomic level. Though the percentage of water in bone is comparatively scarce, bone is permeable and diffusion takes place in bone but at a different rate and extent in its various regions and structures. The extremely rapid uptake of many isotopes into bone is the more direct and objective evidence of bone tissue remarkable permeability.

Space does not permit an exhaustive review of the work that has been done by the use of radioisotopes on the mineral metabolism. Therefore, as in other sections of this article it has been necessary to select perhaps arbitrarily a certain number of contributions for review. For more informations, cf. ARMSTRONG (1952); COMAR and WASSERMAN (1956); MCLEAN and URIST (1955); IRVING (1957); NEWMAN and NEWMAN (1958), MENEELY *et al.* (1958); BAUER *et al.* (1961); COPP and SUIKER (1962); BRONNER (1964); MCLEAN and BUDY (1964).

Though bone is a highly vascularized tissue, the amount of circulating blood which can attain the various sections of the skeleton varies according to the spatial arrangement of the osseous matter, viz., whether spongy or compact bone is concerned. Great differences also exist in the number of vessels per unit volume of bone tissue not only in bones of the various species but even in different sectors of an individual bone. Materials diffusing through the endothelial wall of capillaries and postcapillary veins may penetrate deeply into bone tissue thanks to the network built by bone lacunae and canaliculi, which enclose the osteocytes and their cytoplasmatic processes. This microscopical network permeates the whole bone and opens at the periosteal surface as well as at the surface of all marrow spaces and vascular channels. This network is only partially interrupted at the level of the cementing line bordering the osteons.

R. A. ROBINSON (1960) has proposed the distinction between two major compartments in bone water, viz.: (1) the marrow-vascular-osteocytes space water, or water outside bone matrix, and (2) water in the bone matrix. The latter could in turn be divided in two compartments: (1) one water compartment of the matrix consists of water which is free enough to hydrate inorganic ions and thus participate in their diffusion. This water, according to ROBINSON, is present in the not yet fully calcified matrix and would be displaced by the inorganic phase during progressing calcification; therefore, very little if any free water would persist in fully mineralized structures of bone tissue. The other water compartment of bone matrix (2) consists of water which is "bound" and that therefore does not favour the diffusion of ions through the calcified matrix at least over short periods of time. This compartment of bound water could again be divided into two parts: (1) *water of constitution*, which forms an integral part of bone tissue organic matrix and the water of crystallization of apatite, and (2) the *bound water of the calcifiable bone matrix*, which is postulated as a part of the free water of bone tissue at the beginning of calcification and becomes "immobile" during the mineralization process. This water in fully mineralized bone tissue would be represented by the extremely thin film of bound fluid or "hydration layer" of the apatite crystals (NEUMAN and NEUMAN, 1958).

Thanks to the movement of water and dissolved substances, the minerals, e.g. Ca as a cation and HPO_4 and H_2PO_4 as anions, are carried from the circulating blood to the apatite crystal surface and ions set free from the surface of the crystals may reach the blood. As much as 100% of the plasma Ca may exchange with that of the intercellular fluid and the bone every minute (MCLEAN and URIST, 1955). The blood plasma plus the intercellular fluid forms the *calcium compartment*, which amounts to 20% ca of the body weight; this compartment is said to contain 700 mg of calcium ions in comparison with about 1.200 g of calcium deposited in the whole skeleton in a 70-kg man. The phosphate compartment in the body is larger than the calcium compartment because phosphate ions exchange with the cells while calcium does not or to a very limited extent. The level of Ca in the extracellular fluid is kept constant (from 5.8 to 6.5 mg-%); the level of Ca in the plasma is 10.0 ± 0.6 mg-% in the adult man. The phosphate level is much less constant, e.g. it varies with age and it may undergo large fluctuations in non-physiological conditions (from 0.5 to 16 mg-%). The blood Ca level is kept constant through various regulatory mechanisms: (1) the equilibrium between Ca^{++} and Ca bound to proteins in the serum, (2) the isoionic exchange between skeleton and blood Ca, (3) parathyroid activity with transfer of Ca from bone to blood, and thyroid activity (calcitonin) with transfer of Ca from blood to bone, (4) the intestinal absorption of Ca, which depends only in part on the amount of dietary Ca, (5) the Ca renal excretion, and (6) the Ca intestinal excretion.

Of the positive and negative ions which may enter the body, circulate in the blood and thus reach the skeleton, many show the tendency to be deposited in the bone tissue.

An attempt has been made (MARSHALL and ONKELINX, 1968) to evaluate approximately the time required to radioactive ions of the alkaline earth group to reach the bone crystals embedded in the interstitial highly calcified bone tissue. The coefficient of diffusion for ^{45}Ca, ^{90}Sr and ^{226}Ra in adult dog would be of the order of 10^{-16} cm^2/s; at this rate, according to the authors mentioned, it would take almost one year for an ion to diffuse from a bone canaliculus to the limit of the surrounding matrix which represents the "canalicular territory". This extremely slow diffusion rate would account for the long time required for the fixation of radioactive ions to the crystals of the *old* bone, viz., the sites of the autoradiographical *diffuse component* (p. 823), and for the poor probability that such ions may leave bone unless the area is attained by resorption.

b) Uptake, absorption and excretion of radioactive elements

The intestine is the main route of entrance of radioactive elements in the body, but some may penetrate in soluble form through the respiratory tract or through skin lesions in case of accidents. Absorption takes place mostly in the upper part of the small intestine: a variable part of the ingested radioisotope passes through the alimentary tract unabsorbed. Absorption of soluble radioisotopes, such as those of the alkaline earth group, from the intestinal tract or from the lung may be extremely rapid. On the contrary, the absorption of elements like the lanthanides which form insoluble hydroxides at physiological pH is very small. The intestinal absorption, which in general varies with age and is increased in case of low-Ca diets, permits the passage of radioactive elements into blood; hence they are distributed to the various tissues.

The radioactive material entering bone may be fixed according to various mechanisms (cf. pag. 817) to the organic or the inorganic fraction. In the case of Ca (or Sr, Ra, Ba, etc.) the decrease of the concentration of the element in the blood as a function of time (disappearance curve) seems to follow an exponential course. Mathematical analysis has indicated that such curve represents the summation of at least four separate events. About 70% of the dose disappears from blood within a few minutes; this first rapid loss seems to represent the diffusion of the isotope into the extravascular spaces. The third less rapid loss has been correlated with the bone uptake; most of the injected radiocalcium is found in the skeleton one hour after administration. In mammals the mechanisms by which radiocalcium disappears from the blood are apparently the same for adult and young subjects, but the uptake is quantitatively greater in the skeleton of the young than of the adult animal (twice as great for rabbits, THOMAS *et al.*, 1952; RUBIN *et al.*, 1953).

The rate of uptake varies from species to species; it is, e.g., considerably lower in the cat than in the rabbit or rat (WEIDMANN, 1956). The rate varies considerably also from one kind of element to the other; as said before, the uptake is relatively lower, compared to that of radiocalcium, for the lanthanons and actinides. In the rat, 25% of the parenterally injected light lanthanum, 50 to 65% of the heavy lanthanum deposits in the skeleton. 79% of the plutonium absorbed by the intestine enters the rat skeleton (CARRITT *et al.*, 1947). ^{95}Zr and ^{95}Nb although poorly absorbed by the intestine accumulate in bone to a considerable extent (BÄCKSTRÖM *et al.*, 1967).

While the uptake of radioactive elements, such as Ca, P, Sr, Ra, etc., into bone is a rapid process, e.g. flat and long bones reach the maximum isotope content about 100′ after intravenous injection and this does not decrease significantly during the following 8 to 10 days, the liberation from the skeleton occurs much more slowly. Therefore, while the specific activity of the blood decreases considerably, that of bone keeps almost unchanged.

The Ca absorbed in excess as well as the Ca liberated from the skeleton, e.g. through osteoclastic resorption, may be lost by urinary and fecal excretion. In this respect, not all parts of the bones are equally mobile; trabecular bone is quite mobile in general, cortical bone much less. The radiocalcium of the plasma is excreted into all regions of the gastro-intestinal tract; this Ca mixes with the food Ca and a part at least is absorbed again. The quantity of fecal Ca in relation to body weight is remarkably constant in animals of various age; from radiocalcium kinetics analyses it appears that in bovines (HANSARD *et al.*, 1954) it shows only a trend toward an increase in subjects from 10-day to 190-month old, and it does not change with changes of the dietary Ca (VISEK *et al.*, 1953).

Analysis of the curve of the excretion of Ca by plotting the data for combined urinary and fecal losses indicates that the old animals excrete more radiocalcium than the young but the mechanism of excretion for young and old animals is the same (RUBIN *et al.*, 1953); the excretory output has been found to be an inverse function of the bone uptake of radiocalcium (THOMAS *et al.*, 1952). In man the Ca urinary excretion undergoes only slight changes and no changes take place in the intestinal excretion of radiocalcium at dietary intakes increasing up to ten times the normal (LASZLO and SPENCER, 1956). The intestinal absorption in man is greater for radiocalcium than for radiostrontium but the latter is excreted in larger amount: in fact, Ca seems to move from intestine to blood by active transport and passive diffusion, whereas Sr is restricted to movement by passive diffusion only. An overall discrimination of about 1.6 in favour of Ca in the transfer from blood to bone was observed in the rabbit (KSHIRAGAR *et al.*, 1966). The ratio of $^{45}Ca/^{85}Sr$ intestinal absorption in human beings ranges from 1.9 to 3.5; 40% more of the absorbed dose of ^{85}Sr than of ^{45}Ca was excreted in the urine in 12 days in 50% of the patients studied by SPENCER *et al.* (1960); the ratio of urinary excretion of $^{85}Sr/^{45}Ca$ in terms of absorbed dose averaged 3.7. The quantity of Sr taken up by the skeleton in man is from four to six times greater when the isotope is administered parenterally than orally; the net retention of ^{45}Ca in the human skeleton is about 60% that of ^{85}Sr about 25% four months after treatment (SCHULERT *et al.*, 1959). The avidity of bone tissue for Sr ions is not apparently different from that for Ca ions; however, a larger fraction of the injected dose of Ca than of simultaneously administered Sr is retained by the skeleton in rabbits and rats. This has been attributed in part to a renal discrimination causing a greater relative loss of Sr. In lower vertebrates the situation appears to be different: for example, marine fishes seem to discriminate against Sr relative to Ca, while fresh water fishes lack this discrimination capacity; this different behaviour has been explained by differences in the ion absorption by the gills, skin and gut (ROSENTHAL, 1957).

The ^{85}Sr retention by the rat skeleton as a function of age has been carefully analyzed by SPECKMANN and NORRIS (1956, 1958). Retention of ^{89}Sr and ^{90}Sr is affected also by the diet; fecal excretion of these isotopes is less affected by age and diet than urinary excretion in rabbits. ^{90}Y excretion is greater in old than in young animals and diet seems not to have any effect on the excretion of ^{90}Y in young animals (KIDMAN *et al.*, 1950). By comparing the metabolism of ^{226}Ra and ^{45}Ca in dogs, differences were found in renal clearance rates, plasma level, and skeletal deposition; however, after long observation periods (100 days post-injection) these differences disappear resulting in essentially equal retention of both isotopes.

The few mentioned data should be sufficient to make clear that the biological behaviour of radionuclides in the organism may be various. The metabolic characteristics of high specific activity radioisotopes of seventy elements administered intramuscularly in one tracer dose to rats have been reviewed by P. W. DURBIN (1960) mainly on the base of data collected by the J. G. HAMILTON group at the Division of Medical Physics, Berkeley. In general, the biological behaviour of radionuclides has been found to be characteristic for each group of Mendeljeff periodic table. The following properties apparently determine their behaviour in the mammalian organism: (1) the oxidation state stable at body pH, (2) the solubility of the stable state, (3) the tendency to be incorporated into organic compounds, and (4) the tendency to associate with specific proteins. With few exceptions, the anions — including most of the halogens and the oxygenated and halogenated oxidation states of the elements of group IV, V, VI and the transition and platinum metals — are eliminated quite rapidly from the body chiefly via the kidney. The monovalent cations appear distributed nearly evenly in the soft tissues and excreted through the kidney but with longer persistence in the body than the anions. The bivalent cations, with the exception of Hg, Cd and UO_2, constitute the first major group of bone-seekers and are associated almost exclusively with bone mineral. The tripositive ions tend to associate with protein in the blood, liver and bone; the turnover of the fraction deposited in bone results to be much slower than that of the bivalent elements. The quadrivalent cations, as Sn, Zr, Th and Pu are deposited almost exclusively in the skeleton and held there as long as the tripositive ions.

c) Fixation of radioactive elements in bone

Though the mechanisms of fixation of radionuclides to bone are not yet completely understood, the available evidence indicates that isotopes may be fixed to (or incorporated into) the organic matrix and/or get fixed to the mineral phase of bone tissue.

Fixation to bone organic matrix. It seems to take place in two different ways, viz., through (a) incorporation during the synthesis of the matrix components, and (b) absorption or binding to the laid-down matrix.

The first mechanism (a) is typic of radiosulfate and radiocarbonate, though labeled S and C administered in the inorganic form may also be incorporated into the mineral fraction. Radiosulfate in bone as in cartilage is probably built into the complex mucc polysaccharides, radiocarbonate into collagen proteins. The radioactivity of the ^{3}H-, ^{35}S- or ^{14}C-labeled organic matrix proper seems not to undergo any quantitative changes before and after the calcification process. ^{35}S-sulfate localized in the inorganic fraction of bone probably for heteroionic exchange, seems to be less strongly fixed to bone salt than ^{32}P and ^{45}Ca (ENGFELDT and HJERTQUIST, 1954).

Numerous other bone-seekers which are not normal atomic components of bone become bound to its organic matrix by a sort of colloidal absorption (b). Such would be the case for plutonium and uranium and for many rare earths of the lanthanum and lanthanide series as well as for some fission products. Some of these elements are deposited in periosteum and endosteum, in the uncalcified osteoid and in the regions of small vessels of cortical bone; this is the behaviour of curium, americium, etc. (SCOTT *et al.*, 1948, 1949). A part of the *in vivo* deposited plutonium is incorporated in bone mineral, but at least 50 to 60 % is not removed by acid decalcification (ARNOLD and JEE, 1957). Pu concentrates at the endosteal surfaces and to a lesser degree at the periosteal and endosteal surface of vascular canals; no selective deposition was observed in connection with osteoblastic activity. Other bone-seekers like yttrium are deposited in the sites of active growth beneath the epiphyseal plates but not under the periosteum and endosteum or in the prebone; the uptake of Y seems not to be associated with the normal mechanism of bone matrix formation (RAYNER *et al.*, 1953). Contrary to commun belief that lanthanons have an affinity for the osteoid matrix, it has been shown that ^{91}Y, ^{144}Ce and ^{170}Tm are deposited *in vivo* on bone mineral whenever the latter comes in contact with complexes in blood. *In vitro*, the mineral not the organic phase of bone tissue takes up these rare earths (JOWSEY *et al.*, 1958).

Fixation to the mineral phase. F, P, Pb, Ca, Sr, Ra, Ba, Na, Mg, at least partially Th, and other bone-seekers get fixed to the apatite crystals in various amount. Ca, P, Sr, and Ra have been more widely investigated as to their behaviour. Their distribution in bone follows two fundamental autoradiographic patterns: (a) a lighter diffuse reaction, and (b) limited sites of high concentration ("hot spots"). The latter correspond in general to regions of active calcification of recently laid-down bone tissue (Fig. 18). The persistence of the isotopes in these locations is, however, different for the various elements: Na and Mg are apparently more easily removed than Ca, P, Ra, Sr. This has been assumed as a proof of the different position that the various elements may acquire in connection with the apatite crystal lattice. The same holds when considering the position of one single isotope: its atoms may lie at the surface of the crystals or be more or less deeply buried in the crystal lattice. ^{22}Na a few hours and days after administration appears uniformly distributed in bone tissue. The deposition seems to take place by rapid exchange in the old bone, and accretion in the sites of osteogenesis. After some weeks, an important loss of the deposited ^{22}Na occurs except for the osteons formed at the time of ^{22}Na injection, which retain for several months the radioisotope incorporated (VINCENT, 1960).

The behavior of ^{65}Zn, which has been carefully studied by HAUMONT (1962), appears to be rather different from that of the above mentioned elements. Administered *in vivo*, ^{65}Zn becomes autoradiographically detectable, in primary as well as in secondary bone, in the layers of preosseous tissue about to be calcified; later on, it is buried deeply by subsequent deposition of additional layers of calcifying matrix. ^{65}Zn is not autoradiographically found as a *diffuse* reaction in calcified bone tissue pre-existing to the treatment. The higher concentration of labeled zinc in the skeleton is steadily at the calcification front, although differences in concentration have been observed between, e.g., the periosteal apposition zone and the sites of endochondral ossification. Trauma seems to increase ^{65}Zn uptake in the ends of shaft bones; the affinity of the fractured bone for

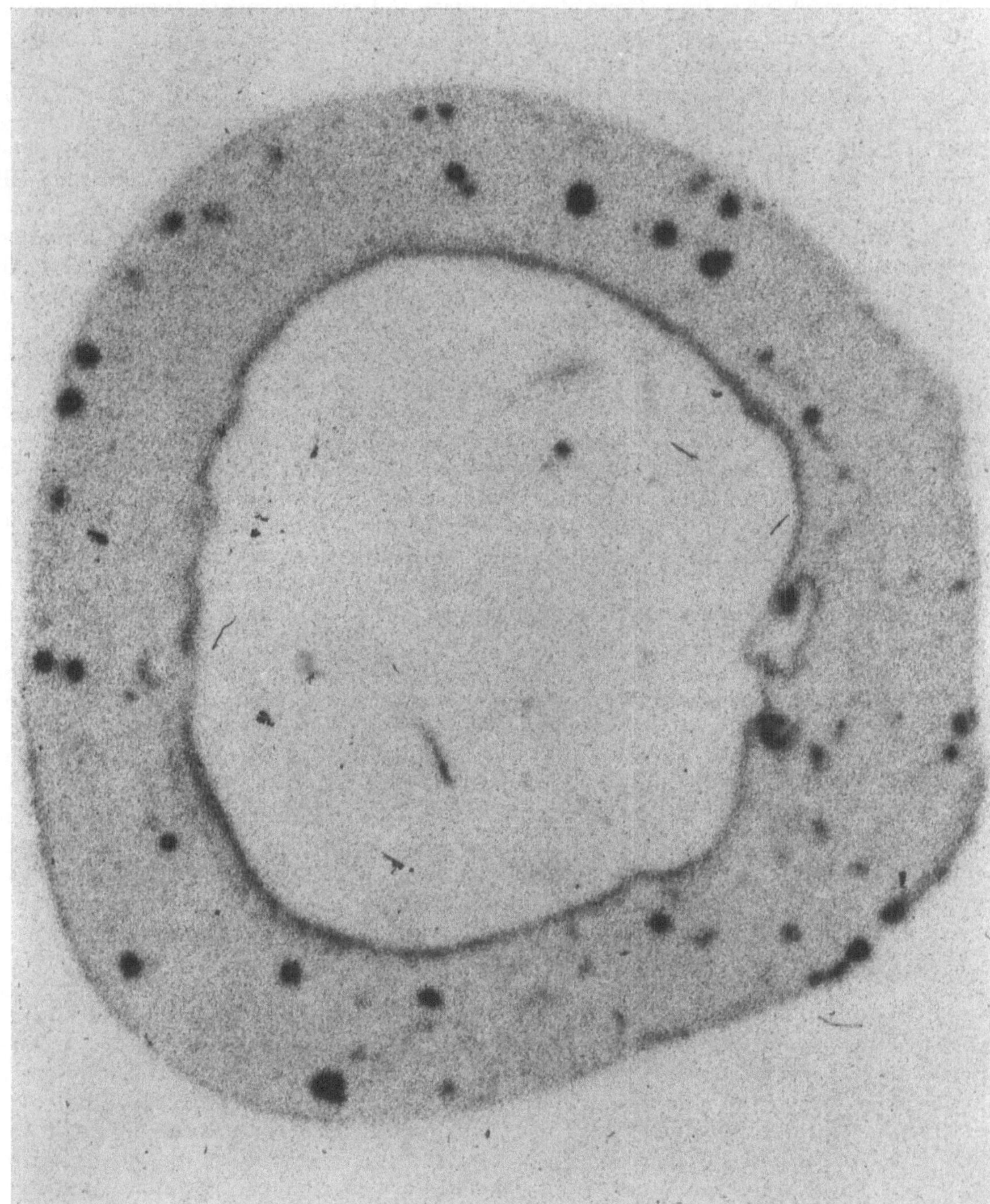

Fig. 18. Autoradiograph of the cross section through the femoral midshaft of an adult dog fourteen days after injection of Ca^{45}. The highest concentration of the isotope is located in osteons formed soon after treatment. The endosteal layer of bone appears less radioactive. A much lower diffuse reaction over the periosteal bone and the old osteons which build most of the compacta. [Courtesy of J. H. MARSHALL *et al.*, Radiat. Res. **10**, 213 (1959)]

^{65}Zn — as well as for ^{45}Ca — is greatly reduced under the influence of Cadmium. In HAUMONT's opinion, Zn would be involved in the mechanism of mineralization as a part of a metalloenzyme.

A full agreement on the size and form of the bone mineral crystals has not yet been reached and, according to W. F. NEUMAN (1960), it cannot be excluded that the crystalline habit of apatite forming in the process of bone matrix calcification may be quite variable. Though the basic structure of bone mineral is that of a hydroxy-apatite, bone salt is not a single, homogenous chemical system (NEUMAN and NEUMAN, 1958). According to the view held by DALLEMAGNE (cf., i.a., HERMAN and DALLEMAGNE, 1961), bone mineral behaves like a homogenous mixture of tricalcium phosphate hydrate and $CaCO^3$, and it contains an apatite phosphate with a Ca/P ratio lower than that of hydroxyapatite. Carbonate is undoubtedly part of bone mineral, probably a separate phase and in varying amount. An intimate relation seems to exist between the collagen fibrils and the bone mineral: the *c* axes of the crystals parallel the longitudinal axes of the fibrils, furthermore the collagen seems to serve as a nucleating center of the crystal seeds (GLIMCHER, 1959). It has been suggested that the organic substratum may preserve the structure and properties of the mineral (DALLEMAGNE and FABRY, 1956; DALLEMAGNE, 1957) and that changes in the collagen structure might induce changes in the physical state of the inorganic phase (ZETTERSTRÖM, 1952).

On the base of modern knowledge of surface chemistry and of experiments performed on synthetic-apatite model system, NEUMAN and NEUMAN (1958) maintain that because the crystals are extremely small and calcium is non-polarizable, strong electric fields are projected away from the crystal surfaces. These fields would give rise to a bound-ion layer, which, in turn, acquires an insulating layer of water, "the hydration shell." Ions diffusing into bone matrix would enter this hydration envelope of the individual crystals and exchange with calcium ions in the surface of mineral crystals. With time these ions would become incorporated to some extent within the crystals probably for diffusion and recrystallization. Exchange between ions in solution and those of the hydration shell is extremely rapid; the exchange between ions in the hydration shell and the crystal surface is fairly rapid, within the crystal lattice is quite slow (NEUMAN and NEUMAN, 1958). FABRY (1958) from studies on the *in vitro* isoionic exchange of synthetic phosphate reached the conclusion that a precise pattern of the different steps in the exchange process cannot be drawn, though the latter takes place at first in surface and attains the crystal interior after a longer contact of the mineral with the fluid phase. More recently it has been hypothesized that the first step in exchange process could be addition of a calcium ion, e.g., radiocalcium, to the surface of bone mineral rather than ejection of a previously bound calcium ion (SAMACHSON, 1967). According to this author, a radioactive ion from surrounding fluid would have more chance of forming a bond with an oxygen than of striking a vacant calcium site. Most of the bonds thus formed would break up immediately, a small proportion only may remain until the neighboring calcium ion is expelled; then, the new ion would slip down to occupy the more stable position made available.

Briefly, a labeled ion may enter the mineral phase of bone tissue through various mechanisms, viz.: (1) new-crystal formation, (2) recrystallization, i.e., dissolution and redeposition of recently formed crystals, (3) surface exchange, (4) intracrystalline exchange, i.e., exchange of surface ions with ions in the crystal interior, (5) crystal growth. For any given bone the extent of new crystal formation and crystal growth seems to be a function of the amount of newly laid-down and progressively calcifying bone matrix. The exchange processes are mainly limited by the degree of mineralization of bone tissue, which is at large a function of its age. Other more general factors such as intake and excretion rate of the labeled ions, vitaminic and hormonal influences may modify the extent and rate of entrance of radioisotopes in bone tissue.

The high concentration of radioisotopes in areas of active bone growth ("hot spots") is interpreted as due primarily to bone salt formation *(accretion)* and laying down of new bone tissue; the specific activity of the new bone tissue has been shown to be the same as that in the blood measured in the large veins (MARSHALL *et al.*, 1959a). When the *accretion rate* and the *bone formation rate* have been studied in the cortex of the adult dog, the former has been found to be two to three times as great as the latter; in the young dog bone shaft the values for the accretion, and the bone formation rate did not differ more than 20% (LEE *et al.*, 1965). In spite of the differences between the two rates in regions where new bone formation was scarce, a strong correlation between the two rates was observed.

Part of the radioisotope uptake may thus be related to crystal formation in rapidly calcifying newly laid-down bone, part to secondary mineralization, i.e., crystal growth in recently formed and not yet fully mineralized bone, and part to ionic exchange. Even in short-term observations, viz., when the animal treated with the isotope is sacrificed a few hours after administration of the tracer, and the autoradiographic distribution of the sites of highest concentration of the isotope reflects the pattern of bone appositional

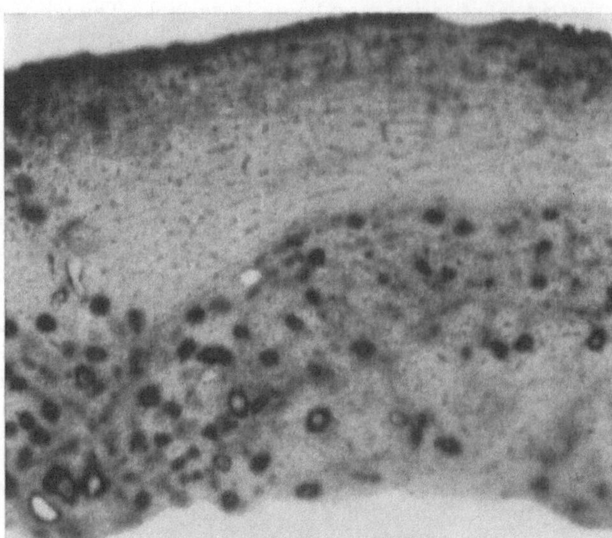

Fig. 19. Autoradiograph from the compacta of the metatarsus of a young adult ox. Undecalcified ground section labelled *in vitro* with ^{45}Ca. Higher concentration of the isotope in recently laid-down bone tissue: outer layer of periosteal bone and osteons. [From R. AMPRINO, Z. Zellforsch. **37**, 240 (1952)]

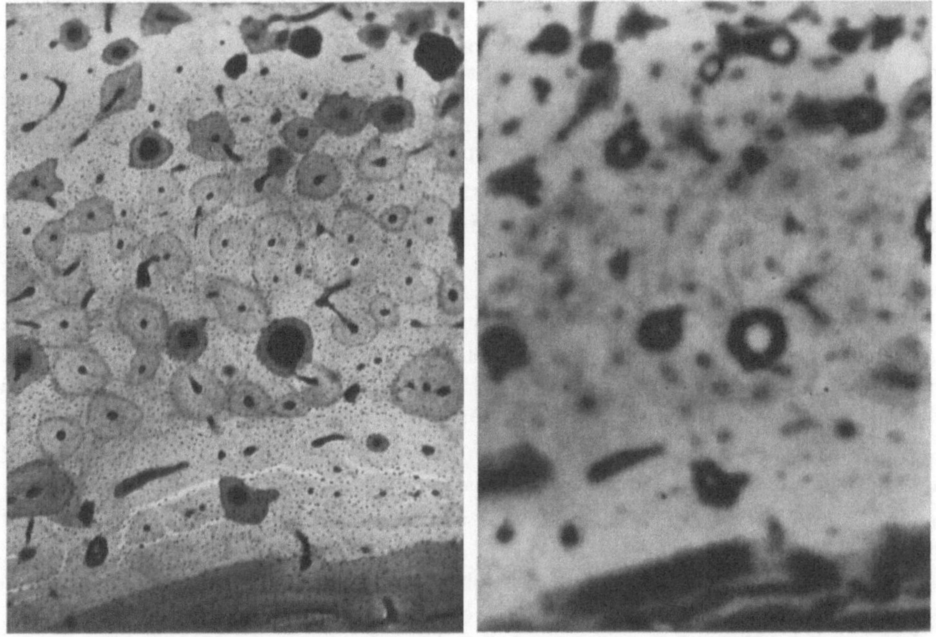

Fig. 20. Microradiograph and autoradiograph after treatment *in vitro* with ^{45}Ca of a cross section of metacarpus compacta of a young growing ox. The radioisotope concentration is higher in the less mineralized more recently formed haversian systems and endosteal bone layers

growth and reconstruction, exchange processes should occur and perhaps even predominate over those due to mineral accretion proper.

Autoradiographs of ground sections of undecalcified bone kept into solutions of radiocalcium show a pattern of distribution of radioactivity which is strikingly similar to that observed in the same type of bone after treatment *in vivo* with the isotope: also *in vitro* ^{45}Ca gets fixed in higher concentration in sites of recently formed bone tissue and of secondary mineralization, viz., in the periosteal and endosteal surfaces, in newly built osteons or fragments of trabecular bone (AMPRINO 1952*a*, 1952*d;* LACROIX 1952)

(Fig. 19, 20). Only processes of exchange not of net transfer of ^{45}Ca to the mineral phase may take place in the *in vitro* experiments. In the regions of recent bone formation the conditions for a rapid diffusion and exchange of ions are more favorable than in regions of long established bone: therefore, in the former the ^{45}Ca fixation rate is higher. In recently formed bone tissue the relative amount of organic matrix in proportion to the mineral fraction is considerably high; the low degree of calcification shown by microradiography in these areas should correspond to the existence there of apatite crystals which are more tiny and whose surface is therefore much greater than in mature bone tissue.

When the organic matrix is removed from the bone sections, the differences in the radiocalcium uptake between recent and old bone tissue disappear: the fixation of the isotope becomes nearly uniform throughout (AMPRINO 1952*b*; DALLEMAGNE *et al.* 1959). This behaviour of bone tissue *in vitro* not only stresses the importance of the organic matrix in the regulation of the ion diffusion and fixation to the mineral phase, but suggests also that in the *in vivo* experiments a large part of the administered isotope which is incorporated in recently formed bone tissue in the first hours after treatment might enter the apatite crystals through exchange process when the specific activity of the isotope in the circulating blood is still high. Another share of labeled ions together with a larger contribution of stable mineral ions takes part into the growth of the crystals in the calcifying areas of bone in the *in vivo* experiments; as a consequence, the radioisotope previously fixed by exchange, and which can be at first readily removed from the bone mineral, becomes deeply buried into the apatite crystals and becomes unavailable for exchange processes. At present, it is generally admitted that *accretion* of bone mineral is the most important way in which dietary calcium is incorporated into the skeleton; this view has been reemphasized by WEIKEL and NEUMAN (1961) on the basis of experiments on young and adult rats fed a diet of constant specific activity for a protracted period to maintain a rather constant blood level of ^{45}Ca. However, the ratio of the amount of radioisotope retained after one administration in the "hot spots", viz., in areas of new bone formation, and of that retained diffusely in the older, highly calcified bone tissue may vary considerably for different radionuclides: a mean ratio of 8.9 for ^{45}Ca, 40.1 for ^{65}Zn and 4.4 for ^{91}Y was observed, e.g., in the cortical bone of the rat, dog and monkey (JOWSEY and ORVIS, 1967).

d) Exchanges between bone crystals and fluid environment

The exchangeable and the non-exchangeable bone fraction. One important limiting factor of the ion-exchange process in the *in vivo* experiments with radioisotopes is the rate of diffusion about the mineral crystals, which depends to a large extent on the amount of "free water" of the matrix (cf. p. 814). In general, the rate of exchange between the fluid phase and the mineral crystal in bone decreases with increasing calcification. Furthermore, the migration of ions is more or less free depending on their hydration and therefore on the volume they occupy: the migration is more difficult for hydrated multivalent cations, easier for monovalent ions and even more so for unhydrated ions.

It has long been recognized that mineral elements are not equally removable from all parts of bone: the mineral of spongy bone seems to be quite mobile, that of cortical bone is only slightly so. Also isotopes when fixed in trabecular bone can be fairly readily removed and pass to blood; when the isotopes are deposited in the old cortical bone removal is almost nil. The fraction of bone in which exchange processes occur and from which mineral can be more easily displaced has been called *labile* or *available* bone and the rest *stable* or *unavailable*.

It is obvious that if all of the Ca ions in the bone mineral were freely exchangeable with those of the blood, the specific activities of blood and bone ^{45}Ca would be equal. But, as mentioned above, after incorporation of ^{45}Ca into bone by accretion as well as by exchange the ^{45}Ca fixed to the growing crystals becomes covered by newly formed mineral and thus removed from direct contact with the fluid phase. In these conditions the removal of the previously fixed ^{45}Ca deeply incorporated within the mineral and its transfer to the blood to maintain the equilibrium conditions is no longer possible (cf., however, p. 810). In the meantime the blood ^{45}Ca is diluted by incoming stable Ca so that shortly after radiocalcium administration the specific activity of the blood ^{45}Ca is lower.

FALKENHEIM *et al.* (1947) found that one fifth of the ^{32}P fixed to bone could be exchanged *in vitro* and maintained that this fraction must represent P on crystal surface; the same was recorded later for ^{45}Ca (FALKENHEIM *et al.*, 1951). NEUMAN and RILEY (1947) using ^{32}P realized that the phase of rapid uptake of isotopes *in vivo* should not be due to bone mineral accretion but to exchange-absorption between the P of the plasma and that on the surface of the bone crystals as previously assumed by HEVESY *et al.* (1940), MANLY and BALE (1939). In fact, bone tissue formation and calcification are slow processes in comparison to the speed of radioisotope uptake in bone, and apparently insufficient to explain the rapid incorporation of the isotope (FALKENHEIM *et al.*, 1951). If the animal given the isotope is kept a longer time before sacrifice, the ^{32}P cannot be easily removed, indicating that it does no longer occupy a superficial position in the crystals (NEUMAN and MULRYAN, 1952). The same results were obtained by SINGER and ARMSTRONG (1951), TOMLIN *et al.* (1955) using ^{45}Ca.

According to DAWSON (1953), 33% of the ^{45}Ca of unashed bone is exchangeable. Approximately 20% of the radiocalcium fixed on bone sections by *in vitro* exchange is quite soluble, as it is lost by simple treatment in distilled water. This fraction is evaluated by DALLEMAGNE *et al.* (1959) to 50% and would be the part adsorbed at the surface or contained in the outer layer of crystals. ARNOLD and JEE (1954) attempted to determine what portion of radiocalcium remains on crystal surface of bone as a function of time following administration of the isotope by submitting to treatment with Ca acetate solutions undecalcified sections of bone from rabbits sacrificed at intervals between one hour and three weeks after isotope injection. One half of the ^{45}Ca fixed in bone seems to be no longer removable through ion exchange as early as one hour after ^{45}Ca administration; these ^{45}Ca ions have apparently been incorporated in a non-exchangeable form of bone mineral. At 24 hours and 21 days after ^{45}Ca administration, the non-exchangeable fraction is increased to 70 and to 85% respectively. Crystal growth and recrystallization process seem thus to remove ions first held in superficial position in the bone crystals to non-exchangeable positions. The rate of this process would be quite rapid. The more recently formed and less calcified osteons appear to belong to this „metabolic" fraction of the skeleton as they are the most sensitive to ionic variations in the inner environment; a fact which has been experimentally tested by VINCENT and HAUMONT (1960) in the compact bone of the cat, dog, monkey. When the immature osteons reach maturity they lose their special reactivity.

All the mentioned processes of diffusion, exchange, crystal growth, recrystallization and new-crystal formation, decrease in rate and quantity with age. HANSARD *et al.* (1954) in cattle have found that the percentage of exchangeable ^{45}Ca is relatively high in the 6-month animal, somewhat lower in the 18-to 36-month subjects and considerably lower in the aged individuals. The age of the bone structures seems thus to be a basic determinant of bone reactivity. The progressive calcification by displacing the water of hydration inhibits diffusion and exchanges; the progressive growth of the crystals by relatively reducing their surface would also limit the rate of ion exchange. The old unreactive bone structures would constitute the metabolically inert, unavailable skeleton which in the adult animals is evaluated at about two thirds of the total. Young reactive bone tissue is continuously supplied through reconstruction; but how great is the part of the skeleton available at any time for exchanges has not yet been determined. A few examples of the attempts made in this direction will be reported. BLACK *et al.* (1953) evaluated the size of the labile pool in an adult dairy cow given ^{32}P: this bone fraction included 1% of the bone phosphorus, viz. about 15 times the all phosphorus of the circulating plasma. This labile fraction seems to be autoradiographically associated with the systems of osteons of cortical bone and in general distributed over the whole trabecular bone. In adult rats given continuously ^{45}Ca in the food for many weeks to keep at a constant level the blood ^{45}Ca, TOMLIN *et al.* (1955) estimated that the exchangeable fraction of cortical bone was so small as to be near the limit of detection with the technique used ($< 0.2\%$); in the age period between four to six weeks, approximately 14% of the diaphyseal bone present at four weeks of age (i.e., at the beginning of ^{45}Ca administration) had been renewed by exchange, and this figure increased to a maximum of about 24% by the 16th week (Tomlin *et al.* 1953).

In general, the exchangeable fraction of bone has been evaluated as short-term exchange, viz., exchange which has a short time constant and therefore the skeleton attains radioactive equilibrium with blood within a few hours after injection of the isotope. J. H. Marshall (1960) has distinguished the *short* from the *long-term* ion exchange depending on whether the time necessary for the attainment of radioactive equilibrium is much shorter or much longer than one week. Marshall *et al.* (1959c) have offered experimental evidence of the fact that over long periods of time loss of the previously deposited isotope occurs even from fully calcified mature bone independently of the intervention of resorption. This long-term exchangeable fraction seems to be represented by a large portion of the whole cortical bone Ca and would correspond in the autoradiographs to the diffuse component (p. 817 and Fig. 18). The loss of ^{45}Ca from the cortical bone of ^{45}Ca injected dogs has been autoradiographically estimated the 10 to 20% in areas not undergoing resorption. For dogs treated with ^{226}Ra the loss reached one half four years after treatment. In radium injected human beings, 90% of the radioactivity of stable cortical bone seems to be lost after 25 to 30 years (Marshall, 1960). This long-term exchange would involve surface exchange, intracrystalline ion diffusion and perhaps recrystallization.

According to Rowland (1961), the loss of ^{226}Ra by exchange "is of such a magnitude as to imply that, at least during the first year after its deposition, direct bone resorption is of little consequence in the removal of Ra from the skeleton of adult dog". Also Lloyd (1965) from a comparison of the autoradiographic measurements of ^{45}Ca concentration — in "hot spots" and "diffuse components" — with chemical assays made on matched whole bones, concluded that loss of activity in young adult rabbits takes place mostly by exchange, resorption playing a relatively minor role.

In man, bone resorption rates would fall in the range of 0.3 to 3% per year between the ages of 20 to 60 (Rowland, 1964). These values, however, are admittedly at least one order of magnitude lower than the results obtained by kinetic studies with ^{47}Ca and ^{85}Sr (p. 828). Rowland (1961) postulates that the rate of loss by exchange of alkaline-earth isotopes from microscopic deposits in bone is closely related to the rate of loss of the isotope from the entire skeleton. This author maintains that it is thus feasible to calculate, from terminal observations of microscopic dose levels, back to the dose that existed in such locations in previous times by means of total-body retention data (Rowland, 1962).

e) Removal of radioactive elements from the skeleton

The mobilization of radionuclides deposited in bone is becoming a problem of increasing concern because of the potential exposure of large fractions of the world population to the bone-seeking transuranic elements and fission products. Many attempts have been made to reduce the radioisotope skeletal burden in animals and man as a sector of the protective measures against the hazard of internal radiations. This problem may be approached from several aspects, viz., regulation of absorption, reduction of the skeletal accumulation or mobilization of the radioactive element after it has been incorporated in the skeleton. In a careful study on calcium and strontium metabolism Gran (1960) concludes that the best protective measure against an excessive accumulation of ^{90}Sr in the human skeleton appears to be a liberal calcium supply in the diet; this treatment should be of special value in the periods of life in which the rate of Ca intestinal absorption is high and in the regions where the daily intake of calcium is in general poor. Among the many substances tested on laboratory animals, a few only have shown a significant efficacy: e.g., sulphates administered to rats directly before or after ^{85}Sr contamination minimize the intestinal absorption of the isotope, i.e., a reduction of 40 to 60% of the average radiostrontium retention was observed (Volp and Roth, 1966). Analogous action without appreciable effect on calcium absorption is exerted by sodium alginates (cf. Triffitt, 1968). Inactive strontium chloride and Mg salts are also able to decrease the retention of radiostrontium in the rat skeleton if given half an hour before or soon after administration of the isotope (cf. Nelson *et al.*, 1963).

The isotopes leave spontaneously the skeleton at a rate so tremendously low — the renal clearance for Ra is less than 1% in 24 hours in humans — that any intervention bound to accelerate this process would be helpful. When the isotope has reached the skeleton and is deeply buried into the mineral, i.e., irreversibly fixed in the non-exchangeable fraction of bone, none of the chemical agents yet tried to remove the radioactive material has proved satisfactorily effective or unharmful.

The problem of radionuclides removal should be viewed in terms of skeletal kynetics taking into account the uneven distribution of radioisotopes in bone and the fact that a connection probably exists between sites of radioisotope concentration and harmful effects (p. 832).

As the exchange processes are not sufficient to insure a rapid removal from the areas of higher concentration, no other alternative is possible than that of favoring the osteoclastic resorption or, in general, the demineralization of the skeleton. Excellent articles on the practical measures for removal of bone-seeking radioactive elements from the body have been published: cf. i.a., Schubert (1955). Useful informations will be found in other reviews, e.g., Comar and Wasserman (1956); Engström *et al.*, 1958; Copp and Suiker, 1962. Only a few data will be reported here.

Regimens designed to favor bone resorption have been used in connection with chemical and hormonal treatment. A low-P diet is said to increase the urinary excretion of radiocalcium and radiostrontium and to reduce their retention in bone (Cramer and Copp, 1951; Ray *et al.*, 1956); but, according to Ito *et al.* (1958*a*) Ca and P deficiency while increases the removal of radiostrontium from bone would not increase its urinary excretion. Low-Ca diet, parathormone treatment, administration of NH_4Cl and citrate apparently have no significant effect on the excretion of plutonium, yttrium, cerium and a very slight effect on strontium excretion in rats (Copp *et al.*, 1947). Some evidence has been offered that citric acid and parathyroid hormone mobilize the mineral cations from deep areas of bone removed from direct contact with the blood (Elliott and Talmage, 1958).

Intravenous injection of calcium gluconate or oral administration of NH_4Cl in man seem to increase radiostrontium excretion; for ammonium chloride treatment the excretion is higher in low-Ca diet patients. The effect of the two mentioned substances administered simultaneously seems to be additive; NH_4Cl is as effective fifteen days after as in the early phase of radiostrontium uptake (Spencer *et al.*, 1958).

An extensive series of studies performed by the Montefiore Hospital group in New York (cf. Laszlo, 1955), illustrates the profound effect of chelating agents upon the disappearance rate of isotopes from the blood plasma, their urinary excretion and their removal from the body (cf. also Rubin, 1953). In therapeutic doses, these agents reduce the biological half-life of radioisotopes in the human body: e.g., administration of sodium EDTA in man delays the entry of radiostrontium in bone and favours the elimination of the fraction already deposited in the skeleton (Spencer *et al.*, 1958). EDTA is effective when administered a few days after exposure in removing plutonium, lanthanum, yttrium, and in general the rare earths and the trivalent transuranic elements. Diethylenetriamine pentacetic acid seems to be more effective than ethylendiamine tetracetic acid for the removal of deposited plutonium (Smith, 1958), ^{90}Y, ^{140}La (Rosoff *et al.*, 1961) and increases the excretion of thorium (Schubert and Fried, 1960); it can remove americium and enhance its urinary excretion when administered a few hours after exposure in rats (Sowby and Taylor, 1960). According to Ito *et al.* (1958*b*, 1958*c*), sodium calcium citrate and sodium tricarballylate exert probably their activity of enhancing the excretion of radiostrontium and of reducing its skeletal accumulation through a chelating mechanism. Both the artificial kidney and ion-exchange column afford additional means for radioactive elements removal (Looney *et al.*, 1957).

f) Biological half-life of bone-seeking radioactive elements

The retention of long-lived radioactive elements in the skeleton may be as long as to cover the entire life-span of the individual. Therefore, it would be useful to know exactly for each period the average concentration of the bone-seeker in the skeleton and the rate of its elimination. Such analyses could be carried out fairly easily in short-lived mammals but they would represent a very exacting task in the case of long-lived animal species. Especially for man, predictions on retention and related quantities must rely on extrapolations based on data recorded over relatively short intervals. These extrapolations have in general been made on the base of the assumption that the retention of radioactive elements in the skeleton decreases exponentially with time. A derived constant, the *biological half-life* is currently used as a fundamental parameter of the retention; the half-life value is especially useful in the calculation of permissible daily intakes of radioisotopes, of permissible body burdens, etc.

Given the various rates of bone formation and resorption in the skeleton at the various periods of life and in different animal species, the rate of elimination of a given radioactive element from the skeleton varies in subjects of different age and in the various mammals. On the other hand, different radioactive elements are eliminated at different rates in a given animal. Accordingly, the biological half-life of the bone-seeker taken up by the skeleton undergoes significant variations in the mentioned conditions. Such variations may be especially striking in cases of skeletal disorders which are accompanied by changes from the normal of the skeletal turnover. Furthermore, for each radionuclide there is a specific physical radioactive rate of decay; therefore, when an isotope enters the metabolic pool of its stable counterpart or of a stable atom whose metabolic behaviour in the organism is similar, its *effective half-life* is a function of its metabolic rate of disappearance from the body, an organ or a system *(biological half-life)* and its physical rate of decay *(physical half-life)* (cf. TULLIS and JOHNSON, 1958). The effective half-life is derived by combining the two disappearance rates according to the formula:

$$\text{effective half-life} = \frac{\text{physical half-life} \times \text{biological half-life}}{\text{physical half-life} + \text{biological half-life}}$$

In general, it can be assumed for each animal species that the biological half-life of a given isotope is shorter in young growing subjects than in the adult. The value of the biological half-life varies considerably from species to species and in pathological conditions affecting the skeleton: for instance, values of the order of 50 ± 7 days and of about 400 days were calculated for the half-life of ^{45}Ca administered endovenously as sodium salt of ^{45}Ca-EDTA in the skeleton of normal adult humans and of the rabbit. In cases of hypocalcemia in man a half-life of 350 days was computed (HUNZIGER and ORTELLI, 1956). BRONNER *et al.* (1956) have derived a half-life value of 261 days for ^{45}Ca in the period of 18 to 59 days following injection of one tracer dose of the isotope in a young adult man. However, the value of the biological half-life for many bone-seekers is much higher than that for ^{45}Ca, is shorter for radiostrontium; in humans given simultaneously ^{45}Ca and ^{85}Sr the ratio ^{45}Ca/^{85}Sr in bone decreases gradually to reach a value of two or more in two to four months. In rats, radiostrontium is more readily eliminated than plutonium, curium, yttrium; the biological half-life of the former has been evaluated to be of the order of three to four months, for the other elements the half-life ranges from one to three years (COPP *et al.*, 1947). Also the heavy lanthanons show an half-life time of about 2.5 years in the rat (DURBIN *et al.*, 1956).

In some special cases of temporary mineral storage in the skeleton, e.g., the medullary bone forming during the egg-laying in pigeons, the rate of turnover and therefore the biological half-life of the injected bone-seeker may vary considerably in the various bones of the skeleton; an interesting fact which shows that, in some special cases at least, the skeleton does not respond as a physiological unity (DALLEMAGNE *et al.*, 1950). In pigeons injected estrogens a ^{45}Ca half-life of 75 days was found in comparison to that of 45 days in the untreated control animals (GOVAERTS *et al.*, 1951).

The traditional concept of an *exponential decrease* in the retention in the skeleton of soluble and readily diffusable bone-seekers seems not to be fully correct. First NORRIS and KISIELESKI (1948) suggested that the pattern of retention for Ca, Sr, Ra, Ba and also for ^{14}C in laboratory animals, ^{239}Pu and Uranium in man, may be better described in terms of a *power function.* The value of the power function has been further appraised by NORRIS *et al.* (1958), and mathematical treatments have been proposed to derivate relationships useful in the determination of permissible daily intake levels and body concentrations of bone-seekers, or to calculate integrated radiation dosages from deposits of radioactive elements in bone. Furthermore, according to the authors mentioned, "the power function indicates clearly that, in its area of application, the concept of "biological half-times" is completely fallacious and may result in gross errors both actually and conceptually". In a study of Ca and Sr metabolism of the rabbit, carried out with measurements of the various parameters over long time intervals compared with the life-span of the species, LLOYD (1964) concluded that only the multi-exponential and the modified power function models provided the best fit to the data over the whole time period. Even these models, however, are considered by the author unsatisfactory for extrapolation to times beyond the range of experimental verification. Thus, the biological retention of alkaline earths can be described in terms of a power function or as a summation of exponential rate processes. For instance, the retention of ^{85}Sr following continuous intake in normal man seems to be well described either by a three component exponential function of time or by the integrated form of the sum of an exponential function and a power function of time (cf. Rundo and Lillegraven, 1966). As Comar and Wasserman (1964) put it, the power function model would be more advantageous for long time predictions, while it offers little clarification of the number and of the nature of the processes involved, and the fit is usually poor at short time intervals.

4. Exploration of the skeletal metabolism by means of radioisotopes

In the last 15 to 20 years radioisotopes have been used as a means of dynamic approach to the study of the kinetics of mineral ions in the organism, and particularly to and from the skeleton. ^{32}P, ^{45}Ca, ^{85}Sr have been more widely applied. At the beginning of this trend of researches, the concentration changes of the ^{45}Ca blood serum recorded at various time intervals from the intravenous administration of the isotope was used to draw curves of the ^{45}Ca disappearance rate from the blood. The mathematical analysis of such curves allowed the distinction of various phases in the disappearance process (p. 815). The rate of the turnover of ^{45}Ca in the blood was then calculated. By the aid of calculations based on blood disappearance curves and on observations of uptake of ^{45}Ca by the bones of experimental animals, attempts were made to computate the rates of bone accretion, resorption and exchange processes in the skeleton. Such analyses have been extended also to the study of the skeletal metabolism in man; by compartmental analysis with the use of models to interpret the isotope data, evaluations of the rates of movement of the isotope between the blood, extracellular fluid and skeleton have been made. This kind of analysis has aroused considerable interest among biologists and clinicians, and various abstract models have been proposed with the aim of reproducing the kinetics of tracer's distribution in the body and of determining indirectly bone formation rates. The number of compartments which appear to represent conveniently calcium metabolism may vary according to various authors; obviously, compartments have not a clear and precise anatomical or physiological counterpart. Models vary from one compartment system to several compartments in exchange with the blood and with each other. Only a few data will be reported in the following, and the reader will find comprehensive accounts on the theoretical bases, the methodological approaches and the limitations of compartmental analysis in articles and reviews appeared in the last decennium: *i.a.*, Bauer *et al.* (1955*a*), Robertson (1957), Solomon (1960), Aubert et Milhaud (1960), Bauer *et al.* (1961), Nordin (1962), Aubert *et al.* (1963), Heaney (1963), Heaney *et al.* (1964), Ray *et al.* (1965), Ray and Mueller (1965), Tomlinson *et al.* (1967) etc.

a) Metabolic tracer techniques

Quantitative studies of the mineral turnover of the skeleton can be made only if bone resorption and formation and the extent of the exchange processes may be measured. Prior to the introduction of radiotracers in biological and medical research, the balance between bone salt formation and resorption was obtained by computing the difference between calcium intake and excretion, assuming that the extracellular calcium content (i.e., less than 1 % of the total body calcium) does not undergo significant changes with time. However, calcium balance does not reflect the metabolic level, while there can be cases, at least in pathological conditions, in which great variations may occur in bone mineral metabolism though bone formation and resorption proceed at equal rates so that the calcium balance is zero. Even in these cases, the application of the radiotracer technique provides an adequate tool for investigation. The study of ^{45}Ca turnover is in fact a more sensitive indicator of bone metabolism than metabolic balance studies and calcium tolerance tests long used in patients and normal individuals (Bellin and Laszlo, 1953).

Two methods have been applied for the evaluation of bone salt accretion and resorption in the skeleton of small mammals, mostly rats. The first general method (1) is based on a combination of the old balance analyses and respectively of radiotracer techniques. The radiocalcium is administered for a few days with the diet and the intake of stable calcium and ^{45}Ca determined. When the animal is sacrificed, the radiocalcium retained in the skeleton is measured. The bone salt accretion is represented by the amount of skeletal radiocalcium divided by the specific activity of the diet ($^{45}Ca/^{40}Ca$). The value of bone salt resorption is obtained from the difference between the bone salt accretion and the net bone increase computed by means of conventional gross methods of bone growth measurements.

The second general method (2) is based on the calculation of the skeleton accretion rate by comparing the body retention, excretion and blood activities following a single tracer doese of radiocalcium. This method has been elaborated first by G. C. H. Bauer and his associated (Bauer, Carlsson and Lindquist, 1955*a*). According to these authors, skeletal calcium is distributed in two fractions, the smaller one of which only is in equilibrium with calcium in the body fluids. Administered radiocalcium is taken up by the skeleton through exchange and new bone salt formation. When after injection of the radiotracer an equilibrium has been attained between radiocalcium concentration in the body fluids and the exchangeable fraction of bone, all radiocalcium entering the skeleton should be incorporated in the non-exchangeable fraction, viz., it should contribute to bone accretion. If the tracer does not leave the non-exchangeable fraction and return into circulation during the experimental period, an estimation of bone exchangeable fraction and of the rate at which radiocalcium is removed from blood for the bone salt accretion may be made. The calculation of these two variables must be based on the data of the integrated blood specific activity, the body retention and the specific activity of the blood at two different time intervals from the radiotracer injection (cf. references on the methods of calculation in Bauer *et al.*, 1958).

Bauer *et al.* have applied their method not only for researches on the bone mineral metabolism of rats in various experimental conditions but also as a routine diagnostic procedure for analyses of the rate of bone formation in the entire skeleton and in localized bone lesions in man. The general validity of the assumptions on which the method is based has been questioned on theoretical and experimental grounds, and even the metabolic model applied on the kinetic analysis has been challenged. One of the more commun criticisms has been that bone retains tracers by a mechanism which is a true measure of bone formation and by at least two other mechanisms which seem independent of new bone formation; by the methods used in kinetic studies it does not appear possible the distinction of the tracer retained by each of the three mechanisms whereas most kinetic studies are based on the assumption that tracer retention by long-term exchange (cf. p. 823) and by secondary mineralization is quantitatively insignificant or is constant at different times. In spite of the criticism aroused, the method has been largely applied and numerous values for the skeletal accretion in rat, farm animals and in man, as determined in this way, are now available (cf. i.a., Bauer *et al.*, 1955*b*, 1956, 1957*b*; Bronner and Harris, 1956; Rich, 1957; Wassermann, 1958; Sternberg, 1966). When the values obtained have been compared to similar data recorded by the use of other methods, a rather good agreement between the two series has in general been found. As an example of application of the Bauer-Carlsson method the data related to the calcium metabolism in the two tibiae of a young rat are reported (Table 1).

Table 1

	Whole tibias	Ends	Shafts
Ca content, mg	66	36	30
Net increase, mg Ca per hour	0.04	0.02	0.02
New bone deposition, mg Ca per hour	0.17	0.14	0.03
Resorption, mg Ca per hour	0.13	0.12	0.01
Exchangeable fraction, mg Ca	2.0	1.7	0.3

(From G.C.C. Bauer, A. Carlsson and D. Lindquist 1955a.)

In a kinetic analysis of the distribution of ^{35}S in man, BAUER and RAY (1958) make use of the following compartment model

$$\begin{array}{c} \downarrow \\ X \rightleftharpoons B \rightleftharpoons Y \rightleftharpoons Z \\ \downarrow \quad \downarrow \\ U \quad A \end{array}$$

where X and Y represent the organic fluids, B the vascular space in which the isotope is introduced, U the urine, Z the exchangeable, and A the non-exchangeable fraction of bone. The validity of the model has been proved by elaborating the experimental data with an analogic computer [see, however, the limitations pointed out by BERGNER (1959) and the work of STOCLET (1960*a*, *b*)].

According to BAUER (1960), in the normal adult man new bone salt is formed at a rate of about 0.5 gm Ca day; a corresponding amount is resorbed. For a calcium skeletal content of 1000 to 1500 gm, the renewal rate would be 0.05%/day. In the newborn the skeleton would be renewed at a rate of 1%/day or higher. As the author points out, these data reflect overall values while the rate of bone accretion is different in various skeletal pieces: higher in long bone metaphyses, in the vertebrae, in flat bones than in the long bone shafts. The bone accretion rate studied in humans with clinically normal skeletal metabolism rises with increasing age to a maximum during early adolescence, to decline slowly to a level of about 0.5 gm Ca/day (BAUER *et al.*, 1957*b*). In normal infants the percentage of bone salt added through accretion in the proximal part of the tibial shaft was found to be 0.05%/hr, i.e., one-fifth as great as in the tibia of young rats; the rate of net gain in bone mineral was estimated as approximately 0.01%/hr, i.e., one-fifth of the accretion rate. The accretion rate changes with age both in rats and men, and the proportion of net increase to accretion seems to be of the same order in man as in rats (BAUER *et al.*, 1961). According to these authors, the amount of bone exchangeable calcium would not undergo any great changes with age varying from 3 to 6 g in both infants and adults; from BRONNER and HARRIS data (1956) it appears that the exchangeable calcium would represent 1% of the total body calcium in adolescents and about 0.5% in young adults.

It is not yet possible to decide whether these values give a true picture of the bone salt accretion and renewal. Some data available from the recent literature do not fully agree with those reported above; for instance, HEANEY and WHEDON (1958) estimate that the normal rate of bone formation is approximately 9 mg Ca/kg/day (9.1 ± 3.9 mg Ca/kg/day) in adult man; the same level (9.4 ± 1.07) was found in 6 out ot 7 patients with osteoporosis, a much reduced rate of bone formation resulted in one patient with uncomplicated hypoparathyroidism and a greatly elevated rate in two patients with ostheitis deformans.

b) External counting methods

By injecting γ-emitters and by the use of scintillation counters for the measurement of radioactivity, external evaluations of the distribution of activity of the radiotracer deposited in the skeleton can be made (BAUER *et al.*, 1958; BAUER and WENDEBERG, 1959). If the countings are carried out at sufficiently long intervals, e.g. several hours or even a few days after administration of the tracer when serum and bone have reached, according to the mentioned authors, an equilibrium condition, the activity ratio between two skeletal locations should indicate relative bone salt accretion rates.

The tracers used have been ^{85}Sr (65-day half-life) and ^{47}Ca (about 5-day half-life). Attempts have also been made with ^{140}Ba, ^{22}Na or ^{24}Na, but the latter cation proved not to be suitable for studies on bone mineral metabolism, and with radiogallium.

In patients with no special osseous localizations, BAUER and WENDEBERG made the measurements over the thigh and knee, representative of compact and spongy bone regions respectively. In cases with localized skeletal lesions the radioactivity was recorded over the lesion and over the corresponding site of the healthy controlateral bone. The counting rate over normal thigh rises to a peak a few minutes after intravenous injection of the isotope then declines during a one to two-week period. The counting rate over the knee in general reaches a peak several hours post-injection (Fig. 21). ^{85}Sr activity has been found to decline at a faster rate than ^{47}Ca activity. Significant differences from unity in the right/left counting rate ratio were recorded only in pathological cases. The counting rate over fractured bone is uniformly higher than over the corresponding sound bone (Fig. 22). The mineral accretion rate in a fracture region increases within a week and it further increases during the first month to reach a peak value at 6 to 8 months after fracture. In patients studied 5 to 10 months after fracture the mean accretion rate in the fracture region was estimated 15.5 ± 7.2 times at least that of the control bone. The accretion rate increases also in the entire fractured leg some months after fracturing,

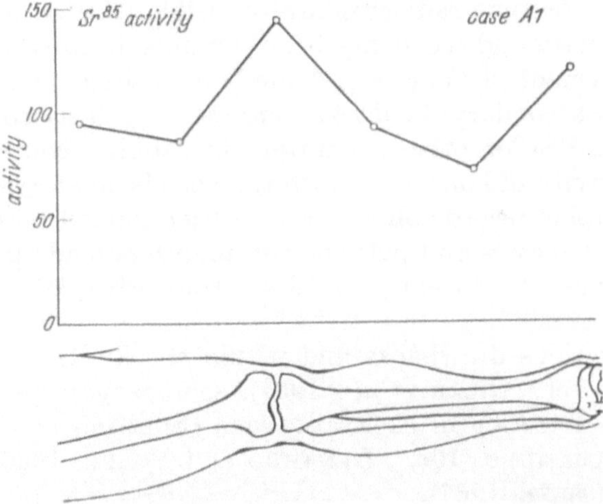

Fig. 21. External counting of radioactivity over the leg of a 9-year boy with clinically normal skeletal metabolism 12 days after injection of ^{85}Sr. On the ordinate the activity in arbitrary units, on the abscissa the location of the counter during the recording. [Courtesy of G. C. H. BAUER and B. WENDEBERG, J. Bone Jt Surg. B **41**, 558 (1959)]

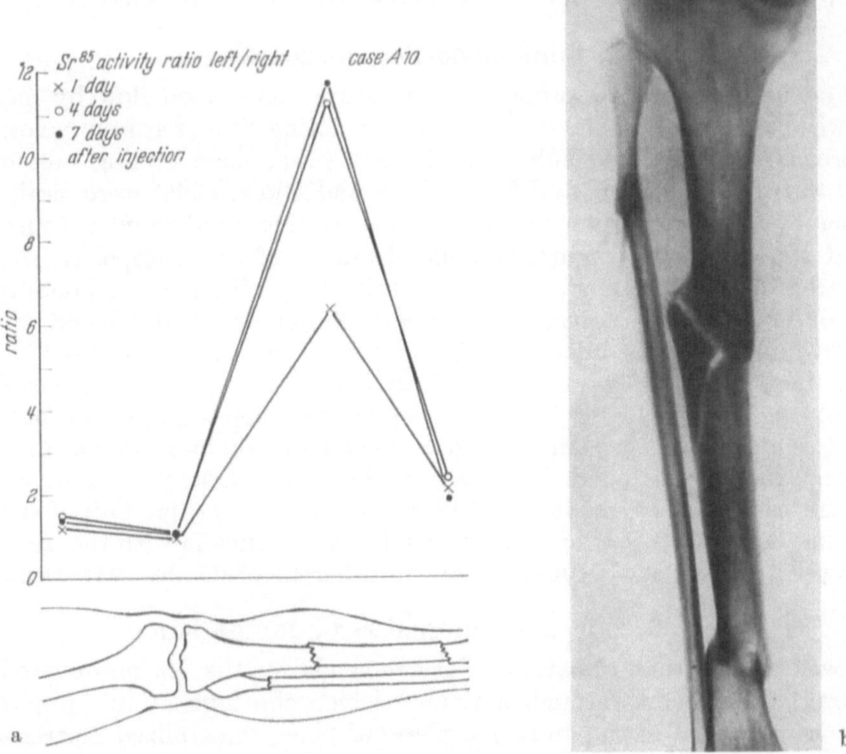

Fig. 22a and b. External counting of radioactivity over the leg of a 27-year man injected with ^{85}Sr. Two transverse fractures (cf. radiograph) of the left tibia one year before investigation healed three months before radioisotope treatment. [Courtesy of G. C. H. BAUER and B. WENDEBERG, J. Bone Jt Surg. B **41**, 558 (1959)]

e.g., 3.8 ± 1.3, and 1.6 ± 0.5 in the knee and thigh region of the fractured leg in patients studied 5 to 10 months after fracturing. No differences in the radiotracer uptake or in the accretion rate were observed between normally healing fractures and fractures showing delayed or non-union (WENDEBERG, 1961). An interesting and promising aspect of the method proposed by BAUER and associated is that some skeletal lesions which determine an increase of the bone accretion rate can be detected by means of external counting technique before they become radiographically visible (BAUER and WENDEBERG, 1959); this is the case of primary and secondary bone tumours, of infectious processes, arthroses, lymphomatous involvment of bone, metabolic bone diseases (e.g., Gaucher's and Paget' disease), osteoporosis secondary to disease processes such as rheumatoid arthritis, etc.

After injection of ^{85}Sr or other γ-emitters in rabbits, continuous recording of the variations of radioactivity of bone areas with time has been accomplished by MACDONALD (1958, 1960). The graphic records obtained have been named *radioisotope osteograms;* the use of γ-scintillation detectors and pulse height analyzers made possible the simultaneous recording on separate charts of the fate of two or three (^{85}Sr, ^{140}Ba, ^{140}La) distinct isotopes injected.

In spite of the various drawbacks and within the limits of application outlined by various investigators (cf. KOLÁŘ *et al.*, 1967), *scintigraphy* has now become a useful, practical tool in the detection of skeletal lesions (FLEMING *et al.*, 1961; RAPKIN, 1964; WENDEBERG and YAMAMURO, 1965; DENARDO and VOLPE, 1966; ESTEBAN *et al.*, 1967; FREY *et al.*, 1967; BESSLER, 1967).

Recently, short-lived isotopes have enabled bone photoscanning with reduced radiation dose. Simple methods of producing such isotopes, e.g., ^{87m}Sr and ^{18}F in a nuclear reactor and of preparing them for injection have been devised (SPENCER *et al.*, 1967; MCCREADY, 1967). Also the short-lived ^{68}Ga has been used. With these isotopes the best scans were obtained approximately one hour after administration to the patient.

5. Bone blood-flow measurement

The first indirect method proposed to measure bone blood flow by means of radioisotopes was based on the bone clearance of circulating ^{45}Ca (FREDERICKSON *et al.*, 1955). This approach was amplified subsequently, and other bone-seeking radioisotopes (^{85}Sr, COPP and SHIM, 1965) or ^{42}K and ^{86}Rb (KANE and GRIM, 1966) were used. In a method more generally applicable when blood-flow must be measured simultaneously in different bones and under various conditions, bone clearance of the isotope, *viz.*, the volume of blood cleared of the isotope by bone, is obtained by dividing the bone uptake by the average concentration of the isotope in one milliliter of arterial blood integrated over the first five minutes after injection. The rate of bloodflow is expressed as milliliters of blood per minute per 100 g wet bone (SHIM *et al.*, 1967). By this method it has been found that, e.g., the rates of blood-flow of various bones in the rabbit and dog are remarkably similar, i.e., they amount to an average of about 10 ml per minute per 100 g of wet bone, marrow included. The rates of the entire skeletal blood-flow in these two species were estimated as about 5 to 10% of the resting cardiac output. Other methods of measuring bone blood-flow are based on a dilution principle with the use of ^{51}Cr-tagged red blood cells (WHITE *et al.*, 1964), or still on different principles (VAN DIKE *et al.*, 1965).

6. Effects of internal radiation on bone

It is well known that radiation injury depends on the *ionization* produced by the passage of the radiations through a tissue. Given the high atomic number of several elementar constituents of the inorganic phase of bone, mineralized matrix absorbs more energy than soft tissues. The ionization at the interface between soft and mineralized tissue or inside soft tissue filled cavities within bone (e.g., osteocytes, content of vascular channels) is much higher than it might be predicted from the dose expressed in roentgens (SPIERS, 1949, 1950). When estimating the dose of radiation received by bone tissue one must therefore take into account, beside the chemical and physical characteristics of the radioactive element, also these two factors, viz., (a) the atomic number of the bone salt, and (b) the size and location of the soft tissue within bone. Relatively simple methods have been proposed also for the calculation of the geometrical functions involved in the evaluation of the absorbed dose in soft tissue cavities in bone containing *alpha*-emitters (HOWARTH, 1965).

If, as generally assumed, damages are exerted on the bone cells directly, or indirectly through injury of small blood vessels, the peculiar distribution of the osteocytes in bone may minimize the effect of radiation in comparison with other tissues in which cells are more closely packed; in other words, fewer cells are more intensely irradiated in a given volume of bone than of any parenchimal tissue (VAUGHAN, 1956).

Among the most hazardous radioactive elements which can attain the human skeleton are strontium, radium and mesothorium. Internal deposition of the latter two may occur as a result of occupational exposure and in patients whom have been treated with radium

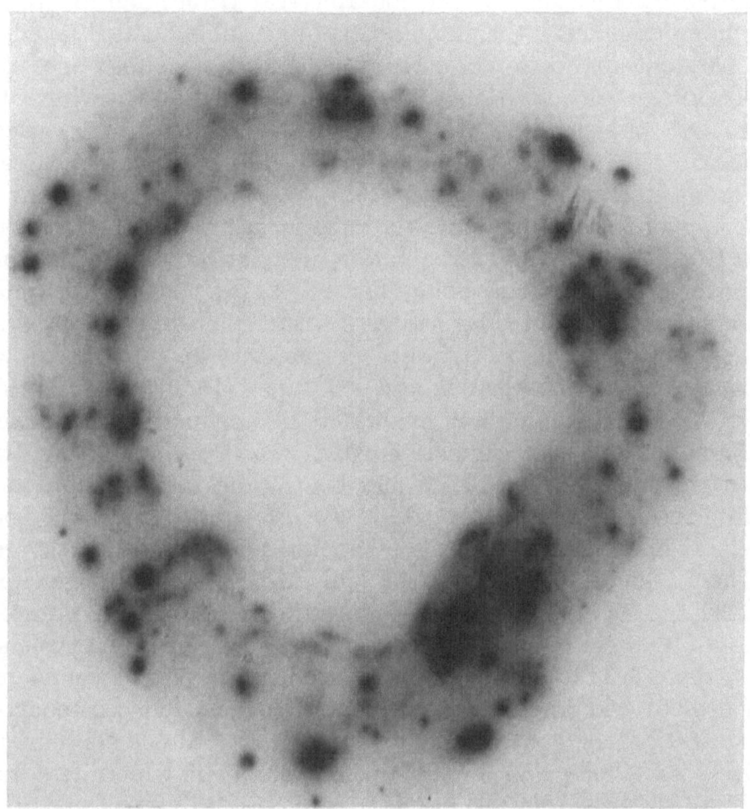

Fig. 23. Autoradiograph of the tibia cross section of a man 84-year old who had been carrying Ra during 36 years (terminal burden 10 μC). Patchy distribution of high concentration sites over a diffuse uniform activity component. [Courtesy of R. E. ROWLAND and J. B. MARSHALL, Radiat. Res. 11, 299 (1959)]

preparations. Radiostrontium, which is a component of the radioactive fall-out, may enter the body through contaminated drinking water and food. Other isotopes, e.g., ^{95}Zr, ^{95}Nb, etc., are absorbed preferably through the lungs; the two mentioned constitute during the first year about 20 % of the total activity of fission products aged from a few days to one year, and their fixation to bone is considerable.

The non-uniform concentration of the isotopes in bones, which in turn depends upon the length of the period of uptake and the age at the time of exposure, is a factor of the degree of non-uniformity of radiation dose received by a given structure. The radiation dose at any point in bone does not, however, depend solely on the concentration of the isotope at that point unless the linear dimensions of the deposits of radioactive material in the bone structures are comparable to the range of the radiation emitted. In human material examined by HINDMARSH *et al.* (1957) in the case of Ra and its daughter products the maximum range of the *alpha* particles in bone ($\sim$ 35 μ) was less than the shortest linear dimensions of the radioactive deposits autoradiographically recorded; in the case of ^{90}Sr the maximum range of the *beta* particles from its daughter product ^{90}Y (about

6 mm in bone and about 1 cm in soft tissues) was much greater than the linear dimensions of radioactive deposits. For ^{226}Ra the maximum dosage non-uniformity factor is, therefore, the same as the ratio of the highest concentration to the average concentration if the total amount of the Ra fixed to bone were distributed uniformly throughout the skeleton. The non-uniformity factors for three cases of radium poisoning with total body burden of 1.2, 1.3 and 10 μg at death studied by LLOYD (1961) was calculated to be in the range 13 to 40. The corresponding non-uniformity factor for an hypothetical deposition of ^{90}Sr in the ^{226}Ra sites was evaluated in the same patients as having a maximum value of 6.

Areas of active calcification, as the metaphyseal trabeculae of growing long bones, the trabecular bone in general, the subperiosteal and subendosteal layers and the regions of the cortex in which calcification of osteons occurs are the sites of greater concentration of most bone-seeking radioactive elements. Not always, however, greater damages are to be found in soft tissue adjacent to these areas; bone reconstruction may in fact determine redistribution of the isotope before or after it has developed its damaging effect. Therefore, a lesion may be found in an area of bone which does not show radioactivity at the time of the control, since the radioactive material may have been removed (HOECKER and ROOFE, 1951). Given the patchy distribution of the sites of higher concentration of radioactive elements in bone (Fig. 23, 24), a chemical estimate of the total skeletal content of any element does not give a true picture of the hazard to which the individual is exposed or of the radiation dose received by given bone constituents. In one Ra patient studied by HINDMARSH and VAUGHAN (1956), the radiation dose received by an osteocyte in a 5 μ lacuna was evaluated by means of *alpha*-track counts to up 0.46 rad/day though the mean skeletal burden was less than 0.3 μg Ra. The authors estimate that if the same burden of Ra had been uniformly distributed throughout the skeleton the dose received by an osteocyte in a 5 μ lacuna would have been 0.03 rad/day.

A high skeletal burden of radioactive elements may determine severe blood or bone alterations. The former, i.e., anaemias or leukemias, preceed in general the second in human cases. Changes in bone are induced more slowly and are represented by osteites (1) and bone tumours (2). The more susceptible bone cells seem to be the chondroblasts and the osteoblasts; therefore radiation dysplasias are more severe in young growing subjects: retardation of growth and fractures may ensue. However, also osteocytes death contributes to the alterations of bone; osteocytes death is a direct consequence of radiation but may be due also to plugging of the vascular channels which determine interruption of blood supply (VAUGHAN, 1956; JEE *et al.*, 1958). According to JEE and ARNOLD (1961), the loss of osteocytes in cortical bone of ^{239}Pu treated dogs results solely from the disruption in the vascular supply and not from direct irradiation death. Osteoclasts seem to be very radioresistant: they have been found to survive an irradiation dose of 280 rep/day (ARNOLD and JEE, 1957) and to maintain the ability to resorb bone in an intense field of irradiation.

Though a precise estimate of the relation of dosage to the degree of bone damage seems impossible to assess, in general the severe damages are caused by the higher doses. Even isotopes with a short half-life when administered in generous amount may exert deleterious effects: 0.1 mc/gm of body weight is a sufficient dose of ^{35}S to arrest growth in weaned rats and to determine severe alterations and destruction of the cartilage (RUBIN *et al.*, 1957). Repair of a bone lesion may occur only after action of the lower doses of radioisotopes with a short half-life.

(1) Radiation osteodysplasia has been experimentally induced in laboratory mammals following injection of various radioactive bone-seekers. According to VAUGHAN and JOWSEY (1956), the microscopical radiological changes in the upper third of the young rabbit tibia following a single intravenous injection of 500 to 1000 μC/kg of ^{90}Sr are represented by (a) an excess of calcified cartilaginous remnants under the epiphyseal plate: the osteogenic sarcoma appeared to develop in this region, (b) persistence of epiphyseal bone with only moderate excess of cartilage remnants, (c) abnormal growth

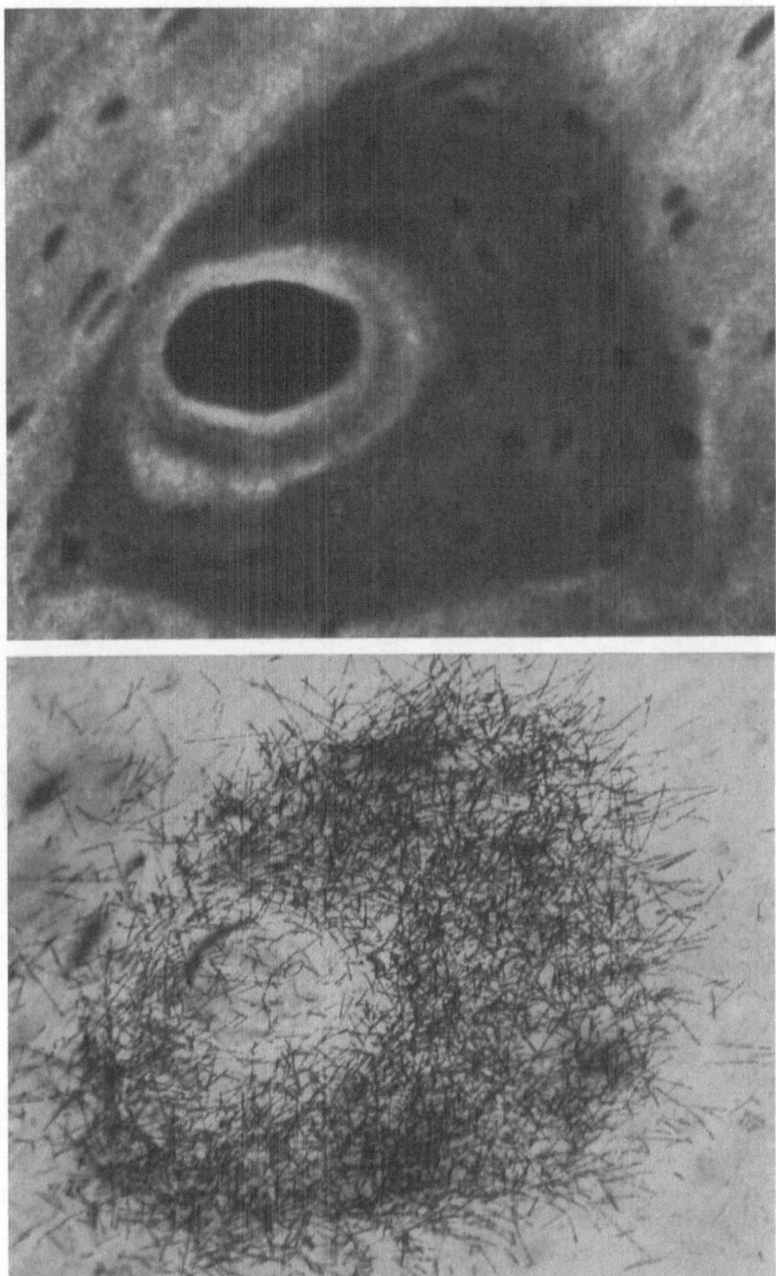

Fig. 24. Microradiograph and α-track autoradiograph at high magnification of an osteon of the compacta of a 56-year old man who had been carrying Ra for 24 years (terminal burden 3.6 μC). High activity in a relatively low calcified osteon. The neighboring older bone tissue contains comparatively little Ra. [Courtesy of R. E. ROWLAND and J. B. MARSHALL, Radiat. Res. 11, 299 (1959)]

of periosteal bone adjacent to unresorbed periosteal bone containing high concentration of ^{90}Sr in the diaphysis, (d) irregular bone formation in the cortex. The bone formed after Ra treatment in mice is atypical and fibrous, many empty lacunae are found; after Pu treatment the newly formed bone is fibrous and empty lacunae are fewer but the trabeculae of spongiosa become more and more compact (BLOOM and BLOOM, 1949). The histological changes of bones occurring in dogs after the administration of four *alpha*-emitters (Pu, Ra, mesothorium and radiothorium) have been analyzed by JEE *et al.*

(1957). The retained dose level of each isotope apparently determines the predominant pattern of changes; radiothorium resulted to be nine times as effective biologically as plutonium. The main changes observed in bone are: (a) reactions to *alpha*-radiations of endosteal and bone marrow cells: complete destruction of the marrow elements and substitution with a fibrous and gelatinous bone marrow, fibrosis on the surface of the endosteal and trabecular bone, excessive endosteal bone formation; (b) disturbances of normal bone growth and reconstruction: changes of bone renewal may be expressed by an excessive number of resorption cavities, formation of abnormal haversian systems, resorption of the periosteal surface with fibrosis, fractures which do not form bony union; (c) formation of osteogenic sarcoma. The extensive resorption is probably stimulated by

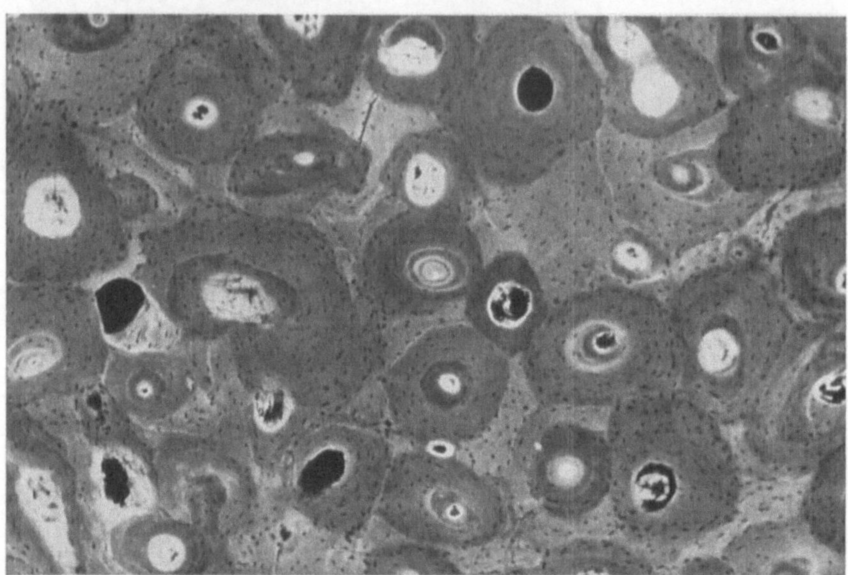

Fig. 25. Microradiograph of the tibia cortex of a man who had been carrying Ra for years. Highly Roentgen-ray absorbing material is plugging more or less completely a large number of haversian channels. The lacunae of osteocytes are preserved throughout. [Courtesy of R. E. ROWLAND, J. B. MARSHALL and J. JOWSEY, Res. **10**, 323 (1959)]

the presence of a large volume of devitalized bone, although not the whole of the latter undergoes resorption (JEE and ARNOLD, 1961). The fractures are believied to depend primarily on alterations in the quality of the matrix of devitalized bone (JEE and ARNOLD, 1960). JEE and ARNOLD (1957), ROWLAND *et al.* (1959) and HINDMARSH *et al.* (1959) have studied the changes in the mineral distribution in compact bone of Ra treated dogs and humans by means of microradiography: highly calcified osteons, hypercalcified plugs in vascular channels, filling of bone lacunae and two unusual types of resorption have been described (Fig. 25, 26).

(2) Osteogenic sarcomas were experimentally induced following injection of the *alpha*-emitters radium, plutonium, uranium. The latent period for Ra chloride and mesothorium treatment has been evaluated of the order of about one year for rabbits and rats. Various kinds of tumors, mainly osteogenic sarcomas, were found in mice receiving endovenously the *beta*-emitter radiostrontium. The incidence of bone tumors seemed to be roughly proportional to the dose in the range from 5.0 to 0.05 mc ^{89}Sr/gr body weight. The latent period was longer than 200 days. In a study of carcinogenesis in female mice it has been observed that gestation and lactation determine increase in the latent period of bone sarcoma, and a reduction in the total number of skeletal tumours in comparison with the unmated controls; instead, the frequency of leukemia appeared increased (NILSSON, 1967). The influence of lactation on the induction of bone tumours has been

attributed to the decreased retention of radiostrontium in lactating animals (NILSSON *et al.*, 1967). As now, it seems that *beta*-emitters are about ten times more effective than *alpha*-emitting isotopes in the production of tumors. Osteogenic sarcomas were induced in rats even with high doses of radiocalcium (BARNER *et al.*, 1958). Osteogenic sarcomas and also other kinds of tumors associated with more or less severe osteodysplasia were observed in Ra dial painters. The dose of radiation necessary for tumor development appeared to be variable in a series of cases of Ra poisoning studied by AUB *et al.* (1952); the body burden varied from 9 μg to 0.8 μg and the latent period from 26 to 12 years.

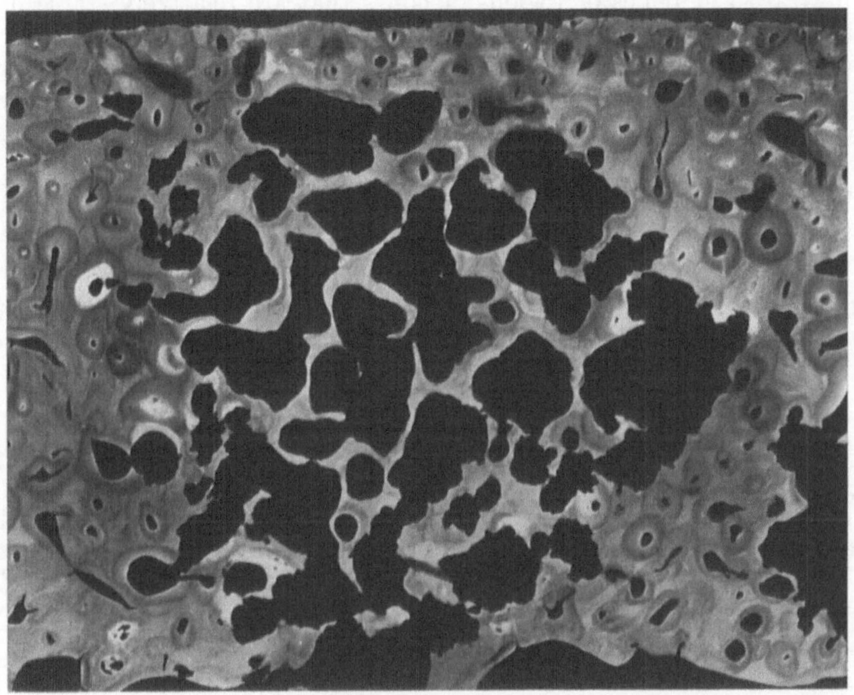

Fig. 26. Microradiograph of the femoral cortex of a man who had been carrying a heavy Ra burden for several years. A multilocular site of bone destruction. Hypermineralization of a few osteons and of their remnants in the areas neighboring the lesion. [Courtesy of R. E. ROWLAND, J. B. MARSHALL and J. JOWSEY, Radiat. Res. **10**, 323 (1959)]

In general, it seems that the time required for tumor development is longer when the overall skeletal burden of Ra is low than when it is high.

Quantitative studies of more than 450 humans who carried skeletal deposits of ^{226}Ra and ^{228}Ra for periods up to about 50 years have been presented as dose versus response relationship (EVANS, 1966). For residual skeletal burdens from about 0.5 to 60 μCi ^{226}Ra, the fractional incidence of osteogenic sarcoma and carcinoma of the paranasal sinuses or of the mastoids was about 40%, and it appeared to be independent of residual body burdens. For residual skeletal burdens less than 0.5 μCi ^{226}Ra, no clinical significant symptoms or discernible life span shortening were observed.

As to the sites of tumour formation in connection with the concentration of radioactivity in bone tissue, no rule can be formulated. This can be readily realized on account of the redistribution that radioactive atoms undergo in most regions of the skeleton. For instance, in ^{239}Pu injected adult beagles, 93.9% tumours arose from spongy regions of bone and only 6.1% from regions of cortical bone: the Pu concentration, however, varied extremely from bone to bone and within individual bones (JEE *et al.*, 1962). According to ARNOLD and JEE (1959), and others, the *diffuse* component (p. 823) may be more important than the *hot spots* in trabecular bone for the production of tumours at the high dose levels. In fact, many of the hot spots in trabecular bone may be resorbed and a substantial amount of the removed activity is redeposited diffusely. The redistribution, in turn, depends to some extent on the degree of the radiation damage incurred, especially on account of the altered circulation which results from direct irradiation of blood vessels. RUSHTON *et al.* (1961) observed that in weanling rabbits given one injection of ^{90}Sr, the sites of induced osteogenic sarcoma were similar in long bones and the mandible, *viz.*, sarcoma seemed to arise in osteogenic connective tissue associated with bone surface in which active deposition or resorption occurred at the time of injection (cf. also MAC PHERSON *et al.*, 1962). However, very high radiation doses may also accumulate, and tumours may arise in bones or regions of bones that are relatively stable, i.e., in which little redistribution took place of the radioelement deposited at first when the isotope concentration in the blood was high. In this connection, interesting observations were made by VAUGHAN and WILLIAMSON (cf. 1966) in their studies of the incidence of tumours arising from tissues adjacent to regions of bone whose turnover rate was extremely different, in groups of rabbits given an injection of various amounts of ^{90}Sr in different age periods from 2 days after birth.

References

ABBOTT, J., and H. HOLTZER: The loss of phenotypic traits by differentiated cells. J. Cell Biol. **28**, 473—487 (1966).

AMPRINO, R.: Autoradiographic analysis of the distribution of labeled Ca and P in bones. Experientia (Basel) **8**, 20—22 (1952*a*).

— Further experiments on the fixation in vitro of radiocalcium to sections of bone. Experientia (Basel) **8**, 380—382 (1952*b*).

— Rapporti fra processi di ricostruzione e distribuzione dei minerali nelle ossa. I. Ricerche con metodo istoradiografico. Z. Zellforsch. **37**, 144—183 (1952*c*).

— Rapporti fra processi di ricostruzione e distribuzione dei minerali nelle ossa. II. Ricerche con metodo autoradiografico. Z. Zellforsch. **37**, 240—273 (1952*d*).

— Autoradiographic research on the S^{35}-sulphate metabolism in cartilage and bone differentiation and growth. Acta anat. (Basel) **24**, 121—163 (1955).

—, and A. ENGSTRÖM: Studies on X-ray absorption and diffraction of bone tissue. Acta anat. (Basel) **15**, 1—22 (1952).

—, e G. GODINA: La struttura delle ossa nei vertebrati. Ricerche comparative negli anfibi e negli amnioti. Comm. Pontif. Acad. Sci. **11**, 329—464 (1947).

ARMSTRONG, W. D.: Phosphorus metabolism in the skeleton. In: Phosphorus Metabolism II, ed. by W. D. MCELROY and B. GLASS, pp. 698—731. Baltimore: Johns Hopkins Press 1952.

— J. SCHUBERT and A. LINDENBAUM: Distribution of radioactive carbon administered as carbonate in the body and excreta of mature rat. Proc. Soc. exp. Biol. (N.Y.) **68**, 233—240 (1948).

ARNOLD, J. S.: Metabolism of bone as studied by radioautographic distribution of calcium, plutonium and radium. Amer. J. Physiol. **167**, 765 (1951).

—, and W. S. S. JEE: Double tracer radioautographic studies of Ca^{45} and Ra^{226} bone disposition. Radiat. Res. **1**, 5 (1954a).

ARNOLD, J. S., and W. S. S. JEE: Ion exchange and recrystallization in fixation of Ca^{45} in the rabbit skeleton. Proc. Soc. exp. Biol. (N.Y.) **85**, 658—663 (1954*b*).

— — Bone growth and osteoclastic activity as indicated by radioautographic distribution of plutonium. Amer. J. Anat. **101**, 367—418 (1957).

— — Autoradiography in the localization and radiation dosage of Ra^{226} and Pu^{239} in the bones of dogs. Lab. Invest. **8**, 194—204 (1959).

— — and K. JOHNSON: Role of radioautographically detected bone growth and remodelling in Ca^{45} excretion and redistribution. XIX. Intern. Physiol. Congr. Abstracts of Communication 1953, pp. 174—175.

— — and K. JOHNSON: Observations and quantitative autoradiographic studies of $Calcium^{45}$ deposited *in vivo* in forming haversian systems and old bone of rabbit. Amer. J. Anat. **99**, 291—313 (1956).

ASLING, C. W., and L. E. NELSON: Autoradiographic localization of growth hormone-induced proliferation in bone and certain soft tissues. In: Radioisotopes and Bone, ed. by F. C. MCLEAN, P. LACROIX, and A. M. BUDY, pp. 191—195. Oxford: Blackwell Sci. Publ. 1962.

AUB, J. C., R. D. EVANS, L. H. HEMPELMANN and H. S. MARTLAND: Late effects of internally-deposited radioactive materials in man. Medicine (Baltimore) **31**, 221—329 (1952).

AUBERT, J.-P., F. BRONNER, and L. J. RICHELLE: Quantitation of calcium metabolism. J. clin. Invest. **42**, 885—897 (1963).

—, et G. MILHAUD: Méthode de mésure des principales voies du métabolisme calcique chez l'homme. Biochim. biophys. Acta (Amst.) **39**, 122—139 (1960).

BÄCKSTRÖM, J., L. HAMMARSTRÖM, and A. NELSON: Distribution of Zirconium and Niobium in mice. Acta radiol. (Stockh.) **6**, 122—128 (1967).

Barnes, L. L., G. Sperling, C. M. McCay and C. E. Brown: The production of osteogenic sarcomas in rats with radioactive calcium. Arch. Path. (Chicago) **66**, 529—535 (1958).

Bauer, G. C. H.: The importance of bone growth as a factor in the redistribution of bone salt. I. Redistribution of radio-active calcium in the skeleton of rats. J. Bone Jt Surg. A **36**, 375—380 (1954a).

— The importance of bone growth as a factor in the redistribution of bone salt. II. Redistribution of radio-active phosphorus in the skeleton of rats. J. Bone Jt Surg. A **36**, 381—386 (1954*b*).

— Rate of bone formation in a healing fracture determined in rats by means of radio-calcium. Acta orthop. scand. **23**, 169—191 (1954*c*).

— Kinetics of calcium and strontium metabolism in man. In: Bone as a Tissue, ed. by K. Rodahl, J. T. Nicholson and E. M. Brown jr., pp. 118—127. New York: McGraw-Hill Book Co., Inc. 1960.

—, and A. Carlsson: Post-fracture bone salt resorption studied in rats. Acta orthop. scand. **25**, 83—88 (1955).

— — and D. Lindquist: Evaluation of accretion, absorption and exchange reactions in the skeleton. Kgl. Fysiograf. Sällskap. Lund Förh. **25**, 1—16 (1955*a*)

— — — A comparative study on the metabolism of Sr^{90} and Ca^{45}. Acta physiol. scand. **35**, 56—66 (1955*b*).

— — — Bone salt metabolism in human rickets studied with radioactive phosphorus. Metabolism **5**, 573—581 (1956).

— — — Metabolism of Ba^{140} in man. Acta orthop. scand. **26**, 241—254 (1957*a*).

— — — Bone salt metabolism in humans studied by means of radiocalcium. Acta med. scand. **158**, 143—150 (1957*b*).

— — — Use of isotopes in clinical studies of skeletal metabolism. In: Radioaktive Isotope in Klinik und Forschung, Bd. III, herausgeg. von K. Fellinger u. H. Vetter, S. 25—39. München: Urban & Schwarzenberg 1958.

— — — Metabolism and homeostatic function of bone. In: Mineral Metabolism, vol. I/B, ed by C. L. Comar and F. Bronner, pp. 609—676. New York: Academic Press 1961.

—, and D. Ray: Kinetics of strontium metabolism in man. J. Bone Jt Surg. A **40**, 171—186 (1958).

—, and B. Wendeberg: External counting of Ca^{47} and Sr^{85} in studies of localized skeletal lesions in man. J. Bone Jt Surg. B **41**, 558—580 (1959).

Bélanger, L. F.: A method for routine detection of radiophosphates and other radioactive compounds in tissues. The inverted autograph. Anat. Rec. **107**, 149—160 (1950).

— Autoradiographic visualization of the entry and transit of S^{35} in cartilage, bone, and dentine of young rats and the effect of hyaluronidase *in vitro*. Canad. J. Biochem. **32**, 161—169 (1954).

Bélanger, L. F.: Autoradiographic studies of the formation of the organic matrix of cartilage, bone and the tissues of teeth. In: Bone structure and metabolism. Ciba Foundation Symposium, ed by G. E. W. Wolstenholme and C. M. O'Connor, pp. 75—88. London: J. A. Churchill Ltd. 1956.

—, and C. P. Leblond: A method for locating radioactive elements in tissues by covering histological sections with a photographic emulsion. Endocrinology **39**, 8—13 (1946).

Bellin, J., and D. Laszlo: Metabolism and removal of Ca^{45} in man. Science **117**, 331—334 (1953).

Bergner, P. E. E.: Dynamic aspects of a method in tracerkinetics. Exp. Cell Res. **17**, 328—335 (1959).

Bernstein, D. S., and P. Handler: Effects of parathyroid extract on sulfate metabolism of cartilage and bone matrix of rachitic rats. Proc. Soc. exp. Biol. (N.Y.) **99**, 339—340 (1958).

Bessler, W.: Resultate mit Sr^{85} Skeletszintigraphie. In: Radioisotope in der Lokalisationsdiagnostik, herausgeg. von G. Hoffmann und K. E. Scheer, S. 431. Stuttgart: F. K. Schattauer 1967.

Black, A. L., M. Kleiber, A. H. Smith and N. P. Ralston: Mobility of skeletal phosphorus in a mature dairy cow as determined with radioactive phosphorus. Proc. Soc. exp. Biol. (N.Y.) **82**, 248—252 (1953).

Bloom, M. A., and W. Bloom: Late effects of radium and plutonium on bone. Arch. Path. (Chicago) **47**, 494—511 (1949).

Bloom, W., J. H. Curtis and F. C. McLean: The deposition of C^{14} in bone. Science **105**, 45 (1947).

Böstrom, H.: Chemical and autoradiographic studies on the sulfate exchange in sulphomucopolysaccharides. Ark. Kemi **6**, 43—57 (1953).

—, and B. Månson: Factors influencing the exchange of the sulfate group of the chondroitin sulphuric acid of cartilage *in vitro*. Ark. Kemi **6**, 23—37 (1953).

—, and E. Odeblad: The influence of cortisone upon the sulphate exchange of chondroitinsulphuric acid. Ark. Kemi **6**, 39—42 (1953).

Bohr, H. H.: Studies on fracture healing. J. Bone Jt Surg. A **37**, 327—337 (1955).

— On the uptake of radioactive Calcium and Strontium in the skeleton of normal and rachitic rats. Acta orthop. scand. **30**, 237—250 (1961).

—, and S. G. Dawids: The effect of cortisone and anabolic steroids on the retention of radioactive Calcium and Strontium in rats. Acta endocr. (Kbh.) **47**, 223—230 (1964).

Boni, M., e A. Rampoldi: Ricerche con l'isotopo radioattivo del solfo (35-S) sulla cartilagine di accrescimento. Ortop. Traumat. Appar. mot. **26**, 45—59 (1958).

Boyd, G. A.: Autoradiography in biology and medicine. New York: Academic Press Inc. 1955.

BRONNER, F.: Effects of parathyroid extract on Ca and sulphur metabolism. Fed. Proc. **16**, 158 (1957).
— Effects of parathyroid extract on metabolism of sulphate in immature rats. Amer. J. Physiol. **198**, 605—608 (1960).
— Parathyroid effects on sulfate metabolism: interrelationships with calcium. In: The Parathyroids, ed. by R. O. GREEP and R. V. TALMAGE, pp. 123—138. Springfield: Ch. C. Thomas 1961.
— Parathyroid effects on sulfate and calcium metabolism. Trans. N. Y. Acad. Sci., S. II, **24**, 265—272 (1962).
— Dynamics and function of Calcium. In: Mineral Metabolism, vol. II/A, ed. by C. L. COMAR and F. BRONNER, pp. 341—444. New York: Academic Press 1964.
—, and R. S. HARRIS: Absorption and metabolism of calcium in human beings studied with calcium[45]. Ann. N. Y. Acad. Sci. **64**, 314—325 (1956).
— — C. J. MALETSKOS and C. E. BENDA: Studies in calcium metabolism. The fate of intravenous injected radiocalcium in human beings. J. clin. Invest. **35**, 78—88 (1956).
BUDY, A. M.: The use of radioisotopes in Orthopaedics. Part II. Application of radioactive tracer techniques to bone. J. Bone Jt Surg. A **45**, 1073—1083 (1963).
CAMPO, R. D., and D. D. DZIEWIATKOWSKI: A consideration of the permeability of cartilage to inorganic sulfate. J. biophys. biochem. Cytol. **9**, 401—408 (1961).
— — Turnover of the organic matrix of cartilage and bone as visualized by autoradiography. J. Cell Biol. **18**, 19—29 (1963).
CARLSSON, A., and D. LINDQUIST: Comparison of intestinal and skeletal effects of vitamine D in relation to dosage. Acta physiol. scand. **35**, 53—55 (1955).
CARNEIRO, J., and C. P. LEBLOND: Role of osteoblasts and odontoblasts in secreting the collagen of bone and dentin, as shown by radioautography in mice given tritium-labeled-glycine. Exp. Cell Res. **18**, 291—300 (1959).
CARRIT, J., R. FOYXELL, J. KLEINSCHMIDT, R. KLEINSCHMIDT, W. LANGHAM, A. SAN PIETRO, R. SCHATFH and B. SCHNAP: The distribution and excretion of plutonium administered intravenously to the rat. J. biol. Chem. **171**, 273—283 (1947).
CARTIER, P. H., B. DE BERNARD and I. LAGRANGE: Studies on the repair of fractures using P^{32}. In Ciba Foundation Symposium on Bone structure and metabolism, ed. by G. E. W. WOLSTENHOLME and C. M. O'CONNOR, pp. 148—160. London: Churchill Ltd. 1956.
COHEN, J., and C. J. MALETSKOS: ^{45}Ca in the study of bone grafts in dogs. In: Radioisotopes and Bone, ed. by F. C. MCLEAN, P. LACROIX and A. M. BUDY, pp. 127—148. Oxford: Blackwell Sci. Publ. 1962.
— — J. H. MARSHALL and J. B. WILLIAMS: Radioactive calcium tracer studies in bone grafts. J. Bone Jt Surg. A **39**, 561—577 (1957).
COLLINS, E. J., O. S. CARPENTER, and V. F. BAKER: Influence of adrenal steroids on radio. calcium metabolism in young beagle dogs. Acta endocr. (Kbh.) **42**, 348—354 (1963).
COMAR, C. L.: Radioisotopes in biology and agriculture. Principles and practice. New York: McGraw-Hill Book Co., Inc. 1955.
— W. E. LOTZ and G. A. BOYD: Autoradiographic studies of calcium, phosphorus and strontium distribution in the bones of the growing pig. Amer. J. Anat. **90**, 113—129 (1952).
—, and R. H. WASSERMAN: Radioisotopes in the study of mineral metabolism. In: Progress in nuclear energy, S. 6, vol. I, pp. 153—196. London: Pergamon Press 1956.
— — Strontium. In: Mineral Metabolism, vol. II/A, ed. by C. L. COMAR and F. BRONNER, pp. 523—572. New York: Academic Press 1964.
COPP, D. H., D. J. AXELROD and J. C. HAMILTON: The deposition of radioactive metals in bone as a potential health hazard. Amer. J. Roentgenol. **58**, 10—16 (1947).
— E. C. CAMERON, B. A. CHENEY, A. G. DAVIDSON, and K. G. HENZE: Evidence for Calcitonin — A new hormone from the parathyroid that lowers blood calcium. Endocrinology **70**, 638—649 (1962).
—, and S. S. SHIM: Extraction ratio and bone clearance of Sr^{85} as a measure of effective bone blood flow. Circulation Res. **16**, 461—467 (1965).
—, and A. P. SUIKER: Study of calcium kinetics in calcium- and phosphorus-deficient rats with the aid of radiocalcium. In: Radioisotopes and Bone, ed. by P. LACROIX and A. M. BUDY, pp. 1—16. Oxford: Blackwell Sci. Publ. 1962.
CRAMER, C. F., and D. H. COPP: Effect of mineral deficient diet on excretion of radiocalcium and radiostrontium. Amer. J. Physiol. **167**, 776 (abstract) (1951).
CURRAN, R. C., and J. S. KENNEDY: The distribution of the sulphated mucopolysaccharides in the mouse. J. Path. Bact. **70**, 449—457 (1955).
DALLEMAGNE, M. J.: Propos sur les sels osseux. Acta physiol. pharmacol. neerl. **6**, 469—478 (1957).
— CH. A. BAUD et P. W. MORGENTHALER: Autoradiographies de coupes d'os compact après marquage aux isotopes *in vitro*. Essai d'interprétation. Histochemie **1**, 185—189 (1959).
—, et C. FABRY: Le problème des sels osseux. Acta chir. belg. et Acta orthop. belg. Suppl. **1**, 75—114 (1956).
— J. GOVAERTS et J. MELON: Influence de la folliculine sur le métabolisme calcique du pigeon, étudiée a l'aide du radiocalcium. Arch. int. Physiol. **58**, 157—187 (1950).
DAVIES, D. V., and L. YOUNG: The distribution of radioactive sulphur (^{35}S) in the fibrous tissues, cartilages and bones of the rat following its administration in the form of inorganic sulphate. J. Anat. (Lond.) 88, 174—183 (1954).

DENARDO, L. G., and J. A. VOLPE: Detection of bone lesions with the Strontium-85 scintiscan. J. nucl. Med. **7**, 219—236 (1966).

DILLA, M. A. VAN, B. J. STOVER, R. L. FLOYD, D. R. ATHERTON and D. H. TAYSUM: Radium (RA^{226}) and Radon (Em^{222}) metabolism in dogs. Radiat. Res. **8**, 417—437 (1958).

DIXON, A. D.: Studies of the growth of the upper facial skeleton using radioactive calcium. J. dent. Res. **40**, 204—216 (1961).

—, and D. A. N. HOYTE: Autoradiographic and alizarin techniques in the study of skull growth. J. Anat. (Lond.) **93**, 589 (1959).

DUDLEY, R. A., and B. M. DOBYNS: The use of autoradiographs in the quantitative determination of radiation dosages from Ca ^{45} in bone. Science **109**, 327—328 (1949).

DURBIN, P. W., M. H. WILLIAMS, M. GEE, R. H. NEUMANN and J. G. HAMILTON: Metabolism of the lanthanons in the rat. Proc. Soc. exp. Biol. (N.Y.) **91**, 78—85 (1956).

DUTHIE, R. B., and A. N. BARKER: An autoradiographic study of mucopolysaccharides and phosphate complexes in bone growth and repair. J. Bone Jt Surg. B. **37**, 304—323 (1955*a*).

— — The histochemistry of the preosseous stage of bone repair studied by autoradiography. The effect of cortisone. J. Bone Jt Surg. B **37**, 691—710 (1955*b*).

DZIEWIATKOWSKI, D. D.: Radioautographic visualization of sulphur-35 disposition in the articular cartilage and bone of suckling rats following injection of labeled sodium sulphate. J. exp. Med. **93**, 451—458 (1951*a*).

— Isolation of chondroitin-sulphate-S^{35} from articular cartilage of rat. J. biol. Chem. **189**, 187—190 (1951*b*).

— Radioautographic studies of sulphate sulphur (S^{35}) metabolism in the articular cartilage and bone of suckling rats. J. exp. Med. **95**, 489—496 (1952).

— Sulphate-sulphur metabolism in the rat fetus as indicated by sulphur-35. J. exp. Med. **98**, 119—128 (1953).

— Effect of age on some aspects of sulphate metabolism in the rat. J. exp. Med. **99**, 283—298 (1954*a*).

— Vitamine A and endochondral ossification in the rat as indicated by the use of sulphur-35 and phosphorus-32. J. exp. Med. **100**, 11—24 (1954*b*).

— Vitamine A and endochondral ossification in the rat as indicated by the use of sulphur-35 and phosphorus-32. J. exp. Med. **100**, 25—32 (1954*c*).

— Synthesis of sulphomucopolysaccharides in thyroidectomized rats. J. exp. Med. **105**, 69—74 (1957).

— Autoradiographic studies with S^{35}-sulphate. Intern. Rev. Cytol. VII, ed. by G. H. BOURNE and J. F. DANIELLI, pp. 159—193. New York: Academic Press 1958.

— Sulfur. In: Mineral Metabolism, vol. II/B, ed. by C. L. COMAR and F. BRONNER, pp. 175—220. New York: Academic Press 1962.

DZIEWIATKOWSKI, D. D., F. BRONNER, N. DI FERRANTE and R. M. ARCHIBALD: Some aspects of the metabolism of sulphate-S^{35} and calcium-45 in the metaphysis of immature rats. Influence of β-estradiol benzoate. J. biophys. biochem. Cytol. **3**, 151—160 (1957).

ELLIOT, J. R., and R. V. TALMAGE: Removal of Ca^{40} and Ca^{45} from bone by citrate as influenced by the parathyroid. Endocrinology **62**, 709—716 (1958).

ELLIS, S., J. HUBLE', and M. E. SIMPSON: Influence of hypophysectomy and growth hormone on cartilage sulfate metabolism. Proc. Soc. exp. Biol. (N.Y.) **84**, 603—605 (1953).

ENGFELDT, B., A. ENGSTRÖM and H. BOSTRÖM: The localisation of radiosulphate in bone tissue. Exp. Cell Res. **6**, 251—253 (1954).

— — and R. ZETTERSTRÖM: Renewal of phosphate in bone minerals. II. Radioautographic studies of renewal of phosphate in different structures of bone. Biochem. biophys. Acta **8**, 375—380 (1952).

—, and S. O. HJERTQUIST: Biophysical studies on bone tissue. X. The *in vivo* and *in vitro* uptake of radioactive isotopes and ionic exchange reactions in bone tissue. Acta path. microbiol. scand. **35**, 205—216 (1954).

—, and R. ZETTERSTRÖM: Biophysical and chemical investigation on bone tissue in experimental hyperparathyroidism. Endocrinology **54**, 506—515 (1954).

ENGSTRÖM, A., R. BJÖRNERSTEDT, C.-J. CLEMEDSON, and A. NELSON: Bone and Radiostrontium. New York: Wiley 1958.

ESTEBAN, J., D. LASS, and S. PEREZ-MODREGO: Detection of metastases in the skeleton with radioactive colloidal gold. Brit. J. Radiol. **40**, 181—183 (1967).

EVANS, R. D.: The effect of skeletally deposited *alpha*-ray emitters in man. Brit. J. Radiol. **39**, 881—895 (1966).

FABRY, C.: L'échange isoionique de phosphates de calcium avec le calcium radioactif. II. L' échange du phosphate synthétique de rapport Ca/P 2.14. Bull. Soc. Chim. biol. **40**, 993—1002 (1958).

FALKENHEIM, M., E. E. UNDERWOOD and H. C. HODGE: Calcium exchange: the mechanism of absorption by bone of Ca^{45}. J. biol. Chem. **188**, 805—817 (1951).

FITTON JACKSON, S., and J. I. RANDALL: Fibrogenesis and the formation of matrix in developing bone. In: Bone structure and metabolism. Ciba Foundation Symposium, ed. by G. E. W. WOLSTENHOLME and C. M. O'CONNOR, pp. 47—64. London: J. A. Churchill Ltd. 1956.

FLEMING, W. H., J. D. MCILRAITH, and E. R. KING: Photoscanning of bone lesions utilizing strontium-85. Radiology **77**, 635—636 (1961).

FOSTER, G. V., A. BAGHDIANTZ, M. A. KUMAR, E. SLACK, H. A. SOLIMAN, and I. MACINTYRE: Thyroid origin of calcitonin. Nature (Lond.) **202**, 1303—1305 (1964).

FREDERICKSON, J. M., A. J. HONOUR, and D. H. COPP: Measurement of initial bone clearance of Ca^{45} from blood in the rat. Fed. Proc. **14**, 49 (1965).

Frey, K. W., A. Sonntag, M. S. Scheybani, D. Krauss, and P. Fuchs: Knochen-Szintigraphie mit Strontium-85. Fort. Röntgenstr. **106**, 206—215 (1967).

Friberg, U., and N. R. Ringertz: An autoradiographic study on the uptake of radiosulphate in the rat embryo. J. Embryol. exp. Morph. **4**, 313—326 (1956).

Frost, H. M., A. R. Villanueva and H. Roth: Measurements of bone formation in a 57 year old man by means of tetracyclines. Henry Ford Hosp. Med. Bull. **8**, 239—254 (1960).

Gaillard, P. J.: Bone culture studies with calcitonin. Abridg. Proc. 4th Europ. Symp. on Calcified Tissues, p. 32—33. Amsterdam: Excerpta Medica Found. 1966.

Garrett, E. R., R. L. Johnston, and E. J. Collins: Quantification of normal and adrenal steroid affected calcium metabolism in the young dog. J. Pharmacol. exp. Ther. **145**, 357—366 (1964).

Geschwind, I. I.: Hormonal control of calcium, phosphorus, iodine, sulfur, and magnesium metabolism. In: Mineral Metabolism, vol. I/B, pp. 387—472, ed. by C. L. Comar and F. Bronner. New York: Academic Press 1961.

—, C. H. Li and H. M. Evans: The effects of hypophysectomy and of growth hormone on the uptake of radioactive phosphorus by tissues. Arch. Biochem. **31**, 168—182 (1951).

Glick, D.: A critical survey of current approaches in quantitative Histo- and Cytochemistry. In: Intern. Rev. Cytology, ed. by G. H. Bourne and J. F. Danielli, vol. II, pp. 447—474. New York: Acad. Press. Inc. 1953.

Glimcher, M. J.: The molecular biology of the mineralized tissues with particular reference to bone. Rev. modern Phys. **31**, 359—393 (1959).

Glücksmann, A., A. Howard and S. R. Pelc: The uptake of radioactive sulphate by cells, fibres and ground-substance of mature and developing connective tissue in the adult mouse. J. Anat. (Lond.) **90**, 478—485 (1956).

Gordon, G. S.: A direct action of parathyroid hormone on dead bone in vitro. Acta endocr. (Kbh.) **44**, 481—489 (1963).

Govaerts, J., and M. J. Dallemagne: Influence of folliculin on bone metabolism, studied by means of radiophosphorus, P^{32}. Nature (Lond.) **161**, 977 (1948).

— —, and J. Mélon: Radiocalcium as an indicator in the study of the action of estradiol on calcium metabolism. Endocrinology **48**, 443—452 (1951).

Gran, F. C.: Studies on calcium and strontium-90 metabolism in rats. Acta physiol. scand. **48**, Suppl. **167**, 1—109 (1960).

Greulich, R. C.: Entry of radio-carbon from labeled bicarbonate into the organic matrix of growing bones and teeth. Anat. Rec. **115**, 312—313 (1953).

— An autoradiographic study of organically bound carbon-14 in growing epiphyseal cartilage and bone. J. Bone Jt Surg. A **38**, 611—626 (1956).

Greulich, R. C., and U. Friberg: Histochemical studies of sulpho-mucopolysaccharides in the organic matrices of mineralized tissues. Exp. Cell Res. **12**, 685—689 (1957).

—, and C. P. Leblond: Radioautographic visualization of radio-carbon in the organs and tissues of newborn rats following administration of C^{14}-labeled bicarbonate. Anat. Rec. **115**, 559—585 (1953).

Hammarström, L., A. Nilson, and J. Ullberg: Distribution of radiostrontium in developing bones and teeth. Microradioautographic study with 85-Sr. Acta radiol. (Stockh.) **3**, 183—192 (1965).

Hansard, S. L., C. L. Comar and G. K. Davis: Effects of age upon the physiological behaviour of calcium in cattle. Amer. J. Physiol. **177**, 383—389 (1954).

— — and M. P. Plumlee: The effects of age upon calcium utilisation and maintenance requirements in the bovine. J. animal Sci. **13**, 25—36 (1954).

Harbers, E.: Autoradiographie als histochemisches Untersuchungsverfahren. In: Handbuch der Histochemie, Bd. I, Teil 1, herausgeg. von W. Graumann und R. Neumann, S. 400—598. Stuttgart: G. Fischer 1958.

Harris, W. H.: A microscopic method of determining rates of bone growth. Nature (Lond.) **188**, 1038—1039 (1960).

Harrison, H. F., and H. C. Harrison: The uptake of radiocalcium by the skeleton: the effect of vitamine D intake. J. biol. Chem. **185**, 857—867 (1950).

Haumont, S.: Le Zinc dans le tissu osseux. Bruxelles: Ed. Arscia 1962.

Heaney, R. P.: Evaluation and interpretation of calcium-kinetic data in man. Clin. Orthop. **31**, 153—183 (1963).

— G. C. H. Bauer, F. Bronner, J. F. Dymling, F. W. Lafferty, B. E. C. Nordin, and C. Rich: A normal reference standard for radiocalcium turnover and excretion in humans. J. Lab. clin. Med. **64**, 21—28 (1964).

—, and G. D. Whedon: Radiocalcium studies of bone formation rate in human metabolic bone disease. J. clin. Endocr. Metab. **18**, 1246—1267 (1958).

Henneman, D. H.: In vitro C^{14}-glycine and C^{14}-arginine metabolism by whole bone and metaphyseal fragments. Abr. Proc. 4th Europ. Symp. Calcified Tissues, pp. 102—103, ed. by P. J. Gaillard, A. van den Hooff, and R. Steendijk. Amsterdam: Excerpta Med. Foud. 1966.

Herman, H., and M. J. Dallemagne: The main mineral constituent of bone and teeth. Arch. oral Biol. **5**, 137—144 (1961).

—, and L. J. Richelle: Le calcium échangeable de la substance minérale de l'os étudiée à l'aide de ^{45}Ca. VII. Activité comparée de fractions d'os total de densité différente. Bull. Soc. Chim. biol. (Paris) **43**, 273—282 (1961).

HEVESY, G.: Radioactive indicators. New York: Interscience Publishers, Inc. 1948.
— H. B. LEVI and O. H. REBBE: Rate of rejuvenation of the skeleton. Biochem. J. **34**, 532—537 (1940).
HINDMARSH, M., M. OWEN and J. VAUGHAN: The relative hazards of strontium-90 and radium-226. Brit. J. Radiol. **31**, 518—533 (1957).
— — — A note on the distribution of radium and a calculation of the radiation dose non-uniformity factor for radium^{226} and strontium^{90} in the femur of a luminous dial painter. Brit. J. Radiol. **32**, 183—187 (1959).
—, and J. VAUGHAN: The distribution of calcium in certain bones from a man exposed to radium for thirty-four years. Brit. J. Radiol. **29**, 71—80 (1956).
HOECKER, F. E., and P. G. ROOFE: Studies of radium in human bone. Radiology **56**, 89—98 (1951).
HOWARTH, J. L.: Calculation of the *alpha*-ray absorbed dose to soft tissue cavities in bone. Brit. J. Radiol. **38**, 51—56 (1965).
HUNZIGER, W. A., u. G. A. ORTELLI: Retention und Austausch von Calcium aus Ca^{45}-Dinatrium-Aethylendiamintetraacetat. In: Radioaktive Isotope in Klinik und Forschung, herausgeg. von K. FELLIGER u. H. VETTER, Bd. II, S. 76—84. München: Urban & Schwarzenberg 1956.
HURWITZ, S.: Bone composition and Ca^{45} retention in fowl as influenced by egg formation. Amer. J. Physiol. **206**, 198—204 (1964).
— Calcium turnover in different bone segments of laying fowl. Amer. J. Physiol. **208**, 203—207 (1965).
IRVING, J. T.: Calcium metabolism. London: Methuen & Co. Ltd. 1957.
ITO, Y., K. TAKAMURA, and H. ENDO: The effect of growth hormone on the incorporation of labeled sulfate into the chick embryo femur in tissue culture. Endocr. jap. **7**, 327—335 (1960).
— S. TSURUFUJI, S. ISHIBASHI, M. ISHIDATE, Z. TAMURA and H. TAKITA: Detoxication and excretion of radioactive strontium. III. Effect of tricarballytic and lactic acids. Pharm. Bull. (Tôkyô) **6**, 34—36 (1958).
— — M. SHIKITA and S. ISHIBASHI: Effect of phosphorus deficient diet with excess of calcium or strontium on the excretion of radiostrontium and its possible mechanism. Pharm. Bull. (Tôkyô) **6**, 115—116 (1958*a*).
— — — — Detoxication and excretion of radioactive strontium. IV. Effect of sodium calcium citrate and the mode of action of citrate. Pharm. Bull. (Tôkyô) **6**, 287—290 (1958*b*).
JEE, W. S. S., and J. S. ARNOLD: Rate of individual Haversian system formation. Anat. Rec. **118**, 315 (Abstract) (1954).
— — Microradiographic studies of cortical bone of chronic toxicity dogs. Semiannual Progress Report, Radiobiology Laboratory, University of Utah College of Medicine, Salt Lake City, Utah, pp. 56—61, Sept. 1957.
JEE, W. S. S., and J. S. ARNOLD: The effect of internally deposited radioisotopes upon the blood vessels of cortical bone. Proc. Soc. exp. Biol. Med. **105**, 351—356 (1960).
— — The toxicity of plutonium deposited in skeletal tissues of beagles. I. The relation of the distribution of plutonium to the sequence of histopathologic bone changes. Lab. Invest **10**, 797—825 (1961).
— — R. S. MICAL, B. BIRD, O. FRENDENBERGER and M. LOWE: Bone: histopathologic and autoradiographic studies. Annual Progress Report, Radiobiology Laboratory, University of Utah College of Medicine, Salt Lake City, Utah, pp. 74—97, March 1958.
— P. OTTOSEN, R. MICAL and M. LOWE: Bone: histopathologic and autoradiographic findings. Annual Progress Report, Radiobiology Laboratory, University of Utah College of Medicine, Salt Lake City, Utah, pp. 86—114, March 1957.
— B. J. STOVER, G. N. TAYLOR, and W. R. CHRISTENSEN: The skeletal toxicity of Pu^{239} in adult beagles. Hlth Phys. **8**, 599—607 (1962).
JODREY, L. H., and K. M. WILBUR: Autoradiograms of irregular surfaces. Proc. Soc. exp. Biol. (N. Y.) **77**, 80—82 (1951).
JOHNSTON, P. M.: Isotopes in studies on the metabolism of bones and teeth. In: Künstliche radio-aktive Isotope in Physiologie, Diagnostik und Therapie, herausgeg. von R. H. SCHWIEG u. F. TURBA, 2. Aufl. Heidelberg: Springer 1961.
JONES, D. C., and D. H. COPP: The metabolism of radioactive strontium in adult young and rachitic rats. J. biol. Chem. **189**, 509—514 (1951).
JOWSEY, J.: Age changes in human bone. Clin. Orthop. **17**, 210—218 (1960).
— W. CAFFERTY, and J. RABINOWITZ: Analysis of distribution of Ca^{45} in dog bone by quantitative autoradiographic method. J. Bone Jt Surg. A **47**, 359—370 (1965).
—, and A. L. ORVIS: Comparative deposition of ^{45}Ca, ^{65}Zn and ^{91}Y in bone. Radiat. Res. **31**, 693—698 (1967).
— M. OWEN and J. VAUGHAN: Microradiographs and autoradiographs of cortical bone from monkeys injected with 90-Sr. Brit. J. exp. Path. **34**, 661—667 (1953).
— R. E. ROWLAND, and J. H. MARSHALL: The deposition of the rare earths in bone. Radiat. Res. **8**, 490—497 (1958).
— —, and F. C. MCLEAN: The effect of parathyroidectomy on haversian remodeling of bone. Endocrinology **63**, 903—908 (1958).
KANE, W. J., and E. GRIM: Blood flow to bone: a quantitative method and its validation. J. Bone Jt Surg. A **48**, 1008—1009 (1966).
KEMBER, N. F.: Cell division in endochondral ossification. J. Bone Jt Surg. B **42**, 824—839 (1960).
KIDMAN, B., M. L. TUTT and J. M. VAUGHAN: The retention and excretion of radioactive strontium and yttrium (Sr^{89}, Sr^{90} and Y^{90}) in the healthy rabbit. J. Path. Bact. **62**, 209—227 (1950).

KIEHN, C. L., H. L. FRIEDELL and W. J. MAC INTYRE: Study of the vitality of tissue transplant by means of radioactive phosphorus. Plast. reconstr. Surg. **3**, 335—339 (1948).

KNESE, K. H., u. A. M. KNOOP: Elektronenoptische Untersuchungen über die periostale Osteogenese. Z. Zellforsch. **48**, 455—478 (1958).

KODICEK, E.: Metabolic studies on vitamin D. Ciba Foundation Symposium on Bone structure and metabolism, ed. by G. E. W. WOLSTENHOLME and C. M. O'CONNOR, pp. 161—174. London: Churchill Ltd. 1956.

—, and G. A. THOMPSON: Autoradiographic localization in bones of [1α—^{3}H] cholocalciferol. In: Structure and function of connective and skeletal tissue, pp. 369—372. Proc. Advanced Study Inst., St. Andrews. London: Butterworths 1965.

KOLÁŘ, J., V. BEK, L. JANKO, L. VYNÁNEK, A. BABICKY u. D. DRÁPELOVÁ: Zum Sinn und Grenzen der Knochendiagnostik mit ^{85}Sr. Fortschr. Röntgenstr. **106**, 216—224 (1967).

KOPRIWA, B. M., and C. P. LEBLOND: Improvements in the coating technique of radioautography. J. Histochem. Cytochem. **10**, 219—223 (1962).

KSHIRAGAR, S. G., E. LLOYD, and J. VAUGHAN: Discrimination between Strontium and Calcium in bone and the transfer from blood to bone in the rabbit. Brit. J. Radiol. **39**, 131—140 (1966).

LACROIX, P.: Autoradiographies du tissu osseux spongieux. Experientia (Basel) **8**, 426 (1952).

— Radiocalcium and radiosulphur in the study of bone metabolism at the histological level. Radioisotope Conference vol. 1, pp. 134—137. London: Butterworth's Scientific Publications 1954.

— The histological remodeling of adult bone. An autoradiographic study in bone structure and metabolism. Ciba Foundation Symposium, ed. by G. E. W. WOLSTENHOLME and C. M. O'CONNOR, pp. 36—44. London: Churchill Ltd. 1956.

— Ca^{45} autoradiography in the study of bone tissue. In: Bone as a Tissue, ed. by K. RODAHL, J. T. NICHOLSON and E. M. BROWN, pp. 262—279. New York: McGraw-Hill Book Co., Inc. 1960.

LANGENSKIJÖLD, A., T. RYTÖMAA, and T. VIDEMAN: An autoradiographic study with ^{35}S-sulphate in the growth in diameter of epiphyseal cartilage in rabbits. Acta orthop. scand., Suppl. No 106, 3—25 (1967).

LASZLO, D.: Biological studies on calcium, strontium, lanthanum and yttrium. Intern. Conf. on the peaceful uses of atomic energy. A/Conf. 8/P/21, U.S.A./1955.

—, and H. SPENCER: Newer techniques in the study of calcium metabolism in man and effects of hormones thereon. In: Hormones and the aging process, ed. by E. T. ENGER and G. PINCUS, pp. 175—200. New York: Acad. Press Inc. 1956.

LAYTON, L. L., with the technical assistance of D. F. FRANKEL and S. SCAPA: Quantitative differential fixation of sulphate by tissues maintained *in vitro*. I. Sulphate fixation as a function of age for embryonic tissues. Cancer (Philad.) **3**, 725—734 (1950).

LEA, L. M., et R. PONLOT: Sur les autoradiographies au Ca^{45} des os longs en croissance. Les mécanismes de l'apposition osseuse souspériostée. Arch. Biol. (Liège) **69**, 455—465 (1958).

—, and J. VAUGHAN: The uptake of ^{35}S in cortical bone. Quart. J. micr. Sci. **98**, 369—375 (1957).

LEBLOND, C. P., and R. C. GREULICH: Autoradiographic studies of bone formation and growth. In: The Biochemistry and Physiology of bone, ed. by G. H. BOURNE, pp. 325—358. New York: Acad. Press. Inc. 1956.

— P. LACROIX, R. PONLOT et A. DHEM: Les stades initiaux de l'ostéogénèse. Nouvelles données histochimiques et autoradiographiques. Bull. Acad. roy. Méd. Belg. **25**, 421—443 (1959).

— G. V. WILKINSON, L. F. BÉLANGER and Y. ROBICHON: Radio-autographic visualisation of bone formation in the rat. Amer. J. Anat. **86**, 289—341 (1950).

LEE, W. R., J. T. MARSHALL, and H. A. SISSONS: Calcium accretion and bone formation in dogs. An experimental comparison between the results of Ca^{45} kinetic analysis and tetracycline labeling. J. Bone Jt Surg. B **47**, 157—180 (1965).

LEMAIRE, R. G.: Calcium metabolism in fracture healing. J. Bone Jt Surg. A **48**, 1156—1170 (1966).

LINDQUIST, B., A. M. BUDY, F. C. MCLEAN and J. L. HOWARD: Skeletal metabolism in estrogen-treated rats studied by means of Ca^{45}. Endocrinology **66**, 100—111 (1960).

LLOYD, E.: The distribution of radium in human bone. Brit. J. Radiol. **34**, 521—528 (1961).

— The assessment of radioactive body burdens of the alkaline earths. In: Assessment of Radioactivity in man, vol. II, pp. 329—343. Vienna: Intern. Atomic Energy Agency 1964.

— Quantitative autoradiography of Ca^{45} in bone. In: Calcified Tissues. Proc. 2nd Europ. Symp., pp. 11—22. Liège: Coll. des Colloques de l'Université de Liège 1965.

LONTIE, P.: Comment se distribue dans le squelette le radiocalcium administré au lapin adulte. Rev. belge Path. **23**, 118—125 (1953).

LOONEY, W. B.: Late effects (twenty-five to forty years) of the early medical and industrial use of radio-active materials. Their relation to the more accurate establishment of maximum permissible amounts of radio-active elements in the body. Part I. J. Bone Jt Surg. A **37**, 1169—1187 (1955).

— C. J. MALETSKOS, M. HELMICK, J. REARDON, J. COHEN and W. GUILD: The artificial kidney and ion-exchange resins as possible methods of removing radio-elements from the body. Radiology **68**, 255—256 (1957).

LOTMAR, R.: Der Einbau von ^{35}S in die Kostalknorpel von Meerschweinchen unter Einfluß verschiedener Glucocorticoide. Experientia (Basel) **16**, 303—304 (1960).

LOTZ, W. E., R. V. TALMAGE and C. L. COMAR: Effect of parathyroid extract administration in sheep. Proc. Soc. exp. Biol. (N.Y.) **85**, 292—295 (1954).

MACDONALD, N. S.: Kinetic studies of skeletal metabolism by external counting of injected in radioisotopes: the radioisotope osteogram. J. Lab. clin. Med. **52**, 541—558 (1958).

— The radioisotope osteogram: kinetic studies of skeletal disorders in humans. Clin. Orthop. **17**, 154—166 (1960).

— P. C. LOVICK and L. I. PETRIELLO: Healing bone fractures and simultaneous administration of radioisotopes of sulphur, calcium and yttrium. Amer. J. Physiol. **191**, 185—188 (1957).

MACINTYRE, I., J. A. PARSONS, and C. J. ROBINSON: The effect of thyrocalcitonin on blood-bone calcium equilibrium in the perfused tibia of the cat. J. Physiol. (Lond.) **191**, 393—405 (1967).

MACPHERSON, S., M. OWEN, and J. VAUGHAN: The relation of radiation dose to radiation damage in the tibia of weanling rabbits injected with Strontium-90. Brit. J. Radiol. **35**, 221—234 (1962).

MANLY LEFEVRE, M., and W. F. BALE: The metabolism of inorganic phosphorus of rat bones and teeth as indicated by the radio active isotopes. J. biol. Chem. **129**, 125—134 (1939).

MARSHALL, J. H.: Microscopic metabolism of calcium in bone. In: Bone as a Tissue, ed. by K. RODAHL, J. T. NICHOLSON and E. M. BROWN, pp. 144—155. New York: McGraw-Hill Book Co., Inc. 1960.

— J. JOWSEY and R. E. ROWLAND: Microscopic metabolism of calcium in bone. IV. Ca^{45} deposition and growth rate in canine osteons. Radiat. Res. **10**, 243—257 (1959*a*).

— — — Microscopic metabolism of Calcium in bone. II. Quantitative autoradiography. Radiat. Res. **10**, 213—233 (1959*b*).

— — — Microscopic metabolism of calcium in bone. V. The paradox of diffuse activity and long-term exchange. Radiat. Res. **10**, 258—270 (1959*c*).

—, and C. C. ONKELINX: Radial diffusion and power function retention of alkaline earth radioisotopes in adult bone. Nature (Lond.) **217**, 742—743 (1968).

— V. K. WHITE and J. COHEN: Microscopic metabolism of calcium in bone. I. Three dimensional deposition of Ca^{45} in canine osteons. Radiat. Res. **10**, 197—212 (1959).

MARTIN, N. D., and E. S. SLATER: Direct tissue radioautography technique applied to teeth. Science **113**, 721—722 (1951).

MCCREADY, V. R.: Clinical radioisotope scanning. Brit. J. Radiol. **40**, 401—423 (1967).

MCLEAN, F. C., and A. M. BUDY: Radiation, Isotopes, and Bone, pp. 1—216. New York: Acad. Press 1964.

MCLEAN, F. C., and M. R. URIST: Bone. An introduction to the physiology of skeletal tissue. Chicago: Chicago University Press 1955.

MERSEELY, G. R., W. L. ALSOBROOK, J. M. MERRIL, O. J. BALCHUM, R. L. WEILAND and C. O. T. BALL: Metabolism of the major mineral elements of the animal body. In: Radiation Biology and Medicine, ed. by W. D. CLAUS. Reading: Addison-Wesley Publisher Co. Inc. 1958.

MILCH, R. A., D. P. RALL and J. E. TOBIE: Fluorescence of tetracycline antibiotics in bone. J. Bone Jt Surg. A **40**, 897—910 (1958).

MILHAUD, G., W. REMAGEN, A. GOMES DE MATOS et J. P. AUBERT: Étude du métabolisme du calcium chez le rat à l'aide de calcium-45. I. Le rachitisme expérimental. Rev. franç. Ét. clin. biol. **5**, 254—261 (1960*a*).

— — — — Étude du métabolisme du calcium chez le rat à l'aide de calcium-45. II. Action de la cortisone Rev. franç. Ét. clin. biol. **5**, 354—358 (1960*b*).

MUELLER, W. J., R. SCHRAER, and H. SCHRAER: Calcium metabolism and skeletal dynamics of laying pullets. J. Nutr. **84**, 20—26 (1964).

NELSON, A., C. RÖNNBÄCK, and L. ROSÉN: Further attempts to influence the elimination of radiostrontium. Acta radiol. (Stockh.) **1**, 129—139 (1963).

NEUMANN, W. F.: Chemical dynamics of bone mineral. In: Bone as a Tissue, ed. by K. RODAHL, J. P. NICHOLSON and E. M. BROWN, pp. 103—117. New York: McGraw-Hill Book Co. Inc. 1960.

—, and B. J. MULRYAN: The surface chemistry of bone. VI. Recrystallization *in vivo*. J. biol. Chem. **195**, 843—848 (1952).

—, and M. W. NEUMANN: The chemical dynamics of bone mineral. Chicago: Chicago University Press 1958.

—, and R. F. RILEY: The uptake of radioactive phosphorus in the calcified tissues of normal and choline-deficient rats. J. biol. Chem. **168**, 545—554 (1947).

NILSSON, A.: Influence of gestation and lactation on radiostrontium-induced malignancies in mice. I. Acta radiol. (Stockh.) **6**, 33—52 (1967).

— A. NELSON, C. RÖNNBÄCK, A.-M. SJÖDÉN, G. WALINDER, and O. HERTZBERG: Influence of gestation and lactation on radiostrontium-induced malignancies in mice. Acta radiol. (Stockh.) **6**, 129—144 (1967).

NORDIN, B. E. C.: Analysis of methods for interpretation of tracer data in bone. In: Medical Uses of Ca^{47}, p. 57. Vienna: Intern. Atomic Energy Agency 1962.

NORRIS, W. P., and W. KISIELESKI: Comparative metabolism of Ra, Sr and Ca. Cold Spr. Harb. Symp. quant. Biol. **13**, 164—172 (1948).

— S. A. TYLER and A. M. BRUES: Retention of radioactive bone seekers. Science **128**, 456—462 (1958).

ODEBLAD, E.: Matrix theory of quantitative apposition autoradiography. Acta radiol. (Stockh.) **45**, 323—339 (1956).

Odell, R. T., C. B. Mueller and J. A. Key: Effect on bone grafts of radioactive isotopes of phosphorus. J. Bone Jt Surg. A **33**, 324—332 (1951).
Okada, T. S.: Autoradiographic study of cartilage differentiation in organ culture. Experientia (Basel) **16**, 160 (1960).
Osborne, J. C., and K. Kowalewski: The uptake of radiosulphur in the fractured humerus in the rat. Surg. Gynec. Obstet. **103**, 38—40 (1956).
Owen, M.: Sr^{90} dosimetry in rabbits. In: Some aspects of internal irradiation, pp. 409—421, ed. by T. F. Daugherty, W. S. S. Jee, C. W. Mays, and B. J. Stoyer. Oxford: Pergamon Press 1962.
— Cell population kinetics of an osteogenic tissue. I. J. Cell Biol. **19**, 19—32 (1963).
— Cell differentiation in bone. In: Calcified Tissues. Proc. 2nd Europ. Symp., pp. 11—22. Liège: Coll. Colloques de l'Université de Liège 1965.
—, and S. Macpherson: Cell population kinetics of an osteogenic tissue. II. J. Cell. Biol. **19**, 33—44 (1963).
— J. Jowsey and J. Vaughan: Investigation on the growth and structure of the tibia of the rabbit by microradiographic and autoradiographic techniques. J. Bone Jt Surg. B **37**, 324—342 (1955).
Pelc, S. R.: Autoradiograph technique. Nature **160**, 749—750 (1947).
— The stripping-film technique of autoradiography. Int. J. appl. Radiat. **1**, 172—177 (1956).
—, and A. Glücksmann: Sulphate metabolism in the cartilage of the trachea, pinna and xiphoid of the adult mouse as indicated by autoradiographs. Exp. Cell Res. **8**, 336—344 (1955).
Ponlot. R.: Le radiocalcium dans l'étude des os. Préface par P. Lacroix. Paris: Masson & Cie. 1960.
Plumlee, M. P., S. L. Hansard, C. L. Comar and W. M. Beeson: Placental transfer and deposition of labeled calcium in the developing bovine fetus. Amer. J. Physiol. **171**, 678—686 (1952).
Prockop, D. J., O. Pettengill, and H. Holtzer: Incorporation of sulfate and the synthesis of collagen by cultures of embryonic chondrocytes. Biochim. biophys. Acta (Aust.) **83**, 189—196 (1964).
Ramsden, E. N.: A review of experimental work on radio-yttrium comprising 1. The tissue distribution, 2. The mechanism of deposition in bone, and 3. The state in the blood. Int. J. Radiat. Biol. **3**, 399—410 (1961).
Rapkin, E.: Liquid scintillation counting 1957—1963: a review. Int. J. appl. Radiat. **15**, 66—87 (1964).
Ray, R. D., D. La Violette, H. D. Buckley and R. S. Mosiman: Studies of bone metabolism. I. Comparison of the metabolism of strontium-90 in living and dead bone. J. Bone Jt Surg. A **37**, 143—155 (1955).
Ray, R. D., and K. H. Mueller: The use of radioisotopes in Orthopaedics. Part III. Experimental and clinical studies. J. Bone Jt Surg. A **47**, 417—425 (1965).
— — B. Sankaran, E. Mensen, and T. Schwartz: Metabolic diseases of bone (kinetic studies). Med. Clin. N. Amer. **49**, 241—258 (1965).
— D. E. Stedman and N. K. Wolff: Bone metabolism. III. The effect of various diets on the mobilization of strontium from the rat skeleton. J. Bone Jt Surg. A **38**, 637—654 (1956).
Rayner, B., M. Tutt and J. Vaughan: The deposition of ^{91}Y in rabbit bones. Brit. J. exp. Path. **34**, 138—145 (1953).
Rich, C.: The calcium metabolism of a patient of a renal insufficiency before and after partial parathyroidectomy. Metabolism **6**, 574—582 (1957).
— Distribution of calcium given by sustained intravenous infusion. J. clin. Endocr. **20**, 147—156 (1960).
—, and J. Ensinck: Effect of sodium fluoride on calcium metabolism of human beings. Nature (Lond.) **192**, 185 (1961).
— —, and H. Fellows: The use of continuous infusions of $calcium^{45}$ and $strontium^{85}$ to study skeletal function. J. clin. Endocr. **21**, 611—623 (1961).
Richelle, L. J., and F. Bronner: The calcium exchange reaction of bone *in vitro*. Effect of parathyroid extract. Biochem. Pharmacol. **12**, 647—659 (1963).
Rigal, W. M.: The use of tritiated thymidine in studies of chondrogenesis. In: Radioisotopes and Bone, ed. by F. C. McLean, P. Lacroix, and A. M. Budy, pp. 197—225. Oxford: Blackwell Sci. Publ., 1962.
Robertson, J. S.: Theory and use of tracers in determining transfer rates in biological systems. Physiol. Rev. **37**, 133—154 (1957).
Robinson, R. A.: Chemical analysis and electron-microscopy of bone. In: Bone as a Tissue, ed. by K. Rodahl, J. T. Nicholson and E. M. Brown, pp. 186—250. New York: McGraw-Hill Book Co., Inc. 1960.
Rosenthal, H. L.: Uptake of Ca^{45} and $strontium^{90}$ from water by fresh-water fishes. Science **126**, 669—670 (1957).
Rosoff, B., S. Ritter, K. Sullivan, H. Hart and H. Spencer-Laszlo: Effect of chelating agents on the removal of yttrium and lanthanum from man. Hlth Phys. **6**, 177—182 (1961).
Rowland, R. E.: Microscopic metabolism of Ra^{226} in canine bone and its bearing on the radiation dosimetry of internally deposited alkaline earths. Radiat. Res. **15**, 126—137 (1961).
— Skeletal retention of the alkaline earth radioisotopes and bone dosimetry. In: Some Aspects of internal Irradiation, pp. 455—467, ed. by T. F. Daugherty, W. S. S. Jee, C. W. Mays, and B. J. Stover. Oxford: Pergamon Press 1962.

ROWLAND, R. E.: Resorption and bone physiology. In: Bone Biodynamics, ed by H. M. FROST, pp. 335—351. Boston: Little, Brown & Co. 1964.

—, and J. H. MARSHALL: Radium in human bones: the dose in microscopic volumes of bone. Radiat. Res. 11, 299—313 (1959).

— — and J. JOWSEY: Radium in human bone: the microradiographic appearance. Radiat. Res. 10, 323—334 (1959).

RUBIN, M.: Application of chelating agents. In: Metabolic Interrelation. Trans. of the fifth Conference, ed. by E. C. REIFENSTEIN jr., pp. 344—354. New York: Josiah Macy jr. Found. 1953.

— K. C. BRACE, H. GUMP, R. SWARM and J. R. ANDREWS: The radiotoxic effects of S^{35} in growing cartilage. Consideration of radioactive sulphur (S^{35}) as a possible radiotherapeutic agent in chondrosarcomas. Radiology 69, 711—719 (1957).

— R. D. THOMAS, T. A. LITOVITZ and C. F. GESCHICKTER: Dynamics of calcium metabolism. Metabolic Interrelation. Trans. of the fifth Conference, ed. by E. C. REIFENSTEIN jr., pp. 53—71. New York: Josiah Macy jr. Found. 1953.

RUF, F.: Über Stoffwechseluntersuchungen mit Radiophosphorus und Radiocalcium im Knochen, insbesondere während der Knochenbruchheilung und in Knochenspüren. In: Radioaktive Isotope in Klinik und Forschung, herausgeg. von K. FELLINGER u. H. VETTER, Bd. 1, S. 212—221. München u. Berlin: Urban & Schwarzenberg 1955.

RUSHTON, M. A., M. OWEN, W. HOLGATE, and J. VAUGHAN: The relation of radiation dose to radiation damage in the mandible of weanling rabbits. Arch. oral Biol. 3, 235—246 (1961).

RUNDO, J., and A. L. LILLEGRAVEN: Uptake and retention of radioactive Strontium in normal subjects. Brit. J. Radiol. 39, 676—685 (1966).

SACKS, J.: Tracer techniques: stable and radioactive isotopes. In: Physical Techniques in biological Research, ed. by G. OSTER and A. W. POLLISTER, vol. II, pp. 1—56. New York: Acad. Press Inc. 1956.

SAMACHSON, J.: Mechanism for the exchange of the calcium in bone mineral. Nature (Lond.) 216, 193—194 (1967).

SCHUBERT, J.: Approaches to treatment of poisoning by both radioactive and non-radioactive elements encountered in atomic energy operations. Geneva Conference Paper, No. P/845 (1955).

—, and W. D. ARMSTRONG: Rate of elimination of radioactive carbon administered as carbonate from the tissues and tissue components of mature and growing rats. J. biol. Chem. 177, 521—527 (1949).

—, and J. F. FRIED: Chelating agents in the treatment of poisoning by polymerizable radioelements. Nature (Lond.) 185, 551—552 (1960).

SCHULERT, A. R., E. A. PEETS, D. LASZLO, H. SPENCER, M. CHARLES and J. SAMACHSON: Comparative metabolism of strontium and calcium in man. Int. J. appl. Radiat. 4, 144—153 (1959).

SCOTT, K. G., H. AXELROD and J. G. HAMILTON: The metabolism of curium in the rat. J. biol. Chem. 177, 325—335 (1949).

— D. H. COPP, H. AXELROD and J. G. HAMILTON: The metabolism of americium in the rat. J. biol. Chem. 175, 691—703 (1948).

SHETLAR, M. R., R. M. BRADFORD, W. JOEL, and R. P. HOWARD: Effects of parathyroid extract on glycoprotein and mucopolysaccharide components of serum and tissue. In: The Parathyroids, ed. by R. O. GREEP and R. V. TALMAGE, pp. 123—143. Springfield: Ch. C. Thomas 1961.

SHIM, S. S., D. H. COPP, and F. P. PATTERSON: An indirect method of bone blood-flow measurement based on the bone clearance of a circulating bone-seeking radioisotope. J. Bone Jt Surg. A 49, 693—702 (1967).

SIMMONS, D. J.: Cellular changes in the bones of mice as studied with tritiated thymidine and the effects of Estrogen. Clin. Orthop. 26, 176—189 (1963).

SINGER, L., and W. D. ARMSTRONG: Retention and turnover of radiocalcium by the skeleton of large rats. Proc. Soc. exp. Biol. (N. Y.) 76, 229—233 (1951).

SIRI, W. E.: Isotopic tracers and nuclear radiations. New York: McGraw-Hill Book Co., Inc. 1949.

SKIPPER, H. E., C. NOLAN and L. SIMPSON: Studies on the hazard involved in use of C^{14}. III. Long term retention in bone. J. biol. Chem. 189, 159—166 (1951).

SOLOMON, A. K.: Compartmental methods of kinetic analysis. In: Mineral Metabolism, vol. I, pp. 119—168, ed. by C. L. COMAR, and F. BRONNER. New York: Acad. Press Inc. 1960.

SOWBY, F. D., and D. M. TAYLOR: Removal of internally deposited americium by chelating agents. Nature (Lond.) 187, 612 (1960).

SPECKMANN, TH. V., and W. P. NORRIS: The retention of $strontium^{85}$ in rats as a function of animal age at injection. Quarterly Report of Biological and Medical Research Division Argonne National Laboratory, ANL-5597, 77—78 (1956).

— — $Strontium^{85}$ retention by the rat as a function of age at injection. Semi-annual Report of Biological and Medical Research Division Argonne National Laboratory, ANL-6093, 82—87 (1958).

SPENCER, H., D. LASZLO and M. BROTHERS: $Strontium^{85}$ and $calcium^{45}$ metabolism in man. J. clin. Invest. 36, 680—688 (1957).

— M. LI, J. SAMACHSON, and D. LASZLO: Metabolism of strontium-85 and calcium-45 in man. Metabolism 9, 916—925 (1960).

— J. SAMACHSON, B. KABAKOW and D. LASZLO: Factors modifying radiostrontium excretion in man. Clin. Sci. 17, 291—301 (1958).

SPENCER, R., R. HERBERT, M. W. RISH, and W. A. LITTLE: Bone scanning with ^{85}Sr, ^{87m}Sr

and ^{18}F. Physical and radiopharmaceutical considerations and clinical experience in 50 cases. Brit. J. Radiol. **40**, 641—654 (1967).
SPIERS, F. W.: The influence of energy absorption and electron range on dosage in irradiated bone. Brit. J. Radiol. **22**, 521—533 (1949).
— Calculation of ionization near bone surface. Brit. J. Radiol. **23**, 743 (1950).
STERNBERG, J.: Effect of tetracyclines on the turnover of Calcium-45 in young rats. Int. J. appl. Radiat. **17**, 497—512 (1966).
STILLSTRÖM, J.: Grain count corrections in autoradiography. I. Int. J. appl. Radiat. **14**, 113—120 (1963).
— Grain count corrections in autoradiography. II. Int. J. appl. Radiat. **16**, 357—363 (1965).
STOCLET, J. C.: Les échanges calciques rapides analysés par le Ca^{45} chez le rat. C.R. Acad. Sci. (Paris) **251**, 1834—1836 (1960*a*).
— Les échanges calciques entre plasma sanguin et divers organes, étudiés chez le rat mâle et femelle à l'aide du Ca^{45}. C. R. Acad. Sci. (Paris) **251**, 1934—1936 (1960*b*).
STRANDH, J.: Chemical and biophysical studies of microscopic structures in compact bone. Acta Univ. upsalien. **3**, 1—16 (1961).
—, and A. BENGTSSON: The uptake of phosphorus in microscopic bone structures in compact bone. Acta Soc. Med. upsalien. **66**, 49—63 (1961*a*).
— — The uptake of calcium in microscopic bone structures in compact bone. Acta Soc. Med. upsalien. **66**, 95—103 (1961*b*).
—, and K. SOLHEIM: The change with age of the uptake of phosphorus in microscopic bone structures. Acta Soc. Med. upsalien. **68**, 135—140 (1963).
TALMAGE, R. V.: Studies on the influence of parathyroid hormone on bone cell modulation. Abr. Proc. 4th Europ. Symp. Calcified Tissues, ed. by P. J. GAILLARD, A. VAN DEN HOOFF and R. STEENDIJK, pp. 99—100. Amsterdam: Excerpta Med. Found. 1966.
—, and J. R. ELLIOTT: Removal of calcium from bone as influenced by the parathyroids. Endocrinology **62**, 717—722 (1958).
— W. E. LOTZ and C. L. COMAR: Action of parathyroid extract on bone phosphorus and Ca in the rat. Proc. Soc. exper. Biol. (N.Y.) **84**, 578—582 (1953).
THOMAS, R. O., T. A. LITOVITZ, M. I. RUBIN and C. F. GESCHICKTER: Dynamics of calcium metabolism. Time distribution of intravenously administered radiocalcium. Amer. J. Physiol. **169**, 568—575 (1952).
TOMLIN, D. H., K. M. HENRY and S. K. KON: Autoradiographic studies of growth and calcium metabolism in the long bones of the rat. Brit. J. Nutr. **7**, 235—252 (1953).
— — — The interstitial metabolism of calcium in the bones and teeth of rats. Brit. J. Nutr. **9**, 144—156 (1955).
TOMLINSON, R. W. S., M. WALL, S. B. OSBORN, and J. ANDERSON: Radiocalcium studies in normal subjects. Calc. Tiss. Res. **1**, 197—203, (1967).
TONNA, E. A.: The cellular complement of the skeletal system studied autoradiographically with tritiated thymidine (H^3TDR) during growth and aging. J. biophys. biochem. Cytol. **9**, 813—824 (1961*a*).
— An autoradiographic evaluation of the aging cellular phase of mouse skeleton using tritiated glycine. J. Geront. **19**, 198—206 (1964).
—, and E. P. CRONKITE: Histochemical and autoradiographic studies on the effects of aging on the mucopolysaccharides of the periosteum. J. biophys. biochem. Cytol. **6**, 171—178 (1959).
— — Use of tritiated thymidine for the study of the origin of the osteoclast. Nature (Lond.) **190**, 459—460 (1961*a*).
— — Cellular response to fracture studied with tritiated thymidine. J. Bone Jt Surg. A **43**, 352—362 (1961*b*).
— — Utilization of tritiated histidine (H^3HIL) by skeletal cells of adult mice. J. Geront. **17**, 353—358 (1962*a*).
— — Changes in the skeletal cell proliferative response to trauma concomitant with aging. J. Bone Jt Surg. A **44**, 1557—1568 (1962*b*).
— — The effects of extraperiosteal injections of blood components on periosteal cell proliferation. J. Cell Biol. **23**, 79—87 (1964).
TRIFFITT, J. T.: Binding of calcium and strontium by alginates. Nature (Lond.) **217**, 457—458 (1968).
TULLIS, J. L., and H. A. JOHNSON: The biological significance of some important internal emitters. In: Radiation Biology and Medicine, ed. by W. D. CLAUS, pp. 341—368. Reading: Addison-Wesley Publishers Co., Inc. 1958.
UEHLINGER, E.: On the influence of thyroxine, thiouracil, cortisone, estrogen and testosterone on endochondral ossification utilizing autoradiography. In: Proc. 3rd Europ. Symp. Calcified Tissues, ed. by H. FLEISCH, H. J. J. BLACKWOOD, and M. OWEN, pp. 243—245. Berlin: Springer 1965.
URIST, M. R., N. S. MAC DONALD and J. JOWSEY: The function of the donor tissue in experimental operations with radioactive bone grafts. Ann. Surg. **147**, 129—145 (1958).
VAN DYKE, D., H. O. ANGER, U. YANO, and C. BOZZINI: Bone blood flow shown with F^{18} and the positron camera. Amer. J. Physiol. **209**, 65—70 (1965).
VAUGHAN, J.: The effects of radiation on bone. In: The biochemistry and physiology of bone, ed. by G. H. BOURNE, pp. 729—765. New York: Acad. Press Inc. 1956.
—, and J. JOWSEY: Preliminary report on lesions in the skeleton of young rabbits following a single injection of ^{90}Sr (500—1000 c/Kg). In: Progress in Radiobiology, pp. 429—433. Edinburgh: Oliver & Boyd 1956.
—, and M. OWEN: The use of autoradiography in the measurement of radiation dose-rate in rabbit bone following the administration of Sr^{90}. Lab. Invest. 8, 181—193 (1959).
—, and M. WILLIAMSON: Variation in "turnover rates" in different parts of the skeleton in

relation to turnover incidence due to 90 Sr deposition. In: Abr. Proc. 4th Europ. Symp. Calcified Tissues, ed. by P. J. Gaillard, A. van den Hooff, and R. Steendijk, pp. 102—103. Amsterdam: Excerpta Med. Found. 1966.

Vincent, J.: Recherches sur la constitution du tissu osseux compact. Arch. Biol. (Liège) **65**, 531—569 (1954).

— Recherches sur la constitution de l'os adulte. Thèse Université Louvain, Editions Arscia, Bruxelles 1955.

— Autoradiographies au Na^{22} de l'os compact de Cercopithèque. Bull. Acad. roy. Méd. Belg., VI. sér. **25**, 283—295 (1960).

—, et S. Haumont: Identification autoradiographique des ostéones métaboliques après administration de Ca^{45}. Rev. franç. Étud. clin. biol. **5**, 348—353 (1960).

Visek, W. J., R. A. Monroe, E. W. Swanson and C. L. Comar: Determination of endogenous fecal calcium in cattle by a simple isotope dilution method. J. Nutr. **50**, 23—33 (1953).

Volf, V., and Z. Roth: Retention of Strontium-85 in rats. III. Effect of increasing the doses of sodium and barium sulphates and role of the time factor. Acta radiol. (Stockh.) **4**, 481—493 (1966).

Wasserman, R. H.: Quantitative studies on skeletal accretion in laboratory and domestic animals. 2nd U.N. Intern. Conf. peaceful uses atomic energy, A/Conf. 15/8/816 (1958).

Weidmann, S. M.: Studies on the skeletal tissues. 4. The renewal of inorganic phosphate in bones of various species of small mammals as a function of time. Biochem. J. **62**, 593—601 (1956).

Weikel, G. H., and W. F. Neuman: Incorporation of dietary radiocalcium into skeleton of rats. Metabolism **10**, 83—90 (1961).

Wendeberg, B.: Mineral metabolism of fractures of the tibia in man studied with external counting of Sr^{85}. Acta orthop. scand., Suppl. **52**, 1—79 (1961).

Wendberg, B., and T. Yamamuro: Mineral metabolism in primary bone tumours studied by external counting of 85-Sr. Acta orthop. scand. **36**, 21—34 (1965).

White, N. B., M. M. Ter-Pogossian, and A. H. Stein: A method to determine the rate of blood flow in long bone and selected soft tissues. Surg. Gynec. Obstet. **119**, 535—540 (1964).

Whitehead, R. G., and S. M. Weidmann: The effect of parathormone on the uptake of P^{32} into adenosine-triphosphate and bone salts in kittens. Biochem. J. **71**, 312—318 (1959).

Woods, K. R., and W. D. Armstrong: Action of parathyroid extracts on stable bone mineral using radiocalcium as tracer. Proc. Soc. exp. Biol. (N.Y.) **91**, 255—258 (1956).

Yagoda, H.: Radioactive measurements with nuclear emulsions. New York: J. Wiley, & Sons Inc. 1949.

Young, R. W.: Regional differences in cell generation time in growing rat tibiae. Exp. Cell Res. **26**, 562—567 (1962*a*).

— Cell proliferation and specialization during endochondral osteogenesis in young rats. J. Cell Biol. **14**, 357—370 (1962*b*).

— Autoradiographic studies on postnatal growth of the skull in young rats injected with tritiated glycine. Anat. Rec. **143**, 1—7 (1962*c*).

— Histophysical studies on bone cells and bone resorption. In: Mechanisms of hard Tissue Destruction, ed. by R. F. Sognnaes, pp. 471—496. Washington: Amer. Ass. Adv. Sci. 1963.

— Specialization of bone cells: In: Bone Biodynamics, ed. by H. M. Frost, pp. 117—142. Boston: Little, Brown & Co. 1964.

Zetterström, R.: Removal of phosphate in bone minerals. I. Renewal rate of phosphate in relation to the solubility of the bone minerals. Biochim. biophys. Acta **8**, 283—293 (1952).

Namenverzeichnis — Author Index

Die *kursiv* gesetzten Seitenzahlen beziehen sich auf die Literatur

Page numbers in *italics* refer to the bibliography

Sachverzeichnis

(Deutsch-Englisch)

Bei gleicher Schreibweise in beiden Sprachen sind die Stichwörter nur einmal aufgeführt

Subject Index

(Englisch-Deutsch)

Where English and German spelling of a word is identical, the German version is omitted